McAlpine's
MULTIPLE SCLEROSIS

For NDC (1918–1986)

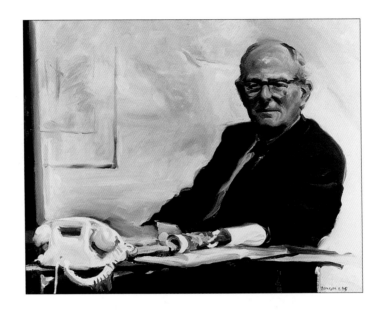

Portrait by Howard Morgan. Reproduced by permission of Harveian Librarian, Royal College of Physicians of London.

Commissioning Editor: Susan Pioli
Project Development Manager: Louise Cook
Project Managers: Cheryl Brant (Elsevier), Gillian Whytock (Prepress Projects)
Editorial Assistant: Nani Clansey
Design Manager: Jayne Jones
Illustration Manager: Mick Ruddy
Illustrators: Antbits Illustration
Marketing Manager: Dana Butler

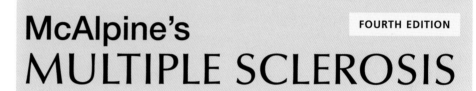

McAlpine's
MULTIPLE SCLEROSIS

FOURTH EDITION

Alastair Compston PhD FRCP FMedSci
Professor of Neurology, University of Cambridge, Cambridge, UK

Christian Confavreux MD
Professor of Neurology, Hôpital Neurologique, Hospices Civils de Lyon and Université Claude Bernard, Lyon, France

Hans Lassmann MD
Professor of Neuroimmunology, Center for Brain Research, Medical University of Vienna, Vienna, Austria

Ian McDonald PhD FRCP FMedSci
Professor Emeritus of Clinical Neurology, Institute of Neurology, University College London, London, UK

David Miller MD FRCP FRACP
Professor of Clinical Neurology, Institute of Neurology, University College London, and Consultant Neurologist, National Hospital for Neurology and Neurosurgery, London, UK

John Noseworthy MD FRCPC
Professor and Chair, Department of Neurology, Mayo Clinic College of Medicine, Rochester, MN, USA

Kenneth Smith PhD
Professor of Neurophysiology and Head of Neuroinflammation Group, King's College London School of Medicine at Guy's, London, UK

Hartmut Wekerle MD
Professor and Director, Max Planck Institute of Neurobiology, Planegg-Martinsried, Germany

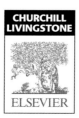

CHURCHILL LIVINGSTONE

ELSEVIER

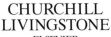

CHURCHILL
LIVINGSTONE
ELSEVIER

© 2006, Elsevier Inc. All rights reserved.

First published December 2005

First edition 1985
Second edition 1992
Third edition 1998

ISBN 044307271X

EAN 9780443072710

British Library Cataloguing in Publication Data
A catalogue record for this book is available from the British Library

Library of Congress Cataloguing in Publication Data
A catalogue record for this book is available from the Library of Congress

Notice
Medical knowledge is constantly changing. Standard safety precautions must be followed, but as new research and clinical experience broaden our knowledge, changes in treatment and drug therapy may become necessary r appropriate. Readers are advised to check the most current product information provided by the manufactacturer of each drug to be administered to verify the recommended dose, the method and duration of administration, and contraindications. It is the responsibility of the practitioner, relying on experience and knowledge of the patient, to determine dosages and the best treatment for each individual patient. Neither the Publisher nor the editors assume any liability for any injury and/or damage to persons or property arising from this publication.

The Publisher

ELSEVIER your source for books, journals and multimedia in the health sciences
www.elsevierhealth.com

Working together to grow
libraries in developing countries
www.elsevier.com | www.bookaid.org | www.sabre.org

ELSEVIER   BOOK AID International   Sabre Foundation

The publisher's policy is to use **paper manufactured from sustainable forests**

Printed in China
Last digit is the print number: 9 8 7 6 5 4 3 2

Contents

Contents

Preface to the fourth edition

Although this book has its origins in the work written by Douglas McAlpine, Nigel Compston and Charles Lumsden in 1955, not one word survives from the original version of *Multiple Sclerosis* and very few from any of its successors – *Multiple Sclerosis, a Reappraisal* (1965 and 1972) and *McAlpine's Multiple Sclerosis* (1985, 1991 and 1998). Much has been published on multiple sclerosis in the last 7 years, from which several new concepts have (re)emerged on the nature of the illness and its pathogenesis and treatment. As a result, our book is significantly restructured and each chapter largely rewritten from the last edition (1998). We see knowledge on this unpredictable and unsettling neurological disease of young adults as falling into five categories: the story of how the evidence supporting contemporary concepts of the disorder was gathered; the cause and course of the disease; its clinical features, and laboratory methods used in making the diagnosis; the pathogenesis; and the management and treatment of multiple sclerosis. We have responded to constructive criticisms offered by readers of the last edition by combining some chapters and adding others, especially to the section on treatment. Each of the last four parts ends with a brief chapter that aims to identify and debate the issues that we consider unresolved or most open to individual opinion. Because *McAlpine's Multiple Sclerosis* is intended to be more than just a mere compendium of what has been published elsewhere, by ourselves and others, throughout we declare a personal position on many topics. Especially in suggesting ideas on the origins of multiple sclerosis; on the issue of heterogeneity and complexity; in debating the relative contribution of genes and the environment in causation and distribution; on the primacy and independence of the inflammatory and neurodegenerative contribution to the pathogenesis; and in reviewing the status of disease-modifying treatments, we do not expect our conclusions to be accepted uncritically. Despite careful editing, it will not be difficult for the reader occasionally to identify passages in different chapters dealing with these and other topics that appear ambiguous. Whilst endeavouring to avoid duplication, we aim to make each chapter complete in itself, and there are therefore a few instances of overlap and repetition.

The style of *McAlpine's Multiple Sclerosis* and its predecessors has been for a limited number of authors to cover as many aspects of the subject as possible. Originally Charles Lumsden wrote on the human and experimental neuropathology, and Douglas McAlpine and Nigel Compston covered everything else. Subsequently, the pathology of multiple sclerosis was described by Roy Weller (1985), Ingrid Allen (1991) and Hans Lassmann (1998) who has revised his analysis for the present edition, basing this account on a personal series of biopsy and autopsy cases using the sophisticated battery of histological and molecular techniques now available. This use of pathological anatomy to inform concepts of the pathogenesis is classic but still highly productive. Charles Lumsden also summarized knowledge on the immunology of multiple sclerosis in the early editions (1955, 1965 and 1972); and this topic was later covered by Richard Batchelor (1985), Alastair Compston (1991) and Hartmut Wekerle (1998) who, in the present edition, describes clinical and experimental immunology as it relates to multiple sclerosis and animal models of the disease, placed in the context of how the immune system works generally in health and disease. In the original edition, Nigel Compston and Douglas McAlpine dealt with the geography and aetiology of multiple sclerosis. These aspects were later discussed by Donald Acheson (1965, 1972 and 1985), Christopher Martyn (1991) and Alastair Compston (1991, 1998 and this volume). Douglas McAlpine revised his initial analysis of the natural history for the 1965 and 1972 editions, and these topics were later described by Bryan Matthews (1985 and 1991) and by George Ebers (1998). Now, we welcome Christian Confavreux who combines access to a natural history cohort that has been scrutinized in detail over many years with a detailed analysis of the extant literature, drawing out lessons for the pathogenesis of multiple sclerosis and identifying comparators for disease modifications attributable to treatment. Bryan Matthews (1985, 1991 and 1998) had taken on the mantle of clinical description from Douglas McAlpine: together, perhaps more than any other section, their contributions gave the book its particular style and reputation. Because these matters do not much change, the clinical description written by Ian McDonald retains some passages from the older text. Bryan Matthews also wrote on the pathophysiology (1985) but this topic was extensively updated by Ian McDonald (1998), based on his own original work on the pathophysiology of multiple sclerosis carried out over several decades. In this edition, Ken Smith brings his expertise in experimental neurophysiology to the account of how function alters, for worse and for better, in the face of factors that compromise and then restore saltatory conduction in the central nervous system. Ian McDonald's chapters on diagnostic methods (1998) and Bryan Matthews's account of the differential diagnosis (1985, 1991 and 1998) are now written by David Miller, who combines extensive clinical experience of multiple sclerosis with expertise and innovation in imaging techniques. Our account of treatment, condensed into a single narrative in 1998, is expanded to five chapters. Gone are the shrill cries of a hawkish analyst seeking to steer a course between fact and fiction in the early days of the 'licensed therapies'; rather, John Noseworthy brings common sense and measured tones to this crucial topic, neither shirking an opinion nor risking analyses unsupported by detailed assessment of the available evidence. Thus, for the fourth edition of *McAlpine's Multiple Sclerosis*, the number of authors has increased to from six to eight, and four contributors are new to the book. Each brings expertise on several aspects of the basic or clinical science of multiple sclerosis, and everyone has contributed to more than one chapter.

The team met in March 2002 to plan the book. First drafts of the chapters were circulated amongst co-authors early in 2004. After editing and revisions, the working versions were distributed to all members of the team, one of whom critically reviewed each chapter – acting as surrogate reader and critic. We met again in October 2004 to review progress (see below). Over the next 4 months, further revisions were made and the final versions of each chapter were re-edited by May 2005. Copy-editing, redrawing of illustrations to achieve a uniform style, scrutiny of page proofs and the insertion of information contained in approximately 250 articles published during 2005 were all completed by late August. The final proofs were checked in September. The c. 6600 references appear as a single alphabetical list at the end of the book. Multiple citations to a given topic also appear alphabetically in the text rather than in chronological order of publication. Thus, the first named are not necessarily the original contributors to that area of research or clinical description. Aspects of every scientific book are out of date before the volume appears. This edition of *McAlpine's Multiple Sclerosis* includes material that the authors consider to be relevant appearing in the literature within 3 months of its publication in November 2005.

McAlpine's Multiple Sclerosis has benefited from the help of many people. Susan Pioli and Louise Cook at Elsevier provided continuous support and encouragement throughout the entire period during which the book was being written. Gillian Whytock and her team at Prepress Projects were meticulous in their attention to detail and ability to juggle the many late insertions and alterations during production; together with the illustrators, design team and typesetters, they have provided a book that matches the aesthetic aspirations of the contributing authors. We thank the following for helpful discussions and the provision of material for inclusion in the various chapters: Fahmy Abdoul Enein, Janice Anderson, Nagui Antoun, Jean-Claude Baron, Ben Barres, Jan Bauer, John Benedikz, William Blakemore, Anthony Bowen, Helene Breitschopf, Simon Broadley, Adolfo Bronstein, Peter Brown, Wolfgang Brück, Herbert Budka, Mary Bunge, Siddharthan Chandran, Olga Ciccarelli, Alasdair Coles, Juliet Compston, Polly Compston, Mark Daly, Gerard Davies, Mervyn Eadie, Celia Ennis, Kryshani Fernando, Virginia Forbes, Peter Forster, Robin Franklin, Jan van Gijn, Sabine Golde, Simon Hickman, John Hodges, Romana Höftberger, Reinhard Hohlfeld, Eric Bond Hutton, Helen Kellar-Wood, Ulrike Köck, John Kurtzke, Angela Kury, Alexandra Kutzelnigg, Kurt Jellinger, Gillian Lee, Marianne Leiszer, George Lowis, Claudia Lucchinetti, David MacManus, Marco Miretti, Katherine Miszkiel, the Multiple Sclerosis Society of Great Britain and Northern Ireland, Colin Mumford, Richard Nicholas, Malcolm Nicholson, France-Isabel Pairel, Charles Poser, Christine Purdy, Waqar Rashid, Stephen Reingold, Colin Renfrew, Neil Robertson, the Royal College of Physicians of Edinburgh, the Royal College of Physicians of London, Jaume Sastre-Garriga, Stephen Sawcer, Steven Scherer, Manfred Schmidbauer, Neil Scolding, Maria Storch, Patricia Sutherland, Cory Teuscher, Pentti Tienari, Alan Thompson, Edward Thompson, John Trowsdale, Sandra Vukusic, Alastair Wilkins, Tarek Yousry and John Zajicek. Katrina Dedman went beyond mere secretarial duties in her dedicated collation of texts, typing of various sections, decoding aberrant handwriting, formatting and retrieving references, and endless checking of details.

We aimed to write a book summarizing everything of importance relating to multiple sclerosis from the time the disorder was first experienced and recognized to mid-2005, and to make

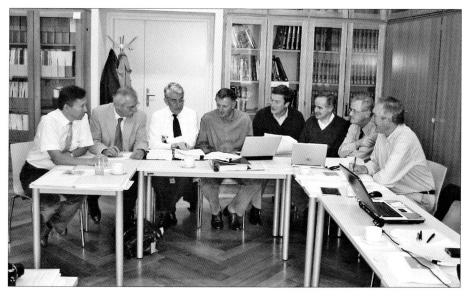

Author planning meeting held at the Center for Brain Research, Medical University of Vienna, Vienna, in October 2004. From left: Christian Confavreux, Hans Lassmann, Ian McDonald, Alastair Compston, John Noseworthy, David Miller, Hartmut Wekerle and Kenneth Smith.

this synthesis useful both for the interested lay person and for the fully informed professional. For those who have the illness, care about someone who is affected, do their best to alleviate the sufferings it brings from various perspectives, or have invested much effort in seeking to understand and solve the problem, we hope that the book is considered to be interesting, balanced, comprehensive and – in showing that the dividend from existing efforts is substantial, and the route to eventual solution charted, even if the pathway can still only be 'seen through a glass darkly' – optimistic. How our efforts are received, and for how long they remain valuable as a record of knowledge on multiple sclerosis is for the reader to judge and the present generation of basic and clinical scientists to influence. For some of us, this edition of *McAlpine's Multiple Sclerosis* has occupied every single moment not spent doing other things during the last 3 years. To borrow (in all humility) from Edward Gibbon (1737–1794) on laying down his pen after completing *The Decline and Fall of the Roman Empire* in 1788:

I will not dissemble the first emotions of joy on recovery of my freedom; but a sober melancholy was spread over my mind, by the idea that I had taken leave of an old and agreeable companion, and that whatsoever might be the future of my history, the life of the historian must be short and precarious.

Alastair Compston
Cambridge
September 2005

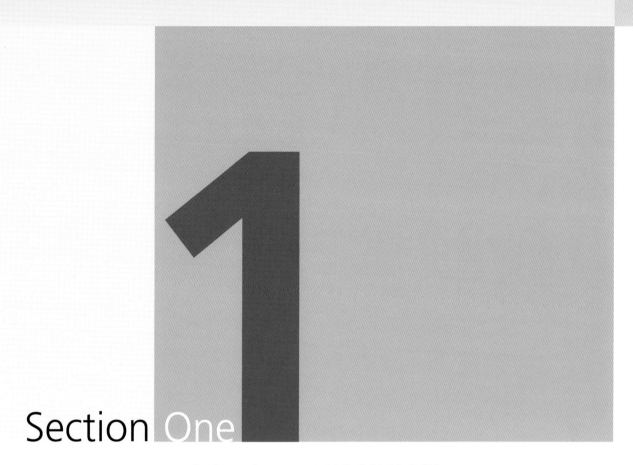

Section One

THE STORY OF MULTIPLE SCLEROSIS

Chapter 1 The story of multiple sclerosis
Alastair Compston, Hans Lassmann and Ian McDonald

The story of multiple sclerosis

1

Alastair Compston, Hans Lassmann and Ian McDonald

THE EVOLVING CONCEPT OF MULTIPLE SCLEROSIS

Multiple sclerosis was first depicted in 1838. The unnamed patient was French, the illustrator a Scotsman. In the six decades that followed, French and German physicians provided a coherent clinicopathological account of the disease. By the beginning of the 20th century, a disease that only a few years earlier had merited individual case reports had become one of the commonest reasons for admission to a neurological ward. Now, multiple sclerosis is recognized throughout the world, with around 2.5 million affected individuals incurring costs in billions of dollars for health care and loss of income. But these crude statistics conceal the harsh reality of a frightening and potentially disabling disease. In writing, in musical expression, or through images on canvas, talented individuals have portrayed the personal experience of multiple sclerosis. They speak for the many denied these cultural conduits for expressing the hopes and fears of young adults facing an uncertain neurological future.

As multiple sclerosis became better recognized in the early part of the 20th century, ideas began to formulate on its cause and the pathogenesis. Research over the last 50 years has illuminated the mechanisms of tissue injury, and the therapeutic era – which will surely culminate in the application of successful strategies both for limiting and repairing the damage – has now begun. For the patient, multiple sclerosis threatens an apparently infinite variety of symptoms, but with certain recurring themes, and an unpredictable course. For the neurologist, multiple sclerosis is a disorder of young adults diagnosed on the basis of clinical and paraclinical evidence for at least two demyelinating lesions affecting different sites within the brain or spinal cord, separated in time. For the pathologist, multiple sclerosis is a disorder of the central nervous system manifesting as acute focal inflammatory demyelination and axonal loss with limited remyelination, leading to the chronic multifocal sclerotic plaques from which the disease gets its name. For the physiologist, it is a condition in which the disease processes produce a remarkable array of abnormalities in electrical conduction. For the clinical scientist, multiple sclerosis is the prototype chronic inflammatory disease of the central nervous system in which knowledge gained across a range of basic and clinical neuroscience disciplines has already allowed rational, if not fully effective, strategies for treatment. For all these groups, multiple sclerosis remains a difficult disease for which solutions seem attainable yet stubbornly elusive. What follows is not a conventional history of achievements in the field of multiple sclerosis but is intended as background to the chapters that follow. It is the story of multiple sclerosis.

NAMING AND CLASSIFYING THE DISEASE: 1868–1983

Few would disagree that the serious study of human demyelinating disease began with the studies of Jean-Martin Charcot (1825–1893) at the Salpétrière in the last three decades of the 19th century. Charcot referred variously to his disease as *la sclérose en plaques disseminées*, *la sclérose multiloculaire* or *la sclérose generalisée*. These names were translated in the New Sydenham Society edition of his lectures (which spread his influence amongst the English-speaking world) as *disseminated (cerebrospinal) sclerosis*. This name was preferred to *insular sclerosis* or *lobular* and *diffuse sclerosis*, under which the first cases had been reported in England, Australia and the New World. It was in Germany that the term *multiple Sklerose* was used from the outset (with variations including *multiple inselförmige Sklerose*, *multiple Hirnsklerose* and *multiple Sklerose des Nervensystems*). This term was occasionally used elsewhere but *disseminated sclerosis* soon became the accepted name amongst English-speaking physicians, even though *sclérose en plaques* persisted in France (and translated in Italian as *sclerosi in plache*). According to Pierre Marie (1853–1940) *polynesic sclerosis* was preferred by some authorities (Marie 1895). Consistency of nomenclature began in the 1950s with the formation of lay patient support organizations. Consensus was eventually achieved with the publication of *Multiple Sclerosis* written by Douglas McAlpine (1890–1981), Nigel Compston (1918–1986) and Charles Lumsden (1913–1974) (Figure 1.1A–C; McAlpine *et al* 1955), since when the condition has universally been known as *multiple sclerosis*. The group of investigators assembled around McAlpine met informally at a 'Disseminated Sclerosis Club' to which others interested in the disease were invited. Apart from McAlpine, those known to have attended included Sydney Allison (1899–1978), Malcolm Campbell (1909–1972), Nigel Compston and John Sutherland (1919–1995).

Douglas McAlpine came from a prominent industrialist family in Great Britain. He had a distinguished military career in both world wars, serving as a neurologist in the Middle East and India, and was appointed in 1924 to the consultant staff of the

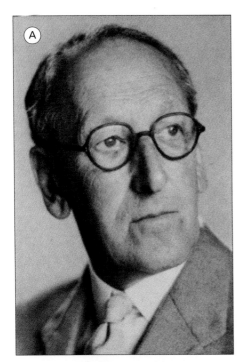

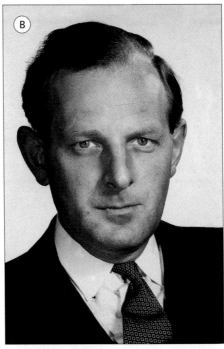

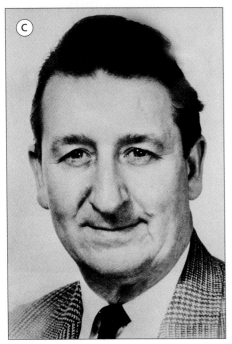

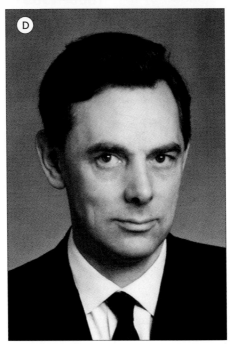

Figure 1.1 (A) Douglas McAlpine (1890–1981); (B) Nigel Compston (1918–1986); (C) Charles Lumsden (1913–1974); (D) Bryan Matthews (1920–2001).

Middlesex Hospital, London, where one of the neurology wards is named after him. After receiving the International Federation of Multiple Sclerosis Societies' first Charcot award, McAlpine wrote to one of his co-authors:

...the Charcot Award has come my way. Special praise was given in N.Y. to our first book. Without your constant help it would never have seen the light of day ... your letter shall be kept as a memento of our happy time together. You made me see light in matters that were then (and still some are) beyond my ken...

Receiving his medical education in Cambridge and at the Middlesex Hospital, Nigel Compston graduated in 1942 and served in the Royal Army Medical Corps. Despite the close association with Douglas McAlpine, which culminated in the publication of *Multiple Sclerosis*, his subsequent career was as a general physician at the Royal Free Hospital in London, where the clinical haematology ward is named after him. He was for many years treasurer of the Royal College of Physicians of London. His memorial in the College garden (after Wren) is: *Si monumentam requiris, circumspice* (if you need a monument [to the man] look around you).

Educated at Aberdeen University, Charles Lumsden learned the techniques of tissue culture and immunocytochemistry (with Elvin Kabat, see below) in the United States during the late 1940s after serving, amongst other places, in the Faroe Islands with the Royal Army Medical Corps. He applied laboratory methodologies to the study of demyelinating disease, publishing the first papers on experimental autoimmune encephalomyelitis from the United Kingdom. As Professor of Pathology in the University of Leeds, Lumsden was vigorous in his defence of pathology as the primary discipline of medicine. A shrewd but shy man, who painted and played the violin with distinction, he acquired the reputation for seldom changing his opinion since his position was not often wrong.

McAlpine accumulated clinical records on 1072 cases of multiple sclerosis, of whom a proportion were consecutive examples seen at onset, and these formed the basis for his clinical descriptions and classification of the disease. In summarizing features of the clinical course, McAlpine, Compston and Lumsden emphasized a number of special features – the symmetry of bilateral lesions, paroxysmal manifestations of demyelination, the predictable evolution of individual lesions according to anatomical principles, the variety of words used by patients to describe motor and sensory symptoms, early disappearance of the abdominal reflexes, the frequency of pupillary hippus (as distinct from the Marcus Gunn pupil, which curiously was not mentioned despite having been described in 1904), and occasional upper limb wasting (illustrated by Oppenheim in his textbook, first published in 1894) with absent tendon reflexes (also with Horner's syndrome in the case of patient WJ). Throughout, McAlpine and Compston relate their analyses to the lives and experiences of individual patients, placed in social context and identifiable to any archival scout by their initials and case numbers. McAlpine and Compston used classical neuroanatomical principles of fibre organization within the spinothalamic tract and dorsal columns to explain the march of sensory symptoms as inflammation (and demyelination) spread laterally through the laminations, and vertically to involve neighbouring segments. The authors dealt at length with features of the natural history that had not previously been described in such detail, pointing out the systematic reduction in relapse rate with time, the interval between the presenting and first subsequent attack depending on mode of presentation, the relationship between age at onset and the progressive course from onset, and aspects of prognosis – observations that were summarized in a much reproduced cartoon depiction of the course of multiple sclerosis (see Figure 1.2). Their differential diagnoses, organized by syndrome, addressed the complex relationship between cervical spondylosis and spinal cord demyelination, the nosological status of Devic's disease and acute disseminated encephalomyelitis (each considered distinct from but easily confused with multiple sclerosis) and emphasized the need for diagnostic caution in the context of a family history, especially when this involved a stereotyped phenotype amongst affected individuals.

In conversation, Nigel Compston was never in doubt that he carried the main burden of collating this information and writing the first manuscript version of *Multiple Sclerosis*. McAlpine was responsible for subsequent editions, working with Lumsden and (Sir) Donald Acheson, an epidemiologist later appointed Chief Medical Officer to the Department of Health in the United Kingdom. Soon after publication of the second edition (1972)

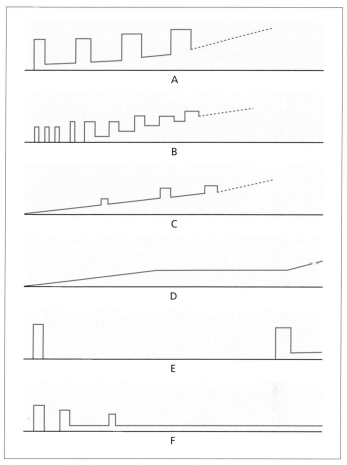

Figure 1.2 (A) Relapses with early and increasing disability. (B) Many short attacks, tending to increase in duration and severity. (C) Slow progression from onset, superimposed relapse, and increasing disability. (D) Slow progression from onset without relapses. (E) Abrupt onset with good remission followed by long latent phase. (F) Relapses of diminishing frequency and severity; slight residual disability only. From McAlpine *et al* (1955) with permission.

McAlpine approached one of us (WIMcD) with a view to him taking over the role of clinical author. McDonald felt that the time was not right. After the death of both McAlpine and Lumsden, the publishers handed over editorship of *Multiple Sclerosis* to Bryan Matthews (1920–2001) for the 1985 edition with Acheson, Richard Batchelor and Roy Weller. Matthews also saw through the press a second edition of *McAlpine's Multiple Sclerosis* (1991) with (Dame) Ingrid Allen, Christopher Martyn and the present editor. He contributed to the third edition published in 1998.

Quintessentially whimsical and dry to the point of dehydration, Bryan Matthews brought natural charm and personal diffidence to his dealings with patient and profession, securing the admiration and deep affection of both fraternities (Figure 1.1D). Matthews combined rich clinical experience of neurological disease with original research contributions; these credentials together with a marvellous literary style made famous his writings on neurology. He is most often quoted for his world weary but nonetheless affectionate opening to *Practical Neurology*:

there can be few physicians so dedicated to their art that they do not experience a slight decline in spirits on learning that their patient's complaint is of dizziness

The son of the Dean of St Paul's, and brought up in a strict household with a nanny who doubled as a lion tamer, Matthews was educated at Marlborough College and at Oxford. Appointed in 1954 as the only neurologist in a large area of England (based in Derby), he gained unrivalled first-hand experience of neurological disease and provided expertise in neurophysiology and neuroradiology. Later, he held academic appointments in Manchester and, as professor of neurology, in Oxford. He it was who perceived the need for surveillance of Creutzfeldt–Jakob disease (CJD) (his only comment during examination of the present editor's PhD thesis was to offer congratulations on incorrectly spelling both parts of that eponymous disorder), and made possible the study of bovine spongiform encephalopathy and variant CJD when these became major public health issues in the 1990s.

John Kurtzke (1988) has reviewed the history of diagnostic classifications in multiple sclerosis. We are also indebted to Charles Poser for additional observations and insights. Diagnostic criteria were originally introduced for epidemiological purposes in order to weight the diagnosis in the absence of pathological proof. In his 1931 survey of north Wales, Allison classified cases as typical; early (in which disseminated sclerosis was nevertheless the most likely diagnosis); impossible to assess through lack of adequate documentation; and doubtful because the symptoms and signs were inconclusive (Allison 1931). But the first attempt at criteria that could be used systematically was provided by Allison and Millar (1954) who classified disseminated sclerosis as: early (few physical signs but a recent history of remitting symptoms); probable (soon changed to early probable or latent: no reasonable doubt about the diagnosis); possible (findings suggesting the diagnosis and no other cause found but the history static or progressive and with insufficient evidence for scattered lesions); and discarded. Ten years later, Poser (1965) surveyed 109 neurologists working throughout the world, but mostly in North America, and found (predictably) that, using these criteria, certain cases presented greater diagnostic difficulties than others. The problems apparently did not reflect local medical cultural differences or the personal experience of individual practitioners. But until the mid-1980s, all surveys of multiple sclerosis continued to use the Allison and Millar criteria with some modifications within categories, including introduction of the term (clinically) 'definite' (Bauer *et al* 1965). Broman *et al* 1965 first sought to integrate the findings on cerebrospinal fluid examination into diagnostic criteria, providing three subclasses within each category of clinically probable, latent and possible multiple sclerosis. Weighting was dependent on typical, normal or atypical changes in an integral evaluation of immunoglobulin concentration, total protein and cell count. The principles developed by Kurtzke in classifying United States army veterans, on which consensus was later reached by a panel of examining neurologists, were formalized by Schumacher *et al* (1965), who categorized definite cases as showing objective evidence for disease affecting ≥ 2 white

matter parts of the central nervous system, occurring in episodes generally lasting >24 hours and separated by ≥ 1 month, or with progression over 6 months, in a person aged 10–50 years at onset, and in whom a competent observer could find no better explanation.

In *Multiple Sclerosis: a Reappraisal*, McAlpine *et al* (1972) focused on the difficult end of the diagnostic spectrum, defining latent probable multiple sclerosis as cases in which there was a history of relapsing–remitting symptoms and physical signs but little or no disability. Probable multiple sclerosis could be diagnosed when the symptoms were relapsing, the signs typical and the spinal fluid abnormal – ideally with normal myelography. Possible multiple sclerosis was used to describe cases with clinical evidence for white matter lesions, and no better explanation than multiple sclerosis to explain the condition. Further modifications adopted by Rose *et al* (1976) were revised definitions for probable multiple sclerosis (two episodes but signs at a single site or a single episode with signs of widespread disease) and possible disease (two episodes with no or few signs). The McDonald and Halliday (1977) criteria added a definition for proven multiple sclerosis (histological evidence from autopsy or biopsy), refined the early probable or latent category (two episodes and a single affected site or a single episode and two affected sites), and tackled in more detail the difficult issues of progressive probable (progressive history with multiple sites affected), progressive possible (progressive history affecting a single site), and suspected multiple sclerosis (one episode at a single site unless the optic nerves were affected). They introduced evoked potentials for the first time as paraclinical tests to aid in diagnosis. Further revisions suggested by Bauer *et al* (1980) were restriction of clinically probable multiple sclerosis to patients with a relapsing history but insufficient signs, or plenty of signs but only a single episode – the early probable and latent categories of McDonald and Halliday (1977) – with abnormal spinal fluid, and no better explanation. Clinically possible multiple sclerosis amounted to the history and signs of one episode affecting a single site but without spinal fluid information – and, still, no better explanation.

Against this background, the Poser committee introduced criteria that were widely accepted and provided a gold standard until the end of the millennium (C.M. Poser *et al* 1983). They incorporated information available from laboratory investigations within the categories of clinically definite and probable multiple sclerosis. These criteria gained widespread acceptance. The Poser criteria did not deal with suspected cases, and investigators therefore assigned this status to all patients thought to have demyelinating disease but without clinical symptoms, signs or laboratory evidence for >1 lesion. The evolution of these criteria for diagnosis and classification of the clinical course coincided with a busy phase of epidemiological studies in multiple sclerosis. Because cases were differently described, comparisons of these morbidity statistics are rather difficult. Adapting from the Allison and Millar classification to the Poser criteria does not materially affect estimates for the total number of identified cases, but differences do arise when surveys are restricted to the categories of definite and probable (Poser) and probable and early (Allison and Millar) cases, since the proportion in the suspected and possible categories needing exclusion differs significantly between the two systems. Some surveys have used the Poser criteria but ignored features such as age at presentation (normally between 10 and 59 years), many of the laboratory investigations now available for documenting the anatomical distribution of lesions, those providing evidence for mechanisms and consequences of the disease process, and the exclusion of conditions that mimic multiple sclerosis (see Chapter 8). Paty and Ebers (1998) added the concept of pseudorelapses, representing transient increases in the intensity of pre-existing symptoms occurring in the context of fever or other conditions known to alter the safety factor for conduction of the nerve impulse, but with rapid reversion to the previous status. New diagnostic criteria have recently been proposed and subsequently updated (McDonald *et al* 2001; see Chapter 7). These make use of laboratory investigations without discarding clinical context and common sense but strive to bring forward the point of diagnosis in the interests of informed prescribing and best clinical practice, whilst still minimizing the risk of erroneous diagnosis. Does any of this help? Much can be said for retaining the position of John Kurtzke (1974):

> *multiple sclerosis is what a good clinician would call multiple sclerosis.*

CLINICAL DESCRIPTIONS OF MULTIPLE SCLEROSIS: 1838–1915

More than any other branch of medicine, the practice of neurology uses the classical method of intuitive conversation, structured examination and selective investigation. This system evolved over several centuries, during which knowledge accumulated on structure and function, localization in health and disease, the reliability of physical signs and laboratory investigations, and nosology. A new knowledge of human anatomy was an early product of the scientific renaissance, which began at Padua where the Republic of Venice had its University. The background was as follows. The great Greek scholar John Bessarion, Bishop of Nicea and later Cardinal, had been sent to the West by the Emperor of Byzantium in 1438 to seek reunification of the Eastern and Western churches as part of a last desperate effort to avoid the collapse of the Byzantine Empire. Though the hierarchy agreed, the people did not and Constantinople fell in 1453. Bessarion, who had brought with him more than 800 manuscripts (over 600 in Greek), remained and gave the manuscripts to the Senate of Venice in 1468. Venice at this time was famous for its independence and the civil and religious freedom it guaranteed. As a result, scholars – both teachers and students – came to Padua from all over Europe. They read the works of Aristotle and Galen, which by the end of the 15th century were appearing in print. These writings enjoyed a new lease of life. Anatomy was as important to the philosophers and artists as it was to the surgeons. Leonardo da Vinci (1452–1519) had performed dissections, better to depict the external form of the body through an improved knowledge of its inner arrangements. But it was the young Flemish anatomist Andreas Vesalius (1514–1564) who provided the major advance with *De Humanis Corporis Fabrica* (Vesalius 1543), published when he was aged 28. Here, he gave the first accurate description and depiction of the human brain. Others borrowed, refined or distorted the details of his neuroanatomy, but the next milestone was the clinical descriptions of Thomas Willis in the mid-17th century.

Willis (1684) referred to his doctrine of the nerves as 'neurology'. Robert Whytt's account of neurology (1765) is psychiatrically flavoured – the distinction between nervous, hypochondriac and hysteric disorders being only the frequency and duration with which patients experience somatic manifestations of emotional states. And not until the 19th century did physicians systematically correlate knowledge gathered from pathological anatomy into systems of neurological disease. John Cooke (1756–1838) wrote a thorough history of contributions to clinical neurology from ancient times to modern (1820–1823) with sections on apoplexy, palsy and epilepsy, and in which he first drew attention to James Parkinson's description of the shaking palsy. Other textbooks in English, French and German soon followed. The contributions to an astonishing range of topics in clinical neurology attributable to Charcot were faithfully recorded and published by his students (1872–1887; translated 1877–1889). But where in all this clinical description does multiple sclerosis make an entry?

The lives of the saints contain reference to the restoration of sight in young women. Without prejudice as to the hagiographical relevance of such occurrences, it is natural to wonder whether some of these individuals may have had optic neuritis. But the scanty evidence precludes a diagnosis. The same is true in our view of the more complex case of St Lidwina of Schiedam (Medaer 1979). The virgin Lidwina fell whilst skating, thereby injuring her ribs and soon developing difficulty with walking. This persisted and other symptoms developed, including asymmetric loss of vision and sensation with bulbar failure, but the illness progressed from onset (with fluctuations relating to contact with Angels – we do not exclude the possibility that these were perhaps the genuine conduits for disease-modifying treatments) until her death aged 53 years in 1433. Margaret Cormack, supported by Poser (1995), has also suggested that the Icelandic saga of St Thorlakr represents an early case history of multiple sclerosis:

> *a woman lost the sight of both eyes and on the next day she lost her speech ... on the third day a candlewick was put around her head and she then recovered the sight of one eye and was able to open both ... on [Sunday] she recovered her speech and on the feast of St Michael ... the sight of the eye that has previously been blind*

Readers of the sagas untranslated favour the view that, in describing patients cured by the holy bishop of Skalholt under the heading of 'miraculum', and in support of his candidature for beatification, these were more probably cases of hysteria (Trygve Holmoy, personal communication 2001). A number of lay descriptions of the plight of individuals with paralytic illness appeared in the following centuries. They are reviewed by J. Murray (2004), who concludes that the cases of Margaret of Myddle (died January 1701) and William Brown, a Hudson's Bay trader of Scottish origin who developed weakness in the legs and visual disturbance in 1811, may well have had multiple sclerosis.

Giovanni Morgagni (1682–1771) first suggested classifications of pathological anatomy (1761), but not until the early 19th century were anatomical and clinical descriptions of neurological disease systematically correlated and illustrated. Charles Poser has brought to our attention a case reported from Leeds in

England having all the features of transverse myelitis, developing 6 days after measles and with full recovery (Lucas 1790). Turning to multiple sclerosis itself, it seems likely that Matthew Baillie (1820) in London and C.P. Ollivier (1824, 1827) in Paris would have included patients with this disorder amongst the cases of paraplegia which they discuss. Baillie (1820), for example, in a paper written to persuade colleagues that in some adult patients paraplegia was due to lesions in the brain wrote:

In adults ... paraplegia, I believe, depends most commonly in a great measure upon a disease affecting the brain itself ... Paraplegia in adults may take place at an early period of life, but more commonly occurs at the middle or more advanced age; it also occurs much more frequently in men than in women. Upon inquiry into the symptoms, some affection of the head will generally be discovered, either some feeling of pain in it, or giddiness... and the vision is often more or less impaired... Sometimes the sight of one eye is almost entirely lost... Sometimes the affection of the brain is marked by a defect in the memory and a want of the ready exercise of the general powers of the mind... Sometimes one or both of the upper extremities are affected more or less with numbness, and with feebleness in their motions... [there is] a sense of numbness in the lower limbs, with an impaired motion in them. At first there is only the appearance of some stiffness or awkwardness in the motions of the limbs, but in time the want of power of motion in the limbs and the inability to preserve the due balance of the body are very much increased, and the person cannot walk without the assistance of one or two sticks.... As the disease advances, the urine passes off more and more in a feeble stream and at length often passes away involuntarily. The bowels... are almost always costive, and at length ... the motions frequently pass off unrestrained by the will. Patients in this complaint will often live for many years, but most commonly the symptoms gradually increase and at the end of a few years they die with their constitutions entirely exhausted. In a few instances recovery takes place.

A convincing case is provided by Ollivier's *Observation XCIV*, which recounts the history of a man who first developed weakness in the legs aged 17, which remitted. He had a further episode aged 20 years, which also resolved. At 25 he again developed weakness of the legs with intermittent impairment of cutaneous sensation. He improved after several months and was able to walk for 45 minutes without resting. By the age of 29 the paraplegia was complete. He was unable to walk and the legs were numb and one or other arm intermittently so. The legs were thin. He was incontinent of urine. Again there was some improvement: he became able to walk alone and regained control of the bladder. The following year while at Digne he noticed that the high temperature of the waters produced much fatigue and an increase in the weakness of the lower limbs. At 31 he developed impaired sensation in the hands. Cold water felt hot. The right arm became weak and writing was difficult. There was then little change until the age of 42 when he gradually developed flexion contracture of the right forearm and hand, which was accompanied by 'very marked rigidity of the muscles'. Three years later the left arm became weak, becoming completely paralysed within about a year. Respiration became difficult and the voice weak. There was little change over the next eight years. At 50 (the year before the publication of Ollivier's book) there was paralysis of the arms and legs with preservation of sensation though he had pain in a sciatic distribution. He had spasms of the limbs, was constipated and micturition was largely involuntary. Nevertheless, his intellectual faculties were preserved, his conversation pleasant, and nothing lost of the gaiety of his character.

An equally persuasive case, and the earliest we have encountered, is that of Thomas Crichton, described by Abernethy (1809) and again by MacKenzie (1840).

Aged twenty three [he] was admitted into St Bartholomew's Hospital on account of a palsy of his limbs ... in the course of six months his lower extremities became affected with occasional twitchings, and he found that he could not distinguish their motions in walking: this increased to such a degree as to make him incapable of taking any exercise. He had, at the commencement of his illness, a confusion on vision, and a constant and violent pain in the head. The former symptom increased so much, that he could discern no object distinctly: a candle, for instance, although held near to him, appeared as large as the moon. The sensation of his lower extremities continued perfect; but the actions of the bladder were no longer under the control of the will; the urine sometimes flowed involuntarily; and, at others, being retained for some hours, with considerable pain. He afterwards began to lose the use of his upper extremities: the left hand and arm were more affected than the right; but there was no difference in the affection of the leg on the same side. His speech, also, became much impaired; he hesitated and faltered considerably, and the tones of his voice were irregular, so that, at length, he could scarcely make himself understood.

We find it difficult to substantiate the claims made on behalf of Richard Bright (J. Murray 2004), Gabriel Andral (W.A. Hammond 1871) or Marshall Hall and John Abercrombie (S.A.K. Wilson 1940) also writing in the 1820s. The first separate work on neuropathology (R. Hooper 1826), attempted a classification (inflammation, tumour, diseased structure and unnatural appearance without tumefaction, and fluid collected around the hemispheres or extravasated) with descriptions of diseases as they affect the meninges, brain, nerves, blood vessels and sinuses. Hooper's *Illustrations of the Morbid Anatomy of the Human Brain and its Membranes* was reissued under a different title in 1828, the author offering those who had already purchased the (1826) loose sheets the privilege of exchange without additional expense. In his otherwise excellent history of neurology, Lawrence McHenry (1969) initiates a serious gaffe in claiming that Hooper's plate 4 illustrates the appearances of multiple sclerosis (citing the 1828 printing). In fact, this is a reference to plate 4 of Carswell's atlas (Carswell 1838; see below) an error that has been extensively copied, notably by Dr J.D. (Jerry) Spillane in his magnificent *The Doctrine of the Nerves* (Spillane 1981). McHenry reproduces a plate showing intracerebral and pontine haemorrhages, and a subdural haematoma but this is from Carswell. That said, not all Hooper's plates were published. The originals together with proof copies of the published versions were purchased at auction by Professor Greenfield of

Edinburgh and eventually found their way into the collection of Sir William Osler (1929). They were bequeathed to the Medical Faculty of McGill University, Montreal, but that archive does not contain any illustration suggestive of the lesions of multiple sclerosis.

It is against this background that the first depiction of the lesions of multiple sclerosis can be considered. Jean Cruveilhier's *Anatomie pathologique du corps humain; descriptions avec figures lithographiées et coloriées; des diverses alterations morbides dont le corps humain est susceptible* is usually found in two volumes bearing the title dates 1829–1835 and 1835–1842, respectively (Cruveilhier 1829–1842). The 40 separate livraisons had started to appear from 1829, which accounts for variation in the date given for publication of Cruveilhier's illustrations of multiple sclerosis. Volume 1 contains livraisons 1–20, and volume 2 numbers 21–40. Livraison 32 plate 2 and livraison 38 plate 5, both in volume 2, depict the lesions of multiple sclerosis. Their publication date cannot have been 1835, as claimed by Charcot and faithfully reproduced by others, and is obviously much later (D.A.S. Compston 1988, Putnam 1938). The rival claim for priority is Carswell's *Pathological Anatomy; Illustrations of the Elementary Forms of Disease* (Carswell 1838) in which plate 4 figure 1 shows 'a peculiar diseased state of the cord and pons varolii', which modern commentators have interpreted as representing the macroscopic appearances of the lesions seen in multiple sclerosis. Charcot wrote (in the English translation by George Sigerson) for the New Sydenham Society:

disseminated sclerosis is mentioned for the first time in Cruveilhier's Atlas d'anatomie pathologique, 1835–42 ... in parts 22 and 23 you will observe representation of the lesions found in disseminated sclerosis and side by side you can read the clinical observations which relate to them... Previous to this epoch, so far as I am aware, there is no trace of disseminated sclerosis to be discovered anywhere. After Cruveilhier, Carswell in the article on atrophy contained in his atlas, 1838, has had lesions depicted which pertain to multiple sclerosis.

The reference by Charcot to parts 22 and 23 does not follow the collation of Cruveilhier's atlas in any of the copies to which we have access. Robert Carswell (1793–1857) studied medicine at the University of Glasgow and was later commissioned by Dr John Thompson of Edinburgh to make a collection of drawings illustrating morbid anatomy, in connection with which he spent 1822–23 at hospitals in Lyon and Paris. He returned to Paris after graduating MD in 1826 and remained there until 1831 by which time he had been appointed to the foundation Chair of Pathology at London University. For a while he studied with Pierre Louis in France, in order to complete the 2000 watercolours of pathological specimens, which he later personally engraved on stone in preparation of his pathological atlas. Carswell (1838) shows consummate artistry in use of the colour spectrum as organs affected by inflammation (pink), analogous tissues (crimson), atrophy (yellow and ochre: with the first illustrations of multiple sclerosis), hypertrophy (brown), pus (yellow and green), mortification (blue-black), haemorrhage (purple), softening (yellow), melanoma (jet black), carcinoma (orange and green) and tubercle (back to red) are pictured and described. We do not know the names of the patients with

multiple sclerosis depicted by Carswell and he never saw them in life. One was under the care of Monsieur Louis in the hospital of La Pitié and the other under Monsieur Chomel at La Charité (Figure 1.3A,B). In his preface to the atlas, dated 15th December 1837, Carswell indicates that he intended 12 fascicles to be included, and implied that these had been produced serially. Instructions to the binders show that the order of production was the reverse of that in which the fascicles would appear in book form so that the section on atrophy, which appears fourth and contains the depictions of multiple sclerosis, was evidently one of the last to be prepared. However, Putnam (1938) has pointed out that this plate has at the foot 'R Carswell ad nat del: Day and Haghe Lith^{rs} to the King' and, unlike illustrations from some of the later fascicles, which are signed 'Drawn on stone by Dr Carswell. A Ducotes. Lithog^r 10 St Martins Lane', it must have been prepared before June 1837 – since that was the month in which William IV died and was succeeded by Queen Victoria. Haghe failed to reverse the disposition of the lesions on the surface of the medulla but was otherwise faithful to Carswell. Plate 4, figure 4 and the corresponding legend depict and describe a brownish patchy external discoloration of the midbrain, pons, cerebellum and spinal cord. In the accompanying text Carswell writes:

I have met with two cases of a remarkable lesion of the spinal cord accompanied with atrophy. One of the patients was under the care of Mr Chomel in the hospital of La Charité; both of them affected with paralysis. I did not see either of the patients but I could not ascertain that there was anything in the character of the paralysis or the history of the cases to throw any light on the nature of the lesion found in the region of the spinal cord. I have represented the appearances observed in one case in plate 4 (figure 4).

The cases illustrated by Carswell were therefore observed by him not later than 1831, may have first appeared in a fascicle produced in 1837, and were published in book form in 1838.

Jean Cruveilhier of Limoges (1791–1874) elected to study medicine under Dupuytren in Paris soon after entering the priesthood. He graduated in 1811. Twice Cruveilhier failed to secure appointments as surgeon to the City Hospital in Limoges, despite meanwhile having taken the chair of operative surgery in Montpellier. He was appointed in 1825 to the professorship of anatomy in Paris. Subsequently he held the first Chair of Pathology in the Faculty of Medicine, provision for which had been made in Dupuytren's will. He remained in Paris, benefitting from material at the Salpétrière and the Musée Dupuytren until the siege of Paris (1870–71) when he moved to his country estate at Succac near Limoges, dying there in 1874 aged 83 years.

The many surviving copies of Cruveilhier's atlas exist either with the livraisons bound sequentially by number, each containing a heterogeneous collection of plates and clinical descriptions, or rearranged by subject with the plates interleaved in varying order presumably at the whim of individual collators (Figure 1.4A–C). The case illustrated in livraison 32, plate 2, figure 1 (Figure 1.4B) had died in the Salpétrière but the name, dates and details are not given. The same is true for another unnamed female patient illustrated in figure 2. In the accompanying text, Cruveilhier uses, for the first time, the term *grise*

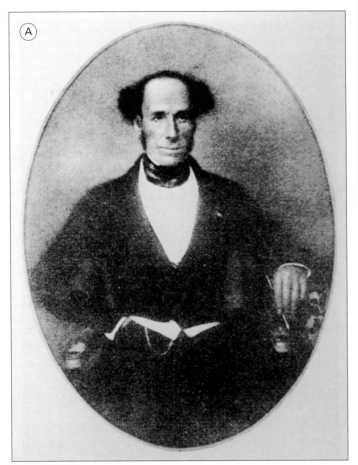

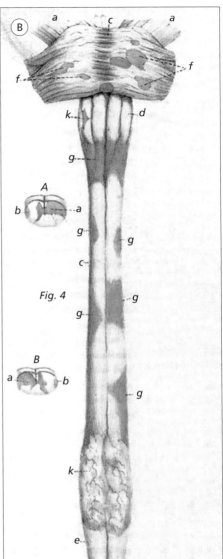

Figure 1.3 (A) Robert Carswell (1793–1857). (B) *f:* Isolated points of the pons varolii of a yellowish-brown colour. *g:* Patches of the same kind on the spinal cord, all of them occupying the medullary substance, which was very hard, semitransparent and atrophied. The atrophy was more conspicuous in some points than in others and is particularly well seen in the figure at *h* where it affects the right olivary body. *k:* Softening of a portion of the cord. *A* and *B* represent transverse sections of the cord to show that the discoloration commences on the surface of the white and extends inwards to the grey substance. From Carswell (1838).

masses disseminées. Cruveilhier's figure 3 shows the case of Madame Gruyer, a 43-year-old embroiderer who had a severe movement disorder, likened to chorea. She spent 2 years as a patient at the Hôpital Necker under the care of Laënnec and 10 years at the Salpétrière. His figure 4 depicts the brain and spinal cord of Darges (aged 37) whose clinical condition was that of a pseudobulbar palsy. In seeking to establish the date of publication of this livraison, some importance should be attached to the case of Femme Cherpin (in whom the lesions illustrated do not resemble those of multiple sclerosis; figure 6). She occupied bed number 8 in St Gabriel ward up until at least 15th September 1838. The text of livraison 32 also mentions another patient alive on 30th November 1838, and cites a publication dated 1839. This dates the appearance of livraison 32 as not earlier than 1839. Livraison 38, plate 5 (Figure 1.4C), illustrates the

case of Josephine Paget who was blind, paraplegic and had severe proprioceptive sensory loss mimicking locomotor ataxia. She was in bed 16 of St Joseph ward at La Charité on 4th May 1840 and died on 20th March 1841. Another patient described in this livraison was alive in August 1841, and Marshall Hall's *Diseases and Derangements of the Nervous System* (M. Hall 1841) is cited in the text. In short, based on the clinical details provided, alternative diagnoses could be suggested for the cases described in livraison 32 whereas the evidence for multiple sclerosis is more compelling for Josephine Paget. Her case history, and hence livraison 38 itself, cannot have appeared until 1841.

Did Carswell and Cruveilhier meet in Paris between 1826 and 1831, after which the former returned to London? It seems coincidental that two pathologists working from the same pool of material in the same city at the same time should

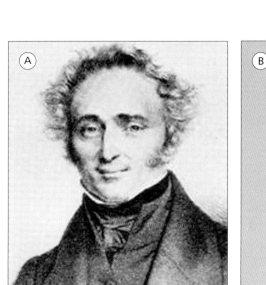

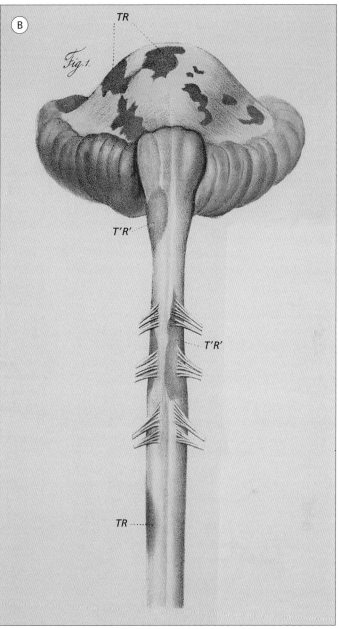

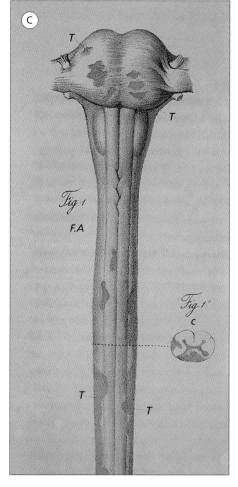

Figure 1.4 (A) Jean Cruveilhier (1791–1874). (B) Reddish grey islets, *TR*, on the protuberantia and cerebellar peduncles. Other reddish-grey islets, *T'R'*, *T'R'*, *T'R'*, on the anterior and lateral aspects of the medulla. Other reddish islets, *TR*, *TR* are visible on the posterior aspects of the medulla: the roots rising at the level of these islets are atrophied. *Fig. 2* shows the posterior aspect of a medulla belonging to another subject; it shows exactly the same change, i.e. a grey transformation by disseminated masses, *TG*, *TG*. (C) *Figs 1 and 1'* show us a new example of this lesion of the medulla which I have described (see livraison xxxii) under the name grey degeneration or transformation of this organ. From Cruveilhier (c.1841).

independently describe the same new disease. Although there is a striking similarity in the distribution of lesions affecting the pons illustrated by Carswell and by Cruveilhier in livraison 38 plate 5, Josephine Paget was alive at the time of publication of Carswell's atlas, so it cannot be the same case illustrated in each pathological work. After Cruveilhier, it is generally held that Frerichs (1849), writing in German, first described pathological features of multiple sclerosis in patients whom he had observed in life. Subsequently, his student Valentiner (1856) reported two cases in which relapse and remission were first emphasized as cardinal features of the disease and the presence of cognitive symptoms also noted. The first patient was a 21-year-old man who presented in 1853. The next year he developed a hemiplegia followed soon after by mental symptoms with a stuporous loss of interest. He died within 2 years of onset and the autopsy showed numerous different sized greyish-red patches with jagged contours. The second case was a woman aged 20 who, in 1850, developed weakness of the right leg that progressed to a paraparesis. She improved but 2 years later developed dysarthria and altered sensation. She died within 3 years of onset, and similar pathological features were noted from which Valentiner concluded:

> to what extent the relative remissions of single symptoms represent a recovery of diseased brain regions cannot be stated as our lack of understanding of the localization of certain central functions as well as of the nature of the disease process forbid any reflection on this.

Charcot was aware of at least three patients with *sclérose en plaques* in whom symptoms had begun in 1855 (see Ordenstein 1868 [*obsérvations* III and VII], Babinski 1885a [*obsérvation* VIII]), and was particularly struck by the clinical appearance of a maid employed in his house whom, initially, he thought had Parkinson's disease (cited by Bourneville and Guerard 1869). Three cases were presented to the *Société Médicale des Hôpitaux* on 9th May 1866. Alfred Vulpian (1826–1887) was the sole author of the report, which appeared in parts, but the third of these makes clear that the paper was read by Charcot (Vulpian 1866). In the first sentence Vulpian reminds his readers that it was Charcot who had described sclerosis of the lateral columns to the society in the previous January (actually it was on 8th March 1865; Charcot 1865). Within a few years, Charcot had gathered together the early descriptions so effectively, adding his own clinical and pathological observations (Charcot 1868a; 1868b; 1877), that the condition was named eponymously after him by Julius Althaus in 1877. However, Charcot must be declared a poor historian. It is a shame that, in the attempt to emphasize his own contributions and those of fellow Frenchmen, published versions of his lectures are disingenuous with respect to the contributions of non-Francophones (see above). These irritations apart, whereas others merely depicted and described aspects of the pathology or made clinical observations, Charcot recognized multiple sclerosis as a distinct entity. He gave it nosological status, made accurate clinicopathological correlations, emphasized its frequency, speculated on the pathophysiology, and always despaired of effective treatment.

Charcot's contributions are in making the story coherent, but on either side of his publications from the late 1860s are not only the important pathological depictions of Carswell (1838) and Cruveilhier (c.1841, with clinical details) but also Rindfleisch (1863) – who described multiple sclerosis as a chronic inflammatory process with three cardinal pathological features: vascular alterations, loss of myelin with preservation of axons and a scarlike 'metamorphosis of the tissue' – and case reports in German (Frerichs 1849; Valentiner 1856) and in English from the United Kingdom (Anon. [Moxon] 1873), Australia (Jamieson 1886; A.K. Newman 1875), the United States (W.A. Hammond 1871; Seguin *et al* 1878) and Canada (Osler 1880). It has been remarked that, despite his emphasis on the disease, Charcot only collected 34 cases throughout his professional career (Sherwin 1957). To us, this seems no mean achievement and it is a mark of Charcot's international influence that a disease that merited individual case reports in the 1870s had become one of the commonest reasons for admission to a neurological ward by the turn of the century – almost certainly an epidemic of recognition rather than the effect of altered biological factors, and a phenomenon that may itself have relapsed and remitted down the years (see Chapter 2).

By 1877, when physicians started to refer to Charcot's disease, the disorder was well known to neurologists working in the United Kingdom and case reports had appeared under the name of 'insular sclerosis' in the *Lancet* on 15th February 1873, 3rd and 17th April and 1st May 1875 (Anon. 1873; 1875a; 1875b; 1875c). All but one of these patients was under the care of Dr Walter Moxon (1836–1886) at Guy's Hospital (the other was communicated to a meeting of the Clinical Society of London by Dr Thomas Buzzard) and presumably Moxon wrote the case reports. In Ireland, a patient of Sir Christopher Nixon was shown at autopsy to have lesions of disseminated sclerosis (Nixon and McSweeny 1893); Tweedy (1894) diagnosed in life a confirmed case of insular sclerosis with extensive lesions in the spinal cord and brainstem. As in the cases described by Moxon, sexual habits and domestic activities were blamed for precipitating the neurological disease.

On 4th December 1867, Dr J.C. Morris presented the case of the late Dr C.W. Pennock to a meeting of the College of Physicians of Philadelphia. From 1843, Pennock had developed progressive disturbances of sensation and motor function in the limbs with sphincter involvement. Silas Weir Mitchell (1829–1914) provided the pathological description of multiple grey lesions (Morris 1868), likely to have been the first description of cortical involvement. A number of cases also appeared in Hammond's *Treatise on Diseases of the Nervous System* (W.A. Hammond 1871). Hammond's account precedes by a number of years the two case reports of Seguin *et al* (1878) and his subsequent description of patients having the combination of severe bilateral optic nerve (or chiasmal) and spinal cord demyelination (Seguin 1880). Seguin is usually credited with describing the first cases from North America and this may be because Hammond allowed confusion to contaminate his otherwise precise clinical observations. The growing awareness of multiple sclerosis as a common disorder of the central nervous system – and the effects of increased access to specialist neurological care, alterations in nosology, and changing concepts of neurological disease amongst females as driving forces in this emancipation of multiple sclerosis in the United States between 1870 and 1950 – are usefully summarised by Talley (2005). Multiple sclerosis was demonstrated at autopsy in Canada by William Osler (1880) and he also diagnosed a number of cases in life.

Evidently, scrutiny of the 786 autopsy records made by Osler at the Montreal General Hospital reveals one definite and two possible examples, providing an estimate for disease frequency (c.1:800) suggesting that multiple sclerosis may not have increased much in incidence over the last 100 years (Ebers 1985a). Dr Alfred Newman (1875) brought the existence of insular sclerosis to the attention of Australian neurologists, retrobulbar neuritis having already been described by MacLaurin (1873). But the first unambiguous Australian case was reported by Jamieson (1886), one of whose patients with 'multiple neuritis' had features that led Frith (1988) to concur with Jamieson that this was a genuine example. After a flurry of further case reports, Flashman and Latham (1915) published a detailed clinicopathological description of multiple sclerosis that set the scene for the experimental and investigative work that has since appeared from Australia.

PERSONAL ACCOUNTS OF MULTIPLE SCLEROSIS: 1822–1998

Down the years artists, poets, authors and ordinary people have left personal accounts of what it is to have multiple sclerosis. These provide telling accounts of the impact made by this quintessentially poignant disease on the sufferer's personal life – appreciation of which by the physician is a prerequisite for sympathetic management. The most comprehensive narrative is also the earliest, contained in two manuscripts archived at the Royal College of Physicians of London. The first is entitled 'The Case of Augustus d'Este'. It was edited and published by Douglas Firth (1948). The second is an unpublished personal diary beginning about 2 years before d'Este's death. Firth was in charge of the Blind School Hospital at Leatherhead in England during the Second World War and it was there, in 1942, that through Firth's interest in old papers he rescued and later published the 72 pages which remained after pilfering and the attentions of rats and human agencies of the diary and almanac written by various secretaries and d'Este between 1822 and 1846.

Augustus d'Este (Figure 1.5A,B) was born on 13th January 1794, inconveniently soon after his parents – Lady Augusta Murray and Prince Augustus Frederick, Duke of Sussex (sixth son of George III of the House of Hanover) – had met in Rome. The further details of that unhappy liaison are described elsewhere (W.I. McDonald 2002) and need not be told here other than to report that the King, acting on the grounds that the union of descendants is invalid without Royal Consent, caused the marriage (conducted in Rome and re-enacted in England during December 1793) to be annulled at the Court of Arches in August 1794, thus making the issue illegitimate. Augustus had a conventional childhood for the times. He was variolated against smallpox using Lady Mary Wortley Montagu's protocol, and suffered green stools, gripings and St Anthony's fire. His mother, with whom he lived, indulged Augustus's every whim and he seems to have behaved, during adolescence and as a young man, in a manner that gave the English aristocracy of the time a deservedly bad name. After studying at Harrow school, where he contracted measles on 26th February 1808, d'Este joined the VIIth Royal Fusiliers in 1812 and eventually reached the rank of Lieutenant Colonel. The case of Augustus d'Este opens thus:

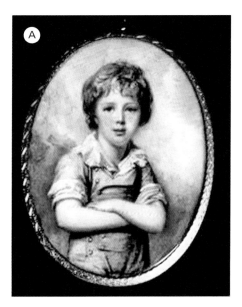

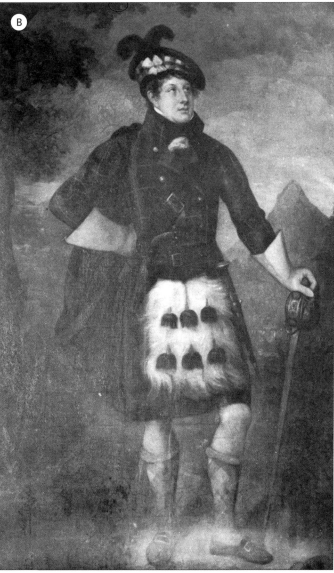

Figure 1.5 (A,B) Augustus d'Este (1794–1848).

illustration continued on following page

Figure 1.5, cont'd (C,D) Examples of the deterioration in d'Este's writing from 1830 and 1848.

1830. —

Whilst at Ramsgate I formed a liaison with a Young woman – I find in my acts of Connection a deficiency of a wholesome vigor – Thinking that possibly some

Page from diary, showing record of time spent in 'walking' and characteristic alterations in writing.

In the month of December 1822 I travelled from Ramsgate to the Highlands of Scotland for the purpose of passing some days with a Relation for whom I had the affection of a Son. On my arrival I found him dead. I attended his funeral – there being many persons present I struggled violently not to weep, I was however unable to prevent myself from doing so. – Shortly after the funeral I was obliged to have my letters read to me, and their answers written for me as my eyes were so attacked that when fixed upon minute objects indistinctness of vision was the consequence – Until I attempted to read, or to cut my pen, I was not aware of my Eyes being in the least attacked. Soon after, I went to Ireland and without anything being done to my Eyes, they completely recovered their strength and distinctness of vision ... In the month of January 1826 ... My Eyes were again attacked in the same manner as they had been in Scotland ... my Eyes again recovered ...

October 17th, 1827. To my surprise I there [in Venice] one day found a torpor of indistinctness of feeling about the Temple of my left Eye. At Florence I began to suffer from a confusion of sight – about the 6th of November the malady increased to the extent of my seeing all objects double. Each eye had its separate vision ... The Malady of my Eyes abated, I again saw all objects naturally in their single state ... Now a new disease began to show itself: every day I found gradually (by slow degrees) my strength leaving me ... At length about the 4th of December my strength of legs had quite left me, and twice in one day I fell down upon the floor ... I remained in this extreme state of weakness for about 21 days ... on the 21st January [1828] I was strong enough to begin a journey from Florence ... to Rome ... On the journey I was able to walk up some steep Hills ... I rode out on horseback most days, and my strength gradually returned. I never was able to run so fast as formerly, nor could I venture to dance.

Thus, on this last occasion, recovery or remission, which had been complete following the first two episodes, was only partial. Further relapses occurred, some with incomplete remission. In 1830, at the time Carswell and Cruveilhier were studying in Paris, d'Este discovered, on a visit to the seaside resort of Ramsgate in southern England, that he was impotent (Figure 1.5C). There were episodes of incontinence. By 1843 he recorded that:

When standing or walking I cannot keep my balance without a Stick... About the 16th of December I returned to London from Brighton in consequence of again considering, that, from the searching quality of the Sea Air, I was gradually becoming less capable of taking exercise.

It is clear by this stage that, after an initial relapsing and remitting course, d'Este was entering the secondary progressive phase of the disease. On 20th January 1846, he recorded:

I have regained some of my Strength ... but then ... I suffer very much indeed from sharp Spasmodic pains in my Feet and Legs ... my Sensations seem to be awful Indicators that some very sad Change has taken place, or is taking place in my System ... For the last 12 months ... my Hands have become slightly sufferers from my Disease

In 1847, d'Este recorded meticulously in a Gentleman's Almanac his determined efforts to keep mobile. His deficit was accumulating. On the 18th and 22nd August he noted:

Alas! Only walk in my Room $14\frac{3}{4}$ minutes ... Alas! Alas! during this week I only walk for 2 Hours and 33 Minutes.

But as all such patients notice, there were variations from day to day. On 1st September he walked for $22\frac{1}{4}$ minutes, on the 2nd for 65 minutes without having to lie down at all during the day, but on the 4th for only 6 minutes. A possible hint of cognitive impairment can be detected when he records on 12th December:

I go to My Sister's Church. A Stranger does Everything – Alas! I cannot follow him. I believe that there was Good in his Sermon.

By this time his handwriting had deteriorated, as can be seen by comparing the working copy of his 'Case' for 1830 (Figure 1.5C) with an entry for 1848 (Figure 1.5D). The last entry was in February and he died in December 1848 aged 54 years having had multiple sclerosis for 26 years – initially with relapses and remissions but with the onset of secondary progression for at least the last decade of his life.

It is significant that historians disagree on the nature of the neurological illness from which Heinrich Heine died in 1856, aged 59 years. Macdonald Critchley (1969) diagnosed neurosyphilis. Schachter (1933) and Ernest Jellinek (1990) consider that Heine had multiple sclerosis. Traditionally, these conditions are the great mimickers of other neurological diseases. Heine was a poet whose work was much used by composers of *lieder* (Brahms, Liszt, Mendelssohn, Schubert, Schumann and Wolf), opera (Wagner) and ballet (Adolphe Adam and Werner Egk). Egk whose 1948 work *Abraxas*, with scenarios based on the writings of Heine, was banned by the Bavarian Minister of Culture after five performances on the grounds of obscenity (Krellmann 1980). Like d'Este, good family connections and a comfortable living enabled him to lead a somewhat erratic social and matrimonial life which, when his medical symptoms began, caused him to conclude that they were due to 'one of those illnesses which Germans suffer who privatize abroad'.

From the age of 35, Heine had intermittent neurological symptoms that can be interpreted as recurrent demyelination affecting the optic nerves and brainstem, followed 10 years later by bulbar symptoms and hemisensory and motor disorders with impaired sphincter function. He was bed-bound for the last 8 years of his life due to progressive tetraplegia with spasms, from which he took solace with increasing doses of opium. He was attended amongst others by Julius Sichel, who had already linked amaurosis with disorders of the spinal cord (Sichel 1837), and provided an early colour illustration of optic atrophy (Sichel 1852–59) but the disc illustrated is not from Heine's fundus.

Until the publication of Augustus d'Este's diary, the best known personal account of multiple sclerosis was *The Journal of a Disappointed Man* published on 31st March 1919 by Bruce Frederick Cummings, who wrote under the pseudonym W.N.P. Barbellion (Figure 1.6). The surname was taken from the Bond Street branch of a London sweet shop chain and the initials

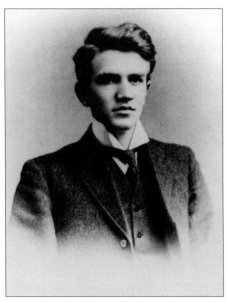

Figure 1.6 Bruce Cummings (1889–1919) (aka W.N.P. Barbellion). Kindly provided by Eric Bond Hutton.

stood for Wilhelm Nero Pilate – the world's three greatest failures (Eric Bond Hutton, personal communication). Despite developing symptoms due to multiple sclerosis in early adult life, and dispirited by the example of his parents who had both had paralytic neurological disorders, Cummings taught himself entomology and obtained a post at the Natural History Museum. The final entries of Barbellion's diary read:

October 12th ... I am only twenty eight, but I have telescoped into those few years a tolerably long life: I have loved and married, and have a family; I have wept and enjoyed, struggled and overcome, and when the hour comes I shall be content to die. October 14th to 29th: miserable. October 21st: self disgust. Finis. [Barbellion died on December 31st (1917)].

In fact, he was far from dead on New Year's Day in 1918. Barbellion had aped Mark Twain in ensuring that news of his death was announced prematurely so that he might enjoy reading posthumous notices of his book. However, his diary was declared 'an acerbic bid for immortality, written by a smart alec rotter', and he only enjoyed his literary fantasy for 18 months, dying aged 30 on 22nd October 1919 at Gerrards Cross. Others have suggested that he accelerated his illness by following contemporary advice to take arsenic and strychnine on a weekly basis. H.G. Wells identified the egoist in Barbellion but – himself an incurable scientific romantic – sympathized with the hopelessness of Barbellion's thwarted scientific dreams:

not for him the Croonian lecture, the listening Royal Society

although Barbellion did publish articles endorsing the statement that, through illness, biological science lost one of its most promising recruits. On 26th April 1913, aged 24, Barbellion first records that his speech and right side are impaired and believes that he must have locomotor ataxy. He saw a well-known nerve specialist (Dr H[ead]), who seems to have had

similar suspicions. Barbellion had what we would easily recognize as symptoms of demyelination but over the next 2 years, despite seeing several neurologists, he remained without a diagnosis until, on attempting to enlist in November 1917, he read on the certificate in the sealed envelope issued by his doctor that multiple sclerosis had been diagnosed at presentation and communicated to his family. He looked up Risien Russell's chapter on the disease in Clifford Allbutt's *System of Medicine*. For Barbellion, learning the true nature of his illness placed him in a detached and rather relaxed state, released (or so he claimed) from his former self-obsession and ambition. Temporarily restored to health, he began again to contemplate a number of zoological projects but he ran from the library, after coming across 'an enormous quarto memoir in the *Trans. Roy. Soc. Edinburgh* on *The Histology of [Disseminated Sclerosis]*' – James Dawson's great work (see below). Increasingly troubled by alternating hemipareses and disturbed sensation in the hands, Barbellion showed good neuroanatomical sense, but a more speculative approach to aetiology, in telling his diary (January 1917) about 'the millions of bacteria gnawing away [his] precious spinal cord'.

Whatever its nature, the process of demyelination did continue and the latter part of Barbellion's diary contains a mixture of nostalgia for his past excursions (literary and field) into natural history, some critical self-analysis, and comparisons between his own condition and that of ordinary healthy people, rehearsing internal and bitter dialogues from which he gained some strength:

I do not envy you your absorption in the petty cares of a commonplace existence.

The real Bruce Frederick Cummings died finally on 22nd October 1919, aged 30 years, at Camden Cottage, Tatling End, Gerrards Cross, in what was once a public house (the Tatling Arms), and is now a Chinese restaurant (Eric Bond Hutton, personal communication).

Ill-health dogged another young scholar and painter in Edwardian England (Figure 1.7). In 1908, Jacques Raverat suffered fatigue and was unable to continue his undergraduate studies at Emmanuel College, Cambridge. He retained his student friendships and eventually married Gwen, Charles Darwin's grand-daughter. Despite manifesting a variety of neurological symptoms – ataxia and spasticity – and finding it increasingly difficult to match the activities of his wife and friends (André Gide, Rupert Brooke and the Keynes brothers, Maynard and Geoffrey), not until 1914 was the diagnosis of *une sclérose disseminées de la moelle épinière* made in his native France. Back in England, he saw Risien Russell (see above), prompting Geoffrey Keynes, who as a medical student had noticed Raverat's gait disturbance at onset in 1908, to write (somewhat confusingly) that he:

was particularly interested to hear of Risien Russell's diagnosis ... I should never have dared to diagnose disseminated sclerosis, because if that's what you've got, you are quite unlike any other case I've ever seen: but then it's rare, obscure, variable and best left to experts to deal with. Typically of course, it ought to be progressive; but not always. Certainly in your case, up to the time I last saw you, there had been no change for better or worse for a long while.

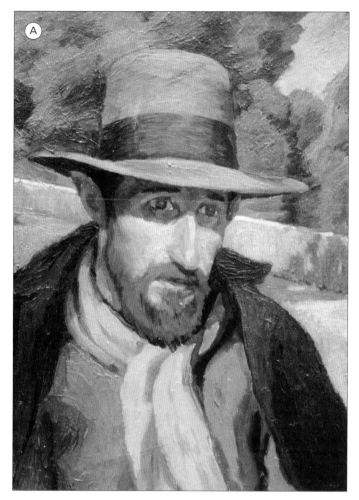

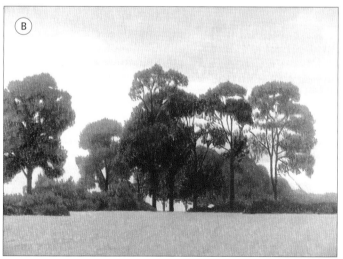

Figure 1.7 (A) Portrait of Jacques Raverat by his wife Gwen c.1924. (B) *Elm Trees and Cornfield* by Jacques Raverat c.1915. From *Gwen Raverat: Friends, Family and Affections*, by Frances Spalding, 2001. Reprinted by permission of the Random House Group Ltd.

By 1915, Raverat's walking had deteriorated. That year, Gwen became pregnant, apparently through artificial insemination (and again in 1919), suggesting that Raverat was impotent. Soon after, he took to using a donkey-driven bath chair. With declining mobility, Raverat admitted to André Gide that he was more absorbed in his painting than before he lost the use of his legs. The next few years were characterized by progressive loss of mobility and stepwise increase in disability during which he also consulted Henry Head but dismissed his advice, 'he wd. only tell me to rest and I am anyhow spending 18 hours out of 24 in bed' and also E.D. Adrian (1889–1977) who, now better known for his contributions to physiology (and Nobel prizewinner for physiology or medicine jointly with Charles Sherrington in 1932), had trained in neurology and was then working at the National Hospital, Queen Square, with shell-shocked patients. In 1922, Raverat lost function in his right hand and started painting with the left without losing effect according to contemporary critics. Raverat reflected on his physical decline to the author Virginia Woolf, complaining about André Gide's lack of understanding for human nature, and adding that he felt:

not of life because I have lost almost every pleasure in the world. Not of death because I am still damnably capable of feeling pain. Please do not repeat this

and comparing his own drawn-out death with the swift demise of his friend Rupert Brooke. Gwen was barely coping with this death-in-life, and the marriage nearly foundered, but events moved swiftly and Raverat developed a series of bladder infections with further increase in weakness and disability. He enjoyed Virginia Woolf's *Mrs Dalloway* read to him from the proofs. But the situation was deteriorating. Whilst Raverat considered:

the condition of my life is such that I have not the advantages of either death or life ... I am still damnably capable of feeling pain. Thank God for morphine

for Gwen the vigil consisted of:

his [objections] to my drawing squiggle-wiggles on the blotting paper while I wait

so that on 6th March 1925 she seized a pillow and terminated Jacques Raverat's suffering (Pryor 2004; Spalding 2001).

The doctor as patient promises special insights into the subjective experience of multiple sclerosis. In her early 20s, Dr Janette Gould sequentially lost vision in both eyes, remembered an episode of weakness in one arm attributed at the time to neurasthenia, and experienced poor balance (J. Gould 1982). The effect of these undiagnosed complaints caused domestic strain and her marriage soon ended in divorce. When her vision again deteriorated, and it was suggested that she might see a neurologist, she recalled the illness, eventually diagnosed as multiple sclerosis, which had affected her late father. She describes the clumsy way in which her own diagnosis was established and eventually communicated, relief only being provided by a sympathetic general practitioner who allowed time for detailed discussion. Six years later, and with many impairments affecting aspects of daily living, she described displacing the reality of the illness with professional and social events. Trips and holidays planned around facilities for the disabled lacked challenge and yet certain sanitary arrangements were unarguably beneficial, allowing Dr Gould periodically to do new things. Her tone is positive, but the catalogue of impairments considerable, and the personal dividend from a few practical adjustments and kindnesses plain to see.

Sandy (Alexander) Burnfield qualified in medicine in 1968 from the London Hospital. However, as he describes in *Multiple Sclerosis: a Personal Exploration*, he had by that time already graduated as a patient having developed optic neuritis 3 years earlier and read the full implications of this diagnosis in the medical school library. As a newly qualified house officer he was confronted by the disease in the neurosurgical and neurological departments, and symptoms soon returned with the development of a useless dominant hand. Burnfield is critical of his initial management and the evasive tone of the neurologist with whom he first dealt, but praises Dr Stanley Graveson (at that time senior neurologist to the Wessex Neurological Centre in Southampton). During the early years of his training as a specialist in psychiatry, he experienced further relapses and developed persistent disabilities, although happily he remains well 40 years after presentation. Still full of optimism, Sandy now considers that he has an unusual optico-spinal form of multiple sclerosis; and his family history illustrates the transitional forms that we describe in Chapter 5 – an affected maternal aunt and maternal second cousin with a great grandmother who used a stick when young, a bath chair when older, and always had a stick to hand in old family photographs. Dr Burnfield considers himself lucky, with lesions confined to the optic nerves and spinal cord, and perhaps with some remyelination (see Chapters 10 and 13); his vision has improved, and a large paracentral scotoma on the right is now just an enlarged blind spot.

His is a beautifully crafted book marking the transition from an initial position of fear and uncertainty to acceptance, adjustment and confidence, describing the cathartic process with dignity. Much of the book is a readable account of the disease for lay persons but Sandy Burnfield orientates his journey with a personal philosophy established in part during psychoanalysis but based mainly on personal qualities, as those who have met him will attest. In chapters on coming to terms with multiple sclerosis, marriage under stress, fulfillment and self-respect, Dr Burnfield has left a personal account that is nonetheless valuable as a general manual for anyone dealing with multiple sclerosis.

Records also tend to be left of the lives of individuals whose contributions to cultural or literary life are curtailed by illness. One such was the British cellist Jacqueline du Pré (1945–1987). Menuhin (1996) has described the early recognition of her talent for the instrument that she wanted to play from the age of four, her precocious success leading to a first solo recital aged 16 at London's Wigmore Hall, and the initial public performance of Edward Elgar's cello concerto – the work with which she was most closely associated and that has, as a result, acquired special symbolism for the plight of the individual with multiple sclerosis (Figure 1.8). Jacqueline du Pré's meteoric rise was not associated with unqualified self-confidence, but this returned after a period of study with Mstislav Rostropovich and led to a brilliant 4-year period of performance with her husband, Daniel Barenboim. In October 1973, at the age of 28, she

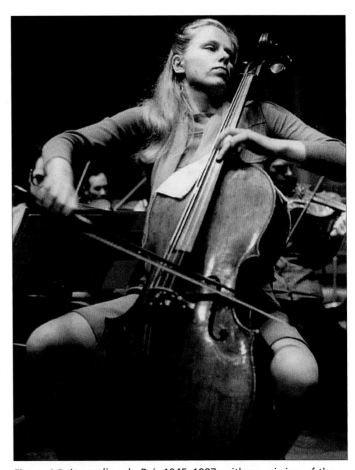

Figure 1.8 Jacqueline du Pré: 1945–1987, with permission of the Multiple Sclerosis Society.

developed symptoms due to multiple sclerosis and the condition soon interfered with her ability to perform. The illness was aggressive, resulting early in the need for a wheelchair, and she died in 1987, aged 42. Jacqueline du Pré is one of many ordinary people in whom multiple sclerosis abbreviated an extraordinary career. Multiple Sclerosis International Federation periodically awards a Jacqueline du Pré fellowship to young and talented investigators from underprivileged countries. Her story has subtly altered public awareness of the illness, at least in the United Kingdom, and recent revelations of the domestic consequences of her illness – described in biographical accounts of her own and her sister's families and in the stage play *Duet for One* and the film *Hilary and Jackie* – have not diminished the iconic status of what her husband considered 'simply one of the greatest musicians ever produced'. On what would have been her 60th birthday, 26th January 2005, BBC Radio 3 in the United Kingdom devoted an evening to the life and music of Jacqueline du Pré, and to increased public awareness of multiple sclerosis. Transcending the abbreviation of a playing career restricted to 10 years of fully active professional performances and recordings, and rising above the technical virtuosity and lyricism of her playing, were moving recollections and commentaries from friends and fellow musicians, and an analysis of her artistry, that continue to motivate those who experience multiple sclerosis and seek to solve the problem.

Also a performer, Vivien Neves, caused something of a stir when in 1971 the London *Times* published a full-page photograph of the *déshabillée* Ms Neves – prompting the *Sun* newspaper, for whom Vivien had regularly appeared, to congratulate its rival on having 'come abreast of the *Times*'. Much witty correspondence followed, for and against this departure from decorum, and the story became national news (in 1971). But in 1979, she developed multiple sclerosis and retired from page three, dying in relative obscurity in 2002.

In a different medium, Peter MacKarrell has left a record of what it is to have multiple sclerosis (MacKarell 1990). As an artist and illustrator, who held academic appointments at Goldsmith's College in south London, his reaction to the development of visual symptoms in 1980 (aged 47) was quickly to embark on a personal, and necessarily lonely, journey externalized in the form of a series of paintings that, in a surreal way (he calls it 'Joycean'), simultaneously depict the painter and his visualized world (Figure 1.9A–G). After a moderately long first remission during which he found difficulty in describing and recording some aspects of the visual experience of optic nerve demyelination, more obvious disabilities accumulated and, by their nature, these inhibited but did not prevent the execution of his works. The rapid evolution of unilateral visual loss over 3 days, and its subsequent recovery, are both depicted. Next, in the Avalon series (named after the boat he took to convalesce in Ireland), he aligned vertical half-circles, the normal left-sided hemifield juxtaposed with his amblyopic right-sided view in order to emphasize the paleness, blurring, bleached reds, impression of a blue filter, and perversions of normal visual illusions familiar to artists. His dominant (left) hand became paralysed early in 1987 and he spent the next several months in hospitals and at a home for the chronic young sick before adaptations allowed continued domestic care. This is where – blind, paralysed and unable to paint – he died towards the end of 1988. That summer, he had dictated a final account of his illness in which he began by summarizing the experience of deteriorating eyesight as 'I saw this' or, in Spanish (for it is taken from Goya), *Yo Lo Vi*. His attitude is one of adjustment and compensation as the gift of a set of coloured crayons brings home the truth that he can no longer distinguish the reds and greens. As conduction slowed in his optic nerves, verbal and other mental processes seemed to quicken. Neatly, MacKarrell elided his disappearing powers of vision with ideas on the sophistication of languages, which sought to distinguish the 11 colours of Burlin and Gray. In the paintings executed after recovering from the first episode of optic neuritis, he recalled deliberately emphasizing those hues, especially red, which he knew from medical consultations and experience selectively to be affected. Later, it proved necessary to modify his techniques still further as cervical cord demyelination forced a sinistral to dextral change in manual activity. However, his final statement, entitled *The Odyssey*, remains optimistic with plans for an active confrontation of deteriorating vision and motor control. A number of MacKarrell's paintings are in collections at Guy's Hospital and the Moorfields Eye Hospital in London.

Many other affected individuals, with and without well-developed artistic talents, have sought to depict the personal experience of having multiple sclerosis or the effect on their perceptions of colour and form; one such is selected from those generously presented by one of our patients (Figure 1.10). A sensitive and dignified account of multiple sclerosis and its impact on the physical activities of a young stage-set con-structor, portrayed in a short film by Emily Richardson of a journey by bicycle 'Coast to Coast' in the north of England, won a millennium award from the Multiple Sclerosis Society of Great Britain and Northern Ireland, and can be viewed at www.samuelmanual.org.uk.

The professional writer as patient offers a special opportunity to describe for others the personal experience of multiple sclerosis. In November 1982, soon after recovering from a phase of low personal confidence, Brigid Brophy (at the age of 53) tripped on leaving a restaurant and was briefly concussed. Several months later, she again noticed difficulty in raising her foot to cross a pavement and realized that the episode could not be dismissed as hapax legomenon (one-off). It was now undeniably a symptom that increasingly interrupted her walking. Encounters with the medical profession proved unrewarding and confrontational with undue emphasis on diet (insufficient protein and too much alcohol), venepuncture on the grand scale, irrelevant replacement of thyroid hormone, and long waits in clinics. Brophy (1987) tells one side of a story cataloguing administrative and clinical frustrations with which doctors are familiar and, with her vulnerable self-esteem, contrived a fictional version in which a figure in authority whose trade is scientific exactitude and for whom veracity is therefore never questioned, undermines an otherwise stable domestic relationship by sowing the seeds of mistrust. Eventually, transfer to a tertiary centre led to evoked potentials, brain imaging and spinal fluid analysis and she learned the diagnosis of multiple sclerosis. Resolutely opposed to research involving animal tissue, Brophy speculates on the cause of multiple sclerosis. Her daughter was tested for the 'genetic trait' at the Bramson Trust in Newcastle (for reference to this work, see Field 1989, and below) and found to be normal. She declares that the solution will emerge from computer modelling of answers to case–control epidemiological questionnaires, and her hunch is that an emotional shock in the 5 years before onset will be shown to be crucial. Soon requiring a wheelchair and other aids to daily living, Brophy deplores the dependence on others that this sporadically 'disgusting' disease imposes, and the slowing of functions that contaminates even those activities that do remain possible for an intellectual who writes. But, in the end, she settles for the Proustian strategy of rerunning remembrances of times past.

Ben Sonnenberg, born in New York in 1936, warns us in the subtitle of his autobiography that nothing had prepared him for the development of multiple sclerosis at the age of 34, although he too had a prolonged prodrome of diagnostic uncertainty despite medical attention (Sonnenberg 1991). On diagnosis, he immediately read the classical and more recent medical literature. By his own account, the conversion from relapsing–remitting disease to secondary progression and the need for two malacca canes did nothing to slacken the pace (or performance) of Ben Sonnenberg's serial approach to relationships with women. But, by 1978, he preferred ground-floor accommodation and soon was using an electric wheel-chair affectionately known as an 'Amigo'. He also read other personal accounts of multiple sclerosis. Sonnenberg is largely dismissive of these efforts but singles out Brigid Brophy's *Baroque-n'-Roll* and Barbellion's *Diary of a Disappointed Man* and *Last Diary*. All three developed metaphors for the poorly understood process affecting their nervous systems. Sonnenberg listened for:

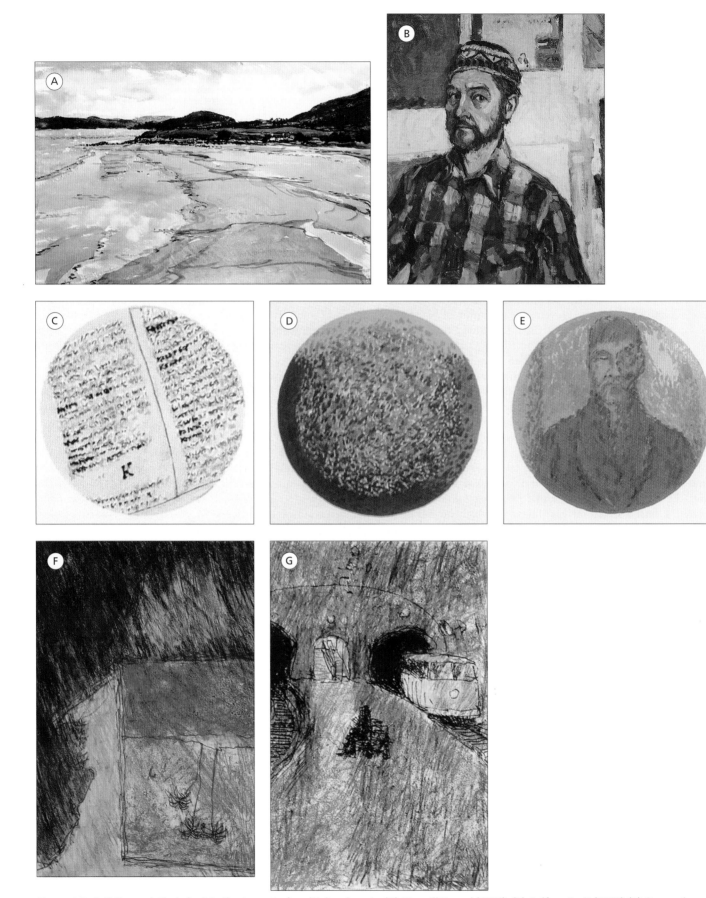

Figure 1.9 Artistic work that depicts the impact of multiple sclerosis. (A) *Stragill Sound* (1976). (B) *Self-portrait* (1978) (C) *Pageswim* (1980). (D) *The grey blanket* (1980). (E) *Portrait of the artist in a maroon dressing gown* (1980). (F) *The travel poster* (1986). (G) *The platform at Uncertain Street* (1986). From MacKarell (1990) with permission.

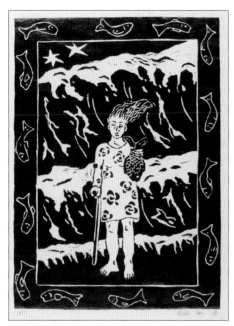

Figure 1.10 Multiple sclerosis: a self-portrait (unsigned).

the silent Virus or the still-as-a-stone Autoimmunity which
being long past [genetically predetermined] can be read like
Linear B only by cryptoanalysts.

And writing in the *Lancet*, Ellis (1998) also rehearses introspective images of a gnawed-at nervous system and the hoped-for
release from inexorable decline through the biology of repair:

ms
it was like his nerves
were dipped in pickling vinegar
piecemeal
starting at the periphery and spotting
in between
and it was changing
like a transforming request
a sensory overload
where some impulses make it
some don't
and that's the story
of his numbness
except that it felt like oatmeal
drying on the skin
only with oats you can see
where the damage is
they say that stress
could have started it
oh he could buy that story
and have pocket change
left over
it was enough to deal with on its own
merits
this moth
eating at the wool of his nerve endings
and the perplexing uncertainty
surrounding repair

THE SOCIAL HISTORY OF MULTIPLE SCLEROSIS

On 1st May 1945 there appeared a classified advertisement in
the *New York Times* that read:

> *Multiple Sclerosis. Will anyone recovered from it please
> communicate with the patient. T272 Times.*

In a letter to one of us (WIMcD) dated 4th May 1999, Ms
Sylvia Lawry (1916–2001) described the response:

> *The ad elicited one response I was hoping for. An anonymous
> letter arrived from a man in Philadelphia whose wife had
> been diagnosed 25 years ago, in Germany. She had never
> been told her diagnosis. She had been completely paralyzed.
> The woman was treated by Professor Otto Marburg. The
> treatment resulted in a reversal of all her symptoms, which
> never recurred. The writer stated that Professor Marburg
> was presently residing in New York, and was on the staff of
> the New York Neurological Institute. My brother and I
> visited with Professor Marburg. I showed him the letter from
> Philadelphia, and he recognized the writer. Professor
> Marburg stated that the medication administered to the
> woman was nicotinic acid, which helped some patients and
> not others. We agreed that my brother would undergo the
> treatment. In his case, it did not help. Information about
> this experience was shared with other respondents to the ad,
> who were mainly persons with MS or their relatives. They
> had urged me to share any positive information resulting
> from the ad. Emphasis on remissions helped to instill hope in
> persons with MS over the years, in the course of my activities.
> The factor of remissions was also encouraging to some in the
> scientific community, that MS was a pioneer field.*

The sharing of information continued. About a dozen of the
respondents to the advertisement met regularly. Already at
the first meeting they began to discuss setting up an organization
to support research. They needed medical advice. Sylvia Lawry
in her untiring searches of the medical literature frequently
encountered the name of Dr Tracy Putnam. At her request he
put together a medical advisory board from prominent neurologists throughout the United States. One of the initial scientific
awards was to Dr Charles Lumsden.

The organization, at this stage called the Association for the
Advancement of Research on Multiple Sclerosis, had four basic
missions:

- to coordinate research efforts on multiple sclerosis in the
  United States and abroad
- to gather statistics on the prevalence and geographic distribution of multiple sclerosis
- to act as a clearing house for information on the disease
- to collect funds to stimulate and support research on multiple sclerosis and allied diseases.

Ms Lawry again exercised her persuasive powers and was
given, free, a tiny room at the New York Academy of Medicine
as an office for the Association. Next she sought publicity for it
and approached Waldemar Kaempffert, the science editor of the

New York Times. He thought the time was not yet right and advised her to recruit a board of directors from lay figures whose names would create public confidence and gain the attention of the press. This she did, when possible selecting individuals who had personal experience of multiple sclerosis. Thus was established a pattern that persists to this day.

It became increasingly clear that there was a widespread need for support services for people with multiple sclerosis. Accordingly she set up local community-based chapters to provide services and to educate patients. They were to raise their own funds, 40% of which were to go to the central support of research. In July 1947, these changes were reflected in a change of name to the National Multiple Sclerosis Society.

Public familiarity with multiple sclerosis was still poor and lay understanding of the needs of sufferers limited. Ms Lawry therefore pressed for wider publicity. The most influential single person whose help she enlisted was Edward Bernays, Sigmund Freud's nephew. He was a pioneer in the public relations industry and an effective moulder of public opinion who numbered amongst his clients General Electric, General Motors and Time Incorporated. He advised her 'keep your eye on page one of the *New York Times*; the people who make page one are those you should go after' (Trubo 2001). This she did to great effect, numbering amongst her supporters politicians (John F. Kennedy), film stars (Shirley Temple Black) and industrialists (Henry J. Kaiser). Bernays joined the Society's national board in 1949 and guided it for the next 40 years, dying at the age of 103.

It soon became clear that similar organizations were needed in other countries. The first was founded in Canada (in August 1948), and the second in the United Kingdom (1953). Others followed and in 1967 the International Federation of Multiple Sclerosis Societies (now Multiple Sclerosis International Federation) was established by Ms Lawry and (Sir) Richard Cave.

In 1952, at the invitation of Lord Howard, Ms Lawry met Cave, a member of the senior legal staff of the House of Lords whose wife suffered from disseminated sclerosis, in the United Kingdom. As a result, the Multiple Sclerosis Society of Great Britain and Northern Ireland was founded in 1953, and Richard Cave served as chairman until 1976. The inaugural meeting was held at the Chenil Galleries in Chelsea, London, on 2nd December 1953 and the guest speaker was the Minister of Health, Mr Iain McLeod. Two consultant neurologists, present to answer questions, preferred to remain anonymous and are identified in the minutes only as Mr A and Mr B. They were Douglas McAlpine and Arnold Carmichael. Nicolson and Lowis (2002) provide an extensively researched account of the Multiple Sclerosis Society of Great Britain and Northern Ireland, setting out its turbulent early history and revealing social and ethical tensions that were ripe as biomedicine evolved in the second half of the 20th century. At first, the only members of the Society were Cave and McAlpine, who was asked to form a medical panel. He soon co-opted Charles Lumsden. Ambiguities immediately arose. The Society devolved responsibility for all opinions on treatment and 'cures', and granted complete autonomy, to the self-appointed medical panel group, who remained anonymous and unaccountable. Officers of the Society thereby granted deference to the 'magic circle of the great and the good at the top'.

They remained uninformed on methods and procedures underlying funding decisions and, unlike the Canadian and United States Societies, accepted the avuncular position of the medical panel that it should gently encourage but not directly sponsor research. In theory, this remained the province of the Medical Research Council. In the event, the panel's early excursions into research funding soon proved controversial. Lumsden received the first grant – supplementing his support from the National Multiple Sclerosis Society of the United States. There were immediate objections to the medical panel favouring 'yet another bio-chemist chasing up yet another nebulous round the corner cure'.

Cave successfully headed off this first of many attempts to reinvest power in the General Council. For a while, the medical panel remained self-regulating and isolationist with respect to non-neurological membership. But time and again, the society's leadership was caught up in accusations of professional arrogance (justified as determination to avoid discredit through support of fringe therapies and quackery), and pressure for lay representation to support what affected individuals saw as the priorities. The problem was McAlpine's refusal to admit members to the medical panel of whom he did not approve, its failure to espouse treatment-related research, and the desire to control sporadic outbursts of regional funding it had not approved. Together, the style led to increasing criticism of the medical panel and the establishment of splinter groups. The generous and sustained support of Lumsden was no less uncomplicated. Such was the consistency and security of his funding, that the Society asked Lumsden to take his next best idea to the Medical Research Council. He agreed but in fact continued to request funds from a local branch of the Society. This was promptly vetoed by the medical panel. Attempts to settle the matter by an explanatory address to the Yorkshire branches misfired due to the patronizing attitude of the medical panel chairman, now Dr Henry Miller, who caricatured Lumsden's work as 'high falutin' research which neither you nor I could understand'.

He used dismissive language and was insensitive with respect to the sentiments of his audience. It has been suggested that, in these last few months of his life, the balance of Miller's mind may have been disturbed (Nicolson and Lowis 2002). His legendary commitment to 'good living' may also have led to a less than restrained evening's work. Understandably, patients admired Lumsden's optimistic rhetoric – feeding an impatient constituency who were only too happy to support his ideas on the pathogenesis and opportunities for immune desensitization, as set out in the reissue of *Multiple Sclerosis: A Re-appraisal* (Lumsden 1972). One concluded:

[in] this complete run-through, we could see no logical step had been omitted and we realized ... that the cause of M.S. is no longer really a problem and the essential causes of the demyelination and sclerosis are understood.

History may conclude that, in seeking to resolve these tensions and head off criticism through the appointment of Professor Ephraim (E.J.) Field to its first research Unit, the Society moved from the frying pan into the fire. Responding to the request for government commitment to basic research relating to multiple sclerosis, the Medical Research Council took over funding for the Unit set up in 1958 under Field's directorship in

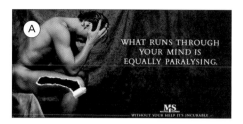

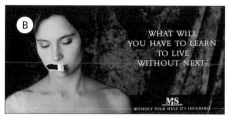

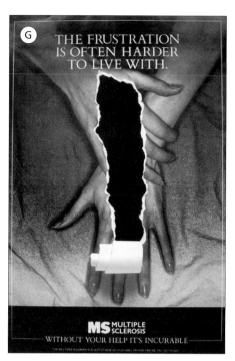

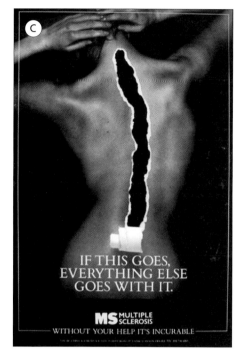

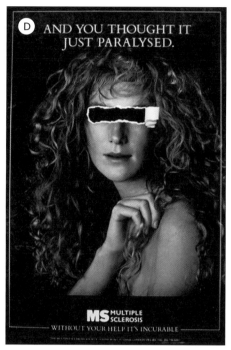

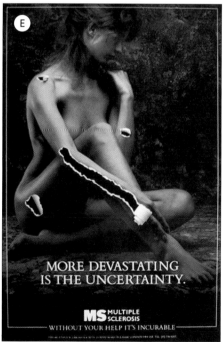

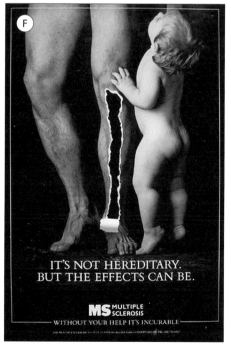

Figure 1.11 Posters from the Multiple Sclerosis Society of Great Britain and Northern Ireland 'Tear Campaign' (1987–1991), with permission of the Multiple Sclerosis Society.

Newcastle. Things soon went wrong – not on the basis of the notorious work claiming to have identified an electrophoretic abnormality of red blood cells that enabled the affected children of probands to be identified presymptomatically, and the disease prevented by dietary manipulation – but because of complaints from within the Unit concerning Field's personality and style of management. He was dismissed as director in 1973 and subsequently sought to discredit the mental stability of the secretary at the Medical Research Council (Sir John Gray). Field's cause was taken up by politicians and discussed in the national newspapers. 'The Prof' was caricatured as a brilliant if somewhat irascible medical research worker with little time for the dullards he encountered in Newcastle. Attempts to limit the perceived damage failed and a ginger group formed within the society – known initially as the Multiple Sclerosis Action Group – from members of the Newham branch, under the leadership of Mr John Simpkins. Later they left the Society altogether, becoming Action Research for Multiple Sclerosis (ARMS). Their activities were also doomed to failure through commitment to expensive therapy centres and research on hyperbaric oxygen – based on the unlikely theory of fat embolism as the precipitating cause of tissue injury in multiple sclerosis (James 1982). Matters came to a head at the Annual General Meeting in 1975 when Cave elected to break up a heated debate between Field and Professor Alan Davison (1925–1993) on the grounds that 'we cannot debate medical matters in front of a lay audience'. 'Why not?' came the vigorous riposte from that lay audience. Unpublished correspondence addressed to Cave from a member of the General Council reveals the depth of feeling:

> Professor Field is a dreadful man, to my mind, the issue he was fighting [for] was not MS research but for the advancement of his own career and for this he was prepared to exploit the fear of MS sufferers.

In response to public outcry, the Society tried to coax Field back, but although supported by the Bransom Trust, he never re-entered mainstream multiple sclerosis research prior to his death in 2002. The Trust itself was eventually wound up in July 2003 after the death of Field's long-term assistant Greta Joyce. Can Field be vindicated as a brilliant clinical scientist but a difficult man? His brother is perceptive concerning E.J. Field's character traits. Dr Leopold Henry Field recalls how (with genuine wit but little attention to factual detail) E.J. Field had dubbed the only useful contribution of an eminent professor of neurology as having been successfully to organize the Christmas party; and he quotes another clinical neurologist as considering that Field 'fiddled' his results. Responding to the suggestion that although Field did not enjoy easy personal relationships, no informed observer would dismiss his work as lacking all quality, Dr Leopold Field confirms that Alfred (for that was his name within the family) had little time for those he regarded as of lesser intelligence. As a schoolboy, E.J. Field matriculated in Latin from scratch to standards required for medical school entry in 6 weeks, rising at 5 a.m. and sitting with gloves and overcoat in the unheated family kitchen to study, but then chose to live at home in Newcastle, and use his state scholarships to support a widowed mother rather than take up a place at the University of Cambridge. Dr Field concludes (L. Field, personal communications):

> put quite simply, the maturity of his personality did not match his IQ … I would certainly have liked his brains but the personality was a problem.

In a long and probing conversation with one of the two leading figures in contemporary experimental neuropathology whom he trained, neither affection nor admiration could easily be discerned.

Following the Field affair, Cave felt it best to resign in 1976 despite receiving general support from a special meeting of the Society, chaired by an ex-Lord Chancellor (Lord Dilhorne), and overseen by the Bishop of Nottingham whom Cave encouraged to 'instil into a number of militant members of the Society, a few gifts of the Holy Ghost, at any rate for the afternoon'.

Sir Richard Cave was succeeded as chairman by Mr Gilbert Macdonald, who had worked in the pharmaceutical industry and brought a sympathetic attitude to scientific expertise alongside modern management skills. The Society evidently needed both. Over this long period, the real aims of the Multiple Sclerosis Society had been skilfully administered by its secretary and chief executive officer, who gradually brought about a commitment to medical research, making the Multiple Sclerosis Society of Great Britain and Northern Ireland (with the equally meritorious National Multiple Sclerosis Society of the United States) the default funder for work that laid the modern foundation for our understanding of the disease. John Walford joined the society in February 1954 and, when he retired in 1994, £30 million had been committed to research and a further £55 million to welfare (Figure 1.11A–G, showing the 'tear campaign' that ran from 1987 to 1991). This was an astonishing legacy, but old attitudes die hard and not all difficulties encountered by the Multiple Sclerosis Society – and the community it serves – have been of merely historical interest. As recently as 1998, the Medical Research Advisory Committee was summarily disbanded by the then chief executive on the grounds that it was overly comfortable in its support of committee members and not in tune with members' real needs for research focused on treatment and management of the disease. Fortunately, however, the Society now again continues to support biomedical research to a level surpassed only, amongst other national bodies, by the Multiple Sclerosis Society in the United States. Nevertheless, the early history of the Multiple Sclerosis Society has had a habit of repeating itself, illustrating why, for this disease more than any other, progress towards an understanding of disease mechanisms and treatment may have been somewhat stifled – and, as a result, giving multiple sclerosis research a reputation for espousing maverick lines of enquiry.

THE PATHOGENESIS AND CLINICAL ANATOMY OF MULTIPLE SCLEROSIS: 1849–1977

The earliest accounts of the causal mechanism of what may reasonably be interpreted as multiple sclerosis reflect the prejudices of physicians at the time: constipation (Abernethy 1809) and onanism (Ollivier 1827). Their conjectures are untouched by the developing ideas about measurement in medicine (see below). More likely explanations were proposed by the middle of the century. Based on their research traditions, various schools addressed the problem of multiple sclerosis but from somewhat different perspectives. The Austro-German school, working mainly under the influence of the famous pathologists Rudolph Virchow (1821–1902) and Karl von Rokitansky (1804–1878), focused their studies on structural changes in the nervous tissue, seeking to explain the nature of the lesions and cause of the disease on the basis of its cellular pathology. In contrast, the French school, dominated by Charcot, was mainly interested in the problems of clinicopathological correlation, trying to understand the diversity of clinical signs and symptoms on the basis of the nature and localization of lesions.

The German school

Frerichs (1849) had to wait for pathological examination of the cases he observed in life and described clinically until Valentiner, his pupil, reported the abnormal firmness or leathery consistency in irregularly circumscribed parts of the white matter, rarely involving the grey matter of the cord, and with a poverty of blood vessels. The patches were almost normal in colour or milky white, dull and occasionally greyish-red. There was a loss of nerve elements. Frerichs' cases had experienced exacerbations and remissions, alternately affecting each side of the body and with selective involvement of the lower limbs, disturbance of mobility outweighing that of sensibility, major manifestations in the spino-medullary junction, and psychiatric symptoms. His patients were young persons otherwise in good general health.

Soon after, Rokitansky (1857) described connective tissue proliferations in the cord, pons and medulla producing progressive paraplegia. He called the pathological substrate *graue Degeneration* (grey degeneration) and stressed its similarity to connective tissue scars in other organs. Seven years later, Rindfleisch (1863) confirmed Rokitansky's primary observations but, in addition, provided the first detailed description of the basic pathological features of multiple sclerosis plaques. He concluded his description by summarizing the findings:

So much about the histological detail on the grey degeneration. We have to recapitulate that three types of changes occur in parallel, first the alterations of blood vessels, secondly the atrophy of the nervous elements and third the metamorphosis of the connective tissue.

He describes the three different pathological changes in detail, pointing out that multiple sclerosis plaques are centred on one or more blood vessels and that these vessels are surrounded by round cell infiltrates. Correctly he concludes that this is the reflection of chronic inflammation. Regarding tissue atrophy, he emphasizes that the process starts with demyelination:

... I mention here, that under the microscope the axons ('Axenzylinder') primarily lose their myelin and can then be traced some distance into the lesion as thin threads, which only contain the axon.

He further describes that the lipid material is taken up by cells and degraded. Finally the third element of pathology is described as connective tissue metamorphosis, which, as dis-

cussed by Rokitansky before, leads to the formation of scar tissue (*narbige Verdichtung*).

Fromann (1864) illustrated the occurrence of demyelination (Figure 1.12) and astrocytosis, collective wisdom having been summarized by Leyden (1863) who recommended that multiple sclerosis and chronic myelitis should be considered as the same disorder. Leyden emphasized that women are affected more often than men, with age of onset usually in the third decade, almost always without a family history and with exposure to dampness or psychic events as major provocative factors. For Leyden, the prognosis was generally poor with occasional pleasant surprises.

Otto Marburg (1906) presented an extensive description of acute multiple sclerosis and his is the first detailed clinical and

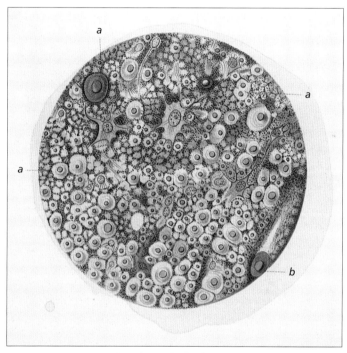

Figure 1.12 Cross-section through the fibrillary degenerated tissue in the vicinity of normal (areas). The original septae are still visible and surround part myelinated and part naked axons. Sometimes they surround empty holes or rare cross-sectioned fibrils. The septae are in the majority – and in particular at their crossing points – enlarged and contain rows of dense granules that can be identified as cross-sectioned fibrils. The fibrils, which are densely packed in the inner spaces of the septae, as well as those which are derived from the granules and grow into the holes of the meshwork, are missing. The eight large distinctly outlined cells appear as homogeneous and shiny masses; also their processes are – as far as they could be delineated – shiny, and only in the periphery of the cells were there fine ill-defined processes in continuity with the surrounding granulated fibrils. A number of nuclei are freely located in the tissue, which is surrounded by a small rim of protoplasm held together by fine granulated septae. The discernible nuclear fibres originate in part from the nuclei or sometimes are just found adjacent to them. At the upper edge of the figure there is an elongated fibril, which originates from the adjacent nucleus. *b*: Blood vessel with thickened vascular wall; *a*: a similar vessel is seen at the left upper edge of the figure. From Fromann (1864).

pathological account of fulminating cases leading to death within 1 year. Marburg emphasized that the disease process in these patients mimics, in all essential respects, components of the more chronic case, but he also identified distinguishing features. He depicted a convincing example of concentric sclerosis, later described by Balo (1928) as *encephalitis periaxalis concentrica*, and showed that the disease process is not confined to the brain and spinal cord, drawing attention to demyelination of the peripheral nervous system in all three of his cases. He defined the basic lesion of multiple sclerosis as an inflammatory process, which is associated with 'discontinuous (that is, segmental) lysis of myelin with relative preservation of axons followed by a proliferation of glia cells and vessels'.

Marburg suggested that the dissolution of myelin is accomplished by a soluble mediator, but that the fragments of myelin are taken up by phagocytes. The final result of this process is described as the replacement of the damaged tissue by a fibrillary network of glia cell processes. Marburg also recognized the abundance of nerve fibres with very thin myelin sheaths (he specifically mentions fibres with thin myelin sheaths that can only be seen after osmic acid impregnation) and discussed whether these reflect incomplete demyelination or remyelination. He observed acute axonal pathology with reactive change and the presence of thin atrophic nerve fibres (see below). In these and many other respects, his ideas were ahead of their time and Marburg anticipated many features of the pathogenesis of multiple sclerosis described throughout this book.

The French school

Charcot made many contributions to the clinical neurology of *sclérose en plaques*. He left a brilliant account of the clinical symptomatology; delineated the cerebral, spinal and mixed cerebrospinal forms (Figure 1.13A–H); and formulated views on the pathogenesis. Apart from these fundamental clinicoanatomical correlations, he developed many ideas concerning mechanisms and pathophysiology, provided the first attempts at measurement, and threw down a therapeutic gauntlet to his successors. Charcot took the view that overgrowth of glia strangles the myelin sheath, sometimes leading to degeneration of the axis cylinders (Figure 1.14A–C). He suggested that the naked axis cylinders might again clothe themselves with myelin and thus effect a *restituto ad integrum*, to quote from J. Dawson (1916) (see below). Amongst the manifestations of cerebral involvement was amblyopia, on which he wrote (quotations in English are from the New Sydenham Society translations of Charcot's lectures, 1877):

Amblyopia is a persistent and frequent symptom of cerebrospinal disseminated sclerosis but it rarely issues in complete blindness. This is worthy of notice since patches of sclerosis have been found after death occupying the whole thickness of the nerve trunk, in the optic nerve, in cases where during life an enfeeblement of sight simply had been noted. This discrepancy between symptom and lesion constitutes one of the most powerful arguments to show that the functional continuity of the nerve tubes is not absolutely interrupted although these, in their course through the sclerosed patches, have been despoiled of their medullary sheaths and reduced to axis cylinders.

Charcot also wrote on the cognitive manifestations of multiple sclerosis:

Most of the patients affected by multilocular sclerosis, whom I have had occasion to observe, have presented at a certain stage of the disease a truly peculiar facies. The look is vague and uncertain; the lips are hanging and half open; the features have a stolid expression, sometimes even an appearance of stupor. This dominant expression of the physiognomy is almost always accompanied by a corresponding mental state which deserves notice. There is marked enfeeblement of the memory; conceptions are formed slowly; the intellectual and emotional faculties are blunted in their totality. The dominant feeling in the patients appears to be an almost stupid indifference in reference to all things. It is not rare to see them give way to foolish laughter for no cause, and sometimes, on the contrary, melt into tears without reason. Nor is it rare, amid this state of mental depression, to find psychic disorders arise which assume one or other of the classic forms of mental alienation.

Charcot described the triad of nystagmus, dysarthria and ataxia resulting from involvement of brainstem–cerebellar connections although his functional anatomy of this region was not sophisticated:

One symptom which doubtless struck you all from the first on seeing the patient enter ... was certainly the very special rhythmical tremor by which her head and limbs were violently agitated whilst she was walking. You have likewise noticed that when the patient sat upon a chair, the tremor disappeared ... from her upper and lower limbs, but only partially from the head and trunk ... In complete repose ... you will be able to assure yourself of the utter absence of all trace of tremor in the different parts ... To cause the rhythmical agitation again to appear throughout the body, it will suffice to make the patient rise from her seat ... You can see that, in the several acts prescribed by the will, the tremor increases in direct ratio with the extent of the movement executed. Thus, when the patient wishes to lift a glass full of water to her lips, the rhythmical agitation of the hand and forearm is scarcely noticeable when taking hold of the object; ... but ... at the moment when the goal is being attained, the glass is ... dashed with violence against the teeth, and the water is flung out to a distance.

On spinal disease, Charcot described the characteristic weakness, spasticity, ankle clonus (spinal epilepsy) and loss of sensibility, referring to the case of Josephine Paget originally described by Cruveilhier:

We should not, however, forget that some of the symptoms of ataxia are found ... when the sclerosed islets in certain regions of the cord spread over a certain height of the posterior columns. A case, the history of which may be found recorded at length in Cruveilhier's Atlas of Pathological Anatomy may be cited as an example of this class. It is the case of the patient Paget. In order to grasp and use a pin she required to have her eyes open, otherwise the pin dropped from her

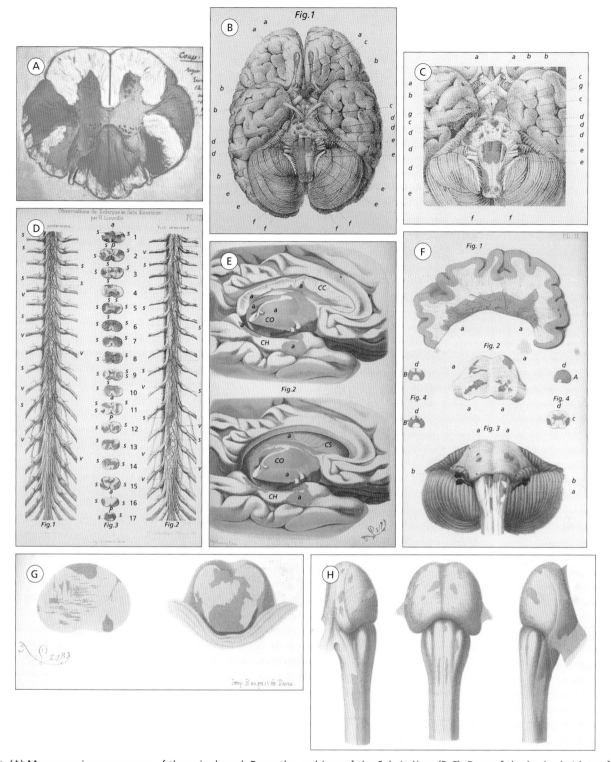

Figure 1.13 (A) Macroscopic appearance of the spinal cord. From the archives of the Salpétrière. (B,C). Base of the brain. *b*: Islets of sclerosis along the optic nerves; *b'*: healthy portion of one of the optic nerves. Patches of sclerosis, disseminated over different parts of the protuberantia, some superficial, others deep seated. Surface slightly depressed at these points. The nerves emerging from the pons appear healthy. From Charcot (1886). (D) Anterior and posterior aspects of the spinal cord (the dura mater is divided and thrown back at either side). *s*: Patches and islets of sclerosis, irregularly disseminated, various in form and dimensions, irregular, isolated or partially united by connections visible on the surface. They predominate here especially in the dorsal region. No 1 from the superior portion of the cervical region immediately beneath the bulbus rachidicus to ... No 5 ... superior dorsal region ... No 14 superior portion of the dorso-lumbar enlargement and No 17 ... terminal cone. From Charcot (1886). (E) Multiple sclerosis. Upper figure: Inner aspect of the left hemisphere, *A*; sclerotic patches occupying the corpus callosum, *CC*; the optic tract, *CO*; the convolution of the hippocampus, *CH*. Lower figure: In this figure, the corpus callosum was lifted up to show the ventricular wall. *CS*: corpus striatum. The other letters have the same significance as in the upper figure. From Charcot (1886). (F) *Fig. 1*. *a.a*: patch of sclerosis arising on the lateral ventricular wall. Superior wall. *Fig. 2*: Section of the protuberantia, the superior half seen from the inferior aspect. *a.a.a.a*: nuclei of the sclerosis. *Fig. 3*. *a.a.a*: Patches of sclerosis; one of them cuts the left olivary body into two parts. *b.b*: Black coloration of the epidemia by silver nitrate. *Fig. 4*. *A.B.B'C*: sections of the medulla. (*d.d* anterior part) *A*. Above the brachial enlargement. *B.B'*. The middle of the medulla. *C*. Three centimetres above the termination of the medulla. Observation *II*: multiple sclerosis. From Ordenstein (1868). (G,H) Multiple sclerosis. Pons and medulla, anterior and left and right lateral surfaces. Sections of the pons. The grey areas represent the plaques of sclerosis. From Charcot (1886).

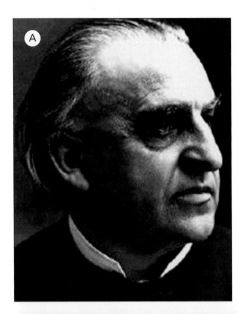

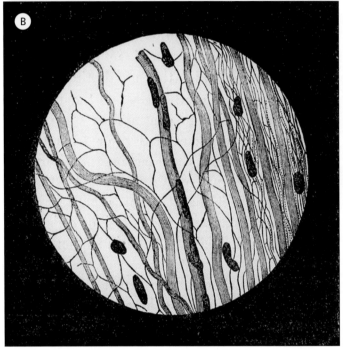

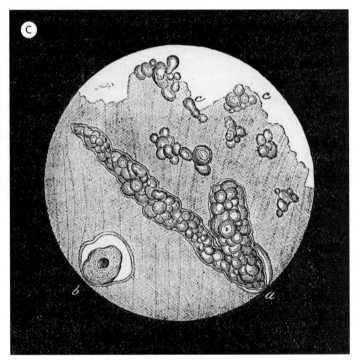

Figure 1.14 (A) Jean-Martin Charcot (1825–1893). (B) Fresh preparation, taken from the centre of a patch of sclerosis, coloured with carmine, and dilacerated. In the centre is seen a capillary vessel, supporting several nuclei. To the right and left of this are axis cylinders, some voluminous, others of very small diameter, and all deprived of their medullary sheaths. The capillary vessel and the axis cylinders were vividly coloured by the carmine; the axis cylinders present perfectly smooth borders, without ramification. Between them are seen slender fibrillae of recent formation, which form on the left and in the centre a sort of network resulting from the entanglement or anastomosis of the fibrils. These are distinguished from the axis cylinders, 1° by their diameter, which is much smaller; 2° by the ramifications which they present in their course; 3° by taking no coloration from carmine. Nuclei are scattered about; some of them appear to be in connection with the connective fibrils; others have assumed an irregular form, owing to the action of the ammoniacal solution of carmine. (C) Patch of sclerosis in the fresh state: *a*, lymphatic sheath of a vessel distended by voluminous fatty globules; *b*, a vessel divided transversely. The adventitious coat is separated from the lymphatic sheath by a free space, the fatty globules which distended the sheath having disappeared; *c*, fatty globules, gathered into small groups, dispersed here and there over the preparation. From Charcot (1868b).

fingers. On a postmortem examination, it was found that one of the sclerosed patches occupied a considerable extent of the posterior columns in the cervical enlargement of the cord.

We can admire Charcot for two other aspects of his contribution to *sclérose en plaques* – the attempt to measure deficits, and to explain their origins in terms of disordered physiological mechanisms (Figure 1.15A–D). He documented the amplitude and range of tremor, distinguishing this from the effects of mercury and Parkinson's disease, and used handwriting to document these clinical features. On pathophysiology he wrote:

I have expressed the opinion that the axis cylinders deprived of medullary sheathing in the midst of the foci of sclerosis plays an important part. The transmission of voluntary impulses would still proceed by means of the denuded axis

cylinder but it would be carried on irregularly in a broken or jerky manner and would thus produce the oscillations which disturb the due execution of voluntary movements.

Here is a sophisticated prediction of the pathophysiology of impulse conduction in demyelinated axons, eventually elucidated both in the peripheral and central nervous systems in the 1960s (W.I. McDonald 1963; W.I. McDonald and Sears 1970; see Chapter 13), but it is an analysis that lacks the anatomical precision of circuitry in the motor system.

Charcot's first student, Ordenstein, was put to work on the clinical distinction between *sclérose en plaques* and Parkinson's disease (Ordenstein 1868). Part two of his thesis concerns the history, pathological anatomy, symptomatology, aetiology, prognosis and therapeutics of the disease. Four cases are documented. These identify 1855 as the year in which Charcot first recognized the clinical manifestations of multiple sclerosis. Alexandrine C. became aware during pregnancy of difficulty in using her legs. She may have had symptoms for the previous 2 years but the diagnosis was established clinically at the Salpêtrière in 1863. Ordenstein also identifies *'femme B'*, a patient of Charcot's who died in 1867, as the seventh case described in the entire literature; she had autopsy-proven *sclérose en plaques* with extensive demyelination in the cerebrum and spinal cord and had also presented in 1855 with weakness in the legs, followed in 1857 by sensory symptoms and loss of vision. Figure 2 from Ordenstein's thesis is the first depiction of the lesions of *sclérose en plaques* from Charcot's laboratory (see Fig. 1.13H). Bourneville and Guerard (1869) completed the clinical description and provided additional illustrations. Later, Bourneville collated and saw through to publication Charcot's lectures on neurological and general medical disease, Joseph Babinski (1857–1932) wrote his medical thesis, *Étude anatomique et clinique sur la sclérose en plaques*, in 1885. Babinski emphasizes hemiplegia as a manifestation of multiple sclerosis. The work also contains an elaborate depiction of early multiple sclerosis lesions, showing the interaction of macrophages with demyelinated nerve fibres (see below). Babinski is the young physician catching the swooning Blanche Wittmann in the much reproduced painting by Pierre Brouillet of Charcot demon-strating hysteria at La Salpétrière during one of his Tuesday lectures.

Gilles de la Tourette (1886) described the gait in neurological disease and depicted the footprints of ataxic patients with *sclérose en plaques* (Fig. 1.15C). But the last of Charcot's pupils to write at length on multiple sclerosis was Pierre Marie (1853–1940) who gave four lectures on the subject to the Faculty of Medicine in 1891 (Marie 1895). More than his predecessors, Marie sought to classify and record the typical disturbance of gait – distinguishing spastic from cerebellar components. On hemiplegia, he was lavish in his praise for the thesis of Blanche Edwards (1858–1941), preferring her account to that of Joseph Babinski (1885a). In chapter 2 of *Sclérose en plaques avec hemi-plegie*, Ms Edwards describes cases from the literature in which recurrent hemiplegia dominated the clinical features of multiple sclerosis, quoting in detail one of five instances known to Charcot, and seven of fifteen under the care of Pierre Marie (B.A. Edwards 1889). She describes rapid onset and recovery, sometimes with aphasia and in the context of pyrexia, but showing a natural history unlike the persistent disability seen with stroke or locomotor ataxia. Her cases had associated deficits affecting eye movements and cerebellar pathways. Whether the clinical separation of cerebellar and hemiplegic deficits under-going evolution at that time in the Paris school was fully in place,

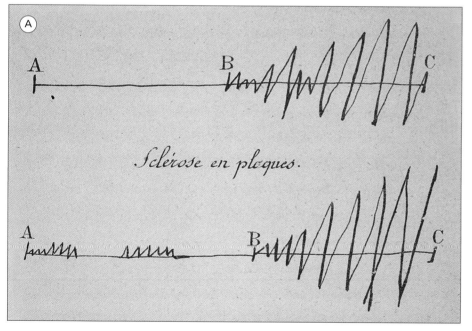

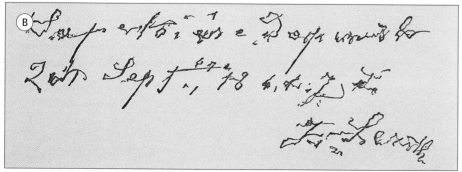

Figure 1.15 (A) Tremor. AB: In all the schemes, periods of rest are illustrated. BC shows the period that accompanies a voluntary movement (writing, carrying a glass to the mouth, etc.). (B) Example of handwriting in a patient with *sclérose en plaques*. From Charcot (1887, 1872).

illustration continued on following page

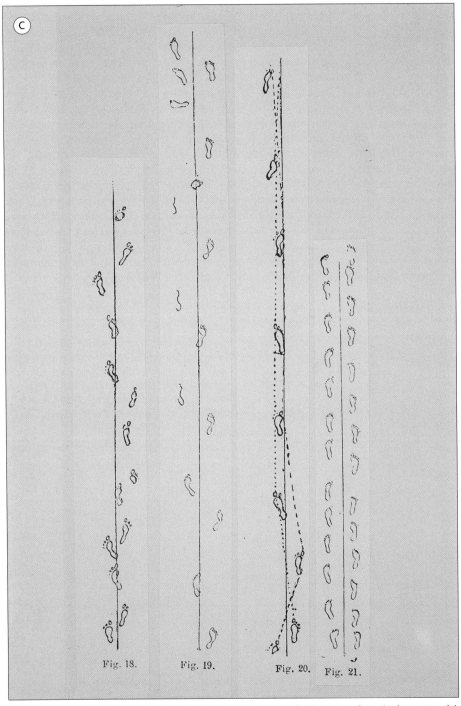

Ⓒ

Fig. 18.   Fig. 19.   Fig. 20.   Fig. 21.

Figure 1.15, cont'd (C) Bilateral unsteady gait. Figs 18 and 19: unsteady gait due to multiple Ménière's sclerosis. Fig. 20: unsteady gait; experimental drunkenness. Fig. 21: unsteady gait being giddyness due to Ménière's disease treated with quinine sulphate'. From de la Tourette (1886).

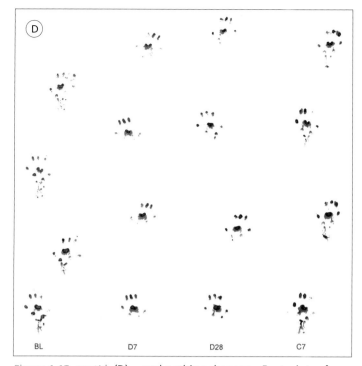

Figure 1.15, cont'd (D) ...and nothing changes... Footprints of one experimental autoimmune encephalomyelitis animal at three different time points (BL, D7, D28) and of one control animal at time point D7. During baseline measurements, the experimental animal puts down the entire foot. After the cytokine injection, the heel was not visible any more on the prints due to slight tiptoeing. In the control animal, which received an injection of phosphate-buffered saline (PBS) only after the sensitization procedure, such tiptoeing was not observed during the entire time course. From Buddeberg *et al* (2004) with permission.

allowing reliable distinction between these anatomical pathways, is uncertain but Edwards leaned much on pathological verification. To us, many of these accounts read more like the paroxysmal manifestations of multiple sclerosis than the hemiplegia that undoubtedly does occur in multiple sclerosis – and, as such, representing the first description of this physiologically exquisite manifestation. Edwards noted a prior description by the English physician, Dyce Duckworth (physician to St Bartholomew's Hospital in London) in the *Lancet* of hemiplegia attributed clinically to insular sclerosis affecting the corpus striatum (Duckworth 1885). But again, the clinical accounts suggest that some at least were patients with disease of brainstem–cerebellar connections (Duckworth acknowledged that the localization might be in the medulla spinalis). G.R. (aged 21) from Wiltshire presented with a spastic weak right leg and severe action tremor of the right arm preventing all skilled movement but had no facial weakness or bulbar symptoms; the prognosis was deemed poor and the case was considered to be untreatable.

Marie was no less thorough in his descriptions of upper limb tremor and sensation, dealing at length with the special senses, hearing and vision, and distinguishing disorders of acuity and colour vision – largely borrowed from Uhthoff (1889) – from those of eye movements. He referred both to external and internal ophthalmoplegias. Marie had been awarded the Civrieux prize of the Academy of Medicine in 1885 for his account of disordered bladder, bowel and sexual function in multiple sclerosis, although he considered these to be rare manifestations. He was strong on the bulbar and visceral manifestations, predating Kinnier Wilson (1928) by several decades on the description of impulsive laughter (which Charcot had himself mentioned, see above), and allowed glycosuria as a sign of demyelination in the floor of the fourth ventricle. More than others writing at that time, Marie recognized the variable symptoms at onset, delineating a number of stereotyped presenting syndromes and documenting the subsequent clinical course, including the category of benign multiple sclerosis. He made the distinction between progression from onset and its development later in the course of the illness. In fact, his account of primary progressive multiple sclerosis is faultless, noting the later age of onset, the worse prognosis, the relative absence of histological (or clinical) involvement of the cerebrum, and the more frequent axon degeneration.

The English school

Although descriptions of the pathology and clinical symptomatology of multiple sclerosis were available in continental Europe, it is a mark of the originality of Charcot's contribution in bringing this disorder to general attention that there is no mention of diseases recognizable as multiple sclerosis in standard textbooks prior to 1868. Almost one entire volume of *A System of Medicine* (1868), edited by Russell Reynolds (physician to the National Hospital in London), is devoted to neurology. Although there are descriptions of chronic sclerosis of the cord, these cases are not suggestive of multiple sclerosis – at best, the series may have included some examples of primary progressive disease. In *On the Use of the Ophthalmoscope in Diseases of the Nervous System and of the Kidneys*, Sir Clifford Allbutt (1871) described R.B. (case 103; referred by Mr Sedgwick of Boroughbridge in Yorkshire) as having chronic disease of the spinal cord manifesting as paralysis, altered sensation and impaired bladder control with reduced central vision and pale optic discs, but he offered no diagnosis. The same is true of William McKenzie in *A Practical Treatise on Disease of the Eye* when he discusses the case of Thomas Crichton (see above: MacKenzie 1840).

That situation changed when Moxon (1875) described eight patients, some of whom had already featured in the *Lancet*, and provided the first detailed description of multiple sclerosis in the English language (Figure 1.16A,B). In his definitive account, Moxon combined clinical and autopsy observations in two patients and described at length the intention tremor of the head and upper extremities, the weakness that may precipitate pressure sores, paraplegia in flexion or extension, nystagmus with dysarthria, impaired control of the sphincters, exaggerated reflex activity, pathological laughter and crying as a manifestation of incipient dementia, and death from pulmonary or bladder infection. The historian George Trevelyan has remarked that:

the poetry of history lies in the quasi-miraculous fact that once on ... this familiar spot of ground walked other men and women ... thinking their own thoughts but now all gone, one generation vanishing after another, gone as utterly as we ourselves shall shortly be gone like ghosts at cock-crow.

Moxon's account of these patients brings the patients back to life, epitomizing the intimacy of the medical encounter. Emily

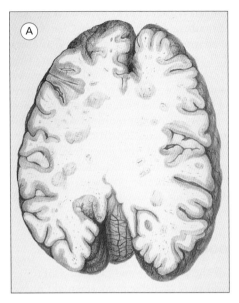

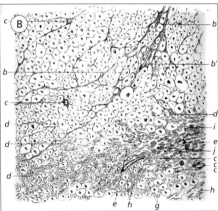

Figure 1.16 (A) Section of the brain showing insular sclerosis. The whole brain is shrunken looking, as will be seen by observing the very uneven elevation of the convolutions and their narrowness, and the depth and width of the sulci between them. The centrum ovale majus, which the section reveals, shows many patches of the colour of the grey matter of the brain, or paler or mottled. These patches are insulated and are scattered very irregularly. (B) Portion of a section of the spinal cord, hardened, stained with carmine, and cleared with alcohol and oil of cloves, showing insular sclerosis. Opposite *a* is healthy texture of the cord, showing the more or less circular sections of the nerve fibres, in each of which the axis cylinder is seen. Scarcely anything is between the fibres here. *bb:* Part of a medullary ray with offsets from it; at *b'* the ray is thickened from early sclerotic change. *cc:* Capillary vessels. These are seen to be closer together in the sclerosed part of the specimen. *dd:* The advancing edge of the sclerosis; nucleated tissue passing in between the individual fibres and separating them from each other; *e:* the sclerosed substance itself; at *ff* the axis cylinders of the nerve fibrils can be seen when their medulla is all destroyed; at *gg* round, and *hh* elongated, nuclei; the latter belongs to the new fibrous tissue, of the former many represent 'granule-cells', the fatty grains of which have been removed in the process of preparation. *i:* The shaded round bodies are amyloid corpuscles. From Moxon (1875).

B. confides to one of the attendant nurses her assumption that the shock of finding her husband in bed with another woman had precipitated the episode of ataxic quadriparesis with which she presented in August 1872 and which Dr Moxon had no difficulty in distinguishing from paralysis agitans. However, for poor Emily, there was to be no relief and she died in January 1873 after accumulating many other deficits, having been ill for <6 months. At autopsy, there were 40 white matter plaques, some the size of 'hemp-seed', affecting the cerebrum, pons and medulla – appearances that had on earlier occasions been confused with *heterotopia cerebri*. Histology showed destruction of the medullary fibres, replacement by fine connective fibrils and granular corpuscles. The case of Emily B. was described again in detail in the *Lancet* of 3rd April 1875. Edward M. featured on 1st May. He was ataxic and paralysed but also showed visual failure and prominent sensory symptoms. Emily B. (aged 25), Matilda P. (aged 23), James P. (a veterinary surgeon, aged 33), Sarah H. (a servant, aged 37), George N. (a clerk, aged 35), Albert F. (a splint cutter for matches, aged 24), Harriet B. (a servant, aged 38, also described in the 3rd April 1875 issue of the *Lancet*) and Edward M. (a footman, aged 32) were all admitted to Guy's Hospital over a 2-year period from January 1873. They described distortions of movement and sensation, suffered the alternating anxieties and hopes of the neurologically ill, died or became disabled, and are now remembered only for their clinical histories and lesions in the cerebrum, pons, medulla and spinal cord. Although Guy's Hospital and William Moxon can take credit for priority in the description of multiple sclerosis in the English language, not all its physicians were unaffected by Charcot's other disease – historical revisionism. Sir Samuel Wilks, writing in 1878, was at pains to point out that:

> *I myself had observed years ago scattered patches of deposit in the cerebrospinal centres, but had failed to associate them with any special form of malady; subsequently Charcot described this sclerosis, disseminated throughout the cord, with the prevailing symptoms which accompany it.*

James Dawson (1870–1927) summarized everything of significance prior to his time and left the greatest pathological account of multiple sclerosis in the English language (J. Dawson 1916). He assigned priority to Cruveilhier (c.1841) for the first depiction (wrongly), Frerichs (1849) for the initial clinical description, Rindfleisch (1863) for formulating ideas on the aetiology, and Vulpian (and Charcot: 1868a; 1868b) for pulling the whole story together. Reviewing the histology of nine personal cases (L.W., a kitchen maid, aged 28; C.S., aged 22; Mrs G., aged 30; J.W.; S.S., a nurse aged 44; C.G., a baker's shopwoman, aged 24; J. McN., a cabinet maker, aged 42; M.R., a typist, aged 33; and L.H., aged 30), Dawson devoted the majority of his text to L.W. She was admitted to hospital in Edinburgh under the care of Dr Alexander Bruce on 4th April 1910 with a 2-year history of weakness and tremor in all four limbs, dysarthria and sphincter disturbance. In hospital (29th May) she had an episode of brainstem demyelination (deafness and tinnitus, right facial palsy, numb left arm, right lateral rectus weakness, tongue deviation to the left and dysphagia). In August, she lost vision in both eyes, developing increasing bulbar failure and died from septicaemia on 5th September 1910. Dawson described the features of early and established lesions in the spinal cord and cerebrum, offering an analysis of their evolution through stages of fat granule cell myelitis (in the cord) to glial hyperplasia. He devoted text to the unusual lesions, including *Markschattenherde* (shadow plaques), and those appearing in grey matter and around the ventricles, optic nerve, peripheral nerves and roots. Next, he turned to an analysis of the changes to be observed in each cellular element of the nervous system – nerve cells and their axons, neuroglia, blood vessels and lymphatics. Form, symmetry and the distribution of lesions were all addressed. After listing the tragic accumulation of lesions throughout the brain and spinal cord of poor L.W., Dawson attempted a clinicopathophysiological correlation. Weakness in the legs was consistent with the extensive spinal cord gliosis; intention tremor with lesions in the superior cerebellar peduncles and red nuclei; disordered eye movements with the periaqueductal plaques; and extensive cranial nerve palsies with involvement of the pons and medulla. Dawson showed that old (sclerotic lesions) were characterized by complete absence of myelin (Weigert stain), dense fibrillary tissue (glial stain), persistence of axis cylinders (silver stain), numerous blood vessels (diffuse stains), no active myelin degeneration (Marchi stain) and an abrupt transition to normal tissue. In acute lesions, the differences were infiltrated blood vessels, active demyelination with fat granule cells, and transitional zones shading into normal tissue. He illustrated the text with 22 colour and 434 black-and-white figures in 78 plates (Figure 1.17A–F).

The section on the pathology of multiple sclerosis and related demyelinating processes that appeared in the first edition of *McAlpine's Multiple Sclerosis* was written by Charles Lumsden (McAlpine *et al* 1955). Lumsden immediately struck a gloomy note in his account by concluding that demyelination might be arrested but never reversed. He went on to emphasize the error rate in autopsy series of patients diagnosed as having multiple sclerosis during life, the symmetry and confluence of plaques, the invariable involvement of the cerebrum irrespective of clinical phenotype, the sparing of peripheral nerves and absence of pathological change outside the nervous system, the nature of shadow plaques (which he considered to be areas of partial demyelination), and the frequency of secondary Wallerian (axonal) degeneration. Lumsden characterized acute plaques as those with preserved myelin sheaths, albeit with interspersed fat-laden microglial cells and some degree of axonopathy. Chronic plaques featured a rim of active myelin removal by microglia, an intermediate zone of gliosis and an acellular core with parallel arrays of astrocytic fibrils and preserved axons. Lumsden speculated on the possibility of intact axons undergoing remyelination with consequential restoration of function. However, he also emphasized the absence of oligodendrocytes both from the rim of acute lesions and in chronic plaques, and he considered it unlikely that surviving oligodendroglia might proliferate. Lumsden had his own way of revising books and he entirely replaced the 1955 version in 1965 and again in 1972. Now, multiple sclerosis was considered an autoimmune disease in which exposure of myelin following various biological accidents induced antimyelin antibody formation leading to plaque formation. The 1972 version contains, in addition to its revision of the pathological anatomy, a definitive account of the chemical pathology of multiple sclerosis. It is said that hard work on this edition took its toll, and Lumsden had several periods of illness prior to his early death in 1974.

Evolving concepts in the pathogenesis of multiple sclerosis: the vascular hypothesis

Rindfleisch (1863) first emphasized the change around blood vessels that has so dominated ideas on the pathogenesis of multiple sclerosis from that time:

If one looks carefully at freshly altered parts of the white matter in the brain, one perceives already with the naked eye a red point or line in the middle of each individual focus, the transversely or obliquely cut lumen of a small vessel engorged with blood. In the spinal cord the ... grey foci (in a transverse section) intervene in a wedge-shaped manner in the substance of the anterior columns from the periphery... The shape and position of these correspond exactly to the supply territory of each blood vessel. All this leads us to search for the primary cause of the disease in an alteration of individual vessels and their ramifications; an assumption which is completely confirmed by microscopic examination. All vessels running inside the foci, but also that traverse the immediately surrounding but still intact parenchyma are in a state characteristic of chronic inflammation... Their walls are enormously thickened by the accumulation of nuclei and cells in the adventitia.

Following Rindfleisch (1863), Marburg (1906) stressed the vascular orientation of lesions, considering the *Körnchenzelle* to be small perivascular round cells that take up myelin debris. In the opinion of these authors, multiple sclerosis was therefore an inflammatory demyelinating disease possibly mediated by a soluble myelinotoxic factor and with relative sparing of axons. But for Charcot, it was primarily a disorder of glia with secondary changes in blood vessels. As he said of Rindfleisch:

It is evident, however, that this explanation only sets the difficulty a little further back. Besides, the predominant part accorded to the vessels in the evolution of the morbid process is anything but demonstrated.

His own view was that:

undoubtedly, the multiplication of nuclei and the concomitant hyperplasia of the reticulated fibres of the neuroglia constitutes the initial, fundamental fact, and necessary antecedent; the degenerative atrophy of the nerve elements, is consecutive and secondary; it had already begun when the neuroglia gave way to the fibrillary tissue, though the wasting, afterwards, proceeded with greater rapidity. The hyperplasia of the vascular parieties plays merely an accessory part.

Against this background of claim and counterclaim for the inaugural event leading to tissue injury, Dawson summarized controversies on the causation and epitomized these as the 'exogenous' or 'endogenous' schools but substituted the terms 'inflammatory' and 'developmental', respectively. He assembled teams who preferred either inflammation or developmental abnormalities as the pivotal abnormality, and listed the (mainly contemporary) onlookers whose views he took to be undecided

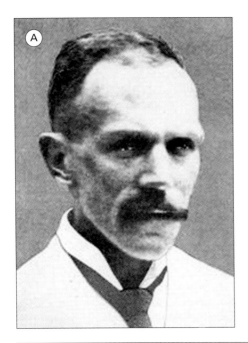

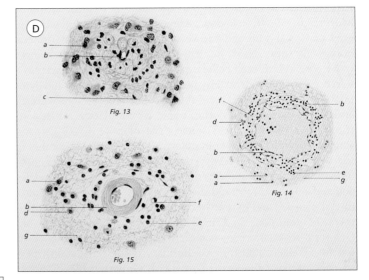

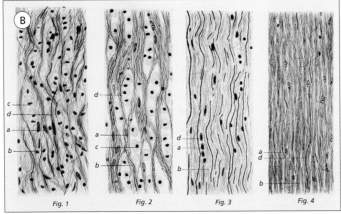

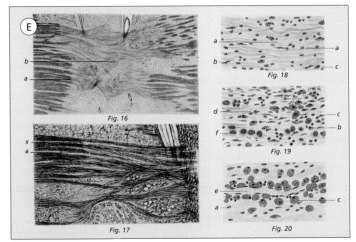

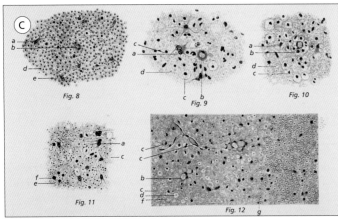

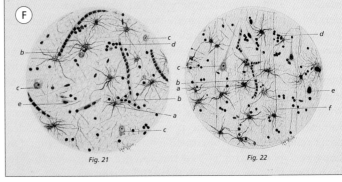

Figure 1.17 (A) James Dawson (1870–1927). (B) *Figs 1–4*: Successive stages in the evolution of a sclerotic area in the posterior columns of the cervical spinal cord. Sections cut in longitudinal direction of the nerve fibres show increasing glia fibril formation. *a*: Glia nuclei; *b*: glia fibrils; *c*: fat granule cells; *d*: persistent axis cylinders. *Figs 1 and 3*: Ford-Robertson's methyl violet stain; *Figs 2 and 4*: palladium methyl violet. (C) *Figs 8–12*: Successive stages in the evolution of a sclerotic area in the posterior columns of the cervical cord. *a*: Glia nuclei; *b*: blood vessel; *c*: fat granule cell; *d*: myelinated nerve fibre; *e*: finely granular glia tissue; *f*: naked axis cylinder; *g*: transition to normal tissue. (D) *Figs 13–15*: Sequence of changes in the blood vessels. *a*: glia nuclei; *b*: blood vessel; *c*: fat granule cell; *d*: cell containing blood pigment; *e*: lymphocyte-like cells; *f*: plasma cells; *g*: glia tissue; *h*: connective tissue cell. (E) *Figs 16 and 17*: Persistence of axis cylinders across a demyelinated area in the pons. *a*: line of transition between myelinated and demyelinated fibres; *b*: median raphe where axis cylinders intersect. *Figs 18–20*: Stages in the demyelination of an area and in the evolution of the fat granule cell. *a*: Small glial nuclei; *b*: transition forms between *a* and *b*; *c*: fat granule cell; *d*: nerve fibre; *e*: blood vessel; *f*: proliferated glia nuclei. (F) *Figs 21 and 22*: Glia changes in a completely demyelinated area in the cortex. *a*: Proliferated glia cells with protoplasm and processes differentiated into fibrils; *b*: capillaries with glia fibrils attached to their outer membrane; *c*: ganglion cells; *d*: small glia cells forming nests around the remains of ganglion cells; *e*: degenerated ganglion cells; *f*: retained axis cylinders. Note that the normal cytoarchitecture of the tissue is preserved. From Dawson (1916).

or uninterpretable. Within the framework of inflammation, he considered as unproven the question of whether the process was targeted against neuroglia, parenchyma, blood vessels or the lymph circulation. In turn, developmental disorders might represent deficiency of the nerve elements (anlage) or multiple gliosis.

Dawson identified Charcot and most of his school as subscribing to the view that multiple sclerosis results from an inflammatory affection of neuroglia that delineates zones within each plaque and surrounds the central blood vessel. Redlich (1896) and Huber (1895) were considered to have broadly similar ideas but saw the insult as a toxin- or microorganism-induced primary degeneration of the myelin sheath with secondary inflammation and blood vessel changes. This is also our reading of Charcot's final position. Dawson himself favoured the formulation of Rindfleisch (1863), who assigned priority to the blood vessels, proposing a sequence in which a chronic irritative condition of the vessel wall alters the nutrition of nerve elements, leading to atrophy with metamorphosis of the connective tissue producing monster glia (Deiters or Rindfleisch cells). In reviewing the history of ideas on the pathology of multiple sclerosis, Dawson indicated that the vascular view was shared by Dejerine (1894), R.T. Williamson (1894, 1908) and Marie (1884, 1895), who suggested that infections initiate the changes in blood vessels but also emphasized the contribution of axon degeneration. The developmental school was headed by Adolphe Strumpell (1853–1925), who drew an analogy with disorders in which congenital abnormalities are invariably associated with secondary gliosis. Strumpell (1896) considered that exogenous insults act upon an intrinsically weakened system. Bramwell (1903) also saw multiple sclerosis as a developmental disturbance. Dawson's team of 'don't knows' included practically everyone who wrote on the pathology of multiple sclerosis between 1903 and 1916, when he himself laid his thesis before the Royal Society of Edinburgh. Amongst this contemporary group was Bielschowsky (1903), who discussed preservation of axis cylinders (nerve fibres) and suggested that the vascular process is directed at nerve fibres more uniformly than glia; he also speculated upon the possibility of regeneration. Curiously, Dawson neglected Marburg's (1906) important monograph identifying shadow plaques but did refer to *Markschattenherde*, which he considered to be evolving lesions, and mentioned three hyperacute cases with an accelerated clinical pattern of relapses, rapid accumulation of deficits and characteristic histological features. In concluding his magisterial account, Dawson returned to the inflammatory versus developmental debate. He noted that E. Müller (1910), the most articulate teacher from the developmental school, proposed that the participation of the blood vessels within the lesion is secondary and that the glial proliferation is more than reparatory, but he had difficulty with the notion of 'multiple gliosis' (reminiscent of Charcot) as the essential process.

Dawson summarized his ideas on plaque formation around brain inflammation to include a sequence of events that, although not disease-specific, produced recognizable clinical characteristics when directed at glia, leading to degeneration of the myelin sheath with fat granule cell formation, and a reactive change in glia involving cell proliferation with fibril formation culminating in sclerosis. The whole process was triggered and modified by exogenous factors whose influences fluctuated, causing the characteristic relapses. Remissions depended more on rerouting of synaptic connections – for us, plasticity – than remyelination.

In providing a definitive analysis of the vascular hypothesis, Fog (1965) started with Borst (1903), who had collected the entire extant European literature, and proposed that plaques have a relationship with blood vessels. This was consistent with the views of Siemerling and Raecke (1911), Schob (1907), who wrote on cortical plaques, and Putnam and Adler (1937). That is not to say that each of these authors was signed up to the notion of an inflammatory mechanism, but merely that – both in the brain and spinal cord – lesions developed in the vicinity of one or more small arteries, veins or capillaries. Fog acknowledged that Marburg (1906; 1933) noted exceptions from this general rule and that G. Steiner (1931) and Hallervorden and Spatz (1933) preferred an interpretation for the anatomy of plaques reflecting an influence of noxious substances diffusing from the ventricular fluid but, nevertheless, Fog felt secure in his own position:

the pathologic–anatomic changes in the central nervous system in multiple sclerosis and disseminated encephalomyelitis may be the result of circulatory disturbances, especially of the venous drainage, but this disturbance may be intermittent and vary in degree.

Fog (1965) mapped the distribution of spinal lesions and concluded that these always evolve longitudinally around the radicular veins in white matter tracts without crossing the territory of neighbouring vessels in the transverse plane so that eventually their distribution is a faithful representation of the venous plexuses (Figure 1.18A–C). Neatly side-stepping rather a large number of neuropathology textbooks written before the early 1950s as not sufficiently interested in the details, Fog assigned authority to McAlpine *et al* (1955) for taking seriously the perivenous doctrine of the distribution and origin of plaques even if 'veins and venules do not determine the subsequent evolution of the form of the plaque'.

Fog (1965) reported in detail on two cases, R.H. and E.W.H., who died aged 50 and 31 years, having had symptoms and signs of multiple sclerosis described in meticulous clinical detail, for 18 and 6 years, respectively. He provided a block-by-block account of the pathology. Thirty-nine of 43 plaques contained a central vein that determined their shape and course – Dawson's fingers. He went further, and allowed that lesions were also associated with the presence of neuroglia (not distinguished as astrocytes or microglia), concluding that the periphlebitis of multiple sclerosis (and the retina) required

the venous wall + neuroglia complex ... multiple sclerosis is a condition of periphlebitis cerebrospinalis et retinalis

but whether this involved preformed lesions of a purely cytological nature, or reflected abnormality of a functional, perhaps enzymatic nature, he knew not.

It seems that even now this debate is not settled, leaving room for a steady stream of eccentric proposals. An Austrian doctor has made available an electronic version of his critical analysis of contemporary concepts on the aetiology of multiple sclerosis suggesting that the perivenous lesions are caused by widening of

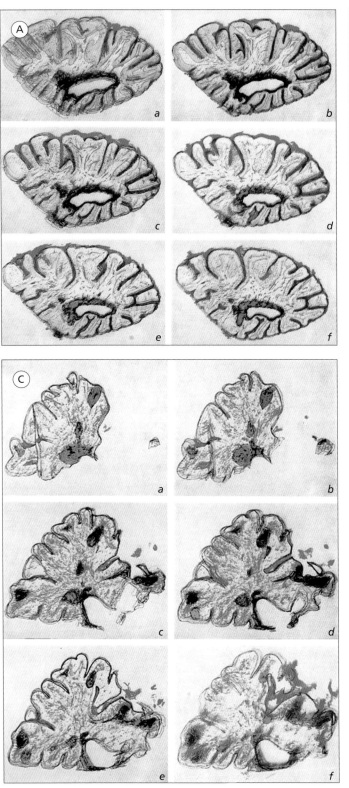

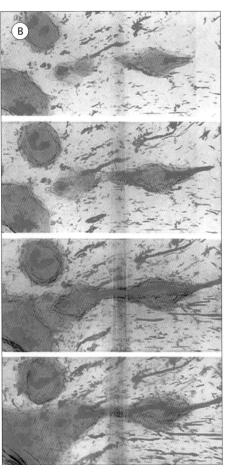

Figure 1.18 (A) Periventricular plaque (Block VIII, 6/58 F). Stereoscopic photographs. Acetate foil. Hemispheral sections. *a*: 155–179; *b*: 185–209; *c*: 212–239; *d*: 242–272; e: 275–296; *f*: 299–320. The great periventricular plaque (*a*) leaves the periventricular, subependymal gliosis (*b*), and decreases in size (*c,d,e*), along the longitudinally running veins, which are directed towards the central part of the white matter (*d,e,f*).
(B) Stereoscopic photographs. (Plaque 4, 'Key-drawing' 3, p. 49, Block 6/59 13 S). Drawings, Wild's method. Several sheets of acetate foil have been superimposed in series. Each photograph represents several sheets. The isolated plaques lie along central vessels belonging to the periventricular veins (lower left on photographs). (C) Periventricular plaque. (Plaque 9, 'Key-drawing' 3, p. 49, Block 6/59 13 S). Stereoscopic photographs. Acetate foil. Hemispheral sections. *a*: 487–475; *b*: 472–457; *c*: 418–394; *d*: 391–367; e: 364–346; *f*: 343–298. The periventricular plaque with a central prolongation upwards (*a*) leaves the subependymal region (*d*) and decreases in size along the longitudinally running transversely cut veins (*e,f*). The prolongation from *a* decreases in size towards the central white matter in the same way, along the veins (*b,c,d*). The longitudinal arrangement of the plaques [green] and the vessels is evident, especially in *f*. From Fog (1965) with permission.

venous foramina in the skulls of affected individuals. We find this hypothesis less than compelling and are sparing our readers further details or advertisement of the website. As late as 2003, the ideas of Charcot have been resurrected (though without identifying them as such). According to Behan *et al* (2003), the notion of multiple sclerosis as a focal inflammatory and autoimmune disease is based on erroneous extrapolation from animal models. Rather, multiple sclerosis is a neurodegenerative and clinically progressive trait in which expression of a gene on chromosome 17 (amongst others), influenced by sunlight and vitamin D activity, promotes generalized astrocyte proliferation with secondary damage to the blood–brain barrier and metabolic defects. Plaques represent focal areas of maximum compromise and not structural, functional and metabolic lesions radiating out in directions determined stochastically and by boundaries within the central nervous system from a nidus of the disease process. Central to this revolutionary formulation is the analysis that 'lesions of MS have... scant or even absent inflammatory reactions ... such infiltrates lack aggressiveness'.

But to quote the alleged authorities for that position, Dawson (1916) considered that:

I am not in agreement with Müller's view that the areas in disseminated sclerosis arise solely on the basis of an increasing glia hyperplasia ... there is overwhelming evidence that the great majority have arisen on an inflammatory basis.

Lumsden (McAlpine *et al* 1955) had once initially taken the position that:

there is ... little inflammatory cellular reaction even during the acute phases of plaque development ... the disease is a toxi-degenerative process

but his last word was:

it is a disorder of the myelin sheath–oligodendroglial cell complex. The evidence that this is ... due to specific anti-myelin antibodies is ... almost inescapable ... small to moderate numbers of plasmacytotoid lymphocytes are regularly present at all stages of actively demyelinated plaques.

And building on Dawson, Adams (1977) provided an unambiguous exposition of the important role played by infiltrating lymphocytes in the pathogenesis of multiple sclerosis:

I have put forward evidence that perivenous cuffing may precede formation of the perivenous plaque and that a probing finger of lymphocytic infiltration (Dawson's finger) pushes along the vein in advance of demyelination.

Evolving concepts in the pathogenesis of multiple sclerosis: evidence for axon degeneration

The role of axonal pathology, and the history of this recognition (Kornek and Lassmann 1999), have recently been revisited as part of the need to understand the natural history of multiple

sclerosis (Figure 1.19A–D). Charcot had described axon loss in some lesions of *sclérose en plaques* (1868b) and linked these to clinical disability:

Generally one of the lower limbs is first and solely affected. The other limb is seized, sooner or later, in its turn; the paresis advances with extreme slowness ... but at last the day comes when ... they may be confined to bed ... This resistance of the axis cylinders ... may account for the slowness with which the paretic symptoms advance in disseminated sclerosis and for the long space of time which elapses before they give place to complete paralysis and permanent contracture.

The problem of axonal loss in multiple sclerosis was very clearly defined by Otto Marburg in 1906 with the following account:

The statement, that axons remain relatively intact is also true for the cases of acute MS. The emphasis in this sentence, however, is not in the word intact but in the word relative, since the fact is more and more appearing, that in multiple sclerosis more axons are destroyed than generally believed.

But Lumsden identified Putnam (1936) as the originator of the concept that there is substantial axon degeneration in the pathology of multiple sclerosis:

The persistence of axons is such a cardinal point in the pathologic picture that many articles on the subject leave the impression that all are intact in all sclerotic plaques. This is certainly not the case, and modern pathologists who have made intensive studies of the disease (for example, Dawson, Spielmeyer, Jakob, Hassin and Bertrand) all agree that axons are seldom undamaged and are often completely destroyed and that secondary degeneration is common.

Clearly, Putnam did not know the literature since there are many very complete descriptions on this topic before Dawson (see Kornek and Lassmann 1999).

That position was modified by Greenfield and King (1936), who found severe destruction (around 80% loss) of axon cylinders in <10% plaques. They also put paid to the notion most clearly articulated by Erben (1898), who had proposed axonal regeneration as the mechanism of clinical remission in multiple sclerosis. Charcot's early awareness of axonal pathology – a variable mixture of demyelinated fibres with increased diameters dispersed by expanded extracellular, large axonal swellings in the plaque centre, thin axons surrounded by glial scar formation, and axonal loss in a minority of patients and lesions – was brought into focus by Marburg (1906), who catalogued the prevalence of these features. Focal axonal swellings predominate in early and acute lesions, followed by disintegration of the whole axon. Other fibres, however, merely showed an even thickening of their calibre. Marburg also addressed in detail the question of secondary tract degeneration and concluded that this is to be found in some tracts normally connected to lesions:

When secondary degeneration is defined by the complete destruction of nerve fibres in the direction of their projection, then the position of Müller has to be endorsed, when he claims its rare occurrence.

He then cites and reports examples of lesions in defined systems, with and without secondary tract degeneration. Marburg's final conclusion on this topic, in a study that described in detail toxic primary demyelination in the peripheral nervous system, was:

In light of my description it is not difficult to interpret the process at the nerve fibre. It completely complies with the picture of the periaxial Neuritis of Gombault...

In line with the parallel development of German and French schools of clinical pathology, Fromann (1878) described axonal transections with swellings at the border of the lesions in multiple sclerosis, and distanced himself from axonal preservation as one criterion for neuropathological definition of the disease although he had been the first to illustrate demyelination in his earlier monograph (Fromann 1864; Figure 1.12). By 1914, Siemerling and Raecke (1914) considered that the sequence of

pathological changes was sufficiently clear to allow the conclusion that a decrease in the number of axons and reduced axonal diameter in surviving fibres characterized chronic plaques, but that most axonal injury occurred early in the disease. This conclusion, reached after much painstaking neuropathological description, had been anticipated by Babinski (1885b), who correlated the extent of inflammation with the degree of axonal loss. Fraenkel and Jakob (1913) described the association with macrophage infiltration. Interestingly, the recognition of axonal injury in multiple sclerosis lesions more or less vanished from the clinical and neuropathology literature after the late 1930s. In part this can be explained by the fact that the issue was settled among neuropathologists, and there was little to be added to existing descriptions. In the clinical literature this topic was, however, nearly completely forgotten and only rediscovered when magnetic resonance techniques revealed quantitative injury or loss of axons.

No work has so influenced neurologists in the English-speaking world as Russell Brain's *Diseases of the Nervous System*, which first appeared (Brain 1933) 3 years after he wrote, on the grand scale, a masterly review for the *Quarterly*

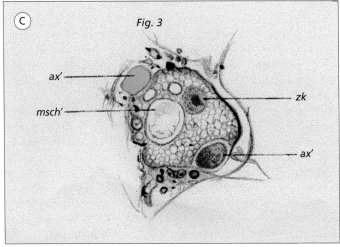
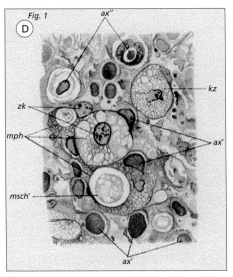
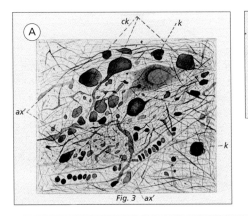
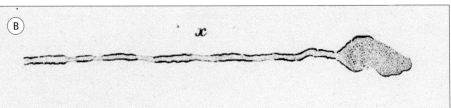

Figure 1.19 (A) Swollen and transected axons in a cervical cord lesion, illustrated by Doinikow (1915). *ax'*: swollen axis cylinders; *ek*: Endkugeln (endballs); *k*: isolated balls. (B) Partly demyelinated axon with terminal retraction ball, illustrated by Carl Fromann (1878). The nerve fibre is depicted from the border of a cerebellar lesion. (C,D) Two illustrations of axons, associated with macrophages in a thoracic cord lesion: *insch*: *Markreste* (myelin debris); *ax'*: swollen demyelinated axon in close contact to macrophages; *ax"*: swollen axon with altered myelin sheath; *kz*: *Körnerzelle* (debris containing macrophage); *zk*: *Zellkern* (cell nucleus); *mph*; macrophage; *gla, glst, ggla*: glia cells, illustrated by Fraenkel and Jacob (1912). From Kornek and Lassmann (1999) with permission.

Journal of Medicine on clinical and pathological aspects of multiple sclerosis (Brain 1930). We can usefully trace the evolution of prevailing views on the pathogenesis and other aspects of the disease through the many editions of this book. Drawing heavily on the observations of Dawson (1916), Brain first describes a sequence in which perivascular infiltration of lymphocytes and plasma cells is followed by phagocytosis of myelin, fibroglial overgrowth and some axonal loss. He notes shadow plaques, now thought to indicate remyelination. In discussing the distribution of lesions throughout the nervous system, Brain emphasizes the co-location of plaques and rich vascular networks around the ventricles, under the pial membranes and in the spinal cord. Dr Brain restates the doctrine of neurobiology inherited from Santiago Ramón y Cajal (1852–1934) and his students Pío del Río Hortega (1882–1945), and Wilder Penfield (1891–1976) (see below), describing the morphological and anatomical arrangements of fibrous and protoplasmic astrocytes, assigning a phagocytic role to microglia but confessing to ignorance on the function of oligodendrocytes. He points out that the early vascular lesion indicates invasion of the nervous system by a systemic and infective factor capable of provoking the astroglial reaction that he regards as the essential pathogenic feature of the disease. However, Russell Brain argues that factors distributed in the cerebrospinal fluid could as easily gain access to the brain parenchyma through the Virchow–Robin spaces, as could material crossing the vessel walls.

By the second edition (Brain 1940), Brain's reading of the pathological papers of Dawson (1916), Putnam (1936; Putnam and Adler 1937) and Greenfield and King (1936) presents a much clearer view of the sequence of perivascular lymphocytic infiltration, lipid ingestion by fat granule cells, myelin degeneration, fibroglial proliferation, and some axonal loss leading to formation of the sclerotic plaque. Russell Brain had further reconsidered his views on demyelinating disease when he returned to the topic in 1951; he wished to emphasize that axon cylinders were often involved in the disease process and he felt ambivalent about the conclusion that myelin destruction was necessarily the primary change. He sensed a growing belief that progress in understanding demyelinating diseases would result from studies of the experimental model first mentioned in his second edition (Brain 1940). Although intravenously injected antibodies recognizing constituents of the nervous system would not reproduce the pathological features of postinfectious encephalomyelitis, Brain accepted as proven the claim that the human and experimental diseases were allergic.

THE LABORATORY SCIENCE OF MULTIPLE SCLEROSIS: 1913–1981

Charcot measured clinical deficits and speculated on their physiological basis but he lacked clear ideas on the neuroanatomical basis for disability. In his magisterial work on the histology of the central nervous system published (in Spanish) between 1899 and 1904 (English translation of the French edition [1909–1911] published in 1995), Cajal applied the neuron doctrine to circuitry underlying motor control and showed the connectivity of Purkinje cells in the dentate nucleus of the cerebellum with input from contralateral corticopontine fibres and output to the opposite cortex via the red nucleus through the superior cerebellar peduncle. But despite clinical measurement of disordered function in defined circuits, the pathways affected by multiple sclerosis and other neurological disorders remained inaccessible to laboratory measurement.

Neurophysiological techniques, developed over a number of years, culminated in the introduction of evoked potentials for measuring conduction, initially in the human optic nerve but subsequently in other central sensory and motor pathways (see Chapter 13 for further details and additional historical perspectives). The exploration of human brain function by evoked potential methods originates with the observations of George Dawson (1912–1983). Before that, Richard Caton (1842–1926), working in Liverpool, had first extended knowledge on the electrical basis for nerve action, discovered by Luigi Galvani (1737–1798) in 1791 and developed by Emil du Bois Raymond (1818–1896) in 1848, to the brain (Caton 1875). Hans Berger (1873–1941) later recorded this activity through the intact skull and the technique was perfected by E.D. Adrian, who also developed methods for recording electrical activity from peripheral nerves. Intracellular recordings later led to elucidation of the conduction of the nerve impulse by Sir Alan Hodgkin (1914–1998) and Sir Andrew Huxley. The group of Martin Halliday and Ian McDonald moved electrical exploration of conduction in the central nervous system into clinical practice, showing the reduced amplitude and delay of the pattern-evoked visual potential in the evolution of acute optic neuritis (Halliday *et al* 1972: Figure 1.20A,B). Subsequently, the prevalence of abnormal visual evoked potentials was described in multiple sclerosis (Halliday *et al* 1973a). Distinctions were made from the reduced amplitude with preserved latency that usually (though not invariably) characterizes compression of the anterior visual pathway (Halliday *et al* 1976); and the important observation was made that, with time, there may be a return towards normal in latency of the evoked potential. This is seen much more frequently in childhood than in adult optic neuritis, suggesting an enhanced potential for remyelination and restoration of normal conduction velocity in the juvenile demyelinated optic nerve (Kriss *et al* 1988).

The discovery by Tom Sears and Hugh Bostock in the 1970s (Bostock and Sears 1976, 1978) that conduction can be restored in persistently demyelinated axons opened the way for an understanding of the early rapid recovery that may be seen after individual episodes of demyelination. It also provided a basis for understanding the mechanism of the long delays in visual evoked potentials. Thus, by the 1970s, sufficient lines of evidence were in place from clinical, pathological and experimental studies to show that adult nervous systems have the capacity for adaptation, plasticity and endogenous remyelination. Work could then begin on the development of strategies for enhancing and supplementing these repair mechanisms (see below).

The most direct method for examining body fluids that reflect brain activity was the introduction of lumbar puncture in life. (Domenico Cotugno [1736–1822] removed fluid from cadavers.) First used at the Middlesex Hospital in London by Walter Essex Wynter (1860–1945) to treat children with tuberculous meningitis (described by Robert Whytt in 1768), the procedure was routinely applied in neurology by Heinrich Iraneaeus Quincke (1842–1922) from 1891. He measured the pressure and examined the chemical constituents of cerebrospinal fluid. Charles Albert Lange (1883–1959) described qualitative features of the

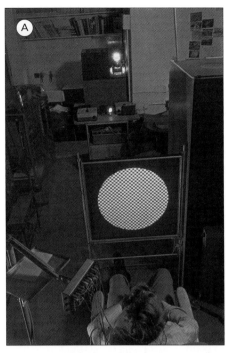

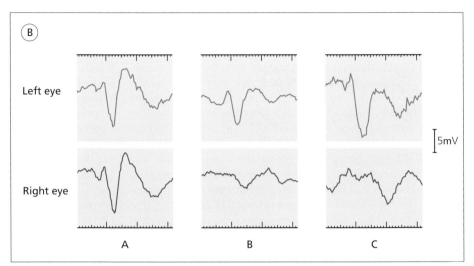

Figure 1.20 (A) The original system used to record visual evoked potentials. (B) *A*: Pattern evoked responses, recorded from a midline occipital electrode from the left and right eye of a healthy subject. *B,C*: Two patients recovering from acute attacks of optic neuritis in the right eye with onset (*B*) 4 weeks and (*C*) 3 weeks previously. Time scale: 10, 50 and 100 ms. Note the delayed peak of the response from the affected eye and its smaller peak-to-peak amplitude. From Halliday *et al* (1972) with permission from Elsevier.

protein content. He published observations on the colloidal gold curve in cerebrospinal fluid of patients with a variety of inflammatory brain diseases (Lange 1913). Lange received his medical degree from Hessische Ludwigs Universität Medizinische Fakultät, in Hesse, Germany, in 1907, emigrated to the United States in 1935 and worked at the department of health in Albany, New York, until retiring in 1951.

Elvin Kabat (1914–2000) provided the first physicochemical characterization of immunoglobulin G and, on return to Columbia University from Sweden in 1941, adapted this to demonstrate intrathecal antibody synthesis in multiple sclerosis (Kabat *et al* 1942: Figure 1.21A,B). Later, he defined the framework and complementarity-determining regions of antibody providing the molecular basis for therapeutic humanization of monoclonal antibodies (see Chapter 18). The paretic Lange curve reflects the presence of cathodic oligoclonal bands (Professor Edward Thompson, personal communication), now forming part of diagnostic criteria for multiple sclerosis. In the modern era, no one did more to illuminate the role and specificity of oligoclonal antibody detected in the cerebrospinal fluid of patients with multiple sclerosis than John Whitaker (1940–2001). One of the most personable and charming individuals in the multiple sclerosis clinical science community, John studied medicine at the University of Tennessee College of Medicine, becoming chairman of neurology at the University of Alabama at Birmingham from 1985 (and president of the American Neurological Association, 1995–97), with a devoted following of patients and loyal professional colleagues.

These markers of an antibody response focused attention on the concept that multiple sclerosis is an inflammatory and – in all probability – autoimmune disorder. That story began with the courageous and successful vaccination of Joseph Meister,

bitten by a rabid dog, by Louis Pasteur in 1885. Thereafter, the experience of injecting brain extracts to treat rabies (Remlinger 1928; Uchimura and Shiraki 1957), or more frivolously to support failing organs (a case reported by Seitelberger *et al* 1958), was complicated by the development of paralysis or even death. Debate ensued on the immune mechanisms involved and what in the inoculum was so neuroprovocative. The ability to reproduce many features of post-vaccination encephalomyelitis and the recognition of a comparable clinical disorder – acute disseminated encephalomyelitis by Hurst (1941) – provided a stimulus for the development of animal models. This led to the development of experimental autoimmune encephalomyelitis in monkeys – fed bananas for breakfast, bread for lunch, hot milk for supper, and raw carrots or roasted peanuts as treats (Figure 1.22; Rivers *et al* 1933; Rivers and Schwentker 1935). Experimental autoimmune encephalomyelitis has since been supported by researchers and funding organizations on an industrial scale (see Chapter 11), with modified protocols allowing extension to species other than primates, and eventually reproducing an increasingly comprehensive catalogue of clinical, natural history and pathological features of the human disease but proving something of a tease with respect to the successful screening of definitive therapies. Nevertheless, experimental autoimmune encephalomyelitis has taught essential lessons on antigen recognition by T cells and cellular immunity, on autoimmunity in general, as well as on the basic mechanisms of inflammation-induced tissue injury in the brain. Most influential was the demonstration that experimental autoimmune encephalomyelitis could be adoptively transferred (Lipton and Freund 1953) and that this was attributable to cells (Paterson 1960) not serum (Chase 1959). Subsequent work established the principle of strain specificity, taken to indicate genetic susceptibility

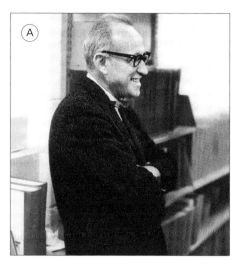

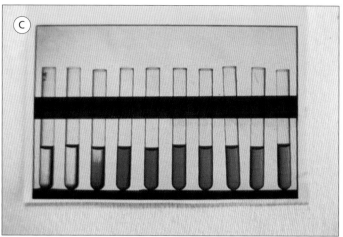

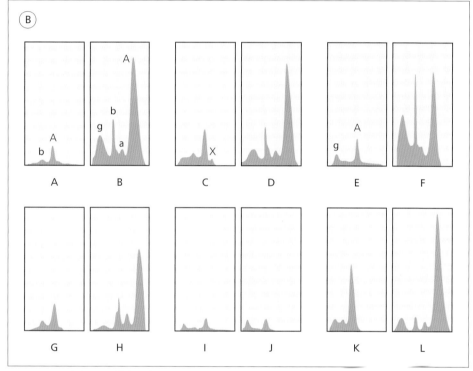

Figure 1.21 (A) Elvin Kabat (1914–2000). (B) Electrophoretic patterns. *A,B*: Idiopathic grand mal (normal), spinal fluid and serum. *C,D*: Anxiety state (normal), spinal fluid and serum. *E,F*: Lymphopathia venereum, spinal fluid and serum. *G,H*: Multiple myeloma, spinal fluid and serum. *I*: Multiple sclerosis, spinal fluid. *J*: Neurosyphilis, spinal fluid. *K*: Diabetic neuritis, spinal fluid. *L*: Left frontal cystic astrocytoma, cyst fluid. From Kabat *et al* (1942) with permission. (C) The paretic Lange curve (kindly provided by Professor Edward Thompson).

(Olitsky and Yager 1949), documented the histological and ultrastructural features (Lampert and Carpenter 1965) and established the relative importance of T lymphocytes (J.F.A.P. Miller 1961; Jankovic *et al* 1962). For many years experimental autoimmune encephalomyelitis was considered an autoimmune disease, mediated by a single immune cell population (Th1 cells), directed against a single antigen (myelin basic protein; Kies *et al* 1960). Extrapolating this simple concept of the pathogenesis to multiple sclerosis suggested many therapeutic options – some (such as Copolymer I) proving partially effective but the majority not becoming established treatments for multiple sclerosis. The reason is that, even in experimental autoimmune

encephalomyelitis, the focus on a purely T-cell-orientated process directed solely against myelin basic protein ignores the contribution of other immune mechanisms, such as demyelinating antibodies (Bornstein and Appel 1961) and different brain antigens, such as proteolipid protein (Waksman *et al* 1954). Later it became clear that autoimmune encephalomyelitis can be induced by several different T-lymphocyte populations; that it can be modulated by additional antibody reactions; and that nearly every central nervous system protein is a potential candidate for an encephalitogenic T-cell response. Now the model is again much closer to multiple sclerosis but the lesson that therapeutic intervention targeting a single mechanism may not be

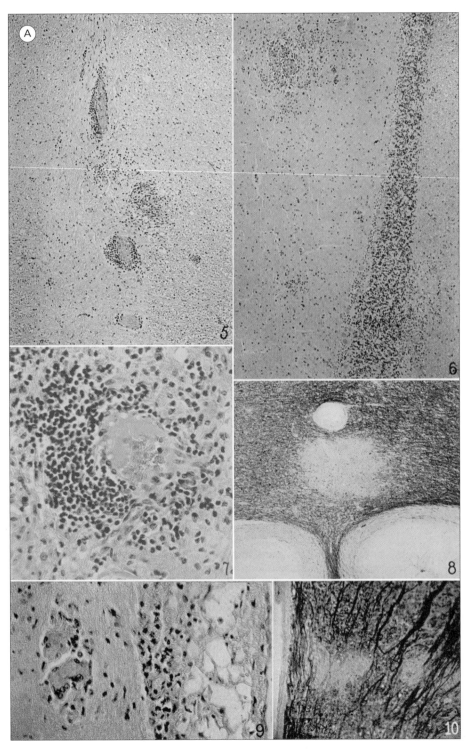

Figure 1.22 Histological features of experimental autoimmune encephalomyelitis. (A) *Fig. 5:* Lesions in the pons of Monkey 30. H & E, ×63. *Fig. 6:* Lesions in the cerebellum of Monkey 30. H & E, ×63. *Fig. 7:* Perivascular infiltration in the pons of Monkey 30. H & E, ×250. *Fig. 8:* Demyelination in cerebellum of Monkey 30. Modified Weigert stain, ×37. *Fig. 9:* Giant cells in cerebellum, and thickened cerebellar meninges infiltrated with mononuclear cells. Monkey 30. H & E, ×250. *Fig. 10:* Demyelination in pons of Monkey 30. Modified Weigert stain, ×37.

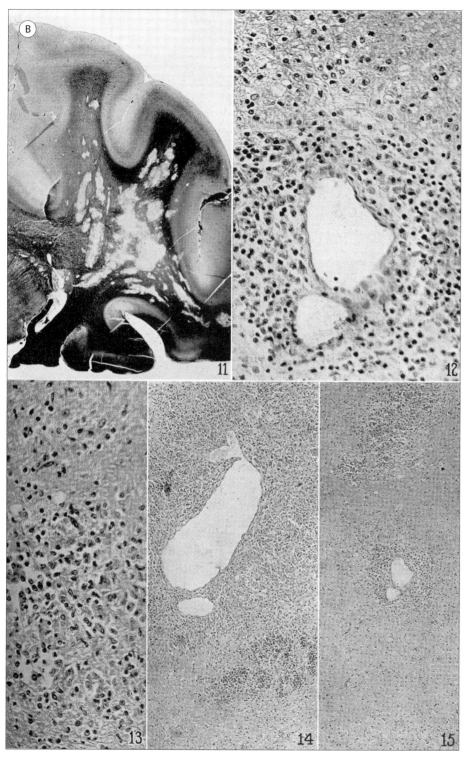

Figure 1.22, cont'd (B) *Fig. 11:* Demyelination in the right parietal lobe of Monkey 31. The picture is suggestive of Schilder's disease. Modified Weigert stain, ×37. *Figs 12–15:* Lesions in the right parietal lobe of Monkey 31. Note the perivascular distribution. H & E, ×250 and ×63. From Rivers *et al* (1933) with permission.

sufficient is still not entirely learned. The current status of experimental autoimmune encephalomyelitis and useful insights into the evolution of knowledge from 1933 are provided by Lawrence Steinman (2003): charting the efforts of three Nobel laureates, his account also highlights the work of 38 named investigators, many working in the current era, who have contributed to knowledge on the merits and demerits of experimental autoimmune encephalomyelitis as a useful and representative model of multiple sclerosis. Ending with a metaphor drawn from reggae ballad music that plays on the rivers theme ('Many rivers to cross but just where to begin' by Jimmy Cliff), Steinman congratulates experimental autoimmune encephalomyelitis on its 70th birthday and wishes it well for the centenary celebration in 2033.

Until 1850, the main methods available for printing anatomical illustrations were woodcuts in which a relief of the image was carved on pear or boxwood. Alternatively, metal plates were engraved with line drawings and printed separately from the text. Lithography, invented and patented by Senefelder in 1799, produced the image with water-repellent grease on stone or metal and inked the contrasting dampened and greased surfaces. This was the first technique suitable for multiple reproductions of the same image (or text) and coloured illustration (first used in Gaspare Aselli's *De lactibus, sive lacteis venis*, which appeared posthumously in 1627). Photography was developed by Niepce and Daguerre (daguerreotypes) and by Fox Talbot, in 1839 and 1840, respectively. It was used sporadically in medical texts from the 1850s. The first neurological photograph depicts the mummified brain of a Muscovy slave exhibited at the 1867 *Exposition Universelle* and published by Thaddee Zulinski. In 1873 Guillaume Duchenne (1806–1875) and Jules Bernard Luys (1828–1897) published a photographic atlas dedicated to neuroanatomy. Charcot placed great emphasis on medical illustration and was responsible for much of the material appearing in the *Iconographie Photographique de la Salpêtrière* (Bourneville and Regnard 1876–1880) and the *Nouvelle Iconographie de la Salpêtrière* (1884–1912). Photographs of Charcot's cases appear in the later writings of Pierre Marie (1853–1940) and other students during the early 1890s. By this time, photographs were more often being used to depict clinical and histological features of neurological disease, although this practice was not fully adopted prior to the introduction of X-rays. We believe that the first photographs dealing with multiple sclerosis were the series showing spinal cord pathology in volume three of the *Nouvelle Iconographie de la Salpêtrière* (Blocq and Londe 1890) and showing the gross and microscopic appearance of extensive symmetrical demyelination in the dorsal root entry zone of the cervical cord (Figure 1.23). Not until 1905 was a clinical photograph published of an individual with multiple sclerosis (Scherb 1905). This patient developed an isolated cerebellar syndrome in 1898 with disturbances of posture whilst walking and sitting, which, despite formidable alcohol intake, was considered by the authors to be a *forme fruste* of *sclérose en plaques* (Figure 1.24).

Definitive textbooks on neuroradiology began to appear within a few years of the demonstration by Wilhelm Roentgen (1845–1923) of the X-ray of the bone in his wife Bertha's hand. It was an imaginative next step to adapt this technique using substances, including radio-opaque dyes, introduced in and around the brain and spinal cord to define their structure by silhouette. In 1918, Walter Edward Dandy (1886–1946) outlined the outer and inner contours of the brain using air introduced directly into the ventricles or lumbar sac. Jean Athanase Sicard (1872–1929) replaced air with iodinized oil and produced images of the spinal canal by myelography in 1921. The most colourful of these early pioneers was Antoni Caetano de Abreu Egas Moniz (1875–1955), who after signing the Versailles treaty for Portugal in 1918, returned to neurology and introduced arteriography (1927). He was best known for pioneering frontal

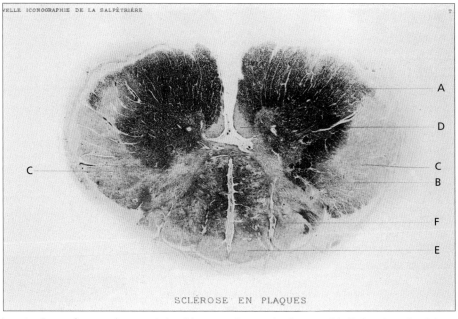

Figure 1.23 Multiple sclerosis. Area of great change. *A:* healthy part; *B:* marginal area with little sclerosis; *C:* lateral fascicles showing considerable change; *D:* sclerotic area of Türck's fascicle; *E:* posterior part of Goll's cord in very changed state; *F:* significantly thickened posterior septum. From Blocq and Londe (1890) with permission.

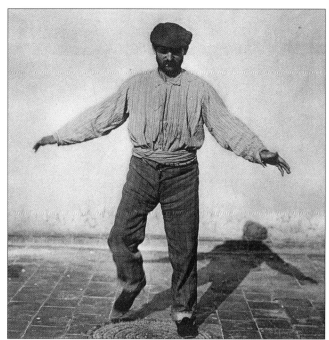
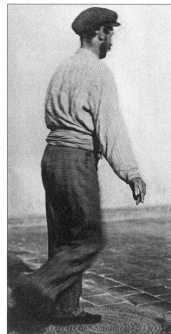
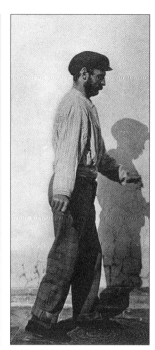

Figure 1.24 Crude multiple sclerosis or Babinski's cerebellar syndrome. From Scherb (1905) with permission.

leucotomy and other forms of psychosurgery (receiving the Nobel prize in 1949 but nearly losing his life at the hands of a gun-crazed schizophrenic patient in his office). Even when neuroradiology was introduced, the procedures offered limited information, showing only the grossest abnormalities, and failing to depict most processes that affect tissue integrity. Neurologists trained exclusively since the early 1970s must find it hard to imagine the confidence needed accurately to localize structural lesions as the sufficient basis for surgical exploration using nothing more than clinical analysis.

Although low-resolution radioisotope brain scans had on rare occasions shown large cerebral lesions in cases of multiple sclerosis, radiological techniques capable of routinely identifying the lesions of multiple sclerosis with some consistency were not available until the invention of computerized axial tomography (CT) by Godfrey Hounsfield (1919–2004) in 1971 (Figure 1.25A). The idea came to Hounsfield on a country walk. With a background in electronics and radar, it occurred to him that readings from a large quantity of measurements taken randomly of objects in a closed box would reveal their shape when processed. It was a small step to add the principles of using an X-ray beam and sensitive detectors rather than film, constrained to slices that were then reconstructed into a three-dimensional image. Although Hounsfield was working for Electric and Musical Industries (EMI), where better to apply this technique than in the brain? The first picture of a cerebral cyst was displayed in April 1972 – to a standing ovation from 2000 conference attendees (*Times*, 18th August 2004). Hounsfield received the Nobel Prize in Physiology or Medicine in 1979. The situation changed even more dramatically with the application of nuclear magnetic resonance to biological structures, for which Paul Lauterbur and (Sir) Peter Mansfield received the Nobel Prize in Physiology or Medicine in 2003 (Figure 1.25B). The application of magnetic resonance imaging (MRI) to multiple sclerosis came early (I.R. Young *et al* 1981; Figure 1.25C,D). This technique has subse-

quently been routinely applied to the diagnosis of multiple sclerosis, the understanding of its pathogenesis, and the assessment of treatment. No procedure has so revolutionized the everyday practice of medicine and opened up methods for studying normal and abnormal structure as the introduction of computerized axial tomography, although its low sensitivity in detecting areas of demyelination and the preclusion of repeated scanning due to radiation exposure have limited its role as a tool in diagnosis and monitoring multiple sclerosis. The subsequently developed techniques for depicting structure and function of the brain using magnetic resonance imaging have, in contrast, proved uniquely valuable in both diagnosis and monitoring the disease course. And even those who witnessed this transition would not have imagined the possibilities (revisiting the glorious age of 18 and 19th century phrenology) for demonstrating functional brain activity during a host of behavioural activations, real and imagined. If award of the Nobel Prize in Physiology or Medicine is about ingenuity, step-changes in knowledge, promotion of human health, and opening up unimagined opportunities for illuminating medicine – motives that inspired Vesalius and Willis – the recognition of Sir Godfrey Hounsfield (and Allan Cormack) in 1979 for their unrivalled contribution in the latter half of the 20th century is surely not contested.

DISCOVERY OF GLIA AND REMYELINATION: 1858–1983

Microscopes were developed in the 1640s and a range of histological stains, suitable for distinguishing cell types within intact tissue, became available during the 19th century. Virchow pioneered the modern concept of the cell theory – every cell is derived from a pre-existing cell – but the nervous system was thought to be an exception and comprised a reticular network rather than an aggregate of individual cells. It was Camillo

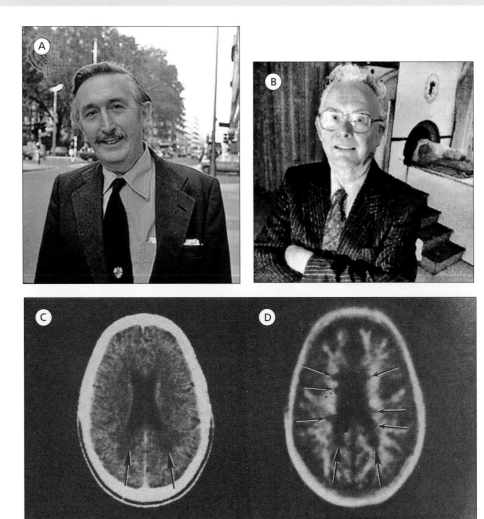

Figure 1.25 (A) Sir Godfrey Hounsfield (1919–2004). (B) Sir Peter Mansfield. (C) Comparable CT and (D) MRI scans (in patient 10) at mid-ventricular level. The two posterior periventricular lesions seen on the CT scan are also seen on the MRI scan (large arrows). In addition six smaller lesions are seen on the MRI scan at the lateral margin of the lateral ventricles (small arrows). The sharply defined area on the medial margin of the left posterior horn is a circular artefact. Parts A, C and D from I.R. Young *et al* (1981) with permission from Elsevier.

Golgi's (1843–1926) silver stain and the use to which this was put by Cajal that culminated in definitive studies of the cellular architecture and organization of the central nervous system. From this work emerged the neuron theory, for which Cajal and Golgi were jointly awarded the 1906 Nobel Prize in Physiology or Medicine. Golgi's first work on glial cells appeared some time before and his final position was that 'true glial cells are nothing more than displaced and transformed neuroepithelial cells'.

Working in the kitchen of the private asylum at Abbiategrasso, Golgi discovererd his silver nitrate 'black reaction' for identifying nerve cells. But, paradoxically, Golgi remained convinced of the reticular theory and he disagreed publicly with Cajal on the neuron doctrine when they gave their 1906 Nobel lectures in Stockholm. As Cajal, the dominant figure in neuroscience, reflected: 'what a cruel irony of fate to pair, like Siamese twins united by the shoulders, scientific adversaries of such contrasting character'.

Cajal's work is relatively unread in the original but translations have appeared in recent years. He described accurately the distinguishing features of neurons and glia within discrete regions of the brain and spinal cord; he characterized their local organization, supplementing the descriptions with beautiful drawings based on Golgi's silver stains; and he consolidated the neuron doctrine. Preceded in this work by Jan Purkinje (1787–1869), Wilhelm His (1831–1904) and Fridtjof Nansen (1861–1930: neuroscientist, Arctic explorer and humanist), Cajal perfected Golgi's method and advanced his discoveries through the study of developing nervous systems in order to overcome the limitation of poor silver staining of myelinated fibres (Figure 1.26A–G). He showed histologically the variability of dendritic arborizations and axon terminations, established that axon cylinders end freely but form contacts, and conceived that the nerve impulse is conducted between axons, dendrites and the cell body of neighbouring neurons. Everything we know about structure, function and physiology in the nervous system at the cellular level, in health and disease, stems from the concept that organization is through the connectivity of functionally independent neurons and their processes. Cajal extended his studies on cellular architecture of the nervous system to a functional analysis declaring the axipetal polarization of dendrites whereas the axon shows somatofugal and dendrofugal transmission of activity away from the cell body and towards its terminals, solving at a stroke, to quote Sherrington, the great question of the direction of the nerve currents in their travel through the brain and spinal cord. In time, no part of the brain and spinal cord went unexplored.

Virchow first described neuroglia ('nerve glue') and assigned two functions – mechanical support of nerve cells and tissue repair (Virchow 1854). Three further activities were proposed before the end of the 19th century – nutritional support of neurons (Golgi 1894), engulfment of cellular debris (Bevan Lewis 1897) and isolation of nervous conduction – originally suggested by Cajal's brother Pedro (Cajal 1913; W.F. Robertson 1897). Oligodendrocytes were not recognized as a distinct macroglial subpopulation until many years after Virchow's original description, due to the lack of specific histological stains. W.F. Robertson (1899) reported the presence of small, process-bearing cells throughout both grey and white matter that stained selectively using a platinum impregnation technique. Believing them to be derived from mesoderm, he named these mesoglia but, in retrospect, this was the first description of the oligodendrocyte (Figure 1.27A; Penfield 1924). Cajal (1913) described a 'third element' of the nervous system (in addition to neurons and neuroglia), which he considered to be analogous to peripheral nerve Schwann cells. del Río Hortega, his most creative pupil, was nevertheless chased out of the Cajal laboratory in 1920 (although discreetly supported by his teacher thereafter) and then moving from Spain to Paris, Oxford and Argentina following the 1936 Spanish civil war. del Río Hortega (1921; Figure 1.27B) distinguished two cell types within Cajal's third element (first, neurons; second, astrocytes; third, mesodermal cells), which he named microglia (see del Río Hortega 1939). He identified oligodendroglia as being of ectodermal origin, and

placed these within Cajal's second element as partners for astrocytes. He established that microglia function as immune cells and have macrophage-like functions within the central nervous system (although even now their origin remains controversial). del Río Hortega (1921) renamed oligodendroglia as oligodendrocytes and described these as perineuronal or interfascicular, with four further types based on variations in cell morphology. Although the biological significance of this classification remained obscure, del Río Hortega's contribution includes the recognition that oligodendrocytes make the myelin sheath that surrounds axons in white matter of the central nervous system.

In fact, the role of neuroglia in myelin synthesis had been appreciated before del Río Hortega's discovery of the oligodendrocyte, Virchow (1854) having introduced the term myelin and described sheaths around nerve fibres. Apart from Cajal's (1913) suggestion that his third element was the central nervous system equivalent of Schwann cells, Hardesty (1904) depicted neuroglia as directly involved in myelin synthesis and, with the illustration of spiral projections from oligodendrocytes extending towards developing myelin sheaths in white matter from young animals, Penfield (1932) was able to conclude that oligodendrocytes 'have to do with the elaboration and maintenance of myelin'.

Despite del Río Hortega's contribution, the technical difficulty of demonstrating cytoplasmic connections between oligodendrocytes and myelin maintained uncertainty concerning the nature of myelinogenesis. Hypotheses included the suggestions that myelin in the central nervous system is produced by astrocytes, by axons, or by fusion of multiple vesicles within oligodendrocytes. Eventually, Bunge et al (1961) provided electron micrographs of developing white matter showing oligodendrocytes that extend processes continuous with the outer aspect of the myelin sheath. They produced the now classical cartoon

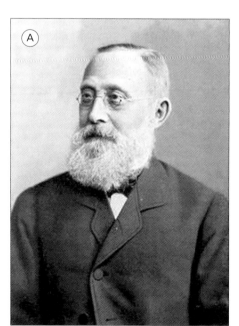
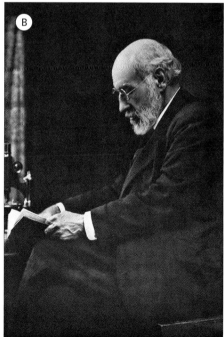
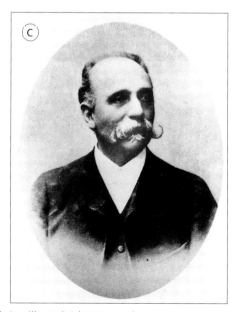

Figure 1.26 (A) Rudolph Virchow (1821–1902). (B) Santiago Ramón y Cajal (1852–1934). (C) Camillo Golgi (1843–1926).

illustration continued on following page

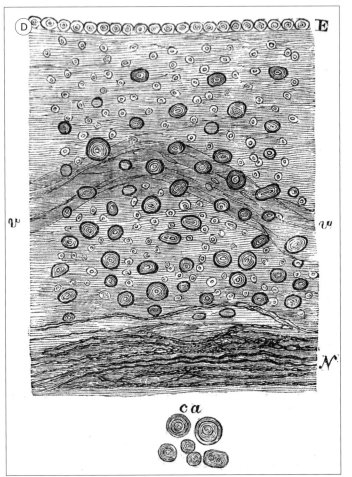

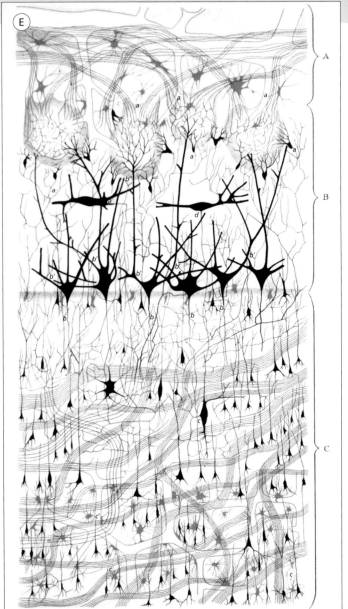

Figure 1.26, cont'd (D) Ependyma ventriculorum and neuroglia from the floor of the fourth ventricle. *E:* epithelium; *N:* nerve fibres. Between them the free portion of the neuro-glia with numerous connective-tissue-corpuscles and nuclei, at *v* a vessel. In addition, numerous corporea amalycea, which are moreover represented separately at c.300 diameters. From Virchow (1858). (E) The individual elements depicted in this figure were drawn point by point with greatest possible accuracy with the help of a 'camera clara' [lucida] developed by Oberhäuser. This drawing shows a piece from a vertical section of an olfactory bulb of a dog at a magnification of approximately 250 times. The three layers of this organ are marked by letters *A, B, C* at the margin of the figure. *A* indicates the superficial layer of the bulb, the layer of peripheral nerve fibres. It consists in essence of nerve fibre bundles, which are derived from the mucosa. These bundles cross each other, traverse to the glomerula, into which they insert and split into fine ramifications. In between these bundles a small blood vessel is visible, which sends several ramifications perpendicularly inwards. *B* depicts the middle layer, the grey matter. The glomerula olfactoria located at its peripheral border, at its inner border are large nerve cells, oriented in a row. The main nerve process (*b, b, b, b*) (the axon) of these cells is invariably directed towards the inner layer of the bulbus. In contrast the protoplasmic processes (*b', b', b', b', b*) project towards the glomerulus, into which they insert and ramify in a complicated manner. This ramification is in this picture only depicted in one process (*b''*). Towards the centre of layer *B* two large spindle-shaped nerve cells are shown, which have a nervous process stained in blue, that forms ramifications and declines into the layer of the nerve fibres. In the vicinity of the glomeruli some small nerve cells are seen. Their processes, which are directed towards the glomeruli, appear to be protoplasmic with a single one, which projects in the opposite direction and shows features of a nervous process. *C* defines the inner layer, the layer of nerve fibres, which originate from the tractus. In the empty spaces between crossing fibres are small elements with predominant pyramidal shape, which are potentially nervous in nature. In the middle of the layer one can see two cells, which appear to be neurons according to their size and shape as well as to the presence of a process (stained blue), that apparently represents a nervous process. The fibrils, which originate from ramifications of this process, merge with the bundles, which arise from the tractus. The complicated ramifications of the nerve fibres have been omitted from this drawing for simplification. The nature of their course and ramification can be estimated in the periphery of layer *C*. There some of the fibres give rise to bundles, they ramify in a complicated manner and traverse in a tortuous course the border to the white matter. They then reach the grey matter, which they cross, and finally they can be followed as delicate microfibres in the glomerula. The stroma of neuroglia cells is depicted as accurately as possible regarding their number and their relation to vessels only in the deep portions of layer *C*, where the star-like neuroglia cells are most abundant. In the other portions they are only shown in the border area between the white and grey matter, in the glomerula and in the layer of the peripheral nerve fibres. (They are depicted in red.) From Golgi (1894).

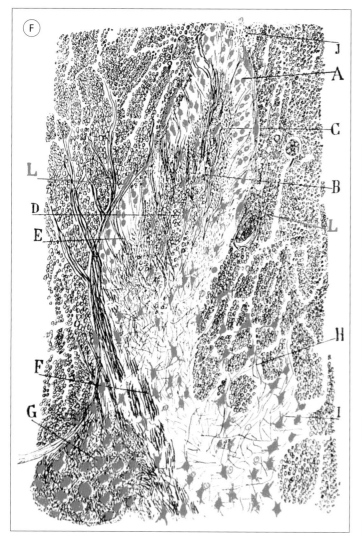

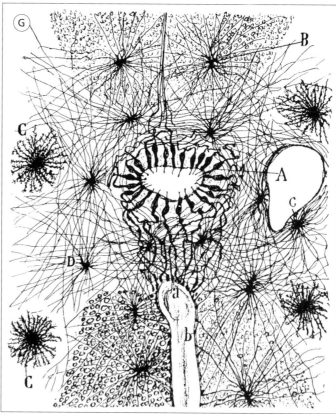

Figure 1.26, cont'd (F) Section of the dorsal horn of the adult human spinal cord. Weigert–Pal method and carmine. *A:* substantia gelatinosa; *C:* fine longitudinal fibres of the dorsal horn head; *D:* other large fibres; *E:* small myelinated bundles for the head of the horn; *F:* fascicles of sensory-motor collaterals; *G:* column of Clarke; *H:* interstitial nucleus. From Cajal (1899–1904). (G) Neuroglia of the central grey region and neighbouring portions of the white matter in the spinal cord of an 8-day-old infant (Golgi method). *A:* ependymal cells; *B:* neuroglia of the white matter; *C:* neuroglia with short processes; *b:* terminal swellings of neuroglial fibrils. From Cajal (1899–1904).

of one oligodendrocyte synthesizing myelin along short segments of several neighbouring axons (Figure 1.28A,B), in a manner similar to the way in which Geren (1954) had shown a few years earlier that the Schwann cell ensheathes the peripheral nerve axon. Subsequent ultrastructural studies have established that a single oligodendrocyte can myelinate internodal segments of 30–50 axons.

Asking whether structural repair occurs in demyelinated lesions is not a new question. In his medical thesis, Babinski (1885a) posed the question in chapter 3 of the section on pathological anatomy: 'Les tubes nerveux de la moelle peuvent-ils se régénérer après d'avoir été detruits?' In fact, his account dealt more with contemporary concepts of regeneration of nerve fibres than remyelination but the answer was staring him in the face since one of the lithographic illustrations to his thesis shows thin layers of myelin surrounding axons that are closely associated with fat granule cells removing myelin debris (Figure 1.29A–C). For Babinski, this was a demyelinating lesion; for us, it is a remyelinating acute inflammatory plaque. Marburg (1906)

also described the unusually thin myelin sheaths and discusses the possibility that they represent remyelination:

It has been postulated that it [remyelination] may occur and there are some observations, which may argue in favour for this view. I just point to the very thin fibers, which appear grey after osmic acid impregnation.

But he left open whether these appearances are due to incomplete demyelination or remyelination. Marburg's student Schlesinger described for the first time large plaques with uniformly thin myelin sheaths (Schlesinger 1909) and gave them the name *Markschattenherde* (shadow plaques). Despite their careful depictions and thoughtful analyses, neuropathologists were also slow to realize the significance of the shadow plaques, which Schlesinger (1909) and Dawson (1916) had both assumed to be evolving areas of demyelination.

Against this background, the topic of remyelination makes no serious progress until the demonstration by Richard and Mary Bunge (Bunge *et al* 1961) of myelin repair occurring in cats

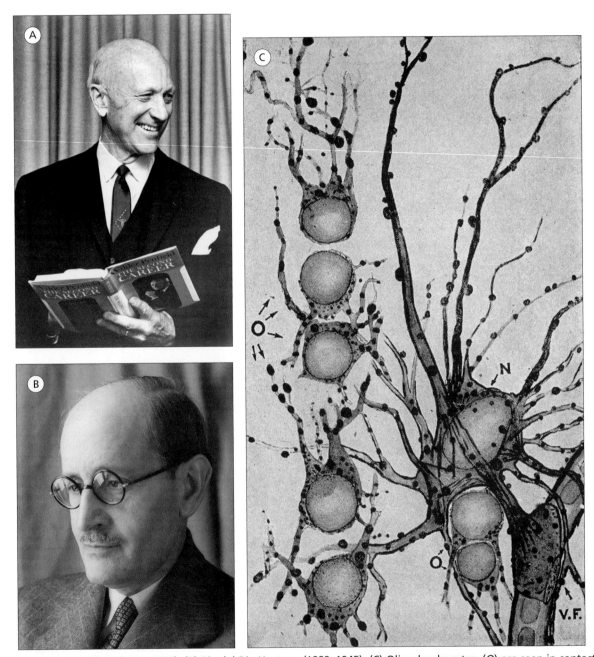

Figure 1.27 (A) Wilder Penfield (1891–1976). (B) Pío del Río Hortega (1882–1945). (C) Oligodendrocytes, (*O*) are seen in contact with the processes of a neuron (*N*) an astrocyte is shown with processes extending towards oligodendrocytes and contacting a blood vessel (at *V.F.*). From Penfield (1924) with permission of the curator of the Wilder Penfield Archive.

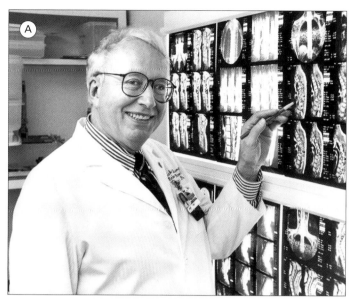

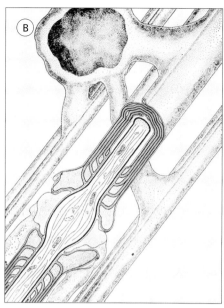

Figure 1.28 (A) Richard Bunge (1932–1996). (B) Illustration of both known and hypothetical aspects of the mature myelin sheath and its relationship to a glial cell. The unit or plasma membrane is designated as two lines separated by a space except in the mitochondria where it is represented by a single line. The inner mesaxon, formed as a glial process completes the inital turn around an axon and starts a second, is retained after myelin formation is completed. Some cytoplasm of the glial process is present here. On the fully formed sheath exterior, a bit of glial cytoplasm is also retained. In transverse section, this cytoplasm is confined to a loop of plasma membrane but, along the internode length, it forms a ridge which may be continuous with a glial cell body. When viewed transversely, the sheath components are oriented in a spiral, only the inner- and outer-most layers ending in loops; in the longitudinal plane, every myelin unit terminates in a separate loop at both ends of the internode. Within these loops, glial cytoplasm is also retained. Bunge *et al* believe that this cytoplasm, contained within the expanded lateral edges of the spiralled glial process, is a continuous cord helically wound around the axon, like cable about a spool. The outer loop, inner mesaxon and sheath endings at a node are illustrated and evidence for a spiral arrangement of myelin lamellae is presented. The connection between a glial cell body and a mature sheath has not been demonstrated. From Bunge *et al* (1961) with permission.

following demyelination induced by cerebrospinal fluid barbotage. After removal of myelin by macrophages, new compact myelin lamellae formed around axons. They commented upon, but did not draw particular attention to, the fact that the myelin lamellae were inappropriately thin for the axon diameter. The Bunges concluded, on the basis of electron microscopy, that the remyelinating cell is an oligodendrocyte. Furthermore, they demonstrated ultrastructural features of the remyelinating cell that distinguished this from a mature oligodendrocyte and, on morphological grounds alone, suggested the involvement of a precursor cell that is bipotential and able to differentiate either into the reactive astrocyte or myelinating oligodendrocyte – antedating by 20 years the formal demonstration of bipotentiality *in vitro* (Raff *et al* 1983). This reactive macroglia was thought equivalent to the spongioblast and so the concept was also advanced of the need for a remyelinating cell to have stem cell properties. Finally, Bunge *et al* (1961) proposed that the reactive macroglial cell is derived from a mature oligodendrocyte, thus starting the debate on dedifferentiation in the oligodendrocyte lineage as the basis for remyelination and repair.

Perier and Gregoire (1965) published the first electron microscopic studies of multiple sclerosis plaques, demonstrating axons partially or completely surrounded by thin myelin lamellae, which they considered to be evidence for remyelination (Figure 1.30). Confirmation that their observations did indeed represent spontaneous remyelination had to await experimental studies. Richard Gledhill, Barry Harrison and Ian McDonald

showed that compression of the cat spinal cord produced lesions in the posterior columns that repair with terminal cytoplasm-filled loops, attached to the axolemma by transverse bands, having short (67–85-mm) internodes and uniformly thin myelin (Gledhill *et al* 1973; Figure 1.31). These are the morphological criteria that have since reliably been used as evidence for remyelination: myelin embedded in a satellite cell with a continuous membrane from the surface of the cell around the axon, back to the surface again, and compacted but inappropriately thin for the corresponding axon, and with a short internode.

Ken Smith and his colleagues provided experimental proof that remyelination restores conduction and made neurophysiological correlations with the histological features (K.J. Smith *et al* 1979; 1981; see Chapter 13). At 1 month, areas of the spinal cord demyelinated with lysophosphatidyl choline were remyelinated by oligodendrocytes and conduction through the lesion was restored but with a reduced safety factor (Figure 1.32). Therefore by the late 1970s it was clear that spontaneous remyelination can follow demyelination in the central nervous system, both experimentally and in the context of multiple sclerosis, and that remyelination restores secure saltatory conduction. The stage was then set for an era of experimental studies aimed at exploring the neurobiology of remyelination and the implications for restoration of structure and function in demyelinated lesions. These preclinical attempts at repair also needed accurate anatomical localization of defined clinical syndromes and the ability to assess their functional deficits.

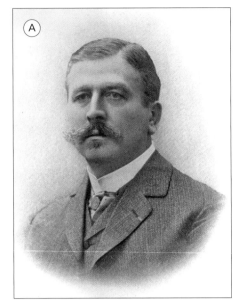

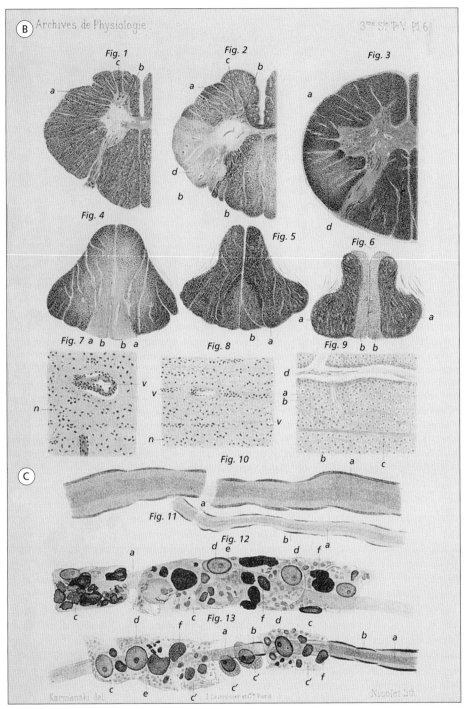

Figure 1.29 (A) Joseph Babinski (1857–1932) kindly provided by Professor Jan van Gijn. (B) *Fig. 1*: Multiple sclerosis. Axial section at the upper thoracic level. Left side: the cord is normal on this section. *a*: myelin sheaths in the cord mantle; *b*: myelin sheaths in the neuropil of grey matter; *c*: nerve cells. Enlargement 6 diameters. *Fig. 2*: Multiple sclerosis. Axial section at the cervical level, done 5 cm above the section shown in *Fig. 1*. Left side: the sections shown on *Figs 1 and 2* belong to the same cord. *a,b,c*: as in *Fig. 1*. *a′*: posterior part of the lateral funiculus comprising the entire area of the crossed pyramidal tract, completely devoid of myelin. Enlargement 6 diameters. *Fig. 3*: Descending sclerosis secondary to a destructive lesion of the internal capsule.: myelin sheaths of the cord mantle; *d*: crossed pyramidal tract affected by sclerosis; numerous persisting myelin sheaths. Enlargement 6 diameters. *Fig. 4*: Locomotor ataxia, cervical region. Only the posterior funiculi are shown on this sketch. *a*: fasciculus cuneatus of Burdach showing sclerosis; *b*: fasciculus gracilis of Goll showing sclerosis and almost entirely devoid of myelin. Enlargement 6 diameters. *Fig. 5*: Multiple sclerosis, upper cervical region. Only the posterior funiculi are shown. This section and the section shown on Fig. 1 of Plate I belong to the same cord. *a*: fasciculi cuneatus of Burdach are normal; *b*: fasciculi gracilis of Goll are mildly sclerotic in their posterior part. Enlargement 6 diameters. *Fig. 6*: Ascending sclerosis secondary to dorsal Pott's disease, cervical region. Only the posterior funiculi are shown. *a*: fasciculi cuneatus of Burdach are normal; *b*: Fasciculi gracilis of Goll are sclerotic and contain numerous normal myelin sheaths. Enlargement 6 diameters. *Fig. 7*: Multiple sclerosis. *n*: nuclei; *v*: vessel. Enlargement 60 diameters. *Fig. 8*: Descending sclerosis. *n, v*: as in *Fig. 7*. Enlargement 60 diameters. *Fig. 9*: Multiple sclerosis, transverse section. The drawing represents part of the nuclei gracilis of Goll shown in *Fig. 1* of Plate I. *a*: axons; *b*: connective tissue; *c*: posterior median sulcus of the cord; *d*: vessels. Enlargement 100 diameters. (C) *Figs 10 and 11*. Normal myelin tubes of the medulla seen in longitudinal section. *a*: Axis cylinder; *b*: myelin sheath; *a*: axis cylinder stripped by a break in the myelin sheath. Enlargement × 1000 diameters. *Fig. 12*. Multiple sclerosis. Distorted myelin tube seen in longitudinal section. *a*: Axis cylinder; *c*: cells surrounding the axis cylinder; *d*: nuclei of these cells; *e*: protoplasm of these cells; *f*: myelin balls. Enlarged × 1000 diameters. *Fig. 13*. Multiple sclerosis. Myelin tube, whilst normal on one side, is in the process of modification on the other side. *a, c, d, e, f*: As in the preceding figure; *b*: myelin sheath; *c*: migratory cells whose protoplasm does not contain myelin debris. Enlargement × 1000 diameters. From Babinski (1885a; 1885b).

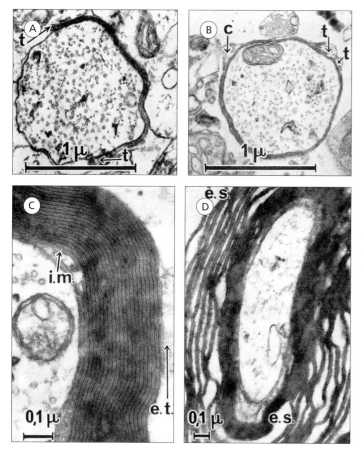

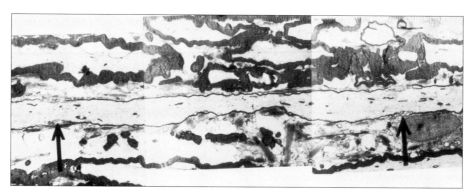

Figure 1.30 (A) An axon containing numerous tubules is half surrounded by a flattened glial cell process from which cytoplasm has been expelled except at the level of the two terminal tongues (*t*). (B) Another axon completely encircled by a flattened glial cell process from which the cytoplasm has been expelled except in one place (*c*) and at the level of the two terminal tongues (*t*) whose apposition constitutes the precursor of the future mesaxon. These pictures suggest abortive remyelination. (C) Large magnification of a normal myelin sheath in the region outside the plaque. The regular periodicity, with its alternating lines of different densities, is well seen. The internal mesaxon (*i.m.*) and part of the external tongue (*e.t.*) can be identified. At the left is the axon containing typical tubules and a mitochondrion. ×114 000. (D) Exceptional appearance of an orderly disruption of a myelin sheath, a cleavage taking place at the level of one out of every two intermediate dense lines. Such a cleavage corresponds to a penetration of extracellular space (*e.s.*) inside the myelin sheath. The axon is relatively normal except that it contains an empty membraneous profile probably corresponding to an altered mitochondrion. ×64 000. From Perier and Gregoire (1965) with permission.

Figure 1.31 One-month lesion. An axon approximately 5 μm in diameter is covered by an inappropriately thin myelin sheath. The arrows mark nodes. The internodal distance is 76 μm. From Gledhill *et al* (1973) with permission.

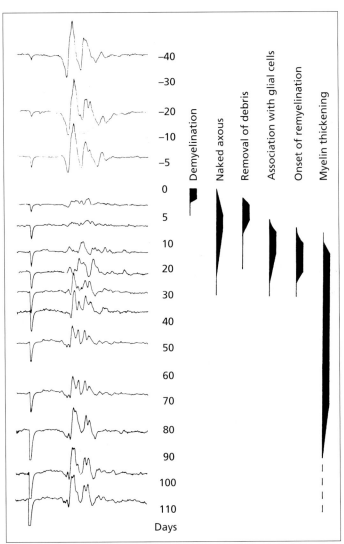

Figure 1.32 Temporal relationship between the compound action potentials recorded through the lesion and the sequence of histological events at the lesion. The block and subsequent restoration of conduction correlate with the periods of demyelination and remyelination, respectively. From K.J. Smith *et al* (1981) with permission.

THE AETIOLOGY OF MULTIPLE SCLEROSIS: 1883–1976

The earliest systematic studies of multiple sclerosis in populations, defined demographically, were made in the first two decades of the 20th century, in continental Europe, the United Kingdom and the United States. The efforts of 19th-century investigators were directed at describing variations in the clinical presentation of multiple sclerosis. Their work highlighted the need for an epidemiological approach to the disease, and the period 1900–1950 saw a gradual evolution of the methods required for accurate definition of population-based statistics (see Chapter 2). Every survey demonstrated the unpredictable clinical evolution of the disease in individuals and the variability of its time course in populations.

The incidence of multiple sclerosis at Manchester Royal Infirmary was $43/10^5$/year between 1892 and 1902 when

Richard Williamson (1862–1937) held the post of medical registrar (R.T. Williamson 1908). At first, epidemiological studies merely provided snapshots of the frequency of multiple sclerosis. They did not aim to achieve an accurate enumeration of cases. (Sir) Byrom Bramwell (1847–1931) had studied multiple sclerosis from 1903, identifying 100 cases amongst 5825 (1.7%) hospital attendants with neurological disease. He noted that the disease appeared to be more common in the north of England than in New York (Bramwell 1903). Whilst aware of some potential confounders, he concluded that the differences were real. Bramwell (1917) first provided evidence on the natural history of the disease, although the patients who formed the basis for his survey had already received various medications, and he headed the section on disease duration 'results of treatment' in 200 cases of disseminated sclerosis. Of these, 106 were known to have died; 64 were alive, but the majority of these were deteriorating, and the clinical status of 30 was unknown. The duration of disease (including living cases) was just over 12 years. Fourteen of 170 had lived >25 years from diagnosis (the longest was 37 years) and 3/170 had died within 1 year. In the fatal cases, life expectancy was <5 years in 21%, <10 years in 51% and <20 years in 87%.

The second publication from the Association for Research in Nervous and Mental Diseases (ARNMD) contained a summary of recent presentations dealing with epidemiological and other aspects of multiple sclerosis. The discussion was recorded verbatim, and a summary presented of the ARNMD Commission under the presidency of Henry Alsop Riley. The contributions of Charles Davenport, Pearce Bailey, Llewellyn Barker, Israel Weschler and Charles Dana were at that time influential in shaping contemporary thoughts on the aetiology of multiple sclerosis and in stimulating surveys of the disease. Davenport (1921, 1922) mapped the frequency of defects found in men drafted into the United States army and showed that the maximum rate for multiple sclerosis was in the states of Michigan and Minnesota (each $18/10^5$), followed by Wisconsin. He noted that these high rates were in states bordering the Great Lakes. Case material was recruited from three military camps and, although the number of affected individuals remained small (only 15 for the whole of Michigan), he rejected idiosyncratic neurological diagnostic habits as the explanation for this pattern. Davenport identified a number of other disorders clustered in these geographical areas and suggested the link between goitre, chorea, varicose veins, varicocele and various heart defects with Scandinavian ancestry. He presented his results in an interesting chart that showed a gradient in frequency of multiple sclerosis from $1/10^5$ in Indians, to $2/10^5$ in mountain regions, $6/10^5$ in coloured agricultural communities from the south, $10/10^5$ in German and Austrian districts, $16/10^5$ in the Scandinavian section, and $29/10^5$ in Finns. Davenport had already drawn attention to the noticeable differences between racial groups at a meeting of the New York Neurological Society in 1902.

At that time, distinction from ataxic paraplegias, diffuse degenerations and spastic paraplegias was imprecise, but by 1921 Davenport already suspected that many of these patients did in fact have multiple sclerosis. He obviously held some of his neurological colleagues in scant regard and dismissed, on the grounds of diagnostic idiosyncracy, the claims of Van Wart who, in 1905 (not referenced) had evidently claimed a rate for multiple sclerosis of $44/10^5$ neurological cases in Louisiana. Davenport recognized that many confounding factors were being introduced and that the main variation between studies related to selection of the denominator rather than variations in numerator. In particular, he noted a racial predilection for the use of certain clinics. However, he was impressed by the survey carried out by Miss Louise Nelson, who took statements concerning the birthplace of 70 foreign-born patients with multiple sclerosis from the records of the Montefiori Home and related the absolute number of cases to at-risk individuals from different racial groups. She (and Davenport) saw at once the lower than expected rates for Russians and Italians, the slight increase for Irish and the even higher rates for English, Germans, Swedes and Norwegians. Since Davenport could not see any reason why Scandinavians should have preferentially decided to use the Montefiori Home, and taking his subsequent analysis of the distribution of multiple sclerosis in the United States by racial origin, he concluded that Scandinavians are at especially high risk of the disease (Figure 1.33A,B). Davenport took the trouble to visit the Swedish hospital in Brooklyn but found no cases of multiple sclerosis resident or listed in the records – although he did note that the hospital had a very low frequency of neurological case material in general. He recognized that native Africans are not completely protected from the disease even though the rates were low; and he pointed out that the disease is infrequent in Japanese.

The volume of ARNMD devoted to multiple sclerosis ended with the conclusions of the learned commission:

In the United States it seems to occur more in the region of the great lakes, at least among young males, while in Europe it prevails more in northern parts than in Italy and about the Mediterranean sea. It is not a familial disease and it is not inherited, there being rare and doubtful exceptions; but in the ancestry, there is often evidence of a neuropathic stock. Acute infections may immediately precede the disease in a small percentage (10 or 12%) and it occurs no more frequently in persons who have had the usual children's infections and fevers than those who have not had them. Further laboratory studies of the use of prolonged and intensive field work including some of the methods suggested by ecology are necessary to give us a knowledge of the real cause of multiple sclerosis. Which cause we do not now know.

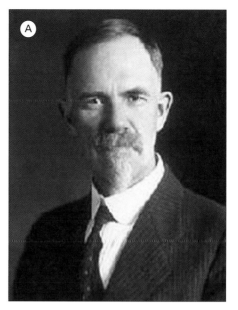

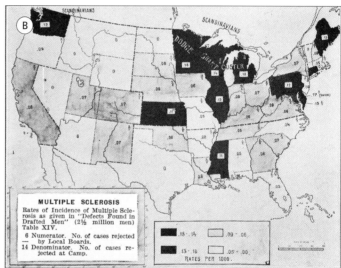

Figure 1.33 (A) Charles Davenport (from 1904, director of the Biological Laboratory, Cold Spring Harbor, Long Island). (B) Distribution of multiple sclerosis in North America by state. 'Dodge', 'Grant' and 'Custer' in the Great Lakes region are the names of camps at which the drafted men from those localities were mobilized. From Davenport (1921) with permission.

Although carefully conducted regional surveys were performed from the late 1920s, information on the epidemiology of multiple sclerosis did not materially increase until the 1950s. Bing and Reese (1926) documented the frequency of the disease in the Swiss cantons, providing rates between 1918 and 1922 of around $36/10^5$ but with variation from 3 to $74/10^5$. The systematic study of multiple sclerosis in populations within the United Kingdom began in 1929 when Sydney Allison personally studied 40 cases while working at Ruthin Castle in Denbighshire (north Wales) supported by one of the first grants for multiple sclerosis research from the Medical Research Council (Figure 1.34A,B). He derived a point prevalence of $13/10^5$ (R.S. Allison 1931). By 1949, 70% of his patients had died but only two survivors had deteriorated between the surveys and one deceased case had had symptoms for 43 years, providing an early example

of benign multiple sclerosis (R.S. Allison 1950). Prompted by Sutherland's survey comparing the frequency of multiple sclerosis in Orkney/Shetland with that in the Western Isles, and Kay Hyllested's impression that the disease was relatively uncommon in the Faroes, Allison visited these islands with Hyllested and Mogens Fog in 1962. They recorded prevalences of $153/10^5$ (62 cases) and $48/10^5$ (17 cases) in Orkney/Shetland and the Faroes, respectively, with a 12% familial frequency in each location. Their conclusion was that Orkney and Shetland are exceptional and the Faroes unremarkable in their relative frequencies of multiple sclerosis. But never one for an elaborate hypothesis, Allison denounced the extravagant speculations that epidemiological studies of that era excited, in his presidential address to the Royal Society of Medicine (1963):

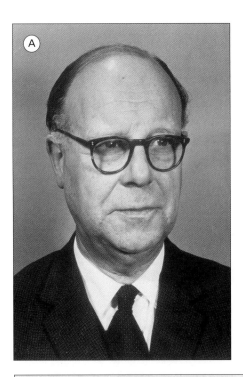

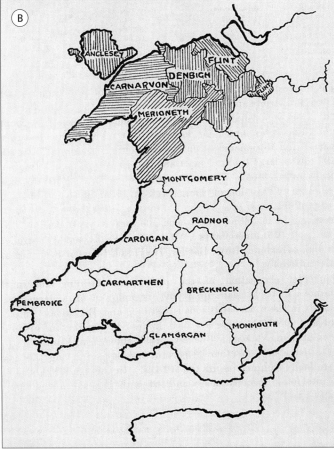

Figure 1.34 (A) Sydney Allison (1899–1978). (B) The area covered by the first epidemiological study of multiple sclerosis carried out in the United Kingdom.

the Hippocratic doctrine of airs, waters and places may have been eclipsed by the discovery of bacteria, viruses and development of the sciences of genetics and immunology but ... caution is necessary in hypothesis building until we can be satisfied that the foundations ... dull prosaic essential facts relating to the true incidence and prevalence of disease ... are secure.

Allison spent several years at sea as a young doctor, writing later on the lessons from naval life for preventive medicine in *Sea Diseases* (Allison 1943). His work in Belfast is commemorated by an annual lecture and prize awarded by the Ulster Medical Society.

In 1930, Russell Brain, reporting on cases seen at the Hospital for Epilepsy and Paralysis, Maida Vale, and the London Hospital was advocating the use of population- rather than hospital-based denominators. He reasoned that the prevalence of multiple sclerosis could be estimated by multiplying rates for incidence or mortality by duration (Brain 1930). In 1940, Brain revised his figure for prevalence to $20/10^5$, noting that urban cases are more common than rural, that the disease rarely occurs in childhood and that only 7% of patients develop multiple sclerosis after the age of 50 years. Incorrectly, Brain reversed the 3:2 sex ratio in favour of men. By 1955, he had updated his figures for prevalence to 1:2400 ($42/10^5$) for England and Wales and 1:1570 for Scotland ($64/10^5$) – establishing the latitudinal differential for the United Kingdom that remains unexplained to this day. The first mortality figures for multiple sclerosis published from the United Kingdom in 1927 showed a national rate of $1.75/10^5$/year (I.G.H. Wilson 1927). Isabel Wilson studied 688 persons who died with multiple sclerosis in the United Kingdom during 1925, noting regional variations from a high in Peterborough to a low in Buckinghamshire, but her main concern (picking up on an idea proposed by James Dawson) was to show, on the basis of differential mortality rates amongst farm workers, that the disease was caused by leptospiral infection. She preferred as vector for the distribution of multiple sclerosis, not *Homo scandinavicus* (see below) but *Rattus norvegicus*. Wilson carried out the first case–control study and showed a higher frequency of presumed exposure to water (on the basis of occupation) amongst 72 patients compared with individuals having other neurological diseases. Sallstom (1942) collected morbidity statistics for multiple sclerosis in Swedish hospitals between 1925 and 1934 and reported a (period) prevalence of $34/10^5$. The steady rise in clinic-based cases was rightly attributed to relaxation in admission criteria and there did not seem to have been a change in annual incidence rates, although these were not directly assessed.

This generation of epidemiologists was not content merely to document numbers of cases but used their surveys to explore aetiological hypotheses relating to the impact of environmental factors such as domicile, climate and soil conditions. The first putative cluster (six cases) was reported from a Berkshire village (Campbell *et al* 1950), blaming lead exposure as the likely cause. Periodically, examples (or anecdotes) implicating specific infections were highlighted, such as the suggestion that multiple sclerosis might be related to swayback. Campbell *et al* (1947) reported on four cases in researchers who had worked in Cambridge in the 1930s on this non-inflammatory demyelinating disease of the central nervous system causing progressive blindness and ataxia in infantile sheep. Reviewing these cases nearly 40 years later – when all four probands were dead – Dean *et al* (1985) provide detailed descriptions and forensic accounts of their admirable attempts to locate notes and tissue from the two individuals who underwent autopsy. Reading these now, the diagnosis of multiple sclerosis seems reasonably secure in all four instances. One had been examined by the elite of London neurology: Sir Charles Symonds, Sir Francis Walshe and Dr Jack Elkington considered case 4 to have disseminated sclerosis; Dr Macdonald Critchley diagnosed human swayback. Post-mortem examination in 1966, with review of the histology in 1981, confirmed multiple sclerosis. Five sheep were inoculated with material from case 4 in Reykjavik, Iceland, but none showed any clinical or histological signs of neurological disease. There were no examples of neurological disease amongst 50 other researchers who worked on swayback in various institutions at that time. Other than commenting on the low probability of four cases linked by occupation and exposure to material from a neurological disorder of sheep developing multiple sclerosis by chance, and the assumption that the explanation lay in common exposure to an environmental agent, the authors offered no new insights.

Cross-cultural studies continued to illustrate differences in geographical (or racial) frequency of the disease. In addition to the work of Davenport, it was assumed that multiple sclerosis was uncommon in Japan (Miura 1911), China (Woods 1929; who believed that 150 of 100 000 patients in Peking had disseminated sclerosis – although he personally had only seen two cases) and India (Sprawson 1927). Fog (1956) has pointed out that these *ex cathedra* opinions on multiple sclerosis in the Orient were based on chance remarks by Miura to Nonne (see Nonne and Holzmann 1911), and by two other Japanese neurologists (Sata and Kuroda) to Siemerling (1924). Against this background, the definitive study of different racial groups began with the influential studies of Geoffrey Dean, appearing from the late 1940s (Dean 1949; Figure 1.35), on the effect of migration to South Africa on the frequency of multiple sclerosis.

Dean arrived in Cape Town on 24th June 1947, toured the country and decided to settle in Port Elizabeth. Struck by the paucity of patients with disseminated sclerosis – which he had been taught to recognize by Sir Henry (later, Lord) Cohen in Liverpool – in the wards at Groote Schuur Hospital, he searched systematically in the other large cities and found only 29 patients: all were white and 15 were immigrants from Europe. Dean founded the South African Multiple Sclerosis Society in 1963, by which stage he had studied the disease for nearly 20 years, concluding that multiple sclerosis is seen in immigrants but is uncommon in native-born whites especially Afrikaners and even less so in mixed race individuals. Later, Dean studied the corollary of that influential epidemiological observation – the increase in frequency in immigrants from the Indian subcontinent, the Caribbean, and Africa to the United Kingdom, and in other informative populations (Dean 2002).

A further milestone in the epidemiology of multiple sclerosis was publication of the second ARNMD volume devoted to the disease, in which Limburg (1950) used mortality statistics to document the distinct geographical distribution of the disease. Mortality rates were greater in temperate zones than the tropics or subtropics and showed higher figures in northern parts of the United States and Italy than in southern regions. A more exten-

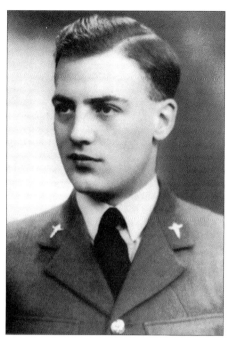

Figure 1.35 **Flying Officer Geoffrey Dean (1943).**

sive survey of mortality for 31 countries between 1951 and 1958, adjusted to the 1950 population of the United States, again showed regional variations but with a trend towards lower rates, reflecting the impact of improved health care following the introduction of antibiotics and other treatments for complications of multiple sclerosis in the early 1950s (Goldberg and Kurland 1962). The ranking of high-frequency countries in these analyses maintained the primacy of Northern Ireland and Scotland, with high rates also in southern Scandinavia and the northern Mediterranean countries, Canada, Australia, New Zealand and the northern United States. As Davenport (1922) had noted, non-whites from the United States had half the rate of caucasians, and low frequencies were reported for Asia, Africa and the Caribbean.

The 'Report to the Northern Ireland Hospitals Authority on the Results of a Three Year Survey on the Prevalence and Familial Incidence of Disseminated Sclerosis' appeared in 1954 (R.S. Allison and Millar 1954). This publication provided the first detailed account of epidemiological methodology, reproduced the charts used to record information, featured the population against which most subsequent standardized prevalence ratios have been compared, and suggested a classification for multiple sclerosis that was widely adopted. Regional rates provided the first substantial increase in estimates for incidence ($2.74/10^5$/year) and prevalence ($79/10^5$), which heralded the modern era (see Chapter 2). The distribution of the disease was commented upon but with no firm conclusion being reached on the urban–rural divide. The story of this and subsequent prevalence surveys in Northern Ireland (see Chapter 2) is summarized by McDonnell and Hawkins (2000).

The individual who has worked hardest to make sense of epidemiological information relating to multiple sclerosis gathered since the 1950s is John Kurtzke (Figure 1.36A,B). His contributions are of lasting importance and are described in detail in Chapter 2. Kurtzke classified the published surveys of prevalence depending upon whether the diagnosis of multiple

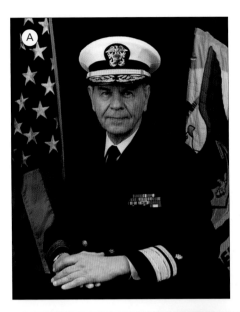

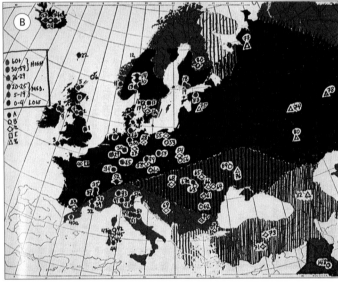

Figure 1.36 (A) John Kurtzke. (B) Point prevalences for multiple sclerosis in Europe to show regional differences in the frequency and the definition of high-, intermediate- and low-risk areas. From Kurtzke (1975) with permission.

Administration into mainstream medicine. Kurtzke, discharged as a pharmacist's mate (2nd class) graduated in medicine, and was put by Harold Wolff to measure the effect of isoniazid in multiple sclerosis. But how would he quantify the effect? Kurtzke applied the rituals of neurological examination as learned at Cornell, and derived a system from which eventually emerged the disability status score and its expanded version, designed to smooth out the Gaussian distribution of the disability status scale and establish a more ordinal measure of disability (Kurtzke 2004). The problem of quantifying severity and progression in multiple sclerosis has long bedevilled study of the natural history in multiple sclerosis. In the last decade, since the possibility of developing effective treatments became more realistic, the need to solve this problem has become more pressing. The issues surrounding quantification in multiple sclerosis are shared with many acute and chronic diseases, and efforts to resolve them have a long history. The growth of understanding in the field of measurement in medicine has been reviewed critically by Tröhler (2000), especially in the 18th century, and by J.N. Matthews (1985) for the last 200 years. They chart the origin of these studies in public health, education and the social sciences from which refined methods for clinical measurement subsequently became commonplace in a range of medical disciplines including neurology. Kurtzke was ahead of his time and the achievement is remarkable. Although as the years have passed, limitations of his scale have become apparent, no alternative has received such widespread support. The Kurtzke Expanded Disability Status Scale (EDSS) has remained the gold standard, albeit with its shine ever so slightly tarnished.

Interpreting the epidemiological pattern: the role of environmental factors

Marie wrote on 'Insular sclerosis and the infectious diseases' (Marie 1884). Noting the freedom needed when interpreting clinical as opposed to experimental results, he considered the anecdotal association of acute infectious disease (typhoid, pneumonia, malaria and the childhood exanthemata) and the onset of multiple sclerosis as sufficient to establish their causal relationship. In fact, he thought it more likely that several organisms were involved, alone or in combination:

the fact, thank God, has been well established viz. that the cause of insular sclerosis is intimately connected with infectious disease.

Marie was prepared to accept that recovery was easily explained on the basis that the essential element needed for nerve conduction, the nerve cylinder, was preserved, and he joined Charcot in concluding that remyelination was responsible for restoring both structure and function. Thereafter, master and pupil differed since for Marie, the disease was triggered by infection, depended on changes in the blood vessels, and resulted in an inflammatory interstitial reaction of the glia.

Section five of Brain's 1930 review dealing with 'experimental transmission and bacteriology' analysed a controversial episode. In 1913, the Englishman William Bullock (who changed his name to Gye, and made important contributions to virology and cancer biology) claimed to have transmitted multiple sclerosis from man to rabbits. Khun and Steiner (1917) reproduced this

sclerosis was confirmed by individual investigators (type A) or assumed from information available in existing medical records (type B). Within these limits, he accepted further variations in methodology and made the influential suggestion that the distribution of the disease fits bands of high, medium and low prevalence. High risk ($\geq 30/10^5$) was found in northern Europe, the northern United States, Canada, southern Australia, and New Zealand; medium risk ($5-29/10^5$) characterized southern Europe, the southern United States and northern Australia; and low risk ($\leq 5/10^5$) areas included Asia, South America and many uncharted regions (1975, 1977).

John Kurtzke's global interest in epidemiological surveys had its origins in his involvement with the neurological misfortunes of United States military personnel in World War Two – 16.4 million men and women on active service by June 1954, attended by 48 000 physicians. Peace brought the Veterans finding using cerebrospinal fluid from patients injected into guinea pigs or rabbits. These apparent successes were matched by as many failures (Marinesco 1919), but it was about this time that general interest in the spirochaete as a potent cause of neurological disease led to the description of this microorganism in tissue removed from patients during life who had multiple sclerosis. These claims culminated in the report by Chevassut (1930) that the organism *Spherula insularis*, designated as viral, could be cultured from the cerebrospinal fluid of >90% of patients with disseminated sclerosis but not controls. In his review, Brain quickly disposed of the spirochaetal theory of disseminated sclerosis but took a more reserved position with respect to Miss Chevassut's findings, suggesting that technical factors may have made it difficult for her directly to visualize the organism in spinal fluid or the nervous tissue itself. He was distinctly lenient on the failure to transfer this organism to monkeys – work that had been reported by (Sir James) Purves Stewart (1930). Notwithstanding uncertainty about the causal role of *Spherula insularis* in disseminated sclerosis, Brain extolled the virtues of using its detection as a diagnostic test. *Spherula insularis* disappeared abruptly from interest following an episode at the Royal Society of Medicine in 1931. Dr Denis Brinton told one of us (WIMcD) that when Carmichael (1931) reported his inability to confirm the findings, Miss Chevassut left the meeting in tears and was not subsequently encountered in neurological circles. In an expanded account of the aetiology, Brain admitted the 'modern tendency to stress constitutional factors' and summarized the evidence on heredity from Curtius' monograph (Curtius 1933; see below). Brain quoted a series, presumably of personal cases, in which exposure to a range of triggers – infections, pregnancy, surgical operations, electric shock, carbon monoxide poisoning and trauma – occurred shortly before presentation. Allowing anecdote to suggest a causal connection between external events and some aspect of disease activity in multiple sclerosis, without the rigour of epidemiological validation, continues to limit progress in advancing ideas on the aetiology to the present day – not least on the topic of trauma and multiple sclerosis (see Chapter 2). It is fundamentally the same problem that confounds the endless reports of apparent success – subsequently not proven – when experimental and often improbable treatments have been assessed in an uncontrolled and unblinded setting.

Squeamishness should not prevent us from mentioning the Schaltenbrand experiment (for a detailed review, see Shevell and Bradley 1994). Georg Schaltenbrand, who died in 1979, trained in neurosurgery with Harvey Cushing and Pearce Bailey in the United States and established the University Clinic in Wurzburg in 1950. He took forward his claim to have transferred multiple sclerosis to monkeys using human cerebrospinal fluid by, in turn, infecting *verblodete Menschen* (imbeciles) with material from these and other primates. One recipient, who had a glioblastoma multiforme, died after the second injection of monkey spinal fluid and was shown to have demyelinating lesions in the conus and peripheral nerves. Later, Schaltenbrand claimed to have produced autopsy-proven demyelination in an individual by injecting cerebrospinal fluid from a patient with active multiple sclerosis. It seems that Schaltenbrand (1943) performed this procedure on up to 45 human subjects, including children with psychiatric disease or idiocy from an institute in Werneck. Inevitably, there has been both exposure (Anon. 1950;

Shevell and Bradley 1994) and defence (Bailey 1950) of Schaltenbrand's work. It shed no light and is one of the darker moments in the history of multiple sclerosis.

Innes and Kurland (1952), writing in the proceedings of the first symposium organized by the National Multiple Sclerosis Society (of the United States of America), summarized all attempts to transmit multiple sclerosis down to 1952. They considered the evidence to be inconclusive. Whilst some of the experiments had produced neuropathological changes, these did not illuminate the problem of multiple sclerosis other than by showing that demyelination has many causes. The donor might or might not have multiple sclerosis. The causative agent might or might not be present. The studies had not involved many recipients and the sampling was sparse. Coincidental events could have been responsible for the reported neuropathological changes. Throughout the 1950s, analogies with research on paralytic poliomyelitis, which culminated in the development of a suitable vaccine, served to strengthen the concept that the geographic distribution, age specificity and socioeconomic predilections of multiple sclerosis could be explained on the basis of age-dependent consequences of infection by a ubiquitous agent. These ideas were sustained by the emerging concepts of slow virus infection, but an organism specific for multiple sclerosis just could not be identified. In 1972, an agent present in tissue extracted from patients with multiple sclerosis was reported to transfer a cytopathic effect to mice (Carp *et al* 1972; Koldovsky *et al* 1975). The Carp agent, serenaded by the *Lancet* as a 'milestone in multiple sclerosis', disappeared from scientific attention when the results could not be reproduced (Carp *et al* 1977). The same fate awaited the human T-cell lymphotrophic retrovirus (Koprowski *et al* 1985) and paramyxovirus SV5 (Goswami *et al* 1987). In Chapters 2 and 12, we update the list of putative but unproven viral triggers for multiple sclerosis based on population serology and viral isolates.

Interpreting the epidemiological pattern: the role of genetic factors

In analysing the evidence for familial clustering, Davenport (1922) had shown that familial cases tend to occur amongst sibships but may also affect first-degree relatives in more than one generation, each pedigree rarely containing more than three affected individuals. He closed with a much quoted summary:

In conclusion, may I be permitted the suggestion that whatever may eventually prove to be the endogenous cause of multiple sclerosis, the factor of heredity cannot be left out of account ... there are probably internal conditions that inhibit and others that facilitate the development of this disease or the endogenous factors upon which it depends and so it comes about that the manifestations or symptoms of the disease differ in different persons; and that they are sometimes very similar in closely related individuals because the hereditary factors of the constitution in which they operate are similar. It seems most probable that such geographical, ethnological and familial distribution as multiple sclerosis shows depends in part upon one or more hereditary factors.

John Sutherland carried out an epidemiological survey of multiple sclerosis in Scotland for his medical thesis submitted to the University of Glasgow in 1950. His interest in the subject was stimulated by Dr D.K. Adams, physician to the Western Infirmary, Glasgow (Sutherland 1989). Sutherland identified 389 cases and examined each personally, showing a difference in the distribution that correlated with the location of Nordic peoples, being higher in the Orkney and Shetland islands and in Sutherland (his family name derives from this region) by comparison with the more Celtic fringe of the Western Isles and mainland (Figure 1.37A–C). Although superficially latitudinal, the gradient therefore appeared to be influenced more by genetic than environmental factors.

The concept of a role for genetic factors in the aetiology of multiple sclerosis, explicit in the writings of Davenport and Sutherland, had earlier been suggested by Charcot on the basis

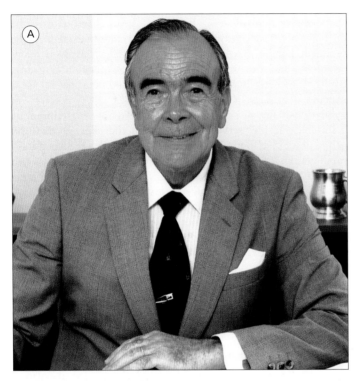

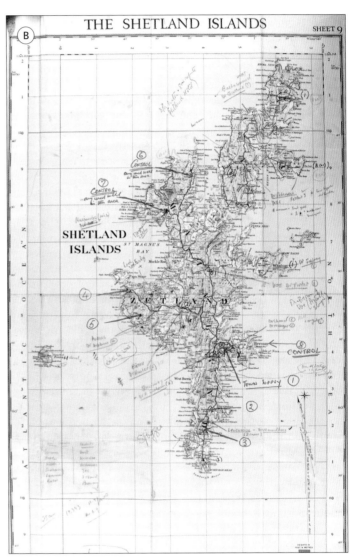

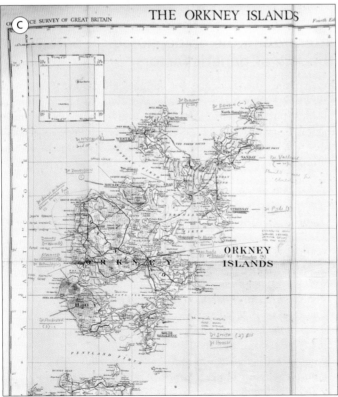

Figure 1.37 (A) John Sutherland (1919–1995). Ordnance Survey maps of (B) Shetland and (C) Orkney Islands, used by John Sutherland to show the names and distribution of cases in the first survey of multiple sclerosis from Scotland and the offshore islands. Kindly provided by Mrs Patricia Sutherland and Professor Mervyn Eadie.

of the occasional family history. The theme re-emerged with a less than convincing report of familial clustering provided by Eichorst (1896), who described a mother–son pair with multi-focal demyelination in the spinal cord demonstrated at autopsy. Cestan and Guillain (1900) made clear the distinction between familial multiple sclerosis and the hereditary spastic paraplegias. Irma Klausner reported on familial risks in 126 affected individuals of whom 31 had a 'nervous' predisposition and two a family history of disseminated sclerosis (Klausner 1901). The first study in the English literature came from Manchester. Two multiplex families were reported. Although concerned that the diagnosis of disseminated sclerosis in three siblings and a paternal cousin in family X might be wrong, Ernest Reynolds had the reassurance of diagnostic confirmation from two eminent London specialists in at least two of these cases (E.S. Reynolds 1904). Family X had a strong history of depressive illness and Reynolds drew attention to the possible association with thyroid disease (goitre). The clinical course in two affected sisters from family Y, each with relapsing–remitting disseminated sclerosis, was markedly different, leading Reynolds to conclude that the recognition of aberrant cases – often diagnosed as hysteria – will lead to increased awareness of familial disease and recognition that the prognosis may be surprisingly benign. By implication, clinical concordance was not a feature of familial disseminated sclerosis. Curtius (1933) accepted 84 reports in the literature of familial multiple sclerosis and performed the first systematic study of recurrence risks in 3129 relatives of 106 probands living in Bonn or Heidelberg. Ten additional cases were identified and the relative risk through having an affected relative was estimated at 40. There were no examples of multiple sclerosis in a control population. In his monograph, Curtius sought to identify aspects of the natural history that might be influenced by genetic background, and he seems to have spotted the apparent association with von Recklinghausen disease (Figure 1.38; see Chapter 3). Curtius' study was criticized for lack of evidence for multiple sclerosis in many relatives on which his conclusions were based. Curtius and Speer (1937) confined their subsequent study to near relatives and, on the basis of four cases amongst 444 relatives, also concluded that siblings had 40-fold population-risk of developing multiple sclerosis.

R.P. Mackay (1950) accepted 177 reported cases occurring in 79 familial pedigrees and added 11 further examples of his own amongst five new families. He emphasized that the commonest relationship between affecteds is sibship, with parental and more distant kinship accounting for 14% and 16%, respectively. Concordant multiple sclerosis in twins was accepted (idem) in five instances. Pratt *et al* (1951) collated 184 familial cases of multiple sclerosis, providing familial recurrence rates in different series between 0 and 9.4%, and reported a familial incidence in their own material of 6.5%, siblings being the main group at risk (0.5%). R. Müller (1953) took Pratt to task for methodological inadequacies but came up with a more or less identical figure in his own survey. Schapira *et al* (1963) found a positive family history in 24/607 (4%) consecutively presenting patients, noticing that females had nearly three times the prevalence of male siblings and that relatives were affected in the order: sisters, mothers, brothers and fathers.

Case reports provided the suspicion that hereditary factors are involved in the development of multiple sclerosis but it

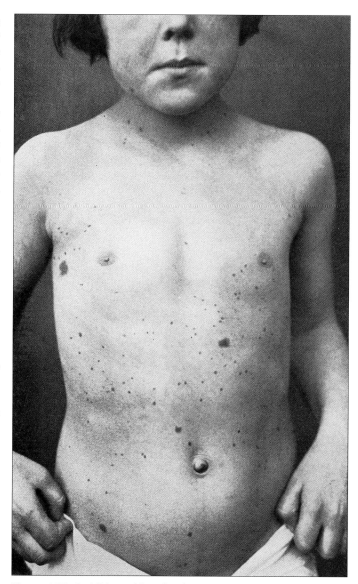

Figure 1.38 A child considered to have von Recklinghausen disease (neurofibromatosis 1) from a pedigree also characterized by examples of multiple sclerosis. From Curtius (1933) with permission.

was necessary to carry out epidemiological studies to establish whether this finding was due to chance. Allison and Millar (1954) reported population-based figures for familial multiple sclerosis, identifying 44/668 families with ≥ 2 or more individuals affected by the disease. Sibships dominated the series (recurrence 1.15%, giving a relative risk of 5–15).

Douglas McAlpine gave a paper on hereditary factors in multiple sclerosis to the 6th International Congress of Neurology, held in Brussels in July 1957 (McAlpine 1957). Reviewing the literature, he reprimanded the authors of many textbooks for ignoring this feature of the disease. In his thoughtful review, McAlpine addressed for the first time many of the issues that have since preoccupied genetic research in multiple sclerosis, and not all of which have been solved. He collated published reports on familial disease and found the rates to be reasonably uniform at 5–10%, although with some variations attributable to methodology, for example a lower figure (2.6%) in the national survey of Denmark conducted by Hyllested (1956). He noticed that the recurrence rate was higher for siblings (1%) than off-spring (≈0.3%). He considered seriously the impact of consanguinity and produced supporting evidence from the surveys of Northen Ireland (Allison and Millar 1954) and Scotland (Sutherland 1956). He noted that Curtius (1933), Garcin (1936) and Pratt *et al* (1951) had each described sibling pairs affected with multiple sclerosis who were reared apart. McAlpine had encountered four examples of conjugal multiple sclerosis and knew of four others; he predicted the importance of studying the recurrence risks in their offspring (see Chapter 3). He summarized the evidence as implicating a genetic factor and considered this to be consistent with either the infective or allergic theories of the aetiology prevalent at the time. Furthermore, McAlpine speculated that the mechanism might involve a genetically determined alteration in the structure of myelin, rendering individuals vulnerable to as yet unidentified factors needed to precipitate demyelination.

The first laboratory studies aimed at identifying the basis for genetic susceptibility were necessarily limited by the few polymorphic systems that could then be studied. Alexander *et al* (1950) and Beebe *et al* (1967) failed to show a distortion in the normal distribution of blood groups amongst patients from New England, whereas McAlpine *et al* (1965) reported a slight excess of group O in a study of patients from six English cities. In an admirably comprehensive survey that combined statistical power with ethnic and regional homogeneity of the participants, C.A. Simpson *et al* (1965) compared blood groups in 507 patients with 94 419 controls, also demonstrating a slight increase in group O, which was not significant. A further study from Newcastle in northern England (J.L. MacDonald *et al* 1976) confirmed this relationship (and also drew attention to the association between multiple sclerosis and homozygosity for the *cde* alleles together with some other minor blood groups). The authors considered that McAlpine's earlier criticism of their work was harsh, but in reappraising the 1965 edition of this book, McAlpine backed off his position with respect to blood groups and susceptibility to multiple sclerosis (McAlpine *et al* 1972). Significantly, MacDonald drew attention to the high frequency of blood group O in populations having a high frequency of multiple sclerosis.

In 1972 an association was described between multiple sclerosis and HL-A3 (now HLA-A3; Bertrams *et al* 1972; Naito *et al* 1972). In the same year, Jersild *et al* (1972) reported an association with the linked allele HLA-B7 but (incorrectly) concluded that this was the weaker (and biologically less significant) association. Jersild *et al* (1973) then looked at the relationship between multiple sclerosis and the HLA-D types, which were defined by mixed lymphocyte cultures. An association was shown with the antigen Ld-7a (later renamed Dw2), present in 70% of Danish patients compared with 16% of controls. Later, the availability of HLA typing led to the first family studies (Alter *et al* 1976; Olsson *et al* 1976), including sibling-pair analyses (Zander *et al* 1976), cross-cultural studies (which hinted at specifically different associations in certain populations: Brautbar *et al* 1976; Saito *et al* 1976), correlations with clinical course and severity (Jersild *et al* 1973), and the assessment of risk in isolated demyelinating syndromes (Platz *et al* 1975; Stendahl *et al* 1976). Winchester *et al* (1975) reported an association between multiple sclerosis and an antigen expressed only on B lymphocytes, designated Ag-7a, and more detailed reports were published in the following year of association with the class II allele HLA-DR2 (Compston *et al* 1976; Terasaki *et al* 1976), which remains the best characterized candidate susceptibility gene for multiple sclerosis.

Douglas McAlpine wrote in January 1977 on receiving a reprint describing the HLA-DR2 association with multiple sclerosis:

> *the intricacies of modern immunology are beyond my comprehension but from your results it is clear that this is proving a field of the greatest importance in MS ... you are right in thinking that your approach is likely to show positive results in some members of MS families. Yes, for long, I have suspected a genetic influence. See the problem of disseminated sclerosis (Brain 1946; 69: 233). I reported 8 examples of familial MS in a series of 142 cases and concluded that the familial incidence was significant but Curtius (1933) was the first to recognize the genetic factor. In our first book (1955) ... we referred to these facts.*

ATTITUDES TO THE TREATMENT OF MULTIPLE SCLEROSIS: 1809–1983

Starting with the first descriptions and clinicopathological correlations in multiple sclerosis, affected individuals and their physicians lamented the difficulty of altering the natural history or, when honesty prevailed, even of masking symptoms. In Chapters 16 and 18, we identify as landmarks in the history of multiple sclerosis, the demonstration that corticotropin alters the rate of recovery from an individual episode, the meta-analysis of azathioprine, and introduction of the interferons. However, failure to make much headway with effective treatment for over 100 years after the first accounts of multiple sclerosis, did not prevent rampant speculation or extensive therapeutic experimentation. As a result, multiple sclerosis soon acquired a regrettable reputation for maverick medicine based on shameless exploitation of its capricious natural history, which flattered the uncritical and those devoted to extrapolation from anecdotal experience.

John Abernethy (1809) offered a variety of treatments to poor Thomas Crichton during his neurological illness (see above):

> *...and as the bowels were deranged, I ordered two grains of Calomel with eight of rhubarb, to be taken twice a week, and some infusion of Gentian, with Senna, occasionally. After using these medicines, for about three weeks, his bowels became regular, the biliary secretion healthy, and his appetite good. He could move his hands and arms nearly as well as ever; and his eye-sight was so much improved that he could read a news-paper; indeed, it was nearly well. The functions of the bladder were completely restored; his speech became articulate; and his general health, in every respect much improved. He remained in the hospital about two months, but with very little amendment in the state of the lower extremities.*

Abernethy was unable to review progress in Thomas Crichton. Within a few years of recovering from his first episode of optic neuritis, Augustus d'Este was in the hands of the quacks. He experienced steel-water in Driburg (on the advice of Dr

Sprangenberg); beefsteaks, fortified wines and linament brushes (Dr Kent); astringent plasters and tepid baths (a Milanese doctor); urethral dilatation and 15 baths a day (Dr Sprangenberg, again); and galvanism:

> *if anything be clear to me ... it is ... that electricity is the most powerful Agent to my injury instead of to my recovery – the air of Brighton I should place in a similar category.*

Repeated versions of bathing in tepid, hot, sea or medicinal waters in many specifically different locations together with shampooing (Drs Brown, Granville, Barlow, Daniell); ingestion of strychnine, metallic salts (especially silver), tonics and aperients (various, including Richard Bright and Dr J.R. Farre); hydropathy at Grafenburg (Dr Praesznitz); cantharides (Sir Benjamin Brodie), and a mere 30 substances ingested in various combinations of tinctures, tonics, soothing drafts, powders and potions (Dr Seymour who visited d'Este on 49 occasions) were all tried (Figure 1.39). When he improved, d'Este believed, as probably did his physician, that some of these ministrations were effective:

> *having [my] weak legs rubbed with brushes and the torpid part of my back ... rubbed ... with a liniment ... succeeded completely.*

On treatment, Charcot came straight to the point:

After what precedes, need I detain you long over the question of treatment? The time has not yet come when such a subject can be seriously considered. I can only tell you of some experiments which have been tried the results of which have, unfortunately, not been very encouraging.

By comparison, his pupil Pierre Marie was much more positive, presumably because he was wedded to the aetiological role of infection and so saw an opportunity for prevention and cure:

> *I have little doubt that ... by the employment of ... the vaccine matter of Pasteur or lymph of Koch the evolution of insular sclerosis will some day be rendered absolutely impossible.*

Although one senses some uncertainty in Hammond's mind on the diagnostic status of the cases he classified as having multiple sclerosis, he was not in doubt that their condition could be improved with hyoscyamus and barium chloride, supplemented with lavish doses of electricity, codliver oil, iron, strychnine, two glasses of wine daily, and a moderate amount of exercise (Hammond 1871). Dr Alfred Newman (1875) acknowledged the hopelessness of identifying effective treatments:

> *the whole armoury of the British Pharmacopaeia has been launched against the disease with uniformly disastrous results.*

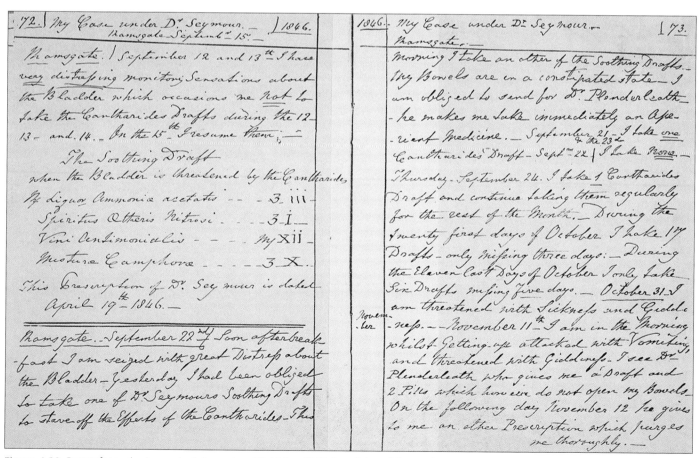

Figure 1.39 Pages from the journal of Augustus d'Esté for 1846 describing visits to physicians and treatments offered for his condition.

Althaus (1877) says not a word on treatment. Gowers (1888) used silver nitrate, quinine, hypodermic arsenic (recommended by Eulenberg), noted that Germans preferred hydropathy and electricity (which he approved for associated peripheral nerve palsies), and advised against pregnancy. Risien Russell (1899) considered the therapeutic prospects in disseminate(d) sclerosis to be gloomy in the extreme – no medicinal agent having the slightest effect in arresting the disease or retarding its progress. Reluctantly, he used silver nitrate or chloride, and arsenic, each to be administered subcutaneously, concluding that solanaine only worked in the symptomatic control of tremor when an erroneous diagnosis of hysteria had been made. Masssage, hydrotherapy and electrical treatment might help spasticity. Adjustments to lifestyle were likely to be more useful, including relocation from cool to sunny climates, elimination of depression, ensured rest, fresh air (in an open carriage or wheelchair) and a diet rich in codliver oil. Infections were so clearly implicated in the causation as to demand prolonged rest from an individual attack, and the possibility of metallic poisoning offered an obvious means of prevention. In time-honoured fashion, Risien Russell concluded with the rousing hope that:

a not very distant future may bring us face to face with a rational and more hopeful means of dealing with so intractable a disease.

In line with contemporary fashion, Bramwell (1917) gave his patients silver nitrate and arsenic to influence the course. He used hydrobromic acid or bromide of potassium for spasticity, and strychnine and iodide of potassium or nux vomica for paralysis, but in no case did it appear to be of the slightest use. Massage, electricity, hydropathy and suspension were of equally doubtful efficacy. Richard Williamson (1908) tried many drugs and found none to be helpful with the possible exception of quinine, which he favoured whilst recognizing that this apparent therapeutic effect could not necessarily be dissociated from the natural history of the disease. In Germany, Strumpell (1931, in English translation) considered rest in hospital to be essential and there he would administer galvanism, carbonic acid baths, friction, iodide of potassium, ergotin, silver nitrate or salvarsan (because of the spirochaetal aetiology), aspirin, arsenic and injections of fibrolysin – all supplemented by gymnastic exercises. Conversely, H. Oppenheim (1911) insisted that hot baths and electrical stimulation should be avoided. Mercury never worked and caused optic neuritis. Silver nitrate and iodide of potassium or Crede's silver ointment were useful treatments. Symptoms could be managed with Veronal for tremor and antiphlogistic-diaphoretic treatment during acute attacks of myelitis or encephalitis. Blood letting could be remarkable in its effects.

No one had very coherent ideas on the mechanisms of action of these agents and few even thought it necessary to speculate. As one of us has pointed out (W.I. McDonald 1983), the rationale for using arsenic was as mysterious to eminent pharmacologists as it was to neurologists of the day. Silver had been known to the Arabs, who considered that nervous diseases were influenced by the phases of the moon, which, in turn, were associated with silver in their system. Gowers (1888) reasoned that since the demyelinating component was more amenable to treatment than the astrocytosis, this was a specific indication for arsenic and silver salts but he offered no explanation for this

didactic view. It has been suggested that W.N.P. Barbellion hastened his own demise through injudicious use of nerve stimulants. He always attributed variations in the natural history of his disease to the mixture of arsenic, morphine and strychnine, which he took regularly from mid-1916. However, he knew this to be merely palliative at best, and after telling his wife, who knew all along, of the diagnosis in November 1916, entertained the hope that:

a physician from London will gallop up hotspur, tether his horse and dash in waiving a reprieve – the discovery of a cure.

Instead, he tried homeopathy and electrotherapy. We are fortunate in having available the encyclopedic collation of treatments that Brickner (1936) identified as having been used prior to 1935. It is a sorry catalogue of thwarted hopes and dashed lives. He rightly identified many of the factors that compromise the scientific evaluation of any new treatment in multiple sclerosis, and the need to time the intervention so as to coincide with a phase of the disease that is actually amenable to treatment. His table, running to 29 pages, lists in alphabetical order substances and methods from antimony to X-ray, almost all of which were somewhere in contemporary use. Trial methodology is conspicuously absent and many studies involved only a trivial number of cases observed for a short period. Brickner welcomed the American Neurological Association's initiative in 1934 to standardize at least some aspects of the protocol for a clinical trial. Surveying what was then therapeutically active, Brickner was particularly attracted to the study of malaria therapy reported by Grosz (1924), who segregated cases depending on clinical course (relapsing and progressive) and used a meaningful functional outcome such as ability to walk. Fever therapy was then very popular, because of its effectiveness in neurosyphilis and the current hypothesis that multiple sclerosis was caused by a spirochaete, and Brickner identified 11 different methods for inducing pyrexia. There were 24 trials of Salvarsan, again reflecting contemporary interest in the spirochaete and multiple sclerosis. Organic arsenicals were not without risk. One of us (WIMcD) recalls a fatal case of the well-recognized acute haemorrhagic encephalitis following their use in the late 1950s. Dreyfus and Mayer (1929) also used malaria therapy in a large number of cases and stratified their analysis according to severity and duration. Mild cases of recent onset responded best to treatment, as expected from the natural history. Brickner also singled out the studies of antimosan and stibenyl by Crecelius (1928), which involved 27 and 6 patients, respectively, studied for up to 5 years. The results seem to us unimpressive, and Brickner himself concluded that any therapeutic effect was short lived. Surgery (including sympathectomy, root section and laminectomy) was in use as a treatment for multiple sclerosis. Parenteral treatments included fibrolysin, haemolytic serotherapy, autotransfusion and implantation of spleen, thymus, thyroid, liver or brain (sadly, no reference is given for this first brain transplant in multiple sclerosis). Brickner (1935) himself had used quinine hydrochloride; and very distinguished neurologists were using sodium salicylate or sulphate, tetrophan and X-rays. Putnam (1939) used Brickner's table of treatments to perform an armchair meta-analysis, claiming that 47% of 1407 treated patients (usually receiving fever therapy, arsenicals or quinine) improved compared with 69% of 133 untreated patients, but he advised caution in drawing the cynical conclusion that medicinal treatment is useless in multiple sclerosis or that the placebo effect is superior.

Fever therapy induced by malaria, typhoid vaccine and other organic or microbial pyrogens, also featured prominently in Brain's account of treatment with no hint of adverse effects. On the other hand, Derek Denny-Brown (1901–1981) summed up fever therapy as being 'seldom beneficial and sometimes disastrous' (Denny-Brown 1952). The study in which Purves Stewart (1930) treated a large number of patients with a vaccine derived from cultures of the putative *Spherula insularis* virus, and which he claimed would arrest the disease, alter the colloidal gold curve and eradicate the organism from cerebrospinal fluid, was cited with the conclusion that removal of the organism from <10% cases placed considerable difficulties in the way of therapeutic enthusiasm for Miss Chevassut's discoveries. The vaccine had been given to 550 individuals in seven trials. Instead, the usual list of metal therapies – arsenic, silver, mercury and antimony – was recommended, and agents such as sodium salicylate or X-irradiation mentioned. Brain concluded that:

the multiplication of remedies is eloquent of their inefficacy.

Sadly, in the first edition of his textbook, he could offer nothing other than tact, judgement, metals and fevers by way of treatment, and even the use of liver had disappointed him. (S.A.) Kinnier Wilson (1878–1937) considered 'the pharmacopeia to have been ransacked for nerve tonics which might influence the course of multiple sclerosis', but he recommended arsenic in the form of Fowler's solution, injections of sodium cacodylate, Crede's silver ointment and other germicidal colloidal metals, including selenium, and aspirin, quinine and mercury. With others, he had used lecithin and fibrolysin but 18 months' treatment terminated in the final rebellion of his hitherto compliant patient. Wilson induced pyrexia with typhoid or paratyphoid vaccines and he used malaria or electrical methods. Surprisingly, these pyrogens did not appear to exacerbate the disease. He was unimpressed by the use of whole liver in comparison with its effect in subacute combined degeneration of the cord.

By 1955, Douglas McAlpine and Nigel Compston did at last have something to say about treatment and management, some of which we would still endorse. They distinguished the needs of the patient early in the illness from problems that arise later. Initially, the requirement was for rest with rehabilitation, taking 3–6 months (ideally) in a sanatorium. For the first time, the authors explained the need for open discussion of the diagnosis, except in the unmarried young adult and those judged to be of 'low moral fibre', and they warned patients not to accept uncritically general accounts of the illness that they may have read. Discussions on marriage and childbearing should be advisory and not proscriptive, but they considered that it made sense to delay pregnancy until the illness has been quiescent for about 2 years. Interest in fever therapy had not waned and we know that Nigel Compston visited Professor Cloake in Birmingham to assess a protocol for its induction with intravenous typhoid A and B vaccine. Cloake noticed a temporary increase in symptoms during the peak of the fever (101°F), which McAlpine and Compston attributed to vasodilatation since they had seen a similar phe-

nomenon with the use of nicotinic acid and NAB (arsenic). Cloake was an advocate of arsenic, which he gave four times annually for the first 5 years and three times thereafter. This work was described in his (the first) Humphry Davy Rolleston lecture to the Royal College of Physicians in 1947 on 'the treatment of disseminated sclerosis by artificial pyrexia and the prolonged administration of arsenic'. The lecture remained unpublished and the then Harveian Librarian, Sir Charles Dodds, and his successor, wrote serially to Professor Cloake between 1953 and 1966 trying to extract a manuscript, but (despite promises of imminent dispatch) with no success. This correspondence closes with an unanswered note of condolences to Philip Cloake's widow, dated April 1969, adding that the College still hoped to acquire the 1947 manuscript should this be found amongst Cloake's papers. It never arrived. McAlpine had himself used arsenic for many years but, in a small uncontrolled trial, Compston (N.D. Compston 1953) was unable to provide any scientific evidence in support of this approach to treatment. Histamine-induced vasodilatation had been used by Horton and Wagener (1948) in patients with optic neuritis, more of whom appeared to regain normal vision compared with the effects of typhoid vaccine, which many had previously received. McAlpine and Compston were unimpressed by the effect of histamine on relapse rate in patients with established multiple sclerosis (Horton *et al* 1944), and they were no more enthusiastic about liver and vitamin B12 or the dietary regimen of Swank (1953) – assembling powerful arguments against the simultaneous use of two or more therapeutic agents, and highlighting the lack of controls and failure to allow for the natural history of the disease in qualifying the putative use of this treatment for multiple sclerosis.

There was short-lived interest in treating multiple sclerosis with intrathecal tuberculin in the late 1950s. It grew out of observations made by Dr Honor Smith (1908–1995) in the course of treating tuberculous meningitis with intrathecal streptomycin. Dr Smith was a devoted, charismatic Oxford neurologist. As the daughter of a Baron, her correct mode of address (which she did not, however, use professionally) was 'The Honourable Honor Smith'. She rode to hounds, appearing for her Saturday morning ward round dressed in hunting garb. Smith and her colleagues reported what they regarded as characteristic changes in the cerebrospinal fluid of patients with multiple sclerosis following the intrathecal injection of tuberculin (H.B. Smith *et al* 1957). They suggested that the administration of tuberculin 'might be beneficial in multiple sclerosis'. H. Miller *et al* (1961a) followed up this suggestion because, as they said:

although the reason for endowing this procedure with any possible therapeutic significance has never been clearly stated, we felt it important that the suggestion should be subjected to carefully controlled assessment...

A large trial was planned but analysed prematurely because of the:

considerable pressure to which neurologists in various parts of the United Kingdom have been subjected by patients who are anxious for them to undertake this form of treatment on the basis of present evidence.

In the event, their study involved 14 patients having lumbar puncture alone, 12 receiving intrathecal saline, and 14 intrathecal tuberculin; a further 10 patients who had received intrathecal tuberculin before the trial began were also studied. Of the total of 50 patients, 7 could not be assessed but their distribution between the groups is not stated. The side effects were distressing:

The '[tuberculin] reaction' was usually accompanied by a constitutional illness with some degree of meningism, and occasional more alarming complications included severe clinical meningitis with troublesome vomiting (four cases), retention of urine (four, including one requiring three weeks' catheterisation), coma (two), dysphagia and dysarthria. In three further patients severe exacerbations of the chronic disease caused some alarm during treatment, and in one of these instances a profound difficulty in walking did not fully recover.

By modern standards this is far from a satisfactory study. Nevertheless, we cannot but agree with the authors' conclusion that:

it seems hardly justifiable to regard the intrathecal administration of tuberculin as a form of treatment for this disease.

The bladder could be managed by altering habits, through the use of atropine and phenobarbitone, and with early use of M&B (sulfonamide) or mandelic acid and hexamine (methenamine) as urinary antiseptics. McAlpine and Compston recommended systems for rehabilitation of traumatic injuries of the nervous system that had recently been introduced by (Sir) Ludwig Guttmann (1952). They could not envisage any circumstance in which it would be valid to terminate a healthy pregnancy in the context of multiple sclerosis but they advised against elective surgery for trivial complaints. It was against this largely historical therapeutic background that McAlpine and Compston were able to introduce their readers to the original results of Glaser and Merritt (1952), Fog (1951) and Miller and Gibbons (1953) who reported on the role of corticotropin in accelerating recovery from relapse in multiple sclerosis, although they found this to be profoundly disappointing by comparison with cases of acute disseminated encephalomyelitis. The combined experience of McAlpine and Compston in 1955 was two treated patients, including one with optic neuritis. A very few cases had been treated with antibiotics (chloramphenicol and penicillin) to control secondary infections. McAlpine and Compston could not reach any conclusions concerning the role of specific disease-modifying agents but they ended their account of treatment with a summary of guidelines adapted from (Sir) Austin Bradford Hill's writings on controls, power, confounding and matching in clinical trials (A.B. Hill 1952). Wrongly, in our view, they considered that the main aim of any treatment should be to reduce the frequency of relapse, ideally demonstrated by comparison between cases or controls but exceptionally through serial observation of individual cases. They felt that influencing disability was a secondary aim in treatment trials, mainly because this was thought to depend absolutely on relapse rate. They advocated the use of follow-up clinics, believing that

so long as these were not advertised as being for people with 'multiple sclerosis' the example of the disabled would not unduly affect the morale of milder cases. They were at pains to point out the need to attend to social aspects of the patient's illness and to involve the family in discussions and decisions.

We have set out above the complex medico-social agenda that surrounded the early years of the Multiple Sclerosis Society of Northern Ireland and Great Britain, and the ambiguous role of Douglas McAlpine (Nicolson and Lowis 2002). Those tensions boiled over in response to action and inaction by the medical panel over the issue of treatment. William Crofton (ex-lecturer in pathology from Dublin who set himself up in London as a private vaccine therapist) declared multiple sclerosis to be a viral disease treatable by vaccination. The vaccine sometimes produced unwanted reactions. One of us (WIMcD) recalls a patient admitted to the National Hospital, Queen Square, in about 1963 with an acute tetraplegia following an injection. A similar though less severe reaction had followed previous exposure. Nevertheless, Crofton had his opinions presented by Lord Brabazon in the House of Lords during 1955. Patients pressed Sir Richard Cave for a rapid response. He deferred to the medical panel. McAlpine answered:

I have spoken to the Medical Defence Union ... [who] advise that if the MSS intend to reply to letters regarding this vaccine, it should seek the advice of Counsel ... the Union would like to see a copy of this letter before it is sent.

Reminded thus of the legal protection under which the medical profession would make up its own mind on what did and did not deserve attention, the Society replied to its members:

unfortunately this Society is unable to comment on the effectiveness of Dr Crofton's treatment, as we cannot usurp medical prerogative ... the best I can do ... is to advise you to contact your doctor and be guided by him in the treatment you undertake.

The request for financial assistance needed by one of its members to attend Dr Crofton was refused – to which the thwarted patient replied:

... that it is very difficult ... for this society to undertake arrangements contrary to established medical and hospital practice involves a misconception so profound as to be ... inexplicable... it is [the conflict of] ... orthodox neglect and unorthodox treatment ... Orthodox members of the profession ... hardly treat their patients at all. I am ... in touch with one of the foremost hospitals in London and have never received any treatment from it ... the Society has made a great mistake in allowing the dead hand of medical negative orthodoxy to fall upon it.

An early applicant for research funding from the Society was (Sir) Ludwig Guttmann, also a member of the medical panel. This was refused, to Cave's embarrassment, on the grounds that his aims were treatment orientated rather than addressing basic mechanisms. Members rehearsed the oft-repeated cry that neurologists were responsible for:

the medical scandal that the treatment of MS has become ... for are they not the experts from the teaching hospitals, who are only too easy to say ... there is nothing more we can do for you.

For his part, Guttmann resigned followed by threats from the medical panel to follow suit, but in their case through pique at such criticism. Nor did this conclude the Society's difficulties with treatment. In the 1960s, Dr P. Le Gac proposed that the lesions of multiple sclerosis were due to rickettsial infection. He recommended long-term antibiotics, physiotherapy, warm sea-water and seaweed baths. The Society's refusal to support this work spawned a new organization, the Multiple Sclerosis Treatments Investigation Group (MSTIG). Predicting that no society that recommends quackery ever succeeds, the Society therefore sought to isolate MSTIG and discredit its empirical rather than rational approach. Eventually, in order to defuse criticism, the Society contracted Professor E.J. Field to confirm that the hypothesis was wrong. This he duly did but MSTIG did not like the choice of investigator:

Professor Field is ... a neurologist ... and the aetiology of this complaint is not his field of work ... the neurologist is unlikely to ... eliminate this condition as its cause does not originate in the neurological field ... this disease is being directed to the wrong specialist for treatment and that is why no progress has been made.

The Society's troubles were not over. Reginald Hawthorn, a Suffolk health farmer, proposed a dietary treatment for multiple sclerosis based on elimination of refined foods, carbohydrates and alcohol. This was taken up by the playwright, Roger MacDougall, who publicized his subsequent spectacular return to health. Again, a spokesman in House of Lords (Lord Willis, a former television playwright best known for the police series *Dixon of Dock Green*), championed the MacDougall diet and reprimanded the Society for not taking this seriously. Dr Reginald Kelly (1917–1990) answered:

I am [carrying out a double-blind trial] ... to acquire scientific evidence as to the value or otherwise of the theories advanced by Robin [sic] MacDougall. This is a very considerable labour but we feel it is imposed upon us, although the pilot trials have not been at all encouraging as to satisfy the clamour of patients.

During the 1960s and 1970s, coherent ideas began to form on the pathogenesis of multiple sclerosis, and impetus from results using corticosteroids in this and other conditions that were then accepted as immune or inflammatory in nature led to the use of various immune suppressants as they became available. W.I. McDonald (1983) has charted the transition from theories on the spirochaetal, spherulitic, bacterial and vasculitic causes of multiple sclerosis to specific therapies since the time of d'Este and provided present-day partners, based on no less flimsy a logic, for many of these apparently absurd treatments.

This situation was common to chronic disease generally. Looking back, we can now see that it was to be expected in illnesses whose courses were subject to wide variations between patients and in the same patient over time. The demonstration of therapeutic effectiveness in this context had to await development of the clinical trial. The story is told in magnificent detail by J.R. Matthews (1995); its application to multiple sclerosis has recently been summarized (W.I. McDonald 2004). The story is simply of the need to quantify and control.

The saga began late in 1821, just a year before d'Este's first symptom, at La Charité Hospital in Paris. Pierre Louis (1787–1872) was interested in tuberculosis, and in *Recherches anatomico-pathologique sur le phthisie* (1825) he argued for the use of numerical method. He applied the calculus of probability recently developed by Pierre-Simon Laplace (1749–1827), who had anticipated that it could be useful in the evaluation of treatment. Louis' views were vigorously opposed by the medical establishment of the day, headed by Cruveilhier and Risueño d'Amador (1802–1849) of Montpellier. They took the view, as did Claude Bernard (1813–1878) in physiology, that certainty could emerge only by a process of induction from the minute observation of individual cases. The issues were hotly debated in the Academies of Science and Medicine in Paris in the 1830s.

The focus moved to Germany in the late 1850s with Gustav Radicke's (1810–1883) publication 'On the importance and value of arithmetic means; with special reference to recent physiological researches on the determination of the influence of certain agencies upon the metamorphosis of tissue; with rules for accurately estimating the same' (translated by F.T. Bond for The New Sydenham Society, 1861). Again, it was the physiologists who, sharing Claude Bernard's view, opposed application of the emerging field of statistics to medicine.

At the end of the 19th century, the controversy moved to London. By this time there had been some acceptance of a role for numerical comparison in medicine. (Sir) Almroth Wright (1879–1940) had argued for the effectiveness of vaccination to prevent typhoid in the Army. But the professor of statistics at University College, Karl Pearson (1857–1936), pointed out flaws in the numerical methods. The major confrontation with Almroth Wright came in 1911 when Pearson's pupil Major (his forename, not a military rank) Greenwood (1880–1949) painstakingly refuted Almroth Wright's claims for the opsonic index, a method Wright had developed that, he claimed, could detect the presence of occult bacterial infection. Greenwood showed that it was invalid. Wright's controversial views had a high public profile and, as the fictitious character Sir Colenso Ridgeon, he was criticized by George Bernard Shaw in his play *The Doctor's Dilemma*. By now, however, the importance of statistics in medicine was gradually being accepted: behind his back, even Wright's colleagues at St Mary's Hospital (where 30 years later Alexander Fleming discovered penicillin) referred to him as 'Sir Almost Wright and Sir Always Wrong'.

Greenwood and his North American colleague Raymond Pearl (1879–1940) continued to promote vigorously the application of statistics to medicine. The next important step came in 1935 with Ronald Fisher's (1890–1962) publication *Design of Experiments*. Here he stressed the importance of randomization in the controlled experiment, a principle developed in his work comparing the yields of different types of grain.

The triumphant summation of work developed over more than a century came in 1948 with the Medical Research Council trial of streptomycin for pulmonary tuberculosis, the disease with which the story of therapeutic measurement had begun (Anon [MRC Committee] 1948). The protocol was devised by

(Sir) Austin Bradford Hill (1897–1991), a pupil of Greenwood. The impact of this study was summed up in a commentary in the Bulletin of the Johns Hopkins Hospital (Marshall 1948):

> *The report [of the trial] merits study not only for the results but for the way the experiment was conducted ... The result is that a rather limited number of cases, only 107 all told, have served to give definitive results which one can interpret with confidence.*

The application to neurology, and in particular to multiple sclerosis, was still some way ahead. The number of participants in the initial trials of corticosteroids for relapse was small relative to variability in the disease. Insistence that the way forward in finding effective treatments for multiple sclerosis would require the use of double-blind placebo-controlled trials involving adequate numbers of patients was the major outcome of an influential meeting organized in 1982 at Grand Island, New York, by the National Multiple Sclerosis Society of the United States (Weiner and Ellison 1983). The first real hopes of that meeting were realized a decade later when the pioneering suggestions of Larry Jacobs (1938–2001) (L. Jacobs *et al* 1981; see Chapter 18) saw completion of a large well-conducted clinical trial showing, not necessarily for the first time, statistically significant effects of pharmaceutical interventions on one aspect or another of the natural history of multiple sclerosis.

Although the therapeutic era has begun, the past is one of clinical charisma and the exploitation of vulnerable patients littering the historical highways and byways of therapeutic endeavour in multiple sclerosis. It has not been a golden road.

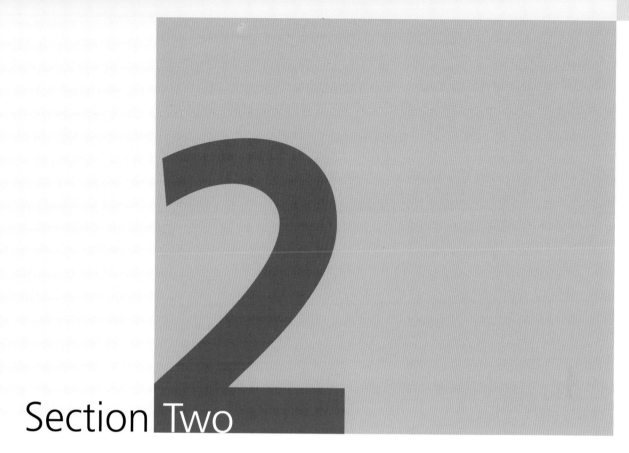

Section Two

THE CAUSE AND COURSE OF MULTIPLE SCLEROSIS

The distribution of multiple sclerosis

2

Alastair Compston and Christian Confavreux

THE RATIONALE FOR EPIDEMIOLOGICAL STUDIES IN MULTIPLE SCLEROSIS

Morbidity statistics for multiple sclerosis have been surveyed in many places, on many occasions and for many reasons. Listing individuals in whom the diagnosis has already been made, or identifying those with one particular feature of the disease, is not a difficult exercise, only requiring clinical resources and limited epidemiological expertise. In practice, the aims of these surveys have varied. Few have proved definitive and method-ological factors have often limited the extent to which useful conclusions can be drawn. This is particularly true when com-parisons have been made between the frequency of multiple sclerosis in different places, or when one area has been surveyed repeatedly over time.

The commonest reason for carrying out an epidemiological survey is to use temporal and geographical gradients, and variations in risk depending on location over defined periods, to generate hypotheses for causation of the disease. In this situation, it is essential to know that claims for reported differences in morbidity statistics are reliable. No studies have contributed more to an understanding of the causation and aetiology of multiple scle-rosis than those charting its global distribution. These epidemi-ological surveys have generated useful hypotheses and spawned secondary research seeking mechanistic explanations for the emerging patterns. But against a background of shifting statistics resulting from methodological variations and, perhaps, genuine changes in disease frequency and distribution both on the global and regional scales, many questions remain unanswered. Even the fundamental issue of whether an explanation for the distri-bution of multiple sclerosis should be forced into purely envi-ronmental or genetic constructs continues to be debated.

Whilst it is interesting to interpret the epidemiology of multiple sclerosis through the social history of populations in which the disease occurs, those that proved informative for epidemiologists working in the early part of the 20th century have been subjected to further changes in structure and distribution, making longitu-dinal or comparative studies difficult to perform and interpret. But despite not yet yielding a definitive account of the aetiology, the effort that has gone into serial identification of cases throughout the world using sound epidemiological principles, supports the concept of an interplay between environmental triggers and genetic susceptibility in the causation of multiple sclerosis. The challenge now is to nail the main factors in each category.

The second application of epidemiological work in multiple sclerosis is in public health medicine. Here, the priority is to assess local needs for the provision of services and allocation of resources. For this purpose, although accurate case definition is a prerequisite, issues relating to disease course and severity in the population as a whole are more important than trawling successfully for each and every affected individual using rigorous clinical and laboratory methods. For these purposes, patterns of disability, impairment and handicap provide the canvas on which the individual needs of prevalent patients are painted.

Lastly, epidemiological scrutiny of a fully ascertained, popula-tion-based register of patients can be used to define the natural history of multiple sclerosis, eliminating the bias inherent in description of the clinical course that inevitably contaminates cohorts derived from specialist clinical teams, groups of patients attending hospital clinics, or extrapolation of individual experience to the population at large. With the need to assess putative treatments that modify the course of multiple sclerosis, detailed description over time of large untreated population-based nat-ural history cohorts has become even more important (see Chapter 4). Putative disease-modifying treatments for multiple sclerosis are now used routinely in many parts of the world. As a result, it is no longer considered ethical to withhold these medications and randomize patients to placebo preparations in clinical trials. The use of historical controls derived from natural history cohorts may therefore be the only comparator available for the assessment of new treatments.

DEFINITIONS AND STATISTICS IN EPIDEMIOLOGY

Although shrouded in the mysteries of professional vernacular, the definitions used in epidemiology are not complex. Statistics are used to protect investigators from believing in their own or other people's hypotheses, arising from random variation and confounding interactions between apparently independent events. Over time and with experience, agreed procedures have been adopted for the assessment of morbidity statistics in mul-tiple sclerosis and for comparisons between factors that aim to distinguish individuals, or groups, having an unusually high or low risk of the disease (Kurtzke 1996).

The term *frequency* lacks precision but is useful in conveying a general impression of how often a particular event has occurred. The *cumulative frequency*, or *lifetime risk*, of multiple sclerosis, is the maximum chance that it will occur at any time during the life of each individual at risk, irrespective of when the condition first manifests. For northern Europeans, an approximate estimate of lifetime risk is 1:400, whereas it is 1:3 for the identical co-twin of an affected individual. Factors influencing the expected frequency of multiple sclerosis can properly be called *risk factors*. *Relative risk* is the product of the proportions of cases and controls with and without a particular risk factor. The *odds ratio* describes the ratio of incidence rates for multiple sclerosis in individuals who have, and have not, been exposed to the same risk factor.

Incidence (or more accurately *cumulative incidence*) measures the number of new events in a defined area over a given period. Events might be new diagnoses, stages reached in the course of the disease, or individual clinical features. The study area can be geographically or demographically defined but anything that deviates too far from a population base is likely to introduce ascertainment bias. The period over which observations are made can be long or short. The former introduces problems through social and age-related alterations in the population at risk. The latter leaves no real time to establish patterns free from natural oscillations in frequency of the disease or defined manifestations. In practice, incidence refers to the number of newly diagnosed patients per 10^5 of the population at risk over one calendar year. Incidence, prevalence and mortality are all ratios of individuals with multiple sclerosis (*numerators*) amongst a population at risk (the *denominator*: see Figure 2.1). Errors in calculating the numerator or denominator will spuriously distort morbidity statistics but the impact will be greater for numerator errors, especially where a group of epidemiological interest has relatively few affected individuals. The odd case omitted, or diagnosed in error, amongst a minority ethnic group studied in a large mixed metropolis will make an enormous impact on estimates for the incidence and prevalence of multiple sclerosis in that community. Although incidence and prevalence can be used to make comparisons between populations, changes in either may arise from predictable cycles in these statistics (*regression to the mean*), and each is dependent on the structure of the population being surveyed (Figure 2.2).

Prevalence defines the number of individuals in whom multiple sclerosis has been diagnosed, or those with a particular feature, in a population at risk on a given occasion. Because it includes all individuals who qualify for the outcome of interest, irrespective of the date of onset, it is numerically larger than incidence. Again, in practice, the event is usually the established diagnosis of multiple sclerosis. Estimates for the prevalence of multiple sclerosis are dependent on diagnostic accuracy. In turn, diagnostic precision depends on the choice and application of criteria for assessing the probability that each individual in the study does have demyelinating disease affecting the central nervous system. Here, there is bound to be an appreciable rate of error since demyelination has an extremely variable clinical phenotype. Prevalence is inevitably dependent on the degree of case ascertainment, and this tends to vary inversely with size and accessibility of the population at risk. It is almost invariable that first surveys underestimate prevalence (and incidence). Higher figures are obtained with second and subsequent assessments due to improved awareness and vigilance amongst both the population at risk and the investigator. It is for this reason that comparisons between neighbouring places and regions cannot

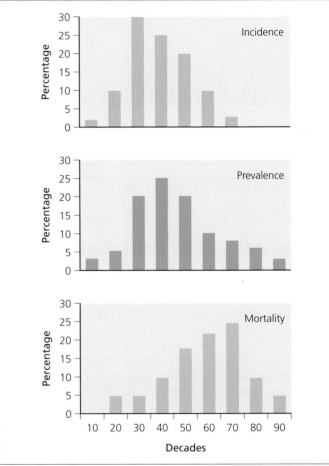

Figure 2.1 Percentage incidence, prevalence and mortality in all affected individuals in a population-based sample by decade. Incidence peaks in the 3rd decade, prevalence in the 4th and mortality in the 7th.

necessarily be used to define variations in the distribution of multiple sclerosis.

The category most likely to escape recognition, especially in first surveys, is the early or benign case. This artefact is especially problematic in areas with relatively underdeveloped health care systems. In this situation, there is also a likelihood that mortality will be higher, tending to reduce the number of individuals with advanced disability. Since duration is short when mortality occurs early, the overall number of prevalent cases will be further reduced. Thus, several factors may combine to favour under ascertainment and low estimates for prevalence in regions with poorly developed medical services. One can only guess at the extent to which this has contributed to apparent geographical gradients in the frequency of multiple sclerosis, and their erosion with serial updating of surveys performed in places enjoying improved health care facilities over time.

One proposed solution to the arbitrary use of *date at diagnosis* as the point of entry into an epidemiological survey is to adjust backwards to the perceived *date at onset* (C.M. Poser *et al* 1992). This is considered appropriate in studies probing the aetiology of multiple sclerosis since it gets closer to the point of origin for the putative risk factor – or so the argument goes.

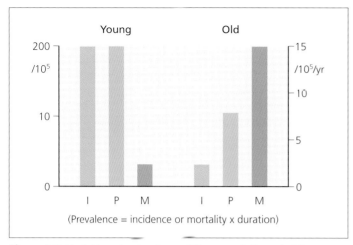

Figure 2.2 Variations in structure of the population at risk (denominator) influence the numerator. Since multiple sclerosis is a disease of young age at onset but long duration, a population with a disproportionate number of young people will show inflated figures for incidence (I) by comparison with mortality (M), whereas a population with an old age structure will show lower prevalence but increased figures for mortality and lower incidence.

Onset, in this context, means the date of first symptoms and so even this statistic does not adjust for the unknown interval between development of the disease process and its first recognized clinical expression. It merely substitutes one imprecise date for another. Proponents of onset-adjusted prevalence argue that it is appropriate retrospectively to include in morbidity statistics those individuals who are later classified as having multiple sclerosis even if their whereabouts and diagnostic status were unknown at the time. They should have been identified and so ought retrospectively to be included. However, all surveys carry incorrectly diagnosed cases and omit individuals who would have been identified in a perfect and fully ascertained study. Assuming that these accumulate at a constant rate, onset adjustment does not improve accuracy in serial estimations of incidence or prevalence.

The denominator, or population at risk, should be demographically based, or selected to suit the hypothesis being tested. Thus, whereas most epidemiological studies will relate to census information for a given location, others will have as their denominator a stratified group – such as patients with the primary progressive phenotype. What must be avoided is bias that loads the probability of any one individual being a case, or having a defined set of clinical features. This is most likely to occur with hospital- or clinic-based samples, where referral is subject to the whimsical nature of access and timing of referral. Attending patients tend to represent the newly diagnosed and more severe end of the clinical spectrum. The occasion on which prevalence is assessed is conventionally a single date (prevalence day) but this can be extended to a period, such as a year. In fact, depending on the outcome of interest, it may be prudent to adopt the *period prevalence* approach so as to ensure that sufficient examples are identified from which to judge the frequency of the event of interest.

Mortality describes the number of individuals with multiple sclerosis, as a proportion of the population at risk living in a defined area, dying over a given period. It does not document individuals with multiple sclerosis as a proportion of those who actually died in the population at that time, but refers to the entire population who could die. More importantly, it can either identify the number dying *from* multiple sclerosis or the number dying *with* multiple sclerosis. With so many uncertainties, and the tendency in most countries for causes of death to satisfy administrative arrangements rather than clinicopathological precision, mortality is operationally a poor statistic for evaluating the epidemiology of multiple sclerosis.

Mortality should match incidence (if each has been accurately assessed and no changes are occurring in aetiological factors determining the frequency of the disease). This is often not the case since it is easier for clinicians and epidemiologists to document new cases than to establish who has died with or from multiple sclerosis. The relative insensitivity of mortality statistics is disappointing since an excess of incidence over mortality in individuals having multiple sclerosis is one way of suspecting that a recent change in aetiological conditions has occurred.

Superficially, mortality also reflects the impact of therapy since improvements in the management of potentially life-threatening complications of multiple sclerosis will reduce death attributable to multiple sclerosis. Conversely, increased longevity merely shifts the balance of mortality from multiple sclerosis to mortality with multiple sclerosis. Longevity upwardly adjusts mortality to a later age without altering the number of people with multiple sclerosis who eventually die from an unrelated cause. It is self-evident that incidence, prevalence and mortality have a close relationship since each relates to a separate phase of the same disease process. In situations where ascertainment has been complete, no changes in survival or diagnostic classification have occurred, and frequency of the disease has not changed, prevalence will be the product of incidence or mortality and disease duration.

Survival refers to the number of patients in a cohort who have not yet reached a defined end point, typically death. It is less easy to measure directly than might be expected. Survival can begin with date of the first symptom, but this often has to be identified retrospectively. Alternatively, onset can be taken as the time of diagnosis, but that may have been influenced by random events and personal attitude relating to medical attendance, over and above patterns of referral and general organization of health care. In fact, disease duration is usually calculated by default on the basis of prevalence and incidence, or taken as twice the interval from mean age of onset to mean age at prevalence (Poskanzer *et al* 1980a) – but this method has wide confidence intervals.

Like all statistics, survival is dependent on full ascertainment of the numerator and denominator. The difficulty lies in the fact that the denominator has continually to be adjusted to account for the shifting number of individuals in the cohort who remain at risk through movement out of the study area and death. Annual rates for survival, based on the number of deaths, are censored for the fraction of each year that those who moved away actually remained within the study area, and hence at risk, allowing the calculation of *cumulative survival*. This approach does not equate to disease duration, or survival from onset, unless the cohort has been ascertained at presentation and is fully prospective. In practice, it is only possible to include cases for assessment of survival from the time at which they first come under observation. (The problems and pitfalls of survival analysis have been amusingly dramatized by John Kurtzke in outlining the fictitious excursions into neuroepidemiology of Halvah Finster and his fistulous disease; Kurtzke 1989.) In order to provide a complete picture on morbidity statistics, in the context of incidence and prevalence in particular locations, some aspects of survival are described in the sections that follow: a more detailed account of survival in multiple sclerosis is in Chapter 4.

Perhaps the factor making morbidity statistics for multiple sclerosis most difficult to establish is the range of age at onset. Without a reliable disease marker, and with such variable modes of presentation, it is difficult to know whether and when an individual is entirely free from the risk of developing multiple sclerosis. This obstacle is partially overcome by calculating *age-* and *sex-specific* rates for incidence, prevalence and mortality. These relate the number of affected individuals to a denominator confined to that proportion of the population at risk, and having the same age and/or sex distribution (to the nearest decade:

Figure 2.3). This goes some way towards dealing with the problem of comparing demographically different populations. Take, for example, the situation of multiple sclerosis in a small rural town attracting people at retirement but offering no employment for the young. The numerator for incidence will be small despite an adequate sample size, whereas prevalence may be proportionately much higher. This is especially likely if the area being surveyed offers excellent facilities for individuals with physical disability. Conversely, an area providing special opportunities for young people, such as a provincial university town, will have a relatively high proportion of individuals at risk, favouring higher statistics for incidence and prevalence but not mortality (Figure 2.2). In general, comparison of age-specific rates for multiple sclerosis in different populations eliminates confounding due to demographic structures.

Major changes in birth rate, or substantial migration over the period in which morbidity statistics for multiple sclerosis are being collected, also affect estimates for incidence and prevalence. The usual way of dealing with these variations has been to relate age-specific rates to a single population, deriving the *standardized prevalence ratio*. Inevitably, the chosen population varies between regions and is rarely agreed. In the United Kingdom, standardized prevalence ratios have been referred to the population of Northern Ireland in the 1960s. Taking equivalence as 100, standardized prevalence ratios are then quoted as >100 or <100. In other disease contexts, an attempt has been made to create a standardized European population for age correction (Figure 2.4: see Waterhouse 1976). Until recently, this reference has not been much used by epidemiologists studying multiple sclerosis.

Confidence intervals provide an additional means of defining the extent to which a given result, or *point estimate*, is likely to be reproducible, and hence valid. Confidence has upper and lower limits. Its range represents possible results consistent with the observations that have been made. Wide confidence intervals invite caution. Narrow ones suggest that the point estimate is likely to be reproducible. The 95% confidence limits are usually quoted. These represent the range for which there is a 95% chance of including the correct value. Although confidence intervals can be used as surrogates for statistical significance, the confidence interval does much more than assess the extent to which the null hypothesis is fully consistent with the results of

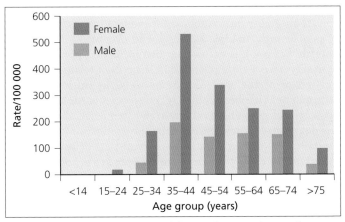

Figure 2.3 Age- and sex-adjusted figures for prevalence of multiple sclerosis in the south Cambridgeshire district of East Anglia in the United Kingdom. Adapted from Mumford and Compston (1993).

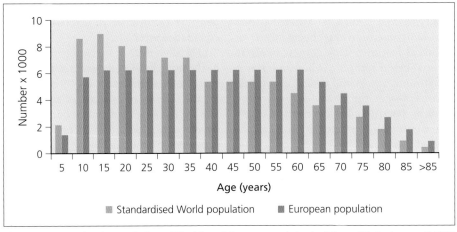

Figure 2.4 Standard populations: World and European. Adapted from Waterhouse (1976).

a particular study. Appropriate use of the confidence interval assumes that the sample studied is unbiased and representative of the population at risk. The method for calculating confidence intervals varies with size of the numerator. For the range represented in most epidemiological surveys of prevalence in multiple sclerosis, the limits are given as:

Upper limit = (numerator/denominator measured in 10^5) × Z
Lower limit = (numerator/denominator measured in 10^5)/Z

where Z is given as: exp (1.96 × [square root of 1/numerator]).

Case–control studies are used to identify risk factors. The contribution of each factor is expressed as an odds ratio or relative risk. These are often used interchangeably, and each is vulnerable to inappropriate selection of controls leading to poor matching between groups. However, matching inevitably excludes assessment of any risk contributed by the matched factor itself (such as age or sex) and events with which it happens to cosegregate. The contribution made by any one factor to the aetiology is the *attributable risk*. This component can potentially be modified, hopefully leading to a reduction in disease frequency. *Confounders* are factors influencing the assessment of another feature because the confounder has its own relationship with the population at risk. Each cofactor then appears to have an independent disease association but only one is biologically relevant.

Matching requires selection for each case of one or more controls from a similar group of individuals at risk who have the same frequency of confounding factors. *Stratification* groups subjects with one shared (and potentially confounding) factor in a particular category. This might be age, a clinical phenotype or a laboratory marker such as genotype. The difficulty with case–control studies in multiple sclerosis is lack of knowledge on potential confounders. In this situation, mismatching may persist – despite best efforts to stratify – through ignorance concerning aetiology of the disease. Matching is an important means of increasing the power of a case–control study. For example, if the hypothesis is that age of infection by Epstein–Barr virus (EBV) in genetically susceptible individuals determines the development of multiple sclerosis, matching both for EBV exposure and identified genetic risk factors will maximize the prospects of showing a difference in risk of multiple sclerosis depending on age at infection. Failure to match may obscure a biologically meaningful difference.

A *cohort study* is one in which the frequency of developing multiple sclerosis is studied in ≥ 2 groups of individuals who differ in their exposure to a putative aetiological factor, which is then assigned a risk. Cohort studies can measure *absolute* as opposed to relative risks and are preferable to case–control surveys. They are difficult to perform in a disease of low overall frequency but can explore several hypotheses simultaneously and relatively quickly. Cases should be representative of all affected individuals. In practice, they tend to be selected from prevalence rather than incidence registers. This runs the risk of introducing survival factors as confounders unless disease duration is uniform.

The threshold for concluding that a given relative risk or odds ratio identifies a factor increasing susceptibility, or conferring protection from the development of multiple sclerosis is, by definition, greater or less than 1. Interpretation depends on the 95% confidence intervals. If these are each >1, there is a >95% chance that the disease is associated with the factor in question. If the intervals straddle 1, the probability is that the factor is neutral. And if the intervals are both <1, the risk factor is considered to be protective. Since very few environmental factors conferring susceptibility or protection (in contrast to variables such as age, sex and race) have survived detailed scrutiny of the epidemiology of multiple sclerosis, it follows that the majority of case–control studies show confidence intervals that include 1, even though the odds ratio may itself be higher.

STRATEGIES FOR EPIDEMIOLOGICAL STUDIES IN MULTIPLE SCLEROSIS

In planning an epidemiological study in multiple sclerosis, the usual practice is to retrieve cases from those already known to be affected. This requires the coordination of lists from various sources. Very few surveys of multiple sclerosis are conducted by making new door-to-door enquiries. In many parts of the world, the diagnostic process is coordinated through hospital clinics to which all individuals with suspected symptoms of the disease are referred. Scrutiny of these departmental records provides the best single source of information when compiling a register of prevalent cases. Many, but not all, can also be identified from records held in primary care (general practice, in the United Kingdom). This is the source best placed to register individuals who have recently entered the area being surveyed, and those with established disease of long duration who may no longer be known to the hospital system. A few prevalent cases may be identified only as residents of homes for the chronic young sick although these rarely yield otherwise unascertained cases. Most epidemiologists find that morbidity registers for diseases that form part of general hospital admission or attendance records are a poor source of information.

The provisional register of prevalent cases must then be revised. Type A studies are those in which each case is assessed personally by the investigator in order to confirm or refute the diagnosis. Type B are those in which the diagnosis is assumed from available paper records. In practice, most studies combine both approaches. The fact that each registered case is domiciled within the study area needs to be ascertained for prevalence day from local health care systems, since movements in and out of the area contribute a significant source of error and will inevitably change between surveys in places providing serial estimations. It is wise to choose an area for which there is contemporary census information on the denominator. L.M. Nelson and Anderson (1995) have debated the relative merits of case finding using various sources in the United States. They conclude that the best yield is to be found through manual sorting of records held in neurology practices, and the files of local services for multiple sclerosis and care of the chronic young sick. They recommend the *capture–recapture* method. Borrowed from zoological and avian practice, this assesses how often the same individuals are identified in serial samples of a population, as the measure of ascertainment.

Serial change in incidence is generally considered a better marker than prevalence for detecting alteration in factors determining the aetiology of multiple sclerosis since these are presumed to be less vulnerable to case ascertainment and changing trends in classification. However, even incidence is not entirely secure.

Raised level of awareness amongst physicians and patients, especially those who are acquainted with or related to patients with multiple sclerosis, increases the recruitment of incident cases. Sudden change in the provision of facilities for the disabled tends to inflate each statistic, as does the arrival of an investigator with a special interest in the epidemiology of multiple sclerosis. Morbidity statistics tend to plateau once ascertainment saturates after a period of steady increase. It follows that differential vigilance and efforts at complete ascertainment will tend to create spurious regional and temporal gradients.

Some questions relating to the epidemiology of multiple sclerosis can only be answered by performing studies in defined locations. It makes little sense to plan a study requiring significant numbers of individuals with a rare manifestation, such as twinning or familial multiple sclerosis, in a community that has a low overall prevalence of the disease. Similarly, ubiquitous but biologically important features may not differ between groups in places where multiple sclerosis is extremely common. The question also arises of whether it is appropriate to perform epidemiological surveys in locations with underdeveloped procedures for medical care. For multiple sclerosis, but not some other disorders, these tend to be regions of low prevalence in which the yield from population surveys is bound to be relatively unrewarding.

Opportunities for identifying risk factors making a significant contribution to the disease, but common in the normal population at risk, are improved in areas of relatively low prevalence. Conversely, risk factors for multiple sclerosis that are not overrepresented in the normal population are identified more easily in high-prevalence regions. Even in these situations, large numbers and extra resources are needed to define the biologically less important risk factors, irrespective of their population frequency. Inevitably, decisions concerning the area to be included in a study represent a trade-off between administrative boundaries for which demographic information is available and a scale sufficient to include enough examples of the factor of interest. Decisions concerning the omission of suspected cases depend on the study aims. For surveys testing biological features, the ideal is to include all individuals who have the disease process even if this is not yet clinically declared. In other contexts, it is essential to restrict inclusions to those with definite disease in order to exclude doubtful cases and prevent contamination of the study aims. These decisions require judgement and knowledge of the disease but inevitably introduce difficulties for regional and cross-cultural comparison of surveys.

Generally, it is unwise to accept as proof the results of a single epidemiological study claiming involvement of any one aetiological factor. Cohort studies require careful selection of participants from a population base in order to avoid recruitment bias. The cohort can only be selected once the research aims have been defined and the population established. Many studies require a system for clinical classification and description of morbidity using well-validated rating scales. Groups defined on the basis of disability, impairment and participation are then selected randomly within diagnostic categories. No rating system addresses all these issues. The Kurtzke Expanded Disability Status Scale (EDSS; Kurtzke 1983a; see Table 6.1) has the merits of widespread use, familiarity amongst clinicians and extensive validation. But it is not ordinal and prevalent cases usually show a bimodal distribution. It is especially insensitive in certain ranges and excessively weighted towards ambulation. Some limitations of the EDSS are circumvented by using life-table analysis of the time taken for patients to reach strategic points on the scale, as part of natural history studies (see Chapter 4), or treatment trials (see Chapter 18). Population association studies often assess the frequency of a technically sophisticated clinical or laboratory marker, not easily applicable to a large sample. The merits of the study then depend entirely on the appropriate selection of cases and controls. Bias or inconsistency for either can invalidate the study. Sociohistorical factors may make for significant differences across even quite small regions, especially when comparing genetic risk factors and environmental exposures. Ethnicity should always be remembered at the planning stage of an epidemiological study. It is, for example, likely to remain an inviolate principle in the assessment of genetic susceptibility, whereas (for example) the potential confounding effect of ethnic heterogeneity is entirely appropriate in a study designed to assess resource requirements for the disabled.

THE GEOGRAPHY OF MULTIPLE SCLEROSIS

In the modern era (for earlier epidemiological work, see Chapter 1), John Kurtzke (Kurtzke 1980a; 1980b; 1983b; 1985b; 1993; 2000) has systematically updated his original landmark overview (Kurtzke 1975) in order to incorporate the results of new surveys. Others have attempted the same (see Bauer 1987; D.A.S. Compston 1990a; Rosati 2001). Earlier editions of this book benefited from the authoritative accounts of Donald Acheson (McAlpine *et al* 1965; 1972; W.B. Matthews *et al* 1985) and Christopher Martyn (W.B. Matthews *et al* 1991). Taking the big picture, Kurtzke concludes that whereas multiple sclerosis was geographically a regional disorder of males in the mid-20th century, subsequent experience shows more multiple sclerosis in places where the disease was already known to occur, diffusion into places where it was hitherto uncommon across even quite narrow confines within single land masses, and a steady increase amongst women and races other than Caucasians. For Kurtzke, the regional increases within Asia have been in the former Soviet Union but not Japan, Korea or China. In Europe, the southern littoral of the Mediterranean and Israel have shown conspicuous increases in prevalence. The same trends are apparent in Central and South America (Mexico, Argentina and Uruguay). But many of these focal trends are based on unpublished data, and hence vulnerable to all the factors that make for serial increase in morbidity statistics independent of an increase in incidence (Kurtzke 2000). A long list of best estimates for the frequency of multiple sclerosis makes dull reading but what emerges from an overview is that the main factor determining patterns in the observed frequency of multiple sclerosis (excluding differences dependent on hospital- or population-based surveys) is when, as much as where, the study was carried out. In following those who have successfully painted the big epidemiological picture on disease frequency and distribution, we have also tried comprehensively to collate studies that variably provide statistics for incidence, prevalence or mortality (Figure 2.5). We have not undertaken the arduous task of calculating confidence intervals for surveys where these

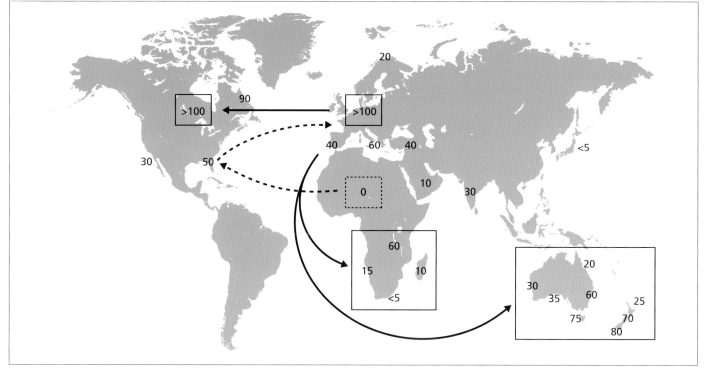

Figure 2.5 Summary of epidemiological patterns in multiple sclerosis. Figures are estimates for prevalence. Solid lines with arrows represent migration vectors of northern Europeans. Open lines with arrows represent migration routes of Africans to the Caribbean and Mississippi delta and to the United Kingdom. In South Africa the numbers refer to English-speaking whites migrating as adults (60), English-speaking whites migrating as children (15), Afrikaners (10) and mixed race individuals (<5), as estimated in the mid-1980s.

are not quoted. Neither, unlike the admirable and pioneering work of John Kurtzke, do we claim to have been encyclopedic in listing each and every epidemiological survey. Inevitably, Europe is disproportionately represented since multiple sclerosis is relatively common and a focus for epidemiological studies (Figure 2.6). For surveys carried out during the heyday of epidemiological studies, readers are referred to two publications acting as important additional sources of primary information, although we suspect that each necessarily took surveys of differing quality in producing overviews. Helmut Bauer summarized the epidemiology of multiple sclerosis in Europe (Bauer 1987) on the basis of presentations held in association with the World Congress of Neurology in Hamburg. The Department of Neurology in Darmstadt celebrated its 20th anniversary with a workshop at which delegates presented recent epidemiological surveys from many parts of Europe (Firnhaber and Lauer 1994).

MULTIPLE SCLEROSIS IN SCANDINAVIA
(Figures 2.7 and 2.8)

The study of multiple sclerosis in Scandinavia has been of considerable importance to those who espouse the genetic doctrine and attribute causation to the Viking gene pool (see C.M. Poser 1994, and Chapters 3 and 5). This region featured prominently in the early studies by John Kurtzke (Kurtzke 1967; 1974; 1975) leading to definition of a Fennoscandian focus. As in most other places, estimates for prevalence outnumber those for incidence. Overall, the trend has been for a steady increase in prevalence,

and for all the usual reasons – improved survival, earlier diagnosis, enhanced vigilance and more sensitive diagnostic criteria. But ascertainment saturation may have occurred allowing morbidity statistics to plateau. The early studies are summarized by Koch-Henriksen (1995).

In the modern era, the systematic study of multiple sclerosis in Denmark began with the pioneering work of Kay Hyllested (Hyllested 1956), initiated at the instigation of Torben Fog, and much dependent on the availability of Danish disease registers. Based on 2140 certain and 341 probable cases, rates were 4.4/10⁵/annum for incidence, and 58/10⁵ for prevalence on 1st October 1949. Age-specific prevalence peaked in the fourth decade and the sex ratio was 1.2F:M. Koch-Henriksen *et al* (1992) used the same Danish Multiple Sclerosis register established by Hyllested to review cases listed on 31st December 1986 whose onset was judged to postdate 1st January 1948. The interval between onset of symptoms and their recognition as manifestations of multiple sclerosis was >5, >10 and >20 years for 51%, 27% and 6%, respectively. The authors knew of 6478 cases incident between 1948 and 1986 (1.4F:M) of whom 83% had clinically definite disease. The ascertainment corrected incidence rate across this period was 4.4/10⁵/year in a population that increased from 4.2 to 5.1 million. Koch-Henriksen *et al* (1992) produced useful lifetime cumulative incidence rates allowing that proportion of the population expected to have developed multiple sclerosis by a given age to be identified (Figure 2.9). At 65 years, 0.31% or 1:314 Danes (1:271 females and 1:372 males) will have developed multiple sclerosis. Incidence rates for the three decades from 1950 were 5.1 (95% CI 4.9–5.3), 3.8

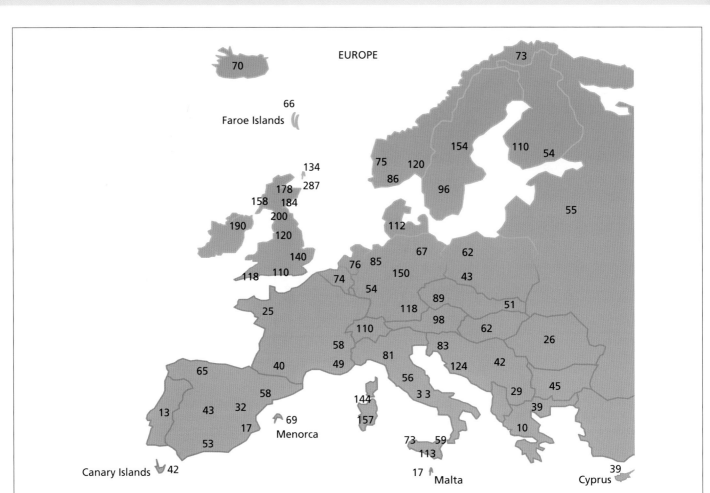

Figure 2.6 Distribution of multiple sclerosis in Europe. Most recent figures are given for prevalence/10^5 population; a 'best guess' is given where local variations exist in the published literature.

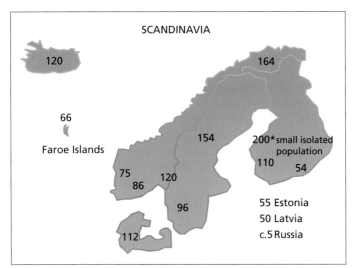

Figure 2.7 Prevalence distribution of multiple sclerosis in Scandinavia. Most recent figures are given for prevalence/10^5 population; a 'best guess' is given where local variations exist in the published literature.

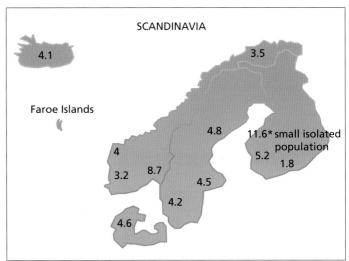

Figure 2.8 Incidence distribution of multiple sclerosis in Scandinavia. Most recent figures are given for incidence/10^5 population/year; a 'best guess' is given where local variations exist in the published literature.

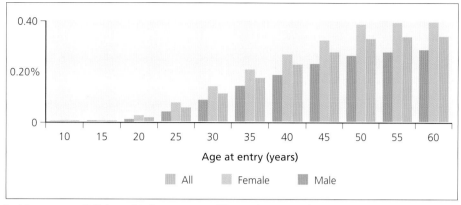

Figure 2.9 Cumulative incidence rates (%) from birth to any specific age by sex and 5-year age entries. Adapted from Koch-Henriksen *et al* (1992). Reproduced with permission from the BMJ Publishing Group.

(95% CI 3.7–4.0) and 4.3 (95% CI 4.0–4.5), respectively. The fall in the second decade (1960–1970) depended on a reduced rate in people aged <35 years but this was followed by an increase for older incident cases, especially females, in subsequent years. The rate for the most recently evaluated quinquennium was 4.6/10⁵/year (95% CI 4.3–5.0; Koch-Henriksen *et al* 1994). After making corrections for the impact of laboratory investigations on the timing of diagnosis, the authors concluded that a change in environmental factors had altered the frequency of multiple sclerosis in the middle decade of their comprehensive survey. We remain to be convinced. By 1993, the number of registered cases on the database, prevalent in 1948 or incident between 1949 and 1993, was 12 070. Crude annual average incidence was 4.99/10⁵/year between 1980 and 1989, and prevalence 112/10⁵ on 1st January 1990 (Koch-Henriksen 1999). Of these 12 070 cases, 6068 had died between 1951 and 1993. Death from multiple sclerosis was registered in 55.4%. As we discuss in Chapter 4, standardized mortality ratios were increased for infectious and pulmonary disease (2.46, 95% CI 2.04–2.94), suicide (1.62, 95% CI 1.29–2.01) cardiovascular disease (1.34, 95% CI 1.22–1.48), and accidents (1.34, 95% CI 1.02–1.71). They were reduced for cancer (0.79, 95% CI 0.70–0.90), perhaps due to incomplete ascertainment and the reduced life expectancy (Koch-Henriksen *et al* 1998). In order to provide an account of survival in the post-antibiotic era, these data were recently reassessed to include only the 9881 cases incident between 1949 and 1996 (and not the cohort prevalent when the Danish register opened in 1948), of whom 4254 had died by January 2000. Multiple sclerosis was associated with a reduction in life expectancy of around 10 years, with 56.4% of deaths attributed to the disease itself and, as before, with an excess standardized mortality ratio for suicide and accidents and protection from cancer. But, as anticipated, the reduction in life expectancy had halved over the period 1948–2000 (Brønnum-Hansen *et al* 2004). Thus, leaving aside minor perturbations, Denmark has seen a two-fold increase in prevalence but stable rates for incidence over the last 50 years, providing clear evidence for the dominant impact of ascertainment and methodology over biological forces in changing the frequency of multiple sclerosis in a community having in place sophisticated nationwide procedures for ascertainment.

A comprehensive analysis of multiple sclerosis over time has also been carried out in Gothenburg, Sweden. The incidence of definite and probable multiple disease dropped progressively from a stable rate of 4.2/10⁵ between 1950 and 1964 over successive 5-year periods between 1974 and 1988 to 2.0/10⁵ (Svenningsson *et al* 1990). Conversely, serial estimates of prevalence showed stable rates adjusted to the population structure of the city at 91, 91 and 96/10⁵ for 1978, 1982 and 1988, respectively (Svenningsson *et al* 1990). These authors point out that the reduction in incidence of multiple sclerosis in Gothenburg, with stable prevalence, over the two 15-year periods 1950–1964 and 1974–1988, coincided with the near complete eradication of measles by vaccination and (by 1990) no measles-vaccinated individual had developed multiple sclerosis in this community. In northern Sweden (Vasterbotten county), onset-adjusted incidence between 1987 and 1997 was 5.2 (95% CI 4.4–6.2) in women and 3.7 (95% CI 2.7–4.9)/10⁵/year (1.4F:M; Sundstrom *et al* 2003). Onset-adjusted prevalence was 154 (95% CI 139–170) in December 1997, with differential rates for women and men of 202 (95% CI 179–228) and 105 (95% CI 89–125), respectively (1.9F:M). Here, the annual increase in prevalence (2.6% compared with rates from Gothenburg between 1990 and 1997) is attributed to a real difference in incidence, compared with southern Sweden, and steady reduction in mortality leading to increased survival. As an approximation to incidence in the population, and to inform the epidemiology of health care needs, G.X. Jiang *et al* (1999) showed rates for first hospital admission of 4.46/10⁵/year (2.19F:M).

There have been rather few epidemiological studies of clinically isolated demyelinating syndromes. Jin *et al* (1998) reported an annual crude incidence for isolated optic neuritis of 1.46/10⁵/year between 1990 and 1995 (4F:M). Age adjustment indicated peaks in the fourth and fifth decades; rates were lower for those not born in Scandinavia; and the conversion to multiple sclerosis correlated with age at presentation.

Another attempt at painting the big Swedish picture on statistics for multiple sclerosis is a review of disability and mortality for 1952–1992 involving, respectively, 11 414 and 5421 cases, referred to equivalent statistics for Parkinson's disease (disability) and motor neuron disease (mortality). Disability attributable to multiple sclerosis and death certification with multiple sclerosis had each risen but showed regional variation (Landtblom *et al* 2002). Subsequently, Landtblom *et al* (2005) compared three sources of information: 1301 hospital admissions from 1925 to 1934, 5425 deaths between 1952 and 1992, and 11 371 disability pension receipts admitted between 1971 and 1994; the prevalence data were most heterogeneous, indicating higher rates, in seven counties surrounding major lakes in southern Sweden and others in regions north of the Bay of Bothnia and around Stockholm.

In western Norway, the incidence for definite or probable multiple sclerosis appeared to increase in Hordaland County from $1.1/10^5$ for 1953–1957 (Larsen *et al* 1984) to $4.9/10^5$ for 1978–1982, before falling to $3.4/10^5$ for 1983–1987 (Grønning 1994; Grønning *et al* 1991). Although incidence for the period 1978–1982 was higher than in the subsequent quinquennium, the relatively long interval from onset to diagnosis (approximately 4 years in most surveys) makes this short-term change difficult to interpret. Hordaland County has also seen a three-fold rise in prevalence from $25/10^5$ in 1963 to $75.5/10^5$ in 1983 (Larsen *et al* 1984). In More, Romsdal County, the average annual incidence changed from $1.9/10^5$ during the period 1950–1954 to $3.8/10^5$ for 1975–1979 (Midgard *et al* 1991). Subsequently, Midgard *et al* (1996a) summarized serial observations of incidence as showing a steady increase to 1975, which became more marked over the next decade but has since declined. Prevalence for definite and probable multiple sclerosis increased from $24/10^5$ in 1961 to $75/10^5$ in 1985 (Midgard *et al* 1991). The Oslo Multiple Sclerosis Registry was used to derive morbidity statistics for eastern Norway based on 794 cases identified by 1999 (2F:M; Celius and Vandvik 2001). Incidence increased over a 20-year period from 3.7 in 1972–1976 to $8.7/10^5$/year in 1992–1996. These incremental changes depended especially on patients with relapsing–remitting disease and females, and were considered by the authors not to have resulted solely from improved ascertainment. Prevalence (based on 579 northern European patients identified by 1995) was $120/10^5$ ($136/10^5$ amongst native Norwegians, originating from throughout the country, and other Scandinavians). These rates are much higher than those reported from a rural area on the west side of Oslo fjord (Edland *et al* 1996). In this survey, prevalence increased from 62 to $86/10^5$ between 1963 and 1993.

In the period 1953–1972, De Graaf (1974) identified cases of multiple sclerosis in the northern counties of Norway, amongst a population of approximately 213 000, of whom Lapps made up ≤10%, the majority being Finns and Nordic people. Cases were classified using the Allison and Millar criteria (see Chapter 1) following personal examination. Annual incidence rates varied from 0.9 to $2.5/10^5$/year but with no temporal trend. Prevalence for all cases was $21/10^5$. Similar incidence rates ($3.0/10^5$/year) were reported from Troms and Finnmark working to a prevalence date of 1st January 1983 (Grønning and Mellgren 1985). Statistics for northern Norway have been updated to 1993 (Gronlie *et al* 2000). Incidence was $3.5/10^5$/year for the period 1983–1992 and, by 1993, prevalence had increased to $73/10^5$. By 1993, there were three individuals with both and three others with one Sami parent, compared with a single parental example in 1983. Nevertheless, regional differences still show lower prevalence in parts with the highest proportional Sami population. Prevalence in Nord-Trondelag County

was $123/10^5$ on 1st January 2000. Age-adjusted incidence increased over the period 1974–1999 from 3.9 to $5.6/10^5$/year (4.6 to 6.3 and 2.2 to $4.4/10^5$/year for females and males, respectively; Dahl *et al* 2004).

The frequency of multiple sclerosis in Vaasa, western Finland, increased steadily from 1964 through 1972 to 1979, by which time prevalence was $93/10^5$ compared with $53/10^5$ in Uusimaa, southern Finland. Incidence rates, updated to 1979, were 3.3 and $2.2/10^5$/year, respectively (Kinnunen 1984). Most changes resulted from increased prevalence in younger age groups. Relaxation of diagnostic criteria or a change in age structure of the population at risk were not thought to be responsible. The authors suggested that the threefold increase in western Norway, matched by a rise in incidence (see above), could not solely be attributed to alterations in demography, survival or ascertainment. They argued that a change had occurred in biological factors determining the frequency of multiple sclerosis. A subsequent update from the same region (Sumelahti *et al* 2001) showed prevalences of 202, 111 and $108/10^5$ in Seinajoki, Vaasa and Uusimaa, respectively, in 1993. Rates for incidence were 11.6 and 5.2 and $5.1/10^5$/year in Seinajoki, Vaasa and Uusimaa, respectively (Sumelahti *et al* 2000). The 1.2-fold increase in Seinajoki (compared with 1983) is attributed to a change in incidence in men; in Uusimaa incidence remains stable in both sexes; and in Vaasa, prevalence is stable but incidence has decreased in both sexes. The authors attribute these changes to environmental conditions rather than differences in case ascertainment. Based on cases dying between 1964 and 1993, survival was >50% at 40 years from onset with an excess of deaths from suicide and neoplasia; complications of multiple sclerosis accounted for 70% of deaths (see Chapter 4; Sumelahti *et al* 2002). A more recent publication qualifies these prevalences: $219/10^5$ (95% CI 190–247) in Seinajoki-south; $136/10^5$ (95% CI 108–164) in Seinajoki-north; and $107/10^5$ (95% CI 90–124) in Vaasa (Tienari *et al* 2004). By comparison, prevalence in neighbouring central Finland in 1993 was lower at $59/10^5$ increasing to $105/10^5$ by 2000. Incidence increased from $3.8/10^5$/year in 1979–1993 to $9.2/10^5$/year in 1994–1998 (Sarasoja *et al* 2004). We discuss the genetic implications of the epidemiological observations from Vaasa in Chapter 3.

The prevalence of multiple sclerosis in the former Soviet Union is now being reported – in many areas for the first time. These statistics must be regarded as preliminary and many of the original reports are only to be found in the proceedings of local meetings published in Russian. The average figures quoted by A.N. Boiko (1994) and A.N. Boiko *et al* (1995) show a gradient of increasing frequency from east and south to northwest, with a low of $<5/10^5$ in Uzbekistan, Kazakhstan, Turkmenistan and Kirghizstan to a high of $>50/10^5$ in Latvia. Within these regions, there appears to be a difference in rate between native populations and Russians, suggesting that, apart from differences in ascertainment dependent on variations in access to specialist medical care, ethnic factors may determine the distribution of multiple sclerosis in the former Soviet Union.

The most parsimonious explanation for geographical and temporal trends throughout Scandinavia is increased survival due to improved symptomatic treatments, consequential shifts in age-specific mortality and more disabled prevalent cases, and a saturation effect of ascertainment. That said, some of the temporal and geographical trends are consistent with real changes in the impact of exogenous factors determining the frequency of multiple sclerosis. Other regions bordering the North Sea have seen a reduction in incidence of the disease (see below for discussion of the Orkney and Shetland islands). The epidemiology of multiple sclerosis relating to islands in the North Atlantic – Iceland and the Faroes – is discussed under the heading of 'Epidemics and clusters of multiple sclerosis'.

MULTIPLE SCLEROSIS IN THE UNITED KINGDOM (Figure 2.10)

We have already described the early history of epidemiological studies of multiple sclerosis in the United Kingdom (see Chapter 1), highlighting the separate activities of Richard Williamson, Russell Brain, Isabel Wilson, Sydney Allison and John Sutherland. Subsequent surveys were carried out in the Western Isles in 1954 (Sutherland 1956) and 1979 (Dean *et al* 1981a), Northumberland and Durham (Poskanzer *et al* 1963), Carlisle (Brewis *et al* 1966), Yorkshire (McCoubrie and Shuttleworth 1978), and Cornwall in 1950 (Campbell *et al* 1950) and 1958 (Hargreaves 1969). From the late 1980s, there was a return to systematic surveying of multiple sclerosis with studies reported from geographically disparate parts of England, Wales, Scotland and Northern Ireland. It is now possible, once again, to review what has been learned concerning the distribu-

tion of the disease and the lessons this provides for a general understanding of the aetiology. Prevalence has risen. Incidence may have reached a plateau or fallen in places previously showing very high frequencies of the disease. The move towards comparability between surveys through the use of standardized diagnostic systems and age- and sex-corrected denominators has eroded but not eliminated the apparent north–south gradient.

Sixty years after Allison (1931) first surveyed multiple sclerosis in the United Kingdom, the frequency was reassessed during 1984–1988 in Wales, this time in the industrial southeast (Swingler and Compston 1988). The tenfold increase in prevalence over 50 years reflects a pattern seen with respect to dissemination of the disease over time in practically every other part of the United Kingdom where serial studies have been performed (Swingler and Compston 1986). Over four decades, the number of newly diagnosed cases of multiple sclerosis showed marked variations in south Wales, the peaks often coinciding with the arrival of a new neurologist but otherwise revealing a slow increase from about 4.8 in 1947 to 8.2/10⁵/year by 1988. The temporal trends arose partly from changes in definition and classification, the availability of laboratory methods for supplementing the diagnosis, and increased clinical vigilance. Mostly, they depended on the steady reduction in mortality that occurred in the second half of the 20th century. Mean duration of disease from onset of symptoms, estimated at 8 years in the early part of that century (Bramwell 1917), had risen to >25 years by the mid-1980s (D.A.S. Compston and Swingler 1989). E.S. Williams *et al* (1991) subsequently reanalysed mortality statistics, calculating annual age- and sex-specific figures standardized to death rates in the United Kingdom for 1974. They found less evidence for the north–south gradient and considered (on the basis of a fall in mortality) that – as in some parts of Scandinavia – the incidence of multiple sclerosis had been falling in Scotland. They considered only those individuals with multiple sclerosis as the underlying cause of death and so underestimated absolute numbers of cases dying with the disease by up to 50%. Whilst confirming the general trend towards a reduction in death rates throughout the United Kingdom, they showed that this was more marked in Scotland and Northern Ireland (39%) than in England and Wales (10%) and highlighted the conspicuous reduction in mortality for Scots aged >65 years. Although the failure to show a correlation between temporal and geographical trends for mortality and prevalence invites the comment that these mortality returns were too crude for useful analysis, the same criticism can be levied at figures for prevalence – traditionally considered the more robust statistic.

The subsequent batch of surveys from new or previously studied parts of the United Kingdom confirms the high overall frequency of multiple sclerosis and, with notable exceptions, continues to show increasing prevalence in each newly surveyed district. Thus, to the previously reported rates of 117/10⁵ in southeast Wales (Swingler and Compston 1988; updated to 120/10⁵ by Hennessey *et al* 1989), 115/10⁵ in the urban area of Sutton close to London (E.S. Williams and McKeran 1986), 99/10⁵ in Southampton (M.H.W. Roberts *et al* 1991) and 178/10⁵ in northeast Scotland (J.G. Phadke and Downie 1987) were added figures of 122/10⁵ for Rochdale in Greater Manchester in 1989 (Shepherd and Summers 1996), 98/10⁵ for Trent in the Midlands (K.W. Allen 1994), 130/10⁵ in southeast Cambridgeshire (Mumford *et al* 1992 – updated to 152/10⁵ by

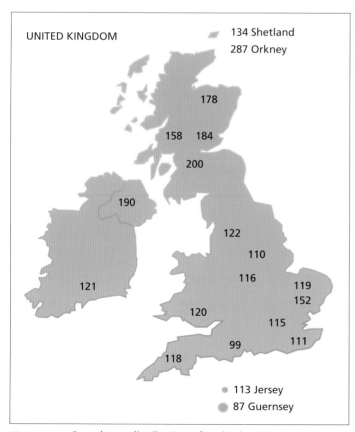

Figure 2.10 Prevalence distribution of multiple sclerosis in the United Kingdom. Most recent figures are given for prevalence/10⁵ population; a 'best guess' is given where local variations exist in the published literature.

N.P. Robertson *et al* 1996a), 119/10[5] in north Cambridgeshire (N.P. Robertson *et al* 1995), 153/10[5] in rural Suffolk (Lockyer 1991), 111/10[5] in the mid-Downs region of Sussex in southern England (Rice-Oxley *et al* 1995) and 113/10[5] and 87/10[5] for Jersey and Guernsey, respectively (G. Sharpe *et al* 1995; these bailiwicks of the Channel Islands come within the administrative boundaries of the United Kindgom but, being 70–100 miles south of the English mainland, are latitudinally comparable to western France, lying 10–30 miles to the west, and may therefore be genetically unrepresentative of southern England). Evidence that Scots have a high risk of multiple sclerosis irrespective of domicile strengthened with the subsequent report of incidence and prevalence rates for the Lothian and Borders regions (southern Scotland), at 12.2 (95% CI 10.8–13.7) and 10.1/10[5]/year (95% CI 6.6–13.6), and 185 (95% CI 175–194) and 201/10[5]/year (95% CI 174–228), respectively. These were equal to contemporary figures for northeast Scotland and the offshore islands (Rothwell and Charlton 1998). This declaration triggered a brief competitive response from Northern Ireland claiming, at 230/10[5] (95% CI 207–256), to have the highest contemporary prevalence rate attributable to Celtic ancestry (McDonnell and Hawkins 1998a) and representing a substantial increase from an earlier estimate for the same location of 137/10[5] (Hawkins and Kee 1988). More accurate figures subsequently emerged of 191/10[5] (95% CI 169–213) using the Poser criteria and 163/10[5] (95% CI 143–183) based on the Allison and Millar classification. Incidence was estimated at 6.5/10[5]/year in the late 1990s (McDonnell and Hawkins 1999). In a more recent comparison within Ireland, the prevalence in Wexford was 121/10[5] (95% CI 101–144) compared with 185/10[5] (95% CI 162–210) in Donegal, Northern Ireland (McGuigan *et al* 2004). Taken together, no one would doubt that Northern Ireland has a relatively high frequency of multiple sclerosis.

After a busy period in the mid-1990s, rather few new epidemiological studies have since been reported from the United Kingdom. One new region of southeast Scotland was screened by Forbes *et al* (1999) providing a rate for prevalence of 184 (95% CI 171–198) and 222 (95% CI 210–240) depending on use of the Poser (727 definite and probable cases) or Allison and Millar (880 early, probable and possible cases), respectively. Use of the capture–recapture method suggested that ascertainment was >93%. Previously reported geographical gradients were considered largely to be methodological and did not hold up after age and sex corrections. A second study, in Fife to the north of Edinburgh, identified 508 patients (2.4F:M) by postal questionnaire providing a standardized prevalence ratio of 178/10[5] (R.M. Grant *et al* 1998). A recent cross-sectional survey of 169 000 Glaswegians showed a prevalence of 145/10[5] and incidence at 5.7/10[5]/year; the crude prevalence in Asians was 63/10[5] (S. Murray *et al* 2004). As in Carlisle, England, when Brewis *et al* (1966) reported on the development of neurological disease between 1946 and 1961, finding a prevalence for multiple sclerosis of 82/10[5], B.K. MacDonald *et al* (2000) prospectively surveyed a population of 100 230 patients registered in 13 general practices in Leeds for neurological diseases. The estimated incidence of multiple sclerosis was 7/10[5]/year (2.8F:M). Lifetime prevalence rates were reported for a subset of 27 658 in whom multiple sclerosis affected 1:500. By chance, a recent conventional prevalence study also comes from Leeds. H.L. Ford *et al* (2002) reported incidence for multiple sclerosis in

792 people with multiple sclerosis (2.3F:M) over the period 1996–9 at 6.1/10[5]/year (95% CI 5.1–7.2). The prevalence changed between October 1996 and 1999 from 93/10[5] (95% CI 86–101: H.L. Ford *et al* 1998a) to 109/10[5] (95% CI 101–116, including 14% suspected cases). Mortality, based on 57 deaths, was 3.2/10[5]/year, reflecting incomplete notifications of mortality and their poor standing as reliable indicators of disease frequency. C.M. Fox *et al* (2004) established prevalence for multiple sclerosis in a first survey from Devon. Using the capture–recapture method to confirm at least 94% ascertainment, they identified 446 cases in a population of 341 796 on 1st June 2001, providing prevalences of 117 (95% CI 106–129) and 118/10[5] (95% CI 105–128), classifying cases using the criteria of either W.I. McDonald *et al* (2001) or C.M. Poser *et al* (1983).

Even now it is difficult to reliably map the distribution of multiple sclerosis across the United Kingdom. Diagnostic criteria, inclusion or omission of suspected cases, quotation of confidence intervals, variable citation of crude and age-adjusted figures, reworking of statistics for time of onset rather than diagnosis, and adjustment to a standardized population must all be taken into account when attempting a reliable overview. Until the mid-1980s, studies of multiple sclerosis in the United Kingdom used the system of classification suggested by Allison and Millar (1954). Adapting to the Poser criteria (C.M. Poser *et al* 1983) does not materially affect estimates for the total number of prevalent cases or standardized prevalence ratios. However, differences do arise when surveys are restricted to definite cases. Readers often fail to separate statistics that do and do not include the fringe of suspected cases. Although differences in numerator are apparent with the recent introduction of revised diagnostic criteria (W.I. McDonald *et al* 2001), comparing the frequency of multiple sclerosis using the Allison and Millar classification with more recent publications is more problematic. For example, the surveys from Northern Ireland and southeast Scotland show differences in prevalence of 28 and 38/10[5], respectively, depending on which classification is used. But the main source of variation lies in the extent to which separate regions have been subjected to the same degree of epidemiological scrutiny.

Previously, the pattern appeared to show a marked difference in frequency between the northeast mainland and offshore islands of Scotland compared with other parts of the United Kingdom. This was most apparent when the estimates for prevalence of multiple sclerosis were being serially updated in northeast Scotland (Downie 1984; Phadke and Downie 1987; Shepherd and Downie 1978; 1980; Sutherland 1956) and in the Orkney Islands (Allison 1963; Fog and Hyllested 1966; Poskanzer *et al* 1980a). Over that period, the highest mainland prevalences were reported for Aberdeen in northeast Scotland, with figures of 127 (95% CI 116–137) in 1970, 144 (95% CI 133–156) in 1973, and 178 (95% CI 166–191) in 1980. Onset adjustment by C.M. Poser *et al* (1992) on these published figures raised the prevalences for northeast Scotland to 117 (95% CI 107–127), 117 (95% CI 107–127) and 139 (95% CI 129–147), respectively. By 1974, when very few other parts of the United Kingdom had been surveyed, the prevalence for Orkney stood at 309/10[5] (95% CI 237–404; Poskanzer *et al* 1980a). S.D. Cook *et al* (1985) documented the annual incidence from 1941 to 1983 and suggested that there had been a steady reduction from 1964. By 1983, the quoted prevalence had also fallen from 309/10[5] in 1974 to 224/10[5] (the figures were 257/10⁵ and 193/10⁵ for probable cases only in 1974 and 1983, respectively).

With the steady rise in prevalence for southern parts of England and the more stable rates in northeast Scotland, there appears to have been a steady reduction in slope of the previously demonstrated gradient in frequency. Without knowing the extent to which surveys of multiple sclerosis in northeast Scotland have saturated prevalent cases, and with continuing uncertainty on whether other parts of the country have yet reached a steady state, it is difficult to predict how much further this gradient will collapse. Forbes and Swingler (1999) assessed the extent to which under-ascertainment, quantitated on the basis of capture–recapture comparisons, is sufficient to account for the latitudinal gradient. However, even after adjustment, they still found higher rates in northern parts of the United Kingdom (>180/10⁵) compared with the south (<160/10⁵). Despite the possibility of waning incidence in Orkney and Shetland, we also retain the view that the northeast of Scotland genuinely has a higher frequency of multiple sclerosis than other parts of the United Kingdom, although a systematic change in prevalence, correlating with latitude throughout the United Kingdom, now seems less likely. If the recent temporal trends are due to altered biological factors that determine the frequency of multiple sclerosis, it follows that these must be environmental, albeit affecting a fertile population, and not genetic. But our preferred explanation is that the epidemiological trends are due to saturation in northeast Scotland, and a catching-up effect elsewhere, resulting from incomplete ascertainment in the early surveys. Therefore, we retain the view that the distribution of multiple sclerosis in the United Kingdom is real and reflects differences in genetic characteristics of the population at risk (see Chapter 5).

MULTIPLE SCLEROSIS IN THE UNITED STATES (Figures 2.11 and 2.12)

The regional frequency of multiple sclerosis in continental North America was first mapped in detail by Limburg (1950) and subsequently by Kurtzke (1993). The highest prevalence is seen in the northwest of the United States (and southern parts of Canada). The lowest figures for prevalence occur in the southeastern states. The combination of a large land mass, and a complex cultural history with substantial and ethnically diverse immigration over the last two centuries, makes it difficult to see clearly the epidemiological picture of multiple sclerosis in North America and to interpret the pattern.

The point that systematic change in prevalence, but not necessarily incidence, is to be expected over time in an area subjected to repeated scrutiny is more than clear in the studies of multiple sclerosis from North America. The surveys from Olmsted County, Minnesota, organized through the Mayo Clinic, are exceptional in terms of the high case ascertainment and sequential assessments of disease frequency made over a period of 100 years (Wynn *et al* 1990). Incidence appeared to remain stable in Rochester at about 3.6/10⁵/year from 1905 to 1974 (men 2.8/10⁵ and women 6.8/10⁵). However, re-evaluation of all patients classified as having possible multiple sclerosis over the period 1905–1984 (Wynn *et al* 1990) revealed a trend towards increasing incidence, especially for women, in whom crude incidence rose from 3.4 to 7.7/10⁵. It remains uncertain

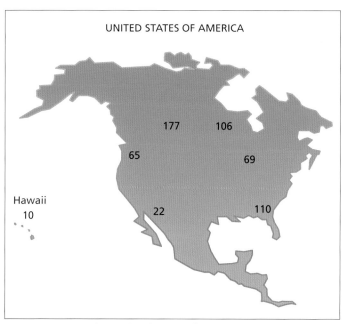

Figure 2.11 Prevalence distribution of multiple sclerosis in the United States. Most recent figures are given for prevalence/10⁵ population; a 'best guess' is given where local variations exist in the published literature.

whether this increase in incidence merely reflects alterations in application of diagnostic criteria and improved ascertainment. These factors, together with improved survival, largely account for the systematic rise in prevalence from approximately 46/10⁵ in 1915 (Percy *et al* 1971) to 108/10⁵ in 1978 (Kranz *et al* 1983), 173/10⁵ in 1985 (Wynn *et al* 1990) and (based on retrospective analysis) 160/10⁵ in 1990 (Wynn *et al* 1990). At the last count, the crude prevalence was 177/10⁵ on 1st December 2000 and incidence was 7.5/10⁵/year over the period 1985–2000. Sex and age adjustment standardized to the 1950 United States Caucasian population showed that the rates have been stable over the last 20 years (Mayr *et al* 2003). The analysis does suggest a small but real increase in incidence from the early 1900s (accounting to some extent for the rise in prevalence) but with interruptions in the otherwise steady rise. Cyclical changes were apparent in the 1910s, 1930s, 1950s and 1980s. Despite the care with which these statistics were gathered, difficulties remain in developing elaborate aetiological hypotheses based on small trends in incidence and, in Rochester, the rate has been steady at 7–8/10⁵ over the last two decades (Weinshenker and Rodriguez 1995). Broadly similar figures are quoted for neighbouring Mower County, Minneapolis (106/10⁵ in 1978; Kranz *et al* 1983). By comparison with other parts of the world, rather few more recent surveys on the epidemiology of multiple sclerosis have been reported from the United States. In northern Colorado, the prevalence was 65/10⁵ in 1982 (L.M. Nelson *et al* 1986). Hopkins *et al* (1991) estimated the prevalence in Galion, Ohio, at 112/10⁵ (95% CI 64–174) on 1st June 1987 amongst a population of 15 161.

The use of defined cohorts has formed the basis for mapping trends in the epidemiology of multiple sclerosis in the United States. John Kurtzke first studied 5305 United States army personnel who served in the Second World War or Korean conflict and were judged by the Veterans Administration to have

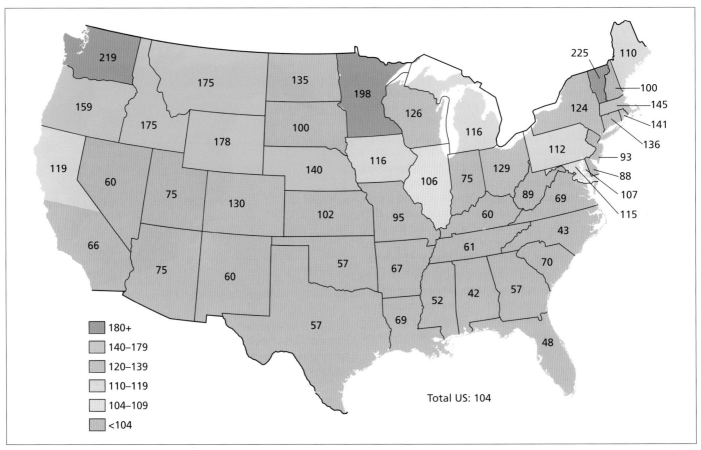

Figure 2.12 Case–control ratios (× 100) for multiple sclerosis by state of residence at entry into active duty for white male veterans of the Second World War. Adapted from Brown JR *et al* (1979). © 1979, reprinted with permission of Lippincott Williams & Wilkins (lww.com).

symptoms of multiple sclerosis recorded during or within 7 years of military service (Kurtzke and Page 1997; Kurtzke *et al* 1979; 1985; 1992; Norman *et al* 1983; W.F. Page *et al* 1993; 1995; Wallin *et al* 2000). The key finding on which all subsequent analyses have been predicated is that prospective incidence series showed high and low rates for multiple sclerosis above and below the 37th parallel, respectively. The gradient is not strictly latitudinal in that it also shows a west–east polarity. Kurtzke has demonstrated an overall distribution for incidence that matches that derived for mortality (Figure 2.12). Comparisons of location at birth and entry into military service, ancestry, demographics and natural history have allowed John Kurtzke and colleagues subsequently to assemble a picture of multiple sclerosis in the United States orientated towards understanding the aetiology from the perspective of epidemiology. From these various opportunities has emerged the principle of an effect on disease frequency of migration between regions of differing risk (see below). W.F. Page *et al* (1993) analysed the distribution of multiple sclerosis in these 5305 veterans with respect to ancestry, having noted differences in frequency of the disease within the northern and southern tiers of high and low risk, respectively. Multiple sclerosis appeared more common in Louisiana, Arizona and southern California – with a high proportion of French and Spanish ancestors – than in other southern states. The authors confirmed the link between Scandinavian (and in some analyses

Scottish, French and Italian but not English or Dutch) ancestry and risk of multiple sclerosis. Ancestry accounted for 45–60% of state-by-state variance and correlated more closely with the risk of multiple sclerosis than univariate analysis of personal ethnicity (W.F. Page *et al* 1995). But, however the issue is approached, the correlation of genetic history and contemporary risk of multiple sclerosis is apparent. Subsequent analysis of the United States veterans cohort drew attention to higher socioeconomic status and years of education as risk factors for multiple sclerosis in whites and black women (Kurtzke and Page 1997), although effects of ethnicity and geography may have confounded this complex multivariate analysis. As discussed in Chapter 4, survival in around 2500 veterans from the Second World War who had developed service-connected multiple sclerosis by 1956 was estimated in 1996 (Wallin *et al* 2000). Median survival times from onset were 43, 30 and 34 years for white females, black males and white males, respectively. Crude 50-year survival frequencies were 32%, 22% and 17%, for these same groups. Reduced survival correlated with male sex (proportional hazard, 1.57), older age at onset (risk ratio, 1.05/year), and high socioeconomic status (risk ratio, 1.05/socioeconomic status category). Factors such as race or place at entry into the military did not influence survival. Standardized mortality ratios showed an excess attributable to multiple sclerosis that declined over the period 1956–1996.

Wallin *et al* (2004) subsequently described 4951 Vietnam era veterans in whom comparisons were made with 9378 matched controls. The cohort is considered representative of contemporary multiple sclerosis in the United States and is additionally useful as a comparator for the previous series of veterans with multiple sclerosis. Differences from the Second World War/Korean conflict series included an increase in the number of women and blacks at risk, as a result of demographic changes within the military. Cases were classified, as before, using the Schumacher and Poser criteria. The main findings were an increase of multiple sclerosis amongst blacks and in women, with partial erosion of the north–south gradient in disease frequency for state of residence at birth or service entry. The possibility exists of confounding effects on these apparently independent findings. Arguing that genetic factors could not have changed over the period during which altered risks for multiple sclerosis were documented in the two series of veterans, the authors promote the primary influence of environmental factors. Others may yet feel that these epidemiological trends illustrate the interplay of altered environmental exposures in populations that have intrinsically different risks. Not least, cultural change has led to significant but geographically uneven Afro-American admixture in this generation.

Hernán *et al* (1999) also adopted the powerful approach of studying a professional group in whom health records made for easy determination of numerator and denominator. They identified new cases of multiple sclerosis amongst the Nurses Health Study (carried out during 1976–1994 on nurses born between 1920 and 1946), and the Nurses Health Study II (carried out during 1989–1995 on nurses born between 1947 and 1964). Based on 181 cases, adjusted incidence rates showed a ratio of 3.5 (95% CI 1.1–11.3) for the northern and 2.7 (95% CI 0.8–8.9) for the middle compared with the southern states, respectively, in the first cohort. However, this gradient was not confirmed in Nurses Heath Study II in which 131 cases were identified providing adjusted incidence rate ratios of 0.8 (95% CI 04–1.6) and 0.9 (95% CI 0.4–1.8) for the northern and middle banded states compared with the south, respectively. This attenuation of the gradient for disease frequency matches the erosion reported for veterans (see above) but has the potential confounder that the age ranges for nurses in the first cohort were 30–74 years, compared with 25–48 years in Nurses Heath Study II. Thus, incidence may not yet be fully declared in the latter.

Taken together, and using a variety of adjustments from the available morbidity statistics, D.W. Anderson *et al* (1992) estimated that there were about 350 000 physician-diagnosed patients with multiple sclerosis in the United States in 1990, compared with 123 000 in 1976. This defines the health care needs, but can anything be learned about aetiology from the patterns defined in the United States? After Davenport (1921; 1922), Bulman and Ebers (1992) re-emphasized the importance of population genetics as a risk factor in North America by correlating the frequency of multiple sclerosis (mapped by Kurtzke) with the distribution of people having Scandinavian ancestry. Of course, social habits shared amongst ethnic communities introduce a potential confounding factor, and the similarities in distribution of multiple sclerosis and ancestry do not amount to evidence *per se* for a genetic mechanism. Our own view is that the distribution of multiple sclerosis in the United States has been shaped by patterns of immigration. High-risk areas in the mid-West were originally mainly populated from northern Germany and Scandinavia. The low-risk areas of the Mississippi delta had a high density of people of African descent. With time, these original groups have moved and mixed thus eroding the differential rates of multiple sclerosis. Despite the genetic stance, this analysis also requires that environmental events triggered the disease process in individuals at risk. It does not exclude geographical and temporal trends in those exposures.

MULTIPLE SCLEROSIS IN CANADA
(Figure 2.13)

The prevalence of multiple sclerosis has been systematically assessed in several Canadian provinces, and some have been serially updated. A first survey of Winnipeg, Manitoba, based on information from case notes and death certificates for the years 1939–1948, reported a prevalence on 1st January 1951 of $40/10^5$ compared with $6/10^5$ in New Orleans (Westlund and Kurland 1953). Two years earlier, the rates in Winnipeg were $42/10^5$ compared with 13 and $41/10^5$ in New Orleans and Boston, respectively (Kurland 1952). Prevalences of 64 and $53/10^5$ were cited from other authors for Rochester and Kingston, Ontario. At reassessment in 1961 (Stazio *et al* 1964), the diagnosis was reviewed in 149 individuals included in the first Winnipeg survey. This exercise was the first to scrutinize diagnostic inaccuracy in detail. Of 112 cases classified as having probable multiple sclerosis in 1951, this degree of certainty held up in only 85. Apart from 3 who were no longer prevalent, 3 others were known not to have the disease, 7 remained as possible cases and in 14 the diagnosis was now thought to be unlikely. In the category of 22 possible cases from 1951, 13 were either known not to have multiple sclerosis or this diagnosis was subsequently considered unlikely. Conversely, of the 15 with dubious diagnostic status in 1951, only 2 had matured clinically and were thought to have multiple sclerosis at follow-up. With

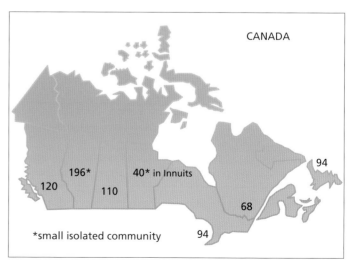

Figure 2.13 Prevalence distribution of multiple sclerosis in Canada. Most recent figures are given for prevalence/10^5 population; a 'best guess' is given where local variations exist in the published literature.

the retrospective application of these corrections, prevalence in 1951 should have been 36/10[5], and the new (1960) prevalence almost identical at 35/10[5]. This is surprising since practically every other serial estimate of prevalence has shown an increased rate, due to improved ascertainment and survival, even when methods and diagnostic criteria are standardized.

Published prevalence rates in Canada have since shown a systematic increase in frequency. This has been most obvious in the study from Saskatoon, Saskatchewan, where estimates for incidence at 4.8/10[5]/year and prevalence of 134/10[5] (Hader 1982) prompted the reaction that Saskatoon should be scrutinized in detail to determine why the frequency was so high. However, it soon became clear that, after allowing for the contributions of improved survival and high case ascertainment resulting from arrangements for the provision of health care, these statistics more accurately reflected the overall prevalence of multiple sclerosis in southern Canada. Subsequent studies, ranging from both coasts of Canada and including the province of Ontario, have shown comparable figures. In British Columbia, the rate was 93/10[5] for probable multiple sclerosis and 130/10[5] for all cases in 1982 (V.P. Sweeney *et al* 1986). Prevalence in Ottawa was 68/10[5] in 1975 (Bennett *et al* 1977) and 94/10[5] in the first survey from London, Ontario, for 1984, at which time 70% of the population was from the United Kingdom and 23% from continental Europe (Hader *et al* 1988). The rate in Saskatoon levelled out at a more representative frequency of 111/10[5] by 1977 (Hader 1982). Conversely, in Newfoundland the first estimate of prevalence was only half that reported for other Canadian centres (55/10[5]; Pryse-Phillips 1986) but this was subsequently adjusted to 95/10[5] in 2001, with stable incidence rates over the period 1994–2001 at 5.6/10[5]/year (Sloka *et al* 2005a). Regional rates were those predicted from contemporary estimates of disease frequency for places in the United Kingdom from which these immigrants had originated (Sloka *et al* 2005b).

Other reports for Canada were provided from southern Alberta where the prevalence in Cardston and Crowsnest Pass was 87/10[5] and 202/10[5], respectively, on 21st June 1989 (G.M. Klein *et al* 1994). Incidence was 4.2/10[5]/year between 1980 and 1989, an increase from 1.3/10[5]/year for 1950–1959 in Barrhead County, and prevalence 196/10[5] in 1990 (S. Warren and Warren 1992). Intensive scrutiny of a smaller area bordering Barrhead County showed comparable figures at 200/10[5] and 7.3/10[5]/year for prevalence and incidence, respectively, suggesting that ascertainment was more or less saturated in the larger survey (S. Warren and Warren 1993). Mortality data relating to multiple sclerosis in the period 1965–1994 were highest in the provinces of Quebec (4.4/10[5]/year) and Ontario (3.9/10[5]/year), intermediate in the western provinces (2.1/10[5]/year), and lowest on the eastern Atlantic seaboard provinces (1.2/10[5]/year; S. Warren *et al* 2003). As expected, rates were higher in females than males, and in those aged >65 years. Taken together, average annual mortality rates fluctuated without any directional trend. These data do not match the distribution of statistics for prevalence, perhaps because of demographic differences in the age and sex structures of the populations at risk throughout Canada. Seven aboriginal people with multiple sclerosis were identified by Mirsattari *et al* (2001) in a study from Manitoba giving a prevalence of 40/10[5] between 1970 and 1996, <50% of the rate expected for Canadians of

northern European origin living in the mid-western provinces. However, the difference may be even greater since five of the seven cases had a phenotype dominated by relapsing spinal cord and optic nerve disease – as seen in several other racial groups with a low overall frequency of multiple sclerosis (see Chapter 5)

MULTIPLE SCLEROSIS IN AUSTRALIA AND NEW ZEALAND (Figure 2.14)

The surveys carried out in Australia and New Zealand over the last 30 years have been especially influential since they have maintained sufficiently consistent methodology over time, allowing temporal and regional comparisons to be made with reasonable confidence. The geographical area under scrutiny is large and incorporates considerable variation in latitude, climate and racial origins. Caucasians have been domiciled in Australasia for over a century, and new migrant groups – Mediterranean and Oriental – have since arrived. However, in other respects the data do not lend themselves to internal comparisons. Four different systems for classification have been used. There has been inconsistency in the choice of denominator within defined geographical regions, for example with respect to the inclusion of aboriginal peoples (notably Maoris in New Zealand). Standardized prevalence ratios have not been adjusted to the same population. The account of morbidity statistics for 1981 (S.R. Hammond *et al* 1987) contains a transcription error from 1961 (McCall *et al* 1968) which, when corrected, reduces the apparent latitudinal gradient.

In the first comprehensive survey in Australia (McCall *et al* 1968), rates for 1961 were based on the Allison and Millar criteria. A south–north gradient in age-standardized prevalence was apparent, ranging from 34/10[5] in Hobart, Tasmania, to 19/10[5] in Perth, Western Australia, and 18/10[5] in Newcastle, New South Wales. By 1981, these rates had risen to 74, 29 and

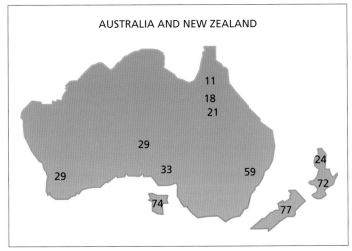

Figure 2.14 Prevalence distribution of multiple sclerosis in Australia and New Zealand. Most recent figures are given for prevalence/10[5] population; a 'best guess' is given where local variations exist in the published literature. Minor differences from figures appearing in the original publications reflect our recalculations.

38/10^5, respectively (S.R. Hammond *et al* 1988). On that occasion, cases were classified using the criteria of Rose *et al* (1976). In surveys carried out by the same investigators (S.R. Hammond *et al* 1987), prevalence in Queensland was 11 and 21/10^5, north and south of the tropic of Capricorn, respectively. These figures compared with prevalences of 7 and 12/10^5 for the same areas in 1961 (Sutherland *et al* 1966), using the World Federation of Neurologists diagnostic criteria. Later, McLeod *et al* (1994) added prevalence figures for South Australia (29/10^5) and reiterated the conclusion that, in the absence of an obvious genetic difference accounting for the sevenfold reduction in prevalence in tropical Queensland compared with Hobart, Tasmania – and despite the lack of any affected Aborigines or Torres Strait Islanders – the main determinant of the Australian gradient was environmental. Using the criteria of Rose *et al* (1976), prevalence in the Australian Capital Territory was 57/10^5 (95% CI 43–74) on national census day in 1996 (R.D. Simmons *et al* 2001). The sex ratio was 2.4F:M. Reclassification using the C.M. Poser *et al* (1983) criteria altered the prevalence to 49/10^5 (95% CI 42–58). Prevalence remained disproportionately high when corrected to the 1981 population by direct comparison with earlier surveys from other parts of Australia. Because disease duration in this cohort was short, longstanding cases may have been missed thereby leading to underestimate of disease frequency. The statistics have been updated for Newcastle, New South Wales, in 1996 with incidence and prevalence at 2.4/10^5/year and 59/10^5, respectively. The increase was attributed to altered incidence in females, aged 20–29 years, and improved survival, also in females (M.H. Barnett *et al* 2003).

S.R. Hammond *et al* (2000a) have again summarized the distribution of multiple sclerosis in five regions of Australia, focusing on individuals who had migrated from the United Kingdom and Republic of Ireland. There is a significantly higher prevalence ratio of multiple sclerosis amongst Australians leaving school at an older age and achieving a higher educational level (S.R. Hammond *et al* 1996). As before, a latitudinal gradient is apparent but the geographical differences are much influenced by the high prevalence in Hobart, Tasmania. Elsewhere, the frequency of multiple sclerosis appears lower than is apparent from contemporary studies in the places of origin within the United Kingdom and Ireland.

In New Zealand, the prevalence of multiple sclerosis was estimated at 69/10^5 in Wellington (south of the North Island) in 1984 (D.H. Miller *et al* 1986a). Comparable figures were reported for the South Island (69/10^5 in Otago and Southland; Skegg *et al* 1987) with much lower rates in northern parts of the North Island (e.g. 24/10^5; 95% CI 18–30 in Waikato). These prevalence studies were consistent with an earlier report of nationwide hospital admission and mortality statistics: both measures suggested that the disease was more common in the South Island and the southern North Island when compared with the northern half of the North Island (Hornabrook 1971). Recently, however, prevalence has been estimated at 50/10^5 (95% CI 40–62) on 15th January 2001 for a northerly part of the North Island (Bay of Plenty: Chancellor *et al* 2003). Fawcett and Skegg (1988) reviewed mortality rates for first admission to hospital in New Zealand excluding individuals with partial or full Maori ancestry. Incidence showed a south–north gradient, decreasing from 6.4/10^5/year in Otago, in the south of the South Island, to 2.7/10^5 in Auckland, which is in the north of the North Island. Age-adjusted mortality varied in parallel from 1.2 to 0.7/10^5. Admissions and deaths were rare in Maoris (20 and 2 cases, respectively). These observed frequencies represented 1.2% of admissions compared with 8.8% expected from the size of the Maori population.

Surveys reporting the frequency of multiple sclerosis in Australia and New Zealand were collated by D.H. Miller *et al* (1990a). The numerators for both countries were compared with an age-adjusted denominator excluding aboriginal peoples only in New Zealand – potentially an important confounder since 16% of the North Island population is of Maori origin. Evidence was presented for a sevenfold difference in frequency between Queensland and Otago. Although the quoted figures were age corrected, results were not adjusted to account for the use of different methods of case classification (usually Allison and Millar or McDonald and Halliday). In New Zealand, the main step in morbidity seems to occur across the North Island. By comparison, Tasmania (Australia) has a much higher prevalence than Waikato even though both are of comparable southerly latitude. Our impression is that the whole Australasian region falls into two clusters: Hobart (Tasmania), Wellington and Otago (South Island) with rates of >75/10^5 and Queensland, Newcastle (New South Wales), Adelaide (South Australia), Perth (Western Australia) and Waikato (North Island) with rates of <40/10^5. Furthermore, multiple sclerosis remains rare in the small community of Aborigines living in mainland Australia and in the Maoris of New Zealand.

Several interpretations of these patterns have been offered. Using the indirect methods adopted by Skegg *et al* (1987) and Swingler and Compston (1986), D.H. Miller *et al* (1990a) argued that the latitudinal gradient is not explained by genetic clines. To us, the methods used do not exclude significant heterogeneity in the distribution of white populations in Australia or New Zealand (Compston 1990b). Sorting ancestry on the number of Mc/Mac prefixes in the telephone directory (as used by Skegg *et al* 1987) does not differentiate Nordic from Celtic peoples, although it is recognized that the predominant settlement of the southern half of the South Island of New Zealand – where multiple sclerosis is common – was Scottish. A proportion of the population from Waikato who declared themselves white nevertheless had up to 50% Maori ethnicity. (In recent times, claiming Maori ancestry has carried social and financial benefits.) More speculative is the suggestion that immigrant groups head for and settle in places having climatic similarities with their homeland, thus tending to maintain localized genetic clines until equilibrium is established. That said, it is worth pointing out that the highest rates for multiple sclerosis seen in Australia are still only half those reported from parts of northern Europe having the same ethnic constitution. This suggests that relative protection is afforded by the environment of the Australian continent for people of European origin.

MULTIPLE SCLEROSIS IN CONTINENTAL EUROPE (Figures 2.15–2.20)

Working versions of geographical differences in the frequency of multiple sclerosis have been subjected to recent revision more in Europe than most other parts of the world. The trend has been for gradual erosion of latitudinal gradients as countries not

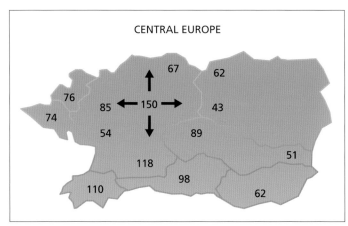

Figure 2.15 Prevalence distribution of multiple sclerosis in central Europe (Belgium, the Netherlands, Switzerland, Austria, Germany, Hungary, Slovakia, the Czech Republic, Poland). Most recent figures are given for prevalence/10^5 population; a 'best guess' is given where local variations exist in the published literature.

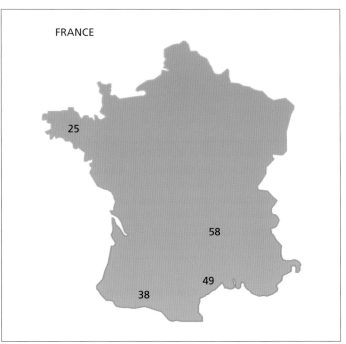

Figure 2.16 Prevalence distribution of multiple sclerosis in France. Most recent figures are given for prevalence/10^5 population; a 'best guess' is given where local variations exist in the published literature.

previously subjected to detailed epidemiological scrutiny, but lying within or adjacent to the high and medium prevalence zones of Kurtzke's 1975 analysis, were studied in detail.

In southern Lower Saxony, Germany, mean annual incidence increased from $2.6/10^5$ to $4.6/10^5$ (S. Poser *et al* 1989b), and prevalence increased from 51 to $118/10^5$, between 1969 and 1989, for all the usual reasons (Poser and Kurtzke 1991). Elsewhere, prevalence ranges somewhat erratically both with respect to latitude (between 49° and 54°N) and time. In 1982, the rate was $67/10^5$ for Rostock (Meyer-Rienecker and Buddenhagen 1988) and $54/10^5$ in Darmstadt (Prange *et al* 1986). In the mid-1980s, it was $62/10^5$ in Stralsund and the Isle of Rugen (Meyer-Rienecker 1994). By the early 1990s, rates of $98/10^5$ were reported from Bochum (Haupts *et al* 1994). In 1992, prevalence was $85/10^5$ and $108/10^5$ (excluding patients with possible multiple sclerosis) in southern Hesse and southern Lower Saxony, respectively (Lauer and Firnhaber 1994, S. Poser 1994). Extrapolation to a large region, based on sampling a proportion of the population at risk, has been used to derive a more contemporary prevalence of multiple sclerosis in Germany of $150/10^5$ (Hein and Hopfenmuller 2000).

In western Poland, prevalence fluctuated between 51 and $43/10^5$ between 1965 and 1981 (Wender *et al* 1985) but the most recent estimate is $62/10^5$ for Szczecin (Potemkowski *et al* 1994). The fall in prevalence between 1965 and 1981 is probably explained by a change in the population structure due to a higher birth rate, artificially expanding that proportion of the population at risk but below the usual age of onset for multiple sclerosis (Cendrowski *et al* 1969, Wender *et al* 1985). Other contemporary surveys include the estimate of prevalence for native Estonians, Russians and other nationalities of 55, 29 and $42/10^5$, respectively, in southern Estonia (Gross *et al* 1993). In

the Czech Republic, prevalence was 51 and $89/10^5$ in east and northwest Bohemia, respectively (Jedlicka *et al* 1994). In Hungary, rates were initially reported as ranging from 32 to $79/10^5$ (Guseo *et al* 1994; Palffy *et al* 1994). However, in Szeged, Hungary, at 31st December 1996 incidence was $7/10^5$/year and prevalence $65/10^5$ (Bencsik *et al* 1998), and prevalence in Csongrad County, Hungary, reported as $62/10^5$ (Bencsik *et al* 2001). The issue of whether Gypsies are protected from developing multiple sclerosis remains important in debating the relative contributions of race and environment in determining risk, since comparisons can be made with the indigenous peoples of central Europe. Palffy *et al* (1994) reported a prevalence of $5/10^5$ amongst a Gypsy population of 22 000 including two autopsy-proven cases. This compared with a frequency of $32/10^5$ in Hungarians. Previously, Palffy (1982) had shown population differences in gene frequency for markers of susceptibility to multiple sclerosis, offering an explanation for the apparent resistance of Gypsies to multiple sclerosis. However, even these carefully conducted studies have examined the frequency of multiple sclerosis in only a small proportion of the Gypsy population of central Europe. On 31st March 1998, the prevalence of multiple sclerosis in two regions of Bulgaria was 45 and $44/10^5$ compared with rates of 19 and $18/10^5$ in Gypsies from the same locations (Milanov *et al* 1999).

In Switzerland, the most recent prevalence was $110/10^5$ for the Canton of Berne (Beer and Kesselring 1994). Using the capture–recapture method and comparing cases identified from 30 multiple sclerosis clinics over a 4-week period and records of the Multiple Sclerosis Society, Baumhackl *et al* (2002) calculated that there were around 7900 affected individuals in Austria providing a nationwide prevalence of $99/10^5$. Whilst this does not reveal regional patterns throughout Austria, an earlier

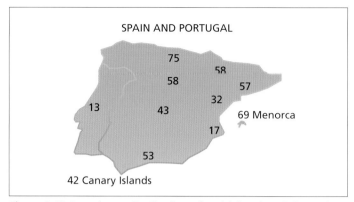

Figure 2.17 Prevalence distribution of multiple sclerosis in Spain and Portugal. Most recent figures are given for prevalence/10^5 population; a 'best guess' is given where local variations exist in the published literature.

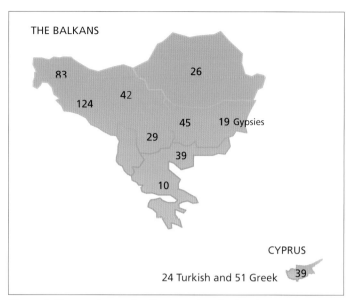

Figure 2.18 Prevalence distribution of multiple sclerosis in Greece and the Balkans (Croatia, Romania, Bulgaria). Most recent figures are given for prevalence/10^5 population; a 'best guess' is given where local variations exist in the published literature.

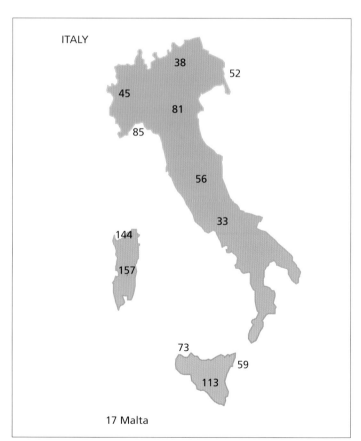

Figure 2.19 Prevalence distribution of multiple sclerosis in Italy. Most recent figures are given for prevalence/10^5 population; a 'best guess' is given where local variations exist in the published literature.

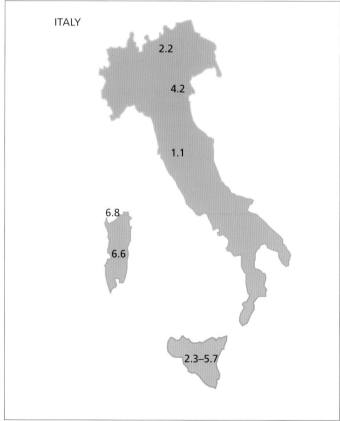

Figure 2.20 Incidence distribution of multiple sclerosis in Italy. Most recent figures are given for incidence/year/10^5 population; a 'best guess' is given where local variations exist in the published literature.

survey had reported a more or less similar rate for Lower Austria (Baumhackl 1995). In the Netherlands, incidence increased from 2 to $5.9/10^5$/year between 1982 and 1992, over which period prevalence rose from $54/10^5$ to $76/10^5$ (Minderhoud and Zwanniken 1994; Prange *et al* 1986). In Flanders, the most recent estimate for prevalence was $74/10^5$ (95% CI 59–89; van Ooteghem *et al* 1994). In general, figures for incidence in other parts of Europe show the same temporal trends, ranging from 0.8 to $3.9/10^5$/year for the regions discussed above and correlating, as expected, with differences in prevalence.

France appeared for some time to be a region having prevalences for multiple sclerosis that were genuinely lower than expected from its geographical location within Europe, if the gradient is latitudinal and not shaped by social and genetic history. Rates for Chalon-sur-Saône (southeast), Avignon (south) and Pyrénées-Atlantiques (southwest) were 58 (95% CI 46–71), 49 (95% CI 39–60) and $38/10^5$ (95% CI 33–44) in the mid-1980s, respectively (Confavreux *et al* 1987; M-P. Roth *et al* 1994a). These figures compare with $25/10^5$ for Brittany in 1978 (Gallou *et al* 1983). But the most recent epidemiological study provides rates for incidence that suggest comparability with other parts of continental Europe. Based on 21 identified cases, Moreau *et al* (2000) showed that the incidence in Dijon, Burgundy, was $4.3/10^5$/year (2.5F:M) between 1993 and 1997.

Morbidity statistics for Spain first reported prevalence rates of $<10/10^5$ (Oliveras De Lariva *et al* 1968). Subsequently, estimates for incidence were $3.7/10^5$/year (95% CI 1.4–6) in Gijon (Uria *et al* 1998), approximately $2.2/10^5$/year in Teruel (Modrego Paedo *et al* 1997), and $3.0/10^5$/year (95% CI 1.8–4.2) in Alcoi (Matias-Guiu *et al* 1994). Corresponding rates for prevalence increased from much lower estimates made in the 1960s to $23/10^5$ (95% CI 25–74) for Gijon (northern Spain), later updated to $65/10^5$ (95% CI 38–92; Uria *et al* 1997); $57/10^5$ (95% CI 40–75) in Barcelona (Catalonia, western Spain); $58/10^5$ in Osana (which lies to the north of Barcelona; Bufill *et al* 1995); $32/10^5$ (95% CI 23–41) in Teruel to the southwest of Barcelona (Modrego Pardo *et al* 1997); $53/10^5$ (95% CI 32–83) in Malaga (southern Spain; O. Fernandez and Bufill 1994; O. Fernandez *et al* 1994); and $17/10^5$ in Alcoi (eastern Spain; Matias-Guiu *et al* 1990; 1994). The most recent wave of surveys includes prevalence for northern Spain (Valladolid) at $58/10^5$ (95% CI 44–76; Tola *et al* 1999). In Bajo Aragon, prevalence rose between 1994 and 2002 from $35/10^5$ (95% CI 20–50) to $75/10^5$ (95% CI 52–97) with a corresponding increase in incidence, between 1984–1993 and 1994–2003, of $3/10^5$/year (95% CI 1.6–4.5) to $4.6/10^5$/year (95% CI 2.8–6.5) representing an increased standardized incidence ratio of 1.4 (95% CI 0.95–2.17; Modrego and Pina 2003). In Calatayud, northern Spain, annual incidence was $2.6/10^5$/year between 1980 and 1989, and prevalence also $58/10^5$ (95% CI 39–78) on 1st April 1995 (Pina *et al* 1998). Incidence in Mostoles, central Spain, was $3.8/10^5$/year (95% CI 2.7–5.3) between 1992 and 1997, and prevalence $43/10^5$ (95% CI 35–54; Benito-Leon *et al* 1998) on 1st February 1998. Incidence was $3.4/10^5$/year (95% CI 2.2–5.3) in the Balearic island of Menorca and prevalence $69/10^5$ (95% CI 50–92) in 1996 (Casquero *et al* 2001).

In the Canary Island province of Las Palmas, prevalence was $6/10^5$ (95% CI 1–22) in the early 1980s (Sosa Enriquez *et al* 1983). This was adjusted to $15/10^5$ (95% CI 8–25) on the neighbouring island of Lanzarote in 1987 (Garcia *et al* 1989). By 15th December 1998, incidence was $2.25/10^5$/year and prevalence had increased in Las Palmas to $42/10^5$ (Hernandez 2002), eliminating the earlier apparent fivefold difference in frequency between the Canary Islands and southern parts of the Iberian Peninsula. The most recent survey (to 31st December 2001) provides estimates of $74/10^5$ (95% CI 56–95) using the criteria of McDonald *et al* (2001), with rates of $62/10^5$ (95% CI 47–79) and $71/10^5$ (95% CI 55–89) adjusted to the standardized world and European populations, respectively (Aladro *et al* 2005). A review of mortality trends in Spain between 1951 and 1997 shows a reduction from 3.1 to $0.6/10^5$/year before and after 1967, respectively, attributable in part to improved life expectancy but also to changes in codification practice (Llorca *et al* 2005).

In considering other regions of Spanish ancestry, Alvarez *et al* (1992) identified 68 cases of multiple sclerosis in Chile and noted that this constituted the largest cohort yet surveyed but did not calculate prevalence. A rate of $4.3/10^5$ (2F:M) was estimated by Callegaro *et al* (1992) for São Paolo in Brazil in 1990. This was updated for 1st July 1997 to $15/10^5$ (Callegaro *et al* 2001). The population is typically Caucasoid and mainly of Portuguese origin but with recent additions of Spaniards, Italians, central Europeans and Japanese.

Whilst momentum is gathering for Iberian epidemiological studies, Greece and the Balkan states have yet to show the same epidemiological commitment. This may explain why their estimates have until recently remained lower. Where available, incidence rates largely correlate with prevalences, being higher in Croatia ($5.9/10^5$/year; 95% CI 4.3–7.8; Sepcic *et al* 1989) and Slovenia ($2.9/10^5$/year; Koncan-Vracko 1994) than in Greece ($1.8/10^5$/year; 95% CI 1.6–1.9; Milonas 1994). Prevalence in Belgrade (Serbia) was $42/10^5$ on 31st December 1996 (1.9F:M; Pekmezovic *et al* 2001). Survival in the same sample has been estimated at 38 years with a 73% probability of 25-year survival for the prevalent population (Pekmezovic *et al* 2002). Prevalence was $83/10^5$ in Slovenia (Koncan-Vracko 1994), $26/10^5$ in Romania (Petrescu 1994), $30/10^5$ (95% CI 27–33) in Bulgaria (Georgiev and Milanov 1994), $124/10^5$ (95% CI 89–169) in Gorski Kotar, Croatia (Sepcic *et al* 1989), and $29/10^5$ (95% CI 27–32) in Macedonia and Thrace, Greece in 1984 (Milonas 1994). Serial update of the prevalence for Evros in northeastern Greece showed increases from $10/10^5$ in 1984, to $30/10^5$ in 1990, and $39/10^5$ on 31st December 1999 (Piperidou *et al* 2003). Because incidence increased between 1974–1978 and 1994–1999 from 0.66 to $2.36/10^5$/year, Piperidou *et al* (2003) conclude that the increase in frequency reflects a change in aetiological conditions over and above the impact of methodological factors.

Multiple sclerosis has been surveyed in three Greek-speaking regions of Cyprus. The coastal areas under scrutiny included more refugees from northern Cyprus (Turkish speaking) than the mountain villages. Overall, the prevalence was $39/10^5$. Only one case of multiple sclerosis was observed in >16 500 refugees from the northern part of the island living in study areas in the south. Trends favouring a higher prevalence in Paphos than Famagusta, or the mountains of Troodos and Kyperounda, were not significant. A tendency towards consanguinity may have determined the relatively high incidence of multiplex families, especially in one village (L.T. Middleton and Dean 1991). In a subsequent assessment, prevalence was higher in the Greek community ($51/10^5$) and among Turkish Cypriots born in Cyprus ($56/10^5$) than in those migrating from mainland Turkey ($24/10^5$; Dean *et al* 1997). These differences were especially marked in men.

In southern continental Europe, Italy stands out as a region that has been studied in great epidemiological detail and, perhaps, consequently has noticeably higher rates than some of its neighbours. Between 1962 and 1982, approximately 30 epidemiological studies were reported from peninsular Italy and prevalence varied from 7 to $27/10^5$. Many of these surveys were based on denominators $>300\,000$ and were carried out in both northern and southern Italy; but standardization to a single population was not usually attempted and demographic differences make the studies difficult to compare. The conclusion, expressed in earlier editions of this book, that Italians have a low risk of multiple sclerosis compared with other Europeans, was first questioned by the findings of Dean *et al* (1976), who showed equivalent admission rates to hospital in London for Italian and English patients. This seemed correct when Dean *et al* (1979) reported that, based on findings from Enna (Sicily), morbidity statistics for Italy might generally have been underestimated. Their work was followed by studies from many other parts of Italy that also upwardly adjusted the overall rates and systematically eroded the latitudinal gradient.

There are several reasons why the study of multiple sclerosis in Sardinians may be of special importance. Disease frequency has been studied repeatedly and determinedly so that contemporary figures for morbidity statistics are fully informative. Sardinia is one of only a few regions where a class II HLA antigen association exists that is specifically different from DR(15)2. The island has a colourful history (see Chapter 5), which could offer explanations for those aspects of its genetic epidemiology that are of general importance for understanding multiple sclerosis.

In Alghero, northern Sardinia, incidence was $4.1/10^5$/year for 1971–1980, with a prevalence of $59/10^5$ (Rosati *et al* 1987). The incidence for native-born Sardinians during 1965–1985 in Sassari (northern Sardinia) was $3.4/10^5$/year (95% CI 2.7–4.2), and serial estimations indicate that this changed from about 1.3–$2.0/10^5$/year before 1977 to around $5/10^5$/year thereafter, with prevalence stabilizing at $69/10^5$ (95% CI 55–86). Surprisingly, no familial cases were identified at that time. Working to the new prevalence day of 1st December 1991, Rosati (1994) estimated prevalence at $103/10^5$ (95% CI 92–115) in Sassari with no difference between rural and urban rates (97 and $108/10^5$, respectively). The frequency of familial multiple sclerosis was now 13%. Incidence was $3.7/10^5$/year (95% CI 3.3–4.1) and quinquennial rates had steadily increased from 1.3–$2.0/10^5$/year around 1962 to $5/10^5$/year, with the highest rate seen in the most recent 5-year period. The most recent updates for Sassari, northern Sardinia, show a steady rise in quinquennial rates for incidence from 2.0 to $6.8/10^5$/year between 1968–1972 and 1992–1997, with prevalence reaching $144/10^5$ (onset adjusted, $150/10^5$) on 31st December 1997 (Pugliatti *et al* 2001a). The rate of increase in prevalence has been steeper in Sassari than Ferrara, northern Italy, commensurate with differential increases in incidence, leading Pugliatti *et al* (2001a) to conclude that the Sardinian focus represents a real increase in disease frequency. Cluster analysis within this well-surveyed region, working to the same prevalence day,

identified a hot spot for multiple sclerosis in individuals resident in southwestern communes between the ages of 5 and 15 years, with evidence for a west–east gradient (Pugliatti *et al* 2001b). This region has a distinct cultural history, being predominantly Logudorese by comparison with Catalan areas showing lower rates.

In Barbagia, central Sardinia, incidence for the years 1961–1980 was $2.9/10^5$/year (adjusted to 3.2 when standardized to the Italian population) based on a numerator of 31 cases. Prevalence in 1975 was $41/10^5$ (95% CI 25–62; standardized prevalence ratio 48.5), and this had risen to $65/10^5$ (CI 44–93; $78/10^5$ standardized to the Italian population) by 1981 (Granieri and Rosati 1982). Serial studies in Macomer suggest that multiple sclerosis was not diagnosed prior to 1952. Between 1952 and 1981, the overall incidence was $6.3/10^5$/year (95% CI 3.4–10.8), with a change from $2.8/10^5$/year for the period 1952–1956 to 10.1, 7, 4.2, 3.9 and $1.8/10^5$/year in sequential quinquennia up to 1981. Prevalence was $62/10^5$ (95% CI 20–143) in 1961, $73/10^5$ (95% CI 30–151) in 1971 and $72/10^5$ (95% CI 31–141) in 1981. The province of Nuoro, central Sardinia, had incidence rates for multiple sclerosis of $4.3/10^5$/year across the period 1955–1995, increasing from 1.95 to $6.6/10^5$/year in the quinquennium 1985–1989 but stabilizing thereafter. Prevalence increased from $103/10^5$ in 1985 to 144 and $157/10^5$ in 1993 and 31st December 1994, respectively (Cassetta *et al* 1998; Granieri *et al* 2000). In a detailed epidemiological survey from the most archaic parts of central Sardinia, the overall estimate for prevalence was $157/10^5$ with variations from 143 to $262/10^5$, the highest regions having an excess of familial cases (Montomoli *et al* 2002a).

In summary, Sardinia had an incidence of around $3.0/10^5$/year in the east, north, central and northwest regions in the 1980s (Granieri *et al* 1983; Rosati 1989; 1994; Rosati *et al* 1986; 1987; 1988) but estimates have since increased to $6.6/10^5$/year in some regions. Although these results have been interpreted as showing that multiple sclerosis was first introduced into the island immediately following the Second World War, with the rise of industrialization and population mixing, the facts are no less consistent with the rival theory that these represent epidemics of recognition rather than the impact of aetiological factors altering the risk of multiple sclerosis. Nevertheless, these figures show that, throughout Sardinia, the main rise in incidence occurred in the 1970s. Cases have all been restricted to those with Sardinian names whose grandparents were born on the island, although some prevalent cases were born elsewhere.

This substantial increase in frequency of multiple sclerosis is not exclusive to Sardinia. In the 1980s, prevalences in the republic of San Marino (Morganti *et al* 1984), the central Sicilian cities of Enna ($53/10^5$) and Caltanissetta ($51/10^5$; Savettieri *et al* 1986), and other parts of Sicily (Monreale $43/10^5$ and Agrigento $32/10^5$; Dean *et al* 1979, 1981b, Savettieri *et al* 1981) were strikingly higher than in neighbouring Malta ($4/10^5$; Vassallo *et al* 1978). As for other parts of the world subjected to serial surveys, more recent estimates show a substantial rise from these figures derived in the mid-1980s. Incidence was $3.3/10^5$/year (95% CI 1.5–6.2) for Monreale over the period 1981–1991 and prevalence was $73/10^5$ (95% CI 44–113) on 31st December 1991 (Savettieri *et al* 1998). Incidence increased to $5.7/10^5$/year and prevalence reached $120/10^5$ by 1995 in Enna, Sicily (Grimaldi *et al* 2001). In the coastal city of Bagheria, the high Sicilian incidence was again demonstrated with an increase from 3.5 to $5.3/10^5$/year between 1985 and 1994 (Salemi *et al* 2000a). Incidence during 1974–1995 in Catania, Sicily, was $2.3/10^5$/year (5% CI 2.0–2.6) with increases from 1.3 to $3.9/10^5$/year across this period, and prevalence on 1st January 1995 of $59/10^5$ (1.2F:M; Nicoletti *et al* 2001). But significantly, the differential between Sicily and Malta persists. An update for Malta on 1st January 1999, based on 63 living cases, showed that annual incidence was $0.7/10^5$/year and prevalence $17/10^5$ ($13/10^5$ for clinically definite disease; 1.4F:M). By contrast, prevalence in the small community of immigrants was $166/10^5$ (Dean *et al* 2002). The case for differences in disease susceptibility based on genetic origins – Maltese speak a Semitic language and have mainly north African Arabic ancestry following the invasion by Habasa in 869/870 AD, whereas Monreale and Enna have strong Norman (northern European) origins – seems strong. A recent genetic analysis of multiple sclerosis in Malta supports this interpretation (see Chapter 3).

An increase in incidence to $2.2/10^5$/year (95% CI 1.8–2.6) was also reported for Ferrara in northern Italy (Granieri and Tola 1994; Granieri *et al* 1985). Prevalence was $27/10^5$ in 1978 (Rosati *et al* 1981). Later, this was corrected to $37/10^5$ and updated in 1981 to $46/10^5$ (95% CI 40–53) based on the identification of 128 cases (Granieri *et al* 1985). The most recent figures are $2.3/10^5$/year (95% CI 2.0–2.6) and 69 (95% CI 61–79) for incidence and prevalence, respectively (Granieri *et al* 1996). Incidence and prevalence have been studied serially in Padova (northeast Italy) over 30 years. In 1970, the rates were $0.9/10^5$/year and $16/10^5$, respectively. Incidence increased from 2.2 to 3.9 to $4.2/10^5$/year over the periods 1980–1989, 1990–1994 and 1994–1999, respectively. Prevalence altered from 18 to 46 to $81/10^5$ (95% CI 70–91) in 1980, 1990 and 1999, respectively (Ranzato *et al* 2003). Here, the authors emphasize the rise in incidence during the 1980s with subsequent stabilization as an indicator that these changes in morbidity reflect the impact of improved diagnostic techniques and reduced latency from onset to diagnosis rather than a real increase in disease frequency. At $2.1/10^5$/year and $33/10^5$ the annual incidence and prevalence of multiple sclerosis in one culturally and genetically isolated Alpine region of northern Italy (Valle d'Aosta) were higher than previously reported but comparable to contemporary studies from neighbouring parts of Italy, with no obvious temporal trends between 1971 and 1985 (Sironi *et al* 1991). Solaro *et al* (2005) surveyed a population of 913 218 people living in the province of Genoa, northwest Italy, to identify 857 affected individuals, providing a rate for prevalence of $85/10^5$ adjusted to Italian standard population; crude (unadjusted) rates were $67/10^5$ (95% CI 60–76) in men and $118/10^5$ (95% CI 108–128) in women. L'Aquila district of central Italy had a prevalence of $56/10^5$ (95% CI 45–62) on 31st December 1996 standardized to the European population (1.9F:M; Totaro *et al* 2000). Standardized mortality rates for Italy between 1974 and 1993 were 4.1 and $5.0/10^5$ for males and females, respectively, with a north–south gradient, excluding Sardinia. Across this period, mortality had reduced in the north but increased in the south, presumably reflecting health care trends superimposed on increased ascertainment and, perhaps, incidence (Tassinari *et al* 2001).

Commenting on the overall picture of the epidemiology of multiple sclerosis in Italy, Rosati (1994) traced the history of Italian epidemiology in multiple sclerosis and lamented the difficulties faced by epidemiologists working within the health care system of the early postwar years – a situation that altered for the better from 1975. Publications on the epidemiology of multiple sclerosis dating from 1980 were considered under the headings of mainland and insular surveys. Prevalences, then ranging from 32 to $69/10^5$, had all increased over time, no longer showing latitudinal gradients or differences between continental Italy and Sicily. By contrast, the figures for Sardinia varied between 59 and $103/10^5$. A centralized survey of incidence (Comi *et al* 1989) based on data for 1971–1980 confirmed this distribution and showed rates, in the 1980s, of 1.1 and $1.9/10^5$/year for the mainland, or Sicily, compared with $4.2/10^5$/year in Sardinia. Others who have scrutinized the frequency of multiple sclerosis in Italy over time (Granieri *et al* 1993) also consider that, with the exception of Sardinia, the apparent gradient in frequency is mainly an artefact arising from differences in case ascertainment between the better and less developed parts of the country. The marked differences in population structure and failure to quote age-corrected figures have also contributed to the creation of a spurious gradient. Studies based on small denominators, so as to maximize case ascertainment, have since shown higher rates than previously claimed, and without regional variations.

With a certain amount of catching up still to occur, we cannot reach a final conclusion concerning the distribution of multiple sclerosis in southern Europe. The trends suggest that, with increased vigilance, estimates for prevalence will continue to rise, but not to the levels seen in northern Europeans. However, we anticipate that some island populations will retain disproportionately high (e.g. Sardinians) and low (e.g. Maltese) figures. Our position is that this reflects differences in genetic susceptibility. Whilst the facts seem clear, others may prefer alternative interpretations and explanations.

MULTIPLE SCLEROSIS IN THE MIDDLE EAST (Figure 2.21)

There are many fewer epidemiological studies from outside Europe, Australia and North America. In serveral of these locations, our figures are taken from Kurtzke (1993), who himself made the calculations using assumptions about factors such as the place of origin and domicile of the index cases. Few of the figures are contemporary and none can be compared with other population-based surveys. Taken together, they give the impression of a low disease frequency in these places. Multiple sclerosis has been studied in Jordan ($7/10^5$ based on 32 cases in Amman; Kurdi *et al* 1977) and Saudi Arabia ($8/10^5$ by comparison between the case ratios for multiple sclerosis and amyotrophic lateral sclerosis; Yaquib and Daif 1988). Using the Schumacher criteria, Hamdi (1975) derived a figure of $3.4/10^5$ for Iraq by estimating the relative frequency of multiple sclerosis (11 cases) compared with motor neuron disease in a hospital-based sample for the years 1967–1969, relating this to a global figure for prevalence of the latter condition. However, this figure represented a threefold increase from an earlier estimate using similar methods (Shaby 1958). The majority of the cases were from northern Iraq where the population is predominantly Kurdish (Indo-European) by comparison with the middle and

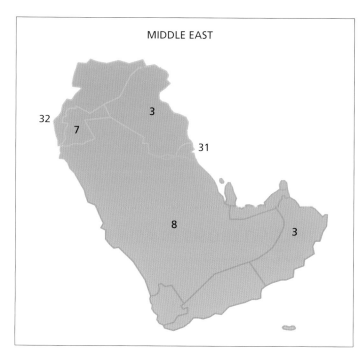

Figure 2.21 Prevalence distribution of multiple sclerosis in the Middle East (Israel, Saudi Arabia, Kuwait, Iraq, Jordan and Oman). Most recent figures are given for prevalence/10^5 population; a 'best guess' is given where local variations exist in the published literature.

southern parts, inhabited more or less entirely by Arabs. It remains uncertain whether this pattern reflects genetic background or administrative arrangements for referral of cases to Baghdad in the 1960s.

By contrast, multiple sclerosis has been carefully surveyed in Kuwait. In the initial survey, prevalence was estimated at $8/10^5$ (Al-Din 1986). In 1988, the previously suspected difference in prevalence between Kuwaitis and Palestinians living in Kuwait was confirmed. Evidence was provided to support the hypothesis that the higher rate in peoples originating from Palestine is genetically determined, resulting from admixture of Caucasian genes as part of that region's turbulent social history. Prevalence was $10/10^5$; 186 of the 201 prevalent cases were Arabs and of these 72 were Palestinians (prevalence $24/10^5$) and 51 Kuwaitis (prevalence $9/10^5$; Al-Din et al 1990). By 2000, incidence had risen to $2.6/10^5$/year from $1.1/10^5$/year in 1993, the main increase being seen in women, with a change in prevalence from 7 to $15/10^5$; by comparison with earlier assessments, prevalence was higher in Kuwaitis ($31/10^5$) than in non-Kuwaitis ($6/10^5$: Alshubaili et al 2005).

Studies of the prevalence of multiple sclerosis in Israel have been particularly influential in developing ideas on the aetiology of multiple sclerosis (Alter et al 1962; 1978; Leibowitz et al 1970). Interpretation is made more complicated by the admixture in recent decades of peoples whose geographical origins were not necessarily in the Middle East. The prevalence for native born Israelis, age-adjusted to the 1960 United States population, was $13/10^5$ in 1965. Kahana et al (1994; see below for studies of migration) updated these figures to 1983. The incidence of multiple sclerosis was $1.4/10^5$/year and prevalence $32/10^5$ for all Israelis. Higher rates were reported for Jerusalem ($2.4/10^5$/year and $61/10^5$, respectively). Karni et al (2003) have

compared the frequency of multiple sclerosis in Jewish and Arab populations of greater Jerusalem. As expected, prevalence had increased in Israelis by December 1995 to $64/10^5$ in European/American Jews, and $52/10^5$ in African/Asian Jews, compared with earlier estimates. The rates for incidence and prevalence in Arabs were again lower ($0.7/10^5$/year and $19/10^5$, respectively) but these observations need to be taken in the context of differential rates amongst Israelis depending on place of birth and African/Asian or European/American Jewish ancestry (see below). Most recently, Tharakan et al (2005) collected cases of multiple sclerosis in Oman, which lies in the eastern Arabian peninsula at 10–30°N and has an estimated population of 1.5 million. Health care is sophisticated and the 34 ethnic Omanis in whom the diagnosis of multiple sclerosis was made between 1990 and 2000 represent a moderately complete sample allowing a minimum estimate of period prevalence at $3/10^5$.

MULTIPLE SCLEROSIS IN AFRICA (Figure 2.22)

The frequency of multiple sclerosis in the African continent has, until recently, been studied in little detail, since it was apparent that this is an uncommon disorder in native peoples from these regions. The continent is populated by African blacks throughout – but especially in the west, central and southern parts – with a significant admixture of Arab ancestry in the north and east, where Asian people are also settled, and white immigrants both to the offshore islands and mainland. It is because of the rarity of the disease amongst African blacks compared with the higher rates seen in immigrants that the study of multiple sclerosis on the African continent, and in African blacks elsewhere, has proved so influential. Despite the overall paucity

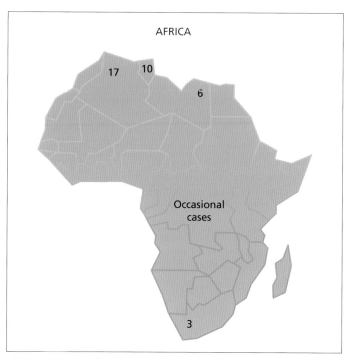

Figure 2.22 Prevalence distribution of multiple sclerosis in Africa. Most recent figures are given for prevalence/10^5 population; a 'best guess' is given where local variations exist in the published literature. For interpretation of South Africa see text and Figure 2.5.

of the disease, there are some reports suggesting a higher than expected frequency of multiple sclerosis in coastal regions of the African continent, in addition to some offshore islands, where social history has perhaps encouraged more genetic admixture than in continental Africa.

Multiple sclerosis has an appreciable prevalence in Libya ($6/10^5$ based on 21 patients in Benghazi, age-adjusted to the population of the former West Germany; Radhakrishnan *et al* 1985) and Tunis ($10/10^5$ based on 73 definite or probable cases; Ben Hamida 1977). Dean (1967) provided morbidity statistics for multiple sclerosis in white South African-born individuals and immigrants to South Africa but did not identify any affected African blacks. Multiple sclerosis was subsequently reported both in mixed race South Africans (Ames and Louw 1977) and in blacks (Bhigjee 1987). In a subsequent survey from Cape Town, the prevalence of multiple sclerosis was $3/10^5$ in pigmented people (B. Kies 1989; Brian Kies, personal communication). Case reports were published, and anecdotes went into circulation, of multiple sclerosis occurring *inter alia* in individuals from Zimbabwe, Kenya, Uganda, Cameroon, Ethiopia and Senegal (Adam 1989; Foster and Harries 1970; Goldstein 1946; Haimanot 1985; Kanyerezi *et al* 1980; Lisk 1991; Mbonda *et al* 1990). In some of these cases the distinction from acute disseminated encephalomyelitis and the exclusion of retroviral infection was assumed rather than proven, and there are uncertainties relating to ethnicity. But with increased world travel, neurologists routinely exposed to cases of multiple sclerosis have encountered patients in Africa meeting diagnostic criteria for the disease. It has been our own experience, mainly based on cases seen at Baragwanath Chris Hani Hospital, Johannesburg-Soweto (through the kindness of Dr David Saffer) that the clinical features are distinct, matching the relapsing Devic's disease phenotype that is rare in Caucasians (see Chapter 5).

It is against this background that Dean *et al* (1994) collated all reports of multiple sclerosis occurring in black South Africans and Zimbabweans. Of the 12 patients, six had disproportionate involvement of the visual system and the frequency of a progressive course from onset was higher than expected in a Western series of cases. A number were lost to follow-up and histological confirmation was not obtained in those who died. Several had evidence for previous, but now inactive, treponemal infection. Nevertheless, the laboratory abnormalities usually associated with multiple sclerosis were present and many had signs rarely having other explanations in Caucasians with neurological disease. Some, especially the cases from Zimbabwe, had a typical history of relapsing neurological symptoms with signs indicating multifocal involvement in episodes. Although not based on an epidemiological study, Kioy (2001) described nine individuals with clinically definite multiple sclerosis amongst 2831 referrals to a private electrodiagnostic clinic (3.5F:M). Two were Asian and seven African Bantus, leading the author to conclude that multiple sclerosis is becoming more frequent in native Africans.

Multiple sclerosis is diagnosed in African Caribbeans (Cruikshank 1973; Cruikshank *et al* 1961). With no cases reported until the 1970s, C. Poser and Vernant (1993) described 11 cases in blacks from Martinique and Guadeloupe who had no evidence for infection by human T-cell leukaemia virus (HTLV)-1. More recently, Cabre *et al* (2001) identified clinically definite multiple sclerosis in 51 individuals of mixed French-African ancestry

living in Martinique, providing a prevalence of $14/10^5$ (95% CI 10–18). The clinical features were broadly equivalent to multiple sclerosis as seen in western Europe but with a lower frequency of oligoclonal bands and higher rate of the Devic phenotype (25%). Leaving those with mixed ancestry, it would be churlish to reject all these cases affecting Africans on the basis of their clinical details. The case for multiple sclerosis, defined by an appropriate clinical and laboratory phenotype, occasionally occurring in African blacks seems good. (We offer an analysis of the origins of multiple sclerosis that leans heavily on the epidemiology and phenotype seen in continental Africa, Asia and the Orient in Chapter 5.)

MULTIPLE SCLEROSIS IN ASIA AND THE FAR EAST (Figure 2.23)

There have been several surveys of multiple sclerosis in India and these show differences in risk depending on ethnicity for individuals living in the same geographical region. The prevalence of multiple sclerosis in Parsees from Bombay and Poona was $26/10^5$ (95% CI 13–40; age adjusted to $24/10^5$) and $58/10^5$ based on 14 and two prevalent cases, respectively, in 1988 (Wadia and Bhatia 1990). These rates are higher than those previously quoted for Indians in Bombay ($1/10^5$; Singhal and Wadia 1975) but comparable to the earlier estimation of prevalence in Parsees from a door to door survey carried out in Bombay (Bharacha *et al* 1988). Multiple sclerosis has also been

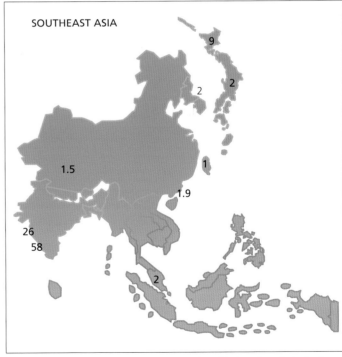

Figure 2.23 Prevalence distribution of multiple sclerosis in India and the Far East (Malaysia, Thailand, China and Japan). Most recent figures are given for prevalence/10^5 population; a 'best guess' is given where local variations exist in the published literature.

reported from southern India (Gourie-Devi and Nagaraja 1982). Reviewing the experience of several decades, Jain and Maheshwari (1985) comment on the greater frequency of multiple sclerosis in northern India, populated by Indo-Europeans, compared with the south, which has a higher density of Tamils and Dravidians. Multiple sclerosis in Chinese and Japanese people is evidently a rare disease with a markedly different phenotype from that seen in the Western world. However, this may be changing. As with the studies in Africans, an additional point of interest lies in the study of the disease amongst Orientals not living in China or Japan. But unlike Africans, who seem to show a changing frequency with relocation to other environments, the evidence suggests that Orientals are not placed at a higher risk of multiple sclerosis through exposure to a novel environment. Y.L. Yu *et al* (1989) studied multiple sclerosis amongst Chinese in Hong Kong and reported a prevalence of $0.9/10^5$ – with a similar clinical phenotype to other affected Orientals. Hung (1982) reported no discernible change in frequency of the disease in Taipei, northern Taiwan, during the 1970s. Prevalence rates for 1975 and 1980 were 0.8 and $0.9/10^5$ in a population of 1.9–2.2 million, respectively. In contrast to other parts of the world, there had been very little change when this region was again surveyed in 2004 ($1.9/10^5$: Tsai *et al* 2004). Hou and Zhang (1992) carried out a door to door survey in the Yunnan Province of mainland China using an 11% sample of the population (just under 0.5 million), identifying only one patient and providing a prevalence estimate of $1.4/10^5$ (95% CI 0–8, age-adjusted to the United States population).

In Japan, neuromyelitis optica was once the common clinical picture but the so-called Western phenotype has increasingly emerged as the expected disease appearance in affected individuals born after the 1960s. Prevalence for all clinical forms was first estimated on the basis of 65 cases identified in ten cities, ranging from latitudes 26 to 44°N, at between 0.9 and $4/10^5$ with a mean of $2.1/10^5$ (Kuroiwa *et al* 1983; see also C.M. Poser 1994). Itoh *et al* (2003) updated an earlier prevalence estimate for Asahikawa, northern Japan, from $2.5/10^5$ in 1975 to $10.2/10^5$ in 2002. As in other series, there had been a change over the 27 years from an optico-spinal to more typically Western phenotype with only 3% of the more recent prevalent population presenting with optic nerve involvement. Houzen *et al* (2003) reported a prevalence of $8.6/10^5$ (2.9F:M) on 31st March 2001 in an area of northern Japan having a stable population at risk and showing very little inward migration or expansion of the denominator, based on postal questionnaire of clinics serving the population. There was a low frequency (16%) of the Devic (optico-spinal) phenotype in the 31 reported cases. An early estimate for the prevalence of multiple sclerosis in Malaysia was around $2/10^5$ (C-T. Tan 1988). Histological confirmation of the diagnosis is claimed for cases from Thailand (Vejjajiva 1982).

Informal conversations suggest that these figures for disease frequency are underestimates. Many neurologists working in Africa, Asia, the Middle East and the Orient have priorities other than documenting numbers of patients with neurological diseases that are rare in their communities. Conferences focusing on the global distribution of multiple sclerosis periodically present an opportunity for bringing these numbers up to date. No such meeting has been held for several years and is overdue.

MULTIPLE SCLEROSIS IN MIGRANTS
(Figures 2.24–2.26)

We have already developed the argument that social and historical events that led people of European, African, Asian, Oriental and Aboriginal stock to mix, move or remain in isolated communities as genetic relics shaped the global distribution of multiple sclerosis. However, especially over the last two centuries, founder populations have been neither geographically nor socially stable and there have been many migrations, involving relatively large numbers of people, which appear also to have influenced the distribution of multiple sclerosis. Migration between high- and low-risk areas has occurred in both directions and involving individuals of all ages. This led to the formal comparison of disease frequency between racial groups living in the same geographical region and, conversely, cohorts of individuals with the same ethnic origins living in different parts of the world. Overall, migration studies emphasize multiple sclerosis as an exogenous disorder, acquired some years before clinical expression and probably in childhood, whereas studies of indigenous peoples provide more compelling evidence for genetic effects on disease frequency and distribution.

One of the earliest and most influential studies of migrants emerged from South Africa in the decades following the Second World War. Arriving by chance in Cape Town, Geoffrey Dean was struck by the markedly different frequencies of the disease in people of African origin and those moving to South Africa during the 20th century (see Chapter 1). Dean (1967) provided annual incidence, prevalence and mortality statistics for multiple sclerosis in white South African-born individuals and immigrants to South Africa. The age-corrected frequency of the disease was highest in immigrants from Europe, lowest in Afrikaaners and intermediate in South African English, both with respect to incidence and prevalence (Kurtzke *et al* 1970b). The absence of multiple sclerosis in African blacks was confirmed but a slightly higher rate was seen in the mixed race population, in whom African and Caucasian genes are shared. However, within the English-speaking white group, there was a marked difference in frequency of multiple sclerosis depending on age at arrival in South Africa. Those moving as adults to South Africa from the areas of northern Europe where multiple sclerosis is common took with them the high frequency of the country of origin, whereas those migrating ≤15 years showed the lower rates characteristic of native-born South Africans. For the 114 northern European immigrants with multiple sclerosis resident in South Africa by 1960, the main risk factor appeared to be migration at ≥15 years (Dean and Kurtzke 1971). Age-adjusted prevalence for persons aged 15–19 years at immigration was $66/10^5$ for those migrating from the United Kingdom, compared with an overall figure for northern Europeans of $51/10^5$, whereas prevalence was $13/10^5$ for those migrating at ≤14 years.

Whilst few would now feel confident about confining risk to a particular calendar age, these studies proved enormously influential in generating concepts on the aetiology of multiple sclerosis. In an earlier edition of this book, we emphasized the danger of developing elaborate hypotheses based on a small numerator and with indirect methods of case ascertainment. The original South African studies depended on only six and 12 identified cases, respectively, in the two most informative groups. Inaccurate

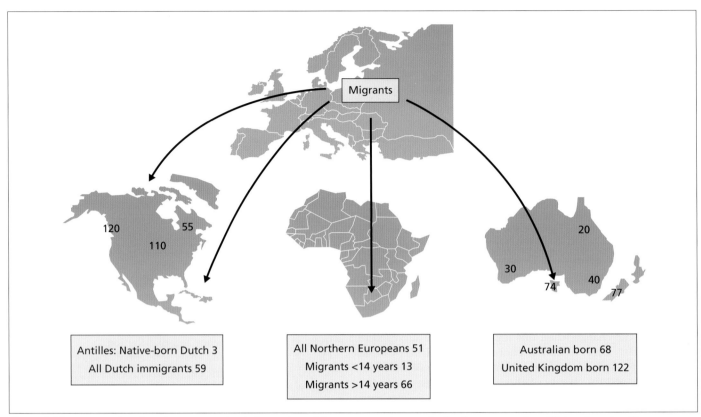

Figure 2.24 Routes taken by migrants proving informative with respect to changes in the frequency of multiple sclerosis with movement from high- to low-risk zones.

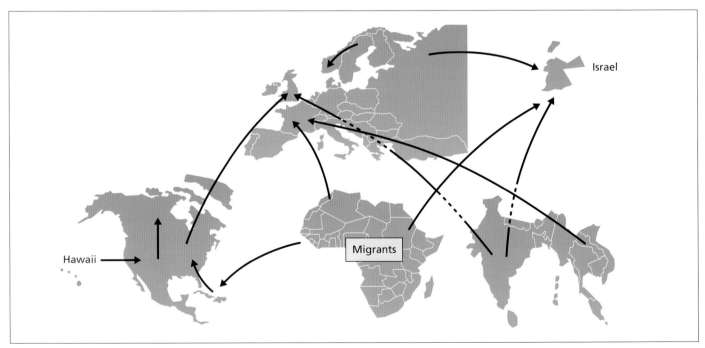

Figure 2.25 Routes taken by migrants proving informative with respect to changes in the frequency of multiple sclerosis with movement from low- to high-risk zones.

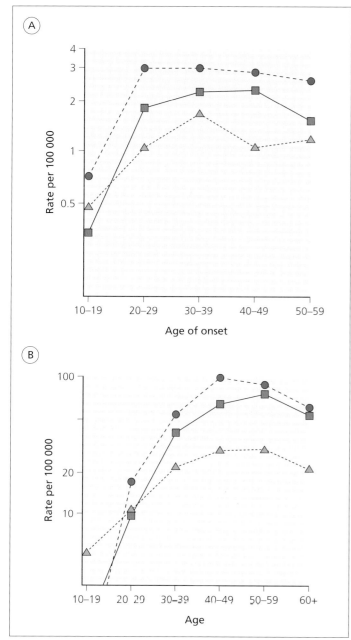

Figure 2.26 (A) Age-specific incidence (/10⁵/year) and (B) prevalence (/10⁵) of multiple sclerosis in Israel (1st January 1981). ● = native-born Israelis whose fathers were born in Europe or America; ■ = native-born Israelis whose fathers were born in Africa or Asia; ▲ = immigrants to Israel born in Africa or Asia. The *y* axis is a logarithmic scale. Adapted from Kahana *et al* (1994). ©1994, reproduced with permission of Springer-Verlag GmbH.

the Antilles, where prevalence for native-born persons was $3/10^5$ compared with $59/10^5$ for Dutch-born migrants (Moffie 1966). Migration of Europeans to Australia and New Zealand has taken place in several phases over the last 150 years. Superficially, this should have provided another opportunity to examine the effect of migration and the ages over which the effects occur. Unlike the African continent, there is no reference rate for prevalence amongst indigenous peoples against which to compare disease frequency in immigrants. Aboriginal people in Australia and New Zealand were rapidly corralled by white settlers, or otherwise disadvantaged. That unglorious history is not our business, but it has reduced the epidemiological opportunity for comparison of disease frequency in diverse ethnic groups occupying the same geographical location. Amongst immigrants to Australia and New Zealand, people originating from groups with a disproportionately high or low risk of multiple sclerosis may, by chance, have settled in particular areas and remained separated from other settlers, thus creating local pockets of susceptibility and resistance. Tasmania stands out as an area of exceptional disease frequency. As a former penal colony, it was initially populated from 1803 by 24 000 individuals, 19 000 of whom were convicts. The present population of 500 000 is descended from the 10 000 founding couples providing a population retaining some genetic isolation. But even here, the prevalence for multiple sclerosis is half that currently ascertained for people of equivalent ethnicity in northern Europe, strongly suggesting that environmental factors have influenced expression of the disease in susceptible individuals. More generally, and in contrast to the findings from South Africa, S.R. Hammond *et al* (2000a) showed that the risk of developing multiple sclerosis was uninfluenced by age at migration – taking 15 years as the point of reference.

Considering migration in the reverse (low to high) direction, no less provocative than the surveys carried out in South Africa has been the study of United Kingdom-born children of immigrants from the Indian subcontinent, Africa and the West Indies (Elian and Dean 1987; Elian *et al* 1990). In claiming that the prevalence of multiple sclerosis in these children approximates to that seen in similar age groups amongst indigenous people, the authors provide powerful ammunition for the environmental doctrine. There are several reasons why the ascertainment of patients prevalent on 1st April 1986, aged >15 years and born in the United Kingdom of parents who were migrants from the West Indies, Africa or Asia, was probably an underestimate. That said, the possibility arises that in accepting the documented diagnosis and not reviewing the evidence, individuals with other diseases may have been included. There would be fewer anxieties about diagnoses in these cases if every patient had been tested for HTLV-I status. Whilst both age at presentation and clinical severity were not typical of multiple sclerosis in white English populations, the authors acknowledge that only the most severe and early onset cases from amongst the cohort at risk were identified in this initial screen, suggesting that the frequency of multiple sclerosis in this group will rise with time. Deaths and significant demographic shifts may have occurred in the immigrant population of London and the West Midlands between the 1971 census and prevalence day in 1986, making the denominator applied to index cases inappropriate. In this respect, it is only partially reassuring that all but one of the 28 West Indian patients was known not to have moved since 1971.

ascertainment or errors of diagnosis affecting a single individual would have significantly altered the conclusions of this study, and at least a 10% error rate for classification is to be expected even in areas surveyed using the most direct methods. That said, the principles first established in studies amongst migrants to South Africa are supported by a number of other surveys. But there are exceptions.

The effect on risk of multiple sclerosis for individuals of Dutch origin migrating to a low-risk region has been reported for

In deriving the denominator, individuals at risk of European ancestry returning from Africa in the 1950s or 1960s were not distinguished from African black immigrants. Census information merely recorded that both parents had been domiciled in one of the New Commonwealth countries. Whereas white repatriates will have spuriously increased the denominator, their affected offspring did not feature in the numerator. However, the effect of these biases was probably small and would have led to the risk of multiple sclerosis in the first-generation children of West Indian, African and Asian immigrants being underestimated. Marta Elian and Geoffrey Dean referred their identification of cases amongst the offspring of New Commonwealth immigrants to age- and sex-specific rates from the 1985 Sutton (Surrey) prevalence study (E.S. Williams and McKeran 1986) and assumed an equal risk for immigrants in order to calculate the number of children expected to develop multiple sclerosis. Much depends on the validity of these expected case numbers. The Sutton study was carried out close to a large urban metropolis where accurate definition of numerator and denominator are more difficult to establish than in population-based surveys and where non-white cases were not excluded. There are difficulties in accepting evidence for an increased risk of multiple sclerosis in the children of immigrants when contemporary figures are not available for the parental generation based on comparable methods of assessment and ascertainment. All the rates cited by Elian and Dean (1987; Elian *et al* 1990) necessarily depend on small numbers and are therefore subject to large confidence intervals. A few errors will have made a large impact on the quoted rates and their interpretation. The authors made little of the greater risk seen for the children of Asian populations by comparison with black populations, although this difference also reflects global trends in the distribution of multiple sclerosis.

To assess the effect of environmental factors in changing the risk of disease for the offspring of non-Caucasian immigrants to the United Kingdom, Dean and Elian (1997) subsequently reported on 76 ethnic Asian individuals with a clinical diagnosis of multiple sclerosis (58 Indians, 17 Pakistanis and 1 Bangladeshi) who were born in the Indian subcontinent, east Africa, Fiji or Malaysia. They showed a higher than expected number of people with multiple sclerosis arriving in the United Kingdom aged <15 years, in each quinquennium under consideration, and this difference was especially marked for females. Conversely, there was no difference in observed and expected age of immigration amongst 60 patients with multiple sclerosis born in the Caribbean.

The danger of extrapolating from studies involving a small numerator in an unusual environment is well illustrated by the study of multiple sclerosis amongst immigrants from Vietnam to Paris, France. Three cases were identified in a cohort of around 3400 persons born of Vietnamese mothers who came to France aged <20 years. However, an essential criterion for immigration was mixed parentage with a French-born father (Kurtzke and Bui 1980). The fact that the cumulative 18-year risk of multiple sclerosis, by 1975, was $89/10^5$ (95% CI 18–260), with an age-specific prevalence of $169/10^5$ (95% CI 94–135) in the third decade, tells us nothing about the shift in risk of multiple sclerosis consequent upon movement of peoples from southern Asia to northern France, because admixture of genes was required in order to establish eligibility for migration. Presumably the majority of Vietnamese not migrating to France did not have French fathers.

As part of a national survey of multiple sclerosis in France, with cases recruited through an appeal on television, Delasnerie-Laupretre and Alperovitch (1992) identified – amongst 8000 cases ascertained overall in France – 246 individuals who had migrated from north Africa in the first quinquennium of the 1960s following the Algerian war for independence. Excluding the 27 patients who had multiple sclerosis before, or at the time of migration, 86% of these 246 probands were European in origin and the remainder Arab or Berber. There was no apparent age- or sex-adjusted difference in frequency or mean age at onset between these individuals and native French cases. Delasnerie-Laupretre and Alperovitch (1992) interpreted this first analysis of north African migration to France as indicating that the provocative exogenous factors are ubiquitous and multiple sclerosis is acquired by the same age irrespective of location. Kurtzke *et al* (1998) subsequently reported on 260 individuals – many presumably also included in the earlier survey – amongst 7507 respondents to a nationwide survey of multiple sclerosis who had immigrated from Algeria, Morocco or Tunisia between 1923 and 1986 (the majority during 1956–1964, and two-thirds from Algeria). Compared with French-born patients, those with multiple sclerosis migrating from north Africa were younger and with an earlier year of onset. Assumptions were made in concluding that prevalence was higher in the immigrants from north Africa developing multiple sclerosis after arrival in France ($77/10^5$; 95% CI 67–87) than those who migrated having already manifested the disease ($17/10^5$; 95% CI 11–24), or native-born French cases (estimated at $50/10^5$). Cabre *et al* (2005) studied the population of Martinique and Guadeloupe, which includes large numbers of individuals who have returned to the West Indies after living for several years in France. Against a crude background prevalence of $15/10^5$ (95% CI 12–18; with higher rates in Martinique than Guadeloupe) and incidence of $1.4/10^5$/year (95% CI 1.0–1.8) on 31 December 1999, there were 33 observed cases amongst migrants whereas 19 were expected (standardized incidence ratio 1.7 (95% CI 1.2–2.4). Incidence was even higher for individuals living in France at <15 years of age (4.1: 95% CI 2.2–6.8). Since the genetic background of the permanent residents and those who spent time in France is similar, these differences are interpreted as reflecting the influence of different environmental conditions in the West Indies and in France.

The studies of multiple sclerosis in United States Army veterans recruited during and following the Second World War, and still under observation by John Kurtzke (see above), provide essential information on which to judge issues surrounding a change in risk of multiple sclerosis with migration between regions of differing prevalence. Kurtzke *et al* (1971; 1985) compared mortality amongst northern-born United States citizens dying in the south, and vice versa. The aim was to compare the frequency of multiple sclerosis in individuals who entered military service from zones differing from those in which they were born. The evidence for a north–south gradient in frequency depended on a mortality rate for southern-born patients dying with multiple sclerosis in the north of $0.7/10^5$/year compared with $0.5/10^5$/year for those remaining in the south. The mortality ratio for veterans born in the high-frequency zones (northern states) and entering service from the middle band dropped from 1.5 to 1.3, compared with 0.7 for those entering middle states but born in the southern states having lower frequencies of multiple sclerosis. Those born in the medium-risk band showed a ratio increase to 1.4 if entering military service in the northern states, and a reduced ratio of 0.7 if relocated before enlistment from the south. However, those born in the south and migrating to either the middle or northern zones showed rates of 0.6 and 0.7, respectively. Taken together, the difference between observed and expected rates showed a significant effect of migration for white males serving during the Second World War that was not apparent in black males or white females (in whom fewer migrations occurred). The gradient in disease frequency associated with state of residence at entry into active service was associated, inversely, with a younger age at onset for the states having higher disease frequencies (Kurtzke *et al* 1992). By contrast, Detels *et al* (1972; 1977) did not report increased rates for mortality or prevalence for southern-born migrants to the northwestern United States (Washington). Kurtzke (1993) has interpreted the apparent high prevalence of multiple sclerosis in Los Alamos County, New Mexico (76/10^5; CI 42–108), as reflecting the immigrant population of non-Hispanic whites in that community because of military activities during and after the Second World War (R.E. Hoffman *et al* 1981).

Against these transcontinental shifts, movement within one relatively small country has previously been associated with alterations in mortality for multiple sclerosis. A reduction was reported in Norway for those moving from high- to low-risk regions with a corresponding increase after migration between low- and high-frequency zones – each compared with individuals having a stable domicile (Westlund 1970). Another informative series of epidemiological studies compared the prevalence of multiple sclerosis amongst Japanese living in Hawaii with inhabitants from the west coast of North America and native Hawaiians. In Hawaii, the prevalence amongst Japanese was 7/10^5 compared with 11/10^5 in Caucasian Hawaiians and 34/10^5 in Caucasian immigrants to Hawaii (Alter *et al* 1971; see also Lauer 1994). These rates were virtually identical for Japanese and Caucasians living in California (7 and 30/10^5, respectively; Detels *et al* 1977) and can be compared with the expected rate of 2/10^5 for native Japanese (Kuroiwa *et al* 1983). Here, the evidence favours a strong protective effect for Japanese irrespective of environment but with some modification of risk on relocation to an area associated with higher rates of multiple sclerosis for the indigenous population.

Israelis are another group in which migration has occurred on a sufficient scale to show important epidemiological principles relating to the risk of developing multiple sclerosis. The original study (Alter *et al* 1962; 1978) in Israeli immigrants showed a difference in prevalence between those migrating from northern Europe (Ashkenazi) and from Asia and Africa (Sephardis). The higher frequency in Ashkenazi than Sephardic Jews also revealed an age at migration effect, in that there were very few affected Ashkenazis in the cohort migrating to Israel before adolescence. Although crude rates retained the difference seen in the parental groups, prevalence in the Israeli-born children of Ashkenazis and Sephardic Jews was the same after age adjustment to the population of the United States. Kahana *et al* (1994) subsequently compared native Israelis whose fathers were born in Israel, Europe or North America, and Africa or Asia, with immigrants (Figure 2.26). Depending on place of paternal birth, prevalence (age-adjusted to the Israeli population of 1960) was estimated at 32/10^5 (fathers born in Israel), 38/10^5 (Europe or North America) and 29/10^5 (Africa or Asia) compared with 14/10^5 in immigrants. Higher rates were observed in Jerusalem (61, 68 and 51/10^5, for these three categories, respectively) than in other parts of the country. In the most recent update of these important Israeli studies, Karni *et al* (2003) reported a lower frequency of disease in Jewish immigrants from Africa/Asia (22/10^5) than in native-born African/Asian Israelis (52/10^5). Rates were similar in native-born and immigrant European/American Israelis (64/10^5 in each, respectively). The implication is that, at least for Ashkenazi and Sephardic Jews, racially determined differences in risk for multiple sclerosis are modified by environment.

Having established from these studies of migration the probability that environmental factors modify inherent risks of multiple sclerosis dependent on ethnicity, it becomes important to establish at what age these influences occur. The studies from South Africa provide a starting point for opening the debate and suggest 16 years as the critical cut-off. The United States veterans' survey also demonstrates that the north–south gradient for place at birth or entry into military service is no longer apparent for place of residence at clinical onset, indicating that acquisition of the disease has occurred earlier, and in all probability during childhood (Beebe *et al* 1967). The study of New Commonwealth immigrants to the United Kingdom is also consistent with an effect of exposure at ≤ 15 years (Dean and Elian 1997). Studies from Norway have shown maximal clustering between the ages of 13 and 20 years, suggesting that events in adolescence correlate with the development of multiple sclerosis in general and age of onset in particular (Riise and Klauber 1992; Riise *et al* 1991).

Kurtzke (1993) considered that matching by age in the study of north African migration to France (Delasnerie-Laupretre and Alperovitch 1992) had introduced a confounding factor since this restricted the study to individuals with the same age at onset. Subsequent observations on altered risks for north Africans in Algeria, Morocco or Tunisia or after arrival in France led Kurztke *et al* (1998) to conclude that multiple sclerosis occurs latently in a small but susceptible proportion of individuals having prolonged exposure to an environmental agent sometime between the ages of 10 and 40 years. Although prevalence rates are lower in Australians than in people of comparable ethnicity in northern Europe (see above), the recent analysis of age range for risk of developing multiple sclerosis in Australians showed (for all ages) that prevalence is similar in Australian-born and United Kingdom-born individuals for all locations except Hobart, Tasmania. Here the prevalence of multiple sclerosis was 68/10^5 in Australian-born compared with 122/10^5 in United Kingdom-born patients. But taken as a whole, there was no significant difference in the frequency of multiple sclerosis in the 331 immigrants from the United Kingdom, aged 29–41 years at prevalence in 1981, who developed multiple sclerosis depending on whether they arrived before (30%) or after (70%) the age of 15 years (S.R. Hammond *et al* 2000a). The key observation that individuals moving as adults to Australia and subsequently developing multiple sclerosis do not have a higher disease frequency than native-born Australians or juvenile immigrants suggests that the risk of exposure spans a much wider age interval than originally proposed from the South African studies.

Clearly, an interval of several years exists between exposure of individuals at risk and the development of clinical symptoms. Typically the environmental event(s) occur in childhood and onset is as a young adult. This situation epitomizes the interplay between genes and the environment in multiple sclerosis. However, exposure may be delayed and the latency prior to development of clinical manifestations can be short or long, making for a wide spectrum both in the age at which susceptibility converts to disease and in the year of onset.

EPIDEMICS AND CLUSTERS OF MULTIPLE SCLEROSIS

Protagonists of the environmental doctrine for causation are naturally enthusiastic about evidence for multiple sclerosis occurring in epidemics. Claims have been made for clusters in the Faroe Islands, Iceland, Orkney and Shetland, and Key West, apart from the more restricted groupings that occasionally feature in regional epidemiological studies (see above).

The most comprehensive survey of multiple sclerosis conducted by John Kurtzke over several decades forms the basis for the claim that epidemics have occurred in islands located in the North Atlantic. The arguments for a point source epidemic in these parts, especially the Faroe Islands, undoubtedly have merit although the evidence is not universally accepted. Others take the view that these are epidemics of recognition, reflecting the arrival of specialist medical services in the islands, rather than a real change in incidence arising from the introduction of transmissible aetiological factors into virgin populations.

In the first survey of Iceland, 168 cases of multiple sclerosis were identified with onset between 1900 and 1975 (Kurtzke et al 1982). Annual incidence rates appeared to rise in about 1922, and then stabilize until a further increase occurred in 1945, heralding a steady decline from the mid-1950s. Average annual incidence rates for 1923–1994 were around $1.6/10^5$/year increasing to $3.2/10^5$/year between 1945 and 1954 and falling to $1.9/10^5$/year between 1955 and 1974. Each quinquennial rate from 1900 was lower than that for 1945–1954, during which age at onset was also younger than before or after this period. These observations led S.D. Cook et al (1980) and Kurtzke et al (1982) to conclude that there had been a postwar epidemic of multiple sclerosis in Iceland, but opinions differ both with respect to the facts and their interpretation. Subsequently, Benedikz et al (1994), for the purposes of assessing the question of an epidemic in Iceland, considered 323 patients with onset of symptoms attributed to multiple sclerosis after 1st January 1900, of whom 252 were still living in December 1989. All but four were born and raised in Iceland and had maternal and paternal families going back several generations. Incidence rates were generally $<1/10^5$ up until the 1930s but then increased to $2.5/10^5$, coinciding with the arrival of two neurologists. With waning enthusiasm, so the analysis goes, there was then a lull until 1945–1955, when incidence increased to $3.3/10^5$/year following the first systematic survey of the disease. With nine neurologists in practice from 1975, incidence peaked at $4.1/10^5$/year, and this rate has since been maintained. Prevalence in Iceland, based on cases ascertained by year of diagnosis, was 33 (95% CI 25–43), 33 (95% CI 26–43), 52 (95% CI 43–63) and $70/10^5$ (95% CI 60–82) in 1955, 1965, 1975 and 1985, respectively.

Onset adjustment changed these rates for 1950 to 1990, by decade, to 50, 52, 62, 85 and $100/10^5$, respectively. The most recent figure for prevalence is $119/10^5$, the slower rate of increase (despite the luxury now of 15 neurologists) suggesting that ascertainment has saturated and steady state is now reached (Benedikz et al 2002).

It is significant that John Benedikz, a neurologist who has worked in Iceland for many years and takes a particular interest in the epidemiology of multiple sclerosis, has questioned whether there has been a genuine increase in incidence. He favours the view that any change in frequency of multiple sclerosis in Iceland during the 20th century reflects improved recognition and the development of more sophisticated diagnostic procedures (Benedikz et al 1991; 1994; C.M. Poser et al 1992). In the era before 1950, case ascertainment was far from adequate, as shown by the long interval between year of onset and diagnosis at that time. Comparisons of disability in the affected cohorts showed an excess of those with severe multiple sclerosis before 1950. The arrival of neurologists in Iceland (two of whom, Kjartan and Gunnar Guomundsson, were prime movers in identifying patients with multiple sclerosis) may have been entirely responsible for the increased number of cases through improved vigilance and recognition. The abrupt reduction in interval between onset of symptoms and diagnosis after 1940 is further evidence for the impact of improved neurological services on case ascertainment.

The 18 Faroe Islands lie in the North Atlantic at latitude 62°N. The population increased from around 15 000 in 1900 to 48 000 in 1990. The islands have had a strong administrative association with Denmark, which has loosened somewhat since 1948. Observations on multiple sclerosis were made originally by R.S. Allison (1963) and Fog and Hyllested (1966). They found fewer cases than expected from comparisons with neighbouring Orkney and Shetland (see Chapter 1). A national multiple sclerosis register was established in 1947 against the background of a long-established health care system, including routine transfer of cases to the Neurology Department of the Rijkshospital in Copenhagen. These and other sources were repeatedly searched for diagnoses of multiple sclerosis by John Kurtzke in his zealous ascertainment of multiple sclerosis in the Faroes, attempting to trace cases from before the Second World War. The Schumacher criteria were used to assign the diagnosis of multiple sclerosis, supplemented by laboratory investigations when these became available. By 1986, 41 cases had been ascertained of whom nine lived abroad for 3 or more years. These were not considered directly to have been part of the epidemic. Neither in the initial survey by Fog and Hyllested (1966), nor in the later assessments by John Kurtzke and colleagues (Kurtzke 1993; 2005; Kurtzke and Hyllested 1979; 1986; 1987; 1988) was any patient identified with an estimated date of onset earlier than 1943. In the initial analysis, there were 16 cases with onset during 1943–1949, and a further 16 developing clinical manifestations during 1950–1973 but none thereafter despite a steady increase in the population. These observations led John Kurtzke and Kay Hyllested to conclude that a 30-year epidemic of multiple sclerosis occurred on the Faroe Islands following the Second World War. The details of this claim were argued in minute detail with comprehensive summaries of the evidence by Kurtzke (1993).

Starting from the premise that multiple sclerosis is acquired at around the time of puberty, John Kurtzke and Kay Hyllested first separated incident cases into those who were pre- and post-pubertal in 1943. This suggested that three epidemics occurred between 1943 and 1973. A fourth was predicted (at approximately a 13-year interval) and was later claimed (Figure 2.27: Kurtzke *et al* 1995). The first was dominated by individuals who were postpubertal in 1943. Conversely, peaks in incidence constituting subsequent epidemics were made up of individuals who were prepubertal at that time. These cases also had a younger age at onset of the disease. John Kurtzke concluded that the critical factor determining the Faroes' experience of multiple sclerosis was occupation by British troops between 1940 and 1945. He proposed that the distribution of multiple sclerosis showed both a temporal and spatial relationship. Villages where individuals lived who contributed to each of the incidence peaks (especially those occurring in the late 1950s and 1960s) within the overall epidemic were also those where troops were billeted. This observation led John Kurtzke to conclude without reservation that the cause of multiple sclerosis (in the Faroes) is a transmissible infection not producing neurological symptoms in the majority of carriers. He argued that the pool of individuals at risk who might have acquired the factor in the early 1940s was that 75% of the population having close contact with British troops. They then represented the source from which others were later affected to create the second phase of the epidemic, and so on. Eventually, the number of susceptible individuals was no longer sufficient to sustain the disease so that the epidemic terminated in the late 1970s. For each case, a minimum exposure of 2 years was needed to acquire the disease.

As a corollary to this argument, it is necessary to suppose that the potency of transmissibility diminished with time. Affected individuals acquired the agent at around the age of 11 years and infected others between, but not after, the ages of 20–25 years (Kurtzke *et al* 1995). Furthermore, susceptibility to infection did not persist beyond the age of 45 years. Overall, about 1:500 individuals exposed to the agent developed clinical manifestations of multiple sclerosis. To some extent the arguments advanced by John Kurtzke have had to be qualified retrospectively through the recognition of additional cases. Updating the story to 1998, Kurtzke and Heltberg (2001) reported prevalence of $66/10^5$ (95% CI 45–93) amongst Faroese age-adjusted to the 1969 United States population. There had been no appreciable change from rates recorded in 1960 ($68/10^5$), 1970 ($62/10^5$) and 1980 ($63/10^5$). Seven new affected individuals with onset at around 21 years were identified between 1986 and 1990 and these have since been accommodated within a fourth epidemic (Kurtzke *et al* 1995). Pulling together a complex story, Kurtzke and Heltberg (2001) conclude that multiple sclerosis is an infectious disease introduced to the Faroese by British troops in the Second World War. The first wave of disease spread from a single individual born in 1919, exposed for 2 years, affected by 1943 and dead by 1971. Twenty others were caught up in the first epidemic, providing a reservoir of the primary multiple sclerosis infection handed on to others exposed for a minimum period of 2 years between the ages of 11 and 45 years. These contributed to the remaining affected individuals grouped in the four subsequent epidemics. Of the 83 cases prevalent at any time, 41 were fully native Faroese and 14 had lived away for short periods. These 55 constitute the epidemic cases; 15 who had lived away for longer and 13 foreign-born cases were

excluded. Median survival has been 29 and 34 years in females and males, respectively. In 'hanging up his Faroese epidemiological boots' in 2001, John Kurtzke settled on the following numbers: epidemic one, 21 – exposed between 1941 and 1944; epidemic two, 10 – exposed between 1945 and 1951; epidemic three, 10 – exposed between 1958 and 1964; epidemic four, 13 – exposed between 1971 and 1977; and a single individual in epidemic five, exposed between 1984 and 1990.

On the nature of the transmissible agent, Kurtzke *et al* (1988) examined the possibility that British troops introduced canine distemper virus, pursuing the hypothesis developed by S.D. Cook *et al* (1978) to explain the epidemiology of multiple sclerosis in Orkney and the Shetland Islands, and in Iceland. In the Faroes, there was no evidence in affected individuals for previous infection by this virus. One patient only had owned a dog with distemper; and there was no correlation between outbreaks of canine distemper and the distribution of residence in incident cases of multiple sclerosis.

Proponents have speculated on dynamics of the transmission hypothesis, whilst accepting the overall concept of an epidemic. Cooke (1990) attached special significance to the absence of individuals, born in 1941–1945, contributing to the second and third phases, and took this to mean that whilst contact with the transmissible agent was universal amongst Faroese, exposure in the first 3 years of life provided absolute protection from the later development of multiple sclerosis. Any differences from the age at exposure analysis based on epidemiological observations elsewhere were attributed to the immunologically naive nature of Faroese encountering the provocative agent during the early 1940s. Sceptics remain to be convinced by any aspect of this analysis. As in Iceland, the availability of improved diagnostic expertise is offered by a resident neurologist (Poul Joensen, personal communication, 1998) to explain the Faroe Islands epidemic, and the lack of such services for the paucity of multiple sclerosis in Greenland. In his part retrospective and prospective survey of neurological disease in the Faroes, 28 cases of multiple sclerosis were identified as causes of disability from 1939 to 1975 – the distribution being 6, 17 and 4 in sequential decades from 1939 and 1 in the 1970s (Joensen 1992). Specific criticisms concerning validity of the diagnoses, exclusions, case ascertainment, definition of epidemics, and the putative role of the British occupation in generating this outbreak of multiple sclerosis (C.M. Poser and Hibberd 1988; C.M. Poser *et al* 1988) are robustly resisted by the main protagonists (Kurtzke 1993; Kurtzke and Hyllested 1988).

In Orkney and the Shetland Islands, the incidence and prevalence of multiple sclerosis were at one time higher, almost by an order of magnitude, than in other regions (Figure 2.28). In presenting their classical study, Poskanzer *et al* (1980a) reviewed certificates located in Edinburgh for deaths attributed to neurological disease in Orkney and Shetland, concluding that the first case of disseminated sclerosis occurred in an Orcadian who died in 1898. A second case was reported 10 years later, and thereafter the diagnosis became more common, coinciding with a general increase in awareness and the adoption of clinical criteria for the diagnosis of multiple sclerosis in neighbouring parts of Scotland. Changes in disease frequency in that era can reasonably be attributed to alterations in nosological fashion. Poskanzer *et al* (1980a) concluded that multiple sclerosis may have been no less frequent an illness in the early years of the 19th century

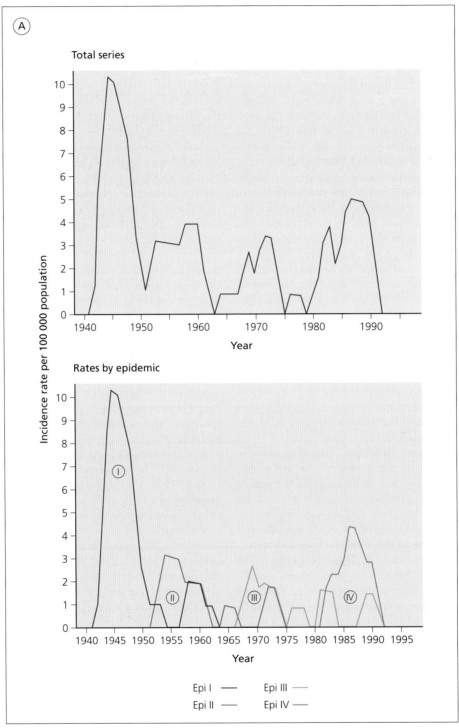

Figure 2.27 (A) Annual incidence (/10⁵) for clinical multiple sclerosis in native resident Faroese, calculated as 3 year centred moving averages, to 1998. Upper panel, total series; lower panel, rates for each of the four epidemics. Adapted from Kurtzke and Heltberg (2001).

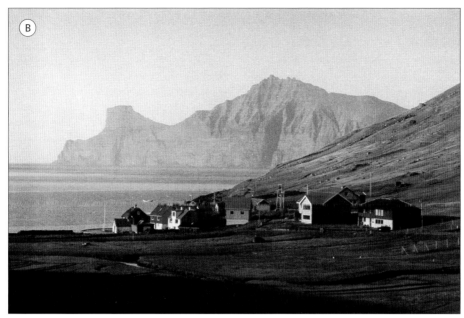

Figure 2.27, cont'd (B) The Faroe Islands from a local picture postcard (c.mid-1990s).

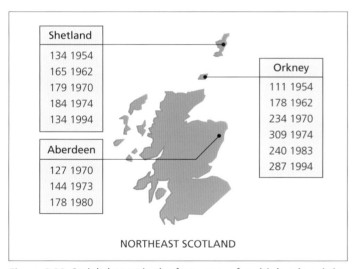

Figure 2.28 Serial change in the frequency of multiple sclerosis in Orkney and the Shetland Islands and northeast Scotland; figures are prevalence/10⁵ population with the year of ascertainment.

than was later apparent. However, as we have indicated, estimates of prevalence carried out on four occasions between 1954 and 1974 showed a steady rise in frequency from $111/10^5$ in 1954 to $309/10^5$ in 1974 for Orkney, and from 134 to $184/10^5$ in Shetland over the same period.

Recognizing that these changes did not necessarily reflect a genuine increase in incidence, Poskanzer *et al* (1980a) defined – as accurately as possible – the date of onset in 66 incident Orcadian and 53 Shetland cases between 1930 and 1969. They concluded that ascertainment would have been reasonably complete between 1940 and 1960, during which annual incidence of the disease was $2.2/10^5$/year in Orkney and $1.6/10^5$/year in Shetland. Quinquennial rates were relatively constant and they attributed a slight reduction towards the end of this period to incomplete ascertainment of undiagnosed cases, made more

obvious by exclusion of individuals with possible multiple sclerosis using the criteria of Allison and Millar. Comparison of incidence and mortality rates confirmed the impression that there had been no significant alteration in statistics for the disease over this period other than those attributable to changes in classification and ascertainment. Several pioneering epidemiologists had previously identified factors tending to maximize the prevalence of multiple sclerosis in surveys conducted on islands (Allison 1963; Fog and Hyllested 1966; Poskanzer *et al* 1976; Sutherland 1956). Over the period of these studies, systematic depopulation in Orkney and the Shetland Islands resulted in an older population, at lower risk of multiple sclerosis. However, given stable incidence, the rise in prevalence was nevertheless attributed to increased survival, from 26 to 40 years in Orkney and 24 to 34 years in Shetland, between 1954 and 1974, together with improved case recognition.

S.D. Cook *et al* (1985) revisited the question of serial change in incidence for multiple sclerosis in Orkney, documenting the annual rate from 1941 to 1983 and claiming a steady reduction from 1964. Between 1941 and 1964, 53 incident patients with probable multiple sclerosis were identified in an estimated cumulative population of 506 541 individuals, whereas only 12 developed relevant neurological symptoms in the comparable group of 320 757 individuals occupying the islands between 1965 and 1982 and showing a different age structure. In a stable population, 33 incident cases would have been expected over this period. The prevalence had also fallen to $240/10^5$ in 1983 for probable and possible cases (compared with $309/10^5$ in 1974). The rates for probable cases were $193/10^5$ and $258/10^5$ in 1983 and 1974, respectively. Disease duration increased to 22 years (providing an estimate for life expectancy, using Poskanzer's method, of 44 years) and, at 52 years, the mean age at the time of prevalence was higher than for any other population recorded at that time. This overall change in disease frequency was attributed to a reduction in the number of older patients, suggesting that prevalence in the sixth decade and beyond had diminished as a result of fewer incident cases in younger age groups.

As part of the systematic attempt to survey multiple sclerosis in the Orkney and Shetland Islands, Stuart Cook and his local collaborators on the islands have serially updated the figures (S.D. Cook *et al* 1988) and last reported a prevalence for probable and definite cases of $287/10^5$ and $134/10^5$ for Orkney and Shetland, respectively, in 1994 (S.D. Cook, unpublished results). These statistics show that there has been significantly less multiple sclerosis in the Shetland Islands since 1965 but this is no longer true for Orkney.

The reduction in frequency of multiple sclerosis seen in northeast Scotland over the same period is reminiscent of epidemiological surveys from other regions that border the North Sea (see above). If these trends reflect a change in biological factors determining the frequency of multiple sclerosis, this can best be attributed, as John Kurtzke has emphasized, to a change in environmental conditions. Population genetics shape the distribution of disease more slowly. The alternative explanation is that the systematic increase in prevalence with time and gradual erosion of the latitudinal gradient in the United Kingdom are due the catching up of more recently surveyed areas with those studied repeatedly over a longer period and already epidemiologically saturated.

It is easy, especially for the individuals concerned, to assume that multiple sclerosis is contagious when a cluster occurs, apparently selecting a group with demographic or social links – for example attendance at the same school, domicile in the same street or membership of the same sports team. With small denominators and a disproportionately high numerator, these claims rarely stand up to detailed scrutiny. Statistical methods usually show that the clusters could as easily have arisen by chance.

Indeed, that was the preferred interpretation offered by Deacon *et al* (1959) to explain an apparent excess of cases in Duxbury, Massachusetts. Having been drawn to the survey by the suspicion of Dr Deacon that too many cases of multiple sclerosis had appeared in the community, the authors identified 16 cases in a population of 4900, of whom 8 were prevalent providing a rate of $224/10^5$ for all probable, and $163/10^5$ for more certain, cases; incidence was $13/10^5$/year (or $6.5/10^5$/year for the cases with physical signs) over the period 1945–1955. At that time, the highest reported prevalence in North America was $64/10^5$ for Rochester, Minnesota (MacLean *et al* 1950), with an incidence of $5/10^5$/year. Perhaps the authors' commendable restraint in claiming a cluster was the disproportionate regional increase in prevalence, rather than incidence, the small sample, the potential impact of even one diagnostic error, the two familial cases, and the awareness that events happen by chance.

Amongst the 10 000 inhabitants of Mansfield, Massachusetts, word of mouth identified 13 probable cases and one possible example of multiple sclerosis, providing a prevalence rate of $141/10^5$ – three times higher than found elsewhere in New England at that time (Eastman *et al* 1973). All were white and 13/14 female. There had been no recent changes in demography. Eight affected individuals lived in close proximity and in a part of town long held to have a 'suspect' water supply.

Koch *et al* (1974) claimed as a time–space cluster, the six cases of multiple sclerosis known to have been born in the small town of Mossyrock, Washington State, between 1916 and 1921, where the population increased from an estimated 100 in 1920

to 415 in 1970. Another case, born in 1942, came to light through enquiry during the survey. A trawl for items of common exposure or comorbidity for infectious disease was suggestive. However, there was no documentary support for the belief, held amongst the cases themselves, that they all had smallpox in 1924; rather it seemed that an epidemic of measles might have occurred at around that time. Dressed up as rates for prevalence and incidence over the 24-year period of $1687/10^5$ and $82/10^5$/year, respectively, these look to be impressive distortions but, to us, the explanation lies in the familial aggregation: one family had two affected siblings; another had three affected siblings, and a first cousin and her son also with multiple sclerosis. In fact, only one case was sporadic.

Cook and Dowling (1982) reported three definite or probable and two possible cases of multiple sclerosis in Sitka, Alaska. Clinical onset occurred between 1967 and 1970. They linked this time cluster to an epidemic of canine distemper virus in dogs occurring in 1965. No cases were known to have been on the island during the period 1949–1979.

Murray (1976) identified ten patients from Nova Scotia living in close proximity during an outbreak of poliomyelitis in 1951. Although he sought a variety of environmental links between these cases, it is significant that six were related, and members of two extended families. A genetic explanation also seems probable for the cluster of 33 cases identified in a small rural community in northern Sweden of whom 21 were linked through kinship (Binzer *et al* 1994). Twenty people working in a New York industrial plant with c.6000 employees exposed to zinc developed multiple sclerosis between 1970 and 1989 (Schiffer *et al* 1994; E.C. Stein *et al* 1987). Here, an assessment of recurrence risks and screening for a number of candidate genes failed to confirm the investigators' hunch that the cluster had a genetic explanation.

An epidemic has been claimed for Key West, a tropical island off the west coast of Florida, where 37 patients with peak onset in and around 1977–1979 were identified in 1984 (prevalence $140/10^5$). The change was not thought attributable to alterations in clinical vigilance or differential migration of symptomatic individuals to a more favourable climate (Sheremata *et al* 1985). Later, S.D. Cook *et al* (1987) checked out the rates of canine distemper on Key West and nearby Stock Island, using the recollections and records of local veterinarians, and claimed a close symmetry between outbreaks of canine distemper in dogs and clustering of multiple sclerosis in these remote parts of south Florida. However, referring to the same group of cases, MacGregor (1991) concluded that the cluster could not be explained by genetic susceptibility and exposure to canine distemper virus or measles. Rather, the vector was considered to be birds and Marek's disease virus the best microbial bet.

Eight of 283 children attending school in a small hamlet (Henribourg, population 75) in Saskatchewan over a 15-year period later developed multiple sclerosis (Hader *et al* 1990). All were affected by one of three measles epidemics to which the community was exposed, and each had consumed well water distributed by ladle from a large crock stationed near the school door. The authors were careful not to overstate the potential significance of this anecdote.

Haahr *et al* (1997) drew attention to eight Danes with multiple sclerosis who lived in a small isolated and stable community. All attended one school over a 7-year period and took part in the same activities, but two were siblings and two others second-degree relatives.

Nine new cases of multiple sclerosis occurred between 1971 and 1990 amongst the 1729 residents of DePue Township, Illinois (Schiffer *et al* 2001). Using various comparators, this was estimated to represent a relative risk of 4.1–17.1 (95% CI 3.1–20.0). No cases were identified before or after these dates. Concern had arisen that morbidity in this mining community was being influenced by exposure to mitogenic trace metals, especially zinc, over this period. Commenting on this report, Park (2002) added triaryl phosphate ester to the list of possible heavy metal culprits. Using a spatial statistic scan, Donnan *et al* (2005) searched a database of 772 cases identified in Tayside, Scotland, between 1970 and 1997 (providing an annual incidence of $7/10^5$/year) for clusters. The general increase in disease frequency showed some evidence for periodicity and peaked in the mid-1990s but with a time cluster between 1982 and 1995 throughout the region, and a spatial cluster in the rural area southwest of Perth between 1993 and 1995. The implication is that these patterns reflect the influence of exogenous aetiological factors, but the impact of changes in scrutiny, as the availability of neurological services has altered, cannot altogether be excluded.

Riise (1997) has brought definitions and common sense to the analysis of these clusters in north Atlantic Islands (Faroes, Iceland, Orkney and Shetland), the United States (Massachusetts, New York, Wyoming, Ohio, Key West and Alaska), Canada (Nova Scotia and Saskatchewan) and Scandinavia. Amongst the post hoc clusters, none is convincing with respect to a specific environmental factor and several seem more closely related to genetic influences. There is statistical evidence for clustering at 21–23 years of age and 2 years prior to onset in the Orkney cases but not Shetland. Conversely, the studies from Hordaland county, Norway, provide evidence for clustering of affected individuals as teenagers (13–20 with a peak at 18 years) but specifically not in the run up to disease presentation (Riise *et al* 1991).

THE ENVIRONMENTAL FACTOR IN MULTIPLE SCLEROSIS

It may seem coy endlessly to refer to those aspects of the aetiology and epidemiology of multiple sclerosis that seem not to be dependent on genetic susceptibility as environmental factors, without being more specific, but, despite much effort, these influences remain unidentified and still somewhat enigmatic. Although many would argue that the environmental contribution is microbial and, in all probability viral, the evidence is limited and alternative hypotheses continue to be explored both within the confines of mainstream multiple sclerosis research and in more maverick circles. Many analysts now conclude that multiple sclerosis does not have a single cause. We discuss later (see Chapter 14) the thorny issue of whether multiple sclerosis is a syndrome resulting from complex genetic traits, multiple causes and mechanistic heterogeneity, in which discrete pathological processes converge on a shared clinical phenotype, or a nosologically distinct but nonetheless complex disorder where definition has become blurred around the edges through confusion with related but recognizably different conditions.

Since it remains an assumption that the environmental factor in multiple sclerosis is microbial, some analysts have sought to implicate altogether different putative risk factors. Often, the evidence is anecdotal and with no attempt to test hypotheses using sound epidemiological principles. The distinction is not always made between factors that may initiate the disease process in multiple sclerosis, those that are claimed to expose latent disease, and events that alter the clinical course in individuals who have already experienced manifestations.

We review 'life events' that have been considered as candidates for affecting the course of the disease in Chapter 4: these include the effects of infections, vaccinations, pregnancy, trauma and stress. Here, these and some other extrinsic circumstances are reviewed for their potential contribution in causing multiple sclerosis – aetiological factors rather than modifiers of the disease process.

Infections

As in many situations where direct leads are lacking, one epidemiological approach is the non-prejudicial trawl for risk factors associated with multiple sclerosis. Hopkins *et al* (1991) examined many candidates – around the general theme of infection and immunity – in a case–control study involving 16 prevalent cases and 61 controls. They showed that a family history of neurological disease, a personal history of allergies, exposure to oral polio vaccine, owning a cat that died from unexplained causes, or completing high school and/or college education were independent risk factors for multiple sclerosis. Blood serology provided no additional clues to the development of multiple sclerosis amongst individuals included in this survey. Evidence for infectivity might be apparent from altered risk amongst those having close personal contact with affected individuals. The answer to the question of whether professionals who frequently meet patients with multiple sclerosis have an increased risk of developing the disease is 'no' but, for methodological reasons, the study by Dean and Gray (1990) cannot be regarded as definitive. Developing the theme that 7 of 307 nurses working in Key West (South Florida) were found to have multiple sclerosis, Dean and Gray (1990) compared expected and observed death certifications for multiple sclerosis in medical practitioners and nurses from the United Kingdom using Office of Population Censuses and Surveys statistics and documentary evidence available from the prospective British Doctors' Smoking Study. In neither case did a trend towards increased risk emerge. However, we do not know the degree of contact between patients and these medical staff. Prospective records of the Danish Multiple Sclerosis Registry identified 60 cases of multiple sclerosis amongst 69 428 nurses registered from 1980 to 1996, where 69 would have been expected, representing a standardized incidence ratio of 0.87 (95% CI 0.6–1.12: Stenager *et al* 2003). The frequency of multiple sclerosis in the spouses of affected individuals (conjugal multiple sclerosis) is no higher than the population risk (Ebers *et al* 2000a; N.P. Robertson *et al* 1997). As we discuss in Chapter 3, the studies of recurrence risk in adoptees, half-siblings and twins also exclude an increased risk of multiple sclerosis through close personal contact with probands.

A survey of risk factors showed seasonal variation in the incidence of optic neuritis and suggested that the subsequent conversion to multiple sclerosis correlated with onset of optic neuritis in the winter or spring (Compston *et al* 1978). Jin *et al* (1999; 2000) have also shown that new episodes of demyelination, especially optic neuritis (ratio 1.84 compared with other disease manifestations; 95% CI 1.13–3.0) cluster in the spring (45% of all such episodes; 95% CI 35–55%), at least in northern Europe. Although this may tell us something about environmental factors causing optic neuritis, the seasonal association within risk of multiple sclerosis is almost certainly confounded by the generally high conversion rate of optic neuritis in adults. Others have shown seasonal variation in symptoms at onset (or during the course) of multiple sclerosis (Andersen *et al* 1993; Goodkin and Hertsgaard 1989). In Japan, 172 exacerbations occurring in 34 individuals with multiple sclerosis clustered in the six summer months but 123 (72%) were in those with optico-spinal disease – making it difficult to generalize these findings (Ogawa *et al* 2004). The increased springtime risk (but not in the winter) is confirmed in meta-analysis of nine studies reporting on optic neuritis (relative risk 1.19, 95% CI 1.16–1.23), six of onset in multiple sclerosis (relative risk 1.45, 95% CI 1.36–1.55) and nine of exacerbations in patients with pre-existing disease (relative risk 1.10, 95% CI 0.7–1.13; Jin *et al* 2000). Marrie *et al* (2000) used the General Practice Research Database to show an increased risk of respiratory infection in 5-, 12- and 52-week periods at risk before first onset of multiple sclerosis. Taken together, these indirect observations do no more than implicate environmental triggers for disease onset in multiple sclerosis but the issue has been more directly studied in the surveys of Sibley and colleagues (see Chapter 4).

Several investigators have attempted to correlate exposure to viral illness in childhood with the subsequent development of multiple sclerosis. Methodology has varied and the results are critically dependent on the choice of controls (for review, see Granieri and Casetta 1997). The picture to emerge from these studies is that the risk of developing multiple sclerosis is increased for individuals affected by a variety of exanthematous and other common viral disorders relatively late in childhood. The studies suggest that a narrow and age-linked period of susceptibility to viral exposure exists in those who are constitutionally at risk of developing the disease. Part of the evidence is provided by population serology but many prefer the interpretation that differences in the titres or distribution of antibodies in case–control series do not relate to specific viral antigens. Rather, these reflect a general enhancement in immune responsiveness. However, one candidate may yet hold some promise.

Compston *et al* (1986) first retrospectively compared historical and laboratory evidence for previous viral exposure in patients with multiple sclerosis and optic neuritis with a cohort of controls screened to have an increased frequency of HLA-DR2, so as to match for at least one marker of genetic susceptibility. Patients with demyelinating disease reported later age at infection by measles, mumps and rubella. Martyn *et al* (1993) subsequently re-analysed these data to show an even more marked effect of EBV infection. Those who reported having infectious mononucleosis at <18 years had a relative risk for multiple sclerosis of 7.9 (95% CI 2–38). Meanwhile, Lindberg *et al* (1991), looking at registries for infectious mononucleosis in Sweden, found a slight excess of multiple sclerosis following EBV infection compared with individuals not reporting exposure. Haahr *et al* (1995) used records from the Danish State

Serum Institute register of EBV infections and the Danish Multiple Sclerosis Registry to identify 16 individuals who developed multiple sclerosis amongst 6853 experiencing EBV infection in the decade 1968–1978 (relative risk 2.8). Median age at infection was 17 years. This did not differ from the age at infection in heterophile antibody-positive individuals not developing multiple sclerosis. Goldacre *et al* (2004) reported an increased risk of multiple sclerosis ≥10 years after hospital admission in Oxford, England, with infectious mononucleosis (rate ratio 14.0: 95% CI 1.5–8.9). High population exposure to EBV makes for difficulty in resolving the disease-related status of these serological observations. Munch *et al* (1998) implicated infection due to an EBV subtype, identified by a 39-bp repeat of the EBNA 6 coding region, in a cluster of eight cases from Fjelso, Denmark. Vaughan *et al* (1996) used more discriminating laboratory markers and showed an enhanced immune response to EBV, involving the glycine/alanine repeat peptide (p62) epitope of EBV nuclear antigen-1, also expressed by other pathogens and cross-reacting with neuroglial cells, in patients with multiple sclerosis previously reported from Norway (Riise *et al* 1991). Subsequently, Marrie *et al* (2000) reported an odds ratio for multiple sclerosis of 5.5 (95% CI 1.5–19.7) for individuals with a clinical history of infectious mononucleosis based on their access to the United Kingdom General Practice Research Database. Hernán *et al* (2001a) confirmed a moderate increase in risk of multiple sclerosis amongst nurses with a history of infectious mononucleosis (2.1: 95% CI 1.5–2.9) especially if the history was confirmed serologically (2.3: 95% CI 1.6–3.5). They also showed that late age at infection by mumps and measles conferred an increased risk of demyelinating disease. H.J. Wagner *et al* (2000) demonstrated universal infectivity by EBV in patients with multiple sclerosis and suggested, on the basis of reduced EBV nuclear antigen-1 antibody, that affected individuals may have defective control of persistent latent EBV carrier state and reactivation. Using samples collected over a 10-year period, Alotaibi *et al* (2004) provided serological evidence for remote EBV infection in 83% of 30 children with multiple sclerosis, compared with 42% of 90 matched emergency department controls and 53 healthy children (p = 0.001). Conversely, exposure to herpes simplex virus was less likely in affected individuals and the effects of cytomegalovirus, parvovirus B19 and varicella zoster were neutral. Ponsonby *et al* (2005) used indirect epidemiological methods to substantiate the hygiene hypothesis, whereby early exposure provides immunological protection, in the specific context of EBV infection: 136 Tasmanian patients, identified from a population-based sample and studied between 1999 and 2001, were compared with 272 matched controls for a history of contact with siblings aged <2 years during their own early childhood (<6 years). Taking 1 year of contact as the reference point, increased exposure correlated with a reduced risk of multiple sclerosis (1–<3 years: adjusted odds ratio 0.57, 95% CI 0.33–0.98; 3–<5 years: 0.40, 95% CI 0.19–0.92; ≥5 years: 0.12, 95% CI 0.02–0.88: p = 0.002). In controls with a history of increased exposure to infant siblings, IgG responses to EBV were reduced and there was a lower probability of infectious mononucleosis. However, in cases, although the reported frequency of mononucleosis and EBV IgG antibody responses were higher, these did not correlate with periods of exposure to younger siblings. Therefore, the simple notion that early contact provides protective immunity, a lower frequency of infectious mononucleosis (at the critical age, later in childhood), and a lower frequency of multiple sclerosis is not directly supported. Large databases in which samples were collected prospectively identify an increased antibody titre to the nuclear antigens of EBV, especially in adults aged ≥ 25 years compared to those aged ≤ 20 years, as a prognostic risk factor for the development of multiple sclerosis (Ascherio *et al* 2001a; Levin *et al* 2005; Sundström *et al* 2006). But, as we discuss in Chapters 5 and 11, the story implicating EBV in the aetiology of multiple sclerosis gains credence from immunological studies showing molecular mimicry with epitopes of myelin basic protein (Lang *et al* 2002).

The list of other microbial agents that have at some time been implicated in the aetiology of multiple sclerosis on the basis of single but unconfirmed isolations is long. The catalogue includes rabies, herpes simplex viridae, scrapie agent, parainfluenza 1, measles, the 'Carp' and 'bone marrow' agents, cytomegalovirus and coronavirus (for a summary of the earlier studies, see R.T. Johnson 1982). Subsequently, the question arose of whether patients with multiple sclerosis had at one time been exposed to human retroviruses. The occasional reports of retroviral genomic material in the central nervous system tissue of patients with multiple sclerosis (Cosby *et al* 1989; Greenberg *et al* 1989; E.P. Reddy *et al* 1989) sustained expectations that a specific cause could be discovered. However, these anecdotes appear no more consistent (Bangham *et al* 1989; Nicholl *et al* 1993; Richardson *et al* 1989) or specific than the serological surveys and periodic viral isolates from cell cultures. Although the nervous system is an important reservoir and site for cytopathic retroviral infection, exhaustive search for evidence of retrovirus using reverse transcriptase activity in blood and cerebrospinal fluid of patients with multiple sclerosis has proved relatively unrewarding (Hackett *et al* 1996). Mogensen (1997) reviewed in detail the question of whether these analyses provide evidence for retroviral infection in multiple sclerosis. Whilst the hypothesis remains tenable, the facts are scanty and, of the newer candidate retroviruses, none appears better supported than its predecessors.

The story began with preliminary reports implicating HTLV-I and HTLV-3 (HIV-1; Koprowski *et al* 1985) in multiple sclerosis. But these were not confirmed (S.L. Hauser *et al* 1986; Karpas *et al* 1986). Sommerlund *et al* (1993) demonstrated retrovirus-like particles in a cell line producing EBV from a patient with a chronic myelopathy attributed to multiple sclerosis. Munch *et al* (1995) demonstrated EBV and a novel retrovirus in a greater proportion of B-cell lines from patients with multiple sclerosis than controls. Against the background of failure to implicate human endogenous retroviruses (HERV) in multiple sclerosis (Rasmussen *et al* 1995), Clerici *et al* (1999) showed enhanced peripheral blood mononuclear cell proliferation and cytokine responses to human HERV peptides in patients with active multiple sclerosis. Trabbattoni *et al* (2000) reported increased production of interleukin-2 and IFN-α, and decreased amounts of interleukin-10 during disease activity, after stimulation of peripheral blood mononuclear cells from individuals with multiple sclerosis with HERV peptides. In a survey of HERV expression in monocytes and brain tissue from individuals with a variety of inflammatory brain diseases, Johnston *et al* (2001) claimed more specific increased expression of HERV-W and HERV-K in brain tissue from individuals with multiple sclerosis

(and selected other disorders). Christensen *et al* (2003) described increased levels of antibody to HERV-H/RGH-2 peptide sequences both in serum and cerebrospinal fluid, and detected HERV-H protease-env splice variant more frequently in mRNA extracts from peripheral blood lymphocytes. Most recently, a mechanistic explanation has been offered through demonstration that increased expression of the HERV-W encoded glycoprotein synactin in astrocytes recovered from acute lesions in multiple sclerosis proved toxic to oligodendrocytes through the release of reactive oxygen species; and antioxidants were effective in protecting oligodendrocytes and limiting the behavioural consequences of tissue injury, in a mouse model of inflammatory brain disease (Antony *et al* 2004).

One component of the HERV-W family is designated 'the multiple sclerosis associated retrovirus' (MSRV). Perron *et al* (1989) had first isolated this retrovirus from the spinal fluid of a patient with multiple sclerosis. Subsequently, this was demonstrated in serum samples from >50% patients in relapse, and extracellular virions were recovered from cerebrospinal fluid containing MSRV *pol* sequence in 5/10 patients with multiple sclerosis but no controls with other neurological diseases (Perron *et al* 1991; 1997). Similarities with paramyxovirus were used to explain serological findings previously reported in multiple sclerosis on the basis of antigen cross-reactivity. Human herpes virus 6 (HHV-6; see below) may trigger expression of MSRV. In collaborative work, Garson *et al* (1998) extended these observations to show that MSRV could be detected in serum from 9/17 (53%) patients, usually untreated, compared with 4/44 controls (7%). Evidence for an association between multiple sclerosis and MSRV continues to accumulate, with differences reported between cases and controls from Sardinia (Dolei *et al* 2002) perhaps correlating with a progressive clinical course (Sotgui *et al* 2002), but whether this is a causal or epiphenomenal relationship still remains unclear.

Immunological methods have been used to provide indirect evidence for virus exposure through, for example, the demonstration of antigen-specific differences in cytotoxic T-cell responses to measles (S. Jacobson *et al* 1985). Wucherpfennig and Strominger (1995) claimed that myelin basic protein-specific T-cell clones from patients with multiple sclerosis are activated by peptides based on those required for class II binding and T-cell recognition and derived both from a bacterium (*Pseudomonas aeruginosa*) and from several viruses (herpes simplex, adenovirus, papillomavirus, influenzavirus and EBV). Since only one pathogen showed sequence homology with the activating peptides, the suggestion is that more than one trigger can activate antigen-specific T cells as part of a non-specific response to infection (see also Chapter 11). An alternative approach has been to use similarities between the pathology and clinical course of virus-induced models of demyelination to support the hypothesis of viral causation in multiple sclerosis. Viral modelling of the pathology and course of human demyelinating disease remains attractive because of the ease with which these systems can be manipulated but the approach does not provide direct evidence for a viral cause in multiple sclerosis. For example, the same sequence of events characterizes the development of tissue injury in visna-maedi as that which occurs with evolution of the plaque in multiple sclerosis. A lentivirus-induced interferon response increases class II histocompatibility antigen expression, amplifying the inflammatory component, whilst also restricting viral replication and leading to persistent infection (Kennedy *et al* 1985). In Theiler's virus infection of the murine nervous system, the initial infection of neurons is followed by direct damage to oligodendrocytes, especially in the spinal cord, producing inflammation and demyelination (Fiette *et al* 1993; Pena-Rossi *et al* 1991). The recognition of genetic restriction in susceptibility to Theiler's virus infection (Bureau *et al* 1993) serves to increase the similarities with multiple sclerosis.

The results of population serology attracted much attention in the 1960s and 1970s but the candidature of organisms implicated through the demonstration of increased antibody titres could not be corroborated using independent techniques. Subsequently, sero-epidemiological studies of *Borrelia burgdorferi* suggested a link with multiple sclerosis. Chmielewska-Badora *et al* (2000) reported an increased frequency of seropositivity in patients with multiple sclerosis (38%) compared with controls (20%). Brorson *et al* (2001) described changes in cerebrospinal fluid and serological reactivity indicating that patients with multiple sclerosis harboured a spirochaetal organism indistinguishable from *B. burgdorferi*. The two organisms attracting most attention since we last reviewed the topic are human herpes virus 6 (HHV-6) and *Chlamydia pneumoniae*.

Sriram *et al* (1999) first identified *C. pneumoniae* in a single patient with multiple sclerosis. This then led to the detection in cerebrospinal fluid of chlamydia in more cases (64%) than controls (11%) and detection of chlamydial genetic material in most patients (97% compared with 18% in controls). There was an excess of anti-chlamydia antibodies (86% in cases vs. 18% in controls). Others could not confirm these findings (Boman *et al* 2000; Saiz *et al* 2001; Treib *et al* 2000). Although individual reports continue to describe an excess of antibodies to *C. pneumoniae* in the cerebrospinal fluid of patients with multiple sclerosis (Hao *et al* 2002; Krametter *et al* 2001; Sotgiu *et al* 2001a), or those with particular features (Contini *et al* 2004), perhaps the most telling study is a comparison between three laboratories of polymerase chain reaction detection rates for *Chlamydia pneumoniae* in the same samples, one being the laboratory that reported the original findings. Whereas Sriram *et al* (1999) found the organism in the majority of patients but few controls, the other two were unable to detect chlamydias in any samples (M. Kaufman *et al* 2002). The story is not settled. Derfuss *et al* (2001) confirmed an increase in intrathecal anti-C. *pneumoniae* antibody synthesis. There was no correlation with disease duration or severity. The oligoclonal bands did not react with *C. pneumoniae* antigen and this could not be identified using molecular techniques. Together, the results suggested a nonspecific polyclonal antibody response rather than implicating an aetiological role for *C. pneumoniae*. A population serology survey using the Nurses Health Study cohort showed an increased odds ratio of 1.7 (5% CI 1.1–2.7) for *C. pneumoniae* seropositivity, especially in patients with progressive multiple sclerosis (7.3: 95% CI 1.4–37.2; Munger *et al* 2003). Grimaldi *et al* (2003) detected sequences of the major outer membrane protein from cerebrospinal fluid in 21% of 107 patients with multiple sclerosis but only 3% of 77 controls. Amongst patients, MRI markers of disease activity and younger age at onset correlated with the presence of *C. pneumoniae* in cerebrospinal fluid samples from patients with relapsing–remitting multiple sclerosis but not those who had entered the chronic progressive

phase. Buljevac *et al* (2003a) correlated peaks in serologically defined C. *pneumoniae* (generally indicating positive polymerase chain reactions for chlamydia) with an increased risk of exacerbation. Dong-Si *et al* (2004) detected C. *pneumoniae*-specific DNA more frequently in the cerebrospinal fluid of individuals with relapsing–remitting multiple sclerosis than those with other neurological disease although the difference narrowed considerably in comparisons with cases having conditions other than multiple sclerosis but nevertheless with abnormalities of the spinal fluid – suggesting that activity rather than disease specificity is the critical trigger to this response.

Nonspecific features supporting the candidature of HHV-6 include the ubiquitous exposure early in childhood, neurotropism, ready reactivation, and the range of cell types that can be infected. But against that general background, Merelli *et al* (1997) failed to detect HHV-6 or HHV-8 DNA in all but a few samples of mononuclear cells from 56 patients with multiple sclerosis. Although HHV-8 could be detected in brain tissue from each of five patients, virus was also recovered from adult but not perinatal stillborn controls. Ablashi *et al* (1998) found that patients with multiple sclerosis had an excess of antibody to early HHV-6 protein (>68% vs. 28% in controls) in comparison with EBV and cytomegalovirus. J.E. Friedman *et al* (1999) reported an excess of HHV-6 structural protein, and antibody to HHV-6 in serum and brain tissue in multiple sclerosis compared with controls. Soldan *et al* (2000) showed increased peripheral blood lymphocyte reactivity of the neurotropic HHV-6A variant. Knox *et al* (2000) identified HHV-6 in 73% of brain and lymphoid tissue samples from patients with multiple sclerosis, especially those showing active demyelination (90%), more often than in controls (13%). In a comprehensive virological screen for HHV-6 infection, Chapenko *et al* (2003) correlated genomic sequences and viral mRNA transcription in peripheral blood mononuclear cells, plasma viraemia, and serum antibodies with clinical, radiological and immunological features of multiple sclerosis. They concluded that HHV-6 is associated with multiple sclerosis, and virus reactivation occurs during periods of disease activity perhaps through modulation of interleukin-12 (IL-12) synthesis. Goodman *et al* (2003) identified HHV-6 genome but not viral antigen in lymphocytes, oligodendrocytes and microglia from all of five biopsies in patients with multiple sclerosis. In pursuing a mechanistic hypothesis, Tejada-Simon *et al* (2003) identified a peptide having identical sequence in myelin basic protein (residues 96–102) and HHV-6 (residues 4–10). Patients had increased antibody titres to both antigens compared with controls and a high proportion of T cells recognized and reacted identically to either the myelin basic protein or HHV-6 derived peptides. But a serological study failed to confirm excess seropositivity for HHV-6 in patients with multiple sclerosis from Kuwait (Al-Shammari *et al* 2003). The most recent reports continue to provide conflicting evidence. Based on an uncontrolled study, Rotola *et al* (2004), reported evidence for HHV-6 (variant A) infection early in the course of multiple sclerosis. Conversely, Tuke *et al* (2004) showed no difference between cases and controls or between plaques and non-plaque regions in post-mortem brain tissue.

Reviewing the evidence from the position of sceptical virus watchers in multiple sclerosis, Swanborg *et al* (2003) conclude that the candidature of neither C. *pneumoniae* nor HHV-6 is yet secure. Review of the literature concerning varicella zoster virus reaches the same negative conclusion on its potential role in the pathogenesis of multiple sclerosis (Marrie and Wolfson 2001). Uncertainty breeds speculation. Those who develop hypotheses about the aetiology and mechanisms of multiple sclerosis exercise the luxury of picking selectively from the entire corpus of knowledge on the disease, any facts that decorate their particular interpretation without necessarily having to test the ideas experimentally. Although often a harmless enough armchair exercise, occasionally the ideas cause distress, undermine mainstream doctrines on the aetiology and mechanisms of tissue injury in multiple sclerosis, require time spent dealing with spurious media interest provoked by the more provocative claims, and distract from serious research. According to Hawkes (2002), multiple sclerosis is sexually transmitted – teenage-onset cases representing examples of child abuse. In the distress that followed this suggestion, the author claimed that his ideas were not intended for lay attention – but agreed to speak on national radio. An institution to which the article was linked dissociated itself from responsibility. Journalists waved the freedom of speech banner. Patients were upset. The Multiple Sclerosis Society was kept busy with enquiries and its professional advisers were required to assemble coherent arguments to offset the implausible. Our own view expressed at the time was that as no new facts were reported, this paper had little if any scientific value. The hypothesis fell down quickly and repeatedly in the face of known facts. The specific claim that multiple sclerosis in young people might result from child abuse seemed mischievous and deeply wounding.

The many unsuccessful attempts to identify causative factors that trigger the disease process leading to demyelination in patients with multiple sclerosis, have fuelled speculation on whether the environmental event is an unusual reaction to a ubiquitous agent or the ubiquitous response to a rare infection (P.G.E. Kennedy and Steiner 1994). The story of searches for a candidate that qualifies as the cause (or one cause) of multiple sclerosis seems much influenced by biomedical fashion and technical opportunities deploying increasingly sophisticated methods of investigation. As each new microbial hare is set running, chased and caught, we seem no closer to incriminating a particular agent.

Noninfectious environmental events

Pursuing reasons for the gender bias in the frequency of multiple sclerosis, Hernán *et al* (2000) used the Nurses' Health Studies I and II (involving 315 index cases from amongst 121 700 aged 30–55 years in 1976 and 116 671 aged 25–42 years in 1989) to show that neither parity nor use of the oral contraceptive pill influence the risk of developing multiple sclerosis, even after adjustment for potential confounding effects. The relationship of pregnancy to multiple sclerosis mainly affects relapse rate in those with established disease (see Chapter 4) rather than the risk of developing multiple sclerosis. There is no evidence that the onset of multiple sclerosis clusters around pregnancy (Birk *et al* 1990; Roullet *et al* 1993; Worthington *et al* 1994). Coming at the problem from the position of whether the higher reported relative risk for multiple sclerosis should be used to modify protocols for hepatitis B vaccination, Tosti *et al* (1999) concluded that much would be lost and little gained in terms of overall public health measures by discontinuing the existing vaccination

programme. Perhaps they need not have worried. Zipp *et al* (1999) did not observe any increase in monophasic demyelinating diseases or multiple sclerosis after hepatitis B vaccination in a cohort of 134 698 individuals enrolled in a United States health care database from 1988 to 1995. Using the Nurses Health Study databases, Ascherio *et al* (2001) showed that the risk of developing multiple sclerosis (and the risk of relapse in individuals with pre-existing disease, see Chapter 4) is not increased after hepatitis B vaccination (relative risk 0.9: 95% CI 0.5–1.6 for any exposure; and 0.7: 95% CI 0.3–1.8 for the previous 2 years) irrespective of the dose or use of recombinant vaccines. But all is not settled. Hernán *et al* (2004) used the General Practice Research Database (GPRD) in the United Kingdom to assess the frequency of immunizations in the 3-year period before onset of symptoms in a cohort of 163 cases incident over a 7-year period compared with 1604 controls. There was an increased risk attributable to hepatitis B (odds ratio 3.1, 95% CI 1.5–6.3) but not tetanus or influenza vaccinations. Commentators have drawn attention to epidemiological deficiencies of this study.

There is a basic human need to explain unexpected illness and everyone feels unreserved sympathy for the person who has multiple sclerosis in their coming to terms with the clinical manifestations and adjusting to their social and domestic implications. It is understandable that an affected person should connect onset or a change in clinical course with life events, such as a recent road traffic accident, but this necessarily raises issues of general importance in which compassion cannot influence the interpretation of evidence. Although the overwhelming majority of medical opinion does not support the conclusion that there is any relationship between trauma and multiple sclerosis, this view is not universally held. The possibility of a relationship between trauma and multiple sclerosis began with the clinical observation that some patients recall an episode of trauma shortly before the onset of symptoms or an exacerbation of pre-existing manifestations of the disease. Clinical anecdotes sustained this belief in an era when evidence-based medicine was poorly developed. Even then, many neurologists concluded that the relationship was coincidental. Since there is consensus that the process leading to tissue damage in the central nervous system that forms the pathological basis for multiple sclerosis is established in childhood, no informed person would now claim that trauma causes the disease. But that leaves unanswered the subsidiary questions of whether trauma allows latent multiple sclerosis to manifest, causes clinically overt disease to relapse, or adversely affects the natural history of the disease (see Chapter 4).

In the 1970s, some patients with multiple sclerosis were advised to have all their amalgam dental fillings replaced on the basis that these contained elemental mercury at about 50% by weight. Mercury is absorbed from amalgam fillings and accumulates in tissues, including the central nervous system. However, we are not aware of any epidemiological evidence that correlates dental management with any aspect of multiple sclerosis, and share the view of the American Dental Association (see *Lancet* 3 August 2002, p. 393) that patients should not have their fillings replaced. Although no difference in number of amalgam fillings (and hence body mercury levels) was found in a case–control study from Leicestershire (England) involving 39 female prevalent patients, McGrother *et al* (1999) correlated dental caries with an increased risk of having multiple sclerosis. Cassetta *et al* (2001) have also formalized the status of this risk factor, showing no significant association between amalgam fillings and the risk of multiple sclerosis. Moving from teeth to industrial exposure, Mortensen *et al* (1998) used the Danish Multiple Sclerosis Register to exclude an effect on the risk of developing multiple sclerosis from presumed solvent exposure by nature of occupation. A national newspaper in the United Kingdom (*Guardian*, 7 June 2003) highlighted the plight of a small community in Scotland where 10 of 600 residents developed multiple sclerosis (period prevalence c.1700/10^5), allegedly due to tributyltin exposure related to protecting the hulls of small ships from overgrowth of barnacles.

In a rambling review, Behan *et al* (2003) claimed that multiple sclerosis is a neurodegenerative and invariably clinically progressive trait driven by the product of a gene encoded on chromosome 17 that is influenced by sunlight and vitamin D activity. We provide a critical analysis of this hypothesis in Chapter 1. But is there substance to the sunshine theory? Acheson *et al* (1960) first linked variations in disease frequency to hours of annual and winter solar radiation taking the position that visible solar radiation protected individuals from developing multiple sclerosis. Lindstedt (1991) related this directly to the latitudinal gradient in disease frequency. Castigating others for not seeing the light with respect to the aetiology of multiple sclerosis, Hutter and Laing (1996) developed the hypothesis that illumination suppresses the immune activation properties of melatonin and the release of inflammatory leukotrienes – making the case for an immunosuppressant effect of environmental light at 2500 lux, and explaining the seasonal onset (winter) of symptoms due to demyelinating disease. Also backing melanin as a marker of the effect, Dumas and Jauberteau-Marchan (2000) proposed that sunlight inhibits the function of cutaneous antigen presentation (Langerhans cells). They suggested that this might account for the rarity of multiple sclerosis in blacks, whereas white immigrants to sunny places possess genes that cannot benefit from the protective effects of sunshine. Conversely, the offspring of these immigrants are advantaged by early exposure to sunlight since this sets their melanocyte and Langerhans cell repertoire more favourably. Mortality returns for multiple sclerosis documented in 24 North American states from 1984 to 1995 showed a negative correlation (i.e. protection) from residential and occupational sunlight (odds ratio 0.24; D.M. Freedman *et al* 2000). Previously, Norman *et al* (1983) had made the valid point that whilst air pollution, ground minerals, solar radiation, temperature, annual rainfall and humidity all correlated independently with birthplace in 4371 veterans having multiple sclerosis, these associations were all eliminated by correction for latitude suggesting that the correlations were confounded. van der Mei *et al* (2001) found a strong inverse relationship between ultraviolet radiation and prevalence of multiple sclerosis in six Australian regions, and offered an immunological hypothesis based on T-cell-mediated immunosuppression to account for these findings. Later, they provided an inverse correlation between exposure to sunshine in childhood and early adolescence, especially during the winter months, and the subsequent development of multiple sclerosis in Tasmania (odds ratio 0.31: 95% CI 0.16–0.59; van der Mei *et al* 2003). These epidemiological data have been used to support the hypothesis that $1\alpha,25$-(OH)$_2$ vitamin D3 exerts an anti-

inflammatory effect mediated through enhanced suppressor cell function (Hayes *et al* 2003). Amongst 187 563 individuals registered with the Nurses Health Study I and II, prospective analysis of dietary vitamin D showed a protective effect of highest compared with lowest intake (age-adjusted relative risk 0.67: 95% CI 0.40–1.12) and for dietary supplementation (0.59: 95% CI 0.38–0.91; Munger *et al* 2004).

Oikonen *et al* (2003) correlated monthly hospital admissions for 1205 exacerbations in 406 patients with multiple sclerosis from southwestern Finland during 1985–1999 with ambient air quality, and correlated relapse rate with high concentrations of inhalable particulate matter (PM10). The confounding effect of PM10s on respiratory infection and relapse rate was not thought responsible for this effect. Bolviken *et al* (2003) mapped gradients in the distribution of multiple sclerosis in Norway with radon in indoor air, and suggested that this is modulated by exchangeable magnesium in the soil and rainfall – each reducing the availability of aerial radon – and showing a negative relationship with multiple sclerosis. Gilmore and Grennan (2003) supported the hypothesis that radon exposure at <15 years is a risk factor for multiple sclerosis. Others have examined the relationship between multiple sclerosis and exposure to ionizing radiation. Based on pooled analysis from two case–control series, Axelson *et al* (2001) reported an odds ratio of 4.4 (95% CI 1.2–2.6) for radiological work and X-ray examinations, noting that five cases in one series had been treated with ionizing radiation.

The possibility that something related to climate may yet be involved is supported by a recent epidemiologically sophisticated survey using 17 874 cases from the Canadian population-based register and 11 502 affected individuals from the United Kingdom, part population-based and part retrospectively identified from death certificates (Willer *et al* 2005). In both countries, being born in November was protective for the development of multiple sclerosis, and (in the United Kingdom) birth in May placed individuals at increased risk – each by comparison with unrelated and sibling controls. Combining these samples and datasets from Scandinavia showed that 8.5% of the 42 045 individuals were born in November compared with 9.1% in May [p corrected (p_c)<0.0001 for each comparison with controls], representing a 13% increase in risk for those born in May (95% CI 5–22%). The effect showed some regional variation, being most apparent in Scotland where the prevalence of multiple sclerosis is high. Despite the very discrete intervals of protection and risk, the authors do not doubt the validity of their findings (based on large numbers, replication and internal consistencies), and consider that these reconcile previous ambiguous findings on season of birth and risk of multiple sclerosis from these same countries (Sadovnick and Yee 1994; Salemi *et al* 2000b; Torrey *et al* 2000; Wiberg and Templer 1994). They offer maternal folate, correlates of infant birth weight, virus infection, and factors predisposing to schizophrenia (which evidently shows a similar effect) – but not signs of the Zodiac – as candidates, preferring seasonal reductions in levels of maternal vitamin D as the most plausible explanation.

With little progress made from the selection of candidate conditions that might account for the environmental factor in multiple sclerosis, less focused screens have been performed in the hope that a general trawl might yield an interesting catch. Such an approach is statistically fraught given the probability of 1:20 factors generating a 'statistically significant' result if considered alone. But, to date, screening populations of patients for antecedent events that can be implicated in the initiation of multiple sclerosis has not identified novel environmental triggers. Souberbielle *et al* (1990) found no difference in past history of specific infections or autoimmune disease in 230 cases and 230 controls although there was an excess amongst cases of hairdressers, and those having professional contact with pathology specimens. The previously reported claim that patients with multiple sclerosis have a greater number of childhood domiciles than controls is refuted by Savettieri *et al* (1991). S. Warren *et al* (1991a) reported a case–control study of environmental conditions at onset and during childhood in 173 Canadian patients with multiple sclerosis. Apart from a family history of diabetes (and multiple sclerosis) in patients with age of onset at <20 years, and some association with rural residence, no aetiological clues emerged from this study. In an exhaustive survey, Kurtzke *et al* (1997) revealed no clues regarding the cause of the putative series of multiple sclerosis epidemics on the Faroe Islands by comparing education, occupation, residences, bathing, sanitary or drinking facilities, domestic architecture or source of heating, diet, contact with animals, most vaccinations (those for smallpox, tetanus and diphtheria were less common), history of exanthematous illnesses, operations, hospitalizations and injuries, and age at menarche. Based on a comparison of 200 recent-onset cases with 202 controls, Ghadirian *et al* (2001) described an increased risk of multiple sclerosis through cigarette smoking, eye disease, a family history of cancer and autoimmune disease, trauma (see below) and contact with caged birds, whereas there was an inverse relationship between disease frequency and contact with cats. The relative

incidence rate for women who smoke is increased and related to duration of exposure, changing from 1.2 (95% confidence intervals 0.9–1.6) in past smokers, to 1.6 (95% confidence intervals 1.2–2.1) in current smokers, 1.1 (95% confidence intervals 0.8–1.6) for 1–9 pack-years, 1.5 (95% confidence intervals 1.2–2.1) for 1–24 pack years, and 1.7 (95% confidence intervals 1.2–2.4) for ≥25 years (Hernán *et al* 2001b). Riise *et al* (2003) also demonstrated an increased risk of multiple sclerosis (relative risk 2.7 for men and 1.6 for women) amongst 22 312 residents of Hordaland County, Norway, who had smoked for ≥15 years. Most recently, Hernán *et al* (2005) compared smoking habits amongst 201 people with multiple sclerosis registered with the General Practice Research Database between January 1993 and December 2000 and 1913 matched controls to show a modest increase in risk (odds ratio 1.3: 95% CI 1.0–1.7) that was more marked for those who had developed secondary progression at a mean follow-up interval of 5.3 years (hazard ratio 3.6 (5% CI 1.3–9.9).

Whether this catalogue includes environmental factors – microbes or conditions unrelated to infectious disease – that do genuinely determine the development of tissue injury in multiple sclerosis must, for now, be a matter of opinion. Many will remain to be convinced that anything of relevance has yet been identified. Others will have greater confidence in the observations made to date: age at infection by EBV; HHV-6; and climate-related alterations in vitamin D status will all have their advocates. But by any analysis, chasing the environmental factor(s) in multiple sclerosis has proved to be an even more perplexing and unrewarding task than practically any other branch of research into this enigmatic disease.

The genetics of multiple sclerosis

3

Alastair Compston and Hartmut Wekerle

GENETIC ANALYSIS OF MULTIPLE SCLEROSIS

The concept of genetic susceptibility was suggested in the early descriptions of multiple sclerosis. Efforts at unravelling this contribution to the aetiology have been sustained, deploying both classic and molecular genetic approaches. Progress has been slow. Milestones in the story include awareness that the condition may be familial (Eichorst 1896), appreciation of differences in gender related and ethnic risks (Davenport 1921; 1922), systematic studies of recurrence risk in families (Ebers *et al* 1986; R.T.C. Pratt *et al* 1951; Sadovnick and Baird 1988), and description of the major histocompatibility complex class I and II associations (Compston *et al* 1976; Jersild *et al* 1972; Terasaki *et al* 1976; Winchester *et al* 1975). Much of this knowledge was in place by the mid-1970s. Surprisingly little further progress has been made over the subsequent 25 years despite the development of strategies for the analysis of complex traits (Risch 1990a; 1990b; 1990c), and the availability of an increasingly versatile range of reagents. The first molecular analysis used restriction fragment length polymorphisms (RFLPs: Botstein *et al* 1980) and appeared in the 1980s (D. Cohen *et al* 1984). Later, the diversity and number of markers began to increase with the availability of microsatellite repeats of di-, tri- and tetranucleotides (Dib *et al* 1996; Gyapay *et al* 1994; Weber and May 1989). Now, it is apparent that the genome is peppered with single nucleotide polymorphisms (SNPs) – theoretically providing a set of markers having properties suitable for detecting all genetic variations, and accounting for the modest increases in susceptibility. As these markers are mapped to sections of the genome adjacent to defined loci, an almost unlimited opportunity arises to screen candidate genes. This luxury of reagents has required new strategies for genetic analysis – sensitive to statistical limitations of genotyping on an industrial scale and the false trails resulting from sampling variance. The pendulum has swung to and from the use of association and linkage as the preferred strategy for detecting these factors (see below). Most studies have focused on the question of disease susceptibility. Some effort has also gone into characterizing genetic effects on clinical features and the disease course, but without unambiguous evidence for the existence of such disease-modifying genes.

Systematic efforts to identify the genetic variants determining susceptibility to multiple sclerosis on the basis of gene maps, and without prejudice as to the number or biological strength of contributory factors, began in the mid-1990s with the advent of whole genome screening for linkage (J.L. Davies *et al* 1994). The first three such screens in multiple sclerosis were published, by agreement amongst the principal investigators, back-to-back in 1996 (Ebers *et al* 1996; Haines *et al* 1996; Sawcer *et al* 1996). When these experiments were conceived, it was generally agreed that an analysis of around 100 affected family members (typically sibling pairs) using about 300 microsatellite markers would provide sufficient power to identify most, if not all, of the susceptibility loci. In fact, none of the screens identified statistically secure linkage, even in the major histocompatibility complex where it was already established on the basis of population associations that a gene must be encoded. In the disappointment that followed, it took some time to appreciate what had gone wrong and to realize that these screens still provided valuable information despite their failure to reveal novel regions of unequivocal linkage. Researchers were forced to accept that the effects attributable to individual loci influencing susceptibility to multiple sclerosis must be smaller than originally assumed. Once this was appreciated, it was quickly realized that association testing would provide a considerably more powerful method for mapping such genes than linkage in affected family members (Risch and Merikangas 1996). Indeed, association is more powerful than linkage in almost every situation (Risch 2000), except where disease results from highly penetrant low-frequency variants – generally known as Mendelian disorders. The problem with setting out systematically to screen the genome for association is the huge number of variants that must be considered (Kruglyak 1999). In the late 1990s, it was clear that only a fraction of the potentially relevant genes had been identified, and that a full list of all functionally relevant variants relating to each was also far from complete. The advent of technology enabling such a screen to be completed (within reasonable time and financial constraints) seemed remote. In 2005, despite exponential growth in the number of identified single nucleotide polymorphisms (SNPs), the position whereby a direct screen of all common/functionally relevant polymorphisms can be undertaken is still some time off. In the vacuum between linkage and direct association screening, application of DNA pooling technology (Barcellos *et al* 1997a) allowed a first pass at screening the genome for association in multiple sclerosis (Sawcer *et al* 2002). Systematic cataloguing of genes and the assignment of their functional properties – culminating in a working draft representing 90% of the euchromatic entire human genome

(International Human Genome Sequencing Consortium 2001; Ventner *et al* 2001) – now provides an opportunity to search an increasingly informative database of mapped genes. Thus, investigators can identify a region of interest on one or more of the 23 chromosomes, varying between 50 and 250 Mb, and immediately identify positional candidates from amongst c.30 000 genes listed on the publicly available Ensembl database, selected both for topography and biological plausibility. The cataloguing of genetic knowledge, access to that information, and the challenge of how reliably to sift the mountain of readily available data are only now being systematically addressed.

METHODS OF GENETIC ANALYSIS

The recognition that multiple sclerosis occurs more frequently in the relatives of people who have the disease, than in those who do not, led to the systematic collection of multiplex families, the determination of recurrence risks for each category of relative, the recruitment of affected and unaffected individuals for genetic studies, and the collection of samples suitable for analysis using modern molecular techniques aimed at mapping and identifying the various susceptibility factors.

Pedigree analysis

Before the advent of molecular genetics, the study of genetic susceptibility in disease was through analysis of pedigrees having more than one affected family member (Figure 3.1). An estimate of genetic risk can be established by determining the frequency of familial cases, and recurrence in defined categories of relatives compared with disease frequency in the population. Familial rates are calculated by comparing proportions and distributions using the chi-squared and log-rank tests, respectively. Recurrence risk within families is expressed as the risk ratio for relatives in different categories compared with the population frequency of disease. The Greek symbol λ is often used to describe the increased risk over and above the population frequency of multiple sclerosis, specified for the category of relative under consideration – conventionally siblings, hence λs. Values for λ can be used as a rough guide to the number of genes conferring susceptibility to multiple sclerosis and their modes of inheritance.

Pedigree analysis depends critically on reliable assignment of disease status amongst family members. Age adjustment is essential given uncertain clinical status in younger family members. For the specific purpose of family studies, the aim is to orientate criteria for inclusion towards biological reality

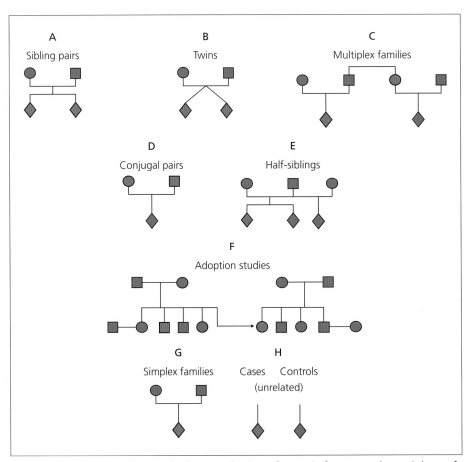

Figure 3.1 Family relationships that can be used to study the contribution of genetic factors to the aetiology of multiple sclerosis. (A) Sibling pairs. (B) Twins. (C) Multiplex families. (D) Conjugal pairs. (E) Half-siblings. (F) Adoption studies. (G) Simplex families. (H) Unrelated cases and controls.

rather than current clinical status whilst nevertheless avoiding the inclusion of doubtful cases. Recurrence risks may therefore need to be estimated under conditions of varying clinical stringency. It is always better to consider these issues when planning the study and not as a defensive position during analysis. A hierarchy for syndromes that may anticipate the subsequent conversion to multiple sclerosis can be proposed. The majority of patients with optic neuritis eventually convert to multiple sclerosis and these cases may be included whereas clinical phenotypes having a lower recurrence risk, such as transverse myelitis, are handled differently.

The use of families for determining the contribution made by genetic factors to susceptibility is best illustrated by the study of concordance in twin pairs, one of whom is already known to have multiple sclerosis (the index case). The expectation is that concordance will occur more often in identical than non-identical twin pairs if there is a genetic contribution to disease causation (Bundey 1991). Although dizygotic twins are genetically no more alike than non-twin siblings, they have closer environmental exposure, before and after birth, potentially leading to non-genetic differences in disease frequency between dizygotic twins and non-twin siblings. Concordance may be quoted as the pair-wise rate: this is the proportion of all pairs in which both partners have multiple sclerosis. It measures genetic contribution to that trait. The proband-wise rate is the recurrence risk in co-twins and this reflects the magnitude of the effect. However, defining probands is not straightforward in concordant pairs since it depends on the method of notification. When twin cohorts are population based, their identification is independent of the disease trait and every affected individual is then a proband even if related to another case. It follows that proband-wise are higher than pairwise rates. Incomplete concordance amongst identical twins has several interpretations. It may occur in Mendelian disorders due to stochastic or chance events. This is designated incomplete penetrance. However, with falling concordance, the role of environmental factors becomes more probable. Approximately 1:80 births are twin. The expected monozygotic:dizygotic ratio is 1:2. Ascertainment bias has probably affected cohorts deviating markedly from this proportion. In practice, where methodology has led to ascertainment bias, the clues are excesses of monozygotic pairs, females and concordant cases.

Pedigree analysis in multiple sclerosis can be extended to include comparisons of recurrence risk in situations that are informative with respect to the relative contribution of genes and the environment in determining disease frequency. Against the yardstick of λs, recurrence risks can be assessed in half-siblings, adoptees and the offspring of conjugal pairs. Since each has to be compared with the population risk, this must first have been accurately ascertained for the demographic group of interest. In multiple sclerosis, the evidence from pedigree analysis effectively excludes single-locus Mendelian inheritance. Multiple sclerosis is assumed to be polygenic. In using affected family members to assess the contribution made by genetic factors to the clinical course and disease pattern, the strategy is to select variables of interest and determine pairwise concordance in a sufficient sample to achieve statistical power. If one disease feature shows excess concordance, affected twin pairs can be used to establish that the effect is genetic and not the result of shared environment. Families with >2 affecteds, and the off-spring of conjugal pairs, are used to assess gene–dose effects. Parent–child pairs can be used to indicate parental imprinting or sex differences in the inherited risk. Potentially, this is confounded by the excess female risk of multiple sclerosis so that the number of mother–daughter should exceed that of father–son pairs. But the main advantage of access to familial cases and their cooperation in genetic analyses of multiple sclerosis is to support molecular genetic strategies for the identification of susceptibility factors.

The analysis of complex traits

Genetic analysis offers the possibility of identifying factors that confer susceptibility to a complex disease such as multiple sclerosis even in the absence of any prior knowledge about the number and nature of the genes involved. Two strategies can be employed – linkage and association (Risch 1990a; 1990b; 1990c; Risch and Merikangas 1996; Risch 2000). Systematic screening of particular chromosomes or even the entire genome may be performed, or markers are selected either on the basis of *a priori* assumptions concerning the nature of susceptibility (candidate genes), or their location within chromosomal regions of interest (positional candidates). Individual markers are rarely informative in every subject tested (single point analysis), in which case information from adjacent markers can be used to estimate the missing data (multipoint analysis). One of the great virtues of genetic analysis is the ease with which evidence derived from independent studies can formally be combined.

Linkage describes the situation in which ≥2 affected relatives share parts of the genome encoding susceptibility genes and nearby markers for a complex trait more often than expected by chance. It has low power but operates over a wide genetic distance. Association is present when people with multiple sclerosis are shown to have a higher frequency of markers informative for alleles increasing susceptibility than unaffected individuals. Association has high statistical power but depends on linkage disequilibrium (see below; a clumsy term, not to be confused with linkage) and therefore operates over short genetic distances. The extent of linkage disequilibrium differs across the genome and between populations. A genetic marker can consist either of a single allele encoded at one locus. Alternatively, it may be a haplotype – a group of alleles encoded at adjacent loci on one particular chromosomal region, and inherited as a block without being disturbed by chromosomal recombination.

Linkage

Linkage has been particularly successful at identifying the genes responsible for monogenic traits, so called because they segregate through families in a pattern that is clearly discernible as following Mendelian laws. In these conditions, the alleles responsible are generally essential to the development of the disease, confer a significant risk when inherited (are highly penetrant), and occur only at low frequency in the general population. Under these circumstances the phenotype of any one individual (affected or unaffected) strongly predicts their underlying disease genotype. Armed with this knowledge, it is possible to perform a linkage analysis by seeking to identify a marker that is inherited through affected pedigrees in the same fashion as the disease. This is a particularly powerful approach.

Unfortunately, in multiple sclerosis, analysis of segregation within families suggests that no particular genotype is essential for the development of the disease, that the risk is conferred by multiple genes, and that each susceptibility allele exerts only a modest effect (each has low penetrance). Large extended pedigrees are uncommon in multiple sclerosis and no discernible model of inheritance can be determined or tested. In this more complex setting, the power of linkage is therefore greatly reduced, and invariably very much less than tests for association (Risch 2000; Risch and Merikangas 1996), although analysis can still be performed using so-called nonparametric approaches (Penrose 1935; Risch 1990a; 1990b; 1990c). These methods are based on the fact that affected individuals within families will tend to share parts of the genome containing susceptibility alleles more often than expected by chance alone regardless of the mode of inheritance. Testing for linkage in this way is thus independent of the underlying model – hence the term nonparametric.

Since cosegregation of a marker and disease within a family can occur by chance, as does excess allele sharing amongst affected family members, evidence for linkage is usually presented in terms of a lod score: this is the logarithm of the odds favouring linkage, being simply the likelihood of observing the data in the presence of linkage divided by the likelihood of observing the data under the null hypothesis of no linkage. In traditional linkage analysis, a lod score of >3 provides strong evidence in favour of linkage, while in nonparametric analysis higher thresholds have been considered necessary (Lander and Kruglyak 1995). Although linkage analysis has only limited power in the context of complex disease when applied to nuclear families, it is expected that large segments of the genome will be shared (since relatively few recombinant events will occur within any one family). As a result, the whole genome can be screened using a relatively modest number of markers making a linkage-based approach extremely efficient. In the early 1990s developments in the human genome project

reached the point where such linkage screens became possible to perform and many such studies have now been completed in multiple sclerosis and other complex diseases. As sibling pairs are generally the most numerous co-affected relatives, and are easy to collect, most of these studies have been based on nuclear families of this type. Under Mendel's laws, a pair of siblings have a 50% probability of inheriting the same paternal allele identical by descent (IBD), and a 50% probability of inheriting the same maternal allele IBD (Figure 3.2). Therefore in the absence of linkage, 25% of affected sibling pairs share both alleles, 50% just one allele (maternal or paternal) and 25% no alleles IBD. Deviation away from this position in favour of excess sharing suggests the presence of linkage. However, determining the actual extent of IBD sharing is not always so straightforward. Because markers are imperfect and do not always uniquely distinguish all four grandparental alleles, simply comparing the genotype of affected siblings – identity by state (IBS) – cannot always identify the extent of sharing IBD (Figures 3.3 and 3.4).

When parents are homozygous, or have the same genotype as each other, the extent of IBD sharing in a pair of siblings cannot be determined unambiguously. This becomes even more uncertain when parental genotypes are unknown, as is often the case for late-onset diseases like multiple sclerosis where parents are not infrequently deceased at the time of study. In this situation, much can be gained from typing other unaffected siblings through which the missing parental genotypes can be more accurately predicted. In multiple affected sibships, several sibling pairs can be considered but various authors have pointed out that the evidence for linkage from each possible pair should be weighted downwards since not all the pairs are fully independent of each other (Payami *et al* 1985; Suarez and Hodge 1979). Since affected sibling pair studies only use information from affected individuals, issues concerning age-dependent penetrance in the unaffected individuals do not arise. The extent of IBD sharing in the gaps between markers can be

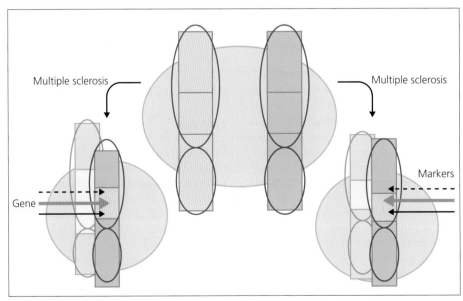

Figure 3.2 Scheme to represent the principles of linkage analysis, with recombination occurring at different chromosomal breakpoints during each meiosis so that some markers are always part of the haplotype shared between affected siblings and others, further removed from the susceptibility gene, are not.

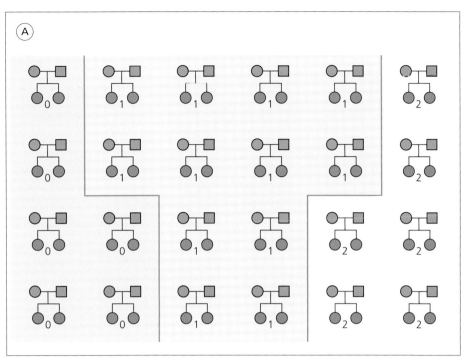

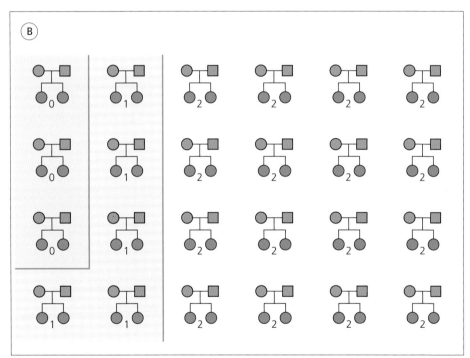

Figure 3.3 Twenty-four sibling pairs typed for a random marker. (A) Distribution of both, either one, or neither allele encoded at this locus is 6/24 (left), 12/24 (middle) and 6/24 (right) as expected from Mendelian principles. (B) Distribution of both, either one, or neither allele encoded at this locus is 3/24, 5/24 and 16/24, respectively, suggesting linkage. Kindly provided by Dr Stephen Sawcer.

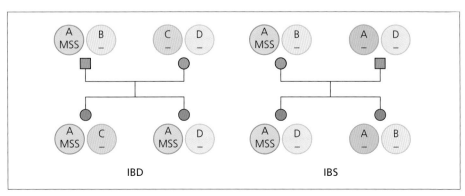

Figure 3.4 Difference between genes present in two affected siblings with multiple sclerosis that have been inherited as part of the same – identity by descent (IBD; lefthand scheme) – and different – identity by state (IBS; righthand scheme) – ancestral haplotypes. A, B, C and D are markers for the four parental haplotypes; *MSS* is the putative susceptibility gene. In the example of IBS, the same haplotype (A) is present in both parents, but only one carries the susceptibility gene for multiple sclerosis (*MSS*).

estimated by allowing for the possibility of recombinant events. The extent to which IBD sharing can accurately be determined is further reduced in these intervals. A variety of computer programs have been developed (Abecasis *et al* 2002; Kruglyak and Lander 1995; Krugylak *et al* 1996) that estimate the extent of IBD sharing using available genotyping data and then compare this statistically with sharing expected in the absence of linkage (Holmans 1993; Risch 1990a; 1990b; 1990c). Many of these programs depend upon estimates of allele frequency, which are generally derived from the data themselves. The proportion of potentially available information about IBD sharing that has been extracted at a particular point in the genome can be also calculated, and provides a useful guide to how well the study has interrogated the available families. In addition, the evidence for linkage supporting particular genetic models can also be tested allowing the creation of exclusion maps. These indicate the extent to which the observed data are consistent with the genetic model under consideration. Regions of the genome where the maximum lod score (MLS) is less than –2 are generally considered to have been excluded from containing a gene conferring the effect tested (Figure 3.5). Stratification is an appealing approach, but its value has been overestimated and the dangers of producing false positive leads underappreciated.

The more markers typed in a linkage screen, the greater the proportion of information extracted and therefore the more powerful the study. However, this is not a linear relationship and additional markers tend to extract decremental amounts of additional information. The number studied is thus a balance between the power desired and the number that can feasibly be typed. When whole genome screening in complex diseases was first employed, the optimal balance was considered to indicate a set of 300–400 microsatellites (E.R. Hauser *et al* 1996). However, as genotyping technology advanced it became clear that denser sets of single nucleotide polymorphism (SNP) markers offer significant advantages (Sawcer *et al* 2004). For a given approach, the number and nature of the families considered primarily determine power. It is now clear that previous estimates for the number of families needed (c.100) were too low and most published studies are therefore underpowered. Datasets of almost 1000 affected family members are still not yielding definitive results (GAMES and Transatlantic Multiple Sclerosis Consortium 2003; International Multiple Sclerosis Genetic Consortium 2005). A theoretical estimate, assuming that susceptibility alleles have a modest frequency and are not rare or ubiquitous, indicates that 1000 sibling pairs are needed to detect a gene conferring λs 1.3, with 5000 pairs needed to identify genes with λs 1.12 (Risch and Merikangas 1996).

Association

Directly testing all variants in the human population for evidence of association would be an ideal way to identify those that determine susceptibility, since these would be certain to be included. However, the full extent of variation is unknown and even the identified variants are too many to study using any currently feasible approach. Fortunately, the evidence suggests that it may not be necessary to test all the variations, and association may be detected indirectly by typing key variants that capture most of the information in their immediate vicinity. Because DNA replication is a high fidelity process, sequence changes

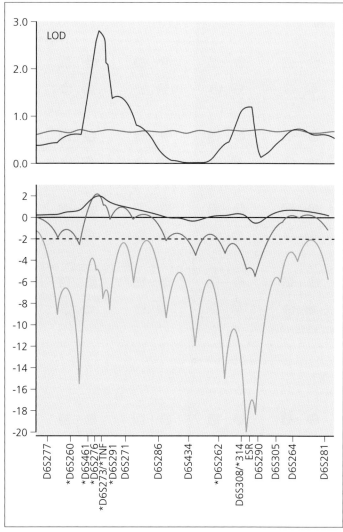

Figure 3.5 Observed multipoint lod scores based on sharing zero, one or two alleles identical by descent for multiple random markers on chromosome 6 (top). Corresponding exclusion map (bottom) for genes conferring susceptibility to multiple sclerosis located on chromosome 6. This shows, for several values of λs, the probability that a susceptibility gene is not encoded at each locus under the model of partial dominance. The indication that, despite a lod score of 4, a susceptibility locus could not be excluded (as seemed likely from previous association studies) was born out by subsequent linkage analysis (see Figure 3.19). Kindly provided by Dr Stephen Sawcer.

(SNPs) are introduced only very infrequently. As a corollary, most copies of a variant allele that is common in the population (those occurring in more than just a few individuals) are likely to have the same ancestral origin. That is, they are likely to be descendants of a single ancestral mutational event, rather than to have arisen as a result of multiple identical mutations at the same locus. When a mutational event occurs it does so on a single chromosome that will be carrying a particular set of alleles at the markers on that chromosome. Each time this chromosome is transmitted to a subsequent generation the allele of interest will be transmitted along with that same set of marker alleles unless a recombinant event splits the haplotype. As recombinant events are more likely to occur between more distantly placed markers than those immediately adjacent to the variant of interest, the size of the haplotype inherited in common by the descendants of the original chromosome is gradually whittled down (Figure 3.6).

Under the common disease/common variant hypothesis, it is likely that variants influencing susceptibility to multiple sclerosis are often to be found in the present-day population and therefore, in most cases, each is related to a common founding event. As a result, allele frequencies at markers close to a susceptibility allele will be distorted in favour of those carried on the original founding haplotype amongst people who have inherited this susceptibility allele – such as affected individuals. Thus, allele frequencies for markers close to susceptibility genes are in a state of disequilibrium between those chromosomes that carry the susceptibility allele (more common in affected individuals) and those without (more common in unaffected individuals). The extent of this disequilibrium varies but is generally greater for tightly linked than more distant markers. This phenomenon is usually referred to as linkage disequilibrium, an apt but perhaps rather confusing term. In the presence of linkage disequilibrium, there is a correlation between marker allele frequencies and the susceptibility allele; these markers can therefore be used as surrogates with which to test indirectly for the susceptibility allele. Detailed analysis of linkage disequilibrium reveals that it is not uniformly distributed across the genome but, rather, shows a high degree of variance. In some places the linkage disequilibrium is intense and almost all the variants in that region show high levels of correlation. Such regions are referred to as 'haplotype blocks' (Daly *et al* 2001), and within these regions just a few common haplotypes account for a high percentage of all variety within the human population. These haplotype blocks vary in size but are generally small with an average size of just 22–44 kb (Gabriel *et al* 2002). In other regions, the level of linkage disequilibrium is low and haplotype diversity is correspondingly high. These regions of high and low linkage disequilibrium tend to alternate and some evidence has emerged that this pattern may reflect the fact that recombination is not a fully random event. At this fine level, there may be a tendency for recombination to occur more frequently at some points than others – hot spots of recombination corresponding to regions of low linkage disequilibrium and the intervening gaps to the haplotype blocks.

Evidence for such hot spots has been found in some parts of the genome (Jeffreys *et al* 2001) but it is not clear whether this nonuniformity of recombination is responsible for the occurrence of haplotype blocks in all regions. Whatever the cause, the existence of these blocks, with their limited haplotype diversity, provides an efficient means for association screening. Within each block, it is possible to select a small sample of SNPs that effectively 'tag' the limited number of common haplotypes (K.P. Johnson *et al* 2001), reducing the number of variants that need to be tested in order to screen for association. This approach is less efficient within the regions of low linkage disequilibrium and is insensitive to the presence of rare variants. Attempts have been made to advantage the search for susceptibility genes using association methods by studying genetically isolated populations – such as Finns and Sardinians – such

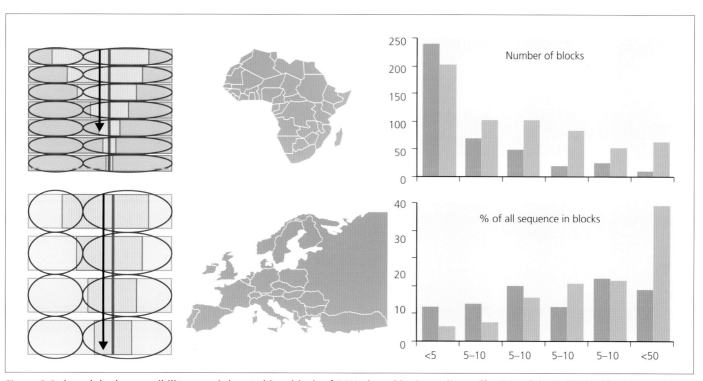

Figure 3.6 An original susceptibility gene is located in a block of DNA shared by immediate offspring of the individual harbouring the polymorphism. With time, recombination whittles down the size of the block shared identically by descent amongst progeny. Eventually the gene is isolated and no longer part of a haplotype block (genetic equilibrium). But this process is incomplete in 'younger' populations and seemingly unrelated individuals may nevertheless share haplotype blocks encoding the susceptibility allele identically by descent from the ancestor (linkage disequilibrium). Against this theoretical background, are shown empirical data indicating the observed number of blocks, and the proportions of the genome accommodated within blocks in an ancient (African; blue) and younger (European; red) population. Adapted from Gabriel *et al* (2002).

populations being expected to have larger blocks of linkage disequilibrium for reasons of population history. In fact, these isolates do not always show more linkage disequilibrium than outbred populations (Eaves *et al* 2000).

Population admixture is another phenomenon known to introduce linkage disequilibrium that could be useful in indirectly mapping genes for complex disease (Terwilliger *et al* 1998). The available epidemiological evidence suggests that racial groups differ significantly in terms of their susceptibility to multiple sclerosis, with Caucasians being most at risk and Africans being relatively protected. On average present-day Afro-Americans have approximately 20% European and 80% African ancestry (M.W. Smith *et al* 2004). Assuming that the racial difference in susceptibility to multiple sclerosis reflects a difference in the risk allele frequencies in these populations it would therefore be expected that Afro-American individuals suffering from multiple sclerosis will show a greater than expected degree of European ancestry in those regions of the genome containing susceptibility genes. Efforts to employ this novel and promising approach are underway.

Much debate in connection with the use of association studies in complex disease has centred around the selection of cases and controls (Figure 3.7; Risch and Teng 1998). It is clear that use of unrelated individuals provides the most power but also that such controls may increase false positives. Unless accurately matched, such studies are susceptible to the perturbations of

population substructure and assortative mating. Aiming to avoid these confounding effects, many investigators use intrafamilial controls, such as the nontransmitted parental alleles of an affected individual – as in a transmission disequilibrium test (TDT) (Self *et al* 1991; Spielman *et al* 1993) – or the genotype of unaffected siblings. Such approaches offer varying protection against confounding effects, depending upon how the analysis is performed, but are invariably much less powerful. When unrelated individuals are used, it is not clear how best to select the controls so as to ensure matching for the relevant factors.

For a given sample, the power of an association test is critically dependent upon the size and nature of the genetic effect being sought, together with the frequency of susceptibility alleles. Power falls off rapidly at extremes of frequency as fewer and fewer of the genotyped subjects prove informative (Risch 2000). The size and nature of genetic effects are unknown but often expressed in terms of the genotype relative risk (GRR), which is the risk conferred by the carriage of a single risk allele as compared with the risk seen in an individual who is homozygous for the wild-type allele (Risch 2000). Experience from other complex traits and available epidemiological data suggest that for risk alleles acting in a multiplicative fashion, the GRR is likely to be <2 for genes conferring susceptibility to multiple sclerosis (Risch 2000). But it is expected that many alleles will confer much smaller risks. Using these estimates, it is easy to see that ≥500–1000 case–control pairs or trio families

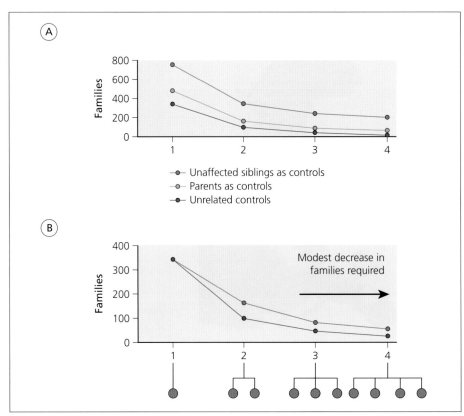

Figure 3.7 (A) The number of simplex families required to demonstrate an association using unrelated individuals, parents or unaffected siblings as controls for genes exerting effects of λs 1 to 4. (B) The number of cases required to demonstrate association with a gene conferring an effect of λs 1–4 obtained from families with 1–4 affected siblings. Kindly prepared by Dr Stephen Sawcer and adapted from Risch and Teng (1998).

(an affected individual and both parents as used in a TDT study) will be necessary to ensure power for even the largest likely effects attributable to moderately common alleles (Figure 3.8; Risch 2000; Risch and Merikangas 1996).

Linkage and association provide different categories of information (Figure 3.9). Assuming a reasonable sample size, any marker distant from a susceptibility gene may be linked but not associated since it will lie outside the block of linkage disequilibrium. A marker lying close to a susceptibility gene may be associated but not be linked if the sample is small. Only the combination of a close marker tested in adequate samples will show both linkage and association. Since it is far from clear that clinical features and variations in the course of multiple sclerosis do not segregate within families, linkage is essentially restricted to the study of susceptibility genes. Association mapping can in theory be used either to reveal susceptibility or disease-modifying genes if appropriate stratifications are employed in designing the study. Meta-analysis of linkage and association screens has been deployed in the expectation that this will reduce the incidence for false positive results and strengthen the candidature of genuine findings in order to select regions for more detailed studies of positional candidates. Combining data sets from ethnically diverse groups necessarily selects for genes conferring susceptibility between populations and obscures the identification of those restricted to particular populations. For a disease that is notoriously variable in its clinical phenotype and in which a case can be made for heterogeneity in the pathogenesis, lumping all cases under the rubric of 'multiple sclerosis' reduces the power to identify any one susceptibility factor and ignores those that may focus the pathological process on defined pathways, shape the clinical course, and (perhaps) determine the response to treatment.

Practicalities of genetic analysis

Unlike Mendelian disorders, the genes responsible for complex traits are probably not mutations coding for aberrant gene products but more frequent polymorphisms that exert only a relatively minor effect on function. A mutation is a genetic variation in the coding sequence of a gene occurring in <1%, and a polymorphism the least common allele occurring in >1% of the population. Polymorphism defines the extent to which a particular gene or chromosomal marker is informative. Not all polymorphisms are functional. Whilst it is logical to conclude that only the functional ones matter, this does not restrict analysis to just those variants affecting the coding regions since those in promoters and modifiers may also have important effects on the behaviour of genes. Most strategies for the identification of susceptibility genes assume that susceptibility is not determined by rare alleles, since the power to find such variants is very low.

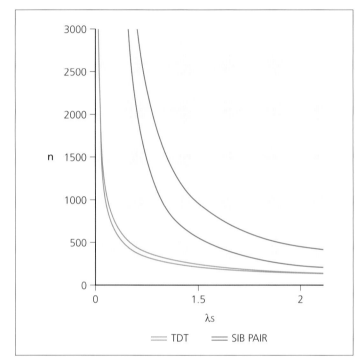

Figure 3.8 Number of families required to provide 80% power of detecting genome-wide significance for a susceptibility gene using linkage (sibling pair analysis) and association (transmission disequilibrium testing). A gene conferring an effect of λs 1.5 requires 100 sibling pairs or 300 simplex families to demonstrate the effect. Adapted from Risch and Meringas (1996).

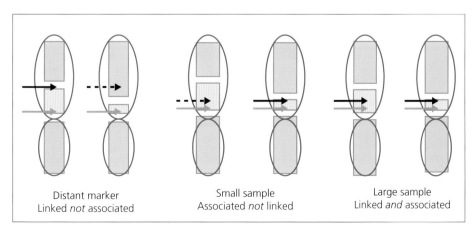

| Distant marker | Small sample | Large sample |
| Linked *not* associated | Associated *not* linked | Linked *and* associated |

Figure 3.9 Markers placed distant from a susceptibility gene may be linked but are unlikely to be associated since these lie outside the block of linkage disequilibrium. Markers lying close to a susceptibility gene may be associated but only linked if the sample is large (given the low statistical power of linkage in affected family members).

At first, the selection of candidate genes represented a compromise between common biological sense, using contemporary ideas on the pathogenesis, and the availability of reagents for defining gene polymorphisms. Much effort was therefore inevitably first directed at phenotypic markers of the major histocompatibility complex (MHC), defined serologically and by cellular typing methods. This was a lucky break since the MHC was quickly implicated and clearly does encode a susceptibility gene for multiple sclerosis. The ability to study genotypes rather than phenotypes opened the possibility of studying many new genomic regions as candidate loci for susceptibility in multiple sclerosis. After the initial studies using restriction fragment length polymorphisms (D. Cohen *et al* 1984), the availability of microsatellite markers, widely distributed across the genome but usually in the intervals between coding regions and made up of repeats involving two or more nucleotides, increased the range and diversity of genotype definition. Now, SNPs provide a sufficient density of markers in and around genes to offer a more definitive approach for indirect screens (Figure 3.10). These occur on average every 1000 base pairs and have a low mutation rate, thus favouring association studies. Progress has been rapid, with the public SNP consortium quickly reporting over 1.4 million unique SNP markers (Sachidanandam *et al* 2001) and the private sequencing effort identifying more than 2.1 million (Subramanian *et al* 2001; Venter *et al* 2001). Now it is estimated that the number of SNPs in the human genome (defined by a rare allele frequency of $\geq 1\%$ in at least one population) is likely to be at least 15 million (Botstein and Risch 2003). The first tranche of 2.5 million are mostly from the 90% that constitute common variants within the population. The 10% of rare alleles will take more effort to identify. The expectation is that the whole genome will soon be characterized for the size, distribution and diversity of haplotype blocks within populations, and the common variants within each block defined using a very few htSNPs (Daly *et al* 2001; Gabriel *et al* 2002).

The genotyping load involved in screening the genome for association is daunting; many thousands of markers will need to be studied in many thousands of individuals. One tactic is not to type individual samples but rather to study pooled DNA (Barcellos *et al* 1997a; Sham *et al* 2002). Although rigorous quantification of DNA samples is necessary when constructing such pools, this one-off effort is relatively small compared with the actual typing. Pooling introduces additional sources of error over and above sampling variance, and thereby reduces the effective sample size of the cohorts being considered (B.J. Barratt *et al* 2002). The number, spacing and type of markers chosen are critical because the central requirement for association mapping is that linkage disequilibrium will only be revealed by markers lying within the relevant haplotype blocks. To date, the greatest technical hurdle for whole genome association screens has been in achieving sufficient marker density to detect the disease association. To increase efficiency, a two- or three-stage approach is generally considered optimal whereby initial screens are conducted using DNA pooling, and then only those sites yielding positive results confirmed using individual genotyping (Barcellos *et al* 1997a; Sham *et al* 2002). Since the number of true loci is likely to be small in comparison with the number of candidate loci, many nonassociated regions are excluded from further study by an initial screen with pooled DNA. Several different methods for determining marker allele frequencies and detecting disease associations have been published (A. Bansal *et al* 2002; Mohlke *et al* 2002).

In the context of pooled DNA, microsatellites present technical challenges due both to stutter artefacts and preferential amplification, which vary significantly between markers (Barcellos *et al* 1997a). Each marker needs to be carefully characterized in advance, using individual typing to identify the number of alleles and potential polymerase chain reaction-related artefacts. Although a time-consuming process, the use of mathematical methods for correction of these artefacts has also been suggested in order to obtain more accurate microsatellite allele frequencies (Perlin *et al* 1995; Setakis 2003). Replicating pool construction, polymerase chain reaction and signal detection improves the 'signal to noise' ratio and becomes more necessary with large pools, but reduces the efficiency that pooling seeks to achieve (B.J. Barratt *et al* 2002). The next

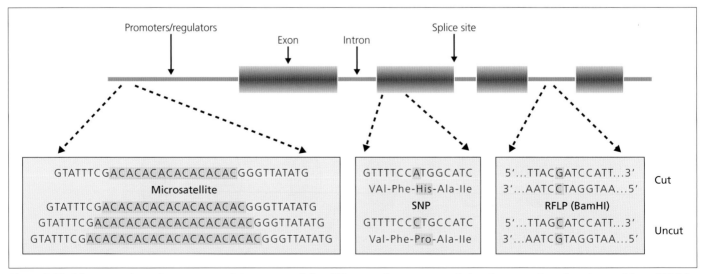

Figure 3.10 Scheme to show the anatomy of the gene and the differences between restriction fragment length polymorphisms (RFLPs), microsatellite repeats and single nucleotide polymorphisms (SNPs). Kindly prepared by Dr Stephen Sawcer.

generation of linkage disequilibrium screens for disease genes will require much larger sample sizes and the use of very dense SNP maps. These can also be typed using pooled DNA but are subject to preferential allele amplification artefacts (Sham *et al* 2002). Since it is now clear that a realistic genome-wide association study may require >500 000 SNP markers, perhaps closer to a million, it follows that future screens will need to employ a multicentre approach and perhaps also a multidisease effort to maximize efficiency and resources. Anticipating these developments, several international consortia have been established for studying the genetics of multiple sclerosis and other putative autoimmune diseases compared with a large generic cohort of controls.

After the initial systematic screen, which excludes candidate genes from most regions of the genome, the next step is to replicate any positive findings in a second sample. Much depends on the care with which the initial screen and this replication are carried out. Lander and Krugylak (1995) have provided guidelines aiming to steer a course between spurious claims for linkage to several thousand markers, and not missing important clues to the location of genuine susceptibility genes through being overly cautious. These initial theoretical limits on statistical analysis have rightly erred on the stringent side. Using simulations of real families, Sawcer *et al* (1997) provided study-specific estimates for expected lod scores under the null hypothesis of no linkage. An MLS of 1.8 was found to have an expectation of one false positive per genome screen. This may be an underestimate where the density of markers has been selectively increased around a region of provisional linkage.

Once regions of interest are provisionally mapped, the next aim is to identify the functional polymorphism. How to reach that position is less clear and several parallel strategies have been suggested. Additional markers are used to try and identify with more accuracy that part of the chromosome where the susceptibility gene is located. If the results continue to support the involvement of this genomic region, more affected relative pairs and more closely spaced markers are applied until thresholds are reached for the identification of secure loci using statistical criteria for genome-wide significance. But the juice that can be squeezed out of the linkage lemon is limited for genes of small biological effect. The alternative tactic is to exploit the greater sensitivity provided by tests of association, narrowing the region of interest with tagged SNPs to identify the haplotype associated with multiple sclerosis. Since clinical heterogeneity within and between patient groups may account for the lack of replication observed between screens, future association studies will increasingly incorporate clinical and other stratifying elements to target specific genetic effects.

At some point, mapping must end and the combination of linkage and association be declared sufficient to concentrate the search for positional candidates within regions of interest. This strategy has worked in an increasing number of disorders. Conversely, many genes are mapped but have no assigned function or apparent relevance to disease. Paradoxically, the number encoding components of the nervous, immune and signalling systems is such as to make practically any region suggestive with respect to sensible candidates for multiple sclerosis. Thus, it is easy to generate enthusiasm for a candidate gene study in multiple sclerosis and somewhat more difficult to nail the culprit.

RACIAL SUSCEPTIBILITY

As discussed in Chapter 2, multiple sclerosis is a relatively common disorder of young adults in northern Europe, continental North America and Australasia, but it is much less prevalent in the Orient, the Middle East, Africa, continental South America and India. But with a growing number of surveys that can reliably be compared, previous evidence for gradients within areas of high frequency (Compston 1990b; Kurtzke 1975) now seems less secure. Nevertheless, the frequency of multiple sclerosis is higher, for example, in southern Scandinavia than the north, in northeast Scotland and the Orkney and Shetland Islands than other parts of the United Kingdom, in Sardinia compared with mainland Italy, and in Sicily but not Malta. In several other parts of the world, the frequency of multiple sclerosis has been shown to differ between geographically discrete but ethnically isolated groups. Commentators have wrestled with these observations in seeking to understand why multiple sclerosis has this characteristic geographical distribution. Our preferred interpretation of these global epidemiological patterns is that racial susceptibility largely determines the distribution of the disease. Specifically, multiple sclerosis is common where the population frequency of northern European genes is high.

Our starting point for a genetic formulation of the distribution of multiple sclerosis is the observation that multiple sclerosis appears concentrated in northern Europeans (Figure 3.11). Rosati (2001) concludes that the disease is unexpectedly uncommon in Saamis, Turkmen, Uzbeks, Kazakhs, Kyrgyzis, native Siberians, North and South Amerindians, Chinese, Japanese, African blacks, and New Zealand Maoris. Against this backdrop of varying European, Indian and Oriental prevalence, multiple sclerosis is disproportionately common in Sardinians, Parsees and Palestinians. Despite the recent description of cases amongst Saami (Gronlie *et al* 2000: see Chapter 2), there remains a south–north gradient in the frequency of multiple sclerosis in Scandinavia. This correlates with the density of Nordic people and Lapps. The same is said to be true for the Yakutes in northern Russia (Popov 1983). The most persuasive example of multiple sclerosis occurring at high frequency in a group having unusual genetic characteristics remains the offshore islands of northeast Scotland where the frequency was at one time higher than in any other region (see Chapter 2). More specifically, the geography of multiple sclerosis in Scotland has been linked to the relative distribution of Nordic (high rates) and Celtic (lower rates) peoples (Sutherland 1956). These and other genetic histories are still marked by differences across relatively small geographic distances in Europe (Menozzi *et al* 1978; Ryder *et al* 1978). More specifically, genetic clines for markers of susceptibility to multiple sclerosis correlate with distribution of the disease (Swingler and Compston 1986; and see Cavalli-Sforza *et al* 1994). Our ideas on the origins of multiple sclerosis are fully set out in Chapter 5.

The epidemiological surveys of Charles Davenport (see Chapter 1) had emphasized that multiple sclerosis is more prevalent in those parts of the United States with a high density of Scandinavian immigrants. Davenport (1922) mapped the frequency of multiple sclerosis, as one of the defects found in drafted men, and showed that maximum rates for this diagnosis were in the states of Michigan, Minnesota and Wisconsin. Taken with his earlier analysis of the distribution of multiple sclerosis

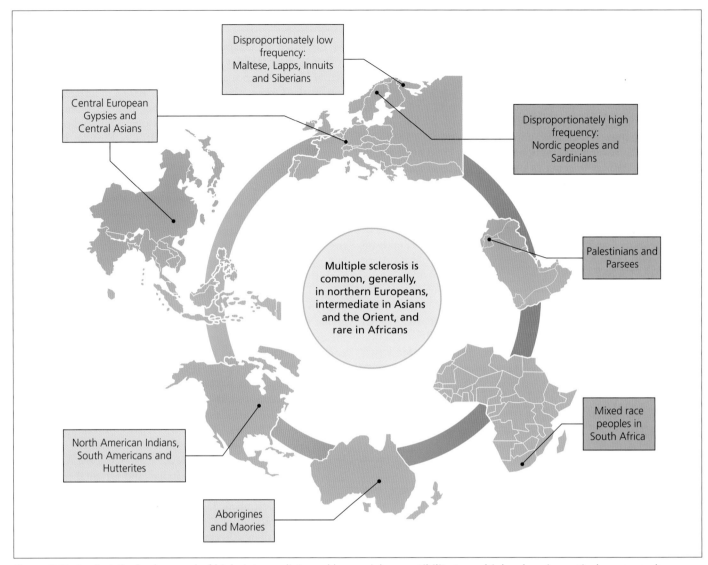

Figure 3.11 Against the background of high, intermediate and low racial susceptibility to multiple sclerosis, particular groups show unusually high or low frequencies.

by racial origin (Davenport 1921), he suggested that Scandinavians are especially at risk of multiple sclerosis. That said, he found no cases resident in the Swedish Hospital or listed in its records. Subsequent analysis supports Davenport's analysis. Bulman and Ebers (1992) showed that the regional frequency of multiple sclerosis matches patterns of migration from Europe, the highest rates occurring in areas populated by people of Scandinavian ancestry and the lowest correlating with the distribution of black immigrants (Figure 3.12).

Multiple sclerosis occurs in Innuits at one-twentieth the frequency seen in other Canadians living in the same areas and it is also a rare disease in the Indian tribes of North America. In fact, the majority of Amerindians with multiple sclerosis have a European ancestor (Hader *et al* 1985). In Canada, the gradient of disease frequency appears to move west to east. The explanation offered is the higher density of Nordic (Scandinavian and Scottish) people in western Canada by comparison with the French-speaking eastern seaboard and Newfoundland. There is, however, one exception to the relationship between frequency

of multiple sclerosis in Canada and northern European ancestry. The Hutterites (a socially isolated religious community originating from southern Germany) appear to be protected from multiple sclerosis despite living in parts of North America and Canada where the disease is otherwise common. The original group of Lutherans, followers of Gaacob Hutter, moved from Germany in the 19th and 20th centuries and established closed communities where social mixing and marriage outside the group remain rare to this day (Hostetler 1974). Hutterites live in parts of Canada and North America having a high prevalence of multiple sclerosis yet, when last reported, only six cases had been identified in their communities. The individual pedigrees were analysed from extensive genealogical records covering eight generations. The six cases included two brothers, two first cousins, male and female, another male and female, all representing two of the three endogamous groups of Hutterites, linked to two common ancestors through lines of descent dating to 1723 (Hader *et al* 1996). Whereas, for example, the Orcadians represent a group in whom genes conferring suscep-

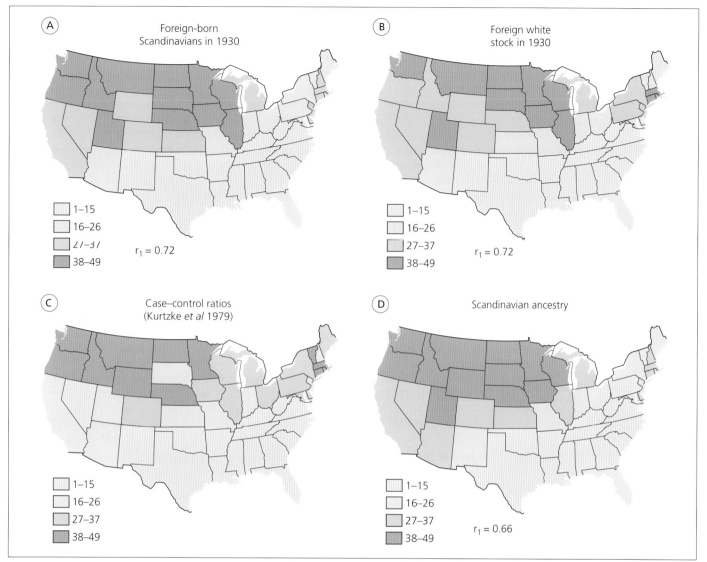

Figure 3.12 The United States are ranked by four different groups (1–15, 16–26, 27–37 and 38–49) in a reverse order for ratios of ethnic origin. (A,B,D) Compiled using the United States census data for the years given; (C) compiled using Kurtzke's case–control ratios from the United States Second World War veteran multiple sclerosis population. The north–south and west–east gradients are seen in (A) for the distribution of foreign-born Scandinavians in 1930, in (B) for foreign white stock (1930) and in (D) for Scandinavian ancestry (1980). The recent migration from the northern to the southern United States has not altered the distribution of individuals of Scandinavian origin. Adapted from Bulman and Ebers (1992).

tibility to multiple sclerosis appear to be highly concentrated, so chance has presumably excluded these factors from the Hutterites of North America.

In Australia and New Zealand, multiple sclerosis is rarely diagnosed in Aborigines or Maoris but occurs commonly amongst whites (S.R. Hammond *et al* 1988; D.H. Miller *et al* 1990a; Skegg *et al* 1987). Using the number of 'Mcs/Macs' in the telephone directory, Skegg *et al* (1987) showed that multiple sclerosis is common in parts of New Zealand where people of Scottish ancestry are to be found. 'Mcs' were not classified on the basis of Celtic or Nordic origin, thus omitting the distinction made by Sutherland in the 1950s.

The higher frequency of multiple sclerosis seen in English-speaking whites in South Africa, compared with Afrikaners (Dean 1967), also suggests a subtle difference in susceptibility between those who migrated from England and Holland. As

discussed in Chapter 2, the change in frequency of multiple sclerosis seen in African blacks, forcibly relocated to the southeastern part of the United States, and in the first-generation offspring of West Indian immigrants to the United Kingdom (Elian and Dean 1987; Elian *et al* 1990) implies that the racial protection of Africans is modified by environment. However, the same alteration in risk is not seen amongst Japanese migrants living in Hawaii or the west coast of North America (Alter *et al* 1971; Detels *et al* 1972; 1977). However, not only does the frequency of multiple sclerosis alter with time; so also may phenotypic expression of the interplay between genes and the environment. Although the epidemiological evidence may not allow too penetrating an analysis, and differences in the degree of Caucasian gene admixture may be influential, the facts suggest that whereas resistance may be relatively more difficult to dislodge in Orientals than Africans, the clinical features of multiple sclerosis may be changing in Japanese with an increasing prevalence of the Western phenotype, and reduction in the more traditional neuromyelitis optica. Again, we draw on this evidence in formulating ideas on the origins and evolution of multiple sclerosis in Chapter 5.

Within central and southern Europe, the study of two other groups has, at one time, proved informative with respect to the question of genetic susceptibility. In Hungary, Palffy et al (1994) reported the prevalence of multiple sclerosis amongst Gypsies to be one-sixth that in other Hungarians, and the frequency was half in a similar comparison from Bulgaria (Milanov et al 1999: see Chapter 2). Sardinians have a higher frequency of multiple sclerosis than other southern Europeans. They also have a specifically different class II major histocompatibility complex association (see below). A corollary to the study of multiple sclerosis in Sardinians is the difference in frequency of the disease in Sicily and neighbouring Malta (Dean et al 2002: see Chapter 2). The social history of these two Mediterranean islands differs in many important respects and this may explain the apparent difference in frequency of multiple sclerosis despite their geographic proximity. The Maltese speak a Semitic language and their surnames indicate a prominent north African influence dating from the main Arab influx with the invasion by Habasa in 869/870 AD and in the 12th century.

GENDER DIFFERENCES IN SUSCEPTIBILITY

Apart from surveys assessing highly selective populations, multiple sclerosis is almost always more common in females than males. The reported figures vary but a sex ratio of 2F:M is usual, irrespective of ethnicity (Confavreux et al 1980; Svenningsson et al 1990; Weinshenker et al 1989a). This ratio differs with age at onset. In children, the excess of females is more marked than in adults – perhaps approaching 3F:M (Duquette et al 1987). Conversely, multiple sclerosis presenting in or after the fifth decade more commonly affects males, and tends to follow a primary progressive course (see Chapter 4). The principle of distinct age-adjusted sex ratios was first recognized by Hyllested (1956) and has been apparent in most subsequent population-based surveys.

It seems unlikely that the excess amongst females has a simple genetic explanation. Many putative autoimmune diseases are more common in females. Although the reasons are not well understood, one hypothesis is that this arises from interactions between endocrine factors and the immune system. More recently, attention has turned to an explanation based on microchimerism (Willer et al 2002). This refers to the stable presence of a small number of non-host cells, usually stem cells or their progeny. Predictably, they are most prevalent in parous women where the physiological role may be to restrict maternal immunological responses against the fetus. Clearly, a variety of other potential mechanisms for becoming exposed to allogeneic cells exists, in both sexes. Microchimerism may increase the risk of autoimmune disease in parous women. It has recently been studied in the context of multiple sclerosis. Basso et al (2004) compared 64 704 Danish women who changed partners in fathering children, and so were at risk of microchimerism, with 86 624 who did not. With access to 213 index cases from these 151 328 women, there was no difference in risk depending on number of men fathering their offspring. The odds ratio for

being diagnosed at ≤2 years of the index pregnancy was higher for women with >1 partner (1.80: 95% CI 0.92–3.51 vs. 0.90: 95% CI 0.64–1.28) raising the possibility that microchimerism may accelerate the timing of diagnosis, or possibly the onset of multiple sclerosis.

Some have claimed that the excess of females with sporadic multiple sclerosis is less apparent in familial cases, especially large multiplex families (Weitkemp 1983), but this is not supported by recent descriptions (Dyment et al 2002a; Modin et al 2003). There is a slightly increased number of same-sex compared with unlike-sexed sibling pairs in the normal population and a tendency for same-sexed pairs to share a closer environment than other siblings. Given the excess of female probands, corrections must be made when assessing preferential risk for male or female offspring of an affected parent but these are worth resolving since the emerging patterns may illuminate genetic mechanisms of inherited risk, and possibly provide clues to the nature of those susceptibilities. The sex ratio of unaffected offspring in patients with the disease does not differ from the normal population.

Weitkemp (1983) reported an increase in the number of same-sex sibling pairs and more distantly related doublets but not parent–child combinations. This would be consistent with an interaction between gender and genes conferring susceptibility to multiple sclerosis. Others have not found this disturbance in sex distribution amongst familial cases (Chataway et al 2001; Hupperts et al 2001; Robertson et al 1996b; Sadovnick et al 1991a). Against the background of no apparent effect on recurrence risk for male and female relatives of affected individuals, we discuss below the related issue, suggested by more recent studies of half-siblings, of a maternal parent of origin effect in susceptibility to multiple sclerosis (Ebers et al 2004).

FAMILIAL MULTIPLE SCLEROSIS

The analysis of pedigrees with familial multiple sclerosis has a long history. In the early 1950s, Pratt et al (1951) collated families from the literature but it soon became clear that, for any meaningful interpretation, ascertainment bias had to be eliminated by performing population-based surveys. In the modern era, the cohort of cases presenting sequentially to the Multiple Sclerosis Clinic in Vancouver has been studied prospectively for family history and recurrence risk amongst defined categories of first- and second-degree relatives over a number of years (Sadovnick and Baird 1988; Sadovnick et al 1988; 2000). Similar studies were subsequently reported from the East Anglian region of the United Kingdom (N.P. Robertson et al 1996a) and from Flanders, Belgium (Carton et al 1997). Overall, familial recurrence amongst 2163 probands was 17.2%, and 432/44 563 first- and second-degree relatives included in these population-based series were also considered to be affected. Recurrence risks in individual categories of relatives, derived by meta-analysis, are shown in Figures 3.13 and 3.14 and Table 3.1.

The Canadian series

The study of recurrence risks in Canada has benefited from nationwide cooperation in the identification of cases through a network of 17 clinics. In British Columbia, the overall frequency

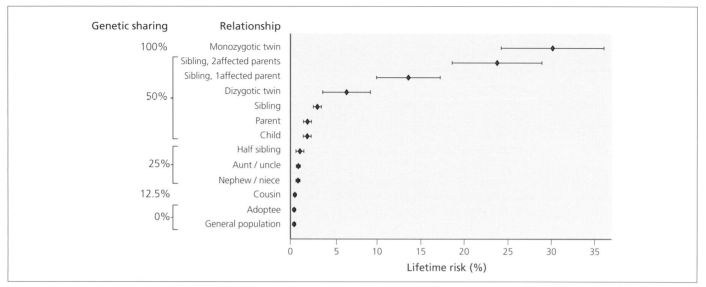

Figure 3.13 Recurrence risks for multiple sclerosis in families. Age-adjusted recurrence risks for different relatives of probands with multiple sclerosis. Pooled data from population-based surveys. Estimated 95% confidence intervals are shown. Figures on left show the degree of genetic sharing between relative and proband. Kindly prepared by Dr Simon Broadley and adapted from Compston and Coles 2003 with permission from Elsevier.

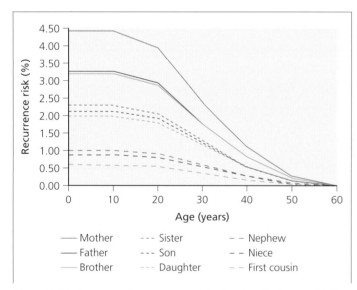

Figure 3.14 Age-specific recurrence risks for developing multiple sclerosis in the relatives of probands with multiple sclerosis for use in counselling; the risk is highest for a young sister and almost negligible for any relative who has reached the age of 50 years and remains unaffected. Kindly provided by Dr Neil Robertson.

of a family history of multiple sclerosis was 20% for first-, second- and third-degree relatives (V.P. Sweeney *et al* 1986). Crude figures may appear misleading and only prove reliable when, as a group, the category of at-risk relatives has reached an age beyond which multiple sclerosis is no longer likely to develop. However, where age of onset is known for the index case but only some affected relatives, age adjustment can be used to estimate maximum likelihood for the development of multiple sclerosis in all at-risk relatives (Cupples *et al* 1991). For parents in the Canadian series, crude and age-corrected recurrence rates were each 2.9%, whereas for the younger nieces or nephews,

many still at risk but unaffected, the crude rate rose from 0.4% to >2% with age correction. The highest age-adjusted figure was seen in sisters of affected females (5.6 + 1.1%). Overall, rates for siblings (3.8 + 0.9% for male and 4.0+ 0.7% for female probands) were higher than for children (2.5 + 1.7% for sons and 2.6 + 1.2% for daughters, respectively) and second- or third-degree relatives (Sadovnick 1994; Sadovnick and Baird 1988; Sadovnick *et al* 1988).

There were no examples of parent–son affected pairs in the first report from Canada (Sadovnick and Baird 1988; Sadovnick *et al* 1988). The updated sample contained the expected number of mother–son pairs and only father–son combinations continued to be under-represented (Sadovnick 1994). Fewer transmissions occurred overall through affected fathers than mothers but this reflected the smaller number of affected males. There was a trend towards higher risk for the relatives of female than male patients but not in the individual categories. Although the Vancouver sample has the double strengths of being population based and numerically large, the reported absence of father–son affected pairs has not been confirmed in other series (Robertson *et al* 1996b; Warren and Warren 1994). Sadovnick *et al* (1998) used 1896 index cases and 8878 first-degree relatives to show that gender, an affected parent and younger age at onset in the index case correlated with an increased risk for siblings. The same referral network was subsequently used to identify a further 1083 index cases, 2166 of their parents and 3112 siblings (Sadovnick *et al* 2000). The same characteristics in probands were associated with increased recurrence risks in siblings. These results suggested an effect of genetic loading in determining absolute risk and anticipation for age at onset. Leaving aside the higher risks in twins, the clinic-based Vancouver experience indicates a lifetime risk of 0.2% for the entire population, and an increase to 3% for first-degree and 1% for second-degree relatives. This represents relative risks for developing multiple sclerosis of 20 for first-degree and 5.5 for second-degree relatives of affected individuals.

Table 3.1 **Crude and age-adjusted recurrence risks for relatives of male and female probands with multiple sclerosis**

Relative category	No.	Crude risk (%)	Age-adjusted risk (%)	95% CI
Father	12/612	1.96	1.99	1.03–3.48
Mother	13/625	2.08	2.11	1.12–3.60
Parent	25/1237	2.02	2.05	1.33–3.02
Brother	18/679	2.65	3.24	1.92–5.12
Sister	25/668	3.74	4.39	2.84–6.48
Sibling	43/1347	3.19	3.82	2.77–5.15
Son	1/560	0.18	0.58	0.01–3.25
Daughter	2/496	1.01	3.19	1.03–7.43
Child	6/1056	0.57	1.83	0.67–3.97
Nephew	3/885	0.34	0.98	0.20–2.87
Niece	7/885	0.79	2.29	0.92–4.72
Nephew/niece	10/1770	0.56	1.64	0.78–3.01
Paternal uncle	5/665	0.76	0.81	0.26–1.89
Paternal aunt	7/583	1.20	1.25	0.59–2.61
Maternal uncle	4/655	0.61	0.66	0.25–1.76
Maternal aunt	5/687	0.73	0.78	0.25–1.83
Aunt/uncle	21/2580	0.81	0.87	0.54–1.33
Paternal first cousin	11/1558	0.71	0.88	0.50–1.57
Maternal first cousin	12/1843	0.65	0.87	0.45–1.53
First cousin	23/3401	0.68	0.88	0.56–1.32
Total	128/11391	1.12	1.54	1.28–1.83

From Robertson et al (1996) with permission.

The suggestion of an effect of birth order amongst siblings, ≥1 of whom later developed multiple sclerosis, remains ambiguous. Isager *et al* (1980) found an inverse relationship with birth order whereas Alperovitch *et al* (1981) reported an association with multiple sclerosis in older siblings. Cripps *et al* (1982) studied 175 sporadic cases but found no effect of birth order. The lack of clustering for birth order amongst an additional 36 affected sibling pairs provided further evidence against common environmental exposure as an aetiological factor in multiple sclerosis. In a separate study of 164 sporadic cases of multiple sclerosis from London, Ontario, there was no difference in birth order or family size compared with matched spouse controls (Gaudet *et al* 1995a). Although not a methodologically powerful approach to the problem, this was considered by the authors to argue against the impact of an infection occurring in adolescence or early adulthood. Gaudet *et al* (1995b) also failed to show a birth order effect for multiple sclerosis amongst 88 multiplex families in which 99 co-affected siblings of 88 probands and 205 younger unaffected siblings were studied. Two more recent Swedish studies address the issue of birth order in multiple sclerosis. Comparing 4443 cases with 24 194 matched controls, Montgomery *et al* (2004) showed reduced adjusted odds ratios for individuals from families having either ≥3 younger or ≥3 older siblings compared with singletons (0.8: 95% CI 0.7–0.92 for younger, and 0.83: 95% CI 0.72–0.96 for older siblings) but the protective effect of being a different sex twin compared with an only child seems counter-intuitive (0.59: 95% CI 0.37–0.95). Ahlgren and Andersen (2005) found no effect of birth order in 211 cases or in a cohort of incident cases born between 1915 and 1929. There seems to be nothing in this story.

The United Kingdom series

In the United Kingdom, Roberts and Bates (1982) carried out a genetic analysis of multiple sclerosis in the northwest of England. They identified 12/1290 first-degree, 7/3318 second-degree and 14/2647 third-degree relatives of probands who also had multiple sclerosis. Subsequently, Robertson *et al* (1996b) screened the western part of East Anglia. Pedigree information was obtained from a cohort of 674/890 (76%) index cases, providing 11 391 relatives of whom 128 were also considered to have multiple sclerosis. The highest age-adjusted recurrence rate was for sisters (4.4%) and brothers (3.2%). There was a slightly lower recurrence risk in parents (2.1%) and offspring (1.8%; sons 0.6% and daughters 3.2%). For female probands, the parental age-adjusted rate was similar for mothers and fathers (combined 1.8%). The highest risk was for sisters (5.1%) but despite age adjustment, the rate for offspring did not rise above 0.8% (sons 0%; daughters 1.7%). The combined adjusted risk for nieces and nephews was 1.3%. For male probands, parental rates were slightly higher (3.2%) but lower in sisters (2.5%) and brothers (3.6%) than for female index cases. Surprisingly, the offspring of male probands had a higher age-adjusted risk (4.9%; sons 2.5% and daughters 7.1%) than was seen in female affecteds. Overall, risk reduced from 2.8% (relative risk 9.2) in first-degree relatives to 1.02% (relative risk 3.4) and 0.9% (relative risk 2.9) in second- and third-degree relatives, respectively, compared with a background age-adjusted risk in this population of 0.3%. There was no preferential recurrence for maternal or paternal relatives. Robertson *et al* (1996c) found additional cases in 33% of 166 families with affected sibling pairs.

The genetic analysis of multiple sclerosis in small populations of special interest has included the Orkney Islands, where 51 patients were compared with controls for consanguinity, kinship and familial recurrence (Roberts 1991; Roberts and Roberts 1979). Consanguinity was increased both in cases and controls, reflecting general features of this island population. Kinship coefficients also did not differ. There was a comparable degree of intertwined families amongst affected and normal individuals, arguing against the recent introduction of a single dominant or codominant gene. The recurrence risks were much lower than has since been reported (see above) for more outbred cohorts (1:164 for sibships; 1:47 for parents; 1:223 for second-degree relatives; and 1:275 for third-degree relatives). In the Shetland Islands, Roberts *et al* (1983) later compared 31 prevalent cases with controls for consanguinity, kinship and familial recurrence. The patients with multiple sclerosis did not differ from the general population except in having a slightly higher frequency of affected relatives (5/1291 vs. 1/534). The findings in both Orkney and Shetland also led Derek Roberts and colleagues to conclude some years ago that the genetic component of susceptibility to multiple sclerosis could only be explained by a polygenic model with a significant contribution from environmental factors. Roberts (1991) assessed all patients with multiple sclerosis in Orkney (alive in 1974 or who had died between 1958 and 1974). The closer relatedness of parents in patients than matched controls suggested that genes inherited from each parent influence susceptibility to multiple sclerosis. This conclusion anticipated the results of studying multiple sclerosis in the offspring of conjugal pairs (see below).

Continental Europe

Wikstrom *et al* (1994) studied a small rural area of western Finland where 29% of 51 probands had a family history of the disease and the recurrence risk amongst siblings was 2.5%. Although small, the study may be informative since these are the families from southern Ostrobothnia in which the gene for myelin basic protein is implicated (see below). Binzer *et al* (1994) reported a high frequency of multiple sclerosis ($253/10^5$) in a small rural district of northern Sweden. Twenty-two of 33 (67%) patients had ties of kinship as did others known also to be affected within the same region. However, where close-knit communities intermarry, chance associations may occur and the prevalence in this area of Sweden is not significantly higher than in other intensively studied isolated communities.

M-P. Roth *et al* (1994b) studied 7802 relatives of French patients identified by advertisement on television. One hundred and seventy had an affected parent made up as 72 mother–daughter, 48 father–son, 37 father–daughter and 13 father–son pairs. Carton *et al* (1997) reported recurrence risks for multiple sclerosis in 22 351 relatives of 674 individuals with multiple sclerosis from Flanders, in whom documentary evidence for the recurrence of multiple sclerosis was available. The frequency of a family history was 15%. Eighty-five of 104 probands from multiplex families had one, 14/104 two, and 5/104 three affected relatives. Almost 20% of families chose not to participate in the study. The authors observed an age-corrected recurrence risk for parents of 1.6% (±0.3%) with figures for siblings, children and uncles/aunts of 2.1 (±0.4%), 1.7 (±0.7%) and 0.7

(±0.1%), respectively. Since the prevalence of multiple sclerosis in this region of Belgium was at that time $88/10^5$ (95% CI 77–99), these recurrence risks are 10–12 times higher for first-degree and threefold for second-degree relatives. Montomoli *et al* (2002b) reported a higher recurrence risk (4.7%) for siblings of index cases from a high prevalence and genetically homogeneous region of Sardinia, representing a risk ratio of 31 compared with the general population. The highest recurrence risk was for siblings of young onset female probands. A more detailed evaluation of 2971 siblings of 901 Sardinian patients (Marrosu *et al* 2002a), identified 59 affected siblings (2%) and correlated recurrence risk with young age at onset (relative risk 2.3) and the presence of other affected family members (relative risk 2.9). In one village, a founder effect was observed in that all 11 cases were descended from three ancestors with no other affecteds amongst the remaining 2346 inhabitants.

Magnetic resonance imaging abnormalities have been used to assess clinically unaffected family members of individuals with multiple sclerosis. S.G. Lynch *et al* (1990) reported changes in four relatives aged <40 and in six aged >50 years. Tienari *et al* (1992a) showed that 6/16 (38%) clinically asymptomatic siblings of patients with multiple sclerosis aged <50 and 8/11 (78%) >50 years had abnormal scans but, using stringent criteria, only 3/27 were considered to show unequivocal evidence for demyelination. Pursuing the other characteristic laboratory feature of multiple sclerosis, Haghighi *et al* (2000) identified ≥2 oligoclonal bands in 9/47 (19%) healthy siblings of index cases with clinically definite multiple sclerosis but only 2/50 controls. To a large extent, these immunological abnormalities reflected an enhanced intrathecal immune response to measles. Their interpretation was that enriched immune responsiveness to infections is inherited but with only a small proportion of affected individuals expressing the clinical phenotype of multiple sclerosis. The issue of comorbidity with other conditions, including autoimmunity, is discussed in Chapter 6.

Models of genetic inheritance

In many complex traits, it has become increasingly clear that the estimate of heritability is confounded by contaminating series with large families resulting from Mendelian inheritance but having the same phenotype as members of less extended multiplex families. Overall, this seems not to be a problem in the specific situation of multiple sclerosis since such pedigrees are rare. When they do occur, extended pedigrees having the clinical features of multiple sclerosis offer an opportunity to assign modes of inheritance – at least in those families, even if generalizations are not appropriate. Modin *et al* (2003) reported a family in which five individuals – the index case, three of her siblings and her daughter – were diagnosed with definite multiple sclerosis. This is easily outdone by Dyment *et al* (2002a) who identified a family having 15 members affected in four generations suggesting autosomal dominant inheritance with reduced penetrance modified by the class II major histocompatibility locus (see below). Clinical characteristics (sex ratio, age at onset, symptoms, imaging features and clinical course) were indistinguishable from sporadic disease. Montomoli *et al* (2002b) favoured the effect of a single dominant gene with extremely low penetrance as the basis for the high recurrence risk amongst siblings in their study from Sardinia (see above).

Pedigree analysis for the Vancouver cohort excluded a single Mendelian gene (with dominant or recessive mode of inheritance) and made unlikely X-linked recessive or dominant effects and maternal inheritance (Sadovnick *et al* 1988; 1991a). Taken with the expected number of affected maternal and paternal uncles of male and female cases, and of concordant father–daughter pairs, the Canadian survey has also been interpreted as excluding mitochondrial or placental transmission and the presence of a Y-linked resistance gene. Increasingly complex models become more difficult to exclude since they are designed to accommodate atypical situations, and a recessive gene with a dominant mode of inheritance cannot be excluded. The United Kingdom series of familial multiple sclerosis excludes all but a polygenic mode of inheritance. The increased frequency of multiple sclerosis observed for second- and third-degree relatives, compared with the remainder of the at-risk population, supports the interpretation that genetic factors influence recurrence. Individuals outside the nuclear family are less likely to have shared the same environmental factors. Others (D. Lord *et al* 1990) wrestled with the family pedigree data concluding that multiple sclerosis occurs in individuals who are homozygous for a recessive gene and carry a dominant X gene showing reduced penetrance – as originally suggested by Pratt *et al* (1951).

To some extent, these attempts to model the genetics of multiple sclerosis from pedigree analyses into an oligogenic structure are doomed in a situation where all the pointers are towards polygenic inheritance with epistatic and multiplicative effects. The point is well made by Lindsey (2005), who simulated recurrence risks for first- and second-degree relatives under a variety of genetic models, concluding that the best fit is for genes encoded at ≥6 interactive loci, the abnormal alleles being common and exerting dominant effects; heterogeneity is not fully excluded.

Twin studies

Many surveys have studied multiple sclerosis in twins (Bammer *et al* 1960; Bobowick *et al* 1978; Cendrowski 1968; Ebers *et al* 1986; French Research Group on Multiple Sclerosis 1992; Heltberg and Holm 1982; Kinnunen *et al* 1987; 1988; Legras 1934; Mackay and Myrianthopolous 1958; 1966; Mumford *et al* 1994; Sadovnick 1982; Sadovnick *et al* 1993; Thums 1951; Uitdehaag *et al* 1989; Willer *et al* 2003; A. Williams *et al* 1980). Some have produced conflicting results, perhaps due to small sample size, and several have been criticized for biased case ascertainment (for review, see Bundey 1991; McFarland 1992). In particular, recruitment by national advertisement or announcement at public meetings has identified cohorts with an excess of female twins and concordant pairs (Mackay and Myrianthopolous 1958; 1966; A. Williams *et al* 1980) – features often characterizing studies dependent on response to public appeal or recall of individuals on hospital-based registers. Monozygotic pairs are often over-represented since their twin status is more likely to be known to the family and physician than is the case for dizygotic pairs. Because they are concerned about the disease, concordant twins are better motivated to participate in genetic studies. Discordant pairs stand a greater chance of including one individual who is poorly disposed towards research and confronting the possibility of personal illness. Other surveys have

drawn on national registers of twins (Heltberg and Holm 1982; Kinnunen *et al* 1987; 1988) or military personnel (Bobowick *et al* 1978) to identify a series for analysis, again introducing the potential for systematic bias if ascertainment is incomplete.

The early studies

Thums (1951) identified 96 patients with multiple sclerosis who had a living twin. He was able to study 13 monozygotic and 30 dizygotic pairs. One monozygotic pair was concordant whereas all the dizygotic twins were discordant. Methods for establishing zygosity and the precision with which multiple sclerosis was diagnosed were not discussed. Mackay and Myrianthopoulous (1958) collected twin pairs by appeal through the news media and obtained a sample biased in favour of monozygotic pairs, same-sex dizygotic twins and females – problems that were recognized when presenting an 8-year follow-up of the study (Mackay and Myrianthopoulous 1966). They found no difference in the concordance rate for multiple sclerosis in monozygotic (23% in 39 pairs) and dizygotic twins (21% in 29 pairs). Twenty-two percent of cases had other affected relatives (21 cases amongst 2900 at-risk relatives) and these families were particularly common when monozygotic twins were concordant for multiple sclerosis. Of these, 67% of families with concordant co-twins had additional cases compared with 10% of families having monozygotic twins discordant for multiple sclerosis. Mackay and Myrianthopolous (1966) favoured a recessive genetic model as the explanation for clustering within families but did not consider polygenic inheritance.

Cendrowski (1968) found no concordance for multiple sclerosis in three dizygotic twin pairs identified in an epidemiological survey of 300 patients. He reviewed 13 previous studies and calculated that 35/234 (15%) dizygotic twins were concordant for multiple sclerosis but we know nothing about the basis for selection of these patients. In an earlier study, Cendrowski *et al* (1969) reported significantly higher concordance for multiple sclerosis in monozygotic (24/90; 27%) than dizygotic pairs (11/85; 13%) but the methods of ascertainment were not population based.

A. Williams *et al* (1980) collected 12 monozygotic and 12 dizygotic twin pairs where the proband had definite multiple sclerosis. Concordance rates for multiple sclerosis were 50% and 17%, respectively. This study was the first to use laboratory markers as an index of subclinical disease in the clinically unaffected co-twin. The presence of oligoclonal bands would not be regarded as diagnostic of multiple sclerosis, but it may nevertheless be important that four monozygotic and eight dizygotic unaffected twin partners had qualitative cerebrospinal fluid abnormalities (X-H. Xu and McFarlin 1984). This cohort of twins was subsequently used to achieve genetic matching in studies designed to assess the relative contribution of germline and somatic mutations resulting in altered immunological behaviour (Utz *et al* 1993). A. Williams *et al* (1980) also made an important point with respect to age correction by emphasizing that two-thirds of monozygotic but no dizygotic pairs aged ≥50 years were concordant.

Population-based studies

With some variations in methodology, six of the more recent studies approximate to a population-based series of multiple sclerosis in twins (Bobowick *et al* 1978; Ebers *et al* 1986, updated in Sadovnick *et al* 1993 and Willer *et al* 2003; French Research Group on Multiple Sclerosis 1992; Heltberg and Holm 1982; Kinnunen *et al* 1988; Mumford *et al* 1994; Stazi *et al* 2002). Five of these surveys are consistent in demonstrating a higher clinical concordance rate in monozygotic (approximately 25%) than dizygotic pairs (about 3%). The French and Italian studies are exceptional in showing no significant difference between monozygotic and dizygotic twin pairs.

Bobowick *et al* (1978) estimated the frequency of multiple sclerosis in 16 000 male twin pairs registered through military service. There were 16 affected probands in 15 pairs. Nine sibships were examined and concordance was present in one monozygotic but no dizygotic pairs. The purpose of this survey was to identify epidemiological risk factors and assess whether the prevalence of trauma, infection, surgery, allergy and animal exposure differed between affected and unaffected individuals.

Heltberg and Holm (1982) took advantage of the Danish registers of twins and patients with multiple sclerosis to identify 47 twin pairs with ≥1 individual affected by multiple sclerosis in whom the living co-twin was personally examined. Four of 19 monozygotic and 1/28 dizygotic pairs were concordant. The more recent study from Scandinavia (Kinnunen *et al* 1988) sought to establish concordance for multiple sclerosis using sickness insurance and hospital discharge registers in all same-sex pairs identified from amongst 13 064 twin pairs of known zygosity on the national register. Eleven monozygotic pairs with a proband having multiple sclerosis were identified but only seven could be studied. Two pairs were concordant, one on the basis of clinical evidence supported by magnetic resonance imaging (MRI). None of six, from amongst ten identified dizygotic pairs with an affected proband, was concordant for the disease. Although the sample was small, these twins were carefully assessed using clinical and laboratory findings. Zygosity was established using red cell markers. In a less than convincing study, Bergkvist and Sandberg-Wolheim (2001) studied viral antibody titres in three monozygotic twin pairs, discordant for multiple sclerosis but still aged <31 years, and failed to identify discriminating differences revealing genetically determined humoral immune abnormalities in multiple sclerosis.

The definitive Canadian study (Ebers *et al* 1986) included 27 monozygotic and 43 dizygotic pairs identified from 5463 patients attending ten multiple sclerosis clinics. Given the level of case ascertainment through the clinic network, this approximates to a population-based study. At first estimate, concordance rates were 26% and 2.3% in monozygotic and dizygotic twins, respectively, compared with 1.9% in 4582 siblings identified from two centres. The Canadian series was updated after 7 years, showing that 8/26 (31%: one case was excluded after review of the diagnosis) were concordant monozygotic pairs compared with 2/43 (5%) dizygotes (Sadovnick *et al* 1993). Mean ages were 48 and 54 years, respectively. Two of 14 monozygotic and 1/7 dizygotic (clinically unaffected) co-twins had MRI abnormalities consistent with the diagnosis of multiple sclerosis. When the clinical and radiological results on a further group of 19 monozygotic and 23 dizygotic twins (the second series) were also included, the overall concordance rates were 17/45 (38%) and 3/66 (5%), respectively. Four monozygotic twins who were clinically discordant and did not have MRI lesions consented to lumbar puncture and no oligoclonal bands

were detected. The most recent update included 370 twin pairs who had reached a mean age of c.60 years making it improbable that the clinical status of co-twins will subsequently change. The sample is considered to include c.75% of all prevalent Canadians who have multiple sclerosis and are a twin (Willer *et al* 2003). Twinning was not found to affect prevalence and was not associated with a higher recurrence risk in non-twin siblings. Proband-wise concordance rates were 25% (SE ±4%) in monozygotic twins, compared with 5% (±3%) in dizygotic pairs and 3% (±0.6%) in non-twin siblings. The excess concordance in monozygotic twins depended mainly on the contribution of like-sexed female pairs in whom the proband-wise concordance rate was 34/100 (34% + 5.7%) compared with 3/79 (4% ± 3%) for female dizygotic pairs. Conversely, there were no differences in males depending on zygosity, although the sample size was smaller. Despite having twice the recurrence rate, the risk to dizygotic twins was not significantly different to non-twin siblings – as in previous studies. Spitsin *et al* (2001) screened 124 pairs of these twins and eight others for blood levels of uric acid, pursuing the logic that low levels might contribute to tissue injury through failure to scavenge peroxynitrite. As in their previous studies of sporadic cases, low levels of uric acid were associated with multiple sclerosis but this was independent of zygosity or clinical concordance.

In the British Isles survey (Mumford *et al* 1994), neurologists were requested to ask all patients with multiple sclerosis during a 2-year period 'are you a twin?', and, if so, to notify the central register in Cambridge. This method was intended to avoid confounding variables that had adversely affected recruitment in other studies, including bias towards monozygosity and clinical concordance. One hundred and forty-six pairs were identified, from all regions of the British Isles, with a mean age among index cases of 42 years (range 15–75; 40 and 44 years for monozygotes and dizygotes, respectively). The sex ratio was 3.4F:M. Based on the known prevalence of multiple sclerosis in the United Kingdom, and the frequency of twinning in the normal population, approximately 15% of all individuals with multiple sclerosis living in the British Isles, who have a twin, were thought to have been recruited.

After exclusions, the co-twin was assessed clinically in 105/110 pairs. Fourteen (13%) were judged to have multiple sclerosis, of whom nine (9%) were already known to be affected. Four (4%) were suspected of having multiple sclerosis, in only one of whom had the diagnosis not previously been considered. Molecular confirmation of zygosity showed 44 monozygotic (42%) and 61 dizygotic twins (58%). This represented a 10% correction rate based on the twins' own perceptions. Not all surveys have required zygosity to be based on laboratory methods and it is generally held that <6% of assignments are incorrect when anthropomorphic characteristics and the impression of individual twin partners are used to assign zygosity (Bundey 1991). Combining the categories of definite, probable and suspected multiple sclerosis, clinical concordance for monozygotic twins was 11/44 (25%) and 2/61 (3%) for dizygotes – or 9/44 (20%) and 2/61 (3%) after exclusion of co-twins with suspected disease. Thirty-three of 61 (54%) dizygotic twins, including both concordant pairs, were the same sex, giving concordance rates of 6% and 0% for dizygotes of the same and different sex, respectively. In 11/105 twin pairs (10%) it was possible to interview and examine one or more non-twin siblings from the same family but none had symptoms or signs suggestive of multiple sclerosis.

Fifty-five asymptomatic co-twins in the British Isles survey were studied by MRI (Figure 3.15). Abnormalities were detected in 6/15 (40%) monozygotic and 20/40 (50%) dizygotic co-twins compared with 8/40 (20%) healthy controls, whose mean age was 41 (18–72) years. Amongst the asymptomatic co-twins aged <60 years, abnormalities were seen in 6/15 (40%) monozygotic and 13/33 (39%) dizygotic co-twins compared with 7/37 (19%) controls. All lesions detected in controls were small and none of these scans fulfilled criteria for abnormalities typical of multiple sclerosis (Thorpe *et al* 1994a).

In the third contemporary survey, from France (French Research Group on Multiple Sclerosis 1992), 54/116 twin pairs were identified amongst a cohort of 7942 patients recruited for other purposes by public appeal on television. They were drawn from a population with a much lower prevalence of multiple sclerosis than in Canada or the British Isles. Only 1/14 monozygotic and 1/40 dizygotic pairs were concordant using clinical criteria. Twelve clinically unaffected co-twins had radiological or electrophysiological abnormalities consistent with demyelination but, as with the clinical findings, their frequency was independent of zygosity. However, confidence intervals for rates relating to monozygotic twins in the Canadian (26, 95% CI 13–43%) and French surveys (6, 95% CI 0–17.1%) overlap, as do the dizygotic rates (5, 95% CI 0–11%; and 3, 95% CI 0–8%, respectively). The difference in these results may therefore be due to sampling.

Most recently, a cohort of 1.3 million Italian twin births has been accessed for probands with multiple sclerosis (Stazi *et al* 2002). Two hundred and sixteen pairs were identified amongst 34 549 probands providing twin rates of 0.62% for the population as a whole. This compares with 1.23% in the Canadian sample. Five of 59 (8.4%) monozygous pairs were concordant

for multiple sclerosis compared with 3/157 (1.9%) nonidentical twin pairs. Comparison of cohorts from Sardinia and continental Italy showed concordance for identical twins of 1/8 (12.5%) and 4/51 (7.8%), compared with 0/10 and 3/147 (2%) in nonidentical twin pairs, respectively. The authors draw attention to the discrepancy between results of this and the French study, each involving populations with a prevalence of c.50/10^5 compared with the rates in Canada and the United Kingdom where multiple sclerosis is about twice as frequent.

Several conclusions can be drawn from the twin and family studies. Concordance in monozygotic pairs exceeds the rate in dizygotes and non-twin siblings. That a significant proportion of monozygotic co-twins in all cohorts are not concordant for the disease, despite having reached an age beyond which multiple sclerosis rarely presents, emphasizes that genetic factors increase susceptibility but only in the context of appropriate environmental conditions. The genes that confer susceptibility are therefore not sufficient for developing multiple sclerosis. The difference in recurrence risk between twins, and first- and second-degree relatives, suggests the independent or epistatic effects of >1 gene. In fact, the difference is a better measure of how many genes are involved in susceptibility to multiple sclerosis than the overall extent of the genetic effect. The trend for affected pairs to be female, over and above the sex bias in multiple sclerosis, suggests a contribution of gender independent of genes. The low concordance rate in monozygotic pairs indicates a significant independent or modifying effect of the environment on expression of genetic susceptibility.

Multiple sclerosis in adoptees and half-siblings

Adopted individuals who subsequently develop multiple sclerosis, and probands who have adopted children, provide an

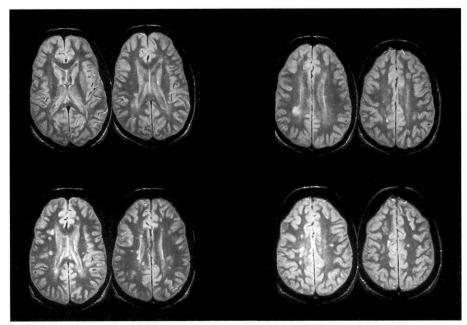

Figure 3.15 Magnetic resonance imaging in a proband with multiple sclerosis (top row) and his clinically unaffected monozygotic twin (bottom row). Both show abnormalities consistent with multiple sclerosis. The co-twin developed clinically definite disease 3 years after this scan was performed. Kindly provided by the NMR Group, Institute of Neurology.

unusual but informative resource for studying the extent to which familial clustering is a consequence of shared genes or environmental contact. Considering individuals with multiple sclerosis adopted at <1 year, and those with multiple sclerosis who through adoption have nonbiological siblings or children, Ebers et al (1995) compared the frequency of multiple sclerosis in the nonbiological parents (n = 470), siblings (n = 345) and children (n = 386) of 238 index cases. The observed recurrence risks were 1/470, 0/345 and 0/386, respectively. These were similar to prevalence (1:1000) and lifetime risks (1:500) for the at-risk (Canadian) population. Conversely, expected rates were 9, 11 and 6, respectively, after age correction based on the study of recurrence risks in biological relatives of index cases (approximately 1:20 for siblings and 1:50 for parents and children; see above). The identification of only one affected individual (a parent) amongst these 1201 relatives of adoptees matches that expected (1.2) on the basis of population risks for northern Europeans, assuming no environmental effect. This parent already had multiple sclerosis at the time of adoption. Thirty-four of the adoptees provided information on 46 of their biological parents and 59 knew details of 127 biological siblings, from whom they had been separated at <1 year of age. Multiple sclerosis was known to have developed in four and one, respectively. These rates are substantially higher than those observed in the nonbiological relatives, supporting the conclusion that (at least in these families) genetic factors are the main determinant of recurrence.

Half-siblings also prove instructive with respect to the nature of familial clustering. Potentially, they identify effects that might influence recurrence, such as breast feeding and maternal genomic imprinting. Having one parent in common, half-siblings share a proportion of parental genes and divide more or less equally into those reared together and apart, at least during the period thought critical for the development of multiple sclerosis. Working from a database of c.16 000 patients with multiple sclerosis, Sadovnick et al (1996a) studied 939 affected individuals who had (between them) 1839 half-siblings and 1395 full siblings on whom clinical assessments could be made. The age-adjusted risk for half-siblings (1.3%, SD 0.6) was significantly lower than for full siblings (3.5%, SD 0.5). The risk did not differ for maternal (of whom more were identified for the usual sociodemographic reasons) and paternal half-siblings. There was no difference in risk for half-siblings reared together (1.2 ± 0.4%) and apart (1.5 ± 0.5%). As with the studies of twins, other first-degree relatives and adoptees, the evidence strongly favours genetic factors as the basis for familial clustering.

The Canadian resource of familial cases has since been used to assess parent of origin effects in half-siblings. Ebers et al (2004) identified 1752 index cases amongst the register of 20 653 affected individuals who had ≥1 maternal or paternal half-sibling, of whom 1567 could be studied. Together, they had 3436 half- and 2706 full siblings. Pedigree analysis compared the recurrence risks (crude and age-adjusted) for full siblings and half-siblings raised together and apart, stratified for maternal and paternal shared parentage. Relatedness, not shared environment, determined the risks being higher in full (3.1: 95% CI 2.4–3.8) than half-siblings (1.9: 95% CI 1.4–2.4). These were uninfluenced by living together (1.8: 95% CI 1.0–2.6) or apart (2.0: 95% CI 1.3–2.7). Given the possibility of under-ascertainment of paternal half-siblings, the recurrence risk appeared higher in the context of affected mothers (2.4: 95% CI 1.6–3.1 vs. 1.3: 95% CI 0.7–2.0). Given the similar recurrence risk in full and maternal half-siblings, these results suggest a significant effect of maternal genes (obvious candidates would be mitochondrial), genetic imprinting or environmental factors over-represented in mothers.

Conjugal multiple sclerosis

Although it would be expected that conjugal multiple sclerosis should occur in proportion to the population risk of the disease (1:600 partners and hence 1:360 000 couples), certain artefacts spuriously influence these statistics. Most obvious is the increased chance of two affected individuals meeting through having the disease, and subsequently marrying. However, there may be disincentives for such unions, for practical reasons. Conjugal disease also applies to the situation where the spouse of an individual who is affected at marriage, also later develops the disease. Most informative are those situations in which two unaffected individuals marry and each subsequently develops multiple sclerosis. Even in this situation, there is obviously a tendency, even in very cosmopolitan societies, for individuals of the same socioeconomic group and ethnicity to marry. If both partners are from groups with a higher than average frequency of multiple sclerosis, conjugal pairs will tend to be more common, by chance, than in mixed marriages or low-risk groups.

Until recently, the literature on conjugal multiple sclerosis amounted to 24 pairs and largely consisted of single case reports, with only four publications describing a few examples (Fredrickson et al 1992; Hyllested 1956; McAlpine et al 1955; Schapira et al 1963). The apparent rarity of conjugal multiple sclerosis has been used as an argument against infection as a major aetiological factor, a conclusion supported by the similar age at onset reported by individuals with conjugal multiple sclerosis (Schapira et al 1963). Although the single case reports provide little information, Finelli (1991) and Fredrickson et al (1992) reported similarities in disease course. An extended family history was also present in one family described by Fredrickson et al (1992). Since conjugal multiple sclerosis is self-evidently rare, systematic surveys are impractical but two large surveys have now been completed.

Robertson et al (1997) identified 58 conjugal pairs as part of a regional population-based survey (n = 4), in response to repeated national appeals from practising neurologists (n = 47), from branches of the Multiple Sclerosis Society (n = 5) or by self-referral (n = 2). Thirteen pairs were excluded, leaving 45 in whom course concordance, timing of onset amongst affecteds, and recurrence risks in children could all be assessed. In 33/45 couples, each affected individual had developed clinical manifestations of multiple sclerosis after first meeting. The prevalence was 0.3/10^5 (95% CI 0.1–1.2), based on the subset of pairs identified in one region of the United Kingdom a population already known to have a prevalence of 133/10^5. Since 79% of this population sample was married, there was no excess of observed over expected cases of conjugal multiple sclerosis (0.1/10^5; 95% CI 0–1.1, or 0.8 conjugal pairs in the population of 668 700). After correction for age and disease duration, and anticipation of diagnosis in the second affected through enhanced awareness, there was no clustering for year at onset.

There was no concordance for disability or mode of presentation. Together, these statistics indicate that, in this context, neither susceptibility nor the clinical features of multiple sclerosis are influenced by contagious environmental factors.

The 45 couples had 86 children. Their mean age was 23 years at the time of the study. Clearly the possibility of additional clinical developments lay ahead. Five of 86 (6%) were already clinically concordant for multiple sclerosis and four (5%) had a history of otherwise unexplained neurological symptoms. Six of 39 (15%) children had abnormalities on MRI (Figure 3.16). Of these, 4/39 (10%) were known to have multiple sclerosis, 1/39 (3%) had suspected disease and the other was clinically normal. Three of 39 (8%) had imaging abnormalities that did not meet criteria for the diagnosis of multiple sclerosis. One had experienced neurological symptoms and two were clinically normal. Thus, around 14% of offspring had multiple sclerosis or an unexplained neurological illness. However, recurrence risks for family members other than offspring were no higher than expected from population-based figures (Robertson *et al* 1996b; Sadovnick and Baird 1988; Sadovnick *et al* 1988). Affected offspring of conjugal pairs tended to have a younger age at onset

(25 years) than those with a single affected parent (28 years) or no family history (31 years), but these small differences may have been confounded by the structure of the study – picking out those with early age at presentation. However, it remains possible that the risk for developing multiple sclerosis is inherited from both parents and shows anticipation.

Subsequently, Ebers *et al* (2000a) identified 23 conjugal cases amongst the spouses of 13 550 northern or central European probands living in Canada, giving a crude risk of 0.17% (95% CI 0.1–0.2). Based on the population prevalence, 20 would have been expected amongst this population whereas 27 were observed after age correction. Allowing for improved ascertainment through enhanced awareness, this frequency again indicates that close physical contact does not increase the risk of multiple sclerosis. Six of 49 offspring were clinically affected (3F and 3M) providing a crude recurrence risk of 12% compared with 0.7% for the children of a single affected parent. After age correction, the recurrence risk for offspring of conjugal pairs was 31% (±11%) – about the same as for monozygotic twins – compared with 2.7% (±1.1% for a single affected parent). Critical of Robertson *et al* (1997) – on ethical grounds and through the introduction of ascertainment bias – Ebers *et al* (2000a) chose not to request magnetic resonance imaging in their juvenile offspring. However, in an unrelated sample, Fulton *et al* (1999) screened for radiological abnormalities and also found white matter lesions in clinically unaffected relatives of a conjugal pair with one affected son, one set of monozygotic sisters, and one sibling pair. Helpfully, Ebers *et al* (2000a) summarized implications for models of genetic inheritance in multiple sclerosis from the conjugal pair series concluding that genetic susceptibility factors overlap and interact between many affected conjugal cases and the general population – arguing for lack of disease heterogeneity – and further parking the concept that individual risk in multiple sclerosis is determined by an infectious agent.

On the related issue of genetic loading through having two parents with increased susceptibility to multiple sclerosis, the Canadian clinic-based network has been used to identify 24 index cases whose parents were related, of whom 22 had 67 siblings (Sadovnick *et al* 2001). Six also had multiple sclerosis, providing a recurrence risk of 9% and supporting the concept that several interacting genes increase the risk of multiple sclerosis.

Genetic influences on clinical course

Clinical analysis of the course and concordance for other features of the disease within pedigrees can be used to gauge the influence of genetic factors in determining the clinical phenotype of multiple sclerosis. The Multiple Sclerosis Genetics Group (1998) described a lower frequency of the primary progressive phenotype in 89 multiplex families than in 425 cases without a family history. However, in most series, familial and sporadic cases follow a typical clinical course and with no correlation between clinical phenotype of the index case and other affecteds (Amela-Reris *et al* 2004; Weinshenker *et al* 1990). In a large population-based sample having a familial recurrence rate of 20%, Ebers *et al* (2000b) studied disability amongst 206 familial cases studied for a mean of 25 years from diagnosis. These had the expected sibling recurrence rate (3.5%). Time for affected individuals in first-only, second- or third-degree and

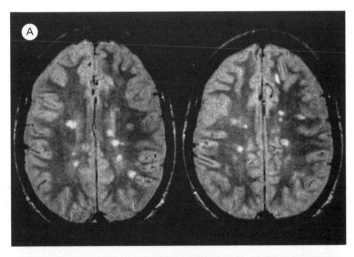

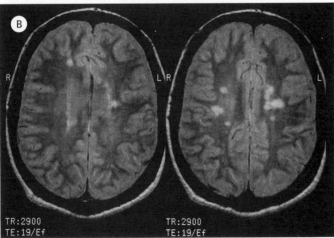

Figure 3.16 (A) Magnetic resonance imaging (MRI) in a clinically affected child of parents with conjugal multiple sclerosis. (B) MRI in the clinically unaffected child of a conjugal pair. From Robertson *et al* 1997 with permission from Elsevier.

mixed pedigrees to reach points 3, 6, 8 and 10 on the Kurtzke EDSS did not differ from each other or 836 sporadic cases. However, onset was earlier and the usual female predominance no longer seen in families with the most cases, and so presumed to have a high genetic load. This study therefore provides no evidence for genetic effects on initial symptoms or the clinical course of multiple sclerosis. Barcellos *et al* (2002) used 184 multiplex families to show concordance for optic neuritis and/or spinal cord involvement as first and second manifestations of multiple sclerosis.

It has been argued that clustering by age at onset is a feature of monogenic disease and clustering by year at onset suggests the contribution of environmental factors; clustering neither by year nor age suggests random exposure to an environmental factor. Perhaps these comparisons offer too crude a method for assessing the relative contribution of genes and environmental factors in determining the development of multiple sclerosis in individuals. The pairs are prone to sampling bias; and concordance for year at onset is confounded by the tendency for earlier recognition of symptoms in the second individual affected in the pair as a result of heightened awareness of the possibility of multiple sclerosis. Evidently, the greatest dividend has been provided by studying pairwise concordance in affected family members. To date, the results of these analyses appear ambiguous with respect to whether genetic factors influence the pattern and course of multiple sclerosis. But with large numbers of siblings, and partial elimination of artefacts inherent in such situations, useful statistical trends may emerge.

In the British Isles survey of twins (Mumford *et al* 1994), one proband had benign relapsing–remitting disease, whereas the monozygotic co-twin had primary progressive multiple sclerosis. Each of the typical phenotypes was represented in the pedigree containing 15 affected members described by Dyment *et al* (2002a). There was no formal analysis of clinical concordance in the initial Canadian series of twins and many concordant pairs had different course classifications but, by comparison with non-twin siblings, the authors commented on the pairs being clinically more alike (Sadovnick *et al* 1993). Doolittle *et al* (1990) evaluated 48 sibling pairs from 44 families and reported clustering with age at onset – the initial symptom occurring within 5 years in 30/48 pairs compared with 16/48 controls. Bulman *et al* (1991a) studied 99 sibling pairs and showed a significant correlation for age at onset in siblings and an even stronger correlation in concordant monozygotic twins, although the impact of recruitment bias was not considered. In a smaller study, Koch-Henriksen (1989) failed to demonstrate clustering for age or year at onset in 22 sibling pairs. Robertson *et al* (1996c) assessed 210/405 families notified as having affected sibling pairs and reported 166 families containing 343 affected individuals (155 pairs and 11 trios, providing 177 pairs). After appropriate correction, there was no correlation between age and year at onset. Mode of presentation and disability, corrected for artefacts that arise from similarity of siblings with respect to duration of disease and age at assessment, showed no correlation, suggesting that individuals with familial multiple sclerosis can neither take comfort nor necessarily be concerned about the pattern of disease in an affected relative. Robertson *et al* (1996c) did, however, show a correlation with disease course, even after exclusion of pairs with primary progressive multiple sclerosis, and affected siblings tended to be same-sex.

Brassat *et al* (1999) showed a correlation with disability, measured by the progression index (a derivative of disability and duration), in 87 siblings with multiple sclerosis but not disease course or age at onset. Trojano *et al* (1999) demonstrated concordance in 36 sibling pairs for age at onset, progression index and sensory symptoms at onset but not year at onset or disease course. S.J.S. Chataway *et al* (2001) also assessed pairwise concordance in 262 co-affected siblings from 250 index cases with multiple sclerosis. Whilst neither age nor year at onset showed significant adjusted intraclass correlation coefficients, 81/262 (31%) affected siblings were concordant for presenting symptom. Clinical course was identical in 50% (0.17: 95% CI 0.08–0.26) and measures of disability (0.11: 95% 0.04–0.19), progression (0.09: 95% CI 0.01–0.18) and handicap (0.08: 95% CI 0.02–0.14) were also significant. Thus, within a sibship, clinical presentation tended to be different but, once established, concordance for the long-term course appeared to be probable as did disability and handicap. Conversely, Oturai *et al* (2004) showed concordance both for clinical course and age at onset in 136 Scandinavian sibling pairs with multiple sclerosis.

Hupperts *et al* (2001) studied 245 concordant parent–child pairs retrieved from a nationwide register of familial multiple sclerosis. There was no distortion in the random distribution of male–female pairings and neither sex nor line of inheritance influenced disability, age at onset or course. However, disability was highest in the male offspring of affected fathers, who more commonly followed a primary progressive course. Conversely, onset occurred earlier in the children of affected mothers. The high further familial recurrence rate (31%) suggested a genetic loading effect in these families and interaction between independently segregating genes (epistasis).

In Sardinia, Cocco *et al* (2004a) assessed age at onset in 41 pairs of familial patients from two generations and 78 affected sibling pairs, each compared with three couples of sporadic patients matched for age. There was a progressive decline in age at onset across five decades that was not considered to have a genetic explanation given the observation that the younger member of affected relatives in successive generations showed similar anticipation to sporadic cases, and there was an effect of birth order on age at onset.

In an attempt to resolve the ambiguity of whether there are important familial effects on the course or features of multiple sclerosis, Hensiek *et al* (2005) sacrificed the safety of a population-based cohort and went for power in numbers, evaluating 1083 families with ≥1 person affected by multiple sclerosis. There was concordance for age at onset for all families (correlation coefficient 0.14; p < 0.001), as well as for affected siblings (correlation coefficient 0.15; p < 0.001), and affected parent–child pairs (correlation coefficient 0.12; p = 0.03) when each was evaluated separately. Concordance was present within affected siblings (correlation coefficient 0.17; p < 0.01) but not the parent–child group (correlation coefficient – 0.09; p = 0.61) for year of onset. The clinical course was similar between siblings (κ 0.13; p < 0.001) but not affected parents and their children (κ 0.03; p = 0.47).

This familial influence on the natural history could be attributed to an effect on disease progression, either from onset or after a period of relapsing–remitting multiple sclerosis. However, despite the expected link between progressive course and severity, there was no concordance for disease severity within any of the considered family groups (correlation coefficients: all families analyzed together: 0.02; p = 0.53, affected sibling group: 0.02; p = 0.61, affected parent–child group: 0.02; p = 0.69). Furthermore, there was no apparent effect of anticipation or genetic loading.

These findings provide evidence for a familial influence on clinical expression of multiple sclerosis, which is more likely to reflect genetic than environmental conditions. The data support the suggestion that the analysis of genetic studies should be stratified in order to separate effects that increase the risk of multiple sclerosis from those that determine the pattern of tissue injury and its clinical expression as disease progression.

It would be hard to take away from the existing literature a clear position on whether age or year at onset, clinical features or patterns of the disease course cluster within families. The samples used to inform these questions are not ideal. The studies are prone to confounding effects of ascertainment. The results remain ambiguous. Resolving these issues has a significance that goes beyond the important application of counselling affected individuals who look to the proximity of multiple sclerosis in an affected first-degree relative as a prognostic indicator. A whole industry of molecular genetic studies has been predicated on the fact that genes shaping the clinical course of multiple sclerosis exist and can be found by stratified case–control studies. If so, these features should be concordant in affected pairs. Without that evidence, continued efforts to account for influences that may not exist could be seen as misguided. For us, the jury is still out.

CANDIDATE GENES IN MULTIPLE SCLEROSIS

In situations where a genetic contribution to the aetiology is apparent but the number, nature and location of genes conferring that effect are unknown, it is reasonable to make a few inspired guesses as to their identity based on a working knowledge of the pathogenesis. Where possible, we have followed the convention of annotating genes in italics and capitals, whereas loci, individual alleles, haplotypes and gene products are in lower case roman script. Traditionally, this convention has not been adopted for the HLA system and genes within its extended haplotype; these are usually presented in upper case but not italicised. The system is clearly imperfect, and we have not resolved all the stylistic ambiguities. The first, and some might say the only, candidate gene to be identified is encoded within the major histocompatibility complex – hereafter described interchangeably as the MHC or HLA (human leucocyte antigen) region – on chromosome 6q21.1-21.3.

The major histocompatibility complex

Although the allelic associations with HL-A3 and B7 were described >30 years ago (Jersild et al 1972), the modern era seeking to unravel the molecular nature and meaning of this serological association began with the first restriction fragment length polymorphism studies of multiple sclerosis (Cohen et al 1984). The work of several decades, involving progressively more sophisticated techniques for analysis of this region, has not unambiguously identified the locus or the allele(s) responsible for the effect, or resolved the nature of this association. The

obvious candidates are either DR(2)15 or DQ6 (Haegert et al 1993; Hillert and Olerup 1993; Spurkland et al 1991a) but the region could encode ≥1 gene and allelic heterogeneity may be present at each locus. As the HLA region has systematically been dissected using serological, cellular and molecular typing methods, revealing increasingly complex arrangements, so the pattern of associations with multiple sclerosis has been refined and strengthened. The allelic association with HL-A3 (now HLA-A3) was soon shown to be secondary to a class I association with HLA-B7. In turn, this was shown to result from linkage disequilibrium to the class II alleles HLA-DR2 and DQw6 (Heard et al 1989a; Olerup et al 1987; Vartdal et al 1989). These alleles are now reclassified as the DR15 and DQ6 subtypes of DR2 and DQw6, respectively. They are the phenotypic expression of the DRB1*1501, DRB5*0101 (DR15) and DQA1*0102, DQB2*0602 (DQ6) genotypes, and correspond to the cellular typing allele Dw2 (Olerup and Hillert 1991). Despite the consistent evidence for a population association, it proved difficult to confirm linkage of HLA genes and susceptibility to multiple sclerosis. Only with the availability of substantial numbers of families (Ebers et al 1996; Haines et al 1996; Sawcer et al 1996) was the earlier inconclusive evidence for linkage, based on studies involving fewer families (Ebers et al 1982b; Kellar-Wood et al 1995), finally resolved. As argued above, this suggested an effect conferred by a gene(s) identical to DR(2)15 or DQ6, or in linkage disequilibrium with the class II region. Because the strength of the association was relatively weak, the assumption has been that the responsible gene(s) exerts a relatively small biological effect.

Structure and function of HLA genes and their products

The HLA complex consists of 3600 Mb of DNA mapped to chromosome 6p21.3 (Figures 3.17 and 3.18). It has been entirely sequenced (MHC Sequencing Consortium 1999). Two hundred and twenty-four genes are located in the MHC at an unprecedented density – 1:16 kb. The (sex-averaged) recombination rate across the MHC is 0.49 cM/Mb, but with three recombination hotspots (Mungall et al 2003). It is predicted that 128 genes are expressed, of which 40% are likely to have products influencing immune function. Most of the pseudogenes are in the class I and II regions with very few in class III. The polymorphisms (peaking around DP, DQ and HLA-B and -C) are the most extensive seen anywhere in the genome and are considered to be the tombstones of 'long-standing battles for supremacy between the immune system and infectious pathogens' (Le Souef et al 2000). Sequence information suggests that the class I and II regions are more extensive than suggested by previous serological analyses. Even so, the classic HLA loci encode only a minority of genes found in the MHC region since this accommodates an additional 120 genes (Beck and Trowsdale 2000). Diversity probably results from recombination between existing alleles or gene conversion events. Linkage disequilibrium across this region is extensive due to the low rate of recombination. In regions that do not span classic HLA loci, linkage disequilibrium is comparable to all other parts of the genome and the number of common haplotypes is no different from elsewhere. Walsh et al (2003) genotyped 201 reliable, polymorphic and evenly spaced SNPs (1:20 kb) in 136

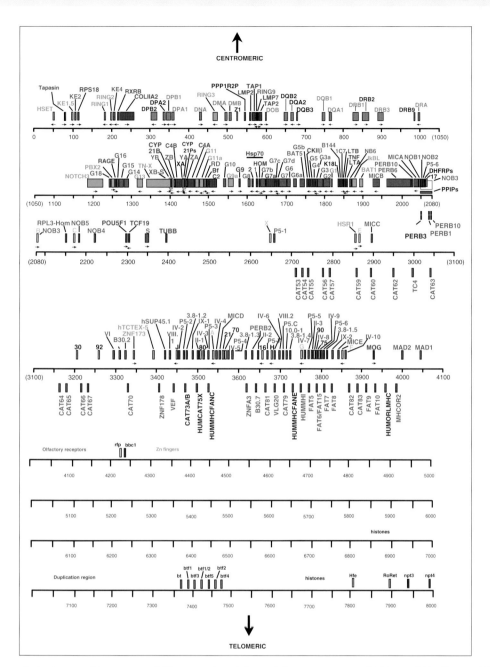

Figure 3.17 Gene map of the human histocompatibility complex. Adapted from Horton *et al* 2004 and kindly provided by Professor John Trowsdale. © 2004, reprinted with permission from Nature Publishing Group (www.nature.com/nature).

independent chromosomes. These were also genotyped for 9 HLA genes, 2 TAP (see below) genes and 18 microsatellites. Markers were genotyped in 18 multigenerational European pedigrees to allow direct assessment of chromosomal phase and, thus, simple reconstruction of haplotypes. Using these SNP data, haplotype patterns of the region were identified and mapped for genetic and physical distance. Although not a complete account of haplotype diversity, this provided a first step towards a comprehensive characterization of the patterns of common variation in the MHC.

After the disease associations were first catalogued in the early 1970s, it became clear that the functional role of HLA gene products is to present peptide to T cells. Antigen is processed under the influence of proteosome gene products and exported to the cell surface in association with peptide transporters (Spies *et al* 1990; Trowsdale *et al* 1990). From there, it is exposed to helper T cells held in the cleft of class I or II molecules and recognized by the heterodimeric T-cell receptor (Bjorkman *et al* 1987; Davies and Bjorkman 1988). Class I molecules present peptides of nine amino acids digested from intracellular antigens. Class II molecules present peptides of 12–24 amino acids derived from the extracellular environment after breakdown in endosomes.

The many class I and II HLA molecules consist of heterodimeric chains with extracellular, transmembrane and intracellular domains. Polymorphism within the class I molecule is determined by amino-acid variations in short sections of the α1 (three sites) and α2 (four sites) extracellular domains. The

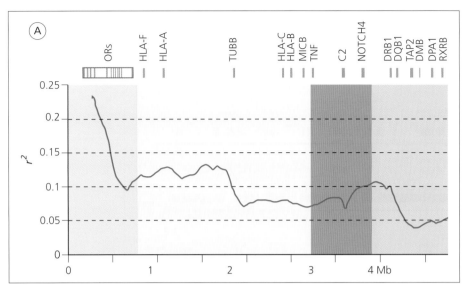

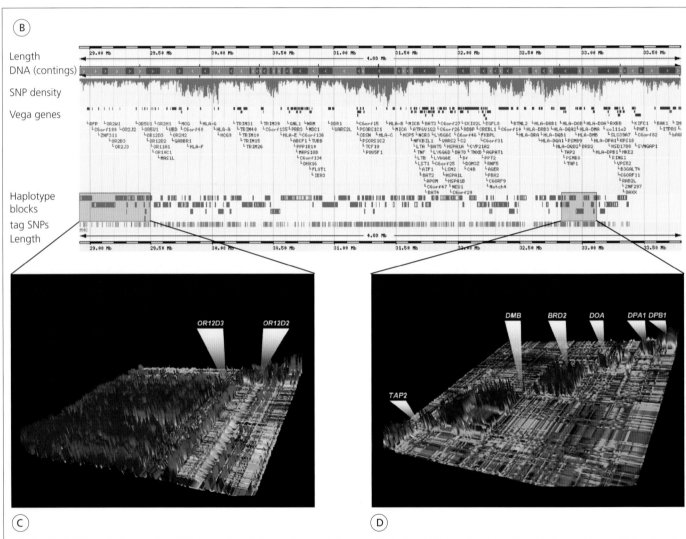

Figure 3.18 (A) Sliding window plot of average r^2 (an estimate of linkage disequilibrium) across the MHC. Average r^2 was calculated from 25 kb to 250 kb in 500-kb sliding windows, at 50-kb increments. MHC extended class I, class I, class III and class II regions (blue, yellow, orange and green, respectively) present comparatively distinct variation patterns of long range linkage disequilibrium, reflected in the haplotype block analysis. (B–D). Linkage disequilibrium structure across the MHC. (B) Distribution of haplotype blocks as viewed in the GLOVAR genome browser. Haplotype blocks are represented as red bars, each comprising a number of SNPs (red marks) located according to map position. The distribution of tag SNPs is indicated by a green track under the red marks. (C) High resolution view of 720 kb of the extended class I region containing a high cluster of genes in linkage disequilibrium interrupted by a single recombination hotspot between *OR12D3* and *OR12D2*. This long range region contains 13 contiguous haplotype blocks. (D) View of linkage disequilibrium structure in the class II region with high linkage disequilibrium regions separated by recombination hotspots mapped to between *TAP2* and HLA-DMB, BRD2 and HLA-DQA, and HLA-DQA and HLA-DPA1. From Miretti *et al* 2005. © 2005, reproduced with permission from The University of Chicago Press.

polymorphic class Iα gene product forms a heterodimer with β2 microglobulin. This is invariant and encoded on chromosome 15q15.3. Class II polymorphisms result from amino acid sequence alterations in the β chain. There are nine β chain genes but the product of only one is used in the assembly of each class II molecule, joining with an invariate α chain. The situation differs for DQ, which has two variable α and β chains. HLA-DP encodes pairs of two α and two β chains but only one of each is expressed. The region contains a number of pseudogenes, identified by molecular analysis but not expressed. Analysis of the HLA system at the genotypic level has allowed better definition of the previously identified cellular and serological specificities. The DRB β chain polymorphisms, which determine the DR15 and DR16 subtypes of DR2, themselves contain three and two different genotypic sequences, respectively, creating further splits in these specificities (Dupont 1992). Genotyping adds to the complexity, revealing at least 315 DRB1, 22 DQA1 and 53 DQB1 alleles (Marsh et al 2002). Usually, the DR and DQ specificities show extremely tight linkage disequilibrium extending across the entire HLA region to include class I, II and III loci. The specificity of allelic distribution within these common haplotypes differs between populations. For example, Klitz et al (2003) listed 75 distinct DRB1-DQA1-DQB1 haplotypes amongst 3798 identified in 1899 individuals.

The tertiary structure of class I and II molecules is broadly similar. Each contains a platform made up of eight parallel β strands with a right-angled pocket constructed from two α helices where most polymorphic residues of the molecule are located (Bjorkman et al 1987; Davies and Bjorkman 1988). Variations in the amino acid structure of the two polymorphic extracellular domains mainly occur in the peptide-binding portion of the α helices (J. Brown et al 1993). These molecules are assembled in the endoplasmic reticulum, glycosylated and associated with β2 microglobulin (for class I) or the invariant class II β chain, respectively. The class I molecules associate with antigen brought to the endoplasmic reticulum by peptide transporter gene products (TAPs), but the presence of the class II invariant chain prevents peptide binding until the molecule disassembles in the acidic environment of the endosome, from where it is exported to the cell surface. Products of the DM locus are required for intracellular aggregation of antigen with class II product and its subsequent processing. Peptide is presented to helper T cells in association with class II molecules, and cell–cell interaction is assisted by a variety of adhesion molecules. Cytotoxic T cells recognize peptide associated with class I products and use the accessory molecule CD8. Helper T cells recognize peptide presented by class II molecules and with accessory binding from CD4. Many other costimulatory molecules are involved (see Chapter 11).

HLA DR associations with multiple sclerosis

DRB1*1501, DRB5*0101 (DR15) and DQA1*0102, DQB2*0602 (DQ6) are the genotypic and phenotypic expression of Dw2, respectively. The relative risk for multiple sclerosis in DR(2)15 Caucasian heterozygotes is <5 but much higher (>10) in homozygotes (Barcellos et al 2003; Beall et al 1995; Kellar-Wood et al 1995). The conclusions reached by these independent studies are supported by meta-analysis (Rasmussen et al 2001a).

The original view that DR(2)15 is a marker of susceptibility to multiple sclerosis only in Caucasians has required modification. Hillert (1994) emphasized that the specifically different disease associations seen with the DR classification alone are no longer apparent when Dw types are compared in parallel. That said, associations are more easily demonstrated in northern Europeans, irrespective of domicile, than in other populations. The evidence is provided by studies involving northern Europeans (Kellar-Wood et al 1995; D.H. Miller et al 1989a; Olerup and Hillert 1991; Olerup et al 1989; Spurkland et al 1991a) but also American blacks (Dupont et al 1977), Faroese (Jersild et al 1993), Russians (Boiko et al 2002; Sudomoina et al 1998), Spaniards (Clerici and Fernandez 1992; Lopez Larrea et al 1990; Uria et al 1993), Mexicans (Alvarado-de la Barrera et al 2000); Italians (Ballerini et al 2004; La Mantia et al 1990), Chinese (Serjeantson et al 1992); Palestinian Arabs (Al-Din et al 1986), Iraqis (Shinar et al 1998), Israelis (Kwon et al 1999), Iranians (Amirzargar et al 1998; Kalanie et al 2000), coloured South Africans (Fewster and Kies 1984), Japanese (Hao et al 1992; Spurkland et al 1991b), Martinicians (Quelvennec et al 2003), non-Parsi Indians (Kankonkar et al 2003), and Asian Indians living in the United Kingdom (Kelly et al 1995a). Of course, even now, there are discrepancies in this catalogue relating to defined populations – notably, Chinese (Kelly et al 1995b) and Hungarian Gypsies (Kalman et al 1991; Takacs et al 1990). More generally, this analysis is in marked contrast to earlier claims for specifically different associations in specific populations. These had suggested an association with HLA-B12 in Asian Indians (Wadia et al 1980), with DR4 in Jordanians (Kurdi et al 1977), Japanese (Naito et al 1978) and Mexicans (Gorodetsky et al 1986), and with Dw3 in Maltese patients with multiple sclerosis (Elian et al 1987). These findings have either not been confirmed in new cohorts of comparable ethnicity, in related groups (Al-Din et al 1986; Hao et al 1992; Spurkland et al 1991b) or, if the specifically different association has been confirmed, an equally strong population association is also found to exist with DR(2)15 (Naito et al 1978).

Surprisingly, in the Orkney Islands, multiple sclerosis is associated with neither HLA B7 nor DR(2)15. Although the frequency of these antigens in Orcadian patients is no lower than in affected individuals from other parts of the United Kingdom, the lack of an association arises from the fact that the frequency of HLA B7 and DR2 in the normal population is >50% (Poskanzer et al 1980b). This has been interpreted as indicating that genes conferring susceptibility to multiple sclerosis are so over-represented in the normal Orcadian population as to leave little room for a disease association (Compston 1981). Conversely, Faroese patients with multiple sclerosis show the expected class II association with DR2 (DR15/DQ6; Jersild et al 1993).

However, Sardinians are the population that stands out as an exception to the rule that multiple sclerosis is DR(2)15 associated (Marrosu et al 1988; 1992). The at-risk population has a higher frequency of DR3 (DRB1*0301, DQA1*0501, DQB1*0201) and DR2 (DRB1*1601, DQA1*0502, DQB1*0102). The DR3 haplotype includes B18 rather than B8, as in other European populations apart from the Basque people, and also differs at the 21-OHDA/C4B loci. DR3 may be preferentially transmitted to affected women through the paternal line (Marrosu et al 2004). The DR2 and DR4 haplotypes have different structures and population frequencies from those seen in other Europeans. There is no increase in DR2 amongst Sardinian patients with multiple sclerosis (5%) compared with controls (7%). Rather, the association is with a specifically different HLA phenotype (DR4) and genotype (DRB1*0405-DQA1*0301-DQB1*0302). The most recent analysis indicates much complexity. Five DRB1-DQB1 haplotypes are associated with multiple sclerosis in Sardinians. These are: DRB1*0405-DQB1*0302; DRB1*1501-DQB1*0602; DRB1*0301-DQB1*0201; DRB1*1303-DQB1*0301; and DRB1*0405-DQB1*0301 (Marrosu *et al* 2001). In some genetically isolated populations, the stronger association is with the ancestral haplotype A3-B18-DR3 (Bitti *et al* 2001). The frequency of DQB1*0301 is reduced in Sardinian patients with multiple sclerosis. In a useful comparative study, La Mantia *et al* (1990) restated the DR(2)15 association amongst patients from all parts of Italy, where adequate studies had been performed, except in Sardinia. In the Canaries, the primary association is with DR15 and DQ6 but a secondary association exists with DR4 (DRB1*0402/0404: Coraddu *et al* 1998). The DR4 association is not seen in southern Spain (O. Fernandez *et al* 2004). In Turkey, there is an allelic association with both DR2 (DBR1*1501, DQA1*0102, DQB1*0602) and DR4 (DRB1*04, DQA1*03, DQB1*0302: Saruhan-Direskeneli *et al* 1997). Thus, there is a DR4 flavour to the association in some southern Mediterranean populations. But this Mediterranean DR4 haplotype is not identical to that seen elsewhere in Europe – the associated genotype being DRB1*0405 in Sardinia and DRB1*0402/0404 in the Canaries – thus presenting opportunities to narrow the region by identifying the segments shared between populations. Overall, the relationship with DR(2)15 makes it difficult to identify secondary allelic associations. But studies involving large numbers of cases, or stratification for DR(2)15, have revealed a subsidiary relationship between multiple sclerosis in northern Europeans and DR(17)3 and DR(13)6 (DRB1*1302), conferring susceptibility and resistance, respectively (Haegert *et al* 1990; 1996; Olerup and Hillert 1991).

HLA linkage

Until recently, evidence for an effect of class II MHC alleles based on linkage studies appeared to conflict with the results of population associations. Affected sibling pair analyses showed no evidence for a bias in sharing of inherited haplotypes (Alter *et al* 1976; Clerget-Darpoux *et al* 1984; Haile *et al* 1981; G.J. Stewart *et al* 1981; Visscher *et al* 1979). Compston and Howard (1982) collated the literature available at the time, with cavalier disregard for case ascertainment and publication bias, concluding that there was more in favour than against evidence for linkage of HLA to susceptibility in multiple sclerosis. But although any genuinely associated allele must also be linked, it took some time to show that this is indeed the case. Once they were completed, the whole-genome screens (see below) revealed that confusion had arisen from the low power of these undersized linkage studies. Thus, the initial failure to demonstrate linkage in population-based studies can be considered a type 2 statistical error. The recent confirmation of linkage in the full-genome screens was to be expected once sufficient power was applied, and epidemiologically authoritative samples used. In 2005, the lod score for linkage of 6p21 to multiple sclerosis in a single large study of multiple sclerosis in populations of northern European origin is 11.7 (International Multiple Sclerosis Genetics Consortium 2005).

But to rehearse the story, linkage was not reliably demonstrated without the evidence from whole-genome linkage screens that were more adequately powered and – by their nature – allowed comparison between the MHC and other parts of the genome (see below). The twin sample collected by Kinnunen *et al* (1988) proved relatively uninformative with respect to HLA linkage since the majority of DR2 identical pairs were not clinically concordant and most discordant pairs were DR2 identical. Ebers *et al* (1982b) showed no deviation in the expected distribution of haplotypes shared identically by descent in 40 affected sibling pairs, on the basis of established parental haplotypes. The study was subsequently updated to include 48 pairs but with no change in result (Sadovnick *et al* 1991a). Govaerts *et al* (1985) included 20 sibling pairs in a study of HLA and multiple sclerosis. The DR2 association was confirmed but with no evidence for distortion in the random distribution of parental haplotypes. Working with sporadic and familial cases of multiple sclerosis and with appropriate controls derived from within and outside these families, Kellar-Wood *et al* (1995) showed association but no linkage of the DR(2)15 allele to multiple sclerosis using a probabilistic method of assigning haplotypes in affected sibling pairs (Holmans 1993). In a sample of 115 affected sibling pairs, index cases had the same frequency of DR(2)15 as 93 unrelated sporadic patients with multiple sclerosis. Comparison of all affected individuals (familial and sporadic) with 130 unrelated controls showed the expected association with DR(2)15/DQ6. Within families, this association was confirmed comparing index cases and unaffected siblings. DR(2)15 showed transmission disequilibrium. But despite these associations, the 115 sibling pairs showed no evidence for linkage of disease susceptibility to the DR locus even in families with the DR15 allele. Conversely, Hillert *et al* (1994) showed that all other affecteds also had DR(2)15 in nine Swedish multiplex families in which each index case was positive for Dw2. Although not epidemiologically reliable, the study provided evidence for linkage of multiple sclerosis to this class II allele and the balance of evidence subsequently shifted back in favour both of association and linkage to HLA.

Linkage analysis in 49 multiplex families from Sweden showed positive lod scores for the DRB1 locus in families with the Dw2 haplotype (lod 2.08) but not without (lod 0.95). DR(2)15 was associated with multiple sclerosis in a comparison of unrelated cases (44%) and controls (18%) and there was transmission disequilibrium within families (Fogdell *et al* 1997). Tienari *et al* (1993) assessed association and linkage to DQA1*0102 and DQB1*0602 alleles in 21 Finnish families with multiple sclerosis. Compared with controls, DQA1*0102-DQB1*0602 showed an increased frequency in patients with multiple sclerosis and their unaffected parents. However, the multiple sclerosis associated alleles were often transmitted to affected individuals on different parental haplotypes, providing evidence for identity by state because of the high overall frequency and parental homozygosity for DQA1*0102 and DQB1*0602. Conversely, identity by descent analysis showed little evidence for linkage. Exclusion of families with a parent homozygous for DQA1*0102, provided a lod score for DQA1 of 6.4 (compared with 5.4 for DQB1). The haplotype transmission test indicated that the DQA1*0102 allele was selectively inherited by affected but not unaffected offspring. Voskuhl *et al* (1996) studied 29 affected sibling pairs from only nine families. There was biased transmission of the DR2/DQw1 allele to affected but not unaffected offspring, and two haplotype sharing was increased. Not surprisingly, Karni *et al* (1999a) were unable to demonstrate linkage in 13 Israeli families, selected for having a low frequency of DR(2)15, in whom there was a disease association with DRB1*1303. Marrosu *et al* (2000a) concluded that HLA makes a small contribution to familial aggregation in multiple sclerosis based on the lower than expected proportion of affected 57 sibling pairs showing zero HLA haplotype sharing, given the *a priori* expectation based on estimates for λs.

Is the multiple sclerosis association primarily with DR or DQ?

Apart from its constituent class I and II genes, the MHC includes a plethora of additional polymorphic loci (MHC Sequencing Consortium 1999) whose alleles offer themselves as candidates for susceptibility to multiple sclerosis. But the extensive linkage disequilibrium within the region has made it difficult to reconcile which locus (loci) encodes the disease susceptibility gene(s). Many alleles at the DR/DQ loci are part of distinct haplotypes. DR(2)15 is often linked to DQ6 as part of the DRB1*1501, DRB5*0101, DQB1*0602 haplotype, and usually associated with DRB5*0101. It is reasonable to conclude that the class I associations are secondary to linkage disequilibrium with class II, and that the latter is statistically stronger and biologically more relevant. This underlies our decision not to catalogue the many studies showing associations between multiple sclerosis and HLA-A3 and -B7, characterizing the literature of the 1970s and 1980s.

That said, Fogdell-Hahn *et al* (2000) have argued on the basis of stratified analyses that HLA-A3 exerts an effect (odds ratio 2.1) over and above the influence of DR(2)15. Ligers *et al* (2001a) showed linkage to HLA even in 58/542 affected sibling pairs in whom DR(2)15 was not represented in the family. This suggested that the susceptibility effect contributed by class II is not necessarily encoded at the DR locus. Subsequently, Harbo *et al* (2004) studied a large sample of affected sibling pair and sporadic cases from Scandinavia and the United Kingdom to show a complementary or, perhaps, independent effect of class I on the susceptibility to multiple sclerosis conferred by DR(2)15; the relative risk in the presence of DR(15) and A3 was 15 compared with 7 and 3, respectively, when these alleles were present alone. Using an extended 5-cM (14-Mb) haplotype analysis of the MHC involving 13 microsatellite markers and DRB1/DQB1 allele typing, Rubio *et al* (2002) also found that genes encoded within the extended class I region confer susceptibility to multiple sclerosis, independent of class II but with epistatic effects. They failed to demonstrate any contribution from the class II (TNFa) region (see below). In a subsequent analysis, the telomeric extent of this Tasmanian haplotype included association with the C282Y allele. This was not seen in a separate cohort of non-European cases from Victoria indicating that the extended haplotype is a population marker in Tasmania but not a susceptibility factor for multiple sclerosis (J.P. Rubio *et al* 2004).

In studying boundaries of the multiple sclerosis-associated haplotype in multiple sclerosis, Olerup *et al* (1990) found no evidence for extension to the DP or DQA2 loci, which lie centromeric to DR, and the effect mapped telomeric to DP. Hillert and Olerup

(1993) later showed that, on its centromeric side, the multiple sclerosis-associated haplotype does not extend to C4/CYP21 within the class III region. Bennetts *et al* (1999) showed tight linkage disequilibrium taking the haplotype beyond DM to the promoter of the DRA locus. On the centromeric side, the balance of opinion favours the view that the TAP alleles do not increase the risk of multiple sclerosis and the susceptibility haplotype therefore does not extend as far as the TAP2 locus.

Hauser *et al* (1989) concluded, on the basis of analysing MHC haplotypes in cases and controls, that the DR(2)15 allele is itself the risk factor for multiple sclerosis and not merely a population marker. That is also the conclusion from a recent high density family-based SNP association screen of the MHC in 1185 individuals with multiple sclerosis from Canada and Finland (Lincoln *et al* 2005). However, those who report an association between multiple sclerosis and DR(2)15 usually also find an increased frequency of DQ6 (Kellar-Wood *et al* 1995; Spurkland *et al* 1991a; Tienari *et al* 1994). Therefore, it is not easy to resolve the question of which gene exerts the greater influence on susceptibility since DR(2)15 and DQ6 are in such tight linkage disequilibrium in Caucasians (Haegert and Francis 1993; Hauser *et al* 1989; Hillert and Olerup 1993; Olerup *et al* 1987; Spurkland *et al* 1991a). Polymorphisms of either gene could directly influence peptide binding and so independently alter immune responsiveness. Francis *et al* (1987a) reported a stronger association with DQ6 than DR(2)15 in Caucasians from northeast Scotland. In arguing that this favoured DQ as the primary susceptibility factor, they drew attention to the high frequency of DR2 in some populations where multiple sclerosis is uncommon. However, they did not comment on the prevalence of DR2 subtypes in these other populations. Heard *et al* (1989b) were ahead of the game in the RFLP era, and used pooled DNA from patients and controls to screen for DP, DQ and DR genotypes. One RFLP appeared to associate with multiple sclerosis independently from the DRβ gene association. Another suggestion has been that heterodimers formed by DQ α and β chains, encoded on the same (*cis*) or different (*trans*) chromosomes, combine within the individual to form a unique susceptibility molecule (Spurkland *et al* 1991a), but the evidence is not conclusive (Olerup and Hillert 1991; Tienari *et al* 1994).

In patients from Iceland, DR2 (DRB5*0101-DQA1*0102-DQB1*0602; DRB1*1501, which is in strong linkage disequilibrium, was not tested) increases susceptibility to multiple sclerosis (relative risk 2.4). DR13 (DRB1*1302-DQA1*0102-DQB1*0604) and DR7 (DRB1*0701-DQA1*0201-DQB1*0201) are both protective [relative risks (RR) 0.33 and 0.12, respectively] – DR13 in all patients and DR7 only in DR2-negative individuals (Haegert *et al* 1996). Specific alleles within these haplotypes conferred susceptibility (DRB5 and DQB1) and protection (DRB1 and DQA1). The effects are considered to be the consequence of specific sequence variations of Phe and Ile at position 67, respectively. Thus, the primary susceptibility association appears to be with DR, whereas the protective effect is conferred by the DQ locus. Hao *et al* (1992) reported that the relative risk for developing multiple sclerosis in Japan was higher in the presence of DQB1 (RR = 4) than DR2 (RR = 2.6). In their study of Asian Indians and Afro-Caribbeans with multiple sclerosis living in the United Kingdom, Kelly *et al* (1995b) reported an increased frequency of DR2 in Asian Indian cases (RR = 2.4; 95% CI 1.1–4.9) with a DQB1*0602 association

(RR = 3.7; 95% CI 1.1–12.3). Although the frequency of DR2 was increased, there was no association in the Afro-Caribbean patients. Compared with Caucasians, only a minority of patients in these ethnic groups have the DRB1*1501-DQA1*0102-DQB1*0602 multiple sclerosis-associated genotype. Multiple sclerosis is rare in Gypsies despite a high population frequency of DR2. The DR2 subtype present in Gypsies is not DR15 (Kalman et al 1991) nor has DQ6 been detected (Takacs et al 1990). DQ6 is evidently not in linkage disequilibrium with DR15 in Gypsies and neither antigen is present at high frequency in patients or controls.

Kelly et al (1995b) attempted to establish the relative importance of the DR and DQ associations by comparing their frequencies in 111 Caucasian patients from the United Kingdom and nine affected Chinese from Shanghai, with controls. The lack of either DR or DQ associations with the Chinese patients led the authors to conclude that neither is necessary for the development of multiple sclerosis, but the sample was small. In Chinese from Hong Kong, the Dw2 haplotype showed a different genotypic configuration and only DQB1*0602 was associated with multiple sclerosis (Serjeantson et al 1992; Spurkland et al 1991b), if correct, shifting attention towards DQ as the primary susceptibility locus – at least in Chinese.

The DQB1*0302 association with multiple sclerosis (Marrosu et al 1988; 1992) and negative relationship with DQB1*0301 in Sardinia can be interpreted as indicating a primary association with DQ since these alleles are each in linkage with DR4. Marrosu et al (2001) examined an 11-Mb interval of the MHC with 19 microsatellites and SNPs for 12 candidate genes. Independent peaks of transmission disequilibrium were detected at DR and DQ, representing the known multiple sclerosis-associated specificities. Haegert et al (1993) failed to show that the residue change at position 26 in DQB, associated with multiple sclerosis in French Canadians, is also relevant in Sardinian patients with the DQB1*0201, DQB1*0302 and DQA1*0301 genotypic associations. Seeking to resolve the issue of whether entirely separate linkage disequilibria and specifically different multiple sclerosis associations exist, Haegert et al (1993) compared patients and controls of differing ethnicity in Canada. An association with DQB1*0602 and DQA1*0102 was confirmed in all groups, although the leucine change at position 26 in DQB distinguished French-Canadian patients from mixed ethnic Canadians, Swedish patients and Sardinians. Coraddu et al (1998a) compared DR and DQ allele frequencies in controls with patients with multiple sclerosis from the Canary Islands. They showed an association with DR(2)15. Amongst individuals with the DRB1*1501 genotype, all controls but only some cases were also positive for DQB1*0602 and DQA1*0102 suggesting a stronger susceptibility effect of DR than DQ. In patients from peninsular Italy, the relative risk conferred by the presence of DRB1*1501 is 1.5, compared with 2.5 and 2.9 for DQA1*0301 and DQB1*0502, respectively (Ciusani et al 1995). The extended DRB1*1501, DQA1*0102, DQB1*0602 haplotype has a relative risk for multiple sclerosis of 3.3. In southern Spain, the association extends across the DR2 haplotype but, of DRB1*1501/DQA1*0102/DQB1*0602, only DQB1*0602 maintains the association in a logistic regression model (O. Fernandez et al 2004). Multiple sclerosis in the Paisa community of Colombia, South America, is also primarily associated with DQA1 (Arcos-Burgos et al 1999). Further resolution of

which gene within the extended haplotype confers the effect on susceptibility to multiple sclerosis will involve fine mapping and the detection of disease-specific sequences. To that end, Boon et al (2001) provided evidence based on haplotype sharing implicating a 51-kb interval in which the only known functional gene is DQ. Hence, that is their preferred candidate. Using the admixture approach in African-Americans, Oksenberg et al (2004) studied 336 affected individuals, 357 unaffected family members and 310 controls to confirm the class II MHC association. Narrowing the interval by examining the relative strength of associations at separate loci, showed that DR(2)15 is associated with multiple sclerosis independently from the extended DR-DQ haplotype, indicating a primary effect of the DR locus. That was also the conclusion of a study from Martinique showing a primary association between susceptibility to multiple sclerosis and DRB1*1503 (not 1501) and with no increase in DQB1*0602 after DR(2)15 stratification (Quelvennec et al 2003). More recently, the approach of subtracting differences in the genome of 605 African-American individuals with multiple sclerosis and 1043 matched controls suggests that a genetic contribution to susceptibility has been 're-inserted' into the admixed population from European (that is, Caucasian) ancestry, thus newly identifying a susceptibility locus on chromosome 1 (Reich et al 2005).

Genes encoded at the closely linked DP locus are evidently not associated with multiple sclerosis. An exception may be the optico-spinal form of multiple sclerosis in Japanese (see below). The original report of an association between DP alleles and multiple sclerosis (DPw4: Moen et al 1984) in Norwegian patients initially was supported by studies from Sweden (in comparisons with Danish controls; Odum et al 1988), Japan (Odum et al 1989) and in Chinese (DPw1, despite absence of the expected DQB1*0602 high-risk allele: Dekker et al 1993). The putative associations conferred a lower relative risk than the neighbouring DR and DQ loci (Moen et al 1984; Odum et al 1988; 1989). Although there was no association, Ciusani et al (1995) reported higher frequencies of DPB1*0301 and DPB1*0201 in Italian cases than controls (24% vs. 11% and 40% vs. 28%, respectively). But in many contemporary studies, DP associations have not been confirmed in a variety of populations (Begovich et al 1990; Fugger et al 1990a; Howell et al 1991; Middleton et al 1992; Morling et al 1992; N.I. Roth et al 1991; Spurkland et al 1991a; 1991b).

Is there a disease-specific class II mutation in multiple sclerosis?

The balance of opinion is that HLA-associated susceptibility to multiple sclerosis is not explained by the presence of a disease-specific mutation distinguishing DR15/DQ6 alleles in patients and controls. Class II alleles in patients with multiple sclerosis are structurally no different from those found in unaffected individuals (Cowan et al 1991a). Three alleles of DR15 (DRB1*1501, *1502 and *1503) have been studied at the sequence level and >90% of British patients with multiple sclerosis carry a DRB1*1501 allele that is identical in sequence to that observed in the general population (Cullen et al 1991). Starting from the observation that the DRB1*1501/DRB1*0400 genotype provides a higher relative risk (9.14) than DRB1*1501 (2.47) and DRB1*0400 (no primary association) alone, Ghabanbasani et al

(1995) proposed that susceptibility depends on conformational changes resulting from the presence of histidine and alanine residues at positions 13 and 71, respectively, in the DRB1 chain. Vartdal *et al* (1989) had earlier claimed that patients with multiple sclerosis from Norway share sequences of the DQβ chain more often than controls. They argued that this amino acid sequence might occur within the DR2, DR4 and DR6 phenotypes, thus accounting for differences in population associations with multiple sclerosis. Subsequently, Spurkland *et al* (1991a) described a disease-associated alteration in the glutamine residue at position 34 of the DQα chain that, when combined with DQB1 sequences, conferred a relative risk of 13 for developing multiple sclerosis. Haegert and Francis (1992) described a leucine residue at position 26 on DQα associated with multiple sclerosis. M. Allen *et al* (1994) reported a base pair change in valine at position 86 of the DRB chain associated with multiple sclerosis. Others have not identified disease-specific DR2 sequences in comparisons of cases and controls (Francis *et al* 1987a; 1991; Olerup and Hillert 1991; Sinha *et al* 1991). Teutsch *et al* (1999) attributed the DR(2)15 effect to the valine/valine genotype rather than glycines at residue 86. Greer and Pender (2005) showed a negative association between the presence of alleles containing glutamic acid at residues 71/74 of the DRβ1 chain and relapsing–remitting multiple sclerosis from onset compared with cases with primary progressive disease or controls; and there was a positive association with the presence of this residue in DR(2)15 negative patients with the primary progressive phenotype. But the concept of a disease-specific motif is challenged by Zipp *et al* (2000a), who demonstrated several multiple sclerosis-associated variations in molecular structure of the class II antigen binding groove but only within the context of the DR(2)15 allele.

Susceptibility and resistance

Until recently, the possibility of a protective effect conferred by class II alleles has been repeatedly assessed, but without clear evidence favouring a particular allele. In the Norwegian series (Spurkland *et al* 1991a), there was a deficiency of DR7-DQB1*0201, as also noticed by others (Gogolin *et al* 1989; Olerup and Hillert 1991). Spurkland *et al* (1991a) also suggested that in Caucasian DR4-positive patients with multiple sclerosis, there is an excess of DQ8 (DQB1*0302) compared with DQ7 (DQB1*0301). This seems true for a number of other groups of patients (Cullen *et al* 1991; Haegert and Francis 1992; 1993; Spurkland *et al* 1991a) but does not stand up to stringent statistical analysis. Three other haplotypes, encoded by DRB1 and DQB1, have been shown to be significantly under-represented in patients with multiple sclerosis and these could represent protective alleles (M. Allen *et al* 1994). Whilst it is inevitable that a study achieving Hardy–Weinberg equilibrium (i.e. identifying the vast majority of variations present in the population) will find a deficiency of other alleles in the presence of a positive association, the expectation is that these will be equally distributed across those prevalent in the population. Several studies have reported a reduction in frequency of DR1, perhaps indicating protection effect rather than reciprocal effects of the increase in DR15 (Pina *et al* 1999; Weinshenker *et al* 1998). For example, Luomala *et al* (2001a) described a protective effect of DR1 (odds ratio 0.3) in Finnish patients with multiple sclerosis; and

Laaksonen *et al* (2002) also reported a specific reduction in DRB1*13-DQB1*0603 in association with the expected excess of DR(2)15 in family-based tests involving patients from Finland.

At the molecular level, in addition to their demonstration of increased risk associated with specific amino acid substitutions at positions 13 and 71, Ghabanbasani *et al* (1995) demonstrated a protective effect of serine and phenylalanine at positions 13 and 47 of the DRB1 chain, respectively, and phenylalanine at position 25 of the DRA1 chain. Allcock *et al* (1999) added alleles of the inhibitor of kappa B-like (IκBL) protein, encoded in the MHC, to the extended haplotype compared in 218 cases and 274 controls. After stratification for DR(2)15, they found a reduced frequency of TNFa-11 and the C allele of *IKBL*, and proposed that these were linked to a gene conferring resistance to multiple sclerosis and modifying the susceptibility effect of the DR(2)15 linked gene. This seems improbable, given the clear evidence from other studies for an increased frequency of TNFa-11 in most other studies (see below). However, Miterski *et al* (2002a) also reported an association with *IKBL* and disease susceptibility whereas an NF-κB promoter polymorphism conferred protection for the development of multiple sclerosis.

Dyment *et al* (2005) genotyped 4347 individuals from 873 multiplex families for DRB1, confirmed the association with DRB1*15 (odds ratio 2.5), and then focused on those families in which DR(2)15 was not present in the parents. Evidence for linkage, through excess haplotype sharing, was still present: more detailed analysis revealed a further association with DRB1*17 and a protective effect of DRB1*14 (odds ratio 0.31). Conversely, DRB1*8 was preferentially associated in the DRB1*15 positive families (odds ratio 2.39). Similar perturbations in transmission were demonstrated for DRB1*01 and DRB1*10, both of which conferred a degree of susceptibility effects and resistance in DRB1*15-positive and -negative individuals, respectively.

Other chromosome 6 genes

The genes for transporters associated with antigen processing of peptides in association with class I HLA products (*TAP1* and *TAP2*) map within the MHC. A class II restricted TAP gene has also been described (Ceman *et al* 1992; Mellins *et al* 1991) and may map to the previously designated DM locus. It has not been studied as a candidate for susceptibility to multiple sclerosis and other autoimmune diseases. However, there is no association with alleles of the HLA-DMA and B loci in Italian patients with multiple sclerosis even after stratification for HLA-DRB1*1501 (Ristori *et al* 1997). Proximity of the TAP loci to other HLA regions that may encode susceptibility genes for multiple sclerosis makes it sensible to stratify results for these alleles, some of which are known to be in linkage disequilibrium (Carrington *et al* 1993).

Liblau *et al* (1993) studied large multifunctional protease (*LMP*) 2 and seven TAP gene polymorphisms. None were associated with multiple sclerosis. Kellar-Wood *et al* (1994a) determined the frequency of TAP1 and TAP2 polymorphisms in 173 patients with multiple sclerosis and 128 unrelated controls whose DR and DQ types were known. Unambiguous allele assignment was not always possible but, allowing for these uncertainties, analysis of genotype and phenotype frequencies also revealed no differences between patients and non-HLA matched controls, even after DR stratification. Vandevyver *et al* (1994a) examined two TAP1 and three TAP2 polymorphisms in

65 unrelated patients with secondary progressive multiple sclerosis but found no difference in allele frequency compared with 66 controls, before or after DR2 stratification. Spurkland *et al* (1994) extended their evidence for the lack of an association with DP alleles to the TAP2 locus, located close to DQ on its centromeric side, supporting the conclusion that HLA-associated susceptibility maps telomeric to the TAP2 locus. Bennetts *et al* (1995) showed no primary association but strong linkage disequilibrium between TAP211*01 and DRB1*1501 in a group of 100 patients with multiple sclerosis from Australia. There was no increase in any one TAP allele frequency in patients who did not independently express class II alleles associated with multiple sclerosis. In a study from Canada, Bell and Ramachandran (1995) also failed to demonstrate an association with any of five TAP1 or TAP2 alleles. Moins-Teisserenc *et al* (1995) showed that 56/104 (54%) patients and 12/55 (22%; RR = 4.2) controls typed for the I/J polymorphism determined by a silent mutation at position 1158. However, the association with multiple sclerosis was no stronger with TAP2-J than DRB1*1501. They suggested that this silent TAP2 mutation might itself be in linkage disequilibrium with an as yet unidentified biologically relevant allele encoded in the same genetic region. Despite these negative findings, Middleton *et al* (1994) reported a significant association between multiple sclerosis and the TAP2 alleles (determined by a valine substitution at position 379 and aspartate at 565), conferring a relative risk of >13 when combined with DR15. However, the high frequency of DR15 in this cohort (95%) makes it difficult to dissociate the relative contributions of these alleles, acting independently or epistatically.

Allelic studies of heat shock proteins (HSPs), encoded at three polymorphic loci adjacent to the class II HLA region, provide no evidence for an association with multiple sclerosis in Italian (Cascino *et al* 1994) or Japanese patients with or without DR(2)15 stratification (Niino *et al* 2001a). There were no significant differences in frequency at the triallelic HSP70-1 locus or at the biallelic HSP70-2 and HSP70-Hom loci in a comparison of 190 patients with 156 controls stratified to include only those homozygous for DR15 or DR3 (H. Kellar-Wood, unpublished observations). Genes involved in the alternative pathway of the complement cascade map to the class III region of the MHC. Despite early suggestions that Bf alleles (Fielder *et al* 1981) and the C4-A4/B2 haplotype (Schroder *et al* 1983) are associated with multiple sclerosis, these associations were not confirmed (British and Dutch Multiple Sclerosis Azathioprine Trial Group 1988a; Bulman *et al* 1991b; Franciotta *et al* 1995). Papiha *et al* (1991) described a reduced frequency of Bf(*)F allele and an increase in Bf(*)F1 amongst patients from northeast England, considered secondary to the Dw2 (DR15) association through linkage disequilibrium seen in cases (especially those with progressive disease) but not controls.

The genes for tumour necrosis factor, TNF – α and β, are encoded in the MHC at 6p21.1-21.3. Both are polymorphic. In terms of nomenclature, it is confusing that the TNF-α and β (lymphotoxin) products are encoded at the TNFa and TNFb loci. TNFa11 and TNFb4 are in linkage disequilibrium with DR(2)15. The issue is whether these loci exert independent effects on susceptibility to multiple sclerosis. Roth *et al* (1994c) showed no primary allelic association with TNFa (13 alleles), TNFb (5 alleles) or TNFc (2 alleles). All distortions in the distribution of TNF gene polymorphisms were attributed to the effect of linkage to DR genes. Specifically, the slight over-representation of the TNFc1-n2-a11-b4 haplotype in multiple sclerosis appeared secondary to the association with DRRB*1501, DQA1*0102, DQB1*0602. An effect of TNFa11 secondary to DR(2)15 was subsequently confirmed in a further French sample (Lucotte *et al* 2000). Sandberg-Wollheim *et al* (1995) had also demonstrated an allelic association with TNFa11 and TNFa4 but neither association was independent of DQA1*0102-DQB1*0602/DR2. Mycko *et al* (1998a) implicated the combined TNF G+A and lymphotoxin-a C+C genotypes in susceptibility to multiple sclerosis. He *et al* (1995) studied a biallelic polymorphism in the TNFa promoter region, known to influence levels of TNF-α. There was no population association with multiple sclerosis or optic neuritis and the high production allele was, if anything, under-represented in patients with demyelinating disease. A small study of affected Italian sibling pairs failed, as expected, to demonstrate linkage to the TNFa locus (Trojano *et al* 1999). Wingerchuk *et al* (1997) also found no disease association with the TNF2 allele. A comparison of TNFa allele frequency showed an increased frequency in German but not Cypriot patients with multiple sclerosis (Maurer *et al* 1999). Conversely, Fernandes-Filho *et al* (2002) found that the 2.2 polymorphism of lymphotoxin was associated with multiple sclerosis in Norwegians, whereas TNFa alleles were not. Weinshenker *et al* (1999) found no association between multiple sclerosis and TNF-R1 – one of the two widely distributed receptors for TNFa and lymphotoxin. However, an association is reported between multiple sclerosis and the 1668*T-G polymorphism of TNF-RII (Ehling *et al* 2004). The association between the C-25 allele of *NOTCH4*, located 0.4 Mb telomeric to DRB1 and separating this from the TNFa locus, is also explained on the basis of linkage disequilibrium (Duvefelt *et al* 2004).

But others have interpreted the TNF story differently. Kirk *et al* (1997) showed that the TNFa 118-bp and TNFb 127-bp alleles are associated with multiple sclerosis in patients from Northern Ireland with transmission disequilibrium in 28 informative meioses. Subsequently, McDonnell *et al* (1999b) confirmed that both associations also characterized primary progressive multiple sclerosis but neither was independent of the DR(2)15 association (here seen both in relapsing–remitting and primary progressive multiple sclerosis, see above). M.A. Armstrong *et al* (1999) were unable to show differences in TNF-α synthesis by mononuclear cells depending on heterozygous or homozygous status for TNFa118 compared with other patients. On the basis of haplotype information from their cohort, they consider the TNFa association to be independent of DR2 susceptibility to multiple sclerosis. Epplen *et al* (1997) reported an independent protective effect of TNFa3 and TNFa5 alleles on susceptibility to multiple sclerosis, not explained by linkage disequilibrium to the DR locus. Fernandez-Arquero *et al* (1999) showed independent effects contributed by DR(2)15 and TNFa but with evidence for epistasis – the presence of both alleles conferring a risk greater than the sum of each. de Jong *et al* (2002a) associated an independent TNFa allele (C1_3_2*354: odds ratio 2.0: 95% CI 1.2–3.1) linked to DR3 in Dutch patients with multiple sclerosis, but with evidence for an epistatic interaction with DR(2)15 (odds ratio 8.7: 95% CI 2.7–29). There was a protective effect of TNFa*107 (odds ratio 0.5: 95% CI 0.3–0.9). The same conclusion was reached in a comparison of DR/DQ (in which the stronger association was with DQA1, see above) and microsatellite markers of TNFa in patients with multiple sclerosis from Colombia, South America (Palacio *et al* 2002).

Zipp *et al* (1995) compared the production of lymphotoxin, TNF-α and IFN-γ by T-cell lines (CD4+) obtained from patients with multiple sclerosis and controls, specific for myelin basic protein and tetanus toxoid. More lymphotoxin and TNF-α but not IFN-γ were produced after antigen stimulation of DR(2)15-positive than -negative individuals (either cases or controls). This functional effect was independent of TNF alleles, suggesting that the mechanism of DR15 susceptibility relates to DR(2)15-linked differences in cytokine production. Huizinga *et al* (1997) showed that the low TNF-α secretor genotype was under-represented in a population of patients with severe multiple sclerosis. Sotgiu *et al* (1999) linked the DR4 association with multiple sclerosis in Sardinians to high TNF-α production but this was not directly attributed to functional properties of the TNFa allele in linkage disequilibrium with DRB1*0405 (DR4). Arguing that differences in the production of reactive oxygen radicals by activated microglia might define individuals at risk of inflammatory injury of myelinated pathways, Nagra *et al* (1997) claimed that the high producer *Sp/Sp* phenotype is more prevalent in young-onset females with multiple sclerosis. However, typically these were benign cases and the association of *Sp/Sp* with a relatively poor prognosis awaits confirmation. Our position is that the tight linkage disequilibrium makes it impossible to distinguish a separate contribution to susceptibility from the TNF locus from that exerted by class II based either on the association and linkage data or functional properties of alleles at these two loci.

Effects on the course and clinical features of multiple sclerosis

HLA stratification for clinical phenotype and course is inextricably tied up with the issue of disease heterogeneity. The majority of surveys investigating HLA class 2 alleles and disease course fail to confirm specifically different associations with any one clinical phenotype. Haile *et al* (1981) and Ho *et al* (1982) first distinguished HLA linkage only in families with DR2-positive affected individuals. Later, Barcellos *et al* (2002) also showed that DR linkage (and concordance for early onset) are confined to families where DR(2)15 is present in affected and unaffected individuals. HLA typing in the large family described by Dyment *et al* (2002a) makes the same point. The presence of DR15 is associated with younger age at diagnosis and female gender in northern Europeans but does not distinguish features relating to disease course, outcome, specific clinical features or paraclinical investigations (Figure 3.19) (Celius *et al* 2000; Hensiek *et al* 2002; Masterman *et al* 2000). The same is true for Arabs (Al-Shammari *et al* 2004). Others have drawn attention specifically to the preferential association of DR15 with age at onset (Shinar *et al* 1998; Weatherby *et al* 2001). But the association has not been reproduced in other large series of European cases (Ballerini *et al* 2004). Taken together, the evidence favours an effect of DR15 on susceptibility rather than modifying the course of (sporadic) multiple sclerosis. It follows that a cohort with this factor will demonstrate earlier age at onset than other patients. Conversely, an association between HLA-DR13 and a benign disease course has been reported from northeast Italy (Perini *et al* 2001). Zivadinov *et al* (2003a) compared 100 patients with 122 controls, demonstrating disease associations with DRB1*15 (DR15), DRB1*03, DQB1*02 and DQB1*03 but no segregation with clinical severity or magnetic resonance markers of inflammation and tissue destruction. T_2-weighted lesion load did correlate with DRB1*04, B7; T_1-weighted lesion load with B7 and DRB1*12; and brain parenchymal fraction with DRB1*12. Weinshenker *et al* (1997) showed three disease-specific sequence changes in the TNFa gene in patients with multiple sclerosis but these affected noncoding regions. Variant alleles showed no correlation with severity or clinical course.

The most ambiguous issue has been whether there is a specific genetic association with primary progressive multiple sclerosis. The original claim was that DR4 confers susceptibility and DQ7

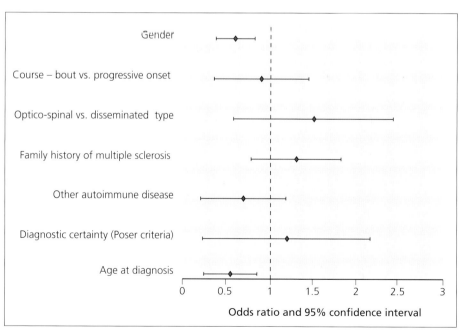

Figure 3.19 Clinical associations with DR(2)15 in multiple sclerosis. Odds ratios and 95% confidence intervals are shown for each characteristic. Adapted from Hensiek *et al* (2002).

resistance to this phenotype in Scandinavian patients (Hillert *et al* 1992a; Olerup *et al* 1989) but these genetic observations were not confirmed (Francis *et al* 1991; Spurkland *et al* 1991a). Support for the original finding was provided by a subsequent study from Spain. de la Concha *et al* (1997) reported an association between DR4 subtypes carrying a valine amino acid substitution at position 86 in the DRβ chain with the primary progressive phenotype. Rasmussen *et al* (2001b) reported an increased frequency of a class II transcriptional regulator (CIITA) promoter allele, acting independently of DR(2)15, in patients with primary progressive multiple sclerosis. In Israel, primary progressive multiple sclerosis has been associated with DRB1*0801-DRA1*0102/DRA1*0401-DRB1*0602 (Kwon *et al* 1999). But others find no significant difference in frequency of DR4 depending on clinical course (McDonnell *et al* 1999c; Weinshenker *et al* 1998). Self-evidently, consensus has not been reached and definitive studies are still needed.

Braun *et al* (1996) sequenced the TNF promoter region in 21 patients with primary progressive and 29 with relapsing–remitting/secondary progressive multiple sclerosis, compared with 22 controls. They found point mutations in 3/21 of the primary progressive group and a slightly higher frequency of heterozygosity in all patients compared with controls. Maurer *et al* (1999) also found no correlation between the presence of TNFa alleles and disease progression.

This situation may be different in locations where multiple sclerosis is clinically distinct. Previously, the phenotype in Japan was characterized by the optico-spinal form of multiple sclerosis. Now, through changing recognition or genuine alterations in disease features, the Western type of multiple sclerosis is increasingly described. Throughout Japan, optico-spinal multiple sclerosis is associated with DPB1*0501 whereas the frequency of DRB1*1501 is increased in the Western type (Fukazawa *et al* 2000a; Ma *et al* 1998; Yamasaki *et al* 1999), although Fukazawa *et al* (2000b) also claim an increased frequency of DPB1*0301 in patients with the Western phenotype. Others have suggested that the optico-spinal form of multiple sclerosis in Japanese is associated with DRB1*0802 (DR8: Ono *et al* 1998). Kikuchi *et al* (2003) emphasized correlation of the Western phenotype with DR(2)15, positive oligoclonal bands and high magnetic resonance lesion load, whereas the same clinical features but absence of oligoclonal banding and relatively few magnetic resonance lesions were associated with DR4. It may be significant that the DR(2)15 association in Japanese with the Western phenotype does not extend to TNFa (Ma *et al* 1998), perhaps narrowing the interval within which the susceptibility effect lies.

The issue of whether the clinical course of multiple sclerosis is influenced by HLA background has been studied ever since the association was discovered. Jersild *et al* (1973) first suggested that Dw2 determines a more severe course. This was confirmed by others (Duquette *et al* 1985; Engell *et al* 1982). Conversely, Madigand *et al* (1982) proposed that the presence of DR3 correlates with a poor prognosis. van Lambalgen *et al* (1986) associated DR(3)17 with progressive disease in males, often clinically more severe, whereas DR(2)15 was over-represented in females with a relapsing course. But the early consensus was that clinical phenotype is probably unaffected by HLA type (British and Dutch Multiple Sclerosis Azathioprine Trial Group 1988a). This cautionary position was supported by Runmarker *et al* (1994a) reporting on patients studied over

a period of 25 years. They showed that DR15/DQ6 did not influence the prognosis although DR17/DQ2 and DR1/DQ5 were over-represented in the quartile with most severe disease. No effect on disease course was identified in patients from Spain with DR(2)15 (Pina *et al* 1999). Studying a population-based sample of patients from Denmark, Schreiber *et al* (2002) also failed to show an effect of DR(2)15 on the clinical course of multiple sclerosis, as did Villoslada *et al* (2002) in Spanish patients. However, the last word has not been heard. Barcellos *et al* (2003) identified fewer individuals with benign and more with severe multiple sclerosis amongst individuals homozygous for DR2.

The identification of associations with multiple sclerosis triggered several studies aiming to link specific laboratory features or putative components of the pathogenesis to HLA type. The design of these studies followed trends in contemporary ideas on mechanisms of tissue injury in multiple sclerosis. Evidence linking Dw2/DR(2)15 to reduced IFN-α production (Salonen *et al* 1982), increased intrathecal immunoglobulin synthesis (Dejaegher *et al* 1983), and enhanced immune reactivity to measles (Greenstein *et al* 1984; Salmi *et al* 1983; Stewart *et al* 1977) – with or without specificity for multiple sclerosis and based on case–control or twin studies – was not confirmed at the time these studies were first performed (Eldridge *et al* 1978; Ilonen *et al* 1977; Lamoureux *et al* 1983; Vervliet *et al* 1983; Zander *et al* 1982).

The most intensively investigated feature of multiple sclerosis for which a laboratory marker has been sought is the conversion from clinically isolated demyelination to definite multiple sclerosis. Clinically, the risk after optic neuritis is highest in the first 5 years but the proportion of cases with widespread demyelination increases steadily with time (see Chapter 6). Actuarial analysis of the available series offers conversion rates varying from 40 to 80%. DR2 is present in a higher proportion of patients with optic neuritis who subsequently develop multiple sclerosis than isolated cases (Compston *et al* 1978; Francis *et al* 1987b; Hauser *et al* 2000; Hely *et al* 1986a; Kelly *et al* 1993; Kheradvar *et al* 2004; Soderstrom *et al* 1998) but the relative risk is low and HLA typing is not useful as a prognostic guide in clinical practice. Sandberg-Wollheim *et al* (1990) made the point that even at late follow-up, 44% of patients with abnormal MRI scans, most of whom had oligoclonal bands from presentation and were DR(2)15 positive, had not developed clinical evidence for widespread demyelination many years after the initial episode of optic neuritis. Hauser *et al* (2000) confirmed the increased risk of conversion to multiple sclerosis in the Optic Neuritis Treatment Trial for individuals with DR(2)15, especially in those with abnormal magnetic resonance imaging at baseline.

In addition to 33 patients with acute unilateral optic neuritis, Kelly *et al* (1993) studied 23 with an isolated cord lesion and 14 with brainstem demyelination. Conversion rates to multiple sclerosis after a mean interval of 5.3 years (range 43–84 months) were 20/33 (61%), 8/23 (35%) and 7/14 (50%), respectively. There was the expected association between these isolated demyelinating syndromes and the presence of DRB1*1501 and DQA1*0102. Both alleles were associated with conversion to multiple sclerosis. This cohort also showed that the presence of multiple white matter abnormalities on MRI at presentation was a more significant risk factor for multiple sclerosis than DR or DQ type.

Other candidate genes

The last few years have seen an exponential increase in studies on candidate genes in multiple sclerosis. The reasons are straightforward. Reagents are available for marking many new functional polymorphisms. It is not hard to present a hypothesis for the putative involvement of any immunoactive, neurobiological or cell signalling molecule in a disease such as multiple sclerosis. The laboratory methods for their detection are readily available and require no great investment. With a little organization, samples from cases and controls can be collected. But despite the huge catalogue of activity, rather little secure knowledge has been gained. Here, too, the reasons are straightforward. The guessing may have been off target, and the pathogenesis of multiple sclerosis may yet have some surprises in store. The strategies are conceptually simple but need sample sizes that require more commitment than has sometimes been deployed. Less than stringent statistical analyses have often allowed false encouragement, with enthusiasm having to be tempered once larger or replicate studies were completed. And yet some of the leads still seem genuine with enough hints of consistency across the component studies to justify continued scrutiny of those regions, or meta-analysis of existing results.

Most studies have been uninformative and the extent to which publication bias has alerted readers to the apparent survivors remains to be established. Assessment of the situation is not helped by the policy of some journals not to publish negative gene screen studies. Others have been commendably indulgent. These candidates fall into several categories: molecules and cytokines involved in mediating interactions between immune cells; chemokines and cell adhesion molecules; assorted inflammatory mediators; other immunologically active molecules; growth factors, their receptors and molecules involved in the signal transduction pathways; and a miscellaneous group of candidates for which the logic underlying their selection is less easy to discern. Each candidate has often been considered both as a susceptibility and disease-modifying factor.

Our approach to this plethora of data is to cover the vast majority of the studies, describing in the text those candidates for which something is still running and tabulating the many apparent casualties (Table 3.2). Readers are asked to consult both text and table since our distribution of putatively positive and negative results is necessarily inconsistent, faced with many mixed messages and difficulties in deciding on the status of a given candidate often studied on many occasions and using cohorts that are not necessarily comparable. Other categories of candidates are grouped for consistency and convenience. In documenting these studies, we do not endorse many of the claims for associations based on undersized studies, with subgroup analyses and insufficient attention to statistical detail. That said, we anticipate that subsequent evidence may make it appropriate to restore the status of some candidates relegated to the list of 'no evidence for an effect on susceptibility or the course of multiple sclerosis' and to relegate some others.

T-cell receptor genes

Ten years ago, the candidates most actively screened related to the T-cell receptor (TCR). This was logical since these are the receptors for antigen presentation by MHC class II molecules (Figure 3.20). Now, attention has moved on to additional accessory molecules, especially CTLA4.

T lymphocytes are classified on the basis of their surface markers, some of which nonspecifically act as adhesion molecules during antigen recognition (see Chapter 11). A broad classification refers to the type of antigen receptor present on any one T-cell clone. This receptor is a heterodimer containing either paired α and β chains or paired γ and δ chains. The

text continued on page 154

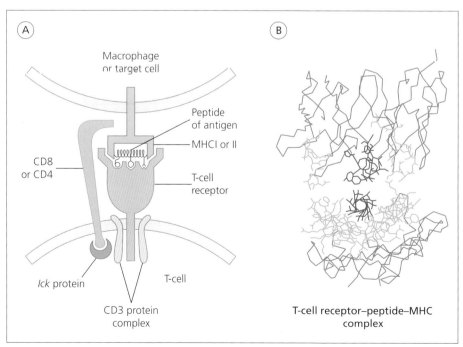

Figure 3.20 (A) Schematic to show the structure of the trimolecular complex. (B) Crystal structure of antibody binding in the cleft of a class II molecule. Adapted from Björkman 1997. © 1997, with permission from Elsevier.

Table 3.2 **Negative candidate screens in multiple sclerosis**

Author	Association	Linkage	Clinical stratification	Candidate	Locus	Comment
Growth factors						
McDonnell *et al* 1999c	Northern Ireland population	–	–	*TGFB1* *TGFB2*	19q13 1q31	Negative screen
A.J. Green *et al* 2001		United States families		*TGFB1* *IL11*	19q13 19q13.3-4	Weak evidence for TGF-β1 linkage in DR(2)15-positive families; weak association with TGF-β1 low producer and benign disease
Weinshenker *et al* 2001	Canadian population and families	Canadian multiplex families	–	*TGFB1*	19q13	Negative screen
Kuhlmann *et al* 2002	German population	–	Relapsing–remitting	*BAX* *BCL2* *BCLx* *P53*	19q13.3-4 11q13.1 20pter-p12.1 8q23.1	Negative screen
Rasmussen *et al* 2000	United Kingdom population	–	Relapsing–remitting, and primary progressive	*HRES1* retro element	1q32-42	Negative screen even with DR(2)15 stratification
Mertens *et al* 1998	–	French multiplex families	–	*TGFB1* *TGFB2* *TGFB3* *TGFBR1* *TGFBR2* *TGFBR3* *FGF1* *FGF2* *FGFRe* *FGFR1* *FGFBR2* *PDGFA* *PDGFRA* *PDGFB* *ERBB* *ERBB2* *ERBB3* *ERBB4* *NT3* *TRKC* *IGF1* *IGF1R*	19q13 1q31 14q24 9q33 3p22 1p32 5q31 4q25-27 4p16 8p12 10q25 7p22 4q11 22q12 7p12 17q11 12p 2q34 12p13 15q24 12q33 15q25-ter	Marginal effect for TGF-β3 after DR(2)15 stratification
V. Hoffmann *et al* 2002	German population	–	Disability and course	*CNTF*	11q12.1	Negative screen even after DR(2)15 stratification
Ban *et al* 2005	United Kingdom population	–	–	*BDNF*	9q22.1	Negative screen
J. Chataway *et al* 1999b	United Kingdom families	–	–	*APOB* *APOC2* *APOH* *MAP1B* *NF1* *NF2* *TIMP3*	2p23-24 19q13 17q22 5q13 17q11.2 22q12 22q12	Negative screen
C.W. Kirk *et al* 2000	Northern Ireland population	–	–	*APOC2*	19q13	Negative screen

Table 3.2 **Negative candidate screens in multiple sclerosis, cont'd**

Author	Association	Linkage	Clinical stratification	Candidate	Locus	Comment
Gervais *et al* 1998	French population	–	–	*APOE*	19q13.2	Negative screen
Ferri *et al* 1999	Italian population	–	Disability and course	*APOEE2–4*	19q13.2	Negative screen
Pirttila et al 2000	Finnish population	–	–	*APOEE2–4*	19q13.2	Negative screen
Savettieri *et al* 2003	Italian population	–	Disability and progression	*APOEE4 APOE* promoter	19q13.2	Marginal inverse effect of ε2 and severity in relapsing–remitting and primary progressive cases
Weatherby *et al* 2000a; 2000b	United Kingdom population	–	Course and disability	*APOE* alleles	19q13.2	Negative screen in relapsing–remitting and primary progressive cases
Masterman *et al* 2002b	Swedish population	–	Course and severity	*APOEE2–4*	19q13.2	Some effect of ε4 in narrowly defined quantiles of severity
Zwemmer *et al* 2004	Dutch population	–	Course and severity	*APOE* alleles	19q13.2	Negative screen but trend to association with ApoE-ε2 in meta-analysis
Zakrzewska-Pniewska *et al* 2004	Polish population	–	Course and severity	*APOEE2–4*	19q13.2	Myeloperoxidase G/G allele associated with severity
Niino *et al* 2003b	Japanese population	–	Course and severity	*APOE* alleles	19q13.2	Negative screen. Low population frequency of ε4
Santos *et al* 2004	Portuguese population	–	Course and severity	*APOEE4 SCA2*	19q13.2 12q24	Negative screen
Al-Shammri *et al* 2005	Kuwaiti population	–	–	*APOE* alleles	19q13.2	Slight increase in ε2 and some effect of ε4 in females with severe disease
Miterski *et al* 2000	German population	–	–	*SCA2*	12q24	Negative screen
Cytokines and other immune molecules						
Epplen *et al* 1997	German population	–	–	*IL1A* *IL1RA* *IL2* *IL2RB* *IL5RA* *IFNA* *IFNB* *IFNG* *IRF1* *IRF2* *CD3D* *FGF1*	2q13 2q14 4q26 22q11 3p24 9p22 9p22 12q24 5q31 4q35 11q23 5q31	Negative screen
Semana *et al* 1997	French population	French families		*IL1RA*	2q14-21	Negative screen
de la Concha *et al* 1997	Italian population	–	Relapsing–remitting, and primary progressive	*IL1RA*	2q14-21	Negative screen

table continued on following page

Table 3.2 **Negative candidate screens in multiple sclerosis, cont'd**

Author	Association	Linkage	Clinical stratification	Candidate	Locus	Comment
H.M. Schrijver et al 1999	Dutch population	–	Relapsing–remitting, and primary and secondary progressive	IL1B IL1RA	2q14-21 2q14-21	Faster rate of progression in IL-1Ra 2+/IL-1β 2– individuals
Ferri et al 2000	Italian population	–	–	IL1A IL1B	2q13-21 2q13-21	Negative screen
Hooper-van Veen et al 2003	Dutch population	–	Course and severity	IL1A IL1B IL1RA	2q13 2q14-21 2q14-21	Negative screen
Feakes et al 2000a	United Kingdom families	–	Disability	IL1RA	2q13-21	Negative screen
Niino et al 2001b	Japanese population	–	Course and disability	IL1B IL1RA	2q13-21 2q13-21	Negative screen
Fedetz et al 2002	Spanish population	–	–	IL2 promoter	4q26-27	Negative screen
Feakes et al 2000b	United Kingdom families	–	–	IL2	4q26-27	Negative screen
Fedetz et al 2001	Spanish population	–	Course and disability	IL6	7p21-15	Negative screen
S. Schmidt et al 2003	German population	–	Relapsing–remitting, and primary and secondary progressive	IL6	7p21-15	Negative screen
Teutsch et al 2003	Australian population and families	–	–	IL7R	5p12-14	Marginal increase in GTG haplotype
Doncel et al 2002	Spanish population and families	–	–	IL10	1q31-32	Slight increase in IL-10G12
Pickard et al 1999	United Kingdom population	–	Course and disability	IL10 promoter	1q31-32	Negative screen
Maurer et al 2000	German population	–	Course and disability	IL10 promoter	1q31-32	Negative screen
Myhr et al 2002	Norwegian population	–	Course and disability	IL10 promoter	1q31-32	Trend towards increased severity and low IL-10 expression allele
B. He et al 1998	Swedish population and families	Swedish families	–	IL2 IL4 IL4R IL10 IFNG TGFB1 TGFB2	4q26-27 5q23-31 16p11.2-12.1 1q31-32 12q24.1 19q13 19q13	Slightly positive lod scores for IFN-γ, IL-4R and TGF-β2
Reboul et al 2000	–	French sibling pairs	–	IL2 IL2RA IL2RB IL2RG IL4 IL4RA	4q26-27 10p15 22q13 Xq13 16p12 16p12	Trend towards IL-2Rβ linkage after DR(2)15 stratification

Table 3.2 Negative candidate screens in multiple sclerosis, cont'd

Author	Association	Linkage	Clinical stratification	Candidate	Locus	Comment
				IL10 *IL10R* *IL12P40* *IL12P35* *IL12RB1* *IL12RB2* *TGFB1* *TGFBR1* *TGFBR2* *TGFBR3* *IFNG* *IFNGR1* *IFNGR2* *CALB1* (vitamin D binding protein)	1q31-32 11q23 5q33 3q25-26.2 19q13 1p31 19q13 9q33 3p22 1p32 12q13 6q23-24 21q22 4q12	
McDonnell *et al* 2000	Northern Ireland population	–	Relapsing–remitting, and primary and secondary progressive	*IL1A* *IL2* *IL2R* *IL4* *IL9* *IL10*	2q13 4q26-27 10p15 16p12 5q23-31 1q31-32	Negative screen
Luomala *et al* 2003	Finnish population	–	Severity	*IL10* *CCR5Δ32* *CTLA4* *TNFA* promoter	1q31-32 3p21 2q33 6p21.3	Negative screen but IL-10AG genotype protective for severity
J. Chataway *et al* 1999a	–	United Kingdom families	–	*C6* *C7*	5p13.1 5p13.1	Negative screen
Kikuchi *et al* 2002b	Japanese population	–	–	*ADRB2* (β_2-adrenergic receptor)	5q31-32	Marginal increase in Gly at codon 16 in secondary progressive cases
Niino *et al* 2002a	Japanese population	–	Age at onset and severity	*ADRB2* (β_2-adrenergic receptor)	5q31-32	Marginal increase in Gly at codon 16 in secondary progressive cases
Savettieri *et al* 2002	Italian population	–	–	*AF1* (estrogen receptor 1)	6q24-27	Negative screen
Vandenbroeck *et al* 1999	Sardinian population and families	–	–	*IFNA* *IFNB*	9p21 9p21	Negative screen
Bergkvist *et al* 1996		Swedish families		*IFNA* *IFNB*	9p21 9p21	Negative screen
Wansen *et al* 1997	Finnish population	Finnish families	–	*IFNG* *IL1RA* *IL1B*	12q14-15 2q14-21 2q14-21	Negative screen
Luomala *et al* 2001b	Finnish population	–	Disability	*IL1RA* *IL1A* *IL1B*	2q13-21 2q13-21 2q13-21	Trend towards increased IL-1Ra allele 2 in women
Epplen *et al* 1997	German population			*IFNA* *IFNB*	9p21 9p21	Negative screen
Bergkvist *et al* 2004	–	Swedish families	–	*IFNG* *IFNGR* *IFNABR* *JAK1* *STAT1* *STAT3*	12q24 6q23-24 21q22.1 1p32.3-31.3 2q32.2-32.3 17q21	Negative screen

table continued on following page

Table 3.2 Negative candidate screens in multiple sclerosis, cont'd

Author	Association	Linkage	Clinical stratification	Candidate	Locus	Comment
Schrijver *et al* 2004	Dutch population	–	Course	*IFNG* *IFNGR1* *IFNGR2*	12q24 6q23-24 6q23-24	Progressive course and more atrophy associated with IFNγR2 allele Arg64
Sriram *et al* 2003	United States population	United States families	Treated with IFN-β	*IFNAR1* *IFNAR2*	21q22.1 21q22.1	No pharmogenetic effect. Weak association between 16469A/T SNP and response to IFN-β
Leyva *et al* 2005	Spanish population	–	Response to treatment with IFN-β	*IFNAR1* *IFNAR2*	21q22.1 22q21.1	Slight increase in frequency of 18417 and 11876 SNPs
Vandenbroeck *et al* 2000b	European populations and familiies	–	–	*IFN* regulatory factor-1	14q11.2	Negative screen
Dai *et al* 2001c	Nordic population- and family-based association	Nordic families	Disability	*IFNG* intron 1	12q24	Negative screen
Kantarci *et al* 2000c	Canadian population	–	Course and disability	*MPO* (myelo-peroxidase)	17q23	Negative screen
Cascino *et al* 1998	Italian population	–	–	*FAS*	10q24	Negative screen in three diseases
Q.R. Huang *et al* 2000	Australian population	–	No	*APO1/FAS* (CD95)	10q24	Trend towards association of Mva 1*2 allele and interaction with TCRβ V8s1*1/1*2
Dai *et al* 2002	Swedish population	–	Course and disability	*CD40* ligand	Xq26	Negative screen
Vorechovsky *et al* 2001	Swedish population	–	–	*CD45*	1q31	Negative screen
Barcellos *et al* 2001	United States population and families	United States families	–	*CD45*	1q31	Negative screen
Miterski *et al* 2002b	German population	–	Course and disability	*CD45*	1q31	Negative screen
Nicholas *et al* 2003a	United Kingdom population	United Kingdom families	–	*CD45*	1q31	Negative screen
Cocco *et al* 2004a		Sardinian families	–	*CD45*	1q31	Weak association after DR(15)2 stratification
Teutsch *et al* 2004b	Australian population	–	–	*CD80* *CD86* *CTLA4*	3q13.3-q21 3q21 2q33	Negative screen including meta-analysis of CTLA4 but CD28-372G allele associated with susceptibility
Kantarci *et al* 2004	United States population	–	–	*CD95* *CD95L*	10q24.1 10q24.1	Negative screen but trend to association of CD95 G and C homozygotes in women
Kroner *et al* 2005	German population	–	Course and severity	*TCR4* (toll-like receptor 4)	9q32-33	Negative screen

Table 3.2 **Negative candidate screens in multiple sclerosis, cont'd**

Author	Association	Linkage	Clinical stratification	Candidate	Locus	Comment
A. Weber et al 2004	German population	–	–	*TRAIL* (TNF-related apoptosis-inducing ligand)	8p21	Negative screen
Weinshenker et al 2000	Canadian population	–	Course and disability	*B71*	3q13.3-21	Negative screen
C.G. Haase et al 2002	German population	–	Course	*ITGA3* (G-protein β3) *CCR5Δ32*	3p21	Trend towards association of Δ32 CCR5 and GNB3 825T polymorphisms with primary progressive disease
Bennetts et al 1997	Australian population	–	–	*CCR5Δ32*	3p21	Negative screen
Silversides et al 2004	Northern Ireland population	–	–	*CCR5Δ32*	3p21	Negative screen
Miyagishi et al 2003	Japanese population	–	–	*CCR2*	3p21	Negative screen but protective effect on susceptibility from –641 allele
Schweer et al 2001	German population	–	–	*CHAMD8* (α2-macroglobulin) *RP6* (lipoprotein receptor related protein)	19p13.12 12p11.2-13.3	Negative screen even after DR(2)15 stratification
Agundez et al 1995	Spanish population	–	–	*CYP2D6*	22q11.2-qter	Negative screen
Landtblom et al 2003	Swedish population	–	–	*CYP2D6* Glutathione *S*-transferase	22q11.2-qter 12p12.3-12.1	Negative screen
Modin et al 2001	Nordic population and families	Nordic families	Disability	*NOS1*	12q24	Negative screen
Tajouri et al 2004	Australian population	–	Gender and clinical course	*NOS1*	12q24	Negative screen
Blanco et al 2003	Spanish population	–	Course and disability	*NOS2A*	17q11.2	Negative screen
Tajouri et al 2004	Australian population	–	Course	*NOS2A*	17q11.2	Negative screen
Bugeva et al 2005	Australian population	–	–	*NOS2A*	17q11.2	Trend towards association in DR(2)15 positive patients
Luomala et al 1999	Finnish population	–	–	*ICAM1*	10p13	Negative screen
Cournu-Rebeix et al 2003	French families	–	Severity	*ICAM1R*	10p13	Negative for susceptibility and severity but ICAM associated with susceptibility not severity
Marrosu et al 2000b	Sardinian families	–	–	*ICAM1*	10p13	Negative screen even after DR(2)15 stratification

table continued on following page

Table 3.2 **Negative candidate screens in multiple sclerosis, cont'd**

Author	Association	Linkage	Clinical stratification	Candidate	Locus	Comment
Sciacca *et al* 2000	Italian population	–	Disability	*PECAM1*	17q23	Negative screen
Nelissen *et al* 2002	Belgian population	–	–	*PECAM1* *MMPG* (Gelatinase B)	17q23 20q11-13	Negative screen
Steckley *et al* 2000	Canadian population and families	Canadian families	–	Vitamin D-receptor *YP24A1* (25(OH)D3 1α-hydroxylase)	12q13-14 12q13	Negative screen
Yeo *et al* 2004	United Kingdom families	–	–	Vitamin D receptor	12q13-14	Negative screen
Niino et al 2002b	Japanese population	–	Age at onset	Vitamin D binding protein	8p11	Negative screen
Caillier *et al* 2003	United States population	–	Course and progression	*SPP1* (osteopontin)	4q11-q21	Negative screen but severity weakly associated with 1284A SNP
Hensiek *et al* 2003b	United Kingdom population	–	Rate of progression	*SPP1* (osteopontin)	4q11-q21	Negative screen
Caillier *et al* 2003	United States population	–	Course	*SPP1* (osteopontin)	4q11-q21	Trend towards severity and 1284A allele
Comabella *et al* 2004	Spanish population	–	–	*SLC11a1* (natural resistance-associated macrophage protein 1)	2q35	Negative screen
Criswell *et al* 2005	United States families	–	–	*PTPN22*	1p13.2	Negative screen
Begovich *et al* 2005	United States population	–	–	*PTPN22*	1p13.2	Negative screen
Other candidates						
Hinks *et al* 1995	United Kingdom population	–	–	*EVI2A* (ecotropic viral integration 2A)	17q11.2	Negative screen
Broadley *et al* 2001b	United Kingdom families	–	–	*NOTCH3*	19p13.2-13.1	No mutations in 93/745 index cases sequenced for exon 3

α/β or γ/δ T-cell receptors are encoded by members of the immunoglobulin gene superfamily. Their products are highly variable glycoproteins associating noncovalently with five other invariant molecules, collectively making up the CD3 complex. The majority of circulating T cells (>95%) express the α/β receptor. The 39–46-kDa α chain and 40-kDa β chain are linked through disulphide bonds with additional interactions contributing to the tertiary structure. As with genetic organization of immunoglobulins, the T-cell receptor has variable (V), joining (J) and constant (C) regions, and diversity (D) segments also occur within the β chains. The V, D and J regions constitute a highly variable domain whilst the C region encodes a 138–179 amino-acid product embedded in the cell membrane. The J region of the T-cell receptor is slightly larger than its counterpart on the light and heavy chains of immunoglobulins but these molecules share many conserved sequences. The T-cell receptor γ/δ chains are more prevalent on T cells during ontogeny leading to the suggestion that the α/β receptor is derived from a γ/δ progenitor. All T-cell receptors appear to use the same accessory molecules during cell–cell contact.

The β chain gene complex lies on chromosome 7q32 and occupies 600 kb (Toyonaga *et al* 1985). The V, D, J and C-α regions are polymorphic at the germline level and include >50 variable gene segments at the centromeric end of the locus. Conversely, there are only two C-β segments and these are highly homologous. The α chain locus is on chromosome 14q11 (Collins *et al* 1985) and the δ chain gene lies between the V and J regions of the α chain gene. The general principle of diversity in the V and J segments is maintained for the α chain. These segments occupy approximately 185 kb, whereas the single C segment is smaller. The γ chain occupies only 180 kb and has fewer V genes. It is encoded at a locus on chromosome 7p32.

T-cell receptor α and β gene polymorphisms have been studied using both population association and linkage studies. These efforts straddle the RFLP, microsatellite and SNP eras. Given the functional interactions, stratification for DR(2)15 has often featured in the analyses. Martell *et al* (1987) first reported a significant increase in frequency of a V region α chain allele in DR15-positive patients with multiple sclerosis compared with controls. This preliminary evidence was supported by Oksenberg *et al* (1988; 1989), who described association with a polymorphism corresponding to Vα and Cα sequences. Sherritt *et al* (1992) also reported that a Cα gene conferred suscep-tibility after stratification for HLA class II. However, the consensus from subsequent population studies is that polymor-phisms within the variable or constant regions of the α chain locus do not contribute to susceptibility in multiple sclerosis (Eoli *et al* 1994a; Hashimoto *et al* 1992; Hillert *et al* 1992b). Family studies have also failed to demonstrate linkage to T-cell receptor α chains. The samples have been small, varying from 14 to 82 families (Eoli *et al* 1994a; Hashimoto *et al* 1992; Lynch *et al* 1992) but, taken together, these studies provide no evidence for a contribution to susceptibility from genes within the T-cell receptor α locus on chromosome 14.

Evidence relating to the β chain remains more ambiguous. The initial population association studies implicated a β chain variable region gene probably mapping within the V region itself and showing epistasis with DR4 (Beall *et al* 1989; 1993; Charmley *et al* 1991; Wei *et al* 1994). These results were not confirmed, perhaps due to differences in the definition of alleles using RFLPs in studies from France (Martell *et al* 1987), North America (Oksenberg *et al* 1988), Scandinavia (Fugger *et al* 1990b), northern Spain (Martinez-Naves *et al* 1993), Belgium (Vandevyver *et al* 1994b) and Northern Ireland (Droogan *et al* 1996), including patients with primary progressive multiple sclerosis (Hillert *et al* 1991). It may not be right to derive a single opinion from these pioneering studies struggling with allele definition, and they illustrate the considerable difficulty of assigning disease suscep-tibility genes based on population studies involving relatively small numbers of cases and controls. The story with respect to family linkage studies has left much the same uncertainty. Some early studies provided evidence for linkage (Seboun *et al* 1989); others did not (Lynch *et al* 1991; Wansen *et al* 1997; N. Wood *et al* 1995a). Twins (from the United States and French samples) have been examined for T-cell receptor gene sharing depending on zygosity and stratified for concordance. These studies showed a disease association with Vβ11 but no association between Cβ, Vβ and Vγ region alleles, or their haplotypes, and concordance in dizygotic and monozygotic twins (Briant *et al* 1993; Roth *et al* 1994d; Utz *et al* 1993).

Studying T-cell receptor genes in isolation may be biologically less meaningful than considering the effect of extended haplotypes and DR stratification. These manoeuvres led to identification of an effect on susceptibility of the Vβ8.1/11 (2-1 alleles)-Cβ haplotype in individuals with DR(2)15, further supporting the evidence for gene complementation (Beall *et al* 1993) with protection conferred by Vβ8.1/11 (1-2 alleles)-Cβ (Hockertz *et al* 1998). Further manipulations suggested that recessive inheri-tance of the T-cell receptor Vβ11 1 allele in DR(2)15-positive, and a Vβ7 1-1/1-2 homozygous haplotype in DR(2)15-negative individuals increased the risk of conversion from relapsing to progressive disease (Hockertz *et al* 1998). Stratifying for DR/DQ increased the evidence for linkage in several other series, either with an effect of DR(2)15/DQ6 (N.W. Wood *et al* 1995a) or DRB1*0301 (Epplen *et al* 1997). Conversely, others have observed a neutral effect of DR(2)15 stratification on the Vβ8 association (Buhler *et al* 2000; Hillert *et al* 1991; Vandevyver *et al* 1994b), or have lost the preliminary evidence for an asso-ciation (Martinez-Naves *et al* 1993).

The most recent published report of this epistatic effect, using a total of 267 families with ≥2 affected siblings typed for 14 RFLPs at the TCRβ locus confirmed no primary linkage or transmission disequilibrium but with DRB1*15 stratification the BV25S1*1-BV26S1*1-BV2S1*1 haplotype was associated with multiple sclerosis – although not after correction for multiple comparisons (Dyment *et al* 2004a). The associated haplotype was typed in an independent sample of 97 nuclear families with a single DRB1*15-positive affected proband. Again, there was no preferential transmission of the BV25S1*1-BV26S1*1-BV2S1*1 haplotype. There were no effects of stratification for clinical course.

Based on these results, one interpretation is that – within the context of the trimolecular complex – susceptibility to multiple sclerosis is conferred by DR15 whereas progression may depend on alleles encoded within the T-cell receptor locus, specificity depending on the class II MHC background. As a refinement, the primary susceptibility determinant is considered to be the class II HLA genotype, in the context of which germline T-cell receptor polymorphisms confer an additional risk despite not being independently associated with susceptibility. This level of complexity could prove to be correct and seems more probable than even more elaborate hypotheses generated to accommo-date results still needing confirmation and clarification. An alter-native view is that a large number of genes with independent and epistatic effects are involved in conferring susceptibility to multiple sclerosis. If one is within the T-cell receptor locus, its contribution may be so small that only with a study recruiting a very large number of affected sibling pairs, and using highly polymorphic markers, could the effects be demonstrated. What remains clear is that existing studies have failed thus far to prove that a gene within or linked to the T-cell receptor β locus confers susceptibility, or influences the course of multiple scle-rosis. If a susceptibility gene lies within this locus, its contribu-tion to the pathogenesis must be small or the effects largely conditioned by the related MHC class II association.

Cytotoxic T-lymphocyte antigen 4 (CTLA4)

A number of accessory molecules are involved in docking antigen-presenting cells to T-helper lymphocytes during induction of the immune response. Some are known to be polymorphic and so offer themselves as additional candidates following the doctrine of an immunological pathogenesis in multiple sclerosis. Two such molecules are CTLA4 (CD152) and CD28. Ligers *et al* (1999) reported population- and family-based associations with homozygosity for the G49 allele of *CTLA4* in relapsing–remitting multiple sclerosis. This was confirmed by Harbo *et al* (1999). Homozygosity of the AA allele of exon 1 was then primarily associated with increased severity in Japanese patients with relapsing–remitting or secondary progressive multiple sclerosis (Fukazawa *et al* 1999a). Kantarci *et al* (2003a) used population- and family-based methods to show an association but no linkage between homozygosity for the AT8 allele, or the extended haplotype in which it most usually occurs, and susceptibility to multiple sclerosis. They summarized the available literature and provided an overall odds ratio of 1.28 (95% CI 1.01–1.63) for susceptibility to multiple sclerosis in the context of this CTLA4 profile but with no effect on disease course or clinical features. Conversely, Maurer *et al* (2002) and Masterman *et al* (2002a) working with the groups that originally first claimed an association to susceptibility in relapsing–remitting multiple sclerosis, then suggested that the closer relationship was with primary progressive disease. Alizadeh *et al* (2003a) identified a single nucleotide polymorphism strongly associated with susceptibility to relapsing–remitting multiple sclerosis in French and Iberian family-based association studies, stratified for DR(2)15. Although there was no association with susceptibility to multiple sclerosis, Bilinska *et al* (2004) reported a fourfold increased risk of secondary progression in Polish patients with relapsing–remitting multiple sclerosis who had genotypes for the CTLA4-AA and AG alleles. Malferrari *et al* (2005) claimed an association between the two locus CTLA4-T/G combination and susceptibility to multiple sclerosis in Italians. An association is reported with the CTLA4 +49G allele and the more extended +49 A/G*G – CT60*G haplotype in Belgian patients with multiple sclerosis (Suppiah *et al* 2005). Kroner *et al* (2005) studied programmed death (PD)-1, a member of the B7/CD28 superfamily of costimulatory molecules, and correlated the presence of a functional polymorphism that acts to inhibit IFN-γ production *in vitro*, with primary or secondary disease progression concluding that the polymorphism influences progression by inducing a partial defect in PD-1 mediated inhibition of T cell activation.

Against this background, Rasmussen *et al* (2001) found no association with *CTLA4* in European and Shanghai Chinese patients with multiple sclerosis. Dyment *et al* (2002b) were unable to demonstrate linkage or association to susceptibility or the clinical course with a microsatellite marking exon 1 of *CTLA4* in Canadian patients. van Veen *et al* (2003a) found no association with susceptibility or the clinical course of multiple sclerosis and CTLA4 or CD28 polymorphisms in Dutch patients with multiple sclerosis. Bocko *et al* (2003) showed no association in Polish cases with multiple sclerosis, and Roxburgh *et al* (2005b), in family-based studies, failed to show any association with susceptibility or disease course. Nor is *CTLA4* associated with multiple sclerosis in Japanese patients with the Western phenotype (Fukazawa *et al* 2005). Finally, in their own series and in a meta-analysis of nine published studies, Teutsch *et al* (2004) failed to demonstrate an association between multiple sclerosis and *CTLA4*. But the last word may not have been heard. Ueda *et al* (2003) mapped susceptibility in a variety of autoimmune diseases to a region linked to genes that, in the mouse, reduce production of the CD80/CD86 ligand-binding domain of CTLA4. However, patients with multiple sclerosis were not included in this autoimmunity screen.

Immunoglobulin heavy chain genes

The detection of plasma cells and B lymphocytes within areas of acute demyelination and the high frequency of oligoclonal banding in spinal fluid samples from patients with multiple sclerosis, has prompted the search for allelic associations and linkage to genes that encode variable and constant regions of the immunoglobulin heavy chain V and C regions, and their Fc receptors.

Immunoglobulin forms the antigen receptor for B lymphocytes. The isoforms are glycoproteins and each of the five classes has two light and two heavy chains with molecular weights of 23 kDa and 53 kDa, respectively. Both heavy chain classes may be associated with either κ or λ light chains linked by disulphide bonds. Neighbouring sections of heavy and light chains are arranged in two domains, each of which is just over 100 amino acids long. These provide the antibody molecule with its tertiary structure. Folds are stabilized by internal disulphide bonds forming loops about 65 amino acids in length. Light chains have two, and heavy chains four or five domains. The antigen-binding site is formed by sections of the two shared heavy/light-chain domains. The first adjacent, and unpaired, section of the heavy chain is hinged to allow flexibility, and this is where enzyme digestion splits the molecule into Fc and Fab portions. As with the T-cell receptor loci, this locus encoding immunoglobulin contains several constant (C), variable (V), diversity (D) and joining (J) genes. Somatic rearrangement during B-cell ontogeny enables one V to join one D and J gene and these are spliced to C region genes before transcription (Tonegawa 1983). Heavy chain allotypes occur mainly at the V and C regions of heavy chains. These confer minor differences in function but mostly serve as population markers of uncertain biological significance. Antigen is bound at the complementarity-determining regions. Genes encoding these portions of the antibody molecule are located in clusters along the chromosome. The heavy chain locus contains 100 V genes, approximately 20 D and 4 J gene segments. The heavy chain gene clusters have been mapped to chromosome 14q32; the λ chain is at 2p12 and the κ chain at 22q11. Functional heavy and light chain V regions are produced from one each of the V_H, D_H and J_H segments. No diversity segments are involved in the production of light chains. At first, immunoglobulin isotypes were recognized serologically. The nine specificities have since been sequenced. The C region is encoded by four exons and the J region (located 5′ to the C region), by a cluster of nine genes of which three are pseudogenes. The diversity segments are arranged in tandem repeat units of 9 kb containing 13 gene segments of which one is a pseudogene. Separate components of the heavy chain gene map from the centromere in the order C-J-D-V, occupying 4 Mb. The light chains of κ type (60%) are encoded on chromosome 2p12 and contain a large number of V segment genes adjacent to five J and one C exon. Many are pseudogenes. The λ chain is encoded on chromosome 22q11 mapping from the centromere in the order V-J-C. Unlike the κ chain, several C region alleles exist but some are pseudogenes. In common with the κ chain, there are a large number of V gene segments. This is to be expected since only the V regions of antibody contribute to diversity. It is advantageous to associate a large number of V genes with a restricted C region since the latter is devoted to nonspecific properties such as complement fixation and receptor binding.

The polymorphic nature of immunoglobulin heavy and light chains has made possible their assessment as candidates for susceptibility in multiple sclerosis. At first, these studies described serologically defined specificities but molecular analysis has since been used to supplement the earlier work. Pandey *et al* (1981) studied 70 patients with multiple sclerosis from the southeastern United States. Nine allotypes were identified and used to construct five haplotypes. The Gm1,17,21 haplotype was associated with multiple sclerosis. Homozygosity further increased the relative risk. Sandberg-Wollheim *et al* (1984) described increased susceptibility in association with Gm1,21 in patients from Sweden. Propert *et al* (1982) then suggested that the Gm3,5,13,14 haplotype is protective for multiple sclerosis. Blanc *et al* (1986) described a different Gm allotype association (in which Gm3,23,5,10,11,13,14 conferred susceptibility to multiple sclerosis, with a modest reduction in Gm 1,3,17) in a study from the Haute Pyrénées region of France. Salier *et al* (1986) stratified Gm allotypes for HLA antigens in a separate French population. Despite the absence of a primary Gm allotype association, the relative risk was increased for individuals who typed both for HLA DR2 and G1m1. The study does not carry conviction since there was a negative effect of this Gm allotype and HLA B7, despite the tight linkage disequilibrium that exists between HLA B7 and DR2 in Europeans. Also, little credence can be given to the complex analysis of disease severity depending on Gm–HLA phenotype interactions. The suggestion was that heterozygosity for Gm1 (Gm1/Gm3) interacts with HLA B7 to increase susceptibility, whereas Gm3 homozygosity is an independent marker of disease severity (Salier *et al* 1986). Sesboue *et al* (1985) also analysed Gm allotypes in French patients with multiple sclerosis and correlated disease severity with increased intrathecal immunoglobulin synthesis and Gm3 homozygosity. Here again, epistatic effects were claimed with DR2 and B7. Francis *et al* (1986) found no independent Gm allotype or phenotype association with multiple sclerosis but susceptibility was increased for individuals with both Gm3,5,10,11,13,14 and DQ1. Hillert (1993) failed to demonstrate an allelic association for three polymorphisms encoded within the C region in cases from Sweden and Norway. Nor was there any correlation between disease course and severity, or an interaction with HLA. Berr *et al* (1989) reported an association between the Km(1) allotype and both older age at onset and disease progression in multiple sclerosis.

With the availability of molecular analyses, Gaiser *et al* (1987) used RFLPs marking the immunoglobulin heavy chain region to detect polymorphisms in the gamma region and reported a negative association between the presence of a 5.9-kb fragment generated following *Bst*E11 restriction endonuclease digestion and multiple sclerosis. The study mixed patients from southern California with those from France and made comparisons with controls from northern California. Analysis of Californian cases and controls showed a significant association but not after corrections were made for multiple comparisons. Walter *et al* (1991) performed a comprehensive analysis of the V and C heavy chain regions using concordant sibling pairs as the index cases for comparison with unrelated and family controls. They reported an association with the V_H2-5 polymorphism. Thereafter, evidence for the association was strengthened by Hashimoto *et al* (1993), who implicated a 3.4-kb allele encoded in the H2 gene region but without linkage in 33 Canadian sibling pairs. Yu *et al* (1993) analysed 40 families with pairs or trios of affected siblings for immunoglobulin allotypes and RFLPs but failed to find either linkage or association. Negative results were also obtained in Norwegian patients (Raknes *et al* 2000). Wansen *et al* (1997) provided no evidence for linkage in 21 multiplex Finnish families using a microsatellite marker 5′ to the IgG-V_H-J region. N. Wood *et al* (1995b) did not confirm the V_H2-5 allelic association with multiple sclerosis reported by Walter *et al* (1991) but provided some evidence for linkage in 124 families with affected sibling pairs. The tentative suggestion that the V_H2 locus may be important in the pathogenesis of multiple sclerosis was at first supported by two whole-genome screens (Feakes *et al* 1998; Giedraitis *et al* 2003: see below) but the status of 14q in general and the immunoglobulin heavy chain locus in particular remains highly provisional.

The other side of the Gm allotype candidate coin is variation in structure of the Fc receptor (FcR). FcγR targets immune complexes to effector cells. Myhr *et al* (1999) showed no effect on susceptibility but proposed that homozygosity for the FcγRIIIB NA2 or FcγRIIA histidine alleles was associated with benign multiple sclerosis in Norway. However, Breij *et al* (2003) showed no association between either susceptibility or the clinical course and three FcγR alleles in a large case–control comparison from the Netherlands.

Cytokines and chemokines

Crusius *et al* (1995) associated allele 2 of the interleukin-1 receptor antagonist (*IL1RA*) with multiple sclerosis (odds ratio 2.2; 95% CI 1.1–4.6). Homozygosity for the A1 allele was also shown to be associated in Italian patients (Sciacca *et al* 1999). However, W-X. Huang *et al* (1996) compared these same alleles in Swedish patients and failed to confirm the putative IL-1Ra association. Nor did Semana *et al* (1997) find an association with the same IL-1Ra allele in population- and family-based studies from western France. But, seemingly, the IL-1Ra allele 2 is associated with relapsing–remitting multiple sclerosis after DR(2)15 stratification in Spanish patients with multiple sclerosis (de la Concha *et al* 1997). de Jong *et al* (2002b) described a twofold increase for familial recurrence risk in the Netherlands for multiple sclerosis in the context of increased ratios of IL-1β:IL-1Ra and IL-10:TNF-α production. C.L.A. Mann *et al* (2002) studied *IL1A*, *IL1B* and *IL1RA*, demonstrating an association between allele 2 of the *IL1RA* and disability both in relapsing–remitting and primary progressive multiple sclerosis in patients from the United Kingdom. H.M. Schrijver *et al* (1999) showed that the combination of IL-Ra allele 2 and absence of the IL-1β allele 2 were associated with increased rate of progression, but not susceptibility, in Dutch patients with multiple sclerosis. Later, they reported that this genotype is associated with high production of IL-1Ra (H.M. Schrijver *et al* 2003). It was necessary for Kantarci *et al* (2000a) to consider only the three most common IL-1Ra alleles in concluding that alleles 2/3 were associated with a benign clinical course in multiple sclerosis in patients from North America. This effect was lost with analysis of the full dataset, and there was no association with susceptibility. Others, using population- and family-based tests of association, have been unable to demonstrate a relationship between susceptibility to multiple sclerosis and the biallelic *IL1B* gene, alleles of its receptor antagonist for which linkage disequilibrium exists (IL-1Ra2 and IL-1β2), or regulatory factors.

Matesanz *et al* (2001) studied the *IL2* gene and claimed an association with secondary progressive multiple sclerosis in Spanish patients, but without a functional effect on *IL2* production. Several authors have claimed association or linkage between *IL4* and multiple sclerosis. Vandenbroeck *et al* (1997) suggested that the *IL4B1* gene polymorphism is associated with later age at onset of disease. Kantarci *et al* (2003b) reported an association between homozygosity for polymorphisms in the *IL4* promoter and susceptibility to multiple sclerosis but not age at onset. Hackstein *et al* (2001) suggested that the association between a functional polymorphism of the *IL4R* gene resulted in reduced IL4 activity, a preponderance of Th1 activity and enhanced production of myelin-associated glycoprotein antibody in German patients with multiple sclerosis.

The IL-6 A5 allele has been linked to benign multiple sclerosis in Sardinian families, with increased severity in individuals having the larger sized alleles (>A6: Vandenbroeck *et al* 2000a). Using a two-stage strategy in which many genes were screened and those suggesting an association then replicated, Z. Zhang *et al* (2005) reported a modest association with lymphocyte activation gene-3 (*LAG3*; encoded at 12p13) and *IL7R* (at 5p13) in 672 Swedish cases compared with an equivalent number of controls. Against a background of generally negative studies, Almeras *et al* (2002) correlated the presence of three *IL10* promoter polymorphisms with disease severity, and others with a mild clinical course. Homozygosity for the functional B polymorphism of the *IL12B* gene was shown to protect from the development of multiple sclerosis in Dutch patients but without an effect on disease course (van Veen *et al* 2001).

Miterski *et al* (1999) demonstrated an association between the IFN-α 07 allele and German patients with multiple sclerosis and, extending the susceptibility haplotype to include the nearby IFN-α10 and IFN-α17 loci, identified additional susceptibility alleles, some of which were functional polymorphisms. Association with the *IFNB* gene was excluded. In a complex design involving cases and controls from Sardinia, North America and Northern Ireland, Kantarci *et al* (2000b) claimed (after several manipulations and stratifications showing inconsistency across the three contributing datasets) a gene dose effect of the CA$_{12}$ allele of the *IFNG* gene in protecting males from developing multiple sclerosis – homozygotes showing a stronger effect than heterozygotes. Later, Kantarci *et al* (2005) showed an association between the *CAn allele and susceptibility to multiple sclerosis in males from the United States and Northern Ireland but not Belgium whereas, again, the CA12 allele appeared protective, but only in the United States population. Goris *et al* (1999) subsequently showed this effect to be most marked in females. They went on to examine additional candidates – IL-22 and IL-26 – thought likely to be in linkage disequilibrium but concluded that the *IFNG* gene itself remained the best candidate (Goris *et al* 2002).

Chemokines and cell adhesion molecules, such as intercellular adhesion molecules (ICAMs), influence inflammation by increasing the migration and parenchymal homing of activated immune cells to sites of inflammation. Mycko *et al* (1998b) reported an association between susceptibility to multiple sclerosis and *ICAM1* exon 6 allele T. There was no interaction with DR(2)15. Fiten *et al* (1999) studied five monocyte chemotactic protein 3 (*MCP3*) polymorphisms in Swedish patients with multiple sclerosis. Curiously, when cases were stratified for DR(2)15, there was a protective effect of the A4 allele interacting with DR(2)15-positive, and the A2 allele with DR(2)15-negative cases – even though the entire cohort showed no allelic associations. Nelissen *et al* (2002) confirmed the association with MCP-3 A2 (and A3) in Belgian patients. In Russians, the same chemokine receptor allele showed an association with early age at onset in DR4-positive patients with multiple sclerosis (Favorova *et al* 2002). Sellebjerg *et al* (2000a) reported that a nonfunctional polymorphism of matrix metalloproteinase-9 was associated with less disease activity although there was no effect on susceptibility in Danish patients with multiple sclerosis. Fiotti *et al* (2004) correlated susceptibility to multiple sclerosis and earlier age at onset with the presence of ≥22CA repeats of the matrix metalloproteinase-9 (*MMP9*) gene. There is one report of association between the G/A polymorphism at position 403 of the RANTES (regulated upon activation T cell expressed and secreted) chemokine in multiple sclerosis in North Americans of European origin, especially in cases with less severe disease but early age at onset (Gade-Andavolu *et al* 2004). Goertsches *et al* (2005) created haplotypes for the disintegrin-like and metalloproteinase domain with thrombospondin type 1 modules (ADAMTS14) family of metalloproteinases using a panel of SNPs in Spanish patients with relapsing–remitting multiple sclerosis: specifically different associations were identified in patients with relapsing–remitting and primary progressive multiple sclerosis compared with controls but there were no correlations with disease severity. Barcellos *et al* (2000) described later age at onset in patients with the CCR5 Δ32 deletion. Homozygosity for Δ32 has been associated with primary progressive multiple sclerosis in Finns (Pulkkinen *et al* 2004) and progression to disability with one or more copies of the Δ32 allele in Israelis (Kantor *et al* 2003). However, many other screens have proved negative (Table 3.2).

Defects of the pro-apoptotic Fas/Fas ligand (FasL) pathway have been proposed as one mechanism of T-cell autoimmunity in multiple sclerosis (see Chapter 11). Zayas *et al* (2001) reported a reduced frequency of the Fas allele B in Spanish and North American patients with multiple sclerosis, some having a positive family history. Something seems wrong here since, paradoxically, the B allele is found in association with the MHC susceptibility haplotype DRB1*0501-DQB1*0602. van Veen *et al* (2002) described a protective effect of the Fas-670*G allele in patients with multiple sclerosis from the Netherlands, but with no effect on disease course. Schrijver *et al* (2004) claimed a weak association between susceptibility to multiple sclerosis and the presence of a TGFβ allele that strengthened with subgroup analysis of males and correlated with MRI indices of accelerated brain atrophy.

Osteopontin has been identified by microarray screening as a potential inflammatory mediator in the lesions of multiple sclerosis. Inevitably it was soon examined as a candidate susceptibility gene. Niino *et al* (2003a) showed that the C/C genotype in exon 6 was increased in Japanese patients with multiple sclerosis whereas the G/G variant of exon 7 associated with older age at onset. There were no effects on disease course or progression. Plasma platelet activating factor acetylhydrolase gene (*PAFAH1B1*) polymorphisms (encoded at 17p13.3) were first shown to be associated with severity in the optico-spinal form of multiple sclerosis in female Japanese patients (Osoegawa *et al* 2004); later a different allelic association was reported between susceptibility and the Western phenotype of multiple sclerosis in Japanese (Osoegawa *et al* 2005). Others have not reproduced these results (see Table 3.2).

Molecules that mediate inflammatory processes or participate in cell signalling have been studied as candidate genetic susceptibility factors. CD45 (protein-tyrosine phosphatase receptor type C) is a polymorphic transmembrane molecule involved in T-cell antigen receptor signalling and is encoded at 1q312-32. Jacobsen *et al* (2000) studied a point mutation of CD45-(*PTPRC*) and showed this to be associated in three of four populations (from Germany and North America), linked in three informative multiplex families, and present amongst affected family members in a fourth. Subsequently, Ballerini *et al* (2002) identified the same point mutation in a minority of Italian patients with multiple sclerosis but in no controls. Vyshkina *et al* (2004) reported preferential transmission of the G allele of *CD45* in family-based association studies, although this allele was only present in a minority of families (7/136). The involvement of *CD45* has not been confirmed in four subsequent screens or meta-analysis (Gomez-Lira *et al* 2003: see Table 3.2). An SNP mutation in *CD24*, implicated in the pathogenicity of autoreactive T cells, is associated with susceptibility and the rate of disease progression in a population- and family-based study from the United States (Q. Zhou *et al* 2003).

Although the evidence indicates that polymorphisms for molecules involved in oxidative stress are not directly involved in susceptibility to multiple sclerosis, C.L.A. Mann *et al* (2000) showed an association with homozygosity for the glutathione S-transferase *MGST1* AA genotype – expected to promote nitric oxide synthase inducibility – and disability after 10-year disease duration.

Luomala *et al* (2000) studied the plasminogen activator inhibitor-1 (*SMARCA3*) promoter and showed an association with susceptibility to multiple sclerosis in females (odds ratio 2.3; 95% CI 1.04–5.23). The associated allele correlates with low PAI-1 production consistent with reduced proteinase inhibition and hence enhanced cell migration through extracellular matrix. In a study of Italian patients, Chiocchetti *et al* (2005) showed a protective effect of the osteopontin-A haplotype and with a reduced rate of conversion to secondary progression with less disability. Pursuing the reason for an increased frequency of multiple sclerosis in females, Niino *et al* (2000a) reported an association between susceptibility and the PvuII allele of the oestrogen receptor gene, whereas the XbaI polymorphism was more frequent in patients with early age at onset. Kikuchi *et al* (2002a) showed independent associations of the [P] oestrogen receptor allele and DR(2)15 in Japanese patients with the Western phenotype. DR(2)15 stratification markedly increased the [P] allele association (odds ratio 16; 95% CI 4–64) in females. Progression index and severity at >5 years were also associated with the [P] oestrogen receptor allele. The vitamin D

receptor has been studied as a candidate, either on the basis that multiple sclerosis is less prevalent in regions characterized by high exposure to sunlight, or because vitamin D has an immuno-suppressive effect (see Chapter 2). Fukazawa *et al* (1999b) described an association between the vitamin D receptor b allele, especially in homozygotes, and susceptibility to multiple sclerosis in Japanese with the Western phenotype. Niino *et al* (2000b) performed a more extensive genotypic analysis of the vitamin D receptor gene and correlated the (Bsm) b and (ApaI) A haplotype with susceptibility, especially after DR(2)15 stratification. In Israel, disease severity is reported to be associated with the M694V mutation of the gene for familial Mediterranean fever (*MERV*) in non-Ashkenazi patients with multiple sclerosis (Shinar *et al* 2003). Turning attention to possible targets for the autoimmune process in multiple sclerosis, van Veen et al (2003b) reported that the CRYAB polymorphism of αB crystallin predisposes to primary progressive multiple sclerosis.

Re-analysis of 32 candidate genes/microsatellite markers after stratification of probands into DR15-positive and -negative groups revealed some clustering into one or other group (A. Hensiek, unpublished observations). As expected, markers located on chromosome 6, close to the HLA region, showed a significant result in the DR(2)15-positive group. Others, however, such as myeloperoxidase, *TMP3*, *IL1R*, spinocerebellar ataxia 1 (*SCA1*) and *APOB* seemed to cluster mainly in DR(2)15-negative individuals. But with the application of Bonferroni correction for multiple testing, none of the results outside the HLA region achieved significance levels, implying that there are no significant HLA interactions for any of the loci selected in this survey. Barcellos *et al* (2004) had a somewhat better dividend from a nonprejudicial screen of 34 candidate genes selected because of their involvement in immune responses. (In this instance, the 33 negative candidates, after statistical correction, are not listed in Table 3.2.) Inevitably most were negative but the promoter for nitric oxide synthase 2A (*NOS2A*: encoded at 17q11) showed transmission distortion both in North American families of European descent and in African-Americans, after statistical correction for multiple testing. These associations were further supported by evidence for linkage of the $(CCTTT)_n$ polymorphism in affected family members.

Structural genes of myelin and growth factors

The myelin sheath contains the products of several genes encoding glycoproteins. Proteolipid protein is involved in apposition of the myelin membrane. It is encoded on the X chromosome. Mutation of the gene causes Pelizaeus–Merzbacher disease. There are no known disorders of the human central nervous system resulting from genetically determined defects of myelin-associated glycoprotein, myelin oligodendrocyte glycoprotein, or 2′,3′-cyclic nucleotide 3-phosphodiesterase but several studies have sought to implicate one or other of these genes in susceptibility to multiple sclerosis. Myelin basic protein is the major structural component of myelin, comprising 35% of myelin proteins in central white matter. It is required for normal compaction of myelin. Biochemical analysis of human myelin has shown several isoforms (18.5, 21.5, 17.2 and 20.2 kDa). The myelin basic protein gene at 18qter consists of seven exons spread over 40–45 kb. Variants are generated from alternative splicing. Exon 2 encodes a sequence of 26 amino acids present in the larger isoforms (21.5 and 20.2 kDa). The 17.2-kDa protein lacks the 11 amino acids encoded by exon 5. Variations in transcription and alternative splicing suggest that the myelin basic protein gene is under the control of enhancers and promoters acting with regulatory factors to control transcription rate. The discovery that isoforms of myelin basic protein arise from alternative splicing of the seven exons has led to the suggestion that defects in the gene or its promoter might alter the gene product or its transcription, leading to aberrant myelination or failure of remyelination.

D.D. Wood *et al* (1996) provided indirect support for the hypothesis that mutations in structural genes for myelin may contribute to disease susceptibility in multiple sclerosis. Normal-appearing white matter from a patient dying with the Marburg variant showed biochemical changes consistent with a genetically determined alteration in charge, the less cationic protein being unable to form compact lamellae and so having a much reduced capacity for remyelination. Boylan *et al* (1987) had previously reported on a region of highly repetitive DNA located 5′ to the first exon of human myelin basic protein containing the promoter region. They identified 11 alleles showing Mendelian inheritance. Sequence analysis showed that this region consisted of a tandem repeat tetramer (TGGA) located 5′ to the first exon and constituting approximately 1 kb of DNA. Subsequently, Boylan *et al* (1990) described ten RFLP alleles contained within the first exon of the main gene ranging in length from 2.05 to 2.15 kb. An association study showed excess alleles in the 2.14–2.15 range. However, precise allele definition was limited with such a small difference in size, especially in individuals who were homozygous for individual alleles. Tienari *et al* (1992b) used a tetranucleotide repeat sequence from the same 5′ regions to amplify five alleles within this segment in cases and controls from Finland. They reported an allelic association with the 1.27 allele (relative risk 3.3 for heterozygotes and 9.2 for homozygotes). Comparisons between familial and sporadic cases, and individuals with different modes of clinical presentation or clinical course, showed no difference in the pattern of allelic association. By extending this work to 21 multiplex families, they also provided evidence for linkage based on 197 genotypings in 59 affecteds and 138 unaffected individuals (maximum lod score 3.42), adopting an autosomal dominant model with penetrance variously estimated at 5%, 38% and 75%. This case material from Vaasa, Finland, shows unusual clustering, raising the possibility that the families are not necessarily representative of multiple sclerosis seen elsewhere in the Western world. The effect can be traced to a subset of individuals with common ancestry and does not hold up in the larger cohort (Pihlaja *et al* 2003). But opportunities now exist for tracing the genealogy of this isolate, linking it to other regions through population history and so seeing more clearly the ancestral origin, and apparently explaining one particular route to increased disease susceptibility.

Studies of structural genes of myelin have mostly otherwise been uninformative. Ibsen and Clausen (1995) detected three alleles of a sequence adjacent to the myelin basic protein gene promoter and reported a disease association with homozygosity for the 1.45-bp allele with a corresponding reduction in frequency of the 1.32-bp allele. These authors offered technical explanations for discrepancies with respect to myelin basic protein gene susceptibility and multiple sclerosis that they and others had studied. Guerini *et al* (2000) showed significant differences in the distribution of myelin basic protein polymorphisms. Homozygosity for the 354-bp allele was associated with relapsing–remitting multiple sclerosis. Subsequently, this association in Italians was extended to a cohort of patients from Russia but, in both populations, the allelic association with myelin basic protein was only detected after the stratification of cases for DR4 and DR5 (Guerini *et al* 2003). Against this background, the balance of evidence is against a structural gene of myelin conferring susceptibility to multiple sclerosis outside the genetic isolate of western Finland.

N.W. Wood *et al* (1994) showed no evidence for linkage or association in affected sibling pairs and unrelated controls. The failure to demonstrate linkage in multiplex families from Salt Lake City (J. Rose *et al* 1993), the lack either of an association or linkage in a small number of affected sibling pairs from Italy (Eoli *et al* 1994b), the absence of a population association in Northern Ireland (Graham *et al* 1993) and Denmark (Nellerman *et al* 1995), and further negative studies from France (Coppin *et al* 2000) and Sardinia (Cocco *et al* 2002) – involving newly defined and existing polymorphisms – has shifted the balance of opinion towards the view that a polymorphism of the myelin basic protein gene does not contribute generally to susceptibility in northern European patients with multiple sclerosis.

Although most effort has gone into assessing myelin basic protein as a candidate gene for susceptibility to multiple sclerosis, Thompson *et al* (1996) excluded an effect of 2′,3′-cyclic nucleotide-3′-phosphodiesterase (CNPase). They sequenced *CNP* in patients with multiple sclerosis and controls and found nine mutations, but none of these was disease specific with the possible exception of a T→C transition at position 4306. This was present in 2/54 cases but no controls. The gene for myelin oligodendrocyte glycoprotein lies telomeric to the MHC. In a study from southwest France, M.P. Roth *et al* (1995) found no difference in allele frequency between 169 patients with multiple sclerosis and 173 controls, concluding that variations in this myelin gene do not confer susceptibility to multiple sclerosis. Although a slight increase in frequency of a 1.9-kb RFLP was reported by A.A. Hilton *et al* (1995) in Australian patients, polymorphisms in the human myelin oligodendrocyte glycoprotein gene do not reproducibly discriminate patients with multiple sclerosis from controls (D. Rodriguez *et al* 1997). Subsequently, Gomez-Lira *et al* (2002) defined new polymorphisms. One sequence was found only in patients with multiple sclerosis, but infrequently, and the Val→Leu mutation at position 142 in exon 3 was under-represented, suggesting a protective effect. Ohlenbusch *et al* (2002) sequenced the myelin oligodendrocyte glycoprotein gene in 75 children with multiple sclerosis but there were no associations with any of the identified polymorphisms. D'Alfonso *et al* (2002) showed no association with myelin associated glycoprotein polymorphisms in a large population-based association study from Italy.

There may be comorbidity between neurofibromatosis 1 and primary progressive multiple sclerosis (see Chapter 6). If so, this is not explained by mutation of the oligodendrocyte myelin glycoprotein gene, embedded within intron 27b of the NF-1 gene (Hinks *et al* 1995; M.R. Johnson *et al* 2000). More generally, B. He *et al* (1998) found no linkage between multiple sclerosis and genes for myelin associated glycoprotein, CNPase, oligodendrocyte myelin glycoprotein gene or proteolipid protein. Seboun *et al* (1999) fared no better in screening 102 sibling pairs for linkage to the genes for myelin basic protein, proteolipid protein, myelin associated glycoprotein, myelin oligodendrocyte glycoprotein, CNPase or oligodendrocyte myelin glycoprotein; each was uninformative with respect to susceptibility.

More than 35 growth factors or genes encoding structural components of the nervous system have been assessed as candidates. Most have proved uninformative (see Table 3.2) but some observations merit description. Giess *et al* (2002) stratified patients with multiple sclerosis for a null mutation conferring reduced function of ciliary neurotrophic factor, normally produced in response to injury and providing potent differentiation and survival effects on oligodendrocytes. They showed earlier age at onset and more severe motor involvement and proposed that this was due to poor regenerative potential following disease activity. The report remains unconfirmed (Hoffmann *et al* 2002) and, clearly, the interpretation makes many assumptions concerning the pathogenesis and genetics of multiple sclerosis. But the main candidate repeatedly suggested as a gene influencing the course of multiple sclerosis rather than susceptibility is apolipoprotein E (ApoE) – a ligand for lipid transport, produced by glial cells and involved both in normal neuronal metabolism and the response to injury. Several neurological disorders appear to be associated with specific ApoE polymorphisms. Evangelou *et al* (1999) first associated the ApoE-ε4 allele with disease severity in multiple sclerosis, explaining this finding on the basis of impaired plasticity and repair after inflammatory disease activity. There followed confirmatory reports of an effect of ApoE-ε4 on disability from Israel (Chapman *et al* 1999; 2001), Austria (Fazekas *et al* 2001), Denmark (Hogh *et al* 2000) and the United States (S. Schmidt *et al* 2002) – both the latter two groups also showing an effect on susceptibility – whereas others have not confirmed the association (see Table 3.2). Kantarci *et al* (2003c) refined the association between multiple sclerosis and ApoE, working from a population base to examine a range of polymorphisms, age at conversion to secondary progressive disease and gender effects. Whilst not entirely settling the issue of an effect of ApoE-ε4 on disease severity, they focused on the e2 allele and concluded that this had a protective effect on severity, but only in women. Others have also described a protective effect of the ApoE-ε2 allele on disease severity but not confined to women (Ballerini *et al* 2000; Savettieri *et al* 2003; 2004; S. Schmidt *et al* 2002). An alternative approach has been to consider radiological markers of atrophy as an intermediate phenotype. Enzinger *et al* (2004) correlated the frequency of T_1 'black holes', and rate at which T_2-weighted lesions converted, with ApoE-ε4. Against this background, Barcellos *et al* (2005) collated the existing literature performing meta- and pooled analyses of data relating to between 2900 and 4000 cases and a comparable number of controls to show that alleles encoded at ApoE do not influence susceptibility to multiple sclerosis, or predict disease course: only in the subgroup analysis of males with two copies of the ApoE-ε4 allele was increased disease severity observed. The ApoC locus (19q13) has been less studied. Zouali *et al* (1999) claimed an effect on susceptibility, but not disease course or progression, for the ApoC-1 allele in six French patients. Gade-Andavolu *et al* (1998) added evidence for an association between the gamma-aminobutyric acid A3

($GABA_{A3}$) receptor and multiple sclerosis to their previous claim for an association with the dopamine D2 receptor gene – suggesting that both mediate their effects through release of prolactin. There are no associations with the prolactin gene or its receptor in Italian patients with multiple sclerosis (Mellai *et al* 2003).

The presence of phenocopies is a major concern in the analysis of complex traits where diagnosis depends on pattern recognition of symptoms, signs and laboratory investigations occurring in the absence of a test for the disease. Although there were no individuals having an excess of triplet repeats for *SCA2*, J. Chataway *et al* (1999a) claimed that the 22-kb allele occurred at a higher frequency in cases than controls reported in the literature. This result prompted an assessment of transmission disequilibrium in family trios supporting an association between multiple sclerosis and the 22-kb allele. A second data set showed similar findings although the evidence for association weakened (S. Sawcer, unpublished observations). One interpretation of this finding is that, in individuals who have a tendency for autoimmunity as a result of the interplay between genetic susceptibility and environmental factors, the inflammatory process may be focused onto a particular system or pathway within the brain and spinal cord in those who have genetic polymorphisms exposing that pathway to tissue injury. In the case of *SCA2*, individuals with the normal 22-kb allele polymorphism may have disproportionate inflammatory demyelination of the spino-cerebellar pathways – similar to involvement of the anterior visual pathway in Harding's disease (see below and Chapter 6). However, the association with SCA2 alleles has not been confirmed (see Table 3.2).

Mitochondrial genes

Recognition that the clinical phenotype of multiple sclerosis, typical imaging features and the presence of oligoclonal bands in spinal fluid may occur in association with pathological mutations of mitochondrial DNA has prompted detailed assessment of mitochondrial genes as candidates for susceptibility factors in multiple sclerosis. Harding *et al* (1992) reported on eight women presenting with bilateral sequential optic neuropathy and later developing symptoms consistent with demyelination outside the visual system. MRI abnormalities typical of demyelination were present in seven patients who were scanned (Figure 3.21). All eight cases had matrilinear relatives affected by Leber's hereditary optic neuropathy, and the 11 778 mutation. In a subsequent review of Leber's hereditary optic neuropathy, Riordan-Eva *et al* (1995) reported that 45% of 24 females with the 11 778 mutation had a multiple sclerosis-like illness. Harding's disease has since been reported in males (Bhatti and Newman 1999; Buhmann *et al* 2002; Olsen *et al* 1995; M. Tran *et al* 2001). Horvath *et al* (2000) screened 39 individuals from 12 families with Leber's disease. Two females had symptoms and signs consistent with the diagnosis of multiple sclerosis (and 11 778 and 14 484 mutations, respectively). Cerebral magnetic resonance abnormalities were not present in any of the remaining 37 family members.

Mutations of mitochondrial DNA are either pathological or normal variations. Neither type has been shown to be associated with multiple sclerosis in systematic screening of unselected patients. However, this has brought to light further cases

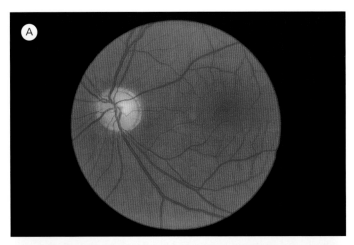

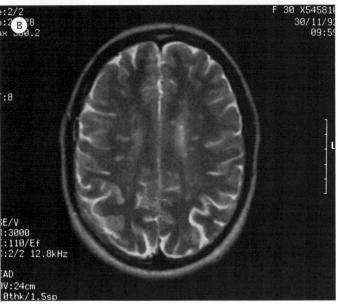

Figure 3.21 (A) Optic fundus from case 1 first describing a multiple sclerosis-like illness in women harbouring a mutation of mitochondrial DNA (Harding's disease). Reproduced with permission from Harding *et al* (1992). (B) Cerebral white matter lesions in another individual with Harding's disease: bilateral involvement of the anterior visual pathway, additional neurological symptoms and a pathological mitochondrial DNA mutation at position 3460.

diagnosed as having multiple sclerosis in whom disproportionate involvement of the visual system is associated with a mutation of mitochondrial DNA. Kellar-Wood *et al* (1994b) found no mutations at the 11 778 mitochondrial DNA site in 307 unrelated patients with multiple sclerosis, randomly selected with respect to clinical presentation, although one harboured a mutation of uncertain significance adjacent to position 11 778. The frequency of mutation at site 13 708 was 13% in cases compared with 11% in a local control population of blood donors. These results seemed to exclude a contribution towards susceptibility in multiple sclerosis at the common sites for pathological mutations of mitochondrial DNA in Leber's hereditary optic atrophy. Vyshkina *et al* (2005a) also screened patients with multiple sclerosis and found a variety of associated haplotypes encoded by mitochondrial and nuclear genes determining components of complex 1 (*NDUFS5* at 1p34.2-p33; and *NDUFS7* and

NDUFA7, both at 19p13), irrespective of clinical phenotype. However, in screening patients with severe visual failure complicating a demyelinating disorder of the central nervous system, 3/20 had mitochondrial DNA mutations involving the 3460 (2) and 11 778 (1) sites, respectively. All were women and none had a family history of ophthalmic or neurological disease. Although the nonpathogenic mutations at positions 4216, 4917 or 13 708 were over-represented, their presence did not correlate with the degree of visual failure. Kalman *et al* (1997) selected 22 patients with prominent optic nerve involvement, 20 of whom met criteria for clinically definite multiple sclerosis. None had the 14 798, 11 778 or 3460 mutations of mitochondrial DNA. Mojon *et al* (1999a) found no pathological (3460 or 11 778) mutations of mitochondrial DNA in 103 Swiss patients. As expected, nonpathological mutations were detected. In Italy, Franciotta *et al* (2000) adopted the same approach. First, two individuals from a group with severe bilateral optic neuritis were shown to have nonpathological mutations at positions 4216, 4917 and 13 708. Both subsequently developed multiple sclerosis. Then, an unselected group of 101 patients with multiple sclerosis was screened. There were no pathological mutations, and no excess amongst patients of nonpathological variants occurring alone or in combinations. Ohlenbusch *et al* (1998a) sequenced mitochondrial DNA from 13 children with multiple sclerosis and 20 controls and found no pathological mutations although nine nonpathological changes (at positions 4216, 4917 and 13 708) were detected in a total of five children, perhaps indicating that these act as secondary predisposing factors in individuals who are already at risk. Since disproportionate visual involvement characterizes demyelinating disease in Japanese, Nishimura *et al* (1995) screened 80 patients from Japan, of whom 18 were women with bilateral visual failure. The 11 778 mutation of mitochondrial DNA was not detected. None of the 11 778, 14 484 or 3460 mutations was present in 20 Korean patients with multiple sclerosis (Hwang *et al* 2001). Most recently, the same low yield of pathological mutations from screening patients with disproportionate involvement of the anterior visual pathway was seen in Iran (Houshmand *et al* 2004).

In view of the evidence that a mitochondrial encoded peptide, the N-terminal portion of NADH dehydrogenase subunit 1, acts as a transplantation antigen in mice, Chalmers *et al* (1995) sequenced the corresponding region of human mitochondrial DNA in 87 patients with multiple sclerosis, 10 with Leber's hereditary optic neuropathy and a multiple sclerosis-like illness, and controls. No disease association emerged. A few base pair changes were identified but these were considered to be harmless polymorphisms. Subsequently, Chalmers *et al* (1996) selected nine families with evidence for maternal transmission but again failed to demonstrate base pair changes in the protein and RNA coding sequences of mitochondrial DNA. Kalman *et al* (1996) sequenced the entire mitochondrial DNA in three patients with multiple sclerosis. As expected, deviations from a reference sequence were identified. Eight variants within ribosomal, transfer or protein encoding regions were compared in an association study. One in *ND5* (part of the mitochondrial genome) and another in the cytochrome-C region were marginally more frequent in cases than controls but neither occurred at sufficient frequency to warrant serious consideration as a susceptibility gene for multiple sclerosis. The study of multiple sclerosis in children concluded that sequence variations in the genes for coenzymes 1–3, ATPase 6 and 8, cytochrome-C, ND1-6, ND4L, rRNA and tRNA do not increase susceptibility to multiple sclerosis (Ohlenbusch *et al* 1998b; Wilichowski *et al* 1998).

Harding's disease therefore represents true disease heterogeneity in that a specific genotype determines a characteristic phenotype that nevertheless meets diagnostic criteria for multiple sclerosis. What remains unresolved is whether the mutation of mitochondrial DNA directs the process of brain inflammation onto a particular site – constituting selective tissue vulnerability, as we originally proposed and others have supported (Harding *et al* 1992; Vanopdenbosch *et al* 2000) – or merely represents the chance occurrence of relatively mild multiple sclerosis and Leber's hereditary optic neuropathy (Kalman *et al* 1999). In our opinion, the latter seems unlikely given the number of cases of Harding's disease and the rarity of isolated Leber's hereditary optic neuropathy in women. More generally, visual involvement in multiple sclerosis may be associated with the haplotype K and J of mitochondrial DNA but only in northern Europeans (Kalman *et al* 1999; Mayr-Wolfart *et al* 1996; Reynier *et al* 1999). It remains possible that this observation is confounded by overlapping mitochondrial genetic susceptibility to the independent disorders – Leber's hereditary optic neuropathy and multiple sclerosis (Kalman *et al* 1999). Severe optic neuropathy occurring in the context of the Devic phenotype amongst Caucasians is not associated with mutations of mitochondrial DNA (Cock *et al* 1997; Kalman and Mandler 2002). In Chapter 5 we offer a highly speculative hypothesis on the use of mitochondrial DNA as population markers for susceptibility to multiple sclerosis, related to the origins and evolution of the disease.

SYSTEMATIC GENOME SCREENING

Even if the most favourable spin is placed on the evidence from studies of candidate genes in multiple sclerosis, the contribution they make still falls short of that implicated by the pedigree analysis of recurrence risk in families. It follows that other genes remain to be identified that contribute to susceptibility in multiple sclerosis. Individually, their biological effect cannot be predicted but everything points to several exerting small effects rather than one highly significant factor. In fact, the largest contributor may already have been identified through the studies on HLA and multiple sclerosis.

Linkage genome screens

For this reason, and following the approach used in studies of diabetes mellitus (J.L. Davis *et al* 1994), three groups of investigators first undertook a systematic search of the genome in the mid-1990s aiming to define the number and location of additional susceptibility genes. Genotyping was completed on cohorts of between 75 and 225 multiplex (usually affected sibling pair) families, together involving >1000 individuals, for each of between 257 and 443 microsatellite markers. These loci had an average spacing of around 10 cM. This density was thought to provide each screen with enough power to identify regions encoding a major susceptibility gene. The markers were considered to have sufficient polymorphism to make a high proportion of the available families fully informative.

In order to achieve economies, the principle of these genome screens was to amplify fluorescently labelled microsatellite repeat sequences using the polymerase chain reaction and measure the product size automatically using an Applied Biosystems 373A sequencing system with GENESCAN software. Sets of markers were chosen to give products of differing lengths so that these could be loaded onto the same lane of an electrophoresis gel and genotyped simultaneously. The use of different fluorescent dyes for markers with similar product sizes increased the number of simultaneous genotypes read from a single lane and compared with standards of known size. Further analysis by GENOTYPER sifted the many peaks, filtered stutter bands, defined the product size range for each allele multiplexed on the gel, and produced a file ready for analysis. These genetic analyses were predicated on the assumption that multiple sclerosis is one disease. The resource needed to map and identify susceptibility genes increases substantially in the presence of heterogeneity. In 1996, this was not considered. Nor could it have been in the absence of genotypic or phenotypic markers for different types of disease.

In their first-stage screen, Sawcer *et al* (1996) used 311 microsatellite markers in 143 sibling pairs. Nineteen autosomal regions showed a maximum lod score at or above the level associated with a nominal 5% significance, defined by computer simulation. For the X chromosome, results were stratified on the basis of gender with independent linkage analysis in same-sex and non-same-sex pairs. Six regions had values above a maximum likelihood score of 1.8 corresponding to the level expected by chance only once per screen. These were located at 1cen, 5cen, 7p, 12p, 17q and 22q. This screen has since been serially updated, including extra markers applied to regions of interest and with the addition of new families (Chataway *et al* 1998; Hensiek *et al* 2003a; Sawcer *et al* 1997). At the conclusion of stage two, exclusion mapping under the assumption of no dominance variance excluded genes with λs5 and λs2 from 93% and 55% of the genome, respectively, whereas small effects λs(1.2) could not be excluded at any point. The mean genome information extraction was 60%, and <3% had an information extraction of <25%. The least informative parts of the genome were those between markers and at the telomeres. Conditioning for DR(2)15 (or an extended DR(2)15-linked haplotype also encoding alleles of TNFa and the DQ locus) showed that the regions of interest on 1p, 17p, 17q and X clustered in families with DR(2)15, whereas the nonsharing group was associated with 1cen, 3p, 5cen, 7p, 14q and 22q (Corradu *et al* 1998b). New regions of interest were found at 5q and 13p (DR(2)15 sharing) and 16p and 20p (DR(2)15 nonsharing). In the most recent analysis (Hensiek *et al* 2003a), 353 markers were used for the final analysis of 226 multiplex families, new data coming from 242 markers not previously typed in the 97 families forming the second set.

The highest maximum likelihood score value (3.1) was observed on chromosome 14 in the area encoding the variable region of the immunoglobulin heavy chain. Four additional regions (1p, 6p, 17q and Xq) had maximum likelihood scores suggestive of linkage (>1.8). All five had already been identified in previous reports (Chataway *et al* 1998; Sawcer *et al* 1996), although the new typing across the genome increased the peak maximum likelihood score at Xq to 2.54. Stratifying these data on the basis of DR(2)15 sharing suggested genetic heterogeneity with linkages on chromosomes 7 and 17 now appearing to reflect loci acting independently of DR(2)15 (Figure 3.22).

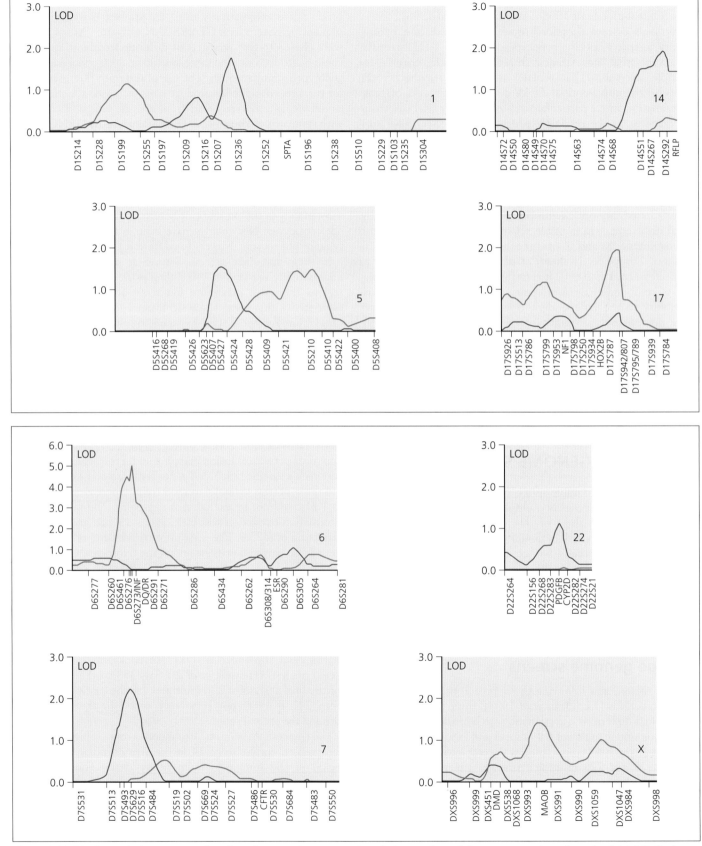

Figure 3.22 Maximum lod score at each point where markers were placed along selected chromosomes, based on the initial United Kingdom whole-genome linkage screen. The blue line indicates results in families where both affected siblings are identical by state for DR(2)15 and the red line those families where there is non-sharing for DR(2)15. Adapted from J. Chataway *et al* (1998).

Haines *et al* (1996) also identified 19 regions of interest on 14 chromosomes in their linkage study involving 75 families (52 included in the first set providing 81 sibling pairs and a further 23 having 45 sibling pairs subsequently added for the study of chromosome 6). These were genotyped for 443 markers providing a 9.6-cM map. The affected relative pair method was adopted to make best use of the more extended pedigrees in 16/52 (31%) of these families. This screen identified 6p21 as a linked region in both sets. The next best lod score was at 7q21-22, reasonably close to the TCRβ locus at 7q35. For the majority of chromosomal regions, this group confined their analysis to the first set of 52 families (81 sibling pairs), setting thresholds for the different statistical tests employed. Regions of interest, other than 6p and 7q, were at 11p, 12q and 19q. These families were then used to show that the contribution to linkage from 6p21 was entirely accounted for by the DR locus, suggesting that the gene responsible is DR(2)15 itself (Haines *et al* 1998). Support was subsequently provided for the 19q linkage in an independent population association (Barcellos *et al* 1997b), especially in families also linked to DR(2)15 (Pericak-Vance *et al* 2001). Serial updating based first on 266 affected individuals in 98 families continued to support linkage at 6p21, 6q27 and 19q13 with additional support for effects encoded at 12q23 and 16p13 (Haines *et al* 2002). Later, the addition of 90 families from France analysed with the existing 98 United States cohort investigated seven regions of interest and confirmed provisional linkage to 1p34, 3p14, 6p21 and 19q13 with reduced evidence implicating 2p, 3q, 5q and Xp (Pericak-Vance *et al* 2004). The second generation full genome screen of 456 affected relative pairs from the United States and France implicated 1q, 6p, 9q and 16p, with less evidence implicating 3q and 5q in the joint population and 18p and 1p and 22q in the United States and French cohorts, respectively. HLA stratification raised the status of 13q and 16q in the combined DR(2)15 population, 2q in the same United States group, and 6q in the French DR(2)15-negative patients (Kenealy *et al* 2004).

In the Canadian series, Ebers *et al* (1996) studied 100 sibling pairs with 257 markers, providing a 15.2-cM map. Subsequent sets, providing 44 and 78 additional sibling pairs, were studied at HLA but the lod score at this locus only reached 0.65. Family-based tests of association did, however, show distortion for a locus outside HLA, suggesting a modest susceptibility effect in this area. In the first cohort of families, a lod score of >4 was present for a locus on chromosome 5. This survived the second but not the third set, which, conversely, provided evidence against linkage with a lod score of <3. The combined lod score for all 222 sibling pairs was 1.6. Overall, regions of interest were identified on chromosomes 2p16, 3p14.1-12, 5pter-14, 11q22-23 and Xp21.1-11.4. The study was updated to include 105 best markers from the three original screens tested in 219 sibling pairs (Dyment *et al* 2001). No markers met criteria for significant linkage. The best supported were at 6p21 and 17q22. Most recently, the study has been repeated to include 552 sibling pairs from 442 families, screened initially with 498 microsatellite markers at an average spacing of 7 cM in 219/552 sibling pairs and then with additional markers in regions of interest in a further set of 333 affected sibling pairs (Dyment *et al* 2004b). Overall, there was more sharing amongst clinically concordant than nonconcordant pairs but this was attributable to the non-DR(2)15 individuals. Linkage was detected at 6p21

(lod 4.4) with suggestive results at 1p, 2q, 5p, 9q, 11p, 12q, 18p, 18q and 21q (lod scores ≥1). Replication analysis involving all 552 affected sibling pairs confirmed 2q27 (lod 2.27), 5p15 (lod 2.09), 18p11 (lod 1.68), 9q21 (lod 1.58) and 1p31 (lod 1.33) as regions of interest, with less evidence at 17q (lod 1.67) where there was association with the marker D17S789. Taken together, the study confirms the supremacy of DR(2)15 but suggests genetic heterogeneity between HLA and other genetic loci.

The region of interest at 5p is close to one of several shown to encode murine experimental autoimmune encephalomyelitis susceptibility genes (see below). This clue led Kuokkanen *et al* (1996) to screen human regions syntenic to the murine genes (1p22-q23, 5p14-12 and Xq13.2-22) in the 21 Finnish families (which may not be fully representative of multiple sclerosis genes by comparison with other northern Europeans: see above). Of these, evidence for linkage was provided only for the markers at 5p (lod score 3.4 for a recombination distance of 10 cM) and the scores were negative at 1p and Xq. Subsequently, Kuokkanen *et al* (1997) reported the more detailed analysis of a genome-wide screen in 16 families using 328 markers. This revealed no statistically significant regions of interest, although positive lod scores were obtained at 6p21 (MHC) and 5p14-12. Increasing the density of markers raised the lod scores in several additional regions (4cen, 11tel and 17q), whereas others (2q32 and 10q21) were unchanged. When all 21 families were typed across regions of interest, the highest lod score (2.8) was at 17q22, as in the previously reported United Kingdom screen.

Exclusion mapping in these screens suggested that despite the prevailing overall estimate of λs at around 40, there is no major susceptibility gene in multiple sclerosis. The next step was to integrate everything into a single meta-analysis. By eye, the task did not look promising – and so, generally, it proved (Becker *et al* 1998; Wise *et al* 1999). The importance of HLA was confirmed but, of the other new regions of interest, several were clearly unique to each screen and so could have been false positives. A first formal meta-analysis was completed in 1998 but not published until 2001 (Transatlantic Multiple Sclerosis Genetics Cooperative 2001). This showed the highest lod scores at 3p21, 5q11, 6p21, 6qtel, 12p13, 16p13, 17q11 and 17q22.

These studies were followed by screens in families from Italy (Broadley *et al* 2001a), Sardinia (Coraddu *et al* 2001), and Turkey (Eraksoy *et al* 2003a), and by surveys of comparable size from Scandinavia (Åkesson *et al* 2002) and Australia (Ban *et al* 2002). Each was small but, although failing to provide statistically unequivocal linkages, more regions of potential interest were identified than expected on the basis of chance alone. Collectively, they have added significantly to the data set available for meta-analysis. This has now been updated to include all ten screens together with 42 new sib pair families from the United Kingdom (Table 3.3) (GAMES and the Transatlantic Multiple Sclerosis Genetics Cooperative 2003). Raw genotyping data were combined from all published genome linkage screens in multiple sclerosis providing linkage analysis of 719 families. One thousand two hundred and eighty-one distinct (fully independent) markers were employed across the nine populations. Some regions were enriched for markers either because they were candidate regions (chromosome 6p21) or because provisionally positive results had been obtained (chromosome 17q21-22).

Table 3.3 **Regions of interest in whole-genome linkage screens**

Country	Chromosome																						
	1	2	3	4	5	6	7	8	9	10	11	12	13	14	15	16	17	18	19	20	21	22	X
United Kingdom	1cen				5cen	6p21	7p							14q			17q22		19q				Xp
United States						6p21	7q				11p	12q							19q				
Canada		2p16	3p14								11q22												Xp21
Meta-analysis 2001			3p21		5q11	6p21 6qtel						12p13				16p13	17q11 17q22						
Finland																	17q22						
Italy	1q42 1q44	2q36			5q33	6pter 6q22				10cen					15q21								
Sardinia	1q31									10q23	11p15												
Scandinavia	1q11 1q24	2q24 2q32	3p26 3q21	4q12		6p25 6p21 6q21			9q34	10p15 10p12	11p15	12q21				16p13	17q25					22q12	Xp22
Australia		2p13		4q26		6q26																	Xp11
Turkey													13q					18q23					
Meta-analysis 2003		2p14				6p21				10p15	11pter					16p13	17q21					22q13	
High density re-analysis 2005					5q33	6p21											17q23						

Together, the map was based on a weighted average of 359 microsatellite markers per family (range 257–453) giving an average marker separation of 10.2 cM. Simulations indicated that, with this map density and family structures, lod scores of 2.2 and 2.9 represent suggestive and significant linkage thresholds, respectively. The identification of four peaks with scores ≥2.1 exceeded the number expected by chance alone. Evidence of significant linkage was observed only on chromosome 6p21. Six non-MHC regions – identified as of interest but less well supported by the linkage data at 2p14, 10p15, 11pter, 16p13, 17q21 and 22q13 – yielded scores >2.0.

Recognizing that existing screens had only extracted a modest proportion of the available information from multiplex families (generally <50%) and invariably included substantial genotyping error rates (≥0.5–1%), and that a data set of c.1000 families might yet prove sufficient to demonstrate linkage outside 6p21, the International Multiple Sclerosis Genetics Consortium (2005) typed available families from Australia, Scandinavia, the United States and the United Kingdom, using a more reliably typed high-density SNP-based linkage screening panel. In total, 2709 individuals from 730 multiplex families were typed for 4506 SNP markers from the Illumina BeadArray™ linkage mapping panel version 3. Together, these families provide 945 informative affected relative pairs; and the panel of markers achieved a mean information extraction at >79% with an estimated genotyping error rate of 0.002%. We consider these to be the most reliable linkage data and they are shown, chromosome by chromosome, in Figure 3.23 and summarized in Table 3.3. The only unambiguous result relates to the HLA region at 6p21, which now has a maximum likelihood score of 11.7; again, the next highest scores were at 17q23 (2.45) and 5q33 (2.18), and ordered subset analysis suggested that there may be an additional locus at chromosome 19p13. However, this screen uses many families shared across the previous larger surveys so that, assuming genotyping accuracy, the same result is to be expected, and these cannot be regarded as fully independent samples or replicate studies.

The study of large pedigrees carries the promise that a gene of general interest might be identified. Vitale *et al* (2002) studied a Pennsylvania family of Dutch origin in whom multiple sclerosis has behaved as an autosomal dominant trait. HLA stratification of a genome-wide screen demonstrated linkage to 12p12 (lod 2.71), conditional also on the presence of DR(2)15/DQ6. Family members with one or other susceptibility allele were

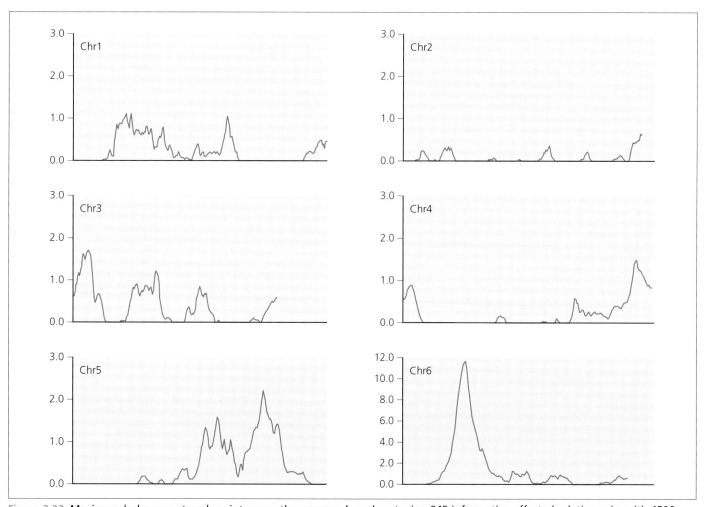

Figure 3.23 Maximum lod scores at each point across the genome based on typing 945 informative affected relative pairs with 4506 SNP markers from the Illumina BeadArray™ linkage mapping panel version 3. The horizontal axis is proportional to the length of the chromosome; and the vertical axis represents the probability that a gene occurs at that locus. The different colours used for each chromosome are for visual effect only. Note that the scale is adjusted on chromosome 6 to accommodate the high lod score by comparison with other chromosomes. Adapted from International Multiple Sclerosis Genetics Consortium (2005).

illustration continued on following page

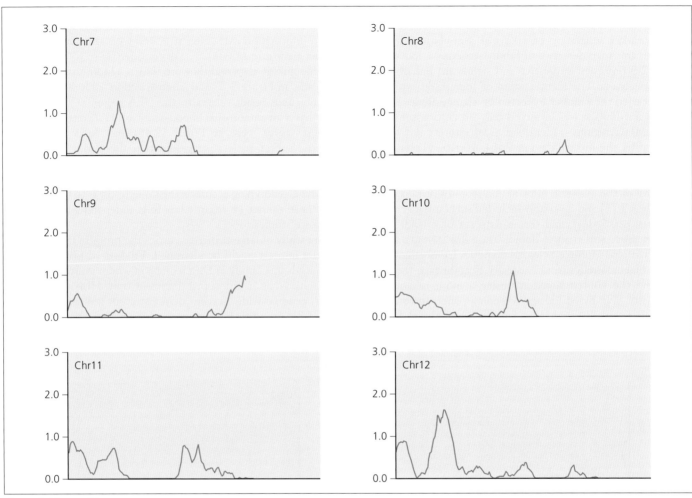

Figure 3.23, cont'd

unaffected. B.P. He *et al* (2002) performed a whole-genome screen on 22 patients from an isolated part of northern Sweden with a high incidence of multiple sclerosis, linked through genealogical records to a common ancestral couple. Five individuals from four nuclear families were screened using 390 microsatellite markers. This identified a candidate susceptibility haplotype, further tested for association in a more extended sample and leading to the identification of a 10-cM interval at 17p11 as the most promising region in this community. However, there was no evidence for HLA linkage or association. Modin *et al* (2003) screened five affected individuals from a consanguinous family with an average of 608 successful genotypes per family member. The highest lod score was at 9q (2.29) and 4/5 affecteds were homozygous for a 43-cM haplotype spanning this region. The remaining case and all unaffecteds were heterozygous – consistent with the interpretation that, in this family, 9q encodes an autosomal recessive gene for multiple sclerosis.

Others have looked at the whole-genome screens and explored selected regions of interest in more detail, hoping to consolidate their status based on mapping, but without picking out positional candidates. The consequences of saturating a region with a much higher density of microsatellite markers than used in an initial linkage screening phase were set out by Feakes *et al* (1999). At that time, the strategy paid a price for increased information extraction by introducing a higher geno-

typing error rate such that a density much higher than 2.5 cM proved unrewarding. The linkage peak on chromosome 17q, originally identified in the United Kingdom screen, is now supported by additional positional screens from Denmark (Larsen *et al* 2000), Canada (Dyment *et al* 2001; 2004b) Finland (Saarela *et al* 2002) and Iceland (Giedraitis *et al* 2003) although a French study found no evidence for linkage to chromosome 17 (Fontaine *et al* 1999). A series of generally small linkage studies in various populations have provided additional support, but falling well short of proof, for effects conferred by several other regions of interest:

- 2p, 3q, 7p and 22q in Italians (D'Alfonso *et al* 1999)
- 3p, 7p, 7q, 12p and 12q in Swedish patients (C. Xu *et al* 1999; 2001; Y. Dai *et al* 2001)
- 5p in Danish cases (Oturai *et a* 1999)
- 7q 21-22 in a mixed European sample (Vandenbroeck *et al* 2002, who suggested protachykinin-1 and plasminogen activator inhibitor-1 as positional candidates; Villoslada *et al* 2004)
- 14q24-32 in Icelandic cases having common ancestry (Giedraitis *et al* 2003)
- 9q in samples from France (Lucotte *et al* 2002) and Finland (Reunanen *et al* 2002) – but only in DR(2)15-negative families (unlike the studies from North America)

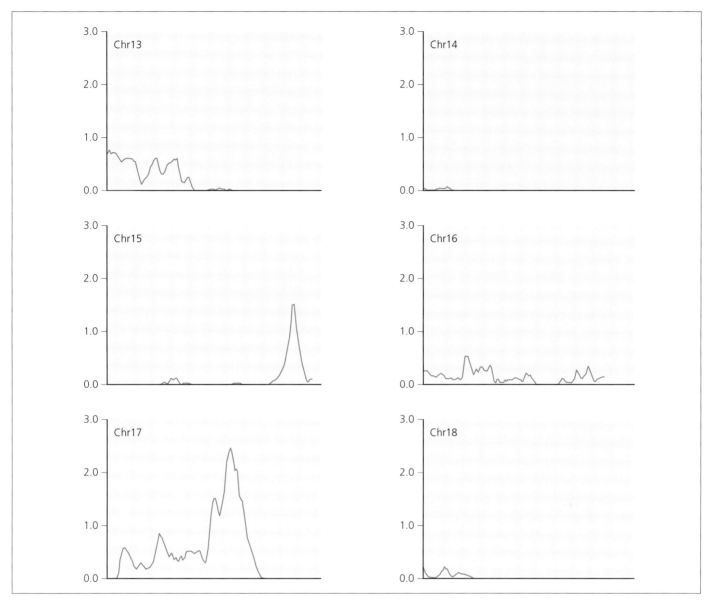

Figure 3.23, cont'd

illustration continued on following page

- 10p15 in a combined Scandinavian, Italian, Sardinian and United Kingdom sample of 449 families (lod 2.5 using a set of 13 markers placed across the region of interest: Åkesson *et al* 2003).

An alternative has been to use regions of interest as a shortcut to the identification of positional candidates, and often using the higher power of association to resolve the interval encoding the susceptibility effect. J. Chataway *et al* (1999b) tested 10 candidates from the various regions of interest emerging from the United Kingdom genome screen using family-based association methods. Of these, only myeloperoxidase, mapping to 17q.23, showed weak evidence for association. This was not confirmed in a Swedish sample (Nelissen *et al* 2000). K.Z. Dai *et al* (2001) picked the T-cell regulator gene SH2D2A as their candidate at 1q21 and showed population and family-based association with reduced *in vitro* T-cell activation amongst carriers of the short (associated) alleles. Cunningham *et al* (2005) selected preprotachykinin-1 (TAC1) as their preferred candidate encoded within the region of interest at 7q21-22 and showed an association with an intron-I SNP. M.B. Mann *et al* (2002) chose phenylethanolamine *N*-methyltransferase as the most promising positional candidate at 17q12-21.2, identified in two whole-genome screens, claiming an association between susceptibility and epistasis between the GG and AA alleles of two regions of the gene promoter. Vyshkina *et al* (2005b) demonstrated altered transmission of haplotypes for β chemokines and chemokine ligands mapping to a 1.85Mb segment of 17q11. On the basis of its role in axonal function, Liguori *et al* (2004) studied synapsin 3 (*SYN3*, encoded at 22q12) as a positional candidate for susceptibility in multiple sclerosis. They described a protective effect on susceptibility of the C polymorphism (odds ratio 0.49: 95% CI 0.35–0.68) forming part of the synapsin 3C 691/A 196 haplotype, and younger age at onset in those with the C 691 allele. To date, the most promising follow-up of provisional linkage from whole-genome screening has been with loci encoded on

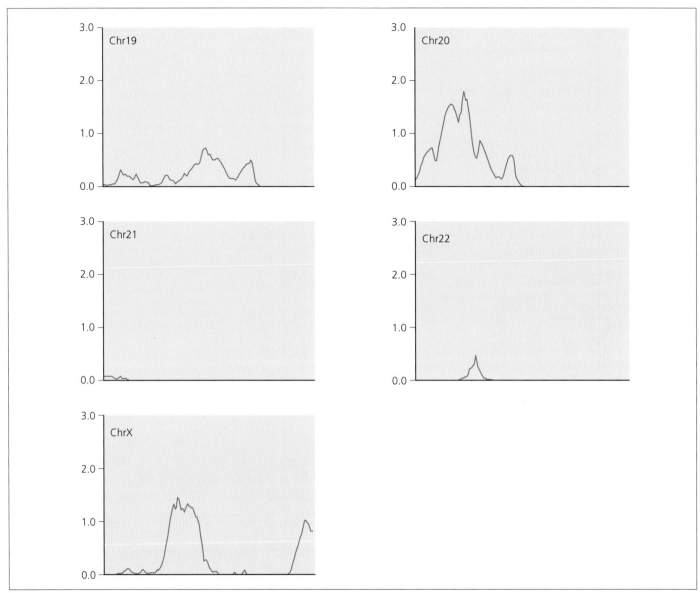

Figure 3.23, cont'd

17q (see above for study of *NOS2A*: Barcellos *et al* 2004). Studies in Finnish families from the southern Ostrobothnia region of western Finland mapped one effect to a 38-Mb region at 17q21-24, and two SNPs from within a noncoding region of protein kinase A (*PRKCA*) have been associated in population- and family-based tests (Saarela *et al* 2003). In a population study from the United Kingdom, Barton *et al* (2004) also reported an association with SNPs marking the *PRKCA* promoter in patients with multiple sclerosis, unclassified for clinical course, but this could not be confirmed.

Association genome screens

The problem with setting out systematically to screen the genome for association is the huge number of variants that must be considered (Kruglyak 1999). A first pass at screening the genome for association in multiple sclerosis was completed in 2002, based on a 0.5-cM map of microsatellite markers and using DNA pools derived from cases with multiple sclerosis, unrelated controls and trio families (affected individuals and their parents). It is worth briefly rehearsing the background to that experiment. In the late 1990s, it was clear that only a fraction of the known genes were identified, and that a full list of all functionally relevant variants relating to each was far from complete. It was also clear that technology enabling such a screen to be completed (within reasonable time and financial constraints) was not realistic. In 2005, despite a provisional full sequence of the human genome and exponential growth in the number of identified SNPs, the position is still not reached where a direct screen of all common/functionally relevant polymorphisms can be undertaken. In the vacuum between linkage and direct association screening, Barcellos *et al* (1997a) suggested that pooling DNA from individuals contributing to a group of interest, such as 'cases' or 'controls', and typing these pools for around 6000 microsatellite markers might efficiently identify at least some of the loci involved in susceptibility to multiple sclerosis.

The Genetic Analysis of Multiple Sclerosis in EuropeanS (GAMES) coordinated whole-genome screens for association in 19 populations from throughout Europe and Australia. Screens were completed in population- and family-based samples from the United Kingdom (Sawcer *et al* 2002; Yeo *et al* 2003), Australia (Ban *et al* 2003), Belgium (Goris *et al* 2003), Finland (Laaksonen *et al* 2003), France (Alizadeh *et al* 2003b), Germany (Goedde *et al* 2002; A. Weber *et al* 2003), Hungary (Rajda *et al* 2003), Iceland (Jonasdottir *et al* 2003), Ireland (Heggarty *et al* 2003), Italy (Liguori *et al* 2003), Poland (Bielecki *et al* 2003), Portugal (Martins *et al* 2003; Santos *et al* 2003), Sardinia (Coraddu *et al* 2003), Scandinavia (Harbo *et al* 2003), Spain (Goertsches *et al* 2003) and Turkey (Eraksoy *et al* 2003b). Each GAMES screen was based on a sample size of approximately 200 cases and 200 controls. Together, GAMES screened 9629 individuals (3376 cases, 3409 controls and 948 trio families comprised of the proband and both parents) from these 19 European nations, mostly with high frequencies of multiple sclerosis, for 6000 microsatellite markers. Nearly all of the screens identified suggestive results from at least some randomly selected microsatellites mapping to 6p21 (encoding the MHC) and, in most populations, these markers clearly emerge as among the most promising (Figure 3.24). Thus (although the lod score has since risen with the application of a higher density screen, see below), the class II region of the MHC shows independent linkage and association with randomly selected markers (albeit with a high *a priori* probability of association given previous reports and the known linkage disequilibrium). (Two screens, Australia and the first German cohort, included only DR(2)15-positive patients.) The TNFa marker was included in the study as a positive control, confirming the ability of this strategy (pooled DNA tested in cases and controls) to identify microsatellites in linkage disequilibrium with a susceptibility locus. Other HLA microsatellites represent positive results

(D6S1615 and D6S2444), albeit with a high *a priori* expectation of showing an association because of the known linkage disequilibrium in this region of the genome. That said, the fact that TNFa and D6S1615 were not shown to be significantly associated in every sample is not unexpected. The individual results are summarized in Table 3.4. These associations are provisional and many will not be confirmed. That said, even the most pessimistic analyst would concede that the experiment involved more markers than had ever been previously considered in multiple sclerosis. Many can now be safely excluded, even if it may take some considerable time to disentangle the genuinely associated from the false positive markers.

The hypothesis was that there would be ubiquitous genes, present in every population at risk of multiple sclerosis. These would be the easiest to find and some might also determine susceptibility to other autoimmune disorders. Also present would be domestic genes, exerting effects restricted to individual populations; these might be found because the size of each constituent population was thought to provide adequate power. But because samples contributing to the pools were not stratified for clinical course or particular features – merely requiring confirmation of multiple sclerosis and allowing partial admixture of relapsing–remitting and primary progressive cases – the study was never designed to do more than detect susceptibility genes, leaving any that might influence the clinical course for subsequent studies. Overall, the samples came from patients with representative features of the disease but the Icelandic cohort had a surprisingly high proportion of benign cases (61%). There was variable inclusion of familial cases.

As an indirect screen for association, GAMES was crucially dependent on the assumption that at least some of the markers tested had alleles in linkage disequilibrium with variants influencing susceptibility to multiple sclerosis. A refinement of that hypothesis assumed that these alleles were over-represented in the European population (given the high disease prevalences: see Chapter 2) and almost certainly were mutations occurring beyond the population bottleneck that constitutes the genetic history of the European population. Put another way, this assumption requires that the majority of susceptibility alleles at a given locus have arisen from a common ancestor and, moreover, that recombination, mutation and gene conversion have not whittled down the nonrandom association with alleles at flanking markers. Association is most likely to be revealed in the context of extensive linkage disequilibrium and is therefore dependent on variables that can never be known or accurately predicted ahead of identifying the disease-associated loci. Factors such as the precise history of flanking recombinant events, as well as the age and frequency of mutation, will all influence the extent of linkage disequilibrium. As it turns out, knowledge of linkage disequilibrium in the human genome has greatly increased since GAMES was designed. It is now clear that the number of markers employed was insufficient and a significant weakness of the design. On the other hand, since it is likely that several loci influence susceptibility to multiple sclerosis, the probability that all of them were badly placed between flanking markers would represent extreme bad luck.

The GAMES experiment was also constrained by the extent to which allele frequency differences can be detected by typing pooled DNA samples, especially when amplification of every microsatellite was limited to a single polymerase chain reaction

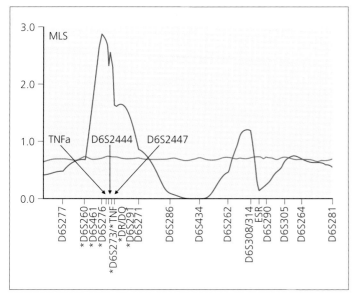

Figure 3.24 Linkage and association with three markers in linkage disequilibrium between multiple sclerosis and the MHC. Adapted from GAMES and the Transatlantic Multiple Sclerosis Genetics Cooperative (2003).

Table 3.4 **Top-ranked markers in whole-genome screens for association completed as part of GAMES (Genetic Analysis of Multiple Sclerosis in EuropeanS)**

Country/ region	Chromosome										
	1	2	3	4	5	6	7	8	9	10	11
Australia						* HLA +ve cases					D11S1765 D11S1986
Belgium		D2S394		D4S418	D5S107 D5S2056	D6S1615 D6S2444 D6S265 TNFa	D7S630	D8S1113		D10S1214 D10S579	D11S1986
Finland	D1S2664 D1S2797 D1S394	D2S142	D3S1611	D4S1535		G511525 SA-99 TNFa		D8S1988		D10S1753 D10S1790	D11S4465 D11S898
France						D6S265 TNFa	D7S1824				
Germany 1	D1S1590 D1S1608 GGAA30B06	D2S1345	D3S3591	D4S2394	D5S2044	* HLA +ve cases		D8S1469		D10S210	
Germany 2		D2S1384 D2S387	D3S1556			D6S1630 D6S2444 TNFa					D11S4195
Hungary		D2S338	D3S1283 D3S3571		D5S2045 D5S502	D6S275 D6S424	D7S2516 D7S630	D8S1762	D9S1853	D10S1669	
Iceland	MYCL1	D2S1396	D3S1588 D3S2404	D4S1647 D4S2394 D4S2414		G511525 SA-99			D9S152 D9S746		
Ireland		D2S1779 D2S319 D2S347	D3S2432	D4S3005	D5S2029 D5S2494	D6S1615 TNFa					D12S1998
Italy		D2S367									
Poland		D2S2153	D3S3568			D6S2444	D7S2521				
Portugal 1				D4S426	D5S1464	D6S2444 TNFa	D7S630			D10S1423	D11S1333 D11S4046
Portugal 2	D1S1725 D1S2770 D1S2816 D1S398 D1S435 D1S518	D2S1346	D3S2459	D4S1645 D4S2417 D4S2629 D4S3256	D5S1466 D5S1725 D5S2494 D5S2500 D5S816	D6S1034 D6S1284 D6S1646 D6S1707 HO16369 SA-99	D7S1824 D7S684	D8S1113	D9S284 D9S52	D10S199	D11S1392 D11S1986
Sardinia		D2S391 D2S408		GATA87B03		D6S271 D6S344	D7S1818		D9S2		
Scandinavia	D1S2724		D3S3683			D6S1652 D6S2447 D6S273	D7S2445		D9S147E D9S1799		
Spain	D1S2852 D1S398 D1S533				D5S1953	D6S1017 D6S1955 D6S2444 G511525 HO16369 SA-99	D7S1818		D9S157 D9S1868 D9S303	D10S1795	
Turkey	D1S2781	D2S149	D3S4018		D5S1453 D5S1505 D5S676	D6S460			D9S1847		D11S4207
UK					D5S112	D6S1615 D6S2444 TNFa				D10S1769	

Table 3.4 Top-ranked markers in whole-genome screens for association completed as part of GAMES (Genetic Analysis of Multiple Sclerosis in EuropeanS), cont'd

Country/ region	Chromosome												Not mapped
	12	13	14	15	16	17	18	19	20	21	22	X	
Australia	D12S313		D14S306		D16S3027		D18S52	D19S190 D19S219					
Belgium			D14S1005	D15S209 D15S659		D17S113 D17S1879			D20S473	D21S1270			
Finland	DD12S395		D14S306				D18S857	D19S247		D212049S			D1S1631
France	D12S1064		D14S1426 D14S605							D21S2051			
Germany 1								D19S932				DXS101	
Germany 2	D12S1724					D17S796		D19S420				DXS8037	
Hungary			D14S281		D16S3097		D18S1127	D19S921	D20S891 D20S892			DXS6807	D1S2677
Iceland	D12S2074			D15S644 D15S817		D17S1848 D17S975		D19S246			D22S417		D3S3509 D6S1689
Ireland	D12S398	D13S1325 D13S792	D14S741	D15S1022 D15S1040	D16S752	D17S907		D19S903				DXS1044	D4S432 D6S1014
Italy													
Poland				D15S649									
Portugal 1													D11S1914 D4S2921
Portugal 2	D12S77 D12S84	D13S1492 D13S1493		D15S1025 D15S644 D15S822	D16S2624	D17S1820	D18S51	D19S413 D19S591 D19S593				DXS1187	D6S1282
Sardinia	D12S1653				D16S420								
Scandinavia												DXS1153	
Spain	D12S1653 D12S1344	D13S1236 D13S777			D16S2613		D18S52	D19S921		D21S1435	D22S692	DXS981	
Turkey	DD12S2075							D19S902					D8S1837
UK													

in each pool, and with no attempt to type individual samples. It was known that many microsatellites emerged artefactually in the list of most extreme markers showing apparent evidence for association in individual screens (Table 3.4). The failure of many to survive the repeat analysis performed after each initial GAMES screen was adjusted using adapting factors (Yeo *et al* 2003) was, in retrospect, not surprising. These refinements do not overcome additional sources of variance introduced by pooling. Therefore the list of best markers identified in each screen still contains a significant number of false positives.

By eye, seven groups observed associations at 19q13, which has previously been implicated by several independent groups and meta-analyses (see above). In addition, a signal at 5p15 in Turkish families was associated (Eraksoy *et al* 2003a) and provisionally linked in an independent data set derived from the same population (Eraksoy *et al* 2003b). More formal meta-analysis of these data considered each case–control cohort with and without adapting factors (Yeo *et al* 2003). Markers were ranked for evidence of association based on the average allele frequency difference seen across the populations (Setakis 2003). For the two laboratory sites at which typing was performed, a total of 5530 and 4378 markers were analysed, respectively. Casualties were those not performing in a significant number of case–control cohorts. The top markers for each analysis were then typed in individual samples. This left a list of 18 associated markers, surviving the analytical algorithm. As expected, five are encoded within the MHC region. Individual genotyping of the remaining 13 non-MHC markers identified the three most strongly associated markers as D17S1789, D19S552 and D20S894 (Table 3.5). Marker D20S894 maps 46.3Kb from the Jagged 1 gene (*JAG1*) immediately under one of the strongest linkage signals identified in the recently completed high density multiple sclerosis linkage screen (see above). Jagged 1 is involved in the differentiation of oligodendrocyte precursors and its expression has recently been correlated with remyelination in the lesions of multiple sclerosis (see Chapters 10 and 12). Eighty-five SNPs were typed in the 937 family trios; although none showed unambiguous evidence for association when analysed individually, 55 of the top ranked were mined for associated haplotype patterns, one of which was associated with multiple sclerosis even after stringent statistical correction. Permutation analysis indicates that the susceptibility effect maps to the interval between markers rs910118 and rs6040079. Marker D11S1986 lies in the 3′ untranslated region of the *POU2AF1* gene, a transcriptional co-activator involved in the regulation of IgG gene expression in B-cells. Twenty-eight SNPs were typed in 937

Table 3.5 Summary of meta-analysis results based on individual genotyping data for the six markers showing nominally significant results in one or more data set (p-values)

	Case–control		Trio family	
	Combining raw genotypes	Combining p-values	Combining raw genotypes	Combining p-values
D17S1789	0.12	0.01	0.58	0.16
D19S552	0.02	0.09	0.29	0.0009
D20S894	0.25	0.04	0.56[a]	0.56[a]
D6S265	4.69E-13	1.16E-05	5.93E-06[a]	5.93E-06[a]
D6S273	1.98E-19	4.02E-16	3.50E-08[a]	3.50E-08[a]
TNFa	4.11E-34	2.78E-21	2.77E-14	1.52E-12

a These results are based on the analysis of a single data set (the UK trio families).

family trios. Again, although no individual marker was associated, haplotype pattern mining revealed one that was associated with multiple sclerosis after statistical correction. Permutation analysis indicates that the susceptibility effect maps to the interval between markers rs7952176 and rs1123066. *PSMC4* (proteasome 26S subunit ATPase 4), *MAP3K10* (mitogen-activated kinase kinase kinase 10) and *AKT2* (v-akt murine thymoma viral oncogene homolog 2) lie within 250kb of the D19S552 marker. Sixty-nine SNPs were typed in 937 family trios but none showed even nominal significance and even the most associated haplotype pattern (involving the seven markers between rs339512 and rs2304186) only achieved a nominal p-value of 0.002 and thus did not survive stringent statistical correction. Taken together, these data suggest that *JAG1* and *POU2AF1* influence susceptibility to multiple sclerosis.

The next generation of linkage disequilibrium screens for disease genes will require much larger sample sizes and the use of very dense SNP maps. It has been estimated that the number of SNPs in the human genome (defined by a rare allele frequency of ≥1% in at least one population) is likely to be at least 15 million (Botstein and Risch 2003) with 10 million SNPs in the public domain, two immediate strategies seem probable. Association studies will be carried out in many populations guided by the linkage screens (Transatlantic Multiple Sclerosis Genetics Cooperative and the GAMES group 2003; International Multiple Sclerosis Genetics Consortium 2005) and availability of gene maps from which to select plausible positional candidates that can be studied using the public database of SNPs, or those identified domestically. The challenges of study design, statistical analysis, definition of intermediate phenotypes and epistatic interactions are not trivial (Carlson *et al* 2004). In situations where no candidate pops out of the database, it is a relatively simple strategy (but not cheap) to screen a region of interest with a sufficiently dense SNP map to narrow the interval within which the susceptibility factor lies, using multipoint association mapping. But what if linkage, being relatively underpowered, has missed the crucial regions of interest? Here, the immediate preferred strategy is to apply the emerging 'Hap-Map' to multiple sclerosis (Figure 3.25). This returns to the issue of population origins and diversity within the genome. The assumption is that, depending on age of the population (and so more for Europeans than Africans), the genome retains a degree of linkage disequilibrium and the number of conserved haplotypes within each block is limited. Once each haplotype is sequenced, defining SNPs are identified that tag each section of linked variants – five, six or however many are revealed per block. The hope is that every susceptibility gene will be encoded within one of the defined haplotypes. Very few, perhaps only one, tagging SNPs are needed to distinguish that haplotype from the remaining blocked variants. This (or these) tagging SNP(s) then serves as a marker of disease susceptibility without the need to test every allele at each locus within the DNA trapped in that particular block. Just how many markers will have to be used in order to screen the genome remains a matter of conjecture: informal estimates vary between 100 000 and 1 million, depending on the depth of information required and whether the population of interest is 'genetically' young or ancient – that is, retaining more or less linkage disequilibrium. By mid-2005, the Hap-Map project had mapped 1.2 million markers, representing one single nucleotide polymorphism for every 660 basepairs, and an updated analysis appeared late in 2005, based on 269 DNA samples from four populations in which all variations in ten 500-kilobase regions had been exhaustively detailed, allowing a better understanding of the haplotype structures of the human genome and providing optimism that tagging-SNPs will indeed prove useful and versatile in exploring genetic associations with disease (The International HapMap Consortium 2005). Several experiments that approximate to a high density screen of the genome for association in multiple sclereois are planned for 2005–2006, using (in the first pass) 100 000–500 000 SNP chips. The first was announced in an extravagant press release from a pharmaceutical company. They used samples from 900 cases (from Sweden, France and the United States) and 900 controls, and screened for 100 000 SNPs; the claim that 80 genes for multiple sclerosis had been identified is taken to mean that, using a non-stringent statistical analysis with minimal correction for multiple testing, the top ranked markers included 80 that sit close to or within genes that suggest themselves as candidates on the basis of having something to do with pathways involved in inflammatory processes and mechanisms of neurodegeneration (Daniel Cohen, personal communication).

Deploying the Hap-Map remains an indirect approach. It is economical yet considered adequate and thorough in screening for the relevant variants. The use of tagged SNPs reliably

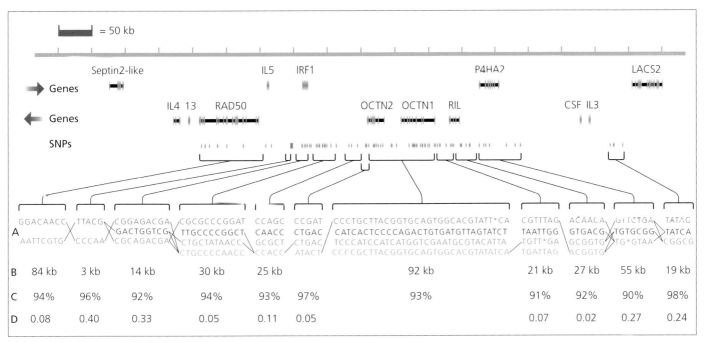

Figure 3.25 (A) Common haplotype patterns in each block of low diversity. Diagonal lines indicate locations where >2% of all chromosomes are observed to transition from one common haplotype to a different one. (B) Percentage of observed chromosomes that match one of the common patterns exactly. (C) Percentage of each of the common patterns among untransmitted chromosomes. (D) Rate of haplotype exchange between the blocks as estimated by the Hidden Mazkov Model (HMM). Several markers at each end of the map were excluded as they provided evidence that the blocks did not continue but were not adequate to build a first or last block. In addition, four markers fell between blocks, suggesting that the recombinational clustering may not take place at a specific base-pair position, but rather in small regions. Adapted from Daly MJ *et al* 2001. Reproduced with permission from Nature Publishing Group (www.nature.com).

marking the extent of diversity across the genome in defined populations brings whole-genome association screening within the range of what can already be achieved using current resources and technology for high-throughput genotyping. But it assumes that common diseases arise from common variants since the Hap-Map may not catalogue all the rare alleles. Self-evidently, it falls short of a direct screen in which each and every variant is studied in all affected individuals and controls.

LESSONS FROM GENETIC STUDIES OF EXPERIMENTAL AUTOIMMUNE ENCEPHALOMYELITIS

It has been recognized for a long time that the induction and expression of experimental autoimmune encephalomyelitis differs markedly between individual outbred animals, and between inbred strains. As in multiple sclerosis, the combination of susceptibility and regulatory genes may govern the complex genetics of experimental autoimmune encephalomyelitis; and the elucidation of animal genetics may therefore directly illuminate the problem of human demyelinating disease. However, the loci conferring susceptibility to these experimental conditions are not necessarily syntenic with those responsible for altering susceptibility to multiple sclerosis.

The strategies for identifying these factors involve classic and molecular genetics. However, animal models offer additional possibilities, which include specific breeding, mutagenesis and the construction of transgenic animals. But, these advan-

tages come with a price. In general, most experimental work uses inbred strains, mainly of rodents. These strains have been derived by brother–sister matings over numerous generations. As a result, each individual member of an inbred strain of mouse or rat resembles the other members much as do monozygotic twins. Thus, apart from epigenetic modifications, each inbred strain of animals genetically corresponds to one outbred (human) individual. Human and rodent immune reactions are often very different in their responses to a given stimulus. Of most importance is the constraint that, to date, all published models of multiple sclerosis require immunization with strong adjuvants, a procedure that differs drastically from the apparently unprovoked development of human disease. Unfortunately, there is no natural rodent variant that develops a spontaneous disease resembling multiple sclerosis – such as one comparable to the non-obese diabetic mouse that mimics human type 1 diabetes mellitus.

Classic 'forward' animal genetics compares response profiles between different strains or mutants and then seeks to identify the gene(s) responsible for these differences. A further elaboration of forward genetics uses mutagenesis of male sperm cells as the basis for creating numerous mutant progeny to screen for somatic changes. This is followed by the identification of these mutated genes (Appelby and Ramsdell 2003; Vinuesa and Goodnow 2004). 'Reverse' genetics creates transgenic mice with altered expression of known, individual genes, expressed in the immune system or within the central nervous system (T. Owens *et al* 2001). The phenotypic effects of transgenes are examined in a second round of investigation.

Reverse genetics: transgenic mouse strains

While classic, forward genetics starts with a phenotypic trait and then tracks the relevant gene, reverse genetics goes in the opposite direction. The strategy first modifies a gene and later looks for the corresponding biological effect – the phenotype caused by that gene modification. Modern molecular technology allows a particular murine gene to be changed, replaced with another or deleted. In the simplest situation, transgenes are inserted randomly into the host genome. Depending on the particular promoter, transgenes can either be expressed globally in all tissues, or targeted to selected tissues. An individual host gene can be cut out of the chromosome (gene deletion, or 'knockout' transgenics), while a more elaborate technology first cuts out a host gene and then replaces it with one copy of the transgene (gene replacement, or 'knock-in' transgenics). In the transgenic models described so far, the artificial gene is expressed throughout the lifetime of the animal. In 'conditional' transgenic animals, however, the timing of transgene expression can be controlled by using drug-sensitive promoters. After undisturbed development, gene deletion or transgene expression are freshly induced by the administration of a trigger – usually an antibiotic or hormone.

A large number of transgenic mice (and rats) have been screened for inducibility of experimental autoimmune encephalomyelitis. Many are listed in Table 3.6 but, still, the reader may miss many interesting genes, and for several reasons. First, there may be no available knockout strains since the gene may have an important role in organ development and, being incompatible with survival and reproduction, the manipulation proves lethal. Second, many transgenic mice show normal susceptibility to experimental autoimmune encephalomyelitis, and such 'negative' studies rarely reach publication. Taken together, the data obtained from screening transgenic, especially knockout, mice for experimental autoimmune encephalomyelitis have proved informative. In some cases, such as studies of *IL6*, the findings have cemented the expected role of genes, in this case of a proinflammatory cytokine. In other situations, such as with

Table 3.6 Effect of gene disruption on experimental autoimmune encephalomyelitis and central nervous system pathology

Target gene	Phenotype
IL4	No effect on experimental autoimmune encephalomyelitis induction or progression (Bettelli *et al* 1998) Increased severity, increased proinflammatory cytokine expression (Falcone *et al* 1998a)
IL6	Resistant to actively induced and transferred experimental autoimmune encephalomyelitis (Eugster *et al* 1998; Mendel *et al* 1998; Samoilova *et al* 1998)
IL10	Experimental autoimmune encephalomyelitis exacerbated, accelerated (Bettelli *et al* 1998; Eugster *et al* 1998; Falcone *et al* 1998; Mendel *et al* 1998; Samoilova *et al* 1998)
IL12	Resistance to experimental autoimmune encephalomyelitis induction (Segal *et al* 1998) No effect (Becher *et al* 2002; Gran *et al* 2002)
IL23	IL-23 produced in central nervous system is centrally involved in experimental autoimmune encephalomyelitis (Becher *et al* 2003; Cua *et al* 2003)
IFNG	Experimental autoimmune encephalomyelitis exacerbated; chemokine dysregulation, neutrophil invasion (Krakowski and Owens 1996; M. Tran *et al* 2000a; Willenborg *et al* 1996)
TNFA	Experimental autoimmune encephalomyelitis delayed, leucocyte traffic affected (Rimington *et al* 1998)
LTA	Experimental autoimmune encephalomyelitis inducibility either not affected, or experimental autoimmune encephalomyelitis not inducible (Suen *et al* 1997)
ICBR (caspase-1)	Reduced incidence and severity of experimental autoimmune encephalomyelitis, defective Th1 induction (Furlan *et al* 1999)
MCP1	Mice deficient in CCR-2 are resistant to experimental autoimmune encephalomyelitis in some, but not all strains (Fife *et al* 2000; Gaupp *et al* 2003; Izikson *et al* 2000)
MIP1A	No effect on experimental autoimmune encephalomyelitis induction, progression or severity (M. Tran *et al* 2000b)
IP10	Lower threshold for expression of disease (R.S. Klein *et al* 2004)
CCR3	No effect on experimental autoimmune encephalomyelitis inducibility (Haskell *et al* 2001)
CSF3	Resistance to clinical and histological experimental autoimmune encephalomyelitis (McQualter *et al* 2001)
SPP1 (osteopontin)	No chronic progression, frequent remissions (Chabas *et al* 2001; Jansson *et al* 2002)
PLAT (tPA)	Delayed onset of experimental autoimmune encephalomyelitis but then increased severity and delayed recovery (W. Lu *et al* 2002)
PRF1 (perforin)	Enhanced severity, chronic relapsing course (Malipiero *et al* 1997)
NOS2A	Enhanced severity and frequency (Fenyk-Melody *et al* 1998; Sahrbacher *et al* 1998)

Table 3.6 **Effect of gene disruption on experimental autoimmune encephalomyelitis and central nervous system pathology, cont'd**

Target gene	Phenotype
CNTF	Increased oligodendrocyte apoptosis and fewer progenitors (Linker *et al* 2002)
NFKB	Lower disease incidence, clinical score, and central nervous system inflammation (Hilliard *et al* 1999)
MMP9	Decreased susceptibility (mice younger than 4 weeks of age) (Dubois *et al* 1999)
FCGRII	Enhanced inducibility of clinical and histological experimental autoimmune encephalomyelitis (Abdul-Majid *et al* 2002)
CD5L	Delayed onset and decreased severity of experimental autoimmune encephalomyelitis (Axtell *et al* 2004)
CD200	Accelerated onset and increased intensity of experimental autoimmune encephalomyelitis (Hoek *et al* 2000)
CD40	No experimental autoimmune encephalomyelitis, no CD4 T-cell activation (Grewal *et al* 1996)
SPN	Reduced and delayed clinical and histological disease severity (Ford *et al* 2003)
BF	Reduction of clinical experimental autoimmune encephalomyelitis; but infiltrates around microvessels (Nataf *et al* 2000)
ICOSL	Enhanced inducibility of clinical and histological experimental autoimmune encephalomyelitis (Dong *et al* 2001)
CD28	Resistance to active induction, not to passive transfer of experimental autoimmune encephalomyelitis (Chitnis *et al* 2001)
TNFSF4	Milder clinical experimental autoimmune encephalomyelitis and reduced central nervous system inflammation (Aboul-Enein *et al* 2003)
TNFSF4L	Mild decrease of experimental autoimmune encephalomyelitis susceptibility (Ndhlovu *et al* 2001)
B7H3	Experimental autoimmune encephalomyelitis onset several days earlier (Prasad *et al* 2004)
SELL (L-selectin)	Central nervous system infiltrates, but no demyelination nor clinical experimental autoimmune encephalomyelitis (Grewal *et al* 2001)
SELPLG (P-selectin)	Slightly accelerated onset of experimental autoimmune encephalomyelitis and increased infiltrate formation (Graesser *et al* 2002)
ICAM1	Paradoxical enhancement (Samoilova *et al* 1998b)
ITGB7 (β7 integrin)	Slight attenuation transfer of experimental autoimmune encephalomyelitis (Kanwar *et al* 2000)
RTN4 (Nogo A)	Partial protection from experimental autoimmune encephalomyelitis induction (Karnezis *et al* 2004)
AF1 (estrogen receptor)	Loss of oestrogen protection from experimental autoimmune encephalomyelitis (H. Liu *et al* 2003; Polanczyk *et al* 2003)

IFNG, the results were unexpected. Instead of nonresponsiveness, *IFNG* knockout mice display a paradoxical enhancement of inducibility. Such observations may lead to the discovery of new gene functions. In less fortunate cases, however, they merely reflect artefacts due to changes in cellular regulation that have arisen during development to compensate for the loss of an important gene. Thus, redundancy of function has undermined the dividend from creating so many transgenic animals for entirely plausible candidate targets. The new generation of conditional gene knockouts, involving gene deletion during adulthood, is expected to resolve many of these problems.

Classic genetics: from gene locus to gene sequence

In its simplest form, the classic genetics approach compares the response of different inbred strains of rodent to a particular encephalitogenic stimulus. Experimental autoimmune encephalomyelitis can be induced by active immunization, passive transfer of pathogenic cells, or (occasionally) by infection with encephalitogenic microbes (see Chapter 11). Depending on the genetic makeup of inbred strains, one and the same stimulus may trigger clinical disease at different frequencies and intensities, or with different clinical phenotypes and contributions of inflammation, demyelination, neuronal depletion and axonal damage. Susceptibility genes affect the rate of disease appearance following a standard induction protocol, while other genes may influence the character of the emerging disease.

There are several ways to identify genes that control susceptibility to experimental autoimmune encephalomyelitis. One strategy uses quantitative trait analysis of intercross and backcross breedings: two inbred strains with distinct responsiveness are crossed; subsequently, the resulting hybrids are further crossed with other hybrids of the same litters (F2 intercross) or with parental animals (backcross). Individual F2 or backcross animals, which carry parental genes in different distributions, are examined for their responsiveness to experimental autoimmune encephalomyelitis (EAE), and these finding are correlated with both parental response patterns. The resulting candidate

EAE genes are mapped to specific chromosomes by linkage to genetic markers (distinguishing both parental strains) with known chromosomal localization.

The breeding studies allow the distinction and relatively crude localization of putative susceptibility genes, but there is no way to extend these investigations to more detailed genetic or immunological analyses. Such studies require the elaborate and immensely cumbersome establishment of congenic recombinant sets of inbred strains. These are genetically identical except for a circumscribed chromosomal segment, which encodes one particular gene or gene cluster; recombinant congenic strains share only a section of a larger gene cluster, such as the MHC. The generation of congenic strains requires long-term breeding programmes in order to achieve a stable strain. Eventually, the chromosome fragment of interest contains the gene of choice but this is embedded in a variable stretch of neighbouring genes.

The combination of linkage studies and congenic strain analyses has produced a highly complex picture, with many different genes affecting the reactivity of experimental autoimmune encephalomyelitis at many stages of the disease process (Table 3.7). As with the genetic studies of multiple sclerosis, the most clear-cut regulatory influence comes from the MHC, in particular from its class II region. It has been known for many years that the classic encephalitogenic autoantigen, myelin basic protein, is readily recognized by mice and rats of certain MHC haplotypes, ignored by other specificities, and has intermediate response patterns in yet others. The class II region of the MHC is profoundly involved in generation of the T-cell repertoire, and in the actual presentation of a particular (auto)antigen to mature T lymphocytes. In addition, however, the MHC contains genes that may influence an autoimmune response by additional mechanisms. For example, *TNFa* and the gene that encodes myelin oligodendrocyte glycoprotein map within the MHC.

An excellent example of a susceptibility gene for experimental autoimmune encephalomyelitis is the gene (*EAE28*)

Table 3.7 Identification and mapping of genes conferring susceptibility to experimental autoimmune encephalomyelitis

EAE gene	Rodent chromosome	Extent (cM)	Markers flanking interval	Sex specificity	Traits	References
EAE1	17	23	H-2		Incidence	Many sources
EAE2	15	10.6–14.8			Incidence	Sundvall *et al* 1995
EAE3	3	29–52	D3Mit29–D3Mit105		Incidence, modifier of chronicity	Butterfield *et al* 1998; Encinas *et al* 1999; Sundvall *et al* 1995
EAE4	7	40–50.3	D7Mit233–D7Mit39		Incidence, spinal cord histopathology	D. Baker *et al* 1995; Butterfield *et al* 1998; 1999
EAE4B	7	≈53	D7Mit253		Overcomes Eae2 protection	Encinas *et al* 2001; Jirholt *et al* 2002
EAE5	17	24.5–33.3	D17Mit10–17Mit150		Incidence	D. Baker *et al* 1995; Encinas *et al* 1999
EAE6A	11	0.25–13	D11Mit72–D11Mit294		Severity	D. Baker *et al* 1995; Encinas *et al* 1999
EAE6B	11	19–28	D11Mit307–D11Mit140		Duration	D. Baker *et al* 1995; Encinas *et al* 1999
EAE7	11	44–58	D11Mit194–D11Mit98		Severity, monophasic subtype, Idd4	D. Baker *et al* 1995; Encinas *et al* 1999
EAE8	2	99–107	D2Mit25–D2Mit200		Incidence, severity, weight loss	D. Baker *et al* 1995; Encinas *et al* 1996; 1999
EAE9	9	22–42	D9Mit22–D9Mit8		Duration, spinal cord suppuration, pertussis toxin, Idd2	D. Baker *et al* 1995; Blankenhorn *et al* 2000; Encinas *et al* 1999
EAE10	3	64.1–79.4	D3Mit14–D3Mit147		Onset	Encinas *et al* 1999
EAE11	16	21–41	D16Mit110–D16Mit140	Male	Incidence, brain histopathology, onset	Butterfield *et al* 1999; Karlsson *et al* 2003

Table 3.7 **Identification and mapping of genes conferring susceptibility to experimental autoimmune encephalomyelitis, cont'd**

EAE gene	Rodent chromosome	Extent (cM)	Markers flanking interval	Sex specificity	Traits	References
EAE12	7	16	D7Mit227–D7Mit25	Female	Relapsing–remitting subtype	Butterfield *et al* 1999
EAE13	13	37	D13Mit66	Male	Monophasic subtype	Butterfield *et al* 1999
EAE14	8	16–33	D8Mit3–D8Mit31	Female	Incidence	Blankenhorn *et al* 2000
EAE15	10	4–19	D10Mit80–D10Mit214	Male	Brain histopathology	Butterfield *et al* 2000
EAE16	12	3–19	D12Mit56–D12Mit2		Spinal cord histopathology	Butterfield *et al* 2000
EAE17	10	44	D10Mit3–D10Mit42	Female	Severity index, spinal cord demyelination	Blankenhorn *et al* 2000
EAE18	18	Syntenic			(= Eae25?)	D. Baker *et al* 1995
EAE19	19	26–53	D19Mit19–D19mit33	Male	Brain demyelination	Butterfield *et al* 2000
EAE20	3	5–23	D3Mit36–D3mit6		Spinal cord demyelination, Idd3	Butterfield *et al* 2000; Encinas *et al* 1999
EAE21	2	30–69	D2Mit269–D2mit17	Female	Brain histopathology	Butterfield *et al* 2000
EAE22	11	49–71	D11Mit38–D11Mit168	Female	Brain histopathology	Butterfield *et al* 2000
EAE23	11	32–44	D11Mit155–D11mit194	Male	Spinal cord histopathology, Chronic subtype, onset	Butterfield *et al* 2000; Karlsson *et al* 2003
EAE24	8	≈10	D8Mit3–D8Mit4		Central nervous system inflammation, paralysis (= Eae14?)	Encinas *et al* 2001
EAE25	18	41–54	D18Mit81–D18Mit3	Male	Spinal cord histopathology	Blankenhorn *et al* 2000
EAE26	5	45–59	D5Mit41	Male	Acute disease, CD8	Karlsson *et al* 2003
EAE27	1	81–88	D1Mit33	Female	Relapsing–remitting	Karlsson *et al* 2003
EAE28 BPHS / HRH1	6	49	D6Mit54–D6Mit216		Incidence; experimental allergic orchitis; pertussis toxin induction for histamine sensitization	R.L.Z. Ma *et al* 2002; Sudweeks *et al* 1993
EAE29 SHS	6	Distal	D6Mit105–D6Mit216		Incidence; natural induction for histamine sensitization	Fillmore *et al* 2003

Kindly provided by Dr Cory Teuscher.

Table 3.8 **Natural mouse mutants used for studies of central nervous system autoimmune responses**

Allele	Classic name	Gene	Experimental allergic encephalomyelitis phenotype
Lpr	Lymphoproliferation	*TNFRSF6*	Acute and transferable
Gld	General lymphoproliferative disorder	*TNFSF6*	Acute and transferable
Me	Motheaten	*HCPH*	Acute and transferable
Xid	X-linked immunodeficiency	*BTK*	Acute and transferable
Nu	Nude	*FOXN1*	Acute and transferable
Scid	Severe combined immunodeficiency	*PRKDC*	Passive, no active experimental allergic encephalomyelitis
Bg	Beige	*LYST*	Acute and transferable
Lps	Lipopolysaccharide response	*TLR4*	Acute and transferable
Sf	Scurfy	*FOXP3*	Acute and transferable

Adapted from Appleby and Ramsdell (2003).

encoding the histamine receptor H1. The histamine receptor is centrally involved in active induction of experimental autoimmune encephalomyelitis by immunization with autoantigen and suitable adjuvants. It has been known through classic back-cross studies that a particular gene mapping to mouse chromosome 6 governs the inflammatory response to *Bordetella pertussis* toxin. This gene is polymorphic, with some mice responding mildly to the bacterial product, and others reacting by a precipitated histamine response, hence the designation *Bphs* (*Bordetella pertussis histamine*). Investigators then produced a series of congenic mouse strains with varying overlapping portions of high-responding *Bphs* chromosome segments grafted on a low-responding chromosome. The controlling segment ultimately contained just one suspect gene, that encoding *Hrh1*, the gene for histamine receptor H1. Subsequent molecular cloning established that indeed a variation of just three amino acids distinguished histamine receptors of high- and low-responding mice. The analysis of transgenic knockout mice confirmed the conclusion (R.L.Z. Ma *et al* 2002).

Enhanced forward genetics: naturally occurring and artificially induced mutants

One productive way to search for autoimmune or other genes makes use of sporadically occurring, spontaneous mutant rodents. Indeed, over the years, geneticists have compiled a panel of inbred mice that all feature immunological abnormalities. These include the unprovoked production of autoantibodies, overproduction or lack of immune cell populations and, in some cases, generalized or organ-specific autoimmune diseases. Detailed genetic studies showed that some of these variant mice had mutations restricted to one particular gene (Table 3.8), whereas others displayed numerous aberrant genes distributed over several chromosomes.

Spontaneous mutations are not very common in regular mice, but their frequency can be increased dramatically by artificial mutagenesis. Several national and international mutagenesis programmes have been established to induce scientifically usable mutations under controlled laboratory conditions. The basic strategy is to treat male mice with the frighteningly effec-

tive chemical mutagen ethyl nitrosourea, which produces multiple changes in the animal's DNA. Treated males are allowed to mate, and their potential offspring are screened for pathological gene expression. Among a universe of genes, mutations relevant for (auto)immunity are determined either by screening untreated animals for their immunological characteristics (*inter alia* immunoglobulin isotypes, autoantibodies and immune cell composition: Vinuesa and Goodnow 2004), or for their responses to immunization against foreign or self antigens. So far, the input of this laborious strategy into autoimmune research appears to be limited and indirect. One published report describes a deficit of circulating B lymphocytes due to a mutilated transcription factor NF-κB (Miosge *et al* 2002). We suspect that information on other autoimmune mutants may yet be slumbering in the electronic archives of the centres involved.

CONCLUSION

Given the very considerable investment of time and resources aimed at illuminating the genetics of multiple sclerosis, it is reasonable to ask why relatively little progress has been made since the mid-1970s when associations with alleles of the major histocompatibility complex were identified. Was the hypothesis wrong? Seemingly not, based on the evidence from classic genetic studies in families. Rather, estimates for the size of the effects have clearly been over-optimistic, and needed scaling down with increasing experience. The development of appropriate statistical methods has not kept pace with the accumulating volume of data requiring analysis. Study design has been inconsistent and not always appropriate, with linkage and association studies both usually proving to be under-powered. The extent to which genotyping errors and poor information extraction have undermined linkage analyses (Sawcer *et al* 2004) and the artefacts introduced into association studies by the use of pooled samples (Yeo *et al* 2003) have proved rate limiting and were only appreciated in retrospect. The phenotype of multiple sclerosis is complex. Although it can be argued that lumping cases will prioritze the discovery of those factors that drive the ubiquitous processes of inflammation and degeneration, disease heterogenicity – if it exists – will have reduced the power of non-stratified samples. But what stratifications make best sense? Genetic factors contribute to the individual and population risk of multiple sclerosis and it is often assumed that these and other factors influence the course and features of multiple sclerosis, but the supporting evidence is scanty. Therefore, selecting cases for clinical features and patterns of the disease course may not be especially advantageous. There is an obvious appeal in selecting for study those populations in which multiple sclerosis is most frequent, on the assumptions that these are the groups with over-representation of the risk factors. But that tactic might have proved counter-productive, as studies of the HLA associations in Orkney and Shetland indicate. Indeed, the suggestion that genes conferring susceptibility to multiple sclerosis arose, and are selectively represented, in the high-risk northern European population is an assumption that may be incorrect. These polymorphisms could have been introduced with the founder populations of Europeans, filtered and concentrated by the subsequent turbulent history of genetic

stratification in those groups but still more easily found in individuals retaining an ancient disease phenotype (see Chapter 5). Thus, failure to select the most informative populations for study – based on understanding the genetics, epidemiology, clinical neurology and origins of multiple sclerosis – may have held back progress in resolving the nature of genetic susceptibility.

Eventually, six main categories of susceptibility gene can be predicted: genes that determine susceptibility to the process of inflammation across a range of disorders – the *autoimmune* genes; those that determine the specificity of that process for the development of multiple sclerosis – the *ubiquitous* genes; those that are relevant for the pathogenesis in isolated populations – the *domestic* genes; those that determine particular phenotypes – the *pleotropic* genes; those that determine variations in the clinical course – the *modifying* genes; and those that cluster to provide specifically different (heterogeneous) contributions to the pathogenesis – the *epistatic* genes.

The natural history of multiple sclerosis

4

Christian Confavreux and Alastair Compston

Many authors have collected large numbers of cases and described the overall course and prognosis of multiple sclerosis (R.S. Allison 1950; Amato *et al* 1999; Bonduelle 1967; Bonduelle and Albaranès 1962; V.A. Clark *et al* 1982; Confavreux *et al* 1980; 1998a; 2000; 2003; Fog 1966; Fog and Linnemann 1970; Goodkin *et al* 1989; Kantarci *et al* 1998; Kremenchutzky *et al* 1999; Kurtzke 1956; 1965b; 1970; Kurtzke *et al* 1968a; 1969; 1970a; 1973; 1977; Leibowitz and Alter 1973; McAlpine 1946; 1961; 1964; McAlpine and Compston 1952; McDonnell and Hawkins 1998b; D.H. Miller *et al* 1992a; Minderhoud *et al* 1988; R. Müller 1949; 1951; Percy *et al* 1971; J.F. Phadke 1987; J.G. Phadke 1990; Pittock *et al* 2004b; S. Poser 1978; S. Poser and Hauptvogel 1973; S. Poser *et al* 1986; Riise *et al* 1988; 1992; Riser *et al* 1971; Runmarker and Andersen 1993; Runmarker *et al* 1994b; A.J. Thompson *et al* 1997; Thygesen 1949; 1955; Trojano *et al* 1995; Wallin *et al* 2000; 2004; Weinshenker *et al* 1989a; 1989b; 1991a; 1991b; 1996).

With such a richness of material, our knowledge in this field is materially greater than for any other chronic disease. Simply stated, multiple sclerosis develops early, and runs a protracted clinical course so that life expectancy is barely reduced. The clinical features are extremely variable and the prognosis unpredictable. Nothing seems to be entirely similar or fully predictable. A detailed knowledge of the overall course and prognosis is therefore desirable for the physician wanting to understand the disease and make it comprehensible to the individual patient facing decisions on personal, family, social or professional involvements and commitments. But there has been a real dividend from recent efforts to define and validate features that predict the future course and, as a result, authoritative data on the natural history are now available. However, these features apply more consistently to groups than to individual patients. Nevertheless, this knowledge allows inferences reliably to be drawn regarding the pathophysiology of the disease; it provides information needed by public health services wanting to calculate disease costs and decide on investments in health care resources; it guides health insurance companies with respect to disability and life expectancy calculations; it sets the pharmaceutical industry agenda for investment in research and development programmes; and it plays an essential role in the evaluation of efficacy in clinical trials. That said, more work is still needed to characterize the natural history of multiple sclerosis and, especially, to resolve whether or not the so-called 'disease modifying agents' do in fact really modify the course of multiple sclerosis.

METHODOLOGICAL CONSIDERATIONS

Several authors have discussed the qualities required for an epidemiologically ideal natural history cohort of patients with multiple sclerosis (Ebers 1998; Sackett *et al* 1985). Keys to success are population sampling, clinical assessments and techniques for data analysis.

Population sampling

An essential prerequisite for obtaining relevant information concerning the natural history is to deal with a source population that can be considered representative of the disease as a whole. Ideally, this means that all examples of the disease living in a well-defined geographical area have been ascertained and included in the cohort. As a result, the sample is population based and fully representative of variations in the disease, within the confines of definition and classification. But hospital- and clinic-based series, although open to referral bias – tending towards over-representation of more severe cases (S. Poser *et al* 1982a; Weinshenker and Ebers 1987) – may also prove representative if the hospital clinic attracts the majority of prevalent patients. For a disease with such a long duration as multiple sclerosis, most cases are likely to attend a specialist centre at least once during the course of their illness. Where this reference centre is especially influential within and beyond the area under study, the probability of a sufficiently representative sample is high. That said, complete ascertainment has always been a challenge in multiple sclerosis. Benign cases tend not to visit neurological departments. Taking this limitation to extreme, the evidence from autopsy series (Engell 1989; Georgi 1961; Gilbert and Sadler 1983; McKay and Hirano 1967), and examples of imaging abnormalities suggestive of multiple sclerosis in asymptomatic individuals (McDonnell *et al* 2003), emphasize that some affected individuals remain blissfully unaware of their disease status throughout life. Even if they are identified, such cases cannot be included in registers using current diagnostic classifications of multiple sclerosis because overt clinical manifestations are mandatory for diagnosis (W.I. McDonald *et al* 2001; C.M. Poser *et al* 1983). Although the effect is small, this bias leads to an overestimation of disease severity.

Another key point is accuracy of diagnosis. There is no diagnostic test for multiple sclerosis. Naming the illness depends on the sum of objective criteria that make the neurologist more or less confident of this formulation. The safeguards are enshrined in the diagnostic algorithms of C.M. Poser *et al* (1983) and W.I. McDonald *et al* (2001). We discuss their merits and demerits, and the separate contributions made to paraclinical investigations in illuminating anatomical and mechanistic aspects of the disease process, in Chapter 7.

There is a minimum sample size below which statistical analysis is underpowered, taking into account variations in the clinical course and features of multiple sclerosis. It is difficult to be dogmatic on where this lower limit stands, but studies based on only a few hundred cases are not likely to provide definitive results with narrow confidence intervals. Conversely, although more is better, increasing the sample size should not be at the expense of accuracy, homogeneity and frequency of assessments. One solution is to pool results from different sources; this is best achieved when observations have been made using protocols that are sufficiently compatible to be managed on the same database. The *European Database for MUltiple Sclerosis* (EDMUS) system provides a good example (Confavreux *et al* 1992). However, an alternative for creating the critical mass of patients needed to address specific questions is to combine cohorts of patients, despite these having been described using different standards. This strategy is being followed at the Sylvia Lawry Centre for Multiple Sclerosis Research in Münich (Noseworthy *et al* 2003).

Last but not least, a cohort can only be considered as appropriate for studying the natural history of the disease when the patients under consideration have not received disease modifying treatments. With the advent and widespread prescribing for the beta interferons, glatiramer acetate and, more recently, mitoxantrone, this is increasingly not the case in multiple sclerosis. The number of cohorts that allow accurate characterization and description of the natural history in sufficient numbers of patients with multiple sclerosis is limited. Because the existing data are possibly the last that will become available, they deserve detailed consideration.

Clinical assessments

Ideally, follow-up should be from disease onset until death for all patients included in the database. In practice, this goal is unattainable because the duration of multiple sclerosis is such that results are invariably analysed long before all patients have reached this end point. Modern statistical methods make it possible to take account of patients with varying durations of follow-up but they only provide estimates and these are likely to deviate somewhat from the true position. Furthermore, difficulties may arise in identifying all members of an inception cohort because it may not be possible to date the onset of multiple sclerosis except in retrospect. Restricting the population under study to patients seen from clinical onset introduces its own systematic bias towards more severe cases, since presentation and diagnosis may both be delayed in individuals with benign forms of the disease – as is clearly shown in the London, Ontario, cohort (Weinshenker *et al* 1989a). This solution is therefore not entirely satisfactory.

Follow-up should be prospective, and made at regular and frequent intervals. Ascertainment of relapses in multiple sclerosis is positively correlated to the frequency of neurological assessments (Fog and Linnemann 1970; Lhermitte *et al* 1973;

U. Patzold and Pocklington 1982). Clinical assessment every 3 or 6 months enables accurate and comprehensive ascertainment of relapses. This is the schedule followed in modern phase III therapeutic trials during the overall study period. Conversely, this ideal is unrealistic for large cohorts of patients seen over a much longer period. Assessment intervals may vary between studies, not only from one patient to another but also for a given individual. It is commonplace for individuals to attend at close intervals during 'hot' periods corresponding to the diagnostic phase, a period of increased disease activity, or when new therapeutic opportunities become available, whereas visits become less frequent at other times. But many other factors determine the frequency of routine visits – the level of health care resources, the willingness of the patient to attend neurological appointments, and availability of the physician. As a consequence, structured and standardized follow-up is clearly an unattainable goal in long-term assessment of the natural history in multiple sclerosis.

It is important to be consistent in the use of definitions and scales, even when assessments are made in retrospect, for all the patients seen throughout the study. The importance of training sessions for assessors to reduce inter-examiner variability has been well demonstrated in the conduct of therapeutic trials – a relatively easy task because such studies rarely exceed 2 years. But this control should also be applied to studies of the natural history. Here, the challenge is more demanding because patients are to be followed for several decades and, almost invariably, by different neurologists. In this respect, the adoption of an acknowledged common language facilitates a uniform description throughout the disease, and an electronic database provides for recording, storing and retrieval of information (Confavreux 1994; Confavreux and Paty 1995; Confavreux *et al* 1992; 1996; Weinshenker 1999). An ideal system has to be quick to complete and user friendly, with an attractive design of the paper forms and screen windows. It must not impose any specific technical demands on the user. The focus must be on basic items and a minimal set of obligatory data that are necessary but also sufficient for comprehensive description of the disease. When EDMUS was developed in the early 1990s under the aegis of the first European Concerted Action, several guiding principles were identified in order to facilitate regular and long-term use of the system, and to avoid compromising the recording physician's daily activities. The EDMUS Steering Committee deliberately gave priority to symptoms rather than signs. Data relating to past events – reported in retrospect by the patient, relatives or attending physician – were recorded in the same language as those derived prospectively. The emphasis was on raw descriptive details assessed directly through interview and examination of the patient. This procedure saves time for the user, ensures a uniform encoding of cases by different applicants, and allows automatic updating of the record whenever additional information becomes available. Scores, indices or classifications derived later are not directly entered in the system, but generated automatically by the program. EDMUS is compatible with any future classifications, since the raw data can be manipulated using new analytical algorithms. Thus, by way of example, EDMUS proved versatile when the need arose to incorporate the McDonald *et al* (2001) diagnostic classification. These safeguards of standardization and computerization provide considerable clinical and research opportunities. Medical practice is improved by allowing rapid access to relevant features of patients' records. Research is made more straightforward. Within and among centres using the same standards, selection of appropriate files, exchange of data, and comparison of individual studies are facilitated. Files from various centres can be pooled for common studies. In this way, information from a critical mass of patients becomes available allowing fundamental issues to be researched with sufficient power, but also encouraging new questions that cannot be addressed by a single centre. These considerations are particularly relevant in a disease such as multiple sclerosis, having a relatively low frequency, and in which clinicians and researchers often use inconsistent terminology.

Data analysis

We have made the point that the researcher does not have access to the entire population from onset to death, and therefore has to provide estimates. For a population of patients studied with respect to a given end point – for instance, the next relapse, a given level of irreversible disability or the onset of progression – any individual fits one of three categories (Figure 4.1):

- the end point has already been reached
- the individual is still under scrutiny but has not reached the end point
- the patient has been lost to follow-up since a given date at which the end point had not been reached.

The last two categories make up the group of censored patients. Obviously, the longer it takes for the outcome of interest to be reached as part of the natural history, the lower the proportion of patients who will actually have reached that end point by the time the study is closed, and the lower will be the reliability of estimates offered, in terms of accuracy and precision.

The classical approach is only to analyse observed data – that proportion of patients who have reached the end point when the survey closes. It is the most straightforward approach, but presently is less favoured because it invariably leads to under-estimation of the true interval from inception to end point. Therefore, it overestimates disease severity because patients who have not yet reached this end point by the time of closure, but will do so later, are not taken into account. Much attention must also be paid to the presentation of results when conclusions are based only on observational data. A classical approach is to stratify results. Considering a given disease duration, those patients who are no longer available for follow-up by the neurologist at this time point, because they have died or become homebound or institutionalized and the neurologist does not search for details of current disability, are excluded from the calculations both for this epoch and those that follow. This invariably results in an underestimation for overall severity of the disease. The statement that 'after 30 years of disease, 50% [of patients] still remain in the benign group', that is, with a Kurtzke Expanded Disability Status Scale (EDSS) score ≤4.0 (Benedikz *et al* 2002), illustrates the point. In this Icelandic study, only 108 of the initial 372 (29%) patients were available at 25–29 years of disease duration; 53 / 372 patients were known to have died at the time of the study. Incorporating these deceased patients into the analysed group would have altered the result so that 51% of the patients had reached an EDSS score ≥7.0 or were dead, with only 35% remaining in the benign group after 25–29 years' disease duration. In a study from New Zealand, study outcomes were presented comparatively, with and without such an adjustment, providing an elegant demonstration of why this manipulation, nonetheless incomplete because censored patients are not taken into account, is important in these calculations (Table 4.1; D.H. Miller *et al* 1992a).

Another method for presenting results when using observed disability data at a given time point is to construct a 'progression index', defined as the ratio of the disability score at any time point to disease duration (see Chapter 6 for a more detailed discussion of disability scales: S. Poser *et al* 1982b). In order to gain an impression of disease severity in a given patient, this index assumes a linear correlation between disability and time. In a German epidemiological study, the progression index, using the Disability Status Scale (DSS) as numerator, turned out to be remarkably stable in individuals over several years (S. Poser *et al* 1982b) but this has not always been the case. This concept of the progression index has several shortcomings, as depicted in Figure 4.2. The index value at any one arbitrary time point does not reveal when in the course of that patient's illness the events determining disability occurred. Conversely, in the patient with stable disability, the progression index decreases with time, ranging from infinity at day 0, through values of 2, 1 and 0.5 for years 2, 4 and 8 to 0.2 at year 20 of disease duration, respectively.

A step forward was made with the introduction of survival analyses (D.R. Cox 1972; Kaplan and Meier 1958). These allow a dichotomized event – that has or has not yet happened – to be considered; but also, when the event has occurred, they reflect the time taken to reach that point. Introduction of the time dimension takes account of patients who have not reached the end point at closure of the study, or are already lost to follow-up. For this reason, probabilistic estimates of time intervals such as those produced by the Kaplan–Meier technique provide longer estimates. These are preferable to analyses based strictly on observational data, but they are not necessarily accurate. The

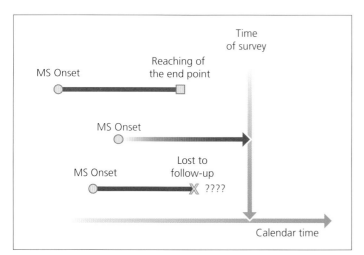

Figure 4.1 Schematic representation of the distribution of patients in a cohort at the time of survey, according to their status with respect to reaching the end point under scrutiny. Top line: patients who have reached the end point before the closing of the survey. Middle line: patients who have not reached the end point at the time of closure. Bottom line: patients who had not reached the end point at the time they were lost to follow-up.

Table 4.1 **Distribution of patients (%) in relation to disability status scale (DSS) scores according to time periods of disease duration (years), among 209 patients with multiple sclerosis. Only observed data are taken into consideration. Importance of adjustment of the data for death. Adapted from Miller *et al* (1992a)**

| | Disease duration (years) | | | | | |
	0–5	6–10	11–15	16–20	21–25	>25
Number of patients	42	50	28	31	27	31
Disability						
Not adjusted						
DSS 0–2	83	46	43	35	30	26
DSS 3–5	14	26	25	32	33	35
DSS 6–10	2	28	32	32	37	39
Adjusted[a]						
DSS 0–2	83	46	41	32	23	14
DSS 3–5	14	26	25	29	25	20
DSS 6–10	2	28	34	39	52	66

a Adjusted percentages after the addition to the DSS 6–10 group of the estimated number of multiple sclerosis-related deaths for a given disease duration within a similar local population of patients with multiple sclerosis.

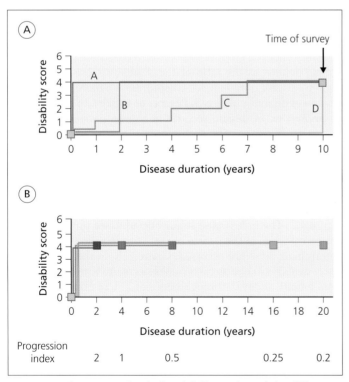

Figure 4.2 The progression index. (A) Illustration of the different time course of disability accumulation in four fictitious patients (A, B, C, D) with a similar progression index of 0.4 at 10 years of disease duration. (B) Illustration of a fictitious patient with a disability score of EDSS 4 throughout the disease course. The longer the disease duration at the time of the survey, the lower the progression index.

proportion of censored patients has a clear influence on these statistics because the higher this proportion, the longer will be the estimated time intervals (Figure 4.3). Life table results can be presented in two ways. The first estimates the survival probability for groups of individuals over time. It aims at illustrating the decreasing proportion of individuals not yet affected by the outcome ('survivors') according to time elapsed since the reference point. The second is the opposite; the results illustrate the cumulative proportion of subjects who have been affected by the outcome of interest over time (Figure 4.4). In both instances, any inaugural episode occurring early or during the course of the disease can be used as the starting point; and any one of several relevant events taken as the 'outcome' or 'dependent variable'. The date of the last examination is used for the patients who have not reached the end point at closure of the survey (censored cases).

Survival analyses maximize the use of information available on every patient in making calculations, but are not ideal for assessing the independent or interactive influence of multiple factors occurring simultaneously. In this situation, the requirement is to stratify the initial population into smaller samples, representing each possible explanatory variable. However, this quickly erodes the power of the initial sample. Therefore, the assessment of a single variable is preferable and multivariate analyses are generally impractical, or very soon reveal their limitations. These considerations led to the development of regression models. The most popular, in studies of the natural history of multiple sclerosis, is the Cox proportional hazards regression model (D.R. Cox 1972). This allows the relationship between a set of covariates and the time to a particular event to be estimated by providing risk ratios for reaching that end point between

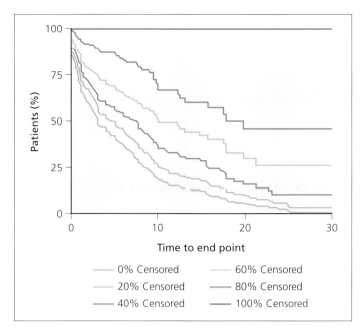

Figure 4.3 Simulation of Kaplan–Meier estimates for the time from inception (such as the onset of multiple sclerosis) to reaching the end point (such as onset of progression) among the 200 patients with multiple sclerosis in a fictitious cohort, according to the proportion of censored patients at the date of the survey. Medians and 95% confidence intervals (years): 0% censored: median 3.0, 95% CI 2.0–4.0; 20% censored: median 4.6, 95% CI 2.9–6.3; 40% censored: median 7.2, 95% CI 5.0–9.4; 60% censored: median 10.1, 95% CI 6.7–13.5; 80% censored: median 17.9, 95% CIs not assessable; 100% censored: not assessable.

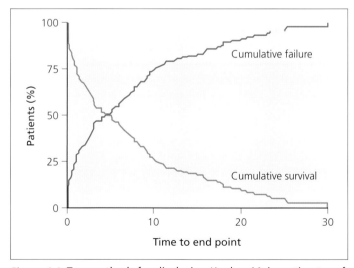

Figure 4.4 Two methods for displaying Kaplan–Meier estimates of the time to reach the end point under study. Blue: cumulative survival – the proportion of individuals (%) still end-point-free, according to the time elapsed since the date of the reference point. Red: cumulative failure – proportion of individuals (%) who have reached the end point, according to the time elapsed since the date of the reference point.

patient groups selected for the different covariates. The proportional hazard model assumes that the risk ratio between two sets of values for covariates is constant over time. Statistical modelling therefore allows for a multivariate analysis and simultaneous weighing of individual factors. It accounts for covariation of the predictors, compensates for censoring, and automatically adjusts for the differences in disease duration (D.R. Cox 1972; Riise *et al* 1988; 1992). The great strength of this method is to allow the weight of each covariate to the event under study to be estimated over time, and the degree of interdependency for each variable to be considered. This method can be used for the whole population under study, and for preselected strata. Other statistical models have been proposed, based upon Markov transitions (Confavreux and Wolfson 1989; Wolfson and Confavreux 1985; 1987) and, more recently, on Bayesian analysis (Bergamaschi *et al* 2001). Whether these are more informative, accurate and precise for individual patients than the Cox model remains to be seen.

It is also important to realize that, by their nature, all the statistical analyses mentioned above only provide probabilities at the population level. The results cannot reliably be applied to the individual. A good example is provided by the relationship between pregnancy and multiple sclerosis (Vukusic *et al* 2004; see below): although the study made it possible to develop mathematical models for the risk of having a relapse in the first trimester of pregnancy, the correct classification was achieved for only 72% of women, even when using the best multivariate model.

The deterministic approach, therefore, also deserves consideration. This differs completely from probabilistic methods, being based upon successive scoring examinations of the individual. These are then plotted on a diagram according to the time of the survey. The mathematical curve best fitting the observed behaviour of the individual can then be identified using a regression analysis. Prediction of the future course of the disease is provided for that individual by extrapolating the regression curve (Figure 4.5). Although it has proved worthwhile (Fog and Linnemann 1970; Patzold and Pocklington 1982), the technique is demanding and of limited application in daily practice, because precise and accurate predictions require long periods of observation and frequent assessments.

Material available for studies on the natural history of multiple sclerosis

Our present knowledge of the natural history of multiple sclerosis is based on long-term studies of cohorts – geographically well defined and subjected to cross-sectional or longitudinal assessments, or both – and on short-term studies that are observational or performed as part of therapeutic trials. Both sources have their merits and demerits but, to some extent, the strengths and weaknesses are complementary. For the long-term natural history studies, precision and reliability of data relating to early phases of the disease are not optimal as, in many instances, these have to be assessed retrospectively. More generally, for the reasons already discussed, precision varies from one patient to another and across different periods of the disease. Conversely, whereas prospective short-term studies may provide precise and robust information regarding the study period, this can seldom be achieved for intervals before and

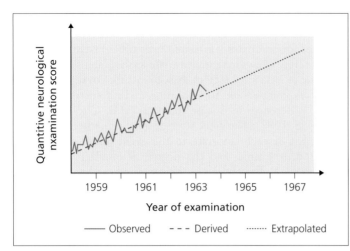

Figure 4.5 Deterministic approach. The successive scoring examinations of a given patient over time allow the best fitting mathematical curve to be derived from the observed curve using regression analysis. Future course of the disease of the individual is predicted by extrapolating the regression curve.

after this brief (and not necessarily fully representative) phase of the disease. Because the period of observation is, by design, limited to several months or years, the value of these studies is restricted to the elucidation only of the short-term course and prognosis. Importantly, such a cohort often provides a narrow representation of the disease in general. Its value can be considered as inversely correlated to the stringency of the inclusion criteria: the more vaguely these are construed, the more variety and breadth creeps into the cohort; the tighter the criteria, the less room there is for variations of the disease spectrum to be included. In practice, we use both sources of information, but as our purpose is to describe the long-term natural history of multiple sclerosis, we focus on the long-term studies in more detail. The number is truly astonishing, many gathered painstakingly in the second half of the 20th century. Perhaps no other disease has been scrutinized in such detail and, as a result, multiple sclerosis stands out as the archetype of chronic diseases, the amazing range of course and prognosis that emerges making it so puzzling to the physician.

The series are listed in Table 4.2 with a summary of the main epidemiological and disease-related features for each. As the table clearly illustrates, many observational natural history studies are based upon more or less complete prevalence material, whereas others rely on samples of patients having contact with a special clinic over a limited period of time (V.A. Clark *et al* 1982; Detels *et al* 1982; Leibowitz and Alter 1970; 1973; Leibowitz *et al* 1964a; 1964b; McAlpine and Compston 1952; R. Müller 1949; 1951; Panelius 1969; S. Poser 1978; Riise *et al* 1992; Visscher *et al* 1984). We do not discard these data because, notwithstanding the reservations expressed above, cross-sectional studies can inform the study of natural history in multiple sclerosis, so long as sufficient source information is available on past medical history to allow researchers the opportunity of constructing a reliable neurological history of the patient. In this situation, the availability of additional longitudinal follow-up (Kantarci *et al* 1998; D.H. Miller *et al* 1992a; Myhr *et al* 2001; Phadke 1987; 1990; S. Poser *et al* 1982a; Trojano *et al* 1995) improves accuracy and makes the study even more informative.

That said, a longitudinal strategy is always to be preferred for reliable assessment of the major outcome criterion – be that relapse occurrence, onset of progression, or time to reach specific landmarks of irreversible disability. In this respect, three cohorts demonstrate features suggesting that they provide reliable information on the natural history of multiple sclerosis:

- a large sample size representative of the population at risk
- prospective long-term longitudinal follow-up with numerous, comprehensive, standardized clinical assessments made at close intervals
- no confounding effects of disease modifying therapeutic interventions
- appropriate statistical analyses, especially the use of survival techniques.

These originate from Lyon, France (Confavreux 1977; Confavreux *et al* 1980; 2000; 2003), Gothenburg, Sweden (Broman *et al* 1981; Eriksson *et al* 2003; Runmarker and Andersen 1993) and London, Ontario (D.A. Cottrell *et al* 1999a; 1999b; Kremenchutzky *et al* 1999; Weinshenker *et al* 1989a; 1989b; 1991a; 1991b). We add to this list, the United States Army Veterans World War II cohort (Kurtzke *et al* 1968a; 1970; 1973; 1977) for its pioneer stance in the field. By contrast, we have discarded from this list the extensive Danish study dealing with progression rates in a sample of very carefully and regularly investigated patients observed over long periods (Fog and Linnemann 1970), because this is based on a highly selected population of patients. Lastly, the most recent studies, developed since patients started to receive disease modifying treatments such as interferon β (IFN-β), glatiramer acetate and mitoxantrone, are considered separately (Amato and Ponziani 2000; Amato *et al* 1999). Because they will repeatedly serve as the major source of information in this chapter, we review briefly the epidemiological and disease-related baseline characteristics of the main long-term natural history cohorts in which longitudinal follow-up is available (Table 4.2).

The United States Army Veterans World War II cohort was set up by John Kurtzke and colleagues based on males diagnosed with multiple sclerosis during Army service between 1942 and 1951 (Kurtzke *et al* 1968a; 1970a; 1973; 1977). It has the strengths of being drawn from a large geographical base, and with prolonged follow-up. But the cohort undoubtedly provides a biased sample. By definition, it is limited to young males. Pre-service onset of multiple sclerosis prevented men from enlisting, whereas disease onset during service may not have been diagnosed as such prior to discharge. The cohort offers opportunities to describe multiple sclerosis from onset. Later, its value deteriorates, because the diagnosis of multiple sclerosis is a cause for medical discharge from service, and for compensation. For men on active duty in the Army, any symptoms interfering with military activities led to early hospitalization. Whenever multiple sclerosis was suspected, a neurological evaluation immediately took place, thus providing clinical and laboratory information at the time of onset, or very close to it. Follow-up information from the Veterans Administration hospitals, as well as other medical records, was usually extensive because disability compensation depended partly on the degree of neurological deficit. For most men with incomplete Veterans Administration follow-up records, special examinations by private

text continued on page 192

Table 4.2 Main series of the long-term course and prognosis of multiple sclerosis: epidemiological and disease-related characteristics

Study	Location	Ascertainment	Follow-up	Population size	Diagnosis classification[a]	Overall course of multiple sclerosis at time of study (%)	Time from onset of multiple sclerosis to initial clinic visit (years)	Duration of multiple sclerosis (years)
Long-term natural history series with cross-sectional and/or some longitudinal assessment								
R. Müller 1949; 1951	Sweden, multicentre	Clinic based	Cross-sectional	810	'Clinically undoubted'	Not available	3 (median)	15.3 (mean)
McAlpine and Compston 1952	London, United Kingdom	Clinic based	Cross-sectional	414	NA	Relapsing–remitting multiple sclerosis 65 / Secondary progressive multiple sclerosis 25 / Progressive onset multiple sclerosis 10	–	11.3 (mean)
Leibowitz et al 1964a; 1964b Leibowitz and Alter 1970; 1973	Israel, countrywide	Hospital/clinic based	Cross-sectional	282	Definite Probable Possible	Relapsing–remitting multiple sclerosis 63 / Secondary or primary progressive 37	–	11.5 (mean)
Panelius 1969	Turku, Finland	Geographically based	Cross-sectional	146	Definite	Not available	–	12.9 (mean)
S. Poser 1978	Germany, multicentre	Hospital/clinic based	Cross-sectional	812	Definite Probable Possible	Relapsing–remitting multiple sclerosis 42 / Secondary progressive multiple sclerosis 40 / Progressive onset multiple sclerosis 18	–	8.7 (mean)
S. Poser et al 1982a	Southern Lower Saxony, Germany	Geographically based	Cross-sectional Some longitudinal	221	Definite Probable Possible	Relapsing–remitting multiple sclerosis 59 / Secondary progressive multiple sclerosis 28 / Progressive onset multiple sclerosis 13	Not available	12.1 (mean)
V.A. Clark et al 1982; Detels et al 1982 Visscher et al 1984	Washington and Los Angeles, USA	Geographically based	Cross-sectional	834–941	Definite Probable	Not available	–	15 (mean)
Phadke 1987; 1990	Grampian region, Scotland	Geographically based	Cross-sectional Some longitudinal	1055	Definite Probable Possible	Relapsing–remitting multiple sclerosis 68 / Secondary progressive multiple sclerosis 23 / Progressive onset multiple sclerosis 9	Not available	1–60 (range)
Minderhoud et al 1988	Groningen, The Netherlands	Clinic based	Some longitudinal	342	Definite Probable	Relapsing–remitting multiple sclerosis 31 / Secondary progressive multiple sclerosis 32 / Progressive onset multiple sclerosis 37	Not available	Not available

table continued on following page

Table 4.2 Main series of the long-term course and prognosis of multiple sclerosis: epidemiological and disease-related characteristics, cont'd

Study	Location	Ascertainment	Follow-up	Population size	Diagnosis classification[a]	Overall course of multiple sclerosis at time of study (%)	Time from onset of multiple sclerosis to initial clinic visit (years)	Duration of multiple sclerosis (years)
D.H. Miller et al 1992a	Wellington, New Zealand	Clinic based Geographically based	Cross-sectional Some longitudinal	209	Definite Probable	Relapsing–remitting multiple sclerosis 65 Secondary progressive multiple sclerosis 30 Progressive onset multiple sclerosis 5	Not available	14.8 (mean)
Riise et al 1992	Europe, multicentre	Clinic based	Cross-sectional	574	Definite Probable Possible	Not available	–	6.6 (mean)
Trojano et al 1995	Bari, Italy	Clinic based	Cross-sectional Some longitudinal	309	Definite	Relapsing–remitting multiple sclerosis 58 Secondary progressive multiple sclerosis 22 Progressive onset multiple sclerosis 19	Not available	9.8 (mean)
Kantarci et al 1998	Turkey, multicentre	Clinic based	Cross-sectional Some longitudinal	1259	Definite	Relapsing–remitting multiple sclerosis 62 Secondary progressive multiple sclerosis 26 Progressive onset multiple sclerosis 12	Not available	8.4 ± 6.7 (mean ± SD) 7 (median)
Myhr et al 2001	Hordaland county, Norway	Geographically based	Cross-sectional Some longitudinal	220	Definite Probable	Not available	4.2 ± 0.3 (mean ± SEM)	14.4 ± 0.2 (mean ± SEM)
Long-term natural history cohorts with longitudinal follow-up								
United States Army Veterans World War II cohort								
Kurtzke et al 1968a; 1970; 1973; 1977	United States	Country based	Longitudinal	527	Definite Probable	Not available	51% seen at onset of multiple sclerosis	72% followed up at 15 years
Lyon, France, multiple sclerosis cohort								
Confavreux 1977 Confavreux et al 1980	Lyon, France	Hospital based	Longitudinal	349	Definite Probable Possible	Relapsing–remitting multiple sclerosis 58 Secondary progressive multiple sclerosis 24 Progressive onset multiple sclerosis 18	4.7 (mean)	9.0 (mean)
Confavreux et al 2000; 2003	Lyon, France	Clinic based Geographically based	Longitudinal	1844	Definite Probable	Relapsing–remitting multiple sclerosis 58 Secondary progressive multiple sclerosis 27 Progressive onset multiple sclerosis 15	6 ± 8 (mean ± SD)	11 ± 10 (mean ± SD)

Table 4.2 Main series of the long-term course and prognosis of multiple sclerosis: epidemiological and disease-related characteristics, cont'd

Study	Location	Ascertainment	Follow-up	Population size	Diagnosis classification[a]	Overall course of multiple sclerosis at time of study (%)	Time from onset of multiple sclerosis to initial clinic visit (years)	Duration of multiple sclerosis (years)
Gothenburg, Sweden, multiple sclerosis cohort								
Broman et al 1981 Runmarker and Andersen 1993 Eriksson et al 2003	Gothenburg, Sweden	Inception cohort Geographically based	Longitudinal	308	Definite Probable Possible	Relapsing–remitting multiple sclerosis 31 Secondary progressive multiple sclerosis 52 Progressive onset multiple sclerosis 17	60% of cases with relapsing-remitting initial course seen from onset of multiple sclerosis	> 25
London, Ontario, multiple sclerosis cohort								
Weinshenker et al 1989a; 1989b; 1991a; 1991b	London, Ontario	Clinic-based Geographically based	Longitudinal	1099	Definite Probable Possible	Not available	197 patients seen from onset of multiple sclerosis	11.9 ± 0.3 (mean ± SEM)
D.A. Cottrell et al 1999a; 1999b Kremenchutzky et al 1999	London, Ontario	Clinic based Geographically based	Longitudinal	1044	Definite Probable Possible	Relapsing–remitting multiple sclerosis 28 Secondary progressive multiple sclerosis 51 Progressive onset multiple sclerosis 21	197 patients seen from onset of multiple sclerosis	24 (mean)
Long-term history series from the therapeutic era								
Amato et al 1999 Amato and Ponziani 2000	Florence, Italy	'Seen at onset' Clinic based	Longitudinal	224	NA	Relapsing–remitting multiple sclerosis 62 Secondary progressive multiple sclerosis 23 Progressive onset multiple sclerosis 15	1.1 ± 0.7 (mean ± SD)	9.8 (mean)

a Whenever necessary, the original criteria used by the authors have been interpreted in order to comply with the C.M. Poser et al (1983) diagnostic criteria. 'Possible' is equivalent to 'suspected' in this classification.
SD = standard deviation.
SEM = standard error of the mean.

neurologists were performed in the period 1960–1962. Original medical records were abstracted by trained researchers. The information in the hands of the Army physician when making the diagnosis of multiple sclerosis was therefore enriched with serial examinations and interval histories gathered during follow-up. The cohort comprises a total of 527 men, among whom 476 were considered to have definite multiple sclerosis according to criteria for space and time dissemination; conversely, 51 were classified as probable because the criterion for dissemination in time was missing. Two distinct groups were considered. One consisted of 293 patients whose inaugural episode occurred before entry to the military, and was distinct from the relapse allowing for diagnosis whilst serving in the Army – an average of 2–3 years from onset. Detailed neurological information was available for the first attack in 10% of cases. The other group consisted of 234 patients whose inaugural episode occurred during military service. Here, neurological data relating to onset were available in 94% of individuals later shown to have multiple sclerosis. The use of medication taken during the 1942–1962 study period is not known, which leads us to think that the treatments were limited to short courses of corticotropin or corticosteroids administered during relapses, only in the latter part of the study.

A Multiple Sclerosis Cohort was established in the Lyon Hospital Department of Neurology in 1957 (Confavreux 1977; Confavreux et al 1980; 2000; 2003). The cohort includes all patients with a diagnosis of multiple sclerosis examined on more than one occasion in the department. This serves as the single referral centre for multiple sclerosis in Lyon City and the Rhône-Alpes region. Lyon is located within the 'département du Rhône', which listed 1 575 000 inhabitants in 1999. The Rhône-Alpes region is made of eight départements (Ain, Ardèche, Drôme, Isère, Loire, Rhône, Savoie and Haute-Savoie) and counted 5 634 000 inhabitants in 1999. Prevalence of multiple sclerosis in the area has been estimated at approximately $50/10^5$ according to the most recent epidemiological study (Confavreux et al 1987). The Lyon Multiple Sclerosis Cohort can be considered representative of patients with multiple sclerosis in this area. Data were computerized in 1976 and, since 1990, entered on the EDMUS software (Confavreux et al 1992). Individual case reports document personal and demographic data, medical history, key episodes in the course of the illness (relapses, onset of the progressive phase, dates of assignment for the successive scores of irreversible disability), biological, electrophysiological and imaging studies, and details of treatment. Observations are entered retrospectively when the patient is first seen at the clinic. Effort is always made to obtain data from the original medical files, especially those relating to the first neurological episode, and on the clinical course and disability. Success is facilitated by cooperation from the regional network of neurologists working in the Lyon area. New observations are then collected prospectively whenever the patient returns, usually on a yearly basis, entered and checked automatically by the system for consistency with older information. By April 1997, a cohort of 1844 patients with definite or probable multiple sclerosis according to the C.M. Poser et al (1983) criteria were included (Confavreux et al 2000; 2003). At that time, the database was locked for the purpose of epidemiological studies. Approximately half of the patients in the cohort had received immunosuppressive drugs, usually azathioprine, at some point during

their disease, mainly the relapsing–remitting phase, and not before the third episode. None of these drugs has ever been shown to reduce progression of irreversible disability in multiple sclerosis, and the inclusion of these cases is considered not to have biased the chosen disability end point measures (D.A.S. Compston and Coles 2003; Noseworthy et al 2000a; Rudick et al 1997b). Betaseron®, the first putative disease modifying agent approved in multiple sclerosis, became available (in France) in February 1996. As a historical aside, the first life table analysis of disability in multiple sclerosis is that reported for the Lyon cohort (Confavreux et al 1980). The disability scale used was appropriate for 1980 (McAlpine and Compston 1952; McAlpine et al 1972). Thus, what are designated 'moderate disability' and 'severe disability' correspond to scores of DSS 4 and 7, respectively (Kurtzke 1961; 1965a).

The Gothenburg Multiple Sclerosis cohort comprised all patients with onset of multiple sclerosis from 1st January 1950 to 31st December 1964, living in Gothenburg, Sweden, at the time of disease onset (Broman et al 1981; Runmarker and Andersen 1993; Svenningsson et al 1990) and satisfying contemporary diagnostic criteria (C.M. Poser et al 1983). The cohort includes 308 patients. Gothenburg is the second largest city in Sweden, with 379 000 inhabitants in 1950 and 431 000 by 1988 (Svenningsson et al 1990). The Sahlgren Hospital Department of Neurology was set up in 1950 and served as the only neurological unit in Gothenburg until 1970 (Broman et al 1981). Almost all neurological patients were referred to the Department because none of the local neurologists had a private practice during this period. After 1970, three part-time neurological outpatient departments were opened, led by neurologists trained at Sahlgren Hospital and maintaining close contacts with the host department. The prevalence of multiple sclerosis ranged from 91 to $96/10^5$ between 1978 and 1988 (Svenningsson et al 1990). The majority of the 308 incident patients were seen early in the disease course: >60% of those with a relapsing–remitting onset attended during the first episode whereas the median time to first examination in the neurological department was 3 years for patients with a progressive initial course of multiple sclerosis. The prognosis of patients seen from onset did not differ from other cases, suggesting that the sample is representative and has the characteristics of an inception cohort. The follow-up has been longitudinal and prospective, extending for ≥25 years from onset in all survivors, with the exception of only four patients (three living abroad) who were lost to follow-up after 13–24 years. Follow-up examinations are mostly carried out by the same neurologists in Sahlgren Hospital, who conducted an average of seven complete neurological examinations on each patient during the follow-up period, and also incorporated data obtained from other neurologists. Primary outcome measures are progression onset for patients with a relapsing–remitting initial course, and reaching DSS 6 for all patients. Data are registered in a specific database. At the times of key analyses, the use of immunological therapies in this population had been limited to short courses of corticotropin in 61 patients. Therefore, although the number of patients included is relatively small, and the study uses a unique scoring system – namely the Regional Functional System Score – and restricts information to DSS 6, 7 and 10 in the database (M. Eriksson et al 2003), the Gothenburg, Sweden, cohort shares several important features qualifying for an appropriate study on the natural history of multiple sclerosis.

The London, Ontario, cohort was established through the multiple sclerosis clinic at the University Hospital in 1972 to provide comprehensive care for patients in the referral area of Southern Ontario (Weinshenker *et al* 1989a; 1989b; 1991a; 1991b). This cohort retains the characteristics of both a tertiary referral centre for the province of Ontario, and a geographically based clinic serving Middlesex County, where an epidemiological study on 1st January 1984 showed a prevalence of $93/10^5$ with near complete ascertainment: 91% of patients were known to be attending the clinic (Hader *et al* 1988). Those patients not registered were mainly the chronic institutionalized individuals, most of whom were already severely disabled when the clinic was established. Patients are followed annually or biennially by neurologists with a special interest in multiple sclerosis. Follow-up is maintained even after patients become institutionalized in nursing homes; and every attempt is made to determine the reason why an individual might have become 'lost to follow-up'. No specific therapies for multiple sclerosis were administered, other than corticosteroids for acute exacerbations, although the clinic has contributed to many therapeutic trials and adopted the prescribing culture now characteristic of centres in North America and Canada. Between 1979 and 1984, the authors reviewed data collected on 1099 consecutive patients evaluated between 1972 and 1984. Information on demographics, clinical course and the progress of disability as a function of time was systematically collected. Data were recorded on standardized forms and entered onto a mainframe computer. They were analysed as a total population but also in two subgroups: the Middlesex County cohort, representing a population-based group for which ascertainment was near complete; and the 'seen from onset' subgroup comprising 197 patients seen by a neurologist ≤1 year from onset. Data on this cohort have been updated to the end of 1996 and the mean duration of the disease at that time reached 24 years (D.A. Cottrell *et al* 1999a; 1999b; Kremenchutzky *et al* 1999).

THE OUTCOME LANDMARKS OF MULTIPLE SCLEROSIS: DEPENDENT VARIABLES

It has long been recognized that the course of multiple sclerosis can be described in terms of relapses, remissions and chronic progression either from onset or after a period of remissions (Charcot 1868b: 1868c; Marie 1884; McAlpine and Compston 1952). Two major outcome measures usefully describe the clinical course and prognosis: the qualitative description, an expression of the interplay between relapses and progression; and the quantitative description, which refers to the accumulation of neurological deficits and is characterized as disability, impairment or loss of social functions. Both can be used in therapeutic trials. Here, we confine our discussion to the role of clinical variables: surrogate markers are covered in Chapter 18.

Course-related dependent variables

Physicians and people with multiple sclerosis know that the cardinal features that characterize the clinical experience of this disease are:

- episodes with full recovery
- episodes with incomplete recovery
- chronic progression.

In general, these phases follow an orderly sequence; but the relationship between episodes and progression is far from straightforward, and a detailed understanding of their interplay is required in order to understand the evolution and dynamics of disability and other outcomes.

Relapses and progression

Relapses – exacerbations, attacks, bouts or episodes – are defined as the first occurrence, recurrence or worsening of symptoms representing neurological dysfunction and marked by subacute onset and a period of stability followed by partial or complete recovery – the whole process lasting ≥24 hours (see Chapter 16). On a small semantic point, it is not strictly correct to refer to the initial episode as a 'relapse'; although this is commonplace, we designate the first experience as the inaugural episode and everything that comes later as a relapse(s). Distinction is made between symptoms attributable only to fatigue, and those associated with fever. Events occurring within a 1-month period are considered part of the same episode (Confavreux *et al* 1992; W.I. McDonald *et al* 2001; C.M. Poser *et al* 1983; G.A. Schumacher *et al* 1965). The experienced neurologist will recognize that, despite these unambiguous definitions, it is not always easy to decide whether particular neurological symptoms do genuinely constitute a relapse. Every specialist is familiar with the difficult issue of resolving the status of worsening paraesthesia, a change in walking, or blurred vision – to name but a few of the very many challenging examples encountered in daily practice. Efforts have been made to rank the level of certainty appropriate for a putative relapse – ranging from highly suggestive symptoms with and without objective features on examination noted by the neurologist, to distinctly atypical or minimal complaints. Ranking can be based on the severity of the relapse with respect to its consequences for daily activities; the impact on objective neurological scores; the decision to administer corticosteroids and hospitalize the patient; and the distinction between new symptoms, those previously experienced and worsening of current manifestations of multiple sclerosis. Paroxysmal neurological symptoms present particular difficulties. Because very many may occur over a short period, confusion can arise as to their status – individually or collectively. Our view is that the onset of these manifestations of multiple sclerosis in isolation may constitute a new episode indicating a focal area of inflammatory demyelination resulting in ephaptic transmission. In the absence of an agreed classification for relapse assessment, it is necessary to take a pragmatic approach and adopt common definitions, both in therapeutic trials and prospective studies for which the study period lasts ≤2–3 years, using standardized clinical assessments performed at regular and close intervals by an assessor who is blinded to the therapeutic intervention and focus of interest in the study. However, this is not realistic for natural history studies where lifelong follow-up is required. In this setting, relapse ascertainment and assessment are generally less reliable, and differ for a given patient over time, and between individuals studied contemporaneously.

Perhaps no term in the lexicon of multiple sclerosis has become so confused as 'progression'. The reason is that, in modern therapeutic trials, the word is used merely to describe a worsening of neurological disability with reference to the baseline. Progression is said to be sustained if confirmed at clinic visits, 3–6 months apart. However, disability worsening, even when sustained at 6 months, does not necessarily equate to an irreversible increase in disability (see below; C. Liu and Blumhardt 2000). Originally, the term was used to define steady worsening of symptoms and signs over ≥6 months (Confavreux *et al* 1992; C.M. Poser *et al* 1983; G.A. Schumacher *et al* 1965), or ≥12 months according to more recent criteria (W.I. McDonald *et al* 2001; A.J. Thompson *et al* 1997). By that definition, once started, progression continues throughout the disease although occasional plateaus and minor temporary improvements may be observed (Lublin and Reingold 1996). The date at which progression starts is invariably assigned in retrospect, once the required 6- or 12-month duration of continuous neurological worsening is confirmed. Herein lies the uncertainty. Relapses can be superimposed on progression, whenever that first manifests (primary and secondary progressive multiple sclerosis). Therefore, it is not helpful to use the word 'progression' both to characterize the worsening of neurological disability attributable to step changes in disability that follow a nasty relapse, and situations in which disability increases systematically over time, even when interspersed with periods of relative stability. For us, this latter is the correct and preferred usage of the term.

The phases of multiple sclerosis

The usual course of multiple sclerosis is characterized by repeated relapses associated, for the majority of patients, with the eventual onset of disease progression. The initial pattern is so characteristic that diagnostic criteria are dependent on the demonstration of dissemination in time. Consequently, it has become commonplace to speak of 'conversion to multiple sclerosis' once the inaugural neurological episode has been followed by a first relapse. By definition, ≥2 distinct neurological episodes must be documented in the course of that patient's illness, the events separated by ≥30 days (McAlpine 1961; W.I. McDonald *et al* 2001; C.M. Poser *et al* 1983). Taken with the phase of secondary progression, this establishes three distinct clinical situations qualifying for the dissemination in time criterion (Figure 4.6). In the relapsing–remitting phase, relapses alternate with periods of clinical inactivity and may or may not be marked by sequelae depending on the presence of neurological deficits between episodes. By definition, periods between relapses during the relapsing–remitting phase are clinically stable. The progressive phase of multiple sclerosis is characterized by a steady increase in deficits, as defined above and either from onset or after a period of episodes, but this designation does not preclude the further occurrence of new relapses. Thus, a full understanding of the natural history requires more than just the two basic contexts of clinical activity to be considered.

The several forms of the clinical course

Patients do not necessarily convert from the relapsing–remitting to the progressive phase: but if they do, the migration is irreversible even though the transition can initially be hard to recognize, especially when the early secondary progressive phase is characterized by continuing relapses. From the first clinical descriptions of multiple sclerosis, it was recognized that the disease may also follow a progressive course from clinical onset.

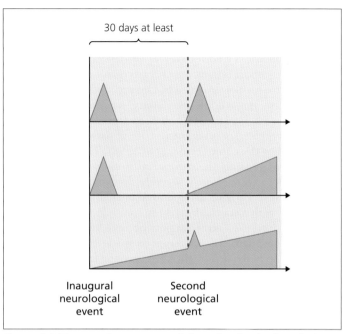

Figure 4.6 Three major patterns of dissemination in time during the course of multiple sclerosis. Top: two consecutive distinct relapses. Middle: inaugural relapse followed by the onset of the progressive phase. Bottom: onset of the progressive phase followed by a superimposed relapse. In these three instances, the time interval required between any two neurological events is ≥ 30 days.

Given this matrix, for many years classification of the clinical course in patients with multiple sclerosis distinguished three categories: relapsing–remitting; relapsing progressive, describing the situation of a relapsing–remitting phase followed by progression; and progressive multiple sclerosis, to cover the eventuality of a progressive course from onset with or without superimposed relapses (Broman *et al* 1981; Confavreux 1977; Confavreux *et al* 1980; Fog and Linnemann 1970; Leibowitz and Alter 1970; 1973; Leibowitz *et al* 1964a; 1964b; McAlpine and Compston 1952; D.H. Miller *et al* 1992a; Phadke 1987; 1990; S. Poser 1978; S. Poser *et al* 1982a; Runmarker and Andersen 1993; Trojano *et al* 1995; Weinshenker *et al* 1989a). At that time, a specific terminology was used by some authors to make the distinction between primary progressive forms with superimposed relapses (the so-called 'relapsing progressive' or 'progressive relapsing' forms, depending on preference) and primary progressive multiple sclerosis without superimposed relapses (the so-called 'chronic progressive' forms). To standardize the terminology used in the description of the pattern and course of multiple sclerosis, and to avoid confusion in communication, an international survey of clinicians involved in multiple sclerosis was performed under the auspices of the National Multiple Sclerosis Society of the USA (Lublin and Reingold 1996). The consensus intended to classify the disease course in four different categories (we regret the use of abbreviations but retain these for clarity of identification):

- *Relapsing–remitting MS (RR-MS)*: 'clearly defined relapses with full recovery or with sequelae and residual deficit upon recovery; periods between disease relapses characterized by a lack of disease progression'.

- *Secondary progressive MS (SP-MS)*: 'initial relapsing–remitting disease course followed by progression with or without occasional relapses, minor remissions, and plateaus'.
- *Primary progressive MS (PP-MS)*: 'disease progression from onset with occasional plateaus and temporary minor improvements allowed'.
- *Progressive relapsing MS (PR-MS)*: 'progressive disease from onset, with clear acute relapses, with or without full recovery; periods between relapses characterized by continuing progression'.

It must be noted that in this classification the presence of superimposed relapses is allowed in cases of secondary progressive multiple sclerosis, whereas primary progressive cases with superimposed episodes are segregated from primary progressive cases without relapses (PR-MS vs. PP-MS). Furthermore, the term 'relapsing progressive multiple sclerosis' is abandoned because the participating clinicians did not agree on its definition and the proposed definitions overlap with other categories. This classification is illustrated in Figure 4.7. Some authors add 'transitional progressive multiple sclerosis' (TP-MS) to this list, in order to identify the few patients with a course that is progressive except for a single relapse at some time (Filippi *et al* 1995b; Gayou *et al* 1997; Stevenson *et al* 1999; 2000). Some authors reserve this term only for cases with a progressive course devoid of superimposed relapses beginning many years after an isolated episode (Gayou *et al* 1997), whereas others allow the single attack before or after the onset of disease progression (Stevenson *et al* 1999; 2000). Because there is no consensus amongst these authors, and the efforts of the National Multiple Sclerosis Society international survey towards standardization and rationalization are sound and deserving of support, our position is that the few cases of transitional progressive multiple

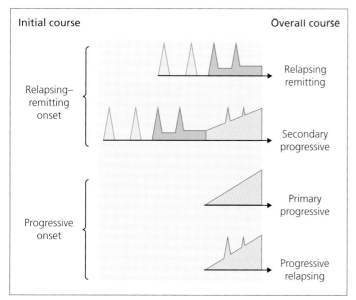

Figure 4.7 Classification of the course of multiple sclerosis. Adapted from Lublin and Reingold (1996). © 1996, reprinted with permission of Lippincott Williams & Wilkins (lww.com).

sclerosis can easily be accommodated within the recommended classification, assignment to the categories of primary or secondary progressive multiple sclerosis being determined by when the single episode occurs (Lublin and Reingold 1996). But we recognize that this can prove confusing to patients seeking not to be classified as having progressive multiple sclerosis when negotiating guidelines for the use of disease modifying therapies that are only prescribed and reimbursed for individuals with relapsing–remitting multiple sclerosis.

Prognosis-related dependent variables

The second dimension in the history of multiple sclerosis is the appearance of disability. This is quantitative and may prove to be transient, partially reversible, or definitely irreversible. A way of describing the natural outcome of multiple sclerosis is therefore to assess the time course to accumulation of disability. We discuss schemes that directly address the rate of progression in Chapter 6; these depend on two closely related scales used in the vast majority of studies that describe the natural history of multiple sclerosis – the DSS (Kurtzke 1961; 1965a) and its more detailed version, the EDSS (Kurtzke 1983a). Until the mid-20th century, standards used to assess the degree of disablement in multiple sclerosis were usually based either upon the capacity to work, or mobility. However, the former criterion is unreliable because it depends on individual fortitude, economic needs, and the nature of employment. The degree of mobility soon emerged as a better standard although it also is subject to potential confounds (McAlpine and Compston 1952). Classifications based mainly on degree of mobility have shortcomings because they do not take account of upper limb function, sensory symptoms, involvement of the bladder and bowel, defective vision, cranial nerve abnormalities, cognitive deficits, mood disorders or fatigue (McAlpine and Compston 1952; Rudick *et al* 1996a). Furthermore, the normal aging process may confound results based on these classifications, in older individuals where comorbidity with musculoskeletal, cardiovascular and respiratory disturbances may introduce complexities. That said, such classifications do reflect the global impairment caused by multiple sclerosis, first manifest as a disturbance in walking. This undoubtedly explains the popularity gained by Kurtzke's scales amongst the community of clinicians with a special interest in multiple sclerosis. Rather few other systems proposed for use in multiple sclerosis have gained acceptance; and, to date, no one fulfils requirements of the international multiple sclerosis community (Hobart *et al* 1996; 2001; Sharrack *et al* 1999). Although new, more sensitive and multidimensional measures have been proposed, particularly for use in clinical trials (Rudick *et al* 1996a; 1997), Kurtzke's scales are not displaced and remain, so far, the 'gold standards' for grading clinical impairment and disability in multiple sclerosis; *de facto*, they now represent reference criteria for any novel system that challenges their status and seeks to remove John Kurtzke from the podium of international approval built on familiarity and usage despite much criticism and exposition of the deficiencies. Of the two, the EDSS is now more commonly used than the DSS, especially in clinical trials (but see also below).

The limitations of the DSS are that the scale is unresponsive, combines impairment and disability, has often been shown to have only moderate inter-rater reliability, is not entirely objective, and is heavily weighted towards ambulation (Amato *et al* 1988; 2004; D.A. Francis *et al* 1991; Goodkin *et al* 1992; Hobart *et al* 1996; 2001; Noseworthy *et al* 1990; Rudick *et al* 1996a; 1997; Willoughby and Paty 1988). It was precisely in order to improve responsiveness that the 'expanded' disability scale was elaborated. However, it soon appeared that what could be gained in precision was lost in reliability. Furthermore, the EDSS was found to provide a ranking that proved too discrete with respect to the well-demonstrated daily fluctuations in neurological signs and symptoms that characterize the course of multiple sclerosis. Administration of the EDSS often proves too complex and time consuming for physicians who do not specialize in multiple sclerosis, and even more so for epidemiological purposes requiring long-term follow-up of very many patients. Therefore, the DSS is often preferred in such settings: for example, only well-identified steps that are easily assessed even in retrospect, such as DSS 4 (limited ambulation but without aid) or DSS 6 (walking with uni- or bilateral support), are important in many epidemiological studies. It is for this reason that the EDMUS Steering Committee decided to design a simplified version of the original DSS allowing similar grading but with more rapid administration and focus on essential points reported directly by the patient, each level having a short, precise and unambiguous description (Confavreux *et al* 1992). In a European multicentre collaborative study involving six centres and 180 patients with multiple sclerosis, agreement was greater for the EDMUS Grading Scale (EGS) than for the EDSS at all intervals (Amato *et al* 2004).

It must be realized that the EDSS is ordinal and categorical but neither quantitative nor continuous. The assumption that disability naturally continues to progress at a similar rate throughout the course of the disease is clearly contradicted by observations made on different samples: the distribution of patients according to DSS score at the last follow-up is bimodal with distinct peaks at DSS 1–2, and DSS 6–7 (Table 4.3) (D.H. Miller *et al* 1992a; Minderhoud *et al* 1988; Weinshenker *et al* 1989a). It follows that the length of time spent by patients at each level of the DSS scale is uneven, being longer for DSS 1–2, and DSS 6–7 (Table 4.4) (Weinshenker *et al* 1991b). Therefore, the progression from one level to the next on the DSS scale cannot be predicted or considered as equivalent. This means that change in the mean DSS, which has often been used in studies on natural history or in therapeutic trials in multiple sclerosis, is not a valid strategy for describing change or comparing groups. Self-evidently, this confusion would not have arisen if letters instead of figures had been proposed to rank the DSS scale. Differences in the proportion of patients changing by a given degree of disability, and the period over which this occurs, are methodologically more acceptable. Ideally, patients might also be stratified by baseline DSS at inclusion (Weinshenker *et al* 1991b). Our position is that, using classifications such as the Kurtzke scales, survival techniques are currently the best means of assessing the time to reach a selected level of disability.

Table 4.3 Distribution (%) of patients in relation to disability status scale at last follow-up examination: data from the literature

Disability status score	Weinshenker *et al* 1989a: n = 1099	Miller *et al* 1992a n = 209
0	–	1
1	17	28
2	14	17
3	11	14
4	6	10
5	3	3
6	19	7
7	18	11
8	8	6
9	2	3
10	1	–

Table 4.4 Time spent at each level of the disability status scale, among 1099 patients with multiple sclerosis. Adapted from Weinshenker *et al* (1991b)

Disability status scale	Patients entering a given disability status score grade (number)	Patients worsening (%)[a]	Time spent at disability status scale grade (mean number of years ± SEM)
1	1037	82	4.1 ± 0.2
2	829	81	2.8 ± 0.1
3	662	82	1.9 ± 0.1
4	536	88	1.2 ± 0.1
5	475	94	1.2 ± 0.1
6	489	60	3.1 ± 0.2
7	306	37	3.8 ± 0.3
8	114	28	2.4 ± 0.4
9	34	41	2.5 ± 0.6

a Percentage of patients who have reached a given disability status scale grade and progressed to the next level of disability during the study period.

THE ONSET OF MULTIPLE SCLEROSIS

The many series that report the natural history of multiple sclerosis provide an excellent basis for describing demographic and disease-related characteristics at the onset of multiple sclerosis, and thereafter. These are summarized in Table 4.5. The reader may (correctly) detect some familiarity in the structure of our accounts on factors detectable early in the illness that correlate with the later course, severity and survival in multiple sclerosis. The influences of gender, age and symptoms at onset on dynamics of the relapsing–remitting phase, disability and time to progression are so interwoven as to create the impression of repetition in one account. But in reality, these interactions reinforce the evidence for coherence in listing features that describe and predict the natural history of multiple sclerosis, at least amongst groups if not the individual patient.

Table 4.5 Main series of the long-term course and prognosis of multiple sclerosis: demographic and multiple sclerosis onset characteristics

Study	Gender: males / females (%)	Age at onset (years)	Initial symptoms of multiple sclerosis (%)		Initial course: relapsing–remitting / progressive (%)
Long-term natural history series with cross-sectional and/or some longitudinal assessment					
R. Müller 1949; 1951	44/56	24 (median)	Optic neuritis Brainstem Motor Sensory Sphincter	20 33 66 33 7	87/13
McAlpine and Compston 1952	35/65	29 (median)	Not available		90/10
Leibowitz *et al* 1964a; 1964b Leibowitz and Alter 1970; 1973	49/51	32.6 (mean)	Visual Brainstem/cerebellar Motor Sensory Motor and sensory Mixed	14 11 38 13 8 12	Not available
Panelius 1969	38/62	28.8 (mean)	Visual Brainstem Motor/coordination Sensory	21 24 33 22	90/10
S. Poser 1978	36/64	31.1 (mean)	Not available		82/18
S. Poser *et al* 1982a	35/65	30 (mean)	Not available		87/13
V.A. Clark *et al* 1982 Detels *et al* 1982 Visscher *et al* 1984	29/71	33 (mean)	Visual Diplopia Other cranial nerves Speech Motor Sensory Incoordination	20 25 20 18 63 61 58	Not available
Phadke 1987; 1990	35/65	30 (median)	Optic nerve Brainstem Cerebellar Spinal cord Cerebral Mixed	11 24 4 42 1 18	91/9
Minderhoud *et al* 1988	40/60	Not available	Not available		63/37
D.H. Miller *et al* 1992a	29/71	32.2 (mean)	Optic neuritis Brainstem Limb sensory Limb motor Limb motor/sensory Cerebellar Cerebral	21 23 27 14 9 2.5 3.5	95/5

table continued on following page

Table 4.5 **Main series of the long-term course and prognosis of multiple sclerosis: demographic and multiple sclerosis onset characteristics, cont'd**

Study	Gender: males / females (%)	Age at onset (years)	Initial symptoms of multiple sclerosis (%)		Initial course: relapsing–remitting / progressive (%)
Riise *et al* 1992	36 / 64	31.7 (mean)	Visual Brainstem Pyramidal Cerebellar Sensory	25 22 35 17 46	88 / 12
Trojano *et al* 1995	44 / 56	26 ± 8 (mean ± SD)	Not available		81 / 19
Kantarci *et al* 1998	36 / 64	27.6 ± 8.8 (mean ± SD) 27 (median)	Optic neuritis Brainstem / cerebellar Motor Sensory Sphincter	20 30 40 43 7	88 / 12
Myhr *et al* 2001	38 / 62	32.5 ± 0.6 (mean ± SEM)	Visual Brainstem / cerebellar Motor Sensory Sphincter Multiple systems involved	16 34 32 34 2 18	81 / 19
Long-term natural history cohorts with longitudinal follow-up					
United States Army Veterans World War II cohort					
Kurtzke *et al* 1968a; 1970a; 1973; 1977	Males only	25 (mean)	Visual Brainstem Motor limb Coordination limb Sensory limb Bowel / bladder Cerebral	31 40 52 44 42 14 13	Not available
Lyon, France, multiple sclerosis cohort					
Confavreux 1977 Confavreux *et al* 1980	40 / 60	31.3 ± 10.1 (mean ± SD) 30.6 (median)	Not available		82 / 18
Confavreux *et al* 2000; 2003	36 / 64	31 ± 10 (mean ± SD) 30 (median)	Isolated optic neuritis Isolated brainstem dysfunction Isolated dysfunction of long tracts Combination of symptoms	18 9 52 21	85 / 15
Gothenburg, Sweden, multiple sclerosis cohort					
Broman *et al* 1981 Runmarker and Andersen 1993 Eriksson *et al* 2003	40 / 60	Not available	Not available		83 / 17
London, Ontario, multiple sclerosis cohort					
Weinshenker *et al* 1989a; 1989b; 1991a; 1991b	34 / 66	30.5 ± 0.3 (mean ± SEM) 29 (median)	Optic neuritis Diplopia / vertigo Acute motor Insidious motor Balance / limb ataxia Sensory	17 13 6 14 13 45	66 / 34
Long-term history series from the therapeutic era					
Amato *et al* 1999 Amato and Ponziani 2000	36 / 64	29.8 ± 9.8 (mean ± SD)	Not available		85 / 15

SD = standard deviation.
SEM = standard error of the mean.

The sex ratio in multiple sclerosis

A female predominance is apparent in all representative studies (Amato and Ponziani 2000; Amato *et al* 1999; Bonduelle and Albaranès 1962; V.A. Clark *et al* 1982; Confavreux *et al* 1980; 2000; 2003; Detels *et al* 1982; Kantarci *et al* 1998; Leibowitz and Alter 1970; 1973; Leibowitz *et al* 1964a; 1964b; McAlpine 1961; McAlpine and Compston 1952; D.H. Miller *et al* 1992a; R. Müller 1949; 1951; Myhr *et al* 2001; Panelius 1969; Phadke 1987; 1990; S. Poser 1978; S. Poser *et al* 1982a; Riise *et al* 1992; Runmarker and Andersen 1993; Trojano *et al* 1995; Visscher *et al* 1984; Weinshenker *et al* 1989a; 1989b; 1991a; 1991b). The usual ratio is two females for one male (2F:M). The highest reported proportion of females is 71% (2.5F:M) in series from North America (V.A. Clark *et al* 1982; Detels *et al* 1982;

Visscher *et al* 1984) and New Zealand (D.H. Miller *et al* 1992a). Similarly, of the 324 living cases in all categories of multiple sclerosis from London, Ontario, and Middlesex County on 1st January 1984, 71% (2.5F:M) were females (Hader *et al* 1988). The lowest proportion reported is 51% (1.04F:M) in Israeli series (Leibowitz *et al* 1964a; 1964b; Leibowitz and Alter 1970; 1973).

Age at onset

It is not always easy to determine the age at which symptoms of multiple sclerosis first develop. Some symptoms, such as paraesthesia, are nonspecific and often so vague as easily to be overlooked. However, there is consensus for peak onset around 30 years of age (Table 4.6 and Figure 4.8) (Amato and Ponziani

Table 4.6 Distribution of patients with multiple sclerosis (%) by age at onset: data from the literature

Age at onset of multiple sclerosis (years)	R. Müller 1951 n = 793	McAlpine and Compston 1952 n = 840	Leibowitz et al 1964a; 1964b n = 266	Panelius 1969 n = 146	Confavreux et al 1980 n = 349	S. Poser et al 1982b n = 1529	Confavreux et al 2000; 2003 n = 1844
<20	22	12	15	11	11	10	12
20–29	46	35	27	48	36	36	37
30–39	24	33	28	31	33	33	30
40–49	7	17	22	9	14	21	15
≥50	1	3	8	1	6		6

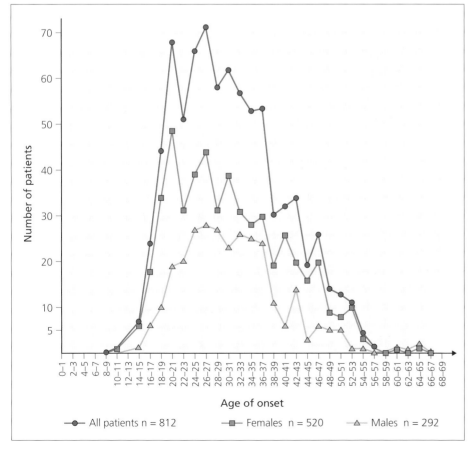

Figure 4.8 Distribution of patients by age at onset of the disease, among 812 patients with multiple sclerosis. Adapted from S. Poser (1978). © 1978, reprinted with permission of Springer-Verlag GmbH.

2000; Amato *et al* 1999; V.A. Clark *et al* 1982; Confavreux *et al* 1980; 2000; 2003; Detels *et al* 1982; Leibowitz and Alter 1970; 1973; Leibowitz *et al* 1964a; 1964b; McAlpine and Compston 1952; D.H. Miller *et al* 1992a; Myhr *et al* 2001; Panelius 1969; Phadke 1987; 1990; S. Poser 1978; S. Poser *et al* 1982a; Riise *et al* 1992; Visscher *et al* 1984; Weinshenker *et al* 1989a; 1989b; 1991a; 1991b). An earlier onset has been found in some series (Kantarci *et al* 1998; Kurtzke *et al* 1968a; 1970a; 1973; 1977; R. Müller 1949; 1951; Trojano *et al* 1995). R. Müller (1949) observed a median age at onset of 24 years in his comprehensive multicentre Swedish study: 22% of cases first experienced symptoms at <20 years. He emphasized that, for the reasons mentioned above, 'the anamnesis should be very carefully recorded in order to obtain more exact information as to the age at the outset of the disease.' This often corrects age at onset to an earlier age by comparison with the spontaneous statements of patients. R. Müller (1949) concluded: 'the explanation of the low age at the outset of the disease in this material is probably only because I devoted more attention to this point than had actually been the case.' For the United States Army Veterans cohort (Kurtzke *et al* 1968a; 1970a; 1973; 1977), the circumstances of enrolment (military service) easily account for the observed low median age at onset (25 years). For the two other series, the explanation is less straightforward (Kantarci *et al* 1998; Trojano *et al* 1995). In the majority of representative series, the distribution of patients with multiple sclerosis by age at onset is bell-shaped, with onset at ≤20 years in around 10%, at ages 20–40 years in 70%, and >40 years in 20% of cases (Bonduelle and Albaranès 1962; Confavreux *et al* 1980; 2000; McAlpine 1961; McAlpine and Compston 1952; 2003; S. Poser *et al* 1982a). In London, Ontario, onset of multiple sclerosis occurred at <20 years in 11%, and at >40 years in 20% of cases, respectively (Hader *et al* 1988). The distribution was less restricted in the study of Leibowitz and Alter (1970; 1973).

Females often appear to have a slightly younger mean age at onset than males (R. Müller 1949; 1950; McAlpine 1961). In London, Ontario, age at onset of clinically definite multiple sclerosis was 29.7 (±10.1) years for females, with a range of 10–58 years, and 31.7 (±11.8) with a range of 6–66 years for males (Hader *et al* 1988). In the Israeli series, the difference was even more marked – mean age at onset with multiple sclerosis being 31.9 years in females and 34.4 years in males. Furthermore, the F:M ratio was found to decrease as age at onset increased (Leibowitz and Alter 1970; 1973; Leibowitz *et al* 1964a; 1964b). Other authors have not considered that gender has a significant impact on age at onset (McAlpine and Compston 1952; Panelius 1969; S. Poser 1978). In the Lyon, France, series (Confavreux *et al* 1980), mean age at onset of multiple sclerosis was higher in females (32.6 years) than males (29.4 years) with a significantly greater incidence of the disease in females aged >40 years at the time of presentation (p < 0.01).

Symptoms at onset

At least in retrospect, symptoms can conservatively be placed in three categories: those affecting the optic nerves, the brainstem, and the long tracts – the latter designating symptoms related to motor, sensory, cerebellar or sphincter disturbances. It must be acknowledged that these categories do not strictly represent anatomical regions in the central nervous system (Broman *et al*

1981). For instance, in addition to the effects on bulbar function, eye movements and motor control, brainstem lesions may also affect the long sensory and motor tracts. Long tract symptoms cannot, in many cases, be referred to a specific part of the central nervous system. We consider it difficult, if not actually erroneous, to force too much precision onto the description and classification of inaugural symptoms and signs in multiple sclerosis, at least in the series for which there is an interval of months or years between clinical onset of the disease and first professional evaluation. For instance, cerebellar symptoms, in many cases assessed retrospectively, cannot always be distinguished from those attributable to involvement of motor or sensory tracts. It is often risky to conclude that gait disturbance is due entirely to ataxia, paraparesis or both – based merely on the interpretation of a neurological interview. Whilst acknowledging that the above classification of symptoms into three categories is imperfect and restrictive, we and others nonetheless consider it to be pragmatic, and an acceptable compromise. For instance, in their comprehensive epidemiological surveys in Norway, Riise *et al* (1988; 1992) changed the classification of initial symptoms for defined categories referable to functional systems of the DSS. For example, 'motor weakness' in the first study was subsequently changed to the 'pyramidal' category. The authors did, however, admit that 'the names used apply to the grouping of symptoms and do not necessarily mean that they can be referred to a specific location or lesion. For instance, "pyramidal function" does not mean that the signs are due only to lesions involving the pyramidal tract' (Riise *et al* 1992). We entirely endorse these conclusions. Their consequences are clear. It is risky and often erroneous to categorize initial symptoms too strictly, at least when the assessment is sometimes made years after disease onset. Data related to initial symptoms must therefore be treated as not very robust in the majority of long-term natural history series. This should be kept in mind when interpreting results on the possible predictive value of initial symptoms for disease outcome.

The different long-term natural history series in the literature show some consensus with respect to the distribution of initial symptoms in multiple sclerosis (Table 4.5). However, detailed comparisons between series are rendered impossible through the use of variations in terminology and the failure by many authors to distinguish the occurrence of symptoms in isolation and in combination. It is difficult to delineate precisely what is intended by the terms 'monosymptomatic, polysymptomatic, monoregional and polyregional' in the studies that adopt these terminologies. That said, an incidence of around 15% for isolated optic neuritis, 10% for isolated brainstem dysfunction, 50% for isolated dysfunction of long tracts, and 25% for various combinations of these features are reasonable estimates for the distribution of initial symptoms in multiple sclerosis (see Chapter 6).

In the rare instances where this issue has been specifically addressed, the influence of gender on symptoms at presentation of multiple sclerosis has been found not to exist (Panelius 1969), or to exert only a marginal effect showing a slightly greater frequency of long tract involvement in men, and of optic neuritis and diplopia in females (Leibowitz and Alter 1973; R. Müller 1949). The latter trend presumably results from the older age at onset of multiple sclerosis in males than females in these series. Indeed, the obvious influence of age at onset has

Table 4.7 Distribution of patients (%) by initial symptoms according to age at onset of multiple sclerosis, among 1096 patients. Adapted from Weinshenker *et al* (1989a)

Age at onset of multiple sclerosis (years)	Optic neuritis	Diplopia / vertigo	Acute motor	Insidious motor	Balance / limb ataxia	Sensory
<20	23	18	6	4	14	46
20–29	23	12	7	6	11	52
30–39	13	11	7	14	15	44
40–49	9	17	3	31	13	33
≥50	6	13	4	47	11	32

consistently been found in all studies that addressed this issue, with a higher percentage of optic neuritis and diplopia in patients with earlier age at onset, and of motor disturbances in the patients presenting later (Leibowitz and Alter 1973; Leibowitz *et al* 1964b; R. Müller 1949; 1951). Table 4.7 shows a further illustrative example from the London, Ontario, cohort.

The initial clinical course

For more than a century, all experts have agreed that multiple sclerosis usually follows an initial relapsing–remitting course, although some individuals progress from onset. Differences emerge amongst series in the literature as to the relative proportions displaying these two patterns (see Table 4.5). Indeed, the frequency of cases with progression from onset has been found to range from 5% (D.H. Miller *et al* 1992a) to 37% (Minderhoud *et al* 1988). The latter figure seems to be an outlier, and may be related to recruitment bias because this Dutch study was mainly devoted to an assessment of year at onset of the progressive phase. The estimate of 34% with primary progressive multiple sclerosis coming from the London, Ontario, cohort is, at first sight, more surprising if one considers the comprehensive sampling (Weinshenker *et al* 1989a; 1989b). Actually, among the subgroup of 197 patients seen from the onset of multiple sclerosis in this series, only 15% exhibited an initial progressive course with or without superimposed relapses, a figure similar to that of the other main long-term longitudinal natural history series (Confavreux *et al* 1980; 2000; 2003; Eriksson *et al* 2003; Runmarker and Andersen 1993). According to the Canadian authors, this disparity could reflect a tendency for patients seen for the first time at a later point in their illness to suppress or forget earlier remitting symptoms when progressive disease subsequently intervenes. It is their experience that a patient may recall a remote first relapse only after several clinic visits (Weinshenker *et al* 1989a). Moreover, when these authors updated details on their cohort in 1996, they had to reassign a significant number of patients with respect to the overall clinical course of the disease (D.A. Cottrell *et al* 1999a; 1999b; Kremenchutzky *et al* 1999). This led to a total of 216 cases with primary progressive multiple sclerosis, as defined. This represented 21% of the total cohort, a figure in agreement with that of the other main longitudinal natural history series (Confavreux *et al* 1980; 2000; 2003; Eriksson *et al* 2003; Runmarker and Andersen 1993). Noticeably,

in all of these longitudinal series, the group of primary progressive multiple sclerosis encompasses cases with and without relapses superimposed on disease progression – that is, progressive relapsing and primary progressive multiple sclerosis according to current definitions (Lublin and Reingold 1996). Taken together, the initial course of multiple sclerosis can be reasonably estimated to be relapsing–remitting in 85% and progressive in 15% of cases (Table 4.5).

It has been appreciated for half a century that men more often show a progressive onset of multiple sclerosis than women (R. Müller 1949; 1951). Symptoms related to dysfunction of long tracts are relatively more frequent in males, whereas optic nerve and brainstem features occur less often in progressive onset than relapsing–remitting multiple sclerosis (Table 4.8) (Confavreux *et al* 1980; McAlpine and Compston 1952; R. Müller 1949; 1950; Riise *et al* 1992; Trojano *et al* 1995). The proportion of progressive onset cases rises steadily with age (Table 4.9) (Confavreux 1977; Leibowitz *et al* 1964a; 1964b; McAlpine and Compston 1952; R. Müller 1949; 1950; Phadke 1990; S. Poser 1978; S. Poser *et al* 1982b; Weinshenker *et al* 1989a). Gender, clinical features, age and the course at onset are interdependent and there is much potential for confounding of contributing factors in these analyses. The strongest correlation between clinical variables and the initial course of the disease is with age at onset. Thus, we can caricature the progressive onset of multiple sclerosis as a disorder of motor deficits occurring in older males. This analysis says nothing concerning

Table 4.8 Distribution of patients (%) by initial symptoms according to the initial course of multiple sclerosis, among 574 patients. Adapted from Riise *et al* (1992)

	Initial course of multiple sclerosis	
	Relapsing–remitting	Progressive
Pyramidal	32	54
Cerebellar	16	23
Brainstem	24	7
Sensory	48	32
Visual	26	17

Table 4.9 Percentages of patients with a progressive initial course of multiple sclerosis according to age at onset: data from the literature

Age at onset of multiple sclerosis (years)	McAlpine and Compston 1952 n = 414	Confavreux 1977 n = 349	S. Poser et al 1982b n = 1529	Weinshenker et al 1989a n = 1099	Phadke 1990 n = 1055
<20	0	3	9	18	3
20–29	5	10	13	19	4
30–39	14	25	27	38	5
40–49	24	24	41	63	14
≥50	29	45		74	27

the contribution to disability of manifestations that are clinically silent but discretely contribute to the accumulation of disability preceding presentation. But whatever came before, the recognition of motor symptoms attributable to multiple sclerosis at onset indicates and predicts a more advanced subsequent course of the disease.

THE OVERALL COURSE OF MULTIPLE SCLEROSIS

Most patients with multiple sclerosis experience changes in their condition that are distinct and hence recognizable – but sometimes only in retrospect – each constituting a pivotal event in the course of the illness. Easiest to recognize are the individual relapses; more elusive, but of considerable significance for the eventual level of disability, is onset of the progressive phase. In recent years, it has become commonplace to refer to a first neurological episode suggestive of multiple sclerosis as the 'clinically isolated syndrome', provided this can reasonably be attributed to the dysfunction of optic nerves, brainstem or spinal cord, with acute or subacute onset followed by recovery, and in the context of paraclinical investigations excluding an explanation other than that of suspected multiple sclerosis (Barkhof et al 1997a; Filippi et al 1994; Morrissey et al 1993a; O'Riordan et al 1998; Tintoré et al 2000). Some physicians restrict this term to situations in which the features are monosymptomatic, but these represent only a proportion of such episodes. Others also allow the term to indicate polysymptomatic presentations not attributable to a single central nervous system lesion, or any initial remitting episode whatever its neuroanatomical complexity. Amongst the subset of 1562 patients with an exacerbating–remitting onset of the disease in the Lyon, France, series, initial episodes were classified as monofocal or multifocal in 78% and 22% of cases, respectively. However, these monofocal initial episodes represent only 66% of the cases among the total cohort of 1844 patients with multiple sclerosis (Confavreux et al 2003). There is no evidence to suggest that the long-term course and prognosis of the disease are determined by the pattern of this initial episode – variously described by authors as monosymptomatic, polysymptomatic, monofocal or multifocal. Quite what they always mean is obscure and, as explained above, in order to avoid confusion, we use the term 'initial neurological episode' to cover these complexities of nomenclature.

Recovery from the initial neurological episode

On average, 85% of inaugural neurological episodes will remit, at least partially. The issue of spontaneous remission from symptoms at onset in multiple sclerosis has been studied in a series of 220 hospitalized male patients: the key predictive factor for remission was duration of the ongoing neurological episode prior to hospital admission (Kurtzke 1956). There was an inverse relationship between duration of the episode prior to admission and the probability of improvement (Table 4.10). The proportion of patients who improved decreased from 86%, when the episode lasted ≤7 days, to no improvement at all for the episodes lasting >2 years before admission. Interestingly, this decrease in the probability of improvement was steady throughout the 2-year interval prior to admission, without any discrete change allowing a recognizable frontier between exacerbation and progression to be established. The outcome of the ongoing neurological episode could not be correlated with age at onset of multiple sclerosis, duration of the disease at admission, age at admission, or symptoms, signs and severity of the neurological episode. However, conclusions regarding the possible lack of influence of age should be treated with caution due to the particular circumstances of inclusion in this Army series.

Table 4.10 Chance of recovery (%) from the first neurological episode subsequent to hospitalization according to duration of the neurological episode, prior to admission, among 220 patients with multiple sclerosis. Adapted from Kurtzke (1956)

Duration of the episode before admission	Probability (%) of improvement of the episode
≤7 days	86
8–14 days	64
15–31 days	38
1.1–2.0 months	18
2.1–6.0 months	14
6.1–12 months	18
1.1–2 years	7
>2 years	0

However, the results – consistent with some earlier observations (R. Müller 1949) – were confirmed and extended in the cohort of 527 United States Army World War II Veterans (Kurtzke *et al* 1973). Here, both duration of the episode prior to admission and its severity as assessed on the DSS scale, showed additive effects: the shorter and more severe the episode, the more likely was improvement at discharge from hospital, a finding consistent with the common experience of physicians involved in the care of people with multiple sclerosis. Significantly, only one patient received corticosteroid treatment during hospitalization.

There is no consensus in the literature on just what should reasonably qualify as incomplete recovery from the first neurological episode. This is particularly difficult to assess in retrospect, by the time disability has accumulated inexorably. Therefore, we are still surprisingly ill-informed on just how good is recovery from the initial attack. For instance, 18% of the 1562 patients with an exacerbating–remitting disease course in the Lyon, France, series (Confavreux *et al* 2003) matched the definition of incomplete recovery – being the persistence of at least a minimum ambulation-related disability or a significant non-ambulation-related problem qualifying for a score of DSS 3 or more after the first neurological episode. Using a similar definition, Trojano *et al* (1995) observed incomplete recovery in 16% of 180 patients with relapsing–remitting multiple sclerosis and in 32% of 69 patients who had matured into the secondary phase during their earlier experience of relapsing–remitting

multiple sclerosis. Using their own criteria, Eriksson *et al* (2003) observed incomplete recovery in 30% of 220 patients with a first acute episode suggestive of multiple sclerosis.

Taken together, these data clearly illustrate the difficulty that the clinician faces in deciding the nature, duration and consequences of early episodes when coming at the problem in retrospect, especially after the onset of secondary progressive multiple sclerosis (Goodkin *et al* 1989).

Development of the second neurological episode

This topic has recently stimulated renewed attention with the advent of possibilities for treatment. The occasion of a second neurological episode is sufficient for establishing that a person in the suspected category has converted to definite multiple sclerosis provided that the second episode involves a new site within the central nervous system (C.M. Poser *et al* 1983). This altered status may provide additional rationale for offering the patient disease modifying therapy.

McAlpine and Compston (1952) first demonstrated that the chance of a second neurological episode is highest immediately following the initial episode with a diminishing risk thereafter (Table 4.11). Their analysis was based upon crude data observed in 354 patients with ≥2 neurological episodes. According to this and other series, 65%, 45% and 25% of patients with a

Table 4.11 Second neurological episode in multiple sclerosis: data from the main series of the long-term course and prognosis in multiple sclerosis

Study	Time from the relapsing–remitting onset of multiple sclerosis to the second neurological episode (years)	Factors predictive of time from the relapsing–remitting onset of multiple sclerosis to the second neurological episode
Long-term natural history series with cross-sectional and/or some longitudinal assessment		
McAlpine and Compston 1952	Observed data 2 (median)	Not available
Myhr *et al* 2001	Observed data 3.5 ± 0.2 (mean ± SEM)	Not available
Long-term natural history cohorts with longitudinal follow-up		
Lyon, France, multiple sclerosis cohort		
Confavreux 1977 Confavreux *et al* 1980	Observed data 2 (median)	Observed data Gender: none Age at onset of multiple sclerosis: none Overall course of multiple sclerosis (relapsing–remitting vs. secondary progressive): none
Confavreux *et al* 2000; 2003	Life table analysis 2 (median)	Not available
Gothenburg, Sweden, multiple sclerosis cohort		
Broman *et al* 1981 Runmarker and Andersen 1993 Eriksson *et al* 2003	Life table analysis *Cases with a 'clinically isolated syndrome' at onset:* 3.25 ± 0.64 (median ± SEM)	Life table analysis Cox regression analysis *Cases with a 'clinically isolated syndrome' at onset:* Gender/age at onset: none Initial symptoms: optic neuritis/sensory, longer; long tracts, shorter; monofocality, none Recovery from first episode: none

SD = standard deviation.
SEM = standard error of the mean.

Table 4.12 **Kaplan–Meier estimates of the time (years) from onset of multiple sclerosis to the second neurological episode, among the 1562 patients with a relapsing-remitting initial course from the Lyon, France, multiple sclerosis cohort. Adapted from Confavreux *et al* (2003)**

Time (years)	0	0.5	1	2	3	4	5	6	7	8	9	10	11	12	13	14	15	16	17	18	19	20
Patients (%) free from second neurological episode	100	81	63	47	37	30	26	22	18	15	14	12	10	9	8	7	6	5	4	4	3	3

	Median time (years)	Patients (%) who did not reach the end point[a]
Time to second neurological episode	1.9 [95% CI 1.7–2.1]	12

a Data on patients who did not reach the end point were censored at the time of the last clinic visit.

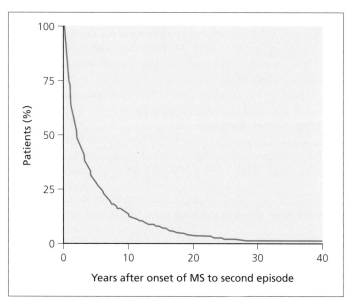

Figure 4.9 Kaplan–Meier estimates for the time (years) from onset of multiple sclerosis to the second episode, among the 1562 patients with a relapsing–remitting initial course in the Lyon, France, multiple sclerosis cohort. Adapted from Confavreux *et al* (2003).

relapsing–remitting initial course of multiple sclerosis remain free from a second neurological episode at 1, 2 and 5 years of disease duration, respectively. A similar distribution was observed in the Lyon, France, series with median time interval of 2 years between the inaugural episode and the first relapse, both when performing the survival analyses early in the course (Confavreux 1977; Confavreux *et al* 1980) and when the cohort was larger and more mature (Table 4.12 and Figure 4.9; Confavreux *et al* 2000; 2003). These results are supported by a Norwegian study showing a 3.5-year mean time to reach the second neurological episode (Myhr *et al* 2001) compared with 4.2 years in the Lyon series (Confavreux *et al* 2000; 2003). That said, given the exponential decay of time to the second neurological episode, medians are to be preferred to means for its description. In fact, only a Swedish study has shown markedly different results (Eriksson *et al* 2003), with a median time to the second neurological episode of 3.25 years, as estimated by survival analysis. In this study, however, the assessments were restricted to cases with a 'clinically isolated syndrome' (see

above) among the cases with an exacerbating–remitting onset of multiple sclerosis. In some of these long-term natural history series, analyses were performed to reveal clinical factors predictive of the time from onset of multiple sclerosis to the second neurological episode. Gender and age at onset of the disease had no effect (Confavreux *et al* 1980; Eriksson *et al* 2003), and neither did the mono- or multifocal nature of initial symptoms, or degree of recovery from the initial episode (Eriksson *et al* 2003; also C. Confavreaux and S. Vukusic, unpublished data) and overall course of multiple sclerosis – whether that is relapsing–remitting or secondary progressive at the time of assessment (Confavreux *et al* 1980). By contrast, visual or sensory symptoms at onset have been associated with a longer time to the second episode, and any spinal cord syndrome with a shorter interval (Eriksson *et al* 2003; Tintoré *et al* 2005; C. Confavreux and S. Vukusic, unpublished data).

A second source of information comes from the placebo arms of randomized controlled trials that specifically enrolled patients with a first neurological episode suggestive of multiple sclerosis – the Optic Neuritis Treatment Trial (ONTT: Beck 1995; Beck *et al* 1992; 1993a), Controlled High Risk Subjects Avonex™ Multiple Sclerosis Prevention Study (CHAMPS: Beck *et al* 2002; Jacobs *et al* 2000) and Early Treatment Of Multiple Sclerosis (ETOMS: Comi *et al* 2001a) therapeutic trials. The cumulative probability according to Kaplan–Meier estimates of developing a second neurological episode qualifying for multiple sclerosis at 2 years was 18% in ONTT, 38% in CHAMPS, and 45% in ETOMS. By definition, only patients suffering from acute optic neuritis were enrolled in the ONTT trial whatever the results of brain MRI, while the CHAMPS trial enrolled patients with a monofocal episode involving the optic nerve (50%), spinal cord (28%) or brainstem / cerebellum (22%) with ≥2 T₂ lesions on brain MRI at entry. In the ETOMS trial, patients were enrolled following either a monofocal (61%) or multifocal (39%) episode with ≥4 T₂ lesions on brain MRI. These recruitment criteria presumably explain observed differences between these trials on the risk of developing a second neurological episode. It is well known that a significant proportion of acute optic neuritis will never convert to multiple sclerosis (Hickman *et al* 2002b). By contrast, recruitment criteria for the ETOMS trial were not restrictive with respect to clinical symptomatology of the initial episode. In this trial, median time to the second neurological episode was close to 2 years, consistent with the interval observed in long-term natural history series. According to the CHAMPS trial, the 2-year cumulative probability of developing a second episode is similar for optic neuritis, spinal cord syndromes, and brainstem/cerebellar syndromes (Beck *et al* 2002). The conversion rate was two times higher for multifocal than monofocal presentations in the ETOMS trial (Comi *et al* 2001a). Lastly, results from the ONTT, CHAMPS and ETOMS trials consistently showed a correlation between T_2 lesion number on brain MRI at entry and the development of a second episode (Beck *et al* 1993a; CHAMPS Study Group 2002; Comi *et al* 2001a; Optic Neuritis Study Group 1997a). The presence of enhancing lesions on the baseline MRI proved the strongest predictor for development of a second episode in CHAMPS (CHAMPS Study Group 2002) but was not influential in ETOMS (Comi *et al* 2001a).

Although usually offering a small sample size, and possibly biased by substantial numbers of patients lost to follow-up, prospective observational studies devoted to patients presenting with clinically isolated episodes have consistently provided results of considerable interest regarding the predictive value of baseline MRI. Although these data are discussed fully in Chapter 7, the story is summarized here in order to supplement the clinically orientated studies under discussion. The presence of multifocal brain MRI abnormalities markedly increases the probability of a second neurological episode within 1–3 years (Barkhof *et al* 1997c; Brex *et al* 2001a; Ford *et al* 1992; Frederiksen *et al* 1991b; Lee *et al* 1991; Martinelli *et al* 1991; D.H. Miller *et al* 1988a; 1989b; Paty *et al* 1988; Tintoré *et al* 2000; 2003), but also after 5 (Morrissey *et al* 1993a), 10 (O'Riordan *et al* 1998) and 14 years follow-up (Brex *et al* 2002). In the National Hospital, London, series of 89 patients, for instance, conversion to clinically definite multiple sclerosis was observed within 5 years in 65% of 57 cases with abnormal baseline T_2 brain MRI (defined as ≥1 lesions compatible with multiple sclerosis) compared with 3% of 32 cases with normal MRI (Morrissey *et al* 1993a). For the 81 patients still followed at 10 years, the corresponding figures were 83% and 11% (O'Riordan *et al* 1998). At 14 years, among the 71 patients still under scrutiny, conversion was observed in 88% and 19%, respectively (Brex *et al* 2002). The T_2 lesion volume on brain MRI at presentation also plays a role, correlating positively with the risk of developing a second episode (Filippi *et al* 1994; Brex *et al* 2002). An inverse relationship between the initial T_2 lesion load and time to development of a second episode has also been demonstrated (Filippi *et al* 1994). Several studies have shown that the presence of gadolinium enhancing lesions on T_1-weighted brain MRI is a stronger predictor than the presence of T_2 lesions for the probability of developing a second episode (Barkhof *et al* 1997a; Brex *et al* 2001a). An extensive analysis of the T_2 and T_1 parameters has also demonstrated that the presence of juxtacortical, infratentorial and periventricular lesions are all independent predictors for the short-term occurrence of a second neurological episode (Barkhof *et al* 1997a). Data gathered from early serial brain MRI add significantly to these predictions. The presence of new T_2 lesions or gadolinium enhancing lesions on a brain MRI performed 3 months after the baseline MRI (Brex *et al* 2001a) or 12 months after the initial episode (Tintoré *et al* 2003) are both predictors for the appearance of a second episode. For instance, among 68 patients presenting with a monofocal episode in the United Kingdom study (Brex *et al* 2001a), the development of a second episode at 1 year was observed in 33% of the 'baseline MRI T_2 positive' patients, 52% of the 'baseline MRI T_1 positive' cases, 57% of the 'repeatedly T_2 positive' individuals (defined by the presence of T_2 lesions on baseline MRI and of new T_2 lesions on the second scan performed 3 months later) and 70% of the 'repeatedly T_1 positive' patients. Information gathered from the second MRI therefore improves the positive predictive value and the specificity of MRI for the development of a second episode. These results are obtained whilst still maintaining sensitivity at >80% for T_2 criteria, but decreasing sensitivity from 61% with the baseline MRI only, to 39% with both brain sets of images using the T_1 criteria. These data served as the rationale for adopting serial early brain MRI as a surrogate for dissemination in time in patients still at the clinical stage of a single neurological episode (W.I. McDonald *et al* 2001).

As discussed in Chapters 3, 7 and 11, typical abnormalities in the cerebrospinal fluid and evoked potentials, sampled at baseline, and the presence of HLA-DR15 antigen are all associated with a shorter time to the second episode. However, their predictive value has been found to be much lower than that of brain MRI features in studies that compared these predictors (Frederiksen *et al* 1991; Lee *et al* 1991; Martinelli *et al* 1991; Morrissey *et al* 1993a; Paty *et al* 1988). Lately, in a study involving 103 patients with an initial monofocal episode, the presence of serum anti-myelin antibodies was associated with an adjusted hazard ratio for developing a second episode of 76 (95% CI 21–285), as compared with the seronegative patients (Berger *et al* 2003). Confirmation of these potentially promising data is required.

Relapse frequency

Despite much heated debate, consensus has not been reached on how often relapses actually occur in the relapsing–remitting phase of multiple sclerosis: estimates range from 0.1 to >1 per year. Such variability is not, in fact, surprising. We have already addressed the difficulties frequently encountered by the clinician in deciding whether the intensity of newly reported symptoms, or an increase in those that already exist, corresponds to recent activation of the disease process. But this judgment also relates to the frequency and timing of assessments. It has been well demonstrated that there are clear-cut differences in estimates of relapse frequency when comparing retrospective and prospective assessments, the latter usually yielding higher figures, and with more frequent scrutiny of the affected person with multiple sclerosis (Fog and Linnemann 1970; Patzold and Pocklington 1982). Therefore, prospective examinations at close intervals would appear the most sensitive strategy for the accurate assessment of relapse frequency. However, matters are not that simple. Indeed, the experience gathered lately from protocols using prospective follow-up of patients at monthly intervals has shown how often clinical assessors are faced with the difficult choice of calling subtle and transitory symptoms given the awareness of daily fluctuations in the experience of symptoms attributable to multiple sclerosis. Suspending judgment before taking a final decision is often wise. Moreover, for the reasons already discussed, prospective assessments at regular and close intervals throughout the duration of the disease for a large cohort of patients are not practical. Ambiguity and inaccuracy are therefore inevitably introduced, from the methodological standpoint, in the ascertainment of relapses in multiple sclerosis. But there is also true variation in relapse frequency – probably for biological reasons. This is clearly seen from the long-term follow-up of many individual patients, and in therapeutic trials recruiting participants with relapsing–remitting multiple sclerosis. Focusing on the untreated group, relapse rate is regularly found to be higher during the one or two years prior to inclusion than during the trial itself. 'Regression to the mean' arises from the fact that patients are often selected during periods of atypical disease activity before resuming their regular habits. Lastly, there are discrepancies in the methods for estimating relapse frequency. Some authors divide the total number of relapses by disease duration (in years) for all the patients in the cohort, whereas others only count relapses occurring during the relapsing–remitting phase of the disease. These sources of variability in evaluating the relapse rate are so influential that it is somewhat risky to compare results between various series; and experience gained from historical controls must not serve as a reference for the study of interest.

The available literature does, however, provide several interesting indicators. In the cross-sectional studies with ensuing retrospective assessment, the relapse rate is usually ≤0.5 per year: rates of 0.39, 0.28, 0.26 and 0.32 per year were observed by McAlpine and Compston (1952), Leibowitz et al (1964a), Panelius (1969), and Myhr et al (2001), respectively. Conversely, in studies with longitudinal prospective assessments, the relapse rate is usually >0.5 per year: estimates of 0.56, 0.86, 1.1 and 0.64 were reported by Fog and Linnemann (1970), Confavreux et al (1980), Patzold and Pocklington (1982), and Goodkin et al (1989), respectively. The results of these prospective studies are fairly consistent with the figure of 2 years for the median time from onset of multiple sclerosis to the second episode, and the same interval before the next in subsequent epochs, during the relapsing–remitting phase of the disease (C. Confavreux and S. Vukusic, unpublished data). It may be concluded that 0.5 or slightly more is a reasonable estimate of the yearly relapse rate in a standard, representative population of patients with relapsing–remitting multiple sclerosis.

Gender and age at onset have consistently been found not to influence the frequency of episodes (Confavreux et al 1980; Leibowitz and Alter 1973; Leibowitz et al 1964a; 1964b; McAlpine and Compston 1952; Panelius 1969), with the exception of a Swedish study in which age at onset correlated inversely with relapse rate (Broman et al 1981). Many authors consider that relapse rate declines with disease duration (Broman et al 1981; Leibowitz et al 1964a; McAlpine and Compston 1952; R. Müller 1949; Myhr et al 2001; Panelius 1969; Patzold and Pocklington 1982). For instance, McAlpine and Compston (1952) found an average relapse rate of 0.4 during the first 5 years of the disease, falling to 0.22 at 20–24 years. This has been challenged by a North American study in which the relapse rate, determined prospectively, was stable during the 3-year follow-up and uninfluenced by overall disease duration (Goodkin et al 1989). The evidence for a stable rate matches our own results, at least when calculations are restricted to the relapsing–remitting phase (Confavreux et al 1980). Furthermore, once the disease has entered its progressive and chronic disabling stage, relapse detection tends to become less prioritized and therefore more easily overlooked, resulting in an under-ascertainment of new episodes.

Onset of progression

Despite the methodological difficulties already discussed, inter-examiner reliability in assessing the onset of progression is reasonable. For instance, in a Dutch study involving 236 patients with primary or secondary progressive multiple sclerosis, agreement between three observers in determining the year of onset for progression was obtained in 62% of the secondary progressive cases and 78% of those with primary progressive multiple sclerosis (Minderhoud et al 1988). In the collaborative multi-centre EVALUED study – involving six European centres, 180 patients with multiple sclerosis and, for each centre, two examiners and 30 patients – inter-examiner reliability was almost perfect with a kappa value of 0.92 when cases had to be categorized according to an exacerbating–remitting or progressive onset (Amato et al 2004). When both examiners had to decide on the development of secondary progression, agreement was again substantial with a kappa value of 0.76. When they had to date the onset of secondary progression, agreement was reached between both examiners within 1 year in 72% of cases.

Our current knowledge on the onset of progression in multiple sclerosis has a reasonably secure evidence base (Table 4.13). Considering a cohort of patients with multiple sclerosis, including those with progression from onset, estimates of the time from onset of multiple sclerosis to progression are reasonably consistent. With calculations based upon observational data only, R. Müller (1949; 1951) found a median time to progression of 10 years. Using survival techniques, median time to progression turned out to be 11 years in the Lyon, France, series (Confavreux 1977; Confavreux et al 1980) and 9 years in the Gothenburg, Sweden, cohort (Eriksson et al 2003; Runmarker and Andersen 1993). In the cases from London, Ontario, the corresponding figure was only 5.8 years (Weinshenker et al 1989a) but it must be remembered that the proportion of cases classified as progressive from onset was unusually high in this cohort. In all these studies, age at onset was a strong predictor of time to progression, as expected from the observation that the proportion of progressive from onset relative to relapsing–remitting multiple sclerosis increases with age at presentation (see above).

The other strategy for addressing the onset of progression is to consider only the population of cases with an exacerbating–remitting onset of multiple sclerosis. This focuses on an issue of utmost importance for many patients and clinicians, because the emergence of secondary progression predicts disability and sets the stage for a less optimistic prognosis from that point forwards. Here, the literature is consistent (Table 4.13). McAlpine and Compston (1952) are to be credited with first clearly demonstrating that 'there is a fairly constant rate of change from a remitting to a progressive course, and a gradual rise in the total percentage of progressive cases as the disease advances'. A similar distribution has been found with analyses restricted to observational data by Broman et al (1981) and with survival analyses in the Lyon, France, series (Confavreux 1977; Confavreux et al 1980; Vukusic and Confavreux 2003b). The median time to secondary progression among the 1562 patients with an exacerbating–remitting onset in the Lyon, France, series was 19.1 years (Table 4.14 and Figure 4.10). From their population of 220 patients presenting with a 'distinct clinically isolated syndrome', Swedish authors observed a median of 19.0 years

Table 4.13 Progression in multiple sclerosis: data from the main series describing the long-term course and prognosis

Study	Time from onset of multiple sclerosis to progression (years)	Factors predictive of time from onset of multiple sclerosis to progression (years)
Long-term natural history series with cross-sectional and/or some longitudinal assessment		
R. Müller 1949; 1951	Observed data *All cases:* 10 (median)	Observed data Gender: male, shorter Age at onset of multiple sclerosis: older, shorter Initial symptoms: optic nerve/brainstem s/sensory, longer; motor, shorter Number of relapses during the first 5 years: greater, shorter
McAlpine and Compston 1952	Observed data *Cases with a relapsing–remitting initial course of multiple sclerosis:* 30 (median)	Observed data Gender: none
Riise *et al* 1992	Not available	Cox's proportional hazards regression model *Cases with a relapsing–remitting initial course of multiple sclerosis:* Gender: none Age at onset of multiple sclerosis: older, shorter Initial symptoms: pyramidal/cerebellar, shorter; visual, longer
Trojano *et al* 1995	Not available	Life table analysis Multivariate analysis *Cases with a relapsing–remitting initial course of multiple sclerosis:* Gender/initial symptoms: none Age at onset of multiple sclerosis: younger, longer Recovery from first episode: complete, longer Time from initial relapse to second episode: none Number of relapses during the first 2 years: none
Myhr *et al* 2001	Life table analysis *Cases with a relapsing–remitting initial course of multiple sclerosis:* 76th percentile: 10 57th percentile: 19	Not available
Long-term natural history cohorts with longitudinal follow-up		
Lyon, France, multiple sclerosis cohort		
Confavreux 1977 Confavreux *et al* 1980	Life table analysis *All cases:* 11 (median)	Life table analysis *All cases:* Gender: none Age at onset of multiple sclerosis: younger, longer *Cases with a relapsing–remitting initial course of multiple sclerosis:* Time from initial episode to second episode: shorter, shorter
Confavreux *et al* 2000; 2003 Vukusic and Confavreux 2003b	Life table analysis *Cases with a relapsing–remitting initial course of multiple sclerosis:* 19.1 [95% CI 17.1–21.1] (median)	Cox proportional hazards regression model *Cases with a relapsing–remitting initial course of multiple sclerosis:* Gender: female, longer Age at onset of multiple sclerosis: younger, longer Initial symptoms: brainstem/long tracts, none; optic neuritis, slightly longer Time from initial episode to second episode: shorter, shorter

table continued on following page

Table 4.13 Progression in multiple sclerosis: data from the main series describing the long-term course and prognosis, cont'd

Study	Time from onset of multiple sclerosis to progression (years)	Factors predictive of time from onset of multiple sclerosis to progression (years)
Gothenburg, Sweden, multiple sclerosis cohort		
Broman *et al* 1981 Runmarker and Andersen 1993 Eriksson *et al* 2003	Life table analysis *All cases:* 9 (median) *Cases with a 'clinically isolated syndrome' at onset:* 19.0 ± 1.6 (median ± SEM)	Life table analysis Cox regression analysis ***Cases with a relapsing–remitting initial course of multiple sclerosis and cases with a 'clinically isolated syndrome' at onset:*** Gender: male, shorter Age at onset of multiple sclerosis: younger, longer Season of onset / year of onset / seen from onset: none Initial symptoms: optic neuritis / sensory / monoregional, longer; long tracts, shorter Recovery from first episode: complete, longer Time from initial episode to second neurological episode:[a] none Number of relapses during the first 5 years of multiple sclerosis:[b] none Disability score at 5 years of multiple sclerosis:[b] higher, shorter Number of affected functional systems at 5 years of multiple sclerosis:[b] greater, shorter
London, Ontario, multiple sclerosis cohort		
Weinshenker *et al* 1989a; 1989b	Life table analysis *All cases:* 5.8 ± 0.3 (median ± SEM)	Not available
Long-term history series from the therapeutic era		
Amato *et al* 1999 Amato and Ponziani 2000	Life table analysis *Cases with a relapsing–remitting initial course of multiple sclerosis:* 70th percentile: 11	Life table analysis Cox regression analysis ***Cases with a relapsing–remitting initial course of multiple sclerosis:*** Gender / age at onset of multiple sclerosis: none Initial symptoms: pyramidal / cerebellar / sphincter / visual, shorter Number of affected functional systems at onset of multiple sclerosis: greater, shorter Recovery from first episode: incomplete, shorter Time from initial episode to second neurological episode: longer, shorter Number of relapses during the first 2 years of multiple sclerosis: none Oligoclonal bands in cerebrospinal fluid at onset of multiple sclerosis: present, shorter Brain MRI at onset of multiple sclerosis: suggestive, slightly shorter

SD = standard deviation.
SEM = standard error of the mean.
a Time to end point (onset of progression) estimated by the survival analysis using the second episode as starting point.
b Time to end point (onset of progression) estimated by the survival analysis using 5 years after onset as starting point.

(Eriksson *et al* 2003). In their series of 190 patients with an exacerbating–remitting onset of multiple sclerosis, Italian authors estimated the 70th percentile time to onset of secondary progression at 11 years (Amato and Ponziani 2000; Amato *et al* 1999), a figure precisely matching those from Lyon, France. Lastly, among their 179 patients with an exacerbating–remitting onset of multiple sclerosis, Myhr *et al* (2001) identified the 57th percentile time to onset of secondary progression at 19 years. It seems reasonable to conclude that 19 years is a reasonable estimate for the median time to secondary progression following an exacerbating–remitting onset in multiple sclerosis.

Age at onset of multiple sclerosis is, by far, the strongest predictor of the conversion to secondary progression (see Table 4.13): the older the age at onset, the shorter the time to onset of progression (Confavreux *et al* 1980; Eriksson *et al* 2003; R. Müller 1949; 1950; Riise *et al* 1992; Runmarker and Andersen 1993; Trojano *et al* 1995; Vukusic and Confavreux 2003b). In contradistinction to these rather consistent observa

Table 4.14 Kaplan–Meier estimates of the time (years) from onset of multiple sclerosis to the onset of secondary progression, among the 1562 patients with a relapsing–remitting initial course from the Lyon multiple sclerosis cohort. Adapted from Vukusic and Confavreux (2003b)

Time (years)	0	0.5	1	2	3	4	5	6	7	8	9	10	11	12	13	14	15	20	25	30	35	40
Patients (%) free of secondary progression	100		99	98	96	93	90	87		84	82	79	76	73		70	67	64	62	60	48	42	33	23	18

	Median time (years)	Patients (%) who did not reach the end point[a]
Time to secondary progression	19.1 [95% CI 17.1–21.1]	68

a Data on patients who did not reach the end point were censored at the time of the last clinic visit.

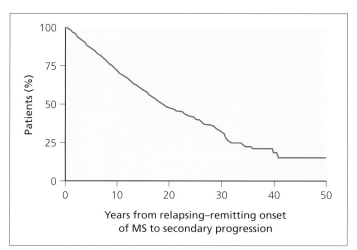

Figure 4.10 Kaplan–Meier estimates for the time (years) from onset to the secondary progressive phase among the 1562 patients with a relapsing–remitting initial course in the Lyon, France, multiple sclerosis cohort. Adapted from Vukusic and Confavreux (2003b).

tions, the cohort from Italy is the only one to conclude that age at onset of multiple sclerosis does not influence time to secondary progression (Amato and Ponziani 2000). The effect of clinical variables, other than age at onset, on the time to secondary progression is weaker or nonexistent. For example, male gender is associated with a shorter time to progression in many series (Eriksson *et al* 2003; R. Müller 1949; 1951; Runmarker and Andersen 1993; Vukusic and Confavreux 2003b) but not in others (Amato and Ponziani 2000; Confavreux *et al* 1980; McAlpine and Compston 1952; Riise *et al* 1992; Trojano *et al* 1995). No study has detected a deleterious influence of female gender on the time to progression. With respect to initial symptoms, most series indicate that symptoms related to the optic nerve, the sensory tracts and, sometimes, the brainstem are associated with a longer time to secondary progression, whereas spinal cord-related manifestations correlate with a shorter interval (Confavreux *et al* 2003; Eriksson *et al* 2003; R. Müller 1949; 1950; Riise *et al* 1992; Runmarker and Andersen 1993; Vukusic and Confavreux 2003b). In a series from southern Italy, initial symptoms had no influence on the time to secondary progression (Trojano *et al* 1995). The Florence, Italy, study led to discordant results, because visual symptoms at onset were associated with a shorter conversion to progression

(Amato and Ponziani 2000). An incomplete recovery from the initial exacerbation has regularly been associated with a shorter time to secondary progression (Amato and Ponziani 2000; Eriksson *et al* 2003; Trojano *et al* 1995). The same is true for the effect of a brief period between onset of multiple sclerosis and the second episode (Amato and Ponziani 2000; Confavreux *et al* 1980; Trojano *et al* 1995; Vukusic and Confavreux 2003b); but this is not observed in all series (Eriksson *et al* 2003). Surprisingly, in the Florence, Italy, study (Amato and Ponziani 2000), a shorter time to the second episode was associated with a longer interval before the onset of secondary progression. R. Müller (1949; 1951) described an inverse relationship between relapse rate in the first 2–5 years of the disease and time to secondary progression. This has not been observed in other series (Amato and Ponziani 2000; Amato *et al* 1999; Eriksson *et al* 2003; Trojano *et al* 1995). In a Norwegian study, the clinical status observed five years after the onset of multiple sclerosis provided additional information: time to progression correlated inversely with disability score and the number of affected functional systems (Eriksson *et al* 2003). Lastly, in the only study that has addressed this issue to date, there is some indication that the presence of IgG oligoclonal bands in the cerebrospinal fluid, or abnormalities on the brain MRI at presentation, are associated with faster conversion to secondary progression (Amato and Ponziani 2000; Amato *et al* 1999).

Taken together, the evidence is that relapsing–remitting multiple sclerosis in males, with older age at onset, involvement of long tracts, a shorter interval between the inaugural episode and first relapse, and incomplete recovery from attacks show a shorter time to onset of progression and more disability at five years.

THE PROGNOSIS IN MULTIPLE SCLEROSIS

Every patient is anxious to know, at various stages throughout the illness, whether the prognosis for disability can be predicted. In fact, details of the time course over which irreversible disability evolves in multiple sclerosis and the eventual outcome do have a reasonable evidence base. But, although the various informative series in the literature show reasonable consistency, it is also worth emphasizing that these conclusions are smoothed out by statistical analysis of populations of patients; and the apparent homogeneity between series conceals extensive individual variation in the course of multiple sclerosis. A third rather unexpected element, but known since the 1970s, is the apparent predictable rate at which disability accumulates.

Accumulation of disability

The long-term follow-up of natural history cohorts from Lyon, France (Confavreux 1977; Confavreux *et al* 1980; 2000; 2003), Gothenburg, Sweden (Broman *et al* 1981; Eriksson *et al* 2003; Runmarker and Andersen 1993) and London, Ontario (Weinshenker *et al* 1989a; 1989b; 1991a) provides useful information on the accumulation of disability. Several other natural history cohorts providing cross-sectional follow-up (Kantarci *et al* 1998; Myhr *et al* 2001), or shorter but nevertheless long-term study of a cohort (Amato and Ponziani 2000; Amato *et al*

1999), have also proved informative (Table 4.15). Each of these series is, in many respects, representative of the disease in an essentially untreated population. The issue of time from onset of multiple sclerosis to assignment of disability landmarks is addressed using life table analysis techniques. Each took DSS 6 to represent a major outcome, describing this as 'assistance required for walking' (Kurtzke 1961) or, more precisely, as the need for unilateral support to walk ≤100 metres without rest. Conversely, they differed in their treatment of other disability milestones. At the lower end of the disability spectrum, the London, Ontario, study (Weinshenker *et al* 1989a; 1989b;

Table 4.15 Time course of irreversible disability in multiple sclerosis. Data from the main series of the long-term course and prognosis of multiple sclerosis

Study	Time from onset of multiple sclerosis to reach selected levels of irreversible disability (years)	Factors predictive of time from onset of multiple sclerosis to irreversible disability
Long-term natural history series with cross-sectional and / or some longitudinal assessment		
R. Müller 1949; 1951	Not available	Observed data Gender: male, shorter Age at onset of multiple sclerosis: older, shorter Initial symptoms: optic neuritis / brainstem, longer; motor / sensory, shorter Initial course: progressive, shorter
Leibowitz *et al* 1964a; 1964b Leibowitz and Alter 1970; 1973	Not available	Observed data Gender: female, slightly shorter Age at onset of multiple sclerosis: younger, longer Initial symptoms: none Initial course: progressive, shorter
Panelius 1969	Not available	Observed data Gender: male, shorter Age at onset of multiple sclerosis: younger, longer
S. Poser 1978	Not available	Observed data Gender / age at onset of multiple sclerosis: none Initial course: progressive, shorter
S. Poser *et al* 1982b	Not available	Observed data Age at onset of multiple sclerosis: older, slightly shorter Initial symptoms: optic neuritis, longer Initial course: progressive, shorter
V.A. Clark *et al* 1982 Detels *et al* 1982 Visscher *et al* 1984	Not available	Observed data Logistic regression analysis Gender: male, slightly shorter Age at onset of multiple sclerosis: older, shorter Residence: Los Angeles, shorter; Washington, longer Initial symptoms: visual / speech / sensory, longer; motor / incoordination, shorter Heat sensitivity: present, shorter Early accumulation of disability: greater, shorter
Phadke 1987; 1990	Not available	Observed data Gender: none Age at onset of multiple sclerosis: younger, longer Familial history of multiple sclerosis: negative, longer Social class: higher, longer Initial symptoms: optic neuritis / brainstem, longer; spinal cord / mixed, shorter Duration of initial symptoms: shorter, longer Initial course: progressive, shorter Time from initial episode to second episode: longer, longer Visual evoked potential latency: normal, longer Cerebrospinal fluid findings: none

Table 4.15 **Time course of irreversible disability in multiple sclerosis. Data from the main series of the long-term course and prognosis of multiple sclerosis, cont'd**

Study	Time from onset of multiple sclerosis to reach selected levels of irreversible disability (years)	Factors predictive of time from onset of multiple sclerosis to irreversible disability
D.H. Miller *et al* 1992a	Not available	Observed data Gender: male, slightly shorter Age at onset of multiple sclerosis: older, shorter Initial symptoms: limb motor, shorter Initial course: progressive, shorter Number of relapses during the first 3 years of multiple sclerosis: none Disability score at 5 years of multiple sclerosis: higher, shorter
Riise *et al* 1992	Not available	Multivariate linear regression analysis *All cases:* Age at onset of multiple sclerosis: older, shorter Initial course of multiple sclerosis: progressive, shorter *Cases with a relapsing–remitting initial course of multiple sclerosis:* Gender: none Age at onset of multiple sclerosis: older, shorter Initial symptoms: pyramidal / cerebellar, shorter *Cases with a progressive initial course of multiple sclerosis:* Gender / age at onset of multiple sclerosis / initial symptoms: none
Kantarci *et al* 1998	Life table analysis DSS 3: 11 (median) DSS 6: 18 (median) DSS 8: 28 (75th percentile)	Life table analysis Cox regression analysis End point = DSS 6 Gender: male, shorter Age at onset of multiple sclerosis: older, shorter Initial symptoms: motor / sphincter, shorter; optic neuritis, slightly longer; polyregional, none Initial course: progressive, shorter Number of relapses during the first 5 years of multiple sclerosis: greater, shorter
Myhr *et al* 2001	Life table analysis DSS 6: 20 (median) DSS 7: 15 (76th percentile)	Life table analysis Cox regression analysis End point = DSS 6 *All cases:* Gender / familial history of multiple sclerosis / initial symptoms: none Age at onset of multiple sclerosis: older, shorter Initial course of multiple sclerosis: progressive, shorter *Cases with a relapsing–remitting initial course of multiple sclerosis:* Gender / age at onset of multiple sclerosis / familial history of multiple sclerosis / initial symptoms: none Time from initial episode to second episode: longer, longer *Cases with a progressive initial course of multiple sclerosis:* Gender / age at onset of multiple sclerosis / familial history of multiple sclerosis / initial symptoms: none
Long-term natural history cohorts with longitudinal follow-up		
United States Army Veterans World War II multiple sclerosis cohort		
Kurtzke *et al* 1968a; 1970a; 1973; 1977	Not available	Observed data End point = DSS 6 and 10 Age at onset of multiple sclerosis / initial symptoms: none Socioeconomic status / month of onset of multiple sclerosis / year of onset of multiple sclerosis: none Number of relapses during the first 5 years of multiple sclerosis: none DSS score at 5 years of multiple sclerosis: higher, shorter Symptoms at 5 years of multiple sclerosis: pyramidal / cerebellar, shorter Number of affected functional systems at 5 years of multiple sclerosis: greater, shorter

table continued on following page

Table 4.15 **Time course of irreversible disability in multiple sclerosis. Data from the main series of the long-term course and prognosis of multiple sclerosis, cont'd**

Study	Time from onset of multiple sclerosis to reach selected levels of irreversible disability (years)	Factors predictive of time from onset of multiple sclerosis to irreversible disability
Lyon, France, multiple sclerosis cohort		
Confavreux 1977 Confavreux et al 1980	Life table analysis DSS 4: 6 (median) DSS 7: 18 (median)	Observed data End point = DSS 4 and 7 Gender / initial symptoms: none Age at onset of multiple sclerosis: younger, longer Initial course: progressive, shorter Time from initial episode to second episode: shorter, shorter Number of episodes during the relapsing–remitting phase of multiple sclerosis: greater, longer Time from initial episode to secondary progression: shorter, shorter
Confavreux et al 2000; 2003	Life table analysis DSS 4: 8.4 [7.8–9.6] DSS 6: 20.1 [18.1–22.5] DSS 7: 29.9 [25.1–34.5] (median [95% confidence intervals])	Life table analysis Cox regression analysis End point = DSS 4, 6 and 7 *All cases and cases with a relapsing–remitting initial course of multiple sclerosis:* Gender: female, longer Age at onset of multiple sclerosis: younger, longer Initial symptoms: optic neuritis, longer; long tracts, shorter Initial course: progressive, shorter Recovery from first episode: complete, longer Time from initial episode to second neurological episode: shorter, shorter Number of episodes during the first 5 years of multiple sclerosis: greater, shorter Time from onset of multiple sclerosis to assignment of DSS 4: shorter, shorter *Cases with a progressive initial course of multiple sclerosis:* Gender: female, longer All of the other clinical variables: none
Gothenburg multiple sclerosis cohort		
Broman et al 1981 Runmarker and Andersen (1993 Eriksson et al 2003	Life table analysis DSS 6: 18 (median)	Life table analysis Cox regression analysis End point = DSS 6 *All cases:* Initial course: progressive, shorter *Cases with a relapsing–remitting initial course of multiple sclerosis:* Gender: male, shorter Age at onset of multiple sclerosis: younger, longer Season of onset of multiple sclerosis / year of onset of multiple sclerosis / seen from onset: none Initial symptoms: optic neuritis / sensory / monoregional, longer; long tracts, shorter Recovery from first episode: complete, longer Time from initial episode to second neurological episode:[a] none Number of episodes during the first 5 years of multiple sclerosis:[b] none Disability score at 5 years of multiple sclerosis:[b] higher, shorter Number of affected functional systems at 5 years of multiple sclerosis:[b] greater, shorter

1991a) and a Turkish study (Kantarci *et al* 1998) focused on DSS 3, describing this as 'moderate dysfunction (monoparesis or mild hemiparesis)' (Kurtzke 1961; Kurtzke *et al* 1973). In Lyon, France (Confavreux *et al* 1980; 2000; 2003), Gothenburg, Sweden (Eriksson *et al* 2003; Runmarker and Andersen 1993) and Florence, Italy (Amato and Ponziani 2000) the investigators favoured DSS 4, describing this as 'relatively severe dysfunction

not interfering with ability to work' (Kurtzke 1961; Kurtzke *et al* 1973) or, more precisely, as limited walking ability without aid or rest for ≥500 metres. When dealing with higher levels of disability, the London, Ontario, and the Turkish studies considered DSS 8, describing this as 'restricted to bed but with effective use of arms' (Kurtzke 1961; Kurtzke *et al* 1973), while the French and Norwegian studies focused on DSS 7, defining

Table 4.15 **Time course of irreversible disability in multiple sclerosis. Data from the main series of the long-term course and prognosis of multiple sclerosis, cont'd**

Study	Time from onset of multiple sclerosis to reach selected levels of irreversible disability (years)	Factors predictive of time from onset of multiple sclerosis to irreversible disability
London, Ontario, multiple sclerosis cohort		
Weinshenker *et al* 1989a; 1989b; 1991a	Life table analysis DSS 3: 7.7 ± 0.4 DSS 6: 15.0 ± 0.3 DSS 8: 46.4 ± 0.1 (median ± SEM)	Life table analysis Multivariate hierarchical analysis End point = DSS 6 (and 8) Gender: male, shorter Age at onset of multiple sclerosis: younger, longer Initial symptoms: optic neuritis, longer; cerebellar / insidious motor, shorter Initial course: progressive, shorter Seen from onset of multiple sclerosis: shorter Time from initial episode to second episode:[a] shorter, shorter Number of episodes during the first 2 years of multiple sclerosis: greater, shorter Disability score at 2 years of multiple sclerosis: higher, shorter Disability score at 5 years of multiple sclerosis: higher, shorter Time from onset of multiple sclerosis to assignment of DSS 3:[c] shorter, shorter
Long-term history series from the therapeutic era		
Amato *et al* 1999 Amato and Ponziani 2000	Life table analysis DSS 4: 12.7 DSS 6: 14.1 (median)	Life table analysis Cox regression analysis Endpoint = DSS 4 and 6 Gender / age at onset of multiple sclerosis: none Initial symptoms: pyramidal / cerebellar / sphincter / visual, shorter; sensory, longer Number of affected functional systems at onset of multiple sclerosis: greater, shorter Initial course: progressive, shorter Recovery from first episode: incomplete, shorter Time from initial to second neurological episode: longer, shorter Number of episodes during the first 2 years of multiple sclerosis: none Oligoclonal bands in cerebrospinal fluid at onset of multiple sclerosis: present, shorter Brain MRI at onset of multiple sclerosis: suggestive, shorter

SD = standard deviation.
SEM = standard error of the mean.
a Time to end point (DSS 6) estimated by the survival analysis using the second episode as starting point.
h Time to end point (DSS 6) estimated by the survival analysis using five years after onset of multiple sclerosis as starting point.
c Time to end point (DSS 6) estimated by the survival analysis using time of assignment of DSS 3 as starting point.

this as 'restricted to wheelchair' (Kurtzke 1961; Kurtzke *et al* 1973) or, more precisely, as an ability to walk ≤10 metres without rest, while leaning against a wall or holding onto furniture. In the Lyon, France, study the emphasis was on irreversible disability; this was assigned only when a given score had persisted for ≥6 months, excluding any transient worsening of disability related to relapse. By definition, when irreversible disability at a given DSS level had been reached, all disability scores during the follow-up of that patient were either equal to or higher than that score. This was automatically checked by the EDMUS software through an appropriate algorithm, and the long duration of follow-up inherent to this natural history study allowed a sufficient period of observation to ensure that, sadly, the disability was indeed irreversible.

The different points of interest regarding disability landmarks in series from the literature inform just about the full spectrum of disability in multiple sclerosis (Table 4.15). The median time from onset of multiple sclerosis to assignment of DSS 3 was estimated at 7.7 years in the London, Ontario, series (Weinshenker *et al* 1989a); and at 11 years in the Turkish study (Kantarci *et al* 1998). Time to DSS 4 has been variously estimated at 6 years (Confavreux *et al* 1980), 8.4 years (Confavreux *et al* 2000; 2003) and 12.7 years (Amato and Ponziani 2000). Perhaps the last figure is overestimated, because the difference in median times to reach DSS 4 and DSS 6 is only 1.4 years in the Florence, Italy, series. Most information is available for DSS 6 and, here, the evidence is generally consistent. The median time from onset of multiple sclerosis to assignment of DSS 6 is 15.0 years in the London, Ontario, series (Weinshenker *et al* 1989a); 18 years in the Gothenburg, Sweden, study (Runmarker and Andersen 1993) and the Turkish study (Kantarci *et al* 1998); 14.1 years in Florence, Italy (Amato and Ponziani 2000); 20

Table 4.16 Kaplan–Meier estimates of the time (years) from onset of multiple sclerosis to the assignment of disability DSS scores, among the 1844 patients in the Lyon, France, multiple sclerosis cohort. Adapted from Confavreux et al (2000; 2003).

Time (years)	0	0.5	1	2	3	4	5	6	7	8	9	10	11	12	13	14	15	20	25	30	35	40
Patients (%) free of																						
DSS 4	100	82	79	73	69	65	61	58	56	52	49	47	44	41	39	37	35	26	17	13	6	0
DSS 6	100	99	98	96	92	89	86	83	80	77	74	72	70	67	63	62	59	50	42	36	28	23
DSS 7	100	100	100	99	98	97	95	93	91	89	87	85	83	81	79	77	75	65	55	50	43	37

	Median time (years)	Patients (%) who did not reach the end point[a]
Time to DSS 4	8.4 [95% CI 7.6–9.2]	44
Time to DSS 6	20.1 [95% CI 18.2–22.0]	68
Time to DSS 7	29.9 [95% CI 25.8–34.1]	79

a Data on patients who did not reach the end point and were censored at the time of the last clinic visit.

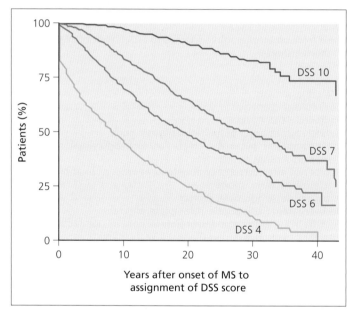

Figure 4.11 Kaplan–Meier estimates for the time (years) from onset of multiple sclerosis to the assignment of DSS 4, 6, 7 and 10, among the 1844 patients in the Lyon, France, multiple sclerosis cohort. Adapted from Confavreux et al (2000; 2003).

years in the Norwegian study (Myhr et al 2001); and 20.1 years in Lyon, France (Confavreux et al 2000; 2003). As for DSS 7, the estimated median time in the Lyon, France, series was variously estimated at 18 years (Confavreux et al 1980) and 29.9 years (Confavreux et al 2000; 2003). In another series Myhr et al (2001) found the 76th percentile time to reach DSS 7 to be 15 years. Our interpretation of this difference over a 20-year period is that, in 1980, the median time was underestimated because the French sample was then exclusively hospital based. Lastly, for DSS 8 the median time was 46.4 years in the London, Ontario, series and the 75th percentile was reached at 28 years in Turkey. Kaplan–Meier estimates for times from onset of multiple sclerosis to assignment of irreversible disability scores of DSS 4, DSS 6 and DSS 7 among the 1844 patients with multiple sclerosis in the Lyon Multiple Sclerosis cohort are

8.4 years (95% CI 7.6–9.2), 20.1 years (95% CI 18.2–22.0), and 29.9 years (95% CI 25.8–34.1), respectively (Table 4.16 and Figure 4.11).

Inter-individual variability

The time intervals offered in the previous section are only global estimates for the prognosis of multiple sclerosis. They allow the archetypal profile of severity to be summarized. The reality is somewhat different. Disease severity may vary considerably from one person to another, as is made clear both to patients and physicians on a daily basis. Considering individuals, the full spectrum of disease is observed – ranging from asymptomatic multiple sclerosis, to benign forms compatible with normal life, so-called malignant variants that prove rapidly disabling, and cases where the condition is immediately life threatening. This variability is represented by the 95% confidence intervals of the time to reach disability landmarks estimated by survival analyses. Self-evidently, they are wide but, thus far, this aspect has not received sufficient critical attention in the literature. The first thorough attempt at documenting and quantifying inter-individual variability in the severity of multiple sclerosis can be credited to Fog and Linnemann (1970). In their prospective longitudinal study of 73 patients followed at 3-month intervals over several years, these Danish authors were able to show how the slope of neurological deterioration, derived from a quantitative neurological examination, could vary from one patient to another. They depicted their observations as a 'fan diagram' (Figure 4.12).

Another approach has been to distribute patients by combining the score of irreversible disability last registered with disease duration to generate a severity classification. This method was applied to the Lyon, France, study (Confavreux et al 1980). 'Benign' forms corresponded to DSS score ≤3 after 10 years, or 4–6 after 15 years of disease duration. 'Hyperacute', 'acute', 'subacute' and 'intermediate' forms corresponded to DSS ≥7 reached within <5, 5–10, 10–15 and >15 years, respectively. With this classification, benign multiple sclerosis represented 14% in the French series whereas hyperacute, acute, subacute and intermediate forms applied to 8%, 8%, 5% and 4%, respectively. A similar classification has been used in a Scottish study, leading to an estimate of 26% benign cases (Phadke 1990). An

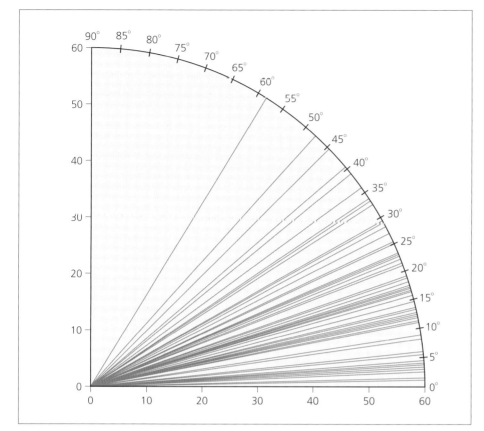

Figure 4.12 Individual slopes of neurological deterioration as assessed from serial quantitative neurological examinations performed at 3-month intervals over several years, among 73 patients with multiple sclerosis. For each patient, the recorded slope has been converted to a linear curve following a regression analysis. Adapted from Fog and Linnemann (1970). © 1970, with permission from Blackwell Publishing Ltd.

inherent limitation to this approach is the great number of 'non-classified' cases (60% in the Lyon, France, series) owing to the limited disease duration at the time of assessment. Self-evidently, some patients initially distributed in the benign group may change course as the disease advances leading to more rapid accumulation of disability. This approach to classification of severity is not therefore satisfactory and should be abandoned, at least when follow-up is short.

The distribution of patients by progression index, calculated for each individual by dividing the DSS score at last follow-up with disease duration (years), was studied in 221 patients with multiple sclerosis in southern Lower Saxony (Figure 4.13; S. Poser *et al* 1982a). The distribution of progression index was linear, notably within the 0–1.2 range, and then reached a ceiling. This did not provide very discriminating results. Benign cases were defined in this study by a progression index of ≤0.2, indicating disability worsening by ≤1 point within a 5-year period. For malignant cases, the progression index was ≥1.4, which equates to a worsening of ≥7 steps within a 5-year period. Applying these definitions, 36% and 2% of the cases could be categorized as benign and malignant, respectively.

Another device for distributing patients at a given level of disability according to severity focuses on the time taken to reach a given milestone (Confavreux 1977; Weinshenker *et al* 1989b). Alternatively, patients are distributed by disability according to given intervals of disease duration. Thus, Achiron *et al* (2003) considered serial EDSS assessments of 1317 Israeli patients with definite relapsing–remitting multiple sclerosis followed at 3–6-month intervals for ≤10 years after onset. As discussed in

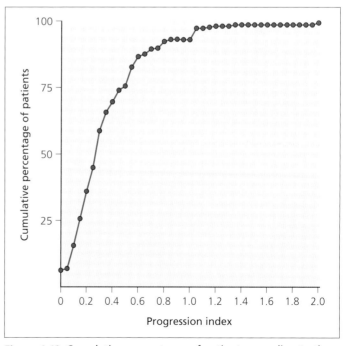

Figure 4.13 Cumulative percentages of patients according to the progression index, among 221 patients with multiple sclerosis from southern Lower Saxony, Germany. Adapted from S. Poser *et al* (1982b). © 1982, with permission from Blackwell Publishing Ltd.

Chapter 6, the most recent approach has been to assign an integral of disability and duration to a particular decile within the distribution observed in a large cohort of cases having equivalent disease durations (Roxburgh *et al* 2005a). Although based upon observational data only and not restricted to the first time a given irreversible level of disability has been assigned during the disease course, both indices allow inferences to be made concerning the estimated median times to reach disability levels. Their results show consistency with those provided by survival analyses in the long-term longitudinal natural history cohorts (see above).

Intra-individual consistency

For any clinician experienced in the management of multiple sclerosis, initially the dominant clinical feature in the majority of patients is the succession of relapses alternating with periods of apparent clinical stability. It may therefore come as something of a surprise to spot that serial quantitative neurological examinations over several years chart steady progression of neurological abnormalities showing, after regression analysis, a linear or curvilinear (with a small inflexion) pattern. This is no less true for cases with a purely relapsing–remitting course than for those with relapses superimposed on disease progression. Again, this was first demonstrated by Fog and Linnemann (1970) in their 73 patients with multiple sclerosis, and later confirmed, using a similar approach, by Patzold and Pocklington (1982) in a study of 102 patients (Figure 4.14). For the majority of patients, it has thus become possible to draw a slope of neurological deterioration that is remarkably stable over many years. According to Fog and Linnemann (1970), once this has been allocated to an individual, it is possible to extrapolate the future course and make prognostic predictions tailored to that individual. Unfortunately, in order to get an accurate and sufficiently precise

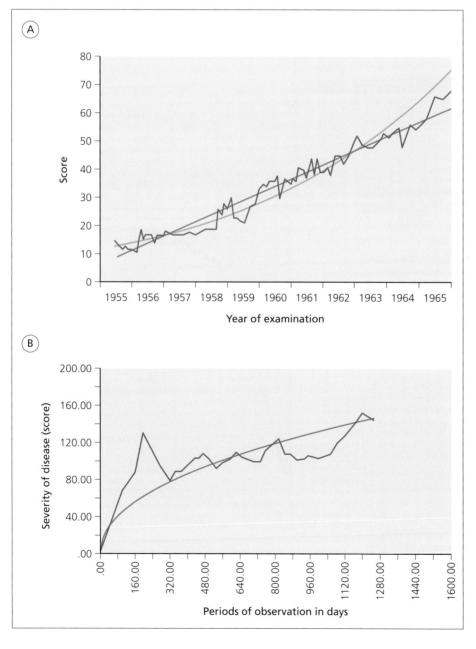

Figure 4.14 Serial quantitative neurological examinations over several years in two individual patients with multiple sclerosis (A and B). In both cases, the observed clinical 'saw-toothed' curve could, after regression analysis, be transformed into mathematical curves. The 'best' fitting curve is selected from the highest correlation coefficient with the clinical curve. Adapted from (A) Fog and Linnemann (1970). © 1970, with permission from Blackwell Publishing Ltd. (B) Patzold and Pocklington (1982). © 1982, with permission from Blackwell Publishing Ltd.

assessment, suitable for reliable predictions, several years of serial examination are necessary, justifiably attracting the criticism that this is now a *post hoc* prognostication, and therefore of limited clinical application.

That said, rather a similar linear evolution has subsequently been observed for the T_2 hyperintense lesion load, the T_1 hypointense lesion load, the ventricular volume and the partial brain volume on brain MRI, and for the cervical area on spinal cord MRI in 41 patients with primary progressive multiple sclerosis followed prospectively for 5 years (Ingle *et al* 2003). In this study, rates of change for MR measures were consistent within individuals but different between patients, in agreement with the intra-individual fixity and the inter-individual variability observed clinically by Fog and Linnemann (1970) and Patzold and Pocklington (1982). Correlations between the clinical changes, as assessed by the EDSS and the Multiple Sclerosis Severity Score, and the MR measures were either absent or weak.

Factors affecting prognosis

The results of the many long-term studies of natural history cohorts provide consistent clues (Table 4.15). Here, we focus on demographic and clinical variables; paraclinical features, including MRI, are discussed in Chapter 7. Our discussion follows the same pattern as for other indices in considering the effects of gender, symptoms at onset, and the initial clinical course on prognosis.

Features at onset

The three long-term longitudinal studies from London, Ontario (Weinshenker *et al* 1989a; 1989b; 1991a), Gothenburg, Sweden (Eriksson *et al* 2003; Runmarker and Andersen 1993), and Lyon, France (Confavreux *et al* 2000; 2003) each found an association between male gender and shorter time to reach disability landmarks. A similar trend has been observed in several cross-sectional studies (Detels *et al* 1982; Kantarci *et al* 1998; D.H. Miller *et al* 1992a; R. Müller 1949; 1950; Panelius 1969) whereas others found no effect of gender (Amato and Ponziani 2000; Myhr *et al* 2001; Phadke 1987; S. Poser 1978; Riise *et al* 1992; Thygesen 1955). Only in an Israeli study did female sex turn out to be associated with worse outcome (Leibowitz and Alter 1970; 1973; Leibowitz *et al* 1964a; 1964b). All studies lead to the conclusion that, when present, the influence of gender on prognosis is weak.

The vast majority of the studies consistently reveal that age at onset of multiple sclerosis is predictive of disability: the older the age at onset, the shorter the time to disability. This has been observed in the long-term longitudinal studies (Broman *et al* 1981; Confavreux *et al* 1980; 2000; 2003; Eriksson *et al* 2003; Runmarker and Andersen 1993; Weinshenker *et al* 1989a; 1989b; 1991a) and other series (Bonduelle 1967; Kantarci *et al* 1998; Leibowitz *et al* 1964a; 1964b; McAlpine 1961; D.H. Miller *et al* 1992a; R. Müller 1949; 1951; Myhr *et al* 2001; Panelius 1969; Phadke 1987; 1990; S. Poser *et al* 1982b; Riise *et al* 1992; Thygesen 1955; Visscher *et al* 1984). Only German (S. Poser 1978) and Italian studies (Amato and Ponziani 2000) concluded that age at onset of multiple sclerosis does not influence the prognosis; the United States Army Veterans World War II cohort provides a similar result but this may reflect the criterion only to enrol military personnel in this series (Kurtzke *et al* 1968a; 1970a; 1973; 1977).

Presentation with optic neuritis is associated with longer time to disability landmarks, whilst onset with a spinal cord syndrome, or motor and cerebellar features, correlates with shorter time to disability (V.A. Clark *et al* 1982; Confavreux *et al* 2000; 2003; Detels *et al* 1982; Eriksson *et al* 2003; Kantarci *et al* 1998; McAlpine 1961; D.H. Miller *et al* 1992a; R. Müller 1949; 1951; Phadke 1987; 1990; S. Poser *et al* 1982b; Riise *et al* 1992; Runmarker and Andersen 1993; Visscher *et al* 1984; Weinshenker *et al* 1989a; 1989b; 1991a). Some authors have not detected a significant influence of initial symptoms on the final outcome (Kurtzke *et al* 1968a; 1970a; 1973; 1977; Leibowitz and Alter 1970; 1973; Leibowitz *et al* 1964a; 1964b; Myhr *et al* 2001). In an Italian study, visual symptoms at onset were associated with a more rapid course of the disease (Amato and Ponziani 2000). For some authors, the greater the number of affected functional systems at onset, the shorter the time to disability (Amato and Ponziani 2000), but others disagree (Kantarci *et al* 1998).

The initial course of multiple sclerosis is the strongest clinical predictor of disability: a progressive course from onset is associated with a shorter time to reach disability landmarks, compared with cases with relapsing–remitting multiple sclerosis. This conclusion is consistent in the essentially cross-sectional series (Amato and Ponziani 2000; Kantarci *et al* 1998; Leibowitz and Alter 1970; 1973; Leibowitz *et al* 1964a; 1964b; D.H. Miller *et al* 1992a; R. Müller 1949; 1951; Myhr *et al* 2001; Phadke 1987; 1990; S. Poser 1978; S. Poser *et al* 1982b; Riise *et al* 1992) and longitudinal series (Broman *et al* 1981; Confavreux *et al* 1980; 2000; 2003; Eriksson *et al* 2003; Runmarker and Andersen 1993;Weinshenker *et al* 1989a; 1989b; 1991a). Using the Kaplan–Meier method of life table analysis for 1844 patients with multiple sclerosis in the Lyon, France, cohort (Confavreux *et al* 2000; 2003), the difference in median interval from onset to reach DSS 4, 6 and 7 between cases with an initial exacerbating–remitting and progressive course, was 11, 16 and 20 years, respectively (p < 0.001, for each comparison: Table 4.17 and Figure 4.15). Taking DSS 6 and 7 as the outcomes, life table analysis of the Norwegian study also shows that patients with an exacerbating–remitting initial course have a much more favourable outcome than those with primary progressive multiple sclerosis (p < 0.001; Table 4.18; Myhr *et al* 2001).

In the Israeli studies, involving 282 patients with multiple sclerosis, the symptoms, course and prognosis appeared remarkably similar in affected individuals from Western Europe and Israel, despite the fact that the latter came from three equally distributed ethnic groups – European, Afro-Asian and native Israeli-born (Leibowitz and Alter 1970; 1973; Leibowitz *et al* 1964a; 1964b). In a large study involving 2934 Australian patients with multiple sclerosis, S.R. Hammond *et al* (1988; 2000b) demonstrated that the course, prognosis and clinical predictive factors were remarkably similar to those observed in populations living in the northern hemisphere; and there were no distinctions between affected individuals from different parts of Australia. Contrasting with this homogeneous clinical pattern in the populations of European origin, whatever the geographical area under consideration, Asian populations affected with multiple sclerosis present several distinguishing features (see Chapters 2, 5 and 6; Kira 2003).

Table 4.17 Kaplan–Meier estimates of the time (years) from onset of multiple sclerosis to the assignment of disability status scale scores among the 1844 patients from the Lyon multiple sclerosis cohort. Influence of the initial course of the disease. A: estimates for the 1562 patients with a relapsing–remitting initial course of multiple sclerosis (see Figure 4.15A). B: estimates for the 282 patients with a progressive initial course of multiple sclerosis (see Figure 4.15B). Adapted from Confavreux *et al* (2000, 2003)

A: Patients with a relapsing–remitting initial course of multiple sclerosis (n = 1562)

Time (years)	0	0.5	1	2	3	4	5	6	7	8	9	10	11	12	13	14	15	16	17	18	19	20
Patients (%) free of																						
DSS 4	100	91	89	84	79	75	71	68	65	61	58	56	52	49	46	44	42	40	38	35	34	31
DSS 6	100	99	98	97	95	93	91	89	86	84	82	80	77	75	71	69	66	63	62	60	59	57
DSS 7	100	100	100	99	99	97	96	95	94	92	90	88	87	85	83	82	80	79	76	73	72	71

	Median time (years)	Patients (%) who did not reach the end point[a]
Time to DSS 4	11.4 [95% CI 10.5–12.3]	52
Time to DSS 6	23.1 [95% CI 20.1–26.1	73
Time to DSS 7	33.1 [95% CI 29.2–37.0	82

a Data on patients who did not reach the end point were censored at the time of the last clinic visit.

B: Patients with a progressive initial course of multiple sclerosis (n = 282)

Time (years)	0	0.5	1	2	3	4	5	6	7	8	9	10	11	12	13	14	15	16	17	18	19	20
Patients (%) free of																						
DSS 4	100	32	28	16	12	9	8	6	5	4	3	2	1	1	1	1	0	0	0	0	0	0
DSS 6	100	98	96	91	82	73	63	57	51	43	37	32	30	27	26	26	25	23	22	21	19	17
DSS 7	100	100	99	98	95	93	89	83	79	75	69	67	61	57	52	48	45	40	40	33	31	28

	Median time (years)	Patients (%) who did not reach the end point[a]
Time to DSS 4	0.0	4
Time to DSS 6	7.1 [95% CI 6.3–7.9]	40
Time to DSS 7	13.4 [95% CI 11.0–15.9]	64

a Data on patients who did not reach the end point were censored at the time of the last clinic visit.
DSS = Disability Status Scale.

Table 4.18 Influence of the initial course of multiple sclerosis on prognosis. Life table analysis showing the probability (%) for patients with multiple sclerosis not to reach the end point according to disease duration (years), among 220 patients with multiple sclerosis. Adapted from Myhr *et al* (2001)

	Disease duration (years)				p value
	5	10	15	19	
DSS 6					
Relapsing–remitting	95	81	72	61	<0.001
Progressive	66	22	10	10	
DSS 7					
Relapsing–remitting	99	91	84	77	<0.001
Progressive	84	61	42	26	

1982). By classifying 1055 patients with multiple sclerosis according to a disease severity algorithm, Phadke (1990) concluded that those with a family history of multiple sclerosis had a more severe course of the disease. By contrast, comparing 143 familial multiple sclerosis patients with 956 sporadic multiple sclerosis patients, Weinshenker et al (1990) were unable to find any difference between familial and sporadic multiple sclerosis with respect to demographic and clinical features, including outcome. Similarly, in a long-term natural history study including 220 patients, a family history of multiple sclerosis did not influence the overall outcome of the disease (Myhr et al 2001).

Time to landmarks and clinical status

Few studies have dealt with the issue of the degree of recovery, perhaps due to methodological difficulties in assessment; but there is agreement that the degree of recovery from the initial neurological episode correlates with an improved prognosis (Amato and Ponziani 2000; Confavreux et al 2003; Eriksson et al 2003; Runmarker and Andersen 1993). Conversely, the criterion of time from onset of the disease to the second neurological episode has received much attention. The usual conclusion is that the shorter this interval, the worse the prognosis (Bonduelle and Albaranès 1962; Confavreux et al 1980; 2003; McAlpine 1961; Myhr et al 2001; Phadke 1987; 1990; Riser et al 1971; Weinshenker et al 1989a; 1989b; 1991a). However, this feature has not emerged as influential when survival estimates are dated from onset of the second episode, as in the Gothenburg, Sweden, study (Eriksson et al 2003; Runmarker and Andersen 1993); and in an Italian series an inverse relationship between time to the second neurological episode and subsequent disability landmarks has been observed (Amato and Ponziani 2000).

Fog and Linnemann (1970) and Patzold and Pocklington (1982) did not find a correlation between relapse frequency and disease progression. In these series, follow-up lasted only a few years, sample size included only 73 and 102 patients, respectively, and progression was indexed to the period of observation rather than to the entire course from onset of multiple sclerosis. In the United States Army Veterans series, Kurtzke et al (1977) were also unable to correlate number of relapses during the first 5 years with disability status at 10 or 15 years' duration. However, assessments were very infrequent during the 20 year follow-up in this series and relapse ascertainment during the initial course not optimal. By contrast, the longitudinal studies from Lyon, France, and London, Ontario (Confavreux et al 1980; 2003; Weinshenker et al 1989a) and what is essentially a cross-sectional study from Turkey (Kantarci et al 1998) have consistently found an association between the number of relapses during the first 2–5 years and subsequent prognosis: the greater the number of early episodes, the shorter the interval to disability landmarks. However, the effect is quite weak, and was not seen at all in the Swedish study when time dependency of the variable was accounted for, and survival analysis estimates of time to DSS 6 calculated using 5 years after onset of multiple sclerosis as the starting point (Eriksson et al 2003; Runmarker and Andersen 1993). Others have also concluded that the number of relapses during the first 2–3 years does not influence the final outcome (Amato and Ponziani 2000; D.H. Miller et al 1992a).

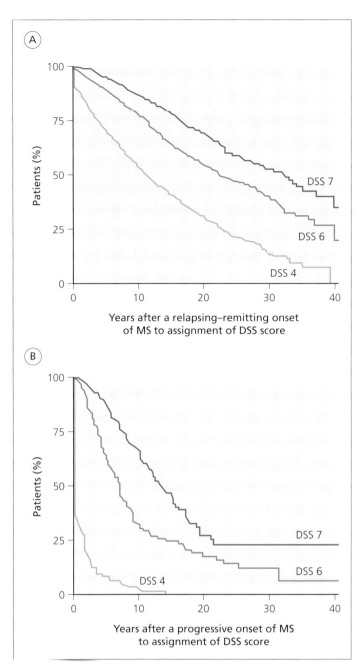

Figure 4.15 Kaplan–Meier estimates for the time (years) from onset of multiple sclerosis to the assignment of DSS 4, 6 and 7 among the 1844 patients in the Lyon, France, multiple sclerosis cohort. Influence of the initial course of the disease. (A) Estimates for the 1562 patients with a relapsing–remitting initial course. (B) Estimates for the 282 patients with a progressive initial course of multiple sclerosis. Adapted from Confavreux et al (2000; 2003).

The potential prognostic influence of many other factors has been explored: socioeconomic status (Kurtzke et al 1970a; Phadke 1990) and the month, season or year of onset (Eriksson et al 2003; Kurtzke et al 1970a; Runmarker and Andersen 1993) but all with negative results. An increase in the subjective intensity of neurological symptoms with exposure to heat (see Chapter 13) has been studied in one series and reported, when present, to be associated with a worse outcome (V.A. Clark et al

John Kurtzke should be credited with first emphasizing the prognostic significance of clinical status at 5 years' disease duration (Kurtzke *et al* 1977): higher DSS scores, the presence of pyramidal or cerebellar signs, and the number of affected functional systems best predict outcome. His study dealt with young soldiers, and the cohort contains almost no cases with a progressive onset. This and the other recruitment biases, already mentioned, may explain why age at onset and initial disease pattern were not shown to influence the clinical course. That said, whenever the possible predictive value of early accumulation of disability has been assessed in other series, much the same conclusion has been reached (V.A. Clark *et al* 1982; Detels *et al* 1982; D.H. Miller *et al* 1992a; Visscher *et al* 1984; Weinshenker *et al* 1989a; 1989b). Moreover, the Gothenburg, Sweden, study has demonstrated that the effect was still present when the time to end point (DSS 6 in this series) was estimated by survival analysis using 5 years from onset as the starting point (Eriksson *et al* 2003; Runmarker and Andersen 1993). Taken together, these observations corroborate, to some extent, the 'individual slope' concept derived from an earlier analysis (Fog and Linnemann 1970).

The literature on assessing the influence of early accumulation of disability on the long-term outcome is reasonably consistent, and supports the conclusion already reached concerning clinical status at 5 years. The time taken to reach higher landmarks of disability correlates with the interval between onset and assignment of DSS 3 (Weinshenker *et al* 1989a; 1989b; 1991a) or DSS 4 (Confavreux *et al* 2003). The same effect was apparent in the London, Ontario, series where the time to DSS 6 was estimated by survival analysis from the point at which DSS 3 had been reached. Conversely, in the Lyon, France, series, the influence of time from onset to DSS 4 was reproduced in the subsequent time to DSS 6 and DSS 7 (p < 0.001, for each) when onset of multiple sclerosis was used as starting point, but vanished when the period of scrutiny was taken forward to assignment of DSS 4 as baseline (Confavreux *et al* 2003).

Time to secondary progression has only been analysed in a single study, perhaps because secondary progression is an end point that occurs relatively late in the course of multiple sclerosis. Using a disease severity classification, we found that shorter times to secondary progression were associated with worse outcomes (Confavreux *et al* 1980). However, survival analyses have not yet been used to assess the prognostic significance of this descriptor.

Multivariate analysis

The list of clinical, imaging and laboratory variables that may bear some predictive value on the time course of disability accumulation in multiple sclerosis is long. Some have a stronger influence than others. None appears to make more than a trivial contribution to the prognosis, and univariate analysis is therefore of little value. To improve the accuracy of these predictions, a logical approach is to combine information provided by the separate factors. But, as it turns out, these combinations of predictors are soon shown to exhibit neither synergistic nor additive effects. Many are interdependent but not additive in their prognostic effect and therefore share predictive influence thus risking the introduction of partially confounding effects. However disappointing hierarchical multivariate analyses may have proved in delivering customized predictions in the clinical setting, some interesting observations have emerged. Those

researchers using crude observational data (V.A. Clark *et al* 1982; Detels *et al* 1982; Leibowitz and Alter 1970; 1973; Leibowitz *et al* 1964a; 1964b; D.H. Miller *et al* 1992a; R. Müller 1949; 1950; Panelius 1969; Phadke 1987; 1990; S. Poser 1978; S. Poser *et al* 1982b; Visscher *et al* 1984) and modern statistical techniques (Amato and Ponziani 2000; Confavreux *et al* 1980; 2003; Eriksson *et al* 2003; Kantarci *et al* 1998; Myhr *et al* 2001; Riise *et al* 1992; Runmarker and Andersen 1993; Weinshenker *et al* 1989b; 1991a) have reached consistent conclusions. The most influential cluster gathers sex, age at onset, initial symptoms and initial course. We rationalize the only exception (Kurtzke *et al* 1977) on the basis of recruitment bias, as already discussed. Older age at onset, early symptoms referable to long tracts, an initial progressive course and male gender are associated with a worse outcome. Conversely, the combination of younger age at onset, optic neuritis as the initial symptom, an early exacerbating–remitting course and female sex are significantly associated with a better prognosis. How the illness starts is the factor most influencing the prognosis. Age at onset comes next in the rankings. Initial symptoms and gender have a marginal or possibly no effect once initial course and age at onset have been considered. A second cluster emerges, gathering features that define clinical status after a reasonable period – 5 years in most studies (V.A. Clark *et al* 1982; Detels *et al* 1982; Eriksson *et al* 2003; Kurtzke *et al* 1977; D.H. Miller *et al* 1992a; Runmarker and Andersen 1993; Visscher *et al* 1984; Weinshenker *et al* 1989a; 1989b). A higher disability score, more affected functional systems, and the presence of pyramidal or cerebellar symptoms all contribute to a worse prognosis. But again to emphasize the point, although highly significant at the statistical level, the prognostic effect of these variables is modest at best, even when combined. Thus, although of undeniable interest in thinking about the generality of patients with multiple sclerosis, application to the individual is of limited value.

Adding currently available laboratory data to the algorithm does not make these predictions any more precise. The expectation that information obtained from MRI examinations of the brain and spinal cord at baseline, and during the early years of the illness, may improve long-term predictions remains to be proven for representative cohorts of patients with multiple sclerosis followed longitudinally over a prolonged period. Simply stated, the clinician remains in the uncomfortable position of being unable to predict prognosis in the individual. More sophisticated models developed to solve this type of problem (see above) have also proven disappointing. They confirm such predictive value as exists for univariate and multivariate analyses; and they provide predictions tailored to the individual by accounting for demographic and disease-related characteristics; but, unfortunately, as illustrated by the London, Ontario, series (Weinshenker *et al* 1991a), the lack of precision renders these models of limited practical value. That said, as expected, the predictive factors for disability accumulation in multiple sclerosis are essentially the same as those that predict secondary progression. Two phenomena seem to be operating – a weak interplay between relapses and prognosis, and a strong connection between age and prognosis (see below).

Benign multiple sclerosis

The previous sections introduced a few distinct features of multiple sclerosis. For instance, with onset at age >50 years, multiple sclerosis is usually characterized by motor and sphincter disturbances, a primary progressive course with few or no superimposed relapses, a lower F:M sex ratio, and more rapid accumulation of disability than in younger patients (Noseworthy *et al* 1983). Here, we focus on one form of multiple sclerosis that evokes strong interest for the affected person, who (understandably) craves reassurance that their condition will follow a benign course. Whilst we can offer group definitions based on the progression index or MSSS (see Chapter 6), the real need is for a catalogue of prognostic features, applicable to the individual, that sustains optimism throughout the duration of the disease.

The existence of benign multiple sclerosis is not disputed: indeed, the reality of the concept is reinforced by the well-known finding of incidental multiple sclerosis at autopsy (Engell 1989; Georgi 1961; Gilbert and Sadler 1983; R.P. McKay and Hirano 1967), and on imaging examinations (McDonnell *et al* 2003). There is also a strong consensus about the archetypal clinical phenotype of benign multiple sclerosis: this is characterized by young females with predominant sensory symptoms and an initial exacerbating–remitting course (Bonduelle 1967; Lehoczky and Halasy-Lehoczky 1963; McAlpine 1961; 1964; R.P. McKay and Hirano 1967; M. Rodriguez *et al* 1994b; D.S. Thompson *et al* 1986). However, working criteria for the definition of benign multiple sclerosis are still debated. According to the results of an international survey undertaken by the National Multiple Sclerosis Society of the United States (Lublin and Reingold 1996), the consensus definition is 'disease in which the patient remains fully functional in all neurological systems 15 years after disease onset'. The boundaries of 'fully functional' are somewhat vague. Furthermore, slightly different definitions are applied, depending on the authors. It is therefore difficult to compare the results from one study with another, and even more problematic to provide a reasonable estimate for the actual frequency of benign multiple sclerosis.

As the architect of many clinicopathological descriptions of multiple sclerosis, Charcot (1872) was the first to suggest that the disease might become completely quiescent or individuals even recover:

Enfin, il n'est pas rare de voir des intermissions complètes qui ont pu faire espérer une guérison définitive [in fact, it is not so unusual to see complete remissions that may even indicate full healing from the illness].

Six decades later, Brain (1936) endorsed the same opinion:

If a remission may last thirty years, why not for a lifetime? The overwhelming number of patients in whom the disease is progressive should not blind us to the probability that the continuous series from the most acute to the most benign forms extends further to include those in whom a first attack is never followed by another.

But it was the seminal work of McAlpine (1961; 1964) that popularized the concept of benign multiple sclerosis. By studying an essentially hospital-based population of 241 patients seen ≤3 years of onset and followed up until ≥15 years of the disease, Douglas McAlpine and his younger colleague were able to demonstrate that 62 patients (26%) were still 'without restriction of activity for normal employment and domestic purpose but not necessarily symptom free' (McAlpine and Compston 1952), after a mean disease duration of 18.2 years. All these patients were able to walk for >500 metres without rest or support from a stick. This would equate with a score of DSS ≤4. The figure of 26% is strikingly consistent with results obtained using survival analysis techniques in long-term follow-up studies of large natural history cohorts. For instance, in the Lyon, France, sample of 1844 patients including those with an initial progressive course, 35% and 26% of the patients had not reached the DSS 4 landmark after 15 years and 20 years of disease duration, respectively (see Figure 4.11). The proportion was 13% at 30 years' disease duration. Considering the subgroup of 1562 patients with an initial exacerbating–remitting course, 42% and 31% still had disability scores <DSS 4 after 15 years and 20 years duration, respectively (Figure 4.15). Furthermore, late reassessment of the Gothenburg, Sweden, cohort after a 37–50-year follow-up by Kaplan–Meier analysis allowed the proportion of benign cases to be estimated at 26% and 21% after 30 and 40 years, respectively (Skoog *et al* 2004). To be classified as benign in this study, patients had not yet entered the secondary progressive phase, and must have retained an EDSS score of ≤4 at the last assessment.

The difficulty arising from the fact that patients with benign multiple sclerosis often escape neurological notice, is well demonstrated by a German study (S. Poser *et al* 1982a). The authors analysed any person suspected of having multiple sclerosis, and living in the geographical area of southern Lower Saxony. There were 221 patients. This group was compared with 1837 cases collected throughout Germany, mainly in hospitals taking part in a national epidemiological programme devoted to multiple sclerosis. There were many individuals in the geographically based series who had never attended a hospital or outpatient department. Although mean disease duration was longer in the Saxony (12.1 years) than the hospital cohort (10.5 years), the percentage of patients unrestricted or minimally affected at the time of the survey was 52% and 26%, respectively. These findings emphasize the high frequency of a benign course in multiple sclerosis likely to escape evaluation in any hospital-based series. Another point deserves comment: it is always difficult, if not risky, to believe that an individual classified as having benign multiple sclerosis will always remain in that category. Indeed, the survival curves show a steady decrease in the proportion of individuals still free from that disability end point, however defined, as the disease advances. This is also illustrated by comparative serial analyses for a given population of patients with multiple sclerosis over time (Hawkins and McDonnell 1999; McAlpine 1964; Pittock *et al* 2004a; 2004b; 2004c). Collectively, these analyses are valuable for discussions with patients and their relatives about the prognosis of the disease, notably at the time of diagnosis. We consider that around 30% of incident patients will prove to have a benign form of multiple sclerosis.

SURVIVAL IN MULTIPLE SCLEROSIS

Lay persons are usually aware that multiple sclerosis is a chronic disabling disease but uncertain whether it is fatal. Not surprisingly, at the time of diagnosis, considerations about life expectancy loom large in the mind of each patient. Recent additions to knowledge concerning when and how the person with multiple sclerosis may die, and factors predicting survival, provide the clinician with an evidence base from which answers both for the patient and their relatives can be derived. Professional perceptions of survival in multiple sclerosis have changed since the 1950s. Earlier surveys had suggested that mean survival from onset was no more than 17 years (Brain 1936; Bramwell 1917; Carter *et al* 1950; Ipsen 1950; Lazarte 1950). Now, this figure is considered to be an underestimate, explained by the series being hospital based and reflecting life expectancy in the pre-antibiotic era.

Lessons from the long-term follow-up natural history cohorts

The issue of survival in multiple sclerosis has been addressed in most long-term follow-up studies of natural history cohorts using both cross-sectional (Table 4.19; Kantarci *et al* 1998; Leibowitz *et al* 1969; D.H. Miller *et al* 1992; R. Müller 1949; 1951; Myhr *et al* 2001; Phadke 1987; S. Poser *et al* 1986; Visscher *et al* 1984) and longitudinal assessments (Broman *et al* 1981; Confavreux 1977; Confavreux *et al* 1980; Eriksson *et al* 2003; Kurtzke *et al* 1969; 1970a; Runmarker and Andersen 1993; Wallin *et al* 2000; Weinshenker *et al* 1989a; 1989b). At their inception, the major objective of these series was to describe the natural history of multiple sclerosis from onset. Therefore, patients were enrolled mainly in the first years of the illness. The duration of follow-up still being limited, the number of deaths relative to the total enrolled population observed in these series was small. For instance, the number of patients dead at closure out of the total number enrolled in the French series was 20 / 349 (Confavreux *et al* 1980), 16 / 1099 in the London, Ontario, study (Weinshenker *et al* 1989a), 49 / 308 in the Gothenburg, Sweden, study (Runmarker and Andersen 1993), and 11 / 220 in the Norway study (Myhr *et al* 2001). The only exception is the United States Army Veterans series, with 127 deceased patients out of 527 young male soldiers (with a median age of 25 years at onset) at closure of the study (Kurtzke *et al* 1970a). Table 4.19 shows that the analyses, whether based upon crude observational data (R. Müller 1949; 1951; Phadke 1987) or survival analyses (Confavreux *et al* 1980; Kurtzke *et al* 1970a; D.H. Miller *et al* 1992), are consistent in showing a median time, from onset of multiple sclerosis to death, of around 30 years. The outlier is Israel where mean time to death, calculated from 52 deceased patients, was 17.4 years (Leibowitz *et al* 1969). The remaining studies provide an estimate for the 90th percentile time to death of 20 (range 15–40) years (Kantarci *et al* 1998; Myhr *et al* 2001; Runmarker and Andersen 1993; Weinshenker *et al* 1989a).

Several of these studies dealing with the issue of clinical factors observed at onset and predictive of death provide consistent results (Table 4.19; Leibowitz *et al* 1969; R. Müller 1949; 1951; Phadke 1987; S. Poser *et al* 1986; Runmarker and Andersen 1993; Visscher *et al* 1984). Gender usually appears noncontributory, although a trend for shorter time to death has emerged for males in some series. With the notable exception of the United States Army Veterans series (Kurtzke *et al* 1970a), for the reasons already mentioned, all the studies conclude that age at onset of multiple sclerosis is a strong predictor of reduced survival: the older the age at onset, the shorter the time to death. Motor, cerebellar or multiple symptoms at onset are

usually associated with a worse prognosis, whereas this is the reverse for optic neuritis or oculomotor manifestations. A progressive initial course has also regularly been associated with a shorter time to death.

Details on the causes of death are to be regarded with some caution because the majority of patients with multiple sclerosis die at home or in institutions for the chronically sick, and not in hospital. Autopsies are seldom performed; this was an issue even for McAlpine and Compston (1952) working at a time when the culture for post-mortem examination was less constrained. Death certificates often prove misleading. For example, death was coded as due to multiple sclerosis in only 53% of 438 instances recorded in 2329 patients with multiple sclerosis from a Californian study (Malmgren *et al* 1983). In a recent study comprising 9881 patients with multiple sclerosis listed in the Danish Multiple Sclerosis Registry, only 82% of death certificates mentioned multiple sclerosis as an underlying or contributing cause of death (Brønnum-Hansen *et al* 2004). The same misclassifications presumably exist for other causes of death. That said, R. Müller (1949; 1951) concluded that 90% of cases died as a result of multiple sclerosis, of whom 5 / 190 had committed suicide. Amongst the remaining 10%, dying from causes unrelated to multiple sclerosis, three individuals had cancer and two suffered from fatal ischaemic heart disease. Of the 121 deaths amongst 476 patients with definite multiple sclerosis in the United States Army Veterans series (Kurtzke *et al* 1970a), 93 (77%) were attributable to multiple sclerosis, 24 (20%) to unrelated conditions, and 4 (3%) of unknown cause. Of the 24 deaths unrelated to multiple sclerosis in this population of young soldiers, trauma, coronary heart disease, cancer and suicide were considered to be the cause of death in 8, 3, 2 and 1, respectively. In his study of 1055 patients, Phadke (1987) registered 216 deaths, 132 of which (61%) were related to multiple sclerosis. Amongst the remaining 84 (39%), cancer and cardiovascular diseases accounted for the vast majority – 25 (12%) and 41 (19%), respectively. No conspicuous over-representation of any one disease, including suicide, has been noted in these deaths unrelated to multiple sclerosis. D.H. Miller *et al* (1992a), in their longitudinal study of 107 individuals with multiple sclerosis, registered 36 deaths. In two-thirds of these cases, death was considered to be related to multiple sclerosis. The two most common remaining causes were cancer and ischaemic heart disease. Nine hundred and twenty-eight patients from the London, Ontario, series could be traced up to 1996 when the survey was closed (D.A. Cottrell *et al* 1999a). By that date, 286 / 928 (31%) had died, 179 (63%) of multiple sclerosis and the remaining 107 (37%) from other causes, notably cardiac disease (12%), cancer (10%), cerebrovascular events (5%) and suicide (2%). The distribution of causes was remarkably similar whether the onset of multiple sclerosis had been relapsing–remitting or progressive.

Lessons from the survival series

Several series have been set up specifically to address the issue of survival in multiple sclerosis (Table 4.20). In fact, with the notable exceptions of the United States Army Veterans study (Wallin *et al* 2000) and the Danish study (Brønnum-Hansen *et al* 2004), most have followed a rather similar epidemiological approach to that of the long-term follow-up studies on natural

text continued on page 226

Table 4.19 Death in multiple sclerosis. Data from the main series of the long-term course and prognosis, and from the main series of survival in multiple sclerosis

Study	Population size	Time from onset of multiple sclerosis to death (years)	Factors predictive of time from onset of multiple sclerosis to death
Long-term natural history series with cross-sectional and/or some longitudinal assessment			
R. Müller 1949; 1951	810	190 patients dead at closure of the survey Adjusted data 81st percentile: 10 62nd percentile: 20	Observed data Gender: none Age at onset of multiple sclerosis: older, shorter Initial symptoms of multiple sclerosis: motor, none Initial course of multiple sclerosis: progressive, shorter
Leibowitz *et al* 1969	282	52 patients dead at closure of the survey Observed data Mean: 17.4	Observed data Gender: male, slightly shorter Age at onset of multiple sclerosis: older, shorter Initial symptoms of multiple sclerosis: cerebellar/multiple, shorter Initial course of multiple sclerosis: progressive, shorter Region of birth: none
Visscher *et al* 1984	941	Not available	Observed data Logistic regression analysis Gender: none Age at onset of multiple sclerosis: older, shorter Residence: Los Angeles, shorter; Washington, longer Initial symptoms: incoordination, shorter; motor, none
S. Poser *et al* 1986	1926	263 patients dead at closure of the survey Excess death rate per 1000 per year = 19.4	Observed data Excess death rate per 1000 per year Gender: none Age at onset of multiple sclerosis: younger, slightly longer Initial symptoms of multiple sclerosis: motor/sphincter/cerebral, shorter; sensory/oculomotor, longer Initial course of multiple sclerosis: progressive, shorter
Phadke 1987	1055	216 patients dead at closure of the survey Observed data Mean: 24.5	Observed data Gender: none Age at onset of multiple sclerosis: older, shorter Initial symptoms of multiple sclerosis: cerebellar, shorter; brainstem/optic nerve, longer
D.H. Miller *et al* 1992a	107	36 patients dead at closure of the survey Life table analysis Median: 29	Not available
Kantarci *et al* 1998	1259	Number of dead patients: not available Life table analysis 95th percentile: 15 89th percentile: 25	Not available
Myhr *et al* 2001	220	11 patients dead at closure of the survey Life table analysis 95th percentile: 15	Not available
Long-term natural history cohorts with longitudinal follow-up			
United States Army Veterans World War II multiple sclerosis cohort			
Kurtzke *et al* 1970	527	122 patients dead at closure of the survey Life table analysis 76th percentile: 20 69th percentile: 25 Median: 35	Life table analysis Age at onset of multiple sclerosis: none
Lyon, France, multiple sclerosis cohort Confavreux 1977			
Confavreux *et al* 1980	349	20 patients dead at closure of the survey Life table analysis 90th percentile: 15 Median: 30	Observed data Gender: male, shorter

223

table continued on following page

Table 4.19 **Death in multiple sclerosis. Data from the main series of the long-term course and prognosis, and from the main series of survival in multiple sclerosis, cont'd**

Study	Population size	Time from onset of multiple sclerosis to death (years)	Factors predictive of time from onset of multiple sclerosis to death
Gothenburg, Sweden, multiple sclerosis cohort			
Broman *et al* 1981 Runmarker and Andersen 1993 Eriksson *et al* 2003	308	49 patients dead at closure of the survey Life table analysis 90th percentile: 22	Observed data Gender: male, shorter Age at onset of multiple sclerosis: older, shorter
London, Ontario, multiple sclerosis cohort			
Weinshenker *et al* 1989a; 1989b	1099	16 patients dead at closure of the survey Life table analysis 88th percentile: 40	Not available
D.A. Cottrell *et al* 1999a	928	286 patients dead at closure of the survey Life table analysis *Cases with progressive onset only* Median: 35	Not available
Series of survival in multiple sclerosis			
Riise *et al* 1988	598	136 patients dead at closure of the survey Life table analysis Median: 27 (from diagnosis of multiple sclerosis)	Life table analysis Cox regression analysis Gender: male, slightly shorter Age at onset of multiple sclerosis: older, shorter Initial symptoms: vertigo, shorter Initial course of multiple sclerosis: progressive, shorter
Wynn *et al* 1990	152	43 patients dead at closure of the survey Life table analysis 76th percentile: 25 (from diagnosis of multiple sclerosis)	Life table analysis Gender: male, shorter Secular trend (1905–1985): none
Midgard *et al* 1995	251	70 patients dead at closure of survey Life table analysis 75th percentile: 20 (from diagnosis of multiple sclerosis?)	Life table analysis Cox regression analysis Gender: male, slightly shorter Age at onset of multiple sclerosis: younger, longer Initial symptoms: paraesthesia, shorter Initial course: progressive, shorter
Wallin *et al* 2000	2489	2059 patients dead at closure of the survey Life table analysis Median: 34	Life table analysis Gender: male, shorter Age at onset of multiple sclerosis: younger, longer Socioeconomic status: lower, longer
Sumelahti *et al* 2002	1614	219 patients dead at closure of the survey Life table analysis 53rd percentile: 40	Life table analysis Gender: none Age at onset of multiple sclerosis: younger, longer Initial symptoms of multiple sclerosis: optic neuritis/sensory, longer Initial course of multiple sclerosis: relapsing-remitting, longer
Brønnum-Hansen *et al* 2004	9881	4254 patients dead at closure of the survey Life table analysis Median: 31	Life table analysis Cox regression analysis Gender: male, shorter Age at onset of multiple sclerosis: younger, longer Initial symptoms: optic neuritis, longer; cerebellar, shorter Year of initial symptoms: more recent, longer

SD = standard deviation.
SEM = standard error of the mean.

Table 4.20 Main survival series in multiple sclerosis: epidemiological and disease-related characteristics

Study	Location	Ascertainment	Follow-up	Population size	Gender: males / females (%)	Age at onset of multiple sclerosis (years)	Initial symptoms of multiple sclerosis (%)	Initial course: relapsing–remitting / progressive (%)	Time from onset of multiple sclerosis to diagnosis (years)	Duration of multiple sclerosis (years)	Overall course of multiple sclerosis at time of study (%)	Diagnosis classification[a]
Riise et al 1988	Hordaland and Vestfold counties, Norway	Geographically based	Cross-sectional Some longitudinal	598	41 / 59	32.7 (mean)	Optic neuritis 15 Diplopia 13 Vertigo 11 Paraesthesia 24 Motor weakness 53 Other 28	79 / 21	Not available	Not available	Not available	Definite Probable Possible
Wynn et al 1990	Olmsted County, USA	Geographically based	Cross-sectional Some longitudinal	152	24 / 76	33 (median at diagnosis of multiple sclerosis)	Not available	Not available	Not available	14 (median) (from diagnosis of multiple sclerosis)	Not available	Definite Probable Possible
Midgard et al 1995	Møre and Romsdal County, Norway	Geographically based	Cross-sectional Some longitudinal	251	44 / 56	33.6 (mean)	Optic neuritis 34 Diplopia 23 Vertigo 19 Dysarthria 6 Ataxia 37 Paraesthesia 49 Motor weakness 52 Bladder 18	85 / 15	5.7 (mean)	18.1 (mean)	Not available	Definite Probable Possible
Sumelahti et al 2002	Southern and Western districts, Finland	Hospital based	Cross-sectional Some longitudinal	1614	34 / 66	31.5	Corticospinal 26 Infratentorial 22 Sensory 33 Unknown 19	76 / 24	4.2 (mean)	Not available	Not available	Definite
Bronnum-Hansen et al 2004	Denmark	Country based	Longitudinal	9881	40 / 60	Not available	Not available	Not available	Not available (mean)	21	Not available Probable	Definite Possible

a Whenever necessary, the original criteria used by the authors have been interpreted in order to comply with C.M. Poser et al (1983) diagnostic criteria. 'Possible' is equivalent to 'suspected' in this classification.

225

history cohorts (see above; Midgard *et al* 1995; Riise *et al* 1988; Sadovnick *et al* 1991b; 1992; Sumelahti *et al* 2002; Wynn *et al* 1990). Therefore, the number of patients dead at closure of the survey was only 136/598 and 70/251 in the Norwegian surveys (Midgard *et al* 1995; Riise *et al* 1988), 219/1614 in Finland (Sumelahti *et al* 2002), 43/152 in the Olmsted County, United States, series (Wynn *et al* 1990), and 145/3126 and 115/2348 (Sadovnick *et al* 1991b; 1992) in the Canadian sample. Median time to death was given as 27 years by Riise *et al* (1988) but this is probably an underestimate because diagnosis of multiple sclerosis was used rather than onset as the baseline for subsequent calculations. In Finland (Sumelahti *et al* 2002) survival was estimated at 40 years from initial symptoms of multiple sclerosis. The other studies estimated the 75th percentile of time from diagnosis of multiple sclerosis to death, at around 20 years (Wynn *et al* 1990; Midgard *et al* 1995).

Wynn *et al* (1990) associated male gender with a significantly shorter time to death whereas this only emerged as a trend, at best, in the Scandinavian studies (Midgard *et al* 1995; Riise *et al* 1988; Sumehlati *et al* 2002). The results of these three studies indicate that younger age at onset of multiple sclerosis, presentation with optic neuritis or paraesthesiae, and an exacerbating–remitting initial disease course are all associated with a significantly longer time from onset to death. From the multivariate Cox regression analyses, Riise *et al* (1988) observed that age at onset of multiple sclerosis is the variable most strongly predicting survival; after correction, the apparent effect of initial course on survival is markedly reduced. But, using a similar technique, Midgard *et al* (1995) concluded that age at onset of multiple sclerosis and initial course of the disease do exert independent effects on survival. The Olmsted County, United States, study (Wynn *et al* 1990) was unable to demonstrate a change in the time to death according to year of diagnosis over the period from 1905 to 1985.

Cause of death has been analysed in several survival studies. Sadovnick *et al* (1991b) attributed death directly to multiple sclerosis in 56 (47%) of the 119/145 (82%) deceased patients in whom information was available. Of the remaining 63 deaths, 29% were suicides, 30% had cancers, 21% suffered acute myocardial infarctions, 11% had strokes and 9% died from miscellaneous causes. Among the population with multiple sclerosis, the proportion of deaths due to suicide was 7.5 times higher and that due to malignancy 0.7 times the rate seen in the age-matched general population. The proportion of deaths due to acute myocardial infarction or stroke was similar in both populations. At conclusion of the follow-up period, 70 Norwegian patients with multiple sclerosis had died (Midgard *et al* 1995): in 54 (77%) instances, death was related to multiple sclerosis, directly or as a contributing factor in 42 and 12 individuals, respectively. In the Finnish study, multiple sclerosis-related causes accounted for 70% of the 219 recorded deaths (Sumelahti *et al* 2002). By comparison with the general population, the proportion of deaths resulting from violence or cancer was higher in the context of multiple sclerosis whereas mortality due to cardiovascular diseases was less frequent.

The United States Army Veterans Study (Wallin *et al* 2000) deserves special consideration for its size, duration of follow-up, and high proportion of patients reaching the end point under scrutiny. It comprises 2489 veterans of the Second World War and the Korean conflict ascertained in 1956 as 'service connected' for multiple sclerosis. They were ascertained for vital status to June 1996 using the Beneficiary Identification and Records Locator Subsystem. At the time of the survey, 2059 (83%) veterans had died. Each patient with multiple sclerosis was matched to a military control referred to year of birth, date of entry into military service, branch of series, and survival throughout the war. Several demographic and disease-related data were systematically recorded: year of birth, sex, race, latitude of residence in the United States (arranged in tiers: north, middle and south) on entry to active duty, socioeconomic status, and age at onset of multiple sclerosis. Nonetheless, there were weaknesses in the study. The population under scrutiny essentially comprises males (96%) and whites (97%), bringing into question the reliability of analyses addressing the possible influence of sex and race on survival, because there is no evidence that women and blacks share the same demographic and socioeconomic profile as white males at entry into military service. Furthermore, for obvious reasons, age at onset of multiple sclerosis (median at around 25 years) was younger than for a general population of patients with multiple sclerosis. Comments on the possible influence of age at onset must therefore be treated with caution, and the estimates of time to death are presumably correspondingly exaggerated. That said, the Veterans study does provide robust estimates for life expectancy in this population of young soldiers. Life table analysis for white males (93% of the total cohort) provides a median time from onset of multiple sclerosis to death of 34 years. From univariate and multivariate analyses, age at onset of multiple sclerosis, sex and socioeconomic status each have independent and significant influences on survival. Younger age at onset, female sex and lower socioeconomic status are associated with enhanced survival. Neither race nor latitude of residence at entry in the army have a significant effect on survival, although they are known to correlate with the frequency (i.e. susceptibility) of multiple sclerosis. Furthermore, this study shows that soldiers with multiple sclerosis generally have reduced survival by comparison with their fellow veterans. White male case survival could be estimated at about 2/3 and 1/3 of that for white male veteran controls by 20 years and 40 years after joining the army, respectively. Using the slightly different comparator of standardized mortality ratios, the study also showed reduced survival in army veterans with multiple sclerosis in comparison with the general United States population.

The national Danish study

The national Danish study makes an especially important contribution to the study of survival in multiple sclerosis (Brønnum-Hansen *et al* 1994; 2004; Koch-Henriksen *et al* 1998; Stenager *et al* 1992). At the most recent update, 9881 patients with multiple sclerosis were registered, amongst whom 4254 (43%) had died during follow-up (Brønnum-Hansen 2004). The cohort takes advantage of the Danish Multiple Sclerosis Registry established on the back of a prevalence survey completed in 1956, and includes information about patients in Denmark with onset of multiple sclerosis from 1949. Virtually all Danish inhabitants with multiple sclerosis are registered on the database, and information is systematically validated and updated. The study is also linked to the Danish Civil Registration System established in 1968, and the Cause of Death Registry comprising data on all deaths since 1943. These two official registers gather data on emigration, death and cause of death for the patients with multiple sclerosis, and for the general Danish population. The recent reassessment included patients whose initial symptoms began in the period 1949–1996, and were logged before 1st January 1997.

Follow-up was scheduled to end in 1999. At that time, the mean duration of observation was 21 years. Of the 9881 registered patients, 40% were males. Mean age at onset of multiple sclerosis was 34.7 years. Median survival time from onset of multiple sclerosis to death was estimated at 31 years (Figure 4.16). The survival curves indicate a median time from onset of multiple sclerosis to death that is about 10 years shorter for patients with multiple sclerosis than for the age-matched general population. The standardized mortality ratio, which is the quotient of the observed death number (in the population with multiple sclerosis) by the expected death number (in the general population) for the period 1949–1999 was 2.89 (95% CI 2.82–2.98). The excess death rate, which is the observed death number less the expected death number per 1000 person-years, was 13.4 (95% CI 12.8–14.0) for the total period of 0–50 years after onset of multiple sclerosis. This rose steadily from 1.8 for the period of 0–1 year, to 24.6 for the interval of 20–50 years after onset of the disease.

Life expectancy was significantly greater in females than males according to the results of the survival analysis (Figure 4.17), the standardized mortality ratios, and the excess death rates. Survival improved significantly during the 50-year period of observation, the median 10-year shorter life expectancy being almost halved during that period (Figure 4.18). This change was independent of the general decline in mortality enjoyed by

Danes since the 1950s and presumably related to improved medical management in the modern era. According to available certificates, 56% of deaths were related to multiple sclerosis. Those unrelated were mainly attributable to cardiovascular diseases (15%), cancer (10%), infectious and respiratory diseases

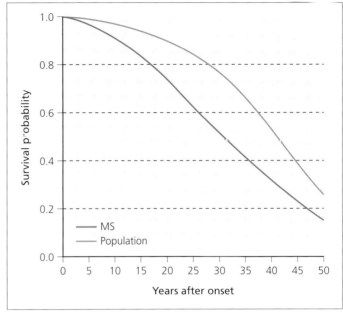

Figure 4.16 Actuarial probability of survival amongst 9881 patients with multiple sclerosis, of whom 4254 had died before the end of follow-up on 1st January 2000, and the matched general population in Denmark. Adapted from Brønnum-Hansen *et al* (2004).

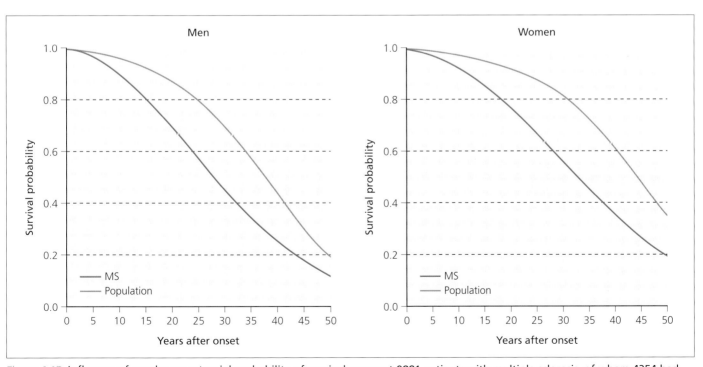

Figure 4.17 Influence of gender on actuarial probability of survival amongst 9881 patients with multiple sclerosis, of whom 4254 had died before the end of follow-up on 1st January 2000, and the matched general population in Denmark. Adapted from Brønnum-Hansen *et al* (2004).

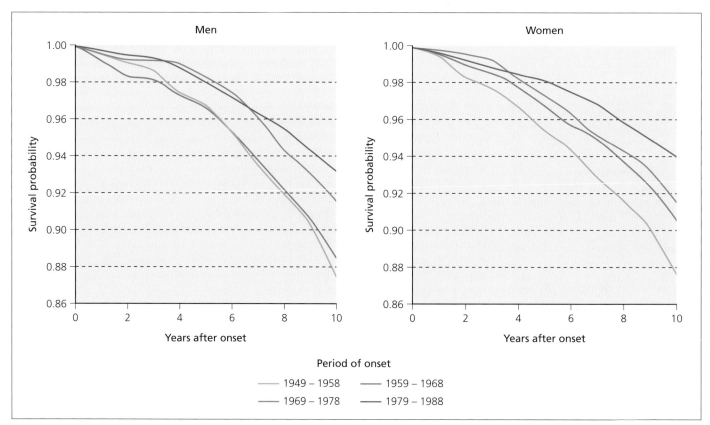

Figure 4.18 Influence of calendar period of onset for multiple sclerosis on actuarial probability of survival amongst 9881 patients with multiple sclerosis, of whom 4254 had died before the end of follow-up on 1st January 2000, and the matched general population in Denmark. Adapted from Brønnum-Hansen *et al* (2004).

(5%) and accidents and suicide (5%). Compared with the general population, there was excess mortality due to cardiovascular disease, infections, respiratory causes, accidents and suicide, but a lower risk of death from cancer.

In summary, a reasonable estimate of the median time from disease onset to death in people with multiple sclerosis is 31 years. This represents a 5–10 year reduction in life expectancy compared with the general population. It seems likely that the modest difference is progressively being eroded with advances in medical management. Female sex, younger age at disease onset, an initial exacerbating–remitting clinical course, and optic neuritis, diplopia or paraesthesiae as initial symptoms are all associated with improved survival. Death is attributable to multiple sclerosis in about two-thirds of patients. It is rare for death to result from involvement of vital centres in the central nervous system. Rather, the reduced life expectancy can be attributed to the bedridden state and its complications in chronically disabled patients. In individuals dying from causes unrelated to multiple sclerosis, the excess is due to suicide compensated by reduced mortality from cancer. Therefore, multiple sclerosis is chronic and disabling but not a fatal disease.

DISEASE MECHANISMS UNDERLYING THE CLINICAL COURSE

For the clinician, the conundrum presented by the clinical course of multiple sclerosis starts with the awareness of at least three different types of clinical evolution, and variable rates of accumulation of disability between patients. Do these patterns indicate the existence of altogether different disorders or are they merely a function of complexity (see also Chapter 14)? Understanding how these patterns come about is fundamental to a sophisticated understanding of multiple sclerosis; and, although this might be considered more the terrain of the expert in physiology or neurobiology, there is much to be learned on this topic from detailed scrutiny of the natural history. Our discussion of mechanisms underlying the disease course in multiple sclerosis necessarily first rehearses, in summary, the experimental evidence.

Inflammation and degeneration

The course of multiple sclerosis may be considered as the expression of two clinical phenomena, relapses and progression, the latter being defined as steady worsening of symptoms and signs over ≥6 months. In turn, this analysis brings into the equation the interplay between two biological activities: inflammation (focal, disseminated, acute or recurrent) and degeneration (diffuse, early, chronic and progressive) (Figure 4.19; for other versions of the same cartoon, see Figures 14.2 and 18.1). There is strong evidence that relapses are mainly the expression of acute focal inflammation occurring within the central nervous system. For each clinical episode, there is an average of ten new MRI lesions (Figure 4.20; see Chapters 7 and 13). One could say that 'multiple sclerosis never sleeps'. This is also one explanation for the strikingly loose correlations with which authorities

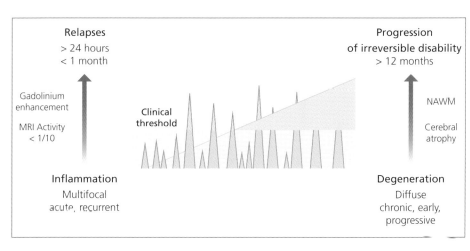

Figure 4.19 Schematic representation of the interplay between relapses and progression, and focal inflammation and diffuse degeneration in multiple sclerosis. NAWM = normal-appearing white matter.

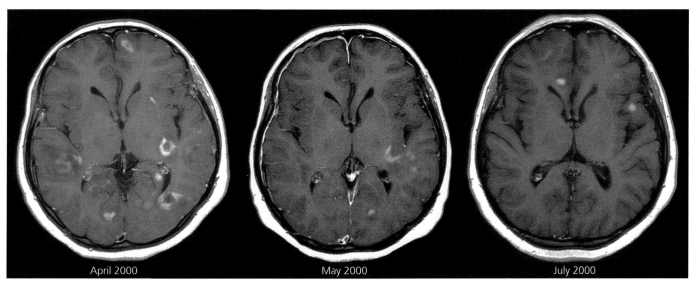

Figure 4.20 Consecutive gadolinium enhanced brain MRI scans from a patient with relapsing–remitting multiple sclerosis. The MRI activity is high despite clinical quiescence during the study period.

working in the 19th century struggled in seeking to match clinical abnormalities to the anatomical lesions observed in their pathological specimens. This so-called *dissociation anatomo-clinique* (clinico-pathological dissociation) was, for these pioneers, a hallmark of *sclérose en plaques* (multiple sclerosis). Relapses are therefore a direct but also a 'filtered' clinical expression of inflammation. This 'filtering phenomenon' may have different origins relating to the complex relationship between injury and repair, plasticity, and the presence of structural abnormality with and without functional perturbations in conduction of the nerve impulse (see Chapters 10 and 13; M. Lee *et al* 2000; Pantano *et al* 2002; H. Reddy *et al* 2000; 2002; Rocca *et al* 2002a; Staffen *et al* 2002). There is also increasing evidence that multiple sclerosis is a neurodegenerative disease, the diffuse and chronic axonal loss correlating with progression and accumulation of disability (see Chapters 1, 10, 12 and 13).

One of the central issues with respect to outcome in multiple sclerosis is the mechanism whereby irreversible disability accrues (Figure 4.21; Confavreux 2002b; Confavreux and Vukusic 2002; Confavreux *et al* 2000). From the clinical perspective, this could simply result from relapses with sequelae.

Under these circumstances, the pattern of accumulation would be stepwise. Alternatively there may be a contribution from superimposed progression. Therefore, it becomes important to reconcile the relative contributions of relapses and progression, and of focal inflammation and diffuse degeneration, in the accumulation of disability. One analysis is that inflammation is directly and exclusively responsible for the initiation of degeneration. This does not necessarily mean that inflammation is also entirely responsible for the perpetuation of degeneration and progression once these have gathered their own momentum (see Chapter 10). But, according to this analysis, relapse and the underlying inflammatory component is the major cause of irreversible disability in multiple sclerosis.

At first glance this assertion is attractive. Among the 1562 patients of the Lyon Natural History Cohort with a relapsing–remitting onset of multiple sclerosis, 274 (18%) did suffer from an initial relapse with irreversible incomplete recovery as defined by a score of DSS ≥3. Among the 1288 patients making a complete recovery, as defined by a score of DSS ≤2, after the initial relapse, 391 (30%) later experienced incomplete recovery from a subsequent episode (Confavreux *et al* 2003).

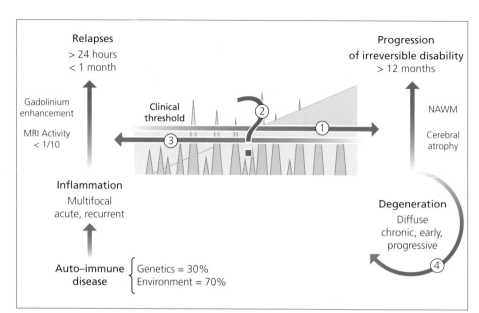

Figure 4.21 Schematic representation of the possible interplay between relapses and progression, and focal inflammation and diffuse degeneration in multiple sclerosis. 1: Relapses and focal inflammation are the major cause of irreversible disability; neurodegeneration follows the phase of active inflammation. 2: Relapses and focal inflammation are not the major cause of irreversible disability; these have independent mechanisms and proceed at different rates. 3: The initial process is neurodegenerative, and damaged tissue stimulates a secondary inflammatory reaction. 4: The initial process is autoimmune with secondary autonomous self-perpetuating neurodegeneration.

A detailed analysis of pooled data from 224 patients with relapsing–remitting multiple sclerosis enrolled in the placebo arms of several randomized clinical trials allows comparisons between EDSS assessments before, at the time of, and after a relapse (Lublin *et al* 2003). The baseline EDSS assessment is defined as the closest measurement preceding the relapse in question. Comparing post-relapse and baseline evaluations, the net increase in the EDSS score was 0.27 (±1.04). This corresponds to 42% of the patients with ≥0.5, and 28% with ≥1.0 increase in EDSS scores. However, the median time between evaluations performed during and after the relapse was only 63 (range 32–140) days.

Similarly, assessment of possible effects from the degree of recovery after the initial episode, time to the next event, and number of attacks during the first years of the disease on the disability accrual process provide consistent results in natural history cohorts. An incomplete recovery from the initial relapse, a short interval between the first two episodes, a high number of relapses overall, or a brisk relapse rate during the first years of the illness are associated with rapid accumulation of irreversible disability (Confavreux *et al* 1980; 2003; Weinshenker *et al* 1989b; 1991a).

However, the real contribution of relapses to disability accumulation is more complex. Evidence from the primary progressive form of multiple sclerosis indicates that progression of irreversible disability may occur without superimposed relapses (Lublin and Reingold 1996), or inflammation defined using standard pathological and MRI criteria. The rate of disability in these cases with progression from onset is similar to that seen in relapsing progressive forms of multiple sclerosis (Confavreux *et al* 2000; D.A. Cottrell *et al* 1999a; Kremenchutzky *et al* 1999).

Informative observations have been made on pooled data from 313 patients with relapsing–remitting multiple sclerosis enrolled in the placebo arms of two large phase III trials of interferon-β1a (PRISMS Study Group 1998) and glatiramer acetate (K.P. Johnson *et al* 1995), assessed at 3-month intervals with a 2-year follow-up (Figure 4.22: C. Liu and Blumhardt 2000). Analyses were performed on the 289 patients with complete EDSS assessments. A significant change was defined as a change of

≥1.0 EDSS points if baseline EDSS was between 0 and 5.0, or ≥0.5 EDSS point change if baseline EDSS was ≥5.5. Patients were distributed into six categories according to the observed course of EDSS scores throughout the 2 years of follow-up:

- 20% exhibited no significant change
- 37% had a fluctuating course with a significant EDSS change but not confirmed at 3 months
- 14% showed an erroneous progression as defined by a significant EDSS increase confirmed at 3 months but not sustained until the end of the observation period
- 15% had a sustained progression with a significant EDSS increase confirmed at 3 months and sustained until the end of the trial
- 8% showed an erroneous improvement with a significant EDSS decrease confirmed at 3 months but not sustained until the end of the trial
- 6% showed a sustained improvement with a significant EDSS decrease confirmed at 3 months and sustained until the end of the trial.

In these series, 29% of the patients could therefore be classified as showing progression in the trial with confirmation at 3 months but, among those who progressed, the EDSS increase was still present at conclusion of the follow-up period in about half the participants. The probability of misclassification at the end of the trial regarding the progression status was 0.52. Applying the more stringent definitions of ≥2.0 EDSS increase and/or a confirmation at 6 months led to essentially the same estimation for the probability of misclassification (range 0.33–0.47). These results clearly show that an increase in disability confirmed at 3 or even 6 months must not be considered as equivalent to an irreversible increase in disability. Interestingly, as discussed above using similar resources, Lublin *et al* (2003) also found a ≥1.0 point EDSS increase relative to baseline in 28% of patients at a median of 63 days after a relapse. This suggests that, in the available placebo cohorts of patients with relapsing–remitting multiple sclerosis, the confirmed disability increases were mainly relapse driven. It seems logical to con-

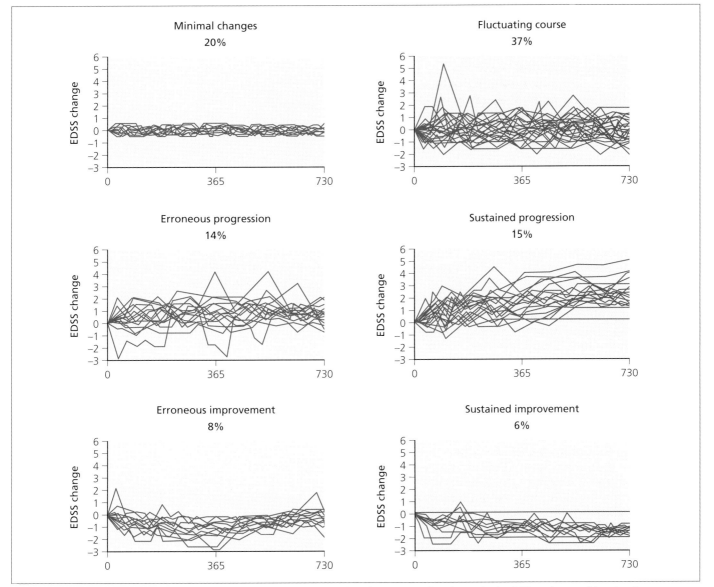

Figure 4.22 Total series of individual plots for EDSS changes from baseline versus days in study, for 289 patients with relapsing–remitting multiple sclerosis enrolled in placebo arms of two phase III trials of interferon-β1a and glatiramer acetate. A significant change is defined as ≥1.0 point EDSS change if baseline EDSS was 0–5.0, or a ≥0.5 point EDSS change if baseline EDSS was >5.5. Patients are distributed into six categories according to the observed course of their EDSS scores throughout the two years of follow-up (see text for precise definitions): minimal changes (20% of the patients); fluctuating course (37%); erroneous progression (14%); sustained progression (15%); erroneous improvement (8%) and sustained improvement (6%). Adapted from C. Liu and Blumhardt (2000). Reproduced with permission from the BMJ Publishing Group.

clude that short-term confirmed increase in disability depends primarily on relapses and is often reversible.

Totally different is the issue of long-term irreversible disability. Lessons from natural history cohorts have been instructive in this respect. For the statistical analysis of the 1844 patients of the Lyon Natural History Multiple Sclerosis Cohort, focus was placed on robust landmarks of disability that could easily be identified through successive neurological assessments as well as by retrospective interview of the patient, whenever necessary. The landmarks were:

- *DSS 4*: defined by walking without aid, although limited, but >500 metres without rest.

- *DSS 6*: walking with unilateral support and limited to ≤100 metres without rest.
- *DSS 7*: home restriction with a few steps still possible holding onto a wall or furniture but limited to ≤10 metres without rest.

Disability was defined as irreversible when one of these steps had been reached and persisted for ≥6 months, excluding any transient worsening related to relapses. This irreversibility was confirmed at any subsequent assessment during follow-up of the patient in subsequent years. From this cohort, the well-known difference between cases with a relapsing–remitting onset and those with progressive disease is again apparent: median time from the onset of multiple sclerosis to assignment of a score of DSS 4, indicating irreversible disability, was significantly longer in the relapsing–remitting than progressive onset cases. The same observation was made for time of onset to assignment of DSS 6 or 7 (Figure 4.23 and Table 4.21). This is in agreement with former analyses of this cohort (Confavreux *et al* 1980) and with results from many other series (Eriksson *et al* 2003; Kantarci *et al* 1998; Phadke 1990; Pittock *et al* 2004b; Runmarker and Andersen 1993; Runmarker *et al* 1994b; Trojano *et al* 1995; Weinshenker *et al* 1989b; 1991a). Nevertheless, progression of irreversible disability from the assignment of DSS 4 to DSS 6 was similar in cases both with a relapsing–remitting and a progressive onset (Figure 4.23 and Table 4.21). This was also true for the progression of disability from DSS 4 to DSS 7, and from DSS 6 to DSS 7 (Confavreux *et al* 2000). This could be interpreted as follows: the rate of progression of irreversible disability from the assignment of DSS 4 is not affected by the presence or the absence of relapses preceding onset of the chronic progressive phase. Confirmation can be found by looking at the influence of current age on the course of multiple sclerosis: age at onset of the progressive phase is similar in primary and secondary progressive multiple sclerosis. It is therefore unaffected by the presence or the absence of relapses preceding disease progression.

The same material allows assessment of the possible influence of superimposed relapses during either the primary or secondary phase (Figure 4.24 and Table 4.22; Confavreux *et al* 2000). Progression of irreversible disability from the assignment of DSS 4 to DSS 6 in the cases with either a primary or secondary progressive course was similar whether or not relapses were superimposed on the progressive phase. Paradoxically, the time from the assignment of DSS 4 to DSS 7, and from DSS 6 to DSS 7, was longer when relapses occurred on the background of progression than when there were no relapses. At the very least, it appears as though the rate of irreversible progression of disability from the assignment of DSS 4 is unaffected by relapses occurring during the progressive phase. Therefore, the evidence is for dissociation between relapses and progression in multiple sclerosis. These results match and extend those from other large studies on the natural history of multiple sclerosis. Data from the London, Ontario, Multiple Sclerosis Cohort show that, by comparison with primary progressive multiple sclerosis, patients with secondary progressive disease take longer to reach end points when survival curves are drawn from the time of disease onset, but a shorter interval when these are taken from onset of the progressive phase (D.A. Cottrell *et al* 1999a; Kremenchutzky *et al* 1999). The same group also showed that the survival curves are almost identical when primary progressive forms with superimposed relapses (progressive relapsing multiple sclerosis) are compared with those without (primary progressive multiple sclerosis *sensu stricto*) with respect to the time from onset to the assignment of DSS 6, DSS 8 and death (Kremenchutzky *et al* 1999). Similar conclusions have been reached by others studying primary progressive forms of multiple sclerosis for the time to DSS 6 (Andersson *et al* 1999).

These results from the Lyon, France, cohort have been reached by dichotomizing the status of relapses as present or not. When analysing the possible influence of relapses at onset and during the early years of the disease, similar results are obtained when the degree of recovery, time to the second

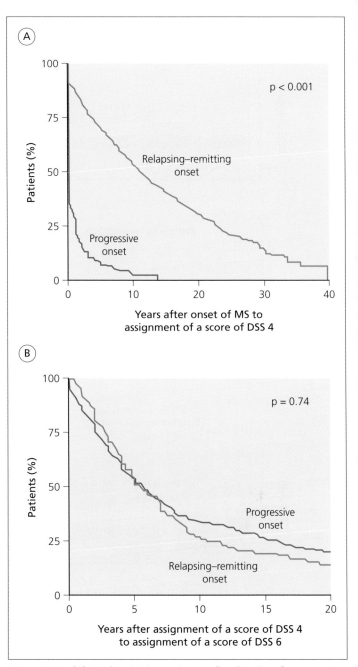

Figure 4.23 (A) Kaplan–Meier estimates for the time from onset of multiple sclerosis to the assignment of DSS 4. (B) Time from assignment of DSS 4 to DSS 6 among 1844 patients according to the initial course of the disease. Adapted from Confavreux *et al* (2000).

relapse, and the number and frequency of episodes are considered (Figure 4.25). For instance, time to a second neurological episode positively influences median times from onset of multiple sclerosis to the assignment of DSS 4, DSS 6 and DSS 7 (Confavreux *et al* 2003). Similar observations have been made in many other series (V.A. Clark *et al* 1982; Confavreux *et al* 1980; Ebers 1998; Fog and Linnemann 1970; Hyllested 1961; Kantarci *et al* 1998; Kurtzke *et al* 1977; Leibowitz and Alter 1973; McAlpine 1961; Midgard *et al* 1995; Minderhoud *et al* 1988; R. Müller 1949; Phadke 1987; 1990; S. Poser and Hauptvogel 1973; 1986; Riise *et al* 1992; Runmarker and

Table 4.21 Kaplan–Meier estimates of the time from onset of multiple sclerosis to the onset of irreversible disability, and of the time course of irreversible disability among 1844 patients with multiple sclerosis, according to the initial course of the disease.[a] Adapted from Confavreux *et al* (2000)

Variable	Relapsing–remitting onset		Progressive onset		p value[b]
	Number of patients (n = 1562)	Median time (95% CI) in years	Number of patients (n = 282)	Median time (95% CI) in years	
Time from onset of multiple sclerosis to assignment of a score of DSS 4	1562	11.4 (10.5–12.3)	282	0.0	<0.001
Time from onset of multiple sclerosis to assignment of a score of DSS 6	1562	23.1 (20.1–26.1)	282	7.1 (6.3–7.9)	<0.001
Time from onset of multiple sclerosis to assignment of a score of DSS 7	1562	33.1 (29.2–37.0)	282	13.4 (11.0–15.9)	<0.001
Time from assignment of a score of DSS 4 to assignment of a score of DSS 6	755	5.7 (4.9–6.4)	271	5.4 (4.3–6.6)	0.74
Time from assignment of a score of DSS 4 to assignment of a score of DSS 7	755	12.1 (10.0–14.2)	271	12.0 (10.1–13.9)	0.70
Time from assignment of a score of DSS 6 to assignment of a score of DSS 7	426	3.3 (2.8–3.9)	169	4.0 (2.9–5.1)	0.48

a Kurtzke Disability Status Scale (DSS) was used to determine the extent of disability.
b p values were calculated using the log-rank test.

Andersen 1993; Thygesen 1949; Trojano *et al* 1995; Weinshenker *et al* 1989a; 1989b; 1991a; 1991b). The originality of the French study is that it assessed the possible influence of the same clinical variables on the progression of irreversible disability from the time of assignment of DSS 4 to DSS 6, and also from DSS 4 to DSS 7 and DSS 6 to DSS 7 (Confavreux *et al* 2003). None of these variables remained predictive of the time course of disability past this point (Figure 4.25). Progression of irreversible disability is seemingly 'amnesic' with respect to the clinical characteristics of relapses that occurred during the initial stages of the disease. More generally, long-term progression of irreversible disability is mainly relapse dissociated and progression driven. These observations are reminiscent of those regarding sex and age at onset of multiple sclerosis in the Gothenburg, Sweden, series: both variables showed a correlation with prognosis when analysed from the onset of multiple sclerosis but not when the analyses were repeated taking 5 years after onset as the starting point (Runmarker and Andersen 1993).

All these observations have been collected using statistical analysis of groups of patients with multiple sclerosis. They are consistent with that claimed for individuals in the 1970s. From his prospective analysis of 73 patients, Fog concluded that the two components of the clinical course of multiple sclerosis are mutually independent. Relapses occur in an unpredictable way. Their frequency varies between individuals but also within a given individual. By contrast, the clinical progression of the neurological deficit can be subjected to mathematical analysis. In an individual patient, it is often very constant in degree and its slope decisive for prognosis. Relapses can be superimposed above the process of progression, but progression apparently pursues its course independent of the individual relapses.

To me at least, it seems strange that such a [steady progression] ... could be explained solely by the summation of single attacks. ... It seems therefore reasonable to believe that the phase of progression represents another biological process than the attack.

Fog and Linnemann (1970)

Course and prognosis: an age-dependent process

The influence of age on the course and prognosis of multiple sclerosis has been much studied, allowing the conclusion that patients with a late onset of disease tend to follow a primary progressive course whereas the majority of those developing symptoms earlier show an initial exacerbating–remitting pattern but with a constant rate of conversion to secondary progressive disease throughout the course of the illness (McAlpine and Compston 1952; A.R. McLean and Berkson 1951; R. Müller 1949; 1951).

More recent studies suggest that age at onset of the relapsing–remitting phase is equivalent in patients later classified either as having relapsing–remitting or secondary progressive multiple sclerosis at the time of study (Confavreux 1977; Confavreux *et al* 1980; Fog and Linnemann 1970; Leibowitz and Alter 1973; S. Poser 1978). In their 73 patients with multiple sclerosis, Fog and Linnemann (1970) found that mean age at onset of the relapsing–remitting phase was 28.5 years, and that this was similar in those remaining with relapsing–remitting multiple sclerosis (27.5 years) or converting to the secondary progressive phase (28.8 years). For onset of the progressive phase, they found a figure of 36.3 years, with no difference between primary (36.3 years) and secondary progressive (36.3 years) forms. In the Israeli series of 266 patients with multiple sclerosis, Leibowitz and Alter (1973) concluded that mean age at onset is 29.4 and 37.4 years for relapsing–remitting and primary progressive cases, respectively. In a cross-sectional study of 812 German patients, age at onset was 28.6 ± 8.9 years for relapsing–remitting multiple sclerosis, 31.2 ± 8.8 years for secondary progressive, and 36.8 ± 9.8 for primary progressive multiple sclerosis (p < 0.001: S. Poser 1978). In a cross-sectional survey of 342 Dutch patients (Minderhoud *et al* 1988), age at onset of the relapsing–remitting phase was the same in 106 individuals with relapsing–remitting multiple sclerosis (28.8 ± 10.8 years) and 108 patients with secondary progressive multiple sclerosis (29.3 ± 8.1 years). Age at onset of the progressive phase was also found to be similar in secondary (37.5 ± 8.3 years) and primary progressive multiple sclerosis (35.7 ± 11.8 years). In the updated London, Ontario, series comprising 1044 cases (D.A. Cottrell *et al* 1999a; Kremenchutzky *et al* 1999), mean age at onset was 28.6 years for cases with an initial exacerbating–remitting course and 38.5 years for multiple sclerosis that was progressive from onset.

At a time when the Lyon, France, cohort contained only 349 patients, multiple sclerosis was considered in the categories of relapsing–remitting and progressive disease (Confavreux 1977; Confavreux *et al* 1980). Mean age at onset was 30.0 years for all individuals. There was no difference in age at onset between patients who maintained the relapsing–remitting course (29.2 years) and those who subsequently converted to secondary progressive disease (31.7 years). Mean age at onset of disease progression was similar whether this occurred in the context of primary (37.3 years) or secondary (38.5 years) progressive multiple sclerosis. Later, the relapsing–remitting phase was itself considered in two stages: pure relapses and relapses with sequelae which, taken with the onset of disease progression, created three phases of the disease for consideration. In practice, these interact in various combinations to generate several different disease patterns, but there is no difference in the ages at onset for pure relapses (29.2 years) and relapses with sequelae (33.9 years). Conversion to disease progression occurs at 38.0 years, with no difference depending on whether this starts *de novo* (37.3 years) or is preceded by a relapsing–remitting phase (38.5 years; Figure 4.26).

Locking the Lyon, France, natural history cohort in April 1997, when it had accumulated 1844 patients, provided an opportunity not only to readdress the possible influence of current age on the course, but now also on the prognosis of multiple sclerosis (Confavreux and Vukusic 2006a). Median age at onset was 29.0 years amongst the 1562 patients with relapsing–remitting multiple sclerosis, 28.7 years in the 1066 patients who continued only to experience episodes, and 29.5 years in those who converted to secondary progression (Figure 4.27). For the 778 patients who experienced disease progression, either from onset or secondary to an earlier relapsing–remitting phase, median age at onset of the progressive phase was 39.1 years. This was no different when the 496 patients with a secondary progressive course were compared with the 282 patients with an overall course progressive from onset: 39.1 and 40.1 years, respectively (Figure 4.27).

In the same series (Confavreux and Vukusic 2006a), the Kaplan–Meier analysis provided estimates for the median age of

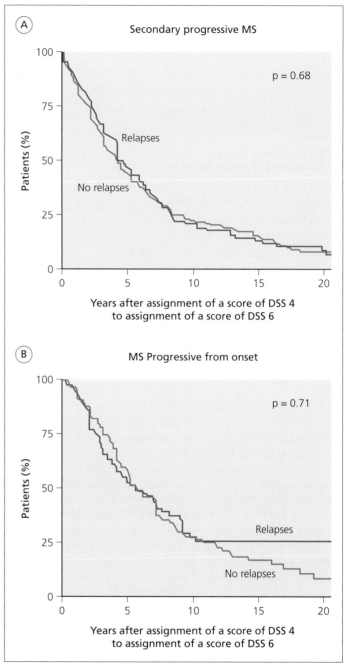

Figure 4.24 (A) Kaplan–Meier estimates for the time from the assignment of DSS 4 to DSS 6 amongst 496 patients with secondary progressive multiple sclerosis. (B) Kaplan–Meier estimates for the time from the assignment of DSS 4 to DSS 6 amongst 282 patients with primary progressive multiple sclerosis. Both graphs are according to the presence or absence of superimposed relapses during progression. Adapted from Confavreux *et al* (2000).

patients at the time irreversible disability scores were reached: 44.3 years for DSS 4; 54.7 years for DSS 6; and 63.1 years for DSS 7 (Table 4.23). The 1562 patients with an exacerbating–remitting initial course were compared with 282 patients having a progressive course from onset with respect to age at the time of reaching irreversible scores of disability. Patients with a relapsing–remitting onset were older than those progressing

Table 4.22 **Kaplan–Meier estimates of the time course of irreversible disability among patients with secondary progressive multiple sclerosis or with progressive disease from onset, according to the presence or absence of superimposed relapses during progression.**[a] Adapted from Confavreux *et al* (2000)

Variable	Progressive course without superimposed relapses		Progressive course with superimposed relapses		p value[b]
	Number of patients	Median time (95% CI) in years	Number of patients	Median time (95% CI) in years	
Secondary progressive multiple sclerosis					
Time from assignment of a disability status score of 4 to assignment of a score of 6	292	4.0 (3.1–4.9)	191	4.4 (3.9–5.0)	0.68
Time from assignment of a disability status score of 4 to assignment of a score of 7	292	7.8 (6.8–8.7)	191	10.0 (7.6–12.4)	0.04
Time from assignment of a disability status score of 6 to assignment of a score of 7	223	2.6 (2.1–3.1)	133	4.3 (3.0–5.7)	0.002
Progressive multiple sclerosis from onset					
Time from assignment of a disability status score of 4 to assignment of a score of 6	163	5.5 (4.5–6.5)	108	5.4 (3.3–7.5)	0.71
Time from assignment of a disability status score of 4 to assignment of a score of 7	163	12.4 (10.2–14.7)	108	11.3 (7.8–14.7)	0.65
Time from assignment of a disability status score of 6 to assignment of a score of 7	104	4.0 (2.8–5.2)	65	3.6 (2.2–5.0)	0.68

a Kurtzke Disability Status Scale was used to determine the extent of disability.
b p values were calculated using the log-rank test.

from onset, for assignment of DSS 4 and DSS 6. However, the differences were only 2.7 and 2.3 years for median ages at assignment of DSS 4 and 6, respectively, for a disease usually encompassing several decades of life. There was overlap in the 95% confidence intervals of these medians for both assignments, but no difference when the two groups of patients were compared with respect to DSS 7 (Figure 4.28 and Table 4.23). Furthermore, patients with a secondary progressive course were younger at the time of reaching DSS 4, DSS 6 and DSS 7 than those with a course progressive from onset (see below). Conversion from the initial relapsing–remitting phase to secondary progression occurs at a constant rate throughout the course of the disease. Considering a cohort of patients with multiple sclerosis studied at a given time, patients with the secondary progressive course represent a subgroup of more rapidly worsening forms of multiple sclerosis within the entire group of patients with exacerbating–remitting disease at onset. Therefore, the actual age at assignment of irreversible disability in patients with an exacerbating–remitting initial course lies between boundaries for this whole group of patients and ages for patients with the secondary progressive course, and closer to ages found in patients with a progressive course from onset. Taken together, it could therefore be concluded that age at time of reaching disability landmarks is not substantially influenced by the initial course of multiple sclerosis, or the mixture of relapses and

progression. This formulation provides further evidence that neurological relapses have essentially no influence on the progression of irreversible disability in the long term.

However, it would be an oversimplification to consider disability in multiple sclerosis as strictly age dependent. Age at onset also influences prognosis: the earlier the onset of the disease, the younger the age at disability landmarks (Confavreux and Vukusic 1980; 2006a). This is well illustrated in Figure 4.29 drawn from the 1980 analysis of the Lyon, France, cohort. Similarly, in a large hospital-based study of 1463 Italian patients with multiple sclerosis (Trojano *et al* 2002), age at onset and current age of the patients both correlated with disease severity – the effect of the former being smaller by comparison. Furthermore, these results, obtained in a cohort of patients, do not contradict the high variability in age at onset of the relapsing–remitting and progressive phases, and times of reaching disability landmarks, observed among individuals with multiple sclerosis. However, the age dependency phenomenon surmounts this variability showing no influence of the initial course on age at disability milestones. The dependency of course and prognosis on current age suggests that mechanisms related to aging play a role in the neurodegenerative process operating in multiple sclerosis. As discussed in Chapter 10, these may operate through unrelated endogenous mechanisms or relate to the complex interplay between injury and repair.

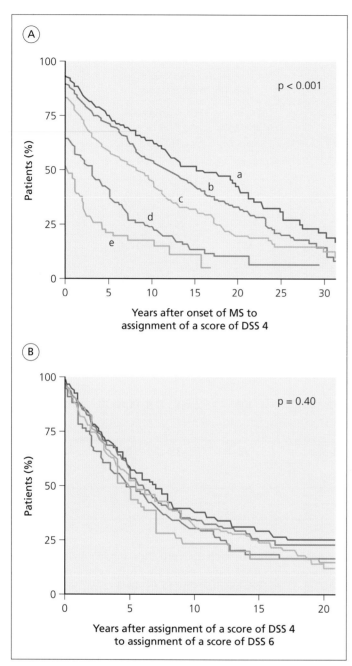

Figure 4.25 (A) Kaplan–Meier estimates for the time from onset of multiple sclerosis to the assignment of DSS 4. (B) Time from assignment of DSS 4 to DSS 6 among 1844 patients according to age of the patient at disease onset. *a*: 0–19 years; *b*: 20–29 years; *c*: 30–39 years; *d*: 40–49 years; *e*: ≥50 years. Adapted from Confavreux *et al* (2003).

To illustrate this point, one might make the comparison with a train having three carriages: the first corresponding to the relapsing–remitting period with recovery; the second to the relapsing–remitting period with sequelae; and the third to the progressive phase (Confavreux 1977). The first traveller – say, a 29-year-old – gets into the front carriage; the next passenger, who is a little late, and aged 34 years, gets in the next accessible carriage as the train moves off; the seriously late traveller, now aged 38 years, just has time to clamber aboard the third carriage and suffers progressive multiple sclerosis.

Alternatively, the metaphor can be constructed along the lines that most travellers get into the first carriage (mean age 31 years) and, as the train stops at different stations, new passengers climb aboard displacing those already settled and relocating them to the second (34 years) and third carriages (38 years). (Whether this formulation tells us more about the behaviour of individuals on the French railway system than multiple sclerosis is a matter for the reader.)

To conclude, disease severity is influenced by age at onset of multiple sclerosis, the benign and severe forms being more frequent in younger and older patients, respectively. But it remains a matter of debate whether, from the patient's perspective, having 'benign' multiple sclerosis from early adult life is necessarily preferable to developing a more 'rapid' form much later (Confavreux 1977; Confavreux *et al* 1980). Clearly, as clinical scientists we wish to deal effectively with all manifestations of the disease without making quality judgments on who has it 'good' or 'bad'.

Primary and secondary progression: differences and similarities

The reasons why progression may start *de novo* or after a period of episodes remains largely unexplained. This has led many neurologists to consider primary progressive multiple sclerosis as a separate entity from other forms of the disease. Recent analysis of the Lyon, France, natural history cohort (Confavreux and Vukusic 2006b) and available data from other sources in the literature has allowed the clinical evidence for and against this hypothesis to be reconsidered.

Secondary progressive multiple sclerosis and relapsing–remitting multiple sclerosis

Table 4.24 shows a difference in the Lyon, France, cohort relating to gender distribution; there are more females amongst 1066 cases with relapsing–remitting disease than in the 496 individuals with secondary progressive multiple sclerosis. By contrast, the two populations are similar in the distribution of initial symptoms during the relapsing–remitting phase, the degree of recovery from the first relapse, and the time from onset to the second neurological episode (Table 4.24). As already discussed, distribution according to age at onset of the relapsing–remitting phase is strikingly similar (Figure 4.27) and in agreement with other series (Fog and Linnemann 1970; Leibowitz and Alter 1973; Minderhoud *et al* 1988; S. Poser 1978). Similarities also emerge from brain MRI analyses. Although the lesion load is usually considered higher in secondary progressive than relapsing–remitting multiple sclerosis, the MRI activity is identical and, to most authors, indistinguishable between these variants of the disease (W.I. McDonald 1994; A.J. Thompson *et al* 1991; Van Walderveen *et al* 1998).

By contrast, the two populations in the Lyon, France, cohort clearly differ in duration of the disease, which was twice as long in the secondary progressive (17.6 ± 9.6 years) compared with the relapsing–remitting multiple sclerosis group (8.7 ± 8.6 years: Table 4.24). Others have reached the same conclusions. In a German study, disease duration at the time of the survey was 6.1 ± 7.2 years in relapsing–remitting and 11.7 ± 8.0 years in secondary progressive multiple sclerosis, a highly significant

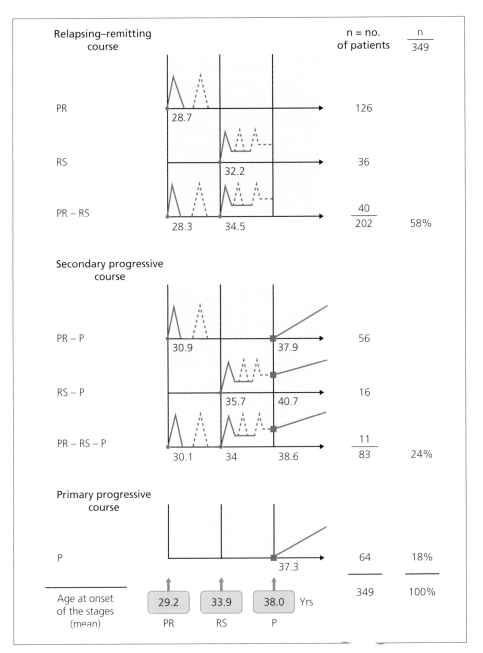

Figure 4.26 Age at onset for the different phases of 'pure relapses' (PR); 'relapses with sequelae' (RS); and 'progression' (P) during the course of multiple sclerosis in 349 patients. Adapted from Confavreux *et al* (1980).

difference (p < 0.001: S. Poser 1978). In an Italian study, corresponding figures were 7.3 ± 5.5 in relapsing–remitting and 14.3 ± 8.6 years in secondary progressive multiple sclerosis (Trojano *et al* 1995). We conclude that patients with an initial exacerbating–remitting course of multiple sclerosis will naturally convert to the secondary progressive phase at a rate of around 2–3% per annum, following an essentially linear curve (see Figure 4.10). The longer the disease duration at the time of the survey, the higher the proportion of cases classified as secondary progressive multiple sclerosis compared with those classified as having relapsing–remitting disease. Although the relapsing–remitting and secondary progressive phases clearly represent two clinical stages of the same disease in patients with bout onset multiple sclerosis, this is an argument in favour of the hypothesis that secondary progressive multiple sclerosis is relapsing–remitting multiple sclerosis that has had 'time to grow older' (Confavreux 1977; Confavreux *et al* 1980).

Primary progressive multiple sclerosis and progressive relapsing multiple sclerosis

By definition, these apparently distinct forms of multiple sclerosis share the progressive onset but differ in that superimposed relapses accompany progressive relapsing but not primary progressive multiple sclerosis (Lublin and Reingold 1996). Among the 218 patients of the London, Ontario, series with an initial progressive course (D.A. Cottrell *et al* 1999a; Kremenchuzky *et al* 1999), 28% exhibited ≥1 distinct relapse during progression, sometimes decades after disease onset, qualifying them for reclassification as progressive relapsing forms of multiple sclerosis (Lublin and Reingold 1996). In 50%, relapses occurred in the first 10 years, and at intervals from onset to 20 years or more for the other half. Relapses were never frequent, and most patients had but a single episode. This was usually mild and followed by good recovery (Kremenchutzky *et al* 1999). Among

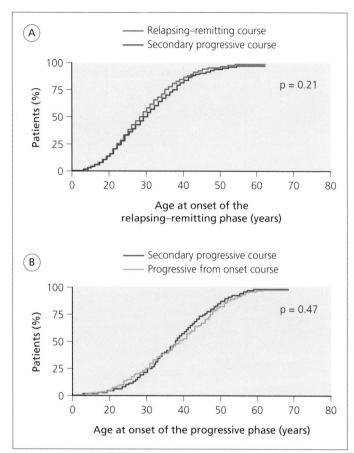

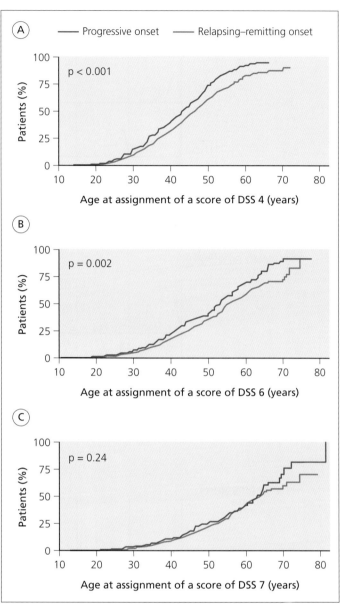

Figure 4.27 (A) Kaplan–Meier estimates for the age at onset of the relapsing–remitting phase of multiple sclerosis. (B) Kaplan–Meier estimates for the age at onset of the progressive phase of multiple sclerosis among 1844 patients with multiple sclerosis, according to the overall course of the disease. Adapted from Confavreux and Vukusic (2006b).

Figure 4.28 Kaplan–Meier estimates for the age at assignment of DSS 4 (A), DSS 6 (B) and DSS 7 (C) amongst 1844 patients with multiple sclerosis, according to the initial course. Adapted from Confavreux and Vukusic (2006a).

the 282 patients with a progressive initial course of multiple sclerosis from the Lyon, France, series (Confavreux and Vukusic 2000; 2006b), 109 (39%) could be qualified thus. Table 4.25 shows that median age at onset was earlier in progressive relapsing (37 years) than in primary progressive cases (41 years; p < 0.02), although this is the only difference that could be observed when comparing these two forms of multiple sclerosis according to demographic and clinical characteristics, such as gender and initial symptoms of the disease. A similar trend for age at onset was found in the London, Ontario, series (Kremenchutzky et al 1999).

The rates at which irreversible disability progresses, calculated from the onset of multiple sclerosis or from assignment of a given disability score, were essentially similar in progressive relapsing and primary progressive multiple sclerosis. In both cases, the Lyon, France, cohort (Confavreux and Vukusic 2000; 2006b) showed median survival times from onset of multiple sclerosis at 0, 7 and 13 years to reach DSS 4, DSS 6 and DSS 7, respectively (Table 4.25). Taking DSS 4 as the baseline, median times to reach DSS 6 and DSS 7 were 5 and 12 years, respectively. From DSS 6, median time to reach DSS 7 was 4 years. These results are consistent with other series. In the London, Ontario, series, there were no differences in time to reach disability

levels assessed by survival analyses from onset of multiple sclerosis when comparing primary progressive and progressive relapsing disease: in both situations, median times to reach DSS 3, DSS 6, DSS 8 and death were 3, 8, 18 and 35 years, respectively (D.A. Cottrell et al 1999a; Krementchutzky et al 1999). No other differences between the two forms of multiple sclerosis could be discerned when calculations were made from assignment of DSS 3 to reach DSS 6, DSS 8 and death (Kremenchutzky et al 1999). In a Californian cross-sectional study based upon telephone interview with a standardized questionnaire – comprising 83 cases with primary progressive multiple sclerosis and 12 with progressive relapsing multiple sclerosis – survival time from onset of multiple sclerosis to reach DSS 6 was 10.2 ± 1.0 years and 10.9 ± 2.6 years in primary progressive and progressive relapsing multiple sclerosis, respectively

Table 4.23 Kaplan–Meier estimates of the age of patients at the time when irreversible disability scores of DSS 4, DSS 6 and DSS 7 were obtained in 1844 patients with multiple sclerosis.[a] Adapted from Confavreux and Vukusic (2006a)

Variable	No. of patients (n = 1844)	Age at assignment of a score of DSS 4			Age at assignment of a score of DSS 6			Age at assignment of a score of DSS 7		
		Median (years)	(95% CI)	p value[b]	Median (years)	(95% CI)	p value[b]	Median (years)	(95% CI)	p value[b]
Overall	1844	44.3	(43.3–45.2)	NA	54.7	(53.5–55.8)	NA	63.1	(61.0–65.1)	NA
Initial course of multiple sclerosis										
Relapsing-remitting	1562	44.8	(43.8–45.9)	Baseline comparator	55.3	(54.2–56.7)	Baseline comparator	62.8	(60.3–65.4)	Baseline comparator
Progressive	282	42.1	(40.2–44.0)	<0.001	53.0	(51.1–54.9)	0.002	63.1	(60.0–66.2)	0.24

a Kurtzke Disability Status Scale (DSS) was used to determine the extent of disability.
b p values were calculated using the log-rank test.

239

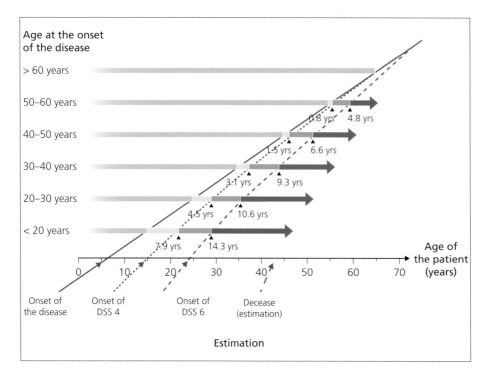

Figure 4.29 Age at onset of multiple sclerosis and age at times of assignment of irreversible disability among 349 patients with multiple sclerosis. Moderate disability = DSS 4. Severe disability = DSS 7. The digits below the horizontal arrows indicate the time (years) to reach the disability landmarks as calculated from the onset of the disease. Adapted from Confavreux *et al* (1980).

Table 4.24 **Comparative demographic and disease-related characteristics of relapsing–remitting cases and secondary progressive cases, among 1562 patients with an exacerbating–remitting onset from the Lyon multiple sclerosis cohort. Adapted from Confavreux and Vukusic (2006b)**

	Relapsing–remitting multiple sclerosis[a] (n = 1066)	Secondary progressive multiple sclerosis[a] (n = 496)	p value
Gender (%)			
Males	32	39	
Females	68	61	0.006*
Age at onset of multiple sclerosis (years)			
Mean ± SD	29.4 ± 9.3	29.8 ± 9.9	0.39**
Median	28.7	29.5	
Initial symptoms of the relapsing–remitting phase (%)			
Isolated optic neuritis	21	22	
Isolated brainstem dysfunction	9	12	
Isolated dysfunction of long tracts	46	47	0.13*
Combination of symptoms	24	19	
Recovery from the first episode (%)			
Complete	83	81	
Incomplete	17	19	0.25*
Kaplan–Meier estimate of the time from onset of multiple sclerosis to the second episode (years)			
Median	1.7	2.3	0.07**
Duration of multiple sclerosis (years)			
Mean ± SD	8.7 ± 8.6	17.6 ± 9.6	< 0.001***

a Defined according to the Lublin and Reingold (1996) classification.
p values are calculated with use of the chi-squared test (*), the log rank test (**), or Student's t test (***).
SD = standard deviation.

Table 4.25 Comparative demographic and disease-related characteristics of progressive relapsing cases and primary progressive cases, among 282 patients with a progressive onset of multiple sclerosis from the Lyon, France, multiple sclerosis cohort. Adapted from Confavreux *et al* (2000) and Confavreux and Vukusic (2006b)

	Progressive relapsing multiple sclerosis[a] n = 109	Primary progressive multiple sclerosis[a] n = 173	p value
Gender (%)			
Males	38	46	0.15*
Females	62	54	
Age at onset of multiple sclerosis (years)			
Mean ± standard deviation	37.3 ± 11.5	40.6 ± 10.7	0.02**
Median	38.1	41.3	
Initial symptoms of multiple sclerosis (%)			
Isolated optic neuritis	1	2	
Isolated brainstem dysfunction	0	1	0.18*
Isolated dysfunction of long tracts	80	87	
Combination of symptoms	19	10	
Kaplan–Meier estimates of the time (median in years)			
From onset of multiple sclerosis to assignment of a disability status score of			
DSS 4	0.0	0.0	0.50**
DSS 6	7.5	6.8	0.37**
DSS 7	13.7	12.8	0.92**
From assignment of a disability status score of 4 to			
DSS 6	5.4	5.5	0.71**
DSS 7	11.3	12.4	0.65**
From assignment of a disability status score of 6 to			
DSS 7	3.6	4.0	0.68**
Kaplan–Meier estimates of the age (median in years) at the time of assignment of a disability status score of			
DSS 4	40.0	43.3	0.003**
DSS 6	52.2	54.7	0.09**
DSS 7	58.7	64.4	0.11**
Duration of multiple sclerosis (years)			
Mean ± standard deviation	10.9 ± 7.4	9.6 ± 8.4	0.20***

a Defined according to the Lublin and Reingold (1996) classification.
p values are calculated with use of the chi-squared test (*), the log rank test (**), or Student's t test (***).
DSS = Kurtzke Disability Status Scale.

(Andersson *et al* 1999) We entirely endorse the position of the Canadian and the Californian studies: these results indicate that progressive relapsing and primary progressive multiple sclerosis are, from a clinical point of view, essentially the same. Therefore, it is appropriate to pool these cases in a single category initially having a progressive course, the only difference being the subsequent experience of superimposed relapses. The occasional confusion between progressive relapsing and secondary progressive multiple sclerosis might account for the slightly earlier onset in progressive relapsing than primary progressive multiple sclerosis. The single report containing preliminary comparative information on brain and spinal cord MRI in these two forms of multiple sclerosis offers no pathological data and lacks firm conclusions (Andersson *et al* 1999).

Secondary progressive multiple sclerosis and multiple sclerosis with a progressive initial course

The variations in clinical pattern between primary and secondary progressive multiple sclerosis have often been compared, and the general consensus is that they are very different. A semantic issue needs to be settled. For several decades, clinicians and investigators involved in the study of multiple sclerosis agreed a single definition for secondary progressive multiple sclerosis and this was eventually adopted in the international survey classification (Lublin and Reingold 1996). The female preponderance expected in a general population of patients with multiple sclerosis is much reduced in cases with an initial progressive course, compared with those with secondary progressive multiple sclerosis (D.A. Cottrell *et al* 1999a; Kremenchutzky *et al* 1999; McDonnell and Hawkins 1996; 1998b; A.J. Thompson *et al* 1997). In the Lyon, France, cohort there was only a trend in that direction, not reaching statistical significance (Table 4.26: Confavreux and Vukusic 2006b). From the clinical perspective, the initial course and symptoms – more often related to dysfunction of long tracts in multiple sclerosis with a progressive onset than in secondary progressive disease – are very different (see data for the Lyon, France, cohort in Tables 4.24 and 4.26). Arguing from the position that age at onset is greater, time to assignment of irreversible disability shorter, prognosis worse (Table 4.26, and see above), MRI characteristics and the pathology are both different (see Chapters 7 and 12; Revesz *et al* 1994), and genetic

Table 4.26 Comparative demographic and disease-related characteristics of secondary progressive multiple sclerosis and cases with a progressive initial course, among 1844 patients with multiple sclerosis from the Lyon, France, multiple sclerosis cohort. Adapted from Confavreux *et al* (2000) and Confavreux and Vukusic (2006b)

	Secondary progressive multiple sclerosis[a] (n = 496)	Multiple sclerosis with a progressive initial course[b] (n = 282)	p value
Gender (%)			
Males	39	43	
Females	61	57	0.32*
Age at onset of the progressive phase of multiple sclerosis (years)			
Mean ± standard deviation	39.5 ± 10.3	39.4 ± 11.3	
Median	39.1	40.1	0.47**
Initial symptoms of the progressive phase of multiple sclerosis (%)			
Isolated optic neuritis	0	2	
Isolated brainstem dysfunction	0	0	
Isolated dysfunction of long tracts	85	84	0.11*
Combination of symptoms	15	14	
Superimposed relapses during the progressive phase (%)			
Yes	40	39	
No	60	61	0.81*
Kaplan–Meier estimates of the time (median in years) from onset of multiple sclerosis to assignment of			
DSS 4	6.1	0.0	<0.001**
DSS 6	12.5	7.1	<0.001**
DSS 7	19.1	13.4	<0.001**
From assignment of a disability status score of 4 to			
DSS 6	4.0	5.4	0.001**
DSS 7	9.0	12.0	<0.001**
From assignment of a disability status score of 6 to			
DSS 7	3.0	4.0	0.09**
Kaplan–Meier estimates of the age (median in years) at the time of assigning a disability status score of			
DSS 4	37.6	42.1	<0.001**
DSS 6	45.5	53.0	<0.001**
DSS 7	53.3	63.1	<0.001**
Duration of multiple sclerosis (years)			
Mean ± standard deviation	17.6 ± 9.6	10.1 ± 8.0	<0.001***

a Defined according to the Lublin and Reingold (1996) classification.
b Denotes the pooling of cases with 'progressive relapsing multiple sclerosis' and of cases with 'primary progressive multiple sclerosis' (Lublin and Reingold 1996).
p values are calculated with use of the chi-squared test (*), the log rank test (**), or Student's t test (***).
DSS = Kurtzke Disability Status Scale.

susceptibility occurs on a different background (see Chapter 3; Masterman *et al* 2000a; Olerup *et al* 1989), the majority of clinicians consider primary progressive multiple sclerosis to be distinct from secondary progressive disease – but that leaves open the issue of whether this arises from complexity or true disease heterogeneity (see Chapter 14).

But the distinctions are not necessarily so clear-cut. In fact, comparing cases from the time that progression becomes manifest (at onset or after a period of episodes) reveals many similarities. Table 4.26 shows that, in the Lyon, France, cohort, age and initial symptoms at onset of the progressive phase were similar in the 496 cases with secondary progressive multiple sclerosis and the 282 cases with progressive disease from onset. The proportion of cases with superimposed relapses during progression was around 40% in both categories. However, the time

course of disability accumulation during the progressive phase of the disease was more rapid and occurred earlier in secondary progressive multiple sclerosis than individuals with a progressive onset. For instance, the median survival time from DSS 4 to DSS 6 was 4.0 years in secondary progressive multiple sclerosis and 5.4 years in multiple sclerosis with progression from onset (p = 0.001). Similarly, median age at reaching DSS 4 was 37.6 and 42.1 years in these two groups, respectively (p < 0.001). This leads to the conclusion that, once clinical progression has started, the rate at which disability accumulates is faster in secondary progressive multiple sclerosis than cases with progression from onset (Confavreux and Vukusic 2000; 2006b). These are not unique observations. From analyses based upon crude observational data, time from onset of progression to reach DSS 7 in a Dutch series was shorter in the 108 cases with secondary

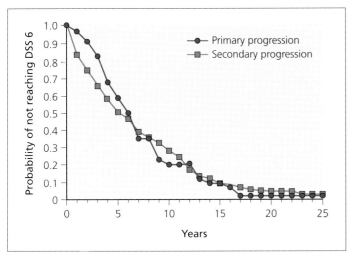

Figure 4.30 Kaplan–Meier estimates for the time (years) from onset of progression to the assignment of DSS 6 among 162 patients with secondary progressive and 36 patients with primary progressive multiple sclerosis. Primary progressive multiple sclerosis denotes here the pooling of cases with 'primary progressive multiple sclerosis' and cases with 'progressive relapsing multiple sclerosis' according to the classification of Lublin and Reingold (1996). Adapted from Runmarker and Andersen (1993). © 1993, reprinted with permission of Springer-Verlag GmbH.

progressive multiple sclerosis than in the 128 cases with progressive disease from onset (Minderhoud *et al* 1988). In the London, Ontario, cohort, the median survival time from onset of progression to reach DSS 6 was 5.5 years in the 538 patients with secondary progressive multiple sclerosis and 9.5 years in the 218 patients with an initial progressive course. For the time to reach DSS 8, the corresponding figures were around 15 and 20 years, respectively (D.A. Cottrell *et al* 1999a; Kremenchutzky *et al* 1999). Conversely, in the Gothenburg, Sweden, cohort (Runmarker and Andersen 1993), median survival time from the onset of progression to DSS 6 was 5.2 years for the 162 cases with secondary progressive multiple sclerosis and 6.0 years for the 36 with progression from onset, but this is not statistically significant (Figure 4.30).

Cases with an initial relapsing–remitting course and cases with an initial progressive course

It serves little purpose to restate the differences regarding sex ratio, age and symptoms at onset or survival times from onset or between disability landmarks because these are essentially similar to what has already been discussed. Our objective here is to compare, within a general cohort of patients having multiple sclerosis, all cases with an exacerbating–remitting onset (i.e. 'relapsing–remitting multiple sclerosis' and 'secondary progressive multiple sclerosis') and those with a progressive onset (i.e. 'progressive relapsing multiple sclerosis' and 'primary progressive multiple sclerosis') with respect to the time course of disability. In the 1562 patients with an exacerbating–remitting initial course and the 282 patients with progression from onset in the Lyon, France, cohort (Confavreux and Vukusic 2000; 2006b), the time from assignment of DSS 4 to reach DSS 6

and DSS 7, and the time from DSS 6 to DSS 7, appeared strikingly similar (Table 4.27). Furthermore, as already discussed, age at time of assigning disability landmarks could be viewed as not substantially influenced by the initial course, be that exacerbating–remitting or progressive.

Therefore, the generally observed more rapid accumulation of disability (Confavreux *et al* 2000; D.A. Cottrell *et al* 1999a; Minderhoud *et al* 1988; Kremenchutzky *et al* 1999), and the earlier age at disability milestones observed in the Lyon, France, series (Confavreux and Vukusic 2006a) in secondary progressive multiple sclerosis compared with individuals with a progressive onset, more probably reflect limited disease duration at the time of the survey. Indeed, the proportion of cases with an exacerbating–remitting onset converting to secondary progression follows a somewhat linear curve during the course of multiple sclerosis. The shorter the disease duration, the fewer the cases with secondary progressive multiple sclerosis within the population of cases having an initial exacerbating–remitting course. The subgroup of individuals with an exacerbating–remitting onset already having converted to secondary progressive multiple sclerosis at the time of any survey, selects the most severe group from the cohort of all cases with an exacerbating–remitting onset. It is therefore not surprising that, the longer the disease lasts, the more estimates for the time course of disability accumulation slow down and approximate to those seen in the population with progressive multiple sclerosis from onset. In the Gothenburg, Sweden, cohort, where the proportion of secondary progressive multiple sclerosis (77% of cases with an exacerbating remitting onset) and the duration of the disease (>25 years) were both high, accumulation of disability was similar in progressive onset and secondary progressive multiple sclerosis (see Figure 4.30; Runmarker and Andersen 1993). Therefore, from a clinical perspective, secondary and primary progression share much more than they differ.

INTERCURRENT LIFE EVENTS

The person with multiple sclerosis is no less exposed to intercurrent life events than any other member of society. These may be natural, such as pregnancy and the puerperium; accidental, as in stress, trauma and infection; or interventional, through vaccinations. The neurologist should be aware of their possible influence on the patient and, in some instances, that person's relatives. Mainly this information provides for accurate and comprehensive counselling but it may also serve medico-legal purposes. Some of these life events can be regarded as experiments of nature, proving informative about disease mechanisms and, sometimes, suggesting new therapeutic strategies.

There is no biological rationale for considering the first clinical episode of demyelination – the onset of multiple sclerosis – as different from the subsequent events, designated 'relapses' once the diagnosis is established. Perhaps, the first episode is more instructive because it lies closer to events that cause the disease process; but it is clear that clinical onset and disease onset are not synonymous, often being separated by many years (McDonnell 2003) or, occasionally, an entire lifetime (Gilbert and Sadler 1983). Here, we leave aside the issues of causation (see Chapter 2) and focus on the possible triggering effect of intercurrent events on the activity of a disease process that is already established, even if not yet clinically overt.

Table 4.27 Comparative demographic and disease-related characteristics of cases with an exacerbating–remitting initial course and cases with a progressive initial course of multiple sclerosis, among 1844 patients with multiple sclerosis from the Lyon, France, multiple sclerosis cohort. Adapted from Confavreux *et al* (2000) and Confavreux and Vukusic (2006b)

	Multiple sclerosis with an exacerbating–remitting initial course[a] (n = 1562)	Multiple sclerosis with a progressive initial course[b] (n = 282)	p value
Gender (%)			
Males	34	43	0.006*
Females	66	57	
Age at onset of multiple sclerosis (years)			
Mean ± standard deviation	29.6 ± 9.5	39.4 ± 11.3	<0.001**
Median	29.0	40.1	
Initial symptoms of multiple sclerosis (%)			
Isolated optic neuritis	21	2	
Isolated brainstem dysfunction	10	0	<0.001*
Isolated dysfunction of long tracts	47	84	
Combination of symptoms	22	14	
Kaplan–Meier estimates of the time (median in years) from onset of multiple sclerosis to assignment of a disability status score of			
DSS 4	11.4	0.0	<0.001**
DSS 6	23.1	7.1	<0.001**
DSS 7	33.1	13.4	<0.001**
From assignment of a disability status score of 4 to			
DSS 6	5.7	5.4	0.74**
DSS 7	12.1	12.0	0.70**
From assignment of a disability status score of 6 to			
DSS 7	3.3	4.0	0.48**
Kaplan–Meier estimates of the age (median in years) at the time of assigning a disability status score of			
DSS 4	44.8	42.1	<0.001**
DSS 6	55.3	53.0	0.002**
DSS 7	62.8	63.1	0.24**
Duration of multiple sclerosis (years)			
Mean ± standard deviation	11.5 ± 9.9	10.1 ± 8.0	<0.001***

a Denotes the pooling of cases with 'relapsing remitting multiple sclerosis' and of cases with 'secondary progressive multiple sclerosis' (Lublin and Reingold 1996).
b Denotes the pooling of cases with 'progressive relapsing multiple sclerosis' and of cases with 'primary progressive multiple sclerosis' (Lublin and Reingold 1996).
p values are calculated with use of the chi-squared test (*), the log rank test (**), or Student's t test (***).
DSS = Kurtzke Disability Status Scale.

Methodological considerations

Many intercurrent life events are suspected of triggering relapses in people with multiple sclerosis but establishing a causal relationship is not always straightforward. There are a number of possible methodological pitfalls. Defining and ascertaining the putative provocative event may be difficult; not for pregnancy and delivery or vaccinations, but more so with trauma, stress and infections (see below), and in deciding with confidence that the patient has genuinely experienced a new relapse. Many episodes are characterized clinically by the worsening of existing symptoms or the reappearance of those formerly experienced by the patient. Here, the distinction has to be made from pseudorelapses in which a variety of mechanisms, other than disease activity, may be responsible for the change in clinical symptoms (see Chapters 13 and 16). It may therefore be appropriate only to consider episodes featuring new neurological manifesta-

tions with respect to the past history of that patient; these more reliably correspond to disease activity in the central nervous system. One solution is to use an acknowledged surrogate marker for relapse. The assessment of MRI activity from new and enlarging T_2 lesions, and gadolinium enhancing lesions on T_1-weighted sequences serve this purpose (W.I. McDonald 1994; McFarland *et al* 1992) but make the study more demanding for the patient; and, for the researcher, more costly and therefore less feasible.

Much attention must also be paid to the protocol design. Prospective studies are considered the gold standard. Ideally, to minimize ascertainment bias, registration of exposure to the event and a new clinical event should be made by two different examiners, blind to the other's observations. Furthermore, patients should not be briefed on the nature and purpose of the study until completion, in order to protect from the potential of that person misconstruing a pseudorelapse for an actual episode, after exposure to the event of interest in the study. All of these objectives are far from easy to achieve in practice. That said, prospective designs reduce the risk of undernotification both for intercurrent events and relapse, especially when assessments are performed at close intervals. Monthly to quarterly assessment of relapse frequency seems to be a good compromise. By contrast, retrospective designs for addressing events such as infection and relapse are much less satisfactory because they introduce recall bias for the putative infection, the status of which can never reliably be ascertained. However, it must be emphasized that there are situations, relating to the epidemiology of multiple sclerosis, for which retrospective protocols represent an excellent choice. The prerequisite is that both the possible triggering event and the clinical outcome can easily be ascertained in retrospect. This is the case for vaccinations, which can reliably be validated from certificates, and for relapses when using pre-established databases containing appropriate descriptors of the disease in individual patients (Confavreux *et al* 2001). Such retrospective protocols offer major advantages. They allow for a quicker answer compared with a prospective protocol, because the research data are available from the outset. Blinding is reliable, thus minimizing association bias – the tendency for patient and examiner spuriously to register a relapse after the possible triggering event.

Ideally, studies that aim to assess the effect of a given event on relapses of multiple sclerosis should be randomized and placebo controlled. This type of protocol can be designed for interventions such as vaccinations. It is, however, unrealistic for natural events – pregnancy and parturition – or episodes of trauma, stress and infection. That is why such studies are mainly observational. Next is the reference population to which events in the group at risk should be compared. Unrelated controls, historical or contemporary, can be selected but for triggering events this may not be ideal. The likelihood of being exposed to the event is never independent of disease activity or disability. A simple example can be offered with respect to pregnancy in multiple sclerosis. This may be because the decision of a woman with multiple sclerosis to become pregnant is bound to be influenced by her level of disease activity. In the two studies on pregnancy and multiple sclerosis using a specific matched group, the control patients had higher annualized relapse rates (0.86 and 0.82) than the pregnancy group during their non-pregnancy phases of the study (0.51 and 0.63, respectively: Roullet *et al* 1993; Sadovnick *et al* 1994). The higher relapse rate in controls from these two examples suggests that the decision to embark on pregnancy is associated with lower than average relapse rates. For this reason, the design in which comparison is made with periods at risk and not at risk for the individual participants is preferred. At-risk periods following exposure to the event of interest are predefined, with the assumption that if a relapse is observed during this period, it can be regarded as associated with the event. Periods not at risk serve as control intervals. The relapse rates during these two epochs are then systematically compared. Such designs, equivalent to a case–control approach (where cases serve as their own controls), have numerous advantages when dealing with acute events such as relapses of multiple sclerosis and transient exposures including vaccinations, infections or obstetric delivery. They avoid the need for control subjects and account for confounding factors that could not be addressed by a classical case–control approach, because of the large variability in clinical characteristics of multiple sclerosis.

The period at risk must be regarded as the limits for an effect – the interval in which a relapse must occur to justify a causal relationship to the event of interest. Over what period to consider exposure potentially relevant requires judgment. The intervals should be set on the basis of plausibility and scrutiny of the available literature. For instance, 2 months was adopted in the study of vaccines and relapses of multiple sclerosis (Confavreux *et al* 2001). For infections, extending the period at risk ahead of the date when the manifestations of infection first became apparent makes sense because of difficulty in precisely dating the onset of many infections (Sibley *et al* 1985). Furthermore, it is well established that virus shedding can occur as early as 13 days before the onset of clinical symptoms (Sibley *et al* 1985). Therefore, it is logical to assess the sensitivity of analyses using varying periods at risk in order to be satisfied that the findings are robust.

Eventually, the investigator has to decide whether an association is coincidental or causal. Biological plausibility must clearly be taken into consideration. Evidence based on anecdotal reports is easily challenged, on the grounds that this introduces bias towards cases exhibiting such an association. That said, these clues should not invariably be discarded without due consideration. Often, it is such anecdotal evidence that suggests a genuine association. It follows that, for physicians and lay people alike, once the suggestions have been duly registered, supportive evidence for the association must be sought from appropriately designed and conducted epidemiological and mechanistic studies. In the event, many alleged associations based on anecdotal reports are refuted by subsequent prospective studies. Lastly, negative studies must also be interpreted properly. It is often said that they can never exclude the putative association. This conclusion can be accepted when the studies are woefully lacking in statistical power; but negative studies may be very informative in providing confidence intervals around the final result. They indicate the range and limits within which the actual magnitude of the association lies with 95% probability.

The possible influence of intercurrent events on the activity of multiple sclerosis is much less easy to establish than a therapeutic effect. Whilst the prospective, randomized, placebo-controlled, parallel groups, double-blind design is ideal, it is not always applicable or even appropriate in an area of research requiring flexibility, imagination and subtlety of approach.

Pregnancy and the puerperium

Multiple sclerosis mainly affects women in their childbearing years, and the issue of pregnancy is therefore a major concern for many affected individuals. Important questions include the effects of pregnancy, delivery, epidural analgesia and breast feeding on the course of the illness; and, conversely, the possible influence of multiple sclerosis on the pregnancy, the delivery and the infant. Understandably, the prospective mother will wonder whether multiple sclerosis may recur in her child, and reflect on the possibility that evolution of her own neurological illness may limit the ability to participate actively in the child's upbringing. Each issue raises anxieties for the young woman with multiple sclerosis wanting to have a child.

For many years, women with multiple sclerosis were actively discouraged from contemplating pregnancy due to the possible deleterious effect of pregnancy on the disease (Douglass and

Jorgensen 1948). But reliable information was lacking and most opinion offered *ex cathedra*. In the early 1950s, the pendulum of opinion swung and pregnancy was stated to be without any adverse effect (Sweeney 1955; Tillman 1950). Since then, a number of studies looking at specific aspects of the potential risks have been published (for review, see Abramsky 1994; Birk and Rudick 1986; Hutchinson 1993), replacing this with a more informed view concluding that relapse rate decreases during the last trimester of pregnancy, but rebounds in the immediate postpartum period. However, important issues were incompletely addressed in these surveys and many findings remained contradictory. The majority of studies enrolled a limited number of patients, and therefore lacked statistical power; they were performed at a single centre so that the results could not be generalized; or the data were gathered retrospectively and so likely to suffer from recall bias. Some surveys had recourse to non-pregnant controls but, as discussed above, women with multiple sclerosis who decide to become pregnant tend to have a more benign course than those who choose not to have children.

Relapses of multiple sclerosis

Pregnancy In Multiple Sclerosis (PRIMS) was the first large prospective study of the natural history in pregnant women with multiple sclerosis (Confavreux *et al* 1998b; Vukusic *et al* 2004). Previously, the only study that could be considered prospective using conventional criteria (Friedman 1987; Rudick 1995) was based on eight women (Birk *et al* 1990). The annualized relapse rate during pregnancy was 0.2, whereas it reached 3.0 during the 3-month post-delivery period (Table 4.28). Four previous studies of pregnancy and relapse frequency in women with multiple sclerosis reported annualized rates for the non-pregnancy period in the range 0.09–0.32 (Ghezzi and Caputo 1981; Korn-Lubetzki *et al* 1984; Millar *et al* 1959; Schapira *et al* 1966) suggesting that the retrospective review was insensitive and not adequate. Presumably the same criticism can be levelled at the study reported by L.M. Nelson *et al* (1988), which used a structured interview screening the past pregnancies of a specific population of women with multiple sclerosis selected for the purpose of a therapeutic trial (Table 4.28). Self-evidently, the

Table 4.28 Natural history literature data on the relapse rate of multiple sclerosis during pregnancy and post partum

Study	Number of pregnancies (number of women)	Annualized relapse rate				
		Pregnancy	1st trimester post partum	Pregnancy year	Internal control	External control
Studies with reference relapse rate <0.5/yr						
Millar *et al* 1959	170 (70)	0.05	0.92	0.26	0.09	0.10
Schapira *et al* 1966	124 (NA)	0.13	0.61	0.25	0.17	0.14
Ghezzi and Caputo 1981	206 (119)	0.22	1.77	0.61	0.32	0.29
Korn-Lubetzki *et al* 1984	199 (66)	0.13	0.82	0.31	0.29	0.28
L.M. Nelson *et al* 1988	191 (111)	0.13	0.92	0.33	Not available	Not available
Studies with reference relapse rate >0.5/yr						
Frith and McLeod 1988	85 (50)	0.30	0.66	0.39	0.53	Not available
Birk *et al* 1990	8 (8)	0.17	3.00	0.88	Not available	Not available
Bernardi *et al* 1991	66 (52)	0.10	0.97	0.32	0.65	Not available
Roullet *et al* 1993	32 (NA)	0.79	1.62	1.00	0.51	0.86
Sadovnick *et al* 1994	58 (47)	0.46	0.97	0.59	0.63	0.82
Worthington *et al* 1994	14 (14)	0.48	1.71	0.79	0.57	0.50
Achiron *et al* 2004	39 (39)	0.58	1.33	0.77	0.79	Not available
De Sèze *et al* 2004	22 (22)	0.22	2.00	0.66	0.61	Not available
Total	**324 (NA)**	0.37	1.15	0.57	0.61	0.79
PRIMS Study						
Confavreux *et al* 1998b	**227 (227)**	0.42	1.22	0.62	0.72	Not available

'Postpartum' refers to the first trimester following delivery.
The pregnancy year includes the 9-month pregnancy and the 3-month postpartum periods.
Internal controls concern the same patients but during outside pregnancy periods.
External controls concern other patients with multiple sclerosis during outside pregnancy periods.
NA = not available.

ability to detect a relapse depends on intensity of the clinical assessments (Fog and Linnemann 1970). We expect a mean relapse rate in young women with recent onset multiple sclerosis of >0.5 per year (Confavreux *et al* 1980; Weinshenker *et al* 1989a). Despite the methodological limitations, these studies did consistently show an increased relapse rate in the first 3 months after delivery. Three of these early surveys (Ghezzi and Caputo 1981; Millar *et al* 1959; Schapira *et al* 1966) also showed a decrease in the number of relapses during pregnancy but with a significantly higher relapse rate overall during the 'pregnancy-year' (9 months of pregnancy and the first 3 months postpartum) by comparison with periods not pregnant in the same individuals, and non-pregnant controls. The fourth study is notable for first recognizing what is now acknowledged to be the true pattern of evolution – that is, relapse frequency decreases during pregnancy and then increases immediately postpartum, but is similar across the pregnancy year to the frequency observed in the same patients out of pregnancy (Korn-Lubetzki *et al* 1984). In other words, pregnancy and childbirth have no net effect on the relapse rate. The single change lies in the chronology of relapses, the latter being deferred to the puerperium.

In the six subsequent studies involving a total of 263 pregnancies, and in which the non-pregnancy period relapse rates were >0.50 per year – suggesting adequate retrospective assessment (Bernardi *et al* 1991; Birk *et al* 1990; Frith and McLeod 1988; Roullet *et al* 1993; Sadovnick *et al* 1994; Worthington *et al* 1994) – relapse rates outside pregnancy were between 0.51 and 0.65 per year; whereas this remained unchanged during pregnancy (0.35 per year), the rate increased during 3 months postpartum (1.05 per year). Across the entire pregnancy year, it was 0.52, much like that observed during periods not pregnant (Table 4.28).

Of these surveys, five allow a more detailed analysis of relapse rate during the separate trimesters of pregnancy and the puerperium (Bernardi *et al* 1991; Frith and McLeod 1988; Korn-Lubetzki *et al* 1984; Roullet *et al* 1993; Sadovnick *et al* 1994). Two reported an increased relapse rate in the third trimester of pregnancy (Frith and McLeod 1988; Roullet *et al* 1993 – this study also reported a significantly higher relapse rate during the pregnancy year in comparison with the control period). By contrast, three others (Bernardi *et al* 1991; Korn-Lubetzki *et al* 1984; Sadovnick *et al* 1994) showed a reduction of relapse rate in the third trimester of pregnancy followed by an increase in the first trimester postpartum compared with the out-of-pregnancy period in the same patients. The increased risk period in the puerperium appeared to stop progressively after 3 months post-delivery. In five of the six reports that have addressed this issue, relapse rates for the 3–6-month postpartum period were no different from baseline rates in non-pregnant periods (Bernardi *et al* 1991; Frith and McLeod 1988; Roullet *et al* 1993; Sadovnick *et al* 1994; Worthington *et al* 1984); the one exception is the Israeli study, in which this rate remained elevated up to 6 months after delivery (Korn-Lubetzki *et al* 1984).

Another way to assess the influence of pregnancy on the relapse rate in multiple sclerosis is to analyse the inaugural episode in the relapsing–remitting form of the disease. This approach supports the provisional conclusions reached by more direct observations. Leibowitz *et al* (1967) found twice as many Israeli patients as controls who had become pregnant during the

year preceding the onset of multiple sclerosis or, for controls, the same year of life. The reverse phenomenon was observed when pregnancy had started 12–24 months before the age at onset, suggesting that pregnancy may precipitate the onset of multiple sclerosis. In a study to which we have already referred, disease onset was in close proximity to the postpartum period in 36 of the 66 women whose 199 pregnancies were considered (Korn-Lubetzki *et al* 1984). A retrospective study of 512 women (S. Poser and Poser 1983) led to the conclusion that the risk of disease onset is increased 2–3 times during the 6 months following delivery compared with pregnancy. Other studies support this finding (L.M. Nelson *et al* 1988). In a prospective study of 63 women with multiple sclerosis from the United Kingdom (Villard-Mackintosh and Vessey 1993), there was no example of disease onset during pregnancy, whereas two women developed symptoms of multiple sclerosis during the first 6 months of the puerperium. The authors conclude that there is no detectable relationship between pregnancy and the onset of multiple sclerosis. More recently, none of 100 Swedish women reported disease onset during pregnancy and the first month following delivery, whereas nine cases were observed during the subsequent 8-month period (Runmarker and Andersen 1995). These authors conclude that the risk of multiple sclerosis developing during pregnancy is significantly reduced and not significantly different from non-pregnancy periods during the postpartum period. However, this study did not specifically examine the 3-month postpartum period, and an effect concentrated in this epoch may have been missed. Taken together, the literature does provide some evidence for an effect of pregnancy deferring the onset of multiple sclerosis into the puerperium.

These clinical data were corroborated by a serial MRI study of the brain using T_2-weighted sequences during pregnancy and the postpartum period in two Dutch women (Van Walderveen *et al* 1994). Although new or enlarging lesions occurred frequently during the months prior to pregnancy, a clear reduction of the MRI disease activity was observed during pregnancy, and stopped altogether during the third trimester of pregnancy. Thereafter, both patients exhibited a return of MRI disease activity to pre-pregnancy levels in the postpartum period; but no clinical relapse occurred during the pregnancy or in the 6 months after delivery in either patient.

The PRIMS study clarified the possible influence of pregnancy and delivery on the clinical course of multiple sclerosis (Confavreux *et al* 1998b; Vukusic *et al* 2004). This was a European multicentre, prospective, observational study conducted through the EDMUS network (Confavreux *et al* 1992). The study was designed without an independent control group. In fact, the ideal controlled study would have been to recruit women with multiple sclerosis and, by random selection, encourage some to become pregnant, and others not, with each cohort followed prospectively over the next two to three years. This is clearly unrealistic. We have already addressed the issue of matched unrelated controls. In the PRIMS study, 269 pregnancies among 254 women were followed up until 24 months after delivery. The mean rate of relapse per woman per year was assessed throughout the study period. The pre-pregnancy rate, 0.7 ± 0.9 per year, decreased during pregnancy, notably in the third trimester, to 0.2 ± 1.0 per year – a two-third reduction. By contrast, the rate in the 3-month postpartum period was increased to 1.2 ± 2.0 per year. Thereafter, from the second

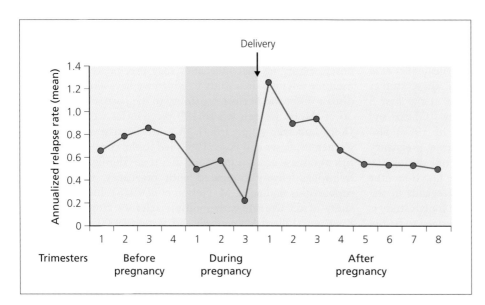

Figure 4.31 Mean annualized relapse rate during the year before pregnancy, the pregnancy and the 2 years after delivery, among 227 women with multiple sclerosis. Adapted from Vukusic *et al* (2004).

trimester onwards and for the following 21 months, the annualized relapse rate fell slightly but did not differ significantly from that recorded in the pre-pregnancy year (Figure 4.31; Confavreux *et al* 1998b; Vukusic *et al* 2004). While the 3-month postpartum period clearly stood out as a high-risk period, only 28% of the cohort had a relapse during that time. Furthermore, the overall effect of pregnancy and the first 3 months of the puerperium (the pregnancy year) on relapse rate was neutral, and similar to the pre-pregnancy rate. The same changes in the frequency of relapses across pregnancy have been more recently observed in smaller and retrospective series (Achiron *et al* 2004b; De Sèze *et al* 2004; Salemi *et al* 2004).

The PRIMS study was also an opportunity to analyse clinical factors that might predict the likelihood of a relapse in the 3 months after delivery (Vukusic *et al* 2004). Clinical predictors were assessed by logistic regression analysis: each relapse experienced during the pre-pregnancy year increased the risk of a postpartum episode by a factor of 1.7; each relapse during pregnancy increased the risk by a factor of 1.8; and patients who had a higher DSS at pregnancy onset were also more likely to have a postpartum relapse (odds ratio 1.3). By contrast, there was no relationship between the occurrence of a puerperial episode and age at onset with multiple sclerosis, age at pregnancy onset, disease duration, total number of relapses before pregnancy, number of previous pregnancies, child gender and (importantly) epidural analgesia or breast feeding. Multivariate models were also used to predict a postpartum relapse, and compared with the observed outcome. In the best multivariate model, only the number of relapses in the pre-pregnancy year, the number of relapses during pregnancy, and disease duration at pregnancy onset independently correlated with the occurrence of a postpartum relapse. When comparing the predicted and observed status, however, only 72% of the women were correctly classified by the mathematical model. Therefore, women with a greater disease activity in the year before and during pregnancy have a higher risk of relapse in the 3 months postpartum. However, this analysis does have its limitations, because there is currently no means of identifying in advance those women with multiple sclerosis who are more likely to relapse, in or out of pregnancy,

for the specific purpose of designing therapeutic trials that aim to prevent subsequent disease activity (Vukusic *et al* 2004).

It is worth pointing out that the decrease in relapse rate during pregnancy is more marked than the effect obtained with any of the licensed disease modifying drugs or oral immunosuppressants (see Chapter 18; Vukusic *et al* 2004). Pregnancy must therefore be viewed as an informative 'experiment of nature'. The protective effect on disease activity is also reproduced in the experimental autoimmune encephalomyelitis model in guinea pigs, rats and rabbits (Abramsky 1994; Evron *et al* 1984). One of the most intense biological features of pregnancy is the high placental and maternal production of sex hormones. Oestrogen and progesterone can suppress experimental autoimmune encephalomyelitis (Trooster 1993; 1994). Pregnancy is also characterized by major immunological changes that reverse with delivery. During pregnancy, there is a shift away from cell-mediated Th1 responses towards enhanced humoral immunity and a Th2 profile (Wegmann 1993). The fetal-placental unit secretes cytokines, such as interleukin-10 (IL-10), that downregulate the production of maternal factors mediating cellular immunity. Immunosuppression could explain maternal tolerance of the fetus. By contrast, delivery might be associated with an inversion of this cytokine balance – similar, in some respects, to the process of graft rejection (Wegmann *et al* 1993). This concept could explain why pregnancy is associated with a spontaneous remission, and the postpartum period with exacerbations in T-cell-mediated autoimmune diseases such as multiple sclerosis and rheumatoid arthritis (Hench 1938). Conversely, B-cell-mediated autoimmune diseases such as systemic lupus erythematosus tend to worsen during pregnancy (Tincani *et al* 1991). A better understanding of the biological mechanisms underlying these pregnancy-related changes in disease activity could usefully illuminate ideas on the pathogenesis and even suggest new treatment strategies.

Short-term disability

Assessing the impact of shifts in the frequency and distribution of new episodes on disability – dependent to some extent on the severity and degree of recovery from the individual relapse – is made difficult by the lack of validated or even widely accepted scales that are sensitive in the short term. The criteria for confirmed worsening of disability are likely to result in misclassification in about 50% of cases even when a minimum 6-month period is required for confirmation (C. Liu and Blumhardt 2000). Two studies have attempted to redress this limitation. Using a scale of doubtful validity, a United Kingdom-based study reported that relapses in the 6 months postpartum were significantly more severe than those occurring during pregnancy (Worthington *et al* 1994). A French group, using the Kurtzke EDSS, also reported more severe relapses in the postpartum period compared with pregnancy but without statistical analysis (Roullet *et al* 1993). In the PRIMS study, there was no evidence of variation in relapse severity between pregnancy and the puerperium, although no direct measures of relapse severity were included (C. Confavreux and S. Vukusic, unpublished data).

The systematic assessment of disability at given intervals during pregnancy and the postpartum period provides another approach, although the low sensitivity of a traditional outcome measure such as the EDSS scale is well known (see Chapter 6; Rudick 1995). Clinical deterioration is usually slow in multiple sclerosis and spans several decades. The first study to tackle the issue of how DSS scores evolve in relation to pregnancy was limited to eight patients. Disability increased systematically from EDSS 2.4 at week 21 of pregnancy to 3.4 at month 6 after delivery (Birk *et al* 1990). The PRIMS study addressed the issue on a much larger scale. The analysis of mean residual DSS showed an increase from 1.1 at 1 year before pregnancy to 2.0 at 24 months post-delivery (Figure 4.32; Vukusic *et al* 2004). The global mean worsening for this 45-month period reached +0.9 DSS points. This is within the expected range of what is known from the natural history of multiple sclerosis in comparable minimally disabled women (Confavreux *et al* 2000; Weinshenker 1989a). Although such observations should be interpreted with caution, because the Kurtzke DSS is cate-

gorical and not quantitative, the mean disability worsening seemed not to occur in steps but was gradual throughout the study period. Despite marked changes in the frequency of relapses observed during pregnancy and the puerperium, accumulation of confirmed disability still evolved without an apparent relationship to these events.

Influence of pregnancy on long-term disability

The impact of pregnancy on the long-term residual disability in multiple sclerosis has been addressed in a number of retrospective or cohort studies. An early observation was that women experiencing the onset of multiple sclerosis after their first conception tended to become more disabled in the long term than those who have not been pregnant (Schapira *et al* 1966). However, the difference is apparent only during the first 10 years of the disease course, and far from reaching statistical significance. Italian researchers found no difference in the distribution of patients according to DSS scores when comparing women with children with those without, after stratification for disease duration (Ghezzi and Caputo 1981). In their study of 72 women with multiple sclerosis having a mean follow-up ≥10 years, S. Poser and Poser (1983) used a progression index (DSS score divided by disease duration) as a measure of prognosis. They found no significant difference in severity between the four groups of patients (all pregnancies before onset; all pregnancies after onset; pregnancies before and after onset; or never pregnant). Similarly, in another survey of 178 women with multiple sclerosis and mean disease duration longer than a decade, no difference was found in the mean DSS score following stratification according to the number of children and adjustment to age at onset and duration of multiple sclerosis (D.S. Thompson *et al* 1986). Long-term disability was similar whether multiple sclerosis started before or after pregnancy. It was significantly lower for women with disease onset during pregnancy but this group contained only ten patients. In a large

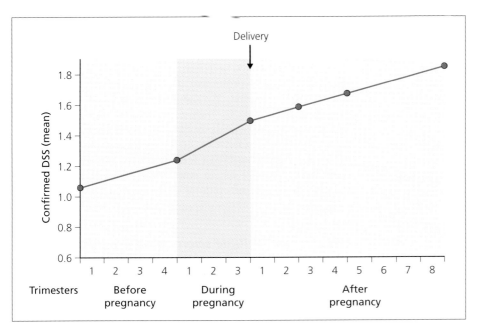

Figure 4.32 Mean confirmed disability, according to DSS, during the year before pregnancy, the pregnancy and the 2 years after delivery, among 227 women with multiple sclerosis. Adapted from Vukusic *et al* (2004).

retrospective population-based Canadian survey of 185 women with multiple sclerosis and a mean disease duration of 15 years, no association could be found between long-term disability and either onset or worsening of the disease during pregnancy and the postpartum (Weinshenker *et al* 1989c). These authors were unable to find any influence on the timing of pregnancies relative to the date of onset, or the total number of full-term pregnancies. Later, a French study involving 32 women with mean disease duration of 10.5 years and full-term pregnancies concluded that pregnancy did not lead to increased disability by comparison with controls (Roullet *et al* 1993). No significant change in the mean EDSS score, measured during the first trimester of pregnancy and 3 years after delivery, was observed in 15 women with multiple sclerosis and full-term pregnancies by Worthington *et al* (1994); they found that the evolution of disability was similar in this group of pregnant patients and nulliparous women who acted as controls.

Two studies have concluded that pregnancy has a beneficial effect on the long-term prognosis in multiple sclerosis (Runmarker and Andersen 1995; Verdru *et al* 1994). Time from disease onset to wheelchair dependence, in the Belgian study involving 200 participants, was 18.6 years for the 40 women with ≥1 pregnancy, and 12.5 years for the 160 women with no pregnancy after the onset of multiple sclerosis (Verdru *et al* 1994). This statistically significant difference persisted after correction for age at onset. But these results must be regarded with caution because the study was restricted to a highly selected population of wheelchair-bound women for whom the dates of onset with multiple sclerosis, pregnancies and wheelchair dependency were all known. Furthermore, the mean age at onset was 11 years younger in the group of women with ≥1 pregnancy than in the group without pregnancy after the onset of multiple sclerosis. In this respect, results of the Swedish and Belgian studies are similar (Runmarker and Andersen 1995; Verdru *et al* 1994). However, the Swedish study was restricted to women with no pregnancy before the onset of multiple sclerosis, and to those with an obvious relapsing–remitting course. Several arbitrary rules were established before making up the matching groups, and these procedures may have introduced confounding effects. Furthermore, the results only reached statistical significance for the lower risk of entering the progressive course in women with a first pregnancy after onset compared with nulliparous individuals. A similar trend was noted regarding the risk of reaching grade 6 on the DSS scale, but this did not reach statistical significance. As acknowledged by the authors, one may wonder if such results are not the result of an interaction bias whereby less disabled and progression-free patients are better motivated to embark on a pregnancy.

Therefore, the current consensus remains that there is no evidence for a significant effect, beneficial or deleterious, of pregnancy on short- and long-term disability in multiple sclerosis. This is somewhat surprising, considering the dramatic increase in the relapse rate during the puerperium. But it must be kept in mind that, overall, relapse rate during the pregnancy year is not different from that observed during the year before pregnancy. Thus, the increased relapse rate in the first trimester postpartum is compensated by reduced clinical activity during the third trimester of pregnancy. We have already discussed the weak correlations between relapse rate and long-term disability in other contexts (Confavreux *et al* 2003).

Influence of epidural analgesia and breast feeding

In a partly interventional study, women with multiple sclerosis breast fed their children less often during the disease (53%) than before developing symptoms (85%), following professional advice given to half of the patients that there was no evidence for breast feeding being harmful (S. Poser and Poser 1983). The first formal study addressing the risk of relapse related to breast feeding was conducted from a structured interview of 111 women with multiple sclerosis experiencing a total of 191 pregnancies (L.M. Nelson *et al* 1988). Women were noticed to have breast fed their child in 50% of instances – a rate considered comparable to that adopted generally in the United States. The postpartum relapse rate was found to be slightly higher in women who breast fed than those who did not. The mean time to exacerbation was similar in both groups. Amongst 15 women with multiple sclerosis, 3/8 who breast fed their infant and 3/7 who did not, suffered a postpartum relapse (Worthington *et al* 1994). Obstetricians and anaesthetists have long been reluctant to prescribe epidural analgesia to women with multiple sclerosis. Anecdotal reports and small series allowed the provisional conclusion that this technique could be associated with a relapse (McArthur and Young 1986; see below).

Against this background, the PRIMS study directly addressed the possible influence of epidural analgesia and breast feeding in multiple sclerosis in a formal and prospective way, although the study was not primarily designed to assess these risks (Confavreux *et al* 1998b). The results were unambiguous: epidural analgesia and breast feeding do not increase the risk of relapse or the level of disability in the postpartum period (Figures 4.33 and 4.34). In this respect, it is important to correct an apparent misreading of the results: women who chose to breast feed experienced less relapses and had milder disability scores in the years both before and during pregnancy, by comparison with women who chose not to breast feed. In the editorial accompanying the original report, it was suggested that 'the finding ... that breast feeding had a beneficial effect by reducing relapses during the course of the study is unexpected' (Whitaker 1998). Nor was it observed. The interpretation of the data on breast feeding by the PRIMS study group is that patients with multiple sclerosis who chose to breast feed had a milder form of the illness from the outset – 12 months before conception – and patients with more active disease decided not to breast feed. It cannot be concluded from the PRIMS data that breast feeding has a protective effect *per se* on disease activity in the postpartum period. We should recall that when the PRIMS data have been used to analyse, by logistic regression analysis and in a multivariate analysis, clinical factors that might predict the likelihood of a relapse in the 3 months after delivery, neither epidural analgesia nor breast feeding proved influential (Vukusic *et al* 2004). A more recent study from Israel also did not find deleterious effects of epidural analgesia and breast feeding in multiple sclerosis (Achiron *et al* 2004b).

Influence of multiple sclerosis on pregnancy, labour, delivery and infant health

Apart from advanced cases of multiple sclerosis with a severe motor deficit, the disease does not appear to influence the course and duration of pregnancy, obstetric labour or delivery.

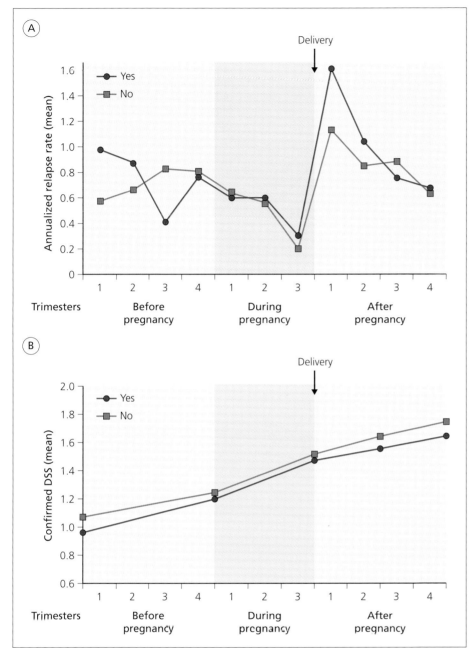

Figure 4.33 (A) Mean annualized relapse rate. (B) Mean confirmed DSS during the year before pregnancy, the pregnancy and the 2 years after delivery depending on epidural analgesia, among 227 women with multiple sclerosis. Epidural analgesia: red line and filled circles. No epidural analgesia: blue line and filled squares. Adapted from Confavreux *et al* (1998b).

The same conclusion applies to the infant in terms of fetal risk of abortion or stillbirth, weight at birth, birth defects, sex ratio, and frequency of twinning (Abramsky 1994; Achiron *et al* 2004b; Birk and Rudick 1986; Confavreux *et al* 1998b; Leibowitz *et al* 1967; McArthur and Young 1986; S. Poser and Poser 1983; S. Poser *et al* 1979a; Roullet *et al* 1993; Sadovnick *et al* 1994; Worthington *et al* 1994).

Pregnancy and multiple sclerosis: a summary

Our position is that there is no medical reason to discourage a woman with multiple sclerosis from contemplating childbirth. Pregnancy is associated with a highly significant decrease in relapse activity and only one-third of women will suffer a relapse during the whole pregnancy period. Conversely, the postpartum is associated with a transient significant increase in disease activity. However, here too, no more than one-third of women will suffer from a relapse during the first 3 months after delivery. Thereafter, the frequency of relapse returns to its pre-pregnancy level. No reliable algorithm is yet available for predicting which patient will experience a relapse postpartum. Although pregnancy and delivery are associated with changes in relapse rate, they do not affect residual disability in the mid and long term. Breast feeding and epidural analgesia have no adverse effect on the disease. Lastly, multiple sclerosis does not itself influence pregnancy, delivery or infant health. Eventually, the decision to contemplate childbearing is most likely to hinge on perceptions of present and future disability, impairment and participation. These are not so easy to predict.

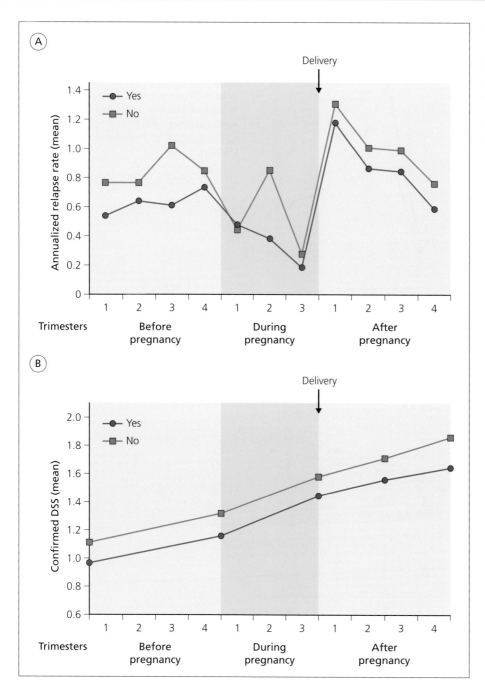

Figure 4.34 (A) Mean annualized relapse rate. (B) Mean confirmed DSS during the year before pregnancy, the pregnancy and the 2 years after delivery depending on breast feeding, among 227 women with multiple sclerosis. Breast feeding: red line and filled circles. No breast-feeding: blue line and filled squares. Adapted from Confavreux *et al* (1998b).

Psychological stress

The possibility that psychological stress may trigger the onset or subsequent activity in multiple sclerosis, first proposed by Charcot (1877), has since been repeatedly proposed (McAlpine 1946). Many patients and physicians are convinced by the putative link. Adding biological plausibility to any evidence for association – if it exists – has generally circled around the concept of neuro-endocrine-immune networks involving connectivity between the hypothalamic-pituitary axis and cytokine production. To us, the link between stressors and molecules that orchestrate and alter immunological behaviour seems easy to state but hard to prove using reasonably rigorous scientific criteria. Of course, psychological stress could alter the blood–brain barrier, vary the Th1 / Th2 cytokine balance, increase T-cell activation against brain proteins, or adjust the hypothalamic-pituitary axis; but all of the supporting data are fragmentary and preliminary (for review see J. Li *et al* 2004a; Mohr *et al* 2004). Furthermore, as discussed in a recent review, the current evidence for an association between psychological stress and activation of multiple sclerosis, at the observational level, is not compelling and the results are often contradictory across different studies (Goodin *et al* 2000). One explanation is that the size effect of any association is small; another that the definition of a stressful event is particularly difficult; and a third, that – judged critically – no relationship exists. The content and personal impact of stressful events cannot easily be standardized, varying (as they do) in origin (e.g. domestic or professional), intensity, duration, frequency and direction of effect (negative or positive). Even this list is not exhaustive. Studies on such ephemeral matters are notoriously prone to recall bias, as the patients, their relatives and physicians naturally tend to relate coincidental adverse life events to changes in the personal experience of multiple sclerosis.

Psychological stress and onset

For reasons that are easy to understand, the question of the possible influence of psychological stress on the onset of multiple sclerosis has been addressed through retrospective studies using a case–control design. The original studies did not find any statistically significant difference in the experience of stress between patients with multiple sclerosis and controls (Antonovsky *et al* 1968; Pratt 1951). Subsequently, positive associations have been claimed. S. Warren *et al* (1982) compared 100 patients with multiple sclerosis with 100 hospital controls matched for demographic variables, psychological stress prior to the onset of multiple sclerosis, and controls of the corresponding age. The two groups did not differ with respect to the happiness of their childhood environment, premorbid ways of coping with life events, or tendency to seek professional help in order to solve an emotional problem. However, patients with multiple sclerosis reported that they were under unusual stress in the 2-year period prior to disease onset more often than controls (79% vs. 54%; p < 0.001). They also experienced three times more stressful life events than controls during this 2-year period. Interview was conducted several years after the clinical onset of multiple sclerosis, and based on information obtained using a questionnaire.

In another study, 39 patients with multiple sclerosis and 40 healthy controls completed a validated, structured interview on stressful experiences (I. Grant *et al* 1989). Patients and controls were matched for sex, age, marital status and socioeconomic position; the study was not blinded. Affected individuals were questioned on stressful experiences over the year preceding the first neurological episode (which had ocurred 2 years earlier on average, with a range of 1–54 months) whereas controls provided information on the year before interview. A greater proportion of patients with multiple sclerosis experienced marked stressful events prior to clinical onset than controls during the year before interview (77% vs. 35%; p < 0.001); the difference was even more noticeable for the 6 months before onset. Less stressful events did not discriminate the groups. A strength of this study was the use of a comprehensive, well-validated, standardized and structured interview; but focusing the interview on a 1-year period represents a limitation. As the authors point out, recall bias increases with interval from life events to retrospective interview. But the effect of this bias may be compensated or even reversed by the 'effort after meaning': for us this is a clumsy phrase seeking to encapsulate the need for individuals who suffer an unfortunate event, such as the appearance of multiple sclerosis, consciously or unconsciously to identify a tangible precipitating trigger and assume a causal relationship; bias is introduced because the patients are more likely than controls to highlight an intercurrent event following such an adverse experience as the clinical onset of multiple sclerosis.

The death of a child must be one of the most stressful experiences imaginable for parents in industrialized countries where infant mortality is low. A nationwide and population-based Danish study examined the possible association between this event and onset of clinical multiple sclerosis (J. Li *et al* 2004a). All 21 062 parents who lost a child at age ≤18 years between 1980 and 1996 in Denmark were included in the exposed cohort studied ≤17 years after bereavement. Each was then matched to 15 other parents who had never lost a child, leading to an unexposed cohort of 293 745 parents. The matching process was based on the family composition at the time of the child's death. The two cohorts were followed for the incidence of multiple sclerosis from 1980 to 1997. Hazard ratios (HR) with 95% confidence intervals were calculated as the measure of association between the exposure and onset of multiple sclerosis, using the Cox proportional hazards regression models. Two hundred and fifty-eight patients with multiple sclerosis were identified, 28 in the exposed cohort and 230 unexposed. Overall, the exposed parents had an increased risk of multiple sclerosis (HR = 1.56; 95% CI, 1.05–2.31). However, the risk remained significant only when the death of the child was unexpected (HR = 2.13, 95% CI 1.13–4.03 for unexpected death vs. 1.33, 95% CI 0.81–2.16 for other deaths), and when follow-up after the child's death lasted >8 years (HR = 1.37, 95% CI 0.78–2.49 for 1–7 years of follow-up vs. 2.25, 95% CI 1.32–3.81 for 8–17 years' follow-up). The strengths of this study are evident: the national system of registries in Denmark allowed for a complete ascertainment of deceased children and for a near complete ascertainment of people with multiple sclerosis over the study period; the focus was on a single well-identified stressor; classifications of exposed and nonexposed parents were unambiguous; diagnostic accuracy and the dating of clinical onset were systematically and appropriately checked in the register; follow-up was complete; data on the exposure and the outcome were collected independently of the research hypothesis; and the sample size was large. But there are nonetheless possible limitations to the study. First, when the study was confined to the 211/258 patients with definite or probable multiple sclerosis, the results were no longer significant (HR = 1.42; 95% CI 0.90–2.24). Furthermore, as the authors recognize, no information was available on lifestyle and occupational factors, physical trauma, infections and family history. It may be hypothesized that, for instance, in subjects with a family history of multiple sclerosis, unaffected family members are disadvantaged by the domestic circumstances (N. Murphy *et al* 1998), leaving children more exposed to events associated with early death, such as trauma, while the parents are more susceptible to develop multiple sclerosis.

Relapse of multiple sclerosis

Only the prospective studies will be considered because the recall bias of retrospective studies cannot easily be reconciled. In the first study, 55 patients with multiple sclerosis were prospectively followed at 4-month intervals for an average of 20 months until a relapse occurred (G.M. Franklin *et al* 1988). At each visit, a standardized structured interview was performed that was sensitive for stressful life events. The 25 patients experiencing a relapse during the study period were compared to 30 who did not; these served as controls. Overall, patients who relapsed did not experience significantly more stressful life events during the 6-month period before that episode than controls

(20.2 vs. 17.2). Extreme stressful life events were marginally more frequent in the patients than controls (p < 0.05). This study is therefore essentially negative with respect to the association between stress and relapse in multiple sclerosis. The prospective design raises its status, as does the collection of data on stress events in advance of possible subsequent relapses.

In a more recent study, 95 pairs of patients with multiple sclerosis, in each of which one was in relapse and the other in remission, were interviewed using a standardized structured questionnaire screening for emotional stressful events (S. Warren et al 1991b). These were more frequent in the 3-month period preceding relapse than in the interval of similar duration prior to interview for patients in remission (57% vs. 28%; p < 0.001). In an Italian study, adopting a rather similar design (Gasperini et al 1995), 89 consecutive patients with relapsing–remitting multiple sclerosis examined in the clinic during a relapse were matched to a patient seen during remission. In the group of patients in relapse in comparison with those in remission, exposure was less frequent – infection, physical trauma, physical overexertion, vaccination and anaesthesia – apart from stressful life events (25% in the relapse group compared with 13% in remission). However, no result was significant, in either direction, but the frequency of exposure was so low for physical trauma, physical overexertion, vaccinations and anaesthesia, as to limit useful conclusions being drawn from this study.

An opportunistic study was carried out in Israel during the first Gulf War (1991) when the Israeli population felt the threat of exposure to missile attacks from Iraq (Nisipeanu and Korczyn 1993). The authors prospectively evaluated a group of 32 patients with relapsing–remitting multiple sclerosis during the screening phase of a therapeutic trial. They found that the number of relapses during the two months of the war and over a comparable period thereafter was significantly lower than expected, based on frequency during the preceding two years, suggesting that not all stress conditions increase the risk of relapses in multiple sclerosis. However, it must be acknowledged that these results could be explained, at least partially, by regression to the mean; typically, this is observed following inclusion of patients in a trial after selection based on a necessary high frequency of a defining entry criterion.

In another study, 23 women with relapsing–remitting multiple sclerosis were followed prospectively for one year (Ackerman et al 2002). They were asked to complete a checklist for stressful events on a weekly basis. A similar procedure was followed for relapses and these were validated thereafter at 4-week intervals by a neurologist blinded to the presence and timing of stressors. During the one-year study period, the patients experienced an average of nine life events (i.e. one every 6 weeks) and 2.6 relapses (one every 21 weeks). Therefore, as many as 49% of stressful life events were associated with a relapse in the subsequent 6 weeks, and 85% of the relapses were preceded by one or more life events in the preceding 6 weeks. The authors were able to demonstrate that a control date selected at random and defined by the absence of relapse in the preceding 6 weeks was associated with a life event during this time window in only 36% of cases. Furthermore, they discovered a 'dose-effect': the higher the rate of life events in a given period, the higher the risk of subsequently developing a relapse. In a subsequent paper, the same authors reported that the risk of stress-related relapses was associated with enhanced cardiovascular reactivity

to acute stress and a higher baseline heart rate (Ackerman et al 2003).

Recently, Dutch authors have enrolled 73 patients with relapsing–remitting multiple sclerosis in a prospective survey with systematic clinical assessments at 8-week intervals. The main objective was to assess the possible association between infections and relapses attributable to multiple sclerosis (see below; Buljevac et al 2002). As a secondary objective, the association between self-reported stressful life events not related to multiple sclerosis and relapses was also explored (Buljevac et al 2003b). During the study period, patients were asked to report in a logbook diary any experience of an emotionally stressful event in the preceding week. Diaries were validated at visits to the clinic. Stressful events directly attributable to multiple sclerosis itself were discarded from the analysis. During the 1.4-year period of follow-up, 70/73 patients (96%) reported ≥1 stressful event, and a total of 457 stressful life events were reported that were unrelated to multiple sclerosis. Overall, 134 relapses occurred in 56 patients, an average of 1.3 per year. Following each stressful event, the risk period for a relapse was set at 4 weeks. Cox regression analysis with time-dependent variables showed that stress was associated with a doubling of the relapse rate (relative risk 2.2; 95% CI 1.2–4.0; p = 0.014) during the subsequent 4 weeks. Infections were associated with a threefold increase in the risk of exacerbation, but this effect was found to be independent of experienced stress. Taken together, the results of these studies are not easy to reconcile, perhaps because of differences in the protocols.

It is only recently that the first prospective longitudinal study of the relationship between psychological stress and disease activity has been assessed using brain MRI (Mohr et al 2000). A total of 36 patients with relapsing multiple sclerosis and ≥1 gadolinium enhancing lesion appearing during the first 24 weeks of enrolment were included. They were evaluated with brain MRI and standardized neurological examination at 4-week intervals for a period of 6–24 months. Disease activity was defined by the presence of ≥1 new gadolinium enhancing lesion not visible on the previous scan. Standardized measures of psychological stress were administered by telephone interview 24 hours before each monthly MRI. Reports were categorized as: major negative events (such as the death of a close family member); conflict and disruption in professional or domestic routine; daily hassles (common events that are irritating or mildly stressful); psychological distress; and positive events (such as an outstanding personal achievement). Stress predictors for the presence or absence of MRI activity on serial scans were analysed by logistic regression analysis for four at-risk intervals: no lag, and 4-, 8- and 12-week intervals after the stressful event. For the entire group of 36 patients, only conflict and disruption in routine correlated with the appearance of new gadolinium enhancing lesions at 8 weeks after the event (OR 1.64; 95% CI 1.22–2.20; p < 0.001). Analyses performed on the subgroup of 17 patients with relapsing–remitting multiple sclerosis generated the same result: conflict and disruption in routine correlated with MRI activity 8 weeks later (OR 1.48; 95% CI 1.03–2.15; p = 0.03). By contrast, among the subgroup of 19 patients with secondary progressive multiple sclerosis, associations involving conflict and disruption in routine were positive at each time point: odds ratios varied between 1.75 and 1.96 but, given the small sample size, showed confidence intervals ranging – for different analyses – from 1.00 to 3.55 for their lower and upper limits, respectively. An association was also found for daily hassles and MRI activity at the week 12 interval (OR 2.16; 95% CI 1.23 3.77; p = 0.006). But there were no significant correlations between stress and clinical relapses of multiple sclerosis for the entire cohort, or the subgroups with relapsing–remitting and secondary progressive multiple sclerosis.

We take these data to indicate that stress is not associated with disease activity in multiple sclerosis. The ascertainment of stressful events, their categorization as exerting positive or negative influences on the individual, and the assessment of intensity were meticulous and made at close intervals. MRI analyses were blind with respect to the clinical events. However, although we find it hard to provide biological plausibility for such a differential effect, the study does suggest an effect of stress depending on clinical course of the disease. Results confined to the subgroup of secondary progressive patients in this study should be treated with caution. These patients were taking part in a placebo-controlled clinical trial of IFN-β1b. The randomization of patients was not known at the time, perhaps leading to a conservative estimation for the association between stressful events and MRI activity due to the inhibitory effect of interferon treatment in multiple sclerosis. However, among the 30 patients with secondary progressive multiple sclerosis eligible for the study, 11 were excluded through not having developed a new gadolinium enhancing lesion on monthly MRI scans during the first six months of potential enrolment. Because these factors might have introduced bias affecting the outcome measure in a direction that cannot easily be predicted, we place more confidence in results for the relapsing–remitting than the secondary progressive group. Indeed, considering the subgroup of 17 patients with relapsing–remitting multiple sclerosis, all took part in a prospective natural history study, and the results regarding a possible association between stressful events and MRI activity were essentially negative.

Meta-analysis

Following a well-described selection process, 14 studies addressing the issue of the association between stressful life events and onset or relapse of multiple sclerosis – most discussed above – have been included in a quantitative meta-analysis (Mohr *et al* 2004), necessarily using a clinical outcome because too few studies have assessed MRI activity as the dependent variable. Of the 14 surveys, 7 were case–control and 7 longitudinal prospective studies. Two examined the onset episode, and 12 dealt with relapses of multiple sclerosis. This meta-analysis led the authors to conclude that stress and clinical activity are significantly associated, with a high degree of consistency between individual studies – whatever the design, methods or sample characteristics. They acknowledged that the size effect, although statistically significant, was modest and results not consistent between groups or individual patients over time. However, the effect was considered clinically meaningful and superior, for instance, to that recently identified in a meta-analysis of efficacy for IFN-β used as a disease modifying drug to reduce relapse frequency in multiple sclerosis (see Chapter 18; Filippini *et al* 2003a). However, the inherent limitation of meta-analysis is the pooling of data having uneven quality. For instance, for 40% of the subjects included by Mohr *et al* (2004),

the stress measure was obtained through an unvalidated questionnaire or interview. In many studies, data on the exposure (stress) and the outcome (onset or relapse of multiple sclerosis) were not collected independently. Not surprisingly in these studies, association between stress and activity in multiple sclerosis has always been found (Gasperini *et al* 1995; I. Grant *et al* 1989; S. Warren *et al* 1982; 1991b). Overall consistency of results does not necessarily ensure accuracy because the same biases will tend to reproduce the same biased, and hence erroneous, results.

Stress and multiple sclerosis: summary

Taken together, our position is that the most persuasive evidence is provided by anecdotal cases or retrospective studies but each is vulnerable to recall bias, especially in the context of disease activity in a chronic debilitating disease, known to be intermittently active as part of its natural history. Conversely, the more rigorous and reliable prospective studies, notably those using an objective outcome measure such as MRI enhancement, provide no compelling data. Some studies suggest that only the more modest stressors – such as conflict, disruption in daily routine or minor hassles – act as activators of multiple sclerosis (Mohr *et al* 2000). Reaching a measured position on interpretation is not made easy by the strikingly discordant results obtained in studies using the same methodology. At one extreme, the threat of missile attack in Tel Aviv during the first Gulf War was found to reduce the risk of relapse (Nisipeanu and Korczyn 1993), and bereavement had no significant influence on MRI and clinical activity (Mohr *et al* 2000). Conversely, others have claimed that losing a child increased the later risk of developing multiple sclerosis (J. Li *et al* 2004a); yet, specificity is undermined by the additional observation that this stressful event was also associated with an increased risk of myocardial infarction, cancer and overall mortality but not stroke or an autoimmune disease such as inflammatory bowel disease (J. Li *et al* 2004a; 2004b).

Despite consistent and confident statements in the literature that psychological stress and disease activity in multiple sclerosis are linked, a more critical reading suggests that the association is, at best, weak and with a modest effect size.

Physical trauma

The Association of Research into Nervous and Mental Diseases (Barker 1922) reached the following conclusion on the relationship between trauma and multiple sclerosis:

> In a small percentage of cases [multiple sclerosis] appears to be excited by trauma, but trauma cannot itself cause it, but may apparently awaken a disease process already potentially existent.

Three lines of evidence are used to inform the debate on whether trauma can trigger clinical manifestations of multiple sclerosis in someone who has the disease process, or alter the course in individuals who have already experienced symptoms. These are the anecdotal experience of individual neurologists, epidemiological observations, and experiments addressing a mechanistic hypothesis.

It is logical to start by assessing the probability of coincidence, that is, estimating how often accidental injury and the onset of multiple sclerosis, a further manifestation of pre-existing disease, or a change in clinical course would be expected to occur together by chance. If the independent rates of the two events are known, it is a simple step to estimate the chance that they will occur together within a given interval. The suggestion has been made that, in this context, the critical period is 3 months. An issue arises with respect to the location and severity of trauma considered as a potential trigger for multiple sclerosis. Most medico-legal attention, and such scientific evidence as can be brought to bear on the subject, relates to the spine in general and the cervical cord in particular. Surveys completed at the beginning and end of the 1980s indicate that the annual frequency of head injury in adults living in the United Kingdom is 1:50 (Jennett 1996). Although not every injury will be of a type considered potentially relevant in the context of multiple sclerosis, the proportion in any 3-month period is 1:200 or 0.005%. Substituting the figure of 1:90 for spinal cord injury (Anon. 1995), the proportion at risk is 1:360 or 0.003% of the population for each 3-month period.

The next step is to estimate the number of individuals developing clinical manifestations of multiple sclerosis, and those experiencing new relapses or a change in clinical course over any 3-month period. Based on morbidity statistics and the natural history of multiple sclerosis (see above and Chapter 2), annual incidence rates for the United Kingdom vary between 5 and $10/10^5$ depending on location. Simply stated, and taking the lower estimate, this means that at least 625 individuals in a population of 50 million (roughly the population of the United Kingdom) will first develop clinical manifestations of multiple sclerosis in each 3-month period. The annual relapse rate is about 0.5 for all patients, although higher for those (around 40%) in the relapsing–remitting phase. The number of individuals experiencing a new episode every 3 months amongst the 80 000 prevalent patients (of the United Kingdom) is therefore at least 4000. The annual conversion rate from relapsing–remitting to progressive disease and the loss of independent walking is around 2%, or 1200 individuals.

Assuming that these patients have the same risk of injury as the unaffected population, and that the age-specific breakdown for each event is roughly aligned (i.e. the decades when the incidence of multiple sclerosis peaks – the 20s and 30s – are also those in which injuries are most prevalent), it follows that:

- The number of newly affected individuals also reporting an accident causing neck injury in any 3-month period is 0.003 × 625 = 1.8, i.e. 1–2 every 3 months or 4–8 in any one year.
- The number of individuals with established multiple sclerosis experiencing a new episode within 3 months of a relevant accident is 0.003 × 4000 = 12 every 3 months or 48 in any one year.
- The number of individuals with established multiple sclerosis converting from the relapsing–remitting to the progressive phase within 3 months of a relevant accident is 0.003 × 1200 = 3.6, i.e. 3–4 every 3 months or 12–16 in any one year.

Epidemiological studies of trauma and multiple sclerosis

The next step is to assess whether what actually happens deviates from this expectation. This is where the epidemiological studies are relevant. The existing studies have their strengths and weaknesses but, taken together (and with the possible exception of electric shock, discussed in more detail below), they do not show an association between disease activity in periods when individuals known to have multiple sclerosis, or first developing clinical manifestations of the disease, are at risk after trauma. Therefore, the epidemiological studies provide no evidence in support of the hypothesis that a causal relationship exists between trauma and multiple sclerosis, and are consistent with the alternative explanation that the temporal coincidence is due to chance. So what is the evidence?

McAlpine (1946) described trauma within a month preceding the onset of multiple sclerosis in 8/142 patients studied between 1937 and 1946 (work that he acknowledged was disrupted by the war), concluding that the number studied was:

> too small to be of statistical value ... A further study is called for since they would seem to indicate the possibility of abnormal reflex or sympathetic activity in the cord in response to peripheral trauma.

McAlpine's conclusion was that the main aetiological factor in multiple sclerosis is virus infection. The same emphasis on an infective aetiology was reached by D.K. Adams et al (1950), who also described accidental or surgical trauma in 41/389 individuals and a history of trauma preceding an exacerbation 'in a considerable number of cases'. Their method of case retrieval was not described and the report lacked controls or statistical analysis.

McAlpine and Compston (1952) reported that 36/250 (14%) patients with multiple sclerosis described episodes of trauma (excluding surgical but including dental) in the 3 months prior to onset of their first symptom. In 22/36, there was a correlation between the site traumatized and the subsequent localization of neurological symptoms. Thirteen of 250 (5.2%) control patients interviewed in a hospital ward had a comparable history. Twenty-nine of 58 patients suffering a total of 80 traumatic episodes during the course of the illness experienced a new episode within 3 months of the traumatic event. The relapse rate in the 3 months following these 80 episodes was 0.43 compared with 0.39/year (i.e. >4 times higher) in 393 unselected patients with multiple sclerosis. McAlpine et al (1955) later concluded that:

> from this evidence there would appear to be little doubt that trauma to a limb or any part of the body, slight or severe, including operation, may occasionally precipitate the disease in a predisposed person or may cause a relapse. This view gains support from the fact that in a significant proportion of cases with a history of trauma shortly before the onset, the site of the trauma would appear to play a part in determining the localisation of the initial symptoms.

By 1965, McAlpine had qualified but did not reject these conclusions on the grounds that the results lacked statistical proof (McAlpine et al 1965). The design did not fully weight incidents that were not followed by new symptoms or consider the severity of trauma; and the possibility existed of recall bias in a retrospective survey of events occurring at the time of disease activity by comparison with those that were not. Understandably, the McAlpine and Compston (1952) series is often used in support of the claim that trauma triggers the clinical expression of multiple sclerosis. However, a number of retrospective but controlled studies carried out since the early 1950s have shown no association between trauma and the onset of multiple sclerosis. Some leave open the question of an effect on clinical course of the disease in those with pre-existing manifestations.

Bamford *et al* (1981) failed to show a relationship between trauma and onset of multiple sclerosis in their retrospective case series. This was followed by a more systematic study of trauma and disease activity in 170 patients studied prospectively by questionnaire (monthly) and physical examination (3-monthly) for 8 years (Sibley *et al* 1991). Defining either the 3- or 6-month period following each event as at-risk, only electrical trauma showed an association with new episodes (defined as the occurrence of new manifestations lasting >48 hours, in the absence of fever, or an exacerbation of old symptoms if there was a change in neurological examination). All other forms of trauma were negatively correlated both with clinical exacerbations and disease progression. Although not a prospective study of multiple sclerosis first manifesting in individuals who have experienced trauma but of new events or later progress in those with pre-existing disease, the distinction between a first and later episode is not of biological importance. The initial analysis used one-tailed and paired t tests; the final analysis quoted p values based on chi-squared statistics. The power of the study was not given but can be estimated by calculation of relative risks. These are:

- all forms of trauma, 1.1 (95% CI 0.8–1.4)
- head injury, 1.08 (95% CI 0.54–2.14)
- electrical injury at 3 months, 3.4 (95% CI 1.2–10)
- electrical injury at 6 months, 2.2 (95% CI 0.8–5.8).

Siva *et al* (1993; see also Kurland 1994) identified trauma in the year preceding onset in 3/223 incident patients from the Mayo Clinic series. This seems a low number but cannot be interpreted in the absence of controls, as pointed out by numerous correspondents to the journal where the report was published. However, the Mayo series of around 3587 persons with head trauma studied prospectively contains 819 within the age range at risk of developing multiple sclerosis of whom two did develop the disease, after intervals of 3 and 15 years, respectively. Five of 942 undergoing cervical or lumbar disc surgery had multiple sclerosis but, in 4, symptoms of the disease had developed 4–15 years before surgery. Disease exacerbations occurred no more frequently in the 6 months after than the 6 months before limb fracture. First, a retrospective analysis was made of disease activity in 122 individuals prevalent in Olmsted county on 1st December 1991 together with 42 comparable patients (i.e. 164 in total) taking a 6-month period at risk. Next, retrospective analyses were made of prospectively gathered health records held at the Mayo Clinic matching 225 individuals incident for multiple sclerosis in Olmsted county between 1905 and 1991 with 819 individuals with head injury between 1935 and 1984 and 942 who underwent lumbar disc surgery between 1950 and 1979. Siva *et al* (1993) combined three studies, and Sunku and Kurland (1994) added 561 seen with cervical radiculopathy between 1976 and 1990 but showed no association with multiple sclerosis – with or without surgery to the cervical spine.

Whilst these surveys approximate to the ideal, in that they look prospectively at the number of individuals showing clinical manifestations of multiple sclerosis in a population-based sample considered at risk through having experienced the putatively provocative event (trauma), they inevitably contain very few individuals with multiple sclerosis in the prospective series. Their power is further diminished by the low number of injuries because the definition required head injury with physical signs, concussion, post-traumatic amnesia or skull fracture and hence excluded many examples of trauma not resulting in bone injuries and confined to soft tissue injury. Wilcoxon sign and rank sum tests were used to analyse these data but recalculation of relative risks with confidence intervals confirms that none of the results is statistically significant. That said, the studies have relatively low power to show an effect.

Two additional contemporary studies are either small or methodologically open to criticism. Neither provides evidence supporting a relationship between trauma and manifestations of multiple sclerosis (Alter and Speer 1968; Gusev *et al* 1996). Discussion of the article by Chaudhuri and Behan (2001) describing a series of cases identified through personal referral might be considered not to belong in an analysis of epidemiological studies dealing with the relationship between trauma and multiple sclerosis. The authors report 39 cases in which a relationship was proposed between trauma and multiple sclerosis. Twenty-four were considered not to have had previous manifestations of multiple sclerosis. Their first symptoms developed between 12 hours and 12 weeks after the traumatic episode. The expression of symptoms was maximal at 2–3 weeks after injury. Fifteen cases had pre-existing manifestations of multiple sclerosis. In each, the clinical course was judged to have deteriorated within 1–12 weeks of injury, with a mean maximum interval of 1–2 weeks. Using an arbitrary (and unvalidated) scale, applied retrospectively, there was no correlation between outcome and the severity of injury. The ApoE4 allele, associated with a poor outcome from head injury, was under-represented in 27/39 tested (70%) compared with historical controls (15%), suggesting to Chaudhuri and Behan (2001) that their patients were destined to follow a benign course as part of the natural history. The authors listed five possible mechanisms (increased permeability of the blood–brain barrier, increased production of proinflammatory cytokines, increased production of nitric oxide synthetase, synergistic effect of psychological stress, and direct axonal injury) as potential mechanisms for the reported effect, preferring, in their summary, a sequence involving stress-related release of proinflammatory cytokines and nitric oxide.

Most experts consider Sibley *et al* (1991) to be the best available epidemiological survey dealing with events triggering activity in multiple sclerosis. It has been criticized on the grounds that the survey is not directly concerned with the most frequent context of whiplash and cervical cord demyelination. (This hypothesis was not under discussion when the study was planned.) Although designed to answer the more general question of a relationship between trauma and multiple sclerosis, the study does have sufficient power to address the specific issue of neck injury and cervical cord demyelination. It has been suggested that a less stringent classification of new episodes might have produced a different result, but looser definitions would have counted a number of episodes resulting from transient changes in conduction through pathways with a reduced safety factor for transmission of the nerve impulse, of doubtful significance with respect to disease activity. The association with electrical injury has been cited as evidence in support of a general relationship between trauma and multiple sclerosis. In the initial analysis, electrical injuries were grouped in the category of burns (although none did in fact produce burns). The annualized exacerbation rate for burns was 0.39 and 0.43 in the periods at risk and not at risk, respectively. Electric shock was reported in 19 instances by 17 patients. Four of these episodes were followed within 3 months (range 1–65 days) by an exacerbation. Three received shocks from domestic appliances. One was adversely affected by a medical instrument designed to provide electric current for the relief of pain due to multiple sclerosis (transcutaneous electrical nerve stimulation). Clearly electrical trauma is not an issue in most cases and this finding in isolation does not materially alter the lack of evidence for the general hypothesis. The statistical significance has 95% confidence intervals >1 only for the 3-month analysis. This is lost if the episode of injury caused by the transcutaneous electrical nerve stimulator is removed. The statistical approach has not included correction for multiple comparisons.

Thus, in terms of design, definition, power and analysis, the studies are not easily compared. However, none provides evidence supporting the hypothesis that a causal relationship exists between trauma and multiple sclerosis, and each is consistent with the alternative interpretation that the temporal coincidence is due to chance. But protagonists of a causal relationship also offer the indirect effects of stress, triggered by trauma, and its physiological consequences as a possible mechanism. Few would disagree that severe trauma to the head and neck with multiple injuries to the affected individual and third parties constitutes psychological stress that would trigger a number of physiological responses. Although a mechanistic hypothesis can be stated based on interactions between workings of the neurological, immunological and endocrine systems, we have already concluded that there is no direct supporting epidemiological evidence that underpins this explanation for a relationship between stress and clinical activity in multiple sclerosis.

The American Academy of Neurology has issued an analysis of the relationship between multiple sclerosis and physical trauma or psychological stress through its therapeutics and technology assessment subcommittee (Goodkin et al 1999). The survey is particularly useful as a source of published material on case–control, cohort and uncontrolled studies, as well as expert opinion and anecdotal evidence. The panel accepted that a hypothesis linking trauma to disease activity in multiple sclerosis could reasonably be proposed based on changes in the blood–brain barrier as the necessary basis for debating the epidemiological evidence. Taking the liberal position of a one-year interval between trauma and any neurological consequences, and confining their scrutiny to injuries of the head and spine, the committee considered that the best available studies provide strong evidence from case–control or cohort studies excluding anything more than a modest effect of trauma on exacerbations of pre-existing multiple sclerosis in the 3 months after trauma. In fact, the evidence was considerably more supportive of no effect than even this modest relationship. Despite low statistical power, the resoundingly negative result of the population-based Mayo Clinic series is seen as particularly strong evidence against a causal relationship. The evidence against an effect of stress, based on the available studies, is seen as marginally less damning even though the mechanistic hypothesis linking stress to disease activity in multiple sclerosis is even less plausible than for trauma.

Mechanistic interpretations

It could be argued that, without supporting epidemiological evidence, it is hardly necessary to examine putative mechanisms – however interesting that might be as an academic exercise. The core of the proposal linking trauma to a change in the natural history of multiple sclerosis is that whiplash injury of the cervical spine leads to alteration in permeability of the blood–brain barrier, locally and at diffuse sites. This enables substances present in the circulation of individuals having the potential to develop multiple sclerosis to reach the abluminal surface of blood vessels and cause clinical manifestations of the disease. One criticism of this hypothesis linking trauma to multiple sclerosis is that it does not provide a general theory of the disease that accounts for all lesions, in all patients, in all places and on all occasions. It is self-evident (and beyond dispute) that most plaques are not precipitated by trauma. Why therefore propose an entirely different sequence of events for demyelination on those rare occasions when there is temporal and anatomical convergence? Even the protagonists offer a causal relationship of trauma to multiple sclerosis as an explanation for ≤0.1% of lesions. Demyelination is a nonspecific pathological response of the nervous system to a variety of insults. Demonstrating that this has occurred at some point following trauma does not of itself indicate that multiple sclerosis has been precipitated.

Patients with multiple sclerosis are described in whom stereotactic brain surgery was used as symptomatic treatment for tremor. The surgical lesions were subsequently shown to be associated with active demyelination in the needle tracts. Gonsette et al (1966: written in French and so mostly read secondhand in review articles) and Hasler et al (1975) found fresh lesions in some but not all patients with multiple sclerosis undergoing stereotactic thalamotomy for relief of upper limb tremor. Some areas of abnormality illustrated as related to brain surgery were not centred on the needle track. Much also has to be taken on trust that the lesions described by these authors, not subjected to rigorous histological analysis and occurring in patients without detailed presurgical assessments (before magnetic resonance imaging was available) who died from multiple sclerosis (in some instances more than a year later), were not part of generally active disease in which histological sampling elsewhere in the nervous system would have shown comparable changes. These details apart, there is a difference between direct trauma of brain tissue by a surgical procedure and soft tissue injury that may, or may not, indirectly distort parts of the central nervous system. It is notable that other neurosurgical procedures in patients with multiple sclerosis do not appear to be complicated by fresh plaques, further suggesting that these may relate to the clinical problems for which the procedures were themselves being carried out rather than the intervention itself.

A key component of the evidence offered in support of a link includes histological analyses of the cervical cord in multiple sclerosis, and correlations between the distribution of plaques and compression points from cervical spondylosis or distortions of the ligaments supporting the cervical portion of the spinal cord. Thus the hypothesis hinges on local rather than generalized effects of trauma on properties of the blood–brain barrier. Brain and Wilkinson (1957) advanced the specific hypothesis that:

the effect of cervical spondylosis upon the spinal cord may be to make it more susceptible to the lesions of disseminated sclerosis at that level ... This may [have been] a chance finding, but it is more likely that the site of the demyelination was associated with the presence of the spondylotic bars ... relapse of the symptoms after trauma would seem to be due to further compression with consequent venous dilatation in a cord already damaged by demyelination.

Oppenheimer (1962; 1978) made observations on the cervical spinal cord – a part of the nervous system chosen for its high prevalence of multiple sclerosis lesions – in 18 patients. The cervical region is also, by definition, the site of cervical spondylosis and cervical myelopathy. David Oppenheimer observed that the lesions of multiple sclerosis are twice as common in the cervical region as elsewhere in the spinal cord, occurring invariably at the 7th cervical level, and showing a fanlike appearance related to the lateral columns. He made three (not fully independent) suggestions to explain these observations: a local rise in venous pressure, focal inflammation and mechanical distortion. Because there was no reason to conclude that the first two would locate to the lateral columns, he preferred the interpretation that mechanical stresses play a part in determining the site of lesions, through forces transmitted via the denticulate ligaments which lead to vascular leakage. David Oppenheimer suggested that fluid with the potential to cause demyelination leaks through the traumatized barrier.

Oppenheimer (1978) anticipated that if, in the context of cervical myelopathy, plaques did not accumulate maximally opposite the sites of spondylitic bars, the specific theory advanced by Brain and Wilkinson (1957) would lose its force. David Oppenheimer's own pathological studies showed a discrepancy between the site of plaques and spondylitis in three cases. He ended by concluding that:

too little is known about the mechanical effects of lateral bending and twisting movements of the neck to justify speculation on the stresses set up in the cord during these movements.

Kidd *et al* (1993) used magnetic resonance imaging to show the maximum distribution of cervical cord lesions at different levels from the sites of compression by spondylitic bars. David Oppenheimer's pathological observations did, however, lead him to offer a more general hypothesis concerning the anatomical localization of plaques affecting the cervical cord in multiple sclerosis. His observations relate to chronic and not acute trauma and the hypothesis does not explain why other parts of the central nervous system are also preferentially affected in multiple sclerosis (the anterior visual pathway and the periventricular white matter). One of the mechanisms that Oppenheimer rejected in discussion of his work (focal inflammation) does in fact better account for the overall distribution of lesions in multiple sclerosis. Bryan Matthews (1991) summarized the situation as follows:

a hypothesis can be constructed linking onset or relapse of multiple sclerosis up to six weeks after concussive head injury but thereafter with rapidly diminishing probability. Minor injury to the spinal cord could be held similarly responsible The hypothesis is based on the unproven primary role of breach of the blood brain barrier in the pathogenesis of the plaque. It is impossible to answer what would have happened if there had been no injury. Neurologists will form their own opinions but would hope to avoid making pronouncements unsupported by evidence.

Our present view is that a complete reading of the literature provides no epidemiological evidence in support of a relationship between trauma and the cause of multiple sclerosis. Trauma does not precipitate latent multiple sclerosis. Nor does it change the activity, course and prognosis in patients with established multiple sclerosis. That position is reached using the following logic:

- The frequencies of trauma and disease activity in multiple sclerosis make it certain that these will occasionally occur together by chance.
- Epidemiological studies do not show an association between trauma and disease activity or the course of multiple sclerosis.
- Colocalization of lesions due to multiple sclerosis and cervical spondylitis, or in patients undergoing direct brain needling, does not establish causality.
- Opening of the blood–brain barrier is necessary but not sufficient for establishing the cascade of events that culminates in the pathological features of multiple sclerosis.

Approached from the rigorous attitude of medical science in assessing evidence, there is no evidence for a causal relationship between trauma and multiple sclerosis. That position is not materially altered if the same questions are asked from the perspective of civil law on a balance of probabilities.

Anaesthesia and surgery

No epidemiologically robust studies of multiple sclerosis and anaesthesia or surgery have been performed and, again, the evidence is mostly anecdotal. Ridley and Schapira (1961) reported a complete absence of exacerbations in the month after surgery in their group of 40 patients studied for this and other forms of surgical trauma. Baskett and Armstrong (1970) detailed four cases in which surgery coincided with disease activity in multiple sclerosis. One elected for sterilization on learning of the diagnosis and suffered a perioperative relapse. The second also had an elective procedure for tendon rearrangement in a spastic leg due to pre-existing multiple sclerosis. The third required surgery for a fractured femur. The fourth relapsed after removal of a breast lump but not following the subsequent mastectomy. The authors rightly drew no firm conclusions about the relationship between general anaesthesia, surgery and multiple sclerosis. In their part retrospective and part prospective surveys, Bamford *et al* (1981) and Sibley *et al* (1991) found that patients with multiple sclerosis had more surgical procedures than controls, through complications of the disease, but relapse rate in the period at risk and rate of progression were uninfluenced. In fact, the period following minor or major surgery was relatively safe (annualized exacerbation rates 0.14 and 0.18 in the period at risk compared with 0.23 and 0.29 at other times).

Data on the possible influence of anaesthesia in multiple sclerosis are still scarce. Siemkowicz (1976) reviewed 16 anaesthetics in 11 patients already known to have multiple sclerosis given over three years, in 5 of whom relapses occurred in the perioperative period. In each, the procedure was either for drainage of abscess or was obviously complicated by infection, which (from what is known both in terms of the effect of pyrexia on the symptoms of multiple sclerosis and the role of infection) provides an alternative explanation for the relapse. This also was the author's conclusion because none of the patients who was not pyrexial after an anaesthetic reported a change in symptoms. Bamford *et al* (1978a) reported on 100 patients with multiple sclerosis questioned about their experience with anaesthesia during the course of the disease. General anaesthesia was performed in 42 patients on 88 occasions. Original medical files were available for 33 patients, allowing data linking anaesthesia and the course of multiple sclerosis to be validated. One patient experienced a relapse in the month following anaesthesia and laparoscopy for tubal ligation. Another, with progressive multiple sclerosis, noted an acceleration in her disability progression following hysterectomy. Spinal or caudal anaesthesia was performed in 14 patients on a total of 18 occasions, including three women undergoing five obstetric deliveries. The only adverse event was a relapse in one patient during the first month postpartum. Local anaesthesia was reported by 98 patients, usually on more than ten occasions; this was mainly for dental procedures and, in 46 patients, dental records were available for validation of the history. No consistent deleterious effect was noticed on the course of multiple sclerosis. The authors reached the same conclusion when they analysed the specific effect of any one anaesthetic agent whatever its mode of delivery. Bamford *et al* (1978a) considered that the rare associations observed between anaesthetic procedures were coincidental and not causal, being consistent with the natural history of the disease. Their only reservations concerned spinal anaesthesia, due to insufficient experience of this procedure at the time. Data gathered subsequently as part of the PRIMS study (Confavreux *et al* 1998b) are reassuring. These are anecdotal data and we are not aware of any structured study devoted to the issue of anaesthesia in multiple sclerosis. We consider that anaesthesia is safe in people with multiple sclerosis and the same is true for surgical procedures. There is no need to let potential effects on activity and the clinical course of multiple sclerosis influence decisions on the need for anaesthesia and surgery.

Infections

Pierre Marie first drew attention to the onset of multiple sclerosis occurring in the wake of febrile infections: typhoid fever, smallpox, erysipelas, pneumonia, measles, scarlet fever, whooping cough, dysentery, diphtheria and syphilis (Marie 1884). He was in no doubt that microbes caused the disease (see Chapter 1) but many unsuccessful efforts have since been made to rediscover the guilty agent(s). Subsequently, the concept of a chronic organ-specific autoimmune disease is preferred

to the formulation of multiple sclerosis as an infectious disease. The contemporary evidence implicating specific microorganisms in triggering the disease process is summarized in Chapter 2. Here, we discuss the role of infections in precipitating disease activity.

Infections and relapses of multiple sclerosis

Anecdotal evidence suggested the possibility of an increased risk of relapse following infection. With the availability of epidemiological studies specifically designed to address this issue, the current consensus is that infections do trigger relapses in multiple sclerosis. In fact, many of the studies show methodological limitations and the relationship may have been overemphasized. Only a minority of infections produce clinically recognizable symptoms (T. Chang 1971). In the most influential study, the frequency of infections in patients with multiple sclerosis was half that observed in age-matched healthy controls; and the frequency was inversely related to disability (Sibley *et al* 1985). Even taking into account that only common viral infections were considered in this study, the facts seem counterintuitive. Self-evidently, the duration and severity of infections vary. Not every event that follows infection necessarily indicates an effect on the underlying disease process; exposure may promote a variety of indirect processes that interfere with electrical properties of the central nervous system (see Chapter 13). A possible solution to the problem of under-ascertainment might be to supplement clinical observations with serial serological studies; but this merely introduces the dilemma of how often and when to take the samples, and what panel of microbiological agents should be screened (Andersen *et al* 1993). Infections, new episodes and pseudorelapses, related to fever or transient cytokine release (see Chapter 13), must each be independently ascertained and correlated using double-blind procedures in order to minimize ascertainment bias and the declaration of spurious associations. Retrospective designs expose recall bias for the ascertainment of infections, and these are difficult to correct. The most appropriate design compares periods at risk and not at risk in which patients serve as their own controls; this was used in the definitive study instigated by Bill Sibley in the United States.

Initially, Sibley and Foley (1965b) followed 34 patients with multiple sclerosis over a period of 3 years; 33/69 relapses (48%) were associated temporally with a common infection. However, the authors were concerned that the association may have been overestimated because patients were aware of the objectives. Therefore, the same group set up a much larger study, in which infection was only one of several factors investigated, and care was taken to avoid any preconception of results amongst participants (Sibley *et al* 1985). One hundred and seventy patients with clinically definite multiple sclerosis were contacted monthly for ascertainment of viruslike infections and clinical relapses, with objective assessment every 3 months, over a mean of 5.3 years. Relapses were defined as new neurological symptoms associated with appropriate change in neurological examination, lasting >48 hours and not associated with fever; viruslike infections were classified on a clinical basis as respiratory, with ('flu') or without ('cold') fever, enteric or herpetic (genital or oral). Periods at risk were defined as the interval covering 2 weeks before and 5 weeks after the infection. All other times on the study were considered not at risk. The rate of relapse was found to be 2.8-fold higher in the at-risk period compared with the control intervals, whatever the level of disability and overall relapse frequency (Table 4.29). This study provided strong evidence for an association between common viruslike infections and relapses in multiple sclerosis. However, among the 771 documented infections, only 67 (8.7%) were associated with a relapse; and there was no link between bacterial infections (mostly of the urinary tract) and disease activity.

In a more limited study of 60 ambulant patients with relapsing–remitting multiple sclerosis followed for a mean of 31 months (Andersen *et al* 1993), the relative risk of relapse was only 1.3 (p = 0.047), using a time window of 4 weeks for the at-risk period (Table 4.29). No significant association was found using the 7-week time window previously adopted by Sibley *et al* (1965). Patients were contacted monthly and examined every 2 months. They knew the objectives of the study. Upper respiratory and gastrointestinal (but not urinary) tract infections were considered.

Two other small studies, each embedded within a placebo-controlled trial of IFN-β and with short follow-up, deserve cautious interpretation. Panitch (1994) examined 30 patients with relapsing–remitting multiple sclerosis every 3 months, and whenever a relapse occurred, during 2 years of the pivotal phase III trial in which patients received either placebo or IFN-β1b at doses of 1.6 or 8 million IU subcutaneously every other day (IFNβ Multiple Sclerosis Study Group 1993). Patients kept daily logs of upper respiratory infections. The at-risk period was defined as encompassing 1 week before and 5 weeks after the onset of upper respiratory tract infections. The relapse rate was 2.5-fold higher in the at-risk period by comparison with control intervals (Table 4.29), irrespective of treatment. The frequency of new or recurrent symptoms, and the severity, duration and response to corticosteroids were similar whether or not the relapses occurred during at-risk periods. However, seemingly no specific effort was made to maintain patients blind to the objectives of the study or to validate infections mentioned in the daily logs. Furthermore, the relapse rate during the 2-year study period was 1.79 per year, which is unusually high given that a proportion of patients were receiving medication that is considered capable of lowering relapse frequency.

S. Edwards *et al* (1998) studied 41 patients with either relapsing–remitting or secondary progressive multiple sclerosis randomly assigned either to placebo, or IFN-β1a at a dose of 6 or 12 MIU by subcutaneous injection three times weekly, and observed prospectively for 15 months (monthly for first 9 months, and then every 3 months). Participants recorded disease activity attributed to multiple sclerosis and episodes considered to represent infections, in a specially designed diary. Blood samples were taken at monthly intervals during the first 9 months and assayed for the presence of antibodies to influenza A, influenza B, respiratory syncytial virus, adenovirus, cytomegalovirus and enterovirus. MRI was used to assess the number and size of gadolinium enhancing lesions. The period at risk was defined as 2 weeks before and after the onset of upper respiratory tract infections. The relapse rate was 2.0-fold higher in at-risk compared to periods non-at-risk (Table 4.29). The severity of relapses did not differ depending on when they occurred. By focusing on the subgroup of serologically confirmed infections, the relative risk for relapse was found to be 3.4-fold higher following exposure compared with intervals not at risk. Infections had no consistent influence on MRI activity. Taken together, these results must be regarded with caution. As the authors indicate, over-reporting by patients of upper respiratory tract viral infections seems likely, because the average rate of such infections was high (2.4 per year) and only 12.5% could be serologically confirmed. Over-reporting of relapses is also possible: the rate was 1.88 per year although two-thirds of the patients were allocated to IFN-β1a. Apparently, individual relapses may have been counted more than once during the 4-week period at risk because only 19 infections were reported by the authors to have been associated with relapses whereas a total of 27 relapses occurred during periods at risk. No sensitivity analysis was performed by changing the location and duration of the time window encompassing the onset of the infection. Symptoms of gastrointestinal or urinary tract infections were not taken into account, perhaps resulting in classification bias for the periods at risk and control intervals. MRI results are difficult to interpret because two-thirds of the patients were randomized to active treatment with IFN-β1a and the code was not broken at the time associations between infections and relapses were analysed.

Recently, Dutch authors have enrolled 73 patients with relapsing–remitting clinically definite active multiple sclerosis in a prospective survey incorporating systematic clinical assessments at 8-week intervals for a mean follow up of 1.7 years (Buljevac *et al* 2002). Symptomatic infection of any type or a

Table 4.29 Literature data on infections and relapses of multiple sclerosis

Study	Number of patients	Time window of exposure to the infection	Relapse rate / year		Relative risk	p value (chi-squared test)
			Period at risk	Period not at risk		
Sibley *et al* 1985	170	−2 to +5 weeks	0.64	0.23	2.8	<0.001
Andersen *et al* 1993	60	−1 to +3 weeks	1.70	1.29	1.3	0.048
		−2 to +5 weeks	1.51	1.33	1.1	0.20
Panitch 1994	30	−1 to +5 weeks	2.92	1.16	2.5	<0.001
Edwards *et al* 1998	41	−2 to +2 weeks	3.27	1.62	2.0	0.004
Buljevac *et al* 2002	73	−2 to +5 weeks	2.05	0.97	2.1	<0.001

putative relapse attributable to multiple sclerosis triggered an additional visit within 3 days. For confirmed infections or a clinical relapse, an additional visit was arranged 3 weeks later. Furthermore, for confirmed infections, three serial MRI examinations were performed at 3-week intervals with T_1 sequences and gadolinium injection. Relapses were graded as 'major' or 'minor', according to change in the EDSS score; and as 'short', 'long' or 'sustained', depending on whether the EDSS score returned to baseline at ≤3 weeks, >3 weeks or ≥3 months. The main analysis involved the 7-week period at risk, previously defined by Sibley *et al* (1985). A total of 167 infections and 145 relapses were recorded. By comparing the period at risk with control intervals, the relapse rate ratio was 2.1 (95% CI 1.4–3.0; $p < 0.001$: Table 4.29). A sensitivity analysis was performed by changing the location and the duration of the time window encompassing the onset of infection: –2 to +2 weeks, +1 to +4 weeks, +1 to +8 weeks, and +3 to +5 weeks. This led to essentially similar results. The relapse rate ratio increased to 2.7 (95% CI 1.5–4.8; $p < 0.001$) when considering 'major long' relapses only. It reached 3.8 (95% CI 1.8–7.9; $p < 0.001$) for the subgroup of 'major sustained' relapses. Thus, the more severe and long-lasting the relapse, the stronger the association with infection: more transient symptoms, coinciding only with the elevation in temperature, would be expected in the context of pseudorelapses. Overall, 46/167 infections (28%) were associated with a relapse during the 7-week period at risk. Urinary tract infections were not associated with an increase in relapse frequency.

The strengths of this study are evident: regular survey visits at close intervals and, in case of any suspected infection or relapse, near immediate additional visits systematically arranged to control for memory biases; infections of any kind (upper respiratory, gastrointestinal and urinary tract) considered; and fever-related neurological episodes excluded as events registered in the study. However, there are possible sources of bias: assessments of infections and relapses were not made by independent masked assessors; no effort was made to perform a sensitivity analysis restricted to relapses featuring neurological manifestations that were new for that patient; the duration and severity of infections were not considered; when a risk period that was not overlapping the infection was considered, no significant association was observed; and power could have been enhanced by introducing a case crossover design that increased the number of control periods.

But the MRI results are puzzling. When comparing the three serial MRI examinations performed after any confirmed infection, the percentage of active scans and the mean number of enhancing lesions per scan remained unchanged. This observation held whether or not the infection was associated with a relapse; whether or not the patient was receiving IFN-β or methylprednisolone; and when a relapse was linked to the infection. One may argue that the increase in MRI activity could have occurred prior to the first infection-related scan. The authors refer to a personal series of nine patients with multiple sclerosis examined at monthly intervals during 8 months, again with no significant change in MRI activity related to the eight infections that occurred during that study period.

Can these seemingly contradictory clinical and MRI data be reconciled? Buljevac *et al* (2002) propose that infections could lead to relapses through a mechanism that is independent of blood–brain barrier dysfunction. Although lesions due to multiple sclerosis can be detected before overt dysfunction of the blood–brain barrier (Filippi *et al* 1998a; 1998b), it remains to be shown that this applies to any one lesion.

For us, the results reported by Buljevac *et al* (2002) raise more questions than answers. Were the study restricted to clinical results, it would be regarded as confirming the association between infection and relapse in multiple sclerosis. This interpretation carries biological plausibility: secretion of proinflammatory cytokines such as IFN-γ, and interaction of the host immune system with viral superantigens (Woodland 2002) are mechanisms accepted as resulting in immune activation leading to relapses of multiple sclerosis. However, the MRI data introduce uncertainties. Generally, the correlation between clinical and MRI activity is well established (Youl *et al* 1991b). The observations offered by Buljevac *et al* (2002) require this relationship to be compromised making it necessary to arbitrate on the relative reliability of MRI data and clinical evaluations.

Specific infections and relapses of multiple sclerosis

By systematic sampling for a panel of antibodies to common respiratory pathogens (influenza virus A, B and C; parainfluenza virus 1, 2 and 3; respiratory syncytial virus; adenovirus; reovirus; Coxsackie virus B1–6; *Mycoplasma pneumoniae*; Epstein–Barr virus; and herpes simplex virus 1 and 2), before the study and every 3 months during the first year, Panitch (1994) was unable to find fluctuations in titre correlating with clinical relapses. Similar results were obtained by S. Edwards *et al* (1998) when testing an equivalent panel of organisms. However, no effort was made in these studies to perform blood sampling in temporal relationship to the infections. This critique cannot be offered on the Swedish work of Andersen *et al* (1993), in which a significant correlation was found between the rise in adenovirus, but not influenza virus, titre and relapse: however, the number of participants was small (seven and six, respectively). In a group of 19 patients with multiple sclerosis followed monthly for one year, active viral replication of Epstein–Barr virus was observed in 73% of patients experiencing relapses during the study period, but in none of the patients with clinical stability, suggesting a role for Epstein–Barr virus as an activator of the disease process (Wandinger *et al* 2000).

The Dutch prospective study of 73 patients with relapsing–remitting multiple sclerosis followed up at 8-week intervals for a mean of 1.7 years also tested the relationship between relapse and serologically defined *Chlamydia pneumoniae* infection (Buljevac *et al* 2003a). Among the 73 patients, 48 did not show evidence of infection during follow-up, 15 exhibited ≥1 serologically defined acute infection, and 10 had a serologically defined chronic infection with *Chlamydia pneumoniae*. In the subgroup of the 15 patients with serologically defined acute infections, the relapse rate ratio was 3.1 (95% CI 1.3–6.7; $p = 0.006$) when comparing infection and noninfection periods. The majority of infections occurred without clinical symptoms of infection. Interestingly, the increased risk of relapses was still observed for the subgroup of chronic *Chlamydia pneumoniae* infections. Furthermore, in the serologically defined acute infections, the alteration in serology specific for *Chlamydia pneumoniae* was usually not accompanied by a rise in anti-*Chlamydia trachomatis*, anti-staphylolysine and anti-mycoplasma antibodies.

Lately, in a pilot observational study of 16 patients with relapsing–remitting multiple sclerosis enrolled on the occasion of a well-documented upper respiratory tract infection and followed for 5.5–12 months, 78% of the 9 infections due to picornaviruses and 17% of the remaining 12 infections (p = 0.01) were associated with a relapse during the period at risk beginning 2 weeks before and lasting until 5 weeks after the infection (Kriesel *et al* 2004). In this study, no consistent association was found between the index infections and influenza A and B, respiratory syncytial virus, adenovirus, parainfluenza types 1–3 and coronaviruses.

The current consensus is to accept that an association exists between infections in general and relapses of multiple sclerosis. This conclusion is well documented in the prospective observational studies. However, it must be stressed that only one study has followed a satisfactory methodology and taken all infections into account (Buljevac *et al* 2002). However, as discussed above, the association between infections and clinical disease activity observed was not supported by MRI outcomes, reducing confidence in the apparent association. There is no evidence that any one pathogen is specifically associated with relapses of multiple sclerosis. It is not hard to offer a mechanistic hypothesis for this generic increase in risk but the issue of whether disease activity associated with specific infections merely reflects secondary immune dysregulation – the audience rather than actors in the drama of multiple sclerosis (Hunter and Hafler 2000) – is unresolved.

Seasons

A correlation between seasons and the frequency of relapse has produced conflicting results. A higher frequency was found in warmer months in Cleveland, Ohio (Sibley and Foley 1965a). Similar results were found in Arizona when 178 patients and 82 controls were followed prospectively for 5 years (Bamford *et al* 1983). Conversely, the incidence of relapse was found to be higher in the winter and spring months in Switzerland (Wuthrich and Rieder 1970). Episodes were more frequent in the spring, medium in the summer and autumn, and lowest in winter when a population-based and prospective incidence survey was conducted in Stockholm County, Sweden, on 147 patients suffering from an inaugural episode of monosymptomatic optic neuritis (Y-P. Jin *et al* 1999). The higher frequency was found during the autumn and winter months in another area of Sweden (Andersen *et al* 1993) and during the coldest (January and February) and the warmest (July and August) months in Japan (Ogawa *et al* 2004). A peak for the incidence of relapses, though not statistically significant, was found in September compared with the rest of the year in the Netherlands (Buljevac *et al* 2002). Lastly, no significant seasonal change could be observed in other areas (Goodkin and Hertsgaard 1989; Koziol and Feng 2004; Panitch 1994; Schapira 1959). Interestingly, seasonal fluctuation of gadolinium enhancing magnetic resonance imaging lesions has been reported from 202 brain MRI examinations performed in 53 patients with relapsing multiple sclerosis (Auer *et al* 2000). There was a clear biphasic fluctuation of disease activity over the year, the mean number of lesions being five times higher in spring than in autumn. By contrast, a large analysis of 1320 brain MRI scans from 120 patients with relapsing–remitting multiple sclerosis

who were part of the untreated arm of a phase III study of glatiramer acetate did not show significant seasonal fluctuations in the number of active MRI lesions (Rovaris *et al* 2001d). A similar conclusion was reached in a group of 24 patients, also with relapsing–remitting multiple sclerosis, included in the placebo arm of a trial using cladribine and involving monthly MRI examinations for one year (Koziol and Feng 2004). The same observation was made in a group of 28 patients with multiple sclerosis (Killestein *et al* 2002c). However, in this study, seasonal fluctuations were observed for the ability of T cells to secrete proinflammatory cytokines such as TNF-α and IFN-γ, with maximum values observed during the autumn. These results confirm those previously obtained in 60 patients with chronic progressive multiple sclerosis showing significantly increased *in vitro* IFN-γ production in autumn and winter by comparison with spring and summer months (Balashov *et al* 1998).

Given the possible difference in seasonal distribution of relapses depending on location, a meta-analysis performed to characterize and quantify seasonal variation in first episodes of optic neuritis or multiple sclerosis, and relapses in individuals with established disease, is helpful (Y-P. Jin *et al* 2000). The authors selected nine reports on inaugural optic neuritis, six dealing with the onset of multiple sclerosis, and nine describing relapses providing appropriate data on the season of the neurological episode. They found a fairly homogeneous pattern with a decreasing frequency in the occurrence of episodes from spring to winter. The size effect was limited, however, as there were only 1.45 times more inaugural episodes in spring than in winter. The difference was even less marked for inaugural optic neuritis and relapses of established multiple sclerosis. We take this meta-analysis, performed with caution and including relevant available data from various countries, to show that the influence of seasons on disease activity, although statistically significant, is nevertheless extremely modest and – as presently understood – of limited value in elucidating factors that trigger the disease process. Furthermore, assuming that there might be a link between cytokine secretion and disease activity, the higher risk observed for relapse occurrence in spring is not consistent with the increased autumn IFN-γ secretion observed in the two studies that have addressed this issue (Balashov *et al* 1998; Killestein *et al* 2002c).

Vaccinations

Since the pioneer work of Louis Pasteur, immunization with vaccines containing neural tissue is recognized as having the potential to cause multifocal inflammatory and demyelinating lesions of the central nervous system. Such phenomena are usually monophasic and self-limited, as in acute disseminated encephalomyelitis. Modern vaccines no longer contain neural tissue derivatives but homologies can exist between microbial and neural epitopes. This molecular mimicry may allow specific immune competent cells activated by the vaccine to respond autoaggressively against the host nervous system. It may also be hypothesized that stimulation of the immune system can activate autoreactive clones through a bystander effect. Because autoimmunity is considered pivotal in the pathogenesis of multiple sclerosis, it is reasonable to suggest that vaccinations might trigger the onset or relapse of multiple sclerosis (Palffy and Merei 1961). This concern was lately revived, especially in France, by the anecdotal reports of a temporal association between vaccination and disease activity following an extensive immunization programme against hepatitis B.

Consideration also has to be given to the possibility that vaccines might not only provoke inflammatory demyelinating diseases of the central nervous system *de novo*, but also trigger the inaugural clinical expression of demyelination in individuals with subclinical disease, provoke a relapse in individuals with established multiple sclerosis, and induce transient physico-chemical changes sufficient to block the nerve conduction in existing but asymptomatic lesions. But, as with all risk factors, coincidental temporal association also needs to be excluded.

The onset of multiple sclerosis

There have been many case reports of multiple sclerosis first presenting after vaccination: influenza is most often implicated (Bakshi and Mazziotta 1996; Bienfang *et al* 1977; Cangemi and Bergen 1980; De la Monte *et al* 1986; Hull and Bates 1997; C.M. Poser 1982; Rabin 1973; Ray and Dreizin 1996; Rosenberg 1970; Waisbren 1982; W.R. Warren 1956; Yahr and Lobo-Antunes 1972), but other vaccines have also been blamed (Behan 1977; S. Holt *et al* 1976; Joyce and Rees 1995; Kazarian

and Gager 1978; Klie *et al* 1982; Mancini *et al* 1996; H. Miller *et al* 1967; Pathak and Khare 1967; Riikonen 1989; Sibley and Foley 1965b; Stevenson *et al* 1996; Topaloglu *et al* 1992). However, there have been very few systematic studies devoted to vaccines in general as risk factors for multiple sclerosis or other central nervous system demyelinating episodes (Table 4.30). The most comprehensive account is the United States case–control study conducted in three large health maintenance organizations (DeStefano *et al* 2003). Potential cases were identified in the automated database with a first diagnosis of multiple sclerosis or optic neuritis between 1995 and 1999. Eligible cases needed to be registered in the database for ≥1 year before diagnosis. Paper medical records were reviewed to confirm case status and determine the onset of clinical events. The index date was taken as the first clinical manifestation of neurological symptoms or signs in each case, and that date was also used for the corresponding controls. Up to three controls from the database were matched to each case. Exposure to vaccinations was ascertained from an automated database, paper medical records and telephone interviews. When a vaccination was reported in the telephone interview but not also captured in the automated database, it was categorized as a 'self-reported vaccination'. Odds ratios were estimated from conditional logistic regression. The study involved 440 cases, of whom there

Table 4.30 Literature data on any vaccination and multiple sclerosis

Study	Number of patients and health status	Assessment of exposure to any vaccination	Time window of exposure to any vaccination before the neurological episode	Odds ratio (95% CI)
Case–control studies with occurrence of first demyelinating episode or onset of multiple sclerosis in cases vs. controls				
Touzé *et al* 2000	121 first demyelinating episodes 121 neurological controls	Telephone interview Copy of vaccination certificate: 17%	60 days 61–180 days	1.4 (0.5–4.3) 2.1 (0.7–6.0)
DeStefano *et al* 2003	440 multiple sclerosis or optic neuritis 950 controls	Automated database Paper medical records Telephone interview Vaccination certification: 35–70%	1 year: Tetanus Influenza Any time: Tetanus Influenza Measles, mumps, rubella Measles Rubella	1.2 (0.7–2.0) 0.8 (0.5–1.4) 0.6 (0.4–0.8) 0.8 (0.6–1.2) 0.8 (0.5–1.5) 0.9 (0.5–1.4) 0.7 (0.4–1.0)
Hernán *et al* 2004	163 multiple sclerosis 1604 controls	Automated database	3 years: Tetanus Influenza	0.6 (0.4–1.0) 1.0 (0.5–2.0)
Relapse of multiple sclerosis				
A.E. Miller *et al* 1997	49 multiple sclerosis, influenza vaccinated 54 multiple sclerosis, placebo injected	Per protocol	6 months	2.0[a]
Confavreux *et al* 2001	643 multiple sclerosis Case crossover design	Automated database Paper medical records Telephone interview Copy of vaccination certificate: 94%	2 months: Any vaccine Tetanus alone Combined tetanus Influenza	0.7 (0.4–1.3) 0.7 (0.2–2.5) 0.2 (0.1–1.0) 1.1 (0.4–3.1)

Multiple sclerosis according to C.M. Poser et al (1983).
a Crude relative risk estimated from available data in the original manuscript.

were 332 with multiple sclerosis and 108 with isolated optic neuritis; 950 controls were included in the analysis. Vaccination against tetanus, which included tetanus toxoid and combined tetanus and diphtheria toxoid vaccines, was the most common inoculum in cases (155/440; 35%) and controls (449/950, 47%). Self-reported vaccinations ranged from 30% (for tetanus) to 65% (for measles, mumps and rubella) of the events. The analyses indicated that having ever received one of the vaccines of interest did not increase the risk of multiple sclerosis or optic neuritis (Table 4.30). In these analyses, all the odds ratios were <1.0; this decrease reached statistical significance for tetanus vaccination (OR 0.6; 95% CI 0.4–0.8). These results did not alter when self-reported episodes were excluded from the analyses, or when the interval between vaccination and the index date was taken into consideration. The authors concluded that the vaccines commonly administered to adults are not associated with an increased risk of developing multiple sclerosis or optic neuritis.

Relapse of multiple sclerosis

Despite the theoretical concerns mentioned above, small observational studies on the safety of influenza vaccination in patients have nonetheless been reassuring (Bamford *et al* 1978b; L.E. Davis *et al* 1972; De Keyser *et al* 1998; Kurland *et al* 1984; Sibley *et al* 1976). For instance, in a group of 180 patients with relapsing–remitting multiple sclerosis, the risk of relapse was significantly higher after a flulike illness (33%) than after an influenza vaccination (5%) over a 6-week period following the event (De Keyser *et al* 1998). Furthermore, in a double-blind placebo-controlled study of safety for swine influenza virus vaccination in patients with multiple sclerosis, the rate of clinical relapse was the same (4/33 patients) for the vaccine- and placebo-treated groups over a 3-month follow-up period (L.W. Myers *et al* 1977). In a multicentre, prospective, randomized, double-blind trial of influenza immunization, A.E. Miller *et al* (1997) enrolled 103 patients with relapsing–remitting multiple sclerosis free of disease modifying agents for ≥6 months. During

the 28 days following inoculation, 3/49 vaccinated patients and 2/54 placebo patients experienced relapses. Over the subsequent 6-month follow-up period, 11 vaccinated patients and 6 placebo patients experienced one relapse each (annualized relapse rate, 0.45 and 0.22, respectively). Mean time interval to the first relapse was 91 days in the vaccine group and 55 days for the placebo group. None of these differences was statistically significant. The authors conclude that influenza vaccination is safe for patients with multiple sclerosis.

The risk of triggering disease activity after any vaccination in patients already affected with multiple sclerosis and free of relapse for ≥12 months was explored in a formal way by the VACCIMUS (VACCines In MUltiple Sclerosis) study coordinated through the EDMUS network (Confavreux *et al* 2001). The computerized EDMUS databases were used to select patients having a relapse between 1993 and 1997 that had been confirmed at neurological consultation, but were free of any new events in the previous 12 months. These data were validated using the patients' medical case records. In a second, independent step, the patients were interviewed on the telephone about all vaccinations received during the entire study period (1992–1997) but were aware neither of the specific hypothesis being tested nor the date assigned to the relapse of interest (to which the interviewer was also blinded). A total of 643 patients were enrolled of whom 96 (15%) had been vaccinated in the 12 months prior to the index relapse. Written confirmation from vaccination certificates was obtained in 94% of these cases. Analyses were conducted using a case-crossover design (Maclure 1991). Exposure to a vaccine in the 2 months preceding the index relapse (the period at risk) was compared with exposure during four 2-month control periods, each patient serving as his/her own control (Figure 4.35). The relative risk of a relapse associated with exposure to any vaccination during the previous 2 months was 0.71 (95% CI 0.40–1.26; Table 4.30). Results were similar for specific vaccinations against tetanus alone (RR 0.75; 95% CI 0.23–2.46); tetanus associated with poliomyelitis or diphtheria (RR 0.22; 95% CI 0.05–0.99); influenza (RR 1.08; 95% CI 0.37–3.10); and hepatitis B (RR 0.67; 95% CI

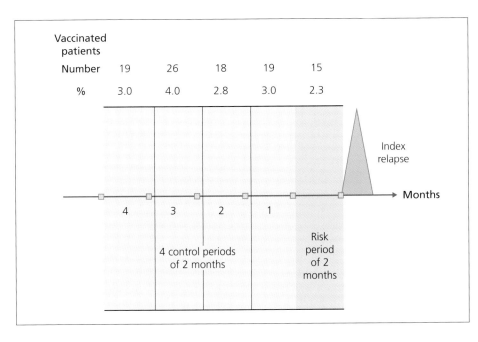

Figure 4.35 Vaccinations and the risk of relapse in multiple sclerosis. Number and percentage of patients with ≥1 vaccination in the successive 2-month periods before the index relapse among 643 enrolled patients. A given patient may have received ≥1 vaccines within ≥1 of the 2-month periods. The relative risk is calculated from the proportion of patients vaccinated during the 2-month period at risk and that of patients vaccinated during the 2-month control periods. Adapted from Confavreux *et al* (2001).

0.20–2.17). These results remained identical (varying between 0.68 and 0.79) when duration of the at-risk and control periods was varied from 1 to 3 months; when all reported vaccinations were included, even if they were not confirmed; and when the analysis was restricted to the patients having only one vaccination during the 12 months preceding the index relapse. The evidence suggested no increase in the risk of relapse following any vaccination, hepatitis B vaccination included, in patients with multiple sclerosis who had been free of a new relapse for ≥12 months.

These results are consistent with the lack of MRI evidence for disease activity in patients with multiple sclerosis following influenza (Michielsens *et al* 1990; Salvetti *et al* 1995) and Calmette–Guérin bacillus (BCG) vaccination (Ristori *et al* 1999). They are also in agreement with the demonstration in patients with multiple sclerosis that influenza vaccination is followed by an increase in the number of influenza-specific, compared with myelin-specific, T cells in peripheral blood (Moriabadi *et al* 2001).

Hepatitis B vaccination

The issue of hepatitis B vaccination and multiple sclerosis has excited particular public attention and deserves special consideration. The failure to eradicate hepatitis B infection by immunization campaigns directed at high-risk groups (health care and laboratory professionals; travellers to endemic regions; patients with liver disease and dialysis patients; prostitutes and intravenous drug abusers) led the World Health Organization to promote mass immunization programmes in babies and pre-adolescents in the early 1990s (Kane 1995). But anecdotal cases, especially in France, and small series of cases of first episodes consistent with demyelination or a new episode in a patient with existing multiple sclerosis developing within a few days or weeks after administration of the vaccine were soon reported (Berkman *et al* 1996; Gout *et al* 1997; Herroelen *et al* 1991; Kaplanski *et al* 1995; Mahassin *et al* 1993; Nadler 1993; Senejoux *et al* 1996; Tourbah *et al* 1999; Trevisani *et al* 1993; Van de Geijn *et al* 1994). By July 1996, about 200 cases were known to the French authorities – generating much concern about safety of the vaccine, although post-marketing surveys were reassuring (Duclos 1992; Levy-Bruhl *et al* 1999; B.J. McMahon *et al* 1992; Niu *et al* 1996; F.E. Shaw *et al* 1988).

Three case–control studies in adults were therefore set up in 1994, at the initiative of the French Agence du Médicament, to address the issue of a possible link between hepatitis B vaccination and the onset of multiple sclerosis (Fourrier *et al* 1999; Sturkenboom *et al* 1999; Touzé *et al* 2000). All three reported nonsignificant increases in the risk of multiple sclerosis after hepatitis B vaccination, with odds ratios within the range 0.9–1.8. Touzé *et al* (2000) included 121 patients with a first episode of demyelination occurring between July 1993 and December 1995, and 121 age- and sex-matched controls seen at the same time. The index date was determined by the onset of neurological symptoms for the case, and this served as a reference for the corresponding control. The patients were interviewed about vaccinations using a written questionnaire and through telephone conversations. Overall, 15 patients with a neurological episode and 9 controls (12% vs. 7%; p = 0.21) reported ≥1 injection of hepatitis B vaccine within a 180-day period preceding the index date. The risk (odds ratio) for a first

demyelinating episode of the central nervous system following any vaccination, as estimated by conditional logistic regression, was 1.4 (95% CI 0.5–4.3) for an exposure within the 60 previous days, and 2.1 (95% CI 0.7–6.0) for exposure within 61–180 days at risk. For hepatitis B vaccination, the figures were 1.7 (95% CI 0.5–6.3) and 1.5 (95% CI 0.5–5.3), respectively. There was therefore a small, but not statistically significant, association between any vaccination, hepatitis B vaccination included, and the development of multiple sclerosis. These results have wide confidence intervals that straddle unity. Furthermore, the reliability of the primary data is questionable, because vaccination certificates were obtained in only 17% of the patients and recall bias is likely to have occurred in retrospective reporting for the remainder – the French population being fully aware of the controversy at the time data were collected for the study. Furthermore, prior to interview, participants had been explicitly informed of the study objectives.

The next study was conducted in 18 departments throughout France and followed a similar design, but aimed to use two controls per case (Fourrier *et al* 1999; Touzé *et al* 2002). In the event, 236 examples of a first demyelinating episode and 355 matched controls were available for evaluation. During the phone interview, 64% of the cases and 71% of the controls referred to a vaccination certificate, but it seems that these were not made directly available to the researchers. Within the 2-month period preceding the index date, 13 cases (5.5%) and 12 controls (3.4%) reported hepatitis B vaccination. Corresponding numbers for the 2–12-month period at risk, were 26 cases (11.0%) and 42 controls (11.8%), respectively. The adjusted odds ratio for a first neurological episode was 1.8 (95% CI 0.7–4.6) for exposure to hepatitis B vaccination ≤60 days prior to the index date, and 0.9 (95% CI 0.4–2.0) for an exposure within the 2–12-month period. These values altered to 1.4 (95% CI 0.4–4.5) and 1.0 (95% CI 0.6–1.9), respectively, when the analyses were restricted to patients referring to a vaccination certificate during the telephone interview. Thus, validation of exposure improved but was still incomplete. Once again, the interviews were conducted in 1998, at a time when the controversy about hepatitis B vaccination was vividly debated in the French media, and the results show wide confidence intervals. Standing back from these data, the authors concede that to test with sufficient power the hypothesis of a multiplication by 1.5 for the risk of a demyelinating event within 2 months of a hepatitis B vaccination would require a sample of 2000 incident cases.

Other studies have been performed outside France. The United Kingdom General Practitioner Research Database (GPRD) was used to identify 481 examples of a first demyelinating episode in cases matched for age, gender and location with up to six controls (Sturkenboom *et al* 1999; 2000). Vaccination histories were collected from the automated database. The risk of a neurological event was 1.5 (95% CI 0.6–3.9) for exposure to hepatitis B vaccination ≤12 months before the index date; and 1.4 (95% CI 0.8–2.4) for hepatitis B vaccination at any time before the index date. In so far as the preliminary publications allow for critical analysis, this study is consistent with the two others provoked by public concern in failing to show a significant effect of hepatitis B vaccination.

In a retrospective cohort study, Zipp *et al* (1999) selected subjects in whom ≥1 year of observation was available after enrolment between 1988 and 1995, and in whom there was no previous record of demyelinating disease, from a United States health care medical insurance database: cases were matched to three or four nonvaccinated controls. This provided 27 229 vaccinated and 107 469 nonvaccinated subjects. For each individual, a systematic search was performed in the database for the occurrence of any central nervous system demyelinating episode (optic neuritis, myelitis, other demyelinating syndrome of the central nervous system, acute disseminated encephalomyelitis, or multiple sclerosis) ≤3 years after hepatitis B vaccination. There were 6 events among the vaccinated, and 25 in the nonvaccinated populations over this 3-year period. The relative risk for a neurological episode in the hepatitis B vaccination-exposed compared with the nonvaccinated group decreased steadily from 1.3 (95% CI 0.4–4.8) to 0.9 (95% CI 0.4–2.1) when the time window following vaccination was increased from 6 months to 3 years. These findings were reported in a research letter, providing limited information on the protocol design and conduct. It seems likely, however, that ascertainment both of vaccination and neurological status were adequate.

The school-based study conducted in British Columbia, Canada, failed to show any increase in cases of multiple sclerosis in 267 412 students who completed vaccination series against hepatitis B virus between 1992 and 1998, at the age of 11–12 years by comparison with the group of 288 657 other students followed in the same area and through the same school system between 1986 and 1992 when hepatitis B vaccination was not available (Sadovnick and Scheifele 2000). There were five examples of multiple sclerosis onset in the vaccinated (1992–1998) and nine in the nonvaccinated (1986–1992) group. It could be argued that the differential follow-up favours the most recently constituted group, many of whom have not reached an age beyond which the risk of developing multiple sclerosis has waned; for this reason, the authors restricted their search for incident cases of multiple sclerosis to adolescents aged 11–17 years in order to match the groups.

More recently, a nested case–control study has been conducted in two large cohorts of nurses set up in the United States in 1976 and 1989, respectively (Ascherio *et al* 2001b). They comprised around 240 000 subjects and, in both, follow-up questionnaires were mailed to the participants every two years. Whenever the diagnosis of multiple sclerosis was reported, this was validated using information obtained from the treating physician, and the date of onset established. Only cases with definite or probable multiple sclerosis were included in the assessment of vaccinations. Each nurse with multiple sclerosis was matched to five healthy controls and one woman presenting with breast cancer from the same source cohort. The date assigned for onset of multiple sclerosis served as reference for information relating to controls. A total of 318 individuals were diagnosed with multiple sclerosis from inception of the cohort to April 1998. In a subsequent step, the vaccination status against hepatitis B was assessed by means of a mailed questionnaire. Only women with a history of hepatitis B vaccination at any time in the past (even after the onset of multiple sclerosis) and for which confirmation could be obtained from a copy of their vaccination certificates were included. This eventually led to the inclusion of 192 patients with multiple sclerosis, 534 healthy controls and 111 women with breast cancer. A total of

32 women with multiple sclerosis (17%), 84 healthy controls (16%), and 15 cases with breast cancer (14%) had received ≥1 dose of hepatitis B vaccine at any time before the index date. The relative risk of multiple sclerosis for women vaccinated against hepatitis B, estimated with the use of conditional logistic regression, was 0.7 (95% CI 0.3–1.8) for the first dose given ≤2 years preceding the onset of multiple sclerosis, and 0.9 (95% CI 0.5–1.6) for exposure to hepatitis B vaccination any time.

Sensitivity analyses confirmed these negative results. The number of vaccine doses received before the index date was similar in patients with multiple sclerosis and controls. The relative risk for multiple sclerosis was similar when the analysis was restricted to women with onset after the introduction into the United States of a recombinant vaccine against hepatitis B (1987). Similar results were obtained when the analysis was restricted to women who declared having been vaccinated against hepatitis B but could not provide a copy of the vaccination certificate. Analyses based on the less reliable information available from self-reporting showed a relative risk for multiple sclerosis of 1.2 (95% CI 0.8–1.7) for hepatitis B vaccination at any time before the onset of multiple sclerosis, and 1.9 (95% CI 1.1–3.3) for a first vaccination ≤2 years before the onset of multiple sclerosis.

In this study, only cases with definite or probable multiple sclerosis but not isolated demyelinating neurological episodes were considered. Although it is unlikely that better validation would have significantly altered the results, little effort was made to validate the vaccination status of women with multiple sclerosis who reported never having received hepatitis B. Self-reporting usually overestimates the extent of vaccination, given public awareness of the controversy on hepatitis B vaccination and multiple sclerosis. In our experience, patients often mistake hepatitis B vaccination for another inoculation. Thus, documentation is all the more desirable. But several features enhance the value of this study: the nested case–control cohort design reduced bias due to inappropriate selection of controls; the response rate to the initial questionnaire was high (95% for cases and 88% for controls); nurses have a high prevalence of vaccination against hepatitis B; confirmation was through access to vaccination records; and consistent results of sensitivity analyses matched the main analysis. A period of 2 years was chosen for the definition of recent exposure to the vaccine; this is rather long and strains the biological plausibility for a causal effect, but carries the advantage of reducing error in determining the date of onset for symptoms of multiple sclerosis.

The other United States nested case–control study already mentioned above (DeStefano *et al* 2003) also showed that hepatitis B vaccination was not associated with an increased risk of multiple sclerosis or optic neuritis (OR 0.9; 95% CI 0.6–1.5; DeStefano *et al* 2003). The authors concluded that case reports linking the onset of demyelinating diseases to recent hepatitis B vaccination probably represent a coincidental temporal association rather than causality. Furthermore, the available data provide no evidence that multiple sclerosis occurring after hepatitis B vaccination shows special clinical features compared with classical multiple sclerosis (Tourbah *et al* 1999).

These apparently consistent results have recently been challenged by the results of a nested case–control study within the General Practitioner Research Database (GPRD) (Hernán *et al* 2004). This uses three million British patients, 5% of the population, enrolled with selected general practitioners who agree to provide demographic and medical information on their patients. In this analysis, cases were selected with a validated first diagnosis of multiple sclerosis established between 1993 and 2000. The index date referred to the onset of first neurological symptoms. Only the 163 cases in whom the index date for first neurological symptoms occurred ≥3 years after registration in the database were selected. These were matched to 1064 controls. Evidence for hepatitis B vaccine, and also tetanus and influenza vaccination, was extracted from the automated database. Conditional logistic regression was used to estimate the odds ratios for onset of multiple sclerosis in the vaccinated subjects. There were 11 cases (6.7%) that received at least one hepatitis B vaccination ≤3 years before the date of first neurological symptoms compared with 39 (2.4%) in controls. The odds ratio for the onset of multiple sclerosis ≤3 years following vaccination was 3.1 (95% CI 1.5–6.3) for hepatitis B vaccination; 0.6 (95% CI 0.4–1.0) for tetanus; and 1.0 (95% CI 0.5–2.0) for influenza vaccination (Tables 4.30 and 4.31). The number of hepatitis B immunizations did not correlate with an increased risk of multiple sclerosis.

The publication of these results revived the controversy in France. However, the study has its limitations. The selection process led to a small sample size yielding only 11 informative cases, further reducing to 3 for vaccination ≤1 year before onset of multiple sclerosis; the 95% confidence intervals are correspondingly wide. Although the index date for the outcome assessment was taken as that on which neurological symptoms first occurred, the date retrieved from computer records was, on average, 24 months later than that recorded on paper records, casting some doubt on the quality of data in the GPRD system. Of the 713 individuals identified within the database as having a diagnosis of multiple sclerosis, only 438 (61%) survived the review of the paper-based medical records to enter the second stage, and only 163 (23%) met the next requirement of having a minimum duration on the database before the onset of multiple sclerosis. Eventually, there were only 11 informative cases (1.5%) who received hepatitis B immunization ≤3 years before the onset of multiple sclerosis. Such drastic culling is fraught with methodological problems and inadvertent bias. Furthermore, so few cases of multiple sclerosis were vaccinated against hepatitis B virus (and this holds also for influenza and tetanus) raising the possibility of incomplete ascertainment of vaccine status in the database. This is not much of a surprise as, for instance, vaccination often takes place in occupational health departments and 'travel clinics'. Quite possibly, only those vaccinations received within the context of general practice were entered into the database. Without cross-validation of database and paper records, the results, which differ markedly from those observed in other studies, cannot be considered as definitive (Naismith and Cross 2004).

The recombinant hepatitis B vaccine is a noninfectious viral vaccine derived from hepatitis B surface antigen (HBsAg) produced in genetically engineered yeast cells (Duclos 2003; Hernán et al 2004). The suggestion that epitopes represented in the vaccine show molecular mimicry with myelin proteins is not confirmed (Gran et al 2000). Therefore, it is unclear how such a vaccine could trigger an immunological process leading to multiple sclerosis. The vaccine contains an adjuvant, aluminium hydroxyphosphate sulfate, also present in other vaccines, such as tetanus vaccine. It is unlikely that this is responsible for the hypothetical adverse effect of hepatitis B vaccination because there are no claims for an increased risk of multiple sclerosis following its administration. Nor can we blame thiomersal, an ethyl mercury preservative used routinely in vaccines, acting directly or through a rise in blood concentrations of mercury (Pichichero et al 2002).

Familial risks

Although this seems to us a somewhat contrived consideration, Touzé et al (2000) recorded the rate of familial multiple sclerosis in patients whose disease appeared after vaccination, hepatitis B included. At 7%, this is lower than generally accepted figures. Conversely, considering the 1110 cases of central demyelinating diseases, 898 of which could be diagnosed as multiple sclerosis, and reported to French national authorities by 31st December 2002, a family history of multiple sclerosis did not appear to affect the risk of initial symptoms in a previously unaffected individual following hepatitis B vaccination (*www.agmed.sante.gouv.fr*).

Vaccination and multiple sclerosis: a summary

Our position is that vaccinations in general and hepatitis B vaccination in particular are not a risk factor for the onset or relapse of multiple sclerosis. The most plausible explanation for the reported examples is coincidence not causality. Therefore, there is *no reason to advise*:

- people with multiple sclerosis to avoid vaccinations, including hepatitis B: it makes sense to wait for a relatively silent period of the disease, free from relapse for 12 months; and patients receiving immunosuppressive drugs should have a higher threshold for avoiding vaccinations with live components
- relatives of patients with multiple sclerosis, notably children, to avoid vaccinations, hepatitis B included
- the general population to avoid hepatitis B vaccination.

This position is endorsed by the American Academy of Neurology (Fenichel 1999; Rutschmann et al 2002), the Institute of Medicine of the USA, the National Multiple Sclerosis Society of the USA (*www.nmss.org*), the World Health Organization (*www.who.int*), the Agence Française de Sécurité Sanitaire des Produits de Santé (*www.agmed.sante.gouv.fr*), the French Conférence de Consensus sur la sclérose en plaques (2001), the Réunion de Consensus sur la vaccination contre le virus de l'hépatite B (*www.anaes.fr*), and individual commentators (Duclos 2003; Expanded Programme on Immunization 1997; Global Advisory Committee on Vaccine Safety 2002; Noseworthy et al 2000a; Poland and Jacobson 2004; Stratton et al 2002). These opinions are supported by the lack of evidence for increased MRI activity in patients with multiple sclerosis following influenza (Michielsens et al 1990; Salvetti et al 1995) and Calmette–Guérin bacillus vaccination (Ristori et al 1999). Although we consider the evidence to be conclusive, it is the case that longitudinal assessment of MRI activity in patients with multiple sclerosis before and after hepatitis B immunization is not yet available. Our position is more reserved on the

Table 4.31 Literature data on hepatitis B vaccination and multiple sclerosis

Study	Number of patients and health status	Assessment of exposure to hepatitis B vaccination	Time window of exposure to hepatitis B vaccination before the neurological episode	Odds ratio (95% CI)
Case–control studies with occurrence of first demyelinating episode or onset of multiple sclerosis in cases vs. controls				
Touzé *et al* 2000	121 first demyelinating episodes 121 neurological controls	Telephone interview Copy of vaccination certificate: 17%	60 days 61–180 days	1.7 (0.5–6.3) 1.5 (0.5–5.3)
Fourrier *et al* 1999 Touzé *et al* 2002	236 first demyelinating episodes 355 neurological controls	Telephone interview Reference to vaccination certificate: 68%	**All patients:** 60 days 2–12 months **Only patients referring to their vaccination certificate during phone interview:** 60 days 2–12 months	1.8 (0.7–4.6) 0.9 (0.4–2.0) 1.4 (0.4-4.5) 1.0 (0.6-1.9)
Sturkenboom *et al* 1999; 2000	481 first demyelinating episodes ?Controls (≤6 per case)	Automated database	12 months Any time	1.5 (0.6–3.9) 1.4 (0.8–2.4)
Ascherio *et al* 2001	192 multiple sclerosis 534 healthy controls 111 breast cancers All hepatitis B vaccinated (any time)	Vaccination certification: 100%	**Analysis using only vaccination certified data:** 2 years Any time **Analysis using only vaccination self-reported data:** 2 years Any time	0.7 (0.3–1.8) 0.9 (0.5–1.6) 1.9 (1.1–3.3) 1.2 (0.8–1.7)
N. DeStefano *et al* 2003	440 multiple sclerosis or optic neuritis 950 controls	Automated database Paper medical records Telephone interview Vaccination certification: 50%	1 year Any time	0.8 (0.4–1.8) 0.9 (0.6–1.5)
Hernán *et al* 2004	163 multiple sclerosis 1604 controls	Automated database	1 year 3 years	1.8 (0.5–6.3) 3.1 (1.5–6.3)
Case–control studies with vaccinated cases vs. non-vaccinated controls, and occurrence of first demyelinating episode or onset of multiple sclerosis				
Zipp *et al* 1999	27 229 vaccinated 107 469 nonvaccinated Outcome = first demyelinating episode	Automated database	6 months 1 year 2 years 3 years	1.3 (0.4–4.8) 1.0 (0.3–3.0) 1.0 (0.4–2.4) 0.9 (0.4–2.1)
Sadovnick and Scheifele 2000	267 412 vaccinated 288 657 nonvaccinated Outcome = multiple sclerosis	School-based vaccination programme	Any time	0.6[a]
Relapse of multiple sclerosis				
Confavreux *et al* 2001	643 multiple sclerosis Case-crossover design	Automated database Paper medical records Telephone interview Copy of vaccination certificate: 94%	2 months	0.7 (0.2–2.2)

Multiple sclerosis according to C.M. Poser et al (1983) criteria.
a Crude relative risk estimated from available data in the original manuscript.

suggestion that some vaccines are protective for the onset and activity of multiple sclerosis. But that said, in a single crossover study involving 12 patients with relapsing–remitting disease, Calmette–Guérin bacillus vaccination has been found to be associated with a 57% reduction in MRI activity (Ristori *et al* 1999) and a 54% reduction in the evolution of new enhancing lesions to hypointense T$_1$ lesions (Paolillo *et al* 2003). Furthermore, tetanus vaccine has consistently been found in large epidemiological studies to be associated with a decreased risk of onset (DeStefano *et al* 2003; Hernán *et al* 2004) and relapse (Confavreux *et al* 2001) of multiple sclerosis (see Table 4.30).

CONCLUSION

Our knowledge of the natural history of multiple sclerosis has made steady progress over the last few decades. Now, the overall course and prognosis are clearly delineated with consistent results available from the different representative cohorts set up since the 1970s. In turn, these registers depend on pioneering efforts developed from the 1950s in northern Europe, the United Kingdom and Germany for collecting cases and issuing statistical descriptions of the clinical aspects and disease morbidity. The progressive acknowledgement of epidemiological standards for comprehensive description of the disease has provided another decisive step, as has the standardization and computerization of medical data, and the adoption of accepted and validated scales describing the course, diagnostic classifications and statistical techniques accounting for censored patients. Several statements can now be made with reasonable confidence:

- Multiple sclerosis is characterized by a relapsing–remitting onset in 85% of the patients contrasting with a progressive onset in the remaining 15%.
- With time, the majority of cases with a relapsing–remitting onset convert to secondary progression, and the median time interval for conversion is around 19 years.
- Relapses persist in around 40% of cases during the progressive phase, be this primary or secondary.
- Clinically detectable relapses have only a marginal effect on the accumulation of irreversible disability.
- For a representative population of patients, it takes a median time of 8, 20 and 30 years to reach the irreversible disability levels of DSS 4, 6 and 7, respectively.
- It takes much longer for cases with a relapsing–remitting onset than those with progressive onset to reach levels of irreversible disability, but median ages at assignment of the irreversible disability levels of DSS 4, 6 and 7 are around 42, 53 and 63 years of age, irrespective of the initial course.
- Onset of the relapsing–remitting and progressive phases, like onset of irreversible disability, is influenced by current age.
- Life expectancy is only marginally reduced by the disease.

These observational data help discussions with patients and their relatives, but also inform health care and insurance systems. They support the adoption of a more comprehensive classification of disease course. They have important implications for understanding disease mechanisms, suggesting that multiple sclerosis is a one stage disorder, with a tight intermingling of acute focal recurrent inflammation and diffuse chronic progressive neurodegeneration from the outset, despite the distinctive clinical course comprising a relapsing–remitting phase followed by chronic progression.

Because the phenotype and course of multiple sclerosis are age dependent, relapsing–remitting disease can be regarded as multiple sclerosis in which insufficient time has elapsed for the conversion to secondary progression; secondary progressive forms as relapsing–remitting multiple sclerosis that has 'grown older'; and progressive from onset disease as multiple sclerosis 'amputated' from the usual preceding relapsing–remitting phase. Times to reach disability milestones, and the ages at which these landmarks are reached, follow a predefined schedule not obviously influenced by relapses, whenever they may occur, or by the initial course of the disease, whatever its phenotype. This leads to a unifying concept of the disease in which primary and secondary progression might be regarded as essentially similar. This formulation resonates with the evidence from genetic analysis of familial multiple sclerosis, which can be summarized

as indicating that one set of genetic factors determines susceptibility but others increase the probability of progression, either from onset or after a period of relapses and remissions (see Chapter 3). From the clinical and statistical position, there are arguments in favour of considering multiple sclerosis as one disease with different clinical phenotypes rather than an entity encompassing several distinct diseases, each having a different aetiology and mechanism – the position of complexity rather than true heterogeneity (see Chapter 14).

It might be considered somewhat provocative to propose a unitary hypothesis when the clinical course is so obviously characterized by a relapsing–remitting phase followed by a progression in the majority of the patients with multiple sclerosis. This unifying concept derived from the statistical analysis of general populations does not preclude considerable variation amongst individuals in the dynamics of neurodegeneration and, in consequence, irreversible disability accumulation. The following position stated more than half a century ago still seems relevant:

Clinical and pathological evidence suggest that the chronic progressive type of the disease does not differ essentially from the more usual remitting and relapsing form, in that fresh symptoms may occur during life, in that lesions of all ages may be found post-mortem. It is not necessary therefore to postulate an alternative hypothesis of causation for these progressive cases.

McAlpine and Compston (1952)

The Lyon, France, cohort demonstrates that the influence of clinical variables observed at baseline, or early thereafter, on the accumulation of irreversible disability is limited to the time from onset of multiple sclerosis to the assignment of DSS 4. The same clinical variables do not influence the course beyond this point and into the upper echelons of disability. Therefore, the natural history of multiple sclerosis is characterized by an initial phase, of variable duration, influenced by these clinical variables; and a second phase, which proceeds independently. This suggests that when a detectable threshold of irreversible disability has been reached, the disease enters a final common pathway, where subsequent accumulation of disability becomes a self-perpetuating process, amnesic to the prior clinical history of the disease.

Interestingly, the period from onset to reaching DSS 4 takes place mainly during the relapsing–remitting phase of the disease, whereas the subsequent accumulation of irreversible disability after the assignment of DSS 4 develops mainly during the progressive phase of the disease. The clinical expression of multiple sclerosis depends, during the first phase, on relapses, which are the clinical counterpart of recurrent acute focal inflammation; during the second phase, there is a contribution from diffuse degeneration and axonal loss manifesting as progression. Clinical progression and neurodegeneration appear tightly linked in a relentless manner, whereas the clinical expression of focal inflammation essentially operates at random. As an aside, we might speculate that the correlation between particular symptoms and disease course is confounded by whether small perturbations in affected pathways do or do not produce symptoms. Some (such as optic neuritis or diplopia) tend to be declared early, whereas others are less likely to be expressed clinically and, when they do manifest, therefore get tarnished with the reputation of being harbingers of a poor prognosis.

The 'amnesic phenomenon' is observed wherever the detectable threshold for irreversible disability is set (Confavreux *et al* 2003; Coustans *et al* 2004), and whether or not the phase of relapses and remissions has passed (Fog and Linnemann 1970; Patzold and Pocklington 1982) and laboratory evidence for neurodegeneration is in place (Filippi *et al* 2003; 2004; Fox *et al* 2000; Ingle *et al* 2003; Rudick *et al* 1999). The clinical expression of disease mechanisms in multiple sclerosis is usually two staged: at first, neurodegeneration is clinically invisible but detectable using laboratory methods that provide more sensitivity; later, diffuse neurodegeneration dominates and this is expressed as irreversible and progressive disability. Thus, the unitary concept is explained by the interplay of recurrent focal inflammation and diffuse chronic progressive neurodegeneration.

The observational data also have important consequences for the elaboration of treatment strategies. It is now clear that immunologically active treatments do not affect the chronic degenerative process operating in multiple sclerosis, despite suppressing acute inflammation. Does this mean that multiple sclerosis is a primary neurodegenerative disease? Not in our opinion: there is too much evidence in favour of primary dysimmune mechanisms, and response to treatments that are sensibly timed. Therefore, even from the epidemiological perspective, we favour the hypothesis of an inflammatory disorder occurring in association with the propensity for neurodegeneration, and a complex postinflammatory interplay of immune mediated insults and loss of tissue integrity that may develop its own momentum.

The dividend from studies of the natural history mainly relates to groups and not the individual patient. We sense that the probabilistic statistical approach has reached its limits when using clinical predictors, and that the elaboration of mathematical models, sophisticated as they may be, will not deliver a comprehensive solution. The same will probably be true for magnetic resonance predictors and biomarkers. Only a deterministic approach, based upon measures performed serially on a given individual, is likely to provide a comprehensive account of the prognosis, allowing an individually tailored extrapolation of the observed slope of deterioration for that individual. This has already proven workable with clinical measurements, demanding as the approach may be both for the physician and patient. However, the approach has clear limitations, because the longer the period of observation, and the closer the clinical assessments, the more precise and accurate the extrapolation. This means that, at present, the answer can only be made available once the disease is already advanced, providing a *post hoc* prognosis of limited practical value. Methods have therefore to be developed that assess whether the bespoke approach can be made informative using all available categories of information.

For all these reasons, we consider it timely to offer a more comprehensive classification of the evolution of multiple sclerosis. The current position has great merits and makes the logical distinction between cases with primary and secondary progression (Lublin and Reingold 1996). However, this classification gathers individuals with and without relapses in the category of secondary progression. It discards progressive relapsing multiple sclerosis and reaches conclusions that are more related to acute recurrent focal inflammation than the timing of progression. Perhaps the distinction between 'primary progressive' and 'progressive relapsing' multiple sclerosis with superimposed relapses seems to derive from a classification bias. Therefore we suggest that multiple sclerosis is categorized as having two types of onset ('exacerbating–remitting' or 'progressive') and three main forms of evolution ('relapsing–remitting', 'secondary progressive' or 'primary progressive'); this results in five subtypes depending on whether or not the progressive phase (itself primary or secondary) develops with or without relapses ('relapsing' vs. 'nonrelapsing'). The scheme is summarized in Figure 4.36.

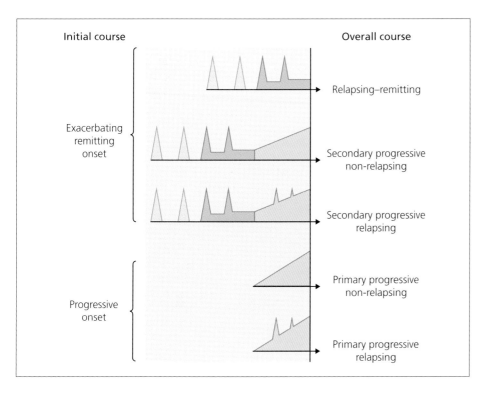

Figure 4.36 Classification of the course of multiple sclerosis. Adapted from Confavreux and Vukusic (2002). © 2002, reprinted with permission of Lippincott Williams & Wilkins (lww.com).

As for the identification of factors that trigger the disease process, without disputing the existence of dramatic, although anecdotal, examples hinting at a close temporal relationship between life events and activity in multiple sclerosis, the scientific evidence supporting most of these claims is not convincing. Standing back from the details, our position is that the evidence is strong for a direct association with the postpartum period; strongly suggestive for an effect of infections; not proven for psychological stress; and unambiguously negative for physical trauma, surgery and anaesthesia, and vaccinations. With so many intercurrent events occurring on a daily basis in the life of people with multiple sclerosis, it is remarkable that any time is left over for periods not at risk.

The origins of multiple sclerosis: a synthesis

5

Alastair Compston, Hartmut Wekerle and Ian McDonald

SUMMARY OF THE PROBLEM

The interplay of nature and nurture, culminating in pathological processes and tissue injury, is reflected by the genetics, epidemiological, immunological and clinical features of many diseases. In general, these tend to be the common scourges of modern medicine, showing geographical variations in frequency and diverse phenotypes, each of which may alter with time. Multiple sclerosis provides a typical example. In common with many other autoimmune disorders, despite much investigative effort and some strong leads, factors accounting for the distribution, origins and mechanisms of the disease remain to be discovered. Much remains enigmatic.

The systematic study of multiple sclerosis in populations, beginning early in the 20th century, showed the condition to be unevenly distributed both within and between countries. Many parts of Europe and North America were repeatedly surveyed. Gradients in frequency were demonstrated in places having generally high prevalences – northern Europe, North America and Australia – compared with other parts of the world. Many analysts picked up on these geographical variations in frequency and formulated ideas on what the distribution might mean. But the facts at their disposal seemed slippery, with morbidity statistics increasing as awareness and vigilance improved, and new diagnostic criteria and definitions were deployed. Especially influential in formulating these opinions were the serial surveys of stable populations, epidemiologically less robust studies of small island populations, and the effects of migration on the distribution of multiple sclerosis. The epidemiologists who pioneered this work soon polarized their interpretation of the emerging patterns around the race versus place – the nature versus nurture – debate. Disease frequency was noted to differ within ethnic groups depending on geography and yet several informative groups, having rich cultural and population genetic histories, retained a low frequency of multiple sclerosis despite domicile in high-prevalence zones. Considerable effort was therefore devoted to the systematic assessment of environmental triggers in the hope that a discrete causative event would be identified, leading to a simple strategy for eradication of the disease. Nothing turned up and, in the frustration that followed, elaborate new hypotheses were offered seeking to account for the distribution of the disease. Quick to replace the environmental doctrine was the concept of genetic susceptibility. Differential recurrence risks for first-degree biological relatives

of probands and individuals becoming part of families through adoption defined the genetic contribution to susceptibility. But, since two-thirds of the monozygotic partners of probands never develop multiple sclerosis, it was concluded that life events select individuals who actually develop multiple sclerosis from amongst those at risk. Given the concession that, however low the threshold for innate susceptibility, disease processes must still be triggered, this now seems a somewhat sterile debate. For most, there is room both for genes and the environment in considering the aetiology and pathogenesis of all complex traits, including multiple sclerosis. This interplay is, of course, the stuff of evolution – not just of disease processes but of speciation and diversity in general.

Here, we stand back from the catalogue of facts laid out in Chapters 2 and 3 and try to see the big picture – loosening the gaze on detail, and peering through the glass darkly. Having rehearsed the facts, as far as they go, we allow ourselves to suggest a specific hypothesis – far from proven, and not accommodating every detail, but open to testing (Compston 2004; Cox et al 2005). Nowhere else in this book do we stray so far from established fact, detach ourselves from the granite of scientific observation – and speculate. Specifically, we argue that European relapsing–remitting multiple sclerosis is the manifestation of a more ancient immunogenetic fault, introduced with the genetic baggage of migrating populations and leading to autoimmunity as their progeny struggled to survive a changing environment. The ancient phenotype was neuromyelitis optica, until recently still the most common disorder in these older populations; transitional phenotypes exist marking the change to relapsing–remitting multiple sclerosis, now common in the northern European and related populations. In the sections that follow, we set out the evidence supporting each component of this story; and conclude with the hypothesis that attempts to explain how multiple sclerosis – as described throughout this book – came about.

THE GEOGRAPHY AND PHENOTYPE OF MULTIPLE SCLEROSIS

Taken at face value, the epidemiological evidence – as we discuss in Chapter 2 – would suggest that, within Europe, multiple sclerosis is more common in southern Scandinavia than the north, in the Orkney and Shetland Islands than the Faroes or Iceland, in Italy (especially Sardinia) than Greece or Spain, in

Sicily compared with neighbouring Malta, and in isolated parts of Finland. In North America, there is a diagonal gradient in frequency with rates highest in the midwest and lowest in the Mississippi Delta. A latitudinal gradient exists for the white Australian population, which shows higher rates in the south than the north. Multiple sclerosis has a frequency in the Far East one-twentieth of that seen in northern Europe. The rate is intermediate in India and Asia but even lower in Africa. But is this geographical pattern clear? And, if no longer opaque, is it stable?

The frequency of multiple sclerosis is considered to have fallen in some places (Orkney, Denmark, southern Sweden, western Norway and Sardinia) and it is rising in other locations. The extent to which the latter is an artefact of ascertainment, or biologically driven, and the difficulty of making comparisons that are not confounded by the catching up of newly surveyed regions, with saturation in those that have been repeatedly scrutinized, cannot immediately be resolved. For John Kurtzke, the doyen of neuroepidemiologists, whereas multiple sclerosis was geographically a regional disorder of males in the mid-20th century, subsequent experience shows that the condition has become more frequent in places where it was already known to occur; has diffused into places where it was previously uncommon, even within quite narrow geographical confines; and shown a steady increase in women, and in races other than Caucasians. Meta-analysis of all surveys in multiple sclerosis where age and sex corrections can be made to the standardized European population, suggests that the perceived differences in distribution may in fact be artefacts of varying demographic structures in the populations at risk (Zivadinov *et al* 2003b). With this manoeuvre, the north–south geographical gradient for age- and sex-adjusted prevalence lessens, and that for age-corrected incidence disappears altogether. Our position is that this reductionist approach, whilst admirably cautious and statistically valid, nevertheless ignores some useful clues to the aetiology of multiple sclerosis. Perhaps, it throws the baby out with the epidemiologically pristine bathwater. We remain of the view that there are geographical differences in the frequency and distribution of multiple sclerosis; and that, although not to be compared uncritically, these nevertheless provide useful insights into the origins and aetiology of the disease.

We have made the point that classifications and diagnostic criteria necessarily change the boundaries of case definition, and so directly affect both local estimates for disease frequency and inter-regional comparisons. Sitting alongside the debate on whether multiple sclerosis is heterogeneous from the perspective of pathology (see Chapters 10 and 14) is the broader issue of where the limits of case definition should be set. In Chapter 6, we describe the relapsing–remitting and primary and secondary progressive forms of multiple sclerosis, Harding's disease, and neuromyelitis optica (Devic's disease). The nosological status of Devic's disease, neuromyelitis optica (monophasic or relapsing), optico-spinal multiple sclerosis and so-called 'Western' relapsing–remitting multiple sclerosis has never been satisfactorily settled. We find these lumped or split, more or less according to whim. The recent pathological characterizations and availability of a serum biomarker are clear votes for the splitters (see Chapters 11 and 12). But we suspect that the relationship may be more complex. Cases of 'multiple sclerosis' seen in Africa, Arabia, Asia and the Far East are often examples of relapsing neuromyelitis

optica. That impression is also apparent from the published series (see Chapter 6). For us, the neurology and pathogenesis of neuromyelitis has a significance that goes beyond mere transcultural neurological nosology.

Eugène Devic (1858–1930) described the combination of myelitis and bilateral optic neuritis. The prognosis was poor and autopsy showed a single spinal focus of acute necrotic myelitis together with optic nerve lesions (Devic 1894; Gault 1894). Later, the term neuromyelitis optica was introduced to describe this disorder. The clinical, radiological and pathological features – as currently formulated – are described in Chapters 6, 12 and 16 (Figure 5.1). Epidemiological studies of demyelinating disease have tended to separate neuromyelitis optica (as originally defined) from multiple sclerosis – whilst noting that the latter often has a specifically different phenotype with disproportionate involvement of the spinal cord and optic nerves in Asian populations. Lumping neuromyelitis optica (monophasic or relapsing) with the Asian (optico-spinal) phenotype of multiple sclerosis allows the frequencies of demyelinating disease confined to the optic nerves and spinal cord and relapsing–remitting multiple sclerosis, as seen in the West, to be compared. The result is rather striking (Figure 5.2). During the second half of the 20th century, it became clear that demyelination – when it occurred in Africa, Asia, the Far East and Aboriginal populations – was typically optico-spinal whereas, at that time, relapsing–remitting multiple sclerosis matching the phenotype seen in northern Europeans was distinctly uncommon (see Chapter 6 for details and references). But the pattern may be changing. Now, at least in Japan, the optico-spinal pattern is seen less frequently whereas the Western features are on the increase (Kira 2003). And for Afro-Caribbeans, born in the French West Indies (Martinique), the frequency of optico-spinal multiple sclerosis changes from 47% in non-migrants to 27% in those living for ≥ 1 year in France before the age of 15 years (Merle *et al* 2005).

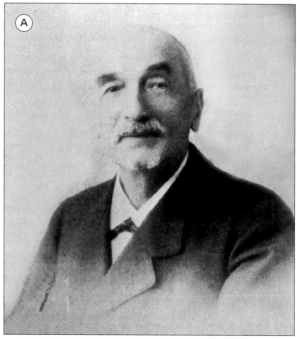

Figure 5.1 (A) Eugène Devic (1858–1930).

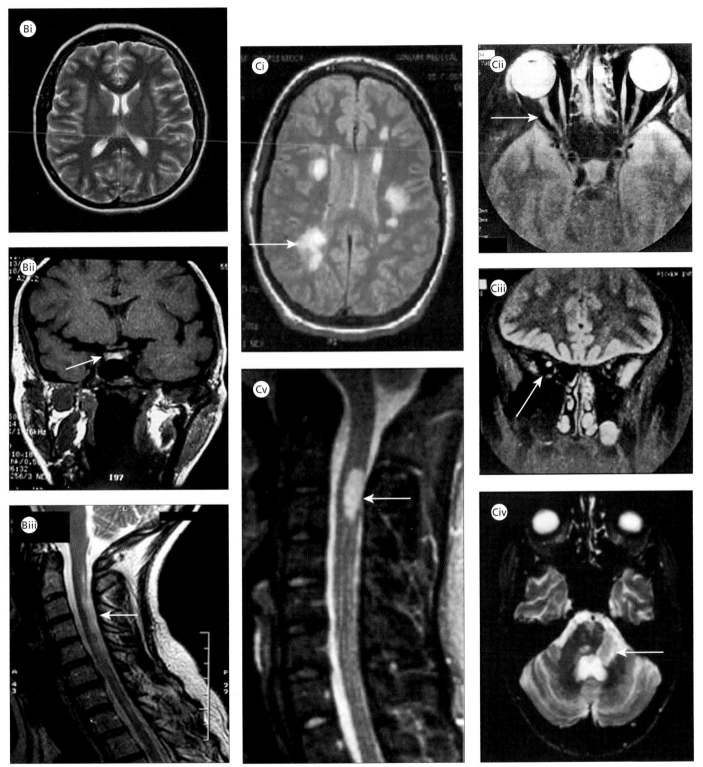

Figure 5.1, cont'd (B) Typical MRI features in relapsing neuromyelitis optica, with normal cerebrum (i), abnormal optic chiasm (ii) and a long linear spinal cord lesion (iii). (C) MRI abnormalities in relapsing–remitting multiple sclerosis affecting the cerebrum (i), optic nerve (ii and iii), cerebellar peduncle (iv) and spinal cord (v).

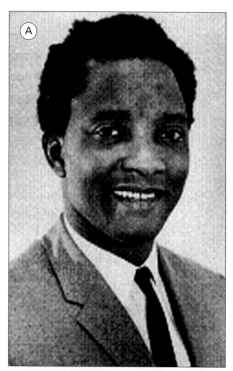

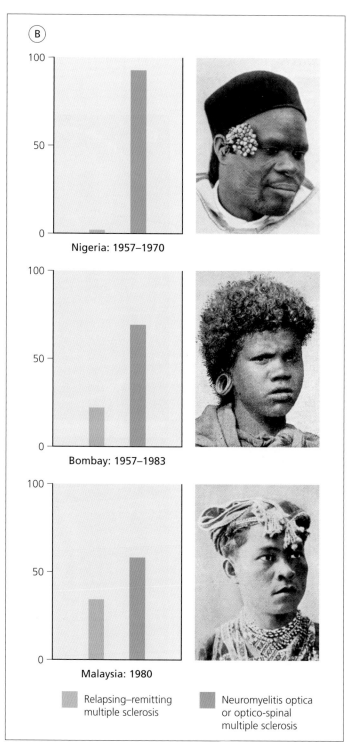

Figure 5.2 (A) Ben Osuntokun (1935–1995): the first African neurologist, who established the frequency of neuromyelitis optica and relapsing–remitting multiple sclerosis in black Africans. (B–E) The relative frequency of relapsing–remitting multiple sclerosis and neuromyelitis optica or optico-spinal multiple sclerosis in Africa, India, Asia, the Far East, aboriginal populations of North America and South America, admixed African–French and African–Americans and northern Europeans.

Nigeria: 1957–1970

Bombay: 1957–1983

Malaysia: 1980

Relapsing–remitting multiple sclerosis

Neuromyelitis optica or optico-spinal multiple sclerosis

Thus, alterations in definition and recognition may have contributed to the changing clinical and epidemiological pattern of multiple sclerosis in Japanese, and the confusion of watching a moving target may not be completed. But is there something more to learn from these clinical patterns: might the diseases have a common ancestry – their different immunopathology, clinical phenotype and disease course reflecting evolution of the disease process?

THE ENVIRONMENTAL FACTOR IN MULTIPLE SCLEROSIS

Populations are not stable, geographically or socially, and migrations involving relatively large numbers of people are known to have affected the distribution of multiple sclerosis. The take on these studies has been to regard multiple sclerosis as an acquired disorder triggered by environmental conditions.

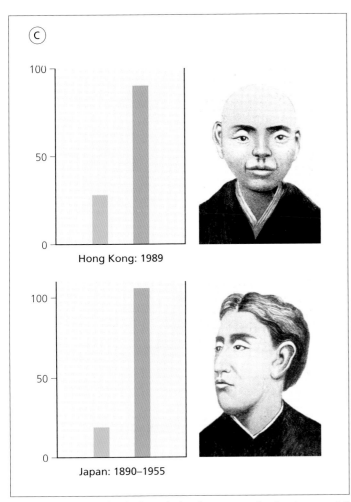

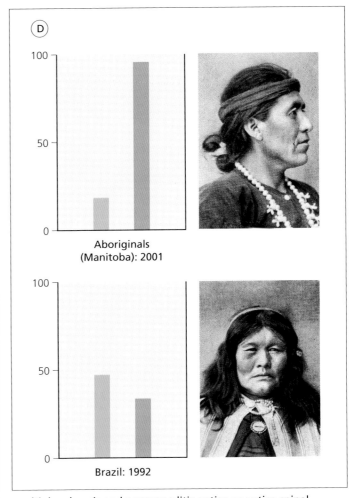

Figure 5.2, cont'd (B–E) The relative frequency of relapsing-remitting multiple sclerosis and neuromyelitis optica or optico-spinal multiple sclerosis in Africa, India, Asia, the Far East, aboriginal populations of North America and South America, admixed African–French and African–Americans and northern Europeans.

Surveys in migrant northern Europeans support the environmental doctrine of causation in multiple sclerosis since, with the exception of Canada, parts of the world colonized from northern Europe show prevalence rates that are lower than the countries of origin. The Australian epidemiological studies reporting on a large geographical area with a relatively homogeneous population mix provide a good example. The distribution of migrants from the United Kingdom and Ireland shows the same latitudinal gradient as for the entire population but with a bias introduced by the high prevalence for multiple sclerosis in the cohort from Hobart (Tasmania); that location apart, the rates are lower than for contemporary studies from the United Kingdom but with no differences dependent on age at migration, taking 15 years as the point of stratification (S.R. Hammond *et al* 2000a). This survey updates the landmark studies from the 1960s, carried out in South Africa, Israel and Hawaii (see Chapter 2). No less influential is the evidence provided by migration in the reverse direction, indicating that Africans and Asians experience a marked increase in risk through being brought up in Greater London or the West Midlands region of the United Kingdom (Dean and Elian 1997). Thus, the studies of migration – moving in low to high, and high to low directions

– provide powerful evidence for the environmental doctrine of causation.

John Kurtzke has been the main proponent for the occurrence of point source epidemics of multiple sclerosis (Chapters 1 and 2). Sceptics prefer the position that these merely follow cycles of increased ascertainment due to local enthusiasm rather than genuine changes in incidence arising from the introduction of transmissible aetiological factors into virgin populations. The fact that all the better documented examples have occurred in small island communities in the north Atlantic can be seen to support either view. Based on the putative epidemic of multiple sclerosis in the Faroes, Kurtzke (1993) concludes that multiple sclerosis originated in Scandinavia (central Norway or the south-central lake district of Sweden) in the early 18th century and diffused across the Baltic states and northern Europe including the British Isles over the next 100 years. From there, it was exported to North America and Australasia, to southern Africa and Italy. It is an attractive hypothesis but whereas for Kurtzke the factors being distributed are germs, for others they are genes.

Rarely in the history of research in multiple sclerosis is there not a hot current microbial favourite for the cause of the disease

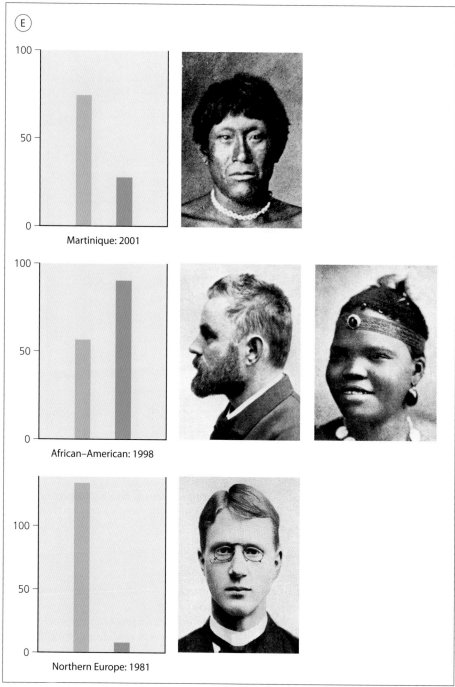

Figure 5.2, cont'd (B–E) The relative frequency of relapsing–remitting multiple sclerosis and neuromyelitis optica or optico–spinal multiple sclerosis in Africa, India, Asia, the Far East, aboriginal populations of North America and South America, admixed African–French and African–Americans and northern Europeans.

based either on population serology, identification of particles in one tissue or another, recovery of defined organisms from body fluids, or unbridled speculation from the armchair. None has stood the test of time; most have disappeared from interest often due to the subsequent recognition of technical artefacts as each tarnished microbe is displaced by new and more compelling germs eager to take their place on the rostrum (see Chapter 2). In the face of these difficulties in pinning the cause of multiple sclerosis on any one organism, some commentators have argued that the disease may have several causes – a floral

approach to the aetiology. But since the search for an environmental cause of multiple sclerosis remains stubbornly unproductive, sceptics point out that, in contrast to the interpretations offered by geneticists, who now have some toe-holds, proponents of the environmental doctrine are still searching for something other than the smoking epidemiological gun in consolidating evidence for a microbial or physical agent as the dominant cause of multiple sclerosis. Frustrated by the low dividend from systematic searches for candidate infectious agents using sophisticated methods for virus detection, alternative

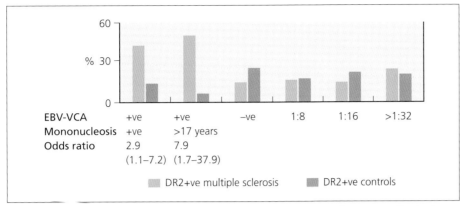

Figure 5.3 The reported age at infection by infectious mononucleosis, and distribution of serum antibody titres to Epstein–Barr virus, in HLA-DR2-matched individuals with multiple sclerosis and DR2-positive controls. EBV-VCA, Epstein–Barr virus – viral coat antigens. Adapted from Martyn *et al* (1993).

theories have therefore been advanced involving the role of climate, diet, geomagnetism, sunlight, air pollutants, radioactive rocks and toxins to account for the global pattern of the disease. We do not find these compelling.

Epidemiology suggests a third factor in the cascade of aetiology and pathogenesis: age at which the exposure to a critical trigger occurs in the susceptible individual. The circumstantial epidemiological evidence supporting (and qualifying) the 'hygiene' hypothesis, and the more specific information relating to Epstein–Barr virus infections are discussed in Chapter 2. Studies on the molecular evolution of Epstein–Barr virus suggest that the two types (EBV-1 and -2) arose from recombination between a proto-Epstein–Barr virus strain and an unknown member of the lymphocryptovirus (and perhaps a third organism), creating genome sequences of the two present-day viruses (McGeoch 2001). Patients with demyelinating disease report later age at infection by measles, mumps, rubella and, especially, Epstein–Barr virus infection compared with controls selected for the same frequency of HLA-DR2 so as to match for at least one marker of genetic susceptibility (Figure 5.3; Martyn *et al* 1993). Infectious mononucleosis after the age of 18 years carries a relative risk for multiple sclerosis of 7.9 (95% CI 2–38). The hypothesis has some support from molecular immunology. Although confined to the study of a single T-cell clone harvested from the blood of an individual with multiple sclerosis, Lang *et al* (2002) describe T-cell receptor specificity for a residue of myelin basic protein (amino acids 85–99) seen in the context of DRB1*1501 restriction, and an epitope of Epstein–Barr virus (residues 627–641) in association with DRB5*0101 (Figure 5.4). Four T-cell receptor peptide contacts were identical for myelin basic protein and Epstein–Barr virus. Thus, there is molecular mimicry.

GENETIC SUSCEPTIBILITY AND MULTIPLE SCLEROSIS

Migration does not just involve the movement of people. Gene transfer and population stratification also follow. Failure to define the environmental cause of multiple sclerosis therefore led others to interpret the distribution of the disease as a function of racial susceptibility and population migrations. Coming at the issue of ancestry from various directions (physiognomy, social history and surname – amongst other indirect clues), commentators have argued for nearly 100 years that the distribution is explained by the fact that multiple sclerosis is a Nordic disease: credit should go to Davenport (1922) for the original observation; to Sutherland (1956) for the first systematic demonstration of differential rates depending on ancestry in the same geographical region; to C.M. Poser (1995) for tying this hypothesis into the rich history of the Viking sagas; and to Skegg *et al* (1987) for the amusing trick of mapping multiple sclerosis to the density of surnames with the prefix 'Mc' in the telephone directories of New Zealand. Each of these commentators concluded that the frequency of multiple sclerosis tracks the dissemination of northern European genes. The increased risk of multiple sclerosis in people moving out of Africa to the United States correlates with the admixture of Caucasian genes into the black community (Chakraborty *et al* 1992). Evidence supporting the hypothesis that susceptibility genes show much the same geographical patterns as the distribution of multiple sclerosis is provided by the clines for markers of susceptibility (Cavalli-Sforza *et al* 1994).

Much information gathered from a variety of epidemiological and genetic sources provides evidence for a contribution from genetic factors in determining susceptibility to multiple sclerosis. Many chromosomal regions of potential genetic interest have been identified, but the genes responsible for susceptibility are not identified, and few of these provisional claims have been confirmed (Chapter 3). Without identifying these factors, little progress can be made in resolving their number and location within the genome, how the products function and interact with the putative environmental factors, and whether heterogeneity determines specifically different disease mechanisms and clinical phenotypes amongst the 'syndrome of multiple sclerosis'. As commentators pointed out in 1996, multiple sclerosis geneticists 'have entered the wood but must now sort out a few trees'. Fifty-two years after James Watson and Francis Crick elucidated the structure of deoxyribonucleic acid, and several decades since Fred Sanger showed how to sequence the stuff, genetic lumberjacks cannot claim poor access to a set of well-honed tools.

The only convincing genetic association and linkage to multiple sclerosis is with HLA-DR(2)15. Our analysis of the MHC, which has been studied for over 30 years, is that the gene

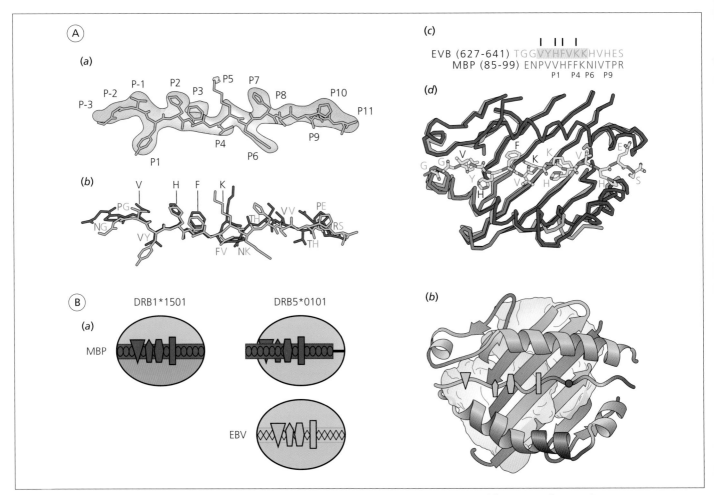

Figure 5.4 (A) Structural comparisons. *(a)*, The Epstein–Barr virus peptide is drawn in green with F_o - F_c omit map shown as a semitransparent surface contoured at 2s. *(b)*, Superposition of Epstein–Barr virus (green) and myelin basic protein (red) peptides based on MHC class II structures. Solvent-exposed residues critical for Hy.2311 TCR recognition are labelled in black. *(c)*, Alignment of Epstein–Barr virus (627–641) and myelin basic protein (87–99) in their MHC class II binding registers. Anchor residues and solvent-exposed residues required for Hy.2E11 stimulation are outlined in yellow, and vertical bars indicate importance to T-cell recognition. *(d)*, Superposed Ca traces of the HLA-DRB5*0101-Epstein–Barr virus (green), HLA-DRB1*1501-myelin basic protein (red) and HLA-DRB5*0101-myelin basic protein (blue) complexes. Differences in B64–B67 are due to lattice contacts in the HLA-DRB5*0101-Epstein–Barr virus crystal and reveal an inherent flexibility in this region of the MHC class II structure. (B) The T-cell receptor recognition surface. *(a)*, Symbolic representations of the DRB1*1501-myelin basic protein, DRB5*0101-myelin basic protein and DRB5*0101-Epstein–Barr virus complexes. The critical peptide residues are represented as a triangle (valine), rectangle (lysine), pentagon (histidine) and hexagon (phenylalanine). *(b)*, Ribbon representation of the HLA-DRB5*0101-Epstein–Barr virus complex, coloured according to differences in the structural superposition with HLA-DRB1*1501-myelin basic protein. Regions in green show least variation, whereas those in red show the greatest changes. The Ca positions of P-1 valine, P2 histidine, P3 phenylalanine and P5 lysine are represented as in (a), and P7 histidine is depicted by a sphere. The putative T-cell receptor binding footprint is represented as a semitransparent surface in pink and blue for the α and β chains, respectively. Structural mimicry is particularly strong within the T-cell receptor α chain binding footprint, in line with observations on the primary importance of this region for T-cell receptor binding. Adapted from Lang *et al* (2002).

conferring susceptibility to relapsing–remitting multiple sclerosis is the class II DR product itself. This makes a relatively small biological contribution to susceptibility but may nevertheless be the most influential factor in the genome. It follows that the remainder are many, also small in their effects and likely to remain hard to track. But even this association has some nuances of interpretation. To varying degrees, the association holds up in practically all populations (see Chapter 3 for details). In the Orkney Islands, multiple sclerosis is not actually associated with either HLA-B7 or DR2. Although the frequency of these antigens in Orcadian patients is no lower than in affected individuals from other parts of the United Kingdom, the lack of an association arises from the fact that >50% of the population are HLA-B7/DR2 positive. This has been interpreted as indicating that genes conferring susceptibility to multiple sclerosis are so over-represented in the normal Orcadian population as to obscure the disease association (Compston 1981). Parts of the southern Mediterranean appear to show specifically different MHC associations – with DR4 not DR(2)15. This applies to populations from Sardinia, Turkey and the Canary Islands, but this Mediterranean DR4 haplotype is not identical across these populations. In Japan, the Western phenotype is associated with

DR(2)15 and, conversely, optico-spinal multiple sclerosis with DR8 (see Chapter 3). Could these be the populations and phenotypes in which finally to resolve mapping that part of the MHC haplotype necessary for susceptibility to multiple sclerosis: are these alternative susceptibility factors responsible for disease phenocopies; or is the explanation more complex?

GENETICS AND THE EUROPEAN POPULATION

Because we attach much importance to the genetic origin of northern Europeans, the stochastic arrival of susceptibility genes for multiple sclerosis in the founder population, and their allelic expansion and distribution through genetic drift and population growth, some genetic history is required. A popular analysis has been to link regions where multiple sclerosis occurs at high frequency to the population genetics of those places. But on how large a canvas should this picture be painted? With the rare exceptions of genetic isolates, most groups have been exposed to prolonged periods of genetic admixture and selection, and have eroded their potential for studies in genetic epidemiology. Nevertheless, we have declared the opinion that multiple sclerosis is a disease of high frequency in northern Europeans. So who are they; and can the focus be narrowed on a more restricted gene pool from within northern Europe?

Asia, the Far East, the Americas, Australia and into Europe are the routes taken by man and woman coming out of Africa. Contemporary analyses of human origins deploy a combination of ephemeral, archaeological, linguistic and molecular genetic analyses of mitochondrial or Y chromosome markers to chart these movements (Mellars 2004; Renfrew 2002; Sykes 1999). Broadly, the patterns are internally consistent, with minor variations in the proposed routes and patterns of dispersal. Phylogenetic dendrograms have been improved by networks allowing the appearance of genetic mutations to serve as temporal and spatial markers of migration and population genetics (Herrnstadt *et al* 2002; Richards *et al* 1996). The original lineage of *Homo sapiens* (L) arose from *Homo erectus* in Africa 150 000 years ago. L1 re-emerged, expanded but remained mainly in Africa and the Mediterranean, including Sardinia, from 100 000 bp with displacements by L2/L3 from 80 000 years ago (Figure 5.5). L3 left Africa for Arabia via the Yemen in 50 000 bp. Her descendants, N and M, made it to Australia, Asia and Turkey by 30 000 bp, and from Asia to North (25 000 bp) and South America (14 000 bp). Mitochondrial markers identify discrete subpopulations of N and M in European, Indian, African, Asian (and American) and Australian populations.

Europe was settled in the Palaeolithic (40 000 bp) and this group is marked by mitochondrial DNA haplogroups U5, H, V, I, W, T and K. Survivors chilled out during the last Ice Age (20 000 bp) in Iberia, the southern Mediterranean and the Ukraine, eventually giving rise to 70–80% of European descendants. With retreat of the ice (15 000 bp), repopulation occurred in the Neolithic period (10 000 bp) from Iberia (haplotype V) and the Ukraine. But in came a new wave from Anatolia carrying mtDNA haplotype J (originating from N) around 8500 years ago, drifting thereafter with the movement of farming as hunter-gatherers ate their way into northern Europe, and gaining a further contribution of the H, T and K haplogroups. Their

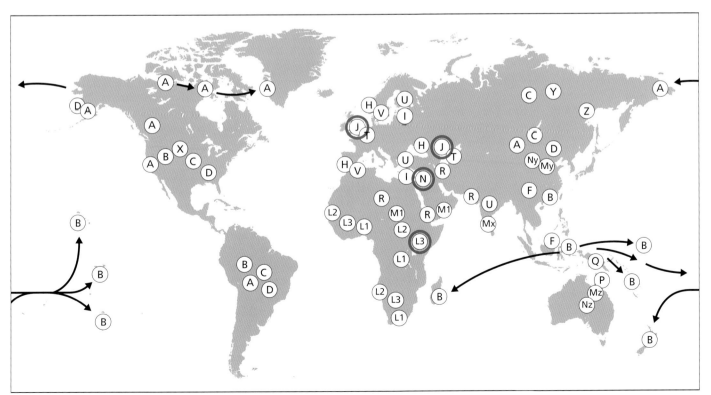

Figure 5.5 Mitochondrial markers for populations emerging from Africa and migrating to Europe in the Palaeolithic and Neolithic. The bold circles identify the haplogroups J and N from which they orginate. Kindly provided by Dr Peter Forster.

descendants represent 20% of the present population. The linguistic markers of these European founders are Finno-Ugrian, proto-Indo-European (Neolithic arriving with the Anatolian wave and haplogroup J) and Basque (Palaeolithic ice-age survivors marked by haplogroup H), respectively.

The main suspect for distributing the genes conferring susceptibility to multiple sclerosis has always been the Nordic peoples. It follows that Nordic gene pools preferentially harbour alleles increasing susceptibility to multiple sclerosis. The style of Norse raiders was to assimilate themselves more or less into the way of life of the local inhabitants, as a result of which the subsequent social and genetic histories of the two populations merge. The migrations of proto-Europeans from northern Europe allowed the races of Scandinavia – Vikings and Goths – to populate parts of northern Britain, Normandy, Sardinia, Sicily and southern Italy. The Celts also moved throughout central Europe from their strongholds in Gaul and visited northern Italy and Greece as well as extensively colonizing Britain. They reached the Faroe Islands and Iceland but were forcibly displaced from many places by Norse invaders, remaining dominant within the United Kingdom only in parts of Wales, the West Country and the fenlands of East Anglia (Keane 1920). C.M. Poser (1995) has charted the travels and influence of Vikings throughout Europe and Asia, seeking to show by historical association that multiple sclerosis has remained a common disease in those parts where Viking genes were liberally distributed. The relationships of these and other migrations to the gene pools of present-day Orcadians and Sardinians are of particular interest given the unusually high prevalence of multiple sclerosis in these populations. In fact, there is also striking congruency for the geographical distribution of other autoimmune diseases, including type 1 diabetes mellitus (Chapter 3).

John Sutherland established differential prevalence rates for multiple sclerosis in Scotland during the early 1950s (Sutherland 1956). These mapped more closely to the distribution of Nordic people than to any geographical gradient. Orkney and Shetland have no Palaeolithic history. They were populated from meso- or early-Neolithic mainland Scotland, tweaked by the Norse interests of the 5th and 6th centuries AD imposing *elite dominance*, and again from Scotland in the 15th century. In asking 'who are the Orcadians?', Roberts (1986) re-evaluated the historical and archaeological evidence that told of a succession of peoples in Orkney of Neolithic and then megalithic origin, followed by Picts, Celts, the Norse and the Scots. Genetic analysis confirmed considerable distance from Iceland, Northern Ireland and the Gaelic fringe of western Europe, and with proximity to Scandinavia and countries bordering the North Sea. Although there were surprising differences from modern gene frequencies for a population generally believed to be of Norwegian ancestry, Roberts assumed that the Scandinavian founder group in the Orkneys also (by chance) had unusual gene frequencies. These have been maintained, whereas present-day Scandinavians have progressively achieved equilibrium with other Europeans, shifting gene frequencies away from their original profile. Roberts considers the Orcadians to be an extreme ultra-European population. According to this analysis, the population is a genetic isolate in which equilibrium has still to be reached despite settlement by Scandinavians more than a millennium ago. Roberts and Papiha (1979) used polymorphic systems

encoded at 23 loci to show that the high inbreeding coefficients characterizing Orcadians are not associated with a greater degree of inbreeding or homozygosity amongst patients with multiple sclerosis than controls. The same high gene frequencies are present in affected and unaffected family members. These are therefore population markers of increased risk rather than disease associations – consistent with the earlier conclusions of Roberts and Roberts (1979) that susceptibility to multiple sclerosis in Orkney is determined by multiple genes, none of which was introduced recently into the population.

Although the origins of Finns may be different from other northern Europeans, study of this population may yield further insight into the genetic origins of multiple sclerosis. Here, the evidence is for an even smaller founder population passing through a bottleneck around 4000 bp and with traces preserved in the contemporary haplotype distributions, especially in small isolates (Laan *et al* 2004; Sajantila *et al* 1996). Whether this knowledge helps directly with our understanding of disease origins is less clear. Evidence continues to accumulate favouring linkage and association with the myelin basic protein gene locus in the community of southern Ostrobothnia – but not elsewhere. The region consists of three parts. Coastal Vaasa was populated from Sweden starting from the 13th century, the northeastern region from eastern Finland in the 16th century, and the Seinajoki region by small groups of immigrants from Satakunta and Pirkanmaa during the 13–15th centuries. The frequency of multiple sclerosis is threefold higher in Seinajoki than the two other parts of southern Ostrobothnia. The archaeological evidence suggests Viking origins. Of the group emigrating to the United States between 1850 and 1923, noted by Charles Davenport to have the highest frequency of multiple sclerosis amongst Scandinavians, half (c.225 000) came from southern Ostrobothnia (P. Tienari, personal communication).

In posing the question 'who are the Sardinians?', Cavalli-Sforza *et al* (1994) describe human settlement dating back 9000 years to the late Palaeolithic with successive intrusions over the last 300 years. Phoenician invasions occurred in the 9th century BC and were followed by visits from Carthaginians (500 BC), Romans (238 BC: they never thought much of the Sardinians, Cicero describing them as '*Sardos uenalis, alium alio nequiorem* – Sards are all for sale, each more corrupt than the next'), Vandals (455 AD), Ostrogoths (525 AD), Byzantines (534–850 AD), and Vikings (860 AD). Thus, the bloodstock of the founders owed much to Carthage and, hence, to Phoenicia. Later invasions by Saracens, Pisans (1258 AD) and Spaniards preceded the established Kingdom of Piedmont. Casula (undated) has traced the history of Sardinia in more detail. The first settlers from the north were from Etruria on the Italian mainland. The west was occupied by travellers from the Iberian peninsula, arriving via the Balearic Islands, and the south was settled by Africans. It was in response to assaults on the coastal communities later established by Phoenicians that a more systematic government of Sardinia was established by Carthaginians in all parts except Barbagia in the northeast. With the conclusion of the first Punic (Carthaginian) War, Sardinia became a province of Rome. After about seven centuries, this influence waned and there were successive invasions from the Vandals of Africa, Byzantines, Islamized Berbers and a series of dynasties from the Italian mainland, notably Genovese and Pisans. The region of Barbagia resisted these changes. A shift towards Iberian dominance occurred in the 14th century. Juame II of Aragon eventually formed the kingdoms of Sardinia and Corsica in 1323 AD. A return to Italian influence occurred with the Treaty of London early in the 18th century, formalized most recently with establishment of the Italian Republic in 1946.

It is remarkable that these successive invasions failed to penetrate the inland regions, remaining as coastal settlements, so that gene mixture amongst aboriginal Sardinians has been limited. Genetic analysis of multiple sclerosis in Sardinians shows heterogeneity with respect to the HLA associations, correlating with – and providing a marker for – preferential clustering of the disease in the more archaic and genetically less disturbed parts of the island (Sotgiu *et al* 2001b). Linguistic data also support the isolation of central Sardinians from the rest of Italy. The surviving language is from the Romance subgroup of the Indo-European family with some words suggesting a pre-Indo-European legacy. Closer relationships exist between Sardinians and Irish, Icelanders, Scandinavians and Anglo-Saxons than with peninsular Italians. The genetic distance of Sardinians from most present-day Europeans is second only to Lapps and exceeds that of Basques. It is reflected by an unusually high frequency of certain blood groups, thalassaemia variants that are otherwise rare, and distinctive HLA phenotypes. These features are explained on the basis of several millennia of genetic drift in a small but isolated island population founded by as few as 1000 pre-Neolithic individuals, the subsequent invasions inflicting successive political and administrative systems and a modified language but leaving rather less genetic trace. A less mysterious origin of Sardinians is suggested by the study of mitochondrial DNA markers indicating that the people of Sardinia were an early mainland European group (Sajantila *et al* 1995).

Thus, the northern European population – in which multiple sclerosis is a common disease – that subsequently came to be distributed across Europe in rather defined and specific directions, can be seen to have originated from a small group of founders marked by particular mitochondrial (J and T) and other population markers. The relevance of this post-Neolithic history is that multiple sclerosis in general and the optico-spinal form in particular is associated with haplogroup J/T in northern Europeans (see Chapter 3; Kalman *et al* 1999; Mayr-Wolfart *et al* 1996; Reynier *et al* 1999) but not in the Palaeolithic survivors represented by present-day Basque people, in whom the frequencies of haplogroups J/T are reduced (Otaegui *et al* 2004). Is it too glib to suggest that optico-spinal multiple sclerosis was the prototypic demyelinating disease reaching Europe with the Neolithic migration, carried not in saddlebags but tucked in the genes, and then distributed as the population of Europe expanded and dispersed?

As we discuss in Chapter 3, pathological mutations of mitochondrial DNA are not associated with multiple sclerosis in systematic screening of unselected patients. Thus, haplogroup J and T appear to be population markers but do not harbour a pathological mutation. If the mitochondrial genetics trail goes cold, where then should the search for genes that do determine susceptibility to multiple sclerosis be focused? When polymorphisms that increase susceptibility to disease arise in a founder group, these will initially be located amongst a large group of linked genes. This block is subject to recombination during subsequent meioses and is gradually whittled down as the population expands. It follows that the progeny of this founder will share segments of DNA identical by descent over several generations. But in time, this linkage disequilibrium degrades. Susceptibility genes can then no longer be identified by association mapping. The population is now in linkage equilibrium. For younger populations, or more recently introduced alleles, the degree of linkage disequilibrium may be sufficient to use markers remote from the disease-promoting polymorphism to track the genetic basis for susceptibility. It follows that the ancient susceptibility genes for multiple sclerosis will be hard to identify by association mapping. Conversely, susceptibility genes represented in the younger European population may still be trapped in large blocks of linkage disequilibrium and easier to find. Although the loss of founder mitochondrial DNA markers is significant, those that are transmitted survive longer as population markers than nuclear genes. Since they provide traces of ancestry over more prolonged periods than nuclear genes, it may therefore be easier to identify a mitochondrial DNA population marker than the nuclear genes putatively introduced with that founder group (Heyer 1995).

Starting with the founder alleles that arrived, by chance, in the proto-European population, systematic filtration of high-risk groups would have culled individuals and genotypes not well suited to surviving the waves of infectious disease, and (conversely) selecting others for their immunological advantages. Identification of the events that drove these changes in genetic makeup of the emerging European population remain shrouded in the mists of microbial history but the answer must lie in one or more public health upheavals of the 12–17th centuries resulting from infectious disease and wars (de Vries *et al* 1980). For example, the Black Death is estimated to have killed >30% of the entire population of Europe in the second pandemic that spread from Siberia to Western Europe in the 1330s; and many subsequent generations took a similar toll from later epidemics until well into the 17th century (Porter 2004). It has been suggested that the price paid for survival is autoimmunity, and the major suspect for having got the genetics wrong (in that respect) is the MHC. Its many polymorphisms are considered to be the tombstones of 'long-standing battles for supremacy between the immune system and infectious pathogens' (Le Souef *et al* 2000). It follows that some susceptibility genes may straddle several disorders supporting the same core inflammatory mechanism even if other factors – genetic, environmental or stochastic – shape the particular phenotype. Thus, it turns out that an allele of the T-cell regulator *CTLA4* increases susceptibility to Graves' disease, autoimmune hypothyroidism and type 1 diabetes (Ueda *et al* 2003).

Although certainly too simplistic a concept, the classical Th1/Th2 paradigm illustrates how small a change might underlie a shift in disease phenotype. The argument goes that multiple sclerosis is driven by cytokines of the T helper-1 (Th1) type, whereas the immunological and pathological features of neuromyelitis optica might reflect T helper-2 (Th2) dominance. It is not hard to imagine a small perturbation in the cytokine milieu rapidly redirecting the path of Th cell differentiation. Perhaps, then, the original expression of autoimmunity to myelin was neuromyelitis optica mediated by Th2 autoimmunity. A key event in transition to the European multiple sclerosis phenotype was a shift in the cytokine response towards a Th1 type. This scheme resonates with the opposite finding in marmoset experimental autoimmune encephalomyelitis that abrogating the Th1 pole of the immune response successfully halts cell-mediated demyelination, only to be followed by a lethal antibody-mediated demyelinating disorder (Chapter 11).

But, if there was a genetic time bomb waiting to go off, what set the fuse? Standing back from the genetic, population history and epidemiological observations on multiple sclerosis, Fredrikson and Hansen (1989) remind us that if multiple sclerosis was a new European disease in the early part of the 19th century, this coincided with the intensive development of trade with the Far East, the Industrial Revolution and mass movement of soldiers within the Napoleonic theatre of battle in Europe. There was every opportunity for a naive but susceptible European population newly to encounter a microbial trigger for multiple sclerosis. Whilst it is possible that a specific and novel microbial challenge occurred that led to the appearance of multiple sclerosis at that time, perhaps a cultural change altered the natural history of an older infectious disease, thereby exposing a window of autoimmune opportunity through changes in age at infection and with markedly different biological consequences – the hygiene hypothesis, so well established for enterovirus infection and paralytic poliomyelitis. And might that agent have been Epstein–Barr virus?

MULTIPLE SCLEROSIS: AN EVOLUTIONARY HYPOTHESIS

We end with a synthesis of these ideas dressed up as a hypothesis (Compston 2004; Cox *et al* 2005). Multiple sclerosis did not begin with wandering Vikings distributing their genetic material throughout Europe and, through their descendants, to other parts of the globe. It evolved from a disease already present in more ancient populations and leaving traces in the present-day spectrum of disease. That disease was neuromyelitis optica, and its pathology was characterized by deposition of antibody and complement – a Th2 type of immune profile. Humoral mechanisms acting against a particular genetic background targeted the disease process to the optic nerves and spinal cord producing long necrotic lesions carrying a poor prognosis for functional recovery. The disease was never common but, by chance, the susceptibility factors were brought to Europe with the small founder group that contributed to the repopulation of northern Europe after the last Ice Age – around 10 000 bp. That founder group is marked by the mitochondrial haplogroup J/T and traces of the association remain. Thereafter, genetic drift and selection pressure from waves of epidemic disease favoured the emergence of high immune response genotypes clustered within the major histocompatibility complex. Now, a Th1 immune response enhancing T-cell and memory responses dominated, overriding the monophasic optico-spinal specificity, exposing new and more ubiquitous antigens, increasing the frequency of episodes and thereby altering the course and phenotype. The lesions were smaller, more sharply defined and (individually) of less immediate functional significance. Transitional forms, such as relapsing neuromyelitis optica evolved and, in time, thus arose relapsing–remitting multiple sclerosis. Its frequency increased during the 19th century and beyond due to population expansion, increased awareness and (perhaps) a genuine increase in incidence. The triggers were infectious disease, with Epstein–Barr virus playing a particular role – its impact emerging most floridly with cultural change consequent upon expansion of the population and industrialization in the 19th century.

Thus, multiple sclerosis did not have its origins in the Northern Mists and Viking longships; rather, these Nordic travellers were innocent carriers of genes that conferred susceptibility – distributors and concentrators but not creators of the risky alleles. We recognize that our hypothesis is taken to the limits of safety by the emerging evidence that, in parts of the Far East where serial observations have been performed, the pattern of demyelinating disease may be changing – with emergence of the Western phenotype and a relative reduction in the proportion of optico-spinal disease. It has been pointed out that this switch from optico-spinal to relapsing–remitting multiple sclerosis follows cultural changes and industrialization in Oriental peoples (Kira *et al* 1999). Our position is that these social shifts exposed the innate vulnerability of those few individuals harbouring alleles that later underwent concentration and stratification amongst progeny of the Neolithic European founders, if they met the crucial environmental conditions. It follows that migration and radical cultural changes reveal in an accelerated form the collision of genetic, environmental and social risk factors that evolved over 10 000 years to create the modern epidemic of multiple sclerosis in Europe. The intrinsic vulnerability is exposed in individuals at risk encountering a new microbial environment at a crucially altered phase of maturation in their immune repertoire. Thus, the phenotype, immunopathogenesis and histological complexity change whereas the frequency of susceptibility genes continues to determine the prevalence of demyelinating disease in the founder and migrant populations, respectively.

This formulation makes many assumptions but goes further than previous analyses. Several commentators have come close: Cosnett (1981a; 1981b) saw a link between neuromyelitis optica disease and multiple sclerosis in Africa; Cree *et al* (2002) gathered and described much of the clinical epidemiological evidence but did not draw the strands together; Kira (2003) used the experience of multiple sclerosis in Japan to great effect, spotting the Th2/Th1 polarities and elaborating many perceptive points, including the effect of cultural change on phenotype, but preferred to separate the Asian and Western forms of multiple sclerosis. An evolutionary approach to the origins of multiple sclerosis is novel but risky and leaves many issues unexplained. It is testable using the matrix of informative populations, mitochondrial and nuclear genetic markers, and discrete clinical syndromes. The zoological record is in the spectrum of pathology and phenotype; the archaeological record is in the global epidemiology of demyelinating disease.

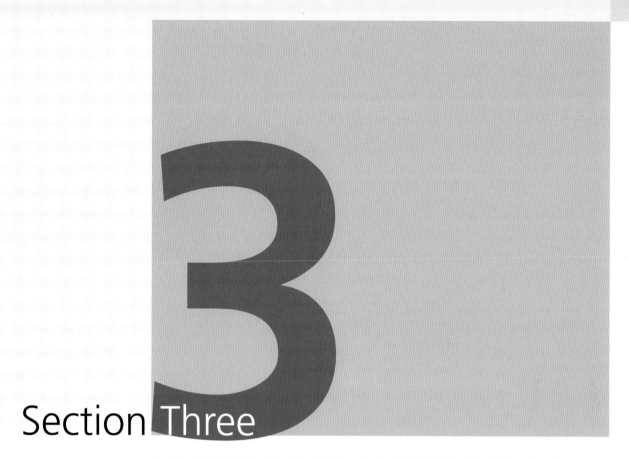

Section Three

THE CLINICAL FEATURES AND DIAGNOSIS OF MULTIPLE SCLEROSIS

The symptoms and signs of multiple sclerosis

6

Ian McDonald and Alastair Compston

An entirely accurate and comprehensive account of the symptoms and signs of multiple sclerosis could only be compiled from a series of geographically diverse population studies of definite cases, minutely observed over the whole course of the disease from first tingle to pathological confirmation. Although we describe the natural history of multiple sclerosis in cohorts observed from onset in Chapter 4, the detailed information needed to catalogue each and every symptomatic experience and their daily variations in intensity is not available, nor can it reasonably be expected. It would, in any event, fail to resolve problems associated with the doubtful case or with delayed diagnosis. In the absence of this information, the mass of published material either lists features encountered at onset and in the course of the disease, or describes single cases and small series of patients with symptoms of particular interest or rarity. In the former, diagnostic criteria are usually stated but detailed description is obviously impossible. Broad headings such as 'visual' or 'brainstem' symptoms are not specific. With individual case reports, doubt may arise as to diagnostic accuracy, particularly if diagnosis is based solely on clinical criteria. However, the autopsy rate in multiple sclerosis is low and it is not possible to confine our consideration to proven cases.

MULTIPLE SCLEROSIS AS A NEUROLOGICAL ILLNESS

The clinical course of multiple sclerosis is as unpredictable as the symptoms that may occur but some patterns can usefully be defined. These are fully discussed in Chapter 4. Eighty per cent of patients present with episodes that recover. The underlying tissue injury may be multifocal or anatomically discrete. Further episodes occur at a random frequency and for an unpredictable period, but average about 0.5/year, decreasing over time. Eventually, a high proportion of patients cease to describe episodic symptoms and the course thereafter is slowly progressive. In about 20%, the illness is progressive from onset. In a prevalent population, approximately one-third of patients are in a quiescent phase of the disease and not significantly disabled; a further one-third are slowly deteriorating; and the remainder are stable but may now be disabled having had the disease for many years (see Chapter 4). The duration of disease from onset or presentation is difficult to assess in a representative population. The previously quoted figure of >25 years now seems to us an underestimate, some individuals succumbing to complica-

tions of disability and infection but most dying from unrelated causes (see Chapter 4).

The most commonly affected sites to produce symptoms are the optic nerves, cervical portion of the spinal cord and brainstem. These will be affected in most patients at some stage in the illness. There is a tendency for old symptoms to recur in subsequent relapses. Many patients report that new symptoms are present on waking. In others, the rate at which a relapse evolves varies from hours to days, with symptoms accumulating in an anatomically coherent way. The rate of recovery is invariably slower than onset and several outcome patterns are recognized. Relapse may occur on an asymptomatic background or complicate existing disability. Recovery from any one episode is often complete but this is not invariable, especially after the first few years, and disability may then accumulate with each new episode. Symptoms which last <24 hours are not usually categorized as signifying a new relapse. Conversely, it is usual to regard manifestations of demyelination developing over several weeks as part of the same episode.

The spinal cord is predominantly involved in most patients with progressive multiple sclerosis, whether this occurs after a period of relapsing disease or from onset. Selective involvement of the optic nerves, cerebrum and brainstem may also progress slowly and account for those patients who present with progressive blindness, dementia, or ataxia. The diagnosis of primary progressive multiple sclerosis should only be made in patients who have been extensively investigated to exclude other disorders. The clinical and laboratory features which distinguish primary progressive multiple sclerosis from other forms of the disease have been re-evaluated (see Chapter 7: A.J. McDonnell and Hawkins 1998b; Thompson *et al* 1997; 2000). Secondary progressive multiple sclerosis tends to affect whichever system has borne the brunt of the earlier disease course. It follows that secondary progression tends to affect the spinal cord, brainstem and cerebellar systems, and cerebrum – with a tendency for visual disabilities to remain stable, albeit at a level of significant reduction in acuity – whereas the hierarchy in primary progressive multiple sclerosis is dominated by spinal cord disease with the syndromes of primary progressive optic nerve, cerebellar and cerebral multiple sclerosis being distinctly less common variants. The onset of secondary progression may be heralded by a severe relapse from which recovery is poor. Once established, progression may be interrupted by further episodes, or proceed without these temporary deviations in clinical activity.

Multiple sclerosis is not necessarily a disabling disease. That said, depending on social and personal circumstances, the ability to participate may be disproportionately reduced in the context of lesions that do not necessarily cause much impairment. Thus, fatigue will affect aspects of daily living that are otherwise well within the physical range of that person with multiple sclerosis. As one of our patients put it (DASC): 'my mind makes appointments for engagements my body is unable to keep.' About 25% of patients have forms of the disease in which only minimal disability accumulates even after many years (Hawkins and McDonnell 1999; McAlpine 1961; 1964; A.J. Thompson et al 1986). Conversely, as the old and contemporary literature reminds us, rare patients may die acutely and early in the course from massive cerebral demyelination or, when the medulla is affected, from respiratory failure (Barnett and Prineas 2004; Marburg 1906). In other cases, relapses occur repeatedly with rapidly accumulating disability producing immobility, lack of protective pharyngeal reflexes and bladder involvement, all of which expose the patient to infection and other consequences of being bed bound. About 5% of patients can be categorized as having this ultra-severe variant of multiple sclerosis, and up to 15% become severely disabled and dependent within a short time (see also Chapters 4 and 12).

Even though the criteria for the diagnosis of multiple sclerosis widely used in clinical practice restrict the ages of onset to between 10 and 50 years, symptoms of demyelinating disease may first occur in children, and in some the illness is already clinically well established in childhood (Boutin et al 1988; Bye et al 1985; Duquette et al 1987). Recent estimates are that 2% of patients with multiple sclerosis present at <10 years and 5% at ≤16 years. These figures are probably confounded by reluctance to make the diagnosis in children. Their presentation is often indistinguishable from that seen in adults, although an encephalopathic form, often mimicking acute disseminated encephalomyelitis but with an otherwise typical subsequent course, is relatively more common in children. At the other extreme, rapidly fatal multiple sclerosis has been described with onset at the age of 81 years (Staugaitis et al 1998).

Establishing the diagnosis, documenting the course, assessing the prognosis and validating the effects of treatment in multiple sclerosis require standardized classifications and measures of disability. We summarized the evolution of these systems in Chapter 1. Diagnostic criteria and the classification of different forms of the disease are discussed in Chapter 7. Here we describe the measurement of severity.

Measurement scales

Three important general questions arise when approaching the problem of selecting or developing a scale with which to measure disease outcome. First, it is crucially important to have a clear idea of what is intended and which outcome is to be measured. Second, there is the issue of whether to choose a generic or a disease-specific scale. The answer depends on the particular aspect of the disease being studied. Third, there is the question of physician versus patient-based assessments. The difference in priorities of the two groups was strikingly illustrated by P.M. Rothwell et al (1997) who studied the perceptions of important determinants of quality of life and found that there was relatively little overlap. Physical functions and role limitations were important to clinicians, whereas mental health and emotional difficulties were more important to patients. There was some overlap for social function, vitality and pain.

There has been much work performed in the past two decades on evaluating scales for use in the assessment of disease. A number of issues have been identified:

- *Scaling*: the first step, one of paramount importance and not easy, is the selection of the items to be measured, which must provide a meaningful and comprehensive index of the disease and how it affects patients. A numerical scale must be assigned which will reflect the changes that are likely to be seen.
- *Acceptability*: the spectrum of health measured must match the distribution of health likely to be seen in the population. In practice, acceptability is determined by examining score distributions and floor and ceiling effects. The mean score should be near the mid-point of the scale.
- *Reliability*: the degree of measurement error must be established by determining inter- and intra-rater reproducibility and consistency of the findings.
- *Validity*: the scale must be shown to measure what it purports to measure. There must be a good correlation with other disability scores and a poor correlation with nondisability metrics.
- *Responsiveness*: the extent to which the scale can detect change must be established.

The Kurtzke scale and its subsequent modification (the Expanded Disability Status Scale [EDSS]: see Table 6.1: Kurtzke 1983a), while encompassing much of the complexity of the condition, apart from cognitive impairment and mood disturbance (Hobart et al 2000), has a number of shortcomings. However, it has stood the test of time and, despite much buffeting from critics, survives. The EDSS is still widely used in natural history studies and therapeutic trials, not least because of its historical significance. However, it shows low inter-rater reliability; is poorly responsive to change; more sensitive in some parts of the scale than others; mixes measures of impairment (what the physician found) with disability (what the patient experienced); and takes no account of the patient's perception of a disease which threatens a huge impact on quality of life. In response to the recognition of these shortcomings, a number of new systems have been proposed recently. Their features are discussed and have been critically reviewed by Hobart et al (1996; 2000) and A.J. Thompson (2002a). None has yet been fully validated although the process has started.

The severity of multiple sclerosis is assessed by a number of scales. Early examples, such as those of McAlpine and Schumacher (see Chapter 1) were simple but lacked sensitivity. Too many patients clustered within a single category of disability. A number of later scales that were straightforward in design proved useful for particular purposes. For example CAMBS attempted a simple, quick, numerical assessment of disability and handicap that combined objective estimates of physical signs and subjective interpretation of handicap, but also documented the extent to which these were attributable to recent relapse and/or disease progression (Table 6.2: Mumford and Compston 1993). The Scripps neurological rating scale (Table 6.3: Sipe et al 1984) has the advantage of being simple

Table 6.1 Expanded Disability Status Scale (EDSS)

0	Normal neurological examination (all grade 0 in functional systems [FS]; cerebral grade 1 acceptable)
1.0	No disability, minimal signs in 1 FS (i.e. grade 1 excluding cerebral grade 1)
1.5	No disability, minimal signs in >1 FS (>1 grade 1 excluding cerebral grade 1)
2.0	Minimal disability in 1 FS (1 FS grade 2, others 0 or 1)
2.5	Minimal disability in 2 FS (2 FS grade 2, others 0 or 1)
3.0	Moderate disability in 1 FS (1 FS grade 3, others 0 or 1), or mild disability in 3–4 FS (3–4 FS grade 2, others 0 or 1) though fully ambulatory
3.5	Fully ambulatory but with moderate disability in 1 FS (1 FS grade 3) and 1–2 FS grade 2; or 2 FS grade 3; or 5 FS grade 2 (others 0 or 1)
4.0	Fully ambulatory without aid, self-sufficient, up and about some 12 hours a day despite relatively severe disability consisting of 1 FS grade 4 (others 0 or 1), or combinations of lesser grades exceeding limits of previous steps. Able to walk without aid or rest some 500 m
4.5	Fully ambulatory without aid, up and about much of the day, able to work a full day, may otherwise have some limitation of full activity or require minimal assistance; characterized by relatively severe disability, usually consisting of 1 FS grade 4 (others 0 or 1) or combinations of lesser grades exceeding limits of previous steps. Able to walk without aid or rest for some 300 m
5.0	Ambulatory without aid or rest for about 200 m; disability severe enough to impair full daily activities (e.g. to work full day without special provisions). (Usual FS equivalents are 1 grade 5 alone, others 0 or 1; or combination of lesser grades usually exceeding specifications for step 4.0)
5.5	Ambulatory without aid or rest for about 100 m, disability severe enough to preclude full daily activities. (Usual FS equivalents are 1 grade 5 alone, others 0 or 1; or combination of lesser grades usually exceeding those for step 4.0)
6.0	Intermittent or unilateral constant assistance (cane, crutch or brace) required to walk about 100 m with or without resting. (Usual FS equivalents are combinations with >2 FS grade 3+)
6.5	Constant bilateral assistance (canes, crutches or braces) required to walk about 20 m without resting. (Usual FS equivalents are combinations with >2 FS grade 3+)
7.0	Unable to walk beyond about 5 m even with aid, essentially restricted to wheelchair; wheels self in standard wheelchair and transfers alone; up and about in wheelchair some 12 hours a day. (Usual FS equivalents are combinations with >1 FS grade 4+; very rarely, pyramidal grade 5 alone)
7.5	Unable to take more than a few steps; restricted to wheelchair, may need aid in transfer; wheels self but cannot carry on in standard wheelchair a full day; may require motorized wheelchair. (Usual FS equivalents are combinations with >1 FS grade 4+)
8.0	Essentially restricted to bed or chair or perambulated in wheelchair, but may be out of bed itself much of the day; retains many self-care functions; generally has effective use of arms. (Usual FS equivalents are combinations, generally 4+ in several systems)
8.5	Essentially restricted to bed much of the day; has some effective use of arm(s); retains some self-care functions. (Usual FS equivalents are combinations, generally 4+ in several systems)
9.0	Helpless bedridden patient; can communicate and eat. (Usual FS equivalents are combinations, mostly grade 4+)
9.5	Totally helpless bedridden patient; unable to communicate effectively or eat/swallow. (Usual FS equivalents are combinations, almost all grade 4+)
10.	Death due to multiple sclerosis

From Kurtzke (1983a) with permission.

but lacked precision in defining degrees of impairment. Normality is scored as 100, and the score diminishes with increasing impairment. Subsequent experience has been limited and the Scripps scale is now mainly of historical interest, along with many others (for review, see Whitaker *et al* 1995a; Willoughby and Paty 1988). Other approaches address severity less explicitly, rather providing standardized protocols and data-bases for describing the history, current status, disability and treatments in individual patients. Inevitably, in the attempt to become comprehensive, they become unwieldy. Although very few clinicians find them convenient for routine use, they serve as important descriptors for patients participating in clinical research.

Of particular interest is the Multiple Sclerosis Functional Composite, as a measure that may prove especially useful in therapeutic trials (Table 6.4: Cutter *et al* 1999; Rudick *et al* 2002; Uitdehaag *et al* 2002). Its development resulted from an international initiative led by the National Multiple Sclerosis Society of the United States. The Multiple Sclerosis Functional Composite comprises timed tests of walking, arm function and cognitive ability expressed as a single score along a continuous scale. The Multiple Sclerosis Functional Composite shows moderately good correlations with the EDSS. It has advantages over the EDSS being continuous, as opposed to ordinal and pro-viding superior inter- and intra-rater reliability. The Multiple Sclerosis Functional Composite provides a good correlation with

Table 6.2 **The CAMBS score**

a) Disability and impairment

– Patient's disability unknown.
1 Fully independent patient with no disturbance of vision, sensation, sphincters, arm function or mobility.
2 Patient with one only of: mild fatigue, visual blurring but able to read, minor sensory symptoms, minor sphincter disturbance, altered arm function or mild difficulty with walking.
3 Patient with one or more of: frequent or permanent assistance with continence, significant visual symptoms preventing reading, inability to use one or both arms, significant pain or dysaesthesiae, requirement for bilateral assistance with walking, significant intellectual impairment.
4 Patient who is wheelchair-bound or has other major disability severely restricting daily activities.
5 Bed-bound or totally dependent on others for all care.

b) Relapse

– Relapse status cannot be assigned.
1 Quiescent or non-relapsing pattern of illness.
2 Subjectively worse than baseline state but improving or objectively unchanged.
3 Subjectively worse than baseline state and continuing to deteriorate.
4 Significantly worse than usual as a result of established relapse.
5 Major deterioration necessitating hospital admission and increased dependency on care-givers.

c) Progression

– No knowledge of natural history of illness up to present time.
1 Apart from any recent acute changes, clinical condition has not changed in past year.
2 Minor deterioration in clinical condition over past year.
3 Significant increase in handicap or disability in past year.
4 Rapid clinical increase in handicap or disability in past year.
5 Devastating progression in past year, i.e. 'malignant' form of disease.

d) Handicap

Ask the patient to mark the line below to obtain a score for handicap.

'Role in Life'

'How severely does your condition affect your ability to perform a normal role in life?'
'Make a mark on one digit on the line below to indicate this.'
'A mark on the figure one would indicate that your condition has no effect on your role in life, your occupation, or your ability to support your family.'
'A mark on the figure five would mean that the condition renders you completely incapable of any useful role in life, and totally prevents you from fitting into your normal social role, e.g. ability to do your job, ability to take a normal part in family life.'
'You may make a mark on any digit on the line.'

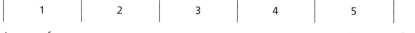

1	2	3	4	5

I can perform a completely normal role in life.

I am completely prevented from holding a normal role in life by my illness.

Overall 'D.R.P.H' Coding: D [ ] R [ ] P [ ] H [ ]

other measures that are specific for disability, including magnetic resonance imaging (MRI) variables (at least in some studies) and patient-reported, disease-related quality of life. It is predictive for clinical and MRI outcome (Rudick *et al* 2002). Encouraging though these results are, problems remain. For example, although (to date) most studies have shown the Multiple Sclerosis Functional Composite to be more responsive than the EDSS, in a trial of corticosteroid treatment the United Kingdom Disability Scale (Table 6.5: Sharrack and Hughes 1999) showed the greatest change, illustrating how the interpretation of outcome can be much influenced by the scale selected (Hoogervorst *et al* 2001).

The importance of patients' perceptions of the impact of multiple sclerosis on quality of life and the effectiveness of treatment has already been mentioned. One consideration is whether patient-based scales can achieve an acceptable level of objectivity and perform well in comparison with other instruments. Recent work on the Multiple Sclerosis Impact Scale (MSIS-29: Table 6.6) suggests that they can (Hobart *et al* 2001; Hoogervorst *et al* 2004). There is no agreed method for determining progression of disability in patients with multiple sclerosis when each patient has had only a single assessment in the course of the disease. Roxburgh *et al* (2005a) have developed an algorithm which relates scores on the EDSS to the distribution of disability in patients with comparable disease durations. Measurements made in the first year did not prove to be reliable indicators of disease but correlations between measurements taken at year 1 and compared 5, 10 and 15 years later indicate that single point assessment data made early in the course can be used to represent disease severity (Figure 6.1). However,

Table 6.3 **Scripps Neurological Rating Scale (NRS) worksheet**

System examined	Maximum points	Degree of Impairment			
		Normal	Mild	Moderate	Severe
Mentation and mood	10	10	7	4	0
Cranial nerves:	21				
Visual acuity		5	3	1	0
Fields, discs, pupils		6	4	2	0
Eye movements		5	3	1	0
Nystagmus		5	3	1	0
Lower cranial nerves	5	5	3	1	0
Motor:	20				
Right upper		5	3	1	0
Left upper		5	3	1	0
Right lower		5	3	1	0
Left lower		5	3	1	0
Deep tendon reflexes:	8				
Upper extremity		4	3	1	0
Lower extremity		4	3	1	0
Babinski: right, left	4	4	–	–	0
(2 each)					
Sensory:	12				
Right upper		3	2	1	0
Left upper		3	2	1	0
Right lower		3	2	1	0
Left lower		3	2	1	0
Cerebellar:	10				
Upper extremity		5	3	1	0
Lower extremity		5	3	1	0
Gait; trunk and balance	10	10	7	4	0
Special category:					
Bladder/bowel/	0	0	–3	–7	–10
sexual dysfunction					
Totals	100				
Neurological Rating Scale score					

Points assigned for each component of the neurological examination are subtotalled, and points for autonomic dysfunction are subtracted, leaving the final (NRS) score.

individual scores on the Multiple Sclerosis Severity Score (MSSS) may alter over time and although differences in mean MSSS (or EDSS) between groups of patients reflect real differences in disease progression, more caution is needed in using the MSSS to predict future disease severity in the individual. By simulating genetic effects on disability (as an example of how the novel scale might be used), the MSSS was shown to be more reliable than other scales available for detecting different rates of disease progression. It will be of considerable interest to see these results confirmed.

The problem of how best to record this information remains unsolved but storage systems need to be versatile without becoming excessively complex. The European Database in Multiple Sclerosis (EDMUS; Confavreux *et al* 1992) has been adopted in Europe, whereas COSTAR (Paty *et al* 1994) is preferred in North America.

Future progress in this important field will depend on the systematic application and head-to-head comparison of existing scales in appropriate clinical contexts, the development of new rationally based scales, and the utilization of more subtle and complex methods of statistical analysis (such as Rasch analysis

and Item Response Theory; reviewed by Hobart 2002). It remains fundamentally important for future research to clarify that scales are reliable (that is, reproducible and free from random error), responsive (sensitive to clinically meaningful change), valid (measure what is intended) and help to inform about the long-term course of the disease. Until a consensus on measurement scales is reached, each investigator must remember that before any study begins decisions must be taken on what precisely it is hoped to show. The relevant scales must be reviewed critically and the instruments chosen must be the most appropriate for the anticipated outcome. The position is well summarized by Hobart and Thompson (2002): 'No instrument has universal usefulness; it is therefore important to identify the strengths and weaknesses of individual measures.'

SYMPTOMS AT ONSET OF THE DISEASE

The symptoms and signs of multiple sclerosis are notoriously variable but in general reflect the extent to which those parts of the central nervous system in which there is a dense concentration of myelinated fibres subserving motor and sensory functions,

Table 6.4 Common naming conventions used for measurement scale or variable across datasets and hierarchy of variables evaluated

Clinical dimension	Test name	Measurement	Metric
Naming conventions			
Arm	Box and blocks test	Mean of right and left arm scores	Number of blocks transferred in 1 min
	Nine hole peg test	Mean of right and left arm scores	Time to insert and remove nine pegs
	Purdue pegboard test	Mean of dominant and nondominant arm	Number of pegs placed in holes in 30 seconds
Leg	Timed walk	A walk of 25 ft (7.5 m)	Time taken in seconds
	Gait test	Gait averaged over two trials	Number of steps per second
	Ambulation index	Scale for assessing ambulation in semi-quantitative terms	Ordinal scale
Cognitive	PASAT – 2 min	Paced auditory serial addition test, 2-min version	Number correct
	PASAT – 3 min	Paced auditory serial addition test, 3-min version	Number correct
	SDMT	Symbol-digit modalities test	Number correct in 90 seconds
Disability	Expanded DSS	Summary measure of functional systems	Ordinal scale

Hierarchy of variables evaluated			
	First choice	**Second choice**	**Third choice**
Arm dimension	Nine hole peg test	Box and block test	Purdue pegboard
Leg dimension	Timed walk	Gait test	–
Cognitive dimension	PASAT (3-min version)	PASAT (2-min version)	SDMT
Visual dimension	Kurtzke functional system	Visual acuity	–

PASAT, paced auditory serial addition test; SDMT, symbol-digit modalities test.

such as the brainstem, cerebellum and spinal cord, are involved (Figures 6.2 and 6.3). The initial manifestations of multiple sclerosis have been analysed in many series. Most are inevitably subject to numerous sources of selection bias and error resulting from the retrospective nature of the enquiry. Even in patients seen and fully documented in what appears to be the first episode of the disease, records may reveal forgotten symptoms of possible but uncertain significance, for example dimly recollected dizziness or paraesthesiae. When the diagnosis is not established until several years after onset, consulting old records will show that the patient's memory is often fallible. It is reasonable to assume that the more time that has elapsed between onset and questioning, the greater will be these inaccuracies. The duration of illness at the time of inclusion in the series may therefore be expected to influence the results of retrospective clinical documentation. Not infrequently earlier episodes are recalled some time after a consultation. One of us (WIMcD) saw an ex-nurse aged about 40 years who, having been questioned about sensory symptoms, later remembered that during her midwifery training (>20 years earlier) she had experienced difficulty delivering babies for several weeks because flexion of her neck led to a surge of paraesthesiae in the trunk and limbs. The combined effect of failure to recall, and the lack of contemporary records, almost certainly explains the considerable difference between the clinical features of initial attacks of multiple sclerosis assigned to soldiers before enlistment and those actually observed during their term of service. The former

were much more likely to be recorded as monosymptomatic, focusing on the core manifestations and often neglecting the many minor complaints that characterized later episodes (Kurtzke et al 1968a).

Comparison between series is not straightforward especially when patients are selected using different methods and criteria. Cases may be based entirely on hospital in-patient material (Shibasaki et al 1981), on men enlisted in the United States armed forces and therefore passed fit for service on recruitment (Kurtzke et al 1968a), or on autopsy series (S. Carter et al 1950). Cohorts approximating to population studies (S. Poser et al 1979b; Shepherd 1979) are inevitably heavily based on hospital records. Diagnostic criteria have varied, 'possible' cases being included (McAlpine et al 1955; S. Poser et al 1979b; Shepherd 1979) or excluded (Shibasaki et al 1981) or only included if considered to be 'strongly possible' (Kurtzke et al 1968a). In the widely cited data of S. Poser et al (1979b; see also R. Kelly 1985), for example, the proportion of definite cases was only 41%. In the otherwise admirable account of symptoms and signs over the course of the disease by Bauer and Hanefeld (1993), the population studied and the diagnostic criteria used are not clearly defined. The headings under which symptoms and signs are listed are often tantalizingly different. Visual failure may be combined with diplopia (S. Carter et al 1950) or symptoms may be vaguely linked as 'affections of the cranial nerves V and/or VII' (S. Poser et al 1979b). Lhermitte's symptom may not be distinguished from other sensory complaints (S. Poser et al

Table 6.5 **Guy's Neurological Disability Scale**

The **Guy's Neurological Disability Scale** is derived from subscales and ranges from 0 (no disability) to 60 (maximum possible disability). The level of disability in each of 12 functional domains is graded according to severity and impact, arranged to represent the following comparable categories on a six point scale.

0   Normal status
1   Symptoms causing no disability
2   Mild disability – not requiring help from others
3   Moderate disability – requiring help from others
4   Severe disability – almost total loss of function
5   Total loss of function – maximum help required

1. Cognitive disability:

0   No cognitive problems.
1   Cognitive problems not noticeable to family or friends.
2   Cognitive problems noticeable to family or friends but not requiring help from others.
3   Cognitive problems requiring help from others for normal daily affairs; patient is fully orientated in time, place and person.
4   Cognitive problems requiring help from others for normal daily affairs; patient is not fully orientated.
5   Patient is completely disorientated in time, place and person.

2. Mood disability:

0   No mood problems.
1   Asymptomatic on current drug treatment.
2   Mood problems present but not affecting the patients' ability to perform any of their usual daily activities.
3   Mood problems affecting the patients' ability to perform some of their usual daily activities.
4   Mood problems preventing the patients from doing all their usual daily activities.
5   Mood problems requiring inpatient management.
x   Unknown (please score as the mean of the cognitive and fatigue disability scores rounded to the nearest integer).

3. Visual disability:

0   No visual problems.
1   Visual problems (blurred vision, diplopia, scotomas) but patient is still able to read ordinary newspaper print.
2   Unable to read ordinary newspaper print.
3   Unable to read large newspaper print.
4   Unable to count fingers if they hold their hand out in front of them.
5   Unable to see hand movement if they move their hand in front of them.

4. Speech and communication disability:

0   No speech problems.
1   Speech problems which do not require the patients to repeat themselves when speaking to strangers.
2   Speech problems which require the patients to repeat themselves when speaking to strangers.
3   Speech problems which require the patients to repeat themselves when speaking to their family and close friends.
4   Speech problems making speech difficult to understand; patient is able to communicate effectively by using sign language or the help of their carers.
5   Speech problems making speech difficult to understand, patient is unable to communicate effectively by using sign language or the help of their carers.

5. Swallowing disability:

0   No swallowing problems.
1   Needs to be careful when swallowing solids or liquids but not with most meals.
2   Needs to be careful when swallowing solids or liquids with most meals; patient is able to eat food of normal consistency.
3   Needs specially prepared food of modified consistency.
4   Tendency to choke with most meals.
5   Dysphagia requiring nasogastric or gastrostomy tube.

6. Upper limb disability:

0   No upper limb problem.
1   Problems in one or both arms, not affecting the ability to do any of the functions listed.
2   Problems in one or both arms, affecting some but not preventing any of the functions listed.
3   Problems in one or both arms, affecting all or preventing one or two of the functions listed.
4   Problems in one or both arms, preventing three or all of the functions listed.
5   Unable to use either arm for any purposeful movements.

7. Lower limb disability:

0   Walking is not affected.
1   Walking is affected but patient is able to walk independently.
2   Usually uses unilateral support (single stick or crutch, one arm) to walk outdoors, but walks independently indoors.
3   Usually uses bilateral support (two sticks or crutches, frame, or two arms) to walk outdoors, or unilateral support (single stick or crutch, or one arm) to walk indoors.
4   Usually uses wheelchair to travel outdoors, or bilateral support (two sticks or crutches, frame, or two arms) to walk indoors.
5   Usually uses a wheelchair indoors.

table continued on following page

Table 6.5 **Guy's Neurological Disability Scale, cont'd**

8. Bladder disability:

0 Normal bladder problems.
1 Asymptomatic on current drug treatment.
2 Urinary frequency, urgency, or hesitancy with no incontinence.
3 Occasional urinary incontinence (once or more during the last month but not every week) *or* intermittent catheterization without incontinence.
4 Frequent urinary incontinence (once a week or more during the last month but not daily) *or* occasional urinary incontinence despite regular intermittent catheterization.
5 Daily urinary incontinence or permanent catheter (urethral/suprapubic) or penile sheath.

9. Bowel disability:

0 No bowel problems.
1 Asymptomatic on current drug treatment or constipation not requiring any treatment.
2 Constipation requiring laxatives or suppositories or faecal urgency.
3 Constipation requiring the use of enemas.
4 Constipation requiring manual evacuation of stools or occasional faecal incontinence (once or more during the last month but not every week).
5 Weekly faecal incontinence.

10. Sexual disabilities:

0 Normal sexual functions or persons who are voluntarily celibate.
1 Reduced sexual interest.
2 Problems satisfying oneself or sexual partner.
3 Physical problems interfering but not preventing sexual function.
4 Autonomic problems interfering but not preventing sexual function.
5 Physical or autonomic problems totally preventing sexual function.
x Unknown (please score as the mean of the lower limb, bladder, and bowel disability scores rounded to the nearest integer).

11. Fatigue:

0 Absent.
1 Occasional fatigue (present some days).
2 Frequent fatigue (present most days).
3 Fatigue affecting the patient's ability to perform some of their usual daily activities.
4 Fatigue preventing the patient from doing all their usual daily activities.
5 Fatigue preventing the patient from doing all their physical activities.
x Unknown (please score as the mean of the cognitive and mood disability scores rounded to the nearest integer).

12. Other disabilities:

0 Absent.
1 Asymptomatic on current drug treatment.
2 Problems, present, but are not affecting the patient's ability to perform any of their usual daily activities.
3 Problems affecting the patient's ability to perform some of their usual daily activities.
4 Problems preventing the patients from doing all their usual daily activities.
5 Problems requiring hospital admission for assessment or treatment.

1979b) or may not feature at all. Cerebellar disturbance may be implied by abnormalities of balance or gait, or by tremor and ataxia, but often no distinction is made from vertigo.

McAlpine (1972), in a review of all previous published reports, found that the incidence of initial symptoms was approximately as follows:

- weakness in one or more limbs 35%
- optic neuritis 20%
- paraesthesiae 20%
- diplopia 10%
- vertigo 5%
- disturbance of micturition 5%
- other <5%.

It was not possible to identify cerebellar symptoms with any certainty from vague descriptions such as 'lack of balance'. His own series (McAlpine *et al* 1972) was large, personally observed and involved cases seen within 3 years of the presumed clinical onset. At 39%, the proportion in whom limb weakness occurred was almost identical to the list above but there was much greater recognition of paraesthesiae as an initial symptom, being present in 40%. Optic neuritis occurred in 29%. The important distinction was made between polysymptomatic (55%) and monosymptomatic (45%) onset. In the former, weakness was present in 50% but in only 26% of those with a single initial symptom. Optic neuritis was more common in isolation, but cerebellar ataxia did not occur without more widespread symptoms. With few exceptions (D.K. Adams *et al* 1950; A.J. Thompson *et al* 1986) subsequent reports have recognized that onset may be polysymptomatic, although the proportion in whom this occurs has varied widely, partly because of differing methods of symptom classification. E.A.C.M. Sanders and Arts (1986) reported monosymptomatic onset in 57%. In contrast, Kurtzke

Table 6.6 Multiple Sclerosis Impact Scale (MSIS-29)

	Not at all	A little	Moderately	Quite a bit	Extremely

- The following questions ask for your views about the impact of MS on your day-to-day life **during the past two weeks**
- For each statement, please **circle** the **one** number that **best** describes your situation
- Please answer **all** questions

In the *past two weeks*, how much has your multiple sclerosis limited your ability to...

	Not at all	A little	Moderately	Quite a bit	Extremely
1. Do physically demanding tasks?	1	2	3	4	5
2. Grip things tightly (e.g. turning on taps)?	1	2	3	4	5
3. Carry things?	1	2	3	4	5

In the *past two weeks*, how much have you been bothered by...

	Not at all	A little	Moderately	Quite a bit	Extremely
4. Problems with your balance?	1	2	3	4	5
5. Difficulties moving about indoors?	1	2	3	4	5
6. Being clumsy?	1	2	3	4	5
7. Stiffness?	1	2	3	4	5
8. Heavy arms and/or legs?	1	2	3	4	5
9. Tremor of your arms or legs?	1	2	3	4	5
10. Spasms in your limbs?	1	2	3	4	5
11. Your body not doing what you want it to do?	1	2	3	4	5
12. Having to depend on others to do things for you?	1	2	3	4	5
13. Limitations in your social and leisure activities at home?	1	2	3	4	5
14. Being stuck at home more than you would like to be?	1	2	3	4	5
15. Difficulties using your hands in everyday tasks?	1	2	3	4	5
16. Having to cut down the amount of time you spent on work or other daily activities?	1	2	3	4	5
17. Problems using transport (e.g. car, bus, train, taxi, etc.)?	1	2	3	4	5
18. Taking longer to do things?	1	2	3	4	5
19. Difficulty doing things spontaneously (e.g. going out on the spur of the moment)?	1	2	3	4	5
20. Needing to go to the toilet urgently?	1	2	3	4	5
21. Feeling unwell?	1	2	3	4	5
22. Problems sleeping?	1	2	3	4	5
23. Feeling mentally fatigued?	1	2	3	4	5
24. Worries related to your multiple sclerosis?	1	2	3	4	5
25. Feeling anxious or tense?	1	2	3	4	5
26. Feeling irritable, impatient, or short tempered?	1	2	3	4	5
27. Problems concentrating?	1	2	3	4	5
28. Lack of confidence?	1	2	3	4	5
29. Feeling depressed?	1	2	3	4	5

® 2000 Neurological Outcome Measures Unit.
Please check that you have circled ONE number for EACH question.

et al (1979) found initial involvement of a single major system (defined as motor, co-ordination, sensory, or brainstem) in only 14%. Visual loss, regarded as a minor system in isolation in this series, was remarkably rare. The most frequent combinations were involvement of all four systems (14%); motor and sensory (12%); motor, co-ordination and sensory (12%); and co-ordination and brainstem (10%).

Paty and Poser (1984), in a series of 461 patients with clinically definite multiple sclerosis, found the first symptom to be visual loss in one eye (17%), double vision (13%), sensory disturbance (36%) and altered balance and gait (from unspecified causes) 18%. Weakness was only mentioned when progressive (10%) but in a minority of patients (6%), the onset was with acute myelitis. The first episode appears to have been mono-symptomatic in the great majority. In the personal experience of Bryan Matthews, onset was monosymptomatic in 70% of patients in two combined series comprising 546 patients with clinically definite multiple sclerosis according to McAlpine's criteria. It was evident, however, that with increasing knowledge and experience, the proportion of patients in whom sensory or paroxysmal symptoms were recognized as initial symptoms notably increased.

Information on the onset of the disease derived from autopsy-proven cases is less informative than might be hoped, being biased by small numbers and selected material. The series of 111 cases collected by C.M. Poser *et al* (1966) was derived from three countries and its unrepresentative nature is suggested by reversal of the usual female preponderance in the cases from Norway and the United States. In histologically proven cases, neither early (Izquierdo *et al* 1986) nor late (Lyon-Caen *et al* 1985) onset of disease is shown to be associated with important differences in initial symptomatology. The latter conclusion, however, is probably an effect of case selection as Hooge and Redekop (1992) found that onset at >60 years is usually with progressive motor weakness.

	0	1	1.5	2	2.5	3	3.5	4	4.5	5	5.5	6	6.5	7	7.5	8	8.5	9	9.5	EDSS
0	0.89	2.94	4.79	6.51	7.76	8.25	8.73	9.18	9.44	9.54	9.62	9.78	9.90	9.94	9.95	9.95	9.99	10.00	10.00	
1	0.64	2.34	4.12	5.75	7.04	7.76	8.38	8.91	9.23	9.42	9.57	9.73	9.88	9.93	9.95	9.98	9.99	9.99	10.00	
2	0.53	1.99	3.65	5.25	6.47	7.21	7.90	8.47	8.83	9.06	9.26	9.50	9.75	9.86	9.93	9.97	9.98	10.00	10.00	
3	0.45	1.73	3.28	4.79	5.98	6.80	7.55	8.14	8.55	8.82	9.05	9.34	9.63	9.78	9.87	9.92	9.97	9.98	9.99	
4	0.33	1.40	2.81	4.23	5.36	6.19	6.95	7.61	8.06	8.37	8.66	9.04	9.45	9.68	9.81	9.88	9.95	9.98	9.99	
5	0.29	1.24	2.54	3.85	4.88	5.73	6.53	7.21	7.69	8.02	8.32	8.80	9.31	9.60	9.77	9.87	9.94	9.97	9.99	
6	0.24	1.10	2.30	3.51	4.51	5.36	6.13	6.79	7.27	7.61	7.95	8.49	9.09	9.46	9.70	9.82	9.92	9.97	9.99	
7	0.23	1.02	2.08	3.14	4.08	4.91	5.70	6.42	6.93	7.29	7.64	8.25	8.93	9.34	9.60	9.76	9.89	9.95	9.99	
8	0.20	0.92	1.90	2.88	3.74	4.48	5.27	6.03	6.54	6.90	7.29	7.96	8.72	9.22	9.55	9.74	9.88	9.95	9.99	
9	0.20	0.86	1.72	2.60	3.38	4.09	4.85	5.59	6.09	6.48	6.90	7.66	8.54	9.09	9.46	9.70	9.86	9.94	9.99	
10	0.19	0.77	1.53	2.34	3.09	3.77	4.51	5.24	5.74	6.12	6.58	7.40	8.32	8.93	9.34	9.61	9.83	9.93	9.99	
11	0.17	0.70	1.38	2.11	2.81	3.42	4.13	4.89	5.40	5.82	6.32	7.18	8.15	8.77	9.22	9.51	9.77	9.91	9.98	
12	0.15	0.64	1.29	1.99	2.65	3.25	3.92	4.63	5.15	5.56	6.06	6.95	7.95	8.63	9.13	9.43	9.72	9.89	9.97	
13	0.14	0.58	1.17	1.83	2.48	3.08	3.72	4.43	4.97	5.38	5.86	6.77	7.84	8.55	9.01	9.34	9.67	9.86	9.96	
14	0.11	0.51	1.07	1.75	2.39	2.96	3.61	4.36	4.92	5.32	5.77	6.62	7.64	8.36	8.84	9.20	9.58	9.82	9.95	
15	0.10	0.46	0.99	1.64	2.25	2.83	3.46	4.21	4.78	5.18	5.58	6.40	7.47	8.20	8.70	9.12	9.53	9.79	9.95	
16	0.09	0.38	0.86	1.42	1.98	2.56	3.20	3.93	4.50	4.87	5.23	6.08	7.24	8.03	8.55	9.05	9.50	9.76	9.94	
17	0.06	0.31	0.76	1.28	1.77	2.31	2.99	3.74	4.28	4.65	5.01	5.85	7.03	7.84	8.39	9.00	9.52	9.79	9.96	
18	0.04	0.24	0.63	1.10	1.54	2.08	2.70	3.36	3.89	4.26	4.60	5.47	6.74	7.63	8.27	8.95	9.49	9.77	9.96	
19	0.05	0.26	0.60	0.99	1.38	1.89	2.49	3.15	3.67	4.06	4.41	5.35	6.68	7.60	8.29	9.01	9.57	9.81	9.97	
20	0.05	0.25	0.59	0.96	1.31	1.73	2.31	2.96	3.45	3.86	4.23	5.15	6.51	7.51	8.25	8.99	9.57	9.80	9.95	
21	0.05	0.29	0.64	1.02	1.40	1.79	2.34	2.95	3.40	3.79	4.16	5.08	6.39	7.40	8.17	8.92	9.52	9.79	9.96	
22	0.04	0.23	0.55	0.92	1.31	1.69	2.21	2.81	3.26	3.66	4.04	4.99	6.35	7.39	8.18	8.89	9.45	9.74	9.95	
23	0.05	0.28	0.61	0.95	1.29	1.67	2.20	2.81	3.24	3.69	4.16	5.13	6.44	7.47	8.24	8.90	9.45	9.76	9.95	
24	0.05	0.25	0.55	0.91	1.29	1.65	2.14	2.73	3.14	3.54	4.01	5.01	6.32	7.37	8.15	8.83	9.41	9.75	9.96	
25	0.05	0.24	0.50	0.80	1.18	1.58	2.05	2.56	2.90	3.28	3.81	4.92	6.28	7.31	8.12	8.80	9.39	9.77	9.98	
26	0.06	0.22	0.49	0.81	1.18	1.57	2.05	2.59	2.96	3.35	3.87	4.95	6.32	7.41	8.22	8.89	9.48	9.80	9.96	
27	0.06	0.24	0.49	0.77	1.13	1.55	2.02	2.53	2.85	3.21	3.74	4.80	6.20	7.33	8.17	8.92	9.56	9.85	9.98	
28	0.05	0.18	0.40	0.71	1.13	1.50	1.87	2.40	2.79	3.07	3.48	4.56	6.00	7.10	7.95	8.79	9.48	9.81	9.98	
29	0.04	0.20	0.47	0.77	1.15	1.48	1.79	2.30	2.75	3.08	3.47	4.40	5.70	6.78	7.68	8.64	9.40	9.76	9.96	
30	0.03	0.16	0.44	0.78	1.14	1.43	1.70	2.27	2.81	3.15	3.48	4.29	5.50	6.57	7.46	8.43	9.27	9.67	9.92	
Years																				

= 1st Decile	= 6th Decile
= 2nd Decile	= 7th Decile
= 3rd Decile	= 8th Decile
= 4th Decile	= 9th Decile
= 5th Decile	= 10th Decile

Figure 6.1 Global Multiple Sclerosis Severity Scores (MSSS) generated from 9892 European patients. The MSSS for an individual patient is ascertained by finding the column corresponding to the patient's Expanded Disability Status Scale (EDSS) and the row corresponding to the number of years since the onset of multiple sclerosis. Deciles are colour coded to show the pattern of disease progression at different disease durations. Adapted from Roxburgh *et al* (2005a).

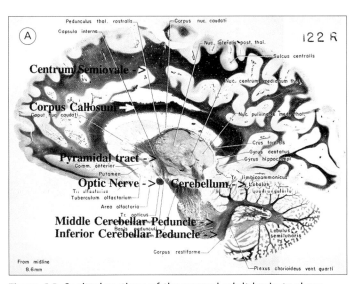

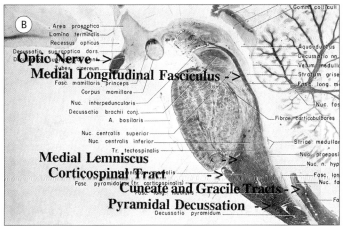

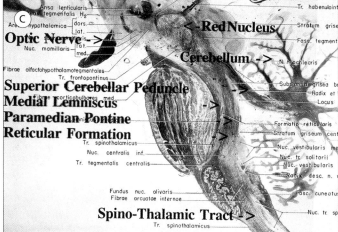

Figure 6.2 Sagittal sections of the normal adult brain to show heavily myelinated areas and pathways commonly affected in multiple sclerosis. (A) 0.6 mm from the midline. (B) 3.4 mm from the midline. (C) 13 mm from the midline. From Singer and Yakovlev (1954) with permission.

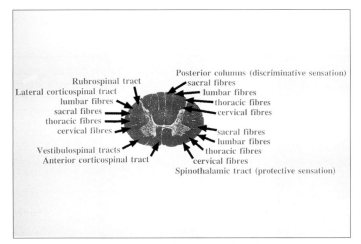

Figure 6.3 Transverse section of the cervical (C5) cord to show heavily myelinated fibre tracts involved in multiple sclerosis. From Tilney and Riley (1938) with permission.

SYMPTOMS AND SIGNS IN THE COURSE OF THE DISEASE

Estimates for the incidence of individual symptoms and signs in the course of multiple sclerosis can only be approximate. Figures obtained from hospital or population series must obviously depend on the duration of disease, which will vary widely between individuals. A further difficulty arises from the remitting nature of multiple sclerosis because important signs may not be registered at the time of examination. Although generally present in the population under scrutiny, their occurrence must be extracted from clinical records that are usually incomplete and hence fallible. Retrospective studies of pathologically confirmed cases, whilst theoretically more reliable, are invalidated by small numbers and the lack of complete information. The evolution and cataloguing of symptoms present in the final years of people severely disabled by multiple sclerosis are seldom well documented.

Despite these obstacles the results in three series (S. Poser *et al* 1979b; Shepherd 1979; Shibasaki *et al* 1981), where comparable, are consistent. The mean time from onset to examination ranged from 8 to 14 years. Weakness, with appropriate reflex changes, was present in approximately 80%. Sensory changes, including paraesthesiae, were noted in a similar proportion. Signs of cerebellar disease, sometimes linked with those of brainstem involvement, were slightly less frequent. Shepherd (1979) did not mention optic atrophy which was found in 44% and 70% in the other two series. Sphincter disturbance was present or had occurred in 56–74%. Signs of cerebral disease, mainly mental disorder, were present in some 30%. The results of Bauer and Hanefeld (1993) are generally in agreement with these other studies but motor and sensory symptoms are given separately for upper and lower limbs. The frequency of individual symptoms and signs, and the assumed sites of involvement, at onset and during the course of the disease, in a large population-based series of cases (from southeast Wales) are shown in Tables 6.7–6.9 (adapted from Swingler and Compston 1992).

It has become apparent that symptomatology, including complaints at onset, may vary between geographical regions. Epidemiological and descriptive clinical studies have noted that demyelinating disease often has a specifically different phenotype in non-Caucasian populations. The most remarkable difference is in the greater frequency of optico-spinal disease in African and Oriental countries. Clearly, this distinction hinges on disease definitions and the nuances of clinical classifications. The clinical boundaries between Devic's disease, neuromyelitis

Table 6.7 Frequency of symptoms in 301 prevalent patients in South Glamorgan who were interviewed (%)

Symptom	Ever?	At onset?	At prevalence?
Weakness	269 (89)	66 (22)	241 (80)
Sensory symptoms	263 (87)	103 (34)	219 (73)
Ataxia	248 (82)	32 (11)	218 (72)
Bladder symptoms	213 (71)	3 (1.0)	188 (62)
Fatigue	171 (57)	5 (2)	144 (48)
Cramps	156 (52)	2 (0.6)	133 (44)
Diplopia	155 (51)	25 (8)	77 (26)
Visual symptoms	148 (49)	38 (13)	98 (33)
Bowel symptoms	126 (44)	0 (0)	112 (37)
Dysarthria	110 (37)	2 (0.6)	74 (25)
Vertigo	107 (36)	13 (4.3)	57 (19)
Facial pain	106 (35)	5 (2)	42 (14)
Poor memory	96 (32)	1 (0.3)	81 (27)
Headache	90 (30)	6 (2)	51 (17)
Mental symptoms	68 (23)	1 (0.3)	49 (16)
Deafness	51 (17)	2 (0.6)	38 (13)
Facial weakness	48 (16)	4 (1)	15 (5)
Dysphagia	40 (13)	1 (0.3)	29 (10)
Sores	36 (12)	0 (0)	21 (7)
Blackout	32 (11)	2 (0.6)	12 (4)
Ageusia	17 (6)	1 (0.3)	5 (2)
Other	31 (10)	3 (1)	24 (8)

Kindly prepared by Dr Robert Swingler.

Table 6.8 Summary of the findings on clinical examination of 301 prevalent patients with multiple sclerosis in South Glamorgan

Sign	Number (%)
Visual function:	
impaired acuity	218 (72.4)
impaired colour vision	180 (59.8)
field defect	78 (25.9)
disc pallor	125 (41.5)
normal	24 (8.0)
Brainstem function:	
nystagmus	145 (48.2)
eye movement disorder	72 (23.9)
facial weakness	27 (9.0)
dysarthria	64 (21.3)
dysphagia	17 (5.6)
other	39 (13.0)
normal	135 (44.9)
Tone and power:	
increased tone	170 (56.5)
monoparesis	20 (6.6)
hemiparesis	13 (4.3)
para- and monoparesis	45 (14.9)
quadriparesis	78 (25.9)
normal power	78 (25.9)
Sensation:	
impaired spinothalamic	148 (49.2)
impaired vibration	135 (61.5)
impaired joint position	185 (38.5)
impaired two point discrimination	116 (42.2)
normal	65 (21.6)
Cerebellar function:	
upper limb ataxia	141 (46.8)
lower limb ataxia	76 (25.2)
combined ataxia	52 (17.3)
normal	109 (36.2)
Tendon reflexes:	
clonus	48 (16.0)
hyperreflexia	178 (59.1)
hyporeflexia	42 (14.0)
normal	42 (14.0)
Cutaneous reflexes:	
absent abdominal	229 (76.1)
unilateral absence	5 (1.7)
upper or lower absence	2 (0.7)
extensor plantar	209 (69.4)
equivocal plantar	38 (12.6)
normal	26 (8.6)
Sphincteric function:	
urinary hesitancy, urgency	116 (38.5)
urinary incontinence	46 (15.3)
bowel dysfunction	23 (7.6)
normal	114 (37.9)
Cerebral involvement:	
mood	80 (26.9)
intellect	40 (13.3)
seizures	12 (4.0)
normal	180 (59.8)

Kindly prepared by Dr Robert Swingler.

Table 6.9 Site of lesions in 301 prevalent patients with multiple sclerosis in South Glamorgan

Sign*	Number (%)
Spinal cord	223 (74)
Visual pathways	277 (92)
Brainstem/cerebellum	166 (55)
Cortex	121 (40)

Kindly prepared by Dr Robert Swingler.
*Spinal cord abnormality is assumed if there is weakness, sensory disturbance in a limb distribution or an extensor plantar response. An abnormality of visual pathways is defined as acuity of 6/9 or worse with correction of refractive error or impaired colour vision or optic atrophy or a field defect. A brainstem/cerebellar disorder is defined as nystagmus, disturbance or extraocular movement, dysphagia or dysarthria. Cortical abnormality includes mood disturbance or intellectual impairment.

optica and optico-spinal multiple sclerosis are indistinct although – as described – clinical symptoms in Devic's disease are restricted to optic nerves and spinal cord. Clinical criteria for diagnosing optico-spinal multiple sclerosis are: main symptoms related to optic nerves and spinal cord; neither cerebellar nor cerebral symptoms and few or absent brainstem signs; and ≥2 neurological episodes. Other distinguishing features of optico-spinal multiple sclerosis, as compared to the Western (or conventional) type of multiple sclerosis, are its higher female to male ratio, older age at onset of the disease, higher frequency of relapses, more rapidly accumulating disability, smaller number of lesions on brain MRI, long lesions extending over many vertebral segments on spinal cord imaging, pleocytosis and absence of oligoclonal bands in the cerebrospinal fluid, and absence of association with the HLA DR15 allele (see Chapter 5).

If Devic's disease (monophasic or relapsing neuromyelitis optica: throughout, we use these terms interchangeably but generally preferring the eponymous 'Devic' to the anatomically descriptive 'neuromyelitis optica') and other relapsing optic nerve and spinal cord syndromes are lumped under the general heading of optico-spinal disease, and compared with relapsing–remitting multiple sclerosis, their geographical distributions are rather striking. Once expertise in clinical neurology became available locally, it emerged that demyelinating disease in Africa, Asia, the Orient and Aboriginal populations is typically optico-spinal whereas (throughout most of the 20th century), relapsing–remitting multiple sclerosis matching the phenotype seen in northern Europeans has been distinctly uncommon. Furthermore, the cerebellar system was almost invariably spared from involvement even in those cases representing an intermediate phenotype (Nakashima *et al* 1999). Osuntokun (1973) first applied sound epidemiological principles to the study of demyelinating disease in Nigeria finding two possible cases of multiple sclerosis, 12 with acute disseminated encephalomyelitis, 95 with Devic's disease and a further 33 either with acute bilateral optic neuritis or transverse myelitis. Thus, 90% of all patients had optico-spinal disease. Each and every study, large and small, from the African continent reinforced this point (Ames and Louw 1977; Cosnett 1973; 1981a; Dean *et al* 1994; Kioy 2001; Modi *et al* 2001; M.H. Silber *et al* 1990; J. Wagner 1956).

Laying aside rigid definitions and looking at the clinical details of the cases described, the high frequency of optico-spinal disease is again apparent in India (Chopra *et al* 1980; S. Jain and Maheshwari 1985; Mathew *et al* 1971; Singhal 1985), Malaysia (C-T. Tan 1988), Korea (Kurtzke *et al* 1968b), China (Arnason *et al* 1982; Tsai *et al* 2004) and Hong Kong (Y.L. Yu *et al* 1989).

More recent series substantiate this observation. A joint study from seven regions identified 263 patients with multiple sclerosis, meeting the Poser criteria, from Hong Kong, Malaysia, Singapore, Korea, Taiwan, India and Thailand: 40% had optico-spinal and 60% Western relapsing–remitting multiple sclerosis and in both groups there were high frequencies of acute cord syndromes with long magnetic resonance (MR) lesions (3.8 ± 2.5 in recurrent optico-spinal cases and 2.9 ± 2.1 segments in Western cases, respectively) and a low rate of oligoclonal banding by comparison with Western series (Chong *et al* 2002). In a series from Oman (Tharakan *et al* 2005), ten of 30 patients had optico-spinal multiple sclerosis and without emergence of the anatomically more distributed phenotype characteristic of multiple sclerosis in Europeans. Our take on cases recently described as 'a central demyelinating disease with atypical features' from Lucknow, India, is that they also fit this category (Pradhan and Mishra 2004). However, the excess of optico-spinal multiple sclerosis is not seen in Iraq (Al-Araji and Mohammed 2005).

The story of Devic's disease and the optico-spinal Asian and Western phenotypes multiple sclerosis has been charted meticulously and over many years in Japan. Again, allowing for a broader definition of Devic's disease than was often adopted at the time, the story is clear. Between 1890 and 1952 there were 124 cases of neuromyelitis optica (72%) and 48 with multiple sclerosis (28%). These ratios have since narrowed but the significant excess of optico-spinal disease is retained (Kuroiwa *et al* 1975; Okinaka *et al* 1958; Shibasaki *et al* 1981) by comparison with northern European populations studied over the same period (Shibasaki *et al* 1981). Kuroiwa *et al* (1982) compared the onset symptoms in 488 cases of multiple sclerosis from six Asian countries with those of 177 cases from Hungary. In the former, visual loss was present at onset in 42% of cases, being bilateral in 16%. Comparable figures for Hungary were 20% and 4%. A similar disparity was found when comparing British with Japanese patients (Shibasaki *et al* 1981). In the former, onset was with monocular visual loss in 21% and with bilateral loss in 3%. In the Japanese patients, the figures were 48% and 22%, respectively. Other notable differences included the incidence of paroxysmal symptoms, girdle sensations, dysphagia, Lhermitte's symptom and transverse myelitis in the course of the disease compared with British patients (Shibasaki *et al* 1981). The point is well made by Fukazawa *et al* (2005), who showed that 21% of 158 Japanese patients with otherwise typical features of multiple sclerosis failed to meet the W.I. McDonald *et al* (2001) criteria through having long spinal cord lesions, and, of these, the majority (21/33) had optico-spinal multiple sclerosis.

Excess of the optico-spinal phenotype is true of the Aboriginal populations of North America in whom five of six (83%) patients showed an aggressive relapsing neuromyelitis optica phenotype (Mirsattari *et al* 2001). In South America, the native population has optico-spinal multiple sclerosis at a high frequency (Arruda *et al* 2001; Lana-Peixoto and Lana-Peixoto 1992; Papais-Alvarenga *et al* 2002). Populations having African and French ancestry in Martinique, also show a higher frequency of optico-spinal multiple sclerosis than occurs in northern Europeans (Cabre *et al* 2001; 2005, Merle *et al* 2005), as does the admixed African–American population (Weinstock-Guttman *et al* 1997) – 17% versus 8% in the most recent analysis (Cree *et al* 2004). This may also be a more severe disease with epidemiological evidence for earlier age at onset, more rapid progression, and more advanced physical and cognitive impairments (Buchanan *et al* 2004). We have already offered a hypothetical explanation for this difference in clinical phenotype in Chapter 5.

INDIVIDUAL SYMPTOMS AND SIGNS

The symptoms and signs listed above as common at onset are also present in virtually every advanced case of multiple sclerosis. In contrast, some features are so unusual as still to prompt single case reports. Until the advent of modern methods, diagnosis in such cases was based on clinical findings – only rarely supported by histological proof. The causal relationship may be strengthened by repeated observation but it is sometimes difficult to distinguish symptoms due to multiple sclerosis from separate conditions occurring by chance or features of associated but distinct disorders. These ambiguous manifestations include, for example, narcolepsy, spasmodic torticollis and the restless legs syndrome.

Motor system

We have already emphasized the frequency of motor disability and impaired mobility in patients with multiple sclerosis. These manifestations of the disease arise from the involvement of several systems involving descending corticobulbar, corticospinal, cerebellar and sensory pathways with added influences from fatigue and motivation (for which an anatomical explanation is less easily offered) and the day-to-day variations in performance to which demyelinated axons in the central nervous system are subject (see Chapter 13).

Limb weakness

Weakness of the limbs is a constant feature of advanced multiple sclerosis. There is little to be gained by attempting to apportion with any precision the number of limbs affected. The commonest distribution is certainly weakness of both lower limbs, usually asymmetric, followed, in decreasing order of frequency, by weakness of one lower limb and one lower and one upper limb, nearly always on the same side. Although patients with severe de-afferentation will declare the useless arm to be 'weak', actual weakness of one arm without leg weakness is uncommon and isolated weakness of both arms is distinctly rare. Thus, motor disability in the limbs is seldom solely the result of weakness but is usually compounded by cerebellar ataxia and, in the arms, by tremor and loss of postural sense.

The initial complaint may be of weakness noticed only after exertion, but gradually increasing thereafter until it is present constantly. Two well-documented cases are described by Ferrari *et al* (1988). In these patients, who had experienced what the authors call 'intermittent pyramidal claudication' for a number of years, there were no abnormal signs on examination at rest, apart from absence of the abdominal reflexes. Weakness, spasticity and extensor plantar reflexes rapidly appeared on exercise but reversed with rest. Acute transverse myelitis is fortunately uncommon in multiple sclerosis, as the prognosis for remission is poor, but lesser degrees of weakness as a result of spinal cord disease often develop rapidly, or even suddenly. Bryan Matthews wrote in earlier editions of his patient who entered the mothers' race at her child's school sports, intending to win, but never finished the 60-yard course.

The diagnostic problem posed by acute or slowly progressive hemiparesis in multiple sclerosis has been partially resolved by MRI. Eight patients are described by J. Cowan *et al* (1990), six with clinically definite multiple sclerosis and two in whom the diagnosis was thought likely, as developing hemiparesis involving the face in all but one. Only a minority, however, were examined by the authors during the hemiparetic episodes and, of these, in only one instance were there no signs of disseminated disease. The most remarkable case was a young man with very frequent brief hemiparetic attacks indistinguishable from transient cerebral ischaemia. Hemiplegia in multiple sclerosis may occur with startling suddenness. A man described to Bryan Matthews how his wife's paralysis, long thought to have been the result of a stroke, came on 'in the time to turn round and close the door.' In Matthews's experience, the commonest form of hemiparesis attributable to multiple sclerosis begins with weakness of one leg, gradually increasing and eventually involving the ipsilateral arm, but not the face. At some point in this slow evolution, the opposite leg is affected, demonstrating that the responsible lesion is evidently in the cervical spinal cord.

A characteristic of many symptoms of multiple sclerosis, most obviously weakness and visual impairment, is aggravation by heat. This is more than simply feeling worse during a heat wave and may be so marked as to cause inability to get out of a hot bath or shower (see Chapter 13: Guthrie 1951; Waxman and Geschwind 1983). This effect is not pathognomonic for multiple sclerosis (D.A. Nelson *et al* 1958) but is certainly strongly suggestive of this diagnosis.

Respiratory weakness

Kurtzke (1970) has drawn particular attention to acute respiratory weakness as a cause of death in multiple sclerosis and believes that this possibility should not be neglected in any patient experiencing sudden deterioration, particularly if the arms are weak. The warning signs are rapid shallow breathing and obvious restriction of respiratory movement. Bilateral diaphragmatic paralysis may, however, occur in the absence of significant limb weakness (Aisen *et al* 1990). Acute ventilatory failure was reported in an acute form of the disease from Japan. A midline medullary lesion was a constant finding in four such cases but the spinal cord was also involved (Yamamoto *et al* 1989). R.S. Howard *et al* (1992) found that in the majority of patients presenting with acute or subacute respiratory distress, the main cause was weakness of the respiratory and bulbar muscles. They emphasized that severe symptoms are not confined to chronic cases of multiple sclerosis but may occur during a relapse early in the disease. In a few patients there was impaired central control of respiration. Chronic respiratory weakness is common in established disease and its effects may be aggravated by the greatly increased energy cost of walking with spastic

legs (Olgiati *et al* 1986). Smeltzer *et al* (1988) found marked respiratory weakness in bedridden or chair-bound patients with upper limb weakness. Abnormal central motor conduction times in response to transcranial magnetic stimulation (sometimes in the absence of overt diaphragmatic weakness) have been described in patients with respiratory weakness attributable to multiple sclerosis (Lagueny *et al* 1998).

Motor pathways

Limb weakness is usually accompanied by the signs of an upper motor neuron lesion but these are also sometimes detected in the presence of normal muscle strength (see Figure 6.4).

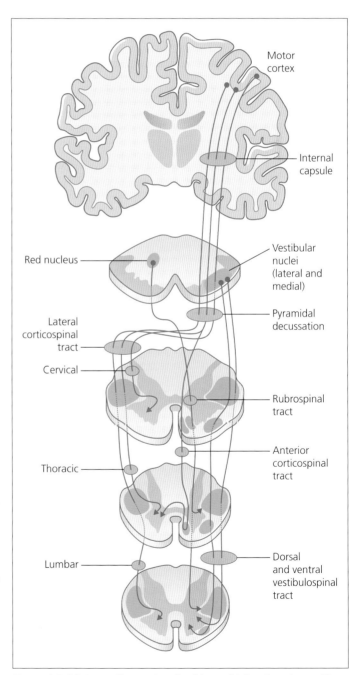

Figure 6.4 Motor pathways involved in multiple sclerosis resulting in weakness and other signs of the upper motor neuron syndrome.

Strumpell (1896) first stressed the importance of examining the abdominal reflexes. He found these to be absent in 67% in a small series, and similar figures were subsequently reported (Shepherd 1979; Shibasaki *et al* 1981). There is nothing remarkable in this but it has been claimed that loss of these reflexes 'distinguishes a high proportion of all cases and is of prime importance at an opening phase' (S.A.K. Wilson 1940). If it were true that the reflexes are frequently lost in multiple sclerosis in the absence of other traditional signs of pyramidal disease, early diagnosis might well be facilitated. There appears to have been no serious study of this claim and the importance still sometimes attached to these reflexes in multiple sclerosis may be regarded as exaggerated. In the form of the disease that begins with slowly progressive spastic weakness of one lower limb, an extensor plantar reflex is also often found on the other side, despite strenuous denial of any relevant symptoms (F.R. Ferguson and Liversedge 1959).

Asymmetry of the tendon reflexes in the upper limbs often affords a useful indication of abnormality. In the lower limbs, tendon reflexes may become clonic, not only on conventional examination but spontaneously – ankle clonus on putting the foot to the ground being the most usual form. In extreme examples, spontaneous patellar clonus may be continuous for prolonged periods, even when posture is not stretching the quadriceps muscles, as when lying flat in bed.

Spasticity

Spasticity, defined as an inappropriate increase in velocity-dependent tonic stretch reflexes, is associated with sprouting of descending motor pathways to form new synaptic connections with spinal neurons, and with denervation hypersensitivity (Figure 6.5). Together, these physiological and structural changes amplify the reactivity of motor segments to sensory input (R.R. Young and Delwade 1981a; 1981b). Spasticity forms only one component of the upper motor neuron syndrome, since damage to descending motor pathways also results in slowness of movement and weakness, but it often dominates the clinical picture. In practice, the concept of spasticity has extended far beyond the resistance to passive movement by which it is usually estimated and includes a complex disorder of voluntary movement and physical changes in muscle and tendons. This, rather than weakness, no doubt accounts for much disability resulting from the upper motor neuron lesion in

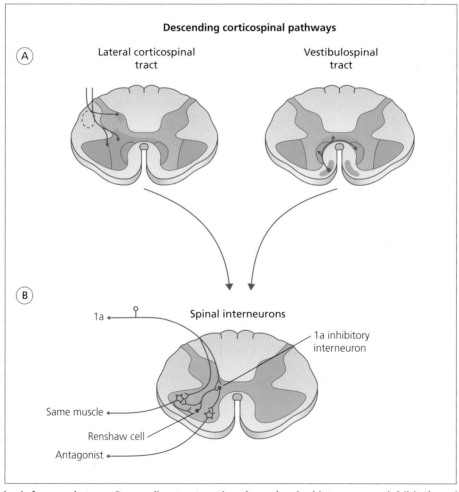

Figure 6.5 Anatomical basis for muscle tone. Descending tracts acting through spinal interneurons inhibit the spinal reflex subserving muscle tone mediated by muscle spindles, 1a afferents and α-motor neurons. The arrangement of (Renshaw cell) interneurons achieves synchronous facilitation and inhibiton of the agonist and antagonist. (A) Influences of descending pathways. (B) Spinal interneurons. The inhibitory Renshaw cell is directly excited by collateral branches of motor neurons and disinhibits antagonist motor neurons by inhibiting 1a interneurons. Adapted from Kandel and Schwartz (1985).

multiple sclerosis, particularly that affecting the lower limbs. Nevertheless, increased tone is an important factor, sometimes resulting in extreme resistance to passive flexion of the knees. Tone is often increased in the upper limb but the flexed spastic arm posture of hemiplegia, typical of stroke, is very uncommon in multiple sclerosis.

In the progressive stage of the disease, increased extensor tone may be exaggerated, manifesting as extensor spasms. These are particularly liable to occur in bed at night or on waking in the morning. They may also be so severe as to eject the patient from a wheelchair. The legs are held rigidly extended, usually for several minutes. These spasms are inconvenient but rarely disabling and seldom painful. The mechanisms of the changes in muscle tone in multiple sclerosis have been reviewed by P. Brown (1994). He points out that normal tone arises from a balance between inhibitory effects on local stretch reflexes (mediated by the dorsal reticulo-spinal tract) and facilitatory effects on extensor tone (mediated by the medial reticulo-spinal and to a lesser extent the vestibulo-spinal tracts). Early in the progressive phase of the disease, when extensor tone and spasms predominate, lesions in the lateral funiculi diminish the inhibitory effects of the dorsal reticulo-spinal tract leading to increased facilitation of the stretch reflex by the medial reticulo-spinal and vestibulo-spinal tract. Later, as loss of the inhibitory influences of the dorsal reticulo-spinal, vestibulo-spinal and medial reticulo-spinal tracts on flexor reflexes occurs, flexor spasms may become prominent. Eventually, when flexor tone dominates, there is a tendency to fall without warning. With increasing disability, the distressing condition of paraplegia in flexion is threatened. In contrast to sudden extension, flexor spasms are frequently painful. Adoption of the flexed posture increases in frequency and becomes permanent, reinforced by contractures in the ilio-psoas and hamstring muscles. It may no longer be possible to sit in a wheelchair. Adductor spasm usually develops during the phase of increased extensor tone but persists into flexion and is an important cause of morbidity. Care of sphincter function is rendered particularly difficult. Flexor spasm increases with persistent stimulation of the reflex by pressure sores or bladder infections, both of which are more likely in these patients. It is not known what proportion of patients with clinically definite multiple sclerosis enter this helpless bedridden state.

In rare instances where complete paraplegia has developed acutely or rapidly, tone in the legs may initially be flaccid, but with retained tendon reflexes and uninterpretable plantar responses, leading to diagnostic confusion. Increased tone develops later, but sometimes only after a delay of some months. (We describe in more detail the pharmacological aspects of treatment for spasticity in Chapter 17.)

Depression of tendon reflexes

Tendon reflexes may be diminished or even lost in multiple sclerosis. This is not surprising given the histological evidence for involvement of the dorsal root entry zone (Garcin *et al* 1962) and the grey matter of the spinal cord. Bonduelle *et al* (1964) noted an absence, sometimes temporary, of one or more tendon reflexes in 13% of patients with multiple sclerosis. Uldry and Regli (1992) described selective absence of tendon reflexes in the upper limb in patients with pain of root distribution.

Muscle wasting: lower motor neuron lesions

Wasting of muscles occurs as a late manifestation of multiple sclerosis, especially in the hands, and in parts subject to pressure palsies as a result of immobility, or when there is interruption of the intraspinal portion of the reflex arc by neighbouring demyelination. At an earlier stage, hand muscle wasting is less common but can be markedly asymmetrical. M. Fisher *et al* (1985) found atrophy of hand muscles in nine of 150 patients. Wasting was unilateral in six and judged to be severe in two patients. Electrophysiological investigation showed no evidence for the denervation that would have occurred with loss of anterior horn cells. In complete contrast, Sheffner *et al* (1992) found electromyographic evidence for denervation in 12 of 13 patients with asymmetrical wasting of hand muscles. In only three could this be attributed to incidental peripheral nerve damage. These two reports are incompatible but it seems unlikely that unilateral severe wasting could result from any cause other than denervation. C. Davison *et al* (1934) reported wasting of the pectoral, glutei, deltoid, sternomastoid and masseter muscles. Motor neuron disease may occasionally develop in someone already afflicted with multiple sclerosis (Confavreux *et al* 1993; Hader *et al* 1986).

Multiple sclerosis and peripheral neuropathy

Since neither is a rare condition, it is not surprising that cases of peripheral neuropathy and multiple sclerosis occasionally co-exist. The literature contains a number of clinical and pathological reports (Dinkler 1904; J. Drulovic *et al* 1998; Lassmann *et al* 1981a; Quan *et al* 2005). Others have described laboratory features of peripheral nerve damage in patients with multiple sclerosis (see Chapter 12). Conversely, there is a high frequency of MRI abnormalities affecting the cerebrum in patients with chronic inflammatory polyneuropathy despite the lack of evidence for disease affecting the central nervous system (Figure 6.6: Mendell *et al* 1987). P.K. Thomas *et al* (1987) described six patients with chronic demyelinating polyneuropathy and unequivocal evidence for multifocal lesions, producing symptoms in the central nervous system, that met the criteria for clinically definite multiple sclerosis. Conditions known to affect central and peripheral myelin were specifically excluded. It seems likely that (at least in these patients) the inflammatory response targeted an antigen shared between central and peripheral myelin. The possibility that these represent the occurrence by chance of two independent conditions affecting the same individual is suggested by the findings of Frasson *et al* (1997) who provided a genetic explanation (duplication of the CMT1a sac junction fragment) for the demyelinating neuropathy affecting two patients with otherwise typical multiple sclerosis.

Fatigue

Excessive fatigue is a common complaint in multiple sclerosis. Although physical disability may contribute, this is not the whole cause since fatigue may afflict those with otherwise rather mild disabilities. Fatigue is, of course, common enough even in the apparently healthy and, in neurological disease, not confined to multiple sclerosis. Parkinson's disease is notoriously tiring even when responding admirably to treatment. The

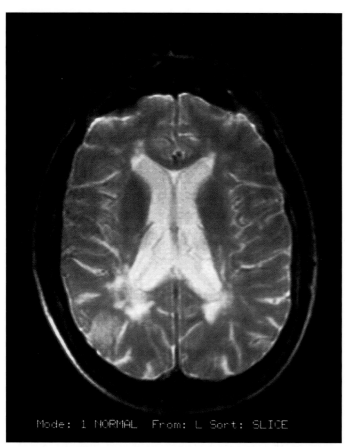

Figure 6.6 MRI showing white matter abnormalities in a patient with laboratory-supported clinically definite multiple sclerosis who also had a severe demyelinating polyneuropathy.

frequency and severity of fatigue is naturally difficult to assess. The usual complaint is of tiredness following ordinary exertion, such as light housework, though a pervasive sense of fatigue unrelated to effort, especially during relapse, is not uncommon. The symptom tends to follow a circadian pattern with most exhaustion being experienced in the early afternoon. Iriarte *et al* (2000) have proposed that fatigue is a complex symptom made up of asthenia (fatigue at rest), fatigability (fatigue with exercise) and worsening of symptoms with effort. In their uncontrolled study, 155 patients (76%) reported fatigue – a figure similar to that recorded by others (Fisk *et al* 1994; Freal *et al* 1984; Reingold 1990). Fatigue is variously rated as the worst complaint in between 14 and 40% of patients (Fisk *et al* 1994; Reingold 1990). In a controlled study (Krupp *et al* 1988), fatigue was present in 28/33 patients but also in 17/32 normal controls. It was not related to depression or degree of disability and in ten patients was claimed to be the first symptom, although retrospective assessment must present insuperable difficulties with accuracy of recall. The adverse effect of heat is the only factor that distinguishes pathological fatigue from the commonplace experiences of normal subjects.

Djaldetti *et al* (1996) made a valiant attempt to quantify fatigue in patients with multiple sclerosis. Deriving a fatigue index based on the ratio of muscle strength decay over time to maximal voluntary contraction, they showed more fatigue in patients with multiple sclerosis having pyramidal tract involvement, especially if implicated in a current relapse, than controls

or a small group of patients with chronic fatigue syndrome. This study emphasizes fatigue as a physical, not a psychological, symptom in multiple sclerosis – as most patients and many physicians would insist. More sophisticated is the physiological analysis of Sheean *et al* (1997) who showed that tiring of sustained muscular effort in healthy individuals is peripheral in origin, whereas patients with fatigue as a manifestation of multiple sclerosis show central failure. This cannot be explained by frequency-dependent conduction block in demyelinated pathways and the authors prefer the explanation that, despite sustained effort, fatigue reflects impaired primary motor cortex drive. The pathophysiology of fatigue is discussed in Chapter 13.

Several studies have explored the relationship between various MRI features and fatigue. The number of patients studied has been small and the results are conflicting (Bakshi *et al* 1999; Colombo *et al* 2000; Mainero *et al* 1999). A recent functional MRI study of 14 multiple sclerosis patients with fatigue, and 14 without, compared with 15 sex- and age-matched controls revealed a distinct activation pattern for cortical and subcortical structures in the patients with fatigue. How such changes might engender the sense of fatigue is unclear (Filippi *et al* 2002a). For the physician, the fact that physiological changes correlate with fatigue should not obscure the possibility that, in the individual patient, there may also be a contribution from depression which is predictive of fatigue (Kroencke *et al* 2000).

The relationship of the so-called chronic fatigue syndrome to multiple sclerosis is somewhat controversial. Since the complaint of fatigue may (understandably) be generalized from the more specific symptom of regional muscle weakness, we are of course always alert to the possibility that a patient in whom chronic fatigue syndrome has been proposed or diagnosed (under various rubrics, including myalgic encephalomyelitis) may have an organic neurological disease, including multiple sclerosis. One of us (DASC) recently made the diagnosis of multiple sclerosis in a woman whose international sporting career had been curtailed, and the next 15 years dominated, by fatigue, long attributed to chronic fatigue syndrome. Fifteen years after onset with an episode of transient hemiparesis, she had few symptoms, other than constipation, or signs, and the diagnosis was clinched by laboratory abnormalities.

Adventitious movements

Apart from tremor and reflex spasms, involuntary movements are an uncommon feature of multiple sclerosis. Fog and Linnemann (1970) described tremor at rest, apparently of Parkinsonian type, in two patients with remission in one instance. Parkinson's disease developing some years after the onset of multiple sclerosis has been reported. Folgar *et al* (2003) reviewed 12 cases, including one of their own. Eight were interpreted as being secondary to multiple sclerosis on the basis of 'conclusive imaging evidence' or an unequivocal response to corticosteroids. Facial masking, seborrhoea and hypokinesia, without tremor or rigidity, occurring in multiple sclerosis is reported to have remitted with intravenous corticosteroid treatment (Vieregge *et al* 1992). Their second case undoubtedly had severe Parkinson's disease but the diagnosis of multiple sclerosis is more doubtful.

Spasmodic torticollis associated with multiple sclerosis was described by Guillain and Bize (1933) and there have been a number of subsequent reports (Klostermann *et al* 1993; Matthews et al 1985; Plant et al 1989). Plant et al (1989) attributed the torticollis in their case to a midbrain lesion shown by MRI. Both the torticollis and the lesion remitted. Monoballism (Thiery and de Reuck 1974), hemiballism (Mouren et al 1966; Riley and Lang 1988) and bilateral ballism (Masucci et al 1989) have all been convincingly attributed to multiple sclerosis in single case reports. Moore et al (1996) describe two siblings with clinically definite multiple sclerosis who each had extensive orofacial, trunk and limb dystonia and blepharospasm in one of the pair. Cervical dystonia is described as the presenting feature of multiple sclerosis (Rüegg et al 2004). Athetosis (Bachman et al 1976) and chorea (Chi-Chen et al 1988; Minagar et al 2002) have also been described, although not always with confirmatory evidence for the diagnosis of multiple sclerosis. The remitting cases reported by Sarkari (1968) may well have had systemic lupus erythematosus. In most of these reports, the movements are extremely persistent. Paroxysmal kinesigenic choreoathetosis has been reported as a presenting symptom in a single case (de Seze et al 2000a). One week after developing a left hemiparesis, the patient developed what might have been designated paroxysmal involuntary movements of the previously affected arm. These were induced by movement and consisted of a tense sensation followed by choreoathetoid movements of the hand lasting 30–60 seconds: MRI showed an extensive lesion in the contralateral posterior internal globus pallidus, posterior internal capsule and anterolateral part of the thalamus, with more distributed brain lesions. Treatment with intravenous methylprednisolone was successful and carbamazepine was not tried; the diagnosis of multiple sclerosis was confirmed by subsequent new episodes.

Myoclonus of different types is described in multiple sclerosis (C.R. Smith and Scheinberg 1990), including intention myoclonus (Hassler et al 1975) and propriospinal myoclonus (Kapoor et al 1992) – the latter associated with a spinal lesion demonstrated by MRI. Palatal myoclonus has been reported in a single case of clinically definite disease (Revol et al 1990), the diagnosis in earlier reports being far less certain. Nocturnal myoclonus affecting the legs is unduly common in multiple sclerosis and may disturb sleep (Ferini-Strambi et al 1994). Simple phonic tic (throat clearing sounds), focal dystonia, blepharoclonus and writer's cramp have been described in single case reports (Coleman et al 1988; Lana-Peixoto et al 2002; Ruegg et al 2004).

The literature on movement disorders in multiple sclerosis is usefully summarized by Tranchant et al (1995), who describe 14 new cases of whom nine had dystonia, three Parkinsonism and two myoclonus, in the context of 135 cases collated from other publications. The authors conclude that paroxysmal dystonias (or tonic spasms), ballism or chorea and palatal myoclonus can be manifestations of multiple sclerosis (and we would add spasmodic torticollis), whereas Parkinsonism, dystonia and other types of myoclonus are coincidental. Overall, our position is that, apart from tremor, involuntary movements are exceedingly rare in multiple sclerosis and not infrequently the result of co-morbidity.

Involvement of the cerebellum and brainstem

Many clinical manifestations of multiple sclerosis arise from demyelination of pathways which converge to travel through the midbrain, pons, medulla and cerebellum. Given the concentration of fibre tracts in this part of the brain and their sympto-matic eloquence, demyelination of structures in the posterior fossa tends to present early and to feature prominently in clinical manifestations of the disease.

Cerebellar symptoms and signs

Symptoms of cerebellar disease are common in multiple sclerosis (Figure 6.7) but in many series the difficulty of distinguishing these manifestations (or their contribution to disordered function) from weakness, spasticity, sensory loss and vertigo, is acknowledged. These difficulties are reflected in clinical practice. To what extent cerebellar ataxia contributes to the characteristic spastic-ataxic gait with stiff legs and feet placed too far apart is necessarily uncertain. Conventional tests of co-ordination are poorly performed by weak or spastic limbs. Kurtzke (1970) thought that the frequency of cerebellar deficit was second only to that of corticospinal involvement, being present in 84% of male patients in a hospital series.

Cerebellar signs at the onset of the disease are distinctly uncommon, although not at the time of first examination, by which stage much else will have happened in the central nervous system of affected individuals, McAlpine et al (1972) found this abnormality in 37% of the series. A patient presenting with a pure cerebellar syndrome is unlikely to have multiple sclerosis, although this can occur (in relative or complete isolation) as one of the progressive syndromes, with paraclinical evidence for more widespread involvement. An alternative diagnosis should be sought and these patients will often turn out to have one or other of the hereditary spino-cerebellar degenerations (see Chapter 8). The early appearance of cerebellar ataxia indicates a poor prognosis and cerebellar signs frequently persist, without significant remission. Impaired control of axial posture is seldom severe enough to be obvious when sitting but certainly contributes to the frequent complaint of poor balance.

Tremor, even for the non-neurologist, is perceived as one of the hallmarks of multiple sclerosis. Indeed, intention tremor is part of the classical triad of Charcot (see Chapter 1). Most neurologists regard this form of intention tremor as common, and the wide-amplitude proximal variant as probably the most disabling. It comes as something of a surprise therefore to find how poorly documented tremor is in multiple sclerosis. Charcot (1875) stated explicitly that rest tremor did not occur. Holmes (1922), who first described the disabling 'rubral' tremor, did not mention multiple sclerosis as one of its causes.

Alusi et al (2001a) have performed a notable service in carrying out a systematic study of tremor in multiple sclerosis, classifying the various types according to the consensus statement of the Movement Disorder Society (Deuschl et al 1998). Since much classificatory confusion has arisen in the past because of the absence of agreed definitions, it is worth quoting the definitions given by Alusi et al (2001a).

- *Rest tremor* is present in a body part that is not voluntarily activated and is completely supported against gravity (ideally resting on a couch).
- *Action tremor* includes any tremor that is produced by voluntary contraction of a muscle, including postural, isometric, kinetic and intention tremor.
- *Postural tremor* is present whilst voluntarily maintaining a position against gravity.

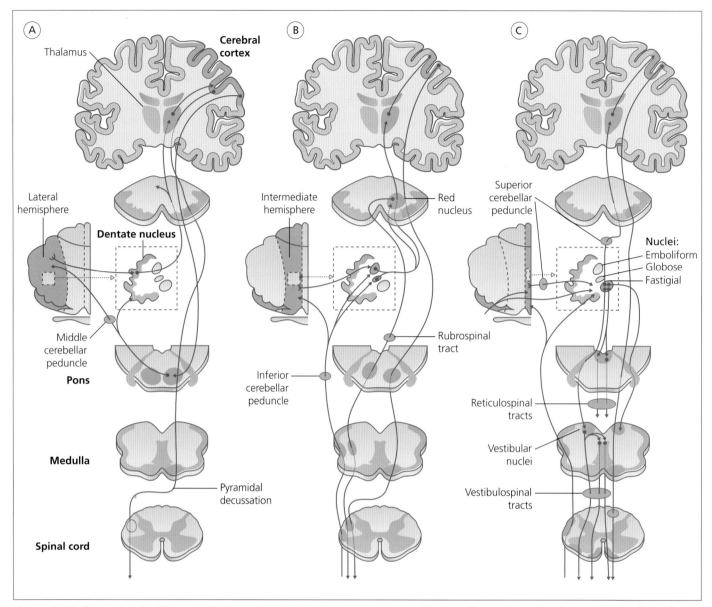

Figure 6.7 Pathways involved in co-ordination providing cerebellar guidance on the intention and success of movement in the limbs. (A) Connections with lateral components. (B) Connections with intermediate connections. (C) Connections with vermis components.

- *Kinetic tremor* occurs during any voluntary movement.
- *Isometric tremor* results from muscle contraction against a rigid stationary object.
- *Intention tremor* during target-directed movement is present when the amplitude increases during visually guided movements towards a target at the termination of movement and postural tremor produced at the beginning and end of a movement is excluded.
- *Holmes's tremor* occurs at rest and during volitional movement but with irregular presentation (in many patients, postural tremor is also present; the tremor often not as rhythmic as other tremors); slow frequency, usually less than 4.6 Hz; and when the timing of a lesion responsible for the tremor can be identified (for example a stroke), a variable delay (typically 4 weeks to 2 years) before first appearance of tremor. It has been labelled in the past under

different names including 'rubral tremor', midbrain tremor, thalamic tremor, myorythmia and Benedikt's syndrome.

Using their classification, Alusi *et al* (2001a) characterized tremor in 100 patients randomly chosen from a multiple sclerosis clinic; being hospital-based, the population characteristics are skewed towards the more severe end of the spectrum. Tremor was reported in 37 patients but was detected in 58. It affected arms (56%), legs (10%), head (9%) and trunk (7%). There were no examples of face, tongue, or jaw tremor. All patients had action tremor, either postural or kinetic (including intention). Rest tremor, Holmes's ('rubral') tremor and primary orthostatic tremor were not seen. What most neurologists refer to as rubral tremor is in fact proximal or distal tremor with a kinetic component, alone or in combination. Only 6% had isolated intention tremor of the upper limb. Twenty-seven per cent of the overall study population had tremor-related disability and this was incapacitating in 10%.

As to the mechanism of tremor in multiple sclerosis, Alusi *et al* (2001a) conclude that it depends on damage to the cerebellum and its connections rather than the red nucleus or midbrain. They acknowledge the difficulty of more precise correlations in view of the multiplicity of lesions in most patients and the scarcity of post-mortem studies on multiple sclerosis patients with documented tremor. Whatever the rubric, and wherever the lesion is placed, there are few clinical syndromes more disabling for the patient, more distressing for their carers or therapeutically more frustrating for the neurologist than the combination of proximal upper limb tremor, titubation and violent shaking of the trunk on attempted change in posture (see Figure 6.2C). Using a population based register from Olmsted County, Minnesota, Pittock *et al* (2004c) identified tremor in 25% and this was disabling in 6/200 (3%) patients.

Dysarthria is uncommon at onset of the disease, being present in 3–5% in the series reported by Shibasaki *et al* (1981). It often emerges later but is not always of cerebellar type (Hartelius *et al* 2000). The classical scanning speech is usually heard in advanced disease and lesser degrees are not distinctive. Cerebellar deficit may cause respiratory impairment. Grasso *et al* (2000) found impairment of a variety of pulmonary function measures in 27/32 patients with severe cerebellar deficit.

Eye movement disorders

The assessment of eye movements is one of the more informative aspects of clinical examination in multiple sclerosis (for a general review of these and other neuro-ophthalmological features, see E.M. Frohman *et al* 2005). Patients use a variety of words to describe visual symptoms and it may be difficult immediately to distinguish involvement of the optic nerves from disorders of eye movement. The term 'double vision' is often used rather loosely to describe a variety of unfamiliar visual sensations. If vision is clear within each eye separately then a disorder of eye movement may be inferred. Some visual symptoms which suggest misalignment of the two eyes, such as ghosting of the image, often turn out to be manifestations of optic nerve disease. Genuine involvement of the central or infranuclear pathways for control of eye movement usually manifests as double vision or defects of ocular stability (oscillopsia) and disequilibrium, making multiple sclerosis one cause of dizziness – the commonest symptom in neurology. Abnormalities evident on clinical examination in asymptomatic patients are also extremely common in multiple sclerosis. Sophisticated methods for recording eye movements reveal a great variety of subclinical abnormalities (Leigh and Zee 1999; Reulen *et al* 1983) and these may prove useful in confirming the existence of multiple lesions.

Representative figures for a complaint of diplopia at onset of multiple sclerosis are 13% in the studies of R. Müller (1949) and S. Poser (1978), 11% and 8% in the British and Japanese patients compared by Shibasaki *et al* (1981), and 22% in the United States Army series (Kurtzke (1970). In cross-sectional studies, diplopia in the course of the disease has been reported to occur in 29% (Bauer and Hanefeld 1993), 35% (Carter *et al* 1950), 39% (R. Müller 1949) and 39% of patients in several European series, compared with 35% in Japan (Shibasaki *et al* 1981).

The separate activities of the six cranial nerves which innervate the 12 ocular muscles and their brainstem nuclei are coordinated to achieve stability of the two eyes, and to allow rapid conjugate deviation to a new position. This must happen in the horizontal and vertical planes, independently and together to produce diagonal movements. Separate mechanisms are needed for vergence movements. These physiological tasks depend on the convergence of several descending supranuclear pathways onto the third, fourth and sixth cranial nerve nuclei, which are themselves interconnected and control a final common pathway for eye movements through the third, fourth and sixth cranial nerves (Figure 6.8A–D).

The sixth nerve nucleus is the main site of exit for the infranuclear pathways subserving horizontal movement. It is linked to the opposite third nerve nucleus through the medial longitudinal fasciculus. The third and fourth nerve nuclei, and their connections across the midline, subserve vertical and vergence movements. The gaze motor commands are integrated in a specialized part of the brainstem which receives the supranuclear inputs. Horizontal movements depend on the paramedian pontine reticular formation which is adjacent to the sixth nerve nucleus and vertical gaze is centred on the rostral interstitial nucleus of the medial longitudinal fasciculus located at the upper pole of the red nucleus.

Saccadic movements are generated from three frontal eye fields (Brodmann areas 6, 8 and 46) and a parietal field (area 39). They are interconnected and influence the gaze centres through crossed direct and indirect (through the basal ganglia) pathways to the superior colliculus. Saccadic movements may be anticipatory, searching, or based on memory. The parietal component seems to be especially important for visuo-spatial responses to seen or heard stimuli. Smooth pursuit movements allow constant tracking of a moving target and originate close to visual area 5 which is concerned with visual motion and connects with the occipital eye field in the inferior parietal lobe from where descending fibres reach the gaze centres by complex routes involving a double decussation in the pons and cerebellum. Saccadic movement is therefore under contralateral and smooth pursuit under ipsilateral hemisphere control. The vestibular input, which is closely related to neck proprioception, acts to keep the eyes stable, gyroscopically, whilst the head is moving and (for horizontal movement) consists of a three-neuron circuit involving the primary vestibular neuron projecting to the vestibular nuclei, from there to the sixth nerve nucleus and thence to the infranuclear pathway.

Within the gaze centres are 'burst' neurons which fire just before and during saccades and initiate movements. 'Pause' neurons fire at all other times and maintain the eyes in a stable position. They are located in the midline caudal pontine nucleus raphe interpositus. These are, in turn, controlled by the neural integrator to produce the step which achieves a new stable position. The vertical gaze centre contains separate neurons for up and down movements. Structures on opposite sides of the brainstem are intimately connected with each other and with the third and fourth nerve nuclei. Up movements depend especially on pathways that traverse the posterior commissure and down movements depend on more ventral parts of the rostral interstitial nucleus. Both are intimately connected with the interstitial

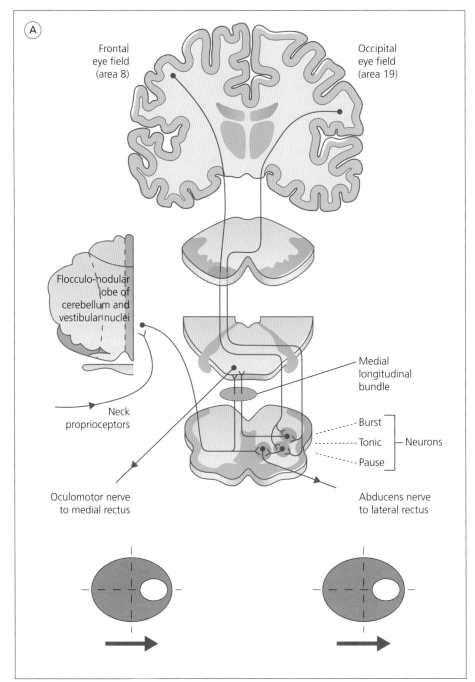

Figure 6.8 (A) Frontal, occipital and reflex pathways converge on the paramedian pontine reflex formation to inhibit existing and initiate new horizontal movements which are co-ordinated by the medial longitudinal fasciculus linking the sixth and third nerve nuclei.

nucleus of Cajal which regulates vertical gaze holding and pursuit. The separate supranuclear influences have differential effects on these neuronal pools. For example, the vestibular and cerebellar inputs selectively control the step change and help to maintain an eccentric position against visco-elastic forces.

From this account it follows that the eyes are aligned on a desired target and can move rapidly to a new position through supranuclear, internuclear, nuclear and infranuclear pathways, some of which are heavily myelinated. As expected, the delicate tonic balance on which these positions depend can easily be disrupted. Abnormal eye movements occur in patients with cerebral, midbrain, cerebellar, vestibular and high cervical cord demyelination. Further details of the mechanism of normal and abnormal ocular motor control are provided by Zee and Leigh (2002).

Double vision is commonly a transient symptom and, at the time of examination, present in a much smaller proportion. Diplopia, subsequently proving to be the onset of multiple sclerosis, is usually the result of a breakdown in the brainstem circuits on which stable fixation and conjugate gaze depend,

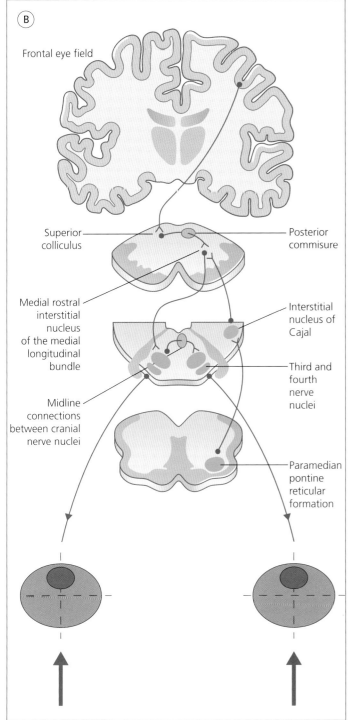

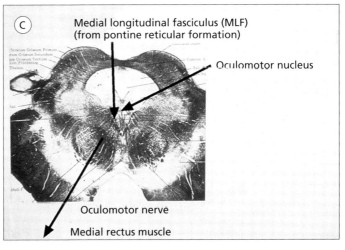

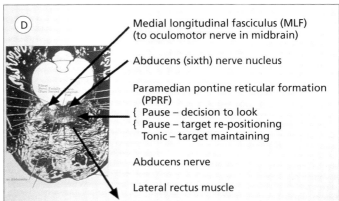

Figure 6.8, cont'd (B) Vertical movements are co-ordinated through connections between the paired third and fourth nerve nuclei; supranuclear innervation is from pathways which reciprocally connect the two interstitial rostral midbrain nuclei of the medial longitudinal bundle at the level of the superior colliculus, and receive an input from the paramedian pontine reticular formation through the interstitial nucleus of Cajal. For simplicity, only one set of pathways is shown. (C) Normal human pons to show the paramedian pontine reticular formation and its immediate connections. (D) Section through the normal human midbrain to show the oculomotor nucleus and its immediate connections. C,D from Tilney and Riley (1938) with permission.

especially internuclear ophthalmoplegia. Onset with an isolated third, fourth, or sixth nerve lesion is seen but these do seem to be rare (Barr *et al* 2000). Only six of 40 patients between the ages of 15 and 50 years presenting in this way were shown later to have multiple sclerosis (Moster *et al* 1984). A rather higher frequency of multiple sclerosis as a cause of sixth nerve palsy (11/45 patients) is reported by Peters *et al* (2002). In eight of these 11 patients it was the sole presenting feature of multiple sclerosis. An isolated fourth nerve palsy is occasionally encountered (Barnes and McDonald 1992; D.M. Jacobson *et al* 1999).

Third nerve lesions are often partial (Ksiazek *et al* 1989; A.G. Lee *et al* 2000; Uitti and Rajput 1986) and complete ptosis is very rare. The incidence of multiple sclerosis was low in the series of 1000 cases of third, fourth and sixth cranial nerve palsies reported by Rush and Younge (1981), but these were not isolated lesions and, in a very high proportion, no cause was found. It is common for ocular palsies in multiple sclerosis to be accompanied by other abnormalities of eye movement.

Uhthoff (1889) first observed the essential feature of internuclear ophthalmoplegia in which the internal rectus muscle does not act fully on conjugate lateral gaze, but does so on convergence. S.A.K. Wilson (1906) gave a fuller description of bilateral weakness of the internal rectus on conjugate gaze with nystagmus, later termed 'ataxic', limited to the abducting eye. The defect of adduction is often that of slow saccadic movement rather than weakness. Complete and incomplete, unilateral and bilateral forms are common in multiple sclerosis (Figure 6.9). They are often asymptomatic but many patients complain of double vision or oscillopsia.

Muri and Weinberg (1985) described detailed clinical methods for detecting the various elements of internuclear ophthalmoplegia. Of 100 consecutive patients with clinically definite disease, 14 had bilateral and 20 unilateral internuclear palsy. Other forms of symptomatic horizontal and vertical gaze palsy, usually partial, may be associated with internuclear ophthalmoplegia, notably the 'one-and-a-half' syndrome (Martyn and Kean 1988), in which there is gaze palsy to one side and impaired adduction to the other (Figure 6.10). Internuclear ophthalmoplegia, while characteristic of multiple sclerosis, is not pathognomonic as it is indicative of a lesion, from any cause, of the medial longitudinal fasciculus that links the third and fourth nerve nuclei. It has been described in many conditions that might be mistaken for multiple sclerosis (see also Chapter 8). Whilst most clinicians would agree that a unilateral internuclear ophthalmoplegia has causes other than demyelination of the medial longitudinal fasciculus, most probably take for granted the probability that bilateral lesions are seldom the result of conditions other than multiple sclerosis. However, this may occur in structural lesions of the brainstem – pontine glioma – and the unwary can be fooled by the bilateral lag in adduction seen in myasthenia gravis. Transient and complex eye movement disorders, including reversible bilateral internuclear ophthalmoplegia, are described in patients taking the immunosuppressant tacrolimus (FK506: M.M.Lai *et al* 2004; Oliverio *et al* 2000). Reflecting on a personal series of 410 inpatients with internuclear ophthalmoplegia seen over 33 years, Keane (2005) considered cerebrovascular disease a more likely explanation (38%) than multiple sclerosis (34%), but 87% of the vascular cases were unilateral, compared with only 27% in patients with demyelinating disease.

Many other abnormalities of eye movement occur in the context of multiple sclerosis but their accurate separation may require physiological recordings (Figure 6.11A–G). Nystagmus is a classical sign of multiple sclerosis. The commonest form is first-degree symmetrical horizontal jerking nystagmus, not resulting in oscillopsia, and not always easy to distinguish from the effects of fatigue or lack of cooperation. Acquired pendular nystagmus is more distinctive. This may be unilateral or, if bilateral, the movements either conjugate or dysconjugate and

resulting in troublesome oscillopsia (Aschoff *et al* 1974; J.J.S. Barton and Cox 1993; Gresty *et al* 1982). A form of pendular nystagmus not visible on unaided inspection can be detected on inspection of the fundus, when the optic disc is seen to be jerking rapidly from side to side over a small range. This should not be confused with latent nystagmus, the other form that may first be seen when looking at the fundus. This is only present when one eye is occluded, as by the ophthalmoscope, and is of sufficiently large amplitude to be visible without the instrument. This phenomenon has no known relation to cerebellar involvement. Vertical up-beating nystagmus is occasionally due to multiple sclerosis (A. Fisher *et al* 1983; Ohkoshi *et al* 1998), and is invariable in the presence of bilateral internuclear ophthalmoplegia. Down-beating nystagmus occurs in idiopathic or paraneoplastic cerebellar degeneration and as a manifestation of the Chiari malformation – one of the potential errors in differential diagnosis (see Chapter 8) – but not infrequently is due to multiple sclerosis. Rare forms of eye movement disorder include convergence-induced nystagmus (J.A. Sharpe *et al* 1975). Periodic alternating nystagmus (J.R. Keane 1974) is a form of spontaneous nystagmus that periodically reverses direction, usually approximately every 2 minutes. In rebound nystagmus, the movement weakens on sustained lateral gaze and there is a transient nystagmus to the opposite side when the eyes return to the primary position. The latter two forms of nystagmus are often missed because the examination is too short. Torsional down-beat nystagmus is associated with internuclear ophthalmoplegia and sixth nerve palsy (E.M. Frohman and T.C. Frohman 2003). Nystagmus often results from disease of the brainstem but symmetrical horizontal gaze nystagmus, frequently seen in multiple sclerosis, is probably of cerebellar origin. The localization of lesions responsible for the various forms of ocular movement disorder in multiple sclerosis is increasingly revealed by MRI (Barnes and McDonald 1992).

Considering all forms, nystagmus was present at the time of examination in 56% of British and 50% of Japanese patients (Shibasaki *et al* 1981). In another series (Bauer and Hanefeld 1993), nystagmus, unassociated with other clinically detectable disorders of eye movement, was found in 28–40% of patients, depending on age, duration of disease and degree of disability. The total incidence of nystagmus was, however, much higher, at 73%, in severely disabled patients.

Probably the commonest observation in patients with multiple sclerosis who have no visual complaint is the replacement of smooth pursuit movements on following the examiner's finger by jerks or saccades. This has no special localizing value but is seen with demyelination of the descending supranuclear occipital pathway (see above) and with involvement of the cerebellar influence on eye movement. It is a reliable sign that may

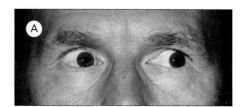
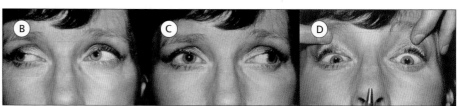

Figure 6.9 Internuclear ophthalmoplegia. (A) Unilateral, gaze to the left (abnormal). (B) Bilateral, gaze to the right (abnormal). (C) Bilateral, gaze to the left (abnormal). (D) Bilateral, convergence (normal).

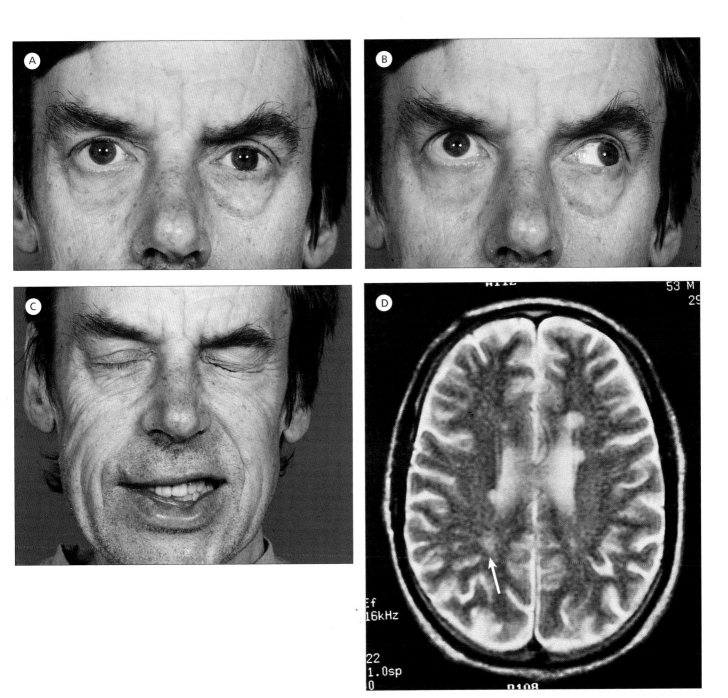

Figure 6.10 One-and-a-half syndrome. (A) Gaze to the right (absent). (B) Gaze to the left (abduction only). (C) Abnormal gaze with associated (partial) right facial palsy. (D) MRI shows the cerebral white matter abnormalities (arrow).

illustration continued on following page

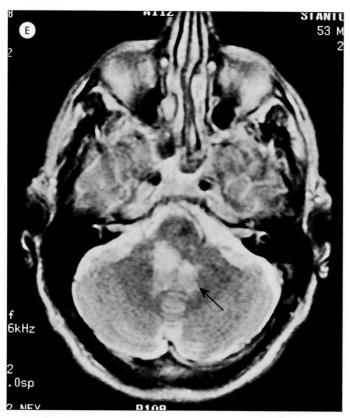

Figure 6.10, cont'd (E) Pontine lesion responsible for the eye-movement disorder (arrow).

identify a second affected site in the patient with spinal cord demyelination or a single previous episode not affecting brainstem–cerebellar connections. Other saccadic disorders include oblique saccades on attempted vertical gaze (E.M. Frohman *et al* 2001) and horizontal monocular saccadic failure (E.M. Frohman and T.C. Frohman 2003). Ocular flutter consists of bursts of horizontal saccadic oscillations without an intersaccadic interval and it is a disabling symptom in patients with multiple sclerosis (Schon *et al* 2001). Opsoclonus, which it has been suggested is the result of selective denervation of pause neurons so that saccadic bursts are constantly active, is similar in appearance and contribution to visual handicap but differs from ocular flutter in that the movements are omnidirectional. Ocular bobbing consists of an initial rapid downward eye movement followed by slow return to the neutral position and denotes cerebellar involvement. The initial deviation may also be upwards (reverse bobbing). Square wave jerks (abrupt displacement from and return to the primary position during central fixation) are seen in association with severe cerebellar deficit. Parinaud's syndrome may be the presenting feature of multiple sclerosis (W.B. Lee *et al* 2003). No doubt our readers have themselves observed variations on the theme of complex eye movement disorders in the context of multiple sclerosis. E.M. Frohman *et al* (2004) describe one such with oscillopsia due to a left-sided rostral midbrain lesion manifesting as convergent-retraction nystagmus in the right eye and divergent-retraction nystagmus in the left eye during attempted upgaze, with features of an internuclear ophthalmoplegia on looking to the right.

Brainstem lesions

Many symptoms are, of course, the result of brainstem lesions. Some are discussed under separate headings (see especially eye movements and cranial nerves) but a few deserve special mention, even though they are rare manifestations of multiple sclerosis. Plaques in the brainstem may occasionally be acutely life threatening. The locked-in syndrome with partial recovery (W.B. Matthews 1991; Seeldrayers *et al* 1987) and lateral medullary syndrome (Bonduelle and Albaranès 1962) have been described. Respiratory failure is only exceptionally the result of involvement of the respiratory centre but temporary paralysis of automatic respiration has been described in proven multiple sclerosis (Bloor *et al* 1974).

Persistent hiccough as a symptom of multiple sclerosis has been described in three patients (McFarling and Susac 1979), all of whom had signs of brainstem lesions in addition to evidence of more widespread disease. Carbamazepine proved to be an extremely successful treatment in one case, but whether hiccough can be included as a paroxysmal symptom (see below) is doubtful. In other cases (Y-Y. Chang *et al* 1994; Funakawa *et al* 1993), remission was achieved with corticosteroids. Hiccough and vomiting, attributed to a brainstem lesion, have been described as the presenting symptoms of multiple sclerosis (Birkhead and Friedman 1987).

Sensory symptoms and signs

Sensory symptoms are common at onset or in early relapse, alone or in combination with other disease manifestations (Figure 6.12). E.A.C.M. Sanders and Arts (1986) noted paraesthesiae as an isolated symptom in 28/127 patients. The sensations were often described as occurring in frequent brief episodes, not easy to distinguish from those regarded as prodromal by Abb and Schaltenbrand (1956). A common pattern is for abnormal sensations, tingling and numbness, to begin in one foot and, in the course of a few days, to spread and involve the whole of both lower limbs, the buttocks and perineum. Loss of perineal sensation is the most obtrusive as the normal sensations of micturition and defaecation may be lost, and genital sensation may also be diminished.

Examination by conventional methods reveals alteration rather than loss of sensation. Pinprick may be felt as distant and cotton wool, while felt, no longer tickles. Such responses may lead to diagnostic error by the inexperienced. Remission is usually complete within a few weeks, but many sharply localized attacks may last no more than a few days. Naturally the symptoms and their spread and distribution are not stereotyped. They depend on the initial site of the lesion and the directions in which it grows. For example the upper limbs and face may be involved. Loss of thermal sensation on the buttocks may be pronounced and motor signs may develop. Despite all these variants, the typical sensory relapse can often be recognized immediately from the patient's description. Rigorous and repeated sensory testing is no longer the style of modern neurology but it is not hard to find sensory differences, many unreported by the patient in advance of physical examination. Thus, loss of vibration sense is common but rarely symptomatic. It usually precedes other manifestations of posterior column involvement such as

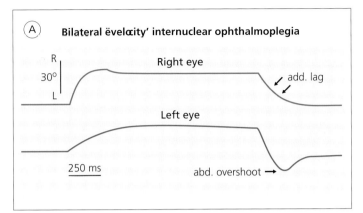

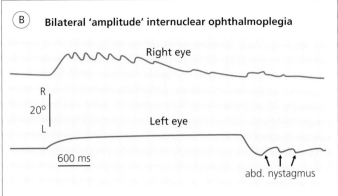

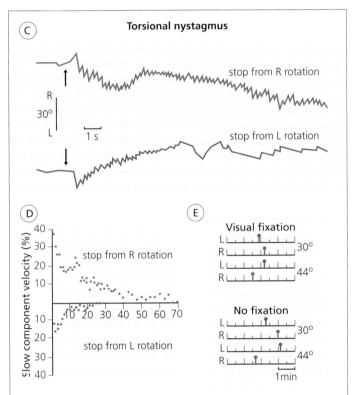

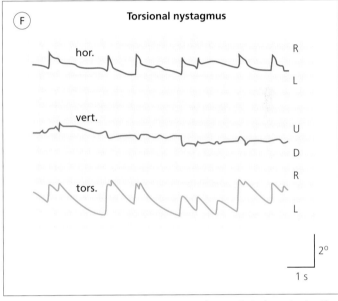

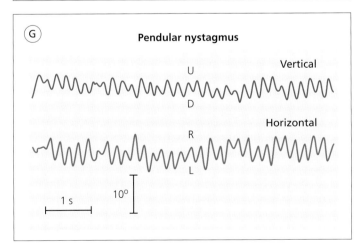

Figure 6.11 (A) Bilateral velocity internuclear ophthalmoplegia: if damage to the medial longitudinal bundle is not complete, there is no actual restriction in the eye displacement. The clinician can diagnose internuclear ophthalmoplegia by the presence of nystagmus (or even a single overshoot as shown) in the abducting eye and/or some lag of the adducting behind the abducting eye (B) Bilateral amplitude internuclear ophthalmoplegia: typical case with severe weakness of adduction during rightwards movement and absence of adduction during leftwards motion. Note abducting nystagmus in both directions. (C–E) Torsional nystagmus: lesions as a result of multiple sclerosis in the floor of the fourth ventricle frequently involve the vestibular nuclei, leading to central nystagmus (often resulting from involvement of the middle cerebellar peduncle) which is right beating or anticlockwise. In (C) post-rotational responses show stronger nystagmus to the left which is also seen in the slow-phase velocity of the nystagmus (D) and on caloric testing with and without visual fixation (E). (F) Torsional nystagmus is illustrated in a patient with a right sixth nerve palsy and a central vestibular syndrome. (G) Pendular nystagmus: there is continuous quasi-sinusoidal oscillation of the eye in both horizontal and vertical planes at 4 Hz. The combination of oscillation in two or three planes results in circular or elliptical ocular trajectories. Kindly provided by Dr Adolpho Bronstein.

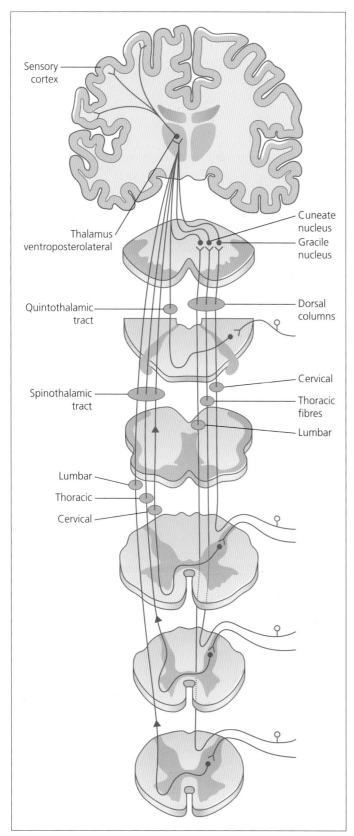

Figure 6.12 Pathways likely to be involved in multiple sclerosis which normally relay protective and discriminative sensation from the limbs.

Labels on figure:
- Sensory cortex
- Thalamus ventroposterolateral
- Quintothalamic tract
- Spinothalamic tract
- Lumbar
- Thoracic
- Cervical
- Cuneate nucleus
- Gracile nucleus
- Dorsal columns
- Cervical
- Thoracic fibres
- Lumbar

altered proprioception; this is much more likely to have been noticed by the affected individual.

The useless hand

One characteristic form of sensory relapse involves loss of positional sense in one or both hands (Figure 6.13A–E). This develops rapidly, the complaint being one of loss of use – the useless hand named eponymously after Hermann Oppenheim. Localization of the responsible lesion to the posterior columns of the spinal cord has been confirmed by MRI (Miller *at al* 1987a). Cutaneous sensation is usually normal and, despite the loss of function, there is no weakness. Although usually preserved, the tendon reflexes may be lost consistent with interruption of the intraspinal reflex arc. Although position sense is demonstrably impaired, sometimes even in the large joints of the limb, this sign is not invariably present. We have seen many patients with inability to use one hand, because of a lesion in the posterior part of the cervical cord, in whom small passive movements could still accurately be detected in the terminal phalanx of the fifth digit (which we consider to be the most reliable method for assessing position sense). The loss of function may more easily be demonstrated by failure to distinguish different coins by touch, or an increased threshold for two-point discrimination. S.A.K. Wilson (1940), noting this discrepancy, drew attention to the much more discriminating task of requiring the patient to place a button through its hole as the best evidence for involvement of the posterior columns. Remission is usual, but not always complete, and the prognosis for recovery of function is generally good.

Persistent dense loss of cutaneous sensation is a rare finding in multiple sclerosis, except in the severely disabled patient or where, exeptionally, there has been a transverse cord lesion. A persistent bilateral sensory level should prompt review of the diagnosis. Hansen *et al* (1996) reviewed abnormalities of thermal sensation in patients with multiple sclerosis. In addition to the expected increased threshold for detecting temperature, a high proportion of patients with definite or probable multiple sclerosis reported a paradoxical experience of warmth in response to a cold stimulus, especially when this followed warmth, providing experimental verification for the perversions of cutaneous sensation which are the everyday experience of many patients with demyelinating disease. In the ambulant patient with moderate disability, cutaneous sensory changes are usually limited to blunting of all forms of sensation asymmetrically in the extremities. This distribution is not easy to explain on anatomical grounds. Vibration sense is nearly always reduced at the ankles if there is any degree of spastic weakness. Postural sense in the toes is also likely to be impaired and loss of proprioception further disturbs voluntary movement, particularly when walking. Sensory symptoms can naturally arise from brainstem lesions, paraesthesiae in the face being particularly common.

Both types of sensory attack described above occur more commonly, but not exclusively, in the early stages of multiple sclerosis. Persistent paraesthesiae are common in established disease, being present in 84% in one series (M.E. Sanders *et al* 1986). The distribution is sometimes closely localized, often in the ulnar two digits in one or both hands, presenting a potential

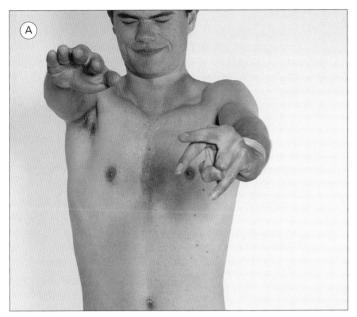

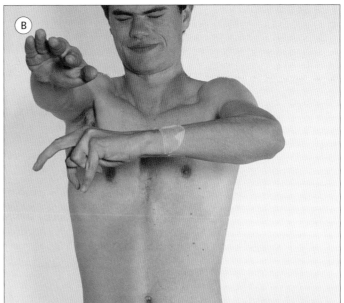

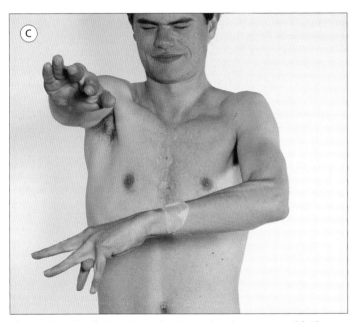

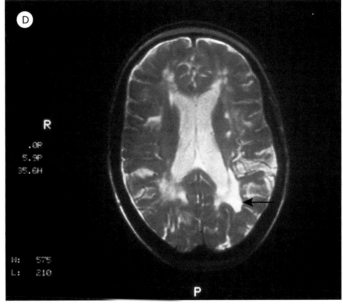

Figure 6.13 (A–C) On attempting to maintain posture with the eyes closed, the fingers develop 'pseudoathetosis' and the affected arm moves towards the opposite axilla. (D) MRI shows the cerebral white matter abnormalities (arrow).

illustration continued on following page

source of diagnostic confusion. Other common symptoms include a constricting feeling around the leg or as a girdle around the trunk. Loss of thermal sensation may be noticed in the bath.

Cortical sensory loss

Sensory changes due to parietal lobe involvement are uncommon but may occur with massive demyelination of the cerebral hemispheres (Graff-Radford and Rizzo 1987). An

example of tactile inattention in an autopsy-proven case with radiological evidence for extensive demyelination in the parietal white matter during life, was given in a previous edition of this book (W.B. Matthews 1991). This 51-year-old woman developed right-sided optic neuritis with partial recovery. In the next 2 years, she sustained a rapid series of severe relapses of multiple sclerosis, including bilateral optic neuritis, paraplegia and cerebellar ataxia, with some remission on corticotropin. A further relapse left her with hemiparesis, hemianopia and tactile inattention.

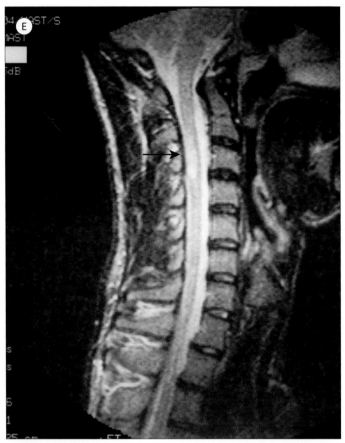

Figure 6.13, cont'd (E) Lesion responsible for the deficit in the cervical cord (arrow).

Restless legs

People with multiple sclerosis, particularly young women, being relatively immobile, are more prone to iron deficiency – an established cause of the peculiarly distressing symptoms of the restless legs syndrome. Unpleasant sensory symptoms relieved by movement suggest this diagnosis but we would not normally attach significance to posture-related sensory complaints in otherwise healthy people.

Pain

Pain is frequently listed amongst the initial symptoms of multiple sclerosis or as occurring in the course of the disease. Shibasaki *et al* (1981) reported pain in 37% of British and 35% of Japanese patients. Similar or higher figures are given for other surveys of clinic patients (Clifford and Trotter 1984; Moulin *et al* 1988; Stenager *et al* 1991). There are wide variations in the reported frequency of pain in the course of the disease, at least in part as a result of differing inclusion criteria. A systematic study was carried out by Svendsen *et al* (2003) who conducted a postal survey of 771 patients with definite multiple sclerosis and 769 individuals from a sex- and age-stratified group from the general population. Pain in the preceding month occurred in 80% of multiple sclerosis patients and 75% of the controls. However, the intensity of pain, the need for analgesic treatment, and the impact of pain on daily life was higher in the patient group. In a postal survey of prevalent patients in King County

(Washington State), 44% (of 442) reported 'bothersome' pain in the preceding 3 months, of whom just over half considered this to have a significant impact on their activities of daily living (Ehde *et al* 2003). Solaro *et al* (2004) categorized pain reported by 1672 Italian patients in a cross-sectional multicentre survey as trigeminal neuralgia (2%), Lhermitte's symptom (9%), dysaesthesia (18%), low back pain (16%) and painful tonic spasms (11%).

In many patients, pain results from disability and not from direct effects of the disease process. Low back pain, sometimes with sciatica, is frequent and can be related to abnormal posture, spasm of the spinal musculature, or osteoporosis linked to immobility and treatment with corticosteroids. The incidence of such pain increases with age, disability and duration of disease. Spasticity is an important factor, including painful flexor spasms.

Pain, apparently as a result of the disease process, is also common and some of its more stereotyped manifestations (headache, trigeminal neuralgia and painful tonic spasm) are discussed elsewhere. Much more troublesome and less well recognized is dysaesthetic limb pain, which is worse at night and aggravated by heat. This may be the presenting symptom, beginning in the feet and gradually spreading up the legs. The pain is persistent and increases on walking. At this stage it may be accompanied by mild spastic paraparesis and loss of vibration sense so that the diagnosis is not immediately apparent. In more advanced disease, similar pain may be widespread on the trunk and limbs. It is one of the most difficult problems encountered in pain-relief clinics and notoriously intractable although the recent introduction of gabapentin may have made some inroads (see Chapter 17). Equally difficult to treat are the rarely seen paroxysms of dysaesthetic pain described below.

Pain of root distribution is less common and should be diagnosed with caution. Such pain has been reported as a presenting symptom of multiple sclerosis in 11 patients (Ramirez-Lassepas *et al* 1992). The distribution was lumbar or lumbosacral in six, thoracic in two and cervical in three. Unfortunately, the cases were not described in detail and the pain was rather obscurely described as paroxysmal, without further explanation. Whether signs of nerve root lesions were observed is not stated. Uldry and Regli (1992) presented a detailed account of four patients with established multiple sclerosis who developed pain and other abnormal sensations in the distribution of cervical nerve roots, accompanied by appropriate physical signs and with MRI abnormalities in the cervical spinal cord. Two had experienced attacks of severe burning pain which resolved rapidly with steroid treatment. Although interest in pain in multiple sclerosis has increased, especially with the improved availability of rehabilitation services, the topic is still unduly neglected.

Lhermitte's symptom and sign

This sensation is undoubtedly a symptom but has more often been called Lhermitte's sign, apparently for the first time by Read (1932), having been described as the initial manifestation of multiple sclerosis by J. Lhermitte *et al* (1924). It is not however confined to multiple sclerosis nor was it first described by Lhermitte. Alajouanine *et al* (1949) corrected the history – '*décrite par Pierre Marie et baptiseé par Babinski*' – in their accounts of head and neck injuries during the First World War (Babinski and Dubois 1918; Marie and Chatelin 1917; Ribeton 1919).

The common form consists of an electric feeling passing down the back to the legs on flexing the neck. Other descriptive terms include tingling, pins and needles and, occasionally, pain. The spread of the sensation may vary. All four limbs may be involved or, rarely, the arms alone. Even more unusually, it may be unilateral or felt as spreading upwards rather than down the spine. The sensation is always brief, estimated as lasting 2 seconds (Kanchandani and Howe 1982). Neck flexion is by far the commonest precipitating cause, although other brusque movements, such as coughing or laughing, may have the same effect. Remission after a few weeks is usual but recurrence is frequent. The symptom has a well characterized physiological substrate (see Figure 6.14; and see Chapter 13, Figures 13.38 and 13.39) but why it occurs in some and not others with cervical cord demyelination is unclear: one of us (DASC) sees annually a patient with Lhermitte's symptom occurring in isolation over many years whose identical twin brother has the same complaint, whereas their sister is affected by severe secondary progressive multiple sclerosis. Occasionally, patients with multiple sclerosis will describe adventitious movements of the legs provoked by flexion of the spine or neck. Although these may have simple explanations in terms of spontaneous muscle spasms, descriptions given by individual patients, or clinical observations, suggest that they are the motor equivalent of Lhermitte's sensory symptom. Another manifestation of cervical cord disease, which is not specific to multiple sclerosis, is increased evidence for pyramidal deficit provoked by neck flexion, and corresponding improvement on neck extension. Presumably these postures subtly enhance or compromise function in partially damaged descending corticospinal pathways. This phenomenon, taught to generations of residents at London's National Hospital, Queen Square, by the late Dr M.J. (Sean) McArdle, is known as Bristow's symptom (or sign) after the patient who pointed it out to McArdle.

Lhermitte's symptom is common in multiple sclerosis. Kanchandani and Howe (1982) found that 38% of their patients with clinically definite disease had experienced the symptom at some stage and it characterizes the first attack in a high proportion. In three patients it was the initial isolated symptom. Paty and Poser (1984) recorded Lhermitte's symptom as an initial complaint in 3% of their series but did not indicate how often it was present in isolation. Al-Araji and Oger (2005) recorded the experience of Lhermitte's symptom in 41% of 300 patients with multiple sclerosis but not one of 100 controls: the symptom usually occurred within the first 3 years, alone (64%) and as a stereotyped complaint, or less commonly in association with other manifestations of the disease. It is much more common in Japanese patients (Shibasaki *et al* 1981). As already remarked, besides trauma, Lhermitte's symptom is not specific for multiple sclerosis and has other causes, including cervical cord compression, radiation myelopathy (Boden 1948) and subacute combined degeneration of the spinal cord (Gautier-Smith 1973). It is unusual but may occur in cervical spondylotic myelopathy.

Disturbances of cognition and affect

A common question from someone trying to come to terms with the idea of having a disease affecting the central nervous system is 'will it affect my mind?' Whatever may seem to be the right reply, the truth is that it probably will. It was already evident to Charcot (1872) that memory is often severely impaired with blunted affect and intellect (see Chapter 1). This encouraged early attempts to identify a specific 'dementia polysclerotica' (Seiffer 1905). Despite the evidence, there was considerable reluctance to accept that mental changes occur except in the terminal stages of the disease. This opinion was supported by misinterpretation of the pronouncement that there is no psychic disorder characteristic of multiple sclerosis (Timme and the Commission 1922) as meaning that, with one exception, no such disorders were likely to occur.

Cottrell and Wilson (1926) wrote a highly influential, but unfortunately misleading, paper, the effects of which can still be detected. They examined 100 unselected hospital patients (but no controls) and by simple questioning decided that 63 had a positive sense of well-being ('euphoria'), while 84 had an unjustified feeling of physical health ('eutonia'). Lability of emotional expression was almost universal. Ten of the patients were severely depressed. These changes were thought to be quite independent of the intellectual impairment that was judged to be present in only two patients. The reputed association of euphoria with multiple sclerosis has proved ineradicably memorable. In contrast, a few years later, Ombredane (1929) found intellectual impairment in 36/50 patients and made the highly pertinent observation that the changes are often not apparent in ordinary conversation or on routine examination, a finding which has often been confirmed (Peyser *et al* 1980; 1990). Dick Pratt made the first systematic attempt to define the spectrum and prevalence of psychiatric features in multiple sclerosis and, with others, ushered in the modern era of cognitive understanding of multiple sclerosis (Pratt 1951).

Cognitive impairment and dementia

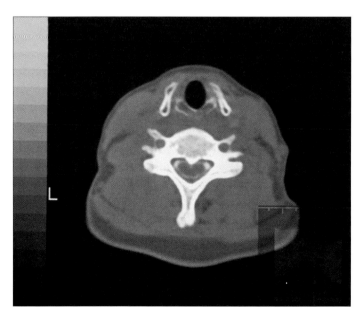

Figure 6.14 CT myelography in a patient complaining only of Lhermitte's symptom as a result of cervical disc protrusion.

It is now accepted that intellectual impairment commonly occurs in multiple sclerosis. In reported series, approximately

45–65% of patients tested are found to have such defects (De Sousa *et al* 2002; Peyser *et al* 1990; S.M. Rao *et al* 1991a; 1991b). These estimates must be approximate since not all authors state the actual number of patients with abnormal test scores but rely on mean figures for the group (I. Grant *et al* 1984). In addition to the usual problem of correct diagnosis, results are influenced by the level of score regarded as abnormal (Van den Burg *et al* 1987). The tests used should not be influenced by reduced manual dexterity or visual acuity. Peyser *et al* (1990) suggested guidelines for neuropsychological research in multiple sclerosis. It is to be hoped that some uniformity in test methods can be agreed as comparison between different reported series is at present difficult.

There is general agreement on the nature and range of the cognitive deficits (Table 6.10). Language, although perhaps not always examined as fully as other functions, is scarcely disturbed even in severely disabled patients (Staples and Lincoln 1979). The ability to perform complex cognitive activities ('multitasking'), attention and executive functions are affected ahead of memory. When present, deficient recent memory is usually the most obvious finding but remote memory is also disturbed (Beatty *et al* 1988; Grafman *et al* 1991; I.Grant *et al* 1984; Litvan *et al* 1988; S.M. Rao *et al* 1984; 1989a). Conceptual reasoning and verbal fluency may also be impaired (Beatty *et al* 1989). These associated abnormalities are typical of subcortical dementia, which is not surprising in view of the major impact of multiple sclerosis on the white matter.

Systematic testing has revealed that impairment of memory and learning ability may occur very early in the course of the disease. Truelle *et al* (1987) found that 55% of patients with disease duration of <5 years and a similar proportion of those with EDSS 0–2 had marked memory impairment. Van den Burg *et al* (1987), in a study of 40 patients with mild disability, found seven to be definitely impaired. Good *et al* (1992) reported that 26/84 patients in remission, free from drugs and with EDSS <6, were intellectually impaired compared with controls. Lyon-Caen *et al* (1986) examined intellect and memory function within 2 years of onset in 21 patients with multiple sclerosis and nine with isolated optic neuritis. Some evidence of cognitive impairment was found in 18 subjects, including six with optic neuritis.

These findings have been extended to include patients presenting with isolated symptoms of the type characteristically occurring in multiple sclerosis (Callanan *et al* 1989). Of 48 patients who had sustained clinically isolated lesions of the optic nerve, brainstem, or spinal cord, only 23% were found to be functioning at or above the level of the 50th percentile of the control group of subjects disabled by other diseases. A further group of 42 patients with acute optic neuritis were examined within 5 weeks of onset (Feinstein *et al* 1992a). Fifty-five per cent of these patients had cerebral abnormalities on MRI. Cognitive function in those without such lesions did not differ significantly from controls, while the group with lesions was significantly impaired in a variety of tests, particularly of attention. In this study, mean results for the different groups were compared and it is not easy to determine, for example, whether any patients with MRI lesions were thought to be functioning normally. However, this is suggested by the observation that a group of socially integrated patients with stable multiple sclerosis was found to function no differently from controls

Table 6.10	**Neuropsychological deficits in multiple sclerosis**
Attention	Visual and auditory attentional deficits, delayed information processing
Memory	Recall more impaired than recognition memory
Executive function	Working memory, verbal fluency, planning, strategy and abstraction impaired
Language	Usually preserved; subtle semantic and circumlocutory naming errors

From Foong and Ron (2003) with permission.

in tests of visuo-spatial problem solving, conceptual reasoning and sorting behaviour (Jennekens-Schinkel *et al* 1989). Neurophysiological evidence for the diffuse impact of demyelination on cognitive performance is provided by Pelosi *et al* (1997) who correlated impairments of working memory with delays in the event-related potential amongst a group of patients with isolated spinal cord demyelinating lesions, some but not all of whom had cerebral MRI abnormalities.

Despite these revelations from formal testing, patients with such clinically isolated syndromes rarely complain of symptoms attributable to cognitive impairment. More generally, although the evidence that cognitive function is often affected very early in the course of the disease is convincing, there is little mention of whether patients are aware of the mild defects found on rigorous testing and whether, at this stage, any disability results. In contrast, severe dementia may occasionally be an early or even the presenting symptom. A.C. Young *et al* (1976) described five patients, in four of whom behavioural or intellectual changes had been the initial symptom. In two, mental changes, not recognized as dementia, had been present for several years before overt evidence of multiple sclerosis appeared. G.M. Franklin *et al* (1989) also emphasized that severe cognitive impairment, out of proportion to physical disability, or even in the virtual absence of other clinical evidence of disease (Hotopf *et al* 1994), may be the presenting feature. Zarei *et al* (2003) have argued on clinical, pathological and MRI grounds for the existence of a syndrome of cortical multiple sclerosis. Their six cases presented with progressive dementia with prominent amnesia, often accompanied by classical cortical features such as dysphasia, dysgraphia and dyslexia. Cortical multiple sclerosis may cause major handicap and multiple sclerosis as the cause is, understandably, easily overlooked. It might reasonably be expected that cognitive abnormalities which reflect the involvement of discrete cortical areas (Figure 6.15) would correlate with topographical evidence from MRI for greatest disease burden at those sites. Working specifically with executive tasks, Foong *et al* (1997) were unable to disentangle the contribution from frontal lobe pathology to the general clouding of intellect, and they found no correlation with regional MRI lesion load (see also below). It must be noted however that the contribution of cortical (grey matter) lesions has not yet been elucidated, since these are rarely detected by standard MRI techniques.

Few longitudinal studies of cognitive function in multiple sclerosis have been published. Mariani *et al* (1991) found no significant deterioration in a small group of patients re-examined after an interval of 2 years. Jennekens-Schinkel *et al* (1990) studied 33/49 patients previously assessed 4 years earlier. Cognitive function, as tested, remained unchanged compared with controls in 76%. Of the remainder, some had deteriorated and others had improved. Feinstein *et al* (1992b) reported a 4.5-year follow-up involving 35/48 patients with isolated lesions originally described by Callanan *et al* (1989). The hazards of this type of study are illustrated by the original presumptive diagnosis of multiple sclerosis proving to be wrong in four instances. In the interval, 19 patients had developed clinically definite multiple sclerosis while the remainder were still classified as having clinically isolated syndromes. On psychometric testing, the only significant difference between these two groups was that visual memory had deteriorated in the former.

Feinstein *et al* (1993a) carried out a detailed study, arduous for all concerned, of 10 patients examined clinically, tested psychometrically and scanned by MRI at frequent intervals for a period of 6 months. Some of the interesting findings are discussed below, but in the present context the result may be summarized as showing that, over this period, patients with stable disease did not deteriorate intellectually and some tended to improve, no doubt as a result of practice. Those with active disease either deteriorated or failed to show the practice effect. Severe cognitive defects occurring acutely in a relapse may, however, remit completely (G.M. Franklin *et al* 1989). Subsequently, Amato *et al* (1995) compared cognitive function in 50 patients early in the course of multiple sclerosis, and after 4 years, with 70 controls. Predictably, the patients performed worse at both assessments. However, whereas defects of verbal memory and abstract reasoning remained stable, linguistic difficulties emerged in the patients with time. In general, these cognitive defects correlated poorly with physical disabilities, disease duration or course but each was a separate predictor of

social handicap. The natural history of cognitive decline has been assesed by Kujala *et al* (1997) who found that patients with impaired cognition continue progressively to accumulate new deficits of memory, learning, attention and visuo-motor performance – independent of concomitant physical deterioration – whereas those with comparable disabilities but normal intellect remain cognitively intact. However, in a recent study, Amato *et al* (2001) re-examined 45 patients and 65 matched controls after 10 years concluding that 'in a sufficiently long follow-up, cognitive function is likely to emerge and progress in a sizeable proportion of patients'. The neurological and cognitive involvement tended to converge. In summary, although early cognitive deterioration is detected at high frequency, there is considerable individual variation and, over a decade, some decline is the rule. Individual variation presumably contributes to the conflict of evidence as to whether cognitive impairment is more severe in primary or secondary progressive multiple sclerosis (Comi *et al* 1995; Foong *et al* 2000).

With time, the impact of cognitive decline is less easy to disguise. The majority of reports on cognitive function in patients with established multiple sclerosis are based on clinic series of patients with varying degrees of disability and duration of disease. Results have been summarized by Peyser *et al* (1990) and the finding that 60% of such patients are found to be impaired has already been cited. The degree of impairment varies widely. Surridge (1969), in a pioneering study of relatively severely disabled patients, found that 41% had mild intellectual loss whereas 14% were moderately, and 6.5% severely, impaired. S.M. Rao *et al* (1991a), in an investigation of 100 community-based patients, found that 43% failed four or more tasks in a battery of tests.

The nearest approach to a population study is that of McIntosh-Michaelis *et al* (1991). Drawn from a population of >400 by alternate sampling, and stratified according to disability, 147 patients were examined at home. Intellect was judged to be reduced in 22% and tests of everyday memory were abnormal in 34%; 33% were impaired on tests of frontal lobe function – mainly planning and verbal fluency – but 55% had no impairment on any of these tests.

These cross-sectional studies cannot answer the question of what chance someone diagnosed in life as having multiple sclerosis has of avoiding dementia. This is what many patients wish to know. The easy assumption that those in a bedridden state will have lost their reason does not seem to have been examined and, indeed, such patients are often deliberately excluded from surveys (S.M. Rao *et al* 1991a) being no longer actively under routine neurological care.

It is probable that cognitive function is more vulnerable in chronic progressive disease (Feinstein *et al* 1992b; Heaton *et al* 1985) than in the relapsing form, although this has not been a constant finding (S.M. Rao *et al* 1991a). Unexpectedly, with few exceptions (Achiron *et al* 2005; Amato *et al* 2001; Feinstein *et al* 1993a; McIntosh-Michaelis 1991), duration of disease has not emerged as a contributory factor (Ivnik 1978; S.M. Rao *et al* 1991a). In most surveys, the degree of disability has been found either not to correlate with mental changes (S.M. Rao *et al* 1984) or to have only a minor influence (S.M. Rao *et al* 1991a). This conclusion may be the result of excluding severely disabled people. McIntosh-Michaelis *et al* (1991) included patients with disability at EDSS ≤ 9.5 and found a strong correlation between

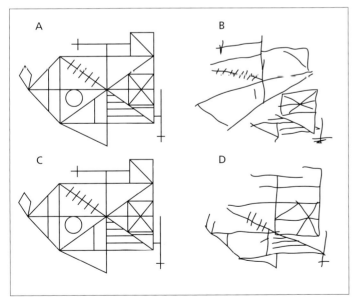

Figure 6.15 (A) and (C) Reye figure drawn normally. (B) Example of severely impaired visuospatial ability in a patient with nondominant cerebral hemisphere involvement by multiple sclerosis. (D) Milder disruption of planning and organization in frontal pathology as a result of multiple sclerosis. Kindly provided by Professor John Hodges.

increasing physical disability and cognitive defect. Intellectual deterioration has not been found to correlate with depression (Good *et al* 1992).

In contrast to the wealth of reports on neuropsychological testing, there is remarkably little systematic evidence on patients' awareness of failing cognitive ability. McIntosh-Michaelis *et al* (1991) found that 44% of their patients were aware of failing memory but, remarkably, only 38% of these performed badly on tests of memory. Thirty-eight per cent reported poor concentration. Relatives and those caring for patients were more aware of the defects, although these were not thought to increase domestic stress.

There is no doubt, however, that cognitive failure does influence disability and participation in the social environment. Patients so affected are less likely to work, take part in social activities, or run their home than those with comparable physical disabilities who remain mentally unimpaired (Jennekens-Schinkel and Sanders 1986; S.M. Rao *et al* 1991b; Staples and Lincoln 1979). Their quality of life is impaired (Benito-Leon *et al* 2002) and, in most situations, there is also no doubt that the difficulties of care are greatly increased.

Cognitive deficits and MRI

It has long been known that dementia in multiple sclerosis correlates with extensive cerebral involvement (Bergin 1957; O'Malley 1966). The advent of MRI led to the hope that the relationship between cognitive deficit and cerebral involvement would be more precisely defined. There is now a large literature on this topic, the striking features of which are variability of the findings and the weakness of their correlations.

However, we should not be surprised, given the lack of pathological specificity for imaging abnormalities. The most frequently sought correlation is with T_2 changes. Yet, it has been known for 20 years that the presence of such abnormalities even in clinically eloquent white matter tracts (such as the pyramidal tract and the optic nerve) is compatible with apparently normal function. This is not surprising either. The changes are the result of local alterations in the properties and relative amounts of intracellular and extracellular water and are thus influenced by gliosis, which is related only indirectly and rather uncertainly to axonal function (see Chapter 13). Moreover, as one of us (WIMcD) has observed, the consequences of previous axonal degeneration (such as after frontal leucotomy) and previous demyelination are indistinguishable so far as the appearance on T_2-weighted images are concerned. That said, there is axonal degeneration in many lesions and so one might expect a broad correlation between severity of cognitive impairment and total T_2 lesion load. This is, in fact, the case (Ron *et al* 1991) and Archibald *et al* (2004) have reported a significant relationship between posterior fossa lesion volume and memory scanning speed. But when it comes to associating defined cognitive deficits with specific T_2 abnormalities, the relationship is weaker. Better correlations are found with changes that more directly reflect axonal loss such as T_1 hypointense lesion load (Camp *et al* 1999; Rovaris *et al* 2000a) and brain atrophy (D. Berg *et al* 2000; Hohol *et al* 1997; Rovaris *et al* 2000a). Newer techniques offer some promise. For example, a greater reduction in the N-acetyl aspartate to creatine ratio in frontal lesions

and normal-appearing white matter has been found using MR spectroscopy in patients with impairment of working memory (Foong *et al* 1999). Comi *et al* (1999) in a multi-parametric MRI study of frontal lobe dementia in multiple sclerosis found a significant correlation between dementia and both T_1-weighted total lesion load and a reduction in the peak height of the magnetization transfer ratio. Neuropsychological deficits have also been found to correlate with changes in magnetization transfer imaging in lesions and normal-appearing white matter, and with fast flair in juxtacortical lesions undetected by conventional MRI (Lazeron *et al* 2000; Moriarty *et al* 1999).

Two other problems should be mentioned which confound interpretation of the relationship between abnormalities on MRI and neuropsychological function. The first is that there are adaptive changes to functional disruption (produced by axonal transection and conduction block – see Chapter 13) which may be compensatory in nature. The remarkable extent of such changes is easily seen in the rather simpler context of the visual and motor systems. Thus, as for other functional systems, the neuropsychiatric deficits observed at any particular time represent the outcome of a balance between impairment and compensation.

The second problem is the present difficulty of determining the extent and nature of abnormalities throughout the specific distributed systems, both subcortical and cortical, which mediate complex neuropsychological functions. The reader is reminded that there is very little *in vivo* information available about cortical lesions (which must make an important contribution to cognitive impairment) because, although common at post mortem, these are rarely seen on MRI. A better understanding of the pathophysiological basis for cognitive impairment in multiple sclerosis must await improved methods for localization and quantification of structural defects, and determination of the pattern and distribution of functional changes (leading either to impairment or to compensation) in the relevant neural systems. Our problems in offering an understanding of mechanisms underlying the next group of symptoms are even greater.

Neuropsychiatric disorders

Controlled studies of the affective state in multiple sclerosis have not unexpectedly shown that depression is more common than euphoria. Surridge (1969) found mild depression in 17% of patients with multiple sclerosis, moderately severe depression in 7% and severe depression in 4%. A further 4% were euphoric and 7% showed marked swings of mood. Depression was no more common in multiple sclerosis patients than in controls with primary muscle disease and it was concluded that the depressed mood is largely a reaction to illness and disability rather than a specific symptom of the disease. Whitlock and Siskind (1980), using control subjects more closely matched for disability, found depression to be much more common in multiple sclerosis and concluded that affective disorder may be a presenting or complicating feature of the disease. This leaves open the question of whether or not depression can be a direct result of cerebral plaques.

Cross-sectional studies have confirmed the frequency of depression in multiple sclerosis and the lifetime prevalence approaches 50% (Minden and Schiffer 1990). Multiple sclerosis greatly increases the risk of psychiatric illness (Ron and Logsdail 1989), including bipolar affective disorder, but the explanation is far from simple. In contrast to dementia, depression correlates better with the degree of stress perceived by the patient than the extent of lesions seen on MRI (Ron and Logsdail 1989). Ron and Feinstein (1992) suggest that the presence of brain damage enhances the effects of environmental factors in causing psychiatric disease. Certainly the majority of those who have studied the problem conclude that depression in multiple sclerosis is the result of depressing circumstances (Baretz and Stephenson 1981; McIvor *et al* 1984; S.M. Rao and Leo 1988). Schiffer *et al* (1983), however, found depression to be commoner in patients with predominantly cerebral rather than spinal disease, the two groups being similarly disabled. More specifically, it is claimed that white matter lesions often affect the arcuate fasciculus in patients with prominent symptoms (Pujol *et al* 1997). The interpretation that depression is reactive and not constitutional in patients with multiple sclerosis is considered by Sadovnick *et al* (1996b) who showed that, whereas the lifetime risk for depression in a cohort of 221 probands is 50% (by the age of 59 years), the recurrence risk in their first-degree relatives is lower than for a reference population of comparable relatives from individuals with primary depressive disorders.

The risk of suicide in multiple sclerosis has generally been held to be low. However, in a population study in Denmark (Stenager *et al* 1992), 58 people with multiple sclerosis were known to have committed suicide over a 30-year period, against an expected figure of 28. Half of these deaths occurred within 5 years of diagnosis. Later, this figure was amended and re-expressed as a standardized mortality ratio of 1.62 (95% CI 1.29–2.01) based on 6068 cases registered between 1949 and 1993 (Koch-Henriksen *et al* 1998). In patients attending clinics in Canada, the suicide rate was 7.5-fold that in a matched population and accounted for 15% of fatalities (Sadovnick *et al* 1991b). Bauer and Hanefeld (1993) reported that 12% of 69 fatal cases of multiple sclerosis were the result of suicide. In Sweden, the incidence of suicide was 90/5052 (1.8%: standardized mortality ratio 2) amongst those with multiple sclerosis dying over the period 1969–1996. The interval from diagnosis was 5.8 years with a particularly high rate in the first year after diagnosis and in young males (Fredrikson *et al* 2003). It is probable that suicide is not infrequently overlooked or concealed. Our own experience (DASC) is limited to three examples. One illustrates the controversial issue of when to name the illness. A patient committed suicide in a public car park on leaving the hospital clinic where she had been told that her symptoms were probably caused by multiple sclerosis (in fact, she was shown to have a brainstem glioma at autopsy). Two others committed suicide after several failed attempts at disease-modifying therapy, including involvement in therapeutic trials, emphasizing the effect of disappointment that can follow a period of heightened expectation sustained by participation in clinical research.

On the vexed issue of euphoria, Minden and Schiffer (1990) emphasize that the definition is far from precise. Euphoria and elation in multiple sclerosis can only rarely be attributed to mania (Kemp *et al* 1977, Peselow *et al* 1981) and, when marked, are associated with dementia and extensive MRI lesions (Rabins *et al* 1986; Ron and Feinstein 1992). The fatuous denial of obvious disability, noted by S.S. Cottrell and Wilson (1926), is entirely distinct from the stoical acceptance of ill-fortune exhibited by many courageous and fully sentient people with multiple sclerosis.

Other forms of psychosis

Early suggestions of a link between multiple sclerosis and schizophrenia (Davison and Bagley 1969) are unconvincing. Occasionally, however, the acute onset of bizarre behavioural symptoms, leading to emergency admission to psychiatric hospital with a diagnosis of schizophrenia, proves to be the initial episode of multiple sclerosis followed by complete remission (W.B. Matthews 1979). Of the nine patients described by Felgenhauer (1990) as presenting with psychotic disorders in the encephalitic form of multiple sclerosis, the diagnosis can be regarded as definite in only two. Onset with acute psychiatric symptoms, in the absence of signs of organic nervous disease, is rare but should not be discounted.

Psychotic illness occurring in the course of the disease was investigated by Feinstein *et al* (1993b). In a large hospital series, only ten such patients could be identified, five with some form of schizophrenia, four with mania and one with psychotic depression. The mental illness had developed later than the onset of neurological disease in every case, although two patients had a past history of less severe mental symptoms. The psychotic symptoms appear to have been transitory. In patients with a history of psychosis there was a tendency for the volume of lesions seen on MRI to be greater than in controls, especially around the temporal horns of the lateral ventricles. The age at onset of psychosis was considerably later than in patients without multiple sclerosis. It was concluded that there is an 'aetiological association' between the pathological process of multiple sclerosis and psychosis, presumably meaning that multiple sclerosis can cause schizophrenia and mania. There are few modern observations on behavioural disorders in chronic multiple sclerosis but clinical experience confirms the occasional presence of paranoid ideas, belligerence, sexual disinhibition and unreasonable behaviour, such as dispersing the family savings, in patients with extensive brain damage. One syndrome that undoubtedly does occur in patients with frontal involvement is a Klüver–Bucy state with hyperphagia and loss of social and sexual reservations. A single male case of acquired sexual paraphilia (disinhibition and an obsessive desire to touch women's breasts) during a relapse is described by Frohman *et al* (2002). MRI revealed a marked increase in the number of enhancing lesions in the right sides of the hypothalamus and mesencephalon.

Hysteria

It is a source of some astonishment that patients with undoubted multiple sclerosis not infrequently develop additional burdens from hysterical symptoms (Aring 1965; Caplan and Nadelson 1980). The signs are usually not difficult to recognize but we have found it best to do no more than note their presence for the guidance of others who may see the patient. These symptoms develop, no doubt, in response to some need that may be detected in the course of enquiry but which can seldom be fulfilled. Caplan and Nadelson (1980) present two instructive case histories of patients with undoubted multiple sclerosis who became incapacitated by nonorganic symptoms. They mention a common feature of such cases – very active involvement in the affairs of the Multiple Sclerosis Society. Often, there is nothing to be gained and perhaps much to be lost in disturbing this way of life, but occasionally hysteria is a major cause of handicap in a patient with an otherwise minimally disabling form of multiple sclerosis and the usual methods of attempting to improve function by physical therapy and encouragement, without confrontation or loss of dignity, may be successful and stable. We deal with the alternative problem of individuals without any evidence for neurological disease presenting features or patterns of illness behaviour which suggest the diagnosis of multiple sclerosis to themselves or others in the discussion of differential diagnosis (see Chapter 8).

Other behavioural disorders

We have seen pathological laughter in multiple sclerosis, so severe as seriously to disrupt the patient's social relationships. From a study of 11 patients with pathological laughter and crying, Feinstein *et al* (1999) suggested that the disorder is mediated by prefrontal cortical dysfunction. Single cases have been reported of association between multiple sclerosis and confabulation (Feinstein *et al* 2000) and episodic hyperlibidinism (Gondim and Thomas 2001). In a postal survey of alcohol and substance abuse in 1374 members of a multiple sclerosis society, 708 provided sufficient data; of these, there was evidence for abuse in 19%. Quesnel and Feinstein (2004), in a study of 140 multiple sclerosis patients, found that one in six drank to excess over the course of their lifetime. There were significant associations with suicidal ideation, substance abuse and a family history of mental illness.

Some unusual cerebral symptoms

Although it is now well known that cortical lesions are common at post mortem, their acute clinical expression is exceptional. Why this should be is unclear. Some of the possible contributing factors have been discussed already and they are considered further in Chapter 13. Over the years, we have encountered a variety of cortical syndromes at presentation or during the course of the disease.

Aphasia

Though rare, aphasia is well documented in multiple sclerosis (Figure 6.16A,B; Kahana *et al* 1971). It usually occurs in the context of massive cerebral demyelination mimicking the presentation of a malignant tumour and in such cases, aphasia is commonly present if the dominant hemisphere is involved. Complete remission may occur (Achiron *et al* 1992a; Hunter *et al* 1987; Mastrostefano *et al* 1987; Sagar *et al* 1982). As already mentioned, dysphasia may be detected in patients presenting with progressive dementia (Zarei *et al* 2003) and may be the principal feature of an acute isolated demyelinating syndrome (Di Majo *et al* 2002). Lacour *et al* (2004) identified 22 patients with acute aphasia amongst 2700 patients registered with three multiple sclerosis centres. In eight, aphasia was the presenting symptom – usually associated with giant plaques on MRI. The prognosis for recovery of speech was good, occurring in 14/22 (64%).

Schnider *et al* (1993) described a severe callosal disconnection syndrome in a patient with multiple sclerosis. She had left-sided agraphia and was unable to name by touch objects placed in her left hand. Memory and the ability to calculate were also impaired. Pelletier *et al* (1992) found evidence for impaired callosal transfer in a group of patients with multiple sclerosis, although it is not clear that this gave rise to significant symptoms. Trinka *et al* (2002) have reported a single case presenting with aphasic status epilepticus. While the MRI and cerebrospinal

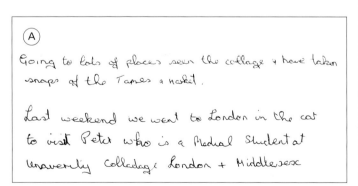

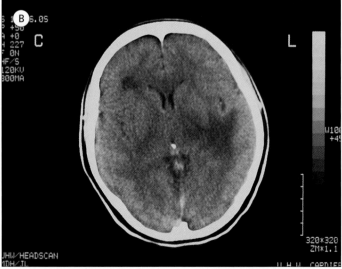

Figure 6.16 **(A)** Example of impaired narrative writing and spelling errors in a patient with a left angular gyrus syndrome as a result of multiple sclerosis. Kindly provided by Professor John Hodges. **(B)** CT scan in a patient with global aphasia (hemiplegia and hemianopia) as a second episode in Marburg-type multiple sclerosis; the first attack had caused a functional transection of the cervical cord and the patient died within 3 years of presentation.

fluid changes were compatible with multiple sclerosis, the formal diagnostic criteria of the International Panel (see Chapter 7) were not fulfilled.

Epilepsy

Early reports of the association between epilepsy and multiple sclerosis are much confounded by doubts concerning the diagnosis of either condition or of a causal connection (W.B. Matthews 1962). Estimates for the frequency of epilepsy at 5% (Hopf *et al* 1970) or even 8% (Trouillas and Courjon 1972) contrast with figures of 1% (Elian and Dean 1977), 2% (Ghezzi *et al* 1990) and 0.6% (Ritter and Poser 1974) in large series that are not greatly different from the accepted figure of 0.5% for the general population. That said, two more recent population-based studies from Sweden (M. Eriksson *et al* 2002) and Sicily (Nicoletti *et al* 2003) report frequencies of epilepsy in multiple sclerosis respectively of 7.8% and 'threefold higher…than in the general population'. Review of 29 published series yielded a prevalence of 2.3% (C.M. Poser and Brinar 2003). All such figures must include some instances of chance association (Kinnunen and Wikström 1986).

Where epilepsy can reasonably be attributed to multiple sclerosis, tonic–clonic convulsion, with or without a focal onset, is the most common form but partial epilepsy may also occur (Cendrowski and Makowski 1972; Gambardella *et al* 2003; Nyquist *et al* 2001). Continuous partial epilepsy (Spatt *et al* 1995; Striano *et al* 2003; S.A.K. Wilson and McBride 1925), and focal (Boudouresques *et al* 1975; Trinka *et al* 2002 – see above) and generalized status (R.S. Allison 1950; Sokic *et al* 2001) have each been described in single case reports.

When epilepsy presents before the onset of overt symptoms of multiple sclerosis, the causal connection may well be in doubt but epilepsy has been reported as the sole presenting symptom (Trouillas and Courjon 1972; Striano *et al* 2003). Epilepsy coinciding with the onset of the disease, or developing later, as in the majority of reported cases (Ghezzi *et al* 1990; Kinnunen and Wikström 1986), is more convincing. Epilepsy occurring in clinical relapse (W.B. Matthews 1962) or in association with otherwise asymptomatic new lesions shown on MRI (A.J. Thompson *et al* 1993a) usually responds well to treatment and does not recur. When associated with progressive disease, particularly deteriorating mental function, or with large unresolving MRI lesions, the fits may prove intractable. Fatal status epilepticus is occasionally the cause of death in multiple sclerosis (Allison 1950).

Multiple sclerosis mimicking brain tumour

There is increasing recognition that multiple sclerosis may present as a mass lesion of the cerebral hemisphere, with rapidly developing hemiplegia, focal or generalized fits, aphasia if the dominant hemisphere is involved, headache and confusion. This may occur at the onset or in the course of established disease (R.J. Abbott *et al* 1982). The mistaken diagnosis of malignant brain tumour is inevitable and the distinction cannot be achieved by imaging techniques alone. Computerized tomography (CT) scanning and MRI may show solid or ring enhancing, space-occupying lesions (Giang *et al* 1992; S.B. Hunter *et al* 1987; Reith *et al* 1981; Sagar *et al* 1982; Youl *et al* 1991a). The

mass lesions shown on MRI have been misdiagnosed as tumour or abscess (see Figure 7.9). Biopsy of these lesions may be difficult to interpret (S.B. Hunter *et al* 1987) and the correct diagnosis may only be made following remission or at autopsy in progressive disease. The issues surrounding biopsy are discussed in Chapter 7. Occasionally a brain tumour may develop in a patient with multiple sclerosis (O.A. Khan *et al* 1997). It is instructive that biopsy material, mostly from cases in which there was difficulty in distinguishing acute plaques of demyelination from brain tumour, has proved enormously important in understanding mechanisms of demyelination and remyelination (see Chapter 12). Remission from symptoms of raised intracranial pressure may be long lasting and may not be followed by recurrent disease, making the distinction from acute disseminated encephalomyelitis especially difficult. In the large series presented by Kepes (1993), description was largely confined to the radiological appearances with little clinical detail.

Altered conscious level

It is rare for the level of consciousness to be disturbed in multiple sclerosis, except as part of terminal coma. Kurtzke (1970) believed that this is sometimes the result of unrecognized respiratory failure, but usually no immediate cause is evident. Bryan Matthews described (in a previous edition) a woman of 26 who died in a coma after a disease duration of only 4 months. Massive demyelination of the brainstem provided a reasonable explanation for the effect on conscious level. The pivotal case of M.H. Barnett and Prineas (2004) followed an equally accelerated course, dying at the age of 14 years after an illness lasting only 9 months. Castaigne *et al* (1966) described recurrent episodes of coma, accompanied by fever, apparently in the absence of infection, in patients with advanced multiple sclerosis. Recurrent stupor for a few days, accompanied by increased signs of brainstem involvement, is occasionally seen in severely disabled patients (Ringel *et al* 1988). Persistent or recurrent hypothermia (Ghawche and Destée 1990; Lammens *et al* 1989; F. Sullivan *et al* 1987; W.B. Matthews 1991) with confusion and stupor have been described in severely quadriplegic patients. Geny *et al* (1992) reported two cases of multiple sclerosis with hypothermia and Wernicke's encephalopathy, responding not to corticosteroids but to treatment with thiamine.

Paroxysmal symptoms

Perhaps no one of the more frequent manifestations is so often misinterpreted – even by experienced neurologists – as the paroxysmal manifestations of multiple sclerosis. Paroxysmal manifestations of multiple sclerosis are the clinical expression of well-defined physiological effects of demyelination on axonal conduction (see Chapter 13). Although several different types of episode are accepted as paroxysmal attacks, they share certain common features: they are brief, often stereotyped for the individual patient and typically occur many times each day over the period of several days or weeks during which each cluster is active. They are often triggered by movement, sensory stimulus, or overbreathing. Almost all are quickly abolished by anticonvulsants and other membrane-stabilizing drugs (see

Chapter 17). M. Eriksson *et al* (2002) found an overall frequency of 8.6% for the prevalence of paroxysmal symptoms at some point during the disease.

The symptoms appear suddenly and continue with great intensity for between days and a few months before remitting completely. Being short and stereotyped, these are often classified as epileptic seizures or transient ischaemic attacks. Conversely, they may be mistaken for new relapses – an astonishing error given the fact that very many may occur within any 24-hour period. Although individually brief, the time-scale of a cluster of paroxysmal symptoms is usually similar to a relapse of multiple sclerosis. Tüzün *et al* (2001) consider that the clusters tend to occur early in the course of multiple sclerosis. It is probable that less frequent attacks may escape recognition. A curious feature is the tendency for individual patients to have more than one form of paroxysm in the course of their disease – ataxia and tonic spasms, akinesia and tonic spasms, and trigeminal neuralgia and itching – each implicating different parts of the central nervous system. There is a racial predilection to paroxysmal symptoms which seem to be more prevalent in Oriental patients with multiple sclerosis (Shibasaki *et al* 1981).

Trigeminal neuralgia

That trigeminal neuralgia might be a symptom of multiple sclerosis was first recognized by H. Oppenheim (1911). Put the other way, there is general agreement that approximately 2% of people with trigeminal neuralgia have multiple sclerosis and 1% of individuals with multiple sclerosis will have trigeminal neuralgia (W. Harris 1950; Ruge *et al* 1958; J.G. Rushton and Olafson 1965). The age of onset is on average 5 years earlier than in the idiopathic form of *tic douloureux* (J.G. Rushton and Olafson 1965) and only rarely is it the first symptom of the disease (Hooge and Redekop 1995; Jensen *et al* 1982).

The nature of the pain does not differ from the idiopathic form except in being more often bilateral (W. Harris 1940) or less frequently triggered (Friedlander and Zeff 1974). The paroxysms have exceptionally been reported to be unusually prolonged (Jensen *et al* 1982). The course of trigeminal neuralgia in multiple sclerosis is not well described. Temporary remission may occur (Olafson *et al* 1966) in response to high-dose corticosteroids. Persistent spontaneous recovery has not been seen in personal cases.

Autopsy has shown plaques in the pons (Garcin *et al* 1960; Olafson *et al* 1966; H. Oppenheim 1911; H.L. Parker 1928) and there may be associated clinical evidence for brainstem disease (Jensen *et al* 1982), but neuralgia is not accompanied by sensory changes in the distribution of the trigeminal nerve, apart from occasional paraesthesiae (J.G. Rushton and Olafson 1965). Trigeminal neuralgia in multiple sclerosis is usually associated with MRI lesions affecting the dorsal root entry zone and without compression of the fifth cranial nerve by ectatic vessels (Gass *et al* 1997). However, we illustrate the exception to that rule in a patient with the unambiguous diagnosis of multiple sclerosis complicated by trigeminal neuralgia associated with multiple white matter abnormalities and a vascular loop compressing the fifth nerve (Figure 6.17A,B). In a recent study of partial trigeminal rhizotomy providing specimens from six patients with multiple sclerosis, a consistent finding was demyelination in the proximal part of the nerve root with clusters of juxtaposed naked axons without intervening glial processes. Such an arrangement is conducive to spontaneous impulse generation and ephaptic cross activation (Love *et al* 2001).

Dysarthria and ataxia

The combination of paroxysmal dysarthria and ataxia in multiple sclerosis was first described by H.L. Parker (1946), but attracted little attention until the much fuller account by Andermann *et al* (1959). The attacks are sudden in onset. Speech is slurred if the patient is talking at the time. This is accompanied by other symptoms, of which the commonest is ataxia, apparently of cerebellar type and usually unilateral, as far as can be determined in the brief period available for examination. Ataxia of gait may lead to falling. Sensory symptoms are also common, with paraesthesiae following a stereotyped pattern, for example involving one side of the face and the digits of the opposite hand. The symptoms can all be attributed to disordered function of the cerebellum and brainstem.

Attacks seldom last for >20 seconds and are usually very frequent. Our former colleague Bryan Matthews recalled a

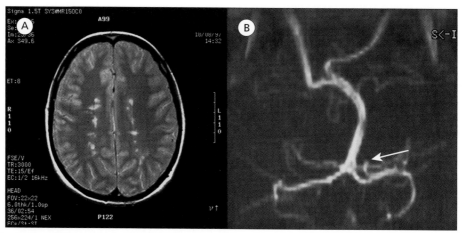

Figure 6.17 (A) Cranial MRI showing lesions consistent with multiple sclerosis and (B) magnetic resonance angiography in the same patient with trigeminal neuralgia indicating a vascular loop compressing the fifth nerve (arrow). Kindly provided by Dr Nagui Antoun.

patient insisting that, throughout the day, an attack occurred 'every alternate minute'. Many attacks appear to be precipitated by walking or talking. One of our patients believed that changing his train of thought provoked an attack. Like other forms of paroxysmal symptoms, attacks are readily induced by over-breathing often after only a few forced respirations.

In Bryan Matthews's personal series of 377 patients, paroxysmal ataxia, with or without dysarthria, occurred in 14 (4%). The paroxysms may occur as the initial symptom of multiple sclerosis (Perks and Lascelles 1976) and in the absence of abnormal physical signs (Twomey and Espir 1980), but are more usual in the course of the disease. It is probable that many instances are overlooked as they may be concealed by a complaint of dizziness, only to be revealed by close questioning and observation.

Tonic spasms

Bryan Matthews made special contributions to these enigmatic manifestations of multiple sclerosis, and first described tonic spasms (W.B. Matthews 1958). He recalled being repeatedly taken to task for using the word 'seizure' in the original description of this phenomenon as a symptom of multiple sclerosis, implying that it is a form of epilepsy but perusal of the discussion to his paper reveals that this was not the view. Epileptic attacks at that time were generally known as 'fits' and one could be 'seized' by conditions other than epilepsy – for example, apoplexy. However, that the term 'seizure' is not entirely inappropriate was dramatically demonstrated to Bryan Matthews by a young man who showed how tonic spasms were induced by using his hand to tie a shoe lace. Sadly, on this one occasion, the spasm led immediately to a generalized epileptic fit, presumably indicating that abnormal transmission had occurred at a cortical level. Although the term paroxysmal dystonia is now popular, 'tonic spasm' is greatly preferable.

These attacks are also often triggered by movement, particularly putting a foot to the ground. The spasm may be preceded by burning or tingling sensations, frequently affecting the limbs and trunk on the side opposite to the muscular spasm. The tonic contraction nearly always begins in one limb and spreads very rapidly to the arm or leg on the same side. Skilled movements such as writing may be interrupted (Figure 6.18A–C). Bilateral spasm is apparently common in Japan (Shibasaki and Kuroiwa 1974) but we have not encountered this variant. The posture adopted shows some variation but often closely resembles that seen in tetany. The face may be contorted involuntarily on the side of the spasm but, as the attack is often extremely painful, grimacing is difficult to interpret. These attacks generally last for no more than 2 minutes but they may be repeated very frequently (80 times in a day being recorded by one patient).

At 4%, the incidence of this symptom in Matthews's series was similar to that of paroxysmal ataxia. It may occur as the initial symptom (W.B. Matthews 1975). It has been reported in association with lesions demonstrated by MRI in the basal ganglia (Lugaresi *et al* 1993), internal capsule (Maimone *et al* 1991a; Spissu *et al* 1999; Waubant *et al* 2001), cerebral peduncle (Spissu *et al* 1999; Verheul and Tyssen 1990), thalamus (Burguera *et al* 1991) and spinal cord (Previdi and Buzzi 1992; Sozzi *et al* 1987). It has been suggested that, in the context of demyelination, the spasms result from ephaptic transmission

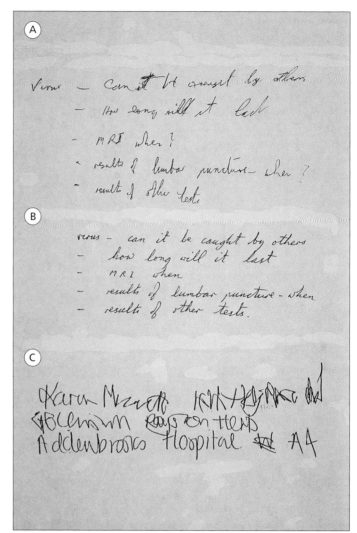

Figure 6.18 Transient disturbance of handwriting in patients with multiple sclerosis experiencing paroxysmal attacks. (A,B) During and outside an episode. '*virus – can it be caught by others – how long will it last – MRI when? – results of lumbar puncture when? – results of other tests*' (i.e. the usual questions of informed patients at the time of investigation!). (C) During an attack. '*Karen********* Royston Herts ****** Addenbrooke's Hospital AA*'.

between a sensory pathway and the corticospinal tract. Apparently this may occur at any level but this is not certain and the pathophysiology is discussed in more detail in Chapter 13. We do not believe that 'paroxysmal dystonia' in multiple sclerosis is a symptom reflecting involvement of the basal ganglia and view this as another paroxysmal disorder of brainstem origin.

Paroxysmal episodes may occur in isolated demyelinating syndromes. Figure 6.19 illustrates the extensive left cerebral hemisphere and right pontine lesions seen at presentation in a man aged 34 years who presented with subacute bilateral visual failure and drowsiness associated with excruciating paroxysmal attacks affecting the left side. These occurred many hundred times each day and were precipitated by each and every attempt at movement. They stopped with the use of carbamezapine. He became comatose, and later locked-in, but survived the acute illness albeit with considerable residual disabilities. The presumed diagnosis was acute disseminated encephalomyelitis.

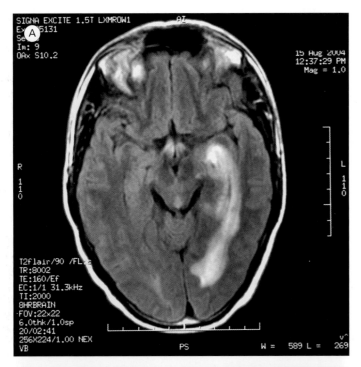

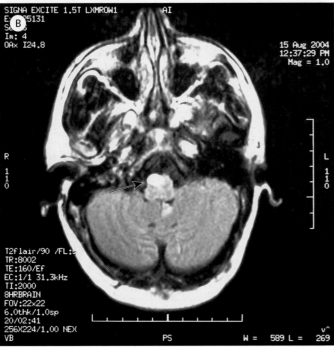

Figure 6.19 (A) Extensive right hemisphere abnormality in acute disseminated encephalomyelitis. (B) Pontine lesion in the same patient responsible for frequent paroxysmal tonic spasms (arrow).

Sensory symptoms and pain

Paroxysmal paraesthesiae, often unpleasant, may accompany dysarthria or tonic spasm but are less easy to identify when they occur in isolation. In a personal case (W.B. Matthews 1975), an extremely disturbing 'quivering' sensation in the right side of the face and right arm, occurring with great frequency in bouts lasting a few seconds, proved to be the first symptom of multiple sclerosis. Segmental burning dysaesthesiae are a common feature of multiple sclerosis in Japan (Yabuki and

Hayabara 1979). Paroxysmal pain characteristically involves a segment of one limb, usually the arm. The timing is different from that of the paroxysmal phenomena described above, as the duration of attacks is longer and the response to treatment with carbamazepine is unconvincing. It is probable that a different form of pathophysiology is involved.

Itching

Paroxysmal itching in multiple sclerosis was first described by Osterman (1976), although itching as an initial symptom was mentioned by McAlpine (1972). Subsequent reports have confirmed the episodic nature of the symptom although, as with pain, it is likely that the underlying mechanism differs from that thought to be responsible for brief paroxysmal symptoms. The attacks last for 20 minutes or longer and respond poorly to carbamazepine.

In Matthews's series of 377 patients, 17 had experienced itching, in one as an isolated initial symptom. Itching affected the upper limbs alone in eight, usually one shoulder region or a localized area of the forearm. The lower limbs were affected in five, most commonly one or both thighs. One patient had itching of the scalp. In the remaining three, more than one area was affected, including the trunk. In nine patients, changes in cutaneous sensation were present in the affected area. Paroxysms are often spontaneous but sometimes seem to be triggered by sensory stimulation or movement. The itching is intense, leading to vigorous but ineffective scratching to the extent of skin excoriation. One patient used a wire brush in an attempt to control the itch.

Diplopia

Diplopia may occur with other symptoms of brainstem disturbance in paroxysmal dysarthria, or as an isolated symptom (Osterman and Westerberg 1975), but it is difficult to recognize. Dysjunctive eye movement (W.B. Matthews 1975) and paroxysmal ocular flutter, responding to carbamazepine, are each described (D.A. Francis and Heron 1985). One of our patients (DASC) developed paroxysmal diplopia, occurring in isolation; each episode was provoked by movement, and these occurred every 2–3 minutes but lasted only a few seconds, during which there was no obvious abnormality of eye movement. The experience was distressing and socially disabling, but the response to carbamezapine was immediate.

Akinesia

Paroxysmal loss of use of one or more limbs is also encountered. This remarkable symptom is exemplified by a young man who complained of frequent sudden episodes of complete inability 'to take a further step'. In observed attacks he would stand quite still for a few seconds before moving on. The attacks were immediately abolished by carbamazepine. The lower limbs are more commonly affected (Castaigne et al 1970; W.B. Matthews 1975), usually simultaneously, but the attacks are so brief that it is not possible to ascertain the nature of this loss of function. Castaigne et al (1970) described a patient with paroxysmal akinesia of one arm triggered by playing the piano, providing a variant of the better known dystonic occupational cramps.

Other forms

Roos *et al* (1991) described a complex pattern of paroxysmal symptoms that they labelled 'kinesogenic choreoathetosis'. These attacks began as sudden freezing when walking but later progressed to include dysarthria and rotational posturing of the head and right limbs, lasting for 50 seconds. Todman (1988) described a young woman with a past history of optic neuritis who presented with paroxysms lasting 20 seconds and occurring every 3 minutes throughout the day. In these attacks there was absence of conjugate gaze to the left and the left eye could not move up or down. In addition, there was mild weakness of the right limbs with an extensor plantar reflex. There were no abnormal signs between the paroxysms. There was a rapid response to anticonvulsant treatment. Nonproductive coughing is a further possible paroxysmal symptom of multiple sclerosis (Jacôme 1985). As a final possible example, we have seen frequent, severely painful extensor spasms of both lower limbs in a patient paraplegic with multiple sclerosis resolve completely with a small dose of carbamazepine, a drug that is ineffective in the treatment of spasticity. A single case of symptomatic hyper-ekplexia (excessive startle reaction to sudden unexpected noise, movement, or touch) has been described in multiple sclerosis (Ruprecht *et al* 2002).

Narcolepsy

At first sight, it might seem rather improbable that narcolepsy could be a symptom of multiple sclerosis but, nevertheless, the two conditions have been reported in the same patient more often than is likely by chance. Ekbom (1966) described a remarkable series of cases of familial multiple sclerosis with narcolepsy and there have been a number of individual case reports (O. Berg and Hanley 1963; Carlander *et al* 2001; Grigoresco 1932; Schrader *et al* 1980; C.Y. Wang *et al* 1998; Younger *et al* 1991). In view of the close association of both conditions with the histocompatibility antigen DR2, it seemed probable that the association had a genetic explanation. Now the evidence is strengthened by the demonstration that narcolepsy, linked to DQB1*0602, is associated with a circulating autoanti-body that enhanced cholinergic activity after passive transfer to mice and is considered a good candidate for mediating injury of hypothalamic neurons responsible for the production of the neuropeptide hypocretin (orexin); hypocretin is involved in the sleep–wake cycles and levels are reduced in the cerebrospinal fluid of narcoleptics (A.J.F. Smith *et al* 2004). Hypersomnia may occur as a transient manifestation of hypothalamic involvement in multiple sclerosis with reduced cerebrospinal fluid hypocretin/orexin-A (as occurs in narcolepsy) during the period of increased sleepiness (Oka *et al* 2004).

Headache

In certain restricted circumstances, headache can be accepted as a symptom of multiple sclerosis – typically in acute optic neuritis or in the rare context of an inflammatory mass lesion affecting the cerebral hemispheres. Less well recognized but nevertheless highly characteristic is the intense posterior headache associated with active inflammatory demyelination affecting structures in the posterior fossa. In most other situations, headache reflects co-morbidity but a striking exception is the report by Galer *et al* (1990) of multiple sclerosis presenting with severe headache and a third nerve palsy. M.S. Freedman and Gray (1989) found that in 44/1113 patients, onset or relapse was heralded by headache that they regarded as of vascular type. Seventeen of these patients had a previous history of migraine. It has been suggested that migraine is unduly common in multiple sclerosis (Watkins and Espir 1966). Rolak and Brown (1990) found that 52% of people with multiple sclerosis had a history of recurrent headache, nearly always antedating disease onset by many years. The headache was not thought to be a symptom of the disease but the result of migraine or muscular contraction. The frequency was, however, much lower in other neurological diseases.

Optic neuritis

That the optic nerves are particularly vulnerable in multiple sclerosis was recognized towards the end of the 19th century by Parinaud (1884) and by Uhthoff (1889), who described both acute optic neuritis and the high incidence of optic atrophy in chronic disease.

Unilateral optic neuritis

The incidence of acute optic neuritis as the initial symptom of multiple sclerosis or as a manifestation of the first attack is well documented, an approximate figure for Europeans being 20%. The frequency of optic neuritis in the course of the disease is much more difficult to estimate because of the retrospective nature of the search for information obtained at an arbitrary interval after onset of the disease. Most such surveys refer to optic atrophy or visual failure and do not comment on identifiable episodes of optic neuritis. A further confounding factor is that symptomless involvement of the optic nerve is extremely common. This is well demonstrated by the frequent finding of abnormal visual evoked potentials in the unaffected eye in patients with unilateral optic neuritis or established multiple sclerosis (Halliday *et al* 1973a; 1973b; W.B. Matthews *et al* 1977; see also Chapters 1 and 13) and by evident optic atrophy in the absence of a history of acute visual loss. Optic neuritis certainly occurs in people with established multiple sclerosis but it is a comparatively rare event in the progressive stage of the disease.

The mean age at which otherwise idiopathic optic neuritis occurs is much the same as that which heralds the onset of multiple sclerosis (Ebers 1985a). The special problem of optic neuritis in childhood is discussed below. Isolated optic neuritis developing >50 years becomes increasingly difficult to distinguish from ischaemic neuropathy (J.F. Rizzo and Lessell 1991) but, when clearly identified, the clinical features and implications do not differ from those of optic neuritis in younger adults (D.M. Jacobson *et al* 1988). The sex distribution is that of multiple sclerosis, with female preponderance (M.M. Cohen *et al* 1979; W.M. Hutchinson 1976; Isayama *et al* 1982).

Optic neuritis occurs with approximately the same frequency in the two eyes (Kurland *et al* 1966; Perkin and Rose 1979; Rischbieth 1968). Bilateral simultaneous optic neuritis must be considered separately as probably having different connotations (see below). Pain may precede or accompany the onset of visual symptoms and has been reported in varying proportions in around 90% of patients, although it is usually mild. The pain is usually described as being 'in the eye', often aggravated by eye movement, and may be felt in the frontal region. It is attributed to stretch of the dural sheath around an inflamed and swollen optic nerve. Presumably its duration, and tendency to precede visual loss, indicate the sequence of inflammation and axonal injury affecting the optic nerve (and other sites in the brain and spinal cord). The pain is occasionally distressingly severe and accompanied by generalized headache. Pain is significantly more common in retrobulbar neuritis, where there is no abnormality of the optic disc (Lepore 1991).

The onset of impaired vision is often described as sudden, though careful questioning almost always reveals that the patient noticed a partial defect that then worsened over hours or days. Quite often, it is first noticed on waking from sleep. Visual loss in one eye, however, may escape notice until the normal eye is fortuitously closed. Precise timing is not always accurate. The defect is certainly often progressive but usually for not more than a week. Documented deterioration for >2 weeks should throw doubt on the diagnosis. The initial visual complaint is usually of blurred vision rather than awareness of the scotoma that may later develop. Visual acuity, as measured on the Snellen chart or equivalent, varies from normality (Frederiksen *et al* 1991a) to complete blindness. In two large detailed studies (Optic Neuritis Study Group 1991; Slamovits *et al* 1991) 3% and 11% of patients had 6/6 (20/20 in the United States) vision and 8% in each series had complete loss of vision. A common finding is acuity of 6/24 or worse. When reasonable acuity is preserved, dulling of colour vision is often remarked upon by the patient.

Several optic disc abnormalities occur in optic neuritis. The optic disc appears normal in about two-thirds of affected eyes (Optic Neuritis Study Group 1991) and shows varying degrees of swelling in the remainder (Figure 6.20A). Fine haemorrhages radiating from the disc (Figure 6.20B) are seen in about 6%. Perivenous sheathing (Figure 6.20C) may be detected but is not specifically related to the optic nerve lesion (Lightman *et al* 1987). As discussed in Chapter 13, retinal grooves or slits attributable to axonal loss in the retinal nerve fibre layer, and corresponding to arcuate field defects, may be seen after single episodes or recurrent optic neuritis (see Figure 13.43).The visual field defect is classically a central scotoma but there is much variation (Bradley and Whitty 1967; Nikoskelainen 1975) and in a large, carefully studied series, a central or centrocoecal scotoma was found on presentation in only 8% (Keitner *et al* 1993). Interestingly, a field defect was found in 69% of unaffected eyes. The pattern may change as the neuritis develops and altitudinal defects are common (W.I. McDonald and Barnes 1992; Optic Neuritis Study Group 1991). With lesions placed at the posterior part of the optic nerve, fibres decussating from the opposite side that loop into the optic nerve before passing into the optic tract may be affected, and the astute observer may be able to detect a junctional scotoma but this is rarely symptomatic.

The afferent limb of the pupillary direct light reflex is interrupted by a lesion of the optic nerve. With gross loss of acuity, the pupil contracts over a small range on exposure to bright light. The Marcus Gunn phenomenon (otherwise known as a relative afferent pupillary defect and detected by the swinging light test) is often present. When the light is shone into the affected pupil, and the normal eye is then covered, the illuminated pupil contracts slightly and then dilates, in response to the exclusion of light from the unaffected eye. This may also be shown by rapidly swinging the light from one eye to the other whereupon the pupil dilates from the position established by consensual contraction already induced by illuminating the normal eye. However, nothing is perfect in neurology and we can offer no sensible explanation for the description of monocular blindness in a patient with multiple sclerosis in whom the direct and consensual pupillary light reflexes were preserved (F. Lhermitte *et al* 1984).

In acute optic neuritis with severe loss of acuity, no response can usually be evoked to pattern reversal stimulation although flash responses may be obtainable. With less severe visual loss, a greatly delayed low-amplitude response can sometimes be obtained, although fixation may be impossible. Occasionally, a normal response can be recorded even in the acute stage when vision is still impaired (W.B. Matthews *et al* 1977; see also Chapters 7 and 13).

It is the rule for good visual acuity to be regained after a first attack of optic neuritis, although there are exceptions. The mean time to reach 6/6 vision, in those who achieved this degree of recovery, was 8 weeks in one series (Perkin and Rose 1979). In another (Bradley and Whitty 1967), 50% of patients had recovered to 6/9 or better by 1 month. The mean time to reach optimal acuity has been found to be 2 months (Earl and Martin 1967). In a detailed prospective study of 20 patients, however, Celesia *et al* (1990) noted that acuity could continue to improve for up to 6 months. Acuity remains ≤6/12 in approximately 14% of eyes and ≤6/60 in 5% (Perkin and Rose 1979). The prognosis for good recovery of vision is influenced by the degree of initial visual loss. Five of 12 patients with loss of light perception recovered normal acuity, but four were left with a dense central scotoma (Slamovits *et al* 1991). Celesia *et al* (1990) also found that severe initial visual loss was followed by permanent visual impairment in 60% of eyes. Factors associated with a good prognosis for eventual recovery are a short lesion on MRI using triple dose gadolinium enhancement, higher VEP amplitude during the acute phase, and early improvement in acuity (Hickman *et al* 2004a).

Recovery of normal acuity does not necessarily equate to full recovery of function, nor complete freedom from symptoms. Contrast sensitivity and colour vision are often not fully restored (Mullen and Plant 1986; Regan *et al* 1977), leading to a common complaint of slight dulling of the visual image. Other residual complaints include intolerance of bright light and difficulty in judging distances. Movement phosphenes, flashes of bright light induced by eye movement (Figure 6.21) may occur in the acute stage of optic neuritis (F.A. Davis *et al* 1976), but more frequently during the recovery phase (see also Earl 1964; Chapter 13).

Uhthoff (1889) described temporary blurring of vision induced by exercise in patients with multiple sclerosis. It is now recognized that this is a manifestation of the adverse effect of a minute increase in body temperature on many symptoms of the disease (see also Chapter 13). It is seldom noticed during the acute phase of optic neuritis but is common during recovery, occurring in 50% in one series, usually within 2 months of onset (Scholl *et al* 1991). It is sometimes the only symptom of optic

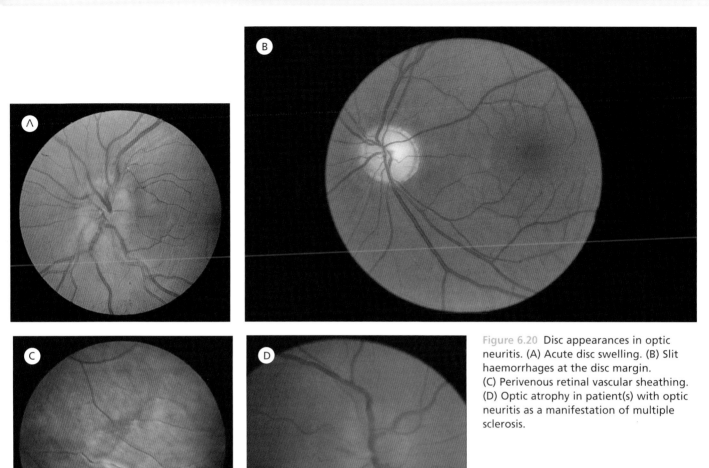

Figure 6.20 Disc appearances in optic neuritis. (A) Acute disc swelling. (B) Slit haemorrhages at the disc margin. (C) Perivenous retinal vascular sheathing. (D) Optic atrophy in patient(s) with optic neuritis as a manifestation of multiple sclerosis.

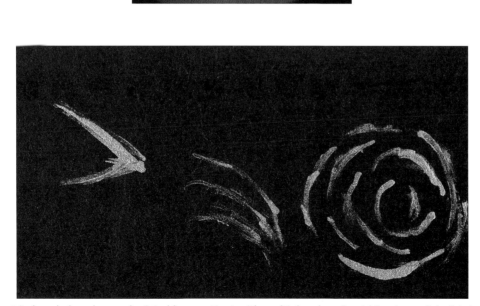

Figure 6.21 Movement-induced phosphenes depicted by a patient with multiple sclerosis wishing to explain this 'unexpected' symptom.

nerve disease, in the absence of a history of previous neuritis. Exercise, a hot bath or meal, smoking and emotional disturbance have all been found to produce this effect. When bilateral, it can be quite disabling as vision may be impaired for as long as 45 minutes after a hot bath or for 20 minutes after a short stroll. Although highly suggestive of demyelinating disease, similar symptoms may occur with other forms of disease affecting the anterior visual pathways (Lepore 1994).

Temporal pallor of the optic disc, either as a sequel to recognized optic neuritis or as a sign of clinically silent optic nerve damage, is frequent in the chronic stages but is often a subjective sign and 'in the eye of the beholder' (Figure 6.20D). Several sources of error contribute to the ambiguity of detecting disc atrophy. The temporal half of the disc is normally paler than the nasal side. The disc in myopic eyes is pale. More important is considerable observer disagreement over this necessarily subjective sign. It should never be cited in isolation as evidence of multiple lesions of the nervous system. In practice, pallor of the nasal side of the disc is a more reliable indicator of pathology than temporal pallor alone. Pallor of the entire disc is also often seen. Exactly what constitutes optic atrophy in lists of signs of multiple sclerosis is difficult to determine. In other contexts, this term is taken to mean impaired vision with pale atrophic discs, but in multiple sclerosis disc pallor is frequent with normal visual acuity. If atrophy is taken to mean simply disc pallor, then this was found to be present following a single attack of optic neuritis in 76% of eyes that had recovered normal acuity (E.A.C.M. Sanders and Arts 1986) and to be twice as common in eyes known to have been affected by optic neuritis as in eyes not so affected (Honan et al 1990). 'Slits' in the nerve fibre layer, best seen close to the disc margin using red-free light, are common following optic neuritis. They represent loss of bundles of axons (see Chapter 13 and Figure 13.43; Frisen and Hoyt 1974; J.A. Sharpe and Sanders 1975), and for the experienced clinician provide a useful sign of optic nerve damage.

Persistent abnormality of colour vision can frequently be detected on testing (Asselman et al 1975; A.C. Harrison et al 1987; Rosen 1965). Subjectively, the complaint is usually loss of brightness but occasionally an inability to match colours, as in a personal case (WIMcD) of an assistant in a shop selling wool for tapestry. Occasional patients do not adjust to the loss of colour vision and find the uniform hues of the changing weather and seasons psychologically disturbing. One of our patients (DASC) sought psychiatric help and sophisticated rehabilitation from visual psycho-physicists to cope with her distress at failing to perceive the greenness of green in springtime grass. We have illustrated and described other subjective experiences of altered colour vision in artists affected by optic neuritis in Chapter 1.

It is not clear how far persistent peripheral defects in the visual fields contribute to continued complaints of fogged vision in the presence of normal central acuity (V.H. Patterson and Heron 1980) and defects in contrast sensitivity are almost certainly more important (Regan et al 1977). Evidence of damage to the anterior visual pathways is not confined to patients with a history of optic neuritis since similar persistent defects are present, although in a smaller proportion, in patients not known to have experienced acute visual symptoms. This is the basis for using visual evoked potentials in the diagnosis of multiple sclerosis. Honan et al (1990) found at least one abnormality of visual function in 92% of patients with a history of optic neuritis and in 73% of those with no such history, but did not relate their findings to the occurrence of symptoms. In a prospective study, Celesia et al (1990) found that visual function, as judged by acuity, returned to normal in 65% of their patients. An afferent pupillary defect may persist after recovery from the acute stage in approximately 50% of eyes (Honan et al 1990). Occasionally patients describe difficulty with depth perception leading to impaired performance in table tennis or golf. Some patients have difficulty in judging the speed of oncoming traffic and thus experience difficulty in crossing the road. The mechanism of these symptoms, possibly related to the Pulfrich phenomenon, is discussed in Chapter 13.

Conversion to multiple sclerosis after optic neuritis

Many attempts to provide answers to the question of how often optic neuritis is a presenting symptom of multiple sclerosis have been seriously flawed. Kurtzke (1985a) was inclined to dismiss all claims claiming a rate of >40%. Criteria for the diagnosis of multiple sclerosis have not been standardized and some surveys have included in the outcome 'possible' cases of multiple sclerosis (Bradley and Whitty 1968; ; D.A.S. Compston et al 1978; Nikoskelainen and Riekkenen 1974; F.C. Rose 1970). The great majority of studies have been retrospective, based on discovering the subsequent course of patients previously known to have attended hospital with optic neuritis (Bradley and Whitty 1968; D.A.S. Compston et al 1978; D.A. Francis et al 1987b). Series reporting rates of progression as high as 85% (Lynn 1959) are frequently cited (for example, Francis et al 1987b; McAlpine 1972) but have never been fully described. Further confusion arises from the inclusion of patients already presenting clinical signs of disseminated disease (W.M. Hutchinson 1976; Landy 1983; Rischbieth 1968). It has been common to report the proportion of patients successfully traced who developed multiple sclerosis, and not of the whole series (Francis et al 1987b). Kurzke's own figure is the lowest rate of progression reported in patients of European origin (13%), but was derived solely from males (Kurland et al 1966), leading to the suggestion that the series may have been contaminated by cases of central serous retinopathy (Ebers 1985a). A prospective study from Japan (Isayama et al 1982) included bilateral simultaneous optic neuritis and this variant is known to have a different prognosis (Hierons and Lyle 1959; Parkin et al 1984).

If conclusions are based solely on studies that have avoided most of the pitfalls outlined above, the available information is much reduced. In the series reported first by M.M. Cohen et al (1979) and later by Rizzo and Lessell (1988), the diagnosis of optic neuritis was clearly examined critically. The study was prospective and very few patients were not traced. At a mean of 15 years, 58% of cases had developed multiple sclerosis (52% of the whole series). Sandberg-Wollheim et al (1990), in a long-term prospective study, found that 33/86 patients had developed clinically definite multiple sclerosis within 7–18 years from the initial episode of optic neuritis and they calculated the risk of progression within 15 years as 45%. This cohort has recently been reassessed (Nilsson et al 2005). It is of great interest that only one more patient has developed multiple sclerosis. Thus, after a follow up of 30 years the overall risk of developing multiple sclerosis is 40%. Actuarial analysis also computed the frequency of multiple sclerosis after optic neuritis in an Australian cohort at 52% (Frith *et al* 2000).

The only possible flaw in these three genuinely prospective studies is that they were of patients attending hospital. Population surveys have recorded lower rates – 17% progression over a mean of 18 years in Rochester, United States (Percy *et al* 1972) and 19% of traced patients over a mean of 9 years in Finland (Kinnunen 1983). Why the results of hospital and population surveys should be so different is far from obvious, but most of the patients seeking advice about recurrent neurological symptoms will be attending hospital and presumably it is the higher rates of progression that are relevant in such cases.

The interval between optic neuritis and the onset of disseminated disease varies from a few weeks to >20 years (Adie 1930; Mackay 1953) or even 37 years (McAlpine and Compston 1952). There is considerable evidence, however, that progression occurs more commonly after a relatively brief interval (Bradley and Whitty 1968; Hely *et al* 1986b; Hyllested 1966; Landy 1983). For example, Sandberg-Wollheim *et al* (1990) found that of the 33 examples of progression to multiple sclerosis in their series, 10 occurred within the first year, seven in the second, and three in the third. Unfortunately, multiple sclerosis continues to develop at a much reduced but approximately steady rate (M.M. Cohen *et al* 1979; D.A.S. Compston *et al* 1978; Francis *et al* 1987b; W.M. Hutchinson 1976; Parkin *et al* 1984; Rizzo and Lessell 1988) and at no point can it be stated that the risk has vanished.

In assessing risk factors, it is now possible to take into account abnormalities on MRI occurring in the absence of new symptoms but having predictive value for subsequent clinical conversion. In practice, these MRI abnormalities become relevant in three situations: the presence of cerebral MRI lesions accompanying an isolated episode of optic neuritis; optic neuritis occurring as the dominant or exclusive manifestation of acute disseminated encephalomyelitis (Dunn *et al* 1986; Kesselring *et al* 1990); and brain MRI lesions developing during the asymptomatic follow-up of the person with optic neuritis. Cerebral MRI abnormalities were seen in 34/53 patients with isolated optic neuritis (Miller *et al* 1988a). Over a mean period of 1 year, 12 developed disseminated clinical disease and a further seven showed new lesions without clinical relapse. In contrast, none of the 19 patients in whom MRI was initially normal developed multiple sclerosis in this period although, in three, new lesions were seen. Five years later, 75% of those with silent MRI lesions, but only 10% with an initial normal scan, had developed multiple sclerosis (W.I. McDonald and Barnes 1992; Morrissey *et al* 1993). We discuss in more detail, and illustrate the role of imaging the optic nerve and cerebrum in optic neuritis (and other clinically isolated syndromes) in anticipating the diagnosis of multiple sclerosis, in Chapter 7.

Abnormalities in the cerebrospinal fluid are also of prognostic value. Stendahl-Brodin and Link (1983) reported that 11/30 patients with isolated optic neuritis had oligoclonal immunoglobulin G in the cerebrospinal fluid. Six years later, nine had developed multiple sclerosis, compared with only 1/19 without oligoclonal bands. In another study (Sandberg-Wollheim *et al* 1990), 25 patients presenting with optic neuritis, who had not developed clinical multiple sclerosis, were examined by MRI 7–18 years later. Nine of the 13 in whom an increased cell count or oligoclonal bands had been found in cerebrospinal fluid at

initial examination had cerebral abnormalities on subsequent MRI. In a subsequent series of 146 patients assessed within 7 years of acute optic neuritis, Söderström *et al* (1998) also identified MRI abnormalities, oligoclonal bands and the presence of human leucocyte antigen (HLA) DR2 as risk factors for the development of multiple sclerosis. The association could not be explained by differences in immune cytokine phenotype (Kivisakk *et al* 1998a). Of the 12 with normal spinal fluid, only two had such lesions. Jin *et al* (2003) have reported a prospective study in which the highest probability (0.66) of developing multiple sclerosis occurred in patients with ≥3 brain MRI lesions and oligoclonal bands in the cerebrospinal fluid at presentation, and the lowest (0.09) in those without these features. Nilsson *et al* (2005) reported that the rate of conversion is significantly increased if inflammatory findings are present in cerebrospinal fluid at onset.

In patients recruited for the Optic Neuritis Treatment Trial (see below and Chapter 16) who underwent spinal fluid analysis at presentation, the presence of oligoclonal bands carried a relative risk of 1.3 (95% CI 1.1–1.7) for developing multiple sclerosis within 2 years, being present in 11 of the 13/89 who converted. However, MRI abnormalities were more discriminating predictors of widespread demyelination in this group. Jetta Frederiksen (1999) is engaged in a prospective, community-based long-term follow-up of 283 patients with acute optic neuritis in which extensive MRI, electrophysiological and cerebrospinal fluid observations are being made from the time of presentation; the patients have been HLA typed. Data are currently available for only 1 year so far and the results are similar to those of other North European investigators. The prevalence was 1.8 per 100 000. In acute monocular optic neuritis (223 cases) the presence of one abnormal paraclinical test at onset significantly increased the risk for development of clinically definite multiple sclerosis. Bilateral acute optic neuritis was much less common (30 cases), especially in women and was less often associated with abnormal paraclinical tests at presentation, in keeping with earlier suggestions that there are causes (including Leber's hereditary optic neuropathy) other than multiple sclerosis for this syndrome.

There is no good agreement on whether the treatment of optic neuritis with methylprednisolone increases the risk of progressive and disseminated disease (Herishanu *et al* 1989; R.W. Beck *et al* 1993a; R.W. Beck 1993b). The effect of intravenous methylprednisolone for 3 days, followed by oral steroids for 11 days, was compared with that of oral steroids for 14 days. In the first group, 8% of patients developed definite multiple sclerosis within 2 years of the attack of optic neuritis, compared with 15% in those given only oral steroids and 17% in the placebo group. The greatest beneficial effect was observed in those with cerebral MRI abnormalities at onset and hence those most at risk. It is not easy to understand how treatment for 3 days, not necessarily started immediately after onset, could exert an effect for 2 years, and the increased incidence of recurrent optic neuritis in patients treated with oral steroids compared with controls is also unexpected. It is not therefore surprising to find that with further follow-up there was no difference in the frequency of multiple sclerosis between those treated with intravenous or oral corticosteroids, or placebo. In the most recent analysis, 30% of the 308 patients enrolled between 1988 and 1991 converted to clinically definite multiple sclerosis but there was no difference in rate between the groups depending on treatment. Visual outcome at 5 years was also no different between groups: 6% of all patients had poor visual recovery; optic neuritis occurred in 28%; this carried an increased risk for multiple sclerosis and was more common in those who did not convert if treated at presentation with oral prednisolone (Optic Neuritis Study Group 1997a; 1997b). MRI lesions at presentation indicated a much increased risk of developing multiple sclerosis. Conversely, all 185 patients with normal imaging appearances, lack of pain, relative preservation of acuity and a swollen disc carried a relatively good prognosis for conversion to multiple sclerosis. The presence of Uhthoff's symptom correlates with an increased risk both of multiple sclerosis and recurrent optic neuritis during a mean of 3.5 years after an initial attack (Scholl et al 1991).

Other factors reported at one time or another to increase the risk of progression include young age of onset (M.M. Cohen et al 1979; Hely et al 1986b; Sandberg-Wollheim et al 1990), female sex (Kinnunen 1983; Rizzo and Lessell 1988), early recurrence of optic neuritis (Sandberg-Wollheim 1990) and the presence of venous sheathing (Lightman et al 1987). Factors found to be without significant effect include relatively advanced age (D.M. Jacobson et al 1988), laterality (Hely et al 1986b), pain (Bradley and Whitty 1968), degree of visual loss and recovery (Bradley and Whitty 1968; M.M. Cohen et al 1979; Kurland et al 1966) and papillitis (M.M. Cohen et al 1979). There has been disagreement on the influence of the month of onset of optic neuritis on subsequent events; some have found optic neuritis in the summer months to be more predictive of multiple sclerosis (W.M. Hutchinson 1976; Taub and Rucker 1954), while others have detected no effect (Bradley and Whitty 1968; Kurland et al 1966; Perkin and Rose 1979). D.A.S. Compston et al (1978) and Nilsson et al (2005) found that optic neuritis in the winter increased the risk of multiple sclerosis (especially in individuals at increased genetic risk through having HLA DR2: see Chapter 3). The same seasonal risk is reported from Japan (Isayama et al 1982). Nilsson et al (2005) also showed an increased risk following recurrence of optic neuritis, in younger patients and those with winter onset.

Recurrent optic neuritis, in the same or opposite eye, is common, but reports do not always distinguish recurrence before and after the onset of disseminated symptoms. Excluding optic neuritis occurring after the onset of multiple lesions, Rizzo and Lessell (1988) reported a recurrence rate of 35% over a mean of 15 years. Francis et al (1987b) found recurrence in 36% of patients traced (representing 25% of the original 146 patients) after a mean period of 12 years. Over the shorter period of 2 years, the recurrence rate in either eye was 20% (R.W. Beck et al 1993a; 1993b). A single attack in each eye is rather more common than two separate episodes in the same eye (Perkin and Rose 1979), but optic neuritis can occasionally occur repeatedly on both sides, especially in the context of Devic's disease. The prognosis for recovery of acuity to 6/9 or better after more than one unilateral episode is reduced to 69% (W.M. Hutchinson 1976; Perkin and Rose 1979).

Recurrent optic neuritis, without known cause, is accepted by Ebers (1985a) as justifying a diagnosis of multiple sclerosis. It was originally reported in two series as increasing the risk of disseminated disease (M.M. Cohen et al 1979; D.A.S. Compston et al 1978) but this was not confirmed on extended follow up

(Francis et al 1987b; Rizzo and Lessell 1988) of each cohort, in conformity with other series (Hely et al 1986b; W.M. Hutchinson 1976). Unfortunately, even when all prognostic indications are favourable, it is never possible to exclude the possibility of progression to disseminated disease sufficient to establish the diagnosis of multiple sclerosis.

Bilateral optic neuritis

A distinction must be made between bilateral sequential optic neuritis and bilateral neuritis with simultaneous onset in the two eyes. We have already made the point that it is relatively common for the second eye to be affected. The interval may be relatively brief. Bradley and Whitty (1967) reported this as occurring within 3 months in 19% of their patients and Hely et al (1986b) in 11% within 4 weeks. It is doubtful whether this pattern of successive attacks influences the risk of developing multiple sclerosis. Kurland et al (1966) and Bradley and Whitty (1967) found no such effect, whereas W.M. Hutchinson (1976) reported a slightly increased risk.

Bilateral simultaneous optic neuritis occurs in acute disseminated encephalomyelitis and is rarely followed by relapse. Hierons and Lyle (1959) reported a series of cases with bilateral optic neuritis and these were reviewed 25 years later (Parkin et al 1984). Of the six adults with acute simultaneous bilateral optic neuritis, one had died with neuromyelitis optica and one was thought to have had early probable multiple sclerosis but died from other causes at the age of 76 years. None of the others developed multiple sclerosis. Twenty patients had bilateral sequential optic neuritis within 3 months and of these seven were known to have developed multiple sclerosis. The numbers are small and it has been suggested that Leber's optic atrophy could not have been excluded at that time (W.I. McDonald and Barnes 1992). A recent follow-up of 23 cases with acute or subacute simultaneous bilateral optic neuropathy revealed that after a mean of 71 months, four were shown by genetic analysis to have Leber's mutation and five had developed multiple sclerosis, the rest remaining undiagnosed (Morrissey et al 1995). The conclusion that simultaneous involvement of the two eyes is less likely to progress to disseminated disease is contrary to that reached by W.M. Hutchinson (1976).

Although progressive decline in visual acuity, unassociated with acute optic neuritis, is documented in multiple sclerosis (Kahana et al 1973; W.B. Matthews and Small 1979), no large longitudinal study has been published. Ashworth (1957) reported nine cases of chronic optic neuritis, and progressive visual failure as the initial presentation of multiple sclerosis has been carefully documented. Onset was unilateral in the five cases described by Ormerod and McDonald (1984), but the other eye was affected later – usually before the onset of disseminated symptoms. The real possibility of diagnostic error in such rare cases was emphasized, especially the need to exclude local structural lesions. Since then, a new syndrome has come to be recognized (see Chapters 3 and 8). This is the multiple sclerosis-like illness associated with mutations of mitochondrial DNA and manifesting as central nervous system demyelination with disproportionate involvement of the optic nerves. Our proposal in the last edition of this book that the condition be known as 'Harding's disease' in memory of the late Anita Harding seems to have found favour. Harding et al (1992) described eight women who presented with bilateral visual loss, six of whom also developed an illness indistinguishable from multiple sclerosis. All had matrilineal relatives with Leber's hereditary optic neuropathy. Visual loss was bilateral, often simultaneous, though sometimes sequential, and was usually rapid, though could be progressive over about a month. The ocular findings were characteristic of an acute optic neuropathy. What was unusual was that in all but one case there was no improvement and the patient remained with severe bilateral visual loss, usually in the range between counting fingers and acuity of 6/60. In one patient examined in the acute phase, there was hyperaemia of the optic disc on the affected side with a small haemorrhage and some retinal oedema. The fully developed fundal features of Leber's hereditary optic neuropathy (hyperaemia of the disc, telangiectasia of the nearby retinal vessels, and dilated and tortuous retinal veins) were not seen in any patient. However, some of the cases were seen before these changes were well known, and others were examined >1 month after the onset of the visual disturbance, by which time the vascular changes of Leber's disease have often resolved. In some patients, the extra-ocular neurological episode preceded the visual loss, whereas it followed the optic neuropathy in others. The early episodes remitted, but secondary progression occurred in two patients. The visual evoked potentials were, as expected, grossly degraded in patients with severe visual impairment; in the patient whose visual acuity recovered to 6/9 (right) and 6/6 (left), the visual evoked potentials were delayed. The cerebrospinal fluid was examined in three of the six patients with disseminated neurological abnormalities. In one it was normal and in the other two there was evidence of increased globulin production. MRI, performed in five of the patients with a multiple sclerosis-like illness, and in the two others with optic neuropathy alone, showed widespread white matter lesions characteristic of (though not specific to) multiple sclerosis.

Although bilateral concurrent optic neuritis is relatively common in Japan, and rarely followed by multiple sclerosis (Isayama *et al* 1982), to some extent this claim relates to the ambiguous nosological status of neuromyelitis optica (Devic's disease: see Chapter 5). Until recently, the diagnosis of Devic's disease (neuromyelitis optica) was reserved for patients with a single episode of spinal cord and optic nerve or chiasmal disease, occurring in either order. Now, it is recognized that both the optic nerve and spinal cord features may recur – sometimes on several occasions – but without clinical involvement elsewhere in the central nervous system. MRI typically shows a long diffuse spinal abnormality, quite unlike the discrete circumscribed lesions of multiple sclerosis, and with high signal in the optic nerves or chiasm but a conspicuous absence of brain lesions. Whilst there is often an excess of white cells, the cerebrospinal fluid is conspicuous for the relative absence of oligoclonal bands (Ghezzi et al 2004; Wingerchuk *et al* 1999). In the original series of cases with Devic's disease, the prognosis was poor and autopsy showed a single spinal focus of acute necrotic myelitis together with optic nerve lesions (Devic 1894; Miyazawa *et al* 2002). Pathologically, the extensive spinal lesions are associated with necrosis and cavitation, acute axonal injury, loss of oligodendrocytes, inflammatory infiltrates and perivascular deposition of immunoglobulin (IgM) and complement. These are the features of a predominantly T helper type 2 immune response

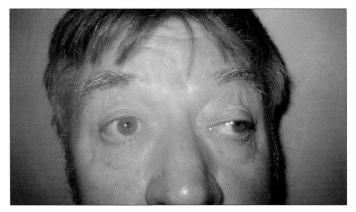

Figure 6.22 Internuclear ophthalmoplegia in a patient presenting with progressive visual failure not associated with a mutation of mitochondrial DNA and attributed to primary progressive multiple sclerosis.

with prominent humoral mechanisms (see Chapter 12: Lucchinetti *et al* 2002). The important therapeutic implication of these analyses is that affected individuals may respond usefully to plasma exchange (see Chapter 16: Weinshenker *et al* 1999b). However, classification remains difficult. Figure 6.22 illustrates asymptomatic (bilateral) internuclear ophthalmoplegia in a patient presenting with severe progressive bilateral visual failure (visual acuities reduced to <6/36 in each eye) but no other presenting features: however, MRI showed multiple white matter abnormalities and the cerebrospinal fluid contained oligoclonal bands; there were no pathological mutations of mitochondrial DNA despite extensive sequencing. Several years later, his balance deteriorated and the diagnosis of primary progressive multiple sclerosis with manifestations confined to the anterior visual pathway and brainstem–cerebellar connections was preferred.

Onset with optic neuritis has been variously reported as adversely affecting the prognosis of multiple sclerosis (Poeck and Markus 1964), linked to a benign course (Kraft *et al* 1981; Phadke 1990; Poser *et al* 1982b), or being without effect (Leibowitz and Alter 1968; Shepherd 1979). E.A.C.M. Sanders and Arts (1986) found the initial course following isolated optic neuritis to be benign but could not detect any long term influence following this mode of onset. They attributed this effect to the relatively long remission after optic neuritis occurring in their series on average 5 years earlier than other presenting symptoms. It is probable that the initial, commonly mild clinical course, does not differ from that following other monosymptomatic forms of onset, such as a brainstem lesion or sensory symptoms (Phadke 1990).

Other lesions of the visual pathway

In a series of papers, Rucker (1944a; 1944b; 1947) gave a detailed description of retinal venous sheathing – periphlebitis retinae – and emphasized the particular association of this abnormality with multiple sclerosis, being present in some 10% of cases at the time of examination. The characteristic appearance is that of a white line on either side of a stretch of vein, not closely approaching the optic nerve head. Haarr (1963) thought that this chronic state was preceded by a more active form in which rounded exudates can be seen around dilated veins

(Fig 6.20C). Single exudates might resolve within a few weeks and the active stage could be observed to persist for up to 2 years, to be followed either by the chronic condition or complete resolution. Engell (1986) in a study of 136 hospital patients and 168 patients at a rehabilitation centre reported that venous sheathing was much more common in active or severe disease, being found in 43% of patients in relapse or with rapidly progressive disease, 5% with slow progression and only 1% of patients with static disease or in remission. He also stated that periphlebitis retinae might persist for a few weeks only, but provided no supporting evidence for this. The chronic changes much more frequently observed are known to persist for up to 2 years (Arnold *et al* 1984) and in one instance for 14 years (Fog 1965).

Histological examination has usually shown perivenous cuffing with lymphocytes and plasma cells (Engell *et al* 1985; P.J. Shaw *et al* 1987), but this appearance is not confined to the active clinical stage, as described by Haarr (1963). In a case where sheathing had persisted for many years unchanged, the cellular response was slight and the main finding was dense collagenous thickening of the venous walls, the arteries being unaffected (Fog 1965). It is certainly tempting to equate these vascular changes with those in recent and chronic multiple sclerosis plaques (Arnold *et al* 1984; Fog 1965). If this is so, it is perhaps surprising that there is so little evidence for remission of periphlebitis retinae. The fact that there is no myelin in the area of the retina affected strongly suggests that the primary lesion is in the vascular endothelium. Why the retinal veins should be selectively affected is not explained. That said, blood vessels in tissues beyond the central nervous system have not been systematically examined.

There are reports indicating that sheathing occurs in 10–40% of patients with multiple sclerosis (Møller and Hammerberg 1963; Orban 1955; Wybar 1952; R.B. Young 1976). Some series have been compared with sex- and age-matched normal subjects, in whom no sheathing occurred. Engell and Andersen (1982), by an ingenious calculation based on the reported incidence and duration of venous sheathing and the duration of multiple sclerosis, concluded that it probably occurred in all cases at some time. Fluorescein angiography will frequently demonstrate leaking of dye from the veins (R.B. Young 1976).

Venous sheathing was found in 6/50 patients with isolated optic neuritis by Lightman *et al* (1987). In four, fluorescein angiography showed leakage at the site of sheathing, but venous leakage also occurred in six eyes in which sheathing had not been detected. In six patients, cells were seen in the vitreous or anterior chamber, in two of whom this was the only abnormality. No additional ocular disease was found. The abnormalities were present bilaterally or solely in the eye contralateral to the optic neuritis in five patients. Sheathing is often missed by the neurologist because it usually occurs at the periphery of the retina and can only be seen with pupillary dilation and the indirect ophthalmoscope. In a personal series (WIMcD) of 50 cases with optic neuritis, sheathing was visible at the posterior pole without pupillary dilatation in only one of six instances (Lightman *et al* 1987).

Periphlebitis retinae is not, however, specific for multiple sclerosis. It is known to occur in association with many infections (notably tuberculosis), and in sarcoidosis and idiopathic pars planitis. Some legitimate confusion may arise with Eales' disease when there are neurological complications. The ocular features

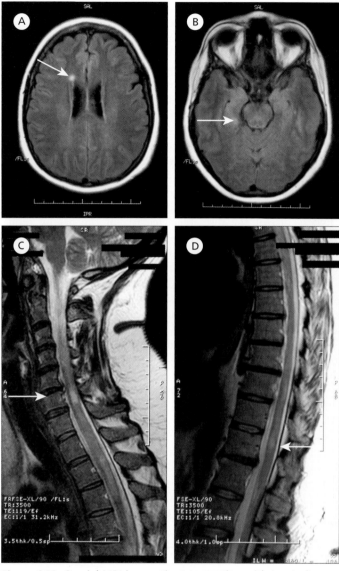

Figure 6.23 Cranial MRI in a patient presenting with 'central serous retinopathy' followed within a few weeks by spinal cord lesions. (A) A single T_2-weighted periventricular lesion; and (B) a lesion in the hippocampus, each at onset. (C) Multiple spinal cord lesions identified on a subsequent occasion. (D) A new spinal cord lesion detected 4 months after presentation, confirming the diagnosis of multiple sclerosis using the W.I. McDonald *et al* (2001) criteria.

originally described were recurrent retinal and vitreous haemorrhage but venous sheathing was later recognized. The association of ocular haemorrhage and abnormal neurological signs was present in 4/17 patients diagnosed as having Eales' disease by White (1961). Abnormalities in the cerebrospinal fluid without clinical evidence of central nervous system disease were found in a further three cases. Although multiple sclerosis had been diagnosed in some of these patients, none satisfied the criteria for definite diagnosis. This is also true of the three patients described by Silfverskiöld (1947) who developed spinal cord lesions during active retinal vasculitis. There was partial remission but after prolonged observation no evidence of multiple lesions. The problem of distinction from multiple sclerosis was discussed by Pépin *et al* (1978). Autopsy has confirmed that neurological symptoms are the result of vasculitis but some perivenous demyelination has also been recorded (Dastur and Singhal 1976). Figure 6.23 shows the cranial cord imaging of a young woman in whom a confident diagnosis of central serous retinopathy was soon followed by symptoms of spinal cord disease. Despite the initial ophthalmological diagnosis, cranial and spinal imaging led to clinical re-evaluation and revision of the diagnosis to multiple sclerosis presenting as optic neuritis.

Uveitis and pars planitis

Inflammation of the uveal tract in multiple sclerosis was first described by Ter Braak and van Herwaarden (1933). In many of the earlier reports, discussed in a previous edition of this book (W.B. Matthews 1991), it is not possible to exclude other causes of ocular disease but an association between pars planitis (inflammation of that part of the ciliary body in contact with the vitreous anterior to the termination of the retina) and multiple sclerosis appears to be established. In terms of frequency and significance for the individual, Bamford *et al* (1978c) found sheathing in 14/127 patients, two of whom also had pars planitis. Sheathing was not related to relapse or degree of disability, but was considerably more common in progressive

disease. Biousse *et al* (1999) found that approximately 1% of 1098 patients attending a multiple sclerosis clinic had uveitis, and 1% of 1530 patients from the uveitis clinic had multiple sclerosis. The ocular and neurological symptoms might occur in either order. In one case they came on together.

Posterior visual pathways

The optic chiasm is a common site for multiple sclerosis plaques but characteristic visual field changes are rarely described, perhaps because they are obscured by the effects of co-existing optic nerve lesions. A small number of cases with bitemporal hemianopia or scotomata, often remitting, have been published (Ashworth 1957; Sacks and Melen 1975; Spector *et al* 1980) but, here, the diagnoses are not always entirely convincing. The optic radiation is also frequently seen on MRI to be involved in multiple sclerosis plaques (R.S.L. Hornabrook *et al* 1992), but hemianopia is only found with extensive lesions (Plant *et al* 1992) and particularly in massive lesions of the hemisphere mimicking brain tumour. Remission is usually complete. The syndrome most usually seen in association with occlusion of the left posterior cerebral artery, or tumours affecting the splenium of the corpus callosum, of alexia with agraphia (and hemianopia)

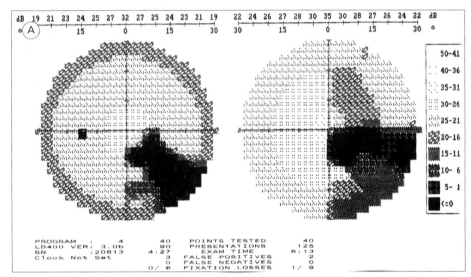

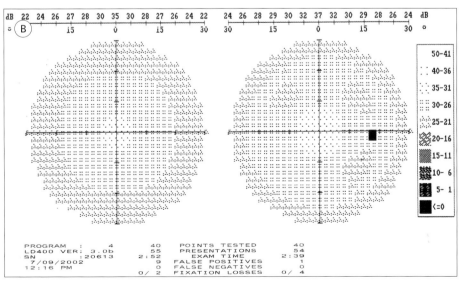

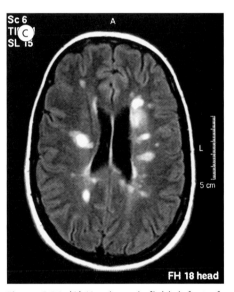

Figure 6.24 (A) Hemianopic field defect of subacute onset with recovery (B) in a patient subsequently developing an acute brainstem lesion with laboratory abnormalities consistent with multiple sclerosis. (C) Cerebral MRI during the initial clinical episode.

is described as the presenting feature of multiple sclerosis (Mao-Draayer and Panitch 2004). Figure 6.24 illustrates the symptomatic right lower quadrantic hemianopia, which later recovered, recorded at presentation in a female aged 46 years with multiple white matter abnormalities on MRI and the presence of oligoclonal bands, who subsequently had a defining brainstem lesion leading to the diagnosis of multiple sclerosis. It is often difficult to decide whether visual perceptual symptoms occurring in patients with multiple sclerosis directly reflect the disease process but Dogulu and Kansu (1997) have shown that brief episodes of 180° inversion of the visual field (upside-down vision) are associated with a pontine lesion. These may represent a further manifestation of paroxysmal symptoms in multiple sclerosis.

Involvement of other cranial nerves

Apart from the optic nerve, which is usually regarded as part of the central nervous system, several cranial nerves may be affected by multiple sclerosis, giving rise to characteristic symptoms. Thomke *et al* (1997) describe an isolated cranial nerve palsy in 24/1489 patients with definite multiple sclerosis (1.6%; one third cranial nerve, one fourth, 12 sixth, three seventh, six vestibular and one cochlear portion of the eighth nerve). Fourteen of 271 (5%) patients seen at presentation had an isolated cranial nerve lesion, and this was the sole manifestation of a new relapse in a further 10/1218 (0.8%) cases. Neurophysiological techniques proved more sensitive in locating the underlying lesion than MRI.

Olfactory nerve

Occasional patients report acute loss of sense of smell. This may occasionally occur in association with widespread symptoms in acute relapse, followed by remission, and has even been reported as the initial symptom (Constantinescu *et al* 1994). Ansari (1976) could find no evidence for symptomless impairment of sense of smell but this may be detected by more sensitive methods (Pinching 1977). The comment by Gowers (1893) that the olfactory pathway is commonly involved in multiple sclerosis is corroborated by recent clinical and MRI studies (Doty *et al* 1998; 1999; Zorzon *et al* 2000). Nearly 40% of patients demonstrate olfactory impairment, and there is a good correlation with lesion load in the olfactory areas of the brain.

Trigeminal nerve

We have already referred to pain as a manifestation of trigeminal nerve involvement. Paralysis of the motor division of the fifth nerve has been described in multiple sclerosis (Gowers 1893; Oppenheim 1914). We have only seen this in isolation (and without any other explanation) in the identical co-twin of a patient examined on behalf of investigators compiling the original Canadian series of multiple sclerosis in twins (DASC: and see Chapter 3). Weakness of jaw muscles was mentioned as a rare event by S. Poser (1978). Trismus has been attributed to multiple sclerosis in a single case but the diagnosis was uncertain (D'Costa *et al* 1990). A complaint of numbness or paraesthesiae in the face is common but sensory loss is often difficult to detect, and the corneal reflex is usually intact. Isolated persistent numbness of the face is more likely to be a manifestation of trigeminal neuropathy than multiple sclerosis.

Facial nerve

Facial weakness is listed in virtually every account of the clinical features of multiple sclerosis but is hardly ever described in detail (Figure 6.25A–C). There is reasonable agreement on the frequency of facial weakness at onset, varying from 1 to 4% (Bonduelle and Albaranès 1962; Kelly 1985), but it is not possible to determine from these reports the important question of how often an isolated facial palsy is the first sign of the disease. Cabrera-Gomez *et al* (2005) describe familial recurrent Bell's palsy in which the proband met criteria for the diagnosis of multiple sclerosis. In a series of 107 Japanese patients of whom 20% had facial palsy within the first 6 years of the illness, 5% had presented with facial weakness (Fukazawa *et al* 1997a). The reported frequency of facial weakness in the course of the disease is far more varied – from 3% (Kurtzke *et al* 1968a), through 10% (Bonduelle and Albaranès 1962; S. Poser 1978) and 20% (Fukazawa *et al* 1997a) to the unrealistic figure of 52% (Carter *et al* 1950). It is seldom possible to determine whether the reported facial weakness has been observed or merely reported by the patients. The weakness is evidently often slight and its type, whether upper or lower motor neuron, difficult to distinguish unless accompanied by other localizing signs. Bonduelle and Albaranès (1962) report that in 15 patients the facial palsy was always peripheral and sudden or rapid in onset. In all but two instances, it was accompanied by other cranial

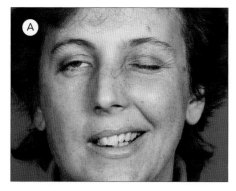
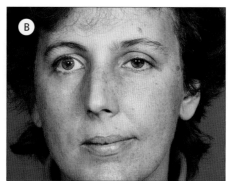
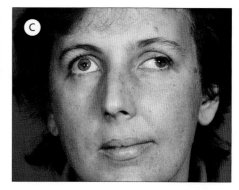

Figure 6.25 (A) Facial weakness during an acute episode of brainstem demyelination as a result of multiple sclerosis. (B,C) Patient also has ptosis and features of one-and-one-half syndrome.

nerve palsies. Bauer and Hanefeld (1993) describe central facial weakness in 8% of their patients and peripheral weakness in 3%.

Whether facial palsy, indistinguishable from idiopathic Bell's palsy, can be a symptom of multiple sclerosis is uncertain. The sophisticated methods of investigation for facial palsy now available do not appear to have been applied in multiple sclerosis. The nearest approach is the report by L. Jonsson *et al* (1991) of a young man with an acute facial palsy, ipsilateral loss of taste and periaural pain. The paralysis was shown to be the result of neurapraxia and was indistinguishable from idiopathic Bell's palsy. There was a past history of remitting sensory symptoms and MRI showed a minute lesion on the appropriate side of the pons, clearing as the facial palsy recovered. Fukazawa *et al* (1997a) showed lesions in the pontine tegmentum ipsilateral to the facial weakness in 84% of patients undergoing MRI.

Disturbance of the sensation of taste in multiple sclerosis is more often related to involvement of the *tractus solitarius* and other central connections of the facial sensory pathways than to facial weakness. It is sometimes seen in association with internuclear ophthalmoplegia. In the 1930s, residents at the National Hospital, Queen Square, in London, were required to pay particular attention to the testing of taste in routine examination of these patients. McAlpine (1972) observed that a complaint of decrease or loss of taste was common in patients with facial paraesthesiae. Hemigeusia has been described as the initial symptom of multiple sclerosis (L. Cohen 1965). In one report (Rollin *et al* 1976) more than 10% of individuals with advanced disease reported hypogeusia, especially in the context of trigeminal pathology. And, in the most convincing case, loss of taste as the presenting manifestation was soon followed by signs of a brainstem lesion with trigeminal sensory loss (Pascual-Leone *et al* 1991).

The term hemifacial spasm has been used imprecisely to describe not only undoubted postparalytic synkinesis and myokymia (Bonduelle and Albaranès 1962), but also spasm of unidentifiable type. Telischi *et al* (1991), however, reported six patients with multiple sclerosis and typical hemifacial spasm. In two, plaques in the region of the ipsilateral facial nucleus were seen on MRI. Facial myokymia consists of rapidly flickering contraction of all the facial muscles but it is nearly always unilateral. Its association with multiple sclerosis was recognized by H. Oppenheim (1917) and emphasized by Andermann *et al* (1961) and W.B. Matthews (1966). The onset is rapid or sudden and is felt by the patient as stiffness of the face. The palpebral fissure is slightly narrowed and the nasolabial fold is deepened by the muscular contraction. The constant rapid flickering or worm-like subcutaneous undulations are unmistakable, although not always remarked upon by the patient. There is no pain. In the personal series of Bryan Matthews, myokymia was observed in 7/377 patients, but it is probably often overlooked.

Electromyography shows that individual motor units are firing in brief bursts at different but almost regular intervals (see also Chapter 13). Remission is usual after a few weeks. Facial myokymia is not pathognomonic for multiple sclerosis as it may occur in intrinsic and extrinsic tumours involving the brainstem, and also in the Guillain–Barré syndrome (Waybright *et al* 1979).

Eighth nerve

While hearing loss can certainly result from multiple sclerosis, its frequency is difficult to estimate as deficiencies are common in control subjects and minor degrees of deafness, particularly if unilateral, may not be remarked upon. For example, in an older series, some degree of hearing loss was found in 46/100 patients, but also in 18/100 controls (Von Leden and Horton 1948). There was marked dissociation between any complaint of deafness and the observed abnormalities. Deafness, clearly due to multiple sclerosis, is rapid or sudden in onset and may affect one or both ears (C. Fischer *et al* 1984). Hearing loss is usually severe and often accompanied by tinnitus and vertigo (Daugherty *et al* 1983). Widespread signs of brainstem and cerebellar disease are usually present, although sudden unilateral deafness with tinnitus has been described as the sole presenting symptom (B. Drulovic *et al* 1993). Sequential bilateral deafness with gadolinium-enhancing lesions at the level of entry of the eighth nerve to the brainstem has been reported (H.J. Barratt *et al* 1988). Central hyperacusis and phonophobia (including the precipitation of unpleasant paraesthesiae by sound) may occur (H. Weber *et al* 2002). Whatever the symptoms in a particular case, clinical remission usually occurs even though residual hearing loss may be detected. However, because hearing loss is an uncommon manifestation of multiple sclerosis, it should alert the clinician to alternative explanations (see Chapter 8) such as retinocochleocerebral vasculopathy (Susac's syndrome).

Vertigo, as distinct from vague dizziness or unsteadiness, is common in multiple sclerosis both at onset and in relapse. The frequency is difficult to estimate owing to overlap with other symptoms in many reported series, but 16% has been cited (Bauer and Hanefeld 1993). In its most alarming form, the dizziness is of acute onset and prostrating, accompanied by vomiting, headache and great difficulty in walking. An attack of this kind is indistinguishable from vestibular neuronitis unless there is accompanying evidence of more widespread disease. Remission is invariable but may take some time. Figure 6.26A,B illustrates the MRI appearances in a patient with vertigo and ataxia as the presenting episode of multiple sclerosis who also had left-sided fifth, facial and eighth nerve lesions at onset, with brainstem demyelination from which recovery was good but incomplete – all associated with severe headache. Positional vertigo, induced by turning in bed or other major changes in posture, may also be caused by multiple sclerosis (Berkowitz 1985; Frohman *et al* 2000) and again cannot be distinguished in isolation from the benign form of this condition. As with many other functions, abnormalities of the vestibular system, apparently unrelated to symptoms, can be detected by refined methods of investigation in a high proportion of patients (Grenman 1985).

Lower cranial nerves

Symptoms arising from disorder of the functions of the lower cranial nerves have been relatively neglected in patients with multiple sclerosis. Dysphagia may occur at any stage of the disease with lesions of the brainstem, but is of particular importance with increasing disability, when bulbar palsy may prove fatal (Bauer and Hanefeld 1993). F.J. Thomas and Wiles (1999) found that 43% of 79 consecutive hospital patients with multiple sclerosis had abnormal swallowing, but barely half complained of this symptom. It did not correlate with nutritional indices. Somewhat lower incidences (24–34%) have been reported (Calcagno *et al* 2002; de Pauw *et al* 2002). Bulbar

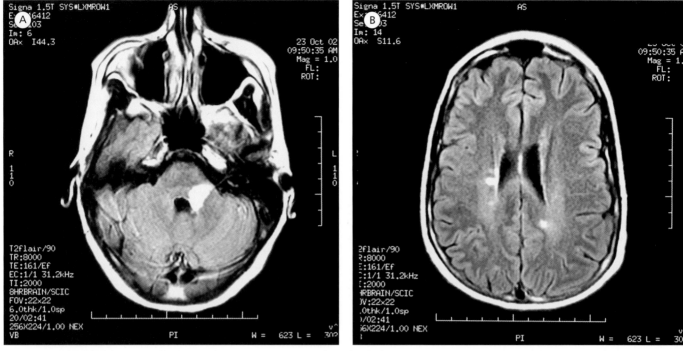

Figure 6.26 (A) MRI showing a brainstem lesion in a patient with multiple lower cranial nerve palsies and intense headache, as part of an isolated (after >2 years) episode of brainstem demyelination but with multiple white matter abnormalities on cranial MRI (B). Kindly provided by Dr Nagui Antoun.

palsy, with its attendant risks, may also occur as part of an acute relapse. Dysarthria is far more common but probably more often the result of cerebellar or corticospinal damage than bulbar palsy. Loss of pharyngeal sensation and the gag reflex are not unusual and glossopharyngeal neuralgia has been reported in a single case (Bauer and Hanefeld 1993). C. Davison *et al* (1934) reported three cases with wasting of the tongue, a remarkable finding that neither we (nor Bryan Matthews) have personally observed in multiple sclerosis.

Autonomic nervous system

Autonomic symptoms rank high in terms of their impact on aspects of daily living, and as reminders to patients and their relatives of what it can mean to have multiple sclerosis. Almost every female patient is aware of her bladder, and very few males eventually escape some impairment of sexual performance. Although these symptoms can often be managed and do not impinge on many domestic roles and professional activities, they are nevertheless a significant cause of morbidity (Hennessey *et al* 1999). McDougall and McLeod (2003) found abnormalities of one or more autonomic function tests (excluding those reflecting bladder, gut, or sexual dysfunction) in more than half of 63 patients with multiple sclerosis. Abnormalities in at least two tests occurred in 18% of patients and were associated with severity of disease. Autonomic dysfunction has been associated with MRI lesions in the hypothalamus, brainstem and spinal cord (see below; De Séze *et al* 2001a). There is evidence that, in broad terms, parasympathetic dysfunction relates to progression of disability, and sympathetic dysfunction to clinical activity (Flachenecker *et al* 2001).

Bladder

Voluntary storage involves bladder distension which stimulates afferent activity in the hypogastric and pelvic nerve fibres. Bladder filling depends on discharges in Onuf's nucleus. This gives rise to the pudendal nerve containing efferent fibres which maintain contraction of the external urethral sphincter and inhibit transmission at postganglionic parasympathetic neurons innervating the detrusor. The result is that urethral pressure exceeds the effect on bladder contents of detrusor contraction and the bladder continues to fill. Voiding occurs with inhibition of sympathetic pudendal nerve firing, which relaxes the sphincter and permits parasympathetic cholinergic contraction of the detrusor (Figure 6.27). Thus, the main function of the sympathetic system is to maintain continence at the sphincter, using α-adrenoreceptors, and to inhibit the detrusor, using β-adrenoreceptors. Storage and emptying require the ability selectively to facilitate and inhibit these spinal reflexes. Upper motor neurons, which originate from the pontine micturition centre and are set by the frontal micturition centre, modulate spinal reflexes so as to favour (at any one time) storage or emptying. With uncoupling of reciprocal arrangements between the detrusor and sphincter, the bladder contracts against a closed sphincter leading to urgency and frequency with hesitancy or incomplete emptying and incontinence – problems which are considerably aggravated by infection and immobility.

Overall, urgency frequency and incontinence are more prevalent in patients with multiple sclerosis, especially women with coexistent stress incontinence, than hesitancy or retention. The term detrusor hyper-reflexia is used to describe a state of impaired storage and this can be demonstrated by cystometry during which

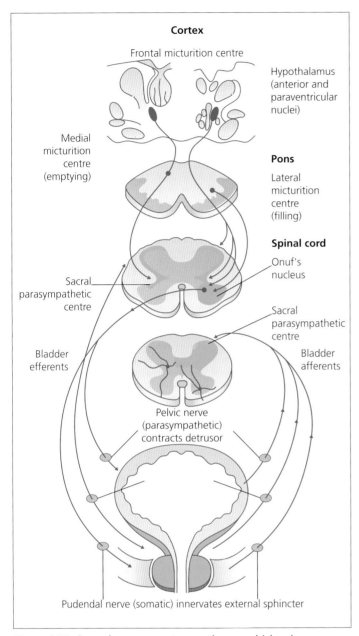

Figure 6.27 Central nervous system pathways which subserve bladder control showing the influence of descending frontal, hypothalamic and pontine micturition centres acting on the sacral parasympathetic nucleus and the motor neuron pool in Onuf's nucleus and their efferents in the pudendal, pelvic and hypogastric nerves together with sites of termination of bladder afferents.

the intravesical pressure (corrected for intra-abdominal changes) rises inappropriately with bladder volume, often with urethral leakage during the procedure. Detrusor sphincter dyssynergia describes the additional component of simultaneous activity of mechanisms which subserve bladder emptying with those that close the sphincter. Often this is associated with incomplete emptying, leaving a significant residual bladder volume.

For many affected individuals, loss of bladder control is the most distressing symptom of multiple sclerosis. Of 297 patients

examined by H. Miller *et al* (1965), 78% had experienced some disorder of micturition and in 52% this had persisted for >6 months at the time of examination. Of these, 60% had urgency of micturition, 10% had been incontinent and 2% had suffered from recurrent retention. In the final analysis of his personal series of 377 patients, Bryan Matthews recorded urgency in 96, hesitancy of micturition in 22, and incontinence in 75. During the earlier course of the disease, 91 had been incontinent. Bladder symptoms at the onset were present in only 13 patients. Betts *et al* (1993) report that of 170 patients with multiple sclerosis referred because of urinary symptoms, 85% had urgency, 82% frequency, 63% urge incontinence, 49% hesitancy and 14% nocturnal enuresis. Only two patients had acute retention. The frequency of abnormal bladder function in multiple sclerosis increases with advancing age, duration of disease and degree of disability (Bauer and Hanefeld 1993).

Isolated instances of retention or incontinence may occasionally be recognized retrospectively as the first manifestations of multiple sclerosis. The common story, however, is for urgency to occur even in mild relapses involving the spinal cord, often followed by remission. After further relapse, urgency and frequency may persist, often accompanied by hesitancy of micturition, severely limiting social activity away from home. Persistent urgency leads to occasional incontinence, becoming increasingly disabling with progressive disease. Nocturia may cause serious sleep deprivation and, in the disabled, exhaustion from struggling out of bed several times each night.

In advanced disease, the nature of the incontinence changes, large volumes of urine being passed without warning and sometimes without awareness, and leading eventually to continuous dribbling. Acute or recurrent retention of urine may occur at any stage of the disease, but is relatively uncommon. Inadequate emptying of the bladder is, however, a very common finding (Betts *et al* 1993). There is often a remarkable disparity between symptoms and the findings on urological investigation. The fundamental defect is nearly always that of varying degrees of hyper-reflexia and dyssynergia between contraction and relaxation of the detrusor and sphincter muscles. An areflexic bladder is exceptional. In general, the presence and severity of disordered bladder function are closely related to the degree of spastic weakness of the lower limbs (Betts *et al* 1993). Secondary impairment of renal function may occur in the progressive phase of the disease (Calabresi *et al* 2002a) but has become a less common complication with more active management of infections and immobility in patients benefiting from rehabilitation services. In a recent clinical, urodynamic and MRI study, Araki *et al* (2003) concluded that detrusor hyporeflexia correlated with pontine lesions, and detrusor sphincter dyssynergia with spinal cord lesions. The pharmacological basis for control of the bladder and the treatment opportunities which this provides are described in Chapter 17.

Bowel

Occasional faecal incontinence has been found to be unexpectedly common in patients with multiple sclerosis, occurring at least once in the previous 3 months in 51% of a large clinic series (Hinds *et al* 1990). Persistent incontinence in ambulant patients is much less common. Constipation, defined as two or fewer bowel movements each week, was reported in 43%. It may be the presenting symptom (Lawthom *et al* 2003). In bedridden patients, persistent constipation requiring manual evacuation is a major problem. Distension of the lower bowel may lead to distressing abdominal bloating. The normal postprandial increase in colonic motility has been shown to be absent in advanced multiple sclerosis (Glick *et al* 1982). Paralysis of gastric motility (Gupta 1984) and functional pyloric obstruction (Graves 1981) have been described in multiple sclerosis, both presenting with vomiting and as the presenting symptom in one case. Wiesel *et al* (2001) have usefully reviewed the pathophysiology and management of bowel dysfunction in multiple sclerosis. They point out that up to 70% of patients complain of constipation and/or faecal incontinence. Both these symptoms are a source of considerable psychosocial disability. The pathophysiological mechanisms are not fully understood, but include involvement of brain and spinal cord resulting in interruption of either or both the central afferent and efferent pathways on which normal bowel function depends. Emotional factors may also contribute.

Sexual function

Sexual function both in men and women is often severely disturbed by multiple sclerosis, but estimates of frequency are distorted by several factors. The psychological effect of having any disease may reduce potency and libido in both affected persons and their partners. Difficulties with sexual function are not uncommon, even in people otherwise in normal health, in those aged >50 years; little difference is reported in this respect between ambulant people with multiple sclerosis and matched normal controls (Minderhoud *et al* 1984). It is, nevertheless, possible to determine that sexual function is often adversely affected by physical effects of the disease. A case–control study of 108 unselected patients with multiple sclerosis, 97 patients with chronic disease and 110 healthy individuals revealed that sexual dysfunction was present in 73% of cases, 39% of chronic disease controls and 13% of healthy controls (Zorzon *et al* 1999).

Erectile impotence was a symptom in 44% of male patients examined by H. Miller *et al* (1965). Vas (1969) found 21/37 ambulant men to be fully potent, compared with 13 who were partially and three totally impotent. A year later, one man had regained potency. In another study (Minderhoud *et al* 1984), 48% of men aged <50 years had major sexual problems, mainly impotence but also difficulties with ejaculation and orgasm. Similar difficulties were found by Bauer and Hanefeld (1993) in 40% of their patients aged <30 years, and these increased moderately with age.

The role of the autonomic nervous system in these problems is shown by the close association with other functional disturbances. There is a clear relationship between erectile impotence and disorders of bladder and bowel and also with loss of thermoregulatory sweating in the lower half of the body (Cartlidge 1972; Vas 1969). Betts *et al* (1994) found that a complaint of erectile failure in multiple sclerosis was always accompanied by urinary symptoms and by signs indicating disease affecting the spinal cord. That said, Zorzon *et al* (2001) make the point that, with time, sexual function changes independently of bladder dysfunction.

Sexual function in women is more difficult to assess, but loss of libido, lack of lubrication and failure of orgasm are common complaints (Lundberg 1981; Minderhoud *et al* 1984; Zorzon *et al* 1999). Hulter and Lundborg (1995) found that established multiple sclerosis had a profound effect on many aspects of female sexuality. In both sexes, alteration in genital sensation, fatigue and spasticity in the lower limbs contribute to sexual difficulties and these difficulties increase with time (Zorzon *et al* 2001). There is a correlation between sexual dysfunction and pontine atrophy determined by MRI (Zivadinov *et al* 2003c; Zorzon *et al* 2003a).

Sweating

Partial, or even apparent total loss of thermoregulatory sweating is common in established disease (Cartlidge 1972; M.J. Noronha *et al* 1968). Despite these severe abnormalities, there is no evidence for distress from failure of heat loss. Hyperthermia has, indeed, been described in multiple sclerosis (Castaigne *et al* 1966; Henke *et al* 2000), but whether as a result of anhidrosis is not clear. Fever, sometimes >41°C, for up to 3 months during relapse has been reported from China (Baoxun *et al* 1981) but, again, the relationship to autonomic dysfunction is unknown. Unilateral hyperhidrosis has been reported (Ueno *et al* 2000).

Horner's syndrome

Bamford *et al* (1980) described Horner's syndrome, pharmacologically localized to a lesion of central or intermediate sympathetic fibres, in three clinically definite cases of multiple sclerosis and stated that it occurred in 2–3% of their patients – a remarkably high proportion. Ptosis may also occur as part of a third nerve palsy and is illustrated as part of the one-and-one-half syndrome in Figure 6.10. Not surprisingly, regional abnormalities of sweating may accompany unilateral Horner's syndrome – the former proving more symptomatic than the pupillary abnormality (Carroll and Zajicek 2004).

Cardiovascular abnormalities

Abnormal cardiovascular responses to many test stimuli can be detected in a high proportion of people with multiple sclerosis (Anema *et al* 1991; Pentland and Ewing 1987; Senaratne *et al* 1984; Sterman *et al* 1985; Thomaides *et al* 1993), but very seldom give rise to symptoms. They progress with time (Nasseri *et al* 1998). Postural hypotension, while found in 13% of patients in one series (Anema *et al* 1991), only rarely results in syncope (Giroud *et al* 1988). Postural dizziness has however been reported in 50% of patients compared with 14% of controls (Flachenecker *et al* 1999). Paroxysmal (Chagnac *et al* 1986) or persistent (Schroth *et al* 1992) atrial fibrillation may occur with acute brainstem lesions. Acute neurogenic pulmonary oedema, unaccompanied by cardiac failure, is a further occasional complication (Chagnac *et al* 1986; Gentiloni *et al* 1992; Summerfield *et al* 2002) and may be the presenting feature (Crawley *et al* 2001). One autopsy case had symmetrical lesions in the dorsal medulla (D'Hooghe *et al* 1989). The importance of assessing cardiovascular function in patients commencing treatment with mitoxantrone has been emphasized in a number of recent publications (see Chapter 18: M. Beer *et al* 2001; Gbadamosi *et al* 2003a; Olindo *et al* 2002).

Hypothalamus

A number of bizarre syndromes have been attributed to presumed involvement of the hypothalamus by multiple sclerosis. These include rapid, fatal, emaciation (Kamalian *et al* 1975), acute depression with hyperthermia (Bignami *et al* 1961), and inappropriate secretion of antidiuretic hormone (Apple *et al* 1978), all combined with more conventional symptoms of the disease. In a study of 53 patients, cortisol release induced by the dexamethasone–corticotropin-releasing hormone test was negatively correlated with the presence and number of gadolinium-DTPA enhancing lesions and positively correlated with ventricular size (E.M. Schumann *et al* 2002). Sleep is often disturbed by the discomforts and inconveniences arising from spasticity, inability to change posture and frequency of micturition (Tachibana *et al* 1994), but there is no evidence for a disorder of circadian sleep regulation in multiple sclerosis (Taphoorn *et al* 1993).

Rare manifestations

Since multiple sclerosis can produce lesions anywhere in the central nervous system, including the cerebral cortex and deep grey nuclei or anterior horn cells, there are very few neurological symptoms and signs which have not occasionally been seen. In recent times, many of these syndromes have been shown to be associated with appropriately placed MRI abnormalities, leaving little doubt as to their causal relationship. Intractable hiccough with cough syncope has been reported in association with cervical cord and medullary lesions (Funakawa and Terao 1998). Unilateral abdominal paralysis in isolation, and unilateral hypoglossal and recurrent laryngeal palsies (one each) have been observed (George Ebers, personal communications). Several of the isolated cranial nerve palsies described above and manifestations outside the central nervous system are equally rare, but it was the opinion of Bryan Matthews that a few cases of optico-ciliary neuritis have been observed in which inflammation of the optic nerve presumably spreads to involve the adjacent ciliary ganglion with resultant temporary loss of pupillary activity.

ASSOCIATED DISEASES

To establish a definite link between multiple sclerosis and a disease in which the cause is better known or more accessible to investigation might well prove a great advance in understanding or, at least, afford an opening to be explored. Unfortunately, associations so far detected are tenuous or with diseases no better understood than multiple sclerosis. Few of the putative correlations have been subjected to rigorous statistical analysis. One obvious method is to screen large series of people with multiple sclerosis for other diseases where the incidences and prevalences are already well known. Difficulty arises from the length of follow-up and high autopsy rate needed to establish an association with a condition having a later age of onset, such as cerebral glioma. This approach was adopted by L.J. Edwards and Constantinescu (2004) who recorded the period prevalence over 1 year of other diseases reported by 658 patients with multiple sclerosis attending a hospital clinic. Listing an excess of asthma, inflammatory bowel disease, type 1 diabetes, pernicious anaemia, autoimmune thyroid disease, uveitis, seronegative arthritis, bipolar disease and melanoma, the emphasis was on autoimmune diseases as the main exemplars of co-morbidity. Another method is to examine series focusing on the other diseases, but accurate identification of those who also have multiple sclerosis in the population from which the series is drawn is seldom precise. The starting point for such investigations is often clinical intuition based on simple observation of a few instances of patients with both multiple sclerosis and the other disease in question. Given these methodological limitations, we anticipate that our choice of material discussed under the heading of associated diseases will raise the odd neurological eyebrow. The boundaries of definition are inexact – as exemplified by the difficulty of where to place Devic's and Harding's diseases, for example – but our broad limits of inclusion and exclusion are explained and justified in Chapter 8, to which the reader is referred.

Autoimmune disease

Multiple sclerosis has many of the aetiological and pathological characteristics of an autoimmune disease and it might therefore be expected that there would be a clustering of other autoimmune diseases in patients with multiple sclerosis and their relatives. There have been frequent case reports on the association with a variety of autoimmune diseases but establishing that the associations are significant has been difficult. Nevertheless, several recent carefully controlled studies do provide convincing evidence for such associations. The risk of autoimmunity is increased in the relatives of probands with multiple sclerosis. An association between multiple sclerosis and inflammatory bowel disease was reported from Canada (Minuk and Lewkonia 1986; Sadovnick *et al* 1989). Midgard *et al* (1996b) found no difference in chronic inflammatory diseases amongst first-degree relatives of 155 patients with multiple sclerosis compared with 200 controls but, at around 48%, the frequency was high in each, perhaps because of the acceptance of the patient's history without confirmation of the diagnoses.

Recently, three surveys have looked at the generality of an increase in frequency of autoimmune disease amongst patients with multiple sclerosis and their relatives. Heinzlef *et al* (1999) studied an unknown number of relatives of 357 French index cases with multiple sclerosis. The cohort was considered to be representative of a population-based sample. Confining the analysis to first-degree relatives, multiple sclerosis recurred in 25 (7%) families and another autoimmune disease in a further 35 (10%). Both multiple sclerosis and another autoimmune disorder occurred in three (1%). They identified recurrence of multiple sclerosis in 55 relatives of the 357 index cases. Eleven of 357 (3%) index cases had another autoimmune disease. Broadley *et al* (2000) assessed the frequency of multiple sclerosis, five definite and three putative autoimmune disorders, and control conditions in the 1315 first-degree relatives of 571 probands, compared with 375 control families. Whereas patients themselves did not have an excess of autoimmune diseases, these were over-represented in family members of individuals with multiple sclerosis. The main effect was attributed to an excess of autoimmune thyroid disease. When the autoimmune diseases were considered individually, the excess of Hashimoto's disease/autoimmune hypothyroidism and Graves' disease/autoimmune hyperthyroidism were each statistically significant (p=0.007 and p=0.0007, respectively). Psoriasis, for which an increased risk in families of patients with multiple sclerosis has been reported in Norwegian families (Midgard *et al* 1996b), showed a similar trend (p=0.05) but no association was observed with inflammatory bowel disease, or atopic asthma. Recurrence risk was especially high in multiplex families. Henderson *et al* (2000) derived an odds ratio of 2.2 (95% CI 1.3–3.7) for recurrence of 11 autoimmune diseases in 722 first-degree relatives of 117 Australian patients with multiple sclerosis. Rates did not differ depending on clinical course. Amongst cases, the odds ratio for autoimmune disease was 1.7 (95% CI 0.9–3.2). An increased familial risk of autoimmunity has also been reported in Italians (relative risk 3.8; 95% CI 2.0–7.1; Zorzon *et al* 2003b). By 2003, The Multiple Autoimmune Disease Genetics Consortium (MADGC: *www.madgc.org*) had identified 200 families in the United States in which two of nine archetypal autoimmune diseases had occurred amongst a nuclear pedigree. Compared with individuals with autoimmune endocrine and rheumatological conditions, it is reported that the relatives of probands with multiple sclerosis with early age of onset, especially the fathers of affected individuals, have an excess of psoriasis (Annunziata *et al* 2003). The failure of Broadley *et al* (2000) to find an increased risk of autoimmune disease in their probands with multiple sclerosis is consistent with earlier larger studies (De Keyser 1988; Wynn *et al* 1990). The data on rheumatoid arthritis were unsatisfactory because of uncertainty about the diagnosis in deceased relatives. The strongest association was with autoimmune thyroid disease, a finding of special interest because of the frequency with which patients being treated with disease-modifying drugs develop Graves' disease (see Chapter 18). The association between multiple sclerosis and type 1 diabetes, originally reported from Canada (Warren and Warren 1982) is rather weak (Broadley *et al* 2000; Lobnig and Chantelau 2002) except in Sardinia where the prevalence of type 1 diabetes is strikingly increased both in patients and their families (Marrosu *et al* 2002b).

An association between myasthenia gravis and multiple sclerosis has been reported on a number of occasions and we have seen it in individual patients in our clinics (WIMcD and DASC). The most recent report describes eight cases from the British Columbia multiple sclerosis and myasthenia gravis clinics (Isbister *et al* 2003). While the study is not population based, and prevalence statistics for myasthenia gravis are not available for British Columbia, the authors reasonably argue that the association is probably not random. However, caution is still needed in view of the negative findings in most other series. There are a few additional reports of an association between multiple sclerosis and inflammatory bowel disease (Kimura *et al* 2000) and ankylosing spondylitis (Hanrahan *et al* 1988; Kahn and Kusher 1979; W.B. Matthews 1968). In each of these examples, the numbers appear greater than expected. However, the retrospective nature of the studies, the lack of suitable controls, and – in the case of inflammatory bowel disease – the negative findings of Broadley *et al* (2000) mean that the associations cannot be regarded as established.

Miscellaneous conditions

From time to time, one sees patients in whom multiple sclerosis co-exists with intramedullary or cerebral tumour: schwannoma (Etus *et al* 2002); meningioma (WIMcD and DASC); oligodendroglioma (Barnard and Jellinek 1967); and astrocytoma (Ho and Wolfe 1981). There may be co-morbidity between neurofibromatosis 1 and primary progressive multiple sclerosis (M.R. Johnson *et al* 2000). Others have extended the phenotype to include neurofibromatosis occurring in the context of relapsing–remitting multiple sclerosis (Perini and Gallo 2001). If there is overlap between neurofibromatosis and multiple sclerosis, this is not explained by mutation of the oligodendrocyte myelin glycoprotein gene which maps to the same locus (M.R. Johnson *et al* 2000). Although the question has been raised whether there is a causal connection between astrocytoma and cycles of proliferation in the plaques of multiple sclerosis, this has not been established; neither has an association between carcinoma and multiple sclerosis (I.V. Allen *et al* 1978). The somewhat ex-cathedra position on the link between astrocytoma and multiple sclerosis taken by Behan *et al* (2003) has been challenged (D.A.S. Compston 2003). Hjalgrim *et al* (2004) looked, reciprocally, at the interaction of Hodgkin's lymphoma and multiple sclerosis. The relative risk for Hodgkin's disease in 11 790 individuals with multiple sclerosis was 1.4 (95% CI 0.63–6.37) and 1.93 (95% CI 1.01–3.71) in their 19 599 first-degree relatives. Conversely, the relative risk for multiple sclerosis was 0.82 (95% CI 0.2–3.27) in 4381 Danes with lymphoma and 2.76 (95% CI 1.44–5.31) in their 7388 first-degree relatives, respectively. The authors prefer the interpretation that this co-morbidity reflects common exposure to environmental conditions. S.H. Mead *et al* (2001) described a family with hereditary spastic paraplegia and epilepsy in which mutation of the spastin gene was present. Two sisters were independently diagnosed with multiple sclerosis but

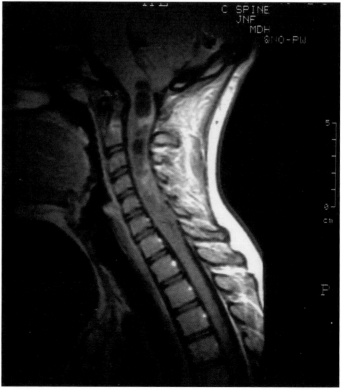

Figure 6.28 Cervical cord ependymoma in a child with multiple sclerosis.

extensive screening of the remaining pedigree failed to reveal clinical or laboratory features of multiple sclerosis. The rare association of a syringomyelia-like cavity with multiple sclerosis (Matsuda *et al* 2001) in patients with severe spinal cord manifestations of multiple sclerosis does seem likely to be causally related in view of the rare but well-documented occurrence of necrosis in severe lesions of multiple sclerosis (Figure 6.28 and see Chapter 12). However, Sotgiu *et al* (2001c) have suggested that mechanisms other than necrosis are involved in cavity formation, including increased cerebrospinal fluid pressure transmitted to the central canal below an area of focal compression cause by a discrete and oedematous plaque.

MULTIPLE SCLEROSIS IN CHILDHOOD

The question of whether multiple sclerosis can present in early childhood has long been controversial. Early reports, mentioned in Chapter 1, in which the frequency of onset at <10 years sometimes approached 10% were dismissed as unreliable by Wechsler (1922). The sources of error in these reports have recently been analysed by Bauer and Hanefeld (1993). Diagnosis was often based solely on clinical evidence and was inadequately supported by necropsy findings. Confusion with metabolic and inflammatory disorders, not recognized at the time, was inevitable and exacerbated by Schilder's description of three different paediatric demyelinating conditions as a single disease. The possibility of the very early onset of multiple sclerosis fell into disrepute, reflected by the exclusion from therapeutic trials of patients with onset at <10 years (Schumacher *et al* 1965). Less justifiably, this criterion was sometimes imposed in epidemiological surveys (Gudmundsson 1971).

At first, the literature was dominated by single case reports, of variable credibility (Arnouts 1959; Bonduelle *et al* 1954; Schneider *et al* 1969). Anecdotal cases of typical multiple sclerosis developing at 3 (Bye *et al* 1985; Hanefeld *et al* 1991) and 2 years of age (Guilhoto *et al* 1995), and even 13 months (Cole *et al* 1995), and 10 months (Ruggieri *et al* 1999; Shaw and Alvord 1987) were reported. Gradually, case series began to emerge (Andler and Roosen 1980; Brandt *et al* 1981; DiMario and Berman 1987; Golden and Woody 1987; Hauser *et al* 1982; Milner *et al* 1990; Selcen *et al* 1996). But careful scrutiny of the diagnoses remains a matter for concern. For example, of the seven cases described by Low and Carter (1956), the diagnosis is only entirely secure in one – a girl aged 6 years at onset of relapsing–remitting disease. In the series of 40 cases from the Mayo clinic (Gall *et al* 1958), onset at <15 years was observed in only eight cases and in some others was retrospectively reported in childhood. The series of eight cases, seven below the age of puberty, reviewed by Isler (1961) seems more convincing.

Recent developments have gone a long way to clarify the incidence and pattern of disease with early onset, but even these larger series present some difficulties. Very few offer more than a handful of cases: 46 children (aged ≤15 years) among a cohort of 810 Swedish patients with multiple sclerosis (Müller 1951); 125/1632 patients from nine Canadian multiple sclerosis clinics (Duquette *et al* 1987); 31/620 patients with multiple sclerosis admitted to the department of neurology in Hannover (Sindern *et al* 1992); 149 cases in a retrospective multicentre Italian study comprising 3375 affected individuals (Ghezzi *et al* 1997); 116/3500 patients followed in the Multiple Sclerosis Clinic of

Vancouver, British Columbia (Boiko *et al* 2002); 83/793 patients followed in the neurological department of Bari (Simone *et al* 2002); and 54 cases identified in a recent prospective multicentre Italian study (Ghezzi *et al* 2002). These series all suffer from epidemiological and methodological limitations: ascertainment is hospital or clinic based and, in one instance (Ghezzi *et al* 2002), inclusion was restricted to cases seen within ≤1 year of onset, factors both known to produce a recruitment bias in favour of more severe cases; and there is overlap of case material between series (Ghezzi *et al* 1997; 2002; Simone *et al* 2002). With the exception of two studies (Boiko *et al* 2002; Simone *et al* 2002), prognosis has been based on crude observational data rather than survival analyses. That said, these series provide useful information and two series, in particular, allow a clearer view of childhood multiple sclerosis to be reached.

Duquette *et al* (1987) reported 129 cases with onset aged <16 years, the diagnosis being considered clinically definite in 100. Although reported in 1987, the cases were ascertained in 1983 and imaging techniques not included in the diagnostic criteria. It is not stated how the age at onset was established, whether by observation or retrospective enquiry. In only eight patients was onset at <11 years. Based on a survey of 4632 people with multiple sclerosis, the onset of symptoms was in the first decade of life in 0.2%. In the series of 19 cases described by Boutin *et al* (1988), four were aged <10 years at onset. MRI was not available in the initial episode but subsequent contact with these cases confirms the validity of the diagnoses. The clinical data and period of follow up were not always adequate for a diagnosis of multiple sclerosis. Most recently, Ghezzi *et al* (1997) described a cohort of 149 Italian children with multiple sclerosis presenting before the age of 16 years, representing 4.4% of affected individuals from the four contributing populations.

Bauer and Hanefeld (1993) identified 129 cases diagnosed as having multiple sclerosis at <18 years appearing in the published literature before 1980, the approximate date at which modern diagnostic techniques became routinely available. Of these, the onset was before puberty (judged to be at the age of 12 years) in only 20. Bauer and Hanefeld (1993) found 176 cases with onset at <18 years published since 1980, but in only 43 did the disease begin aged <12 years. In their personal series, Bauer and Hanefeld (1993) studied 20 cases under the age of 15 years, of whom 11 were aged <10 years at onset. Of these, six were classified as having definite multiple sclerosis, three as probable and two as possible examples.

The frequency of multiple sclerosis appearing at ≤16 years has been in the range of 2.7% (Duquette *et al* 1987) to 5.7% (Müller 1951), with the other series finding 5% (Sindern *et al* 1992), 4.4% (Ghezzi *et al* 1997), and 3.6% (Boiko *et al* 2002). The only exception comes from the Bari study with a figure of 10.5% (Simone *et al* 2002) but, here, the authors acknowledge the probability of overestimation due to recruitment bias in a department of neurology having a special interest in multiple sclerosis with childhood onset. Therefore, the onset of multiple sclerosis at ≤16 years can be estimated at around 4% of all affected individuals. As for onset before the age of 10, the best estimate is around 0.4%. The excess of females has consistently been found to be even higher in multiple sclerosis with a childhood onset than in adult cases (2.5–4.7 F:M for children aged 12–16 years: Boiko *et al* 2002; Duquette *et al* 1987; Ghezzi *et al*

1997; 2002; Müller 1951; Simone *et al* 2002; Sindern *et al* 1992). However, the ratio is much lower in cases, with more boys than girls, when onset is <10 years, and the sex ratio may even reverse (range 0.5–0.8 F:M: Ghezzi *et al* 1997). But there are exceptions to this general trend (Boiko *et al* 2002; Müller 1951).

Clinical features

In general, childhood multiple sclerosis displays the same characteristics as adult onset cases, including movement disorders (Shiraishi *et al* 2005), and the accumulation of cognitive impairments over time (MacAllister *et al* 2005). There is no justification for identifying a juvenile form of the disease. Agreement has not been reached on the subsequent course of the disease in patients within the age group that constitutes the great majority of childhood multiple sclerosis but the impression is for relatively infrequent progression from onset, slower conversion to the secondary progressive phase and, hence, less rapid accumulation of irreversible disability. Sadly, however, lethal or malignant cases do occur in children and these may not come to the attention of the adult neurology department.

Duquette *at al* (1987) found that the initial symptoms were often mild and followed by complete, prolonged remission. Overall, the Italian cohort (which showed the usual high F:M sex ratio and predominant involvement of the optic nerves and brainstem), also followed a relatively benign course (Ghezzi *et al* 1997). In contrast, Bauer and Hanefeld (1993) described the disease as progressing rapidly, before and after puberty. This difference may result from the largely retrospective nature of the former study, the relatively trivial initial symptoms being insufficient to trigger investigation at the time. It is clear, however, that even at this age the disease may sometimes be progressive from onset, although the remitting form is more common.

In a small proportion of cases, perhaps more frequently in very young children, multiple sclerosis may present with acute diffuse encephalopathy. Fever and meningism then accompany varying degrees of impaired conscious level, cerebral oedema and swollen optic discs. Focal motor seizures may occur (Bye *et al* 1985; Septien *et al* 1991) with signs of brainstem involvement. In such cases the distinction from acute disseminated encephalomyelitis can only be made by the later occurrence of remission and relapse or of progressive disease, which may take the form of increasing dementia (Bye *et al* 1985). Even with prolonged observation, these childhood onset cases presenting with an acute or subacute encephalopathy continue to pose diagnostic problems (see Chapter 8). The same is true for cases presenting with massive cerebral MRI lesions and following a relapsing–remitting course (Leuzzi *et al* 1999). As we discuss in Chapter 8, the situation is much complicated by the difficulty in distinguishing childhood multiple sclerosis from acute disseminated encephalomyelitis. But this optimism often proves to be misplaced.

Amongst a small informal series observed by one of us (DASC) are three children in whom the optimistic diagnosis of acute disseminated encephalomyelitis in this situation was preferred to multiple sclerosis on the basis of altered conscious level, epilepsy and headache in addition to optic nerve involvement. One subsequently developed a sub-acute cord lesion, suggesting a second lesion sufficient for establishing the diagnosis of multiple sclerosis, but investigations showed a mass lesion which proved to be a low-grade cystic astrocytoma. The tentative diagnosis of multiple sclerosis was suspended but later she had recurrent optic neuritis with oligoclonal bands and new MRI abnormalities. Histological review confirmed the diagnosis of her cord lesion and the working diagnosis remains childhood multiple sclerosis and astrocytoma. The second made a slow cognitive recovery from the presumed episode of acute disseminated encephalomyelitis occurring at the age of 10 years. A new episode of optic neuritis 6 weeks after presentation (leaving her with significantly reduced vision) and the later development of generalized epilepsy were considered to be part of the original illness, but 4 years later she had an acute episode of vertigo with abnormal vertical eye movements and MRI showed a new lesion in the midbrain (see Figure 6.29). She has now reached adult life with no further episodes of demyelination in the last 8 years. The third, whose older sister developed an aggressive form of multiple sclerosis with onset as a teenager, made a full recovery from her initial episode: for the next 5 years she had no definite new manifestations of central nervous system demyelination but, aged 19, developed Lhermitte's symptom with unpleasant hemisensory symptoms and signs of a spastic paraparesis: repeat MR imaging showed many new cerebral and spinal lesions since the inititial investigations performed in childhood.

In childhood multiple sclerosis, the cerebrospinal fluid cell count is occasionally >100 mm^3 (Arnouts 1959; DiMario and Berman 1987; Issler 1961; Van Lieshout *et al* 1993). An unusual proportion of polymorphonuclear leucocytes may be present (Bejar and Ziegler 1984; Hauser *et al* 1982). The concentration of total protein is usually within normal limits or slightly elevated (Boutin *et al* 1988; Duquette *et al* 1987) but levels >100 mg/100 mL are occasionally reported (Gall *et al* 1958; Matthews 1985; Schneider *et al* 1969). Oligoclonal bands were found in all definite cases by Bauer and Hanefeld (1993).

Multiple hypodense white matter lesions have been shown by CT scanning in a high proportion of cases (summarized by Bauer and Hanefeld 1993). Ring enhancement may be seen (Brandt *et al* 1981). As in adult disease, MRI is much more frequently abnormal than CT scanning and many more lesions are shown. Generally, the features are the same as in adults. Several cases are described, as in adults, where the radiological appearances suggested an apparent mass lesion (Bauer and Hanefeld 1993; Golden and Woody 1987; Rusin *et al* 1995; Van Lieshout *et al* 1993) but with eventual confirmation of clinically definite childhood multiple sclerosis either through follow up or pathological confirmation. Serial MRI is of great value in the distinction from acute disseminated encephalomyelitis (Milner *et al* 1990). MRI features can also be used to predict conversion to multiple sclerosis after an episode of isolated demyelination in childhood. Lesions perpendicular to the corpus callosum and well defined discrete lesions are considered more specific but less sensitive than the application of criteria (proposed by Barkhof *et al* 1997) for the radiological confirmation of multiple sclerosis in adults (Mikaeloff *et al* 2004).

There is evidence that childhood onset multiple sclerosis evolves more slowly than adult onset disease (Simone *et al* 2002), in keeping with the observation that even in adults, those with onset between 20 and 35 years show slower accumulation of disability and severity more than in cohorts with onset between 36 and 50 and 51 and 65 years, respectively (Trojano *et al* 2002).

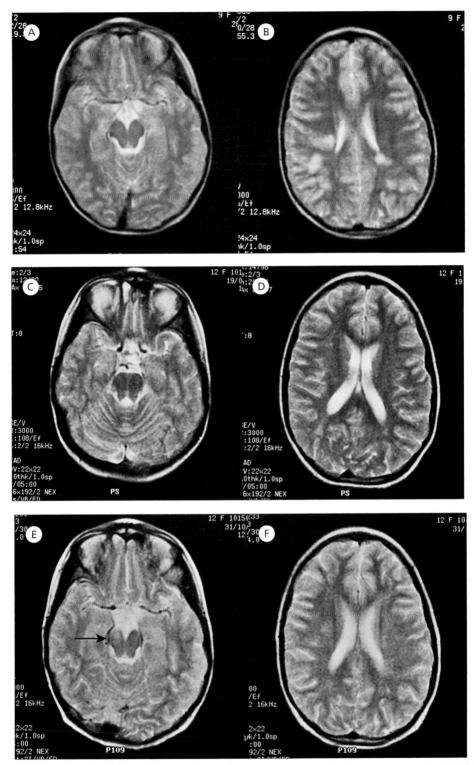

Figure 6.29 Female child with 'acute disseminated encephalomyelitis' at age 8 years. (A,B) MRI abnormality. (C,D) Subsequent images became normal. (E,F) Within 1 month, she had an acute midbrain lesion (arrow).

Optic neuritis

The mean age of onset in reported cases of optic neuritis in children is around 9 years, but it has been observed as early as age 3 (Kriss *et al* 1988), girls being more frequently affected than boys. There are significant differences from the adult form, including the apparently higher frequency (67%) of bilateral simultaneous or closely consecutive attacks (De Leersnyder *et al* 1981; Haller and Patzold 1979; Kriss *et al* 1988; Riikonen *et al* 1988). An uncertain number of cases of unilateral optic neuritis may be missed in young children who show no alteration in behaviour to alert their parents to the possibility of monocular change in vision. Swollen discs, usually bilateral, occur in a similar proportion and headache or pain in the eye and loss of central vision in the majority. Infection or inoculation precede optic neuritis in between 20 and 46% of cases (Meadows 1969; Kriss *et al* 1988). The prognosis for recovery of vision is usually excellent with rapid return to normal visual evoked potentials (Kriss *et al* 1988), although occasional instances of persistent blindness have been reported (De Leersnyder *et al* 1981; Riikonen *et al* 1988). These studies were performed before genetic testing for Leber's hereditary optic neuropathy became available and this may be the correct diagnosis as in some adults with permanent visual loss (Morrissey *et al* 1995). In a retrospective series from the Mayo Clinic (1950–1988), 13% of 79 children, aged <16 years at presentation and reviewed a mean of 19.4 years later, had developed multiple sclerosis. Actuarial analysis indicated conversion rates of 22% and 26% at 30 and 40 years, respectively (Lucchinetti *et al* 1997). Clinical features did not discriminate those who converted from those who did not. There was an increased risk in the context of bilateral sequential or recurrent unilateral optic neuritis, and prior history of infection within 2 weeks of developing the visual loss carried a relatively good prognosis.

All these clinical features indicate, not unexpectedly, that in a much higher proportion than in adults, optic neuritis in children can be attributed to a restricted form of acute disseminated encephalomyelitis. Progression to multiple sclerosis may, however, occur, being reported in 28% in the four series cited above. This figure is remarkably close to the 27% progression after a mean of 8 years previously described (Kennedy and Carroll 1960; Kennedy and Carter 1961). These figures are not strictly comparable with those cited for isolated optic neuritis in adults since patients with signs of disseminated disease were included in all series. In most reports, unilateral optic neuritis was more likely to herald multiple sclerosis but this was not confirmed by Kriss *et al* (1988). In the most recent report of childhood

multiple sclerosis (Bauer and Hanefeld 1993), the initial symptom was isolated unilateral optic neuritis in 2/20 personally observed children.

As Meadows (1969) first noted and Kriss *et al* (1988) confirmed, signs of neurological involvement beyond the optic nerves are not uncommon in the acute phase. One of us (WIMcD) has seen several examples of acute bilateral optic neuritis in childhood with good recovery of vision, in whom, after an interval of weeks or months, there is one or more acute episodes of cerebral dysfunction, including epilepsy, resolving without persistent deficit. These episodes are accompanied by rather large MRI lesions sometimes involving the cortex (Figure 6.30). Long term follow-up is needed on these patients.

CONCLUSION

No account of the symptoms and signs of multiple sclerosis can be other than selective and incomplete. This is emphasized by the increasing recognition that the diagnosis is often not made in life, either because symptoms go unrecognized or because none has occurred or been recorded (Georgi 1961; Castaigne *et al* 1981; Phadke and Best 1983; Gilbert and Sadler 1983; Engell 1989). No symptomatic correlations can be made for the great majority of fleeting cerebral abnormalities seen on MRI and even established chronic demyelination in highly eloquent sites, such as the optic nerve and spinal cord, may be symptomless (Ghatak *et al* 1974; Wisniewski *et al* 1976). The precise mechanisms by which events in the evolving plaque, and their representation by imaging or under the microscope, explain the symptomatic experiences of individual patients are still relatively unexplored but we discuss what is known concerning these aspects of the pathophysiology and pathogenesis in Chapter 13.

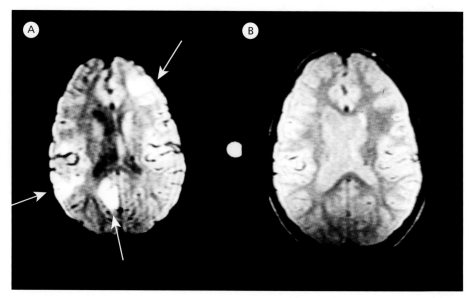

Figure 6.30 (A) T$_2$-weighted MRI during an episode of cerebral symptoms following acute optic neuritis in childhood. (B) The same MRI appearances 2 years later.

The diagnosis of multiple sclerosis

David Miller, Ian McDonald and Kenneth Smith

DIAGNOSTIC CRITERIA FOR MULTIPLE SCLEROSIS

Given the lack of a specific laboratory test for multiple sclerosis, the only certain means of proving the diagnosis is histological examination of tissue obtained from multiple sites within the central nervous system. The neurologist confronted with a patient in whom the diagnosis of multiple sclerosis is suspected must answer a number of questions:

- Is the history compatible?
- Are there multiple lesions in the central nervous system?
- Are the lesions demyelinating in nature?
- Is there an immunological abnormality in relation to the central nervous system?
- Does an alternative and more likely explanation for the clinical and investigative picture seem likely?

In some cases, the clinical picture alone may be sufficient to establish the diagnosis with considerable confidence. Even then, the neurologist often seeks the reassurance of confirmatory results from laboratory investigations, especially when treatments carrying known or unknown risks of long-term adverse effects are being contemplated. However, there is often genuine diagnostic uncertainty, especially early in the course of the disease. A number of schemes for assigning relative certainty to the diagnosis have been used over the years. At first they were based on clinical features alone but, in 1983, a distinguished group of neurologists reached consensus on a classification that, although retaining some weaknesses, gained widespread acceptance in clinical practice, epidemiology and treatment trials (Table 7.1; C.M. Poser *et al* 1983). The Poser criteria had as their gold standard for the diagnosis of multiple sclerosis two or more attacks affecting two or more necessarily separate sites within the central nervous system (including one or other optic nerves) but, for clinically definite disease, also allowed clinical evidence to be replaced by laboratory abnormalities at the second site. Imaging, electrophysiology and cerebrospinal fluid examination were used to supplement evidence for the diagnosis in situations where clinical criteria were not met, either through absence of the second clinical episode or affected site. Not every patient fitted neatly into this classification and the patients with progressive disease proved especially difficult to evaluate. McAlpine *et al* (1955) had distinguished patients in whom a single episode

is followed some years later by progressive disease and called these transitional progressive cases. This category was largely ignored but Gayou *et al* (1997) showed that, amongst 214 consecutively presenting patients, 12 had transitional multiple sclerosis compared with 38 with primary and 55 with secondary progressive disease. Serial assessments of clinical activity and magnetic resonance imaging (MRI) confirmed that transitional progressive multiple sclerosis behaves more like primary than secondary progressive disease.

The issue of working definitions for primary progressive multiple sclerosis was finally tackled by A.J. Thompson *et al* (2000) who argued that there should be clinical progression for at least 1 year and that three levels of diagnostic certainty could be defined – based on a consideration of the findings from cerebrospinal fluid examination, MRI and evoked potentials. To make a definite diagnosis according to these criteria, there must be oligoclonal bands present in the cerebrospinal fluid. In addition, it is required that there is either 'definite' MRI abnormality (that is nine or more brain lesions; or two or more spinal cord lesions; or one spinal cord lesion plus four to eight brain lesions), or 'equivocal' (that is, lesser degrees of) MRI abnormality together with a delayed visual evoked response. In essence, the categories of probable and possible primary progressive multiple sclerosis require lesser degrees of abnormality within this spectrum of potentially informative laboratory investigations (A.J. Thompson *et al* 2000).

Against this background, new criteria have been proposed both for clinical and research purposes. One guiding principle was to bring forward the point at which the diagnosis of multiple sclerosis can be made with sufficient security, in the interests of informed discussions with individual patients, and as the basis for taking decisions on the use of disease-modifying treatments early in the disease course when these are most likely to be useful. The other purpose was to make best use of the accumulated evidence on the predictive value – sensitivity and specificity – of laboratory investigations introduced since 1983, whilst still recognizing that these methods are not universally available or performed to comparable standards (Tables 7.2–7.4 and Figure 7.1) These new criteria, developed by an International Panel, have generally been well accepted (W.I. McDonald *et al* 2001). The main change is that specific MRI features for dissemination in time and space are now incorporated. Thus, if a patient has a single clinical episode characteristic of demyelination accompanied by signs only of the

Table 7.1 Poser criteria for the diagnosis of multiple sclerosis

Category	Attacks	Clinical evidence	Paraclinical evidence	CSF OB/IgG
A. Clinically definite multiple sclerosis				
CDMS A1	2	2		
CDMS A2	2	1	and 1	
B. Laboratory-supported definite multiple sclerosis				
LSDMS B1	2	1	or 1	+
LSDMS B2	1	2		+
LSDMS B3	1	1	and 1	+
C. Clinically probable multiple sclerosis				
CPMS C1	2	1		
CPMS C2	1	2		
CPMS C3	1	1	and 1	
D. Laboratory-supported probable multiple sclerosis				
LSPMS D1	2			+

CSF, cerebrospinal fluid; OB, oligoclonal band; IgG, immunoglobulin G. From C.M. Poser et al (1983) with permission.

Table 7.3 McDonald criteria for multiple sclerosis: MRI evidence for dissemination in space

Three of the following:

- one or more gadolinium enhancing lesions or nine or more T_2 hyperintense lesions if there is no gadolinium enhancing lesion
- one or more infratentorial lesions
- one or more juxtacortical lesions
- three or more periventricular lesions

Notes: (i) one spinal cord lesion can substitute for one brain lesion; (ii) two T_2 lesions plus cerebrospinal fluid oligoclonal bands also constitute evidence for dissemination in space.
From W.I. McDonald et al (2001) with permission.

Table 7.4 McDonald criteria for multiple sclerosis: MRI evidence for dissemination in time.

1. If a first scan is >3 months after the onset of the clinical event, the presence of a gadolinium enhancing lesion is sufficient to demonstrate dissemination in time, provided that it is not at the site implicated in the original clinical event. If there is no enhancing lesion at this time, a follow-up scan is required. The timing of this follow-up scan is not crucial, but 3 months is recommended. A new T_2 or gadolinium enhancing scan at this time then fulfils the criterion for dissemination in time.

2. If the first scan is performed <3 months after the onset of the clinical event, a second scan done 3 months or more after the clinical event showing a new gadolinium enhancing lesion provides sufficient evidence for dissemination in time. However, if no enhancing lesion is seen at this second scan, a further scan ≥3 months after the first scan that shows a new T_2 or gadolinium enhancing lesion will suffice.

From W.I. McDonald et al (2001) with permission.

Table 7.2 McDonald criteria for multiple sclerosis: categories of multiple sclerosis

Clinical presentation	Additional data needed for diagnosis of multiple sclerosis
Two or more attacks; objective clinical evidence of two or more lesions	None[a]
Two or more attacks; objective clinical evidence of one lesion	Dissemination in space demonstrated by MRI[b] or Up to two MRI detected lesions consistent with multiple sclerosis plus positive cerebrospinal fluid[c] or Await further clinical attack implicating a different site
One attack; objective clinical evidence of two or more lesions	Dissemination in time demonstrated by MRI[d] or Second clinical attack
One attack; objective clinical evidence of one lesion (monosymptomatic presentation; clinically isolated syndrome)	Dissemination in space demonstrated by MRI[b] or Up to two MRI detected lesions consistent with multiple sclerosis plus positive cerebrospinal fluid[c] and Dissemination in time demonstrated by MRI[d] or Second clinical attack
Insidious neurological progression suggestive of multiple sclerosis	Positive cerebrospinal fluid[c] and Dissemination in space demonstrated by: (i) nine or more T_2 lesions in the brain or (ii) two or more lesions in the spinal cord or (iii) four to eight brain lesions plus one spinal cord lesion or Abnormal visual evoked potential[e] associated with four to eight brain lesions, or with fewer than four brain lesions plus one spinal cord lesion demonstrated by MRI and Dissemination in time demonstrated by MRI[d] or Continued progression for 1 year

a No additional tests are required (however, if MRI and cerebrospinal fluid are undertaken and are negative extreme caution should be taken before making a diagnosis of multiple sclerosis. Alternative diagnoses must be considered and there must be no better explanation for the clinical picture).
b Must fulfil the Barkhof/Tintoré criteria (Table 7.3).
c Positive cerebrospinal fluid established by oligoclonal bands detected by established methods (preferably isoelectric focusing) different from any such bands in serum or by a raised immunoglobulin G index.
d Must fulfil the criteria in Table 7.4.
e Abnormal visual evoked potential of the type seen in multiple sclerosis (delay with well-preserved wave form).
From W.I. McDonald et al (2001) with permission.

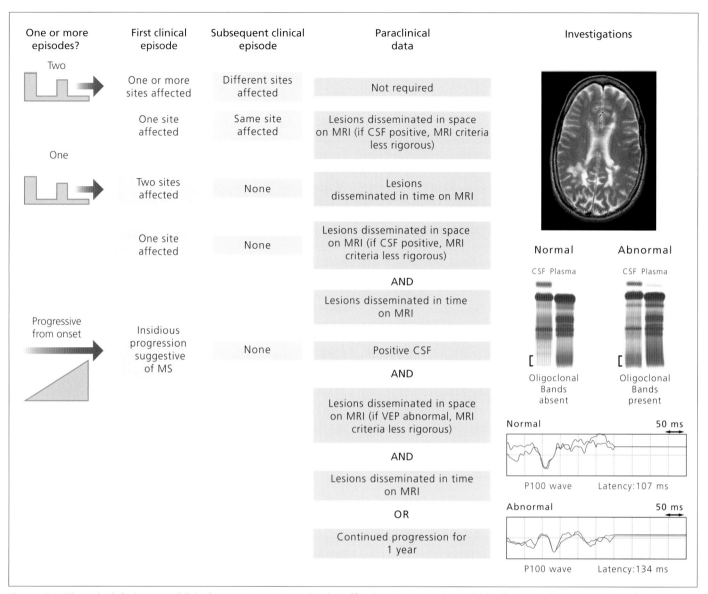

One or more episodes?	First clinical episode	Subsequent clinical episode	Paraclinical data	Investigations
Two	One or more sites affected	Different sites affected	Not required	
	One site affected	Same site affected	Lesions disseminated in space on MRI (if CSF positive, MRI criteria less rigorous)	
One	Two sites affected	None	Lesions disseminated in time on MRI	
	One site affected	None	Lesions disseminated in space on MRI (if CSF positive, MRI criteria less rigorous) AND Lesions disseminated in time on MRI	
Progressive from onset	Insidious progression suggestive of MS	None	Positive CSF AND Lesions disseminated in space on MRI (if VEP abnormal, MRI criteria less rigorous) AND Lesions disseminated in time on MRI OR Continued progression for 1 year	

Figure 7.1 The principle is to establish that two or more episodes affecting separate sites within the central nervous system have occurred at different times, using clinical analysis or laboratory investigations. Patients with an appropriate clinical presentation, but who do not meet all of the diagnostic criteria may be classified as having 'possible multiple sclerosis'. CSF, cerebrospinal fluid; VEP, visual evoked potential. Adapted from Compston and Coles (2002).

symptomatic lesion on examination, the demonstration by MRI of dissemination in time and space allows a diagnosis of multiple sclerosis. If the patient with a single attack has signs of two lesions on examination, MRI evidence for dissemination in time will satisfy the diagnosis of multiple sclerosis. If a patient has two clinical episodes suggestive of demyelination (as with the previous Poser criteria, it is required that at least 30 days separates the two events) but signs of only one lesion on examination, MRI evidence for dissemination in space will achieve a diagnosis of multiple sclerosis. In a patient who has two relapses and signs of two lesions on examination, MRI is not required for diagnosis, as was the case for the Poser criteria (such cases were then designated as clinically definite multiple sclerosis).

The MRI features of dissemination in space in the new criteria have evolved from the previous efforts of several imaging research groups to increase the specificity of MRI findings for

multiple sclerosis (Barkhof *et al* 1997a; Fazekas *et al* 1988; D.W. Paty *et al* 1988; Tintoré *et al* 2000). At an early stage, Fazekas *et al* (1988) suggested that support for the diagnosis of multiple sclerosis provided by T$_2$-weighted MRI required the presence of three or more lesions *and* two of the following three features:

- areas of abnormal signal with a diameter of ≥ 6 mm
- areas of abnormal signal abutting the bodies of the ventricles
- areas of abnormal signal in the infratentorial region.

Subsequently, Barkhof *et al* (1997a) analysed the use of multiple individual features of brain MRI lesions in determining which combination in a multifactorial model was best able to predict conversion from a clinically isolated syndrome to multiple sclerosis. After a mean follow-up of 3 years, they identified a high predictive value for conversion when four features were present:

- one or more gadolinium enhancing lesions
- three or more periventricular lesions
- one or more juxtacortical lesions
- one or more infratentorial lesions.

Tintoré *et al* (2000) proposed a modification of these Barkhof criteria, limiting the requirement to any three of the four features, and substituting the need for one gadolinium enhancing lesion with the alternative of at least nine T_2 lesions. The combined criteria of Barkhof modified by Tintore were adopted by the International Panel as evidence for dissemination in space (W.I. McDonald *et al* 2001; Table 7.3). The Panel included two additional items in its dissemination in space criteria. First, one spinal cord lesion can substitute for one brain lesion. Second, the criteria are satisfied by the combination of two T_2 lesions together with the presence of oligoclonal bands in the cerebrospinal fluid.

The key feature for MRI dissemination in time using these revised criteria is that a new lesion should appear at least 3 months after the clinical onset. This could be a gadolinium enhancing lesion on any scan obtained 3 or more months after clinical onset or, if such a scan does not show any enhancing lesions, the presence of a new T_2 lesion on a subsequent scan will suffice.

The new criteria recommend that they are best applied to individuals aged between 10 and 59 years. They also no longer include the categories of clinically definite or probable multiple sclerosis. Rather, the diagnostic categories are:

- multiple sclerosis – when the criteria are met
- possible multiple sclerosis – for those at risk of multiple sclerosis but for whom diagnostic evaluation is equivocal
- not multiple sclerosis.

Preliminary studies have attempted to validate the new criteria in terms of specificity and predictive value for development of clinically definite multiple sclerosis (discussed below). The criteria have both strengths and weaknesses and these are discussed further in Chapter 9. They are likely to be revised and fine tuned as more experience is gained of their application and indeed modifications to the criteria are expected following the meeting on a reconstituted International Panel in March 2005. Here, we consider the contribution that special or paraclinical investigations can make to the diagnostic process, but start by reiterating that, as in all branches of clinical neurology, laboratory investigations should never replace a full evaluation of the history and clinical examination when seeking to establish the diagnosis.

SELECTION OF INVESTIGATIONS

Three types of investigation may be needed in patients suspected of having demyelinating disease: MRI, evoked potentials and cerebrospinal fluid examination. Their purpose is to document the dissemination of lesions in space and time; to confirm the presence of intrathecal inflammation; and to exclude conditions that mimic demyelination. The starting point for diagnosis in the individual patient is the clinical picture. More than any other feature, this determines the nature and number of investigations required to reach the appropriate level of diagnostic certainty. In essence, the neurologist must ask the questions: which parts of the nervous system should I investigate; and how best can this be achieved?

The diagnosis of multiple sclerosis cannot by definition be made on clinical grounds alone, if there has been only a single episode (for example, optic neuritis). However, the risk of disseminated disease developing later may be estimated from MRI, evoked potentials and cerebrospinal fluid data (see below). Making use of their predictive values may have therapeutic implications, especially as treatments that safely delay the progression of disability are increasingly made available. By applying the most recently published authoritative criteria, such paraclinical investigations can be used to make a diagnosis of multiple sclerosis 3 months after symptom onset (W.I. McDonald *et al* 2001).

A commonly encountered problem is the patient who has had several episodes of neurological symptoms suggestive of multiple sclerosis, but who, on examination, has abnormal signs relating only to the most recent event. In these circumstances, MRI, or occasionally evoked potentials, reveals whether the nervous system has been involved at other sites even though these have not given rise to clinical manifestations. In selecting the parts of the nervous system that should be examined to demonstrate dissemination in space, the neurologist is guided by the history, deliberately choosing those sites that the current clinical assessment indicates not to be involved. For example, for patients with recent onset of symptoms attributable to a spinal cord lesion, we scan the brain and in some instances select visual or auditory evoked potentials. In the context of recent visual loss, brain and possibly spinal MRI – on occasions supplemented by somatosensory and auditory evoked potentials – are appropriate methods for exploring clinically unaffected parts of the nervous system. There is a catch, however. Moving straight to the clinically unaffected nervous system on the assumption that the presenting syndrome is the result of inflammation and demyelination runs the risk of missing a local structural lesion. Therefore, in this example, the cord should also be targeted to exclude other diagnoses.

In cases where the diagnosis remains in real doubt, it is often helpful to answer two questions. First, is there evidence for the pathological process of demyelination? This can be inferred from the presence of a delayed evoked potential with a well-preserved waveform, though considerable caution is needed when this appears distorted (see Chapter 13). Since demyelination, axonal loss and gliosis each occur in multiple sclerosis, it might be hoped that imaging appearances would suggest the diagnosis, but no one morphological component has a specific imaging marker and these tissue-based interpretations cannot therefore reliably be made. Second, is there an abnormality of the immune mechanism in relation to the central nervous system? This is most readily judged from examination of the cerebrospinal fluid which will provide evidence for intrathecal synthesis of oligoclonal immunoglobulin G. This approach is particularly helpful in complex cases where considerable doubt remains about the disease mechanism, and in patients presenting with progressive syndromes attributable to a single site in which, over and above exclusion of a structural lesion, other disease processes could be involved – motor neuron disease, hereditary spastic paraplegia or spino-cerebellar degeneration. In these and other situations, the issue is to get a lead on the underlying disease process despite the relative or complete absence of MRI abnormalities. Examination of the cerebrospinal fluid is also of considerable importance in the investigation of individuals where imaging is likely to be relatively uninformative, such as the older patient with longstanding and previously undiagnosed demyelinating disease or those with genuinely late onset disease, in whom the specificity of MRI white matter lesions is low. There are also occasions when MRI abnormalities are not apparent, or are of a minimal nature such that specific diagnostic criteria for multiple sclerosis are not fulfilled, yet where the presence of oligoclonal bands and delayed visual evoked potentials suggest demyelination, and one is reminded that MRI abnormalities are not required to make a clinical diagnosis of multiple sclerosis. Nevertheless, we do recommend especial caution in making the diagnosis when there are no abnormalities to be seen on good quality images obtained from both the brain and the whole of the spinal cord – such a finding must be very rare in clinically definite disease.

When the clinical picture is not episodic, or does not change while the patient is under observation, the demonstration of new focal lesions on MRI carried out over time may be very helpful in establishing the multiphasic nature of the disease process leading to the diagnosis of multiple sclerosis. Again, the most recent diagnostic criteria for multiple sclerosis allow for the criterion of dissemination in time to be fulfilled by MRI evidence alone (W.I. McDonald *et al* 2001).

In rare instances, the diagnosis of multiple sclerosis will be established by histopathological examination of a brain biopsy. The setting in which this usually occurs is a patient with an acute and fulminant presentation, clinical features indicating a rapidly progressing cerebral hemisphere lesion, and the radiological finding of a large mass lesion or lesions in the cerebral white matter. The suspicion of cerebral tumour or of an atypical inflammatory or infectious process leads to biopsy and correction of the diagnosis to inflammatory demyelination.

It is important again to stress that no one of the routinely used investigations (MRI, cerebrospinal fluid and evoked potentials) provides a result that is pathognomonic for multiple sclerosis. Formulation of the diagnosis depends on giving due weight to each element of the clinical and investigative picture. Herein lies the skill of the neurologist. Having outlined the general approach to the use of investigations, we now describe what they have to offer.

MAGNETIC RESONANCE IMAGING

It is difficult for the younger neurologist to appreciate the changes in practice arising from the introduction of brain imaging in the early 1970s. This has become an enormously important tool in clinical medicine, especially neurology. MRI provides noninvasive high-resolution and relatively artefact-free images of the brain and spinal cord and has the advantages over computed tomography (CT) scanning of not being subject to bone hardening influences, and proving uniquely sensitive in detecting many extrinsic and intrinsic pathological conditions. The value of MRI was recognized by the award of the Nobel Prize in Physiology or Medicine in 2003 to two pioneers of the technique for human imaging: Dr Paul Lauterbur and Sir Peter

Mansfield (see Chapter 1; Gore 2003). In patients with spinal cord disease, the availability of MRI has rendered the earlier, invasive method of myelography obsolete. The opportunities for laboratory evaluation of multiple sclerosis were transformed with the introduction of MRI (I.R. Young *et al* 1981).

Methodology

MRI scanners are large magnets that produce a strong local magnetic field. This is created within the scanner by generating currents in coils surrounding the bore after they are cooled to an extremely low temperature using liquid helium (these are known as superconducting magnets). In body tissues, atoms that contain an uneven number of protons and neutrons have a small magnetic charge (such as ^{1}H, ^{23}Na, ^{31}P). When a subject is placed in the strong magnetic field, slightly more of these nuclei are oriented parallel rather than at an angle to the strong external field and, thus, they generate a net magnetization along the axis of this orientation. By applying radiofrequency pulses, the magnetization of the tissue can be excited to produce a nuclear magnetic resonance (NMR) signal that is detected by an external receiver. Using mathematical methods, such as two-dimensional Fourier transformation, together with additional gradient pulses that alter the local magnetic field in space, it is possible to locate all of the acquired NMR signals in their correct spatial positions, and thereby to produce two- or three-dimensional images.

The ^{1}H protons constitute by far the most abundant nuclei in the body from which NMR signals can be generated. Most protons in tissue are contained in water molecules (although fat protons also produce NMR signals at sites where they are concentrated such as the orbit). After the initial exciting radiofrequency pulse is discontinued, the water protons relax back to their resting state orientated along the strong magnetic field of the scanner. This process is governed by two main NMR properties – T_1 (longitudinal) and T_2 (transverse) relaxation. Thus MRI generates tissue contrast largely as a result of variations in the amount (proton density) of water and its T_1 and T_2 relaxation times. In turn, these are influenced by the macromolecular environment of the water molecules. Additional properties that can influence image contrast on certain MR sequences are diffusion of the protons and magnetization transfer (the latter is the transfer of magnetization between the protons when they exist in different physicochemical states).

Given that the dominant mechanism for differentiating normal and pathological tissues on conventional MRI is the concentration and macromolecular environment of water, it is possible to see that this brings a fundamental strength and weakness of the modality for diagnosis. The strength is a remarkably high sensitivity in detecting pathological abnormalities in soft tissue. The weakness is the limited pathological specificity. An important adjunct in diagnostic imaging is the use of paramagnetic gadolinium-containing chelates as contrast agents. Gadolinium contains seven unpaired electrons and water protons that come within its vicinity experience a marked decrease in their T_1 relaxation rate. Thus areas of contrast enhancement (increased signal) are seen on T_1-weighted scans. Gadolinium chelates do not enter the normal brain because of the tight blood–brain barrier but they will enter regions where this has been made permeable.

Clinically definite multiple sclerosis

It is important at the outset to reiterate that all images depend ultimately on the relative amounts and physicochemical environment of water protons in each area of the brain. The changes produced by disease may be characteristic but, by their nature, cannot be specific for any particular pathological process. It follows that the diagnosis of multiple sclerosis cannot be made on the basis of MRI alone. That said, the form and distribution of MRI abnormalities in multiple sclerosis are such that the appearances in any one case may be highly suggestive. MRI is accordingly of great value in clinical neurology and the assessment of individual patients. Its contribution, taken in the context of the remaining clinical and investigative picture, is often decisive.

Brain T_2-weighted MRI

T_2 contrast is the key feature that gives these approaches a high sensitivity for depicting focal white matter lesions in multiple sclerosis. This may be achieved using spin echo, fast spin echo or fast fluid attenuated inversion recovery (FLAIR) sequences. Multiple areas of high signal are seen in the periventricular region in 95% of patients. The abnormalities may be either discrete and focal (Figure 7.2) or confluent (Figure 7.3). They tend to involve the deep rather than the more peripheral white matter, although focal lesions are common enough in the periphery. The opposite distribution is more characteristic of vascular disease (Figure 7.4: see below), but neither is specific. Juxtacortical lesions (in subcortical white matter and abutting the cortex) are characteristic of multiple sclerosis, being present in about two-thirds of patients (D.H. Miller 1988; Figure 7.5). Conversely, sparing of the subcortical U-fibres is observed in some forms of arteriosclerotic small vessel disease. The rare involvement of the corpus callosum in vascular disease contrasts with the frequent location of lesions at this site in multiple sclerosis (Gean-Marton *et al* 1991; Offenbacher *et al* 1993). Corpus callosum lesions are a useful diagnostic feature best appreciated on sagittal T_2-weighted images, although they can

also be observed on the more frequently acquired axial images (Figure 7.2). Lesions in the posterior visual pathways, most notably the optic radiations, are frequently seen (Hornabrook *et al* 1992; Figure 7.6).

Other common sites of involvement in multiple sclerosis are the brainstem and cerebellum (Barkhof *et al* 1997a; Figure 7.7). Brainstem lesions characteristically abut onto cerebrospinal fluid spaces, both anteriorly and adjacent to the fourth ventricle or aqueduct. In contrast, arteriosclerotic small vessel disease more often produces abnormalities in the central pons or midbrain that evidently do not extend to the parenchymal surface. Lesions of cerebellar white matter are seen in about 50% of patients with clinically definite multiple sclerosis.

Abnormalities of the grey matter, defined by MRI, occur much less often than those present in white matter. In our own series, the basal ganglia are affected in about 10% of cases (Miller *et al* 1997; Ormerod *et al* 1987). The low sensitivity of conventional MRI contrasts with the high frequency of pathological abnormality found in the thalamus post mortem (Cifelli

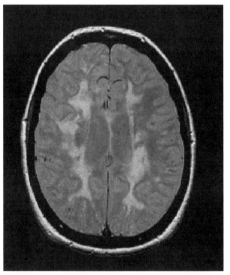

Figure 7.3 Multiple sclerosis. T_2-weighted axial brain MRI shows confluent periventricular abnormalities.

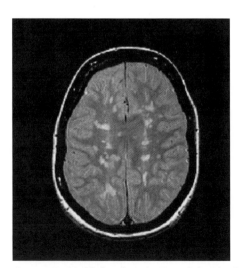

Figure 7.2 Multiple sclerosis. T_2-weighted axial brain MRI reveals multiple periventricular and discrete white matter lesions in addition to involvement of the corpus callosum.

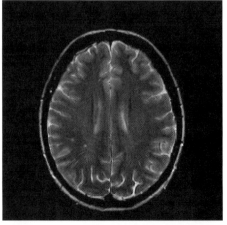

Figure 7.4 T_2-weighted MRI showing subcortical lesions that are characteristic – though not specific – for small vessel disease.

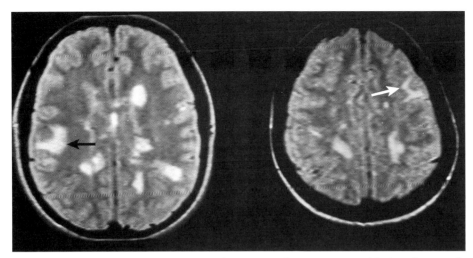

Figure 7.5 Multiple sclerosis. T_2-weighted MRI scans show juxtacortical lesions (arrowed).

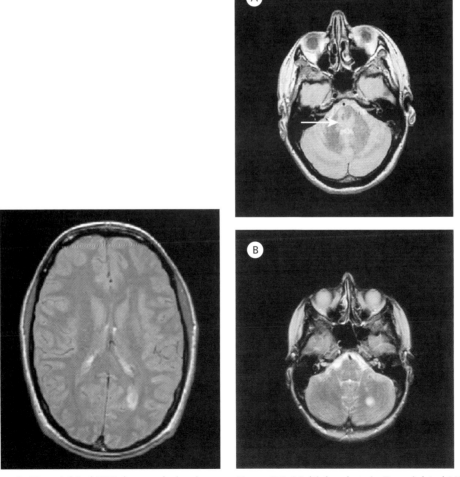

Figure 7.6 Multiple sclerosis. T_2-weighted MRI shows a lesion in the optic radiation.

Figure 7.7 Multiple sclerosis. T_2-weighted MRI scans. (A) Lesion in the brainstem. (B) Lesion in the cerebellar white matter.

et al 2002). Cortical involvement, although commonly demonstrated at autopsy (Brownell and Hughes 1962; D. Kidd *et al* 1999a; Petersen *et al* 2001) is also infrequently recognized on routine scans. In part, this is because of partial volume effects but more likely reflects the fact that cortical plaques of demyelination have proton density and T_2 relaxation measures only marginally different from the surrounding grey matter. Cortical lesions are occasionally seen using gadolinium enhancement (see below). White matter lesions at the cortico-medullary junction are more readily seen using fast FLAIR sequences (Figure 7.8) and such lesions may on occasions extend into the cortical grey matter. The detection of intracortical lesions has been recently found to be improved by the use of a 3D double-inversion recovery sequence (Geurts *et al* 2005), although still only a minority of pathologically detected lesions is visible on MRI. Hypointensity on T_2-weighted images is reported in both cortical and deep grey matter structures in multiple sclerosis (Bakshi *et al* 2001; 2002; Grimaud *et al* 1995; Tjoa *et al* 2005) and has been associated with increasing disability, T_2 lesion load and brain atrophy. T_2 hypointensity may reflect increased iron deposition associated with neurodegeneration.

Although the great majority of brain lesions in multiple sclerosis are <5 mm in diameter, very large lesions occasionally occur and the extent of mass effect may even suggest the differential diagnosis of cerebral tumour (Figure 7.9). The detection of additional typical white matter lesions will give a clue to the correct diagnosis but, on occasion, uncertainty is such that biopsy is performed. A few large lesions exhibit multiple concentric rings of alternating high and low signal. This radiological appearance probably corresponds to the alternating bands of demyelination and myelination reported in Balo's concentric sclerosis (Iannucci *et al* 2000a; Stadelmann *et al* 2005; Figure 7.10). Acute lesions often display a single concentric ring of low signal on T_2-weighted images that correlates with macrophage infiltration and lipid breakdown at the lesion edge, and with gadolinium enhancement on post contrast T_1-weighted scans (see below).

Compared with T_2-weighted spin echo and fast spin echo sequences, the fast FLAIR sequence has the advantage of greater sensitivity in the cerebral hemispheres, especially subcortical white matter (Filippi *et al* 1996). This advantage is offset by it being less sensitive in the posterior fossa (Gawne-Cain *et al* 1997), and spinal cord (Stevenson *et al* 1997). Fast spin echo T_2-weighted sequences have largely replaced conventional spin echo sequences as they enable more rapid scanning of the brain and spinal cord. In the NMR Research Unit at Queen Square, London, the standard diagnostic T_2-weighted imaging sequence now is a double-echo proton-density and T_2-weighted fast spin echo, with which 3-mm axial contiguous slices and whole spinal cord 3-mm contiguous sagittal images can be captured in 6 and 10 minutes, respectively (Miller *et al* 1997). Many centres also add a fast FLAIR sequence because it makes cerebral white matter lesions more conspicuous. A gadolinium enhanced T_1-weighted sequence is also being increasingly used in the diagnostic workup (Fazekas *et al* 1999) and should now be used routinely in patients with single clinical episodes where it may contribute to the earlier diagnosis of multiple sclerosis (W.I. McDonald *et al* 2001).

Spinal cord T_2-weighted MRI

The spinal cord is commonly involved radiologically, whether or not this part of the central nervous system manifests symptoms and signs. Cord lesions are best detected on proton density and T_2-weighted images. In the sagittal plane, the lesions are usually less than one vertebral segment in length and occupy only part of the antero-posterior diameter of the cord (Figure 7.11). Axial scans reveal lesions involving only part of the cross-section of the cord, characteristically asymmetric and extending to the surface, sometimes in a wedge shape (Lycklama *et al* 2003; Figure 7.12). Although involvement of posterior and lateral quadrants is frequently seen, lesions not uncommonly extend into the central grey matter. Acute lesions may display swelling and those present over a period of time are associated with focal atrophy of the cord.

The sequences most often used to depict spinal cord lesions in multiple sclerosis are sagittal T_2-weighted fast or conventional spin echo (Figure 7.11), on occasions complemented by axial T_2-weighted imaging. The latter is useful in confirming an equivocal lesion seen on sagittal imaging. Short tau inversion recovery

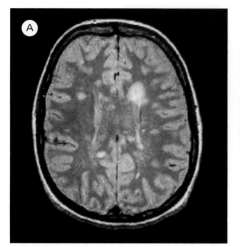 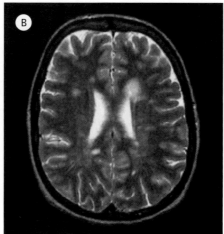 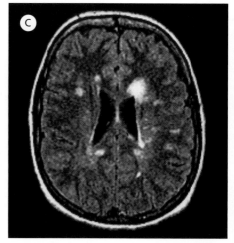

Figure 7.8 Multiple sclerosis lesions depicted using (A) proton density, (B) T_2-weighted, and (C) fast FLAIR sequence. Several subcortical lesions are better seen on fast FLAIR.

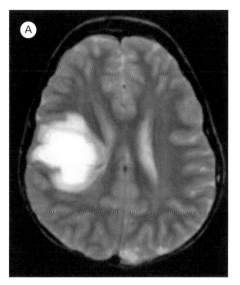

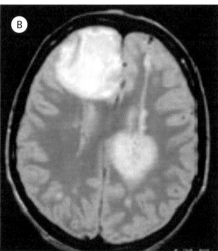

Figure 7.9 Multiple sclerosis. T$_2$-weighted scans showing large cerebral hemisphere lesions with mass effect. Kindly provided by Dr Claudia Lucchinetti.

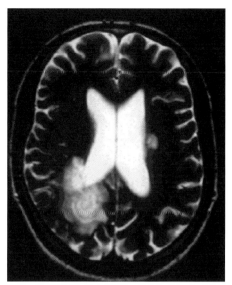

Figure 7.10 Multiple sclerosis. T$_2$-weighted MRI shows a lesion with alternating bands of high and normal signal (Balo's concentric sclerosis). From Kastrup *et al* (2002) with permission.

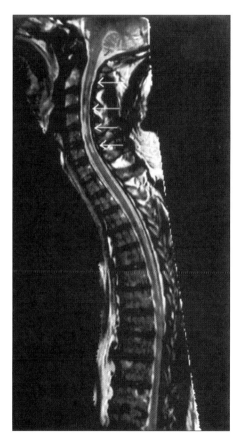

Figure 7.11 Multiple sclerosis. T$_2$-weighted sagittal MRI of the spinal cord shows multiple, small intrinsic lesions (arrowed).

fast spin echo (fast STIR) imaging has a slightly higher sensitivity than fast or conventional spin echo in detecting some cord lesions but this gain is offset by more frequent occurrence of artefacts (Bot *et al* 2000). Fast STIR has not become a part of the standard protocol for detecting spinal cord lesions.

Abnormalities in the cord may be seen when none are detectable in the brain, a finding of particular importance in primary progressive multiple sclerosis where cerebral lesions are less extensive than in other forms of the disease, and may even be absent (Kidd *et al* 1993). Thorpe *et al* (1996b) emphasized the value of cord imaging in 20 patients with clinically suspected multiple sclerosis but normal or near normal brain MRI. All 20 patients exhibited at least one focal cord lesion (median 2; range 1–6). The value of other laboratory investigation in such cases was also emphasized by the presence of cerebrospinal fluid oligoclonal bands in 13/15 and delayed visual evoked potentials in 10/18 subjects. Diffuse hyperintensity on proton density weighted images of the cord may also be seen, more so in primary progressive than in other forms of multiple sclerosis (Lycklama *et al* 1998).

As with the corpus callosum, the cord is rarely involved by vascular disease and, unlike the cerebrum, asymptomatic areas of high signal are very uncommon as an incidental finding with increasing age (Thorpe *et al* 1993). A recent study compared brain and spinal cord MRI in 25 patients with clinically definite

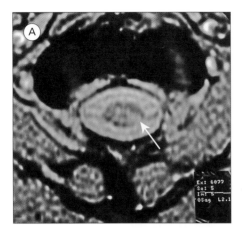 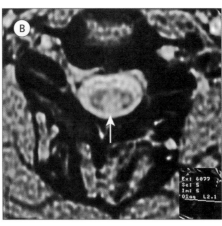

Figure 7.12 Multiple sclerosis. (A) and (B) T_2-weighted axial MRI scans through the spinal cord show two intrinsic lesions that involve only part of the cord cross-section and extend to the surface of the cord (arrows). Kindly provided by Dr Katherine Miszkiel.

multiple sclerosis and 66 with other neurological disorders, including inflammatory conditions (49 cases including systemic lupus erythematosus, Sjogren's syndrome and sarcoidosis) and cerebrovascular disease (17 cases; Bot *et al* 2002). In the brain, MRI revealed abnormalities in 100% of individuals with multiple sclerosis and in 56% of those with other diseases. In the cord, high signal lesions were seen in 92% with multiple sclerosis but only 6% with other diseases.

Gadolinium enhancement

An important step forward in the assessment of multiple sclerosis by MRI was the introduction of gadolinium-DTPA (diethylenetriamine pentacetic acid) and other gadolinium containing chelates as enhancing agents (R.I. Grossman *et al* 1986; Miller *et al* 1988b). Gadolinium-DTPA is normally excluded from the parenchyma of the brain and spinal cord by the blood–brain barrier and so the presence of enhancement indicates an increase in vascular permeability that, in the context of multiple sclerosis and related disorders, occurs in association with inflammation. The standard method for detecting enhancement is to perform a T_1-weighted scan 5–10 minutes after a bolus intravenous injection of 0.1 mmol/kg of a gadolinium-containing contrast agent. Various appearances are encountered in enhancing lesions (Figure 7.13). Some lesions tend to enhance uniformly, and focal homogeneous enhancement may be seen within larger lesions. Other, often larger, lesions show ring enhancement, corresponding with the pattern of inflammation sometimes seen at post mortem. The rings may be complete or partial – the latter, also called an incomplete ring, considered as particularly characteristic for multiple sclerosis (Masdeu *et al* 2000). However, ring enhancement is seen in a number of other pathological conditions, including brain abscess and metastases.

Enhancement is the earliest change detectable by MRI in the development of most new lesions in relapsing–remitting and secondary progressive multiple sclerosis (Figure 7.14; Kermode *et al* 1990; see Chapter 12). Enhancement is almost invariably seen in the relevant pathway at the onset of symptoms. It is also more commonly seen at other sites during clinical relapse (R.I. Grossman *et al* 1986; Kappos *et al* 1999; Smith *et al* 1993) more so than during remission. These sites include the cerebral cortex where, for the reasons given above, unenhanced lesions are difficult to visualize. However, most enhancing lesions occur in cerebral white matter and are as abundant in the subcortical and juxtacortical regions as in deep white matter (M.A. Lee *et al* 1999; Figure 7.13). It is not uncommon to see several areas of enhancement in the white matter at a particular time. Rarely, >100 such areas may be visible (Figure 7.15).

Enhancement lasts on average 4–6 weeks (Figure 7.13; Miller *et al* 1988b). It may, however, disappear more rapidly and in studies of patients undergoing weekly MRI, some new lesions enhance for as little as 1 week (Cotton *et al* 2003; H.M. Lai *et al* 1996). The fact that enhancement rarely lasts more than 2–3 months could be useful in helping to distinguish multiple sclerosis from other conditions such as tumour or neurosarcoidosis, where enhancement (without corticosteroids or other treatment) can be expected to persist. A further helpful feature is the extensive meningeal enhancement often seen in neurosarcoidosis but not as a feature of multiple sclerosis (see Figure 8.19; Lexa and Grossman 1994).

The high frequency of gadolinium enhancement in new lesions is seen in the relapsing–remitting and secondary progressive phases of the disease. However, there is convincing evidence that enhancement is less frequent in those patients with secondary progressive disease in whom superimposed relapses are no longer occurring (Kidd *et al* 1996; Tubridy *et al* 1998b). It is very strikingly more rare in primary progressive disease, in which only about 5% of new lesions enhance (A.J. Thompson *et al* 1991). The implications of this observation for understanding of the pathogenesis are discussed in Chapter 13.

There is evidence to suggest that some lesions which fail to show enhancement using conventional doses of gadolinium, standard sequences and imaging up to 20 minutes after bolus injection, may nevertheless have abnormal vascular permeability (Barnes *et al* 1991; Filippi *et al* 1995b; Silver *et al* 1997). The number of visible lesions may increase by 120% when a triple dose of a gadolinium chelate (0.3 mmol/kg) is combined with magnetization transfer imaging and the scan is delayed for 40–60 minutes after injection. The most important single factor contributing to the increase in sensitivity is the higher dose of contrast. Most additional enhancing lesions are seen in patients who already have some other enhancing lesions using single dose contrast. These methods to increase sensitivity are not relevant diagnostically but may have advantages in clinical trials by reducing the size of the required sample population (Koudriavtseva *et al* 1997; D.H. Miller *et al* 1996; Silver *et al* 1997; 2001). However, even in that context, the gains are

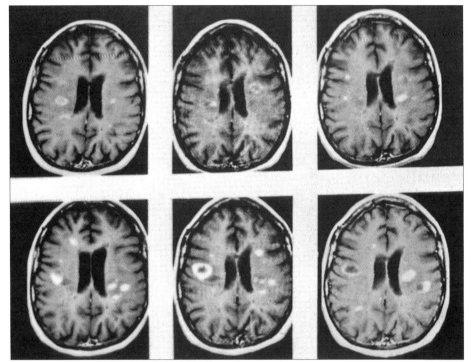

Figure 7.13 Serial monthly gadolinium enhanced T_1-weighted brain MRI over 6 months (starting at the top left and ending at the bottom right) in a patient with relapsing–remitting multiple sclerosis. Several new enhancing lesions appear each month and cease enhancing 1 or 2 months later. Some lesions show homogeneous enhancement while others display ring enhancement.

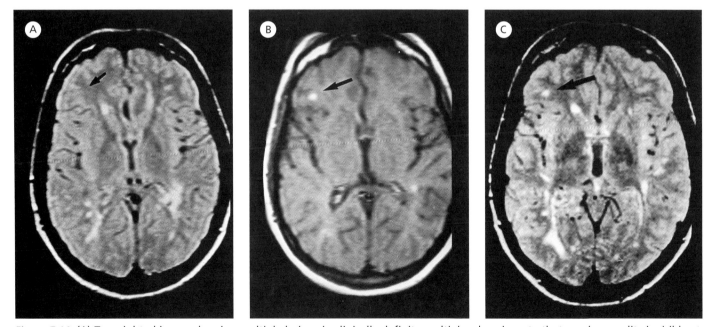

Figure 7.14 (A) T_2-weighted image showing multiple lesions in clinically definite multiple sclerosis; note that no abnormality is visible at the tip of the arrow. (B) Gadolinium-enhanced T_1-weighted image. Note that there are several areas of enhancement, one of which is at the tip of the arrow. This image was taken a matter of minutes following the T_2-weighted images. (C) T_2-weighted image some weeks later, now showing a lesion visible at the tip of the arrow.

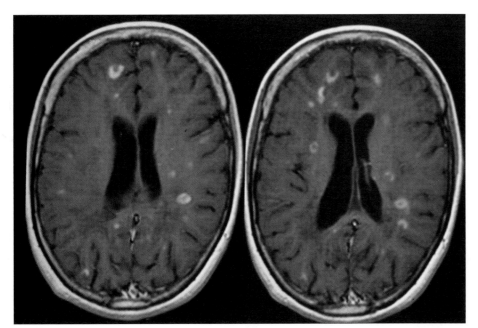

Figure 7.15 Gadolinium enhanced T₁-weighted MRI in clinically definite multiple sclerosis. This patient has >100 enhancing lesions at this time.

modest because the increase in overall sensitivity is offset by a greater variability in activity between patients. There is some evidence that the frequency of gadolinium enhancing lesions is highest in the earliest years of the disease, and may even occur early in primary progressive disease when triple dose gadolinium is used. In a recent study of 45 patients with primary progressive multiple sclerosis and disease duration <5 years, >40% had enhancing lesions (Ingle *et al* 2005).

T₁ *hypointense lesions*

Even though sequences providing proton density and T₂-weighted images are now standard, T₁-weighted inversion recovery images were used first in the assessment of multiple sclerosis (I.R. Young *et al* 1981). However, the overall sensitivity of inversion recovery was subsequently shown to be less than for T₂-weighted MRI. More recently, there has been interest in the appearance of lesions seen on T₁-weighted spin echo images because of their potential for revealing evidence of parenchymal destruction (Van Waesberghe *et al* 1999). Whereas about 20–30% of chronic T₂ lesions are persistently T₁ hypointense on T₁-weighted spin echo sequences in multiple sclerosis (Figure 7.16), such an appearance is less common in the white matter lesions associated with normal aging and small vessel disease (Uhlenbrock and Sehlen 1989). Chronic T₁ hypointense lesions have been correlated with greater axonal loss than T₁ isointense lesions. However, T₁ hypointensity on a single scan that does not allow the age of lesions to be determined should be interpreted with some caution, because T₁ hypointensity is not uncommonly a reversible finding of acute gadolinium enhancing lesions (Bagnato *et al* 2003). Resolution of T₁ hypointensity, when it occurs in such lesions, takes place over several months.

Relationship of abnormal signal to pathology

With the advent of MRI, close similarity between the distribution of areas showing abnormal signal on MRI and the dis-

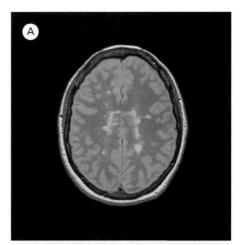

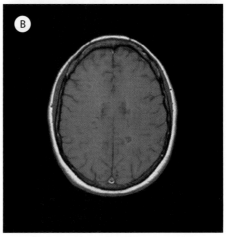

Figure 7.16 (A) T₂-weighted and (B) T₁-weighted MRI in multiple sclerosis. A minority of the T₂ lesions are visible as areas of T₁ hypointensity (colloquially called 'black holes').

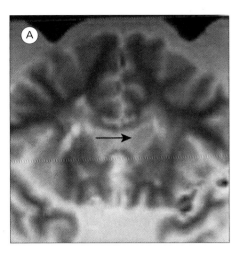

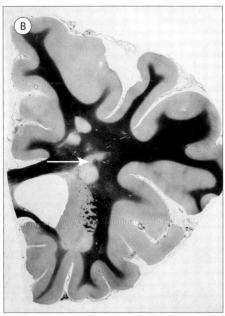

Figure 7.17 (A) T$_2$-weighted image of a formalin-fixed brain from a patient with clinically definite multiple sclerosis. (B) Section of the right hemisphere of the brain in a plane corresponding with the MRI in (A). There is good correspondence between the location of the imaging abnormalities and areas of demyelination (Heidenhein stain). From Ormerod *et al* (1987) with permission.

tribution of lesions at post mortem (see Chapter 12) soon suggested that the former represent plaques. This was more formally demonstrated by scanning formalin-fixed brain and correlating the images with tissue sections subsequently cut in the imaging planes (Figure 7.17; Ormerod *et al* 1987; W.A. Stewart *et al* 1986). More recent studies have indicated that not all MRI visible lesions correspond to classical plaques of demyelination. In some areas, inflammatory changes, such as microglial activation only, have been observed (De Groot *et al* 2001). Other T$_2$ lesions may represent areas of remyelination or shadow plaques (Barkhof *et al* 2003a). As described in Chapter 13, it has become clear that there is more to the interpretation of images than their topography, however important these correlations between imaging and pathology are.

In the early MRI literature, it was frequently reported that lesions could sometimes completely disappear, but this phenomenon is rarely seen with modern high-resolution scanners (A.J. Thompson *et al* 1991). Nonetheless, new lesions are seen to wax and wane in size over a matter of weeks (C. Isaac *et al* 1988; Willoughby *et al* 1989), and quantitative studies have shown, as expected, that at least some of the disappearing element of the lesions depicted on T$_2$-weighted or proton density images is attributable to oedema (Larsson *et al* 1988).

We now know that the residual abnormal signal in lesions originates from alterations in the amount and physicochemical state of extra- and intracellular water in the chronic plaques (Barnes *et al* 1988). Standard T$_2$-weighted MRI does not reveal either normal or pathological myelin and the common practice of referring to regions of abnormal signal as areas of demyelination is plainly wrong, and may even be misleading. Nor does it distinguish the extent of axonal loss in longstanding lesions.

Measures of atrophy

Another finding is the presence of apparently global spinal cord and cerebral atrophy, which may progress over as short a period as 12–18 months (Figure 7.18). It is seen at all stages of multiple

sclerosis and becomes increasingly marked with clinical progression and increasing disability (Figure 7.19; Losseff *et al* 1996a; 1996b; D.H. Miller *et al* 2002). Recent studies have used statistical parametric mapping to segment white and grey matter, indicating that significant atrophy occurs in both types of tissue (Chard *et al* 2002a; Sastre-Garriga *et al* 2005). Grey matter atrophy involves both neocortex (DeStefano 2003) and deep grey matter (Cifelli *et al* 2002). About 45% of normal white matter consists of axons and it is likely that progressive atrophy reflects underlying neuroaxonal loss. Because it correlates with clinical disability, the measurement of spinal cord and brain atrophy holds promise as a method for the assessment of therapeutic efficacy in clinical trials (D.H. Miller *et al* 2002). Progressive grey matter atrophy and ventricular enlargement have been detected during the first 3 years of multiple sclerosis following presentation with a clinically isolated syndrome (Figure 7.20; Dalton *et al* 2004a). Progressive grey matter atrophy also occurs in the early years of both relapsing–remitting and primary progressive multiple sclerosis (Tiberio *et al* 2005; Sastre-Garriga *et al* 2005). It follows that a high priority for therapeutic research in multiple sclerosis should be to find treatments that prevent neuroaxonal loss in the early stages of the disease. Although atrophy can readily be appreciated by visual inspection of scans when severe, more subtle degrees can only reliably be measured using quantitative methods. It is important to note that since atrophy is a feature of many other neurodegenerative disorders, it is not a useful diagnostic feature in everyday clinical practice.

Magnetic resonance spectroscopy

Magnetic resonance spectroscopy is making a significant contribution to our understanding of the pathogenesis of multiple sclerosis (see Chapter 13) but it has not established a place in routine diagnostic practice. Instead of studying water protons, spectroscopy investigates other proton-containing metabolites. Two metabolites of particular interest are *N*-acetyl aspartate and

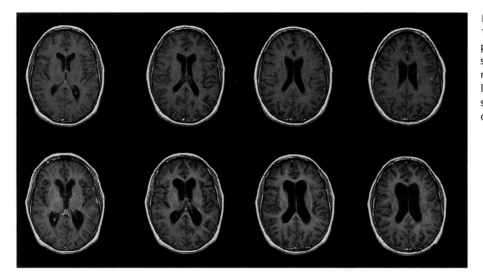

Figure 7.18 Serial T$_1$-weighted MRI over 18 months in a patient with secondary progressive multiple sclerosis showing striking development of atrophy. The top row shows baseline scans at four different levels in the brain and the bottom row shows the scans 18 months later at the corresponding levels.

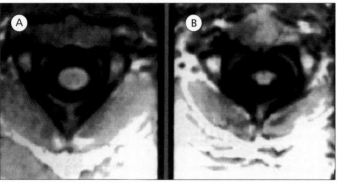

Figure 7.19 (A) Axial T$_1$-weighted through the upper cervical cord showing a normally sized cord in a multiple sclerosis patient with minimal disability (EDSS = 1). (B) Marked cord atrophy in another patient with severe disability (EDSS = 8). From Losseff *et al* (1996b) with permission.

myoinositol (Ins). *N*-Acetyl aspartate is contained almost entirely in neurons and axons, thus providing an indication of neuroaxonal damage and loss, which is thought to be the main substrate of irreversible disability in multiple sclerosis (Davie *et al* 1995; Fu *et al* 1998; Sarchielli *et al* 1999). However, decreases in *N*-acetyl aspartate are sometimes partly reversible (DeStefano *et al* 1997; Narayanan *et al* 2001). Reduction in *N*-acetyl aspartate sometimes reflects reversible mitochondrial dysfunction rather than cell death (R.E. Brenner *et al* 1993). Myoinositol is produced by glial cells. It is elevated in normal-appearing white matter early in multiple sclerosis, perhaps reflecting inflammation extending beyond focal lesions (Chard *et al* 2002b). There are several reasons why spectroscopy has a limited role in routine investigation and in resolving aspects of the differential diagnosis in multiple sclerosis. It is difficult to obtain reproducible spectra; the low signal to noise ratio of the metabolites limits the investigation to large lesions or normal appearing tissues; and broadly similar metabolic changes are seen in a number of different types of lesion. Reduced *N*-acetyl aspartate and increased choline-containing compounds are seen in tumours and leucodystrophies as well as demyelinating multiple sclerosis lesions, the former indicating axonal damage

and the latter an increase in membrane turnover. One case has suggested that the lesions of acute disseminated encephalomyelitis may differ from multiple sclerosis and leucodystrophies in having a normal choline content (Bizzi *et al* 2001).

Magnetization transfer imaging

Magnetization transfer imaging is sensitive to tissue disorganization (Dousset *et al* 1992; 1994; 1995; Grossman 1994). An additional pulse is applied that interrupts the normal exchange of magnetization between freely mobile water protons and those bound to macromolecules, in particular myelin in normal-appearing white matter. Quantitative data from these various sequences are being evaluated and studies to date suggest that, compared with standard T$_2$-weighted lesion measures, they provide a closer reflection of disease progression and disability. The magnetization transfer ratio provides a sensitive measure of disease progression in normal-appearing white and grey matter (Filippi *et al* 1999a) and reveals abnormalities from the early stages of disease (Figure 7.21; G.R. Davies *et al* 2004; Traboulsee *et al* 2003). The lesion magnetization transfer ratio provides an indication of myelination (Barkhof *et al* 2003a; Schmierer *et al* 2004).

The magnetization transfer ratio has not proved to be of much value in differential diagnosis. Multiple sclerosis white matter lesions have been shown to have lower ratios than those caused by vascular disease or oedema (Gass *et al* 1994; Reidel *et al* 2003; Rovaris *et al* 2000b). Abnormalities have been detected in the normal-appearing brain tissue in multiple sclerosis but not in acute disseminated encephalomyelitis (Inglese *et al* 2002a). However, there is overlap between disease groups and controls. Lack of specificity, together with the difficulties of accurate quantification, have prevented the magnetization transfer ratio being used as a reliable and practical diagnostic tool for individual patients.

Functional MRI

Functional MRI (fMRI) investigates regional blood flow changes within the brain in response to specific activation algorithms. A more detailed account of the physiological principles of fMRI

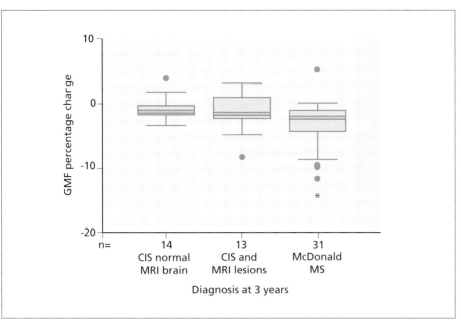

Figure 7.20 Box plot showing the medians, interquartile ranges (box), highest and lowest values (whiskers), excluding outliers (circles) and extreme value (asterisk) for grey matter fraction (GMF) percentage change in clinically isolated syndrome patients divided into those with (n = 13) and without (n = 14) MRI lesions, and individuals who developed multiple sclerosis within 3 years (n = 31). Significant grey matter atrophy was seen in those with a diagnosis of multiple sclerosis. Adapted from Dalton *et al* (2004a).

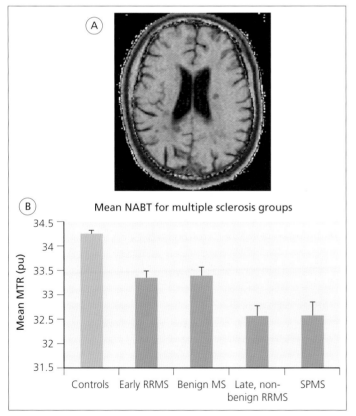

Figure 7.21 (A) Magnetization transfer ratio image of the brain. (B) Mean magnetization transfer ratio derived from histogram analysis of the normal-appearing brain tissue shows abnormalities in all multiple sclerosis clinical subgroups compared with controls, even those with relapsing–remitting disease (RRMS) and <3 years' disease duration. NABT = normal appearing brain tissue; SPMS = secondary progressive multiple sclerosis. From Traboulsee *et al* (2003) with permission.

and pathophysiological insights obtained in multiple sclerosis are provided in Chapter 13. Recent studies have shown that abnormal patterns of cerebral activation are already seen in patients with clinically isolated syndromes (Filippi *et al* 2004; Rocca *et al* 2005) A group of seven patients who had experienced a single episode of optic neuritis exhibited an abnormal and extensive pattern of activation beyond the primary visual cortex in response to a flashing light stimulus administered several years after the clinical episode (Figure 7.22; Werring *et al* 2000b). Another group of 16 patients with a variety of clinically isolated syndromes was reported to exhibit abnormal activation extending beyond the contralateral primary somatomotor cortex in response to a finger flexion extension algorithm, this occurring in spite of an absence of clinical motor dysfunction (Rocca *et al* 2003b). These studies indicate that cortical plasticity is a remarkably early feature in patients with central nervous system demyelination, and one must ask whether such altered and potentially adaptive activation patterns will have a prognostic or even diagnostic role. It seems unlikely that a major role will emerge for diagnosis, since the latter necessarily depends on showing dissemination in space and time of the underlying pathological (that is, structural) process *per se*, although it is intriguing that, in a recent small cohort study of 16 clinically isolated syndrome patients, early diagnosis of multiple sclerosis was more likely to follow in patients who exhibited a widespread and bilateral activation pattern to a unilateral upper limb motor activation paradigm (Rocca *et al* 2005).

Other methods

A number of quantitative MR measures have been used to investigate lesions and normal-appearing tissues. Diffusion weighted imaging has shown increased diffusion in normal-appearing white and grey matter (Cercignani *et al* 2001a; 2000b) and

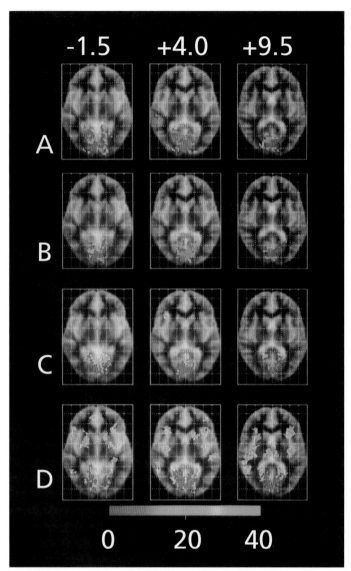

Figure 7.22 Functional MRI elicited response from monocular visual stimulation in healthy controls. (A) Left eye, (B) right eye, (C) patients with previous unilateral optic neuritis when stimulating the clinically unaffected eye and (D) affected eye. In healthy individuals, activation is largely confined to the primary visual cortex. Extrastriate activation is most apparent after stimulating the affected eye of patients. From Werring et al (2000b) with permission.

et al 2004). It is also increased for several weeks in white matter with normal appearance prior to a lesion appearing in relapsing–remitting disease (Wuerfel et al 2004). The increases in perfusion in these studies may reflect altered metabolic activity of the tissues as a result of inflammation during the relapsing–remitting phase. Such techniques offer valuable new windows for exploring and elucidating pathogenic mechanisms, and especially for understanding the nature of abnormalities beyond visible white matter lesions, but they do not currently have diagnostic utility.

A new area of MRI research and development revolves around efforts to achieve cellular and molecular specificity. The field is still at an early stage. MR contrast agents that use ultrasmall particles of iron oxide will produce a marked shortening of T_2 and T_1 relaxation times in regions where they accumulate, because of the creation of marked inhomogeneity of the local magnetic field. Such particles are avidly taken up by reticulo-endothelial cells, and in monocytes and macrophages. In a study of 10 patients with multiple sclerosis in whom ultrasmall particles of iron oxide were injected intravenously, enhancement was seen in 33 lesions in nine patients on T_1 and T_2-weighted images (Dousset et al 2000). All but two of the 33 iron oxide (Sinerem) enhancing lesions also exhibited gadolinium enhancement, indicating the acute inflammatory nature of the lesions with breakdown of the blood–brain barrier. Gadolinium enhancing lesions are reported to contain activated macrophages (Brück et al 1997; D. Katz et al 1993) and collateral investigation in experimental autoimmune encephalomyelitis has shown good correspondence between areas of Sinerem enhancement and macrophage infiltration (Dousset et al 1999). The clinical study also revealed 24 additional lesions that displayed gadolinium but not Sinerem

decrease in fractional anisotropy in white matter tracts (Ciccarelli et al 2001). Anisotropy is high in normal white matter tracts because diffusion is much higher along than across fibres. Thus, a decrease in anisotropy implies structural damage in the fibre pathway. Diffusion tractography is a promising tool for measuring fibre tract integrity by an assessment of their volume and fractional anisotropy (Ciccarelli et al 2003a; 2003b), although at present the measures have limited reproducibility and are confined to only the largest cerebral tracts (such as the optic radiation; Figure 7.23). Increased T_1-weighted relaxation has been shown in normal-appearing grey and white matter (C.M. Griffin et al 2002a). Perfusion is reduced in grey matter in progressive forms of multiple sclerosis (Figure 7.24) but is increased in white matter in relapsing–remitting disease (Rashid

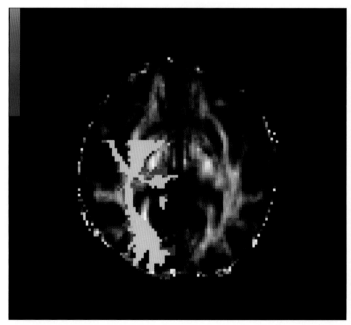

Figure 7.23 Diffusion tractography map generated from diffusion tensor MRI showing the optic radiation (indicated in yellow). Kindly provided by Dr Olga Ciccarelli.

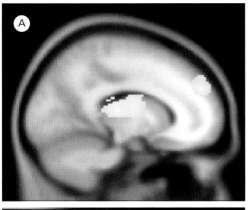

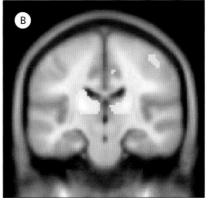

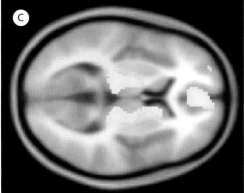

Figure 7.24 (A) Sagittal, (B) coronal and (C) axial co-registered perfusion MRI maps using arterial spin tagging comparing a group of primary progressive multiple sclerosis patients with controls. Areas of decreased perfusion (yellow colour) are noted in deep and cortical grey matter in primary progressive multiple sclerosis. From Rashid *et al* (2004) with permission.

enhancement. Obvious questions arise as to whether the presence of lesions displaying Sinerem enhancement is associated with greater tissue damage because of the presence of activated macrophages or a poorer clinical prognosis. Further studies that investigate such issues are awaited. Other targets for cell-specific MRI in central nervous system inflammatory/demyelinating diseases are T lymphocytes (S.A. Anderson *et al* 2004), and oligodendrocyte progenitors and stem cells (Frank *et al* 2003). Such approaches are currently experimental but have potential for translation to clinical studies with further research and development.

Other imaging and radiological techniques

As technologies available for depicting structure and function in the central nervous system became ever more sophisticated over the last 30 years, their potential application in the context of multiple sclerosis has been evaluated. Although MRI provides the main advance of clinical utility in relation to multiple sclerosis, there follows a brief review of the contributions from other modalities that have been used to image the nervous system in multiple sclerosis.

Computed tomography

Prior to the advent of MRI, CT scanning was sometimes used to demonstrate cerebral hemisphere lesions in multiple sclerosis, visible as multifocal areas of low attenuation in the white matter (Cala and Mastaglia 1976). Active lesions were also depicted as areas of high attenuation after the injection of iodinated contrast

media (Vinuela *et al* 1982), but this was of limited value and the sensitivity of CT scanning was always poor. In the first comparative study of CT versus inversion recovery T_1-weighted MRI in 10 patients with multiple sclerosis, 19 lesions were detected on CT and 131 on MRI (I.R. Young *et al* 1981). The discrepancy in sensitivity between CT and MRI became even more apparent when T_2-weighted imaging was shown to be superior to inversion recovery for detecting multiple sclerosis lesions. High-resolution orbital CT is still useful for investigating patients presenting with undiagnosed optic neuropathies in whom the differential diagnosis may arise between optic neuritis, other inflammatory optic neuropathies or optic nerve compression.

Positron emission tomography (PET)

This modality has been used as a research tool to study multiple sclerosis. Decreased oxygen utilization has been observed in the brain (Brooks *et al* 1984), consistent with loss of neuroaxonal tissue. Another PET study, that used ^{18}F-deoxyglucose to quantify the cortical cerebral metabolic rate of glucose, reported reductions in the cortical and deep grey matter of multiple sclerosis subjects compared with healthy controls (Blinkenberg *et al* 2000). The decrease in glucose metabolism correlated with increasing T_2 lesion load and cognitive impairment. Single positron emission computed tomography (SPECT) studies have also revealed a correlation between decreased regional cerebral blood flow and cognitive impairment (Pozzilli *et al* 1991; Lycke *et al* 1993).

A PET radioligand marker (called PK11195) for peripheral benzodiazepine receptors, which are located on activated

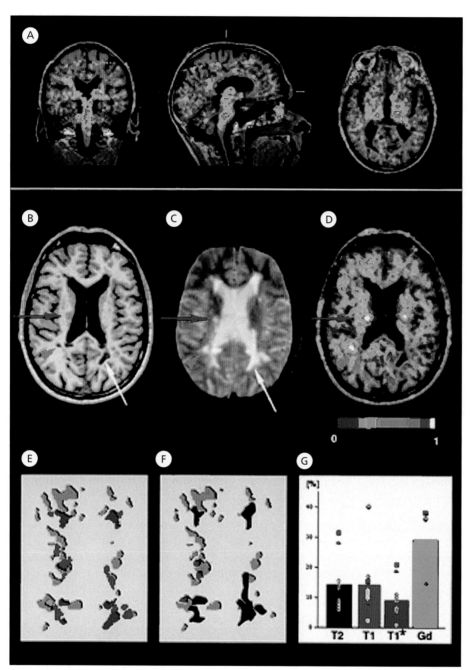

Figure 7.25 MRI and [^{11}C](R)-PK11195 PET. All images follow the radiological convention, i.e. the left side of the image corresponds to subject's right side. (A) Three orthogonal views of [^{11}C](R)-PK11195 images co-registered and overlaid on the MRI of Patient 9, showing spinothalamic tract-associated [^{11}C](R)-PK11195 signals extending through the brainstem and pons into the thalamus. (B–D) T$_1$-weighted (B) and T$_2$-weighted (C) MRI and [^{11}C](R)-PK11195 PET (overlaid on to T$_1$-weighted MRI) (D) of Patient 9 show lesions in all different spin-echo MRI sequences that partially overlap with areas of significantly increased [^{11}C](R)-PK11195 binding (red arrow). The white arrow points to a 'black hole' in an area that appears strongly hypointense in the T$_1$-weighted MRI and has little binding of [^{11}C](R)-PK11195. Note, however, that a similar black hole (yellow arrowhead) adjacent to the right occipital horn of the lateral ventricle shows significant [^{11}C](R)-PK11195 binding. (E–F) Demonstration of the definition of the MRI lesion load masks in Patient 9 (purple, T$_1$-weighted MRI lesions excluding black holes; blue, black hole only; green, gadolinium-enhancing areas; dark grey (in F), T$_2$-weighted MRI lesions; red, areas of overlap between significantly increased [^{11}C](R)-PK11195 binding and MRI-defined areas of pathology); yellow, areas of increased [^{11}C](R)-PK11195 binding and no overlap with any MRI-defined pathology. (G) Average percentage volume of the MRI-defined lesions overlapping with increased [^{11}C](R)-PK11195 binding. The red square represents Patient 8 and the red triangle Patient 6, who were both in relapse at the time of the scans. The yellow diamond represents Patient 9, who had secondary progressive multiple sclerosis. T1*, black holes.

microglia, has revealed increased activity not only in gadolinium enhancing lesions but also in normal-appearing white matter and deep grey matter nuclei (Figure 7.25; Banati *et al* 2000; Debruyne *et al* 2003). While this marker may be of value for monitoring disease course and therapeutic intervention, neither PET nor SPECT currently have a role to play in the diagnosis of multiple sclerosis.

Ultrasonography

Based on the emerging evidence that brain atrophy is a feature of multiple sclerosis, transcranial sonography has been applied to the investigation of ventricular dimensions in multiple sclerosis. In a study of 38 patients who were followed for 2 years, there was a significant increase in the width of the third ven-

tricle (Kallmann *et al* 2004). The measurements of the third ventricle obtained by sonography correlated well with those measured from MRI scans and a correlation was observed between disability and third ventricle width not only in this study but also in an earlier report on 74 patients (D. Berg *et al* 2000). Whilst transcranial sonography has no role in diagnosis, the authors of these studies suggested that it could provide an inexpensive test for monitoring the course of brain atrophy in multiple sclerosis.

Myelography

Myelography was once the only certain method for excluding a compressive lesion in patients presenting with a spinal cord syndrome, but the advent of MRI has rendered this investigation largely obsolete. It should now only be required when MRI is contraindicated (patients with cardiac pacemakers) or impossible to perform (extreme obesity preventing the subject from entering the scanner or the subject having metal implants).

Retinal nerve fibre layer imaging

A relatively recent development has been the introduction of noninvasive measurement of thickness in the retinal nerve fibre layer using optical coherence tomography. This provides cross-sectional imaging of internal tissue microstructure by measuring the echo time delay of back-scattered infrared light using an interferometer and a low coherence light source. It is therefore somewhat analogous to ultrasound imaging except that light is used instead of sound. Using an early model of optical coherence tomography, Parisi *et al* (1999) described thinning of the retinal nerve fibre layer in multiple sclerosis patients who had a previous episode of optic neuritis. More recently, Trip and colleagues (2005) quantified both retinal nerve fibre layer thickness and visual function in 25 patients who had incomplete visual recovery after an attack of unilateral optic neuritis and compared the findings with those seen in 15 healthy controls. The retinal nerve fibre layer thickness was reduced by a mean of 33% in the patients' affected eye compared with healthy controls and in patients there was a significant correlation between the extent of fibre loss and the degree of impairment of visual function. Although the technique is unlikely to have a major role in diagnosis, it has promise as a non-invasive tool to monitor axonal loss and its prevention, in optic neuritis and – possibly – multiple sclerosis.

Clinically isolated syndromes

A central element in the power of MRI as a diagnostic aid is its ability to detect clinically 'silent' lesions as well as those expressed in the acute relapse. Nowhere is this better demonstrated than in the assessment of patients with clinically isolated lesions of the type seen in multiple sclerosis. The responsible symptomatic lesions are also usually readily demonstrated.

Optic neuritis

In optic neuritis, abnormalities of the optic nerve can be detected in the acute stage in >95% of patients (Gass *et al* 1996) if a phased array local coil or a conventional head receiver coil are used, together with an appropriate sequence to suppress the signal from orbital fat such as short inversion time inversion recovery (STIR), or fat suppressed T_2-weighted fast spin echo (Figure 7.26). Coronal imaging with high resolution is the best way of depicting optic nerve involvement. Enhancement is usual during the acute attack (Youl *et al* 1991b). In a large study, Kupersmith *et al* (2002) reported the presence of gadolinium enhancement of the optic nerve in 101/107 patients with acute optic neuritis. When the enhancement was more extensive or involved the optic canal, there were greater visual deficits apparent during the acute stage but the location and length of enhancement were not predictive of visual recovery. Enhancement of the optic nerve was observed in 27/28 (97%) cases using triple-dose gadolinium in a recent study of patients within 4 weeks of the onset of optic neuritis (Hickman *et al* 2004a). The enhancement is usually seen as a homogeneous region within the optic nerve though we have sometimes seen it to be more apparent involving the outer nerve and/or sheath (Figure 7.27). The length of optic nerve lesions ranges from a few millimetres to the whole nerve. There is some evidence that longer lesions, when seen on the STIR sequence, and when they include the intracanalicular portion of the optic nerve, are associated with poorer visual outcome (Kapoor *et al* 1998; Miller *et al* 1988c). Exceptionally, the abnormal signal can extend back to a swollen chiasm (Figure 7.28; Cornblath and Quint 1997). Acute lesions more often display swelling whereas it is not unusual to see a degree of optic nerve atrophy in chronic lesions.

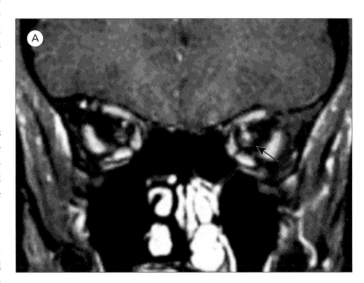

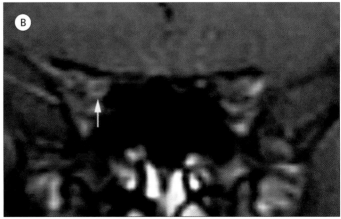

Figure 7.27 Triple-dose gadolinium enhanced coronal T_1-weighted MRI in two cases of acute optic neuritis. (A) Homogeneous enhancement of the left optic nerve. (B) Enhancement of the right optic nerve sheath (arrowed).

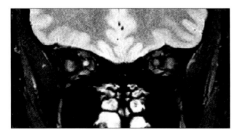

Figure 7.26 Coronal T_2-weighted fast spin echo image through the orbits of a patient with unilateral optic neuritis. High signal is seen in the affected optic nerve.

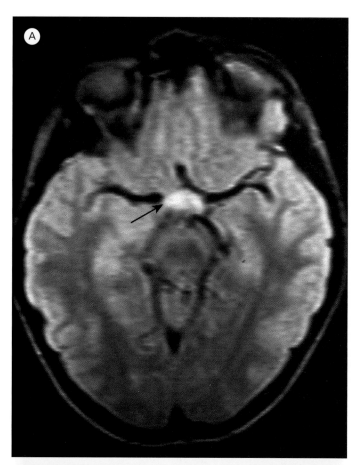

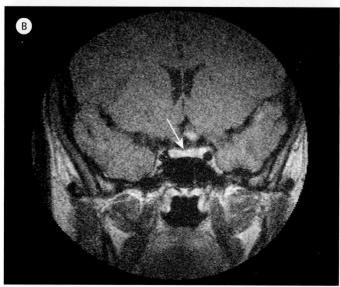

Figure 7.28 Chiasmal involvement in optic neuritis (arrows). (A) T₂-weighted MRI. (B) Gadolinium enhanced T₁-weighted MRI.

In a recent serial study using quantitative measures of optic nerve size, we observed a mean 20% increase in cross-sectional area of the acutely symptomatic nerve and a mean 12% decrease in its area after 1 year, when compared with the clinically unaffected nerve (Figure 7.29; Hickman *et al* 2004b). Magnetization transfer imaging has shown decreases in optic nerve magnetization transfer ratio following an attack of optic neuritis (Inglese *et al* 2002b; Thorpe *et al* 1995). A serial study reported that

magnetization transfer ratio reached its nadir after about 6–9 months and then increased slightly by 1 year, possibly reflecting remyelination (Hickman *et al* 2004c)

Brainstem lesions

MRI detects the causative lesion of isolated brainstem syndromes in about 90% of cases, and provides good anatomical correlation with the clinical features (Bronstein *et al* 1990a; 1990b; Ormerod *et al* 1986). For example, in patients with an acute onset of diplopia and an internuclear ophthalmoplegia, it is usual to find an area of high signal in the region of the medial longitudinal fasciculus. As at other sites, the areas of increased signal almost always persist after full clinical recovery. Most, but not all, acutely symptomatic brainstem lesions exhibit gadolinium enhancement.

Spinal cord lesions

The frequency with which the causative lesion is found in acute or chronic spinal cord syndromes was found to be rather lower in the early studies (64% for the cervical region; D.H. Miller *et al* 1987a), but it is undoubtedly higher using more modern instruments. Reflecting the sites of clinical and pathological predilection, lesions are most commonly seen in the cervical spinal cord, although any part may be affected including, exceptionally, the conus medullaris (Figure 7.30). The spatial resolution of spinal cord imaging is still not good enough to permit detailed correlations between the location of lesions and their clinical expression down to the level of individual white matter tracts. Nevertheless, broad correlations are possible, such as between lesions involving the dorsolateral part of the mid- or lower cervical cord and the useless (deafferented) hand syndrome (see Figure 7.31; D.H. Miller *et al* 1987a), ipsilateral lesions and partial Brown–Sequard syndrome, or posterior lesions and Lhermitte's symptom. A rather surprising finding in spinal cord imaging has been the frequency with which swelling is observed. This was sometimes revealed by myelography in the pre-MRI era but the procedure was infrequently performed in acute myelopathy because of its invasive nature, and was less sensitive than MRI in detecting minor focal changes in size such as are now seen routinely. Swelling is observed in many acutely symptomatic lesions but may persist for several months. The pattern of gadolinium enhancement in cord lesions is similar to that seen in the brain, in that both uniform and ring-like patterns are seen. Occasionally, one sees a rather patchy lesion extending over several segments but, more typically, the lesions are less than one segment in length. It is rare for demyelinating cord lesions to display T₁ hypointensity. In contrast, patients with acute transverse myelitis often exhibit lesions in which there is marked swelling with signal change extending over multiple segments of the cord, sometimes with T₁ hypointensity.

Additional lesions and the risk for multiple sclerosis

There are many reports of clinically silent lesions involving cerebral white matter and spinal cord at the time of presentation with clinically isolated syndromes (Figure 7.32). The frequency varies somewhat, but overall is about 60–70% in the brain (L.D. Jacobs *et al* 1986a; Ormerod *et al* 1987) and 30% in the

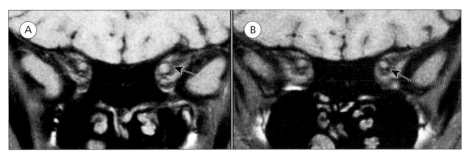

Figure 7.29 Coronal fast FLAIR images through the orbits. (A) During an attack of left optic neuritis and (B) 12 months after the episode of left optic neuritis. The affected nerve is swollen acutely and atrophic 1 year later (arrows).

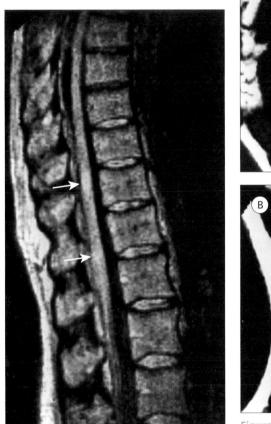

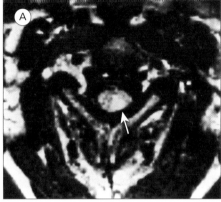

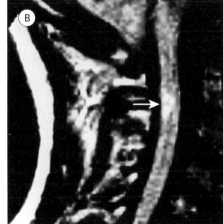

Figure 7.30 T$_2$-weighted MRI showing a conus lesion (lower arrow) in a patient with multiple sclerosis; there is another lesion (upper arrow) two segments higher up.

Figure 7.31 T$_2$-weighted scan. (A) Axial and (B) sagittal MRI showing a posterior cervical cord lesion (arrows) in a multiple sclerosis patient with deafferentation of the upper limb (useless hand of Oppenheim).

spinal cord (Dalton *et al* 2004b; O'Riordan *et al* 1998a). The presence and number of such lesions is of predictive value for the development of multiple sclerosis in the next 1–5 years (Beck *et al* 1993b; Campi *et al* 1995; B. Ford *et al* 1992; Frederiksen *et al* 1991a; Ghezzi *et al* 1999; L.D. Jacobs *et al* 1997; Martinelli *et al* 1991; D.H. Miller *et al* 1988a; 1989b; Morrissey *et al* 1993a; Söderström *et al* 1994a; 1998; Tas *et al* 1995). In a 3-year follow-up study of 52 patients presenting with an isolated acute partial myelopathy, Cordonnier *et al* (2003) confirmed numerous other studies in showing that brain MRI abnormalities are predictive for conversion to clinically

definite multiple sclerosis. Additional predictive features were the presence of sensory symptoms, cerebrospinal fluid oligoclonal bands and posterolateral spinal cord lesions.

The cohort followed for the longest time to date is reported from the National Hospital in London. By 5 years after presentation, 72% of those with additional lesions had developed clinically definite multiple sclerosis compared with 6% of patients without abnormalities at other sites (Morrissey *et al* 1993a). After 10 years, the gap for the whole group had narrowed slightly (83% versus 11%), but the significantly better prognosis for those without cerebral lesions at presentation was

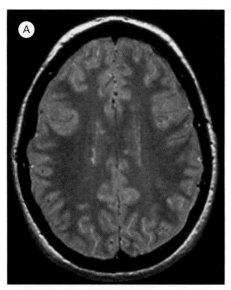

Figure 7.32 T$_2$-weighted MRI of two young adults with clinically isolated optic neuritis. (A) Brain MRI shows periventricular and callosal lesions. (B) Spinal cord MRI shows multiple thoracic cord lesions (arrows).

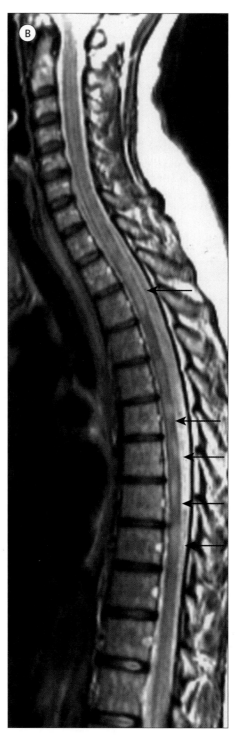

still striking (O'Riordan *et al* 1998). After 14 years, 88% of patients with an abnormal scan had developed clinically definite multiple sclerosis compared with 19% of those with normal MRI at presentation (Brex *et al* 2002). Caution is needed in interpreting the precise proportions converting to multiple sclerosis because about one-third of patients were lost to follow-up. In the North American Optic Neuritis treatment trial cohort, follow-up after 10 years revealed conversion to clinically definite multiple sclerosis in 56% of patients who had an abnormal brain MRI at presentation and in 22% with a normal scan (Optic Neuritis Study Group 2003). Taken together, these

two long-term follow-up studies, of 10 and 14 years duration, indicate that the majority of patients with clinically isolated syndromes and brain MRI abnormalities will develop clinically definite multiple sclerosis (60–80%), whereas a considerably smaller proportion (about 20%) with a normal scan are seen to convert after prolonged follow-up.

The predictive value of the Barkhof/Tintoré criteria (see above) were tested in a group of 309 patients with a first clinical episode followed up for 2 years as part of a therapeutic trial (Barkhof *et al* 2003b). In the placebo arm of the study, the rate of conversion to clinically definite multiple sclerosis was

23% in subjects who had at least two MRI features, 38% in those with three components, and 57% when all four features were present. In a further study, Tintoré *et al* (2001) demonstrated that the original Barkhof MRI criteria, when applied to 112 patients with a clinically isolated syndrome, were more specific for multiple sclerosis (specificity 70%) than either the Paty *et al* (1988) or Fazekas *et al* (1988) MRI criteria (both 51%) or the presence of cerebrospinal fluid oligoclonal bands (43%).

The McDonald criteria proposed two additional modifications to the necessary evidence for dissemination in space. The first allowed the combination of two brain MRI lesions and cerebrospinal fluid oligoclonal bands as sufficient features. However, application of this modification to a cohort of clinically isolated syndrome patients showed them to have a rather low specificity (63%) for developing clinically definite multiple sclerosis after 3 years (Tintoré *et al* 2003). The second modification was to allow one spinal cord lesion to substitute for one brain lesion. Dalton *et al* (2003b) investigated the effect of this change in a group of 115 patients with clinically isolated optic neuritis who underwent combined brain and cord imaging. Although they found that 31 (27%) had clinically silent lesions in the cord, all but four of these individuals had additional brain lesions. Not surprisingly, allowing a cord lesion to substitute for a brain lesion had little impact on the frequency with which multiple sclerosis was diagnosed at follow-up. It follows that there is little if any role for spinal MRI in the routine investigation of patients with isolated optic neuritis, although future reviews of the diagnostic criteria might usefully consider whether spinal MRI findings could be included more effectively than is currently the case.

Serial scanning and the risk for multiple sclerosis

One essential diagnostic criterion for multiple sclerosis is the appearance of new lesions over time. MRI is currently the most powerful method available for obtaining this information, not least because the annual frequency with which new lesions appear, calculated from serial scanning in patients with established relapsing–remitting and secondary progressive disease at monthly intervals, is five- to ten-fold higher than that determined on the basis of clinical relapse – and occasionally much higher. When there is uncertainty about the diagnosis of multiple sclerosis early in its course, it is often worth repeating the scan after 6–12 months. Although not specific for multiple sclerosis, the appearance of a new lesion may be decisive in the appropriate clinical context.

In patients with clinically isolated syndromes, MRI evidence for dissemination in time is incorporated in contemporary criteria for the diagnosis of multiple sclerosis (W.I. McDonald *et al* 2001). These require evidence for a change appearing 3 or more months after the clinical episode (Figure 7.33). This can be either gadolinium enhancement or a new T_2 lesion. Subsequently the predictive value of serial MRI has been reported for cohorts of patients based in London and Barcelona with a clinically isolated syndrome, and followed independently and prospectively from onset. The studies show that either new gadolinium enhancement or T_2 lesions after 3 months (Brex *et al* 2001a; Dalton *et al* 2002a; 2003a), or new T_2 lesions after 1 year (Dalton *et al* 2002a; Tintoré *et al* 2003), carry high specificity for developing clinically definite multiple sclerosis after 3 years. The requirement for dissemination in both space and time increased the specificity for developing clinically definite multiple sclerosis compared with merely requiring evidence for dissemination in space on the first scan. These findings suggest that the new imaging criteria for multiple sclerosis are reliable when applied in an appropriate clinical setting by experienced clinical teams, and that requiring evidence for dissemination in time is, as expected, an important element in ensuring that the diagnosis is accurate. It is nevertheless worth adding that the new criteria (W.I. McDonald *et al* 2001) allow either MRI or clinical evidence for dissemination in space and time to secure the diagnosis of multiple sclerosis. Therefore, some patients can be diagnosed without fulfilling the new MRI criteria for dissemination in time and space. In the study of clinically isolated syndromes by Dalton *et al* (2002b), after 1 year of follow-up, 22 had developed multiple sclerosis by MRI criteria alone, 13 by both MRI and clinical criteria, and three by clinical criteria alone.

MRI lesions and the risk for disability

Filippi *et al* (1994) correlated the amount of affected cerebral tissue at presentation in individuals with isolated syndromes with subsequent disability in those who developed multiple sclerosis during follow-up over 5 years. In the London cohort studied for 14 years, the strongest correlation was between concurrent change in T_2 lesion volume and disability developing during the first 5 years. Thereafter, changes in T_2 volume appeared to make little impact on the future clinical course (Brex *et al* 2002). The strength of the correlation between T_2 volume increased over the first 5 years, and disability at year 14 remained modest (r = 0.61), suggesting that some but not most long-term disability can be related to early lesion load. Those who developed secondary progressive disease had – as a group – larger lesion loads at 5 years than those who exhibited a benign course. However, considerable inter-individual variations were also observed, some patients showing minimal later disability despite exhibiting large early lesion loads, whereas others developed secondary progressive disease in the context of quite small lesion loads at presentation. In another cohort of 42 patients followed for 8 years after onset with a clinically isolated syndrome, disability at follow up was significantly related to total T_2 lesion load and infratentorial lesion load at presentation (Minneboo *et al* 2004). While these findings suggest that treatments that suppress the accumulation of T_2 lesions in early relapsing disease have the potential to modify the long-term course with respect to the development of disability, T_2 load *per se* is not enough to guide treatment decisions in the individual patient. It should also be remembered that mechanisms underpinning the relationship between MRI lesions and long-term disability are not well understood.

Normal-appearing brain tissue abnormalities detected by MRI

Some recent investigations have reported the presence of a variety of quantitative MRI abnormalities in white and/or grey matter with normal appearance in patients with clinically isolated syndromes, or very early in the course of relapsing–remitting multiple sclerosis. The abnormalities include a reduction in magnetization transfer ratio (Griffin *et al* 2002a; Iannucci

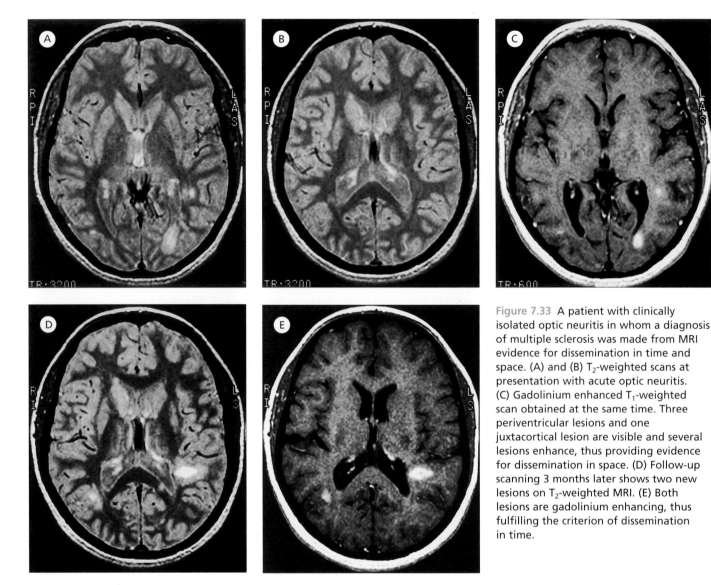

Figure 7.33 A patient with clinically isolated optic neuritis in whom a diagnosis of multiple sclerosis was made from MRI evidence for dissemination in time and space. (A) and (B) T$_2$-weighted scans at presentation with acute optic neuritis. (C) Gadolinium enhanced T$_1$-weighted scan obtained at the same time. Three periventricular lesions and one juxtacortical lesion are visible and several lesions enhance, thus providing evidence for dissemination in space. (D) Follow-up scanning 3 months later shows two new lesions on T$_2$-weighted MRI. (E) Both lesions are gadolinium enhancing, thus fulfilling the criterion of dissemination in time.

et al 2000b), an increase in T$_1$ relaxation time (Griffin et al 2002a; 2002b), increased diffusivity (Gallo et al 2005) and – on MR spectroscopy – a reduction in N-acetyl aspartate (Chard et al 2002a; 2002b; 2002c; Filippi et al 2003) and an increase in myoinositol (Figure 7.34; Chard et al 2002b; Fernando et al 2004). In addition, progressive ventricular enlargement and grey matter atrophy have been detected in patients evolving from a clinically isolated syndrome to multiple sclerosis within 1–3 years (Figures 7.20 and 7.35; Dalton et al 2002b; 2004a). Whilst such studies have collectively emphasized that there is a diffuse and progressive pathological process occurring from the earliest stages of the disease, and by implication raising the potential for some of the quantitative imaging measures having a useful prognostic role (although that can only be determined through follow-up), the abnormalities described are not sufficient to provide diagnostic utility. They are subtle, have not always been reproduced in different centres, are not sufficiently studied in other conditions, and are difficult to implement with adequate quality control on a routine basis.

Other central nervous system disorders

The differential diagnosis of multiple sclerosis and MRI findings encountered in many of these disorders are discussed in Chapter 8. Here, we confine ourselves to the MRI findings encountered in two 'generic' categories of neurological disease that are sometimes difficult to separate by clinical and/or MRI findings from multiple sclerosis: cerebrovascular (small vessel) disease and cerebral tumour.

Nonspecific age-related changes caused by small vessel disease

A common source of difficulty is the presence of small areas of high signal in the cerebral white matter of older patients (see Figure 7.4). With modern high field instruments such changes are seen with increasing frequency in healthy individuals aged >40 years. In our series of 131 apparently healthy individuals aged 17–79 years, more lesions were seen at 1.5 than at

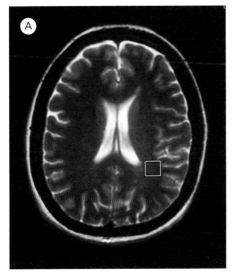

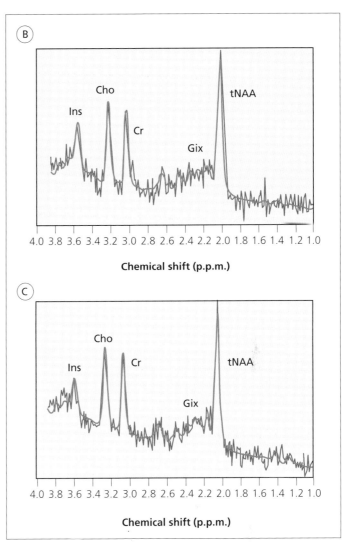

Figure 7.34 (A) MRI shows a voxel of normal appearing white matter. (B) Proton magnetic resonance spectroscopy from normal appearing white matter voxel shows an elevation seen in the myoinositol (Ins) peak in patients with clinically isolated syndromes. (C) Healthy age-matched control spectrum. Cho (choline), Cr (creatinine and phosphocreatinine) and tNAA (total *N*-acetyl aspartate) are also shown. From Fernando *et al* (2004) with permission.

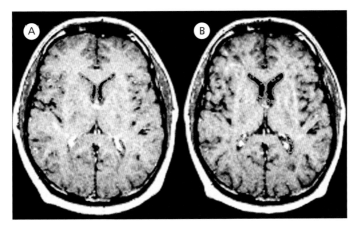

Figure 7.35 T$_1$-weighted MRI scans in a patient who presented with isolated optic neuritis and went on to develop multiple sclerosis during the follow-up year. (A) Obtained at presentation and (B) 1 year later. Significant ventricular enlargement – indicating loss of brain tissue – has occurred during follow-up. The green line indicates the lateral ventricle margins; the measure of ventricular volume was generated using an automated boundary detection method. From Dalton *et al* (2002b) with permission.

0.5 Tesla field strength. In those under 50 years of age, four (4.5%) had multifocal white matter abnormalities. Eight (30%) of those aged between 50 and 59 years had abnormal scans. In the 13 subjects aged 60 or over, seven (54%) had abnormal MRI examinations (D.H. Miller *et al* 1997). These appearances are nonspecific and, although their pathogenesis is not fully understood, they probably reflect small areas of ischaemia in the elderly (Kirkpatrick and Hayman 1987). The characteristics of their location, size and frequency help to make the distinction from the lesions of multiple sclerosis. Age-related lesions tend to be smaller and situated away from the ventricles, often in the subcortical white matter. Sometimes an appearance of multiple small lesions in a linear distribution is seen in the centrum semi-ovale, possibly indicating watershed ischaemia. When periventricular abnormality occurs, it may have a smooth contour – unlike the irregular and asymmetrical appearances associated with periventricular plaques of demyelination. The basal ganglia are quite frequently involved in small vessel disease, whereas MRI-detectable lesions in this location are uncommon (<10%) in multiple sclerosis (D.H. Miller *et al* 1997; Ormerod *et al* 1987). Conversely, although commonly involved in multiple sclerosis, the corpus callosum (Gean-Marton *et al* 1991) and spinal cord (Bot *et al* 2002) are rarely affected by age-related vascular changes. Thorpe *et al* (1993) observed only a single abnormality in the spinal cords of 45 apparently healthy individuals, and none in the 17 individuals aged over 50 years. Thus, MRI of the spinal cord is often helpful when there is diagnostic doubt in the older decades. Several sets of criteria have been devised to help distinguish the imaging appearances of multiple sclerosis and small vessel disease, most particularly those of Paty *et al* (1988) and Fazekas *et al* (1988). It should be noted that the Barkhof/Tintoré and McDonald criteria for multiple sclerosis, although useful in defining the risk for developing clinically definite multiple sclerosis in patients with a single clinical episode of suspected demyelination, have not been tested in a study that compares multiple sclerosis and small vessel disease. Conversely, the Fazekas criteria have been extensively validated in this context. It should be emphasized that although these criteria have proved relatively specific for multiple sclerosis when compared with subjects with small vessel disease, they are not pathognomonic, and some patients with vascular disease are encountered in whom all of the Fazekas criteria features are met.

The abnormalities found in apparently healthy individuals are usually not extensive but occasionally cannot be distinguished from those seen in established multiple sclerosis. The occasional demonstration of multiple lesions in healthy individuals is in keeping with the reports of unexpectedly finding the plaques of multiple sclerosis at post mortem (Ghatak *et al* 1974; Gilbert and Sadler 1983; Phadke and Best 1983).

In contrast to these focal cerebral changes, there are characteristically extensive confluent changes in the cerebral white matter in dementia associated with advanced cerebral vascular disease (Figure 7.36). The condition is sometimes referred to as 'Binswanger's disease' and the imaging appearance is included under the somewhat ill-defined term 'leucoariosis' (Hachinski *et al* 1987). Such confluent changes in the cerebral white matter may also be seen in apparently healthy individuals of advanced years. All these appearances can be indistinguishable from those seen in advanced multiple sclerosis. A feature that aids the

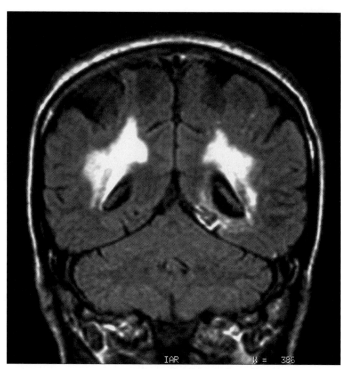

Figure 7.36 Coronal T_2-weighted MRI of a subject with hypertension and dementia. There is extensive periventricular and deep white matter abnormality with sparing of subcortical U-fibres (Binswanger's subcortical arteriosclerotic leucoencephalopathy). Kindly provided by Professor Tarek Yousry and Dr Ralf Jager.

distinction is characteristic sparing of subcortical U-fibres in Binswanger's disease, whereas the lesions of multiple sclerosis frequently involve this region.

Tumours

Intrinsic neoplasms of the nervous system are rarely confused with multiple sclerosis. Occasionally, however, focal swelling of the brain (Figure 7.9) or spinal cord occurring in the context of acute inflammatory demyelination, closely mimics a tumour. The symptoms and signs of raised intracranial pressure may even be present. That such appearances can be the result of multiple sclerosis lesions – sometimes showing necrosis, cyst formation and extensive oedema – has been confirmed histologically (Youl *et al* 1991a). In addition to tumour or demyelination, a large ring enhancing mass lesion will include brain abscess in the differential diagnosis. The presence of other clinical and MRI features of multiple sclerosis point to the correct diagnosis and, in this situation, it is usually appropriate to defer surgery while treating with corticosteroids and performing serial scans to see whether there is sustained regression of the mass with symptomatic improvement.

The need occasionally to biopsy these cases as part of clinical management has, by serendipity, allowed a much improved understanding of the early pathological features of multiple sclerosis and histological validation of the acute imaging appearances (see Chapter 12). A major international research initiative is currently using biopsy or autopsy material to investigate immunopathogenic mechanisms and MRI/pathology correla-

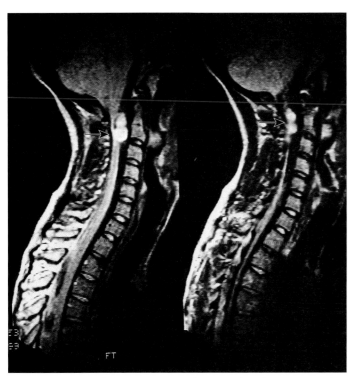

Figure 7.37 MRI of the craniocervical region showing compression of the cord by a neurofibroma (arrows).

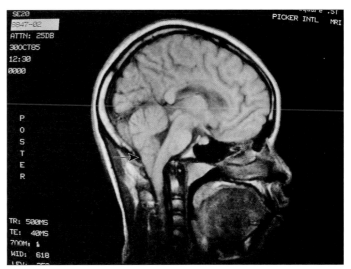

Figure 7.39 Herniation of the cerebellar tonsils demonstrated by MRI (arrow) producing intermittent neurological symptoms misdiagnosed for several years as multiple sclerosis.

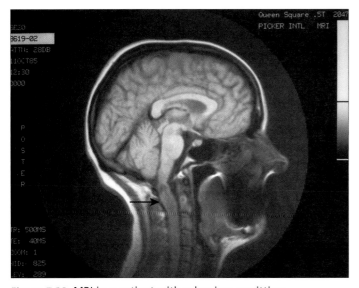

Figure 7.38 MRI in a patient with relapsing–remitting neurological symptoms affecting a single site (the cervical cord) in whom the erroneous diagnosis of multiple sclerosis had previously been made. The lesion was an ependymoma (arrow).

tions. Initial reports have emphasized the occurrence of four types of active lesion in multiple sclerosis (Lucchinetti *et al* 2000). As discussed in Chapter 12, the most prevalent are Types I and II, which respectively exhibit features suggesting T-cell-mediated and T-cell/antibody-mediated demyelination with myelin as the principal target. Type III and IV lesions show features suggestive of ischaemia and a primary dystrophic process

of oligodendrocytes, respectively. These reports emphasize that individual patients exhibit the same, single type of active lesion. It is as yet less clear how this form of lesion staging relates to clinical prognosis or MRI findings, although a more favourable response to plasma exchange has been reported in patients who exhibit Type II lesions (Keegan *et al* 2004). Interpretation of the neuropathological data is complicated by the fact that a large proportion of multiple sclerosis lesions that require biopsy are, inevitably, atypical being unusually large and with aggressive clinical manifestations.

Tumours arising outside (e.g. meningioma and neurofibroma, Figure 7.37) or inside (e.g. ependymoma, Figure 7.38) the neuraxis, and congenital disorder, such as the Arnold–Chiari malformation (Figure 7.39), all of which can simulate primary progressive multiple sclerosis, are readily distinguished by MRI (see Chapter 8 for further clinical discussion of these differential diagnoses).

EVOKED POTENTIALS

The exploration of human central nervous system function by evoked potential methods originates from the observations of Dawson (1947a; 1947b). The impetus to apply these techniques to multiple sclerosis came from two directions. First, was the demonstration that, as in the peripheral nervous system, central demyelination also slows conduction. This slowing serves, in optimal conditions, to distinguish the underlying pathological process from axonal degeneration where surviving conduction is normal or of only slightly reduced velocity (see Chapter 13). Secondly, peripheral nerve conduction studies from the 1960s proved useful in distinguishing demyelinating from degenerative peripheral neuropathies. In 1971, it occurred to one of us (WIMcD) that evoked potential methods might be used in a similar way, and with Martin Halliday an evoked potential study of optic neuritis was undertaken (Halliday *et al* 1972; see Chapter 1). Somatosensory evoked potentials had already been used to a limited extent to investigate the pathophysiology of central nervous system dysfunction in a variety of disorders, including multiple sclerosis (J.B. Baker *et al* 1968; Halliday and Wakefield 1963; Namerow 1968b). The systematic exploitation of evoked potential techniques as diagnostic aids began, however, with the pattern reversal visual evoked potential in optic neuritis, which at once revealed a dramatic increase in latency, detectable in 90% of cases (Halliday *et al* 1972). More modest delays were soon found to be characteristic findings in somatosensory (Desmedt and Noel 1973; Fukushima and Mayanagi 1975; Small 1976; D.G. Small *et al* 1978; Trojaborg and Petersen 1979) and auditory evoked potentials (Chiappa 1980; Eisen and Odusote 1980; Robinson and Rudge 1977). Delays in the motor response evoked by electrical (Cowan *et al* 1984; Marsden 1980; Merton and Morton 1980a; 1980b; Merton *et al* 1982; Mills and Murray 1985; Rossini *et al* 1985) or magnetic (Barker *et al* 1985a; 1985b; 1986; Hess *et al* 1986; Ingram *et al* 1987) stimulation of the cortex were later observed.

Application of evoked potential techniques to the clinical assessment of patients with multiple sclerosis began right away (Halliday *et al* 1973b), and their value was at once apparent. As already pointed out, the principal contributions of evoked potentials have been to answer the questions:

- Is a clinically silent lesion present?
- Is the process of demyelination present?

One selects a pathway for the evoked potential that assesses an asymptomatic region of the nervous system. The result of the examination may of course answer both questions but, if not, a clinically affected part of the central nervous system may then be chosen for interrogation. Although the introduction of MRI from the 1980s has substantially reduced the frequency with which evoked potentials are ordered as diagnostic tools in cases of suspected multiple sclerosis, they are still of use when there is diagnostic difficulty. This applies especially to use of the visual evoked potential. A report of the Quality Standards Subcommittee of the American Academy of Neurology has recently evaluated the utility of evoked potentials in identifying clinically silent lesions in patients with suspected multiple sclerosis (Gronseth and Ashman 2000). They produced the following recommendations.

- Visual evoked potentials are probably useful to identify patients at increased risk for developing clinically definite multiple sclerosis.
- Somatosensory evoked potentials are possibly useful to identify patients at increased risk for developing clinically definite multiple sclerosis.
- There is insufficient evidence to recommend brainstem auditory evoked potentials as a useful test to identify patients at increased risk for developing clinically definite multiple sclerosis.

This sensibly conservative approach has been further tempered by the subsequently published new diagnostic criteria for multiple sclerosis, which rely more heavily on MRI evidence of dissemination in space and time to enable the diagnosis (W.I. McDonald *et al* 2001).

Evoked potentials have been infrequently used to monitor the course of established multiple sclerosis, and the advent of MRI has probably inhibited efforts to investigate serial changes in evoked potential measures. A 2-year study of a mixed cohort of 30 patients with relapsing–remitting or secondary progressive multiple sclerosis showed a modest relationship between changes in disability and visual and motor evoked potential measures but also concluded that a reliable prediction of the course of multiple sclerosis is not possible from the evoked potential measures (Fuhr *et al* 2001). The introduction of evoked potentials has been of great value in understanding the pathophysiology of central nervous system demyelination in patients, and in confirming that the detailed findings from experimental studies are reproduced in humans. We will consider each modality used for evoked potentials in some detail, partly because of their historical contribution to our understanding of multiple sclerosis, and in part because of their remaining utility (Figure 7.40).

Visual evoked potentials

It was a stroke of good fortune that the method of pattern reversal stimulation used by Halliday and his colleagues to study the cortical representation of vision was close to the optimum – as it turned out – needed to demonstrate delays in optic neuritis (Halliday *et al* 1972). The flash evoked potential is much less sensitive to the effects of demyelinating lesions in multiple sclerosis (Halliday *et al* 1972; Namerow and Enns 1972; Richey *et al* 1971; Rouher *et al* 1969) and is not now used in routine clinical practice. It has a small place in helping to determine whether any visual function remains in severely impaired individuals, and in the assessment of an intact visual pathway in individuals with hysterical blindness who elect not to fixate on a more subtle stimulus.

Although there are minor variations between laboratories, the standard technique of stimulation is to use a chequerboard pattern of black and white squares that reverses at 2 Hz and where each square subtends approximately 50 minutes of arc at the retina. The whole stimulus usually occupies 32° of the field. For special purposes, half field and central field (4°) stimuli are invaluable. Further details of the technique are given in standard works of reference (for example, Halliday 1993).

Optic neuritis

The normal pattern reversal induced visual evoked potential is dominated by a large positive wave at approximately 100 ms (P100; Figure 7.41). In the acute stage of optic neuritis, the response is decreased in amplitude or, if the visual acuity is <6/24, it is usually absent. Any surviving response is delayed. As recovery of vision occurs, the amplitude increases and a delayed response with a well-preserved waveform is seen in 90% of patients (Halliday *et al* 1973a). The mean delay is approximately 35 ms (Halliday *et al* 1973a). Delays persist in about 90% of adults, although the latency may decrease after many months, sometimes reverting to normal values (see Chapter 13 and Figure 7.42). In a follow-up study lasting 4 years, W.B. Matthews and Small (1979), found that the latency returned to normal in 19% of subjects. Hely *et al* (1986b) observed a similar rate of recovery. Brusa *et al* (2001) also noted shortening

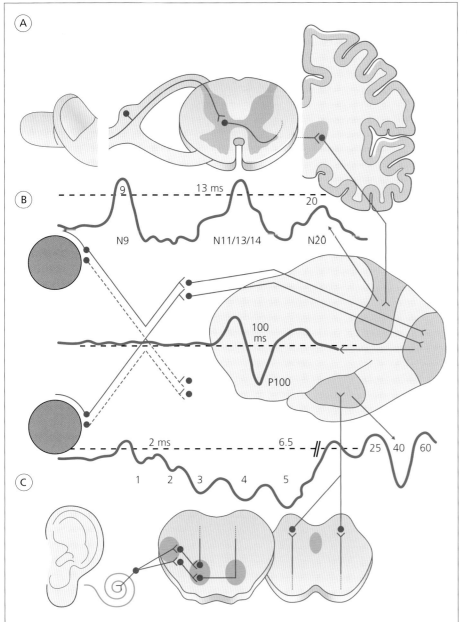

Figure 7.40 Scheme showing the major normal waveforms of the evoked potentials and their sites of origin. (A), Somatosensory, (B) visual and (C) auditory.

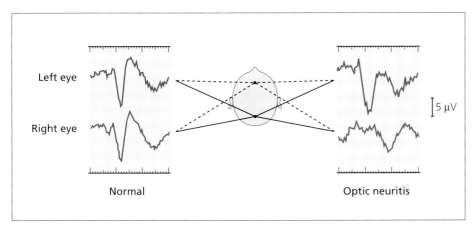

Figure 7.41 Visual evoked potentials to pattern reversal stimulation. On the left are responses from an apparently healthy control and on the right, responses from a patient with acute right optic neuritis. Note the substantial delay in the P100.

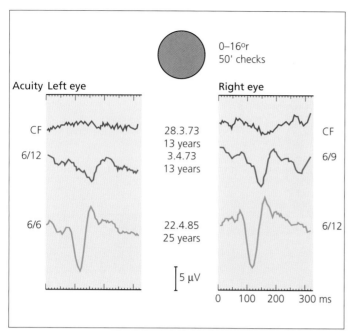

Figure 7.42 Visual evoked potentials to pattern reversal recorded from a girl aged 13 years at presentation, 3 days, 9 days and 12 years after onset of an attack of acute bilateral optic neuritis. Kindly provided by Drs Martin Halliday and Anthony Kriss. Adapted from W.I. McDonald (1986).

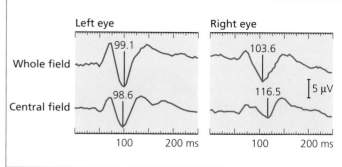

Figure 7.43 Visual evoked potentials to pattern reversal stimulation in a patient with a lesion of the right optic nerve. Top trace. normal response to 'whole' field stimulation; bottom trace. delayed response to stimulation of the central 4°. Kindly provided by Dr Steven Jones.

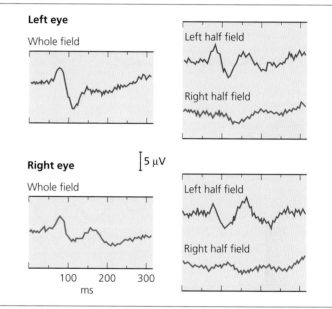

Figure 7.44 Visual evoked potentials to pattern reversal stimulation. Note that the responses evoked from stimulation of the right half fields are delayed compared with those following stimulation of the left half fields. Kindly provided by Dr Steven Jones.

latency of response with increasing years following optic neuritis and proposed that this evolution is compatible with remyelination. After an episode of optic neuritis in childhood, normal latencies are seen in about 50% of patients, perhaps signifying a greater capacity for remyelination in the young (Kriss *et al* 1988; see Chapter 13). Occasionally, the latency from the affected eye remains within normal limits. In these circumstances, the observation of a pathological latency difference between the eyes (>6 ms in our laboratory) may be diagnostically helpful.

When only a small proportion of the fibres subserving central vision is affected, the abnormality may not be detectable within the large response mediated by the normal fibres after full field stimulation. Here, stimulation of the central 4° in isolation may be decisive (Figure 7.43).

Posterior visual pathway lesions

Occasionally, visual symptoms are produced by large lesions involving the optic tract or radiation (Figure 6.24; Plant *et al* 1992; see Chapter 6). Even in the absence of a hemianopia detected by standard clinical methods, delays after stimulating homonymous half fields may be detected to diagnostic advantage (Figure 7.44). Pathologically, demyelinating lesions affect the chiasm in neuromyelitis optica and also in the typical case of multiple sclerosis; however, clinical presentation with a bitemporal hemianopia is exceedingly rare.

Nonorganic visual impairment

The visual evoked potential is often helpful in assessing patients in whom there appears to be a discrepancy in the physical findings suggesting that the abnormality may not be organic in nature. The finding of an evoked potential of normal amplitude, waveform and latency with a visual acuity of 6/24 or less provides strong evidence for nonorganic disturbance. Conversely, when it is uncertain whether any organic abnormality is present and physical examination is normal, the finding of a delay – sometimes detectable only in central field visual evoked potentials – may be invaluable.

Problems of interpretation

In interpreting the results of visual evoked potentials, it is important to be aware that the normal response elicited by stimulation of the paramacular region of the retina in isolation in normal subjects has a latency of approximately 135 ms. Thus, a central scotoma resulting from any pathological process affecting the retina or optic nerve, whether degenerative or demyelinating, may result in an apparent delay which does not necessarily signify the presence of demyelination; it may instead reflect predominant paramacular stimulation.

Another source of confusion is the distorted waveform that can arise in a variety of conditions often – but not invariably – nondemyelinating in nature. In these circumstances, it may be difficult to identify the P100, and accordingly impossible to determine whether there is a true delay attributable to demyelination.

Finally, although compression of the optic nerve usually produces a visual evoked potential of irregular form without a convincing increase in latency of the P100 (Figure 7.45. Halliday *et al* 1976), it must be remembered that a substantial delay with a well-preserved waveform is simply characteristic of the pathological process of demyelination, however it may be caused. For example, a classical delayed response with a preserved waveform is occasionally seen not in optic neuritis but, rather, arising from compression of the anterior visual pathway (Figures 7.46 and 7.47). This finding is in keeping with the experimental

observation of compression-induced focal demyelination in the spinal cord (Holmes 1906) and experimentally in the optic nerve (Clifford-Jones *et al* 1985a; 1985b).

Electroretinogram

Electroretinography is useful as a research tool in the assessment of retinal involvement in demyelinating disease. Various changes have been described at different stages of optic neuritis (Halliday 1993), but they are not of diagnostic help in the investigation of patients suspected of having multiple sclerosis.

Multiple sclerosis

The usefulness of the visual evoked potential in the diagnosis of multiple sclerosis derives from the frequency with which the optic nerve is affected, with or without relevant symptoms, and the usual persistence of the evoked potential abnormality. Overall, this is delayed in approximately 70% of patients suspected of having multiple sclerosis and in up to 90% in some series of patients with clinically definite disease (Halliday 1993).

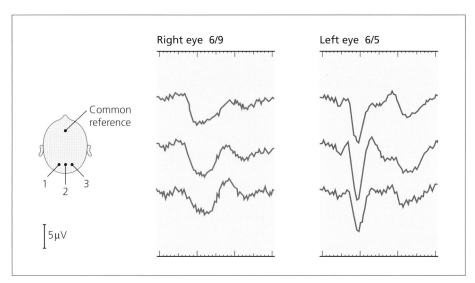

Figure 7.45 Visual evoked potentials after pattern reversal stimulation in a patient with compression of the right intracranial optic nerve by a sphenoid wing meningioma. The waveform is distorted compared with the response from stimulating the left eye. Kindly provided by Dr Martin Halliday.

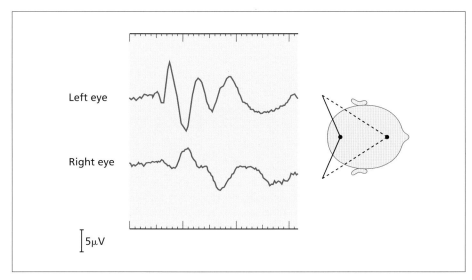

Figure 7.46 Pattern responses from each eye in a patient with a sphenoidal ridge meningioma showing the distortion of normal waveform and the delayed latency of the response from the affected eye. Visual acuity was 6/9 in each eye at the time of the recording. Time scale 10, 50 and 100 ms. From Halliday *et al* (1976) with permission.

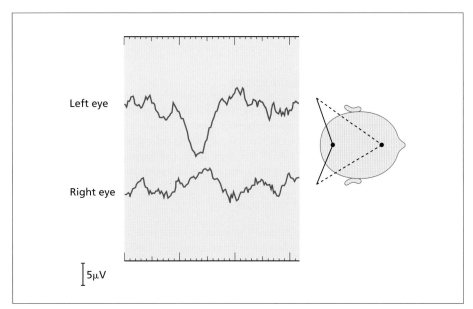

Figure 7.47 Pattern responses from each eye in a patient with pituitary adenoma. VAL 6/6; VAR 6/36. Note the grossly altered waveform of the response from the right eye with loss of the major positive component and a reduction in the overall amplitude. The response from the left eye, which has a reasonably well-preserved waveform, is pathologically delayed. Time scale 10, 50 and 100 ms. From Halliday *et al* (1976) with permission.

As expected, the risk of developing the clinically expressed, disseminated form of multiple sclerosis is increased in those monosymptomatic patients who may present with nonvisual symptoms, if the visual evoked potential is found to be abnormal (see Halliday 1993 for review of the extensive literature). Simply stated, this indicates that a second site is involved but the greater sensitivity of MRI has superseded the visual evoked potential in this setting. Visual evoked potentials are the only electrophysiological diagnostic tests retained in the new diagnostic criteria for multiple sclerosis. A delayed evoked potential does not carry the same status as an emerging MRI lesion in the revised diagnostic criteria (see above; W.I. McDonald *et al* 2001). However, the finding is of particular value when primary progressive multiple sclerosis presents as a progressive myelopathy. In such a context, brain MRI is frequently normal or reveals a paucity of abnormalities but it should be remembered that some genetically determined disorders may be associated with optic pathway and spinal cord involvement, reproducing the clinical and laboratory features of primary progressive multiple sclerosis. Examination of the cerebrospinal fluid achieves special significance in this situation.

In patients presenting with complex clinical pictures in which multiple sclerosis is but one of a number of alternative diagnoses, the finding of a delayed evoked potential is useful in indicating that the pathological process affecting the optic nerve is consistent with demyelination. The cause of the delay is then established from a consideration of the rest of the clinical and investigative picture.

Somatosensory evoked potential

Principles determining the nature of the abnormalities and practical usefulness of the somatosensory evoked potential in the diagnosis of multiple sclerosis are the same as those already discussed with regard to the visual system. The standard method of stimulation is by suprathreshold electrical stimulation of the median or posterior tibial nerves. The response recorded from the scalp over the Rolandic area is dominated by a positive wave at 20 and 40 ms after stimulation of the median

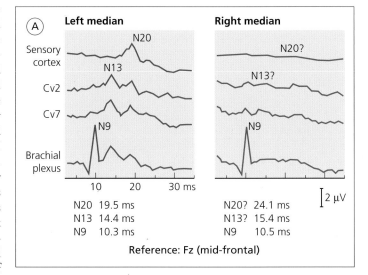

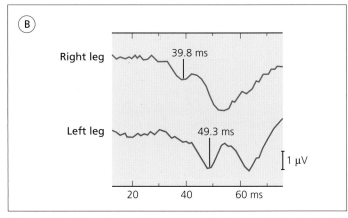

Figure 7.48 Delayed somatosensory evoked potential in clinically definite multiple sclerosis after stimulation of the (A) right median nerve (normal response after stimulation of the left median nerve), (B) left tibial nerve (response following stimulation of the right tibial nerve is of normal latency). Kindly provided by Dr Stephen Jones.

and posterior tibial nerves, respectively (Figure 7.48). Central conduction time is determined by the difference between recordings made over the root entry zones of the cervical and lumbar cord.

As with the visual evoked potential in optic neuritis, the somatosensory response is reduced or absent in the acute phase of demyelinating myelopathy involving the dorsal part of the cord. Given adequate recovery, a delayed response (usually persistent) is found. The choice of the lower or upper limb for stimulation is dictated by clinical needs. When looking for evidence of a cord lesion in an asymptomatic patient, it is best to start with the upper limb somatosensory response both because of the high frequency of plaques in the cervical cord (Oppenheimer 1978) and the greater ease with which this response can be obtained.

The reported frequency of abnormalities in clinically definite multiple sclerosis and in patients without sensory symptoms or signs varies widely. An approximate overall frequency of 80% for clinically definite multiple sclerosis is reasonable, with lower figures for less definite diagnostic categories. Clinically unsuspected lesions may be detected in about 20% of patients being investigated for multiple sclerosis (Small *et al* 1978; Trojaborg and Petersen 1979). Since MRI has now largely replaced somatosensory and auditory evoked potentials as a means of detecting asymptomatic lesions in the diagnosis of multiple sclerosis, the reader is referred to the comprehensive review of Jones (1993) for further details of the variations reported from laboratories investigating different patient groups and using a variety of stimulating and recording techniques.

Auditory evoked potentials

The short latency (≤10 ms) response obtained from scalp electrodes after auditory stimulation by clicks is characterized by five waves, of which I and II originate from the eighth nerve external to the brainstem, wave III from the cochlear nucleus, and IV and V from the region of the superior olivary complex (McPherson and Starr 1993).

In demyelinating disease there is characteristically an increase in latency between I/II and the later waves, the amplitude of which is often reduced (Figure 7.49: Chiappa *et al* 1980; Eisen and Odusote 1980; K. Robinson and Rudge 1977). Abnormalities in the brainstem auditory evoked potentials are rather less frequent than in the visual or somatosensory systems in clinically definite (approximately 50–75%) and suspected (approximately 25%) multiple sclerosis (McPherson and Starr 1993). This investigation is accordingly less useful in the routine diagnostic assessment of patients thought possibly to have multiple sclerosis, especially with the advent of MRI, but can occasionally be of value.

As in the case of the visual evoked potential, end organ damage from whatever cause may interfere with the response as, of course, may conductive deafness, both of which must be excluded before interpreting the results.

In addition to the standard short latency auditory evoked potentials, long latency responses may be elicited by delivering complex harmonic tones. These are more likely to be abnormal than short latency responses in patients with multiple sclerosis (S.J. Jones *et al* 2002), and probably reflect the effects of disseminated central nervous system lesions rather than lesions of the afferent pathway *per se*.

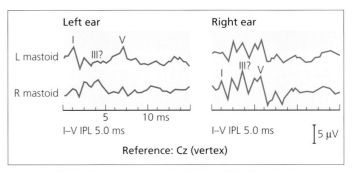

Figure 7.49 Auditory evoked potential in clinically definite multiple sclerosis recorded after click stimulation of each ear. There is an increased latency between waves I and V on left ear stimulation. Kindly provided by Dr Stephen Jones.

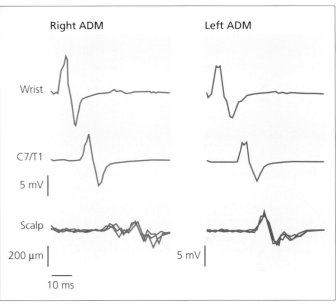

Figure 7.50 Responses recorded from the left and right abductor digiti minimi (ADM) in clinically definite multiple sclerosis after transcranial magnetic stimulation of the contralateral cortex. Note the delay and abnormal waveform in the response from the right (central motor conduction time 9.4 ms) compared with the left (central motor conduction time 6.3 ms) ADM. From Hess *et al* (1986) with permission.

Motor evoked responses

The recording of motor responses to electrical or magnetic cortical stimulation was subsequently added to the repertoire of investigations for the diagnosis of multiple sclerosis. As expected, delays have been demonstrated by both methods (Figure 7.50; Barker *et al* 1986; Cowan *et al* 1984; Hess *et al* 1986; 1987; Ingram *et al* 1987; Mills and Murray 1985; Rossini *et al* 1985). As with afferent evoked potentials, the responses are somewhat variable. This is a consequence of being synaptically mediated. In terms of diagnosis, it must be remembered that there can be a delay in activation of the motor neuron pool in purely degenerative disorders of the cortico-spinal pathway, such as motor neuron disease. Nevertheless, very long delays (of the order of 20 ms) are more likely to result from demyelination

(Thompson *et al* 1987). The diagnostic usefulness of the motor response is limited by the fact that a delay in the response is rarely found in the absence of abnormalities detectable by clinical examination (Hess *et al* 1986; 1987; Murray 1991). Nevertheless, the motor evoked potential has a limited role in the assessment of complex cases. In a study of 19 patients with primary or secondary progressive multiple sclerosis followed up for 1 year, an increasing delay of central motor conduction time was observed in four patients, all of whom also developed new spinal cord lesions on MRI (Kidd *et al* 1998). However, 15 patients in the same study exhibited clinical deterioration indicating that the latter frequently occurs in the absence of a further prolongation of central motor conduction time: the authors took this to mean that clinical progression is more likely the result of increasing axonal loss rather than demyelination.

Other electrophysiological investigations

Although a number of other electrophysiological measures have been applied successfully to detect abnormalities in patients with central nervous system demyelination, none has established a useful role in routine diagnostic practice. In this section, several such techniques are briefly reviewed.

Laser evoked potentials

Laser evoked potentials provide a means for detecting abnormalities in conduction through the spinothalamic tracts. The potentials are elicited by an infrared thulium laser stimulus. The laser beam is directed to produce a painful heat stimulus to the skin of the hand and foot and recordings of the negative and positive evoked potential responses are made at the vertex. An early study revealed absent or delayed responses in 8/12 patients with definite multiple sclerosis (Kakigi *et al* 1992). In a recent analysis, the relative sensitivity of laser evoked potentials was compared with that of standard median and tibial somatosensory evoked potentials in 20 patients who fulfilled standard diagnostic criteria for multiple sclerosis (Spiegel *et al* 2003). Laser evoked potentials were abnormal in 12 (60%) and standard somatosensory recordings were delayed in eight (40%) patients. In seven cases, the abnormalities of spinothalamic function detected using laser evoked potentials were subclinical. Although of interest, because of the apparently greater sensitivity compared with somatosensory evoked potentials, this and other neurophysiological investigations have been largely superseded by MRI as a means for detecting clinically silent lesions.

Ocular microtremor

Using a piezoelectric transducer, abnormalities of ocular microtremor have been studied in patients with multiple sclerosis. In a series of 50 patients, abnormalities were seen in 78%, and were most likely to occur in those with signs of brainstem or cerebellar disease (Bolger *et al* 2000). The frequency of normal (physiological) ocular microtremor was reduced in the multiple sclerosis subjects compared with healthy controls. The investigation has not found a place in diagnosis and would seem unlikely to do so in view of the need to place the monitoring equipment on the sclera.

Vestibular evoked myogenic potentials

This more recently developed neurophysiological technique studies the modulation of tonic electromyographic activity of the sternocleidomastoid muscle in response to a vestibular activation stimulus. It is proposed as a method for detecting brainstem lesions. In a recent investigation of 40 patients with multiple sclerosis, abnormal vestibular evoked myogenic potentials were found in 28 subjects, including four in whom brain MRI was normal (Alpini *et al* 2004). However, in another study of 36 patients with multiple sclerosis, vestibular evoked myogenic evoked potentials were less sensitive than either MRI or visual evoked potentials in detecting abnormalities (Bandini *et al* 2004). Further studies in multiple sclerosis and other disorders will be needed to determine its sensitivity and specificity as a diagnostic tool.

EXAMINATION OF THE CEREBROSPINAL FLUID

Examination of the cerebrospinal fluid obtained at lumbar puncture has had a role in the diagnosis of multiple sclerosis for more than 70 years. Greenfield and Carmichael (1925) showed that a paretic colloidal gold curve in the presence of a negative test for syphilis was characteristic although not, of course, diagnostic for multiple sclerosis. Kabat *et al* (1942) took the next step when they showed that proteins in the cerebrospinal fluid were electrophoretically different from those in serum (see Chapter 1). Further electrophoretic studies followed (Scheid 1944 – see Bauer 1953; Cumings 1953; Felgenhauer 1971), but it was Lowenthal *et al* (1960; Lowenthal 1964) who demonstrated the diagnostic potential of cerebrospinal fluid protein electrophoresis by virtue of bands observed in the gammaglobulin region. Link (1967) showed that these represented immunoglobulin G (IgG); and the group of Dr W.W. Tourtellotte provided evidence that the IgG originated in the lesions of multiple sclerosis (Tourtellotte and Parker 1966; Tourtellotte *et al* 1980). The antigens, however, still await definitive identification. Electrophoresis of the spinal fluid proteins led to a marked increase in sensitivity, but not specificity, in detecting abnormalities. With the advent of other laboratory investigations, in particular MRI, the role of lumbar puncture in the diagnosis of multiple sclerosis is now less important, but it remains of great value in the assessment of complex cases where an important question is whether the disease process is immunologically mediated. In these circumstances, the demonstration of intrathecal IgG synthesis is often crucial in determining the next step in diagnostic assessment, or in supporting a diagnosis of multiple sclerosis when it has been suspected but not definitively established on other grounds.

We discuss the immunological properties of cerebrospinal fluid and the lessons learned for understanding the pathogenesis of multiple sclerosis in Chapter 11. Here, the more pragmatic position is adopted of how the various findings can be used to supplement clinical features in establishing the correct diagnosis of multiple sclerosis in a given case. We consider that examination of the cerebrospinal fluid is particularly valuable in two contexts. In older patients who present some years after first developing symptoms; and in those with a late onset progressive syndrome which may be the result of demyelination, MRI cerebral white matter lesions suggestive of multiple sclerosis may be age related and not the result of inflammatory demyelination. The detection of oligoclonal bands is then highly informative. Second, the examination of cerebrospinal fluid has a role in patients with progressive myelopathy at all ages. The revised criteria for the diagnosis of primary progressive multiple sclerosis require the demonstration of oligoclonal bands (McDonald *et al* 2001). To illustrate this point: in the context of cord flattening due to spondylosis on MRI, and with little or no cerebral white matter abnormalities, the question arises of whether the diagnosis is spondylitic myelopathy, primary progressive multiple sclerosis or comorbidity? Often, the presence of oligoclonal bands will tip the balance of probabilities in favour of demyelinating disease and spare the patient unnecessary spinal surgery with a low dividend for clinical improvement (Figure 7.51).

Cerebrospinal fluid examination is also of value in that findings outside the expected range should lead to a careful reassessment of the diagnosis. Now, we discuss the typical profile basing this account on previous summaries, some especially helpful in that they represent consensus reports (Andersson *et al* 1994; Tourtellotte 1985; Tourtellotte *et al* 1988; Whitaker *et al* 1990).

Cell count

It is common to find a modest pleocytosis of 10–20 cells/cm^3 at the time of relapse. That such counts are also seen during clinical remission is not surprising given the five- to 20-fold greater frequency of lesion activity detected by MRI compared with clinical assessments and the chronic persistent inflammatory reaction in the brains of patients in remission. Cell counts of >50 cells/cm^3 are rare and should raise the suspicion of an alternative diagnosis. In acute disseminated encephalomyelitis and transverse myelitis, the cell count may be considerably higher (>100/cm^3) in the acute phase (Miller *et al* 1956). That said, we have occasionally seen counts of up to 100 cells/cm^3 in patients fulfilling standard criteria for the diagnosis of clinically definite multiple sclerosis. Lymphocytes usually make up 90% and polymorphonuclear cells <5% of the differential count. Cytospin preparations also often contain macrophages and the occasional plasma cell.

Total protein

The total protein is normal in about two-thirds of patients, but modestly elevated (0.5–0.7 g/L) in the remainder. Exceptionally, higher levels are seen and, when there is swelling in the spinal cord with an acute lesion, the level may be >1 g/L. Very high levels of protein (>2.5 g/L) may also be found with the rare combination of central and peripheral demyelinating disease fulfilling standard diagnostic criteria for multiple sclerosis and chronic inflammatory demyelinating polyneuropathy (P.K. Thomas *et al* 1987; see Chapter 6). We have seen such a patient with a total spinal fluid protein of 2.6 g/L who developed the additional complication of secondary raised intracranial pressure.

Intrathecal IgG synthesis

Intrathecal IgG synthesis is highly characteristic of multiple sclerosis. The most widely used means for demonstrating this feature is isoelectric focusing of contemporaneous serum and

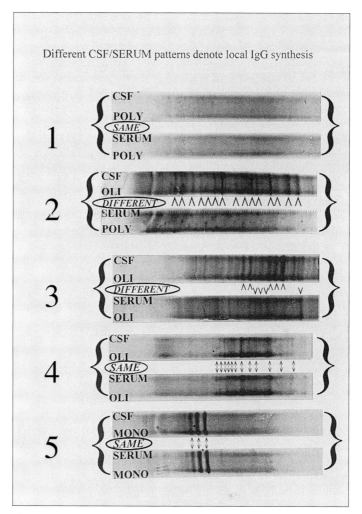

Figure 7.51 Five patterns of isoelectric focusing. Type 1 is a normal pattern from a patient with benign intracranial hypertension. Type 2 is a typical oligoclonal pattern in a patient with clinically definite multiple sclerosis. Type 3 is a 'greater than' pattern, also in a patient with clinically definite multiple sclerosis where there are more bands in cerebrospinal fluid than in the corresponding serum sample. Type 4 is a mirror pattern in which the same bands found in the systemic circulation are passively transferred into the spinal fluid, in this case from a patient with the Guillain–Barré syndrome. Type 5 is a monoclonal paraprotein in serum transferred passively into the spinal fluid in a patient with IgG paraprotein neuropathy. POLY = polyclonal; OLI = oligoclonal; MONO = monoclonal. Cathode is on the right. From Andersson *et al* (1994) with permission.

spinal fluid samples, so that the synthesis of IgG specifically in the central compartment can be estimated. In practice, agarose gels are preferred by some laboratories because of a lower false-positive rate but these offer a less sensitive approach (Lunding *et al* 2002). The demonstration of oligoclonal bands in cerebrospinal fluid but not serum (Figure 7.51), or of additional bands in the cerebrospinal fluid despite abnormalities in serum, provides clear evidence for intrathecal synthesis and carries the implication that an immunological process is active in the central nervous system. Using isoelectric focusing, oligoclonal bands are found in >95% of patients with clinically definite disease (Andersson *et al* 1994). Their absence in a patient suspected of having multiple sclerosis should lead to a careful reassessment of evidence for the diagnosis (Zeman *et al* 1996). The presence of identical bands in serum and cerebrospinal fluid indicates a systemic immune response with passive transfer of immunoglobulin from serum, and is of no diagnostic value. It should also be noted that the frequency of oligoclonal bands in the cerebrospinal fluid of Oriental patients with clinically definite multiple sclerosis is lower (approximately 33%: Y.L. Yu *et al* 1989) than in patients of European origin (>90%; McLean *et al* 1990). It is unclear whether this relates to the higher frequency of optico-spinal presentation reported in Oriental populations (see Chapters 5 and 6).

Oligoclonal bands are sometimes absent at or near the clinical onset of multiple sclerosis, but emerge after follow-up and repeat lumbar puncture. Serial analysis of the cerebrospinal fluid has shown that once present, oligoclonal bands persist in individuals with multiple sclerosis. Disappearance, as may be seen in acute disseminated encephalomyelitis (Kesselring *et al* 1990), makes the diagnosis of multiple sclerosis highly unlikely. The presence of oligoclonal bands in patients with optic neuritis and other clinically isolated syndromes is associated with an increased likelihood of conversion to clinically definite multiple sclerosis in the next 5 years (see Chapter 6).

Several other approaches have been taken to demonstrate intrathecal IgG synthesis. The Link index is the ratio of IgG in cerebrospinal fluid and serum divided by the ratio of albumin in spinal fluid and serum. It correlates with the results of cerebrospinal fluid electrophoresis or isoelectric focusing but is rather less sensitive than these qualitative methods (Andersson *et al* 1994). Quantitative methods have also been developed for intrathecal IgG production (Tourtellotte 1985), but they are technically difficult and are more relevant to research than routine diagnosis (Andersson *et al* 1994).

It must be emphasized again that, as in the case for MRI and evoked potentials, the demonstration of oligoclonal bands present selectively in cerebrospinal fluid is not specific for multiple sclerosis. It tells the physician that there is an intrathecal immunological abnormality. Other clinical and investigative data provide the evidence from which the cause may be determined. Intrathecal IgG synthesis is seen in several other immunological disorders, in acute and chronic inflammation or infection of the brain and meninges, and in the paraneoplastic syndromes (McLean *et al* 1990; see Chapter 8). Although it is claimed that neurosarcoidosis may be associated with oligoclonal bands in the cerebrospinal fluid (McLean *et al* 1990; Zajicek *et al* 1998), a current expert view suggests that such bands may not be found in histologically confirmed disease (Ed Thompson, personal communication). Further study of this difficult topic is clearly needed. Although the number of possible causes for increased intrathecal IgG synthesis is large, it is true to say that amongst individuals of northern European origin living in temperate climates, multiple sclerosis is outstandingly the commonest cause of intrathecal IgG synthesis.

Cerebrospinal fluid oligoclonal IgA and IgM bands also occur in multiple sclerosis (Leary *et al* 2002; Vilar *et al* 2003). A recent report suggests that the presence of cerebrospinal fluid oligoclonal IgM may be associated with a poor long-term prognosis (Villar *et al* 2003). However, this study was small and only 11/29 individuals had IgM bands. A later report from the same investi-gators reported more relapses and disability in 15 patients who had oligoclonal IgM against myelin lipids when compared with 33 patients who lacked such bands (Villar *et al* 2005). Further work is needed to investigate this potential prognostic marker.

Other investigations using blood and cerebrospinal fluid

Because the composition of cerebrospinal fluid reflects aspects of what is happening in the central nervous system parenchyma, several procedures have been developed to analyse many of its normal and pathological constituents, including those that reflect spillover of processes also active in the systemic circulation or specifically located in the central nervous system. Peripheral blood markers of disease activity are more likely to be dominated by systemic immunological or inflammatory events unrelated to events germane to the central nervous system disorder. Potential markers of disease have included measurements of lymphocyte subpopulations (Navikas *et al* 1996a; 1996b), production of cytokines (Peter *et al* 1991), endothelial cell markers (Dore-Duffy *et al* 1995; Minagar *et al* 2001), cholesterol (Giubilei *et al* 2002) and myelin breakdown products, which are also detectable in urine (Whitaker *et al* 1993; 1994). Myelin breakdown products, of course, are detected whenever there is myelin destruction whether this results from primary demyelination or is secondary to axonal degeneration induced by infarction, trauma or chronic degenerative disorders. These procedures do not currently have a role in routine diagnostic assessment of the individual patient. Similarly, measurements of putative biochemical markers of glial proliferation or axonal loss in the cerebrospinal fluid – such as S110b protein, 14-3-3 protein and nonphosphorylated neurofilaments – are likely to demonstrate abnormalities in a number of neurodegenerative and neuroinflammatory disorders in which gliosis and axonal loss occur (Irani and Kerr 2000; De Séze *et al* 2002).

Petzold and colleagues (2002) investigated biomarkers for glial responses in the cerebrospinal fluid of 51 patients with multiple sclerosis. Patients with severe locomotor disability exhibited higher levels of cerebrospinal fluid glial fibrillary acidic protein when compared with less disabled patients and controls. Levels of S100b tended to be higher in relapsing–remitting subjects than in those with secondary or primary progressive disease and post-mortem examination revealed that S100b was higher in histopathologically acute lesions. The authors suggest that there are different patterns of glial activation according to disease course and disability.

Axonal markers may be of more relevance for monitoring disease progression (Martinez-Yelamos *et al* 2001) since axonal loss is the major substrate of irreversible disability in multiple sclerosis. Phosphorylated forms of neurofilament are principal components of the axoskeleton released during axonal injury. In a recent study, two neurofilament heavy chain phosphoforms were analysed from the cerebrospinal fluid of 34 patients with multiple sclerosis and 318 noninflammatory neurological controls (Petzold *et al* 2005). Measures were taken at baseline and after 3 years. An increase in the NfH[S135] was seen in 59% of patients with primary or secondary progressive multiple sclerosis but in only 14% with relapsing–remitting disease. The level of NfHS[135] was also moderately correlated with disability. These results support the notion that progressive axonal loss underpins increasing disability and suggest that the cerebrospinal fluid level of NfH[S135] may be a prognostic marker. Confirmation of these findings in another study is needed.

Recent interest has been shown in the measurement of serum anti-myelin antibodies. While these are present in subjects with multiple sclerosis, there has not been a convincing demonstration of their specificity or sensitivity as a diagnostic tool. A recent study by Berger *et al* (2003) investigated 103 patients with clinically isolated syndromes of the type seen in multiple sclerosis. The subjects were pre-selected by requiring the presence of disseminated white matter lesions on brain T_2-weighted MRI that fulfilled the Fazekas criteria (Fazekas *et al* 1988), accompanied by the presence of cerebrospinal fluid oligoclonal bands. At presentation, 22 had antibodies to both myelin basic protein and myelin oligodendrocyte glycoprotein, 42 had antibodies to myelin oligodendrocyte glycoprotein alone, and 39 did not have antibodies to either of these myelin antigens. During follow-up, further relapses allowing a diagnosis of clinically definite multiple sclerosis occurred in 21/22 (95%) who were positive for both antibodies, 35/42 (83%) who were positive for anti-myelin oligodendrocyte glycoprotein, but in only 9/39 (23%) who were negative for both antibodies. It should be noted that this study cohort was biased by the application of entry criteria that ensured a high *a priori* likelihood of having multiple sclerosis. The most one can infer is that, in those clinically isolated syndrome patients who – from the presence of characteristic multifocal MRI white matter lesions – have a strong probability of developing multiple sclerosis, the absence of anti-myelin antibodies may identify a subgroup in whom the risk is somewhat lower. The remarkable finding of this single study needs to be confirmed in other laboratories and in a broader cohort of unselected patients with clinically isolated syndromes. The subsequent reports that patients with multiple sclerosis and healthy controls have a similar proportion of anti-myelin oligodendrocyte glycoprotein IgG and IgM (Lampasong *et al* 2004) and that anti-myelin antibodies do not correlate with either MRI abnormalities or development of early multiple sclerosis in a cohort of patients with isolated optic neuritis (Lim *et al* 2005) raise doubts whether these laboratory findings will prove to have a sustainable diagnostic value.

More recently, Lennon *et al* (2004) have described a serum marker for the subgroup of patients in whom the clinical phenotype is dominated by optico-spinal multiple sclerosis or neuromyelitis optica. The investigators in this study used indirect immunofluorescence with a composite substrate of mouse tissues to identify a distinctive pattern of IgG staining of central nervous system microvessels, pia, subpia and Virchow–Robin spaces. They called this antibody NMO-IgG and found that it was present in 33/45 (73%) North American patients who had a definite diagnosis of neuromyelitis optica made on the basis of having clinical involvement confined to the optic nerves and spinal cord in association with various combinations of a normal brain MRI scan at first presentation, a spinal cord lesion extending over more than three vertebral segments on MRI investigation, and a cerebrospinal fluid pleocytosis greater than 50×10^6 white cells per litre. The NMO-IgG autoantibody was also identified in 6/11 (55%) Japanese patients with the optico-spinal form of multiple sclerosis and in 16/35 (46%) North

American patients who were considered to be at high risk of neuromyelitis optica in that they had either monophasic or recurrent transverse myelitis with a longitudinally extensive cord lesion or recurrent optic neuritis. In contrast, NMO-IgG was detected in only 2/22 (9%) North American patients with multiple sclerosis in whom the presentation was with optic nerve or spinal cord involvement and in none of 24 patients with classical multiple sclerosis (19 North American and 5 Japanese) who were included as a pathological control group. This study suggests a potentially important role for NMO-IgG testing in the differential diagnosis of inflammatory myelopathies and optic neuropathies – independent confirmation of the findings from other laboratories is awaited.

A STRATEGY FOR THE INVESTIGATION OF DEMYELINATING DISEASE

We conclude with a scheme that we consider to represent a compromise between economy, precision and convenience – both for the patient and neurologist – in investigating the individual suspected of having demyelinating disease. It embodies the principles of the available methods and our clinical experience in their application.

A key aspect in selecting which investigations to perform is their sensitivity to detect relevant abnormalities, and hence their likelihood of providing positive diagnostic information. It is therefore important to note that MRI is more likely than evoked potentials to demonstrate dissemination in space, and that there is a high probability of detecting oligoclonal bands in cerebrospinal fluid in established multiple sclerosis. The study of Beer *et al* (1995) highlights the relative sensitivity of paraclinical tests in their diagnostic classification of 189 consecutive patients referred for suspected multiple sclerosis. At discharge from hospital, 142 individuals received a diagnosis of multiple sclerosis based on the Poser criteria and 47 were classified as not having multiple sclerosis. The authors found that, when taken as single tests, imaging had the greatest reclassification sensitivity (60%), followed by examination of the cerebrospinal fluid (31%), and then visual (28%), motor (19%) and somatosensory evoked (12%) potentials. It was noted that MRI had a lower specificity than the other investigations, emphasizing the importance of applying the more specific rules to define the nature of the required imaging abnormalities, as embodied in the recent diagnostic criteria (W.I. McDonald *et al* 2001). It should be stressed again that no imaging, cerebrospinal fluid or evoked potential abnormality is 100% specific for multiple sclerosis. Undue or exclusive reliance on any of the paraclinical investigations invites misdiagnosis.

In clinical practice, patients present with symptoms attributable to demyelination of the central nervous system in one of three categories:

- individuals with unequivocal relapsing–remitting episodes, originating from separate sites within the central nervous system, in whom demyelination is the most likely pathophysiological explanation for each event (clinically definite or probable multiple sclerosis)
- individuals with a recent clinically isolated episode typical of demyelination, with or without a suspicious past history

- individuals with slowly progressive neurological symptoms which might be due to demyelination.

Clinically definite multiple sclerosis

The patient with episodes disseminated in time, each of which can be attributed to demyelination, requires no investigation prior to establishing the diagnosis of clinically definite multiple sclerosis if presentation occurs between the ages of 20 and 50 years, separate anatomical sites within the central nervous system have necessarily been affected on different occasions, and the clinical phenotype is typical for multiple sclerosis. Nevertheless, it can nowadays be considered as normal practice to confirm the clinically definite diagnosis by demonstrating the presence of characteristic abnormalities in brain MRI. These are expected in >95% of such individuals.

When the criteria for clinically definite multiple sclerosis are not met – perhaps the patient has a typical history of relapsing and remitting symptoms but on examination has signs of only one central nervous system lesion – the first and most appropriate investigation is brain MRI. If this demonstrates typical abnormalities, no further investigation is necessary but some neurologists nevertheless advise cerebrospinal fluid examination to demonstrate intrathecal inflammation. Some still perform multimodal evoked potentials if imaging and spinal fluid are both normal, since multiple sclerosis very occasionally occurs in the absence of MRI or cerebrospinal fluid abnormalities. However, the main priority in such cases is to consider and exclude conditions that can mimic multiple sclerosis, and to establish that there is an organic neurological disease.

It is not uncommon to encounter patients giving a history compatible with, but not strongly suggestive of, multiple sclerosis in whom there are no abnormalities on examination. In this context, the first step is to determine whether any organic abnormality is present. Our approach is to begin with MRI of the brain and, if this is normal, the spinal cord provides complementary evidence excluding a structural abnormality. An important caveat to bear in mind in this context is the nonspecificity of several small subcortical white matter lesions on brain MRI. These are a not uncommon incidental finding in middle-aged adults and may even occur in younger people. Many neurologists will be familiar with radiological reports that have inappropriately suggested demyelination leading to worried and frightened individuals being given an incorrect diagnosis of multiple sclerosis entirely out of clinical context. Conversely, small, well-defined, intrinsic spinal cord lesions do not occur with aging or small vessel disease *per se* and provide more specific evidence for demyelination (Bot *et al* 2002). Examination of visual, auditory and somatosensory evoked potentials can also be useful. Significant delay provides evidence for the pathological process of demyelination although, as emphasized above, this is not specific for multiple sclerosis. Rarely, it may be appropriate to examine the spinal fluid for evidence of inflammation but, when symptoms are thought not to be organic, lumbar puncture is best avoided. Every experienced clinician will recall patients in whom the procedure added little but was later perceived to have been complicated – usually 'causing' intractable backache – and sustaining a variety of nonorganic complaints. Although some of us have occasionally made the diagnosis of multiple sclerosis in individuals whose symptoms and signs did not match the criteria for clinically definite multiple sclerosis, and in whom all three categories of investigation were normal, this would have to be seen as an exceptional situation. In general the diagnosis should be considered less likely as each investigation proves negative.

Other structural lesions, such as meningioma, can present with relapsing symptoms and it is for this reason that investigation is essential, even in the context of a relapsing history, if the previous events have not involved separate sites in the central nervous system. Even when the history does implicate different parts of the nervous system, errors can occasionally arise from the co-existence of more than one disease. It is for this reason that the individual past episodes need to be evaluated carefully before deciding that investigation is unnecessary, even in the patient with a relapsing history.

The age limits of 20–50 years are conservative and a significant number of patients with multiple sclerosis present in childhood or later than the sixth decade. However, outside this age band, the probability of an alternative diagnosis increases and the threshold for investigation of disorders that may mimic multiple sclerosis falls. The diagnosis of multiple sclerosis should always be more carefully considered in ethnic groups in whom it is known to be less common (see Chapter 3).

The isolated demyelinating lesion

The decision to investigate patients with an isolated episode of demyelination and a past history of neurological symptoms depends entirely on interpretation of the previous event. If, in retrospect, this can also be attributed with confidence to demyelination, management is the same as for patients with disease disseminated in time. If the previous episode is of doubtful significance, investigation follows the protocol for patients with a first episode of demyelination. Much therefore depends on interpretation of the past history; making the distinction between significant previous episodes and those that can safely be ignored requires clinical experience. Symptoms that are likely to be relevant in making the diagnosis of multiple sclerosis in the patient with a recent episode of demyelination, but which may not have assumed significance at the time, include unilateral blurring of vision, numbness in an anatomical distribution (such as the lower limbs and trunk as far as the waist) or Lhermitte's symptom, double vision and inability to use a limb, especially if these complaints have been present for several days or weeks. Symptoms from the past history, often mentioned by patients but usually turning out not to be important, include any neurological events lasting <24 hours, patchy numbness relieved by change in posture, giddiness, encephalitis or meningitis, bladder symptoms on straining, psychiatric symptomatology and epilepsy.

The approach to investigation and diagnosis of patients who present with a clinically isolated syndrome typical of demyelination (for example, unilateral optic neuritis, internuclear ophthalmoplegia or partial myelitis) should take account of the recently published new diagnostic criteria for multiple sclerosis (W.I. McDonald *et al* 2001). For the first time, these make it possible to diagnose multiple sclerosis after a single clinical episode using paraclinical investigations to establish dissemination in space and time. As discussed above, since the criteria have been published, further experience has been reported of their application in the context for which they were partially designed – the patient with a clinically isolated syndrome – and, in particular, their ability to predict the development of clinically definite multiple sclerosis. The MRI criteria for dissemination in space and time have a high specificity and positive predictive value for clinically definite multiple sclerosis (Dalton *et al* 2002a; Tintoré *et al* 2003). However, sensitivity of the dissemination in time criteria is low after 3 months follow-up because, at this time point, the criteria require there to be a gadolinium enhancing lesion (Dalton *et al* 2002a). Substitution of a new T_2 lesion for a gadolinium enhancing lesion at this stage increases sensitivity without losing specificity (Dalton *et al* 2003a). Because of the overall robustness of these criteria, we think it is now appropriate to discuss the possibility of multiple sclerosis with young adults who present with clinically isolated syndromes and to offer further investigations designed to refine the probability or actually establish the diagnosis of multiple sclerosis.

The strategy for investigation of clinically isolated syndromes should always include a consideration of other potential diagnoses, often starting with some simple blood tests, for example towards the exclusion of systemic lupus erythematosus, neurosyphilis and Lyme disease. The choice of more specific investigations will depend on the anatomical region involved clinically. In the case of brainstem syndromes, brain MRI is mandatory, as is spinal MRI in patients presenting with isolated spinal cord syndromes. In clinically isolated optic neuritis, there should always be a specialist ophthalmology review, bearing in mind that some conditions – neuroretinitis and central serous retinopathy – may be otherwise impossible to distinguish from optic neuritis. Imaging is not usually required for the diagnosis of optic neuritis, and the decision whether to perform brain MRI is based on the potential for predicting or diagnosing multiple sclerosis. We approach this issue by first explaining that for about 50–60% of people with optic neuritis, the cause is multiple sclerosis. We discuss something of the nature of multiple sclerosis, emphasize its potential to be benign, and then offer to perform brain MRI to refine the prognosis explaining that an abnormal scan implies a 60–80% likelihood of having multiple sclerosis whereas a normal scan reduces that probability to around 20%. In those who opt for investigation, we arrange a T_2 and gadolinium enhanced scan and follow the patient up promptly. If the scan has been performed >3 months after the attack and fulfils the McDonald criteria for dissemination in space and time, multiple sclerosis is diagnosed. If the scan is abnormal but the criteria for multiple sclerosis are not fulfilled, we suggest a repeat T_2-weighted scan between 3 and 6 months after the original study, as this offers the best prospect of establishing MRI evidence for dissemination in space and time (Dalton *et al* 2003a). Not all patients wish to undergo initial or repeat scanning and it is clearly important to respect their wishes at each stage. We also do not recommend repeat scanning beyond these two initial studies since it becomes increasingly likely that the disease will declare itself clinically as much as by MRI in the longer term.

Within the McDonald criteria, the combination of cerebrospinal fluid evidence for oligoclonal bands along with two T_2 brain lesions is sufficient to constitute evidence for dissemination in space. Detection of oligoclonal bands in a patient with a clinically isolated syndrome in whom there is incomplete or absent imaging evidence for multiple sclerosis can be useful in suggesting the likelihood of inflammatory demyelination. Whichever criteria for dissemination in space are used (MRI alone or MRI combined with examination of cerebrospinal fluid) an essential requirement for diagnosing multiple sclerosis using the McDonald criteria is the evidence on MRI of new lesions at least 3 months after the clinical attack. This requirement not only improves specificity of the criteria for developing clinically definite multiple sclerosis (Dalton *et al* 2002a; Tintore *et al* 2003) but also helps to avoid misdiagnosing cases of acute disseminated encephalomyelitis as multiple sclerosis. It should, however, be noted that acute disseminated encephalomyelitis is uncommon in the adult age group, and rarely presents as one of the clinically isolated syndromes typically ushering in the clinical course of multiple sclerosis. If doubt exists in distinguishing the two conditions, serial MRI and cerebrospinal fluid examination may assist: in acute disseminated encephalomyelitis, it would be unexpected for new lesions to develop over a period longer than several weeks and, perhaps, for oligoclonal bands either not to be present at all or – unlike multiple sclerosis – to disappear with follow-up.

This discussion of our approach to investigating patients with optic neuritis and other clinically isolated syndromes addresses only the issue of diagnosing multiple sclerosis. A separate but highly relevant issue arises when there is consideration given to commencing early disease-modifying treatment. Based on evidence that interferon-β delays the time from first attack to development of clinically definite multiple sclerosis in those with abnormal MRI (Comi *et al* 2001a; Jacobs *et al* 2000), it is the practice of some neurologists to initiate therapy after one episode. In these circumstances, MRI abnormalities are taken into account in deciding whom to treat. In countries where guidelines for disease-modifying treatments in multiple sclerosis require that there have been two relapses in the previous 2 years, the issues dictating investigation after single clinical episodes are those relating to diagnosis.

The progressive syndrome

Investigation is mandatory when there is uncertainty about the nature of the presenting episode, and in all patients with slowly progressive symptoms originating from a single anatomical site. The first priority is to assess the affected part radiologically. Formerly, a common error was to restrict examination by contrast myelography to the level at which clinical symptoms were perceived to have arisen, failing to recognize that, in the context of spinal cord disease, motor signs discriminate poorly between different sites of involvement and that sensory levels are necessarily displaced several segments from the affected level because of the lamination of fibres in ascending sensory pathways. This strategic error is less likely with the advent of MRI and the whole of the spinal cord can be readily imaged in a single field of view using phased array receiver coils. In all patients presenting with progressive spastic paraplegia, spinal MRI is mandatory unless it is contraindicated, in which case myelography will still be required.

Even if spinal cord imaging shows an appropriately placed structural abnormality, the clinician still needs to decide on its

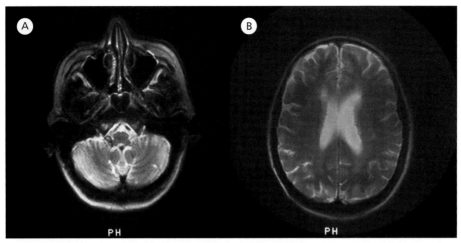

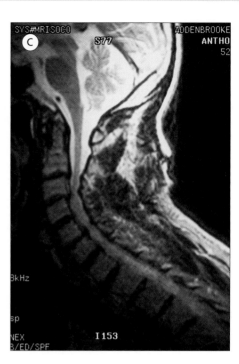

Figure 7.52 (A) T$_2$-weighted image showing few high signal abnormalities in the cerebellum of a patient aged 65 years with a progressive cerebellar syndrome, oligoclonal bands and delayed visual evoked potentials. (B) Periventricular abnormalities in the same patient. (C) Cord flattening as a result of spondylitis in a patient with a primary progressive spinal cord syndrome, oligoclonal bands and delayed visual evoked potentials.

significance. A large extradural tumour or intrinsic swelling arising from astrocytoma or ependymoma can reasonably be taken to account for the presenting symptoms and be managed by neurosurgical and neuro-oncological colleagues in the appropriate manner. However, other structural abnormalities may be detected, such as disc herniation with narrowing of the cervical canal and slight cord compression, which are not necessarily significant – the presenting symptoms and signs of demyelination happening to arise (coincidentally) at a site of minor but insignificant structural damage. Under these circumstances, and always when imaging shows no structural lesion, it is necessary to carry out MRI of the head, seeking to demonstrate white matter abnormalities indicative of multifocal inflammatory brain disease. If cerebral MRI precedes radiological investigation of the clinically affected part, the possibility arises that white matter abnormalities will be demonstrated and the diagnosis of multiple sclerosis made, even when there is a significant coexisting local lesion.

Since it is now known that nonspecific white matter abnormalities almost never occur spontaneously in the spinal cord in otherwise normal individuals, their detection can be taken as evidence for the process of demyelination, although on a single scan this will not distinguish between a monophasic illness and multiple sclerosis. In the context of a progressive spastic paraplegia of at least 1 year's duration, the presence of two or more discrete spinal cord lesions of a type characteristic of demyelination can be used to support a diagnosis of primary progressive multiple sclerosis (W.I. McDonald *et al* 2001; A.J. Thompson *et al* 2000). A combination of one cord lesion and between four and eight brain lesions may also be used to support a diagnosis of primary progressive multiple sclerosis, as may nine or more brain lesions alone – providing that the brain lesions also appear characteristic for demyelination and cord imaging has excluded any other pathological process. Without evidence for cerebrospinal fluid oligoclonal bands to accompany these imaging findings, the most recent diagnostic criteria recommend that the diagnosis of

primary progressive multiple sclerosis should be regarded as probable; when bands are present, it may be classified as definite (A.J. Thompson *et al* 2000).

Analysis of cerebrospinal fluid may also resolve difficult diagnostic situations when imaging both the affected part and the cerebrum fails to provide sufficient information for establishing the diagnosis (Figure 7.52). Evoked potentials may also be delayed in disorders that present with progressive disease at a single site in older patients, and hence run the risk of confusion with multiple sclerosis. In these situations, the demonstration of oligoclonal bands favours the diagnosis of inflammatory brain disease rather than late onset genetically determined or degenerative conditions and can resolve an otherwise diagnostically difficult problem.

Where neuroradiological investigation and spinal fluid analysis exclude a structural abnormality but fail to provide evidence sufficient for the diagnosis of multiple sclerosis, it is appropriate to review the patient after several months and be prepared to repeat all the investigations. Every clinician experienced in the management of neurological disease will have encountered patients in whom competent investigation at presentation failed to detect a structural lesion that subsequently became clinically and radiologically apparent. Likewise, the laboratory evidence for demyelination may only emerge during follow-up.

UPDATING THE MCDONALD DIAGNOSTIC CRITERIA AND THE PROSPECT OF FUTURE REVISIONS

It is inevitable that as further experience is reported in the application of existing diagnostic investigations, and as new diagnostic techniques emerge, internationally accepted criteria for the diagnosis of multiple sclerosis will periodically be amended and updated. Indeed, an International Panel was convened in March 2005 to review the widely accepted criteria that were developed by another panel 4 years earlier (W.I. McDonald *et al* 2001). In a prior review article, three members of the new International Panel had considered the performance of these 2001 criteria based on reports that had emerged in the 3 years subsequent to their publication (Polman *et al* 2005b). While a generally favourable performance had been evident, potential areas for modification and improvement were identified. These included:

- more specific definitions for clinical dissemination in space
- less stringent criteria for MRI dissemination in space
- allowing a new T_2 lesion as early evidence for dissemination in time in patients with single clinical episodes
- greater integration of spinal cord MRI findings
- no longer a requirement for the presence of cerebrospinal oligoclonal bands to diagnose primary progressive multiple sclerosis.

The revised criteria developed by the new Panel were published late in 2005 (Polman *et al* 2005c). They partly address the issues anticipated above and also reaffirm the 2001 criteria in taking the view that multiple sclerosis should not be diagnosed in the absence of any objective clinical evidence for abnormality. The main areas of revision – summarized in Table 7.5 – are in the MRI criteria for dissemination in space and time (for application in patients who present with a relapse onset syndrome) and in the diagnostic criteria for patients with a slowly progressive syndrome.

Although some of the revisions are logical and expected, ambiguities and uncertainties remain:

- Why does the interval for fulfilling MRI dissemination in time differ for a new T_2 lesion (> 30 days) and a gadolinium-enhancing lesion (≥ 3 months)?
- Will the waiver on requiring cerebrospinal fluid abnormalities open the way for more diagnostic errors in patients with progressive myelopathy?
- Why does a gadolinium-enhancing lesion retain its place within the criteria for dissemination in space when in fact it is a measure of lesion activity, not location?
- Can MRI dissemination in space criteria be further simplified when dissemination in time is also unequivocally present?

With regard to the last question, recent experience in one of our centres – where a cohort of patients with clinically isolated syndromes consisting predominantly of isolated optic neuritis has been systematically followed up – suggests that such an approach does indeed improve the sensitivity of an early diagnosis of multiple sclerosis whilst retaining high specificity (Swanton *et al* 2005; Table 7.6).

The reader is advised to review and adopt the amended criteria of the 2005 International Panel (Polman *et al* 2005b). We expect there to be further revisions in the years ahead. The competent neurologist with an interest in demyelinating disease will know the importance of keeping abreast of such developments and will always be aware that the highest levels of accuracy in diagnosis continue to rely on clinical thoroughness and expertise combined with a well informed application and interpretation of the available investigative techniques.

Table 7.5	**2005 International Panel revisions to the McDonald diagnostic criteria for multiple sclerosis**
MRI dissemination in space	Three out of four of the following: 1. one or more gadolinium enhancing lesions or nine or more T_2 lesions if there is no gadolinium enhancing lesion 2. one or more infratentorial lesions 3. one or more juxtacortical lesions 4. three or more periventricular lesions Note: (i) a spinal cord lesion can be considered equivalent to a brain infratentorial lesion; (ii) an enhancing spinal cord lesion is considered to be equivalent to an enhancing brain lesion; (iii) individual spinal cord lesions can contribute along with individual brain lesions to reach the required number of T_2 lesions
MRI dissemination in time	There are two ways to show dissemination in time using imaging: 1. the detection of gadolinium enhancement at least 3 months after onset of the initial clinical event, if not at the site corresponding to the initial event 2. detecting a *new* T_2 lesion if it appears at any time compared to a reference scan done at least 30 days after the onset of the initial clinical event

Diagnosis of multiple sclerosis in disease with progression from onset	1. One year of disease progression (retrospectively or prospectively determined)
	2. Together with two of the following three:
	  a. positive brain MRI (nine or more T_2 lesions or four or more T_2 lesions with abnormal visual evoked potentials
	  b. positive spinal cord MRI (two or more T_2 lesions)
	  c. positive cerebrospinal fluid (isoelectric focusing evidence of oligoclonal bands and/or elevated IgG index)

Adapted from Polman et al *(2005b)*

Table 7.6 Sensitivity, specificity and accuracy of the 2001 McDonald criteria and a set of modified criteria (as defined by Swanton *et al* 2005) after 3 months follow-up of patients with clinically isolated syndromes for conversion to clinically definite multiple sclerosis within 3 years

	True positive	False positive	True negative	False negative	Sensitivity	Specificity	Accuracy
McDonald criteria for multiple sclerosis: brain MRI only	18	3	48	21	46%	94%	73%
McDonald criteria for multiple sclerosis: brain and cord MRI	18	3	48	21	46%	94%	73%
Modified criteria for multiple sclerosis: brain MRI only	29	4	47	10	74%	92%	84%
Modified criteria for multiple sclerosis: brain and cord MRI	30	4	47	9	77%	92%	86%
McDonald criteria for disseminated in space: brain MRI only	30	11	40	9	77%	78%	78%
McDonald criteria for disseminated in space: brain and cord MRI	31	11	40	8	79%	78%	79%
Modified criteria for disseminated in space: brain MRI only	35	13	38	4	90%	75%	81%
Modified criteria for disseminated in space: brain and cord MRI	37	15	36	2	95%	71%	81%
McDonald criteria for disseminated in time	19	5	46	20	49%	90%	72%
Modified criteria for disseminated in time	30	6	45	9	77%	88%	83%

True positive = criteria positive and clinically definite multiple sclerosis.
Sensitivity = true positive/true positive + false negative.
False positive = criteria positive but not multiple sclerosis.
Specificity = true negative/true negative + false positive.
True negative = criteria negative but not multiple sclerosis.
Accuracy = true positive + true negative/true positive + false positive + true negative + false negative.
False negative = criteria negative but clinically definite multiple sclerosis.

McDonald criteria for disseminated in space: three out of the following four features:
 nine or more T_2 brain lesions or one or more gadolinium enhancing lesion
 one or more infratentorial lesion[+]
 one or more juxtacortical lesion
 three or more periventricular lesions

(One spinal cord lesion can substitute for one brain lesion).

Modified criteria for disseminated in space: one or more T_2 lesions(s) in two or more of the following regions:
 periventricular
 juxtacortical
 infratentorial[a]
 spinal cord.[b]

a, excluded in cases of brainstem syndrome; b, excluded in cases of spinal cord syndrome.

McDonald criteria for disseminated in time: one or more new gadolinium enhancing lesion.
Modified criteria for disseminated in time: one or more new T_2 lesion.

Adapted with permission from Swanton et al (2005).

The differential diagnosis of multiple sclerosis

8

David Miller and Alastair Compston

THE SPECTRUM OF DISORDERS MIMICKING MULTIPLE SCLEROSIS

Multiple sclerosis is the commonest demyelinating disease affecting the central nervous system of young adults living in the Western world. The diversity of symptoms and signs which may occur, and the unpredictable course, afford almost unlimited opportunities for misdiagnosis. That said, whilst there are very many disorders with which multiple sclerosis might be confused, these fall into several distinct categories in which the sources of error can be systematized.

The classification of demyelinating diseases (Table 8.1) is based on clinical features, pathological and imaging appearances, and aetiological considerations. The clinical suspicion of demyelination, as a pathological process, is high when a young adult develops one or more neurological episodes consistent with damage to white matter tracts within the central nervous system, especially when these affect the optic nerves, brainstem or spinal cord. However, more or less identical episodic symptoms are also caused by vascular or structural lesions, albeit less frequently. Although there are more likely explanations for intermittent neurological symptoms in children or the elderly, multiple sclerosis can affect people in these age groups. Demyelination is also suspected clinically when neurological syndromes indicating widespread involvement of the central nervous system follow within a few days or weeks of an infectious illness or vaccination (acute disseminated encephalomyelitis). Patients developing clinical evidence for extensive brainstem damage in the context of hyponatraemia, or more usually following its over zealous correction, may develop large confluent areas of pontine or extrapontine myelinolysis. In some young patients with progressive neurological disease, widespread demyelination results from genetically determined disorders of myelin formation (the leucodystrophies). Symptoms as a result of demyelination may also occur following direct viral infection of the central nervous system, especially in immunocompromised individuals. Thus, demyelinating disease may develop abruptly or slowly; unannounced or in the context of a precipitating event; early or late in life; as a sporadic condition; triggered by preceding infection or metabolic circumstances; and as part of a familial disorder.

Pathologically, a simple approach is to distinguish those disorders of myelination associated with perivascular inflammatory cell infiltration from the noninflammatory forms of demyelination (see Chapter 12). Inflammation initially characterizes the focal and multifocal lesions associated with demyelination occurring in optic neuritis, transverse myelitis, multiple sclerosis, Devic's disease, acute disseminated encephalomyelitis and the more specific syndromes that follow vaccination and exanthematous illnesses. Extensive noninflammatory confluent areas of demyelination are seen in the leucodystrophies, progressive multifocal leucoencephalopathy and central pontine myelinolysis. However, even within these two main subdivisions, important differences exist which suggest that several mechanisms of myelin injury contribute to the location, course, prognosis and extent of demyelination. Furthermore, the possibility of inflammation occurring secondary to tissue injury cannot be ignored (see Chapters 12 and 14).

Acute postinfectious encephalomyelitis, acute haemorrhagic leucoencephalitis (Hurst's disease), postvaccinial encephalomyelitis and some cases of subacute necrotizing myelitis, transverse myelitis and optic neuritis can legitimately be included within the syndromes of acute disseminated encephalomyelitis. Balo's concentric demyelination, Devic's disease, and Marburg type or mixed peripheral and central forms of demyelination are usually considered within the context of multiple sclerosis. The commonest forms of leucodystrophy encountered in clinical practice are metachromatic leucodystrophy, adrenoleucodystrophy and Krabbe's disease. The nosological status of Schilder's disease is increasingly insecure. As originally described, it probably included cases of leucodystrophy and subacute sclerosing panencephalitis. It is doubtful that Schilder's disease exists as a distinct disorder, either within or without the spectrum of multiple sclerosis. Accordingly, it is not discussed further here although we retain a brief description of the neuropathology in Chapter 12.

Brain imaging provides a further means of classifying demyelinating disease. Magnetic resonance imaging (MRI) studies show that isolated areas of demyelination actually occur rather infrequently. Thus, many patients with symptoms and signs attributable to a single anatomically placed lesion show multiple central nervous system abnormalities, typically affecting the periventricular white matter. To some extent, the characteristic imaging appearances of acute disseminated encephalomyelitis differ from those seen in multiple sclerosis, primary progressive inflammatory demyelination and the leucodystrophies. However, as pointed out in Chapter 7, these differences do not in themselves provide a reliable means for distinguishing the various conditions. Approaches to classification of the demyelinating diseases and the strategies for distinguishing the separate conditions recognized

Table 8.1 Classification of demyelinating disease

Isolated demyelinating syndromes
Acute haemorrhagic leucoencephalomyelitis – Hurst's disease
Acute disseminated encephalomyelitis
Optic neuritis
Cord lesions
    acute necrotizing myelitis
    transverse myelitis
    chronic progressive myelopathy
    radiation myelopathy
    HTLV-1 associated myelopathy
    monophasic isolated demyelination – site unspecified

Multiple sclerosis
    Relapsing–remitting
    Secondary progressive
    Primary progressive
    Benign
    Malignant or Marburg variant
    Childhood
    Silent multiple sclerosis
    Devic's disease
    Balo's concentric sclerosis
    Combined central and peripheral demyelination

Central pontine myelinolysis
Pontine
Extrapontine

Leucodystrophies
Adrenoleucodystrophy
    X-linked childhood adrenoleucodystrophy
    X-linked adult-onset adrenomyeloneuronopathy
    autosomal recessive neonatal adrenoleucodystrophy
    autosomal recessive Zellweger's syndrome
Metachromatic leucodystrophy
    late infantile
    juvenile
    adult onset
    multiple sulphatase deficiency
Krabbe's disease
    childhood onset
    late onset
Canavan's disease
Alexander's disease
Pelizaeus–Merbacher disease
    connatal form
    late onset
Vanishing white matter disease
Oculodentodigital syndrome

in clinical practice are somewhat merged in the accounts that follow.

From the clinical perspective, the importance of syndromes that can be attributed to focal demyelination (usually of the optic nerve, brainstem or spinal cord) lies in the fact that these are sometimes genuinely monophasic and do not recur or lead to widespread clinical manifestations. Other cases represent the inaugural episode of multiple sclerosis and many strategies have been developed for assessing the risk of conversion to multiple sclerosis following each type of episode, based on clinical features and laboratory (mainly imaging) investigations. These rates vary with the different syndromes, and ages at presentation. Self-evidently, they increase with duration of follow-up, although the number of new individuals developing recurrent demyelination

reduces with time. Since imaging studies have established that a high proportion of patients with clinically isolated demyelinating syndromes have anatomically disseminated lesions at presentation, laboratory markers provide one potential means for stratification and prediction of the long-term outcome. For this reason, particular importance is attached to the concept of temporal dispersion of lesions in the assessment of individual patients. Multiple sclerosis can reliably be diagnosed on clinical grounds only when more than one demyelinating episode, separated by at least 1 month and with clear evidence for recovery between attacks, has occurred and not merely on the basis of anatomically disseminated lesions. Even under these circumstances, many clinicians would reserve judgement until symptoms have been intermittently present for at least 6 months. However, imaging evidence for temporal dispersion following a clinically isolated episode is increasingly being accepted as an alternative way of securing the diagnosis of multiple sclerosis at an earlier stage and in advance of the second clinical event (W.I. McDonald *et al* 2001). The distinction between anatomical and temporal dissemination of lesions is clearly illustrated by the multifocal but monophasic nature of acute disseminated encephalomyelitis by comparison with multiple sclerosis.

With prudence, most potential diagnostic errors can be avoided, and only the more exacting problems need be considered here. Sources of diagnostic difficulty may conveniently be summarized as:

- diseases that may cause multiple lesions of the central nervous system and also often follow a relapsing–remitting course
- systematized diseases causing lesions in separate parts of the central nervous system but usually with symmetrical manifestations and a progressive course
- isolated or monosymptomatic central nervous system syndromes often suggesting a single white matter lesion
- nonorganic symptoms which mimic the clinical manifestations and course of multiple sclerosis.

DISEASES THAT MAY CAUSE MULTIPLE LESIONS OF THE CENTRAL NERVOUS SYSTEM AND ALSO OFTEN FOLLOW A RELAPSING–REMITTING COURSE

Diseases in which multiple lesions affect the central nervous system, and the illness follows a relapsing course, may appear to fulfil the strictest clinical and paraclinical diagnostic criteria, and so are easily confused with multiple sclerosis (Table 8.2). Modern techniques, including brain imaging, are helpful but not necessarily decisive in making the distinction from multiple sclerosis. The ambiguity may only be resolved if positive evidence for the specifically different condition becomes available – usually from laboratory or histological investigations.

Acute disseminated encephalomyelitis

In its classical form, acute disseminated encephalomyelitis is an illness of childhood that is of acute or subacute onset, in which an inflammatory and demyelinating process simultaneously affects multiple parts of the central nervous system, often

Table 8.2 **Diseases causing multiple lesions sometimes with a relapsing–remitting course**

Acute disseminated encephalomyelitis
    acute haemorrhagic encephalomyelitis
    post-vaccinial encephalomyelitis
Systemic lupus erythematosus
Anti-phospholipid antibody syndrome
Primary Sjögren's syndrome
Behçet's disease
Central nervous system vasculitis
    as part of a systemic vasculitis
    isolated central nervous system vasculitis
    systemic sclerosis
    Susac syndrome
Noninflammatory vascular disorders
    CADASIL
Sarcoidosis
Chronic infections
    Lyme disease
    meningovascular syphilis
    Human immunodeficiency virus (HIV) encephalitis
    progressive multifocal leucoencephalopathy
    subacute sclerosing panencephalitis
    Whipple's disease
Primary cerebral lymphoma
Mitochondrial disease

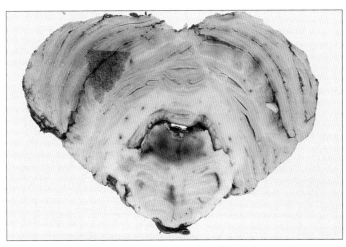

Figure 8.1 Macroscopic appearance of the brain in a patient aged 31 years who died from acute disseminated encephalomyelitis after an illness lasting 10 days; there is diffuse midbrain damage from a combination of demyelination and tentorial herniation as a result of cerebral oedema. Kindly provided by Dr Janice Anderson.

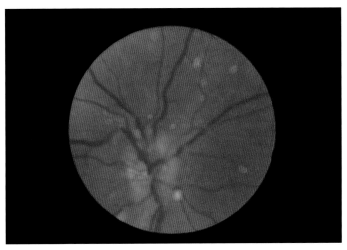

Figure 8.2 Optic disc appearance in a patient with acute optic neuritis associated with *Mycoplasma pneumoniae* infection.

shortly following an exanthematous or infectious illness Although an acute and fulminant presentation may be similar to acute (non-inflammatory) encephalopathy in children or young adults (Reye's syndrome), also occurring as part of several specific metabolic and infectious illnesses, the latter condition is distinguished by the presence of specific laboratory abnormalities, including hyperammonaemia, hepatic dysfunction and hypoglycaemia.

In acute disseminated encephalomyelitis, the cerebrum usually bears the brunt of the illness. Headache, fever and drowsiness sometimes progress to coma within a few days. Convulsions may occur, although these are seen in <20% of cases (Dale *et al* 2000; Hynson *et al* 2001). Focal neurological abnormalities typically include motor, sensory, visual and cognitive syndromes. These usually indicate multiple lesions of the brain but there may be associated brainstem involvement (Figure 8.1). Optic neuritis is common and often bilateral (Figure 8.2.). Occasionally, the peripheral nervous system is also involved. In other cases, the clinical picture is restricted to focal involvement of the brainstem, optic nerves or spinal cord – alone or in combination – and without much in the way of cerebral features. Patients with post-infectious focal inflammation of the central nervous system may be systemically ill with pyrexia and marked meningism. These features occur both in the encephalitic and myelitic forms of the disease. The cerebrospinal fluid shows a mixed polymorphonuclear and lymphocytic or predominantly mononuclear pleocytosis with raised protein and slight reduction in glucose. Oligoclonal bands are often present but, unlike multiple sclerosis, these may subsequently disappear (see below: Kesselring *et al* 1990).

The symptomatology, course and prognosis of acute disseminated encephalomyelitis in adults do not differ significantly from the classical post-exanthematous condition of childhood (McHugh and McMenamin 1987). Although a wider range of causative organisms has been implicated, the individual adult case more usually develops spontaneously or in the context of a non-specific respiratory infection. But even in children, a presumptive diagnosis of acute disseminated encephalomyelitis is often made in the absence of an identified provocative cause, especially in cases of acute cerebellar ataxia. Despite surviving the acute illness, patients may be left with persistent neurological deficits. The prognosis correlates inversely with the rate of onset of disability and overall severity. There is some evidence that outcome is influenced by the early use of high dose corticosteroids but this has not been formally evaluated. Fulminant cases of central nervous system inflammatory demyelination have been treated with plasma exchange (Bennetto *et al* 2004; Keegan *et al* 2002; 2005; Weinshenker *et al* 1999b), and with improvement reported in about 45%.

First described in 1790 (see Chapter 1), the classical accounts of acute disseminated encephalomyelitis and post-vaccinial encephalitis were written several decades ago (Miller and Evans

1953; Miller *et al* 1956). Several hundred cases were reviewed from personal experience or reports in the literature but no attempt was made to separate diffuse from anatomically restricted forms of para-infectious neurological disease, including polyradiculitis. Some cases were probably due to direct viral infection of the nervous system and related disorders that were not then recognized. The Newcastle experience indicated that about 1:1000 children with exanthematous disorders develop acute disseminated encephalomyelitis, the risk being slightly higher with pertussis and scarlet fever than with measles and rubella. The majority of those cases in these series were encephalopathic or multifocal. The encephalomyelitis that complicates rubella does not differ materially from the acute disseminated encephalomyelitis of measles except that it is less frequent and perhaps more severe. There is a late progressive variant, analogous to subacute sclerosing panencephalitis. Postvaricella infectious encephalomyelitis is often indistinguishable from other forms of the disorder but almost 50% of cases show a pure cerebellar syndrome sometimes associated with involuntary movements. This carries a relatively good prognosis with a low rate of persistent disability (Brumlik and Means 1969). Many other specific causes of acute disseminated encephalomyelitis have been described including a large number of bacterial and viral infections (Table 8.3). Toxic causes include injection of herbal extracts (Schwarz *et al* 2000), bee sting (Boz *et al* 2003) and anti-tetanus toxin (Hamidon and Raymond 2003). Prominent basal ganglia involvement, both clinically and with imaging, is often a feature in children with post-streptococcal acute disseminated encephalomyelitis and may be related to a

high frequency of anti-basal ganglia antibodies associated with this infection (Dale *et al* 2001).

Since an illness consistent with acute disseminated encephalomyelitis may later convert to multiple sclerosis, the natural history of childhood onset demyelinating disease has particular clinical poignancy. The natural wish is for a monophasic disorder and the initial preference is usually to diagnose acute disseminated encephalomyelitis. But the reality is that the monophasic nature of acute disseminated encephalomyelitis, defined in its typical form by the absence of subsequent relapse, can only be established with confidence after prolonged observation. Early judgement is invariably difficult. When acute disseminated encephalomyelitis clearly follows specific viral infection or innoculation, particularly in a child, the distinction from multiple sclerosis can be made with some confidence. There are no secure guidelines for distinguishing the encephalopathic presentation of multiple sclerosis from acute disseminated encephalomyelitis developing without preceding infection, especially in adults. Despite following what is essentially a monophasic course, separate sites may be involved sequentially in the acute phase giving the appearance of a temporally disseminated illness. Our position is that the clinical features of acute disseminated encephalomyelitis may evolve over a reasonably short period without it becoming necessary to change the diagnosis to that of multiple sclerosis. For this reason, we remain to be convinced by the claim for co-occurrence of acute disseminated encephalomyelitis and multiple sclerosis in two cases (Ravaglia *et al* 2004). Rather, we prefer the interpretation that these were the encephalitic and myelitic presentations of relapsing–remitting multiple sclerosis, respectively. The

Table 8.3 Infections associated with acute disseminated encephalomyelitis

Childhood exanthematous illnesses[a]	H.G. Miller and Evans 1953; H.G. Miller *et al* 1956; Brumlik and Means 1969
ECHO and coxsackievirus	Tyler *et al* 1986
Adenoviridae	Kesselring *et al* 1990
Herpes simplex 1	Kusuhara *et al* 2002; An *et al* 2002
Varicella zoster and human herpes virus-6	An *et al* 2002
Mycoplasma	Riedel *et al* 2001; Pfausler *et al* 2002
Borrelia burgdorferi	van Assen *et al* 2004
Campylobacter	Orr *et al* 2004
Pasteurella multocida	Proulx *et al* 2003
Plasmodium vivax	Koibuchi *et al* 2003
Streptococcus	Dale *et al* 2001
HIV	Narciso *et al* 2001
Rocky Mountain spotted fever	Wei and Baumann 1999
Influenza virus	Nakamura *et al* 2003
Parainfluenza virus	Au *et al* 2002; Voudris *et al* 2002
Puumala virus	Toivanen *et al* 2002
Hepatitis C virus	Sacconi *et al* 2001
Hepatitis A virus	Alehan *et al* 2004; H. Tan *et al* 2004
Coronavirus	Yeh *et al* 2004

a Including measles, rubella and varicella.

relationship of acute disseminated encephalomyelitis to clinically isolated demyelinating lesions – bilateral optic neuritis and acute transverse myelitis in children and adults, or cerebellar ataxia following childhood varicella – is particularly ambiguous (Tselis and Lisak 1995).

The use of paraclinical investigations often does not resolve the distinction between acute disseminated encephalomyelitis and multiple sclerosis (Dale *et al* 2000; Hahn *et al* 2004; Hartung and Grossman 2001; Hynson *et al* 2001). The recent literature focuses on the role of MRI but this investigation is also not decisive. Although extensive multifocal white matter and grey matter lesions are characteristic of acute disseminated encephalomyelitis (Figure 8.3), the appearances may be indistinguishable from those seen in multiple sclerosis and occasionally MRI can be normal even when the patient presents in an obtunded state (Hollinger *et al* 2002; Murray *et al* 2000). It has been proposed that an abnormal electroencephalogram can aid the diagnosis when the MRI findings are unhelpful (Hollinger *et al* 2002). Kesselring *et al* (1990) studied six adults and six children, developing optic nerve, cerebral, brainstem and cord disease, alone or in combination, following infection by mumps, varicella, *Mycoplasma*, adenovirus and non-specific respiratory infections. Clinical features alone were unhelpful. Oligoclonal bands were found to be transiently present in acute disseminated encephalomyelitis, a finding that contrasts with their persistence in multiple sclerosis. Although multifocal asymmetric white matter abnormalities were not discriminating, some cases of generalized and clinically isolated post-infectious demyelinating syndromes showed extensive and rather symmetric changes in the cerebral or cerebellar white matter and in the basal ganglia (Figure 8.4). Many lesions show gadolinium enhancement in the acute phase (Singh *et al* 1999). This may be homogeneous or ring shaped (Lim *et al* 2003), with individual lesions exhibiting a mixture of enhancing and non-enhancing properties (Tenembaum *et al* 2002) or no enhancement at all (Hynson *et al* 2001). Rarely, the lesions of acute disseminated encephalomyelitis appear cystic on MRI, thus mimicking brain abscess (de Recondo and Guichard 1997; Go and Imai 2000;

Lim *et al* 2003), but large ring enhancing lesions with a cyst-like appearance can also occur in multiple sclerosis. In short, the pattern is not distinguishable with certainty from multiple sclerosis on a single scan.

Rather more useful is the information provided by serial or gadolinium-DTPA (diethylenetriamine pentetic acid) enhanced scans. These suggest that, whereas lesions persisting on T₂-weighted images long after the clinical manifestations have resolved do not provide useful information, the development of new T₂ lesions or the demonstration of new areas with gadolinium enhancement indicates ongoing disease activity typical of multiple sclerosis (Brex *et al* 2001a). If a sufficient follow up interval – probably at least 3 months – has elapsed, the occurrence of new gadolinium enhancing lesions excludes the diagnosis of acute monophasic demyelination (Brex *et al* 2001a; McDonald *et al* 2001). O'Riordan *et al* (1999) showed that only 1/11 patients with acute disseminated encephalomyelitis patients followed up for 8 years exhibited new lesions. This individual was aged 52 years at follow-up and the small cerebral white matter lesion observed might have been due to small vessel disease. There was also a striking tendency for resolution of the T₂ lesions originally detected following the acute monophasic disease: the resolution was partial in seven cases and complete in three (Figure 8.4). In three other examples of monophasic central nervous system demyelination in childhood presenting as hemiparesis (which seem most likely to be cases of acute disseminated encephalomyelitis), the cerebral lesions were extensive and exhibited mass effect during the acute phase but subsequently displayed marked resolution with follow up (Yapici and Eraksoy 2002).

How long to wait before concluding that the diagnosis is one of monophasic demyelination is difficult to establish. The 6 months suggested by Kesselring *et al* (1990) in children may be adequate for purposes of definition but the interval before relapse after an initial attack of multiple sclerosis is clearly often much longer. It has been suggested that new episodes of central nervous system damage may occur 18 months after the initial episode in acute disseminated encephalomyelitis but this freedom

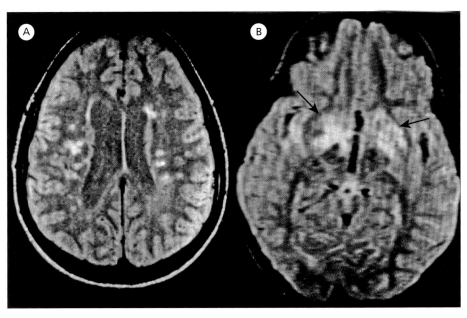

Figure 8.3 Acute disseminated encephalomyelitis. T₂-weighted brain MRI reveals (A) multifocal white matter and (B) grey matter lesions. From Confavreux and Vukusic (2002). © 2002, reproduced with permission of Lippincott Williams & Wilkins (lww.com).

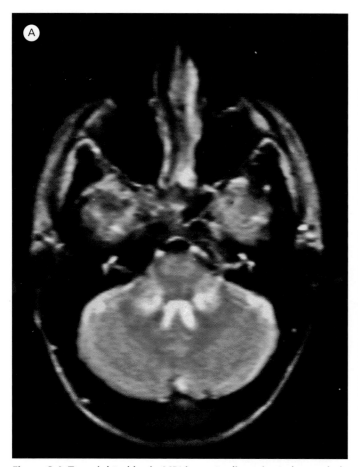
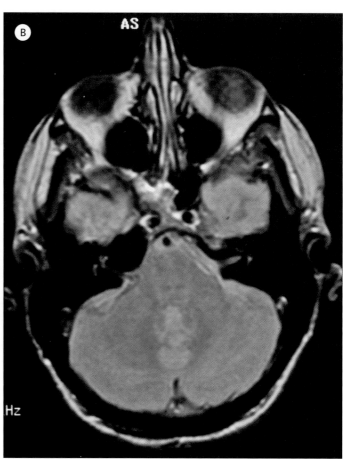

Figure 8.4 T$_2$-weighted brain MRI in acute disseminated encephalomyelitis. (A) The rather symmetrical appearances characteristic of the acute phase. (B) Marked resolution 10 years later.

of interpretation depends on the erroneous assumption that multiple sclerosis does not occur in childhood, and cases of this type would not now be included in a series of patients with acute disseminated encephalomyelitis. The matter is further complicated by the proposal that a syndrome of multiphasic disseminated encephalomyelitis occurs both in childhood (Dale *et al* 2000; Dale *et al* 2000) and in adults (Khan *et al* 1995).

The situation may nevertheless be clearer in children where the *a priori* expectation of multiple sclerosis as the eventual explanation for a first episode of demyelination is lower. Dale *et al* (2000) described 48 children in whom the diagnosis of central nervous system inflammatory demyelination was made through a tertiary referral centre. Of these, 28 were classified as having acute monophasic disseminated encephalomyelitis, 13 had multiple sclerosis and seven were considered to have multiphasic disseminated encephalomyelitis. By comparison with multiple sclerosis, cases of acute disseminated encephalomyelitis showed younger age at onset; a higher likelihood of preceding infection (74% vs. 38%); a greater frequency of encephalopathy (69% vs. 15%), pyramidal tract signs (71% vs. 23%) and poly-symptomatic features at presentation (91% vs. 38%); a greater likelihood of blood leucocytosis (64% vs. 22%) and cerebrospinal fluid pleocytosis (64% vs. 42%); a lower frequency of cerebrospinal fluid oligoclonal bands (29% vs. 64%) and MRI periventricular white matter lesions (44% vs. 92%; Figure 8.5) and more basal ganglia lesions (28% vs. 8%). On follow-up MRI, there was partial or complete resolution of lesions in 90% with acute disseminated encephalomyelitis and no new abnormalities were seen. Whereas partial lesion resolution was also seen in those with multiple sclerosis, all of the latter subjects displayed new lesions at follow-up. Although only 23% of subjects in both groups had optic neuritis, this was always bilateral in cases of acute disseminated encephalomyelitis, and unilateral in multiple sclerosis. The seven cases of multiphasic encephalomyelitis normally had only a single relapse. This occurred within a few months of the original episode and often while treatment with corticosteroids was being electively withdrawn.

A retrospective report on 31 children diagnosed with acute disseminated encephalomyelitis reported a high frequency of prodromal illness (71%) with an impaired conscious state (68%) and ataxia (65%) at presentation. There was a low frequency of cerebrospinal fluid oligoclonal bands (3%) and, although MRI white matter lesions were seen in 90%, there was less frequent periventricular and callosal involvement (both 29%; Hynson *et al* 2001). Grey matter lesions were seen in 61%, including the basal ganglia in 39% and thalamus in 32%. It is notable that gadolinium enhancing lesions were seen in only 29% of children in this study. This rather challenges the notion that enhancement is the rule for acute inflammatory/demyelinating central nervous system lesions. Four children had relapses – in two cases within weeks of the original episode and 2 years after the initial event in the others.

Another recent study reported on 84 children with a diagnosis of acute disseminated encephalomyelitis who were followed for a mean of 6.6 years (Tenembaum *et al* 2002). There was a

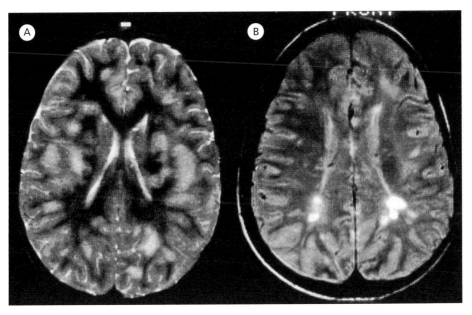

Figure 8.5 T$_2$-weighted brain MRI.
(A) Acute disseminated encephalomyelitis.
(B) Multiple sclerosis. In the former there
are more discrete cerebral white matter
lesions whereas periventricular
abnormalities predominate in the latter.
From Dale *et al* (2000) with permission.

preceding viral illness or vaccination in 74%. The most common presenting features were acute hemiparesis (76%), unilateral or bilateral long tract signs (84%), and mental changes (69%). None of 54 children who had cerebrospinal fluid examination exhibited oligoclonal bands. Brain MRI revealed multifocal grey and white matter lesions, of varying size, in 86% of cases. These were sometimes large and with a mass effect. The thalamus was involved bilaterally in 12%. In two cases (2%), some lesions were haemorrhagic. Of the 27 who had gadolinium enhanced scans, 30% showed open ring enhancing lesions, and in two cases these was a mixture of enhancing and non-enhancing lesions. Follow-up revealed a generally good prognosis with 89% having minimal or no disability (EDSS 0–2.5). MRI revealed marked resolution of abnormalities and no evidence for new lesions. Ten children experienced a single relapse at a median of 2 years after the initial attack. However, MRI did not reveal new lesions at the time of these relapses, nor did the cerebrospinal fluid contain oligoclonal bands. The authors called these cases biphasic disseminated encephalomyelitis.

In a further series of 18 children with a diagnosis of acute disseminated encephalomyelitis (Gupte *et al* 2003), the most common presentations were ataxia (10 cases), headache (8) and weakness (5). MRI lesions were seen in white and grey matter. The cerebrospinal fluid contained oligoclonal bands in only 4/13 (31%). Most children recovered although five had residual deficits. Two had a relapse, on both occasions within weeks of the original episode and shortly after discontinuation of steroid treatment. The authors suggest that the term multiphasic disseminated encephalomyelitis should only be used if there has been a single relapse following close after cessation of steroid treatment for the first attack. Another recent series of 18 children with a diagnosis of acute disseminated encephalomyelitis reported a high frequency of preceding upper respiratory tract illness (72%), onset in winter or spring (88%), motor deficits (77%), asymmetrical cortical grey matter lesions (80%), and subcortical white matter lesions (93%; Murthy *et al* 2002). A large series of children with acute disseminated encephalomyelitis following rubella and varicella has recently been reported from

Moscow (Idrissova *et al* 2003). Cases complicating rubella had an explosive onset with seizures, coma and moderate pyramidal tract signs, whereas those following varicella were characterized by cerebellar ataxia and mild pyramidal dysfunction.

Brass and colleagues (2003) also reported that a number of clinical and MRI features helped to distinguish the acute disseminated encephalomyelitis from multiple sclerosis in childhood. They compared seven children diagnosed with acute disseminated encephalomyelitis (mean age 8.7 years) with 17 diagnosed as multiple sclerosis (mean age 12.4 years) and found the following differences: fever (43% vs. 6%), headache (57% vs. 24%), fatigue (71% vs. 29%), vomiting (57% vs. 0%), encephalopathy (71% vs. 6%), corpus callosum lesions (17% vs. 64%) and periventricular lesions (50% vs. 91%).

The results of a large study organized by the French Neuropaediatric Society and involving 296 children <16 years having a first neurological episode consistent with inflammatory demyelination of the central nervous system between January 1985 and December 2001 has recently challenged this idea (Mikaeloff *et al* 2004a; 2004b). An initial diagnosis suggestive of acute disseminated encephalomyelitis was made in 119 (40%) cases, multiple sclerosis in 96 (33%) and a monofocal episode in 81 (27%). During a median follow-up of 1.9 years, 72/200 (36%) individuals with isolated demyelination at presentation had a second neurological episode qualifying them for the diagnosis of multiple sclerosis: 34/119 (29%) cases initially diagnosed as acute disseminated encephalomyelitis and 38/81 (47%) classified as having an isolated and monofocal episode. Median time from disease onset to the second neurological episode, as estimated by the Kaplan Meier technique, was 1.9 years. It was 6 years for the patients with an onset ≤10 years, and 1 year for those with onset at >10 years. Therefore, the final diagnosis was multiple sclerosis in 168 cases (57%), monophasic acute disseminated encephalomyelitis in 85 individuals (29%), and single monofocal episode in 43 patients (14%). Among the 168 children with multiple sclerosis, median age at onset was 13.1 years and the sex ratio 2.1 F:M. Age at onset in the 85 children finally classified as having acute disseminated encephalomyelitis was 6.4 years and the sex ratio 0.8 F:M. Even with a relatively short period of follow-up, the results of this representative study suggest that multiple sclerosis appears to be more frequent than acute disseminated encephalomyelitis, and half of the cases initially considered to have monophasic demyelination do in fact experience a second neurological episode within 2 years. Monophasic acute disseminated encephalomyelitis occurs predominantly before the age of 10 and in males, whereas multiple sclerosis predominantly develops later and in females. However, these statistics do not help in making a more accurate prognostic evaluation in the individual, at presentation.

Can consensus be reached on whether acute disseminated encephalomyelitis is a disease entity quite distinct from multiple sclerosis, as opposed to a spectrum of syndromes with overlapping transitional cases? Although the pathological hallmark of the former condition is considered to be multifocal lesions of a similar age that exhibit perivenous inflammation with adjacent demyelination and oedema, Lumsden (1970) could find no meaningful pathological distinction between the two conditions. Bauer and Hanefeld (1993) cited cases of relapsing disease following viral or vaccinial encephalomyelitis (see below), arguing against a rigid subdivision. A child who sustained three separate attacks of unilateral optic neuritis in the 3 years following acute disseminated encephalomyelitis induced by influenza vaccine remained symptom free >15 years after the last attack (Matthews 1991). In a recent editorial, Hartung and Grossman (2001), reviewing several recently published series, suggested that acute disseminated encephalomyelitis and multiple sclerosis fall within a common spectrum of inflammatory demyelinating diseases. However, efforts to make this distinction have sometimes foundered through allowing too liberal criteria for acute disseminated encephalomyelitis that include a number of the isolated clinical syndromes typically associated with conversion to multiple sclerosis in young adults. Not surprisingly, when such criteria have been employed many patients have subsequently been re-classified as having multiple sclerosis once further manifestations of demyelination are observed (Schwarz *et al* 2001). The situation is even more problematic when criteria are proposed for distinguishing multiphasic disseminated encephalomyelitis from multiple sclerosis. It has been suggested that relapses involve the same location in the further episodes of acute disseminated encephalomyelitis (Cohen *et al* 2001) but those familiar with multiple sclerosis will recognize that relapses manifesting as recurrence of previously experienced symptoms are not uncommon.

Our view is that monophasic acute disseminated encephalomyelitis exists as an entity separate from multiple sclerosis, although it is only rarely encountered beyond childhood. We recognize that, although there is a combination of clinical and radiological features that favour the diagnosis of acute disseminated encephalomyelitis over multiple sclerosis (Table 8.4), no single manifestation is completely specific. We do not recognize an entity of multiphasic disseminated encephalomyelitis that is distinguishable from multiple sclerosis in adults. When this has been suggested as the diagnosis, there have usually been atypical features for multiple sclerosis (such as encephalopathy or tumour-like lesions on MRI), and we take the view that unusual presentations of a common disease are a more likely explanation than another condition of doubtful nosological status.

Table 8.4 **Features of a monophasic illness that are more characteristic of acute disseminated encephalomyelitis than multiple sclerosis**[a]
Childhood age of onset (especially younger children)
Prodromal infection or vaccination
Polysymptomatic presentation
Impaired consciousness
Pyramidal tract features
Ataxia
Bilateral simultaneous optic neuritis.
Complete transverse myelitis
Raised cerebrospinal fluid lymphocyte count (>50/mm^3)
Low frequency and impersistence of cerebrospinal fluid oligoclonal bands
High frequency of MRI grey matter lesions (cortex and basal ganglia)
Extensive white matter lesions (subcortical > periventricular)
Frequent gadolinium enhancement of lesions in acute phase
Mass effect of lesions on MRI
Marked resolution of new lesions at follow-up
No new lesions at follow-up
No relapses at follow-up (occasionally one during first few weeks)
a No single feature is pathognomonic of acute disseminated encephalomyelitis and on occasions may be seen in multiple sclerosis.

Acute haemorrhagic encephalomyelitis

The hyperacute form of acute disseminated encephalomyelitis (Hurst's disease) is usually preceded by a nonspecific respiratory infection about 10 days before the onset of neurological symptoms. In some cases, there are no prodromal complaints. Young adult males are most commonly affected, complaining initially of headache or dizziness and progressing over hours through stages of disorientation, confusion and drowsiness to coma (Hurst 1941). The rate of progress is such that events usually overtake the detection of focal signs and this form of the disease is frequently fatal, although affected individuals may remain in a persistent vegetative state for several weeks, and some survive with severe disability following treatments which reduce intracranial pressure (C-C. Huang *et al* 1988). The combination of pyrexia and a marked cerebrospinal fluid pleocytosis with a predominantly neutrophil response mimics pyogenic infection of the central nervous system but the course is not influenced by antimicrobial treatment. Pathologically, the disorder is characterized by fibrinoid necrosis and inflammatory infiltration of vessels, oedema, perivenular petechial haemorrhage and macrophage infiltration around vessels in both grey and white matter but without demyelination (Figure 8.6; Hart and Earle 1975; Russell 1955; see Chapter 12). In some cases, the clinical and pathological features of acute haemorrhagic leucoencephalitis are focal, suggesting a rapidly growing tumour or herpes simplex encephalitis. These transitional forms are important in establishing that Hurst's disease is part of the spectrum of acute disseminated encephalomyelitis and they provide evidence for the sequence of events involved in the pathogenesis of multifocal demyelination of the human nervous system. The widespread use of MRI has also revealed that a small percentage of cases with otherwise typical acute disseminated encephalomyelitis exhibit haemorrhagic lesions (Dale *et al* 2000; Tenembaum *et al* 2002).

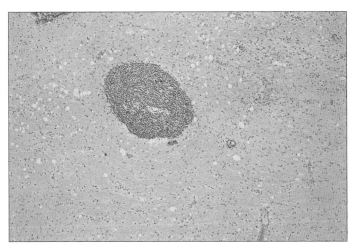

Figure 8.6 Acute perivascular infiltration in the same patient as in Figure 8.1. Haematoxylin and eosin; magnification ×30. Kindly provided by Dr Janice Anderson.

Postvaccinial encephalomyelitis

Postvaccinial encephalomyelitis has become a rare disorder (Fenichel 1982) and the definitive series was collected several decades ago following the need to vaccinate large numbers of individuals against smallpox as part of public health measures. The 62 cases studied clinically and pathologically by de Vries (1960) were collected over 34 years and were necessarily severe. In all, the neurological illness developed within 21 days after vaccination and, where fatal, death occurred at or soon after 13 days. In these hyperacute cases, the pathological findings resemble transitional forms of acute haemorrhagic or disseminated encephalomyelitis and the general principle that demyelination occurs secondary to blood–brain barrier permeability is again borne out. The clinical illness starts with a vaccinial skin reaction and systemic symptoms which merge with the neurological manifestations, typically affecting the cerebrum but sometimes presenting as a myelitic disorder. One of us (DHM) has observed Devic's disease following smallpox vaccination. Despite having a high mortality, subjects with postvaccinial encephalomyelitis may recover spontaneously and completely. It was thought that the risk had gone with the global eradication of smallpox infection and consequent cessation of vaccination programmes. However, a vaccination programme has been reintroduced recently for certain groups in view of concerns about global bioterrorism, raising the possibility that there may be further cases, although they can be largely prevented by administering antivaccinia gammaglobulin at the time of vaccination (Miraville and Roos 2003). It is to be hoped that the series reported from south Wales following the vaccination of 800 000 individuals at risk will never be repeated. Eleven patients developed generalized or restricted forms of encephalomyelitis and several other postinfectious manifestations of neurological disease, affecting either the central or peripheral nervous systems (Spillane and Wells 1964).

One reason for believing that acute disseminated encephalomyelitis arises from immune sensitization to brain antigens is that it may follow the use of rabies vaccine containing central nervous system tissue (Uchimura and Shiraki 1957). This form of the disease behaves much like other cases of acute dissemi-

nated encephalomyelitis and the pathological features are also indistinguishable. However, cases have not been seen since the method for preparing this and other vaccines was altered.

Systemic lupus erythematosus

Although the nervous system is involved in a high proportion of individuals with systemic lupus erythematosus, diagnostic confusion does not arise in the great majority either because there is obvious evidence for systemic disease or the neurological symptoms are unlike those commonly encountered in multiple sclerosis (J.T. Sibley *et al* 1992). The diagnosis of systemic lupus erythematosus should take account of established diagnostic criteria (Table 8.5; Hochberg 1997; E.M. Tan *et al* 1982). A standard nomenclature system for neuropsychiatric involvement has also been developed, but this was more to aid accuracy in clinical research rather than to replace clinical judgement in diagnosing individual patients (Table 8.6; ACR Ad Hoc Committee on Neuropsychiatric Lupus Nomenclature 1999). In a recent report, the most common neuropsychiatric manifestations amongst 128 unselected patients with lupus were neuropsychological impairment (80%, most often mild), headache (57%), depressive mood disorder (47%), poly- or mononeuropathy (30%), anxiety (24%) and seizures (16%; Brey *et al* 2002).

Disseminated relapsing–remitting disease, with symptoms indistinguishable from those of multiple sclerosis, has occasionally been reported (M. Hutchinson and Bresnihan 1983) – a substantial and persistent elevation in erythrocyte sedimentation rate or acute phase protein concentration providing an initial clue to the correct diagnosis.

The presentations most likely to be confused with multiple sclerosis are the various combinations of optic neuritis and myelopathy. Optic neuritis, which is not recognizably different from that seen in multiple sclerosis, may be the initial symptom (Schwartzberg *et al* 1981). Optic neuropathy in systemic lupus erythematosus may, however, take different forms – acute retrobulbar neuritis, ischaemic neuropathy or progressive visual failure (Jabs *et al* 1986). Symptoms of spinal cord disease may be slowly progressive (Fulford *et al* 1972; Provencale and

Table 8.5 **American College of Rheumatology revised criteria for the classification of systemic lupus erythematosus 1982[a] with updating 1997[b]**

Malar rash
Discoid rash
Photosensitivity
Oral ulcers
Arthritis
Serositis
Renal disorder
Neurological disorder
Haematological disorder
Immunological disorder:
    anti-DNA: antibody to native DNA in abnormal titre *or*
    anti-Sm: presence of antibody to Sm nuclear antigen *or*
    positive finding of antiphospholipid antibodies[b]
Antinuclear antibody

A person is considered to have systemic lupus erythematosus if four or more of the 11 criteria are present. NB: this table is an abbreviated summary and the original publications should be referred to for further information. a E.M. Tan et al (1982); b Hochberg (1997).

Table 8.6 **Neuropsychiatric syndromes observed in systemic lupus erythematosus**[a]

Central nervous system

Aseptic meningitis
Cerebrovascular disease
Demyelinating syndrome
Headache (including migraine and benign intracranial
   hypertension)
Movement disorder (chorea)
Myelopathy
Seizure disorder
Acute confusional state
Anxiety disorder
Cognitive dysfunction
Mood disorder
Psychosis

Peripheral nervous system

Acute inflammatory demyelinating polyradiculoneuropathy
(Guillain–Barré syndrome)
Autonomic disorder
Mononeuropathy, single/multiplex
Myasthenia gravis
Neuropathy, cranial
Plexopathy
Polyneuropathy

a From ACR Ad Hoc Committee on Neuropsychiatric Lupus Nomenclature (1999).

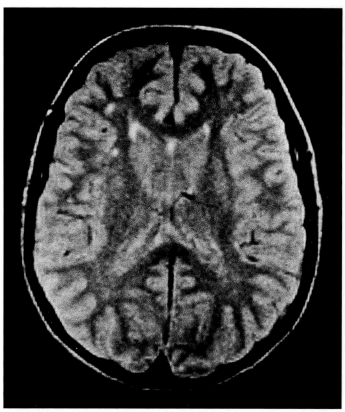

Figure 8.7 T$_2$-weighted image in systemic lupus erythematosus showing the predominantly peripheral distribution of the focal lesions.

Bouldin 1992), recurrent (Tola *et al* 1992; M.Yamamoto 1986) or, more commonly, acute or subacute (Barile and Lavalle 1992; Lavalle *et al* 1990). Optic neuritis can accompany acute transverse myelitis (S. Oppenheimer and Hoffbrand 1986; Simeon-Aznar *et al* 1992) or precede the onset of paraparesis and ataxia (Tola *et al* 1992). Such presentations are inevitably suggestive of Devic's disease or multiple sclerosis, and the results of diagnostic tests do not always reliably allow these distinctions to be made.

Internuclear ophthalmoplegia, even as an initial sign (Cogan *et al* 1987; Hammondeh and Kahn 1982; Jackson *et al* 1986), and unilateral tonic spasms (M. Hutchinson and Bresnihan 1983), both characteristic features of multiple sclerosis, have been described in systemic lupus erythematosus.

When the central nervous system is involved in systemic lupus erythematosus, the cerebrospinal fluid has been found to contain oligoclonal immunoglobulin G (IgG) in 42% of cases (Winfield *et al* 1983). Routine examination of the cerebrospinal fluid occasionally shows levels of total protein and cell counts that are outside the ranges expected in multiple sclerosis (Provencale and Bouldin 1992). However, these distinctions are not necessarily reliable and brain MRI can also show discrete and periventricular white matter lesions, not immediately distinguishable from those of multiple sclerosis (Figure 8.7; Ormerod *et al* 1987). One clue to a vascular rather than demyelinating aetiology is a predominance of subcortical and white matter lesions that extend beyond the periventricular region. Small cortical T$_2$ hyperintensities or foci of cortical atrophy may indicate previous small areas of infarction (D.H. Miller *et al* 1987b). When larger vessels are involved, the areas of abnormal signal conform to the classical territories of arterial distribution (Figure 8.8). Abnormalities are reported using MR spectroscopy and single photon emission computed tomography (SPECT) as the basis for

studies of brain metabolites and perfusion, respectively, in patients with a clinical diagnosis of neuropsychiatric lupus – sometimes even in the absence of visible MRI abnormalities (Handa *et al* 2003).

In cases with acute transverse myelitis, swelling of the cord may extend over many segments in association with increased signal on T$_2$-weighted MRI and gadolinium enhancement (Figure 8.9; D.H. Miller *et al* 1992b). Such extensive cord lesions are rarely seen in multiple sclerosis. Visual evoked potentials may be delayed (Jabs *et al* 1986). Serological tests for systemic lupus are also not wholly discriminating and antinuclear factor – usually but not invariably in a low titre – has been found in approximately 30% of people with multiple sclerosis (Barned *et al* 1995; Dore-Duffy *et al* 1982). In a prospective survey, 22% patients with multiple sclerosis had circulating anti-nuclear autoantibodies, usually in the range of titres 1 : 80 to 1 : 160 (Collard *et al* 1997). These were undetectable in cerebrospinal fluid and had no systemic clinical associations. Concomitant drug treatment might have induced autoantibody production in some patients. Most consider that the occasional presence of autoantibodies in patients with multiple sclerosis is an epiphenomenon indicative of an underlying autoimmune process rather than being directly involved in the pathogenesis (de Andres *et al* 2001). Transverse myelitis in systemic lupus is, however, strongly associated with anti-phospholipid antibodies (Lavalle *et al* 1990; J.H. Kim *et al* 2003).

While transverse myelitis may be the presenting symptom of systemic lupus erythematosus, in the majority of reported cases the onset of neurological symptoms is preceded or accompanied

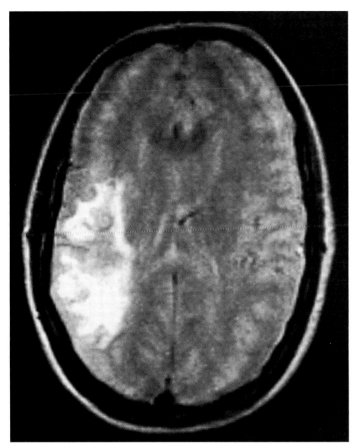

Figure 8.8 T$_2$-weighted image in systemic lupus erythematosus showing an extensive area of infarction.

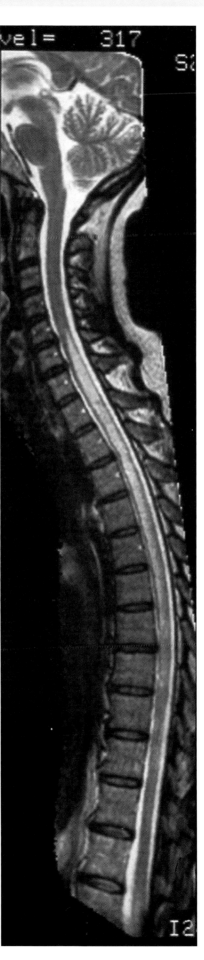

Figure 8.9 T$_2$-weighted image of the spinal cord in systemic lupus erythematosus showing diffuse high signal with swelling.

by evidence for systemic disease, even though this may only be recognized in retrospect (Andrianakos *et al* 1976). It is the concomitant systemic features that often prove crucial in establishing the diagnosis. That said, the distinction between systemic lupus erythematosus and multiple sclerosis sometimes remains in doubt. Pender and Chalk (1989) reported the combination of relapsing spinal cord disease and optic neuritis. The patient described by Devos *et al* (1984) and the three reported by Kinnunen *et al* (1993) almost certainly had both systemic lupus erythematosus and multiple sclerosis. A further intriguing suggestion of a relationship between the two diseases is the occurrence of multiple sclerosis in one identical twin and systemic lupus erythematosus, without nervous system involvement, in the other (F.F. Holmes *et al* 1967). A brother and sister had multiple sclerosis and the former had three children with systemic lupus erythematosus (Sloan *et al* 1987). A woman with multiple sclerosis is described whose mother had systemic lupus erythematosus (Hietaharju *et al* 2001).

Introduction of the term lupoid sclerosis (Fulford *et al* 1972) does not assist greatly in clarification, although any physician experienced in the management of demyelinating disease will recognize the convenience of that description for the patient with relapsing symptoms, at least some of which are unusual for multiple sclerosis, and in whom there is suggestive serological evidence for systemic lupus erythematosus. This combination may be sufficient to prompt the use of immunosuppressive treatments (such as oral cyclophosphamide) not used routinely in patients with conventional forms of multiple sclerosis.

Anti-phospholipid antibody syndrome

Although closely related to systemic lupus erythematosus – and indeed some patients with the latter condition manifest the same immunological abnormalties – there is an identifiable group of patients, usually with a multisystem clinical syndrome, in whom anti-phospholipid antibodies are thought to play a specific pathogenic role. Usually known as the primary anti-phospholipid syndrome, it has also recently become known in some circles as Hughes syndrome in deference to the physician who first reported this association (G.R.V. Hughes 1983). The most characteristic and classical clinical features reflect a disturbance of the blood coagulation system with an increased frequency of both venous and arterial thromboses. Young women are usually affected, presenting with deep vein thromboses, pulmonary embolism or recurrent spontaneous abortion. The most common neurological manifesations are migraine, often with aura, or transient ischaemic attacks affecting the carotid, vertebral or ophthalmic artery territories. The association with migraine may be coincidental, bearing in mind the high prevalence overall of the latter condition in the young adult population. Stroke as a result of cerebral infarction can occur, and is potentially the most significant neurological complication. The typical features are hemiplegia, hemianopia, dysphasia and a variety of posterior circulation syndromes. Movement disorders, especially chorea, are also relatively frequent. In general, presentation with acute neurological episodes suggestive of demyelination is uncommon. Ischaemic optic neuropathy may occur but the clinical features – optic disc swelling and altitudinal field defect with poor recovery – suggest a vascular rather than demyelinating mechanism. Transverse myelitis is reported and, as in cases of systemic lupus erythematosus, the syndrome is often severe with major sensorimotor deficits and limited neurological recovery. Rarely, multiple cerebral infarcts in the anti-phospholipid antibody syndrome can result in a relapsing clinical picture and MRI findings similar to those of multiple sclerosis (T.F. Scott *et al* 1994). B.J. Kelly *et al* (1989) described (unfortunately only in abstract), two patients with the anti-phospholipid syndrome manifesting as venous thromboses and spontaneous abortion who developed clinical features highly characteristic of multiple sclerosis – optic neuritis, transverse myelitis, Lhermitte's symptom, paroxysmal tonic spasms and internuclear ophthalmoplegia.

The diagnosis is based on a characteristic clinical syndrome in combination with typical laboratory abnormalities. Consensus efforts have been made to achieve a uniform set of criteria for achieving a firm diagnosis (Table 8.7; W.A. Wilson *et al* 1999). In some patients there is thrombocytopaenia. Anti-nuclear antibodies may be detectable, especially in patients with coexisting systemic lupus erythematosus, but their presence is not required to make the diagnosis. Disorders of clotting include prolongation of the partial thromboplastin time and the presence of lupus anticoagulant detected using the dilute Russell's viper venom time. The most specific serological association is the presence of a raised titre of anti-phospholipid antibodies directed against cardiolipin. In active disease, these will normally be markedly elevated. Both IgG and IgM antibodies are found and a sustained increase in the IgG form is suggestive of disease activity. Patients with neurological involvement may demonstrate abnormal imaging. Infarction is the basis for

Table 8.7 **Proposed preliminary criteria for the diagnosis of anti-phospholipid syndrome**[a]
Clinical criteria
Vascular thrombosis
One or more clinical episodes of arterial, venous or small vessel thrombosis in any tissue or organ, with confirmation by imaging, Doppler ultrasound or histopathology, except for superficial venous thrombosis.
Pregnancy morbidity
One or more unexplained deaths of a morphologically normal foetus at or beyond the tenth week of gestation
or
One or more premature births of a morphologically normal neonate at or before the 34th week of gestation because of severe pre-eclampsia, eclampsia or severe placental insufficiency
or
Three or more unexplained consecutive spontaneous abortions before the tenth week of gestation, with maternal anatomic and hormonal abnormalities and maternal and paternal chromosomal causes excluded.
Laboratory criteria
Anticardiolipin antibody titre of IgG and/or IgM isotype in blood, present in medium or high titre, on at least two occasions, at least 6 weeks apart
Lupus anticoagulant present in plasma, on at least two occasions at least 6 weeks apart, detected according to the guidelines of the International Society on Thrombosis and Hemostasis (J.T. Brandt *et al* 1995)
a In abbreviated form from W.A. Wilson et al (1999); one or more clinical and one laboratory criteria must be present for a patient to be considered as having definite anti-phospholipid syndrome.

cases of ischaemic stroke and can involve either the anterior or posterior circulation. Other patients display multiple and mainly small cerebral white matter lesions, predominantly in subcortical rather than periventricular regions. The low specificity of this imaging appearance must also be emphasized, especially with increasing age, where asymptomatic white matter lesions are a frequent manifestation of arteriosclerotic small vessel disease. Patients with acute transverse myelitis may exhibit extensive lesions involving multiple segments of the spinal cord and accompanied by swelling in the acute stage.

From the neurological perspective, the diagnosis is often considered but rarely made. There is potential for this disorder, which has a vascular prothrombotic pathogenic mechanism, to produce multifocal relapsing central nervous system involvement such that the diagnosis of multiple sclerosis is considered. A practical difficulty is that mild elevation in the IgG anti-cardiolipin antibody titre is occasionally found in the normal population (Tanne *et al* 1999). It has been suggested that the clinical phenotype in patients with demyelinating disease and anti-phospholipid antibodies selectively affects the optic nerves and spinal cord (Karussis *et al* 1998). In a sample derived from attendance at a rheumatology clinic, 23/26 patients with clinical features suggesting multiple sclerosis (especially transverse myelitis or optic neuritis) had anti-phospholipid antibodies compared with 166/296 of those without these neurological features (Ijdo *et al* 1999). Others have not found a correlation between anti-phospholipid antibodies and a distinct clinical phenotype in groups of patients with multiple sclerosis (Heinzlef *et al* 2002; Roussel *et al* 2000; Sastre-Garriga *et al* 2001). A firm conviction that the neurological syndrome is the result of anti-phospholipid syndrome requires robust clinical and laboratory evidence, and the exclusion beyond reasonable doubt of other potential neurological causes. The proposal that patients with multiple sclerosis should routinely be tested for anti-phospholipid antibodies (Cuadadro *et al* 2000) runs the risk of incorrectly reversing a definite clinical and laboratory diagnosis of multiple sclerosis on the basis of a modest elevation of anti-cardiolipin antibody titre. The abrupt onset and duration of the neurological deficits often suggest a vascular disorder resulting from transient ischaemia rather than demyelinating disease. Non-neurological features indicating a systemic thrombotic disorder, and the history of recurrent sponaneous abortions, should alert the physician to this potential diagnosis. The importance of making the correct diagnosis lies in the fact that, although not without its risks, anticoagulant treatment with warfarin reduces the future risk for stroke and other thrombotic events. When previous thrombotic events have occurred, it has been recommended that anticoagulation should aim to reach an International Normalized Ratio (INR) of 3–4 to obtain an optimal therapeutic effect and reduce the risk of further thromboses (G.R.V. Hughes 2003).

Primary Sjögren's syndrome

Sjögren's syndrome is a relatively common multisystem disorder, most often characterized by a triad of keratoconjunctivitis sicca, xerostomia and another connective tissue disease – usually rheumatoid arthritis. Classification criteria for the condition have been published recently (Table 8.8; Vitali *et al* 2002). It has previously been held that neurological complications are relatively rare. When they occur, they usually affect the peripheral nervous system or trigeminal nerve, often manifesting as sensory neuropathy or ganglionopathy, sometimes confined to the trigeminal territory. It is, however, noteworthy that severe myelopathic syndromes can also be encountered. From the histological perspective, the lesions of Sjögren's disease are not demyelinating but resemble those of paraneoplastic syndromes (Bakchine *et al* 1991). In 1986, however, E.L. Alexander *et al* (1986) re-emphasized earlier reports (Atwood and Poser 1961) that the clinical features of central nervous system involvement might mimic those of multiple sclerosis. They described 20 patients, all of whom had been regarded as having multiple scle-

rosis. In only four had Sicca syndrome been recognized before the onset of neurological symptoms. In the majority, the course was relapsing and remitting, including internuclear ophthalmoplegia and signs of spinal cord and cerebellar disease. Once the suspicion of an alternative diagnosis had been raised, confirmatory evidence was obtained from the obvious systemic abnormalities, involvement of the peripheral nervous system and detection of autoantibodies (anti-Ro and anti-La). Visual evoked potentials were frequently abnormal and oligoclonal IgG usually present in the cerebrospinal fluid. MRI showed small numbers of white matter lesions indistinguishable from those of multiple sclerosis in some patients (E.L. Alexander *et al* (1986). The resemblance to multiple sclerosis was heightened by clear descriptions of optic neuritis (Figure 8.10) as an early or initial symptom of Sjögren's syndrome (Wise and Angudelo 1988). Tesar *et al* (1992) described three patients with optic neuropathy, indistinguishable from optic neuritis, but in whom other neurological and systemic features eventually drew attention to the correct diagnosis. Other case reports emphasize the occurrence of transverse myelitis in Sjögren's syndrome (Manabe *et al* 2000; Wakatsuki *et al* 2000) and a recent study described nine female patients with a previous diagnosis of primary progressive multiple sclerosis in whom the combination of sicca complex symptoms and investigative findings fulfilled the criteria for Sjögren's syndrome (Pericot *et al* 2003).

These reports naturally give rise to concern that many patients thought to have multiple sclerosis are wrongly diagnosed. However, reassessment of large clinic series has, in general, been reassuring with no increase in the frequency of Sjögren's syndrome. Complaints of dry eyes and mouth are almost invariably attributable to medication (Metz *et al* 1988; Noseworthy *et al* 1989a; Sandberg-Wollheim *et al* 1992), although Miró *et al* (1990) revised the diagnosis of multiple sclerosis to Sjögren's syndrome in two of 64 patients on the basis of clinical suspicion and salivary gland biopsy.

Two recent series from a single centre slightly alter this perspective on the easy separation of Sjögren's syndrome from multiple sclerosis. De Séze *et al* (2001b) performed detailed laboratory investigations looking for evidence of Sjögren's

Table 8.8 **Classification criteria for Sjögren's syndrome[a]**
Ocular symptoms: 'dry eyes'
Oral symptoms: 'dry mouth'
Ocular signs: positive Schirmer's or Rose Bengal test.
Histopathology: focal lymphocytic sialoadenitis in minor salivary gland biopsy
Salivary gland involvement: based on unstimulated whole salivary flow or parotid sialography or salivary scintigraphy
Autoantibodies: to Ro (SSA) or La (SSB) antigens
Primary Sjögren's syndrome is defined by the presence *either* of any four of these six items including histopathology or autoantibodies *or* three of four objective (non-clinical) items
a In abbreviated form from Vitali et al *(2002).*

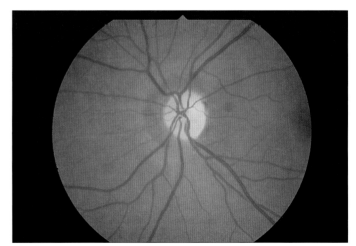

Figure 8.10 Optic disc appearance in a young female with recurrent optic neuritis and other manifestations of demyelination having anti-Ro autoantibodies, skin changes, and a positive family history of Sjögren's syndrome.

syndrome in 60 patients with a presumptive diagnosis of primary progressive multiple sclerosis. Their investigations included a Schirmer test, salivary gland scintigraphy, salivary gland biopsy and investigation for anti-Ro and anti-La antibodies. There was a remarkably high frequency of abnormalities for many of these investigations and, using previously proposed European diagnostic criteria (Vitali *et al* 1996), the authors diagnosed Sjögren's syndrome in ten (16.6%) patients. These findings are difficult to interpret, given that it is unusual to perform such extensive investigations in an older adult population – the mean age was about 50 years – and an age-matched control group was evidently not studied. Delalande *et al* (2004) subsequently reported 82 individuals with Sjögren's syndrome, selected for neurological involvement. Fifty-six of the 82 had disease of the central nervous system – affecting the spinal cord (29 cases), cerebrum (33 cases) or optic nerves (13 cases). Abnormalities of the visual evoked responses (61%) and the presence of oligoclonal bands (31%) were relatively frequent. Seventy per cent of the 58 cases who had MRI scans showed cerebral lesions and 40% met radiological criteria for multiple sclerosis; 75% of the 29 with symptomatic spinal cord disease had discrete cord lesions but MRI was normal in the absence of clinical evidence for spinal involvement. Reassuringly, despite these clinical similarities, most patients (51/82) also had involvement of the peripheral nervous system, and anti-Ro/SSA autoantibodies were detected (sometimes only with serial testing).

Taken together, it would seem that misdiagnosis is rare but that Sjögren's syndrome can occasionally cause relapsing–remitting disease of the central nervous system before onset of the classical sicca syndrome (Ménage *et al* 1993) although usually with simultaneous involvement of the peripheral nervous system. A previous lack of agreed diagnostic criteria for Sjögren's syndrome (Anon. 1992), the serum anti-Ro/La antibodies being neither constant nor specific (as is also true for the diagnostic criteria in multiple sclerosis), has not helped rational debate on this aspect of the differential diagnosis (P.M. Moore and Lisak 1990).

Behçet's disease

Involvement of the central nervous system in Behçet's disease has frequently been reported since the 1950s but, in the majority of cases, the clinical features do not closely resemble those of multiple sclerosis. The more usual manifestations are, for example, meningoencephalitis (O'Duffy and Goldstein 1976), progressive pseudobulbar palsy (Motomura *et al* 1980) or intracranial hypertension (Pamir *et al* 1981). There are rare instances of spinal cord disease, with progressive or partially remitting weakness and sensory change. Brainstem syndromes including ophthalmoplegia and cranial nerve palsies, accompanied by hemiplegia, are not infrequent. The large study by Siva *et al* (2001) – reporting from Turkey, where Behçet's disease is relatively common – provides a particularly useful indication of the frequency of various neurological manifestations. Of 164 patients in whom neurological abnormalities were present, features at presentation included: headache (61.6%), motor symptoms (53.7%), cerebellar symptoms apart from dysarthria (29.9%), brainstem symptoms other than dysarthria (29.3%), dysarthria (22.6%), behavioural symptoms (12.2%), sensory symptoms (11%), alteration of consciousness (7.3%), cognitive

symptoms (2.4%) and other symptoms (9.8%, including seizures, peripheral neuropathy and optic neuritis). The final diagnoses – after imaging and cerebrospinal fluid studies – were: a parenchymal syndrome (neuro-Behçet's disease, 75.6%), venous sinus thrombosis (12.2%), optic neuritis (0.6%), psycho-Behçet's syndrome (0.6%) and indefinite (11%).

The presentation with spinal cord or brainstem features may not be clinically distinguishable from multiple sclerosis (Shakir *et al* 1990). Paraplegia may be sudden in onset (Bergerin *et al* 1980). Optic neuropathy, either in isolation (Kansu *et al* 1989) or associated with disseminated symptoms (Bergerin *et al* 1980), is rare and probably the result of ischaemia. In acute attacks, fever, headache, meningism and a raised sedimentation rate and C-reactive protein are common (Chajek and Fainaru 1975). Motomura *et al* (1980) found that, in contrast to multiple sclerosis, Lhermitte's sign, internuclear ophthalmoplegia and tonic spasms do not occur.

Fifty patients with Behçet's disease who had attended the National Hospital in London over a 10-year period were discussed by D. Kidd *et al* (1999b). The most frequently observed neurological findings were brainstem syndromes, followed by spinal cord or hemisphere lesions, and meningoencephalitis. Optic nerve, vestibulo-cochlear and peripheral nerve involvement was less common. Over an average of 3 years' follow-up, most had only a single neurological episode and made a good recovery. The prognosis was less good in those with recurrent episodes (one-third) or a high cerebrospinal fluid pleocytosis at presentation. Four patients experienced progressive neurological deterioration.

Siva *et al* (2001) also studied prognosis in their large cohort with neurological manifestations. After 10 years, 45% had accumulated severe disability (Expanded Disability Status Scale >6), with early cerebellar features and progressive symptoms each predicting a poor prognosis. A better prognosis was seen in patients whose presentation was with headache or venous sinus thrombosis.

Investigations can be of value in distinguishing these conditions. In Behçet's disease, the cerebrospinal fluid may show a pleocytosis beyond the range seen in multiple sclerosis (Shakir *et al* 1990). Conversely, oligoclonal IgG is rarely present in Behçet's disease. In one study, although seven patients had matching bands in serum and cerebrospinal fluid, none of 35 had oligoclonal bands restricted only to the cerebrospinal fluid (D. Kidd *et al* 1999b). Disseminated white matter lesions are sometimes shown on cerebral MRI (Figure 8.11; Morrissey *et al* 1993b), although such changes are rarely extensive (D. Kidd *et al* 1999b). On the other hand, there may be striking involvement of the brainstem, thalamus and internal capsules (Figure 8.12; Akman-Demir *et al* 2003). Acute lesions in these regions may be large, and accompanied by swelling and gadolinium enhancement resembling the appearances of a tumour. Mass effect may be observed with slow enlargement over months followed by resolution following the use of corticosteroids (Erdem *et al* 1993a; Kermode *et al* 1989). Atrophy can develop later in previously affected regions (Figure 8.13; Akman-Demir *et al* 2003).

Since there is no specific test for Behçet's disease, the diagnosis has to be based on the association of aphthous oral ulceration with genital ulcers, intra-ocular inflammation or defined skin lesions (Table 8.9; International Study Group for Behçet's Disease 1990). A positive pathergy test – in which a small

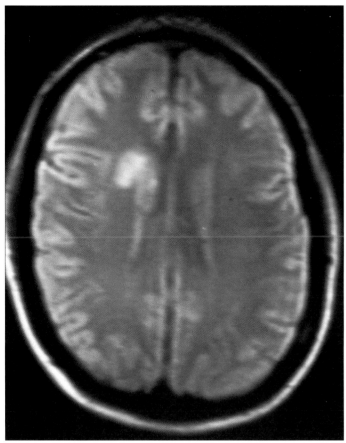

Figure 8.11 T$_2$-weighted MRI in Behçet's disease showing an area of high signal in periventricular white matter.

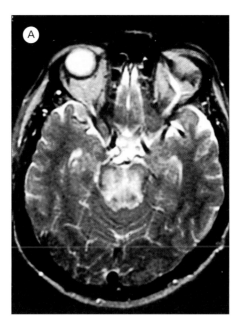

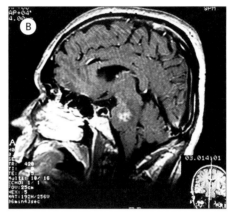

Figure 8.12 (A) T$_2$-weighted and (B) Gadolinium enhanced T$_1$-weighted MRI in Behçet's disease showing an extensive lesion of the brainstem. From D. Kidd *et al* (1999) with permission.

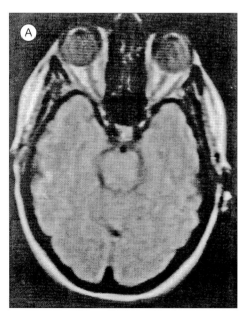

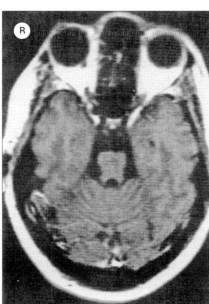

Figure 8.13 Behçet's disease. Serial MRI of an adult female with a brainstem syndrome. (A) T$_2$-weighted scan during the acute phase shows high signal and swelling of the midbrain. (B) T$_1$-weighted scan 5 years later shows midbrain atrophy. Reproduced with permission from D.H. Miller *et al* (1997).

Table 8.9 **Diagnostic criteria for Behçet's disease**[a]
Recurrent aphthous ulcers: on three or more occasions in any one year
and

Any two of the following features:
    genital ulceration
    intra-ocular inflammation: iritis, uveitis or retinal vasculitis
    skin lesions: erythema nodosum, papulo-pustules, folliculitis and acne (post adolescent and not on corticosteroids)
    positive pathergy test

a From International Study Group for Behçet's Disease (1990).

papule or pustule develops at the site of a sterile needle prick – provides additional support for the diagnosis in an appropriate clinical context, although it is neither completely specific nor sensitive. Neuro-Behçet's disease can, however, develop before the appearance of mucosal ulceration (Kozin *et al* 1977) or even in its absence (Lueck *et al* 1993).

Central nervous system vasculitis

Vasculitis can affect the central nervous system as part of a systemic disorder or as an isolated manifestation. Central nervous system involvement can be multifocal and multiphasic and the lesions are inflammatory in nature. There is potential for the clinical and laboratory manifestations of central nervous system vasculitis to overlap with those seen in multiple sclerosis, although it is uncommon that there is serious difficulty in making the distinction. Here, the differential diagnosis of vasculitis has to be considered.

Systemic vasculitis with central nervous system involvement

Involvement of the central nervous system by vasculitis occurs as part of a systemic vasculitic disorder or as an isolated condition. The former category includes polyarteritis nodosa, Churg–Strauss syndrome (in which there is eosinophilia and pulmonary involvement) and Wegener's granulomatosis (in which renal and pulmonary involvement are common). When it occurs, neurological involvement is most often, but not exclusively, confined to the peripheral nervous system: a rapidly evolving and progressive mononeuritis multiplex or symmetrical polyneuropathy is characteristic. Nevertheless, transient ischaemic episodes or strokes can occur in a multifocal pattern in patients with a systemic vasculitis. Oculomotor palsies or visual impairment are seen with the orbital involvement that not uncommonly occurs in Wegener's granulomatosis. Many patients with an active polyarteritis will be systemically unwell and will exhibit a raised erythrocyte sedimentation rate and the presence of anti-neutrophil cytoplasmic antibodies. Such a clinical picture, along with peripheral nerve and systemic non-neurological involvement, means that multiple sclerosis will rarely arise in the differential diagnosis of systemic arteritis. Prompt diagnosis is crucial because vigorous immunosuppression with pulsed corticosteroids and cyclophosphamide have a major beneficial effect in a group of disorders that previously had a high mortality rate.

Isolated central nervous system vasculitis

Isolated or primary central nervous system vasculitis is much more difficult to diagnose since the characteristic serological abnormalities that accompany systemic vasculitic disorders are typically absent. The illness usually evolves over months although more protracted courses spanning years, with fluctuating or even relapsing and remitting symptoms, are occasionally seen. The manifestations often include features not expected in multiple sclerosis: headache, obtundation, meningism, seizures, and stroke-like episodes. In some cases the occurrence of optic neuropathy, myelopathy (which can be acute or chronic) or brainstem involvement may raise the possibility of multiple sclerosis. MRI findings are largely nonspecific, often with multifocal white matter and grey matter lesions, some of which may display enhancement or haemorrhagic features. A rare but characteristic finding is of large numbers of punctate foci of gadolinium enhancement in the white matter (Figure 8.14; Campi *et al* 2001). Such lesions often persist for many months. Intrinsic cord lesions are seen in patients with myelopathic presentation. The cerebrospinal fluid will normally show evidence of inflammation, with a mononuclear pleocytosis, an elevated protein and the presence of intrathecal oligoclonal bands. Cerebral angiography has long been advocated but is rarely useful in diagnosis – segmental narrowing of smaller arteries proving neither specific nor sensitive for isolated central nervous system vasculitis. The crucial diagnostic test is brain and leptomeningeal biopsy to provide a pathological diagnosis.

The diagnostic difficulties associated with central nervous system vasculitis – whether systemic or part of an isolated process – are emphasized by Scolding *et al* (1997) who described eight patients with vasculitis in whom cerebral manifestations dominated the clinical presentation, often without systemic features. Seizures (focal and generalized), stroke-like episodes, acute and subacute encephalopathy, cognitive impairment, movement disorders and cranial nerve palsies were all observed. Many of these syndromes would not ordinarily be confused with multiple sclerosis, but three patients had an illness with relapses and remissions and optic nerve and brainstem involvement, entirely consistent with the symptoms and signs of multiple sclerosis. Of these, two had oligoclonal bands and one had typical MRI abnormalities. Multiple sclerosis was the preferred diagnosis at presentation in all three patients and the correct explanation only emerged when atypical features were analysed in more detail, supplemented by investigations looking for an underlying vasculitis, including the presence of anti-neutrophil cytoplasmic antibodies. Against a clinical background suggestive of multiple sclerosis, the clues in these three cases were seizures, headache, encephalopathy, stroke-like episodes, fever, arthralgia and skin rash. The importance of diagnosing central nervous system vasculitis lies in the prospect that it can be effectively treated in most instances with cyclophosphamide. Corticosteroids are also frequently used, especially to treat acute neurological events.

Systemic sclerosis

Multiple sclerosis has been described in association with systemic sclerosis (Trostle *et al* 1986), but a causal connection was not suggested. The typical case with calcinosis, Raynaud's

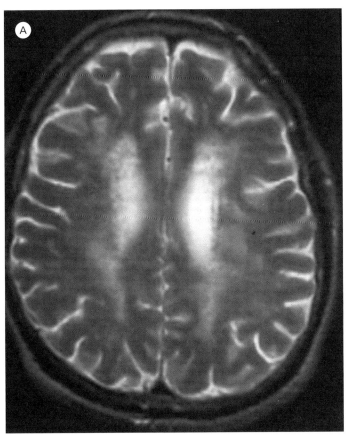

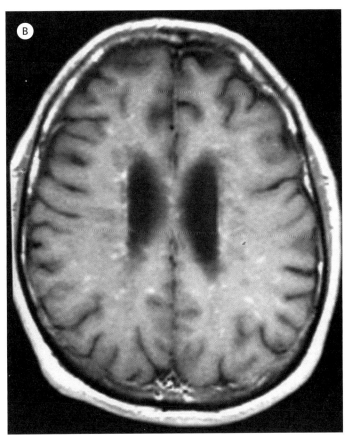

Figure 8.14 (A) T$_2$-weighted MRI in isolated cerebral vasculitis showing multiple lesions. (B) Gadolinium enhanced T$_1$-weighted scan showing multiple areas of enhancement. Reproduced with permission from D.H. Miller *et al* (1997).

phenomenon, dysphagia, sclerodactyly and telangiectasia will not cause confusion. When the nervous system is involved, peripheral nerves are more usually affected, but vasculitic lesions affecting the central nervous system can mimic episodes of demyelination. Averbuch-Heller *et al* (1992) decribed four patients with myelopathy indistinguishable from spinal demyelination.

Susac syndrome

This rare syndrome is defined by the clinical triad of retinal disease, sensorineural deafness and encephalopathy. The pathological basis is a microangiopathy of small vessels in the brain, retina and cochlea. It usually presents in young women and is often monophasic and self-limiting (Meca-Lallana *et al* 1999). Multiple white matter and grey matter lesions may be seen on MRI and confusion with multiple sclerosis or acute disseminated encephalomyelitis occurs if there is clinical evidence for multifocal white matter disturbance (Murata *et al* 2000). A high frequency of central corpus callosum lesions was reported in a recent review of 27 cases along with another 51 described in the literature (Figure 8.15; Susac *et al* 2003); gadolinium enhancement in the parenchyma and leptomeninges was also reported. Essential clues to the diagnosis are deafness (which is an unusual feature of multiple sclerosis) and retinal vascular disease. For this reason, Susac syndrome is discussed more in the ophthalmic than the neurological literature. Recurrences have been

described up to 18 years after the original episode (G.W. Petty *et al* 2001).

Noninflammatory cerebrovascular disease

Less confusion may arise in making the distinction between vascular disease affecting the central nervous system when this does not have the added twist of biomarkers indicating inflammatory brain disease, but the noninflammatory vascular disorders may mimic the clinical features and imaging appearances of multiple sclerosis.

Multiple cerebral emboli in a young adult, notably arising from subacute bacterial endocarditis or atrial myxoma, can present with clinical features resembling those of multiple sclerosis. A more common problem is that of the young woman taking an oral contraceptive who experiences the rapid onset of focal neurological signs – weakness and sensory loss in one upper limb, for example. Unless MRI shows multiple lesions, investigation is unlikely to distinguish between infarction and demyelination. Visual evoked potentials seldom show changes of diagnostic value in the initial attack of multiple sclerosis and cerebrospinal fluid oligoclonal IgG may be present in acute cerebrovascular disease (Roström and Link 1981). In doubtful circumstances, it may seem best to discontinue the contraceptive pill and await events. However, in other circumstances where MRI shows multifocal lesions characteristic for demyelination,

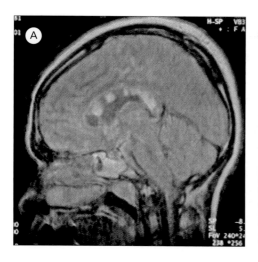

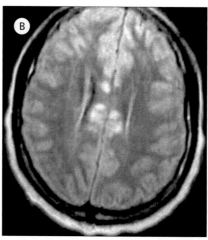

Figure 8.15 (A) Sagittal and (B) axial T$_2$-weighted MRI in Susac's syndrome shows white matter lesions and corpus callosum involvement. From Susac *et al* (2003). © 2003, reprinted with permission of Lippincott Williams & Wilkins (lww.com).

and the cerebrospinal fluid exhibits oligoclonal bands, a more confident diagnosis of demyelinating disease will be made and contraception allowed to continue.

Cerebral autosomal dominant arteriopathy with subcortical infarcts and leucoencephalopathy (CADASIL)

In the last decade, the autosomal dominant disorder known as cerebral autosomal dominant arteriopathy with subcortical infarcts and leucoencephalopathy (CADASIL) has become recognized as a significant cause of stroke and migraine in young adults (Dichgans *et al* 1998). There is usually a positive family history of strokes occurring at a relatively young age. Dementia may develop with disease progression. MRI reveals multifocal or symmetrical white matter lesions that are sometimes very extensive. Brain imaging is often already abnormal in the pre-symptomatic phase. Distinctive radiological features of CADASIL are prominent involvement of the anterior temporal white matter and external capsules (Figure 8.16; O'Sullivan *et al* 2001). This imaging pattern will suggest the correct diagnosis in cases where a multifocal relapsing and remitting or progressive central nervous system syndrome have erroneously led to the suspicion of multiple sclerosis (O'Riordan *et al* 2002). The cerebrospinal fluid does not contain oligoclonal bands. The characteristic small vessel arteriopathy may be diagnosed from a skin biopsy. The disorder is the result of a mutation of *Notch3* located at chromosome 19q12 (Joutel *et al* 1996).

Sarcoidosis

Sarcoidosis is a multisystem granulomatous disorder, with the most frequent clinical manifestations related to intrathoracic disease (especially pulmonary involvement with mediastinal lymphadenopathy). It is generally estimated that about 5% of cases develop evidence for central nervous system involvement. A recent study reported neurological involvement in an unusually high proportion of cases (26%; R.K. Allen *et al* 2003), although many of these patients had peripheral nerve or muscle involvement that would not be confused with multiple sclerosis. The prognosis seems poorer for central than peripheral nervous system involvement (Ferriby *et al* 2001). Diagnosis of neurosarcoidosis is most challenging when there is no evidence for

disease outside the nervous system, and it is sometimes only diagnosed definitively following biopsy of central nervous system or meningeal tissue (Bode *et al* 2001; F.G. Moore *et al* 2001). The manifestations and management of sarcoidosis affecting the nervous system have been recently reviewed (Hoitsma *et al* 2004; Nowak and Widenka 2001; Vinas and Rengachary 2001). These reviews highlight the frequency of nervous system involvement (seen in 5–15% of patients with sarcoidosis); the most frequent clinical manifestations (cranial nerves, meninges, optic nerves and spinal cord); the role of neuroradiological and other laboratory investigations in supporting the diagnosis (whilst noting that there is no pathognomonic non-invasive investigation and that the diagnosis is often only made after granulomatous lesions are demonstrated from biopsy of affected conjunctiva, muscle, lymph node, liver or central nervous system tissue); and the approach to treatment (for which corticosteroids are the mainstay but often associated with adverse effects because of the need for long-term maintenance therapy). Nowak and Widenka (2001) propose the following differential diagnosis when sarcoidosis involves the central nervous system parenchyma: multiple sclerosis, cerebral metastasis, cerebral lymphoma, tuberculosis, fungal infections and high- and low-grade glioma. When there is meningitis, the differential diagnosis proposed is: bacterial meningitis (such as *Borrelia* sp.), tuberculous or carcinomatous meningitis, meningioma, leukaemic infiltration, meningeal lymphoma and meningeal plasmacytoma. To either list could be added isolated angiitis of the central nervous system.

Most forms of neurosarcoidosis do not resemble multiple sclerosis but where the spinal cord and optic nerve are involved the distinction can be extremely difficult. Since sarcoid myelopathy typically presents as chronic progressive paraparesis, resulting from compression, ischaemia or parenchymal disease (Day and Sypert 1976), but occasionally has a rapid or subacute onset (Bogousslavsky *et al* 1982; Nathan *et al* 1976), confusion can arise with both the relapsing–remitting and progressive variants of multiple sclerosis. Lhermitte's symptom has been reported in neurosarcoidosis (Sauter *et al* 1991).

The clinical features of sarcoid optic neuropathy (Figure 8.17) often closely resemble those of demyelinating neuropathy (Beardsley *et al* 1984; Piéron *et al* 1979; Rush 1980), although E.M. Graham *et al* (1986) found that visual loss is usually more gradual. Recovery may follow treatment with corticosteroids

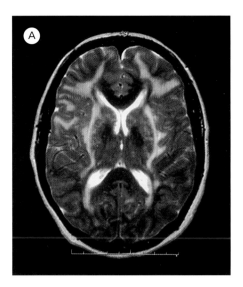

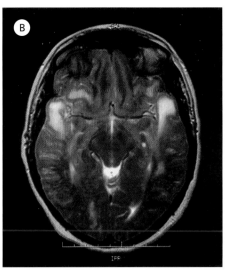

Figure 8.16 T$_2$-weighted MRI in CADASIL. There are extensive white matter abnormalities. Characteristic involvement of (A) the external capsules and (B) anterior temporal white matter. Kindly provided by Professor Tarek Yousry.

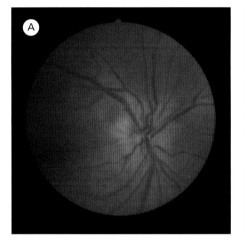

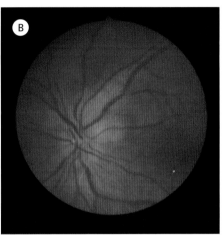

Figure 8.17 Bilateral optic disc appearances showing infiltration in a patient with histologically proven neurosarcoidosis.

but can occur spontaneously (Galetta *et al* 1989). E.M. Graham *et al* (1986) also noticed that although there is improvement with corticosteroid treatment, patients may subsequently become steroid dependent with relapses occurring as the dose is reduced. A particular diagnostic challenge arises when optic neuritis presents as the first symptom of systemic sarcoidosis (DeBroff and Donahue 1993). It was noted by L.P. Frohman *et al* (2003) that characteristic ophthalmic features suggesting a granulomatous optic neuropathy (periphlebitis, uveitis and optic disc granuloma) were only found in a minority of patients whose sarcoidosis presented as an anterior visual pathway disturbance. However, their study did report a high frequency of abnormalities on chest X-ray (72%), gallium scan (93%), cerebrospinal fluid (88%) and anterior visual pathway imaging (70%), and angiotensin-converting enzyme was elevated in 76% (L.P. Frohman *et al* 2003). Whilst this emphasizes the value of such investigations when sarcoid optic neuropathy is suspected, the frequency of abnormalities reported in this study is higher than that observed by other experienced clinicians (J.P. Lynch 2003).

Sarcoid meningoencephalitis inevitably results in symptoms attributable to multiple lesions, including cranial nerve palsies and signs of brainstem disease, which present diagnostic difficulties. However, features such as headache, papilloedema and diabetes insipidus steer the clinical diagnosis away from multiple sclerosis.

Overt systemic sarcoidosis is usually present before the onset of neurological involvement, or is readily found on routine investigation. When there is diagnostic doubt, histological confirmation must be sought from biopsy of accessible suspect lesions or tissue commonly affected by sarcoidosis – gum, conjunctiva, lymph node, muscle and other sites. The Kveim test is unreliable (positive tests have been observed in clinically definite multiple sclerosis) and is no longer available in the United Kingdom given concern about the potential for prion transmission. In about 10% of patients with neurosarcoidosis, there may be no evidence for systemic sarcoidosis (Oksanen *et al* 1985) and, rarely, autopsy indicates that there is no involvement outside the nervous system (Beardsley *et al* 1984).

The cerebrospinal fluid total protein may be greatly raised and oligoclonal IgG is sometimes present (Kinnman and Link 1984; Zajicek *et al* 1999). The cell count is often increased with an excess of neutrophils and eosinophils. Glucose is occasionally reduced. There may be elevation of angiotensin-converting enzyme in the cerebrospinal fluid and serum. Whilst initially this appeared to be a promising diagnostic test (T.F. Scott 1993), further experience suggests that it is a rather nonspecific finding that may also be seen in other inflammatory neurological disorders. Genetic mutations may also be associated with elevated serum levels of angiotensin-converting enzyme (Linnebank *et al*

2003). Tahmoush *et al* (2002) suggest that a level of cerebrospinal fluid angiotensin-converting enzyme >8 nmol/mL/min is suggestive of neurosarcoidosis.

Cerebral MRI sometimes shows white matter and periventricular lesions similar to those of multiple sclerosis (Figure 8.18A; D.H. Miller *et al* 1988d; Lexa and Grossman 1994) but involvement of the cortex or hypothalamus is not expected in the latter condition. The lesions of sarcoidosis can be demonstrated as areas of increased signal and swelling in the optic nerves (Bode *et al* 2001; Engelken *et al* 1992) and spinal cord. Enhanced MRI is especially valuable. It often shows meningeal involvement (Pickuth *et al* 2000), most commonly involving the basal cisterns, pituitary and hypothalamic regions, but also involving meninges overlying the cortex, brainstem, spinal cord and cauda equina (Figure 8.19). Parenchymal granulomatous lesions in the cortex, white matter, brainstem, optic nerves, other cranial nerves, spinal cord, cauda equina and nerve roots may all enhance (Sauter *et al* 1991). Enhancement of meningeal, parenchymal or periventricular lesions was detected in 15/17 (88%) cases in one study where gadolinium enhanced MRI was performed (Lexa and Grossman 1994). Lesions in the

brain or spinal cord sometimes exhibit a mass effect, simulating the appearance of a tumour. Hydrocephalus can also occur. Enhancement of parenchymal lesions in sarcoidosis generally lasts longer than the 4–6 weeks that characterizes the evolution of the enhancing phase of multiple sclerosis lesions, although corticosteroid treatment for sarcoidosis often leads to the resolution of enhancement (Lexa and Grossman 1994). In a minority of cases, the distribution of white matter abnormalities is indistinguishable from that seen in multiple sclerosis, and this observation is in keeping with the post-mortem findings (Figure 8.18).

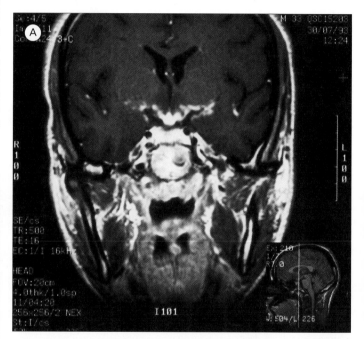

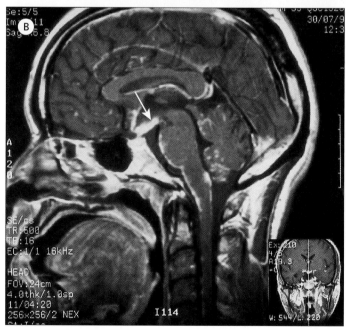

Figure 8.19 Gadolinium enhanced T$_1$-weighted image in neurosarcoidosis. Note the widespread meningeal enhancement. (A) Coronal section and (B) sagittal section showing the optic tract (arrow).

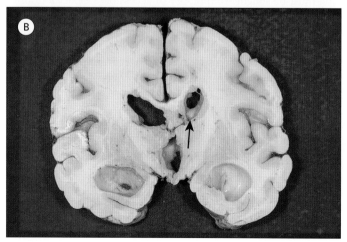

Figure 8.18 (A) T$_2$-weighted MRI in neurosarcoidosis showing multifocal and periventricular abnormalities indistinguishable from those seen in multiple sclerosis. (B) Post-mortem specimen showing involvement of the ventricular lining by sarcoid tissue (arrow). Kindly provided by Dr Trevor Hughes.

Zajicek *et al* (1999) reviewed 68 patients with definite or probable neurosarcoidosis, a definite diagnosis (seen in 12/68 cases, 18%) being dependent on finding sarcoid granulomas on nervous system histology. Twenty-six (38%) patients presented with uni- or bilateral optic nerve disease. This had often first been diagnosed as optic neuritis but carried a worse prognosis for vision – although referral patterns may have inflated the apparent frequency of visual involvement. Nineteen (28%) of the 68 subjects had significant spinal cord disease with neurological involvement at other sites in about half these cases. The spinal cord syndrome produced a picture similar either to subacute transverse myelitis or chronic spinal cord demyelination. However, this and other reports (Prelog *et al* 2003; Zajicek 1990; Kaiboriboon *et al* 2005) illustrate the coexistence of spinal cord and cauda equina involvement in neurosarcoidosis – a clinical syndrome that also occurs in multiple sclerosis as a result of the involvement of the conus medullaris. Neurosarcoidosis presented with brainstem or cerebellar symptomatology, not easily distinguished from multiple sclerosis, in 14/68 (21%) cases. Twenty of 54 (37%) patients had oligoclonal bands and a further ten (18%) showed isoelectrophoretic abnormalities of proteins both in serum and cerebrospinal fluid. White matter abnormalities were present on MRI in 16/37 (43%) patients. Meningeal enhancement with gadolinium best discriminated the appearances from those of multiple sclerosis and was seen on 11/29 (38%) scans (Zajicek *et al* 1999).

A subsequent systematic analysis of spinal fluid samples from patients diagnosed with neurosarcoidosis, based on a stringent set of criteria that required a neurological syndrome compatible with neurosarcoidosis and histological verification of granulomas, suggests that local intrathecal production of oligoclonal bands is a relatively uncommon feature – being seen in only one of 19 cases (Ed Thompson, personal communication). This finding suggests that some cases reported in earlier series – where oligoclonal bands were positive but histological confirmation of the diagnosis was not mandatory – did in fact have multiple sclerosis. A definitive answer is not possible and the chance concurrence of two relatively common disorders cannot absolutely be excluded. Nevertheless, in making the distinction between sarcoidosis and multiple sclerosis, the status of oligo-

clonal bands (usually negative in neurosarcoidosis and positive in multiple sclerosis) is of some diagnostic value.

Although peripheral nerve involvement is seen less commonly than central nervous system involvement, there should be no confusion with multiple sclerosis when it does occur. Focal, multifocal and diffuse neuropathies were reported in a review of 11 cases with sarcoid neuropathy confirmed on nerve biopsy (Said *et al* 2002). Nine also had histological evidence for muscle involvement and there was pulmonary or mediastinal involvement in eight. The biopsies revealed necrotizing vasculitis in addition to granulomas in seven cases.

Infections

A number of specific infections can reproduce the typical presenting features of multiple sclerosis and this potential area of diagnostic confusion becomes even greater with the development of chronic infections – not least because some may trigger autoimmune processes as part of the complex interplay between pathogen and host response.

Lyme borreliosis

In an endemic area (Figure 8.20), acute Lyme disease will usually be recognized from the rash and from the constitutional disturbance, although the history of tick bite may not be forthcoming. Neurological involvement at this acute or subacute, essentially monophasic, stage can resemble multiple sclerosis, with cranial nerve lesions, particularly facial palsy, widespread paraesthesiae due to radicular involvement and signs of spinal cord disease (Bateman *et al* 1987; Pachner and Steere 1985; Pachner *et al* 1989). Optic neuritis has rarely been described (Winyard *et al* 1989). After reviewing published cases, D.M. Jacobson *et al* (1991) concluded that the relationship between optic neuritis and Lyme borreliosis remains ambiguous. However, they make a case for serological testing in isolated optic neuritis in endemic areas, with antibiotic treatment in patients showing a rise in antibody levels on paired sera. Acute transverse myelitis (Rousseau *et al* 1986) and meningoradiculomyelitis (Tullman *et al* 2003) have also been reported.

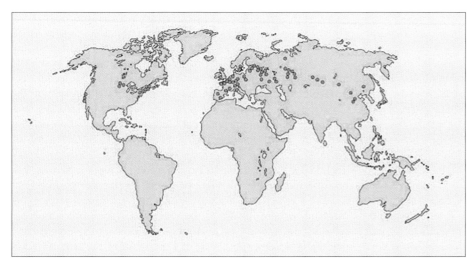

Figure 8.20 **Lyme disease: a global map showing the geographic distribution of the disease.**

Myelitis may reflect primary infection or an early immune-mediated postinfectious response (Lesca *et al* 2002).

Far more difficult diagnostic problems are posed when chronic progressive or relapsing neurological disease develops in what is regarded as tertiary Lyme disease, many years after infection or long after clinical evidence for infection has waned (Ackerman *et al* 1988). Syndromes that have been considered to represent chronic neuroborreliosis include progressive spastic paraparesis (Kohler *et al* 1986), transverse myelitis (Reik *et al* 1986; Weder *et al* 1987), cerebellar ataxia (Benoit *et al* 1986), recurrent cranial nerve palsies (Pachner and Steere 1985) and dementia (Logigian *et al* 1990). Optic neuritis was mentioned but not described by Ackerman *et al* (1988). Optic neuropathy in a case described by Schechter (1986) case was clearly ischaemic. More recent studies have suggested that chronic neurological syndromes may be related to borreliosis through an immunopathogenic mechanism (Hemmer *et al* 1999; Muraro *et al* 2003).

MRI may show disseminated white matter lesions (Logigian *et al* 1990), which result from focal vasculitis and demyelination (Oski *et al* 1996; Romi *et al* 2004), and the cerebrospinal fluid may contain oligoclonal IgG (Finkel and Halperin 1992). Positive serology for *Borrelia burgdorferi* merely indicates past infection and is unlikely to be relevant in the absence of other evidence for infection (Coyle 2002; Coyle *et al* 1993). Investigation of patients diagnosed as having multiple sclerosis in endemic areas has not revealed any excess of positive tests for *Borrelia* (Schmutzhardt *et al* 1988; Coyle 1989). Although the finding of antibodies in cerebrospinal fluid is a more reliable indication of central nervous system involvement (Ackerman *et al* 1988; Finkel and Halperin 1992), it is not possible easily to culture *Borrelia burgdorferi* and there is no reliable assay for active (as against past) infection (Coyle 2002). This creates difficulties of diagnosis in patients presenting with an atypical neurological syndrome and positive *Borrelia* serology. The diagnosis of borreliosis is most unlikely if the patient has not visited or lived in an area where the *Ixodes* tick (the vector that transmits the infection to humans) exists. Conversely, the diagnosis of Lyme disease can reasonably be considered if the patient lives in an endemic area. However, because Lyme disease is endemic in those parts of Europe and North America that are also areas of high prevalence for multiple sclerosis, it is also quite possible that the occurrence of positive *Borrelia* serology in a patient with otherwise typical multiple sclerosis is coincidental. In our view, a confident diagnosis of neuroborreliosis infection should only be made when the patient lives in or has visited an endemic area, has a neurological syndrome typical for borreliosis such as facial palsy, sensorimotor radiculitis or meningitis, and manifests positive *Borrelia* serology in the cerebrospinal fluid. We doubt that there is a chronic progressive or relapsing form of neuroborreliosis infection that genuinely represents part of the differential diagnosis of multiple sclerosis but recognize that this is an opinion not shared universally.

Meningovascular syphilis

Neurosyphilis is now a comparative rarity in countries where multiple sclerosis is prevalent and is therefore more likely to be overlooked on the few occasions when a patient does present with luetic disease. Oculomotor palsies, perhaps combined with hemiparesis, certainly bear a superficial resemblance to multiple

sclerosis, but headache and epilepsy are often prominent manifestations and classical pupillary abnormalities may be present. Cerebrospinal fluid will usually exhibit a lymphocytic pleocytosis with raised protein and IgG and oligoclonal bands. Laboratory diagnosis is based on serological investigation of blood and cerebrospinal fluid (Reik 2002). Nonspecific serological abnormalities are the rapid plasmin reagin (RPR) and venereal disease research laboratory (VDRL) tests, but up to 20–40% of positive blood results are false positives and as many as 25% of subjects with late neurosyphilis may have a negative blood test. A positive cerebrospinal fluid VDRL provides definite evidence for neurosyphilis but again this test may be negative in 30% of cases. More specific and sensitive evidence for syphilitic infection is a positive test for treponemal antibodies, such as the serum fluorescent treponemal antibody absorption test, which is almost always informative but does not distinguish active from past infection.

Syphilitic optic neuritis is usually bilateral, with disc swelling, enlarged blind spots and peripheral constriction of the visual fields (Graveson 1950). Syphilitic myelopathy may be acute or slowly progressive (Siller 1989). Florid manifestations of neurosyphilis are now most often complications of human immunodeficiency virus (HIV) infection.

Human immunodeficiency virus (HIV)

Vacuolar myelopathy related to acquired immunodeficiency syndrome (AIDS) presents as progressive spastic paraparesis and sensory ataxia (McArthur 1987) but, both clinically and pathologically, it more closely resembles subacute combined degeneration than multiple sclerosis (Petito *et al* 1986). Confusion might arise, however, from the frequent association with AIDS-related dementia, the clinical evidence of multiple lesions being supported by MRI findings that can mimic those of multiple sclerosis (McArthur 1987). Oligoclonal bands are rarely present in the cerebrospinal fluid and the more usual MRI appearances of prominent atrophy with hazy or diffuse white matter signal changes, rather than distinct multifocal lesions, are points of distinction.

HIV is one of the many antecedent infections recognized in acute disseminated encephalomyelitis (Table 8.3; Narciso *et al* 2001) and meningoencephalitis may occur during acute seroconversion, within a few weeks of infection. Discriminating between AIDS and multiple sclerosis is rarely problematical. However, J.R. Berger *et al* (1989) described seven men, seropositive for HIV-1, with clinical disease indistinguishable from relapsing–remitting multiple sclerosis. In two, the histopathology at autopsy was that of multiple sclerosis and it is probable that their disease was not directly the result of the infection. More intriguing is the report of fulminating and rapidly fatal leucoencephalopathy as the first indication of HIV infection, with the histological changes of multiple sclerosis (Gray *et al* 1991). These cases suggest that a putatively T-cell-dependent autoimmune disorder like multiple sclerosis can occur in individuals with low or absent T-cell counts. On reflection, this is perhaps not surprising since additional pathogenic mechanisms are likely to be operating in chronic multiple sclerosis, including, tissue damage secondary to microglial and macrophage activation. Also, at least some of the clinical manifestations of HIV infection are now considered to be part of the immune reaction to infection, and HIV-induced macrophage activation in the central nervous system is likely to be a mechanism for the tissue damage that leads to HIV dementia (McArthur *et al* 2003). [Human T-cell leukaemia virus type 1 (HTLV-1) associated myelopathy presents as a chronic myelopathy and is discussed below.]

Progressive multifocal leucoencephalopathy

Progressive multifocal leucoencephalopathy normally manifests in immunosuppressed individuals. In the past it was commonly seen in patients with AIDS but now occurs rarely in HIV-positive individuals treated with combination antiretroviral therapies. It is the result of an infection of oligodendrocytes by activated JC virus, a papovavirus existing in a dormant state in many healthy individuals. Multiple large areas of myelin destruction develop subacutely in the cerebral white matter and less often in the posterior fossa. Clinical manifestations include hemiplegia, dysphasia, hemianopia, seizures and cognitive impairment. MRI reveals extensive and asymmetric lesions in the cerebral white matter, without mass effect, and usually (though not invariably) without gadolinium enhancement. The clinical presentation and radiological picture can be similar to that of the fulminant Marburg variant of multiple sclerosis and diagnostic biopsy may be undertaken that shows characteristic oligodendrocyte inclusions. However, the occurrence of such an illness in the context of immunosuppression should suggest progressive multifocal leucoencephalopathy, and JC virus DNA can be detected in the cerebrospinal fluid (Yiannoutsos *et al* 1999). The prognosis is poor unless the underlying immunosuppression can be reversed. Specific antiviral therapies have to date been largely ineffective. A contemporary focus on progressive multifocal leucoencephalopathy in the context of multiple sclerosis has been stimulated by the report of two cases developing in patients treated with the combination of IFN-β1a and Tysabri (Kleinschmidt-DeMasters and Tyler 2005; Langer-Gould *et al* 2005). One proved fatal whereas the other exhibited partial recovery after treatment was discontinued. Tysabri is a therapeutic humanized monoclonal anti-adhesion molecule antibody showing beneficial effects on the clinical course of relapsing multiple sclerosis (see Chapter 18). These cases raise questions of how the development of progressive multifocal leucoencephalopathy might be related to the impairment of lymphocyte trafficking, and whether such cases might be prevented by laboratory screening to detect preclinical JC virus activation that would lead to early discontinuation of treatment (Berger and Koralnik 2005).

Subacute sclerosing panencephalitis

This chronic measles infection of the central nervous system is rarely seen since the widespread introduction of measles vaccination. It presents mainly in childhood, and the usual picture is of a subacute and relentlessly progressive syndrome with behavioural and locomotor deterioration, leading to obtundation and periodic myoclonic jerks. Such a course is unlikely to be confused with multiple sclerosis. MRI has on occasion shown extensive white matter abnormalities and occasional patients present in late adolescence or as young adults. Usually, there is generalized brain atrophy and areas of focal signal change are not prominent (D.H. Miller *et al* 1990b). The EEG may show periodic high voltage complexes, and the cerebrospinal fluid contains oligoclonal bands specific for measles virus. Antiviral treatments that may be used include isoprinosine, interferon-β and intraventricular interferon-α, but the prognosis is poor.

Whipple's disease

This is an infectious disease caused by the weakly Gram-positive rod-shaped bacillus, *Tropheryma whippelii*. Gastrointestinal involvement leading to a malabsorption syndrome is a frequent manifestation but the central nervous system is also affected. The most common features are brainstem syndromes (oculo-masticatory myorhythmia – rhythmic myoclonic movements of the jaw, lower face, and eyes – is said to be almost pathognomonic of cerebral Whipple's disease), dementia and an akinetic-rigid syndrome. MRI may be normal but generalized atrophy and multifocal white matter and grey matter lesions in the cerebrum or lesions in the brainstem can all occur (Wroe *et al* 1991). Both homogeneous and ring-enhanced lesions have been described, as have multiple peripherally located space-occupying lesions (Figure 8.21). The cerebrospinal fluid may be normal or show pleocytosis (mononuclear cells) with a raised protein and oligoclonal bands. Positive polymerase chain reaction for *T. whippelii* is of diagnostic value but is only available as a specialized investigation in a limited number of laboratories. Whereas the gastrointestinal diagnosis of Whipple's disease is made from small bowel histology, confirmation of neurological involvement may require brain biopsy (Erdem *et al* 1993b; Wroe *et al* 1991). Although the importance of recognizing Whipple's disease lies in the potential for effective treatment, many neurologists will never see a case and, if they should, the most typical clinical presentations are unlikely to be confused with multiple sclerosis. Antibacterial treatments include tetracyclines, co-trimoxazole, cefixime and rifampicin. While stabilization of neurological status is to be expected, some patients appear to worsen despite antibacterial treatment.

Primary lymphoma of the central nervous system

There is some evidence that lymphoma confined to the central nervous system has increased in prevalence over recent years. Primary central nervous system lymphoma can occur in immunologicaly competent individuals and may present as solitary or multifocal lesions (Kuker *et al* 2005). In the latter situation, multifocal lesions of various sizes – some large and with mass effect and others much smaller – may occur in the cerebral white matter. The picture may then resemble demyelination (Figure 8.22). A periventricular predilection is apparent but not universal. There have been infrequent instances when lesions involve the spinal cord. The clinical manifestations are subacute and progressive and include hemiparesis, hemianopia, seizures, obtundation and myelopathy. Lesions often display gadolinium enhancement and there may be initial clinical improvement accompanied by remarkable radiological resolution in response to a course of high-dose corticosteroids. This response may lead particularly to the early suspicion of multiple sclerosis. However, the lymphoma soon recurs and becomes progressive. Cerebral biopsy is required for definitive diagnosis.

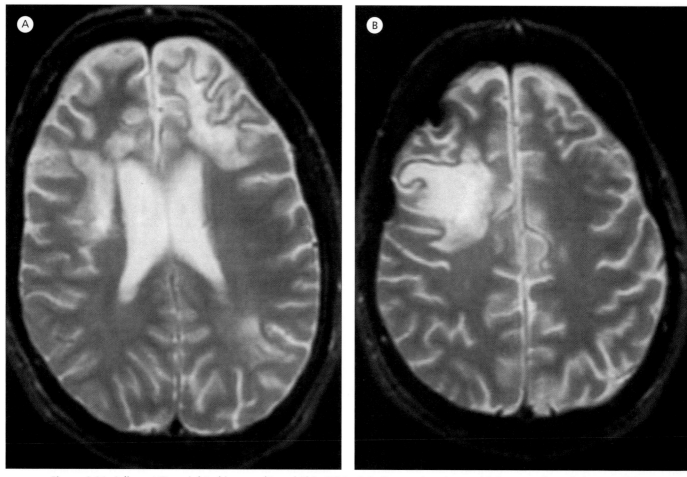

Figure 8.21 Adjacent T$_2$-weighted images (A and B) in Whipple's disease showing multiple parenchymal abnormalities.

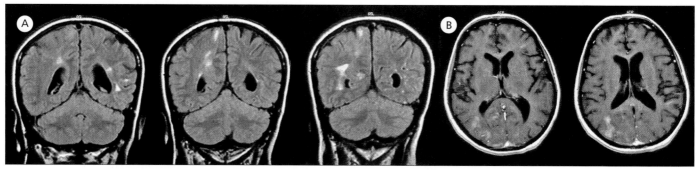

Figure 8.22 A case of biopsy-proven central nervous system B-cell lymphoma. (A) Multiple white matter lesions on T$_2$-weighted images. (B) Some display gadolinium enhancement.

Mitochondrial disease

Some forms of mitochondrial disorder can cause multifocal and relapsing central nervous system syndromes. The best characterized is Mitochondrial Encephalopathy with Lactic Acidosis and Stroke (MELAS). Patients can present at any age with acute hemispheric events suggestive of cerebral ischaemia – typically, hemiplegia and hemianopia – but in addition there may be more generalized encephalopathic features with headaches, seizures and obtundation. The acute episodes tend to occur during times of increased metabolic stress, especially intercurrent infections. T$_2$-weighted MRI reveals large areas of abnormal signal involving

cortex and adjacent white matter that resemble infarction, but do not conform to a single arterial territory. Diffusion weighted MRI has been reported to show increased diffusion during the acute phase (Kolb *et al* 2003; Oppenheim *et al* 2000), and this protocol may therefore be useful in making the distinction from acute infarction in which context diffusion is decreased. Recovery is variable, but there is sometimes complete resolution of the imaging abnormalities. The cerebrospinal fluid and serum may show raised lactic acid. MELAS is the result of a pathological point mutation of mitochondrial DNA (most often at base point 3243). The main differential diagnosis is with cerebrovascular disease rather than multiple sclerosis. Individuals with Leigh's disease, or subacute necrotizing encephalomyelitis, develop a progressive brainstem syndrome with respiratory failure, dystonia, eye movement abnormalities and areflexia. Again, the episodes are usually triggered by intercurrent infection and the disease is more common in children. Thus, it may be considered as an alternative to childhood onset multiple sclerosis but should rarely cause diagnostic difficulties in adults.

SYSTEMATIZED CENTRAL NERVOUS SYSTEM DISEASES

Since multiple sclerosis is a disorder in which oligodendrocytes and their dependent myelin sheaths are primarily affected, its manifestations are mainly confined to white matter tracts. It will therefore occasionally be confused with other disorders which target myelinated pathways in the central nervous system but lack its characteristic clinical course (Table 8.10).

Hereditary ataxias and paraplegias

The classical form of Friedreich's ataxia presents in the first or second decade with progressive ataxia, weakness of the limbs and extensor plantar responses, but absent tendon reflexes. To this picture may be added, in some families, optic atrophy, early dementia and deafness. However, even with such widespread signs, there is seldom a close resemblance to multiple sclerosis. More difficult is the atypical case of sporadic cerebellar ataxia.

The nosology and classification of these spino-cerebellar degenerations, and the group of hereditary paraplegias which are even more likely to be confused with multiple sclerosis, were the special expertise of Anita Harding (Harding 1984). A significant number of individuals within pedigrees having the pure form of hereditary spastic paraplegia show onset between the ages of 10 and 50 years (meeting one criterion for the diagnosis of multiple sclerosis), and there is a high prevalence of sensory and bladder symptoms, all of which can cause considerable diagnostic uncertainty. However, the gait is usually dispropor-

tionately spastic for the degree of weakness, there is often a *pes cavus* foot deformity, and distal amyotrophy. The muscle wasting, and associated neurological features, distinguish the more complicated forms of hereditary spastic paraplegia and make confusion with multiple sclerosis less likely, but difficulties may still arise from the coexistence of spastic paraplegia with optic atrophy and cerebellar signs, including dysarthria and nystagmus. The report of multiple sclerosis in two members of a family with hereditary spastic paraplegia caused by a frame shift of the spastin gene may be coincidental (S.H. Mead *et al* 2001).

Given the occasional familial clustering of multiple sclerosis, and the episodic clinical course of some inherited conditions, a vague history in near relatives of difficulty in walking is often impossible to confirm as evidence of hereditary disease but certain clinical features may be of diagnostic help. Marked asymmetry of physical signs is a strong indication of multiple sclerosis rather than a systematized degeneration, while moderate symmetrical spasticity with preservation of vibration sense is more suggestive of hereditary spastic paraplegia. The distinction from Mendelian inherited disorders of the nervous system (the hereditary ataxias and paraplegias) is made more difficult by the fact that affected sibling pairs with multiple sclerosis sometimes show course and clinical concordance. This is most likely in the context of primary progressive multiple sclerosis, thus making the distinction from hereditary spastic paraparesis particularly tricky (see Chapter 3). Conversely, there may be a poor correlation between onset, severity and clinical features in members of the same pedigree with one or other of the inherited ataxias and paraplegias, especially in those disorders showing genetic anticipation and juvenile forms resulting from triplet repeat expansion in succeeding generations.

The MRI findings in degenerative ataxic disorders are predominantly those of atrophy, although there are no intracranial changes in pure spastic paraplegia (Ormerod *et al* 1994). A variable degree of cerebellar and/or brainstem atrophy is present in all but the earliest stages of hereditary or idiopathic late onset cerebellar ataxia (Figure 8.23), the notable exception being Friedreich's ataxia where atrophy is largely confined to the spinal cord and medulla. Rarely, white matter signal changes are seen in disorders considered to be primarily neurodegenerative. This is not surprising given that gliosis is a pathological feature of these disease processes. Degenerations of grey matter may simulate primary progressive multiple sclerosis. Autosomal dominant cerebellar ataxia is distinguished by the presence of severe cerebellar atrophy and a paucity of white matter lesions (Burk *et al* 1996). Friedreich's ataxia may, however, show nonspecific white matter abnormalities in about 40% of patients (Ormerod *et al* 1994) but specific gene testing will establish the correct diagnosis.

Whilst oligoclonal IgG has occasionally been present in the cerebrospinal fluid, it is likely to be an incidental finding. The more usual absence can help to make the distinction from multiple sclerosis (Ormerod *et al* 1994). Visual evoked potentials are often abnormal in hereditary ataxia (L. Pedersen and Trojaborg 1981) but marked asymmetry would favour multiple sclerosis. In Friedrich's ataxia but not multiple sclerosis, sensory nerve action potentials are absent and ECG abnormalities may be present. Most importantly, identification over the last decade of the genetic basis for Freidreich's and many of the other

---

Table 8.10 Systematized central nervous system diseases

Hereditary ataxias and paraplegias
Leucodystrophies
    adrenoleucodystrophy
    metachromatic leucodystrophy
    globoid (Krabbe's leucodystrophy)
    adult onset dominant leucodystrophy
    vanishing white matter disease
    hereditary adult onset Alexander's disease
    oculodentodigital dysplasia syndrome
Vitamin B12 deficiency
    nitrous oxide-related myelopathy
Cerebrotendinous xanthomatosis
Phenylketonuria
Leucoencephalopathy related to glue-sniffing
Multiple system atrophy
Paraneoplastic syndromes
Coeliac disease
Myeloneuropathy from acquired copper deficiency
Cerebellar ataxia with anti-GAD antibodies
Motor neuron disease and its variants

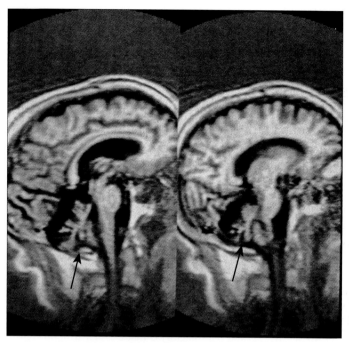

Figure 8.23 Sagittal T$_1$-weighted MRI in a patient with hereditary spinocerebellar ataxia showing marked cerebellar atrophy.

hereditary ataxias allows specific molecular diagnoses to be made (Campuzano *et al* 1996).

The locations of genetic loci for many chronic progressive hereditary ataxias, including Friedreich's (spinocerebellar) ataxia, SCA1–8, SCA10–14, and dentato-rubro-pallido-luysian atrophy are summarized by Opal and Zoghbi (2002). Specific gene mutations for all of these conditions are recognized and mapped to a variety of chromosomes. In several, the mutation arises by a common mechanism of repeat expansion within the disease-causing gene (for example, in Friedreich's ataxia, there is a GAA repeat expansion in intron 1 of the *X25* gene located on chromosome 9q13; in SCA1, -2 and -3, there are CAG repeat expansions within the relevant genes located on chromosomes 6p23, 12q24 and 14q32, respectively). The genetics of hereditary spastic paraplegia are complex; at least 20 loci have been implicated to date (Blumen *et al* 2003; Fink 2002). In eight, the loci encoding these genes are known. The most common cause is a mutation of the spastin gene (*SPG4*) located on chromosome 2p22. This accounts for 40% of cases of autosomal dominant hereditary spastic paraplegia (McDermott *et al* 2003). Both in the hereditary ataxias and paraplegias, there are sometimes distinctive clinical features – in addition to the core ataxia or paraplegia – that associate with abnormalities at specific genetic loci.

Leucodystrophies

The distinction between multiple sclerosis and dysmyelinating disease has long been argued. The changing classifications put forward by neuropathologists and the emerging position on whether or not multiple sclerosis ever occurs in children have informed this debate. Distinctions have now been made between a number of poorly understood developmental disorders of white matter, conditions such as subacute sclerosing

panencephalitis with which they were originally confused, and multiple sclerosis occurring in children and young adults. These genetically determined white matter disorders are reviewed and beautifully illustrated by van der Knaap and Valk (1995; see Figures 8.24 and 8.25). New syndromes continue to be identified, in part aided by the identification of genetic mutations (Schiffmann and van der Knaap 2004). Many of these disorders – including adrenoleucodystrophy, metachromatic leucodystrophy and Pelizaeus–Merzbacher disease – show diffuse white matter changes that are extensive and may reach an extreme degree in advanced cases, extending far out into the gyral white matter (D.H. Miller *et al* 1997). Few are of importance in the differential diagnosis of multiple sclerosis in adults, although some, such as Pelizaeus–Merbacher disease, are disorders of myelination and therefore relevant to a full understanding of demyelinating disease. Even those leucodystrophies which routinely have adult onset forms, or may occasionally present outside childhood, have clinical phenotypes that are unlikely to cause confusion. Table 8.1 provides a classification of leucodystrophies that includes conditions which will be not confused with multiple sclerosis. Table 8.10 provides a smaller list of leucodystrophies that deserve special mention in the context of multiple sclerosis and its differential diagnosis. These are now discussed in more detail.

Adrenoleucodystrophy

This group of disorders is characterized by the accumulation of very long chain saturated fatty acids in all lipid-containing tissues and body fluids, including plasma. They arise from defective very long chain fatty acyl-CoA synthetase activity in peroxisomes (Wanders *et al* 1988) and lead to the accumulation of membrane-like cytoplasmic inclusions in brain tissue (Schaumburg *et al* 1974; 1975). The gene responsible for adrenoleukodystrophy, *ABCD1*, maps to Xq28, close to that for glucose-6-phosphate dehydrogenase deficiency and colour blindness (Aubourg *et al* 1990). It codes for a peroxisomal membrane protein that is a member of the ATP-binding cassette transporter superfamily (Mosser *et al* 1993). All racial groups are affected and the incidence in the United States is about 1 : 16 800 (Bezman *et al* 2001).

The diagnosis is confirmed by detecting markedly elevated very long chain fatty acids in plasma or cultured skin fibroblasts (A.B. Moser *et al* 1999). Three X-linked clinical syndromes share this biochemical abnormality:

- childhood onset adrenoleucodystrophy
- adult onset adrenomyeloneuropathy
- mild adult onset adrenomyeloneuropathy that affects 50% of women who are heterozygous for the X-linked gene.

The adult syndromes presenting with progressive spastic paraparesis are those most likely to be confused with multiple sclerosis. The clinical phenotype of childhood and adult disorders, while usually quite distinct within individuals, may both be seen in the same family (Elrington *et al* 1989).

X-linked childhood adrenoleucodystrophy usually presents between the ages of 4 and 8 years with behavioural disturbance, dementia and epilepsy followed by involvement of special senses and motor systems. Although a significant proportion of

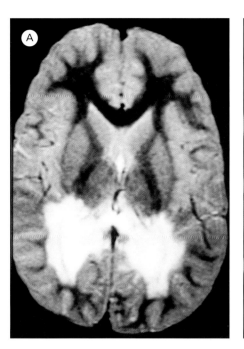

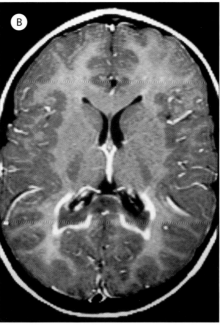

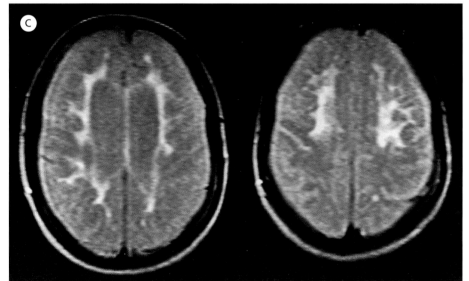

Figure 8.24 (A) T$_2$-weighted MRI of adrenoleucodystrophy in childhood. (B) Gadolinium enhanced T$_1$-weighted image of same patient. Note the extensive enhancement around the trigones. (C) T$_2$-weighted images of metachromatic leucodystrophy.

children later develop adrenal insufficiency, Addison's disease may precede the neurological manifestations by several years (Menkes 1990; Sadeghi-Nejad and Senior 1990) or may occur without nervous system involvement (Josien *et al* 1993; O'Neill *et al* 1982). The cerebrospinal fluid is usually normal (Ménage *et al* 1994), although oligoclonal IgG bands have been described (Dooley and Wright 1985). White matter lesions are usually seen on MRI in childhood adrenoleucodystrophy. These often begin in the posterior hemispheres and advance forwards as the disease progresses (Figure 8.24A). The lesions sometimes display gadolinium enhancement at the advancing edge of the lesion (Figure 8.24B), in keeping with the post-mortem finding of inflammation (H.W. Moser 1997). The MRI white matter lesions become more extensive over time, mirroring the progressive clinical deterioration.

MRI findings vary with age at presentation and to some extent predict the future course (Loes *et al* 2003). If the patient is young and there is initial parieto-occipital or frontal white matter involvement with gadolinium enhancement (the former distribution being more commonly seen than the latter), rapid progression of MRI abnormalities is likely. If abnormalities are confined to the corticospinal tract or cerebellar white matter, a slower evolution occurs: such a pattern is usually seen in adolescents or adults. A reduced *N*-acetyl aspartate to choline ratio in normal-appearing cerebral white matter on MR spectroscopy is also associated with progression of MRI abnormality (Eichler *et al* 2002).

Adrenomyeloneuropathy typically presents in adult men with a slowly progressive spastic paraparesis, impaired vibration and other sensory modalities in the lower limbs, and bladder dysfunction. Clinicians may be alerted to unusual causes for this otherwise common neurological problem by the presence of

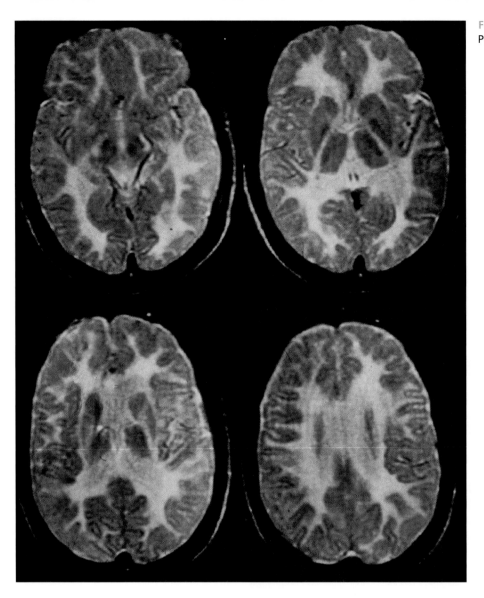

Figure 8.25 T$_2$-weighted MRI in Pelizaeus–Merzbacher disease.

peripheral nerve involvement (J.W. Griffin *et al* 1977), but the specific diagnosis is often overlooked if the very long chain fatty acids are not assayed. Less common clinical manifestations include Klüver–Bucy syndrome, dementia, spinocerebellar degeneration and olivopontocerebellar atrophy (H.W. Moser *et al* 1984; Nakazato *et al* 1989); overall, about 40% who present with the adrenomyeloneuropathy phenotype show various degrees of cerebral involvement (van Geel *et al* 2001). The typical myelopathic presentation can easily be misdiagnosed as a progressive spinal form of multiple sclerosis. Important clues to the correct diagnosis will be a positive family history in brothers or other male relatives in the maternal line, and a previous or concurrent diagnosis of Addison's disease from clinical and/or biochemical manifestations (Rees *et al* 1975). Brain MRI is abnormal in 50% of men with adrenomyeloneuropathy (Ménage *et al* 1994): the most common findings are symmetrical parieto-occipital abnormalities (Figure 8.26), although frontal or cerebellar white matter lesions may be observed. However, none of these epidemiological, clinical, biochemical or imaging clues to

the diagnosis may be present and we recommend that plasma very long chain fatty acids are checked in all patients with an unexplained progressive myelopathy.

Female heterozygotes may develop relatively mild, and occasionally remitting, spastic; limb weakness and sensory loss, but cerebellar involvement is rare (Dooley and Wright 1985; Marsden *et al* 1982; Ménage *et al* 1994; H.W. Moser *et al* 1991). Although adrenal disease is almost never present in carriers, very long chain fatty acids are usually elevated. Brain imaging (in rare instances showing abnormalities of the corticospinal tracts or cerebral white matter resembling those found in males with adrenomyeloneuropathy) or measurement of the auditory evoked brainstem responses may help in diagnosis of the carrier state (Moloney and Masterson 1982; O'Neill *et al* 1983). However, although decreased *N*-acetyl aspartate is demonstrated on MR spectroscopic examination of corticospinal projection pathways in cerebral white matter, indicating axonal damage or loss, brain MRI is normal in a large majority of female heterozygotes (Fatemi *et al* 2003).

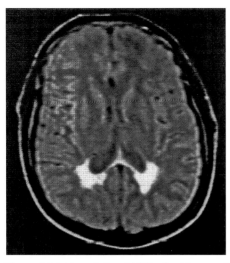

Figure 8.26 T₂-weighted MRI of a 40-year-old male with adrenomyeloneuropathy showing symmetrical parieto-occipital white matter abnormality. From D.H. Miller *et al* (1997) with permission.

Autosomal recessive adrenoleucodystrophy presents in infancy with seizures, hypotonia, retardation, retinal degeneration and hepatic involvement (H.W. Moser 1997; H.W. Moser *et al* 1984; 1991). Females are more commonly affected than males. The pattern of organ involvement and mode of inheritance are similar in neonatal adrenoleucodystrophy and Zellweger's syndrome, the distinction being that the latter is more severe and usually leads to death within 2 years. Both conditions are recognized as disorders of peroxisomal assembly or biogenesis (Raymond 2002), and should be seen as entirely distinct from the X-linked adrenoleucodystrophies.

Metachromatic leucodystrophy

Most autosomal recessive leucodystrophies predominantly affect children. The early adult form of metachromatic leucodystrophy is rare, or perhaps seldom diagnosed, and tends to present with intellectual or emotional abnormalities (Cerizza *et al* 1987). As with many other inherited disorders, onset at >60 years has been described. Presentation with dementia and behavioural disorders is usual (Alves *et al* 1986). Ataxia, paralysis and optic atrophy only develop in the later stages, although the presentation is occasionally with paraparesis or cerebellar ataxia (Hageman *et al* 1995) and the condition can then more easily be mistaken for multiple sclerosis. Clinical evidence for peripheral neuropathy may be revealed by slowed nerve conduction although instances are reported of normal nerve conduction in adult patients (Cengiz *et al* 2002; Marcao *et al* 2005). The full range of clinical manifestations has probably not yet been fully explored. For example, although typically the course is progressive with steady decline into dementia or persistent vegetative state, Sadeh *et al* (1992) describe an apparently unique case with relapsing–remitting metachromatic leucodystrophy. The diagnosis may be confirmed by demonstrating increased urinary sulphatide excretion with a deficiency of aryl-sulphatase A in urine, peripheral blood leucocytes and skin fibroblasts, or by the demonstration of metachromatic material in peripheral nerve biopsies.

Globoid cell leucodystrophy (Krabbe's disease)

Krabbe's disease is an autosomal recessive disorder arising from reduced galactocerebrosidase activity as a result of mutation of the *GALC* gene at 14q24. The late onset of globoid cell leucodystrophy is very rare – almost all cases present at before the age of 5 years and so are almost never confused with (childhood) multiple sclerosis. Grewel *et al* (1991) describe the onset in a 14-year-old boy, not finally diagnosed until the age of 24 years. We know of one case presenting in the third decade and another is recently described who presented with a gait disorder aged 43 years (Brockman *et al* 2003). Four additional cases (two sibling pairs) are described aged 24–35 years, in whom the clinical presentation resembled hereditary spastic paraplegia with prominent MRI signal abnormality in the corticospinal tracts (Figure 8.27; L. Farina *et al* 2000), although in one sibling pair there was striking asymmetry of the clinical and MRI findings. Presentation with spastic paraparesis and brain MRI abnormalities in adults may be associated with a T1835C point mutation (De Stefano *et al* 2000; Satoh *et al* 1997). One of us (DASC) has recently been criticized for failing to make the diagnosis of adult onset Krabbe's disease in a female with a family history both of myotonic dystrophy and 'hereditary spastic paraparesis' in whom a mild spastic gait disorder was associated with a demyelinating peripheral neuropathy and marked asymmetric wasting of the shoulder girdles producing one flail upper limb: here, the confusion was not with multiple sclerosis but in failing to explore all possible causes for familial spastic paraplegia. The clinical picture in Krabbe's disease is typically dominated by progressive intellectual and motor decline with pyramidal, extrapyramidal and cerebellar involvement, together with epilepsy, visual failure and peripheral neuropathy. Visual evoked potentials are delayed but there are no oligoclonal bands in the cerebrospinal fluid. MRI usually shows periventricular and other white matter abnormalities although it can be normal (Bajaj *et al* 2002). MR spectroscopy reveals decreased *N*-acetyl aspartate and increased myoinositol and choline containing compounds in cerebral white matter (Brockmann *et al* 2003) although such findings are not specific for the condition. Examination of peripheral blood leucocytes or skin fibroblasts confirms the deficiency of β-galactocerebrosidase.

Adult onset dominant leucodystrophy

Forms of dominantly inherited leucodystrophy also occur exclusively in adults and may closely resemble chronic progressive multiple sclerosis (Baumann and Turpin 2000; Eldridge *et al* 1984; Schwankhaus *et al* 1994). A report of a large kindred that included 21 affected individuals from four generations emphasized the occurrence of prominent and early abnormalities of the autonomic nervous system including orthostatic hypotension, a finding that would not be expected in multiple sclerosis (Eldridge *et al* 1984). Also unlike multiple sclerosis, MRI shows diffuse, nondiscrete, white matter disease and oligoclonal IgG is not present in the cerebrospinal fluid (Schwankhaus *et al* 1988). It remains uncertain whether all the adult onset dominant leucodystrophies are one and the same disorder, and many are

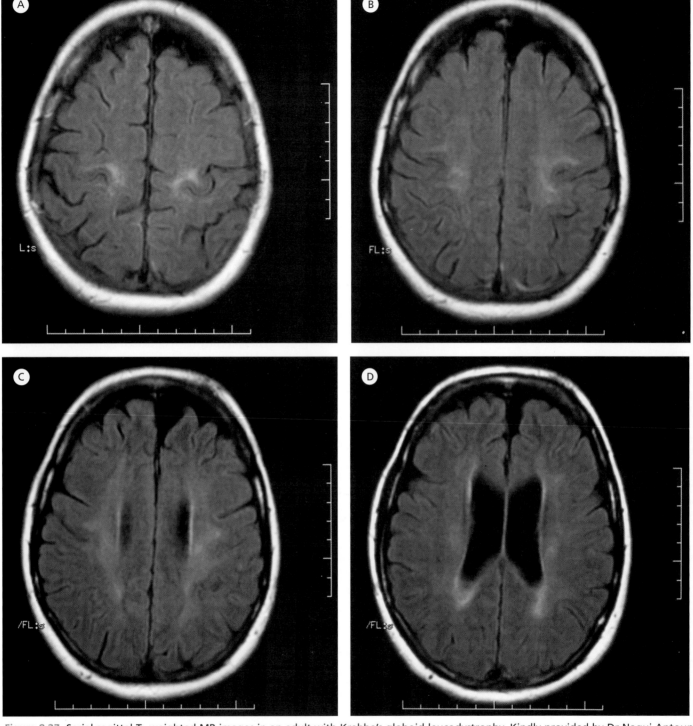

Figure 8.27 Serial sagittal T$_2$-weighted MR images in an adult with Krabbe's globoid leucodystrophy. Kindly provided by Dr Nagui Antoun.

difficult to distinguish from the complicated hereditary spastic paraplegias. An addition to this group is a family with spastic paraparesis, ataxia and mild dementia, presenting in adulthood but with onset in childhood. Diffuse white matter abnormalities were present on MRI, whereas pathognomonic features of the other leucodystrophies were absent (Fukazawa *et al* 1997b). In another recently described family, the prominent manifestations were cerebellar ataxia and dementia associated with extensive MRI white matter abnormalities (Tagawa *et al* 2001). In one of the subjects studied at post mortem, vacuolar changes were observed in the cerebral and cerebellar white matter and brainstem. In another pathologically confirmed case of dominantly inherited adult onset leucodystrophy, MRI showed minimal abnormality of the white matter although there was frontal and corpus callosum atrophy (Letournel *et al* 2003).

A new leucodystrophy has been recently described that is thought to have an autosomal recessive inheritance and presents in childhood or adolescence with progressive pyramidal, cerebellar and dorsal column dysfunction (van der Knaap *et al* 2003). MRI reveals cerebral and cerebellar white matter abnormalities and striking involvement of specific brainstem and spinal cord tracts along with an elevated lactate in white matter.

Vanishing white matter disease

This leucodystrophy has an unusual characteristic in that the clinical presentation is frequently with acute episodes of neurological deterioration. It is an autosomal recessive disorder that most often presents during childhood although onset in young adults is also described (van der Knaap *et al* 1998). Episodes of neurological deterioration, consisting of obtundation, seizures, weakness and ataxia, may occur spontaneously or, more characteristically, in association with an intercurrent infection or minor head trauma. Examination may reveal signs of cognitive, pyramidal and cerebellar dysfunction. MRI shows extensive symmetrical abnormality of cerebral white matter often with marked tissue destruction such that large areas of cavitation are apparent, thus accounting for the diagnostic term that has been assigned. Vanishing white matter disease is attributable to a mutation in any one of the five subunits making up the eukaryotic translation initiation factor gene mapping to 3q27 (van der Knaap *et al* 2002). It is thought that abnormal protein synthesis leading to cell damage occurs at times of increased metabolic demand, such as a rise in body temperature during intercurrent infections. Given the usual age of onset in childhood, and the characteristic radiological appearance, vanishing white matter disease is not likely to be confused with multiple sclerosis. That said, the presentation with acute episodic deterioration may mimic the relapses of multiple sclerosis and it should be borne in mind that episodes at onset do not automatically exclude the possibility of leucodystrophy.

Hereditary adult onset Alexander's disease

Although this leucodystrophy, characterized pathologically by Rosenthal fibres, is more common in childhood, occasional cases are seen in adults. The latter typically present with a progressive spastic paraplegia, pseudobulbar palsy, ataxia, palatal myoclonus and a positive family history suggesting dominant inheritance (R.S. Howard *et al* 1993; Schwankhaus *et al* 1995). MRI reveals profound atrophy of the medulla oblongata and upper spinal cord, but with sparing of the pons. Two recent cases were identified with a mutation in the gene for glial fibrillary acidic protein (Namekawa *et al* 2002). The clinical and MRI picture should not be confused with multiple sclerosis.

Oculodentodigital dysplasia syndrome

This is a rare autosomal dominant disorder in which central nervous system white matter is sometimes involved (Loddenkemper *et al* 2002). The clinical diagnosis is made on the basis of characteristic morphological abnormalities affecting the face, eyes, dentition and digits. The specific findings are a depressed nasal bridge, thin nose with hypoplastic alae and thin, anteverted nostrils, microphthalmos with abnormalities of the iris and microcornea, syndactyly and camptodactyly of the fourth and fifth digits, and hypoplasia of the tooth enamel (Loddenkemper *et al* 2002). Neurological findings include spastic paraparesis, gaze palsy, bladder and bowel disturbance, visual loss, deafness, ataxia

and nystagmus. Diffuse or subcortical high signal in the white matter has been reported on MRI as has basal ganglia hypointensity.

Vitamin B12 deficiency

Confusion between subacute combined degeneration of the spinal cord and multiple sclerosis should only arise in the rare examples with relatively early onset of spastic leg weakness but no signs of peripheral neuropathy. Cervical MRI reveals high signal confined to the posterior columns in a symmetrical manner in some but not all patients (Figure 8.28). A potential cause for confusion with multiple sclerosis is the high frequency of Lhermitte's symptom in subacute degeneration of the cord. This symptom can also result from cord compression (see Figure 6.14; Gautier-Smith 1973). Visual impairment is very uncommon but visual evoked potentials may be delayed in the absence of visual symptoms (Fine and Hallett 1980). Cognitive impairment and diffuse cerebral white matter MRI abnormality are occasionally encountered. In making the diagnosis, it should be noted that the serum vitamin B12 level is usually but not invariably reduced below the normal laboratory range in cases of

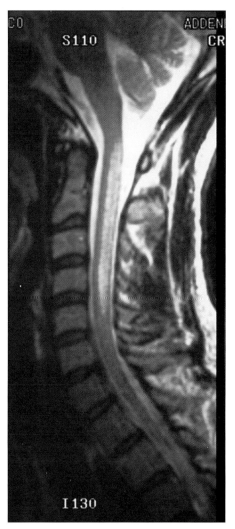

Figure 8.28 T$_2$-weighted MRI in a patient with subacute combined degeneration of the spinal cord showing extensive alteration in the T$_2$-weighted signal from the posterior columns. Kindly provided by Dr Nagui Antoun.

subacute combined degeneration of the spinal cord. When the level is not reduced but the condition is still suspected on clinical grounds, other characteristic biochemical findings that can aid diagnosis are an increase in serum homocysteine and methylmalonic aciduria.

Finally, the presence of a serum B12 level mildly below the normal range may sometimes be seen as an isolated and incidental laboratory abnormality during work up of patients with a neurological disorder. Interpretation of this finding requires liaison with laboratory staff and does not always indicate a causal relationship between the abnormal investigation and the neurological disorder.

Myelopathy due to nitrous oxide toxicity

A number of reports exist of subacute combined degeneration of the spinal cord and a low vitamin B12 level in patients in whom a history emerges of recurrent nitrous oxide inhalation for recreational purposes (Ng and Frith 2002). This has been seen in health-care professionals with access to the agent. Users of nitrous oxide for recreational purposes sometimes refer to the practice as 'nanging'. Signal abnormalities may be seen in the posterior columns on spinal MRI. Nitrous oxide causes irreversible oxidation of the cobalt atom of vitamin B12, making the vitamin inactive. Patients with incipient vitamin B12 deficiency for other reasons are more susceptible to develop this adverse neurological effect of nitrous oxide. Treatment is immediate cessation of nitrous oxide and administration of vitamin B12. A progressive myelopathy affecting the lateral and posterior columns is also described in association with inhalation of heroin vapour, adding to the syndrome of acute myelopathy following insufflation, although the authors speculate that adulteration of the substance with contaminants may also have exposed this addict to nitrous oxide (Nyffeler et al 2003).

Cerebrotendinous xanthomatosis

This rare autosomal recessive metabolic disorder is caused by mutations of the sterol 27-hydroxylase gene. It normally has a non-neurological presentation with tendon xanthomas. Other features include cataracts, elevated serum cholestanol and urinary bile alcohols, and premature cardiovascular disease. The neurological presentation can be with a prominent progressive spastic paraplegia accompanied by symmetrical intrinsic signal abnormalities in the posterior and lateral columns of the spinal cord on MRI (Verrips et al 1999). Bartholdi et al (2004) describe progressive myelopathy in one of two sisters in whom cerebrotendinous xanthomatosis was eventually diagnosed many years after the proband had been treated with a variety of immunosuppressants on the assumption that she had primary progressive multiple sclerosis. Other neurological features include cerebellar signs, peripheral neuropathy, seizures and dementia. MRI may show cerebellar white matter abnormalities and abnormal signal within the dentate nuclei (Clemen et al 2005). Treatment with chenodeoxycholic acid and a statin may prevent further neurological deterioration.

Phenylketonuria

This inherited disorder of phenylalanine metabolism is diagnosed at neonatal screening and prompt institution of a strict diet to avoid hyperphenylalaninaemia will prevent future neurological complications. However, some individuals who do not comply fully with the diet may present with a progressive neurological disorder later in life. The main manifestation is a progressive spastic paraplegia. Patients occasionally have episodes of neurological deterioration that resemble the relapses of multiple sclerosis (A.J. Thompson et al 1990a; 1993b). Additional reported features include cognitive impairment and ataxia. MRI reveals a symmetrical increase in T_2 signal of cerebral white matter with a predilection for periventricular and posterior hemispheric regions (A.J. Thompson et al 1990a). The past history and biochemical findings are, of course, distinctive even if the MRI appearances can be confused with multiple sclerosis (Figure 8.29). The MRI changes are thought to represent dysmyelination and are reversible with re-institution of the correct diet (A.J. Thompson et al 1993b), which also leads to clinical stability or improvement.

Leucoencephalopathy related to glue-sniffing

Inhalation of volatile solvents can result in white matter damage. Toluene is probably the main cause of neurological injury, and people who chronically inhale volatile glues for recreational purposes may develop a progressive and diffuse clinical and radiological leucoencephalopathy (Yamanouchi et al 1995). Pathologically, there is diffuse white matter demyelination. Although visual evoked potentials can be delayed, the diffuse and nonfocal nature of MRI abnormalities together with absence of cerebrospinal oligoclonal bands will be strong pointers against a diagnosis of multiple sclerosis. Diagnostic confusion is more likely if the patient presents with acute and recurrent episodes of neurological disturbance (M.B. Davies et al 2000).

Multiple system atrophy

This progressive neurodegenerative disorder of adults from middle-age onwards should rarely be confused with multiple sclerosis given the typical manifestations of an akinetic-rigid syndrome and autonomic failure. However, cerebellar features are prominent in some patients, and there may also be eye movement abnormalities and pyramidal tract signs that superficially raise the possibility of demyelination. The evolving clinical course should soon establish the correct diagnosis and additional investigations are very helpful in making the distinction. MRI is not expected to display multifocal white matter lesions in multiple system atrophy (unless they are age related), but there may be prominent hypointensity of the putamen on T_2-weighted images, atrophy of posterior fossa structures and a cross-like area of T_2 hyperintensity in the pons (Figure 8.30). The cerebrospinal fluid does not contain oligoclonal bands.

Paraneoplastic syndromes

Subacute paraneoplastic cerebellar degeneration, when associated with gynaecological cancers, presents a stereotyped pattern of severe, rapidly advancing, symmetrical ataxia of the trunk and limbs, and also should not be confused with multiple sclerosis. In other forms, particularly those related to small cell cancer of the lung, cerebellar signs are less prominent and are accom-

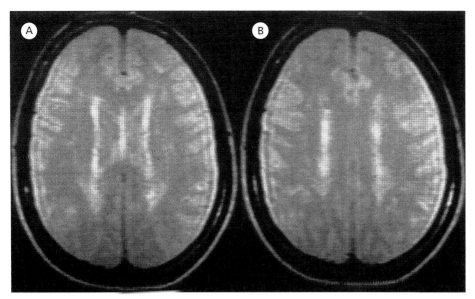

Figure 8.29 T$_2$-weighted MRI scans in a young adult with phenylketonuria showing periventricular abnormality with a posterior predominance. From D.H. Miller *et al* (1997) with permission.

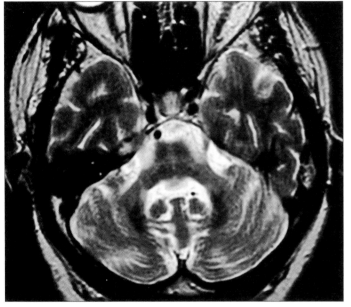

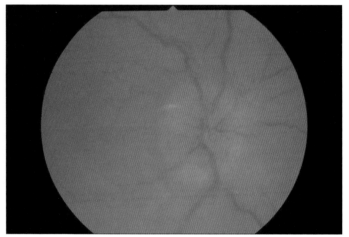

Figure 8.31 Optic disc appearance in a patient with paraneoplastic bilateral sequential visual failure in association with bronchial carcinoma.

Figure 8.30 T$_2$-weighted MRI of a patient with multiple system atrophy. The pons is atrophic and within it there is a cross-shaped area of hyperintensity. Kindly provided by Dr Katherine Miszkiel.

panied by more widespread evidence for cerebral and spinal cord disease (Chabriat *et al* 1994; Henson and Urich 1982; W.P. Mason *et al* 1997; Posner 1986). As the cancer is usually occult at this stage, diagnosis may be difficult, particularly when optic neuritis or other forms of retinal degeneration occur (Figure 8.31; Boghen *et al* 1988; P.R. Rudge 1973; Waterston and Gilligan 1986). Clinical evidence of peripheral nervous disease is often present and should alert clinicians to the possibility of an underlying malignancy.

The cerebrospinal fluid usually shows a lymphocytic pleocytosis and oligoclonal IgG. In pure cerebellar degeneration, imaging shows cerebellar atrophy but in the multifocal forms, MRI is either normal or suggestive of limbic encephalitis. Long lesions involving the spinal cord accompanied by gadolinium enhance-

ment have been reported in cases with myelopathic presentation (Mokri *et al* 1998). Anti-neuronal antibodies are reliably detected in some forms of paraneoplastic disease and their presence often resolves the situation where demyelinating disease is amongst the differential diagnoses. [19]Fluoro-deoxyglucose-labelled positron emission tomography may be useful in demonstrating the occult carcinoma (Younes-Mhenni *et al* 2004).

Coeliac disease

Occasionally, patients with coeliac disease may develop a number of neurological syndromes including spino-cerebellar degeneration, encephalopathy, myoclonus and peripheral neuropathy (Bhatia *et al* 1995; Chin and Latov 2005; W.T. Cooke and Smith

1966). Recently, cases of progressive cerebellar ataxia have been associated with anti-gliadin antibodies (Hadjivassiliou et al 1998). However, as an isolated laboratory finding, it may be difficult to evaluate the significance of these antibodies since they occur in 8–12% of healthy controls (Abele et al 2003; Hadjivassiliou et al 2003). Whilst it is generally unlikely that cases of multiple sclerosis will be confused with the neurological complications of coeliac disease, we have encountered patients in whom intermittent neurological symptoms, consistent with multiple sclerosis and designated as 'demyelinating' have later been attributed to coeliac disease on the basis of a positive test for anti-gliadin antibodies and in the absence of gastrointestinal symptoms. Referral to the gastroenterology service and small bowel biopsy may be needed to resolve the matter.

Myeloneuropathy from acquired copper deficiency

There have been several reports in recent years indicating an association of acquired copper deficiency with a progressive myeloneuropathy (Hedera et al 2003; Kumar and Low 2004; Kumar et al 2003; 2004; Schleper and Stuerenburg 2001). The neurological presentation is seen in adults and resembles that of vitamin B12 deficiency. In some cases, the copper deficiency has been considered secondary to zinc overload (Hedera et al 2003; Kumar et al 2004) and in others to a malabsorption syndrome, sometimes following gastric surgery (Kumar and Low 2004; Kumar et al 2003; Schleper and Stuerenburg 2001). There is a striking reduction in serum caeruloplasmin and copper levels and an associated anaemia or pancytopaenia. Electromyography may reveal an axonal neuropathy and MRI in some cases shows extensive signal change in the posterior cervical cord. Recognition of this disorder is important because copper therapy has been reported to prevent further clinical deterioration.

Cerebellar ataxia with anti-glutamic acid dehydrogenase antibodies

The association between stiff man syndrome and antibodies to glutamic acid decarboxylase (GAD) is well known, and it is unlikely that such a neurological presentation will be confused with multiple sclerosis. More recently, there have been reports of cerebellar ataxia associated with anti-GAD antibodies. In one series of 14 adult patients with ataxia (median age of onset was 51 years) and serum anti-GAD antibodies, 13 were female, 11 had late onset insulin-dependent diabetes mellitus, eight had evidence of autoimmune thyroiditis, 10 had oligoclonal bands, and five of six tested had anti-GAD antibodies in the cerebrospinal fluid (Honnorat et al 2001). The effect of ataxia was more pronounced on the gait than individual limbs and was slowly progressive in most cases. Brain MRI was normal or showed atrophy confined to the cerebellum.

Motor neuron disease and its variants

In a few patients who go on to develop the typical clinical picture of amyotrophic lateral sclerosis (with disseminated upper and lower motor neuron abnormalities), the early presentation may be with a clinically predominant or exclusive upper motor neuron syndrome that leads to the suspicion of demyeli-

nation. It is now recognized that focal areas of pathologically increased signal in the pyramidal pathways are seen in about 70% of patients with motor neuron disease, with increased signal in white matter of the precentral gyrus in a small number of patients (Thorpe et al 1994b; 1996c). Signal change in the cerebral peduncles is often traceable down through the brainstem to the spinal cord (Figure 8.32). It is important to distinguish these pathological features from the areas of relatively high signal seen in the region of the pyramidal tracts in the internal capsule – but not below this level – in about half of normal individuals. The symmetry of these changes and, in motor neuron disease, the absence of other MRI abnormalities characteristic of multiple sclerosis, serve to distinguish the conditions.

A diagnosis of primary lateral sclerosis is sometimes made in patients with a history of progressive spastic tetraparesis extending over several years that have no lower motor neuron degeneration, sensory involvement or family history. Atrophy of the precentral gyrus has been described in some of these patients (C.E. Pringle et al 1992). Central motor conduction is usually delayed (W.F. Brown et al 1992). The reported cases are somewhat heterogeneous and the true nosological status of the condition remains uncertain.

ISOLATED OR MONOSYMPTOMATIC CENTRAL NERVOUS SYSTEM SYNDROMES

In approximately 85% of patients, the first symptoms and signs of multiple sclerosis can be attributed to the effects of a single lesion of the nervous system (Table 8.11). Such symptom clusters are naturally extremely diverse and cannot all be considered individually. With transient symptoms, precise diagnosis may often be impossible. This is perhaps not always desirable in patients who find it difficult to cope with the possibility of further episodes of demyelination. Conversely, many patients who have been reassured during a first or previous episode of demyelination would in retrospect have wished to know at an earlier stage in the illness that multiple sclerosis was a possibility. (We discuss when and what to tell patients in Chapter 15.)

Some symptoms resulting from isolated demyelinating lesions are much more suggestive of multiple sclerosis than others. For example, an acute lower motor neuron facial palsy can be the initial symptom of multiple sclerosis, but other causes (idiopathic Bell's palsy) are more likely. Conversely, acute internuclear ophthalmoplegia in a young woman, without any other detectable cause, is highly suggestive. Symptoms induced or greatly aggravated by exercise or heat should also alert suspicion. Optic neuritis is described in Chapter 6. With the aid of modern imaging techniques it should be possible to avoid most of the diagnostic pitfalls presented by isolated lesions of the central nervous system, provided the indications for their use are recognized. The approach to investigation is described in Chapter 7.

The clinical course of many essentially progressive lesions is occasionally marked by fluctuations, particularly sudden exacerbation and, more rarely, partial or complete remission. A good example is the onset of symptoms as a result of an intracranial meningioma during pregnancy followed by remission in the weeks after delivery. For example, Bickerstaff et al (1958) described unilateral visual loss as a result of pressure on the optic

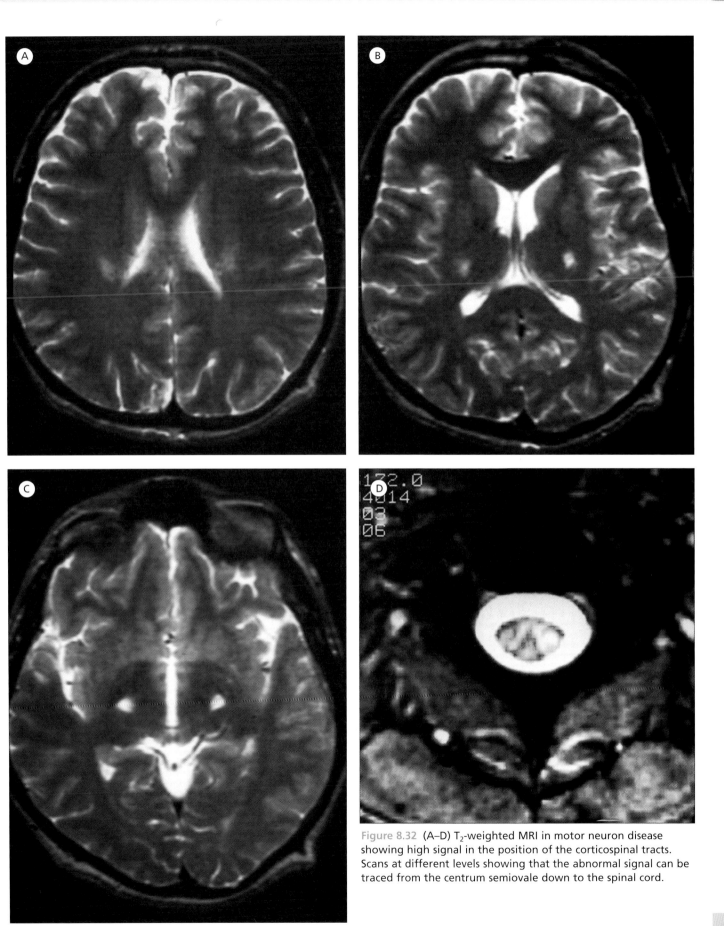

Figure 8.32 (A–D) T$_2$-weighted MRI in motor neuron disease showing high signal in the position of the corticospinal tracts. Scans at different levels showing that the abnormal signal can be traced from the centrum semiovale down to the spinal cord.

Table 8.11 **Isolated or monosymptomatic central nervous system syndromes**
Spinal cord syndromes
Chronic
compression
cervical spondylotic myelopathy
Chiari malformation
spinal dural arteriovenous malformation
HTLV-1-associated myelopathy
noncompressive myelopathy
primary lateral sclerosis
amyotrophic lateral sclerosis
Acute
compression
spinal cord stroke
transverse myelitis
acute necrotising myelitis
other myelitides
Visual failure
Acute
anterior ischaemic optic neuropathy
Leber's hereditary optic neuropathy
central serous retinopathy
neuroretinitis
chronic relapsing inflammatory optic neuropathy
paraneoplastic optic neuritis
other disorders
Chronic
Migratory sensory symptoms
Central pontine myelinolysis

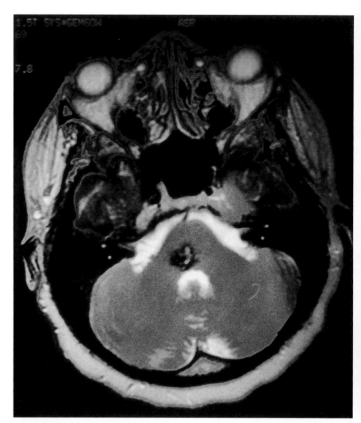

Figure 8.33 T_2-weighted brain MRI showing a cavernous haemangioma of the brainstem. The low signal regions are due to haemosiderin deposition. Kindly provided by Dr Katherine Miszkiel.

nerve from a meningioma, with a central scotoma, occurring during pregnancy with subsequent recovery. This phenomenon can be linked to the presence of female hormone receptors in some forms of intracranial tumour (Poisson 1984). One of our patients (DASC) with olfactory groove meningioma and bilateral papilloedema (in whom the diagnosis of multiple sclerosis did not arise) presented in the puerperium with recurrent headache which developed only on breast feeding.

There is no obvious explanation for the occasional relapsing–remitting course of symptoms attributable to brainstem glioma where the initial symptoms, such as ocular palsies and focal weakness, may remit in a manner indistinguishable from multiple sclerosis (Sarkari and Bickerstaff 1969). A similar remitting course, including the marked day-to-day fluctuations characteristic of multiple sclerosis, has been described in extramedullary tumours located at the foramen magnum (L. Cohen and Macrae 1962).

Vascular anomalies, both arteriovenous malformations and cavernous angiomas, involving the brainstem may present with remitting symptoms and signs diagnosed for many years as multiple sclerosis (Figure 8.33; Sadeh *et al* 1982; Stahl *et al* 1980). Cavernous angiomas are not revealed by angiography but show a characteristic appearance on MRI, with mixed low and signal on T_2-weighted images – the former as a result of local magnetic field inhomogeneity induced by haemosiderin (Requena *et al* 1991). Arachnoid cysts in the foramen magnum may also present with fluctuating symptoms, which often cannot easily be attributed to a single lesion (Lehman and Fieger 1978). Pain is a prominent symptom in reported cases. The symptoms of tumours involving the spinal cord may also fluctuate or remit.

Again, vascular malformations provide the most striking examples. Although less often remarked upon, spontaneous remission is also described for the symptoms and signs of other spinal cord tumours (Hirschbiegel 1967). The presence of a structural lesion, amenable to surgical treatment or some other form of intervention, should be assumed until proved otherwise. Although these patients may turn out to have primary progressive multiple sclerosis (see Chapters 6 and 7), there is no excuse for failing to exclude the structural lesion and this error rightly exposes the unwary physician to medico-legal attention.

Structural and noninflammatory infectious spinal cord syndromes

The principles of how the clinical features and course of anatomically discrete syndromes can be confused with multiple sclerosis, and the issues that arise with respect to overlapping disorders, are well exemplified by consideration of conditions affecting the spinal cord.

Spinal cord compression

The highly important distinction between progressive spinal multiple sclerosis and compression of the spinal cord should now usually be possible without recourse to invasive procedures. Myelography is no longer required unless MRI is contraindicated or not available. In young adults where confusion can easily arise with multiple sclerosis, many causes of compression (neurofibroma, meningioma or prolapsed intervertebral disc) are benign and amenable to surgery if diagnosed in time. Although S. Poser *et al* (1978) attempted to determine whether the spinal form of multiple sclerosis can reliably be distinguished on clinical grounds from other forms of spinal cord disease, they could offer little guidance. In practice, features more suggestive of spinal cord compression than multiple sclerosis are a reproducible and crisp cutaneous sensory level, root pain and segmental muscle wasting. A high index of suspicion is the best safeguard against error.

Investigation must be directed to the site of the lesion (Figure 8.34), and spinal cord MRI is the essential diagnostic investigation (Figure 8.35). It is not permissible to diagnose multiple sclerosis on the basis of progressive paraplegia and delay of the visual evoked potentials, in the absence of clear clinical evidence

for multiple lesions, and until a structural lesion has formally been excluded (Figure 8.36). The report of multiple cerebral white matter lesions on MRI, thought to be consistent with multiple sclerosis, in two patients subsequently shown to have thoracic extramedullary spinal tumours (Salvi *et al* 1992) will not surprise the experienced neurologist. We deal later with the tricky issue of double diagnoses.

Cervical spondylotic myelopathy

The cardinal feature of spondylotic myelopathy is spastic paraparesis, not differing in any important respect from that of multiple sclerosis. The distinction is made even more difficult by the undoubted fact that the two conditions may coexist (Figure 8.37). This was shown conclusively by Brain and Wilkinson (1957) who suggested that damage to the cord caused by spondylosis favoured the formation of plaques in that region. It was believed by D.Oppenheimer (1978) that traction through the denticulate ligaments was responsible for the localization of plaques in the lateral columns of the cervical spinal cord (see Chapters 4 and 12). However, while MRI studies confirm that spondylotic compression and intrinsic cord lesions of multiple sclerosis both have a predilection for the mid-cervical cord, the demyelinating lesions are usually not located at the precise level of the external compression (Kidd *et al* 1993; Thorpe *et al* 1993). Using modern diagnostic techniques, Burgerman *et al* (1992) identified six patients with both conditions, two of whom benefited from surgery.

In view of the known association, it is not entirely realistic to list features thought to differentiate one condition from the other. Patients with spondylotic myelopathy are apt to be older and disturbance of sphincter control is a late symptom. Pain and loss of tendon reflexes in the upper limbs are less helpful in diagnosis than might be expected.

Chiari malformation

Type 1 Chiari malformation, in which ectopic cerebellar tissue passes through the foramen magnum into the cervical canal, may present in adult life in the absence of skeletal deformity of the skull or neck (Figure 7.39). In the majority of individuals with cerebellar ectopia, the clinical syndrome does not resemble multiple sclerosis but is that of syringomyelia or hydrocephalus. In a proportion, however, the predominant signs are cerebellar ataxia, spastic weakness of the limbs and nystagmus, under which circumstances the diagnosis of multiple sclerosis may naturally be considered (Mohr *et al* 1977). The occurrence of trigeminal neuralgia and Lhermitte's symptom and sign increase the resemblance (Banerji and Millar 1974). There has been a report of delayed visual evoked potentials in cerebellar ectopia (W.I. McDonald and Halliday 1977). Internuclear ophthalmoplegia is a feature of the more severe type 2 Chiari malformation, which is unlikely to be mistaken for multiple sclerosis (A.C. Arnold *et al* 1990), but also occurs in type 1 malformations where it may cause diagnostic confusion (Rudick *et al* 1986). The nystagmus is often vertical, and most characteristically down beat – a distinct abnormality of eye movement alerting clinicians to lesions of the foramen magnum, paraneoplastic disease and multiple sclerosis (see Chapter 6). Definitive diagnosis can be established by MRI, and CT/myelography is no longer necessary.

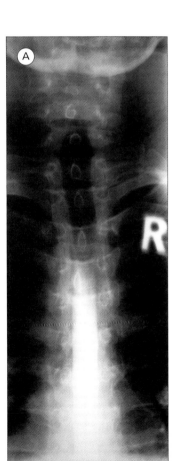
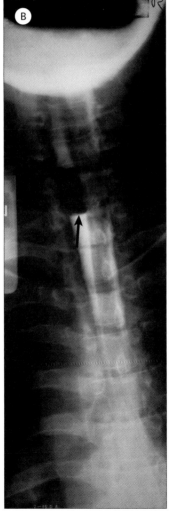

Figure 8.34 Diagnosis of multiple sclerosis corrected in a patient with a slowly progressive spinal syndrome (due to spinal meningioma). (A) Contrast radiology had not been carried up to the level indicated by the clinical history and signs. (B) The lesion was demonstrated once the appropriate level was studied on the myelogram. This is perhaps of historical interest, since nowadays this diagnosis would invariably be made using MRI, but nonetheless makes an important clinical and anatomical point.

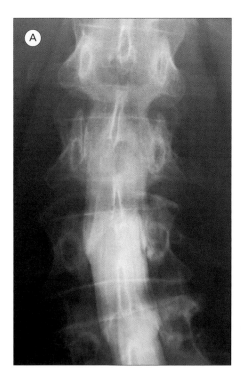

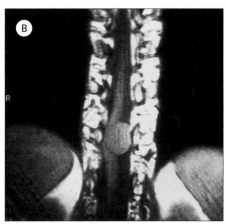

Figure 8.35 Erroneous diagnosis of multiple sclerosis made in the context of a slowly progressive spinal syndrome. (A) Investigation by myelography. (B) Corrected (to spinal meningioma) more easily by access to MRI.

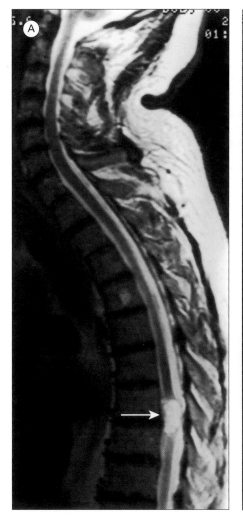

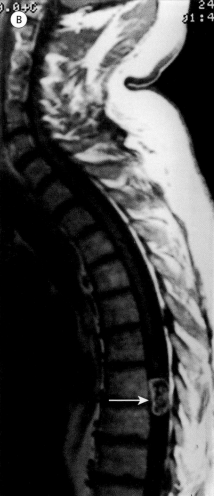

Figure 8.36 (A) T$_2$-weighted and (B) gadolinium enhanced T$_1$-weighted MRI of a meningioma causing compression of the thoracic spinal cord (arrows). Kindly provided by Dr Katherine Miszkiel.

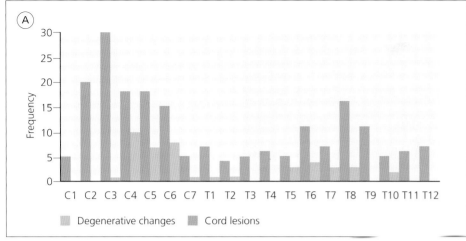

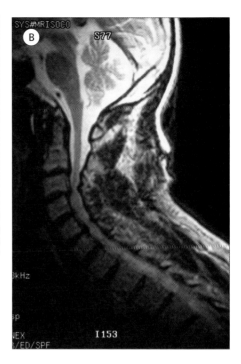

Figure 8.37 (A) Frequency of lesions due to multiple sclerosis adjacent to each vertebral body in the patient population alongside the incidence of degenerative changes (disc protrusion or osteophyte formation). From D. Kidd *et al* (1993) with permission. (B) Narrowing of the cervical canal as a result of spondylosis in a patient with primary progressive multiple sclerosis. Kindly provided by Dr Nagui Antoun. See also Figure 7.52C.

Spinal dural arteriovenous malformation

This condition most often affects middle-aged males. The presentation is with a progressive, often asymmetric, spastic paraparesis, evolving over months to years. There may be some diurnal or exercise-related fluctuation in symptoms. Progressive signs are often preceded by transient episodes of weakness, sensory loss or sphincter disturbance, without accompanying pain (Aminoff and Logue 1974; Cardon *et al* 1992; Dhopesh and Weinstein 1977; Symon *et al* 1984). In addition to pyramidal tract signs, quadriceps wasting and loss of a knee or ankle jerk provides evidence for lower motor neuron involvement at the lumbosacral level. This combination of features is explained by the fact that dural arteriovenous malformations most often occur in the thoraco-lumbar region and involve the conus as well as upper motor neuron fibres. The report that three of 11 (27%) patients with spinal arteriovenous malformations had cerebrospinal fluid oligoclonal bands (O. Cohen *et al* 2000) indicates the potential for incorrect diagnosis if undue significance is attached to spinal fluid abnormalities. However, the crucial diagnostic investigation is a good quality MRI scan of the thoraco-lumbar region. In most instances, multiple small serpiginous signal voids are seen predominantly over the dorsal aspect of the cord (Figure 8.38). These dilated veins are virtually pathognomonic of arteriovenous malformation. Because they are sometimes subtle and not readily visualized, formal spinal arteriography is usually required to confirm the diagnosis (Figure 8.39). Other frequent MRI findings are swelling and increased T_2 signal of the lower cord as a result of venous stasis and oedema, and gadolinium enhancement involving vessels or cord. The malformation is often effectively treated by angiographic embolization or in some instances by surgical removal.

Tropical spastic paraplegia: HTLV-1-associated myelopathy

The clinical features of HTLV-1-associated myelopathy do not resemble those of relapsing–remitting multiple sclerosis but can closely mimic the chronic progressive form of the disease. The age incidence of HTLV-1 myelopathy and the progressive myelopathic form of multiple sclerosis are similar. Mean age at onset of symtoms was 46 years in one series of patients with HTLV-1 myelopathy (J.K. Cruickshank *et al* 1989), whereas the mean age of onset in primary progressive multiple sclerosis is 40 years (A.J. Thompson *et al* 2000). Pain in the back and distally in the legs is common at onset and bladder symptoms occur early. Spastic weakness may initially be unilateral but is eventually symmetrical. Tendon reflexes are increased in the upper limbs but the ankle jerks are sometimes absent. Sensory symptoms in the lower limbs are constantly present. Abnormalities of the cranial nerves are exceedingly rare. There are no remissions but after slow progression the condition may arrest. The condition progresses quite rapidly in a few individuals (Lima *et al* 2005).

The cerebrospinal fluid contains oligoclonal IgG but, in contrast to multiple sclerosis, bands are also present in serum (Link *et al* 1989; C.M. Poser *et al* 1990). A positive serological test for syphilis is common. Adult T-cell leukaemia cells (a result of HTLV-1 infection) are occasionally seen in blood or spinal fluid. Visual evoked potentials are often symmetrically delayed (P. Rudge *et al* 1991). MRI shows white matter lesions in the cerebrum but the brainstem is relatively spared and no lesions are seen in the cerebellum (P. Rudge *et al* 1991). Spinal MRI reveals thoracic cord atrophy (A.K. Howard *et al* 2003). Antibodies to HTLV-1 are present in blood and cerebrospinal fluid.

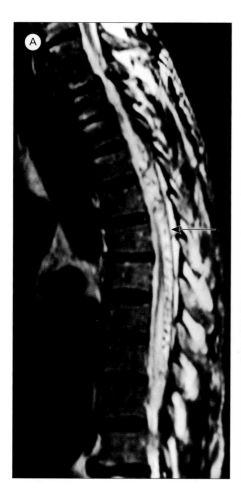

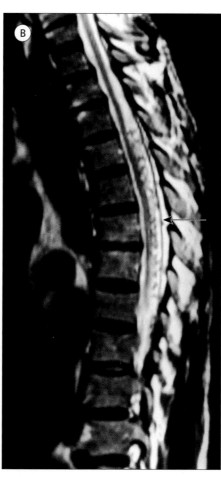

Figure 8.38 T₂-weighted sagittal MRI showing a spinal dural arteriovenous malformation. (A,B) Dilated veins over the dorsal thoracolumbar cord are seen as areas of serpiginous signal void on two consecutive slices. Kindly provided by Dr Katherine Miszkiel.

Myelopathy occurs predominantly in people inhabiting or coming from areas where HTLV-1 is endemic, particularly the West Indies and Japan, but sporadic cases have been reported from many countries (Gessain and Gout 1992). The virus can be transmitted by sexual contact, blood transfusion and intravenous drug abuse (Janssen *et al* 1991), but only a small minority of those infected will develop myelopathy. A condition with some similarities to Devic's disease is described in eight HTLV-1 negative women from the West Indies with recurrent episodes of spinal cord or visual involvement and endocrinopathies. Imaging showed cavitation of the spinal cord with few cerebral lesions and autopsy revealed inflammation and demyelination (Vernant *et al* 1997).

Noncompressive progressive myelopathy

Chronic progressive paraparesis presents a common problem of differential diagnosis and causes such as cervical spondylotic myelopathy, tropical spastic paraplegia and spinal cord compression have been considered above. In countries where multiple sclerosis is prevalent, this is the commonest cause of progressive noncompressive paraparesis. Thus, of 223 Danish patients with spastic paraparesis, either isolated or as part of more widespread disease, 129 (58%) were diagnosed as having multiple sclerosis on first admission to hospital (Hübbe and Dam 1973).

Conversely, only six of 32 undiagnosed cases (19%) were found to have multiple sclerosis on prolonged follow-up. Marshall (1955) reported multiple sclerosis at autopsy in 34% of a similar series of patients. A positive diagnosis at time of presentation is now possible in a higher proportion of patients as a result of the emergence of several key paraclinical investigations over the last 30 years: specifically, evoked potentials, cerebrospinal fluid examination for oligoclonal bands, and MRI.

When they were introduced, it was naturally hoped that the inexpensive and noninvasive techniques of evoked potential recording would reliably indicate disseminated disease in the context of a progressive spinal syndrome. Re-reading this literature shows that in the most extensive assessment of visual evoked potentials in undiagnosed spinal cord disease (Blumhardt *et al* 1982), abnormalities were found in 36% of 64 patients with chronic progressive paraparesis and in 33% of 38 with chronic relapsing myelopathy. It is not known, of course, how many patients actually had multiple sclerosis. Paty *et al* (1979) investigated 72 patients with chronic progressive myelopathy, using evoked potentials, spinal fluid examination and CT brain scanning. Oligoclonal bands were present in 44%, abnormal evoked potentials in 35% and imaging abnormalities (nearly all merely consisting of diffuse atrophy without focal lesions) in 50%. No firm conclusions on the distinction between the group with multiple sclerosis and those with other diseases seemed apparent.

extramedullary tumours. As experience in the use of MRI has increased, criteria for the diagnosis of primary progressive multiple sclerosis have been proposed that incorporate specific brain and spinal cord imaging findings in patients presenting with progressive myelopathy (A.J. Thompson *et al* 2000).

One other condition, first described in the 19th century, to emerge intact from the syndrome of progressive paraplegias is primary lateral sclerosis (Pringle *et al* 1992a). The late onset may prove sufficient to make the distinction from multiple sclerosis but there is overlap with primary progressive spinal demyelination. The absence of a family history or signs of upper motor neuron lesions dating from childhood (*pes cavus*) helps to distinguish this condition from the hereditary spastic paraplegias. Spastic weakness of the legs is soon associated with generalized spino-bulbar involvement, producing pseudobulbar palsy and mimicking motor neuron disease but without muscle atrophy or fasciculations. Smooth following eye movements are often lost and the bladder may be involved, further increasing the similarity to multiple sclerosis. MRI does not show white matter abnormalities, although focal atrophy of the precentral gyrus has been reported on sagittal T_1-weighted images, and (as expected) central motor conduction times are prolonged (Pringle *et al* 1992a). Oligoclonal bands are not present in the cerebrospinal fluid.

The early manifestation of widespread lower motor neuron involvement, both clinically and on electromyography, will usually prevent confusion between the classical form of motor neuron disease, amyotrophic lateral sclerosis and multiple sclerosis. A few cases that evolve to typical motor neuron disease nevertheless have an initial phase in which the manifestations exclusively affect upper motor neurons. In about 70% of patients, MRI reveals symmetrical high signal confined to the corticospinal tracts in the centrum semiovale, internal capsule, cerebral peduncles, pons and upper cervical cord (Thorpe *et al* 1996c). Such findings are unlike those seen in multiple sclerosis and give a clue to the correct diagnosis.

Acute spinal cord compression

It is self evident that when a patient presents with an acute clinically isolated and hitherto unexplained spinal cord syndrome, the first and foremost priority must be to identify any surgically treatable compressive lesion – intervertebral disc protrusion, extradural abscess or haematoma. Immediate MRI should be performed, followed by neurosurgical referral if compression is found. The success of surgical decompression is inversely related to the period during which compression has been present. That said, patients presenting with the Brown-Séquard or conus medullaris syndromes in whom spinal cord compression or central lumbo-sacral disc prolapse are the presumed causes until proved otherwise, not infrequently turn out to have demyelinating lesions. However, to make that diagnosis without first formally excluding a structural lesion is inexcusable.

Spinal cord stroke

Infarction of the cord may result from overt cardiovascular disease – bacterial endocarditis, aortic aneurysm or rupture of an arteriovenous malformation, or a profound drop in blood pressure – but may also occur for no detectable reason, even at

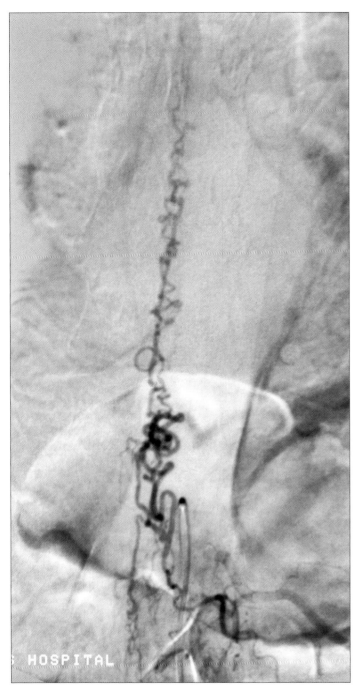

Figure 8.39 Spinal arteriography in a male aged 52 years with a progressive paraparesis and unstable bladder as a result of spinal arteriovenous malformation showing filling through the lower intercostal branches. Kindly provided by Dr Nagui Antoun.

As expected, MRI has proved more informative (Figure 8.40). D.H. Miller *et al* (1987a) showed that 18/29 patients with chronic progressive paraparesis had changes typical of multiple sclerosis on MRI of the head and a further three had single lesions. Of 33 patients with chronic relapsing myelopathy, 25 had typical changes of multiple sclerosis and one had a single lesion. The method was very much more sensitive than recording evoked potentials. It is of interest that of the 130 patients originally referred for this investigation, nine were found to have compressive lesions, including two with

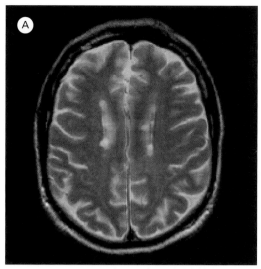

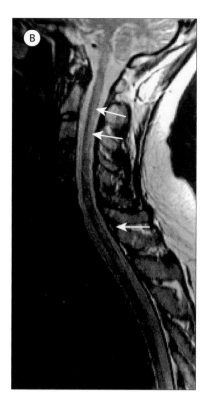

Figure 8.40 T$_2$-weighted MRI in a 40-year-old with a clinically isolated progressive spastic paraplegia. There are multiple cerebral white matter and spinal cord lesions suggesting demyelination. (A) Brain and (B) spinal cord (lesions arrowed).

autopsy (H.L. Lipton and Teasdell 1973). A few cases are the result of fibrocartilaginous embolism after the nucleus pulposus of an intervertebral disc has herniated into an adjacent vertebra. The infarction can be confined to the territory of the anterior spinal artery on one side, resulting in a partial Brown-Séquard syndrome, with sparing of the posterior columns. Multiple sclerosis may also present with any one of these spinal syndromes (D.H. Miller *et al* 1987a), but the onset is usually less abrupt, the neurological deficit less severe and the prognosis for recovery from the episode in question rather better.

Transverse myelitis

An acute or subacute lesion of the spinal cord is a classic presentation of multiple sclerosis and yet this syndrome has other causes which, despite in some situations leaving the patient severely disabled, do not recur. The history of early accounts, starting with Charlton Bastian (1882; 1910), and subsequent clinical descriptions and ideas on the aetiology and pathogenesis are given by Krishnan and Kerr (2005). A comprehensive recent review discusses the presentation, investigation, diagnosis and management of transverse myelitis and offers a set of criteria to distinguish idiopathic cases from those with a recognized cause (Transverse Myelitis Consortium Working Group 2002). Another review considers the differential diagnosis and management of acute myelopathies including transverse myelitis (Kaplin *et al* 2005). The vexed question of Devic's disease is discussed in Chapters 5 and 6, and the ways in which modern imaging techniques have greatly assisted the recognition of compressive lesions is covered in Chapter 7. It is unusual, but not exceptional, for systemic disease manifesting as acute myelitis to occur in the absence of evidence for disease of other organs, although this may not be recognized before the onset of para-

plegia. Systemic lupus erythematosus and the other systemic diseases discussed above, infarction of the spinal cord, and parainfectious myelitis (acute disseminated encephalomyelitis) can all present as myelitis. An association of transverse myelitis with primary biliary cirrhosis has also been reported (Papadopoulos *et al* 2005).

Onset may be acute or subacute in acute inflammatory demyelination of the spinal cord and, from the clinical perspective, the process often ascends or spreads transversely (J.T. Hughes 1978). The diagnosis of transverse myelitis is usually made by exclusion and, as with acute disseminated encephalomyelitis in adults, the precipitating cause is seldom identified. However, clinical and laboratory criteria can usefully distinguish the various causes. The relationship of isolated spinal demyelination to multiple sclerosis is complex, as with more generalized forms of inflammatory central nervous system disease. Cord lesions due to multiple sclerosis are usually partial, sometimes conforming to the Brown-Séquard syndrome, but acute or subacute cord lesions may occur that exactly mimic transverse myelitis. This term is usually reserved for patients in whom the spinal lesion does not recur but the distinction may not be easy in the acute stage. The most reliable indicator is the presence of spinal shock in the acute monophasic lesion (McAlpine 1931). T.F. Scott *et al* (1998) emphasize that symmetry of the motor and sensory manifestations of acute spinal cord disease usefully identifies the patient with transverse myelitis, whereas spinal involvement in multiple sclerosis is usually asymmetric. Defined in this way, they report a low conversion rate from transverse myelitis to multiple sclerosis. Even though a monophasic episode of cord inflammation may result in persistent disability, many patients, including those with severe myelitis, recover fully and without sequelae (Altrocchi 1963; Berman *et al* 1981; H.L. Lipton and Teasdell 1973). MRI

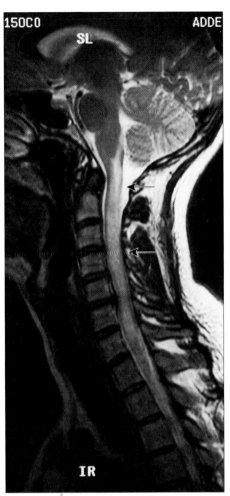

Figure 8.41 Swelling and high T$_2$-weighted signal in the cervical cord and medulla (arrows) from a patient with acute transverse myelitis. Kindly provided by Dr Nagui Antoun.

of the brain sometimes shows asymptomatic areas of abnormal signal in the white matter. The predictive value of such changes for the later development of multiple sclerosis is discussed in Chapter 7. In transverse myelitis, the acute cord lesion is typically extensive, involving multiple cord segments (Figure 8.41), whereas in multiple sclerosis the cord lesions are usually small.

Acute necrotizing myelitis

The original description of necrotizing myelitis was in men, rather older than most cases of transverse myelitis, and with slowly progressive lumbar cord disease occurring in association with chronic respiratory disease (Foix and Alajouanine 1926). The term acute necrotizing myelitis can reasonably be applied to patients developing severe inflammation of the thoracic or spinal cord, in whom flaccid areflexic paraplegia with anaesthesia and loss of sphincter control progresses rapidly over hours (H.I. Hoffman 1955). Inflammation is sufficient to cause severe pain with meningism and systemic symptoms, including pyrexia. The clinical presentation suggests cord compression. Contrast radiology or imaging often reveal a swollen cord with spinal block. Since the cerebrospinal fluid shows a marked polymorphonuclear pleocytosis, raised protein and lowered glucose

concentrations, these patients are frequently thought to have pyogenic or tuberculous infection of the central nervous system and are treated with appropriate antimicrobial therapy. In some cases surgical exploration is undertaken to exclude intraspinal abscess. Because of the possibility of infection, there is often a reluctance to use corticosteroids but the course of acute necrotizing myelitis may be significantly influenced by high-dose intravenous methylprednisolone. Acute necrotizing myelitis has an appreciable mortality but in survivors the systemic features resolve within weeks, leaving significant handicap and disability. One of our patients (DASC), a 14-year-old girl with acute necrotizing myelitis in whom complete functional cervical cord transection was associated with spinal block due to cord swelling, meningism, pyrexia and a marked polymorphonuclear pleocytosis with reduced glucose, eventually made a complete and stable recovery, apart from minor bladder instability, after treatment with high-dose intravenous methylprednisolone. She remains well more than 15 years later. Conversely, another adult female patient with signs of functional cord transection due to acute necrotizing myelitis, made no useful recovery and soon developed acute demyelination of the dominant hemisphere manifesting as aphasia with hemiplegia, followed by brainstem symptoms and other features of the Marburg variant of multiple sclerosis from which she died within a few years of presentation.

Many organisms have been implicated by association in the aetiology of acute necrotizing myelitis (Table 8.12). Acute necrotizing myelitis is also described after rabies vaccination, as a complication of acute lymphocytic leukaemias, lymphoma, hypernephroma and other forms of carcinoma, and in acquired immunodeficiency syndrome (Bassoe and Grinker 1930; Britton *et al* 1985; Grisold *et al* 1980; Lester *et al* 1979; Mancall and Rosales 1964; Ojeda 1984). When acute necrotizing myelitis has occurred in association with tuberculosis (R.A.C. Hughes and Mair 1977), along with pleocytosis and glycorrhaccic changes that often occur in cerebrospinal fluid, it is not surprising that these patients are usually treated with antituberculous therapy, at least until bacteriological results are available.

A syndrome of progressive necrotic myelopathy has been recently described by J.D. Katz and Ropper (2000). Nine adult patients were reported in whom acute or subacute episodes of worsening occurred every few months leading to paraplegia or tetraplegia. There was evidence of flaccid, areflexic weakness, denervation over several spinal segments, and atrophy or cavitation of the cord in the chronic stage (although during acute episodes the cord was swollen and displayed gadolinium enhancement over several segments). In six patients, there were neither cerebrospinal fluid oligoclonal bands nor brain MRI abnormalities but two had prolonged visual evoked potentials. The condition worsened in spite of immunomodulatory therapy, and in two patients in whom pathological data were obtained there was evidence for cord necrosis. The authors suggest that these cases were indistinguishable from a limited form of Devic's disease.

Other forms of myelitis

The majority of patients with transverse myelitis are not systemically ill and the neurological disorder usually evolves over a few days. Onset with back pain and an ascending level is more frequent than in patients considered to have multiple sclerosis (Jeffrey *et al* 1993). Although the premonitory symptoms

Table 8.12 **Infections associated with acute necrotizing transverse myelitis**

Herpes zoster virus	Hogan and Krigman 1973
Herpes simplex virus type II	Wiley *et al* 1987; Ahmed 1988
Tuberculosis	Hughes and Mair 1977
Coxsackie B4 virus	Ku and Lee 1998
Tuberculin skin testing (PPD0 cytomegalovirus)	Jing *et al* 1998 Giobbia *et al* 1999; Karacostas *et al* 2002; Fux *et al* 2003
Mycoplasma pneumoniae	Parisi and Filice 2001; Goebels *et al* 2001
Burkholderia pseudomallei	Haran *et al* 2001
Coxiella burnetii	Waltereit *et al* 2002
Cladophialophora bantiana	Shields and Castillo 2002
Group B streptococcus	Schimmel *et al* 2002
Pneumococcus	Ben-Dov *et al* 2002
Dengue 2 virus	Leao *et al* 2002
Acinetobacter baumanii[a]	Ubogu *et al* 2003
Borrelia burgdorferi	Lesca *et al* 2002
Babesia microti	Oleson *et al* 2003
Hepatitis C virus	Zandman-Goddard *et al* 2003

a Inadvertently delivered through an intrathecal pump.

are often sensory or sphincter disturbance, in the severe case these are followed by devastating loss of mobility. With time, the weakness increases and may spread to involve one or both arms, usually in an asymmetric pattern and showing the flaccid areflexia characteristic of spinal shock. Sensory loss replaces the paraesthesiae and there is often a band of unpleasant hyperaesthesia at the upper sensory level. As in other cases of incomplete focal spinal disease, this may not accurately reflect the site of spinal affection because of lamination of fibres in the spinothalamic pathways. Sphincter control is lost but unlike those with multiple sclerosis, the patient usually has acute bladder retention rather than urgency or urge incontinence.

The need to exclude a structural cause for subacute cord injury occurring as a manifestation of transverse myelitis means that many patients undergo radiological investigation. Jeffrey *et al* (1993) reported that swelling of the cord was sometimes present in patients categorized as having parainfectious myelitis, but not in multiple sclerosis. However, focal cord swelling can undoubtedly occur in multiple sclerosis, usually limited to only one or two segments and diminishing with follow-up, although complete resolution may take several months. Austin *et al* (1992) found MRI of the cord to be abnormal in only seven of 18 adults with transverse myelitis and the abnormality did not correlate with the cause of the myelitis. When the onset is subacute and accompanied by focal swelling of the spinal cord, the distinction from an intrinsic tumour may be impossible without biopsy (Reznik *et al* 1994), although the overwhelming preference, if myelitis is thought most likely, would be to await follow-up and demonstrate resolution of swelling noninvasively by repeat MRI.

D.H. Miller *et al* (1987a) showed cranial MRI abnormalities typical of multiple sclerosis in 15/30 patients with acute myelitis <50 years and although, on a single scan, acute disseminated encephalomyelitis could not be excluded, the majority of patients had a partial cord syndrome that was more suggestive of multiple sclerosis. In a series of 31 patients from the Middle East with no specific cause identified, there was no radiological evidence for involvement outside the spinal cord and none of the patients developed episodes suggesting more widespread demyelination over the ensuing 9 years (Al Deeb *et al* 1997), suggesting that these were examples of restricted postinfectious encephalomyelitis. It is important to analyse the spinal fluid if myelography is used to exclude cord compression, since spurious changes may later be detected. Lumbar puncture should also be carried out in cases investigated by MRI. The spinal fluid shows an increased mononuclear cell count, numerically intermediate between the marked pleocytosis of acute necrotizing myelitis and the abnormalities seen in patients with multiple sclerosis. The total protein is raised and oligoclonal bands may be present but the glucose is usually normal. Multiple sclerosis and transverse myelitis cannot reliably be distinguished on the basis of changes in cerebrospinal fluid but a cell count >100 lymphocytes/cm^3 is less likely in the former, and cerebrospinal fluid oligoclonal IgG is found inconsistently in patients thought to have parainfectious myelitis (Jeffrey *et al* 1993).

The clinical diagnosis of multiple sclerosis will often only be established by subsequent clinical events. However, to complicate matters, there have been reports of recurrent transverse myelitis without other central nervous system manifestations (Kim 2003; Tippett *et al* 1991). Kim (2003) compared 21 patients with recurrent cord relapses in whom a diagnosis of multiple sclerosis had been made with 15 patients having no evidence clinically or on MRI for involvement outside the spinal cord (called idiopathic recurrent transverse myelitis). Compared with the group with multiple sclerosis, the latter differed by having a male preponderance, an absence of oligo-clonal bands, and a higher frequency of relapses and episodes of transverse myelitis. The cases of recurrent transverse myelitis have a number of features in common with Devic's disease apart from the absence of visual involvement, and one can argue that they should fall within the rubric of multiple sclerosis, albeit with an unusual clinical and immunopathogenic phenotype. The eight cases described by Fukuzawa *et al* (2003), in whom there were recurrent episodes of transverse myelitis associated with additional inflammatory episodes involving the cerebrum and brainstem, are – in our view – best regarded as cases of multiple sclerosis.

Unlike acute disseminated encephalomyelitis, transverse myelitis is more common in adults than children, and in women than men. Since the diagnosis is often made by exclusion, with somewhat unhelpful laboratory abnormalities and bacterio-logical findings, the probability arises that a heterogeneous collection of cases has been included in most large series. Berman *et al* (1981), working from a population base in an attempt to avoid selection bias, found that a high proportion of cases originally designated as transverse myelitis had to be excluded from their study. In the remainder, incidence peaked in the second and third decades with a further bimodal increase in patients aged over 70 years. Infection was reported more frequently in younger than older patients. For these two reasons, patients with spinal stroke are sometimes erroneously diagnosed as having transverse myelitis, and this is especially problematic in patients with sensory signs indicating an anterior cord lesion. Formerly, meningovascular syphilis was regarded as an impor-tant cause of acute myelitis whereas the more recent literature is replete with examples of transverse myelitis complicating col-lagen vascular disease.

De Séze *et al* (2001c) reviewed the clinical and laboratory fea-tures and outcome profiles of 79 patients presenting with an acute myelopathy. The patients were classified into six diag-nostic categories: multiple sclerosis (34 examples), systemic dis-ease (13, including cases of systemic lupus erythematosus and Sjögren's syndrome), spinal cord infarction (11), parainfectious myelopathy (5), delayed radiation myelopathy (3), and cases of unknown origin (13). A motor deficit was more frequent and spinal cord MRI lesions were more extensive in the systemic disease and spinal cord infarction groups when compared with multiple sclerosis. The five patients with parainfectious myelopathy all had extensive cord lesions and four exhibited swelling and gadolinium enhancement. All three patients with delayed radiation myelopathy had a long lesion associated with gadolinium enhancement and – in two cases – swelling of the cord. Brain lesions were predictably more common in mul-tiple sclerosis (68%) but were also seen in 31% with a systemic disease. Whereas 88% with multiple sclerosis had oligoclonal bands in their cerebrospinal fluid, these were present in only 17% of the systemic disease group and in none of the patients with spinal cord infarction. Clinical outcome at 12 months was classified as good in 88% with multiple sclerosis, but poor or fair in 91% with spinal cord infarction and 77% with systemic diseases.

A further study compared MRI findings in nine patients with acute transverse myelitis and 13 with myelitis as a manifestation of multiple sclerosis (Bakshi *et al* 1998). In the former group, long lesions involving multiple cord segments were character-istic whereas in the latter group the lesions involved on average only one or two segments of cord. Swelling of the cord was seen equally in both groups. Brain MRI was normal in 78% with acute transverse myelitis but in only 15% with multiple sclerosis.

The series reported by Berman *et al* (1981) is probably repre-sentative with respect to prognosis in acute transverse myelitis. Sixty-eight per cent of patients in whom follow-up information was available made an adequate recovery over the ensuing 3 months. Three died and 14 were left with significant persistent disability. Only one patient subsequently developed multiple sclerosis. Preceding infection was reported in only one-third of patients, the majority of whom had upper respiratory infection, other causes being herpes zoster or simplex virus infection, hepatitis and smallpox vaccination. Kalita *et al* (1998) reported that a poorer outcome of acute transverse myelitis was associated with severe weakness and denervation on elec-tromyography. Devinsky *et al* (1991) described the clinico-pathological findings in nine fatal cases of herpes zoster myelitis resulting from direct infection of oligodendrocytes and occur-ring in association with immune suppression. They emphasized the 12-day interval between appearance of the cutaneous rash and the onset of neurological symptoms, with vertical and hori-zontal spread producing motor involvement and a tendency to spare the posterior columns. Tyler *et al* (1986) listed the fol-lowing viral causes of transverse myelitis in man: picornaviruses, togaviruses, retroviruses, orthomyxoviruses, paramyxoviruses, bunyaviruses, arenaviruses, rhabdoviruses, hepatitis viruses, herpes viruses and poxviruses. Isolated case reports emphasize the occurrence of transverse myelitis after infection with hepa-titis A, hepatitis C (Annunziata *et al* 2005), cytomegalovirus, herpes simplex type 2, toxoplasmosis, schistosomiasis, *Borrelia* and *Coxiella* (see also Lesca *et al* 2002; Waltereit *et al* 2002). Epstein–Barr virus infection has resulted in cases of myeloradi-culitis and encephalomyeloradiculitis with the presence of viral DNA in cerebrospinal fluid suggesting a direct infectious mech-anism. The clinical outcome for four such recently reported cases was variable (Majid *et al* 2002).

Visual failure

There are innumerable infective, toxic or physical causes of optic nerve disease that are unlikely to be confused with multiple sclerosis. Several rare causes due to systemic disease resulting in diagnostic difficulty have already been discussed above under a number of headings.

Anterior ischaemic optic neuropathy

Although anterior ischaemic optic neuropathy is generally held to be easily diagnosed, it may in fact be difficult to distinguish from optic neuritis in the absence of arteritis (Figure 8.42; Rizzo and Lessell 1991) found a considerable degree of overlap between the clinical features of these conditions. Ischaemic optic neuropathy generally affects older people and the sex inci-dence does not show the female preponderance characteristic of multiple sclerosis and optic neuritis. Pain in the eye is more frequent in optic neuritis, and disc swelling is almost invariable in ischaemic neuropathy. The onset of visual loss is usually

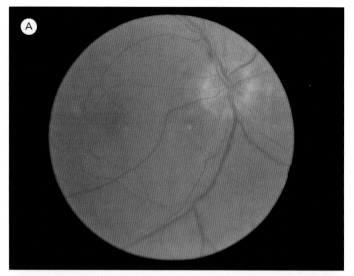

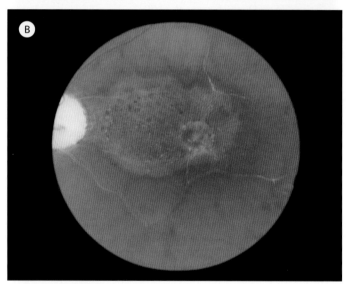

Figure 8.42 (A) Acute optic disc swelling in ischaemic optic neuropathy. (B) Late nerve fibre bundle atrophy following acute embolic ischaemic optic neuropathy.

abrupt, with little progression in ischaemic optic neuropathy, but the initial severity of visual loss is highly variable and not dissimilar in both conditions. A central scotoma is more often found in optic neuritis whereas a sector defect, often altitudinal and with an arcuate component, characterizes ischaemia. That said, the two conditions cannot reliably be distinguished by their visual field defects (W.I. McDonald and Barnes 1992). Much greater improvement of visual acuity is usual after the acute event in cases of optic neuritis.

Leber's hereditary optic neuropathy

Leber's hereditary optic neuropathy occurs predominantly in men. Typically, visual loss evolves synchronously in each eye, progressing more slowly than in bilateral demyelinating optic neuritis. In some patients with Leber's disease, visual loss in each eye occurs consecutively after a brief interval. Pain on eye movement and Uhthoff's phenomenon may each occur but these features are less frequent than in demyelinating optic

neuritis (Riordan-Eva *et al* 1995). A centro-caecal scotoma is characteristic (Nikoskelainen *et al* 1977). Retinal microangiopathy and swelling of the optic disc may be observed in the acute stages of visual failure but are far from constant and seldom persist (Riordan-Eva *et al* 1995), and fluorescein angiography does not show leakage at the disc. Inheritance is strictly maternal and descendants of male patients are not affected. The molecular defect is a pathological point mutation in mitochondrial DNA (Wallace *et al* 1988). Several are described, one in particular (the 14484 point mutation) being associated with relatively good visual recovery: 71% with this mutation had a final visual acuity of at least 6/24 in one large series (Riordan-Eva *et al* 1995). Harding's disease (see *McAlpine's Multiple Sclerosis* 3rd edition, page 135; Harding *et al* 1992) and its relationship to multiple sclerosis are described in Chapters 3 and 6.

Central serous choroidoretinopathy

Optic neuritis may be closely mimicked by central serous choroidoretinopathy. This affects young adults, especially males, causing unilateral blurred vision but only slight loss of acuity and no impairment of colour vision. There is often distorted perception of straight lines, which gives the clue that the problem is of retinal not optic nerve origin. The pupillary light reflex is not affected. Changes at the fovea may be difficult to identify ophthalmoscopically and fluorescein angiography is often helpful. Multiple sclerosis is wrongly diagnosed on the basis of presumed optic neuritis and unreliable soft neurological signs (Krauscher and Miller 1982). The probability that this condition has been confused with optic neuritis in some series, accounting for the lower than expected conversion rate to multiple sclerosis after an episode of visual loss, is described in Chapter 6.

Neuroretinitis

The presentation of neuroretinitis resembles optic neuritis even more closely than central serous choroidoretinopathy. Rapid visual loss is accompanied by pain in the eye or headache. The optic disc is swollen. Some patients report vague sensory or bladder symptoms. The clue to diagnosis is the presence of a macular star, either at onset or within 2 weeks. This condition has been thought not to be related to multiple sclerosis (Parmley *et al* 1987) but the rarity of the disorder is such that there have been no large studies of its natural history.

Chronic relapsing inflammatory optic neuropathy (CRION)

Some patients who present with recurrent episodes of optic neuritis appear, on closer inspection, to have a distinct inflammatory disorder that has recently been designated chronic relapsing inflammatory optic neuropathy (CRION; Hickman *et al* 2002b; D. Kidd *et al* 2003). Characteristic features are acute severe visual loss associated with particularly severe and persistent orbital pain that requires powerful analgesia. The optic neuritis may be unilateral or simultaneously bilateral. Gadolinium enhanced MRI may reveal extensive swelling and enhancement of the optic nerve although this can also be seen in typical cases of optic neuritis. Brain MRI is normal. Spontaneous recovery is unusual but visual recovery may occur with early institution of high-dose intravenous methylprednisolone followed by a tapering dose of oral corticosteriods. Relapse sometimes occurs as the dose is reduced. Long-term immunosuppression is often used to prevent these relapses and modify the course of the disorder. The clinical picture is reminiscent of that encountered in granulomatous optic neuropathy but, in cases diagnosed as CRION, there is no clinical or laboratory evidence for systemic sarcoidosis even after prolonged follow-up (Kidd *et al* 2003).

Paraneoplastic optic neuritis

Both optic neuritis and retinitis occur as paraneoplastic syndromes. Presentation of optic neuritis is with subacute visual loss and disc swelling, accompanied by evidence of retinitis and vitreous cells (Figure 8.31). The disorder is associated with IgG antibody to collapsin response mediator protein-5 (CRMP-5) and most patients are smokers with an underlying small cell lung carcinoma (S.A. Cross *et al* 2003). There is a cerebrospinal fluid pleocytosis with oligoclonal bands, and a variety of associated neurological features indicating a more diffuse encephalo-myelo-radiculo-neuronitis.

Progressive visual failure

Progressive visual failure as the initial and sole manifestation of multiple sclerosis should be accepted only with the greatest reservation (see Chapter 6). Potential pitfalls for the neurologist who assumes that demyelinating disease is the correct explanation for progressive loss of vision are considerable (Ormerod and McDonald 1984). High resolution imaging of the optic nerves and chiasm with CT and/or MRI is mandatory to exclude a compressive lesion. Occasional instances of progressive bilateral (Ormerod and McDonald 1984) or unilateral (Eidelberg *et al* 1988) optic neuropathy do nevertheless occur, albeit uncommonly, in multiple sclerosis. These constitute unusual variants of primary progressive multiple sclerosis.

Sensory symptoms

Patients with the harmless condition of migrant sensory neuritis (named eponymously after Wartenberg) are usually diagnosed as having multiple sclerosis on the basis of disseminated, remitting, sensory changes, but the symptoms are quite distinctive (Matthews and Esiri 1983). They apparently arise from the stretching of cutaneous nerves. The characteristic sequence is of a brief searing pain, clearly perceived as superficial, in a strictly localized area of an extremity, occurring during rapid movement of the limb. This is followed by blunting of cutaneous sensation in the same area. This always involves the distribution of a cutaneous nerve and is never segmental or extensive. The frequently involved nerves are digital, sural, terminal radial and ulnar and the patellar plexus. Remission occurs within a few weeks but further episodes, affecting different nerves, are common and may be interpreted as confirming an erroneous diagnosis of multiple sclerosis. Our former colleague and author of this book let it be known that he was a martyr to this complaint (Bryan Matthews, personal communication).

Surprisingly, it seems that the prodromal sensory symptoms of migraine, undoubtedly relapsing–remitting, can be mistaken for those of multiple sclerosis (T.J. Murray and Murray 1984).

Central pontine myelinolysis

This is a noninflammatory demyelinating disorder that involves the central pontine tegmentum. It is entirely unrelated to multiple sclerosis. Central pontine myelinolysis usually presents in the context of a major electrolyte disturbance, most often hyponatraemia that has been rapidly corrected. There may be evidence of poor nutrition or alcohol abuse and it has been seen in association with hyperemesis gravidarum. Within 10–14 days of over zealous correction of the serum sodium, the patient develops a severe neurological deficit over a few days with quadriparesis and pseudobulbar palsy. This can proceed to the locked-in state. In other instances there are few or no symptoms, the diagnosis being made on the basis of a characteristic MRI abnormality, high signal on T_2-weighted and low signal on T_1-weighted images of the central pons without gadolinium enhancement or mass effect (Figure 8.43). The demyelination is thought to result from rapid osmotic shifts. With appropriate support, including intensive care and assisted ventilation, most patients will make a good recovery. The MR abnormality also resolves. The characteristic clinical and radiological picture should rarely be confused with an acute episode of brainstem demyelination due to multiple sclerosis.

NON-ORGANIC SYMPTOMS

People who fear that they might have multiple sclerosis and who have read or heard of the symptoms to be expected often complain of fluctuating vision, clumsiness and tingling in the extremities. The time course of these symptoms rarely resembles the relapses and remissions of multiple sclerosis. Blurred vision clears on rubbing or resting the eyes, and the ataxia does not usually result in self injury. The sensory symptoms are sometimes unilateral, and, although it has often been thought that they are more likely to affect the left arm and leg, either side may be involved (J. Stone *et al* 2002). More widespread sensory disturbance may also occur. The sensory symptoms often disappear on re-positioning of the limbs. Tingling persists for periods of a few minutes to half a day and recurs at irregular intervals. Sometimes these symptoms are recognizable as the effects of hyperventilation.

Another type of presentation is the persistent and usually multiple non-organic symptoms and signs found in people who think they have multiple sclerosis, sometimes in response to physical or mental trauma, but in whom no neurological diagnosis is made after thorough examination and investigation. It is sometimes stated that urinary or faecal incontinence are reliable indications of organic disease but this has not been our experience. The physical signs, in addition to the usual collapsing limb weakness as a result of fluctuating effort and simultaneous contraction of agonists and antagonists, can be highly elaborate, including spasmodic involuntary movements. The gait is often profoundly ataxic but with inconsistencies and a bizarre appearance that actually requires considerable athleticism to maintain an upright posture. In those with medical knowledge, the extensor plantar reflexes can deceive even the most experienced neurologist (Hankey and Stewart-Wynne 1988). Unilateral loss of vibration sense over the forehead is a particularly useful sensory finding in some patients with a non-organic disorder. The diagnosis of non-organic or functional disorder requires

435

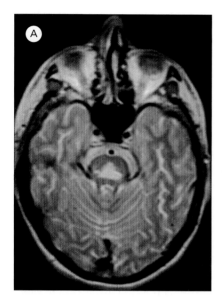

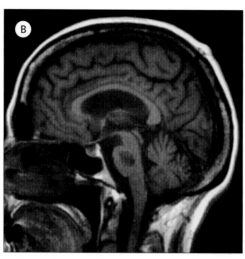

Figure 8.43 (A) T$_2$-weighted and (B) T$_1$-weighted MRI in central pontine myelinolysis show characteristic signal changes in the central pons.

thorough investigation to provide mutual reassurance that there is no associated neurological disorder. The diagnosis of multiple sclerosis becomes unlikely in the presence of normal brain and spinal cord MRI, especially if combined with the absence of oligoclonal bands. But multiple sclerosis will sometimes be diagnosed with confidence and conviction in the absence of laboratory support if the clinical features are considered genuine and appear to have no better explanation. When multiple sclerosis has to be 'un-diagnosed', the situation can be formulated as a somatization disorder and explained to the patient as an abnormality of function with intact structure in the nervous system. These conversations are not easy and often end in distress for the patient apparently denied the prop of an organic explanation for symptoms that are genuinely experienced and seem real enough. Management is difficult, and may involve referral to liaison psychiatry but with uncertain benefits. Prolonged (12-year) follow-up has been recently reported on 60 patients in whom a diagnosis of unilateral functional weakness or sensory disturbance was made (J. Stone *et al* 2003). Of the 42 from whom information was obtained, 35 (83%) reported continued weakness or sensory symptoms and most had limitation of physical function, distress and other somatic symptoms. Patients with sensory symptoms at presentation had a better outcome than those with weakness. Accuracy of the original diagnosis was vindicated and a discrete neurological diagnosis (multiple sclerosis) emerged in only one instance. Assessment is especially difficult in patients who do have multiple sclerosis but in whom the major complaints and disabilities are dominated by elaboration and non-organic manifestations.

HOW ACCURATE IS THE DIAGNOSIS OF MULTIPLE SCLEROSIS?

In the accounts of diseases discussed above are many reports of overlap between the clinical and paraclinical features relied on for the diagnosis of multiple sclerosis. Before the ready availability of MRI it was estimated that approximately 10% of referrals to specialist multiple sclerosis clinics harboured an incorrect diagnosis, with considerable ambiguity in a further 5–10% (Herndon and Brooks 1985). Engell (1988) found that the diagnosis was correct in 485/518 (94%) patients diagnosed as having clinically definite multiple sclerosis in whom necropsy was subsequently performed, but the sample is not free from selection bias. In that series, mistakes included the Chiari malformation (one case), subacute combined degeneration of the spinal cord (one case), spinocerebellar degeneration (two cases), arteriovenous malformation (three cases), stroke or diffuse vascular disease (three cases) and intracranial tumour (seven cases).

Rudick *et al* (1986) describe in detail a series of patients, all satisfying stringent criteria for multiple sclerosis, in whom investigation eventually disclosed a different diagnosis. One patient had been followed for 15 years in a specialist multiple sclerosis clinic. Three were found to have unusual forms of vascular disease and two had spino-cerebellar degeneration. There were single cases of the Chiari malformation, arteriovenous malformation, hysteria, intrinsic spinal cord tumour and benign extramedullary tumour. These authors suggest warning signals (red flags) demanding reconsideration of the diagnosis – for example, absence of eye signs; failure of remission in young patients; and localized disease or atypical clinical features, particularly absence of sensory change or bladder disturbance in the presence of considerable motor disability.

As Herndon (1994) has emphasized, MRI and refined methods of spinal fluid analysis, if correctly applied, have largely eliminated the classical mistake of diagnosing tumours involving the nervous system as multiple sclerosis. Errors are now more frequent in the reverse direction – massive demyelinating lesions of the hemisphere, with resulting oedema, being mistaken for malignant tumours. Uncritical use of MRI may also lead to the erroneous diagnosis of multiple sclerosis in patients aged over 40 years, with inappropriate symptoms and a few (presumed) vascular white matter lesions shown on the scan mainly in a non-periventricular location. In the context of a disease which, at any one time, affects 1 : 800 of the population, it is self-evident that double diagnoses will occasionally occur. These can be diagnostically taxing, especially when multiple sclerosis has already been accurately diagnosed and the second disorder produces symptoms which reliably mimic the manifestations of focal demyelination (Figures 8.44 and 8.45).

In contrast, multiple sclerosis may not have been considered during the life of patients with chronic neurological disease who are subsequently proven histologically to have pathological features of the disorder. Phadke and Best (1983) describe four such cases, three of whom were elderly and thought to have unusual symptoms and signs of cerebrovascular disease. Six much younger patients are listed by H.J. Bauer and Hanefeld (1993), all of them dying from multiple sclerosis within a brief period from onset, in whom quite different diagnoses had been entertained. Multiple sclerosis can surprise even the most experienced neurologist.

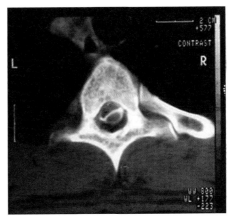

Figure 8.44 CT myelography in a young man with a previous episode of optic neuritis developing a progressive cord lesion as a result of a coincidental spinal neurofibroma.

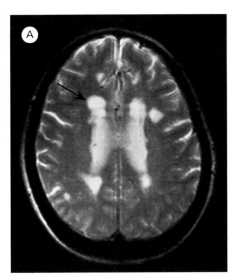
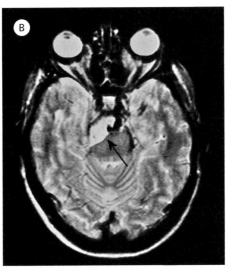
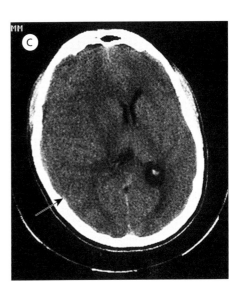

Figure 8.45 (A, B) Adjacent T$_2$-weighted MRI in a patient with white matter abnormalities as a result of central demyelinating disease (arrow) who also has a sphenoid ridge meningioma producing facial pain and ophthalmoplegia. (C) Patient with multiple sclerosis who became drowsy after a fall and had a chronic subdural haematoma (arrow).

Multiple sclerosis in the individual and in groups: a conspectus

9

David Miller, Ian McDonald and Alastair Compston

In the preceding three chapters, we give a broad account of those clinical and investigative aspects of multiple sclerosis that have particular relevance for the early phase of the disease, when – first and foremost – it is essential to make the correct diagnosis. Each chapter stands alone in its coverage of three particular areas: the clinical manifestations of multiple sclerosis (Chapter 6); the judicious use of investigations (Chapter 7); and the differential diagnosis (Chapter 8). Our emphasis is on those aspects that require consideration in groups of patients – in short, the general features of multiple sclerosis. Here, we develop a perspective on how the neurologist should approach the diagnostic process when encountering the individual patient who may have multiple sclerosis. We consider a number of typical and atypical clinical settings, disease subgroups, laboratory investigations that may present ambiguities or uncertainties, and the value of currently accepted diagnostic criteria. In seeking a conspectus, we draw on much relevant information contained in the preceding three chapters.

THE TYPICAL CASE

Whereas a good neurologist will naturally tend to remember better and ruminate more extensively on those cases that have proved diagnostically most challenging, he/she will also have become accustomed to making the diagnosis of multiple sclerosis without difficulty in a substantial proportion of patients. Achieving this clinical aim in a timely and uncomplicated fashion requires a good working knowledge of the typical manifestations of multiple sclerosis, based on regular and sustained exposure to patients with the disorder, supplemented, but not replaced, by access to facilities for investigation. Once made, the neurologist will have in mind a perception of the laboratory abnormalities and pathological processes at work in the newly diagnosed patient that can reasonably be regarded as 'typical'.

Laboratory investigations

Although few neurologists would nowadays choose not to perform a magnetic resonance imaging (MRI) scan when faced with someone who they believe has multiple sclerosis, the diagnosis can be made on clinical grounds alone. Both the previous (C.M. Poser *et al* 1983) and more recent (W.I. McDonald *et al* 2001) diagnostic criteria consider that, in a patient aged 10–59 years, two or more 'typical' relapses separated in time and signs of two or more central nervous system white matter lesions separated

in space are sufficient to establish the diagnosis of multiple sclerosis without the need for supplementary laboratory investigations. However, because such patients will have a ≥ 95% probability of exhibiting characteristic multifocal white matter abnormalities on brain MRI, it makes eminent sense to perform this investigation in all such cases at first presentation. That is our routine practice. Having done so and confirmed the presence of characteristic abnormalities on brain imaging, an argument can be made for only offering additional specific investigations if the clinical manifestations are entirely or predominantly confined to the spinal cord, in which case spinal MRI should be undertaken to detect intrinsic lesions that further support the diagnosis and to exclude another cord pathology. In such 'typical' cases, we no longer routinely resort to cerebrospinal fluid examination because the detection of oligoclonal bands – whilst providing additional support for the diagnosis – will be of limited value in situations where there is already a high level of diagnostic certainty. However, our threshold is low and the situation changes if there is a suspicion that the patient may have an alternative inflammatory or infectious disorder in which cerebrospinal fluid examination provides specific diagnostic information (for example, neuroborreliosis or neurosyphilis), and we recognize that in some geographical regions – e.g. where there is a high prevalence of Lyme disease – cerebrospinal fluid will be routinely obtained. Thus, these considerations are influenced by local neurological experience and the prevalence of alternative disorders. In these situations, it is nevertheless likely that the clinical and/or MRI features will already have alerted the clinician to some feature that is atypical for multiple sclerosis.

The pathological substrate

An understanding of the pathology and pathophysiology of multiple sclerosis (see Chapters 12 and 13) helps to understand the typical clinical and laboratory manifestations of the disease. This knowledge not only assists with diagnosis but also helps the patient to understand what is happening, and to appreciate nuances of the possible prognoses. Patients can be informed – using appropriate language and metaphors pitched so as to be accessible to the individual – that acute relapses are the result of conduction block associated with acute demyelination plus a direct effect of inflammatory mediators; and that subsequent recovery reflects several mechanisms – resolution of inflammation, insertion of sodium ion channels along the internodal membrane of axons, cortical adaptation, and remyelination. This information can be communicated to patients presenting with acute relapses along with encouragement that recovery is likely to be good from the immediate episode. Explanation of this underlying pathophysiology also provides a rationale for discussing the use of acute anti-inflammatory intervention with high-dose corticosteroids – if this is felt to be appropriate – to expedite recovery.

Recognition that an increase in body temperature leads to frequency-dependent conduction block in areas of demyelination helps in understanding the characteristic symptoms such as Uhthoff's phenomenon and exercise-induced lower limb weakness. Such symptoms, when seen at presentation, provide strong clues toward the correct diagnosis. The paroxysmal manifestations of demyelination, such as tonic spasms and trigeminal neuralgia, are also useful pointers to the diagnosis when encountered in young adults. Curiously, these are often not identified even by the experienced neurologist. Conversely, they may be interpreted erroneously as new episodes indicating a high relapse rate.

The realization that progressive multiple sclerosis results from the permanent and ongoing loss of axons helps to explain the nature of the problem to patients with this form of multiple sclerosis at the time of diagnosis. The opportunity then arises to discuss current research strategies aimed at protecting axons and enhancing their long-term survival. A sense of optimism that there will be progress towards developing effective therapies can realistically be transmitted to patients, based on the burgeoning scientific knowledge in understanding mechanisms of axonal and neuronal injury and protection.

Frequent variants of the clinical phenotype

Over the last 10 years, there has been a more consistent definition of multiple sclerosis subgroups – in particular, the designation of relapsing–remitting, secondary progressive, primary progressive and benign forms of the disease. Lublin and Reingold (1996) defined benign multiple sclerosis as those patients who have an expanded disability status scale score of 3 or less after 15 or more years from onset. Using this definition, approximately 30% of subjects who present with relapsing-remitting disease will experience a benign course. The Multiple Sclerosis Severity Scale, which refers the clinical course of the individual to the distributions of severity and duration in a cohort of >10 000 European cases, can be used to define benign disease as those in the lower three deciles, and accelerated multiple sclerosis as individuals grouped in the top three deciles of the derived scores from 0–10 (Roxburgh et al 2005a; see Chapter 6).

This information is important and provides grounds for cautious optimism at the time when bout onset multiple sclerosis is diagnosed. Notwithstanding, it should be understood that patients with minimal disability after 15 years may yet become disabled and/or develop secondary progressive multiple sclerosis in subsequent years. An early clinical course in relapse onset disease characterized by purely sensory relapses or optic neuritis, a long interval between the first and second relapse, a minimal MRI lesion load or normal brain scan, and no significant disability after 5 years from onset can usefully be communicated to patients as markers of a benign course, whilst recognizing that there is no certainty for prognosis. Conversely, entry into the progressive phase – from onset or after a number of relapses – later age at onset (to some extent confounded by the higher frequency of a progressive course), early involvement of motor systems, and a high relapse rate from the outset are all poor

prognostic factors. In short, all progressive forms of multiple sclerosis carry a less favourable prognosis. Cases of multiple sclerosis presenting during adolescence are not uncommon and in general show the typical relapsing–remitting course seen in young adults despite often getting off to rather an explosive start with encephalopathic features. Perhaps there is a dividend for recovery and stabilization from the apparent enhanced ability for remyelination of the juvenile brain and spinal cord. Primary progressive onset at this age is rare. Less commonly, multiple sclerosis presents in younger children, even within the first decade. The course is variable.

Sites involved

Certain clinical features are more characteristic than others when one considers the site affected within the central nervous system. The most frequently encountered primary and secondary progressive syndrome is spastic paraplegia due to spinal cord involvement; progressive ataxia – with or without cognitive impairment – is less often observed and progressive optic neuropathy is rare. The relapse onset form of multiple sclerosis indicates a spinal lesion in about 50% of patients at first presentation, optic neuritis in 25% and a brainstem lesion in 15%. Only in about 5% of patients does the first acute relapse, manifesting as hemianopia or aphasia, indicate a lesion in the cerebral hemispheres.

Spinal cord relapses of multiple sclerosis usually cause a partial myelopathic syndrome and are typically accompanied by small lesions on MRI that occupy only one segment in length, and only part of the cross-section of the spinal cord. Presentation with an acute complete flaccid paraplegia is more likely the result of another disorder such as acute disseminated encephalomyelitis, transverse myelitis, Devic's disease (neuromyelitis optica), and spinal cord infarction – and the MRI cord lesion in other inflammatory conditions is usually extensive in both its longitudinal and transverse extent. Optic neuritis in multiple sclerosis is unilateral in >90% of instances. Bilateral simultaneous optic neuritis brings to mind alternative diagnoses, including acute disseminated encephalomyelitis, Leber's hereditary optic neuropathy or Harding's disease. However, it can also occur in multiple sclerosis: follow-up of 23 adult patients who presented with an undiagnosed acute or subacute bilateral simultaneous optic neuropathy revealed an eventual diagnosis of multiple sclerosis in five (22%; Morrissey et al 1995).

Simultaneous onset with evidence for more than one clinical lesion in the central nervous system white matter is not uncommon in multiple sclerosis (Vitdehaag et al 2005); nor is the development of a second episode within a few days or weeks of the first. Such cases will bring to mind acute disseminated encephalomyelitis, but this is a less commonly encountered disorder in the young adult age group. The formal diagnosis of multiple sclerosis requires unambiguous clinical and/or laboratory evidence for dissemination in space and time according to established criteria (see Chapter 7).

Ethnic variations

Whilst ethnic variations in the prevalence of multiple sclerosis are recognized, and presumably reflect differences in susceptibility to the disease and exposure to risk factors, there is also some evidence that the manifestations may differ somewhat amongst ethnic groups. Thus, the relapsing–remitting pheno-type with entry into the progressive phase defines the disease in Caucasians whereas a specifically different phenotype charac-terizes the condition as it appears in most other racial groups (see Chapters 5 and 6). This variation is most apparent in reports of the disease emanating from Japan. Whereas numerous cases with clinical and laboratory features otherwise typical for 'Western' multiple sclerosis are reported, about 15–40% are described as having an optico-spinal form of disease (Kira 2003). A close inspection of the reports of these cases shows that they have an older age of onset than typical multiple sclerosis; attacks are confined to the optic nerves and spinal cord; brain imaging is often normal or shows only minor abnormalities; the cerebrospinal fluid usually does not contain oligoclonal bands but does show a pleocytosis; and spinal lesions involve many segments on MRI (Kira 2003). This description is similar to what others have called Devic's disease in cohorts reported from the United States and United Kingdom, where it has been noted that such a picture is seen in other nonCaucasian and Caucasian ethnic groups (A. Compston 2004; Cox *et al* 2005; Mandler *et al* 1993; O'Riordan *et al* 1996; Wingerchuk *et al* 1999). Whether all such cases represent variants of multiple sclerosis or a separate disease can be debated. Although a hypothesis is set out in Chapter 5 seeking links between the origin of relapsing–remitting multiple sclerosis and Devic's disease, from a contemporary perspective we take the pragmatic view that the different clinical, laboratory and pathological phenotypes reflect ethnic variations in genetic predisposition and pathogenesis driving subtly different disease mechanisms expressed as distinct phenotypes. This view is reinforced from the Japanese studies: whereas the group with a 'Western' type of multiple sclerosis is associated with an increased frequency of HLA-DRB1*1501 (the same antigen associated with multiple sclerosis in Caucasian populations in Northern Europe and elsewhere), cases of optico-spinal multiple sclerosis are associated with HLA-DRPB1*0501 (Kira 2003; see Chapter 3).

ISOLATED SYNDROMES AND THEIR OUTCOME: JUDICIOUS USE OF INVESTIGATIONS AND CRITIQUE OF THE 2001 McDONALD DIAGNOSTIC CRITERIA

Following the meeting of an International Panel in March 2005, amendments to the existing criteria of W.I. McDonald *et al* (2001) were published late in 2005 (Polmand *et al* 2005b). These address some weaknesses of the 2001 criteria that are discussed in this section. The reader is encouraged to become familiar with and adopt the 2005 revised criteria (see Chapter 7 for our analysis and summary: the main changes from 2001 are summarized in Table 7.5). Nevertheless, although changes in some finer details of the laboratory investigations are proposed, the general approach to the patient who presents with a clini-cally isolated syndrome is expected to follow essentially similar principles to those outlined in this section.

The most significant development in recent diagnostic criteria has been the specific incorporation of laboratory evidence for dissemination in space and time to enable a diagnosis in patients who have only had a single clinical episode of demyelination (W.I. McDonald *et al* 2001). Following the meeting of a newly

constituted International Panel in March 2005, amendments to the most recent criteria of W.I. McDonald *et al* (2001) will soon be published. These are expected to address some of the perceived weaknesses discussed in Chapter 7. The reader is encouraged to become familiar with and adopt these amended criteria when they are published early in 2006. Although changes in some of the finer details relating to use of investiga-tions are anticipated, the general approach to the patient pre-senting with a clinically isolated syndrome is expected to follow essentially similar principles to those already available, and as discussed in this section. The new laboratory criteria are largely – though not exclusively – based on MRI findings. Their appli-cations are discussed in detail in Chapter 7. Here, we analyse the strengths and weaknesses of the new MRI criteria for dis-semination in space and time and propose how imaging and other investigations are best employed in patients presenting with clinically isolated syndromes. Much of this discussion is based on a recent critique, prepared by DHM and several col-leagues on behalf of a European research network (MAGNIMS) that has an interest in magnetic resonance in multiple sclerosis (D.H. Miller *et al* 2004)

Strengths of the 2001 McDonald magnetic resonance imaging criteria

The criteria represent the first constructive effort to address how to use noninvasive surrogates for pathological observation in conjunction with clinical findings (Table 9.1). Biopsy and autopsy studies have shown that the conventional MRI white matter lesions seen on T_2-weighted scans are co-localized with corre-sponding pathological abnormalities (W.A. Stewart *et al* 1986; Ormerod *et al* 1987), although with the exception of a relation-ship between gadolinium enhancement and inflammation (Brück *et al* 1997), conventional MRI findings do not correspond to specific histopathological features. Because MRI shows many clinically silent lesions, and new enhancing lesions are correlated with relapses (Kappos *et al* 1999), inclusion of MRI findings in the new criteria has the potential to increase diagnostic sensi-tivity whilst retaining clinical relevance. As it was already widely used to assist in diagnosis, the inclusion of MRI in the new cri-teria was very timely.

MRI of the brain and spinal cord not only provides evidence for temporal and spatial lesion dissemination supportive of mul-tiple sclerosis but also is a powerful tool to exclude other diseases

---

Table 9.1 **Strengths of the 2001 McDonald diagnostic criteria for multiple sclerosis**
1. Rational new concept based on sensitive *in vivo* method for detecting pathology
2. Requiring MRI within the diagnostic criteria helps exclude other diseases

3. Allows an earlier diagnosis
  – In clinically isolated syndromes, the criteria are specific and accurate in predicting clinically definite multiple sclerosis
  – Potential to benefit from earlier disease-modifying treatment
  – Reduce uncertainty and anxiety for many patients

4. Conservative MRI criteria for dissemination in space and time reduce likelihood of false positive diagnosis of multiple sclerosis (as a result of nonspecific or irrelevant MRI abnormalities)

that might mimic the disease. These include extra-axial structural lesions compressing the spinal cord, optic nerves or cervical-medullary junction at the foramen magnum, and other intrinsic pathologies including infarction, haemorrhage and neoplasia.

In patients with clinically isolated syndromes, Dalton et al (2002a) found that, after 3 months, 20/95 (21%) had developed multiple sclerosis based on the new criteria, whereas only 7/95 (7%) had developed clinically definite disease. After 1 year, the corresponding figures were 38/79 (48%) and 16/79 (20%); and after 3 years they were 29/50 (58%) and 19/50 (38%). Tintoré et al (2003) found that, over the first 12 months, the new criteria more than tripled the frequency with which multiple sclerosis was diagnosed – from 11 to 40%. Our experience is also that the increase in diagnostic sensitivity, using the new criteria, makes its impact in the first year after the clinically isolated syndrome; thereafter, as one would expect, the relative proportion of patients diagnosed with multiple sclerosis through having a second episode increases steadily (Dalton et al 2003a).

An early diagnosis of multiple sclerosis has potential implications for treatment. Randomized, placebo-controlled trials of interferon-β in patients with clinically isolated syndromes and an abnormal brain MRI scan have shown that treatment delays the time to having a second clinical episode and reduces the number of new inflammatory (gadolinium enhancing) lesions seen on follow-up MRI (Jacobs et al 2000; Comi et al 2001a). Inflammation is associated with axonal damage (Trapp et al 1998), and axonal loss is reported to be present in lesions from the early stage of multiple sclerosis, even within the first year (Kuhlmann et al 2002b). Some neurologists would therefore consider treating patients early in the course of the disease – once a diagnosis has been established – with disease-modifying treatments that are able to reduce the frequency of inflammatory lesions.

Very importantly, making a definitive diagnosis allows an informed discussion of prognosis with the patient. Although the initial impact may be distressing, many patients report benefits from receiving the diagnosis (Heesen et al 2003); the relief from diagnostic uncertainty has been associated with a sense of strength to fight the disease and improved well-being, along with a reduction in anxiety (Mushlin et al 1994; Strasser-Fuchs et al 1997). The new MRI criteria provide benefit by reducing uncertainty through earlier diagnosis. As set out in Chapter 15, it is essential to provide patients with adequate and timely support during this diagnostic phase and we have found the early involvement of multiple sclerosis specialist nurses very helpful.

Conservative MRI criteria reduce the likelihood of making a false-positive diagnosis of multiple sclerosis based on nonspecific or irrelevant MRI abnormalities. It is not uncommon to encounter patients with somewhat vague symptoms in whom a diagnosis of multiple sclerosis has been erroneously based on the presence of T_2 white matter lesions. In the general population, cerebral white matter abnormalities due to small vessel disease are frequently found in those aged over 50 years, and sometimes also in younger individuals (Cooney et al 1996; R. Schmidt et al 1991). The requirement for relatively conservative (specific) imaging criteria in conjunction with consistent clinical findings will help to avoid making a false-positive diagnosis of multiple sclerosis.

The potential for a false-positive diagnosis when applying less conservative criteria are highlighted when one considers a recent Report of the Therapeutics and Technology Assessment Subcommittee of the American Academy of Neurology on the utility of MRI in suspected multiple sclerosis (E. Frohman et al 2003). This report proposed that in patients with a clinically isolated syndrome, the finding of a few (at least three) T_2 white matter lesions is a more appropriate predictor of the development of clinically definite multiple sclerosis within the next 7–10 years than the more stringent criteria proposed by the International Panel (W.I. McDonald et al 2001). However, three recent long-term follow-up studies show that the presence of T_2 lesions per se does not guarantee that patients will develop clinically definite multiple sclerosis. First, a 14 year follow-up of mixed clinically isolated syndrome patients with abnormal MRI found that only 88% developed clinically definite multiple sclerosis (Brex et al 2002). Furthermore, one-third of the originally recruited cohort could not be recontacted. Hence, it would be imprudent to assume that all of these patients – about one-half of whom had abnormal imaging at presentation – would have gone on to develop multiple sclerosis. Secondly, a 10 year follow-up of patients with isolated optic neuritis and abnormal MRI reported that only 58% developed clinically definite multiple sclerosis (Optic Neuritis Study Group 2003). Most recently, an 8 year follow-up of another group of patients with mixed clinically isolated syndromes found that only 74% with an abnormal MRI brain scan had converted to clinically definite multiple sclerosis (Minneboo et al 2004). It is clear from these studies that the simple presence of brain lesions in clinically isolated syndrome subjects does not guarantee the development of clinically definite multiple sclerosis, at least over 8–14 years. On the other hand, there is a risk that minimal MRI criteria such as those suggested by the Frohman subcommittee will invite an incorrect diagnosis of multiple sclerosis to be made by less experienced physicians based on nonspecific clinical findings and a few, small, incidental subcortical areas of high signal on MRI.

The increased availability of magnets operating at 3 Tesla – which might increase sensitivity for the detection of nonspecific, subtle white matter changes – has the potential to increase false-positive diagnoses in the future. This is another reason why MRI criteria should be based on characteristics that are relatively specific for multiple sclerosis.

Weaknesses of the new magnetic resonance imaging criteria

The MRI criteria were derived from studies that investigated conversion from a clinically isolated syndrome to clinically definite multiple sclerosis (Table 9.2). They could be perceived

---

Table 9.2 Weaknesses of the new MRI diagnostic criteria for multiple sclerosis

1. The criteria could be perceived as prognostic rather than diagnostic
2. Incomplete incorporation of spinal cord findings
3. Limited specificity of dissemination in space criteria per se in clinically isolated syndromes for development of multiple sclerosis
4. Insensitive dissemination in time criteria at early clinically isolated syndrome follow-up
5. Variable results in different clinically isolated syndromes
6. Only conventional MRI findings are considered
7. Conceptual difficulty with combined cerebrospinal fluid and MRI criterion for dissemination in space

as prognostic rather than diagnostic. No study has so far addressed the specificity of the criteria by systematic comparison of multiple sclerosis with other diseases that have clinical or radiological similarities. The criteria were also based on the findings reported in three relatively small patient cohorts with limited follow-up who were recruited in specialized referral centres and selected as having a 'typical' clinically isolated syndrome (Barkhof *et al* 1997a; Brex *et al* 2001a; Tintoré *et al* 2000). Such subjects are not representative of all multiple sclerosis patients at presentation.

The criteria allow for substitution of one brain abnormality by one spinal cord lesion. It has since been shown that the presence of one cervical cord lesion is useful in differentiating patients with multiple sclerosis from those with systemic lupus erythematosus (Rovaris *et al* 2002a). In a recent MRI study of patients with early multiple sclerosis, the brain MRI criteria proposed by W.I. McDonald *et al* (2001) were not fulfilled in 34% of cases, but this percentage was reduced to 15% and 6% respectively, if substitution by one cord lesion or by an unlimited number of cord lesions respectively was allowed (Bot *et al* 2004). The detection of characteristic intrinsic spinal cord lesions on spinal MRI is very useful where multiple sclerosis is suspected but combined assessment of clinical features, brain MRI, evoked potentials and cerebrospinal fluid remains equivocal (Thorpe *et al* 1996b). Cord lesions are rarely seen in normal individuals (Thorpe *et al* 1993) or in other inflammatory or vascular central nervous system diseases (Bot *et al* 2002; Rovaris *et al* 2000a; 2001a; 2002c). However, these studies are based on patients in whom the diagnosis of multiple sclerosis is already secure. The utility of cord MRI in patients with clinically isolated syndromes (aside from the exclusion of alternative pathology in the case of isolated cord syndromes) hinges on the detection of clinically silent lesions disseminated in space and time over and above what is detected in the brain. In a study of 115 patients with isolated optic neuritis, the inclusion of at least one spinal cord lesion to substitute for brain lesions within the new criteria had remarkably little impact in diagnosing multiple sclerosis (Dalton *et al* 2003a). More work is needed to define how best to incorporate spinal cord MRI into diagnostic criteria.

The criteria have limited specificity for establishing the conversion of clinically isolated syndromes to multiple sclerosis based on dissemination in space *alone*. Although the presence of both gadolinium enhancing and nonenhancing lesions on a single scan intuitively suggests multiphasic disease, the MRI definitions of dissemination in space adopted in the new criteria do not make this distinction, and when they have been applied to a single scan at presentation with a clinically isolated syndrome they have proved less specific than the requirement for at least 3 months definition of dissemination in time (Dalton *et al* 2002a; Tintoré *et al* 2003). The dissemination in space criteria also performed poorly in one large study of a placebo clinically isolated syndrome cohort participating in a clinical trial (CHAMPS Study Group 2002). It therefore appears premature to recommend a diagnosis based on single scan features within 3 months of a clinically isolated syndrome.

The imaging criteria for early dissemination in time may be overly restrictive, because they require that there is a gadolinium enhancing lesion on a 3-month follow-up scan. The dissemination in time criteria are insensitive at early follow-up of individuals with clinically isolated syndromes. Dalton *et al*

(2003a) found that if new T_2 lesions on the follow-up scan at 3 months in patients with a clinically isolated syndrome are allowed as an alternative to gadolinium enhancing lesions, the sensitivity for detecting cases who went on to develop clinically definite multiple sclerosis after approximately 3 years increased from 58 to 74%, whilst the high specificity for clinically definite disease was maintained at 92%. This study also showed a high specificity and sensitivity (both 89%) in patients with any T_2 abnormality at baseline and new T_2 abnormality at 3 months. This suggests the potential favourably to modify and optimize the MRI criteria for both dissemination in space and time once there is a more substantial evidence base available for analysis (Swanton *et al* 2005). Further research could also usefully investigate whether MRI dissemination in time over a shorter interval (new lesions after one rather than the presently required 3 months) might prove sufficient in terms of specificity and positive predictive value for clinically definite multiple sclerosis reliably to be incorporated into future revisions of the diagnostic criteria.

The results vary between different clinically isolated syndromes. One research group has reported that the MRI dissemination in space criteria are less specific in patients with clinically isolated syndromes of the brainstem (Sastre-Garriga *et al* 2003; 2004), when compared with those having isolated optic neuritis or spinal cord syndromes. This difference may in part be the result of the symptomatic infratentorial lesion not being included within the MRI criteria for dissemination in space, and suggests that for patients with brainstem syndromes, some adaptation of the criteria is required.

The currently used MRI criteria only include conventional lesion measures. This is appropriate because, at the present time, other less conventional MRI measures are difficult to quantify and assess in a routine diagnostic work-up. Nonetheless, non-conventional techniques such as magnetization transfer imaging, proton MR spectroscopy, and diffusion tensor imaging have the potential to provide more specific information with respect to underlying disease pathology, and are abnormal very early in the disease, even in the normal appearing brain or spinal cord (Filippi *et al* 1999a; Fernando *et al* 2004; Inglese *et al* 2002b; Rocca *et al* 2000; Rovaris *et al* 2000b; 2002c). To determine whether any of these approaches will emerge as having diagnostic or prognostic utility, careful follow-up studies will be required of prospectively recruited cohorts of patients with clinically isolated syndromes. Such studies will need to ensure scanner stability (Ropele *et al* 2005) and should have the aim of reliably defining normal from abnormal measures in individual patients. This will be challenging because the quantitative extent of abnormalities observed in normal appearing tissues is small.

There is a conceptual difficulty in combining cerebrospinal fluid findings and MRI criteria for dissemination in space within the same scheme. Using the new criteria, if a patient has cerebrospinal fluid oligoclonal bands, only two T_2-weighted MRI lesions are required to constitute evidence for dissemination in space. This recommendation is illogical, because the immunological process detected in the cerebrospinal fluid does not of itself imply any particular number or location of focal lesions within the central nervous system. Furthermore, when applied in a clinically isolated syndrome cohort, this criterion was found to have a low specificity (63%) for development of clinically definite multiple sclerosis (Tintoré *et al* 2003). Whilst lumbar puncture undoubtedly remains a very valuable diagnostic investigation in some circumstances, future studies will need to reconsider how the cerebrospinal fluid findings might more effectively be incorporated in revised diagnostic criteria. The standardization of laboratory methods for cerebrospinal fluid examination in multiple sclerosis diagnosis is also crucial, and was not addressed in detail in the McDonald criteria. A recent expert consensus statement on this aspect is both timely and helpful (Freedman *et al* 2005a). The expert group conclude that the current gold standard – which has the best specificity and sensitivity for the diagnosis of multiple sclerosis – is the qualitative investigation for oligoclonal IgG bands, performed using isoelectric focusing on agarose gels followed by immunoblotting. Such analysis should be performed on unconcentrated cerebrospinal fluid and with a serum sample run in parallel in order to establish that there is intrathecal synthesis – that is, bands confined to the cerebrospinal fluid.

Approach to investigating patients with a clinically isolated syndrome

It must be emphasized that the enhanced status placed on MRI findings in the new diagnostic criteria will only add value when applied to subjects who have had a detailed and competently performed neurological history and examination. Their utility in the face of inadequate documentation or nonspecific clinical findings is not known, but one could easily imagine that they will be less reliable than when the clinical features are clearly described and strongly suggestive of demyelinating disease. The increasing role of MRI in diagnosis also demands high-quality image acquisition, and the scans should be interpreted and reported by an experienced neuroradiologist, who is familiar with the appearances seen in multiple sclerosis and with the specific imaging criteria for diagnosis.

The new diagnostic criteria will be used by some neurologists for the initiation of disease modifying treatments. However, there is to date only limited evidence that the criteria are relevant to treatment response or disease prognosis (Barkhof *et al* 2003b; Beck *et al* 2002). We take the view that establishment of the diagnosis and decisions on treatment are processes that should be separated. The criteria were developed for diagnosis and – based on current evidence – should be used for that purpose alone. The decisions on when and in whom to introduce disease-modifying treatment will be influenced by many other factors (see Chapter 18).

In our view, the investigation of patients who present with a clinically isolated syndrome typical of demyelination should take into account the new criteria because the MRI evidence for dissemination in space and time has a high specificity and positive predictive value for clinically definite multiple sclerosis (Dalton *et al* 2002a; Tintoré *et al* 2003). Sensitivity is also high, provided that a new T_2 lesion is allowed to substitute for a gadolinium enhancing lesion on the initial follow-up scan required to show dissemination in time, and if the first scan was obtained within 3 months from onset of the presenting syndrome.

Investigations should consider other potential diagnoses, and include some simple tests, designed to exclude systemic lupus erythematosus, neurosyphilis, sarcoidosis and Lyme disease. In brainstem syndromes, brain MRI is mandatory, as is spinal cord MRI in patients with isolated cord syndromes. Patients with isolated optic neuritis should see an ophthalmologist because some conditions – neuroretinitis and central serous retinopathy amongst others – are otherwise impossible to distinguish from optic neuritis. Imaging is rarely needed for diagnosis of optic neuritis *per se* and the decision whether to perform brain MRI is based on the potential for predicting or diagnosing multiple sclerosis.

In trying to secure a diagnosis of multiple sclerosis, we recommend the following approach in patients with isolated unilateral optic neuritis and other typical clinically isolated syndromes:

- At the time of diagnosis, it is explained that for about 50–60% of people, the cause is multiple sclerosis. A brief discussion of the nature of multiple sclerosis takes place, including an emphasis of its potential to be mild and nondisabling.
- It is explained that brain MRI can provide a more accurate prediction of multiple sclerosis such that, if the scan is abnormal, the chances of developing clinically definite multiple sclerosis are 60–80% whereas, if it is normal, they are only 20% (Brex *et al* 2002; Minneboo *et al* 2004; Optic Neuritis Study Group 2003).
- In those who opt to have a scan, T_2 and gadolinium enhanced brain MRI are performed in a timely manner.
- If MRI is performed >3 months after the attack, and fulfils the MRI criteria for dissemination in space and time, multiple sclerosis is diagnosed.
- If MRI is normal, the patient is given qualified reassurance and repeat scans are not recommended for as long as the patient remains well.
- If MRI is abnormal but the criteria for multiple sclerosis are not fulfilled, a repeat T_2 brain scan between 3 and 6 months after the original imaging has a significant prospect of providing MRI evidence for dissemination in space and time (establishing the diagnosis of multiple sclerosis) provided that a new T_2 lesion is allowed as evidence of dissemination in time (Dalton *et al* 2003a).
- If the diagnosis is not established after performing the follow-up scan, further imaging is not routinely recommended because the disease will become relatively more likely to manifest clinically in the longer term – most of the gain in diagnostic sensitivity using MRI occurs within 12 months of follow-up (Dalton *et al* 2002a).
- If the diagnosis is not established after performing the follow-up scan but inflammatory demyelination is strongly suspected, it is helpful to examine the cerebrospinal fluid for oligoclonal bands and to perform evoked potentials.
- MRI should be performed to a high standard consistent with modern neuroradiological practice and should be reported by a clinician with extensive experience of the imaging appearances in multiple sclerosis and other white matter disorders.
- Patients need close support from, and ready access to, their clinical team throughout the diagnostic process.

In patients with a less typical presentation, it becomes particularly important to perform appropriate clinical and paraclinical investigations (including MRI) seeking alternative diagnoses or aiming to reveal other features suggestive of multiple sclerosis. The new MRI criteria have not been properly evaluated in these patients. Therefore, it may prove useful to consider additional information potentially available from MRI that could enhance specificity – multifocal homogeneous or ring enhancing white matter lesions and/or corpus callosum involvement are particularly useful findings – as well as using other paraclinical tests. Identification of spinal cord MRI lesions adds specificity, especially in differentiation from other inflammatory or vascular central nervous system diseases (Lycklama *et al* 2003). It is important to ensure good clinical follow-up, which of itself can provide crucial diagnostic clarification. Further MRI examination could also prove decisive when evidence emerges for dissemination in space or time.

COMORBIDITY AND ASSOCIATED DISEASES

The patient with multiple sclerosis is no less vulnerable than anyone else to develop other common neurological problems such as migraine, lumbar and cervical spondylosis, and (in older subjects) cerebrovascular disease. All experienced neurologists will be familiar with cases of double diagnosis, which may even include the co-occurrence of multiple sclerosis with extrinsic or intrinsic cerebral or spinal neoplasms. Some less specific symptoms that occur in multiple sclerosis – fatigue, somatic pain syndromes, and disordered bowel function – may sometimes be the result of disease affecting other body systems and the indiscriminate attribution of nonspecific symptoms to multiple sclerosis may delay detecting other important disorders.

For the patient with multiple sclerosis, it is clearly important that other significant medical conditions are diagnosed correctly and promptly. Effective and timely treatment could improve quality of life and even survival. One should avoid being too ready to attribute atypical or nonspecific symptoms to multiple sclerosis. As a neurologist, it is also important to recognize limitations in being able to recognize and diagnose non-neurological disorders. When there is doubt that a significant new clinical manifestation can be attributed to multiple sclerosis or another neurological problem, this uncertainty should be declared to the patient's primary-care physician, and it will also often be appropriate to recommend or initiate referral to other specialties.

The conditions that are considered genuinely to occur at increased frequency in people with multiple sclerosis, naturally or exposed by treatment, are mostly autoimmune, especially thyroid disease. These and other conditions are listed, and the causal or coincidental nature of the association debated, in Chapters 6 and 18.

SITUATIONS IN WHICH ALTERNATIVE DIAGNOSES SHOULD BE CONSIDERED

There are two self-evident pitfalls in relation to the differential diagnosis of multiple sclerosis: one is making the diagnosis in someone who has another and potentially treatable disorder; the other is failing to make the correct diagnosis in someone who has multiple sclerosis. The consequences of either error can be serious for the patient, in terms of both physical and psychological health, and for the neurologist may result in unwelcome complaints or even medicolegal attention. It is therefore of paramount importance that the diagnostic process is informed from a position of wide experience and working knowledge of the main diagnostic possibilities and their manifestations.

It can be useful to remind oneself of not uncommon clinical settings where there is a pressing need to consider alternative diagnoses. Foremost amongst these is the patient presenting with a clinically isolated spinal cord syndrome, whether it be acute, progressive, recurrent or fluctuating. A simple rule of thumb is that all such patients should be investigated with a spinal MRI scan that surveys the full extent of the cord from foramen magnum to conus. Prior to the availability of MRI, a more selective approach was inevitably required when deciding who should be subjected to the altogether less agreeable investigation of myelography and, as elaborated in detail in Chapter 6, certain features of the spinal syndrome will favour a demyelinating aetiology as against other disorders. A progressive syndrome with a well-defined sensory and motor level and associated segmental or radicular pain will inevitably suggest a compressive lesion. That said, it was well recognized that mistakes were made when there was over-reliance on clinical features alone: cord compression may sometimes present with a fluctuating or partially reversible syndrome. Since MRI is non-invasive – and can be performed in all but a very few individuals – it should always be carried out in the patient with clinically isolated spinal cord disease.

Another situation where alternative diagnoses must be sought is the patient with atypical optic neuritis or progressive optic neuropathy. Atypical features for optic neuritis are severe pain and visual loss with persistent visual failure. One of us (DHM) recently saw a patient with established multiple sclerosis who presented with acute visual loss accompanied by severe ocular pain and vomiting. Understandably, referral from the multiple sclerosis nurse requested consideration for treatment with methylprednisolone for what was thought to be an episode of optic neuritis. The observation of a fixed and dilated pupil triggered immediate referral to ophthalmology where a diagnosis of acute angle closure glaucoma was made. Cases of true optic neuritis in which particularly severe pain and visual loss occur should bring to mind sarcoidosis or chronic relapsing inflammatory optic neuropathy in which context more aggressive steroid treatment may be required. Progressive visual failure as a result of optic neuropathy should always trigger imaging of the anterior visual pathway seeking a compressive lesion. The lesion may be obvious on imaging – a large pituitary adenoma or subfrontal meningioma – but at other times prove very subtle and difficult to detect (for example, a small intracanalicular optic nerve meningioma) unless careful high-resolution MRI with gadolinium enhancement is performed.

Another frequently encountered clinical problem is the patient referred with a suspected diagnosis of multiple sclerosis, but in whom the history is one of multiple, nonspecific and debilitating symptoms. Examination reveals no neurological abnormalities with clear evidence of 'functional' or 'nonorganic' impairments. The situation may have been complicated by an earlier brain MRI scan that revealed a few small subcortical white matter lesions, leading a less experienced clinician to suggest that the patient has multiple sclerosis. Faced with clear evidence for a functional disorder, it is of paramount importance to bring the diagnostic process to as clear a conclusion as possible. One wants to know if there is any evidence for underlying neurological disease, bearing in mind that it is not uncommon to encounter patients with both multiple sclerosis and functional overlay. It is therefore often appropriate to be thorough in performing investigations, and we will routinely include brain and spinal cord MRI, cerebrospinal fluid examination and visual and somatosensory evoked potentials to settle the matter. One is in a much stronger position to conclude beyond reasonable doubt that such a patient does not have multiple sclerosis when all of the investigations are normal, and the ability to make a confident diagnosis of a functional disorder can at least provide some reassurance for the patient and an appropriate direction for future management.

WHEN TO IGNORE 'INCONVENIENT' LABORATORY RESULTS OR CLINICAL FINDINGS: TAKING THE BEST POSITION

As a general rule, when all the clinical and laboratory features point towards the diagnosis apart from a *single* finding that is atypical or inexplicable, it is probably safe to ignore the latter and accept the diagnosis based on a balance of probability. One may encounter a patient in whom the clinical and laboratory findings all point towards a diagnosis of multiple sclerosis but discover, for example, that the vitamin B12 level is slightly low or that spinal cord MRI shows spondylotic changes with mild compression of the spinal cord. While these laboratory findings should be carefully considered in their own right – and in the case of the low vitamin B12 level one may want to investigate further by checking serum homocysteine, urinary methylmalonic acid and serum intrinsic factor antibody, and (possibly) administer a course of vitamin B12 injections – they should not necessarily lead one away from an otherwise confident diagnosis of multiple sclerosis. One of us (DHM) recently encountered a young adult male patient in whom a progressive cerebellar and pyramidal tract syndrome was accompanied by T_2 abnormalities on brain MRI that were typical for demyelination, cerebrospinal fluid oligoclonal bands and characteristically delayed visual evoked potentials. After extensive investigation revealed no alternative diagnosis, it was concluded that the single atypical feature of multifocal calcification in the cerebral white matter did not detract from an otherwise secure diagnosis of multiple sclerosis.

Atypical clinical findings in multiple sclerosis are many and varied (see Chapter 6), and might for example include an absent deep tendon reflex, a third nerve palsy, deafness or hemianopia. When these occur as isolated features within the context of an otherwise typical clinical and laboratory disease, they can be accommodated without the need to invoke additional diagnoses. On the other hand, if there is more than one atypical feature, or at any time the balance of typical versus atypical features is unfavourable, it is prudent to retain an open mind, not to commit to a definite diagnosis, and to consider more rigorously the possible alternative diagnoses. Continued follow-up and a preparedness to reinvestigate are both encouraged when faced with an undiagnosed neurological disorder.

'PATHOGNOMONIC' VERSUS 'UNHEARD OF' FEATURES OF MULTIPLE SCLEROSIS

While the process leading to a final diagnosis of multiple sclerosis – or not, as the case may be – involves the evaluation of many different pieces of information derived from clinical and laboratory assessment, it can be useful to keep in mind specific features that are so distinctive that, in their own right, they direct one strongly towards or away from the diagnosis. While no single feature is totally reliable (for or against the diagnosis), there are some which are so typical or atypical that one some-

times hears these referred to as 'pathognomonic' or 'unheard of' features of multiple sclerosis.

When choosing features that are particularly characteristic for multiple sclerosis, it should first be emphasized that they are most appropriately used in a demographic and epidemiological context where multiple sclerosis is likely to occur. Such clinical features have their greatest specificity in young adults, aged between 20 and 40 years. They also offer more diagnostic value when seen in a geographical location and population in which multiple sclerosis is relatively common and other conditions constituting the differential diagnosis correspondingly less likely. With these caveats, syndromes that are highly suggestive for multiple sclerosis are acute or bilateral internuclear ophthalmoplegia; Lhermitte's symptom; unilateral facial myokymia; a clearly elucidated history of a spontaneously remitting and purely sensory spinal cord syndrome with involvement of the lower limbs and the waist or trunk; deafferentation of one or both hands with predominant posterior column involvement; and unilateral remitting optic neuritis. Even so, such syndromes may rarely be due to another diagnosis; internuclear ophthalmoplegia may occur in systemic lupus erythematosus and the same ophthalmoplegic appearance is seen in myasthenia gravis; Lhermitte's symptom is often a feature of vitamin B12 deficiency and cervical disc prolapse; and optic neuritis may be caused by syphilis and other microbial infections. Also, the 'pathognomonic' syndromes are sometimes seen as isolated episodes of demyelination that never convert to multiple sclerosis. Even after prolonged follow-up, about one-third of young adults with otherwise typical optic neuritis do not develop other features of multiple sclerosis.

In considering the 'unheard of' features, perhaps better called 'red flags' against the diagnosis, the following could be included: a progressive spinal cord lesion with a well-defined sensorimotor level accompanied by segmental and radicular pain; acute complete flaccid transverse myelitis (although this is a feature of Devic's syndrome); acute low back pain with urinary retention and isolated sacral sensory loss (although conus involvement in multiple sclerosis may produce a similar picture, this presentation should always suggest an acute cauda equina syndrome due to a central lumbosacral disc protrusion); isolated epilepsy without other neurological features; isolated dementia without other neurological features (although the cognitive presentation of multiple sclerosis is well described); a progressive spinocerebellar disorder with no focal abnormalities in the brain or spinal cord on MRI (although there may be regional atrophy, e.g. in the cerebellum, in cases of hereditary spino-cerebellar ataxia); prominent lower motor neuron features such as wasting and fasciculation; and a very strong family history of 'multiple sclerosis' with several affected individuals in the pedigree.

No account can safeguard the casual clinician from failing to spot other and perhaps more treatable conditions, or the obsessional differential diagnostician from never being able to come off the fence and name the illness. Common sense must prevail and, as mentioned in Chapter 1, the experienced neurologist is usually pretty good at falling in line with the dictum:

multiple sclerosis is what a good clinician would call multiple sclerosis.

Kurtzke (1974)

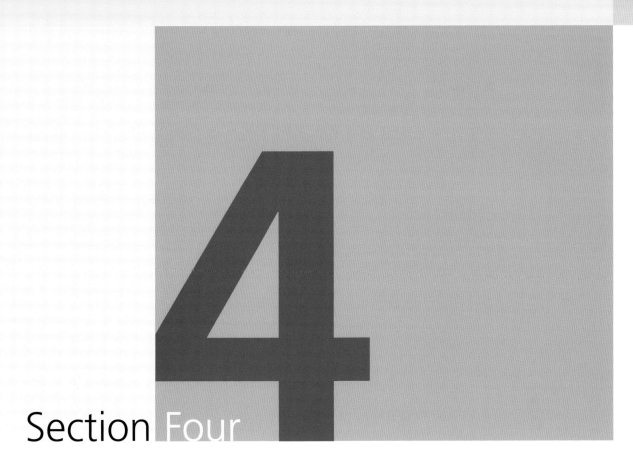

Section Four

THE PATHOGENESIS OF MULTIPLE SCLEROSIS

The neurobiology of multiple sclerosis **10**

Alastair Compston, Hans Lassmann and Kenneth Smith

ORGANIZATION IN THE CENTRAL NERVOUS SYSTEM

Considered as man or machine, everyone would agree that the human central nervous system is an organ of remarkable diversity and sophistication. Although much is now revealed, perhaps it is unreasonable – even philosophically unsound – to expect that the human brain can ever fully understand itself.

The evolution of nervous systems allowed primitive organisms to respond to their environment. The need to sense external threat was met by reflex withdrawal. Then it became expedient to explore the external environment through the development of goal-directed activities. Nervous systems began to control some aspects of the internal environment, contributing to homeostasis. With time, the emergence of protective and discriminative sensation, the special senses, movement and coordination underpinned the development of new motor and cognitive behaviours that further enhanced interaction with the physical and social environment.

Some principles of structure, function and organization in the brain and spinal cord are now revealed. Central to that knowledge are the cell doctrine (perfected by Cajal and Golgi in the 1890s: see Chapter 1; Cajal 1894; Golgi 1894), the integration of facilitatory and inhibitory neuronal circuits dependent on reflex activity (summarized by Sir Charles Sherrington in his 1906 Silliman Lectures to Yale University: Sherrington 1906), and organization around functional systems and regions serving defined properties. In this way, the nervous system discharges its responsibilities to the organism as a whole. The fundamental units consist of neurons and their axonal and dendritic processes embedded in a glial network providing additional structure and function. In their different ways, macroglia (oligodendrocytes and astrocytes) and microglia also contribute to the cellular architecture of the central nervous system (Figure 10.1). Oligodendrocytes synthesize and maintain the myelin sheath that extensively coats nerve fibres in white matter, and underpins saltatory conduction of the nerve impulse. These are terminally differentiated cells with a limited response to injury. It is assumed that they depend for renewal on the availability of precursors. Astrocytes provide architecture for neurons and define anatomical boundaries. They act as a source of growth factors and cytokines, assume many physiological roles including those necessary for conduction of the nerve impulse, and participate in the response to injury. Microglia are bone marrow

derived cells of the macrophage lineage providing the nervous system with a degree of immunological competence. Astrocytes and microglia are each highly reactive cells that play important roles in health and disease, contributing both to tissue injury and to repair.

Communication between interconnected axons and dendrites across synapses is adaptable and forms the basis for plasticity in the central nervous system. The presynaptic membrane has vesicles containing locally active neurotransmitters. These are released in response to the nerve impulse and controlled by calcium influx. The transmitters drift across the synapse, bind to receptors on the postsynaptic membrane, causing direct or indirect opening and closure of ion channels, with effects on conductance across the postsynaptic membrane. Channels gate the passage of sodium, potassium, calcium and chloride ions thereby producing local current (see Chapter 13). The main excitatory neurotransmitter is glutamate whereas glycine and γ-aminobutyric acid (GABA) are inhibitory molecules. Indirect activity of ion channels is mediated through G-proteins and secondary messenger systems including cyclic adenosine monophosphate, inositol phosphates, arachidonic acid metabolites, and protein kinases. It is the binding by neurotransmitters or peptides to postsynaptic receptors and their effect on ion channels that lead to the inhibition or excitation of the postsynaptic neurons. Not all synapses deploy chemical transmission and a few rely on electric transmission.

Because tissue injury in multiple sclerosis involves neuronal and axonal loss, demyelination and oligodendrocyte depletion, remyelination and astrocytosis, the fully informed student of the disease will want to have some working knowledge of how these individual components of the central nervous system develop and, therefore, may regenerate. Simply stated, remyelination and repair are often conceptualized as a re-enactment of the same processes that occur so successfully during development of the normal nervous system. In 2005, the most common question asked by the informed patient attending a specialist in multiple sclerosis must be 'what's new with stem cells?' Therein lies a complex social, ethical and biological set of questions. Whilst patients may not expect the neurologist to recite details of genes and transcription factors that regulate stem cells and their differentiation into glial fates, a reasonable working knowledge of those processes does provide a platform from which the clinical scientist can formulate an answer, steering a course between hyperbole and realisitic appraisal of the

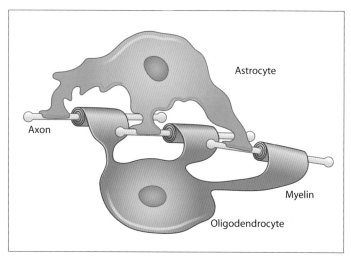

Figure 10.1 Oligodendrocytes and astrocytes interact with axons to establish the cellular architecture of axon–glial interactions.

prospects for a therapy that rebuilds the areas of tissue injury in multiple sclerosis.

Development in the central nervous system begins when the embryonic mesoderm induces the overlying dorsal midline ectoderm to form neuroectodermal cells of the neural plate. This becomes invaginated along its length to form the neural groove, the lips of which eventually fuse so that neuroepithelial cells comprising the neuroectoderm become the neural tube surrounding what will become the ventricle. Neuroepithelial cells lining the ventricle rapidly proliferate, and cells migrate along the neural tube from this layer to form a specialized subventricular zone where further division continues. As the cerebral vesicles enlarge, primitive neuroepithelial cells elongate and eventually migrate, some continuing to span the developing nervous system as radial cells. Others detach and migrate by translocation or free locomotion. These neural precursor cells mature through neuroblast, glioblast and ependymoblast stages, gradually losing the potential for mitosis. Precursors lose their multi-potentiality and develop into cells committed either to neuronal or glial lineages. At first, most cells in the subventricular zone are neuronal and have a low rate of division, whereas the glial lineage has a greater capacity for mitosis and fewer of these cells are found in the germinal zones. In terms of lineage commitment, neural stem cells identified in one region of the developing nervous system acquire different phenotypes depending on the location in which they are allowed to mature. This emphasizes the role of growth and other environmental factors in orchestrating the timing and specificity of maturation in the central nervous system. The need to select survivors from cells that are overproduced in the developing nervous system involves apoptosis (alternatively referred to as programmed cell death). Survival is probable for cells receiving adequate amounts of trophic factors. The lack of a positive signal provided by neighbouring cells is seen as the most likely mechanism of programmed cell death. Apoptosis differs from necrosis in that the cell contents are contained and do not elicit a local inflammatory response, the debris being removed by microglia. It is a feature both of development and pathological processes (Raff 1992). Programmed cell death makes it safe to retain a source of mitotic precursors in the mature nervous system, whilst avoiding uncontrolled growth. This is a more efficient way of allowing cellular plasticity than suppressing the ability to generate new cells. Although long considered incapable of regeneration, the adult mammalian central nervous system can undergo stem-cell-dependent neurogenesis and gliogenesis, thereby (in principle) re-establishing axon–glial interactions needed for remyelination and safe conduction of the nerve impulse. An essential feature of stem cells is proliferation and self-renewal.

Simply stated, the steps in development are the birth of pluripotential stem cells, their commitment to organ-specific fates, and lineage differentiation. These events occur in response to the effects of growth factors and other ligands, acting on specific receptors, followed by signal transduction, gene expression and transcription with the production of molecules that alter cell behaviour and enable interactions with the local cellular environment. However, as more is revealed about the molecular basis of communication between the different types of neurons, macroglia and microglia, it becomes increasingly clear that the expression of receptors and the production of corresponding ligands are not so tightly constrained. Thus, despite emerging down different lineages having defined functions, the separate classes of cells to be found in the central nervous system often share many molecular and neurochemical characteristics, making it less easy to understand the innate organization, and illustrating the general principle of redundancy that makes for safety should one element or another fail. In turn, this presents the neurobiologist with a difficult task in elucidating the many complexities. There is a continued requirement for specific growth factors and cytokines, many produced by astrocytes and microglia, once cell fate is committed. At first sight, it is odd that many of these molecules crop up both in neurobiological and immunological contexts. But the close relationship between injury and repair makes this overlap rather logical. For example, activated immune cells (T and B lymphocytes and monocytes) are a potent source of neurotrophins, mainly brain-derived nerve growth factor (BDNF; Kerschensteiner et al 1999), and enhanced growth factor production may be one consequence of drug treatment (Petereit et al 2003; Ziemssen et al 2002).

In this chapter, we describe the principles of glial development and myelination; mechanisms of oligodendrocyte and axonal injury and demyelination; and repair of axon–glial interactions. The emphasis is on *in vitro* analyses. More detailed accounts of the immunological mechanisms, pathological features, and physiological consequences of these processes are to be found in Chapters 11, 12 and 13, respectively.

CELL BIOLOGY OF THE CENTRAL NERVOUS SYSTEM

From their origins as stem cells, the separate elements of the nervous system must undergo proliferation, migration, differentiation into defined progeny, and survival. Once in place, cell–cell interactions are fashioned and fostered so as to create the cellular architecture that translates structure into function. Each of these steps occurs in response to the intrinsic machinery of the cells participating in the various processes, and they are orchestrated by the molecules that dominate the environment at any one time. The concentrations of these factors are phasic and the net effects often represent a balance of positive and negative – attractive and repellent, facilitatory and inhibitory – forces. The key molecules are growth factors, chemokines and other ligands, their respective receptors, and the signalling pathways they transduce. It is generally the case that proliferation and migration precede differentiation. Indeed, for many cells these are 'either … or' states. Thus, molecules that promote proliferation tend to inhibit differentiation, and vice versa. A major event in development is the switch from a molecular environment, characterized by the availability of ligands, expression of cell surface receptors and activation of signal transduction pathways that are mitotic and pro-migratory, to one in which all of these elements disappear from the local environment to be replaced by a new cast of factors that inhibit proliferation and promote differentiation. Not all the details of these rules are yet fully understood, and much of the information is preliminary, apparently ambiguous and subject to revision. Nevertheless, certain fixed points are reliably established even if further details are bound to emerge in time. Most of the knowledge has been gained from the study of development in rodents; much is based on *in vitro* analyses, and the use of transgenic animals. The characteristics that emerge cannot be assumed also to apply to human cells. The reductionist approach of studying cells *in vitro* offers many opportunities but also has significant limitations. Furthermore, it is often assumed that repair is simply a recapitulation of development; but that working hypothesis is now shown to be too simple and, although developmental biology can set a framework, in the end studies of the human adult nervous system undergoing repair are needed to inform the transition from experiment to application in the context of multiple sclerosis.

Cell survival

Acting together or in sequence, growth factors orchestrate development within the nervous system. Many also support the survival of fully differentiated cells. The need to select survivors from cells overproduced in the developing nervous system involves programmed cell death. The mechanism of culling is apoptosis, and this is especially prominent during development and maturation of the central nervous system. The principle of sculpting definitive structures from an abundance of cells was worked out in the worm, *Caenorhabditis elegans*. The arrangement in invertebrates, such as the fruit-fly, *Drosophila*, is both more complex and less conserved than in other classes, ending with the completion of development. Conversely, in mammals, apoptosis remains active in the adult and contributes to pathological processes. Thus, the worm strategically removes 131 of its full complement of 1090 cells through the balanced activities of *EGL1*, *CED3*, *CED4* (death genes) and *CED9* (a suppressor of cell death). Mammalian homologues of Ced-3 in the worm are caspases, and related molecules, some of which are specific for neurons. In mammals, programmed cell death is orchestrated by the family of caspases, related molecules such as interleukin-1 (IL-1) converting enzyme, and the Bcl-2 family consisting both of anti-apoptotic (Ced-9/Bcl-2-like and Bcl-X) and pro-apoptotic (Egl-1-like, Bax, Bad and Bid) molecules. These are localized at the mitochondrial outer membrane, and the endoplasmic reticulum and perinuclear membrane, acting to stabilize mitochondrial structure and function. Some are expressed transiently

during development to maintain survival whilst trophic support is being established through synaptic connectivity. Others persist both in the brain and/or peripheral nervous system throughout adult life. A few are implicated only in pathological processes. Proteases such as caspase 8 are recruited into apoptosome complexes induced by ligation of death receptors including CD95 (Apo-1/Fas) and tumour necrosis factor (TNF) receptor 1 using the Fas-associated death domain protein (FADD). T cells use this mechanism to remove infected target cells (see Chapter 11). An additional mammal-specific apoptotic mechanism involves formation of a complex including *APAF1* (Apoptotic protease activating factor-1; homologous to CED-4). This transmits apoptotic signals from mitochondrial damage, releasing cytochrome C and activating caspase 9. Caspases cleave proteins supporting the nuclear membrane and cause apoptosis by activation of the endonuclease that digests DNA. Especially in the nervous system, the stimulus to apoptosis (or the brake on its intrinsic activity) is the limiting amount of peptide growth factors. Because the organ is so dependent on apoptosis, defects in the regulatory system affecting caspases or the CD95/TNF-receptor are often expressed as a disorder of the nervous system. For example, failure to apoptose progenitors leads to uncontrolled proliferation of the periventricular zone in Apaf-1 null mice (Cecconi *et al* 1998). Conversely, overexpression of Bcl-2 can compensate for growth factor deprivation and prevent neuronal death from loss of trophic support, and cell injury. Thus, Schierle *et al* (1999) showed that cell death is reduced *in vitro* and *in vivo* by the caspase inhibitor Ac-YVAD-cmk. (For more detailed reviews of neuronal apoptosis see Meier *et al* 2000; Yuan and Yankner 2000.)

Nerve growth factors bind the TrkA, TrkB and TrkC cell surface receptors and set up a cascade of intracellular events through phosphorylation of the cytoplasmic tail of membrane-bound tyrosine kinases. Molecules participating in downstream events are cyclic-AMP response element binding protein (CREB), Forkhead and NF-κB. Prominent amongst the signal transduction pathways is Akt/phosphoinositol 3-kinase, activated by several neurotrophins and by Ras. Activated Akt inhibits pro-apoptotic molecules such as Bad and therefore keeps neurons alive. Various mechanisms and interventions that activate Akt can replace the need for neurotrophin or anti-apoptotic molecules, emphasizing the interplay and redundancy of ligand and receptor-based signal transduction in cell death and survival. Mitogen-activated protein (MAP) kinase activates the extracellular signal regulated protein kinase (ERK) and MAP kinase/ERK (MEK) pathways. These are specifically implicated in a different set of neurotrophin-related survival pathways but may converge on phosphorylation of CREB and Bcl-2. It follows that these anti-apoptotic events are also linked to active phases of neurotrophin-induced cell proliferation. It has long been known that electrical activity and ion exchange events also influence cell survival (Z. Mao *et al* 1999). Growth factor deprivation and MAP kinase/phosphoinositide 3-kinase inactivity lead to cell death, through the release of reactive oxygen species and the activation of c-Jun amino-terminal kinase (JNK), with the collapse of gene transcription and protein synthesis. Paradoxically, acting through the p75 neurotrophin receptor, growth factors may cause apoptotic death in cells stimulated to divide but unable to enter the cell cycle (see below and Chapter 12; Bamji *et al* 1998; Casaccia-Bonnefil *et al* 1996; Muir and Compston 1996).

Stem cells

Stem cells self replicate through asymmetric division, some of their progeny maintaining a further source of proliferative cells and others differentiating down a variety of fate-committed lineages in defined environments. Identification is by surface markers, cell-specific or stage-specific transcriptional factors, or the behaviour of their progeny. Self-evidently, stem cells are plentiful and active – both in terms of proliferation and differentiation – during development. A major advance in neurobiology was the realization that stem cells persist in most, if not all, adult tissues, where potentially they provide a renewable source of lineage-specific cell types.

Embryonic stem cells differentiate through the stage of embryoid bodies to the broad categories of ectoderm, mesoderm and endoderm. The transcriptional repressor factor Bmi-1 is required for self-renewal of stem cells but not for their survival or differentiation (Molofsky *et al* 2003). There follows an orderly development within each of blood, endothelial, muscle and neuronal fate-committed progeny. Transplanted at these primitive stages, the cells will assume the specificity of cell types characteristic of the host environment – including neurons in the brain (Brustle *et al* 1997). These rules of development are governed by the intrinsic properties of stem cells and the chance (or not) of exposure to growth factors and environmental cues to which their evolving and dynamic repertoire of receptors and transcription factors make them sensitive at any one time. To summarize a fiercely complicated story, and one that can only get more cluttered with factors acting to promote and inhibit development, embryonic stem cells proliferate in response to soluble factors such as leukaemia inhibitory factor (LIF), bone morphogenetic proteins (BMP) and Wingless-Int (Wnt). Their differentiation into neural stem cells is promoted by insulin-like growth factor (IGF) and fibroblast growth factor-2 (FGF-2) but inhibited by noggin and chordin. Neural stem cells proliferate in response to FGF-2, epidermal growth factor (EGF) and sonic hedgehog (Shh; K. Lai *et al* 2003).

The principal source of neural stem cells during development is the subventricular zone and overlying ventricular ependyma (Johansson *et al* 1999). Neural stem cells are identified by expression of the cytoskeletal markers nestin and musashi. The most important factors acting on neural stem cells are EGF and FGF-2. There may also be a requirement for IGF-1, without which neither EGF nor FGF-2 induce the proliferation of (murine) neural stem cells. Specifically, EGF acts on neural stem cell proliferation whereas FGF-2 seems to be more important for neural stem cell survival in response to autocrine production of IGF-1 (Arsenijevic *et al* 2001). The distribution of adult neural stem cells is more restricted than in the embryo. Apart from the subventricular zone, they are present especially in the hippocampus (P.S. Eriksson *et al* 1998) and olfactory bulb (Herrera *et al* 1999; Kukekov *et al* 1999) but also in the neocortex (Maglivi *et al* 2000). Activation of the nuclear receptor TLX has been identified as the key event in maintaining the proliferating undifferentiated progenitor status of adult (murine) neural stem cells, suppressing their switch to defined fates (Shi *et al* 2004). However, this analysis is complicated by the fact that mature cells undergo dedifferentiation and act as a renewed source of pluripotential stem cells. Differentiated mammalian precursors may switch between separate lineages. Kondo and Raff (2000)

turned oligodendrocyte precursors back into neural stem cells that were then able to self-renew and differentiate into neurons, astrocytes and oligodendrocytes. Remarkably, neural stem cells can even assume a haemopoietic fate (Bjornson *et al* 1999). In their capacity to dedifferentiate, astrocytes appear, under some circumstances, to be the most dynamic amongst those cell types present in the adult nervous system. It was the selective depletion and reappearance of stem cells in areas populated only by green-fluorescent-protein-labelled astrocytes, and the migration of these nascent stem cells to the olfactory bulb where they differentiated into neurons, that established the stem cell credentials of subventricular zone astrocytes in mammals (Doetsch *et al* 1999; Laywell *et al* 2000). A subsequent interpretation is that the stem cell properties of astrocytes represent a default state of neuroepithelial development from radial glia to mature astrocytes but with the potential for reversing this process (Doetsch 2003). However, as is now evident throughout the whole story of glial neurobiology, caution is needed in unqualified extrapolation of principles derived in rodents to the human central nervous system. In rats and mice, stem cells born in the subventricular zone are distributed – as part of neurogenesis – through the rostal migratory stream. This does not exist in adult humans. Instead, glial precursors are found in a dense ribbon around the lateral ventricle where they may proliferate. They can differentiate into neurons *in vitro* but the message seems to be that, apart from within the hippocampus, the adult central nervous system can replenish astrocytes and oligodendrocytes but lacks the potential and migratory pathway for distributing new neurons (Sanai *et al* 2004).

Nuances of interpretation colour all these observations. One is the dependence on markers that may not be entirely specific for defined fates. It is not easy to distinguish true differentiation of bone marrow stem cells to a neural fate from fusion with pre-existing differentiated host cells – neurons, in the case of the nervous system (Alvarez-Dolado *et al* 2003). Gradually the possible explanations – both biological and spurious – for these changes in cell type have been whittled down by laboratory manipulations or protocols for detection *in vivo*, revealing fusion between differentiated cell types, transdifferentiation between different preformed cell types, transdetermination by recommitting one lineage of stem cell differentiation to another, and dedifferentiation of a mature cell to its own precursor status (for review, see C.M. Rice and Scolding 2004). The issue with respect to applying knowledge on the biology of stem cells to multiple sclerosis is whether their differentiation into the three main defined phenotypes – neuron, astrocyte and oligodendrocyte – is predictable or random, and open to manipulation. The first step is to characterize the survival, migration and differentiation into neurons, astrocytes and oligodendrocytes *in vivo* of neural stem cells under the influence of local environmental cues (Reubinoff *et al* 2001). Reduced expression of the intracellular regulator of cytokine signalling SOCS2, in response to LIF, switches neural stem cell differentiation from a neuronal to a glial fate – perhaps by failing to inhibit growth-hormone-mediated suppression of neurogenesis (Turnley *et al* 2002).

First to appear are radial glia. Differentiation occurs with the asymmetric distribution of cell surface receptors: the progeny of neural stem cells retaining high FGF receptor expression express markers of radial glia, through sustained asymmetric division, eventually form oligodendrocytes and astrocytes (Sun *et al* 2005). These form parallel arrays from the subventricular zone to the subpial brain surface (Cameron and Rakic 1991). Initially, radial glia are bipolar, with a short process connecting the cell body to the adjacent ventricular zone, and a longer process penetrating the developing cortical plate, reaching to the pial surface and terminating in the glial limiting membrane. Outward migration of the cell body then occurs, altering the relative length of the two processes. As movement occurs towards the cortex, the descending process is lost, the ascending one elaborates and the cell begins to resemble the mature astrocyte with randomly orientated processes. The radial network coincides with neuronal histogenesis, suggesting that this serves as a scaffold for nerve cells migrating from their germinal zones towards the developing cortex. Oligodendrocyte precursors may also use radial glia to get around the developing nervous system. The wave of neuronal growth is associated with inhibition of glial proliferation. However, as nerve cells switch from the phase of migration to the establishment of synaptic connections, radial glia recommence their own proliferation and differentiation into multipolar stellate cells (Culican *et al* 1990) expressing a variety of glial antigens including glial fibrillary acidic protein (GFAP), glutamate transporters and adhesion molecules (for review, see Doetsch 2003).

However, radial glia are now also considered to be the main source of proliferative precursor cells in the main zones of neurogenesis – the subventricular zone, hippocampus and olfactory bulb (Doetsch 2003). The distinguishing feature of mature astrocytes is expression of the intermediate filaments GFAP, S-100 and vimentin (Eng and Ghirnikar 1994) but the distinction is blurred given that 'mature' astrocytes replace radial glia as the population of persistent neural precursors in mammals. With expression of the transcription factor Pax 6 in mice, radial glia also generate neurons in the developing cerebral cortex (Heins *et al* 2002). Because of their early appearance in cell development, it is significant that mouse embryonic stem cells can be induced to differentiate into radial glia, retaining an appropriate morphology and expressing appropriate cytoskeletal markers (nestin, RC2 and GFAP: Liour and Yu 2003). One stimulus for the development of radial glia and other members of the astrocyte lineage from stem cells may be BMP-4 (Gomes *et al* 2003), a member of the transforming growth factor-β (TGF-β) superfamily. Without the nuclear receptor co-repressor (N-CoR) of transcription, neural stem cells maintained by culture in FGF-2 spontaneously differentiate into astrocytes. Glial differentiaton can also be induced by ciliary neurotrophic factor (CNTF) acting through phosphatidyl-inositol-3-OH kinase/Akt kinase to phosphorylate N-CoR, whereas this molecular event and astrocyte differentiation are each inhibited by recruitment of protein phosphatase-1 to N-CoR (Hermanson *et al* 2002). FGF-2 regulates the ability of CNTF to induce astrocyte differentiation by facilitating access of the STAT/CRER binding protein to the GFAP promoter, switching methylation between amino acids that destabilize progenitor status and forcing astrocyte differentiation (M.R. Song and Ghosh 2004). Mature astrocytes develop in the context of BMP, LIF, CNTF and signalling through Notch1. It has been suggested that they represent the default stage of development from neural stem cells, appearing when neurogenesis and oligodendrocyte development are restricted in *OLIG1/2* and *NGN2/MASH1* transgenic mice (Q. Nieto *et al* 2001; Zhou and Anderson 2002).

Turning to neuronal fates, factors produced by hippocampal astrocytes are able specifically to regulate neurogenesis from neural stem cells (H. Song *et al* 2002). In primates, the evidence suggests that proliferation occurs *in situ* rather than through cell migration from a remote precursor depot (E. Gould *et al* 1998). Their differentiation to a neuronal fate is promoted by platelet derived growth factor (PDGF) and inhibited by Notch1. Those derived from the (murine) basal forebrain differentiate into GABAergic neurons and oligodendrocytes, populating the cortex and hippocampus (W. He *et al* 2001). New neurons generated in the dentate nucleus of the adult mammalian hippocampus acquire the electrical properties and synaptic activity of fully functional neurons (van Praag *et al* 2002). Retinoic acid also promotes embryonic cell differentiation down the neuronal lineage. In humans, adult subventricular zone cells and occasional cortical cells express markers of neural stem cell precursors. Proliferating neurons are present in the hippocampus of patients given bromodeoxyuridine to assess the mitotic activity in primary tumours outside the central nervous system, and studied at autopsy up to 2 years later (P.S. Eriksson *et al* 1998). With clinical applications in mind, J.H. Kim *et al* (2002) have reproducibly derived dopaminergic neurons from neural stem cells by inducing Nurr1 in cultured embryonic stem cells, retaining behavioural and electrophysiological properties appropriate for cells of midbrain origin and correcting abnormalities in animal models of movement disorders.

A neural fate can be induced in mesodermal stem cells derived from bone marrow or skin (see Figures 10.2 and 10.3; Bjornson *et al* 1999; Cogle *et al* 2004; Joannides *et al* 2004; Liang and Bickenbach 2002; Sanchez-Ramos *et al* 2000; Toma *et al* 2001). After 6 weeks, samples of adult human dermis cultured in EGF and FGF-2 show proliferative cells, expressing markers of neural stem cells (nestin and musashi-1) that can be coaxed into neuronal differentiation by hippocampus-derived astrocyte-conditioned medium – the cells displaying the morphology and neurotransmitter characteristics of GABAergic and glutamate and showing voltage-sensitive calcium transients (Figure 10.3; Joannides *et al* 2004). Stem cells obtained from murine bone marrow, enriched on adult haematopoietic progenitors (CD117-positive), yield cells expressing oligodendrocyte markers after transplantation into the neonatal mouse brain (Bonilla *et al* 2002).

From the perspective of multiple sclerosis, perhaps most interest attaches to the possibility of driving oligodendrocyte development from stem cells. Rodent oligodendrocytes develop from progenitors that also give rise to neurons under the influence of Olig1 and Olig2 (Q.R. Lu *et al* 2001; 2002; Takebayashi *et al* 2002) – both of which are induced by Shh and encode basic helix–loop–helix proteins. Neurotrophin (NT)-3, thyroxine and the related tri-iodothyronine, retinoic acid and glucocorticoids each also stimulate oligodendrocyte differentiation and maturation from stem cells or committed precursors *in vitro*. A protocol that permits the generation of oligodendrocyte precursors and astrocytes, first described by Brustle *et al* (1999), involves sequential EGF and basic FGF exposure of embryonic stem cells aggregated into embryoid bodies, followed by FGF-2 and PDGF. Further modifications, suitable for differentiation of human embryonic stem cells, are provided by Niston *et al* (2005). On growth factor withdrawal, the stem cells differeniate into oligodendrocyte precursors, and subsequently into mature oligodendrocytes, expressing CNPase and

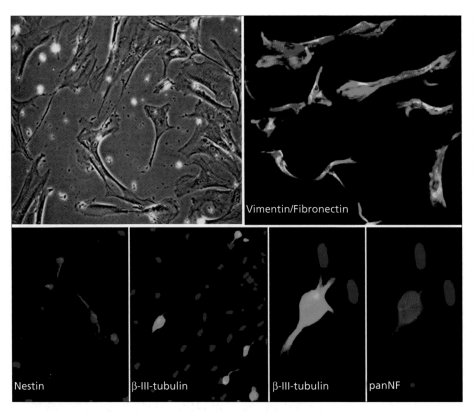

Figure 10.2 Generation of neurons from adult human bone marrow. Adherent bone marrow stromal cells grown in serum co-express vimentin and fibronectin (top panel). Treatment with growth factors epidermal growth factor and fibroblast growth factor results in induction of nestin-expressing neural precursor cells, which upon exposure to astrocyte derived signals differentiate into βIII tubulin and neurofilament expressing cells. Reproduced from Joannides *et al* (2003) with permission.

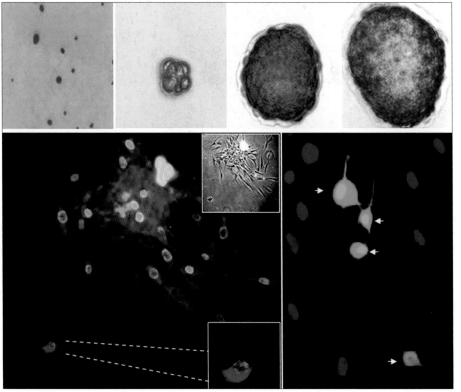

Figure 10.3 Generation of neurons from adult human skin. Skin cells divide and form spheres after treatment with growth factors, epidermal growth factor and fibroblast growth factor (top panel). Spheres contain dividing neural precursors co-expressing nestin (red) and bromodeoxyuridine (green). Neural differentiation of skin derived spheres showing cells expressing βIII tubulin (arrowheads). Reproduced from Joannides *et al* (2004). © 2004, with permission from Elsevier.

O4, and astrocytes in about equal numbers. These cells are able to myelinate naked axons (see below). Embryonic stem cells exposed to retinoic acid were shown to generate oligodendrocytes after culture in medium conditioned by oligodendrocyte progenitor enriched neurospheres (S. Liu *et al* 2000). In EGF-stimulated populations of neural stem cells, additional exposure to FGF-2 steers the differentiation of oligodendrocytes and inhibits neuronal development acting through the FGF-2 and -3 receptors (Reimers *et al* 2001).

MACROGLIAL LINEAGES IN THE RODENT AND HUMAN NERVOUS SYSTEM

Classified broadly into astrocytes and oligodendrocytes, macroglia in the central nervous system are in reality a much more diverse population consisting of several morphological and functional subpopulations of each.

Astrocytes

Astrocytes have diverse functions (Figure 10.4). They provide architecture for neurons, define anatomical boundaries, and are critically involved in maintaining a constant extracellular ionic milieu – a major requirement for neuronal impulse generation and propagation. They act as a source of growth factors and cytokines. Astrocytes influence neuronal energy metabolism through the provision and transport of glucose. They provide a substrate for axonal and dendritic plasticity, and sequestrate toxic substances including excitatory neurotransmitters such as glutamate. They participate in the response to injury (Shao and

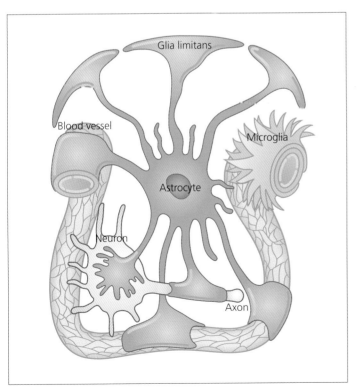

Figure 10.4 Interactions of astrocytes in the central nervous system.

McCarthy 1994; Wilkin *et al* 1990). Finally, they now top the list of central nervous system cells having the potential to re-engage the developmental process and act as stem cells (see above; Doetsch 2003).

The classification of astrocytes has gone through a series of modifications. Originally distinguished as protoplasmic or fibrillary (Andriezen 1893; Cajal 1913; A. Peters *et al* 1976), protoplasmic astrocytes were mainly identified in the grey matter whereas fibrillary cells were most abundant in white matter. These broad classifications became particularly persuasive with the discovery *in vitro* of distinguishing surface markers. Thus, the protoplasmic astrocyte was conspicuous for staining with the surface antibody Ran-2 (Bartlett *et al* 1981) but not the anti-ganglioside antibody, A2B5. Conversely, fibrillary astrocytes were negative for Ran-2 and stained for A2B5. This distinction gained credence with the availability of results from developmental studies of the rodent optic nerve leading to the designation of type 1 and type 2 astrocytes. Here, protoplasmic (type 1) astrocytes appeared to provide cues for oligodendrocyte progenitor cell differentiation. The intimate relationship between astrocytes and axons at the node of Ranvier, and the demonstration of sodium channels at high concentration at the node itself suggested that astrocytes might exhibit major specializations in astrocyte function at this site (Arroyo and Scherer 2000). These cells were designated as type 2 astrocytes (ffrench Constant and Raff 1986). Other soluble and extracellular matrix molecules were identified that were needed to maintain this phenotype, preferentially induce development of the type 2 astrocyte and inhibit differentiation down the default pathway of the oligodendrocyte lineage (Lillien *et al* 1990). Although morphological studies subsequently identified up to nine categories amongst spinal cord astrocytes, all with staining properties of the putative type 2 astrocyte (Black *et al* 1993), there were many unresolved controversies in this classification. In time, the ion channel properties of astrocytes resembling the type 2 (fibrillary) astrocyte were shown to be no different from those of the type 1 (protoplasmic) cell (B.P. Fulton *et al* 1992). In fact, morphological visualization of rat optic nerve oligodendrocytes and astrocytes *in vivo* did not support the existence of a separate type 2 astrocyte population (Butt and Ransom 1989). Furthermore, the morphological and biochemical properties of type 2 astrocytes eventually resembled those of type 1 astrocytes after a period of time in culture (Skoff *et al* 1976). As a result, several distinguishing features came to be considered *in vitro* artefacts, not faithfully replicating the *in vivo* arrangements. However, leaving aside the type 1 (protoplasmic) and type 2 (fibrillary) classification, the concept of astrocyte heterogeneity still seems valid. Regional specialization is apparent from ion channel characteristics (Black *et al* 1993), the expression of cell surface molecules (Kobayashi *et al* 1996), immunological properties (Girgrah *et al* 1991) and the expression of intracellular molecules (P.J. McKinnon and Margolskee 1996).

The oligodendrocyte lineage

Precursor cells which generate oligodendrocytes can be recovered from many parts of the developing nervous system. Studies of the optic nerve and spinal cord have proved especially influential in characterizing cell lineages and the factors that orchestrate proliferation, migration and differentiation.

Oligodendrocyte progenitor

One previously much characterized step in oligodendrocyte development featured the oligodendrocyte-type 2 astrocyte (O-2A) progenitor recovered from the rodent optic nerve, cerebrum and hindbrain (Figure 10.5). Although highly influential, it is now recognized that this cell, capable of developing both oligodendrocyte and astrocyte progeny, was characterized in an entirely artificial milieu, and the direct dividend of knowledge for understanding *in vivo* properties of the oligodendrocyte lineage based on such studies is limited. Tissue culture studies from the laboratory of Martin Raff showed that the O-2A cell is bipolar or tripolar (Raff *et al* 1983). The antigenic phenotype was defined by staining for the ganglioside GD3, the cytoplasmic intermediate filament vimentin, and A2B5 but not galactocerebroside or GFAP (Raff *et al* 1983; 1984). Cells of the oligodendrocyte lineage were also shown to express nicotinic and muscarinic acetylcholine receptors at several stages in their development. Oligodendrocyte differentiation represents the default pathway for the O-2A progenitor *in vitro*. This occurs in the absence of serum-derived signals whereas, in the presence of serum, most cells acquire astrocyte markers whilst retaining progenitor-related gangliosides. A further defining characteristic of the O-2A cell is its capacity for proliferation, self-renewal and motility (R.K. Small *et al* 1987).

Failure to reproduce the staining properties of the O-2A cell *in vivo* soon brought its status into question. However, with time, the use of existing and additional markers, together with advances in knowledge of stem cell development, have revealed what always seemed clear – that the ability to define steps marking cell lineage development depends on the availability of appropriate methods and reagents for their detection, in both the rodent and human central nervous systems. The O-2A cell was therefore an early and pioneering discovery in the much richer and more extensive catalogue now revealed. Many intermediate components are identified. More surprising is the discovery that these intermediate phenotypes are also present in the adult nervous system (see below).

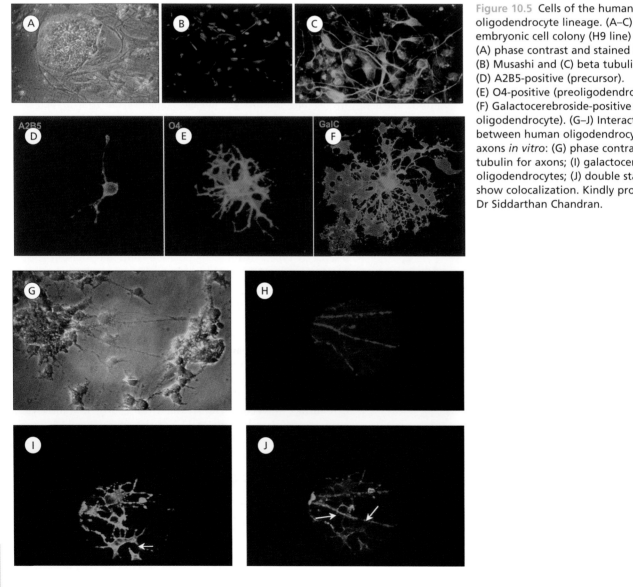

Figure 10.5 Cells of the human oligodendrocyte lineage. (A–C) Human embryonic cell colony (H9 line) under (A) phase contrast and stained for (B) Musashi and (C) beta tubulin. (D) A2B5-positive (precursor). (E) O4-positive (preoligodendrocyte). (F) Galactocerebroside-positive (mature oligodendrocyte). (G–J) Interactions between human oligodendrocytes and axons *in vitro*: (G) phase contrast; (H) beta tubulin for axons; (I) galactocerebroside for oligodendrocytes; (J) double staining to show colocalization. Kindly provided by Dr Siddarthan Chandran.

Tissue prints obtained from sections of fresh optic nerve and other parts of the central nervous system contain A2B5-positive cells that have the morphology of cultured O-2A progenitors. The O-2A lineage cells were identified *in vivo* by exploiting their expression of glutamate receptor channels of the quisqualate/kainate type (B.P. Fulton *et al* 1992). Unipolar and bipolar cells ultrastructurally resembling O-2A progenitors were identified in the developing rat optic nerve. An alternative approach was to identify progenitor cells with anti-NG2 chondroitin sulphate proteoglycan (J.M. Levine *et al* 1993). This appeared to associate closely with the PDGF-receptor, suggesting that NG2 staining is a reliable surrogate marker for the PDGF-signalling pathway (Nishiyama *et al* 1996). Addressing the problem of specific identification of these cells *in vivo*, Pringle *et al* (1992b) showed specificity of *in situ* hybridization labelling the O-2A cell for PDGF-α chain receptor mRNA, and this technique has since been used to identify populations of cells in the spinal cord and ventricular zone during embryonic development (Pringle and Richardson 1993). With time, the most versatile and widely used reagents have proved to be PDGF-α chain receptor and NG2. In the normal adult central nervous system, NG2-positive cells are widely distributed in the brain and spinal cord, showing proliferative and oligodendrocyte precursor cell properties – at least in the adult rat central nervous system (M.R. Dawson *et al* 2003). However, they usually contact the node of Ranvier (Butt *et al* 1999), leading to the suggestion that they should be called *synantocytes*, from the Greek 'to contact' (Butt *et al* 2002). NG2 cells selectively express mRNA only for oligodendrocte proteins (Ye *et al* 2003), and so may be precursors preferentially set to respond to demyelination.

Oligodendrocyte precursor maturation preferentially uses the PDGF-α chain receptor and its PDGF-AA ligand, rather than PDGF-B, in most parts of the nervous system where oligodendrogenesis is possible (Fruttiger *et al* 1999). Proliferation of the oligodendrocyte precursor in response to PDGF-AA requires cell binding to extracellular matrix through aVβ3 integrin with activation of the phosphoinositide 3-kinase signal transduction pathway (W. Baron *et al* 2002; 2005). Proliferation stops when the PDGF-α chain receptor becomes marooned in a plasma membrane lipid raft but the receptor maintains a role in cell survival. This is mediated by PDGF-α chain receptor clustering with α1β6 integrin in response to axonal laminin 2 which acts through the oligodendrocyte phosphoinositide 3-kinase/Akt pathway (W. Baron *et al* 2003). A similar mechanism operates in the signalling of oligodendrocyte survival mediated by PDGF-α (Decker and ffrench Constant 2004). Proliferation and migration of oligodendrocyte precursors are increased by hepatocyte growth factor in association with alterations of the actin and β-tubulin cytoskeleton (Yan and Rivkees 2002). Migration may involve a response to the attractant (netrin-1) and repulsive (semaphorin 3A, which also exerts proliferative effects) receptors that are present on the oligodendrocyte precursors migrating into the embryonic optic nerve (Spassky *et al* 2002). But the process has to be more tightly regulated to achieve a uniform distribution of precursors during development, and prevent everything stacking up around the astrocytic source of trophic molecules. At first, netrin-1 is attractant for progenitors expressing the 'deleted in colorectal cancer' – or DCC – receptor. Later, coexpression of the Unc5 receptor netrin-1 is repellent and so halts the progess of progenitors, thereby achieving a

uniform distribution. Expression of the transcription factor ATF5 is required to suspend differentiation into oligodendrocytes so that adequate distribution of precursors may occur: loss of ATF5 leads to premature differentiation and aberrant migration (Mason *et al* 2005). At this stage of development, migration is also promoted by the high but transient expression of the CXCR4 receptor for the chemokine CXCL12 (Dziembowska *et al* 2005). By manipulating transgenic mice that fail to express the PDGF-α receptor, McKinnon *et al* (2005) emphasise the critical dependence of signal transduction though the phosphotidylinisotol 3-kinase (PI3-K) pathway for cell migration, and of phospholipase Cγ for proliferation; these behaviours occur in response to high and low doses of PDGF-α, respectively. The mitotic effect of PDGF-α is inhibited, and differentiation promoted, by the activity of metabotropic P2X and P2Y receptors that influence intracellular levels of adenosine di- and triphosphate (Agresti *et al* 2005).

Different arrangements are evidently found in the developing spinal cord which, through its dorsal-ventral and caudal-rostral polarities, presents special opportunities to study oligodendrocyte development. As in other parts of the nervous system, development in the spinal cord involves an orderly sequence of migration from germinal centres, concentration at sites of myelination, proliferation and then differentiation. Each step is regulated by signals that facilitate and others that inhibit these processes. Amongst astrocyte-derived molecules that limit the migration of oligodendrocytes *in vitro* are N-cadherin (Schnadelbach *et al* 2000).

During normal development, oligodendrocytes originate from restricted foci within the ventral neural tube under the influence of ventral-midline-derived (notochord and floorplate) sonic hedgehog (Shh) signalling (Figure 10.6; Pringle and Richardson 1993; Orentas *et al* 1999). They share development with motor neurons from a pool of cells whose position is influenced by the transcription factor Pax6 (T. Sun *et al* 1998). The subsequent switch from neurogenesis to oligodendrocyte development is determined by *SOX9*, with some redundancy from other Sox transcription factors (Stolt *et al* 2003). Graded Shh signalling patterns the ventral neural tube by influencing the expression of various transcription factors including the basic helix–loop–helix genes *OLIG1* and *OLIG2* (Q.R. Lu *et al* 2000; Takebayashi *et al* 2000; Q. Zhou *et al* 2000) and *NKX2.2* and *GLI2* (R. Liu *et al* 2003; Qiu *et al* 2001). *OLIG1* and *OLIG2* represent the earliest cell-type-specific genes within the oligodendrocyte lineage and their expression precedes markers of the oligodendrocyte precursor, including PDGF-α receptor and DM20/PLP (Q.R. Lu *et al* 2000). Transgenic studies suggest a hierarchy of cells involved in early development of the spinal cord (Gabay *et al* 2003). Olig1- and Olig2-positive cells are tripotential – differentiating into neurons, astrocytes and oligodendrocytes. These are expressed on radial glia and their deletion leads to failure of oligodendrocyte development but not NG2-expressing cells: Y. Liu and Rao (2004) conclude that the Olig1, Olig2 and Nkx2.2-positive cell is an oligodendrocyte-neuronal precursor, but not the exclusive source of oligodendrocytes (or neurons) in the developing spinal cord. Whereas Olig2-positive cells develop into oligodendrocytes, FGF-2 is required to induce the oligodendrocyte fate in Olig2-progenitors *in vitro* acting through Shh to induce *OLIG2*. Extinction of *OLIG2* commits the cell to become an astrocyte. Factors other than Shh determine cell fate

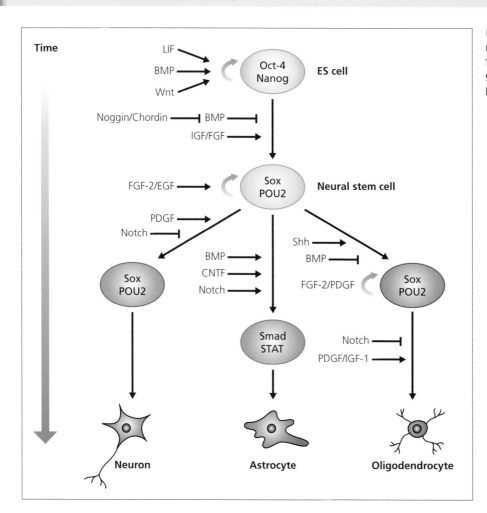

Figure 10.6 Stages in the development of neurons, astrocytes and oligodendrocytes from stem cells, and the influence of growth and transcription factors. Kindly prepared by Dr Siddarthan Chandran.

along the ventral-dorsal axis of the developing spinal cord (Barth *et al* 1999; Ishibashi and McMahon 2002; Liem *et al* 2000; McMahon *et al* 1998; Pierani *et al* 1999;). Some originate from the dorsal cord (Wada *et al* 2000). Conversely, Mekki-Dauriac *et al* (2002) showed that BMPs negatively regulate spinal cord oligodendrocyte specification.

At first, it seemed probable that oligodendrocyte precursors arise exclusively from the ventral ventricular zone under the influence of Shh produced from the floor plate, and that oligodendrocyte development in the dorsal cord only results from a ventral to dorsal migration (A. Hall *et al* 1996; Pringle and Richardson 1993; Pringle *et al* 1998; Timsit *et al* 1995; Warf *et al* 1991; W.P. Yu *et al* 1994). The source has since been localised to the Dbx-1 expressing domain of the dorsal cord (Fogarty *et al* 2005). This analysis does not exclude the possibility that the lack of oligodendrocytes in isolated rat embryonic day 14 (E14) dorsal spinal cord-derived cultures depends on failure to provide signals necessary for the generation of oligodendrocytes from neural precursors already present in the dorsal cord. This seemed possible given the fact that dorsally derived cell populations have the capacity to generate oligodendrocytes *in vitro* upon exposure to notochord or Shh, and following transplantation (Hardy and Friedrich 1996; Orentas *et al* 1999; Trousse *et al* 1995). In addition, dissociated E14 dorsal cultures stimulated with FGF-2 and EGF generate oligodendrocytes following mitogen withdrawal (Chandran *et al* 1998).

The latent oligodendroglial potential of E14 dorsal cord suggests that stimulation and proliferation of a dorsally derived cell may generate oligodendrocytes in response to these and other mitogens, without the need for inward migration of cells from the ventral cord. The FGF-2 pathway to oligodendrocyte development is Shh independent whereas, conversely, inhibition of FGF-2 prevents the effect of Shh on the generation of oligodendrocytes. Perhaps, this is explained by the constitutive effect of FGF-2 on levels of MAP kinase needed for Shh to induce OLIG2 (Kessaris *et al* 2004). There is also a need for Gli3 to interact with Shh in promoting the development of oligodendrocytes, without which there is sustained neurogenesis in the developing spinal cord (Oh *et al* 2005). Chandran *et al* (2003) had earlier characterized the relationship of rat E14 dorsally derived precursors to oligodendrocytes and the role of Shh in mediating oligodendrogenesis following expansion of these precursors in response to FGF-2. Using clonal analysis, embryonic dorsal spinal cord was shown to contain an FGF-2-responsive stem cell, providing evidence for the existence of a Shh-independent pathway for the generation of oligodendrocytes. FGF-2 mediated induction of oligodendrocytes required MAP kinase signalling and inhibition by BMP-4 and Wnt (Shimizu *et al* 2005). Analysis of uncultured and FGF-2-treated embryonic spinal cords from mice homozygous for a null mutation of Shh revealed a hedgehog-independent pathway for the induction of OLIG2 and NKX2.2 genes and oligodendrocytes.

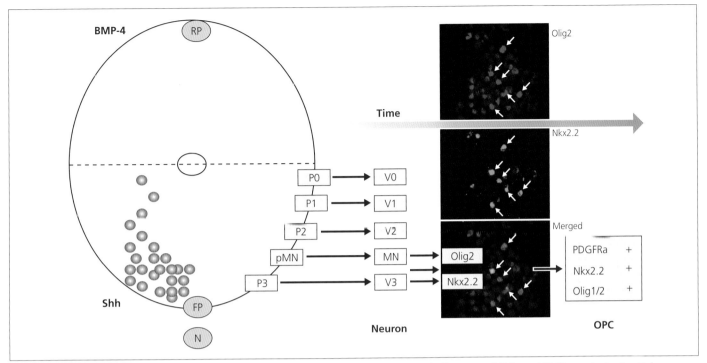

Figure 10.7 Polarity of development in the rat spinal cord showing the competing influences of Shh and BMP on pluripotential precursors. Kindly prepared by Dr Siddharthan Chandran.

Broadly similar results, manipulating the competitive antagonism between Shh and BMP-4 to produce ectopic production of oligodendrocytes in the dorsal cord, have since been demonstrated in Xenopus (R.H. Miller *et al* 2004). Others have shown that the tripotential oligodendrocyte precursor differentiates following stimulation with thyroid hormone (Gregori *et al* 2002). This acts via the p53 and p73 thyroid hormone receptors, whereas PDGF withdrawal signals only through p73 (Billon *et al* 2004). IGF-1 acts to inhibit BMP-4 signalling and thereby induces oligodendrocyte development from neural progenitors (Hsieh *et al* 2004); and migration in the developing spinal cord is inhibited by interactions between the chemokine CXCL1 produced by microglia and the CXCR2 receptor expressed on the oligodendrocyte precursor (R. Filipovic *et al* 2003; Tsai *et al* 2002).

Shh also orchestrates oligodendrocyte precursors generated in the subventricular zone of the forebrain under the influence of *OLIG1/2*, *NKX2.2* and *SOX9/10* (Nery *et al* 2001; Soula *et al* 2001; Tekki-Kessaris *et al* 2001) and populating the cortex in two waves (Ivanova *et al* 2003). This combination also promotes the development of oligodendrocytes from human olfactory epithelium derived progenitor cells (X. Zhang *et al* 2005). But there are differences in the use of transcription factors and, for example, Gli2 seems not to be involved (Qi *et al* 2001). Shh promotes GABAergic and oligodendrocyte lineage restriction by activation of basic helix–loop–helix transcription factors Olig2 and Mash1 with opposition from BMP temporally and spatially regulated by additional ligands and inhibition by noggin (Yung *et al* 2002). In the developing optic nerve, inhibiting glial expression of noggin (normally itself antagonized by BMP) checks oligodendrocyte precursor proliferation and induces an astrocyte fate (Kondo and Raff 2004). Thus, a model emerges in which oligodendrocyte development is compartmentalized in response to the gradient created by competing influences of Shh

and BMP produced at opposite poles of the spinal cord and telencephalon (Figure 10.7).

Preoligodendrocyte and oligodendrocyte

A first step in differentiation of the oligodendrocyte progenitor appears to be expression of the surface molecule marker recognized by the monoclonal antibody O4 (Trotter and Schachner 1989) which stains sulphatide and seminolipid. There is a corresponding loss of vimentin-staining filaments with differentiation. Proliferation and bipotentiality are maintained with the acqusition of O4 (Warrington and Pfeifer 1992) but the cell is no longer motile (Warrington *et al* 1993). At this stage of partial differentiation, it is a pro-oligodendrocyte. This transition is marked by accumulation of the S100B protein that is subsequently lost as the cell becomes a fully differentiated oligodendrocyte (Deloulme *et al* 2004; Hachem *et al* 2005).

The behaviour of A2B5-positive and O4-positive cells differs, reflecting stages in precursor development. PDGF-AA increases the expression of O1 on PDGF-postive cells (but not on those that are O4-positive) except in the presence of FGF-2 when proliferation is also induced. FGF-2 and IGF-1 enhance the expression of O1 by O4-positive (but not A2B5-positive) progenitors. Proliferation of the O4-positive cell requires the addition of PDGF-AA, FGF-2 and IGF-1 (J.L. Mason and Goldman 2002). The role of IGF-1 and FGF-2 may be specifically to trigger the S phase of the cell cycle prior to differentiation (H. Jiang *et al* 2001). IGF-1 enhances FGF-2 induction of cyclin D1, activation of G(1)-cyclin–cyclin-dependent kinase complexes, and phosphorylation of retinoblastoma protein – transcription factors that are involved in the switch from proliferation to differentiation (Frederick and Wood 2004). A major regulator of oligodendrocyte development is the Notch1 receptor which binds its ligand

Jagged1. This interaction induces Hes5 which inhibits the differentiation of oligodendrocyte precursors (S. Wang *et al* 1998). The order of events is disrupted in the absence of Notch1, resulting in ectopic placement of oligodendrocytes, premature differentiation and excessive apoptosis (Genoud *et al* 2002). Other ligands that interact with Notch and influence the development of oligodendrocytes from progenitors include NB-3, a member of the F3/contactin family. The switch from precursor status to terminal differentiation is inhibited (and hence timed) by the helix–loop–helix protein Id2 (S. Wang *et al* 2001), followed by signalling through the FGF-R3 (Oh *et al* 2003). To add further complexities, the proliferative effects on O4-positive cells are inhibited by IL-1β, acting through the p38 MAP kinase signal transduction pathway. This cytokine thereby promotes differentiation and survival of mature oligodendrocytes (Vela *et al* 2002). In the developing human nervous system, there is an interval between the stage of immature oligodendrocyte development and the onset of myelination during which the pioneer cells make multiple contacts with axons and express O1 but not O4 or myelin basic protein (Back *et al* 2002).

The sequential expression of a number of oligodendrocyte- or myelin-specific components follows during subsequent maturation. These include galactocerebroside GalC, the surface expression of which is generally accepted to mark terminal oligodendrocyte differentiation, signalling the loss of both proliferative and migratory potential. Myelin basic protein expression is followed by the intracellular appearance of proteolipid protein and the surface expression of myelin oligodendrocyte glycoprotein, representing the final immunocytochemically identifiable stage of oligodendrocyte maturation. At an ultrastructural level, oligodendrocyte maturation is associated with a decrease in size and an increase in density of organelles and nuclear heterochromatin. Differentiated oligodendrocytes possess a number of characteristic ultrastructural features – narrow, fine processes, cytoplasm containing numerous microtubules and ribosomes, an eccentric nucleus, and an absence of intermediate filaments (McCarthy and De Vellis 1980; A. Peters *et al* 1976).

PDGF is mitogenic for oligodendrocyte progenitors but they differentiate after a defined number of divisions (Raff *et al* 1983). However, FGF-2 indefinitely suspends their maturation and promotes migration. This may explain why FGF-2 administered to rats after the completion of myelination (at P6-9) results in an extensive loss of myelin due to disrupted oligodendrocyte function and myelin protein synthesis (Goddard *et al* 2001). Neuregulins act on oligodendrocyte precursors to promote their proliferation and survival, inhibiting the differentiation of mature oligodendrocytes (Canoll *et al* 1996; Sussman *et al* 2005). They also increase the complexity and branching of membranes produced by cells that have differentiated into mature oligodendrocytes (Raabe *et al* 1997). Amongst growth factors implicated in the terminal differentiation and process outgrowth of oligdendrocytes are those belonging to the CNTF family, with activation of its 130-kDa glycoprotein receptor and downstream Janus kinase signal transduction pathway (Stankoff *et al* 2002a). The activity of CNTF may also involve coexpression of choline acetyltransferase and muscarinic receptors (S.C. MacDonald *et al* 2002). The various isoforms of receptor for thyroid hormone are expressed during the development of precursors to mature oligodendrocytes. Thyroid hormone promotes that differentiation. Transgenic loss of the T3 receptor suspends

precursor differentiation and impairs myelination (Baas *et al* 2002). The edg-2 receptor is expressed coinciding with oligodendrocyte maturation but there is no evidence for an effect of its natural ligand, lysophosphatidic acid (Stankoff *et al* 2002b). Erythropoeitin is implicated in the late stage of oligodendrocyte development, and it also promotes astrocyte proliferation perhaps through autocrine activity (Sugawa *et al* 2002). NB-3 triggers translocation of the Notch intracellular domain acting via Deltex1 and leading to increased transcripts of myelin-associated glycoprotein (Cui *et al* 2004). The switch to oligodendrocyte differentiation and production of myelin membrane can also be triggered by transfecting oligodendrocytes with NT-3 (N. Rubio *et al* 2004) acting through cyclic AMP response element binding protein (CREB) and inhibiting (the anti-apoptotic protein) Bcl-2 (Saini *et al* 2004). Survival factors for cells of the oligodendrocyte lineage include IGF-1, IGF-2, LIF, IL-6 and NT-3 and CNTF (Barres *et al* 1992).

Oligodendrocyte precursors express a repertoire of extracellular matrix molecules at different stages in development. These integrins exert effects by amplifying the signalling of growth factors such as PDGF and neuregulin. One mechanism for this amplification is integrin activation – a conformational change in the integrin induced by the growth factor that increases ligand binding affinity. This interaction provides the mechanism for a fundamental process in neural development – target-dependent survival of newly differentiated cells. As laminins are expressed on the surface of target axons, only those oligodendrocytes that establish contact will amplify signals from the limiting concentration of available growth factors and so survive, while the remainder will undergo apoptosis.

Myelin-forming oligodendrocytes use an α6 integrin-regulated switch in the signal transduction pathway on which they depend for survival from phosphoinositide 3-kinase to MAP kinase on contact with axons (Colognato *et al* 2002). This also checks the ability of neuregulin to inhibit precursor cell differentiation, thereby promoting the availability of mature oligodendrocytes needed for establishing axon–glial interactions (Calaora *et al* 2001; Vartanian *et al* 1999), acting through the erbB2 receptor (S-K. Park *et al* 2001a). Laminin-2 is required for central nervous system myelination in mice activating phosphoinositide 3-kinase and stimulating integrin-linked kinases (Chun *et al* 2003). TNF-α may have the same inhibitory effect on oligodendrocyte precursor maturation (Cammer and Zhang 1999). Knockout of the *ERB2* receptor (through which neuregulin signals) leads to widespread hypomyelination as a result of arrested development of oligodendrocyte precursors, many of which undergo apoptosis, and incomplete oligodendrocyte differentiation (J.Y. Kim *et al* 2003). However, oligodendrocytes and myelination develop normally in the absence of erb3 (Schmucker *et al* 2003) – suggesting some redundancy in the erb/neuregulin system. Oligodendrocyte precursors express metabotropic glutamate receptors (mGluR5; Luyt *et al* 2003). Adenosine released by electrically active neurons may be the signal that inhibits proliferation and triggers differentiation of the oligodendrocyte precursor as it establishes axonal contact (Stevens *et al* 2002). The extension of processes by mature oligodendrocytes involves protein kinase C-mediated expression of matrix metalloproteinase-9 (Oh *et al* 1999). It is inhibited by Sema3 signalling through the collapsing response mediator protein 2 and Unc-33 like protein 2 (Ricard *et al* 2000).

The issue of whether mature oligodendrocytes can dedifferentiate is much debated. Initially, this was proposed as an explanation for the appearance of new myelinating cells in human and experimental lesions. Later, the existence of proliferative and pluripotential precursors in adult nervous systems was seen as an alternative source of remyelinating cells. Now, the possibility that mature phenotypes may slip back through the developmental repertoire reawakens the concept of dedifferentiation. In reaching the conclusion some time ago that oligodendrocytes may dedifferentiate, P.M. Wood and Bunge (1991) compared oligodendrocytes and immature progenitors for their capacity to proliferate, generate new oligodendrocytes and myelinate. They showed enhanced myelination by cells that expressed markers of mature, compared with precursor, oligodendrocytes. Later, Crang *et al* (2004) confirmed that, when cultured with EGF and FGF-2, putatively mature oligodendrocytes underwent cell division (and were able to remyelinate acute lesions). However, their preferred explanation lay in reduced credibility for the markers of maturity rather than the suggestion that mature oligodendrocytes may dedifferentiate. These observational studies have been supplemented by attempts to stimulate cell division in mature oligodendrocytes.

Grinspan *et al* (1993) and Muir and Compston (1996) each reported that mixed cultures of differentiated oligodendrocytes and O-2A progenitors exposed to basic FGF show an increased number of O-2A cells and a decreased proportion of oligodendrocytes. This could be interpreted as indicating dedifferentiation. Since cultures depleted of O-2A cells subsequently showed a rapid return in the number of these progenitors, in contrast to oligodendrocyte-depleted cultures, Grinspan *et al* (1993) concluded that there must be a direct effect of basic FGF on proliferation and dedifferentiation of mature oligodendrocytes to form a new population of oligodendrocyte precursors. However, Muir and Compston (1996) preferred the explanation that fully differentiated oligodendrocytes are capable neither of proliferation nor of remyelination. They interpreted the findings of Wood and Bunge (1991) as indicating that mature dividing cells are merely the progeny of progenitors which have recently divided and then differentiated, giving the appearance of being both mitotic and mature. Furthermore, Muir and Compston (1996) showed that fully differentiated oligodendrocytes stimulated to divide by exposure to basic FGF, transduce the mitotic signal and enter the cell cycle but cannot divide. Therefore, they commit to the default pathway of apoptosis. Subsequently, R. Bansal and Pfeiffer (1997) qualified this observation by showing that, on exposure to FGF-2, rat oligodendrocytes first re-enter the cell cycle without dividing. They then switch off myelin gene expression and alter their expression of FGF receptors. They do not dedifferentiate but may survive (at least for 48 hours) in this nonmyelinating state. More prolonged stimulation *in vitro* leads to apoptosis. Casaccia-Bonnefil *et al* (1996) also showed that mature postnatal rat cortical oligodendrocytes, but not their progenitors or astrocytes, are selectively killed by exposure to nerve growth factor (NGF), binding through the p75 receptor when trkA is not coexpressed whereas no such effect is seen with BDNF or NT-3. The p75 receptor may be upregulated on oligodendrocytes within the lesions of multiple sclerosis. Mature oligodendrocytes increase the expression of pro-apoptotic (Bax and Bad) but not anti-apoptotic (Bcl-2) molecules (Osterhout *et al* 2002). Goddard

et al (1999) showed increased numbers of preoligodendrocytes but gaps in the amount of myelination and myelin proteins achieved by differentiated oligodendrocytes, following injection of FGF-2, whereas IGF-1 had no effect on preoligodendrocytes. The number of mature oligodendrocytes and their ability to myelinate axons in the developing anterior medullary velum were both increased.

Thus, there may be diametrically opposite effects of growth factors on cells of the same lineage depending on the expression of receptors, the signals transduced and their ability to enter the cell cycle. Although it would be premature to extrapolate from these *in vitro* findings to therapy in multiple sclerosis, the observations obviously invite caution in planning for the indiscriminate exposure to growth factors of cells (in this instance mature oligodendrocytes) that cannot respond by cell division and therefore may die by default.

Adult oligodendrocyte progenitor

With development, the highly proliferative ventricular zone, where glial progenitors are born, diminishes in size to leave the subependyma containing cells, which continue to proliferate in response to physiological signals, thereby maintaining a quiescent population of adult stem cells with neuronal and glial potential. Soon after the O-2A oligodendrocyte precursor was identified *in vitro*, it became clear that cells having the properties of oligodendrocyte precursors could also be recovered from the adult rodent nervous system (ffrench Constant and Raff 1986; Wolswijk and Noble 1989). Each expressed the ganglioside recognized by A2B5 but, whereas only the adult cell also stained for O4 (in which respect it resembles the preoligodendrocyte), the neonatal progenitor was characterized by vimentin intermediate filaments. The adult oligodendrocyte progenitor was described as usually unipolar, with a slower rate of migration and a longer cell cycle than the neonatal counterpart (Wolswijk and Noble 1989). It behaved as a stem cell, dividing asymmetrically (at least *in vitro*) to produce one daughter O-2A cell and one oligodendrocyte (Wren *et al* 1992). Adult O-2A progenitors were shown to re-enter a more proliferative phase for a limited period, perhaps by resuming the phenotype, growth factor responsiveness and behaviour of neonatal O-2A progenitors, thereby increasing their rate of division prior to final differentiation and so maximizing the production of oligodendrocytes ultimately derived from the adult O-2A progenitor pool (Engel and Wolswijk 1996; Wolswijk and Noble 1992). This evidence for the presence of fate-committed precursors in the adult nervous system may now seem self-evident given the subsequent expansion of information on adult stem cell biology but it was pioneering at the time.

The same sequence of migration, proliferation and differentiation operates for the adult and neonatal oligodendrocyte precursors. Irrespective of site of origin, cells of the adult oligodendrocyte lineage show a reduction in proliferation with the acquisition of O4 staining. Their growth factor requirements are similar to neonatal cells with a proliferative response to basic FGF, PDGF and NT-3 whereas the CNTF group, IGF family and NT-3 act as survival factors. Although proliferation is arrested in mice that are deficient in cyclin-dependent kinase-2 (CDK2) mice, maturation of oligodendrocyte precursors is not triggered, indicating that signals other than cell cycling from

G(1) to S phase, dependent on cdk2 and cyclin2, are required for differentiation (Belachew *et al* 2002). It has been estimated that around 1% of all mature oligodendrocytes (and also 1% of astrocytes) in the adult (rat) spinal cord are the recent progeny of actively dividing progenitors (Horner *et al* 2000).

Human oligodendrocyte precursors

Useful as have been these studies, it is clear that, with respect to glial lineages, significant differences exist between the rodent and human central nervous systems. Kennedy and Fok-Seang (1986) first showed that a bipolar, A2B5-positive cell could be cultured from human fetal brain. Subsequent analyses indicated that human oligodendrocyte precursors are born in many parts of the central nervous system, including the spinal cord (Weidenheim *et al* 1994; W.P. Yu *et al* 1994) by 7–9 weeks of gestation, and can be identified 2–3 weeks before the onset of myelination. A2B5-positive radial glia with some similarities to the rodent O-2A progenitor were cultured from embryonic (6–9 weeks) human spinal cord. There were no proliferative responses to PDGF or FGF-2 (Aloisi *et al* 1992) but human neurospheres expanded with FGF-2 increase their yield of oligodendrocytes when stimulated with T3 (K. Murray and Dubois Dalcq 1997). Satoh and Kim (1994) found that, while immature oligodendrocytes (from human embryonic brain at 12–15 weeks) appear constitutively to divide in untreated cultures, no significant additional proliferative response is evoked by the addition of PDGF and/or FGF-2. Furthermore, at this stage, no staining is seen with either A2B5 or GD3 antibodies.

Rivkin *et al* (1995) studied human cerebra from 15–18-week fetuses and generated cultures, maintained long-term in serum-free medium, in which large numbers of glia with the morphology and phenotype of O-2A cells differentiated both to preoligodendrocytes and fully differentiated oligodendrocytes over the ensuing weeks. Cells were identified in tissue sections which had the staining properties of progenitors and fully differentiated oligodendrocytes. Culture in serum-containing medium yielded progenitors, oligodendrocytes and cells with the morphological appearance of type 2 astrocytes, and this was taken as evidence for bipotentiality. Proliferation was not demonstrated. As in the rat, oligodendrocyte precursors are born on each side of the spinal cord ventral ependyma above the floor plate, coinciding with the expression of growth promoting factors such as Shh. Their number increases in the ventral and lateral portion of the cervical and then the lumbar cord, thereafter populating the lateral and dorsal regions by the time myelination starts at embryonic day 83 (Hajihosseini *et al* 1996).

Chandran *et al* (2004) compared and contrasted the capacity of neural precursors derived from the developing human and rodent spinal cord to generate oligodendrocytes. The developing human spinal cord showed a comparable ventral-dorsal gradient of oligodendrocyte differentiation potential to the embryonic day 14 rodent spinal cord. However, unlike the rat cord, FGF-2 expanded human neural precursors derived from both isolated ventral or dorsal cultures had no obvious capacity to generate oligodendrocytes following FGF-2 treatment. Candidate growth factors suggested from rodent studies, including FGF-2 and PDGF, did not stimulate proliferation of human oligodendrocyte lineage cells. Seemingly, the (as yet uncharacterized) environment of the demyelinated adult rat spinal cord is not sufficient to stimulate the differentiation of immature human spinal cord cells to form oligodendrocytes. Thus, as expected, there are interspecies differences in the capacity of neural precursors to generate oligodendrocytes (Figure 10.8). That said, H.C. Wilson *et al* (2003) defined human embryonic oligodendrocyte precursors using PDGF-α receptor, A2B5 and NG2 (also present on a proportion of O4-positive preoligodendrocytes). Defined thus, the human precursors responded by proliferation to PDGF, NT-3 and glial growth factor-2 whereas IGF-1 exerted a maturational effect – as in rodents.

A cell of the oligodendrocyte lineage has been identified in the adult human nervous system, expressing O4-related antigens but not galactocerebroside. Unlike its O4-positive/galactocerebroside-negative neonatal rodent counterpart (the preoligodendrocyte), this human cell is neither bipotential nor proliferative *in vitro* (R.C. Armstrong *et al* 1992). The preoligodendrocyte possesses multiple cellular processes and is A2B5-negative.

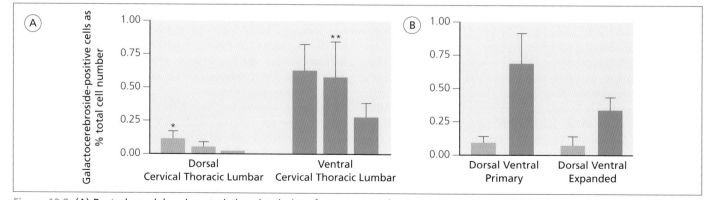

Figure 10.8 (A) Rostral–caudal and ventral–dorsal polarity of emergence of galactocerebroside-positive (oligodendrocytes) in the developing human spinal cord. Dissociated cell suspensions from isolated ventral and dorsal halves of spinal cord were divided into cervical, thoracic and lumbar segments. Cells were stained for galactocerebroside at 7 days post-plating (* p < 0.05, ** p < 0.05). (B) Relative distribution of galactocerebroside-positive cells in isolated ventral and dorsal halves of developing human spinal cord before (primary) and after (expanded) exposure to FGF-2 in neural precursor cultures.

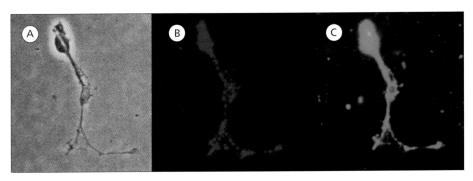

Figure 10.9 Adult oligodendrocyte precursors derived from human temporal lobe white matter. (A) Phase contrast. (B) A2B5-positive. (C) The same cell also stains for PDGF-α receptor. Magnification ×400. From Scolding *et al* (1998b) with permission.

Building on earlier observations concerning the specificity of PDGF-α chain receptor mRNA hybridization for oligodendrocyte precursors, Gogate *et al* (1994) stained cells in the adult human subventricular zone using this technique. However, oligodendrocyte lineage cells expressing PDGF-α chain receptor message failed to proliferate *in vitro*.

Scolding *et al* (1995) studied cells of the oligodendrocyte lineage in cultures prepared from normal-appearing temporal lobe white matter, removed in the course of surgery for drug-resistant epilepsy in adult patients (Figure 10.9). Three per cent of cells were O4-positive/galactocerebroside-negative preoligodendrocytes (R.C. Armstrong *et al* 1992), but a small proportion (1.3%) of oligodendrocyte lineage cells was also observed. These consisted of uni- or bipolar cells positive for A2B5 and negative for galactocerebroside, GFAP and vimentin, and for markers of microglia (p150) and neurons (neurofilament). Bi- or unipolar cells were O4 negative, but in other respects closely resembled the rodent O-2A progenitor both in morphology and immunophenotype. After 5–7 days *in vitro*, the number of cells with the antigenic profile of O-2A progenitors diminished. This was matched by the appearance of A2B5-positive and GFAP-positive cells or (less often) newly derived oligodendrocytes (A2B5 and galactocerebroside positive). Further investigation confirmed that cells with the progenitor phenotype were bipotential *in vitro*. Although the adult human progenitor exhibited a proliferative response when grown on contiguous monolayers of human astrocytes, no proliferation was observed in response to stimuli known to promote rat neonatal O-2A progenitor division – either defined growth factors, including PDGF, FGF-2 and NT-3 (alone or in combinations), or incubation of human progenitor cells with (human) astrocyte conditioned medium, B104 neuronal cell line conditioned medium, or culture on embryonic rat dorsal root ganglion cells – each of which causes rat oligodendrocyte progenitors to proliferate. The growth factor requirements for proliferation of the adult human oligodendrocyte progenitor are still not fully defined.

Taken together, these studies dealing directly with properties of the oligodendrocyte lineage in the human central nervous system may have relevance for multiple sclerosis. The adult human central nervous system does possess cells of the oligodendrocyte lineage able in principle to generate myelinating cells from pools of precursors. There may be regional diversity in this potential but the specific lessons of rodent neurobiology cannot necessarily be extrapolated directly to understanding the human oligodendrocyte lineage.

INTERACTIONS BETWEEN GLIA AND AXONS

Myelination occurs when the membranous processes of mature oligodendrocytes contact and ensheathe axons with a diameter of at least 0.2 μm, and compact to form the myelin lamellae needed for saltatory axonal conduction. The process depends on cell surface and extracellular matrix molecules which promote interactions between myelin and axons (Bartsch *et al* 1993). Differential expression of adhesion molecules, including janusin, tenascin, laminin and fibronectin, is required for stability of the emerging glial neuronal unit (M. Jung *et al* 1993). It is not surprising that, in negotiating stable relationships, several important influences mediated by soluble factors and cell–cell contacts are exchanged between axons and glia.

Oligodendrocyte progenitors need to orientate their processes and maximize points of contact with the nonmyelinated axon. The migration of O-2A cells occurs along established axonal tracts which provide a migration substratum consisting of axons that are aligned in parallel (Colello *et al* 1994; R.K. Small *et al* 1987). Webb *et al* (1995) identified topographical signals for migration and orientation of O-2A progenitors *in vitro*, using microfabricated substrata of varying width and depth. Oligodendrocytes and their precursors aligned preferentially on substrates with a width of 260 nm and depth of 400 nm, approximating to the dimensions of axons found in the developing rat optic nerve. Neurons are less sensitive to topographical information than cells of the oligodendrocyte lineage and, *in vivo*, oligodendrocytes and their progenitors may use smaller topographical cues during pathfinding than neurites. Whilst it has previously been suggested that orientation involves realignments of high-order cytoskeletal actin, confocal microscopy indicates that oligodendrocytes and their progenitors have diffuse cytoplasmic organization of actin and little or no high-order actin arrangement into cables. It remains possible that surface contours lead to local redistribution of surface adhesion and extracellular matrix molecules which orientate these cells during axonal contact, transducing second messengers that affect the cytoskeleton. The movement of migrating cells is influenced by receptor–ligand adhesions with the extracellular matrix and, hence, by discontinuities in substratum adhesiveness (Kiernan and ffrench Constant 1993). Integrins are one of several adhesion molecules determining cell–cell interactions in the developing and postmature nervous system. Variation in their expression regulates the migration and subsequent stability of glia and neurons, and so contributes to the cellular architecture of the central nervous system. R. Milner and ffrench Constant (1994) and C.E. Shaw *et al* (1996) described specific splicing arrangements for integrins (α6 with β1; and αv with β1), both on myelinating oligodendrocytes and their progenitors (by comparison, for example, with Schwann cells which utilize α6β1 during maturation and α6β4 during myelination of peripheral nerves). In addition to the guidance provided by glia for axons during development, a reciprocal role is seen for axons in orientating oligodendrocyte progenitors. The alignment of oligodendrocyte processes coincides with the initial expression of myelin proteins, especially proteolipid protein (Thomson *et al* 2005). For example, Xin *et al* (2005) show that the loss of *OLIG1* (see above) does not affect the development of oligodendrocyte progenitors (see below) but, despite making axonal contact, transgenic mice lacking *OLIG1* fail to regulate transcription of myelin specific genes: as a result, multilamellar wrapping of myelin membranes is not normal, myelination fails and, in the presence of continued glial fibrillary acidic protein expression, there is extensive astrocytosis. Acting through the transcription factor RhoA, LINGO-1 normally prevents oligodendrocyte differentiation and myelination. Manipulations of co-cultures *in vitro* show that inhibition of LINGO-1 results in well developed myelinated axons with defined nodes of Ranvier; and the analysis of transgenic mice confirms the inhibitory role of LINGO-1 and RhoA on myelination.

Influences of axons on oligodendrocyte precursors

Although it is the oligodendrocyte that ultimately synthesizes and maintains myelin around short segments of neighbouring axons, debate continues on which cells within this lineage are primarily involved in myelination (and remyelination). The balance of opinion, taken both from *in vitro* and cell implantation studies, is that the myelinating cell must divide and this emphasizes the pivotal role of oligodendrocyte precursors. From an early stage in the study of myelination *in vitro* it emerged that neurons are mitogenic for cells of the oligodendrocyte lineage (P.M. Wood and Williams 1984). The effect is mediated by both cell–cell contact and soluble mediators. It was first suggested by S.J. Chen and De Vries (1989) that the axonal plasma membrane contains a mitogen for oligodendrocytes. Gard and Pfeiffer (1990) reported that whereas oligodendrocyte precursors respond to medium conditioned with astrocytes, meningeal cells and neurons, preoligodendrocytes respond only to the neuronal stimulus. Guilian *et al* (1991) characterized a growth factor from neuronal cell lines which promotes myelin protein synthesis in mammalian glia. Barres and Raff (1993) showed that electrical activity in axons influences progenitor proliferation. The number of mature oligodendrocytes is matched to local axon density, survival being orchestrated by the number of axons requiring myelination (Burne *et al* 1996). Zajicek and Compston (1994) showed that PDGF, acting through its β-chain, and FGF-2 of neuronal origin stimulate glial progenitor proliferation. Axons appear to be able to replace FGF-2 as a factor that is necessary for the survival of human oligodendrocytes *in vitro* (Whittemore *et al* 1993). In the context of experimental spinal cord axonal injury, interven-

tions that increase the availability of NT-3 and BDNF cause local proliferation of oligodendrocyte lineage cells (McTigue *et al* 1998). NT-3 increases the proliferation and differentiation of oligodendrocyte progenitors and the process formation of mature oligodendrocytes acting through cFos and tyrosine kinases (Heinrich *et al* 1999). Loss of IGF-1 is associated with arrested maturation of oligodendrocytes and failure of myelination (see below; Ye *et al* 2002). The laminin receptor α6β1 integrin expressed on oligodendrocytes enhances the sensitivity of oligodendrocytes to the effects of the neuron-derived growth factors implicated in oligodendrocyte survival (Frost *et al* 1999), especially neuregulin (P.A. Fernandez *et al* 2000). By and large, active proliferation precludes differentiation. Therefore a further effect of axons on the behaviour of the oligodendrocyte lineage is to inhibit maturation. Myelin basic protein expression was shown by R.D. McKinnon and Dubois-Dalcq (1990) to be blocked in progenitors after 48 hours' incubation with FGF-2 of axonal origin. In the neonatal optic nerve, loss of axons blocks the development of oligodendrocytes but leaving abundant NG2-positive glia, whereas axonal transection has neither effect, suggesting that the requirement on axonal signals of glial precursor differentiation and oligodendrocyte survival decreases with maturation (Greenwood and Butt 2003).

Formation of the myelin sheath

Myelin synthesis is triggered when the elongated oligodendrocyte processes make contact with nearby axons and form a cup at the point of contact, extending lengthwise to form a trough whose two lips advance around the circumference of the axon until they meet. One then passes beneath the other to become the inner tongue of the future sheath which rotates many times around the axon to form the multiple membrane layers or lamellae. The developing myelin sheath extends lengthwise in both directions along the axon to form an internodal segment. But at the advancing edge, each layer of the spiral retains a bead of cytoplasm where the two inner leaflets of the surface membrane remain separate. In three dimensions, this bead comprises a ring of cytoplasm around the axon and is termed the lateral loop. Transverse bands, regularly arranged sites of close membrane apposition spaced 10–15 nm apart, later develop between the end of each lateral loop and the underlying axolemma. There are as many lateral loops at the leading edge of the advancing sheath as there are lamellae, and these become stacked in a regular way, those of the outermost lamellae lying outside those of the innermost. The complement of lateral loops at one end of each developing internode almost abuts onto its adjacent counterpart, and together these form the paranodal region next to the node of Ranvier.

During compaction, the cytoplasmic content of all except the inner- and outermost lamellae of the developing spiral sheath is gradually extruded, and the two inner leaflets of the surface membrane lipid bilayer thus become opposed. They then fuse to form the major dense line visible in ultrastructural cross-sections (Figure 10.10). The two outer leaflets of the adjacent layers of the spiral process are also closely opposed, and although they commonly appear to form only a single, less dense intraperiod line, electron microscopy confirms that the intraperiod line comprises two separate leaflets (Raine 1984). Inner and outer tongues of cytoplasm remain where the corresponding

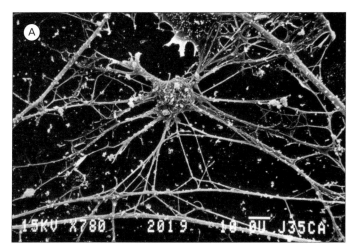

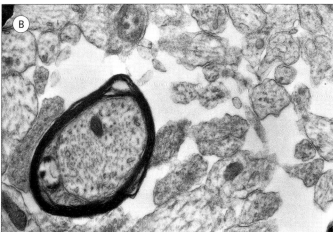

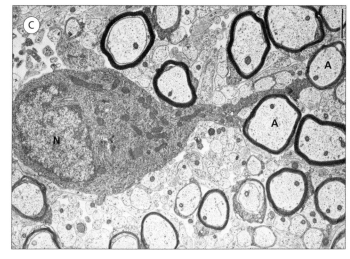

Figure 10.10 (A) Rat O-2A progenitors associate *in vitro* with several bundles of dorsal rat ganglion axons shown by scanning electron microscopy. (B) Formation of compact myelin sheaths around axons shown by transmission electron microscopy. Reproduced from Zajicek *et al* (1992) with permission. (C) One oligodendrocyte myelinates several neighbouring axons.

central and outermost lamellae have not compacted. Radial components visible in ultrastructural cross-sections of myelin probably correspond to stacks of tight junctions arrayed in lines from outermost to innermost lamellae. These are thought to seal adjacent lamellae together and to anchor the outer cytoplasmic tongue.

Compact myelin thereby consists of a condensed lipid-rich membrane wrapped spirally many times around axons to form a segmented sheath. This is interrupted periodically along the course of the axon at the (nonmyelinated) nodes of Ranvier – areas where electrical resistance can be low because of the high concentration of sodium channels, and where depolarization is thereby facilitated. In myelinated axons, the action potential induced by depolarization generates electrical currents, in turn triggering depolarization at the next node of Ranvier. This saltatory conduction is considerably more rapid than continuous propagation of the nerve impulse (see also Chapter 13).

One function of oligodendrocytes, revealed by disruption in mouse models of defective oligodendrocyte development, is the distribution and clustering of sodium and potassium channels at nodes of Ranvier (Figure 10.11; see also Chapter 13; Mathis *et al* 2001). Specifically, oligodendroyte-derived soluble factors induce clustering of the Na(v)1.2 channels whereas successful myelination is required for clustering of the Na(v)1.6 channels (M.R. Kaplan *et al* 2001). With maturation, the diffuse distribution of the Na(v)1.2 channels is rationalized. They are

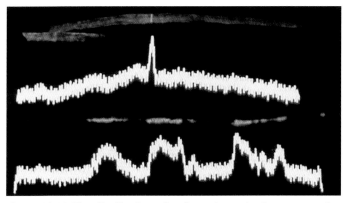

Figure 10.11 The distribution of sodium channels, demonstrated using a sensitive radioimmunoassay, and after nerves were experimentally demyelinated *in vivo* with doxorubicin (adriamycin). From J.D. England *et al* (1991). © 1991, with permission from Elsevier.

retained along the myelinated segments but are replaced by Na(v)1.6 channels at the nodes (T. Boiko *et al* 2001). Coinciding with the onset of myelination, neurofascin (NF155) clusters at the paranodal portion of the myelin sheath and adheres to the contactin-associated protein (Caspr1) that is present on the axons at the forming node of Ranvier (Charles *et al* 2002b).

465

Their expression is regulated by the transcription factor NKxb-2 (Southwood *et al* 2004). It floats on the nodal membrane as part of a lipid raft (Schafer *et al* 2004). In some myelin-deficient rats, the sparse myelin sheaths seem insufficient to establish the normal distribution of paranodal molecules – contactin, Caspr and neurofascin – or the $K(v)1.1$ and $K(v)1.2$ potassium channels, although sodium channels and ankyrin G are appropriately segregated (Arroyo *et al* 2002). Caspr inhibits the interaction of neurofascin with contactin and hence its ability to function at the cell surface (Gollan *et al* 2003). Caspr disappears from demyelinated axons in the lesions of multiple sclerosis, and reappears with remyelination. Wolswijk and Balesar (2003) interpret the distribution spreading out from a normal paranodal distribution as evidence that reduced expression of Caspr precedes and determines the early ultrastructural stages of myelin disruption. Interactions between myelin-forming cells and neurites ready for coating are altered *in vitro* by growth factors. PDGF and, especially, the combination of neuregulin and thyroxine enhance, and LIF inhibits, the process (S.K. Park *et al* 2001b).

Myelin should not be regarded simply as an inert insulating material. Although its dynamic function is poorly understood, it is rich in a number of specific enzymes, including a basic protein kinase and cyclic nucleotide phosphodiesterase, and myelin possesses a variety of membrane ion channels. The commonly drawn distinction between oligodendrocytes and myelin is unhelpful and biologically somewhat artificial. Rather, the parent oligodendrocyte soma continues to support this metabolically active specialized membrane throughout the lifetime of each cell, so that the functional and anatomical concept of an oligodendrocyte–myelin unit arises.

Myelin accounts for approximately 70% of the dry weight of the mammalian central nervous system, and each interfascicular oligodendrocyte, myelinating up to several tens of internodes along neighbouring axons, produces myelin membranes equivalent to 600–700-fold its own cell body surface membrane (Figure 10.12). Myelin is composed of lipid (70–75% dry weight) and protein (25–30%). Around 25% of the lipid is cholesterol and 40–45% is phospholipid, but the remaining 25–30% is galactolipid (Norton and Cammer 1984). Galactocerebroside is the major myelin glycolipid (23%), and both polyclonal and monoclonal anti-galactocerebroside antibodies are specific surface markers of myelin and oligodendrocytes both *in vivo* and *in vitro* (Ranscht *et al* 1982). The myelin membrane also expresses many receptors for growth factors and cytokines. Recent additions to the established catalogue include oestrogen receptor and caveolin-1 – a negative regulator of endothelial nitric oxide synthase (Arvanitis *et al* 2004). Antibodies to the remaining galactolipid (sulphatide) are less specific *in vivo* although they reliably identify oligodendrocytes *in vitro*. Of the minor lipid components of myelin, gangliosides together comprise <1% of total lipid.

Antibodies to myelin-specific proteins are also widely used in immunocytochemical studies. The two major proteins are proteolipid protein (approximately 50% total protein) and myelin basic protein (30–40%). Antibodies to both proteins label myelin sheaths *in vivo*, but are less reliable for oligodendrocyte cell bodies. Mature oligodendrocytes can be identified in cell culture using both antibodies. Myelin basic protein is translated in the myelin sheath whereas proteolipid protein is localized in the cell body. The third main fraction of myelin proteins is the group of Wolfgram proteins, which constitute approximately 5% of myelin by dry weight. The higher molecular weight band (W2) is thought to be tubulin (Norton and Cammer 1984), while the doublet of lower molecular weight (W1) corresponds to the myelin-specific enzyme 2',3'-cyclic nucleotide 3'-phosphohydrolase (CNPase; Sprinkle *et al* 1980). Several other myelin proteins have been described but without necessarily being implicated in myelination. One, however, is highly relevant. Nogo is the best characterized of a series of molecules expressed on the myelin membrane that acts to inhibit axon growth (see below); its role in perpetuating the chronic axonopathy of secondary progressive multiple sclerosis, and the potential for anti-Nogo antibodies to promote axon outgrowth in that phase of the disease remain unexplored. Anti-CNP-ase antibodies can be used to identify myelin and oligodendrocytes both *in vivo* and *in vitro* (S.U. Kim *et al* 1984).

Proteolipid protein and DM20 have roles in formation of the intraperiod line and in maintaining axonal integrity but are also involved in the early stages of axon–oligodendrocyte interaction and in wrapping of the axon. A novel oligodendrocyte-specific protein related to peripheral myelin protein 22 was described by J.M. Bronstein *et al* (1996). Although widely distributed and following a developmental profile similar to proteolipid protein, its role in myelinogenesis and relevance for demyelinating disease remain to be determined. Connexins may also contribute to the stability of adjacent layers during myelin compaction. Antibodies to the minor myelin components, myelin-associated glycoprotein and myelin oligodendrocyte protein, which constitute <1% of the myelin proteins, also label oligodendrocytes and myelin *in vivo* (Linington *et al* 1984). Myelin-associated glycoprotein has an important role in stabilizing the initial glial–axon contact as the spiral process begins in anticipation of compaction. However, myelination proceeds normally in transgenic mice which are deficient in myelin-associated glycoprotein (Montag *et al* 1994).

In addition to its role in axon guidance, netrin-1 is widely distributed on oligodendrocytes and may act over short ranges to maintain axon–glial interactions (Manitt *et al* 2001). A novel myelin protein, designated microtubule-associated protein-2 expressing exon 13, is transiently expressed by embryonic oligodendrocytes during myelination – and by the processes extending from oligodendrocytes successfully engaged in remyelinating the lesions of multiple sclerosis (Shafit-Zagardo *et al* 1999). As part of the growing body of evidence for survival signals exerted by glia on axons (see below), Sheikh *et al* (1999) demonstrated reduced myelin-associated glycoprotein expression and demyelination with axonal degeneration in mice lacking complex gangliosides. Garbern *et al* (2002) showed, both in transgenic mice and in people with null mutations of *PLP1*, that although lack of proteolipid protein does not affect myelination, it is also associated with length-dependent axonal degeneration. Conversely, the expression of polysialylated neural cell adhesion molecule (PSA-NCAM) acts as a repellent signal for axon–glial contact and its expression relates inversely to myelination (Charles *et al* 2000). Aberrant PSA-NCAM expression may account for the failure of demyelinated axons to remyelinate in multiple sclerosis (Chapter 12; Charles *et al* 2002a) and loss of the inhibitory Notch1/Jagged1 signalling in mice also leads to increased myelination and overabundance of myelin genes during development (Givogri *et al* 2002).

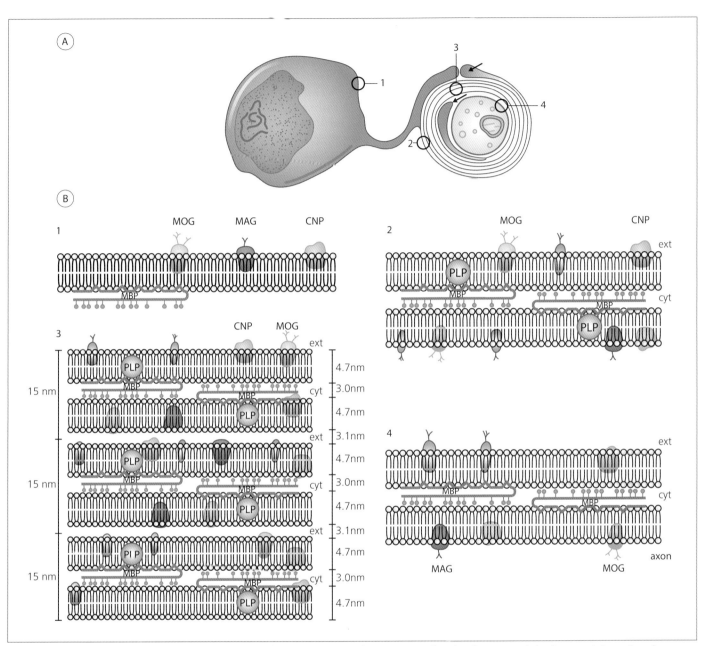

Figure 10.12 (A) Schematic drawing (not to scale) of the relationship between an oligodendrocyte and the internodal myelin of a nerve fibre. Despite being continuous from cell to compact sheath, the membrane is not uniform in either chemical composition or molecular architecture. (The proposed structure and composition of the four zones indicated are described in part B of this figure). Note also that oligodendroglial cytoplasm extends right through the sheath and is identifiable on this diagram as the outer and inner loops (arrows); in paranodal myelin it becomes even more plentiful in the form of the nodal loops (not shown). (B) Schematic representation (not to scale) of the molecular architecture of the central myelin sheath, prepared by Dr Brenda Brankin based on Rumsby (1978), Schwob *et al* (1985) and Brunner *et al* (1989). The occurrence and disposition of proteins in the different zones of the oligodendrocyte–myelin unit is shown. 1. The oligodendrocyte membrane associated zone. 2. The myelin surface associated zone. Highest amounts of MOG are found in this zone. 3. The compact myelin zone; the controversy as to whether MAG is present in compact myelin has not yet been resolved. 4. The myelin/axon interface zone; highest amounts of the cell adhesion molecule MAG are found in this zone. MOG = myelin oligodendroglial glycoprotein; MAG = myelin-associated glycoprotein; MBP = myelin basic protein; PLP = proteolipid protein; CNP = 2',3'-cyclic nucleotide 3'-phosphodiesterase. Adapted from I.V. Allen (1991). © 1991, with permission from Elsevier.

The blood–brain barrier

The central nervous system is separated from the systemic circulation by the blood–brain barrier. This is composed of a layer of endothelial cells abutting a basement membrane interspersed with pericytes around which a continuous covering is provided by the extended foot processes of astrocytes (M. Bradbury 1979) and microglia (Figure 10.13). Unlike most other parts of the microvasculature, tight junctions exist between adjacent endothelia. Whilst highly permeable to water and lipid-soluble molecules, the blood–brain barrier prevents the free passage of most solutes from the systemic circulation into the central nervous system, although essential nutrients (including glucose and certain amino acids and ions) are transported by specific carrier mechanisms, so that the extracellular environment within the brain is not simply that of a plasma filtrate. Blood–brain barrier diffusion is, however, restricted for polar molecules, including proteins, but it is important to note that even in this situation, the blood–brain barrier does not present an absolute impediment. It allows diffusion gradients to develop between the plasma and extracellular space within the central nervous system, which depend upon the size (molecular radius) and the charge (isoelectric point) of the respective molecules. Thus, as an example, the diffusion constant between plasma and cerebrospinal fluid for immunoglobulin G is, on average, 500 : 1. This implies that significant amounts of specific autoantibodies can reach even the normal brain in situations where their peripheral titres are very high.

Certain small and circumspect areas of the rodent nervous system lack continuous tight junctions (the pituitary gland, median eminence, area postrema, preoptic recess, parahypophysis, pineal gland and endothelium of the choroid plexus; Brightman 1991), although the existence and extent of these physiological defects in primates are uncertain. Human fetuses as young as 7 weeks show the presence of tight junctions both between neighbouring choroid plexus epithelial cells and individual cere-

bral endothelia so that, as soon as these cells differentiate, they have well-formed tight junctions (Mollgard and Saunders 1986). Other components of the blood–brain barrier are provided by the basement membrane and perivascular glia limitans. The basement membrane is formed by layers derived both from endothelial cells and astrocytes. It is therefore much thicker compared with basement membranes found in other blood vessels, serving as a molecular sieve that restricts the penetration of molecules depending on their molecular radius and charge. The glia limitans is essentially formed by tight layers of astrocyte processes covered by a basal lamina. Although mammalian astrocytes do not present an absolute obstacle, they are probably essential for the development of tight junctions in the overlying endothelial cells (Janzer and Raff 1987; Tao-Cheng and Brightman 1988). A peculiar membrane specialization is found at the glial vascular interface in astrocyte endfeet, the so-called orthogonal array of particles or assemblies. These may represent high conductance potassium channels (E.A. Newman 1986). Ultrastructural analysis of the developing chick blood–brain barrier reveals a role for aquaporin-4 on the astroglial endfeet, eventually enveloping the endothelium-pericyte layer. Disruption of the blood–brain barrier is associated with reduced expression of aquaporin-4, indicating a close relationship between water transport regulation and blood–brain barrier development (Nico et al 2001). A further component of the perivascular glia limitans is the microglial cell, which has been demonstrated between the astrocyte foot processes of cerebral microvessels (Lassmann et al 1991a).

Pericytes are adventitial contractile cells forming the smooth muscle cells of larger vessels. They may have a role in growth control since they inhibit endothelial cell proliferation in vitro (Risau 1991). In addition, bone marrow-derived macrophages are present in the perivascular space of medium-sized and larger cerebral vessels. In normal brain their main function is to take up and digest material that has passed the blood–brain barrier or been liberated within the central nervous system tissue. In addition, however, these cells have phenotypic features and some functional properties of dendritic cells. These cells seem to be the first line of immunological defence in the central nervous system.

Astrocytes are highly reactive cells. A decade ago, Eddleston and Mucke (1993) valiantly catalogued observations based on in vivo and in vitro studies of astrocytes, listing >100 adhesion, antigen-presenting, calcium-binding, cytokine, cytoskeletal, immediate response, eicosanoid, enzyme, defined epitope, receptor, transport and various miscellaneous markers which are upregulated on astrocytes in response to >300 stimuli. Self-evidently, even this complex matrix of stimuli and responses is now several orders of magnitude greater. Reactivity increases the availability of trophic factors, cytokines, proteases, protease inhibitors, and cell surface and matrix molecules. Several are simultaneously produced by microglia and it has been suggested that these same cytokines produced at different stages in the response to injury and by different cell types mediate both pro- and anti-inflammatory effects. The requirement for extracellular matrix as a stimulus for astrocyte differentiation indicates one mechanism of astrocytic reactivity, since central nervous system damage will invariably expose extracellular matrix molecules such as chondroitin sulphate proteoglycans to drive astrocytic differentiation.

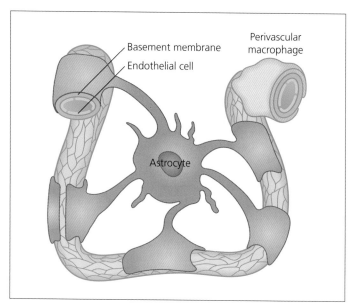

Figure 10.13 Components of the blood–brain barrier. Perivascular macrophages contribute up to 30% of the glial end-feet around the basement membrane.

The emphasis on astrocyte reactivity and its deleterious effects has mainly been considered in the context of axonal regeneration and cell migration (see below). TGF-β1 increases the availability of neurite growth promoting molecules (laminin and fibronectin), limits the infiltration of macrophages and microglia, and acts to organize the formation of a glial limiting membrane made up of reactive astrocytes (Logan *et al* 1992; 1994). Astrocyte proliferation is inhibited by TGF-β (K.E. Hunter *et al* 1993). In the context of multiple sclerosis, Peress *et al* (1996) colocalized all isoforms of TGF-β to astrocytes in areas of chronic demyelination, whereas TGF-β2 predominated in microglia bordering acute active lesions.

It has not proved easy to extrapolate from *in vitro* to *in vivo* observations in the study of reactive astrocytes. Cells in culture behave differently from their resting counterparts in intact tissue. They lose certain features of contact inhibition, and express large amounts of GFAP and other markers indicating reactivity (for review, see V. Wu and Schwartz 1998). Therefore, the biochemical and cellular features of tissue culture observations cannot necessarily be extrapolated to biological systems. However, conditions have been defined that approximate more closely the behaviour of the *in vitro* (reactive) astrocyte to its resting counterpart *in vivo*. These include exposure to certain neurotransmitters (Pennypacker *et al* 1996), but mainly depend on the use of neuronal coculture systems that downregulate astrocyte proliferation and GFAP expression (Guenard *et al* 1996; L-C. Wang *et al* 1994).

The origin of reactive astrocytes is not resolved. Although some have migrated into lesions, and others proliferated locally, most are resting cells with an altered phenotype. Many cellular and molecular markers have been described that are considered specific for astrocyte reactivity (Ridet *et al* 1997) but increasing evidence suggests that the reactive astrocyte is not a single entity (Hatten *et al* 1991; Hoke and Silver 1994). Thus, the characteristic feature of astrocytosis is cell hypertrophy with change from the protoplasmic to fibrillary morphology and usually with proliferation. These changes are accompanied by increased GFAP expression – and this has served as a sufficient marker for the reactive astrocyte. One suggestion is that signalling through FGF-R3 normally inhibits GFAP expression (Pringle *et al* 2003) but it is difficult to identify any astrocyte that does not express GFAP, and its candidature as a marker sits uncomfortably with evidence that *GFAP*-negative transgenic mice show a normal astrocytic response to injury (Pekny *et al* 1995). Rather, the physiological importance of GFAP is suggested by the demonstration of impaired myelin maintenance in GFAP-negative transgenic mouse (Leidtke *et al* 1996).

Astrocyte reactivity in response to destructive tissue injury increases the availability of growth and neuroprotective factors – especially IGF-1 but also PDGF and FGF-2 (Komoly *et al* 1992; Wilczak and De Keyser 1997; D-L. Yao *et al* 1995). Astrocyte proliferation and reactivity generally culminate in formation of the astroglial scar. Made up mainly of hypertrophied astrocytes, this also wraps in fibroblasts and meningeal cells which form a new glia limitans with surviving astrocytes. Scar formation is prominent in response to injury in the adult (Mathewson and Berry 1985) but not the neonatal central nervous system (J.S. Rudge and Silver 1990). Some reactive astrocytes express nestin but these are probably distinct from the nestin-positive multipotential progenitors that also may accumulate at sites of tissue injury (Johansson *et al* 1999). Bush *et al* (1999) targeted GFAP to deplete transgenic mice of reactive astrocytes following physical injury (stab wound) of the forebrain. The complex phenotype included failure to limit the local inflammatory response, increased neuronal degeneration, prolonged permeability of the blood–brain barrier, and increased or disorganized neurite outgrowth. A more refined analysis of injury in mice with conditional deletion of *GFAP* as a means of preventing astrocyte reactivity, converted small self-limiting lesions to areas of persistent blood–brain barrier disruption, intense inflammation and tissue destruction with oligodendrocyte and neuronal depletion, and widespread demyelination (Faulkner *et al* 2004).

Clearly, the damaged brain needs to steer a clever course between promoting reactive changes in astrocytes, which usefully encapsulate the area of tissue injury and provide mediators for the promotion of recovery, whilst avoiding formation of a dense astrocytic scar that may exclude cells and mediators needed to repair neurons and glia. Without knowing in detail the benefits that accrue from astrocyte reactivity during the evolution of tissue injury and repair in multiple sclerosis, the majority of lesions eventually acquire a dense glial scar, giving lesions the hard or sclerotic consistency from which the disease gets its name.

DEMYELINATION

The pivotal role of inflammation, arising from the accumulation of activated T lymphocytes migrating from the systemic circulation, in setting up the cascade of events that culminates in demyelination is central to our concept of the pathogenesis of multiple sclerosis. The notion that inflammation is the engine that drives the many other components of tissue destruction does not go unchallenged. Others consider that the neurodegenerative element is independent and may even be the primary event (see Chapters 1 and 14).

The blood–brain barrier prevents the passage of most large molecules and cells, although specific vesicular and other transport mechanisms provide the brain with essential nutrients and permit a degree of cellular traffic. Cellular infiltration of the central nervous system is described in detail in Chapter 11. In summary, penetration of cerebral vessels, at least by lymphocytes, occurs through channels of endothelial cells and thus represents an active process mediated by endothelia. Cellular transmigration also depends on alterations in the expression of cell surface molecules on activated T cells as well as endothelial cells together with the secretion of enzymes that degrade the extracellular matrix in the subendothelial space. The constitutive expression of specific molecules that determine immunological recognition and cellular adhesion alters under conditions of inflammatory cell activation, amplifying the steady-state cellular surveillance that occurs in health and contributing to the perivenular concentration of inflammatory cells that characterizes most demyelinating diseases (Carrithers *et al* 2000). Thus, migration results from changes on endothelia and activated lymphocytes. Certain addressins highly concentrated on endothelial cells by the action of locally acting cytokines (IL-1 and TNF-α) interact with ligands on the surface of circulating lymphocytes or inflammatory cells. Specific receptor ligand interactions include intercellular adhesion molecule (ICAM)-1 reacting with leucocyte function antigen (LFA)-1, LFA-3 which links exclusively with the T-cell ligand cluster defined CD2, and CD9 which selectively adheres to B lymphocytes. Other adhesion systems, such as complement activation products and CD44, are ubiquitously expressed and nonspecifically enhance contact between circulating and endothelial cells. Soluble adhesion molecules, such as ICAM, inhibit mononuclear cell migration across endothelial barriers. Migration can be actively prevented by blocking antibodies directed, for example, at the α4 chain of integrins. The critical factor in determining propagation of the immune response is that only those cells primed against central nervous system antigen become reactivated and attract, or locally activate, effector cells, whereas those that do not encounter specific antigen leave the central nervous system without consequences or die by apoptosis (Wekerle et al 1986). Cellular traffic across the blood–brain barrier nonspecifically permits a variety of other potentially pathogenic molecules to assemble on the abluminal surface of cerebral vessels, creating the conditions needed for cellular, antibody, complement and macrophage mediated tissue injury. Next in the cascade of events is outward migration of cells from the perivascular space into the tissue. This is largely promoted by local production of chemokines interacting with specific receptors on migrating cells, and by enzymes which degrade tissue barriers and extracellular matrices (Zang et al 2000b). Chemokines specific for T cells are IP-10 and MIG (monokine induced by IFN-γ). Neutrophils respond to Gro-α and IL-8, and T cells and monocytes respond to RANTES (regulated upon activation normal T-cell expressed and secreted), MCP-1 (monocyte chemoattractant protein 1) and MIP-1α (macrophage inflammatory protein 1α). The IP-10 receptor is CXCR3 and CCR5 binds the MIP-1α and RANTES ligands. IL-2 induces the secretion of metalloproteases by T cells and this enhances their ability to adhere and migrate through endothelial barriers.

Toxic molecules for oligodendrocytes

Many forms of injury converge on a few final common pathways and several of these may lead to cell death. In reviewing these mechanisms, mostly elucidated in vitro, we do not infer that demyelination in multiple sclerosis is invariably the consequence of oligodendrocyte depletion – although that undoubtedly does occur. Rather, we review these processes from the general perspective of injury and repair at the single cell level. When neurons and glia are physiologically active, they respond to molecules that bind to receptors, open ion channels and transduce signals across the cell membrane, leading to changes in intracellular calcium and protein kinases, induction of immediate early genes and transcription of cell-specific products. Biochemical systems which subserve physiological functions in health are seemingly hijacked by pathological processes. That said, the entry of calcium and associated intracellular signals shows different temporal and spatial organization when physiological events switch to calcium overload and cell injury. The threat to cell survival and the recovery of cell homeostasis require rapid intracellular reactions leading to protein synthesis. Manipulating these final common pathways may provide one means for protecting cells from injury but attention has also turned to events occurring earlier in the biochemical cascade of cell death, at the cell membrane. Brosnan and Raine (1996) and Ludwin (1997) have summarized the available evidence on

those factors likely to be present in the central nervous system during health or disease known from in vivo and in vitro studies to be capable of injuring oligodendrocytes or disrupting axon–glial interactions. A further review of factors which mediate oligodendrocyte injury, based on in vitro evidence and the study of individual lesions, set in an historical perspective, is given by Raine (1997). Because these molecules exert physiological effects, injure oligodendrocytes and axons, and are the products of inflammatory cells and glia, we also discuss these toxic molecules in Chapters 11, 12 and 13 – inevitably with some overlap and slight repetition.

Oligodendrocytes are almost as susceptible to anoxia and excitotoxic damage (kainate and glutamate) as are neurons. Matute (1998) infused the optic nerve with kainate and observed acute injury of axons with additional damage to oligodendrocytes after more prolonged exposure. Oligodendrocyte depletion and neurofilament dephosphorylation (indicative of axonal stress) are inhibited by AMPA (α-amino-3-hydroxy-5-methylisoxazole-4-propionic acid) receptor antagonists in experimental models but these effects do not directly correlate with the degree of inflammation (Pitt et al 2000). Our position is that much hinges in this study on the analysis of only two representative animals and a similar study on AMPA-R blockade in experimental autoimmune encephalomyelitis showed beneficial effects mainly for grey matter neurons (T. Smith et al 2000). The amount of glutamate released endogenously following spinal cord injury is sufficient to cause local oligodendrocyte depletion (G.Y. Xu et al 2004). The expression of group I metabotropic glutamate receptors (mGluRs) decreases with oligodendrocyte maturation, acting through protein kinase Cα coupled to phospholipase C – making precursors more susceptible than their differentiated progeny (Deng et al 2004). Conversely, group I and II mGluRs are induced by cell activation and altered glutamate homeostasis, dependent on glial activation, perhaps explaining the injury of neurons (dephosphorylation of neurofilament and increased β-amyloid precursor protein) and oligodendrocytes in the lesions of multiple sclerosis (Geurts et al 2003; P. Werner et al 2001). Others have shown that oligodendrocytes are protected from excitotoxicity by IL-6 and a chimeric IL-6/IL-6R derivative acting through gp130 and STAT1/3 signal transduction (Pizzi et al 2004). Building on the demonstration that IGF-1 protects oligodendrocyte precursors from excitotoxic injury signalling through Akt, Ness et al (2004) demonstrated that IGF-1 inhibits mitochondrial injury and cytochrome C release, and prevents caspase-9 induction but does not limit calcium entry nor influence other pro- and anti-apoptotic molecules. In this system, oligodendrocytes are injured by IL-1β in coculture with astrocytes and microglia, perhaps by buffering astrocyte uptake of glutamate. Against this background, it is not so surprising that oligodendrocytes are protected in vivo by AMPA receptor antagonists (T. Smith et al 2000) as are those exposed to TNF-α, suggesting that this cytokine also operates in part through excitotoxic mechanisms (J.L. Takahashi et al 2003; see below). IGF-1 affords relative protection of oligodendrocyte precursors from excitotoxic injury, acting through TrkC and the Akt signal transduction pathway (Ness et al 2002).

Although the effects are to some extent inseparable from excitotoxic mechanisms, inflammatory mediators are also a major source of oligodendrocyte injury. It was originally reported that intravitreal injection of TNF-α leads to demyelination of mouse optic nerve axons (H.G. Jenkins and Ikeda 1992). Butt and Jenkins (1994) labelled optic nerve oligodendrocytes with lucifer yellow and observed the effects of TNF-α on the normal arrangement whereby oligodendrocytes extend approximately 20 processes with an average length of 200 mm. Initially, nerves injected with TNF-α showed swollen myelin processes which then unravelled, eventually losing continuity with the oligodendrocyte cell body. Our interpretation of these local injections of a proinflammatory cytokine is that these mainly provoked Wallerian degeneration. Introduction of this cytokine into the murine spinal cord was initially reported as causing an inflammatory response which reproduced many features of autoimmune encephalomyelitis (R.D. Simmons and Willenborg 1990). However, contemporary studies again suggest that direct injection of TNF-α into the adult rat spinal cord appears only to elicit a mild inflammatory response without oligodendrocyte or myelin injury (see Chapter 13; S.M. Hall et al 2000).

Oligodendrocytes die after exposure to TNF-α from apoptosis acting through TNF-related apoptosis inducing ligand (TRAIL). Although apoptosis inducing (TRAIL-R1 and -R2) and blocking (TRAIL-R3 and -R4) receptors are present, TRAIL itself is not constitutively expressed in the nervous system (Dorr et al 2002). IFN-γ selectively induces TRAIL-1 and promotes oligodendrocyte susceptibility to TRAIL-induced death whereas microglia are rich in TRAIL-3 and so resistant to TNF-α (Matysiak et al 2002). In the context of soluble TNF-α, apoptotic death of oligodendrocytes is mediated through the JNK-3 and not the MAP kinase pathway, resulting in downstream effects on mitochondrial function (Jurewicz et al 2003). Oligodendrocytes possess receptors for TNF-α and Fas, providing a basis for signals which activate both apoptotic and necrotic death pathways (D'Souza et al 1995; 1996a). Death of oligodendrocytes may also occur through Fas receptor activation of p53, both in vitro and in the lesions of multiple sclerosis (Wosik et al 2003). TNF-α but not NGF stimulates p75 and induces apoptosis through upregulation of JNK and NF-κB (Ladiwala et al 1998; 1999). Oligodendrocytes are protected from TNF-α-induced apoptotic death by inhibition of the IL-1β converting enzyme/CED3 caspase family (Hisahara et al 1997) and by IGF-1 (Ye and D'Ercole 1999). The sensitivity of oligodendrocyte lineage cells decreases with maturation, being more marked in those staining for A2B5 and O4 compared with O1 cells and fully developed oligodendrocytes: this differential sensitivity does not correlate with alterations in the expression of TNF-α receptors (Pang et al 2005). Others conclude that oligodendrocytes are resistant to physiological concentrations of soluble TNF-α through growth factor protection. Louis et al (1993) first showed that CNTF protects rodent oligodendrocytes from injury by TNF-α; and the same effect was later observed for human cells (D'Souza et al 1996b). Later, Takano et al (2000) reported protection from TNF-α, acting through the Akt pathway and stabilizing the mitochondrial membrane potential. Transgenic mice deficient in CNTF show increased loss of mature oligodendrocytes, myelin dystrophy and axonal loss with a reduction in recruitment of proliferating precursors in myelin oligodendrocyte glycoprotein induced experimental demyelination – effects which appeared to be mediated through CNTF protection from TNF-α (Linker et al 2002) acting through the Janus kinase (Jak) and other signal transduction pathways

that shift the balance of Bcl-2 proteins in an anti-apoptotic direction (Maier et al 2004). The most parsimonious interpretation of these data is that CNTF acts as a neuroprotective growth factor, perhaps expressed in response to injury, that limits the direct effects of proinflammatory cytokines on cells of the oligodendrocyte lineage. As such, this may be one of the more promising molecules for evaluation as a therapy in multiple sclerosis.

Synergistic effects have been demonstrated for different growth factors in protecting oligodendrocytes from TNF-α-mediated injury (Figure 10.14). The in vitro evidence suggests that IGF-2 and CNTF act through an autocrine loop to block oligodendrocyte toxicity due to TNF-α released by IFN-γ-activated microglia (Nicholas et al 2002). The activity of JNK-stimulated by TNF-α receptor ligation confirms that these factors inhibit TNF-α signalling. Irrespective of activation, conditioned media do not induce JNK activity in oligodendrocytes unless CNTF or IGF-2 activity are neutralized. The TNF-α-containing medium of IFN-γ-treated, but not non-activated, microglia is then toxic for oliogodendrocytes. TNF-α release by the microglial cell line (BV2) is also prevented by ligand binding to the galanin receptor, through a post-translational mechanism (Su et al 2003). Butzkueven et al (2002) showed that LIF protects oligodendrocytes in an immune-mediated model of demyelination by a mechanism which is similar to the effect of CNTF.

The paradox whereby a receptor–ligand system primarily involved in development of the nervous system is borrowed in the context of another biological process is well illustrated by semaphorin and plexin. Acting through members of the plexin gene family, soluble semaphorin 4D (CD100) produced by T lymphocytes collapses oligodendrocyte processes and induces neuronal apoptosis (Giraudon et al 2004). The demonstration of sCD100 in the cerebrospinal fluid of patients with inflammatory brain disease provides circumstantial evidence for the clinical relevance of these observations (see below). Majed et al (2005) showed differential upregulation of semaphorin receptors Plexin-A1 and Neuropilins 1 and 2, in vitro and in vivo, following activation of microglia. Recombinant Sema3A induced apoptosis of microglia in vitro, and production of Sema3A by stressed neurons mediated apoptosis of activated microglia. Together with the in vivo demonstration of enhanced Sema3A production by adult neurons threatened by local inflammation, these results supported a novel semaphorin-mediated mechanism of neuroprotection.

Nitric oxide injures oligodendrocytes in addition to its now well-characterized effect on axons (see below, and Chapter 13). Oligodendrocytes from the developing nervous system may be more susceptible to oxidative mechanisms than mature cells – perhaps because of their enhanced ability to metabolize hydrogen peroxide resulting from increased glutathione peroxidase activity (Baud et al 2004). But, here too, the nitric oxide story is of injury and protection resulting from close interaction between growth factors and cytokines. The Janus-headed molecule TNF-α is another ambiguous character. Merrill et al (1993) showed in cocultures of rat microglia and oligodendrocytes that antagonists of nitric oxide, as well as anti-TNF-α antibodies and TGF-β, each protect rat oligodendrocytes from cell death mediated by nitric oxide, IFN-γ and TNF-α, acting alone or in combination. Death of oligodendrocytes following exposure to IFN-γ and lipopolysaccharide is associated with inducible nitric

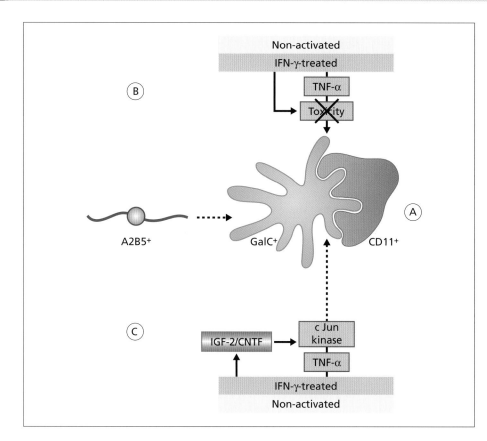

Figure 10.14 (A) Activated microglia kill opsonized oligodendrocytes by cell–cell contact and local release of TNF-α. (B) Oligodendrocytes are not susceptible to soluble TNF-α. (C) However, soluble TNF-α becomes toxic in the absence of IGF-2 and CNTF. These growth factors are produced by microglia and so normally act to inhibit bystander damage of healthy oligodendrocytes. Kindly prepared by Dr Richard Nicholas.

oxide synthase (iNOS) expression and nitric oxide production within the cultures – effects that are specifically inhibited by IL-10 and, to a lesser extent, by IL-4 (Molina-Holgado et al 2001). Reduced iNOS/nitric oxide production by activated microglia in response to parthenolide depends on inhibition of MAP kinase but not NF-κB (Fiebich et al 2002). Catecholamine-induced apoptotic death of oligodendrocytes and oligodendrocyte precursors is mediated by inhibition of intracellular glutathione, resulting in increased reactive oxygen species, and is inhibited by caspases – effects that are more pronounced in precursors than differentiated cells (Khorchid et al 2002). Survival is reduced by exposure to neuregulin, as is the ability of activated microglia to release toxic oxygen species and nitrites (glial growth factor-2; Dimayuga et al 2003). Oligodendrocytes and astrocytes are lysed by the proinflammatory platelet-activating factor acting through caspase-3 (Hostettler et al 2002).

One old story that may yet have some mileage, given the evidence for humoral mechanisms of tissue injury in some multiple sclerosis lesions and in Devic's disease (see Chapters 5 and 12), relates to complement-mediated brain injury. Because they lack a factor (CD59) that normally protects cells from autologous complement injury by regulating assembly of the membrane-attack complex (Wing et al 1992), rat oligodendrocytes and their progenitors activate complement in vitro (Scolding et al 1989a). They are protected by reincorporating CD59 on the cell surface. This effect is reversed by an anti-CD59 monoclonal antibody (Zajicek et al 1992). Human oligodendrocytes express all the lytic complement components of the classical and alternative pathways (Hosokawa et al 2003) but complement activation is evidently not a property of human oligodendrocytes (R.C. Armstrong et al 1992; Zajicek and Compston 1995).

Oligodendrocytes cultured from samples obtained at craniotomy are not lysed by contact with normal human serum, and they do express CD59 (Scolding et al 1998a).

Whether or not this reveals a mechanism of oligodendrocyte injury in vivo must remain in doubt, but the work has revealed a principle of general importance – the possibility of repair in the central nervous system at the single cell level. Cells exposed to sublytic concentrations of complement or T-cell-derived perforin show a transient increase in intracellular calcium during which pores forming in the membrane are gathered into vesicles and shed from the cell surface, thereby restoring membrane integrity and leaving the oligodendrocyte metabolically intact (Figure 10.15; Scolding et al 1989b; Zeine et al 2001). Using microfluorimetry of indo-1 fluorescence to detect calcium levels, A. Wood et al (1993) showed that oligodendrocytes recover from sublytic complement attack coinciding with calcium oscillations whereas nonoscillating oligodendrocytes are rapidly lysed. The coincidence of oligodendrocyte recovery with calcium oscillation suggests that the complex calcium signal following pore formation stimulates protective mechanisms. Calcium ionophores do not produce similar oscillations. T-cell-derived perforin causes increased membrane permeability, identical to that seen following complement attack, and an abrupt rise in cytosolic free calcium (Figure 10.16A; J. Jones et al 1991; Scolding et al 1992). A small amount is released from internal stores but the majority enters from outside the cell. Scolding et al (1995) used a variety of growth factors to protect rat oligodendrocytes from complement attack but were unable to control the rise in calcium or alter the threshold for vesicular recovery. Conversely, inhibiting the intracellular calcium-activated protein calmodulin, using W7, lowered the threshold for com-to destroy foreign invaders. The same mechanisms mediate damage of the host tissue in infectious or autoimmune-mediated inflammatory diseases. As a safety factor in the body's defence repertoire, these mechanisms show redundancy, enabling the organism to eliminate infectious agents or infected cells even when one or more effector pathways of immune defence is blocked. Although conferring a major advantage to the immune system, this redundancy creates major problems for the therapy of immune-mediated diseases. It is, in theory, unlikely that blockade of a single immune effector pathway will confer a major beneficial effect in such a complex disease as multiple sclerosis. As summarized above (see also Chapter 11), multiple different immune-mediated pathways can lead to demyelination and central nervous system tissue damage. However, these *in vitro* studies convey a key message, and one that appears relevant for understanding and limiting the pathogenesis of multiple sclerosis lesions.

First, although exquisite specificity of the immune reaction results from engagement of the specific arm of the immune system, involving cytotoxic T cells and autoantibodies, a great deal of tissue damage in inflammatory lesions is mediated through antigen-independent pathways using the products of activated effector cells, such as macrophages or microglial cells. Most immune-mediated mechanisms of tissue injury affect oligodendrocytes and myelin sheaths more than other constituents of the central nervous system. This may result from the specific metabolic requirements involved in synthesis and maintenance of the elaborate lipid layers of myelin sheaths. Thus, the development of demyelinated plaques in multiple sclerosis does not necessarily imply that this is a disease in which the immune reaction is specifically directed against myelin. On the contrary, these data suggest that any chronic inflammatory process of the white matter can result in a degree of primary demyelination.

Second, for some immunotoxins, such as reactive oxygen species or excitotoxins, the targets are not only mature oligodendrocytes but also progenitor cells. It follows that the specific inflammatory environment in a given lesion may determine the extent of endogenous remyelination occurring once the active phase of tissue destruction is completed.

Third, the same immunotoxin may affect cellular elements of the central nervous system to a differing degree, depending on functional properties of the cells. Nitric oxide and oxygen radicals damage cells directly through the induction of cell membrane damage, and indirectly through mitochondrial injury. Direct toxicity appears to be independent of cell function, but may preferentially affect cells with elaborate cell membranes. Thus, oligodendrocytes appear to be exquisitely vulnerable. Conversely, indirect toxicity through mitochondrial damage will be most deleterious in cells that are under metabolic stress, such as electrically active axons and neurons. This implies that, in patients with multiple sclerosis, the same immune effector pathway may lead to primary demyelination in some situations, and to primary axonal injury in others. This may in part explain differences in the pathology of lesions characterizing relapsing–remitting versus progressive multiple sclerosis.

Finally, the extent and nature of tissue damage in immune-mediated diseases of the central nervous system is also likely to be influenced by genetically determined susceptibility of the target tissue. This could influence the global extent of tissue injury (reflected in disease severity), the type of cells and structures

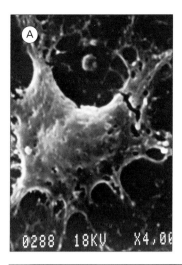
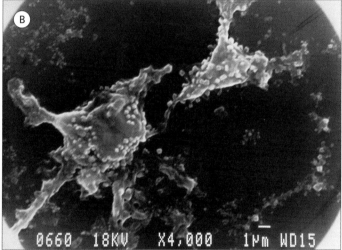

Figure 10.15 Reversible injury of oligodendrocytes by membrane vesiculation. (A) Oligodendrocytes are shown before initiating nonlethal injury with complement. (B) After 3 minutes, numerous vesicular structures brightly stain with anti-C9 antibody and avidin gold appears on the cell and its processes. From Scolding *et al* (1989b) with permission.

plement lysis by blocking vesiculation. Under these circumstances, concentrations of serum from which oligodendrocytes were normally protected by vesicle formation proved lethal (Scolding *et al* 1992). Taken together, the evidence points to a pivotal role for calcium and calmodulin in orchestrating the response of oligodendrocytes to membrane injury. Although a correlation exists between recovery and transient elevation of intracellular calcium in populations of oligodendrocytes, this relationship can better be characterized by calcium imaging of single cells. These studies illustrate that a delicate balance exists between injury and repair, oligodendrocytes showing heterogeneous responses under broadly similar experimental conditions. Individual cells exposed to the same concentration of pore-forming agent differ markedly in the extent to which intracellular calcium increases, the site of entry and whether or not this is associated with a general increase in membrane permeability (Figure 10.16B and C; A. Wood *et al* 1993).

All of these studies show that the immune system is equipped with a multitude of effector mechanisms, designed effectively that are preferentially injured (axons or myelin), or even the location of the lesions within the brain. Perhaps, the best example is selective involvement of the anterior visual pathway in patients with multiple sclerosis harbouring a mutation of mitochondrial DNA (Harding's disease; see Chapter 6).

From all that has been said, it seems clear that the lesions in patients with multiple sclerosis develop in the context of a complex interaction and mixture of different antigen-dependent and -independent mechanisms. The mix of these different factors determines the quality and fate of the lesion. It is likely

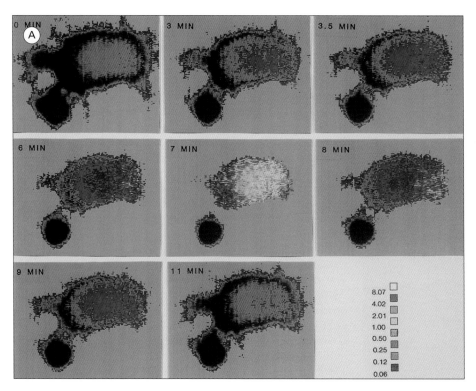

Figure 10.16 (A) Cytosolic-free calcium imaging in oligodendrocytes attacked with perforin. Fluorescence ratio images were calibrated according to the colour scale shown. Numbers represent minutes after addition of perforin. From J. Jones *et al* (1991) with permission. (B,C) Serum-induced $[Ca^{2+}]$ oscillations show variable latencies and patterns following exposure to sublytic concentrations of normal rat serum at 37°C. The oligodendrocyte shown in (B) illustrated oscillations 2 minutes after addition of 1:30 serum, maintained an elevated basal $[Ca^{2+}]$ throughout, and was propidium iodide negative 45 minutes and 2 hours following recording (n=9). The oligodendrocyte illustrated in (C) did not oscillate and became propidium iodide positive only 5 minutes after the addition of 1:30 serum (n=2). Adapted from A. Wood *et al* (1993).

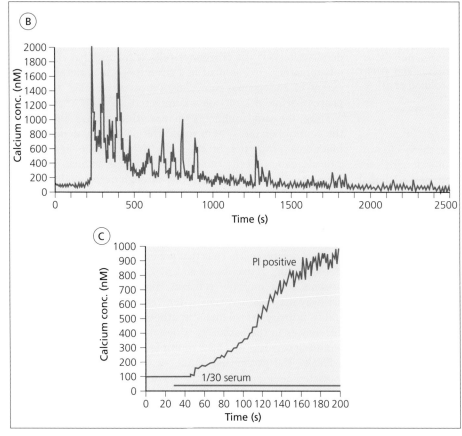

that this environment is, in part, genetically determined and, thus, heterogeneous between patients as well as depending on the type and stage of the disease.

The role of microglia

Infiltrating macrophages or resident microglia produce many of the soluble factors already implicated in oligodendrocyte injury. In addition to their role in development, they also contribute phagocytic properties to cell injury and removal and they are the brain's own and only effective immunological cell. Microglia are distinguished phenotypically from brain macrophages by differential expression of CD45 and CD11. Both cell types play a complex, and in some respects paradoxical, role in development, injury and repair of axon–glial arrangements within the central nervous system. Microglia are similar to astrocytes in changing their morphology and behaviour with activation. The most potent activators *in vitro* and perhaps *in vivo* are products such as bacterium-derived lipopolysaccharide, the T-cell-derived cytokine IFN-γ, and the colony stimulating factors. To a varying extent, these activators lead to the expression of co-stimulatory molecules B7-1/2 and CD40, and they are inhibited by IL-4, IL-10, IL-11, TGF-β1 and NGF – sometimes through autocrine effects on the corresponding receptors (Wei and Jonakait 1999). Activated microglia change their morphology (becoming amoeboid and motile), and release proinflammatory cytokines, chemokines and mediators that orchestrate immune functions.

Microglia and oligodendrocyte survival

Media conditioned by nonactivated microglia increase the number of surviving galactocerebroside-positive oligodendrocytes *in vitro* (Nicholas *et al* 2001a). Survival results from inhi-

bition of endogenous oligodendrocte precursor apoptosis and promotion of oligodendrocyte differentiation which override the effects on maturation of PDGF and FGF-2 (Figure 10.17). These soluble factors act by upregulation of NF-κB in oligodendrocyte precursors. Anti-PDGF antibody abolishes this effect even though PDGF-α chain is expressed at similar levels on both non-activated and IFN-γ-activated microglia, and their conditioned media have similar levels of PDGF-α chain bioactivity. However, the soluble factors produced by nonactivated microglia recruit phosphoinositide 3-kinase to the PDGF-α receptor and synergize with endogenous PDGF-α chain to increase NF-κB activation. These effects are not observed with supernatants from microglia treated with IFN-γ. Therefore, depending on activation state, microglia produce soluble factors that promote oligodendrocyte development through an effect on PDGF-α receptor signalling. These appear not to be any one of the many growth factors known to act on cells of the oligodendrocyte lineage.

Microglia as antigen-presenting cells

The terms professional and non-professional define antigen-presenting cells which initiate antigen-specific primary or only secondary immune responses, respectively. These differences impact on the stimulation required to trigger naive, as opposed to memory, T-cell activation (see Chapter 11). The issue of whether antigen presentation occurs exclusively within the central nervous system, or uses cells (of peripheral or brain origin) that encounter antigen in draining lymph nodes and stimulate lymphocytes before migrating into the central nervous system, is not fully resolved. Microglia (or bone marrow-derived macrophages) are the best candidates for a brain-derived antigen-presenting cell. Astrocytes, cerebrovascular endothelial cells and pericytes are also all capable of restimulating lympho-

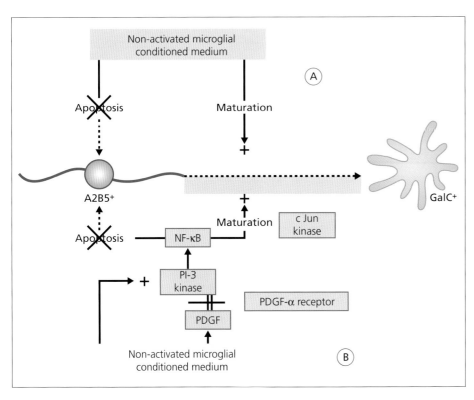

Figure 10.17 (A) Soluble factors released by non-activated microglia increase oligodendrocyte survival by inhibiting apoptosis and promoting differentiation of their precursors. (B) Signalling is through the PDGF-α receptor activating NF-κB. Kindly prepared by Dr Richard Nicholas.

cytes – and there is now experimental evidence that dendritic cells can migrate from the periphery and trigger the local central nervous system immune response (V.H. Perry 1998).

The antigen-presenting role is primarily assigned to the CD45^{high} CD11b/c$^+$ perivascular macrophage rather than the CD45^{low} CD11b/c$^+$ parenchymal microglial cell. Unlike perivascular macrophages, microglia fail to produce IL-2, resulting in limited T-cell proliferation and the promotion of apoptosis. Microglia secrete IL-1 and constitutively express class II major histocompatibility complex (MHC) and the B7 accessory molecules following activation. Costimulation is most effectively delivered through CD28 and B7, and/or CD40 and its ligand. These costimulatory molecules are upregulated on microglia by IFN-γ and lipopolysaccharide under inflammatory conditions. Antigen presentation by microglia to memory T cells results in cytokine release and this reciprocally activates naive microglia, suggesting that presentation of recall antigen creates an environment that propagates the immune response (G.L. Hall *et al* 1999). Agresti *et al* (1998) showed that induction of MHC-class II antigen on microglia involves synergism between IFN-γ and TNF-α. IFN-γ increases the expression of TNF-αR1 acting through the STAT1 signal transduction pathway, and also the interferon regulatory factor 1 (IRF-1). These molecular events allow TNF-α to induce binding of NF-κB to endogenous enhancers of MHC-class II antigen expression. This is increased by TGF-β1 in microglia but not macrophages (Pazmany *et al* 2000). Anti-inflammatory cytokines – especially the T helper type 2-associated products IL-4, IL-10, prostaglandin-E2 and TGF-β1 – downregulate these costimulatory molecules, suppressing proliferation, activation, adhesion, migration, phagocytosis and mediator production. Apoptosis of autoreactive T cells using perforin and the Fas/Fas-ligand pathway also reduces the proinflammatory activitiy of microglia. In many situations, these events lead to apoptotic death of microglia unless these are protected by Bcl-2.

Interactions between microglia and oligodendrocytes

IFN-γ upregulates the expression of a heterogeneous group of molecules on microglia involved in the phagocytosis of opsonized particles. These include the FcR1 (CD64), FcRII (CD32) and FcRIII (CD16) receptors for immunoglobulin; complement components C1q, iCR3, and C5a; and IL-8, TNF-αR1 and the bacterial peptide f-Met-Leu-Phe. Reichert and Rotshenker (1996) showed that, whereas most receptors are expressed by microglia manipulated *in vitro*, others (especially MAC-2 but also Fc) are only upregulated *in vivo* following injury. The activation of microglia by lipopolysaccharide, leading to interactions with oligodendrocytes, involves the toll-like receptor (TLR4) both *in vitro* and *in vivo* (see Chapter 11; Lehnardt *et al* 2002). Microglia expressing these receptors are able to attract and engage target cells (Figure 10.18A).

Receptors for the growth regulated oncogene-α and IL-8, CXCR1 and CXCR-2, are present on oligodendrocytes, enabling the response to migratory and proliferative signals in the inflamed central nervous system (Nguyen and Stangel 2001). The CXCR1 receptor is upregulated by TGF-β1 and this involves inhibition of the Erk transcription pathway (S. Chen *et al* 2002). *In vitro*, significant cell death occurs when oligodendrocytes derived from mixed rat cortical glia are cultured without growth supporting factors. The soluble factors released from these cultures are chemotactic for microglia. This occurs before major cell loss has occurred. Microglial chemotaxis does not result from the release of cellular debris since the effect is not reproduced by osmotic lysis of freshly plated oligodendrocytes. IFN-γ activation increases the sensitivity of microglia to these chemoattractants (Nicholas *et al* 2003a). The stressed oligodendrocyte signals its distress and either summons assistance or suicidally attracts activated microglia. The initial recruitment of microglia by stressed oligodendrocytes could represent part of a survival response engaged by injured cells but this is a potentially dangerous liaison.

Activated microglia mainly kill oligodendrocytes by cell–cell contact. Receptor–ligand interactions then allow microglia to deliver the lethal TNF-α signal to target cells (Figure 10.18B,C; see also Figure 10.14; Zajicek *et al* 1992). The main relevance of complement activation in multiple sclerosis (see above; Scolding *et al* 1989a; 1989b) may be in the breakdown of C3, releasing membrane-bound and fluid-phase products which determine interactions between oligodendrocytes and macrophages or microglia. Their receptors for C1q, C3b (CR1) and iC3b (CR3) bind ligands on target cells. Some are constitutively expressed, whereas others require cytokine activation. van der Laan *et al* (1996) confirmed that uptake of myelin by macrophages is enhanced by opsonization with complement, involves the CR3 receptor, induces a rise in intracellular calcium, and is associated with the production of TNF-α and nitric oxide by these activated macrophages. In practice, however, Fc receptors may be the more relevant vehicle for cell–cell contacts. Of particular relevance to multiple sclerosis is the demonstration that antibody in low concentration, coating the surface of the oligodendrocyte or its myelin sheath, opsonizes the target cell for lytic damage by microglia using their Fc receptors (Scolding and Compston 1991). Demyelinated axons are coated with anti-myelin oligodendrocyte glycoprotein antibody in the lesions of acute multiple sclerosis (Genain *et al* 1999) although these antibodies are directed against linear epitopes that do not induce demyelination *in vivo*. The study used glutaraldehyde-fixed and osmicated material – not ideal for the detection of tissue-bound antibodies, perhaps explaining why these results have not been reproduced using frozen sections, even in experimental situations that are clearly driven by anti-myelin oligodendrocyte antibodies such as experimental autoimmune encephalomyelitis in primates (Hans Lassmann, unpublished observations). The potential role of myelin oligodendrocyte glycoprotein is further suggested by the high prevalence of intrathecal anti-myelin oligodendrocyte glycoprotein antibodies that persist in multiple sclerosis from an early stage in the illness, unlike the evolving pattern of antibody responses to myelin basic protein. van der Goes *et al* (1999) have made a systematic analysis of antibody opsonization of myelin, finding effects of many isotypes and specificities but with a maximal effect of anti-myelin oligodendrocyte glycoprotein Z12 specificity. Macrophages engaged in phagocytosis produce reactive oxygen species and these are also directly involved in the uptake of myelin fragments (van der Goes *et al* 1998). Activated microglia increase their production of TNF-α and nitric oxide after binding immunoglobulin to the Fc receptor, with signal transduction through the phosphoinositide 3-kinase pathway, but these activities then inhibit the phagocytotic properties of microglia

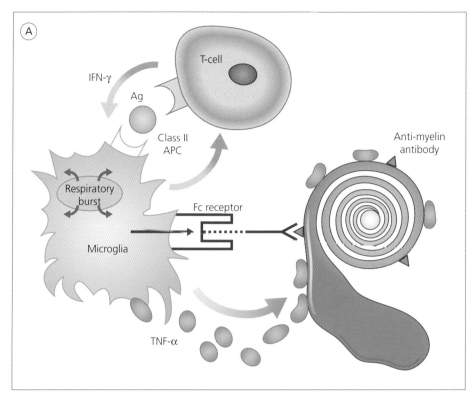

Figure 10.18: (A) Representation of the T cell–microglia interaction in the central nervous system. T-cell-derived IFN-γ is the main pro-inflammatory cytokine; activated microglia undergo a respiratory burst, amplify antigen presentation and produce proinflammatory cytokines. APC = antigen-presenting cell. (B) Scanning electron microscopy to show phagocytosis of opsonized oligodendrocytes by activated microglia: resting microglia and nonopsonized oligodendrocytes do not interact. (C) Activated microglia adhere to and injure oligodendrocytes opsonized with sublethal concentrations of complement. From Zajicek *et al* (1992) with permission.

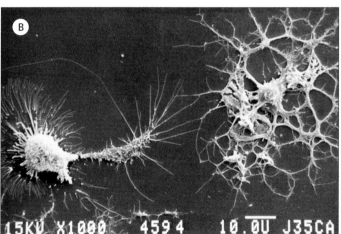

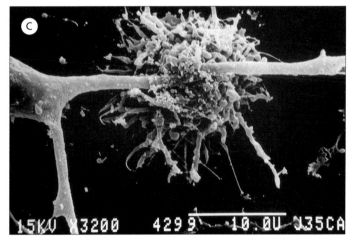

presumably by blockade of the Fc receptor (Stangel and Compston 2001). Astrocytes also protect oligodendrocytes from apoptotic death under defined tissue culture conditions, not dependent on growth factor deprivation, through cell–cell contact mediated by interactions between extracellular matrix laminin-2 and its receptor, α6β1, present on oligodendrocytes (Corley *et al* 2001). Scarisbrick *et al* (2002) showed that expression of a serine protease acting on myelin basic protein and myelin-associated glycoprotein was increased in the lesions of multiple sclerosis, Theiler's murine encephalomyelitis virus and myelin oligodendrocyte glycoprotein induced experimental autoimmune encephalomyelitis in marmosets. Myelencephalon-specific protease reduced the complexity and number of processes seen on immature and differentiated oligodendrocytes *in vitro* and after transfection but did not reduce cell survival.

Analysing this and other evidence, two important principles of injury and survival emerge. The signals transduced by cells during physiological activity are the same as those that become overloaded during pathological events leading to cell injury and death.

AXON DEGENERATION AND RECOVERY OF FUNCTION

The symptoms of inflammatory brain disease are believed to result from the failure of axonal conduction, augmented by a disruption of synaptic processing. No longer is it appropriate to think merely in terms of demyelination as the main consequence of brain inflammation. Rather, symptom onset and recovery must be understood in terms of altered structure and function in the entire myelinated oligodendrocyte–axon unit and its synaptic connections. Nor, given the capacity for plasticity and functional adaptation, is clinical recovery necessarily synonymous with structural repair. Pathological evidence showing the distribution, extent and timing of axonal loss in multiple sclerosis is discussed in Chapter 12, and the physiological consequences of this damage in Chapter 13. Here, we summarize the immunological and biological mechanisms of axonal injury.

Clinical observations and related laboratory and experimental studies indicate that acute cytokine release leads to transient conduction block most likely through indirect mechanisms, involving nitric oxide, in the form of one or more of the reactive nitrogen species. Brief exposure to nitric oxide donors produces reversible conduction block in normal or, especially, demyelinated axons. Hence, one mechanism of onset and recovery must be the arrival and subsequent removal of inflammatory mediators reversing the functional deficit affecting intact myelinated axons. As discussed in Chapter 13, K.J. Smith *et al* (2001c) showed that, amongst a list of candidate molecules, donors of nitric oxide could reversibly impair conduction in normal or demyelinated rat spinal cord axons. Conduction block in pathways affected by multiple sclerosis might also be caused by other inflammatory mediators, and a pentapeptide QYNAD (Gln-Tyr-Asn-Ala-Asp) has been advanced as being able to block sodium channels in human neuroblastoma-glioma NH15-CA2 cells. QYNAD is present in the cerebrospinal fluid from patients with multiple sclerosis at concentrations that are three-fold to 14-fold those found in normal controls (Brinkmeier *et al* 2000). The effects on sodium channels have not been reproduced in other studies (Cummins *et al* 2003; Quasthoff *et al* 2003), but it remains likely that some inflammatory mediators yet to be identified will impair neurophysiological function.

More prolonged exposure to the donors of nitric oxide causes axon degeneration especially if the axons are electrically active. This analysis resonates with contemporary studies of axonal pathology in multiple sclerosis. Immunohistochemical staining for amyloid precursor protein confirms that axonal injury occurs as part of the acute demyelinating lesion (B. Ferguson *et al* 1997). Axonal damage in acute inflammatory plaques is shown histologically (Trapp *et al* 1998) and radiologically through reduction in the neuronal spectroscopic marker, *N*-acetyl aspartate (Davie *et al* 1994). This acute axonal damage mainly occurs in active lesions and correlates with the degree of inflammation (see also B. Ferguson *et al* 1997; Kornek *et al* 2000; Kuhlmann *et al* 2002b; Trapp *et al* 1998). Once axonal injury is established, recovery must presumably partly depend on plasticity: at the axonal level through restoration of conduction following increased insertion of sodium channels along the demyelinated axonal surface; through redundancy and rearrangement of connectivity in specific pathways; and through expansion of cortical receptor fields for a degraded axonal signal. Remyelination of surviving axons may also contribute to restoration of function.

Mechanisms of acute axonal injury

Microglia and astrocytes synthesize nitric oxide via iNOS. The nitric oxide kills neighbouring cells through DNA damage, poly-ADP ribose polymerase overactivation, adenosine triphosphate (ATP) depletion (J. Zhang *et al* 1994), p53 accumulation (Forrester *et al* 1996), and opening of the mitochondrial permeability transition pore (G.C. Brown and Borutaite 2001). Nitric oxide inhibition of mitochondrial respiration leads to ATP depletion in neurons, glutamate release, and excitotoxicity (Bal-

Price and Brown 2001). Energy failure after nitric oxide exposure may similarly contribute to conduction block and axon degeneration in rat dorsal root preparations (K.J. Smith *et al* 2001b). Soluble factors released by activated microglia impair neurons *in vitro*. Effects on neuronal mitochondrial (cytochrome oxidase) activity are blocked by anti-TNF-α antibodies, and cell death is prevented by an intracellular increase of NF-κB (Nicholas *et al* 2001b). Although this neuronal dysfunction is initially reversible, a separate and potentially lethal sequence of events follows more prolonged exposure to microglial soluble factors – mimicking the electrophysiological studies of K.J. Smith *et al* (2001c). In cocultures of rat microglia and embryonic cortical neurons, iNOS-derived nitric oxide appears to be responsible for neuronal death from IFN-γ and lipopolysaccharide-activated microglia. Neurons allowed to mature *in vitro* remain sensitive to nitric oxide but, whereas blocking NMDA-receptor activation with MK801 has no effect on the nitric oxide-mediated toxicity of immature neurons, MK801 rescues 60–70% of neurons matured in culture for 12 days. This increase in protection from toxicity matches increased neuronal expression of NMDA receptors. MK801 also delays the death of more mature neurons caused by the nitric oxide donor DETA NONOate, indicating that one of the deleterious mechanisms initiated by nitric oxide is excitotoxic, most likely through neuronal glutamate release. Thus, similar concentrations of nitric oxide cause neuronal death by two distinct mechanisms: nitric oxide acts directly upon immature neurons and indirectly, via NMDA receptors, on more mature neurons (Figure 10.19; Golde *et al* 2002). The induction of iNOS and the axonal toxicity of nitric oxide are dependent on calcium-mediated toxicity consequent upon uncontrolled influx of sodium through voltage-gated channels (Garthwaite *et al* 2002; K.J. Smith *et al* 2001b). Interactions between CD40 ligand and its receptor on microglia lead to production of TNF-α (J. Tan *et al* 1999) and the death of motor neurons *in vitro* but this also requires prior activation with lipopolysaccharide and release of nitric oxide (B. He *et al* 2002b). Axons are protected by sodium-channel-blocking agents, such as flecainide, phenytoin and lamotrigine, that prevent the conditions necessary for reverse sodium/calcium exchange (Figure 10.20; see Chapter 13; Kapoor *et al* 2003; Lo *et al* 2003).

These findings raise the possibility of axonal protection by existing or novel therapies in the context of inflammatory brain disease. Walker *et al* (1997) demonstrated that calpain-inhibitor 1 (ALLN) increases the stability of iNOS protein in dexamethasone-treated macrophages, implying that corticosteroids reduce nitric oxide by destabilizing the inducing enzyme. Subsequently, Walker *et al* (2001) reported that purified calpain degraded iNOS when translated in cells *in vitro*. ALLN is not specific for calpain but also potently inhibits the proteasome. Inducible NOS was recently identified as a proteasome substrate, itself readily degraded in the presence of calpastatin (Musial and Eissa 2001). Therefore, rather than affecting calpain activity, glucocorticoids may regulate iNOS expression by accelerating proteasome-dependent degradation. Golde *et al* (2003) showed that addition of dexamethasone (1 μmol/L) to activated cocultures of microglia and neurons is neuroprotective. These changes are reversed by the glucocorticoid receptor-blocker RU-486. Furthermore, proteasome inhibitors block iNOS degradation but do not reverse the dexamethasone effect, indicating that the main mechanism of corticosteroid activity on

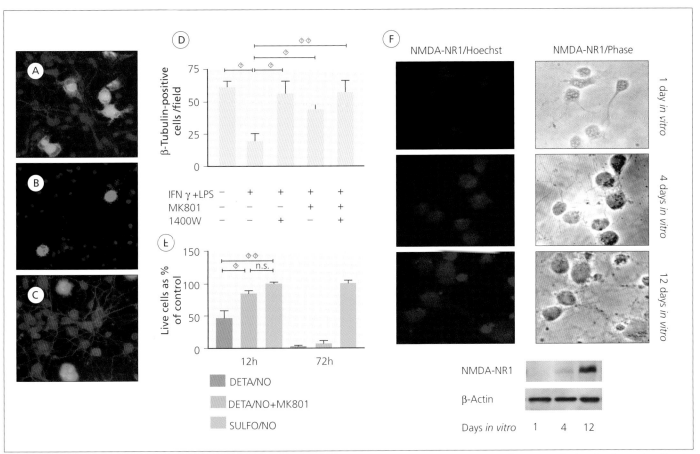

Figure 10.19 (A) Toxic effect of IFN-γ and lipopolysaccharide activated microglia on neurons. Cortical neurons (1 day *in vitro*, visualized with anti-γ-tubulin, red) survive and form long processes after 3 days in coculture with microglia. Addition of IFN-γ and lipopolysaccharide to cocultures of neurons and microglia induces neuronal death after 3 days. (B) IFN-γ and lipopolysaccharide induce significant increase of lactate dehydrogenase release when added to microglia-neuronal cocultures for 3 days, but not in neuronal or microglial control cultures. MTT (3-[4,5-dimethylthiazol-2-yl]-2,5-diphenyltetrazolium bromide) metabolism shows significantly reduced viability only in IFN-γ and lipopolysaccharide-treated cocultures, but not in controls. Reduced ³[H]-GABA-uptake confirms that cell death in activated cocultures is the result of a loss of neurons. (D) Inhibition of iNOS with 1400 W completely abolishes microglial neurotoxicity. (E) DETA/NO, a slowly releasing nitric oxide donor causes dose-dependent neuronal death. Microglial nitric oxide mediates its effect on more mature cortical neurons partially via NMDA-receptor-activation. (F) NMDA-receptor (subunit NR1) expression in cultured cortical neurons. Adapted from Golde *et al* (2002).

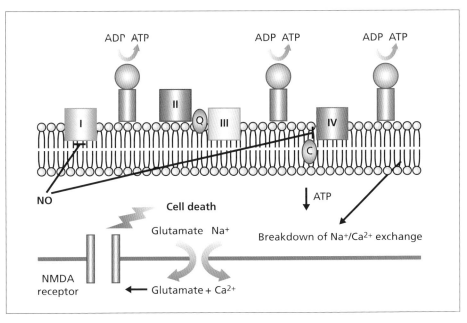

Figure 10.20 The effect of nitric oxide on mitochondrial function, producing energy failure with consequent loss of the sodium/calcium exchange mechanism exposing the neuron to excitotoxic injury through calcium overload. Kindly prepared by Dr Sabine Golde.

iNOS is reduction in protein synthesis rather than gene expression. However, Diem *et al* (2003) have shown that methylprednisolone has an opposite effect, increasing retinal ganglion cell apoptosis in the myelin oligodendrocyte glycoprotein-induced model of experimental autoimmune encephalomyelitis by calcium-dependent inhibition of the neuroprotective endogenous MAP kinase phosphorylation pathways.

Mechanisms of chronic axonal injury

A number of clinical trials have now made the point that the suppression of inflammation in chronic multiple sclerosis rarely does much to limit the accumulation of disability through sustained progression (see Chapter 18). One interpretation of these observations is that axonal loss and inflammation are independent pathologies (Confavreux *et al* 2000). The epidemiological jury may still be out on whether there is a correlation between the early inflammatory load and subsequent clinical course but the experimental evidence supports a direct relationship. Most axonal loss is seen in secondary progressive multiple sclerosis and, in this context, can be explained by two processes. First, acutely transected axons undergo Wallerian degeneration within days, and certainly within the subsequent 18 months (J.H. Simon *et al* 2001), but this seems not to produce a progressive clinical deficit. Secondly, axons that escape injury in the acute phase may later degenerate through a noninflammatory mechanism – one that is nevertheless dependent on prior inflammation – loss of trophic support for neurons and axons normally provided by oligodendrocytes and myelination.

Raff *et al* (2002) reviewed details of the distal degeneration (Wallerian) that follows axotomy and proximal dying back towards the neuronal cell body that is more characteristic of metabolic, toxic and immunological insults. The same process may be used selectively to sculpt exuberant axonal and neurite outgrowth during development, without compromising neuronal survival. Studies in the Wallerian degeneration slow (*Wld*) mouse indicate that loss of the distal axon involves an active process in which a nuclear fusion protein affects the synthetic pathway for nicotinamide adenone dinucleotide (NAD) and ubiquitination. Although Bcl-2 is protective in some experimental models, dying back axonopathy does not necessarily involve apoptosis and caspase-mediated cell death. Perhaps the main lesson from this analysis is the focus on axonal and neuronal injury as independent events that are capable of being dissociated – a principle that seems obvious but perhaps too often neglected. The influence of oligodendrocytes on axonal calibre and function is well described. Oligodendrocytes myelinate axons, increase axonal stability and induce local accumulation and phosphorylation of neurofilaments within the axon (S.T. Brady *et al* 1999; Colello *et al* 1994; Sanchez *et al* 1996). Neuronal function is further influenced by oligodendrocyte-derived soluble factors that induce sodium-channel clustering along axons, necessary for efficient saltatory conduction, and maintain this clustering even in the absence of direct axon–glial contact (see above).

Several models of primary immune-mediated demyelination are associated with axonal injury that cannot entirely be explained by inflammation *per se* (McGavern *et al* 2000). Mouse models in which myelination is disrupted, usually by transgenic methodologies, have established the role of specific myelin proteins and factors produced by oligodendrocytes in determining neuronal and axonal survival. In principle, all myelin mutants resulting in chronic myelin impairment or demyelination are associated with axonal injury. Although some studies have suggested that axonal injury is present only in some myelin mutants (Lappe Siefke *et al* 2003) and lacking in others, such as myelin basic protein-deficient animals (Phokeo and Ball 2000), more detailed analysis has revealed profound axonal injury also in the myelin basic protein-deficient *shiverer* mouse (Loers *et al* 2004). Neurons demonstrate a marked increase in survival when cocultured directly with oligodendrocyte precursors and differentiated oligodendrocytes, and this effect is reproduced using medium conditioned by differentiated oligodendrocytes (Wilkins *et al* 2001). Some attention has focused on IGF-1, as cells of the oligodendrocyte lineage produce IGF-1, and neutralizing antibodies to IGF-1, but not other candidate trophic factors, block the soluble survival effect of oligodendrocytes. Recombinant IGF-1 promotes neuronal survival under identical conditions. These effects act through the phosphoinositide 3-kinase/Akt signalling pathway. Conversely, differentiated oligodendrocytes increase neurofilament phosphorylation and axonal length as the result of an effect of glial cell derived nerve growth factor acting through the MAP kinase/Erk pathways (Wilkins *et al* 2003). Thus, factors released by oligodendrocyte precursor cells and oligodendrocytes induce the activation of at least two intracellular pathways within neurons, and these support different structural and functional properties of the neuron and its axonal appendage (Figure 10.21).

In a different system, X. Dai *et al* (2003) confirmed the trophic effect of oligodendrocytes and their conditioned medium on the survival of cholinergic neurons – effects that were attributable to NGF and BDNF acting through tyrosine kinase pathways. PDGF also protects axons from lysophosphatidylcholine toxicity *in vivo* but it is unclear whether these effects are direct or attributable to oligodendrocyte intermediates (Jean *et al* 2002). Wilkins and Compston (2005) showed that rat cortical neurons exposed to a nitric oxide donor, that normally proves lethal, were protected specifically by oligodendrocyte conditioned medium and by IGF-1, whereas medium conditioned by oligodendrocyte precursors and glial cell derived nerve growth factor, acting through the MAPkinase/Erk pathway enhanced axon survival (Figure 10.22). In addition, p38 MAPkinase signalling pathways were activated by nitric oxide exposure, and inhbition of p38 led to neuronal and axonal survival effects. Oligodendrocyte-conditioned medium and IGF-1 (but not glial cell derived nerve growth factor) reduced p38 activation in cortical neurons exposed to nitric oxide. Furthermore, inhibitors of p38 activated MAPkinase/Erk signalling in cortical neurons. Together, these results indicate that different mechanisms underlie neuronal and axonal destructive and protective processes, and suggest that trophic factors may modulate nitric oxide-mediated neuron/axon destruction via specific pathways. Although the principles are broadly similar, IGF-1-mediated protection of neurons from nitric oxide (Wilkins and Compston 2005), and of oligodendrocytes from glutamate-mediated excitotoxicity (Ness *et al* 2004), differ in the details of which molecules mediate these effects.

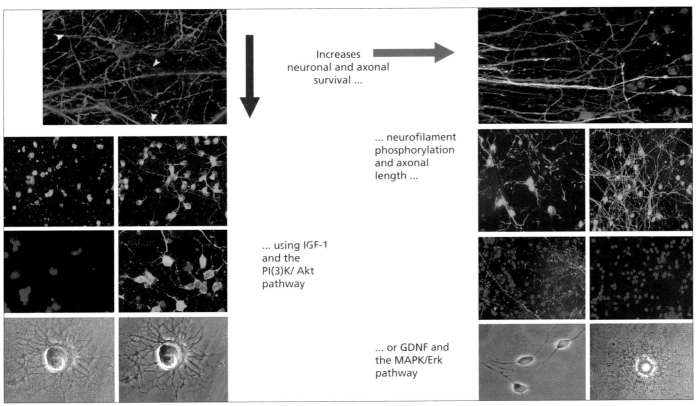

Figure 10.21 Effects of medium conditioned by oligodendrocyte precursors and mature oligodendrocytes increases neuronal survival using IGF-1 produced by oligodendroglia, acting through the IGF-1 receptor present on neurons and with signalling through the phosphoinositide 3-kinase/Akt pathway. Effects of medium conditioned by mature oligodendrocytes increases neurofilament phosphorylation and axonal length using glial cell derived nerve growth factor with signalling through the MAP kinase/Erk pathway. Modified from Wilkins *et al* (2003) with permission.

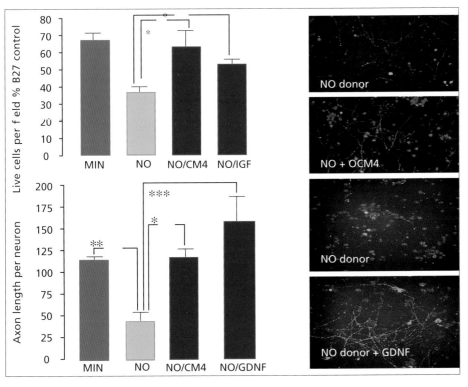

Figure 10.22 Insulin-like growth factor 1 and glial cell derived nerve growth factor protect neurons and axons, respectively, from injury mediated by nitric oxide donors and medium conditioned by activated microglia. MIN = minimal medium; NO = nitric oxide; CM4 = oligodendrocyte-conditioned medium; IGF = insulin-like growth factor; GDNF = glial cell-derived nerve growth factor. Adapted from Wilkins and Compston (2005) with permission.

Axonal regeneration

A marked difference exists in the extent to which axon regeneration occurs in the central and peripheral nervous systems. Characterizing and comparing biological properties of the response to axotomy of central and peripheral nerve fibres has provided many insights into axon regeneration, and led to strategies for manipulating events so as to secure functional recovery in clinical practice. However, with the exception of some success following reimplantation of avulsed peripheral nerve roots into the spinal cord, most of this work remains experimental. Nevertheless, a dividend from the application of these advances in neurobiology, leading to improved outcome after spinal cord injury, is anticipated.

Although the failure of central axons to regenerate following injury to the adult central nervous system can be explained in part by intrinsic growth-limiting properties, several inhibitory effects on axon growth mediated by components of the developing vertebrate nervous system have been identified. In one sense, the lack of axonal regeneration which characterizes adult mammalian nervous systems can be considered as the price paid for needing an inhibitory environment to guide axons during development, for stabilizing arrangements in the postmature nervous system, and for inhibiting uncontrolled axonal exploration. *In vitro* studies indicate that astrocytes, mammalian oligodendrocytes and central myelin each actively inhibit neurite growth. Astrocytes block axon regeneration through a mechanism which induces the normal stop signals on growth cones. Extracellular matrix molecules produced by astroglia which have growth inhibitory properties include tenascin and chondroitin sulphate proteoglycans (Fawcett and Asher 1999; Ramer *et al* 2000). The ability of embryonic growth cones to penetrate their surrounding astrocyte matrix depends on local secretion of proteases in response to FGF-2, IL-1 and TNF-α (Fok-Seang *et al* 1998).

The failure of axon regeneration correlates with the amount of local reactive glial extracellular matrix (marked by proteoglycan expression) and, if axons can traverse that impediment, normal white matter is relatively permissive (Davies *et al* 1997). Chondroitin sulphate proteoglycans are used throughout biology to form barriers. They are upregulated in scar tissue following injury of the nervous system, acting as major factors blocking regeneration of damaged axons. This effect is mediated by protein kinase C, through activation of Rho, and its inhibition enhances axon regeneration *in vivo* (Sivasankaran *et al* 2004). Much of the inhibitory activity of proteoglycans expressed in the context of injury depends on their glycosaminoglycan chains. Treatments that remove these chains reduce the inhibition of axon regeneration. NG2 has been identified as an inhibitory chondroitin sulphate proteoglycan in scar tissue affecting the peripheral nervous system. The glycosaminoglycan chains can be removed by treatment with chondroitinase ABC. *In vivo* experiments have shown the efficacy of chondroitinase ABC in promoting axon regeneration in the brain and spinal cord and correlated these histological effects with behavioural recovery. Chondroitin sulphate proteoglycans are laid down as perineuronal nets in the brain and cord coinciding with the termination of critical periods of plasticity. These coats of inhibitory molecules contribute to the restriction of plasticity in the adult central nervous system. Chondroitinase ABC can restore plasticity in the adult cortex and spinal cord (E.J. Bradbury *et al* 2002; Moon *et al* 2001).

Although some effects are primarily dependent on age and maturation of neurons (Bouslama-Oueghlani *et al* 2003), axon growth inhibition is additionally inhibited by myelin proteins. Nogo (formerly NI-35 and NI-250) is produced by mature oligodendrocytes. A member of the reticulin family, it is produced by oligodendrocytes but not Schwann cells. Products of the *Nogo* gene are therefore intracellular but may act to contain axons within their nerve bundles in health. Nogo signals in association with the neurotrophin p75 receptor and LINGO-1, acting on RhoA to increase the expression of oligodendrocyte myelin glycoprotein (Mi *et al* 2004). After fibre tract injury, Nogo spills from the disrupted oligodendrocyte–myelin unit and acts, unhelpfully, to inhibit neurite outgrowth and axon regeneration (M.S. Chen *et al* 2000; GrandPré *et al* 2000; Prinjha *et al* 2000). Bregman *et al* (1995) showed that anti-IN antibodies placed in the parietal cortex of animals undergoing spinal hemisection partially restore motor function by enhancing recovery of brainstem-spinal or cortico-spinal fibres, and promoting plasticity of surviving serotonergic and adrenergic descending motor neurons. Functional recovery and new connectivity from neighbouring parts of the contralateral cortex are also reported using IN-1 antibody in destructive lesions (Kartje *et al* 1999) and experimental stroke (Papadopoulos *et al* 2002). Another candidate molecule for mediating the growth inhibition of specific axons (embryonic cerebellar and adult dorsal root ganglion cells) is myelin-associated glycoprotein, which is involved in the initial adhesion between the processes of myelinating cells and axons (McKerracher *et al* 1994; Mukhopadhyay *et al* 1994). Myelin-associated glycoprotein and Nogo both appear to bind the same receptor such that anti-Nogo receptor antibody and soluble Nogo-R, each prevent inhibition of neurite outgrowth by myelin-associated glycoprotein (Domeniconi *et al* 2002). However, as with many other aspects of myelin biology, these inhibitions are in turn dependent on specific conditions and mediated by defined signalling pathways. In the acute phase of axonal injury in dorsal root ganglia, a conditioning lesion of the dorsal branch is associated with raised cAMP levels and myelin-associated glycoprotein no longer inhibits growth of the central process, acting though a protein kinase signalling pathway. Only with the return to normal levels of these factors are the inhibitory properties of myelin-associated glycoprotein on central axons restored (Qiu *et al* 2002).

The Nogo receptor mediates the effect of these inhibitory myelin proteins but, in order to enhance axon regeneration, its inhibition must be performed in conjunction with promotion of the neuronal growth programme (Fischer *et al* 2004). Overexpression of GAP-43 in Purkinje cell neurons overrides the effects of myelin inhibitory molecules and enables neurites to sprout, but this may be because they are encouraged to shed their myelin sleeves (Gianola and Rossi 2004). The list is not complete. Oligodendrocyte myelin glycoprotein (Omgp) has recently been characterized as another molecule present on oligodendrocytes that inhibits neurite outgrowth (K.C. Wang *et al* 2002). NG2 chondroitin sulphate proteoglycan, expressed on the surface of oligodendrocyte precursors, also inhibits neurite outgrowth (Z.J. Chen *et al* 2002). Neurons produce plasticity-related gene 1 presumably to space themselves from neighbours during development (Bräuer *et al* 2003).

REMYELINATION

If, as we have argued, the attrition of axons occurs acutely, as a result of the direct effects of inflammation, and chronically through loss of trophic support normally maintained by cell contact and soluble mediators produced by the oligodendrocyte lineage, it follows that immunological and neurobiological components of the pathogenesis each need to be considered as part of a comprehensive strategy for limiting the damage. This analysis goes further, however. The importance of remyelination is given a more enhanced status than the potential merely to restore conduction through previously demyelinated axons. Rather, the emerging evidence indicates that remyelination is essential for axonal survival. Self-evidently, the availability of stem cells and precursors committed to the oligodendrocyte lineage in the adult central nervous system suggests a potential for endogenous repair of surviving axons, re-enacting the developmental process of myelination. As we describe in Chapter 12, this undoubtedly does happen but the extent and durability of these myelin sheaths seem limited – at least in those areas that subsequently become 'lesions'. One can only speculate on the extent to which the central nervous system accommodates other patches of inflammation and demyelination that are never revealed because remyelination has been rapid and complete leaving no trace of a prior area of demyelination, at least upon gross examination. However, we know enough about the fragile nature of oligodendrocyte precursor cell maturation, and its dependence on ideal growth factor and environmental conditions, to guess that a limiting factor in achieving remyelination is failure of the endogenous process at some stage in the complex sequence between the birth of stem cells and the restoration of saltatory conduction through new myelin sheaths.

A number of basic questions arise with respect to the practicalities of repairing demyelinated but viable axons – experimentally and in multiple sclerosis:

- Can surviving oligodendrocytes remyelinate naked axons or must there be a source of precursor cells?
- Are stem cells for glia present in the adult human nervous system? If so, can they migrate from germinal centres to sites of injury?
- Can cells other than oligodendrocytes be used as surrogates for remyclination?
- Will growth factor therapy prove effective and be well tolerated as a means of promoting repair?
- Will endogenous repair or assisted remyelination restore structure and function of the adult human nervous system?
- Given the contribution made by inflammation to axonal regeneration, will suppression of the inflammatory response compromise the repair process?

Some answers are already available.

Endogenous remyelination

The early experimental studies, involving mechanical and gliotoxin-induced demyelination, showed that endogenous remyelination does occur, and it restores conduction in the central nervous system (Felts and Smith 1992; K.J. Smith *et al* 1979). Later, these observations were supplemented by models of focal demyelination in which repair was directed at the defined lesion by stereotaxic cell implantation. These showed that remyelination involves the recruitment of oligodendrocyte precursors into an area of demyelination by a combination of proliferation, migration and differentiation into remyelinating oligodendrocytes. Failure of the process might be attributable to any one of these separate components. In seeking a full understanding of factors that determine the success or otherwise of remyelination, a key issue to emerge was therefore the need to identify the environmental factors that orchestrate these different phases. Thus, the concept arose that some lesions fail to repair through shortage of cells (failure of recruitment) whereas others remain demyelinated because the precursors cannot make the transition to remyelinating oligodendrocytes (failure of differentiation). Several factors that regulate precursor proliferation and migration in development serve similar functions during remyelination, including the growth factors PDGF and FGF-2. The complex biology of oligodendrocyte differentiation, largely studied *in vitro* and using developmental models, is less well understood in the context of remyelination. Repeated insults seem to limit the success of remyelination. It follows that mechanisms of remyelination need to be characterized in informative animal models, and not simply inferred from developmental studies.

As in the lesions of multiple sclerosis, the availability of oligodendrocyte precursors is not the major limiting factor in restricting remyelination in the experimental context. With anti-galactocerebroside antibody-mediated demyelination of the feline optic nerve, small glial cells derived from precursors located outside the lesion differentiate into oligodendrocytes and achieve extensive remyelination. These normally reside in central fascicles of the optic nerve and concentrate early at the margins of the lesion (Carroll *et al* 1998; Jennings *et al* 2002). In other situations, demyelination (with or without inflammation) also provides the stimulus to proliferation of NG2 cells (Di Bello *et al* 1999). Remyelination of a focal lesion is associated with increased expression of the Nkx2.2 transcription factor in those NG2-positive precursors that subsequently differentiate to produce mature myelinating oligodendrocytes – recapitulating what is seen normally in the developing optic nerve (Fancy *et al* 2004; M. Watanabe *et al* 2004). Arnett *et al* (2004) showed selective nuclear expression of *OLIG1* in cells repopulating areas of experimental demyelination and in the NG2-positive progenitors that accumulate around the edge of lesions in multiple sclerosis. Since transgenic mice lacking *OLIG1* have some myelinated axons (see above) but fail to repair the lesions produced by gliotoxins, the suggestion is that the role of Olig1 in differentiation is more closely involved in remyelination, perhaps due to redundancy and compensation at the time of normal development. Oligodendrocyte progenitors showing bromodeoxyuridine uptake, indicating that some cells have proliferated, accumulate in areas of immunologically mediated demyelination of the spinal cord (Keirstead and Blakemore 1999). PDGF and FGF-2 are required for the proliferation of oligodendrocyte precursors appearing early in areas of experimental demyelination prior to remyelination (Frost *et al* 2003). FGF-2 and FGF-R gene expression peak during the initial stage of remyelination on oligodendrocytes and astrocytes, suggesting that their production is under autocrine control (Messersmith *et al* 2000). CNTF produced by astrocytes also increases the availability of FGF-2R and ligand in a virus-induced model of demyelination (Albrecht *et al* 2003). Remyelination is defective in transgenic mice lacking *IL1B*, apparently through reduced astrocyte and macrophage-microglial production of IGF-1 (Mason *et al* 2001).

On the issue of whether or not those cells that are around the lesions can migrate, the evidence suggests that proliferating oligodendrocyte precursors move steadily but slowly in older animals (Blakemore *et al* 2000). This could result in delayed interaction between oligodendrocyte precursors and demyelinated axons, in turn determining failure of remyelination because the conditions required to drive that process have resolved (Blakemore *et al* 2002). Thus, failure to capture a window of opportunity for remyelination, rather than the absolute availability of oligodendrocyte precursors, could be crucial in limiting the extent of remyelination (Chari and Blakemore 2002b).

The next concern is whether those cells that do reach the site of demyelination can proliferate and differentiate. In myelin oligodendrocyte glycoprotein-induced experimental allergic enecephalomyelitis, NG2-positive precursor cells respond to repeated waves of inflammatory demyelination, becoming reactive and displaying markers of differentiated oligodendrocytes but not necessarily engaging the naked axons (Reynolds *et al* 2002). However, these repeated demyelinating insults seem not to diminish the potential for remyelination – again, arguing against exhaustion of the available pool of cells capable of capturing naked axons (Penderis *et al* 2003a). One view is that the reduction in remyelinating potential seen with age is an intrinsic property of oligodendrocyte precursors (Chari *et al* 2003a). In the gliotoxic model, showing age-related remyelination by Schwann cells and oligodendrocytes, comparison of transcription factors serving as markers for precursors indicates that remyelination is preferentially driven by the Schwann cell rather than the oliogdendrocyte component (Sim *et al* 2002a). The age-related difference in remyelination is explained by delay in the migration and differentiation of oligodendrocyte precursors rather than an absolute deficiency in remyelinating cells (Sim *et al* 2002b). There is a delayed production of PDGF-A (determining precursor recruitment), IGF-1 and TGF-β (involved in differentiation, and mainly produced by macrophages) but not of FGF-2 in older animals showing impoverished remyelination (Hinks and Franklin 2000). Delivery of FGF-2 in the engineered CG4 glial cell line enhances the proliferation and migration of oligodendrocyte lineage cells into areas of demyelination without affecting the ability of these line cells to differentiate and myelinate axons *in vitro* (Magy *et al* 2003).

However, although engineering increased expression of PDGF increases the number of oligodendrocyte precursors in immature and adult animals, this manoeuvre does not alter the timing or increase the eventual degree of remyelination (Woodruff *et al* 2004). Others have shown that stereotactic delivery of growth factors may influence remyelination. Thus, glial growth factor-2 has been reported by some to increase remyelination, modify the clinical course and promote the T helper type 2 immunological phenotype in experimental demyelinating disease (Cannella *et al* 1998), although others have not confirmed these features (Penderis *et al* 2003b). Infusion of PDGF and NT-3 into toxin-induced lesions of the corpus callosum increases the number of oligodendrocytes, reduces the extent of demyelination and accelerates remyelination (Allamargot *et al* 2001; Jean

et al 2003). But IGF-1 infusion is not associated with enhanced remyelination despite a few demonstrable effects on TGF-β2 and -3 (Cannella *et al* 2000). Further manipulations include the administration of thyroxine; experimentally, this inhibits proliferation of oligodendrocyte precursors within lesions and promotes their differentiation (Calza *et al* 2002).

Cell implantation using animal cells

Because it maximally recapitulates the range and variety of environmental conditions and local signals on which endogenous remyelination depends, transplantation has been the preferred method for assessing the myelinating potential of macroglia. The results complement evidence available from manipulating repair accomplished by endogenous cells of the oligodendrocyte lineage. Although it was the prospect of clinical intervention that initiated and has since sustained research into remyelination, the main dividend (to date) from experimental studies of glial cell implantation has been an improved understanding of myelination and glial neurobiology. A source of precursor cells able to proliferate, migrate and differentiate in the vicinity of the demyelinated axon is required for successful remyelination. Postmitotic oligodendrocytes neither divide, differentiate nor remyelinate axons (Crang and Blakemore 1998). Cell implantation does not achieve remyelination if division of the cultured cells is inhibited by X-irradiation. Both findings suggest that the origin of the remyelinating cell is a precursor and not a dedifferentiated mature oligodendrocyte. The evidence supporting this fundamental principle of cell-based strategies for enhancing remyelination has been gathered from a variety of *in vivo* experimental sources, complemented by *in vitro* data and observations in the lesions of multiple sclerosis.

Much of the present focus is on the potential for stem cells to replace missing cells of the oligodendrocyte lineage capable of remyelination. Embryonic stem-cell-derived oligodendrocytes myelinate axons *in vivo* in the dysmyelinating *shiverer* mouse, even at some distance from the site of transplantation (S. Liu *et al* 2000). EGF-stimulated neural stem cells delivered by intraventricular and cisternal injection in neonatal *shiverer* mice adopt glial phenotypes and internodal myelinated segments (Mitome *et al* 2001). Cells isolated from the porcine subventricular zone and transplantated into the gliotoxic irradiated lesions (lacking the potential for endogenous remyelination) achieve extensive remyelination if first stimulated to enter the oligodendrocyte lineage by exposure *in vitro* to B104-conditioned medium (P.M. Smith and Blakemore 2000). In other systems, neural precursors survive, differentiate into oligodendrocytes, preferentially populate white matter tracts, and contribute to myelination in a dysmyelinating model of myelin-associated glycoprotein deficiency for at least 6 months (Ader *et al* 2001). Murine stromal bone marrow cells transplanted into the demyelinated rat spinal cord themselves achieve oligodendrocyte and Schwann cell remyelination sufficient to restore conduction (Akiyama *et al* 2002). Embryonic stem cells, first manipulated *in vitro* to promote oligodendrocyte development and then transplanted into dorsal columns, myelinate extensive regions of the rodent myelin-deficient spinal cord and are later found distributed beyond the site of implantation. Intraventricular delivery is associated with even more extensive distribution of the embryonic stem cell oligodendrocyte and astrocyte progeny.

The message is that prior manipulation of donor cells by growth factors and retinoic acid is crucial in steering their behaviour after implantation and avoiding formation of heterogeneous tissue and teratomas (Brustle *et al* 1999).

Further evidence is provided through the use of cells or cell lines that have already acquired fate commitment to the oligodendrocyte lineage. CG4 (oligodendrocyte lineage line) cells injected into the intact ventral horn of the rat spinal cord lesioned in the dorsal column, and with high-dose X-irradiation in advance of cell implantation, migrate into the lesion as progenitors without undergoing differentiation and then remyelinate naked axons (R.J.M. Franklin *et al* 1996). However, without X-irradiation, cell survival is restricted to the inoculation site with no surviving transplanted cells seen elsewhere in the spinal cord. Furthermore, oligodendrocyte precursor proliferation in adult rats is inhibited throughout the white and grey matter by corticosteroids (Alonso 2000). Normal tissue apparently does not favour oligodendrocyte progenitor migration but the reactive change which occurs in and around lesions is sufficient to support both survival and movement of cells, presumably as a result of the local availability of cytokines and growth factors produced by reactive astrocytes and microglia.

The role of inflammation in repair is again emphasized by the demonstration of impaired remyelination in association with reduced numbers of proliferating NG2-positive cells and mature oligodendrocytes in transgenic mice lacking TNF-αR2 and, hence, unable to signal TNF-α (Arnett *et al* 2001). Mice deficient in Rag-1 which lack both B and T lymphocytes show reduced spontaneous remyelination after exposure to lysolecithin, and this effect is more specifically attributed to CD4 and CD8 cells. Depleting experimental lesions of OX-42-positive macrophages using clodronate liposomes, early in the repair process, inhibits oligodendrocyte remyelination but not Schwann cell remyelination, indicating a primary role for macrophage-derived factors during the induction stage of remyelination (Kotter *et al* 2001). Immunosuppression with cyclophosphamide but not cyclosporin-A impairs the extent of oligodendrocyte remyelination in toxin-induced demyelination of the rat spinal cord (P.M. Smith and Franklin 2001). The migration of cells transplanted into the ventricles or administered by intrathecal injection is much influenced by the state of inflammation, indicating that factors released as part of the inflammatory process are chemotactic for remyelinating cells (Ben-Hur *et al* 2003). N-Cadherin is identified as the main initial adhesion molecule acting between axons and myelinating glial cells.

Using the *taiep* rat myelin mutant, characterized by chronically demyelinated axons set in an astrocytic environment but without acute inflammation, Foote and Blakemore (2005) showed that transplanted oligodendrocyte precursors compete unsuccessfully with endogenous cells for access to lesions whereas they do enter areas denuded of host oligodendrocytes; but this repopulation only leads to remyelination in the presence of acute inflammation. Thus, for cells in the proximity of demyelinated axons, the major factor limiting remyelinating in the lesions of multiple sclerosis may be the absence of a local inflammatory response rather than loss of axonal signals.

These structural alterations are associated with restoration of function, assessed electrophysiologically and through behavioural analyses. Experimentally, remyelination restores conduction (K.J. Smith *et al* 1981) and glial cell implantation alters structure and function in the central nervous system (Groves *et al* 1993; Jeffery and Blakemore 1997; P.D. Murray *et al* 2001). Until recently, stereotactic delivery of the remyelinating cell seemed the only possible option. However, the situation may have changed with the demonstration of remyelination and acute neuroprotection following intravenous delivery of neural stem cells. Murine neural stem cells injected intravenously into animals with experimental autoimmune encephalomyelitis express the adhesion molecules needed to adhere to and penetrate the blood–brain barrier (Pluchino *et al* 2003). Evidently, they successfully seek out areas of demyelination and, once in place, some of them differentiate and remyelinate surviving axons. Most of these stem cells, however, remain in an undifferentiated phenotype and appear to stimulate endogenous remyelination, possibly through the production of neurotrophins. This not only achieves structural repair but also restores physiological conduction and motor function in affected animals. Furthermore, remyelination protects axons from the degeneration that otherwise follows demyelination. The important prediction that successful remyelination of focal lesions might directly protect axons is also confirmed in the mouse hepatitis model of demyelination (Totoiu *et al* 2004). Subsequent work from the Italian team provides some clarification of these observations. Again, the movement of neural stem cells across the blood–brain barrier is explained by their expression of VLA-4, binding to VCAM-1 on brain endothelial cells, and the chemokine receptors CCR1, CCR5 and CXCR4. But, whereas in the previous model of chronic injury with predominant neurodegeneration, neural stem cells were stimulated to undergo terminal differentiation and induce – directly or indirectly – axonal protection and remyelination, in the situation of chronic inflammation, these same neural stem cells exert anti-inflammatory properties, on Th1 but not Th2 lymphocytes, and themselves survive the waves of repeated immune attack to which the central nervous system is being exposed (Pluchino *et al* 2005). These results suggest a remarkable set of attributes for cells that have not been manipulated *in vitro*. In recounting the journeys of these *Milanese* stem cells, from intravenous delivery to the nooks and crannies of demyelinated lesions buried deep within the central nervous system, we are reminded of the no less remarkable travels of another Italian explorer – Marco Polo. Whilst providing hope and raising expectations, many practical, clinical, ethical and biological problems remain to be overcome before remyelination can become a reality for individual patients with multiple sclerosis.

Cell implantation using human cells

Despite the good results obtained when reconstructing glial–neuronal interactions by cell implantation using rodent material, until recently results with human cells have been less successful (Figure 10.23). Cells of the human oligodendrocyte lineage transplanted into myelin-deficient rodents were shown to survive, even after prolonged cryopreservation, and myelinate central axons (Seilhean *et al* 1996). More recently, this effect has specifically been linked to the activity of oligodendrocyte precursors and confirmed using an adult source of myelinating cells (Windrem *et al* 2004). Unlike animals injected with ethidium bromide, these *shiverer* mice have normal numbers of astrocytes. This may be important since human oligodendrocyte

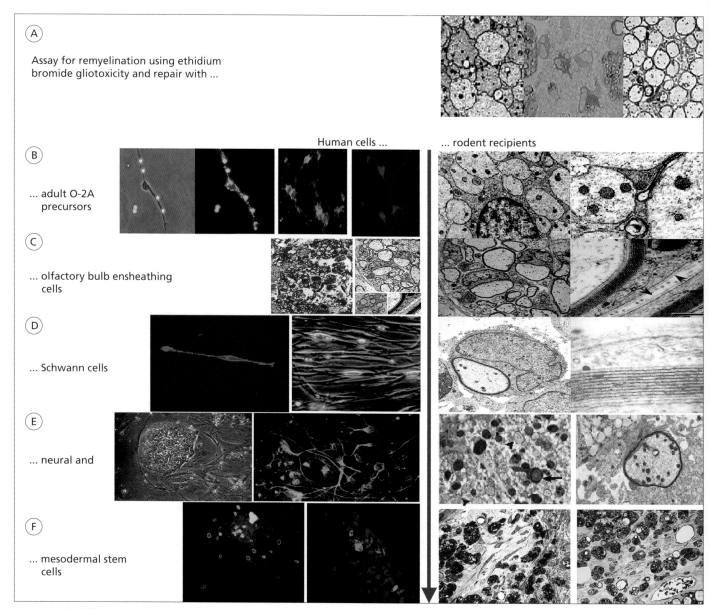

(A)

Assay for remyelination using ethidium bromide gliotoxicity and repair with ...

Human cells ...   ... rodent recipients

(B)

... adult O-2A precursors

(C)

... olfactory bulb ensheathing cells

(D)

... Schwann cells

(E)

... neural and

(F)

... mesodermal stem cells

Figure 10.23 (A) Using the ethidium bromide model of focal demyelination, remyelination is established following cell implantation with rodent oligodendrocyte precursors, a variety of morphological arrangements, all falling short of significant remyelination, are seen with xenogeneic transplantation of human. (B) Adult O-2A precursors. (C) Olfactory bulb ensheathing cells. (D) Schwann cells. (E) Neural stem cells. (F) Mesodermal stem cells. Kindly provided by Professor William Blakemore and Dr Siddharthan Chandran. (A, B, C, D) from Groves *et al* (1993), reproduced with permission of Nature Publishing Group (www.nature.com/nature); S.C. Barnett *et al* (2000); and Brierley *et al* (2001), reproduced with permission from Cognizant Communication Corp.

precursors proliferate and survive in response to astrocyte-derived factors. Transplantation of human glia, using mixed cultures including oligodendrocyte progenitors, into focal demyelinating lesions confirms that oligodendrocyte lineage cells fail to migrate but survive in clumps within the lesion (Targett *et al* 1996). In this situation, oligodendrocytes extend processes which contact rat axons but without the formation of myelin sheaths. Instead, the membranes end in terminal loops where the processes abut onto demyelinated axons. Given their ability to myelinate the central nervous system, human Schwann cells have been evaluated in experimental rodent models of demyelination (Brierley *et al* 2001). Failure to purify the cell implant by immunoaffinity (using human NGF receptor) led to

extensive fibroblast overgrowth and axon degeneration whereas remyelination was achieved using an enriched population. Kohama *et al* (2001) harvested Schwann cells from sural nerve in the amputated legs of patients with vascular disease or diabetes. These cells achieved extensive remyelination at 3–5 weeks after transplantation into the X-irradiation/ethidium bromide-lesioned dorsal columns of immunosuppressed Wistar rats. The remyelinating cells stained for an anti-human nuclear monoclonal antibody. Explants of the remyelinated segments showed improved conduction velocity and frequency response properties. Action potentials conducted over a greater distance into the lesion, suggesting that conduction block had been overcome. Olfactory bulb glia have a permissive role on axon regeneration in adults and form myelin sheaths capable of restoring conduction of the nerve impulse in experimental rodent models of remyelination. Olfactory bulb ensheathing cells have the advantage over Schwann cells of improved migration and the ability to integrate within areas of astrocytosis. Human olfactory ensheathing cells proliferate in astrocyte-conditioned medium *in vitro* and can be identified by expression of the p75 low-affinity NGF receptor. After transplantation in the X-irradiated ethidium bromide gliotoxic lesion of the rat spinal cord, they adopt a remyelinating phenotype and capture a proportion of naked axons with a histological pattern similar to Schwann cell repair (S.C. Barnett *et al* 2000). The remyelinating potential of olfactory bulb ensheathing cells, however, is improved when the cells are cotransplanted with (rodent) meningeal cells (Lakatos *et al* 2003). Clearly, olfactory ensheathing and Schwann cells share the property of low morbidity access as the basis for clinical applications of cell implantation since either could be obtained from the intended recipient and would therefore be suitable for autotransplantation – with all its attendant immunological and ethical advantages. Akiyama *et al* (2001) implanted neural stem cells harvested at surgery from the adult human subventricular zone and expanded in EGF/FGF-2. Although these cells adopted a neuronal or astrocytic fate *in vitro*, transplantation into the demyelinated (and astrocyte-free) spinal cord resulted in extensive Schwann cell remyelination and restoration of nerve conduction.

Recent observations confirm that when oligodendrocyte progenitors are transplanted into recently demyelinated lesions, denuded of astrocytes, the axons are remyelinated both by Schwann cells and oligodendrocytes; but when transplanted into chronically demyelinated lesions, remyelination is achieved by oligodendrocytes alone (Blakemore *et al* 2003). However, even though demyelinated lesions of the central nervous system can be preferentially repopulated by Schwann cells, these are not precocious myelinators mainly because each Schwann cell only captures a single axon and their territory is also limited by host astrocytes. Niehaus *et al* (2000) have related the relative failure of remyelination with disease progression to the presence in cerebrospinal fluid of the anti-oligodendrocyte precursor antibody AN2. But lack of oligodendrocyte precursors is not necessarily the most parsimonious explanation for poor remyelination in the clinical context. The human preoligodendrocyte and its progenitor have each now been identified in the lesions of multiple sclerosis (Scolding *et al* 1998b) but quantitative assessments suggest that, as in experimental contexts, the number and performance of these cells decreases with disease duration both in the brain and spinal cord (Wolswijk 2000; 2002; and see Chapter 12). What this does not reveal is whether lack of remyelination is a function of age and determines chronicity and progression, or merely one marker of the worn out lesion. The close proximity of astrocytes can impair oligodendrocyte remyelination, so that demyelinated axons persist (Blakemore *et al* 2003). The literature is confused on whether progenitors present within persistently demyelinated lesions do (Maeda *et al* 2001) or do not (Wolswijk 1998) express the nuclear proliferation antigen Ki-67, and so can meet the essential criterion for remyelination – that is, cell division.

The presence of PDGF-α receptor/NG2-positive cells (see above) in areas of remyelination in the lesions of multiple sclerosis, other than chronic and persistently demyelinated plaques,

is consistent with their putative identity as oligodendrocyte precursors (H.C. Wilson *et al* 2004). Whatever the state of proliferation, it seems clear that many of these potentially remyelinating cells have not successfully completed the process of engaging and wrapping naked axons (A. Chang *et al* 2002; R. Reynolds *et al* 2002). A minority of cells, seen to proliferate in the lesions of multiple sclerosis, express markers of mature oligodendrocyte differentiation (Schonrock *et al* 1998) but, unlike the situation in development, oligodendrocyte precursors present in the inflammatory lesions of multiple sclerosis do not express growth regulated oncogene-α and the chemokine CXCR2 – thus, in theory, limiting their capacity to proliferate and migrate (R. Filipovic *et al* 2003). Others have found cells expressing surface markers of oligodendrocyte precursors (NG2 and PDGF-α receptor), and the ligand GGF2 with its three receptors (erbB2, -3 and -4) throughout the white matter, including the lesions of multiple sclerosis and coexpressing the proapoptotic p75 neurotrophin signalling molecule (A. Chang *et al* 2000) but not concentrated in areas of active remyelination (Cannella *et al* 1999). The presence of an antibody (AN2) that lyses oligodendrocyte progenitors *in vitro* correlates with disease activity in relapsing–remitting multiple sclerosis but any effect on remyelination is not yet known (Niehaus *et al* 2000). Areas of poor remyelination in multiple sclerosis have been correlated with increased concentration of extracellular matrix TGF-β1 and high expression of Jagged1 on reactive astrocytes, in the vicinity of Notch1 and Hes5-positive oligodendrocyte precursors. Conversely, remyelination was characterized by an absence of Jagged1/Notch1 expression. The implication is that the Notch1/Jagged1 system controls the degree of remyelination in the lesions of multiple sclerosis (John *et al* 2002) but clinical neuroscience often progresses erratically – two steps forward and one sideways. Thus, Stidworthy *et al* (2004) showed in a model of toxic demyelination that, despite expression of Notch1 receptors on oligodendrocyte precursors and widespread availability of Jagged1 from a variety of local cellular sources, remyelination is unaffected. Exploiting the observation that remyelination proceeds more slowly in older animals, they did not demonstrate age-related differences in Notch1/Jagged1 expression. Knocking out *NOTCH1* and inducing demyelination with cuprizone in these transgenic mice also failed to influence remyelination. In another similar study on remyelinating lesions in experimental autoimmune encephalomyelitis, Notch expression was found to be highest in oligodendrocytes and progenitor cells during the phase of active remyelination (Maria Storch, unpublished observations). Thus, the jury remains out on whether persistent Notch1/Jagged1 expression prevents tissue repair in demyelinating disease, and (once again) clinical and experimental observations have proved difficult to reconcile.

Others have shown that an antigen (designated microtubule-associated protein 2+13) present on oligodendrocytes during myelination is re-expressed by cells actively involved in the remyelinating lesions of multiple sclerosis (Shafit-Zagardo *et al* 1999). It is a simple step to suggest that a genetic polymorphism in one receptor or its ligand might determine the success or otherwise of repair, perhaps making the difference between a mild or severe course or, even, no phenotype despite cycles of inflammatory injury. Reactive astrocytes bring cytokines or growth factors that promote repair to experimental demyelinating lesions, and areas of tissue damage in multiple sclerosis (Komoly *et al*

1992; D.-L. Yao *et al* 1995). However, although required for oligodendrocyte development, and normally produced by astrocytes and neurons, neuregulin expression is reduced in the active lesions of multiple sclerosis (Viehover *et al* 2001). Taken together, the findings suggest that the problem in multiple sclerosis is not poor availability of oligodendrocyte precursors but, rather, the environment in which they are struggling to perform. However, the experimental evidence is different. Prolonged exposure to cuprizone does indeed lead to sustained loss of remyelination but this can be overridden by transplantation of oligodendrocyte precursors. In this situation, it is availability, not the environment, that is preventing repair of demyelinated axons (J.L. Mason *et al* 2004). Seemingly, rodent axons – at least those that are normally unmyelinated – never tire of their ability to undergo myelination, remaining receptive throughout life (Setzu *et al* 2004).

Circumstantial evidence for functional consequences of endogenous remyelination in multiple sclerosis is provided by serial studies of evoked potentials showing reduction in latency of the visual response between 0.5 and 3 years after an episode of optic neuritis, either as a result of remyelination or neuronal plasticity, but with rather few effects on visual function (Brusa *et al* 2001). If remyelination is indeed the explanation for these serial changes, there may be a small dividend – in terms either of structural or functional recovery – from strategies for yet more efficient remyelination although the possibility of improving axonal survival may be critical.

Given the potential for endogenous remyelination of the central nervous system by oligodendrocyte progenitors and their progeny, it is reasonable to ask whether enhanced repair might be a dividend from containing tissue injury – the scales being tipped in favour of remyelination once the rate of injury has been restricted. Spontaneous remyelination is much enhanced in animals with Theiler's murine (demyelinating) encephalomyelitis virus treated with immune serum raised by immunization with spinal cord homogenate (M. Rodriguez *et al* 1987). Subsequently, the effect on remyelination was obtained with antibodies directed specifically against myelin basic protein (M. Rodriguez *et al* 1996). The best analysis is that a family of naturally present, autoreactive, immunoglobulin M antibodies able to cross-link cell surface determinants on the oligodendrocyte cell surface acts to promote the normal reparative potential of the central nervous system (Bieber *et al* 2002; Ciric *et al* 2003; Warrington *et al* 2000). This observation raises the question of whether increased remyelination is merely the consequence of successful disease suppression, promoting endogenous repair, or depends directly on immunoglobulin M which binds and stimulates cells of the oliogodendrocyte lineage – as suggested by the coassociation of inflammation and remyelination both in experimental lesions and multiple sclerosis. In this respect it may be significant that the Fcα/μ receptor for immunoglobulin M is also present on cells of the (murine) oligodendrocyte lineage and myelin (Nakahara *et al* 2003). There is no evidence for a direct effect of polyclonal immunoglobulins on proliferation, migration or differentiation of oligodendrocyte precursors *in vitro* (Stangel *et al* 1999). Nor are these functions influenced by drugs that manipulate the immune system in multiple sclerosis (Halfpenny and Scolding 2003). The available evidence suggests that pooled immunoglobulin G and immunoglobulin M fractions protect (rat) oligodendrocytes by

inhibition of antibody-mediated phagocytosis and termination of the immune reaction. The mechanism is induction of apoptosis in infiltrating T cells through nitric oxide and TNF-α-dependent mechanisms rather than by direct stimulation of oligodendrocytes. Hence, enhanced remyelination probably depends on manipulating the relationship between inflammation and repair rather than a direct growth promoting effect (Stangel *et al* 1999; 2000b).

Lessons from experimental neurobiology for multiple sclerosis

We have argued that oligodendrocytes and axons are each injured acutely as part of the inflammatory process but the extent to which a cell can survive the inflammatory process is modulated by its growth factor-dependent state of health. The stressed oligodendrocyte signals its distress and either summons assistance or suicidally attracts activated microglia but encouraging a potentially dangerous liaison. Cell death may occur in response to a state of injury from which protection would be anticipated under more favourable neurobiological conditions. For those cells in the penumbra, caught in the cross-fire of the inflammatory process but whose fate still hangs in the balance, an optimal growth factor environment may be protective, thus reducing the amount of bystander damage. Thus, growth factor availability within and around a focus of inflammation may be crucial in determining the limits and boundaries of each individual lesion.

In debating the merits and demerits of suppressing the inflammatory process, it is important to consider that inflammation supports remyelination (see above) and may also enhance axon regeneration. The story goes that macrophages release IL-2 which transiently removes the inhibitory constituents from oligodendrocytes and astrocytes. The poor regenerative response of the central (compared with the peripheral) nervous system is associated with slower recruitment of macrophages in response to injury (Hirshberg and Schwartz 1995). Neuronal survival in the crushed optic nerve is enhanced if myelin-specific autoimmune T cells are injected locally, perhaps by a mechanism involving transient reduction in energy requirements as a result of reduced nerve activity (Moalem *et al* 1999). The functional advantage of allowing inflammation to enhance axon regeneration was shown by Rapalino *et al* (1998) who observed improved motor recovery in rats made paraplegic by complete spinal cord transection, after transplantation with macrophages first primed *in vitro* against peripheral nerve. Neuroprotection after spinal cord injury is also provided experimentally by systemic immunization with myelin basic protein specific autoreactive T cells (Hauben *et al* 2000b). Functional recovery is associated with reconstitution of nerve fibres across the lesion and restoration of motor conduction. No additional repair is achieved by manipulating growth factors within these lesions. That said, a note of caution is needed. Neuroprotective effects of autoimmune T lymphocytes are not seen in all animal strains. The reason for this discrepancy is unknown. In addition, it appears to be the same T-cell population, which at low numbers mediates protection and at high numbers triggers acute disseminated encephalomyelitis. In addition to these discrete manipulations of axon growth, it is claimed that (experimentally), transplanted stem cells survive and differentiate into neurons, astrocytes and oligodendrocytes with associated improvements in motor function (J.W. McDonald *et al* 1999). Saturating spinal cord lesions with olfactory bulb ensheathing cells or Schwann cells increases the extent of axonal outgrowth and impulse conduction for a limited distance into the transected zone (Imaizumi *et al* 2000). This effect is enhanced if the olfactory bulb ensheathing cells are engineered to produce glial cell derived nerve growth factor (Cao *et al* 2004) but not everyone agrees with the olfactory bulb ensheathing cell story (Boyd *et al* 2004).

In the context of multiple sclerosis, one major goal is to make oligodendrocytes from a readily available source that does not challenge ethical and moral principles, and to show that these will integrate and protect surviving axons at sites of demyelination. To raise the stakes, can areas devoid of functioning axons and myelin be replenished so as fully to reconstruct the normal cellular architecture of the central nervous system? By any standards, research is active in this field. The awareness of stem cell

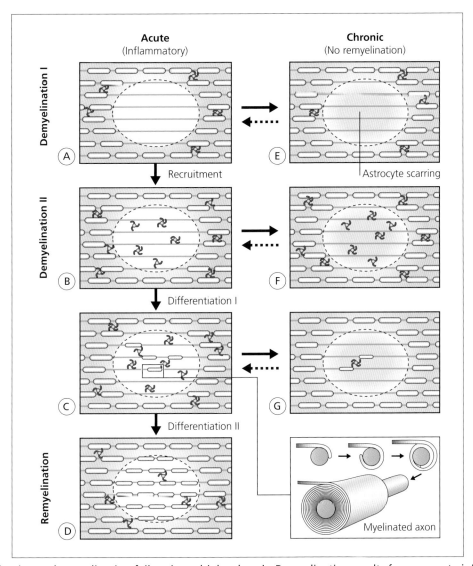

Figure 10.24 Remyelination and remyelination failure in multiple sclerosis. Demyelination results from an acute inflammatory episode in which oligodendrocytes and the myelin sheaths that they make and maintain are damaged. In some instances, there might also be a loss of oligodendrocyte progenitor cells (A), but in other instances they can be preserved (B). The first stage of remyelination requires the recruitment of oligodendrocyte progenitor cells; in (A), this will mean their migration from normal tissue surrounding the lesions, as well as their proliferation, whereas in (B), recruitment will involve predominantly their proliferation. Once recruited, the oligodendrocyte progenitor cells must then engage demyelinated axons as they begin the differentiation phase (C), a process that involves a sheet-like oligodendrocyte process wrapping around the axon in a spiral and eventually compacting to form new myelin sheaths (inset). Once this process is complete, the lesion has been myelinated (D). The momentum for the signalling events that drive this process is associated with the inflammatory response. (E–G) Should there be a failure to create the correct signalling environment, then the process will arrest and the lesion will persist as a chronically demyelinated lesion that is characterized by scarring astrocytes. Depending on the nature of the demyelination process or the stage at which remyelination stops, these lesions will be either deficient in oligodendrocyte progenitor cells (E) or contain oligodendrocyte progenitor cells (F). If the remyelination process stops at the onset of the differentiation phase, then the lesion will contain premyelinating oligodendrocytes (G). According to this schema, for remyelination to occur in the chronic lesions, it is necessary to create an environment that is associated with the acute inflammatory environment in which remyelination proceeds efficiently (broken arrows). Adapted from R.J. Franklin (2002).

biology and its early application to the problem of multiple sclerosis has fuelled high expectations amongst affected individuals and their advocates that the problems of tissue repair and remyelination are now tractable.

Whilst there has been a move away from dependence on embryonic sources of fate-committed progenitors as the preferred strategy for restoring structure and function in diseased tissues, the performance and availability of adult stem cells is less predictable (for review, see C.M. Rice and Scolding 2004). The discovery that adult stem cells can be gathered from one tissue and switch fate to another (Eglitis and Mezey 1997; Y. Jiang *et al* 2002; 2003) provides opportunities in theory for generating precious but otherwise inaccessible cells. The possibilities seem especially attractive for easily obtained and renewable sources such as bone marrow or skin, both of which have been shown to contain stem cells capable of neural fate given appropriate manipulation and stimulation *in vitro*. The conversion of mesenchymal stem cells into progeny with various neural fates offers a potential link between promise and reality; at present, most biological promise would seem to lie with embryonic stem cells maintained and manipulated *in vitro*. These were originally identified in the mouse (M. Evans and Kaufman 1981) but have now also been derived from human embryos (Thomson *et al* 1998). Thus, whilst the longevity and versatility of multipotent adult progenitors may be no less than for embryonic stem cells, only the latter have been shown to survive, differentiate, connect and function after implantation in damaged tissues. Furthermore, they can be manipulated *ex vivo* and used to deliver a payload of passenger molecules to strategic sites of tissue injury, activating cell suicide genes thereafter in order to prevent uncontrolled proliferation – the ultimate altruistic Trojan horse. That said, their commitment to defined pathways of differentiation seems fragile. At the technical level, an alternative is to use nuclear transfer from somatic cells to design viable embryonic stem cell lines (Wakayama *et al* 2001). The harvesting of embryonic stem cells necessarily ends the existence of the donor embryo and – although they have been derived from extra embryos superfluous to the needs of assisted fertilization – the biological possibilities bring the moral and ethical dimensions of such work sharply into focus.

Recent pathological studies have uncovered two features that question whether the application of stem cell biology will make a difference to tissue repair in this disease. In debating why remyelination fails in multiple sclerosis, we borrow a question from R.J. Franklin (2002). First, spontaneous remyelination is already pronounced, in particular at early stages of the disease (see Chapter 12). When this fails, it does so not necessarily through the critical loss of oligodendrocytes or their progenitor cells, but rather because axons are destroyed or may become nonpermissive for remyelination. Thus, transplantation of stem cells, once this becomes feasible and safe, may offer rather a small dividend for improved remyelination and axonal protection and in only a small minority of patients and lesions. However, as recently shown, stem cells may also function as a source of neurotrophic factors, and these might alter the environment of poorly remyelinating lesions to advantage. Self-evidently, any consideration of stem cells as medicines for multiple sclerosis must include the need to prevent further tissue injury as part of the overall strategy for limiting and repairing the damage.

To make compact myelin, the remyelinating cell must proliferate. Despite some suggestion of dedifferentiation in mature oligodendrocytes, it follows that repair depends on a supply of progenitors, or cells that arise even earlier in this cell lineage. Many, if not all, are available in the adult nervous system. Several – especially those defined by PDGF-α receptor, NG2 and the myelin transcription factor 1 (MyT1) – accumulate in and around the demyelinated lesions in experimental animals (Sim *et al* 2002a) and in multiple sclerosis (Scolding *et al* 1998b; Wolswijk 1998; 2000; 2002). Their availability may wane with time and repeated insults, through age-related depletion and targeting of precursors by the disease process itself. However, the best guess is that the lack of remyelination depends more on the failure of oligodendrocyte precursors to perform, than on their absence from the arena of demyelination (Penderis *et al* 2003a). This raises the subsidiary question of whether the failure to engage is through active inhibition, or the lack of cell-based and soluble signals needed for the process of differentiation to proceed. Although individual candidates can be considered (amongst them IGF-1, TGF-β, Notch1/Jagged1, PSA-NCAM, the integrin family, and a variety of transcription factors – as discussed above), the available evidence points more to the need for multiple interacting growth factor influences on oligodendrocyte precursors, so as maximally to realize their potential for remyelination (Stidworthy *et al* 2004). Whatever their individual identities, the coassociation of remyelination with acute inflammation suggests that the infiltrating cells, or those that react within the central nervous system (astrocytes and microglia), not only cause the damage (and the process of clearing degenerate tissue) but also deliver the payload of reparative molecules during a window of opportunity for triggering and completing the repair process (see Chapter 11; Kerschensteiner *et al* 1999). Perhaps no single missing factor determines the failure of demyelinated lesions to repair. Rather, one or more of the multiple steps and signals required for ordered and successful oligodendrocyte precursor proliferation, migration, differentiation and synthesis of compact myelin – and the need for these events to proceed in sequence and with correct timings – goes awry (Figure 10.24). One event may slip up here or there, and another elsewhere and on a different occasion.

The immunology of inflammatory demyelinating disease

11

Hartmut Wekerle and Hans Lassmann

MULTIPLE SCLEROSIS AS AN AUTOIMMUNE DISEASE

Multiple sclerosis is the most important inflammatory disease of the central nervous system (CNS). In contrast to other encephalitides, the inflammatory changes underlying multiple sclerosis do not seem to be direct responses to microbial infection. Instead, they are caused and sustained by autoimmune responses. The central hypothesis is that T lymphocytes with receptors for central nervous system myelin components enter the brain, respond locally to their target antigen, and (indirectly) attack local cells. These autoaggressive T cells trigger an inflammatory cascade that is responsible for all the neurological deficits seen in affected individuals.

This concept takes issue with several time-honoured dogmas of neuroimmunology. How can immune cells mount an attack against one of the body's own tissues? What are the origin and nature of these misguided immune cells? It has been maintained traditionally that the central nervous system is exempt from physiological immune mechanisms. How then can we explain pathological autoimmune responses occurring within the central nervous system? Both sets of questions must be answered convincingly in order to understand the pathogenesis of multiple sclerosis.

First, we explain the general organization of the immune system, then discuss mechanisms that result in autoimmune attack against self, and see which of these mechanisms contribute to the pathogenesis of multiple sclerosis. We consider the central nervous system tissues as an environment for immune reactivity. We examine the global conditions that allow or prevent immune responses in central nervous system tissues, and then specifically describe the changed central nervous system arrangements in the lesions of multiple sclerosis.

The immune system is the body's main defence force. It must protect against the myriad of environmental microbial organisms and also against potentially cancerous cells arising within tissues of high cellular turnover. The immune system works as a formidable killing machine. It is designed to spot, encircle and neutralize any suspicious structure appearing in the body and threatening its well-being. In this context, suspicious means any material deviating from healthy self tissues. If immune cells lose their ability to distinguish suspicious foreign and intact self components, they may attack and damage normal tissues – and

thus cause autoimmune disease. These are not rare and exotic afflictions, but count among the most important problems in clinical medicine. 'Autoimmune diseases together constitute the third-greatest clinical burden, after cardiovascular diseases and cancer' (Nossal 2001). Autoimmunity may affect diverse organs, causing diseases ranging from rheumatoid arthritis, insulin-dependent diabetes mellitus, ulcerative colitis and systemic lupus erythematosus to multiple sclerosis. It should be stressed, however, that the autoimmune concept in multiple sclerosis lacks formal proof. However, it rests on several diverse lines of evidence, which, taken together strongly suggest that immunopathological events, which we presume to be of an autoimmune nature, are responsible for the occurrence and development of the disease.

One of the strongest arguments in favour of an immune pathogenesis for multiple sclerosis comes from the morphology of its lesions. As detailed in Chapter 12, the lesion in multiple sclerosis is characterized by perivascular round cell infiltration, and these accumulating lymphocytes spill into the surrounding parenchyma. Active lesions in multiple sclerosis are almost indistinguishable from areas of inflammation seen in diseases of proven autoimmune pathogenesis, especially models of experimentally induced autoimmune encephalomyelitis (EAE; see below). The second line of evidence supporting the autoimmune hypothesis is genetic and rests on the association of disease susceptibility with polymorphic genes that are potentially involved in autoimmune responses (see Chapter 3). The best-documented example is the major histocompatibility complex (MHC), whose class II products are required for the presentation of autoantigen to T lymphocytes and are, in addition, crucially involved in the development of the immune repertoire. Finally, the autoimmune pathogenesis of multiple sclerosis is endorsed by the relative success of therapies that suppress or modulate the immune response (see Chapter 18). For example, β-interferon (IFN-β) has a favourable effect in reducing relapse rates and decreasing lesion load as assessed by magnetic resonance imaging (MRI). The same is true for Copaxone (copolymer-1), which diverts myelin-reactive T cells from the pathogenic Th1 (T helper 1) profile to the regulatory Th2 (T helper 2) pattern. Finally, some antibodies that blindfold or eliminate activated T cells were found to be beneficial in clinical trials (von Andrian and Engelhardt 2003).

IMMUNE RESPONSES: INNATE AND ADAPTIVE

Evolution has provided two protective immune systems, the innate and the adaptive. Both share the ability to identify a potentially harmful external (or internal) structure, and then mount a response designed to neutralize this threat. At the same time, either type of response must be selective, meaning that the destructive potential must be directed exclusively to the suspected target, while the body's own tissues are completely spared. The two immune systems fulfil their tasks admirably well, although they use radically different principles.

The innate immune response is phylogenetically old. It acts in worms and insects as well as mammals. It is fully preformed in the healthy organism. Its elements are present in the tissues irrespective of microbial threat. In stark contrast, the more modern adaptive immune system formed much later in evolution. It is only found in vertebrates. Adaptive immune responses only offer protection following a first encounter with a microbial target. This contact leads to a maximal response concentrated on the particular microbe, with the generation of killer cells or molecules that neutralize and eliminate the target with maximal efficiency.

Both responses have their advantages and drawbacks. The preformed, innate immune response can act more or less instantaneously against an enemy, but its weapons are quite blunt. Due to good but not perfect self–nonself discrimination, the reaction may create some collateral damage to healthy tissues. In contrast, adaptive immune responses need time to develop fully but, once established, are extremely specific for the pathogen and maximally efficient. To mount an almost ideal defence, both immune systems join forces, forming one coherent two-tiered system of protection that combines and correlates their independent mechanisms. It follows that their regulatory signalling mechanisms are tightly interconnected through bridging cells and soluble molecules.

Innate immunity

Each living organism, from amoeba to human, lives in a sea of microbes that threaten to invade and decompose the organism. This happens after death. The healthy living body, however, is protected by efficient mechanisms that hold back most microorganisms, and quickly inactivate those that have intruded into the organism. Protection comes from robust outer membranes that act as almost impermeable antimicrobial barriers, plus mechanisms of innate immunity that form the first line of defence against those microbes that manage to breach the barriers (see Table 11.1).

In insects, a particular gene, *Toll*, encodes receptor structures that specifically discriminate microbial structures. Toll receptor-mediated recognition stimulates particular migratory cells in the fly haemolymph, 'haemocytes', to swallow small microbes, or encapsulate larger microbes and fungi. Soon after this discovery, Toll-like genes and receptors were found throughout phylogeny, including within the human genome. Indeed, Toll-like receptors are now recognized as the key antimicrobial structures. We now know of an ever-expanding family of Toll-like receptors that recognize different components of microbial organisms (Hoffmann *et al* 1999).

Toll-like receptors bind bacterial membrane components (endotoxin), polysaccharides of bacterial capsule structures, viral RNA and bacterial DNA. They are present in many cell types – but mainly professional antigen-presenting cells (dendritic cells), macrophages, polymorphonuclear leucocytes and all components of the phagocytic system (Akira *et al* 2001). As in insects, activation of Toll-like receptors on vertebrate cells leads to activation, which, in the case of phagocytes, may stimulate phagocytosis and secretion of soluble antimicrobial effector proteins – most prominently defensins and proteases. Both act by perforating the microbial membrane and thus destabilizing the organism.

Members of the Toll-like receptor family are involved in pattern recognition. Globally, they distinguish molecules found on bacteria and viruses but rarely, if ever, on vertebrate cells. Thus, they discriminate microbial structures from self but do not sharply identify the exact nature of a microbial product. They share this recognition strategy with other innate receptors, for example mannoside receptor or C-reactive protein, and thus differ from immune receptors (T- and B-cell receptors), which recognize small circumscripted molecular determinants or epitopes.

If the innate immune receptors act quite bluntly, this is also true for innate effector molecules. Defensins, for example, kill bacteria by inserting holes into their membranes, but at the same time quite often also affect the surrounding host tissue. In addition, the molecules provide chemotactic signals that attract dendritic cells to sites of fresh infection (Yang *et al* 2002).

In general, the relative disadvantage of limited self–nonself discrimination is outweighed by the speed of innate immune reactivity. Responses occur rapidly, almost immediately after bacterial infection, and reach any location of the affected organism. As will be shown later, innate immune responsiveness is almost ideally complemented by adaptive immunity. This is superior in terms of specificity. It is important to note that the rules that operate in immune responses against foreign antigens also pertain to pathological autoimmune responses. Responses of the innate immune system can profoundly influence the course and intensity of autoimmune responses delivered by the adaptive immune system (Bachmann and Kopf 2001).

Adaptive immunity: immune repertoire and immune surveillance

The adaptive immune system is much more powerful and elaborate than its innate counterpart. Its enormous efficiency depends on two qualities – precision of the actual response and immunological memory. Immune responses are highly specific. If, for example, an infectious agent enters the body, the ensuing response focuses exclusively on this microbe, ignoring other potential antigens for the moment. In this way, the immune response can be maximally efficient whilst exerting minimum effort. Morever, typical immune responses leave a specific imprint on the immune system. Thus, they imprint immunological memory. A microbe entering the body for a second time will trigger a much more vigorous immune reaction than on first encounter. The immune system remembers the old microbial acquaintance and responds with a more intense and quicker set of reactions.

The structural basis for immune specificity and memory resides in the clonal diversity of preformed lymphocytes. The

Table 11.1 Comparison of innate immune signalling proteins in *Drosophila* and mammals

	Drosophila	Mammals
Pattern recognition receptors		
Non-signalling	GNBP (3)	CD14, MD-2
LPS	?	TLR4
PG, LP, zymosan	?	TLR2
Flagellin	?	TLR5
Bacterial DNA	?	TLR9
Orphan receptors	18 wheeler, dTLR3–9	Other TLRs
Cytokines and receptors		
TNF-α/TNFR	TNF-like/TNFR-like[a]	TNF-α/TNFR1&2
Spätzle/Toll	Spätzle/Toll	?
IL-1β/IL-1R-related	None	IL-1β/IL-1R (8)
Intracellular signalling components		
Adapters	Tube, dMyD88	MyD88, Tollip
Pelle-like kinases	Pelle	IRAK (4)
TRAF	DTRAF1–3	TRAF1–6
MAP3K	dTAK1, dMEKK	TAK1, TAB1 & 2, NIK, MEKK1–3
Atypical PKC	DaPKC	PKC-ζ and λ, p62
RIP-like proteins	IMD	RIP
NF-κB components		
IBs	Cactus	IκBα, β, γ, ε,
IκB kinases:		
IKKα/β	DMIKKβ (*IRD5*)	IKKα, β
IKKγ	DmIKKγ (*KENNY*)	IKKγ/NEMO/IKKAP
IKKε-like	DmIKKε/dIK2	IKKε/i, TBK/NAK/T2K
NF-κB precursors	Relish	p105, p100
and products	Relish N & C	p50, p52
NK-κB subunits	Dorsal, Dif	RelA/p65, RelB, c-Rel

Both known and putative innate immune signalling proteins are categorized into pattern recognition receptors, cytokines and their receptors, intracellular signalling components, and NF-κB-related kinases and transcription factors. The number of orthologs per genome is indicated in parentheses.

a The Drosophila TNFR-like predicted gene contains a TNFR-like cysteine-rich extracellular domain but does not include a TNFR-related intracellular domain.

Reproduced with permission from Silverman and Maniatis (2001).

immune system is composed of lymphocyte families – clones – each of which is characterized by diverse surface receptors for antigen. Ideally, each clonal receptor can bind and recognize just one antigenic structure. Thus, a foreign antigen intruding into the tissue binds and selects those lymphocyte receptors with the best fit. These cells are activated to multiply and differentiate to effector cells responsible for neutralizing the antigen.

How can a specific immune cell spot its antigen in the body? How can antigen-specific immune cells fulfil their protective mission? The answer is by immune surveillance. At any time there are millions of immune cells, especially of the antigen experienced memory type, roaming through the body's organs, scanning tissues for intruded microbes or for newly arisen tumour cells. However, immune surveillance relies not just on random migration. Patrolling immune cells have antennae for chemical signals that attract them to suspicious areas in a tissue. The attracting signals are chemokines, small molecular proteins secreted by dendritic cells when activated by a microbial structure. Dendritic cells play a pivotal role in linking innate and adaptive immune responses. Activation by microbes happens by mechanisms of innate immunity, while attraction of memory T cells leads to adaptive immunity.

However, dendritic cells are much more than just sensors. They take up bacteria and digest their antigenic structures to make them recognizable by T lymphocytes. Dendritic cells are professional antigen-presenting cells. They offer freshly digested antigen to attracted memory T cells. In addition, having picked up antigen, dendritic cells leave the peripheral tissue and migrate through lymphatic vessels to the nearest immune organ – often a lymph node – there they import and present the antigen to freshly generated naive T cells.

T LYMPHOCYTES

The adaptive immune system relies on two main protagonists, T cells and B cells. Both are practically indistinguishable by morphological criteria, and both lineages also develop from common progenitors residing in the bone marrow. The two differ radically, however, in their function. The main role of B lymphocytes is the production of humoral antibodies, but they play an additional role in presenting antigen to T lymphocytes. T lymphocytes are the main regulatory cells in the immune system, helping B lymphocytes to mount an optimal antibody response and downregulate ongoing immune responses; also, T cells are effector cells in the responses of delayed-type hypersensitivity.

T-cell receptors

There are two classes of T-cell antigen receptors. The majority of T cells use the $\alpha\beta$ receptor (see also Chapter 12). These include most $CD4^+$ and $CD8^+$ T cells, which recognize peptide antigens in the molecular context of MHC class I and class II, respectively. A minority of T cells, whose recognition properties are much less well known, use instead a pair of $\gamma\delta$ T-cell receptors. Both classes of T cell are consistently found in the infiltrates of demyelinating diseases, but whilst lymphocytes using $\alpha\beta$ receptors have been characterized as definitely pathogenic effectors, the role of $\gamma\delta$ T cells remains enigmatic (see below).

Although T- and B-cell (immunoglobulin) receptors share some elementary principles, they differ radically in other respects. Both receptor types are composed of two identical heavy (H) and two identical light (L) chains. Like immunoglobulin genes, T-cell receptors are encoded by C, V and J genes, arranged in a large cluster located on human chromosome 7 (Figure 11.1). The antigen-recognizing surfaces of the $\alpha\beta$ and $\gamma\delta$ T cells are formed by individual combinations of these V, J

and D genes, rearranged and spliced by the recombinase machinery. Further diversification of the T-cell receptor is achieved by inclusion of N region nucleotides. In contrast to B-cellular immunoglobulins, T-cell receptors remain unchanged throughout an immune response. They do not sharpen their affinity by somatic hypermutation upon contact with antigen, and there is no intraclonal class switching of T-cell receptor.

T-cell receptors bind their antigen complex by a surface formed from the complementarity-forming region 3 and a bound antigenic peptide (Figure 11.2). Antigen binding causes a structural change in the T-cell receptor molecule, which triggers a cascade of signals that ultimately arrives in the nucleus and results in T-cell activation – expressed as transcription of activation-related genes. The T-cell receptor chains are anchored in the cell membrane, but they do not have cytoplasmic tails sufficient to import the activation signal into the cell. This is done by a cluster of molecules of the CD3 class, sticking around the T-cell receptor chains and extending long protein domains into the cytoplasm. The CD3 cytoplasmic domains contain a sequence motif termed ITAM (immunoreceptor tyrosine-based activation motif), originally discovered in B cells but also present in T lymphocytes and mast cells (Reth 1989). In response to antigen binding, protein phosphorylation of ITAM and conformational changes of the CD3 cytoplasmic domains lead to the binding and activation of a relay of signal proteins that transport the information into the nucleus (M.M. Davis 2002). Why is T-cell receptor signal transmission so complicated, and why does it involve so many individual components? The answer is that intermolecular cooperation facilitates fine tuning of the signal strength. As will be seen later, it is the strength of the antigenic signal plus additional stimuli that determines the functional character of a newly triggered immune response.

Antigen recognition by T lymphocytes is very different from their B-cell relatives. A mature B lymphocyte can recognize a correctly folded antigen by direct ligation of its membrane immunoglobulin receptor, be it surface bound or in solution. Antigen recognition by the T cell is altogether different. It requires antigen first to be taken up, processed and presented by an antigen-presenting cell. These cells internalize the antigenic protein and split it into small peptide fragments, whose

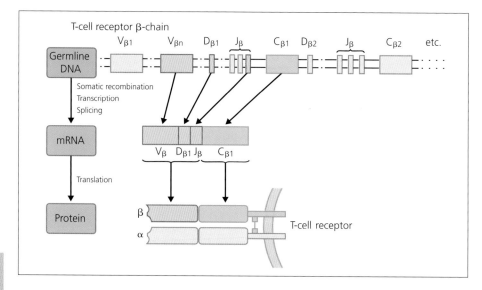

Figure 11.1 Rearrangement of germline genes in formation of the T-cell receptor. The germline DNA encoding the T-cell receptor β chain genes contains 65 (46 functional) variable (Vβ), 13 joining (Jβ; not all are shown), two diversity (Dβ) and two constant (Cβ) segments (Rowen et al 1996). The V domain of the T-cell receptor β chain is encoded by three gene segments, Vβ, Dβ and Jβ. Rearrangement of these gene segments generates a functional exon that is transcribed and spliced to join VDJ to C. The resulting mRNA is translated to yield the T-cell receptor β chain protein. The mRNA coding the T-cell receptor α chain is constructed by similar mechanisms (not shown). Adapted from Hohlfeld (1997).

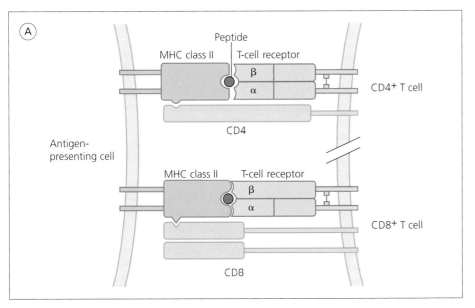

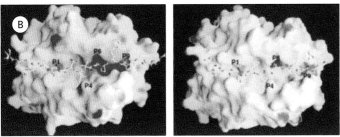

Figure 11.2 (A) Antigen recognition by CD4+ T cells (top) and CD8+ cells (bottom). The T-cell receptor of CD4+ cells recognizes an antigen peptide bound to an MHC class II molecule (such as HLA-DR, -DP or -DQ) on the surface of an antigen-presenting cell. The receptor of CD8+ T cells recognizes an antigen peptide bound to MHC class I molecule (such as HLA-A, -B or -C). CD4 and CD8 act as coreceptors. Adapted from Hohlfeld (1997). (B) Presentation of major encephalitogenic peptides by HLA-DR antigens. Crystallography of HLA-DR2a–myelin basic protein and HLA-DR2b–myelin basic protein complexes. Left is a top view of the HLA-DR2a–myelin basic protein 86–105 complex. Right is a top view of the HLA-DR2b–myelin basic protein 85–99 complex. (A) from Y. Li *et al* (2000). © 2000, with permission from Elsevier.

length may vary between eight and several dozen amino acids. Within the cytoplasm of the antigen-presenting cell, some peptides are bound to molecules encoded by the MHC. Principally, all classic MHC molecules comprise two protein chains, which form a deep and polymorphous cleft. Its molecular shape is determined by the amino acid sequence of each MHC molecule, which is highly polymorphic (see also Chapter 3). During processing, the emerging antigenic peptides compete for binding to the MHC molecule cleft, and the peptide with the best fit wins. The newly formed complex of peptide and histocompatibility antigen complex is then transported to the surface of the antigen-presenting cell for the attention of specific T cells. To be activated, T cells must recognize determinants on the lips of the MHC molecule along with peptide side chains that point out of the groove.

There are, however, two sets of MHC molecules with differing structural details – both in terms of peptide binding characteristics and the sets of T cells to which they present antigen. MHC class I proteins are formed by one polymorphic H chain and one monomorphic L chain (β2-microglobulin). Class I MHC mole-

cules preferentially bind relatively short peptides within the endoplasmic reticulum. Many are derived from endogenous protein components. Class I embedded peptides are presented to CD8+ T cells (Figure 11.2A, bottom), the major T-cell subset containing most of the cytotoxic killer lymphocytes. In contrast, MHC class II proteins can bind longer peptide fragments and do so in a special vesicular compartment distinct from classic lysosomes. Most of the class II bound peptides come from exogenous proteins, which have been taken up by the antigen-presenting cell and degraded intracellularly. Class II restricted peptides are presented to CD4+ T lymphocytes (Figure 11.2A, top, and 11.2B), the cell class comprising helper T cells, along with effector cells involved in cellular hypersensitivity responses (Germain 1994).

In addition to activation by peptide binding, T-cell receptors can be stimulated by 'superantigens'. These microbial products bind to the outside of MHC molecules and the T-cell receptor, rather than binding to its groove and antigen-binding complementarity-determining region 3 (CDR3) surface. Thus, individual superantigens do not distinguish single T-cell clones, which are defined by their peptide–MHC specificity, but bind to V gene-specific structures outside the CDR3. Different superantigens bind distinct panels of Vβ proteins, thus implying that a given superantigen activates all T-cell clones using this segment (Herman *et al* 1991). Activation of T cells by microbial superantigen is of considerable clinical interest because this mechanism may contribute to the pathogenic activation of potentially self-reactive T-cell clones, which persist in the healthy immune repertoire in a dormant state.

Antigen presentation

The immune response is remarkable for its adaptability and specificity. It is flexible. Depending on the nature of a particular immunogen, the response may be mild or violent, use either chiefly cellular or humoral mechanisms, localize to a particular part of the body, and be very short-lived or long-lasting. These properties result from complex but robust intercellular regulation that starts and ends an immune response. The process is initiated by contact of immune cells with the immunogen. In the case of T cells, antigen recognition is not a simple binding phenomenon. Rather, it involves a complex interaction between the recognizing T cells and another player that presents the putative antigen in a recognizable fashion. T cells have receptors that intrinsically are unable to recognize intact foreign or self protein antigen. In order to be recognizable by T cells, proteins must be taken up by antigen-presenting cells, and cleaved into small peptide fragments (usually composed of 10–30 amino acids). The peptides are then bound into specifically shaped folds of MHC class I or class II proteins. The T-cell receptor recognizes the surface formed by the MHC protein and bound antigenic peptide.

The community of mature T cells using the αβ T-cell receptor falls into two major classes, each distinguished by a particular accessory recognition molecule – the CD4 and CD8 coreceptors. CD4 molecules bind to MHC class II proteins. Consequently, CD4$^+$ T cells recognize antigen in the context of MHC class II. These proteins are specialized to pick up exogenous proteins (often bacterial structures), which are processed in particular intracellular compartments. CD4$^+$ T cells participate in responses against particulate microbes (bacteria or fungi) and parasites, either controlling B-cell mediated antibody production or cellular responses of delayed-type hypersensitivity. In contrast, CD8 has an affinity for MHC class I proteins, which preferentially bind intracellular antigens (typically viral products). CD8$^+$ T cells differentiate to cytotoxic ('killer') cells that are pivotal in protection from virus infections and tumour cells.

The immune synapse

Binding of MHC–peptide complexes to specific T-cell receptors is necessary, but by no means sufficient to trigger an immune response. In addition to the T-cell receptor, an impressive number of accessory molecules must participate in productive antigen recognition. Located near the T-cell receptor, they have to bind specific counterparts on the antigen-presenting membrane (Figure 11.3).

The elaborate structure of their intercellular contact area reflects the complexity of interactions between the recognizing T lymphocyte and antigen-presenting cell. This has rightly been dubbed the 'immune synapse'. Like its neurobiological counter-

part, the immune synapse is a highly elaborate structure organized in an amazingly ordered fashion (Figure 11.4). Moreover, both types of synapse are ephemeral. They form when and where needed and resolve after completion of their function. An immune synapse is initiated by the contact between T-cell receptor and MHC–peptide. This process leads to the local concentration of most available T-cell receptors to form a patch on the T-cell membrane, with a symmetrical accumulation of MHC–peptide molecules on the antigen-presenting cell side. During development of the synapse, additional molecules form concentric rings around the contact zone formed by T-cell receptor, MHC molecule and digested peptide. These include costimulatory molecules (which send additional signals for activation) as well as cell adhesion molecules (which stabilize the synaptic adhesion). Other molecules are sorted out of the synapse, such as CD45, a phosphatase, and CD43, a highly sialylated glycoprotein (A.S. Shaw 2001). Synapses are highly ordered not only on the membrane but also beneath the surface. In the case of synapses formed by cytotoxic T cells and their target cells, cytotoxic granules polarize, accumulate close to the contacts made by T-cell receptor, MHC and peptide, and are discharged towards the target, with subsequent cytoskeletal rearrangement of both cells (Dustin and Colman 2002).

A neurobiologist might object to the term 'immune synapse', suspecting a trick metaphor merely reflecting shallow similarity between neuronal and immunological contact interfaces, and representing the attempts of one discipline to stand (we might say 'trample') on the gigantic shoulders of another. As it now emerges, however, the analogies between both types of contact go deeper. Immune and neuronal synapses share remarkable features in common. They both concentrate specific cell adhesion molecules, primary adaptors, and use identical structures such as agrin, a proteoglycan involved in the aggregation and organization of synaptic receptors (A.A. Khan *et al* 2001). Both synapses exchange specific transmitter molecules through a synaptic cleft of around 30 nm (Donnadieu *et al* 2001), and there are also functional similarities. Finally, as in neuronal synapses, immune synapses are notable for their structural plasticity (Dustin and Colman 2002).

Immune synapses are central to the overall functioning of the immune system. Synaptic contacts are essential in the formation of the T-cell repertoire in the thymus, in homeostatic survival of T cells, in helper interactions between CD4$^+$ T cells and B lymphocytes, and in the rejection of infected target cells by CD8$^+$ T cells.

Antigen-presenting cells: professional and facultative

Although the first obvious prerequisite, MHC expression, is met by many cell types, not all are equally competent in presenting antigen to T cells. This is because, whilst MHC class I expression is constitutive in most tissues, this is not the case for expression of MHC class II. However, class II expression is readily induced on many cells by suitable proinflammatory stimuli – γ-interferon (IFN-γ) and tumour necrosis factor α (TNF-α) – even in the 'immune privileged' central nervous system (Wekerle 1994).

Given the relatively modest requirements of T cells, MHC expression may be sufficient for antigen presentation to experi-

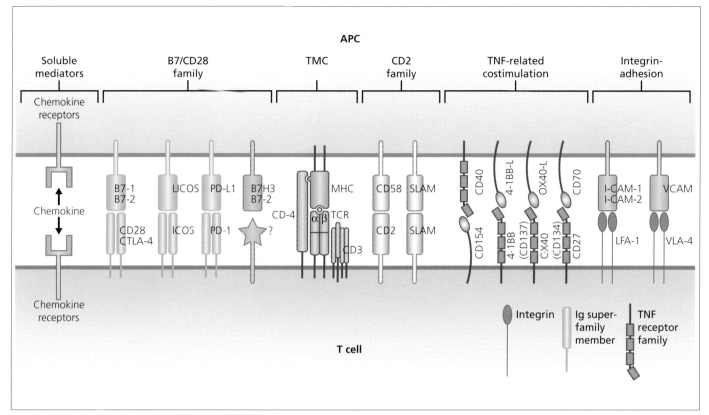

Figure 11.3 Cell adhesion molecule interactions at the interface between a CD4+ T cell (bottom) and an antigen-presenting cell (APC; top). Antigen specificity is conferred by the clonotypic T-cell receptor, which recognizes an antigen peptide (arrowhead) bound to an MHC class II molecule. Signal transduction is mediated by the invariant proteins of the CD3 complex associated with the T-cell receptor. Various additional costimulatory signals are transmitted by interactions between costimulatory molecules and their ligands (B7-1 and B7-2 with CD28, CD2, TNF-α gene families and their receptors, CD40 and CD40-L, and CTLA-4). Binding between cell adhesion molecules (LFA-1–ICAM-1/2, VLA-4–VCAM) stabilizes the contact between T cell and antigen-presenting cell. ICAM = intercellular adhesion molecule; VCAM = vascular cell adhesion molecule; TCR = T-cell receptor; CTLA = cytotoxic T-lymphocyte antigen; LFA = leucocyte functional antigen; VLA = very late antigen; TMC = trimolecular complex; SLAM = signalling lymphocytic activation molecule. Kindly provided by Professor Reinhard Hohlfeld.

enced memory or effector T cells. Naive CD4+ T cells are more demanding. They require – apart from MHC–peptide presentation – an elaborate set of costimulatory elements, some found only on dendritic cells, the professional antigen-presenting cell. Another quite special type of antigen-presenting cell is the B lymphocyte. B cells are much more selfish. They present antigen in order to activate helper T cells, and then receive reciprocal instructions directing the further fate of their own antibody response. Prominent examples are helper T-cell-derived cytokines – IFN-γ, interleukin 4 (IL-4) and IL-10 – which control immunoglobulin isotype switching (see below).

Dendritic cells

Dendritic cells count among the most intriguing elements of the immune system. They are truly multifunctional and pivotal in their performances. They play central roles in shaping the immune repertoire, initiating the response, deciding its character, and bringing everything to a close. Dendritic cells maintain immunological memory and connect innate with adaptive immune reactivity.

The discovery of dendritic cells strictly dates from 1973 (Steinman and Cohn 1973). However, it should be noted that they have made other appearances, depending on location,

wearing different disguises, such as interdigitating cells in the thymus (Kaiserling *et al* 1974) and veiled cells in the blood circulation (Hoefsmit *et al* 1982). Dendritic cells are the professional antigen-presenting cell *par excellence*. They carry out their manifold functions by presenting foreign or self antigen to specific T cells under very different conditions. As professional antigen-presenting cells, dendritic cells have the entire set of MHC antigens and costimulatory molecules required productively to engage any T lymphocyte – naive or memory, CD4 or CD8. Owing to their lineage diversity and functional plasticity, antigen presentation by dendritic cells may result in activation of an immune response, with formation of immune memory, or conversely the establishment of immune nonresponsiveness, or tolerance. Dendritic cells may also decide whether responding CD4+ T cells take the Th1 or the Th2 pathway of differentiation.

Dendritic cells are positioned strategically in practically all healthy tissues with the notable exception of the central nervous system parenchyma. Thus, they are the pioneer immune cells that make contact with a newly arrived pathogen. The antimicrobial response of a peripheral dendritic cell is multifaceted. First, microbial structures are sensed by the dendritic cell's innate pattern receptors (Toll-like or mannoside receptor). The

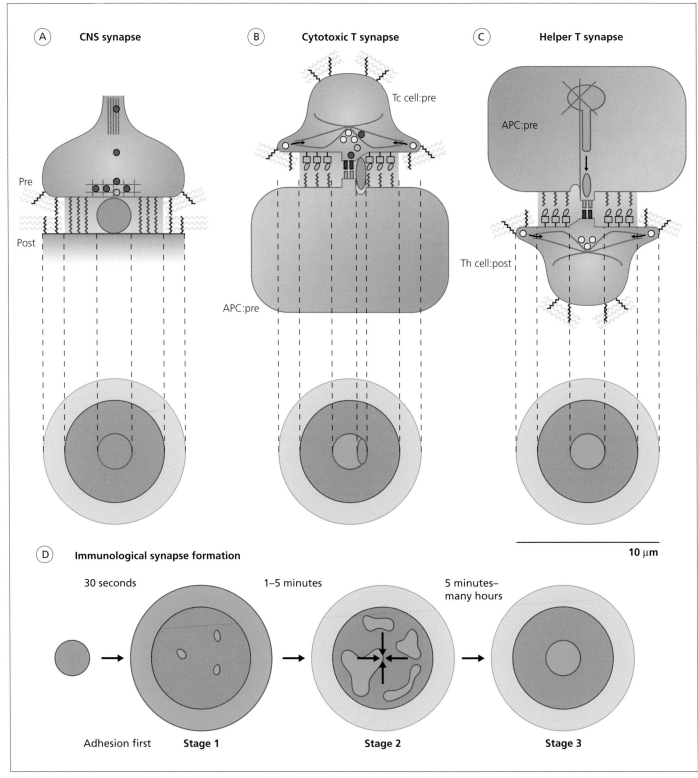

Figure 11.4 Comparison of the immune and neural synapses. Effector immune synapse linking CD8+ T cell with its target. (A) The neural synapse. (B) Inductive immune synapse formed between the CD8+ Tc cell as presynaptic and the antigen-presenting cell as postsynaptic. (C) Inductive immune synapse formed during antigen presentation between the antigen-presenting cell as presynaptic and the CD4+ Th cell as postsynaptic. (D) Diagram of the immune synapse formation. Green represents interactions between the T-cell receptor and peptide–MHC antigen. Red represents LFA-1–ICAM interaction (see Figure 11.3). Blue represents exocytic (secretory) vesicles. Yellow represents CD43 at the boundaries. Orange represents microtubules. Pale turquoise represents material in the synaptic cleft. Adapted from Dustin and Colman (2002). © 2002, with permission from Science.

dendritic cell responds to the stimulus by releasing chemotactic and proinflammatory soluble factors. These attract recirculating elements of the immune system, most prominently antigen-experienced memory T cells. At the same time, dendritic cells undergo further differentiation. They engulf and process the foreign structure, rendering it recognizable by T cells. Attraction of memory T cells and recognition of antigen on the dendritic cell are crucial aspects of immune surveillance.

The function of a dendritic cell is not exhausted by peripheral antigen presentation to memory cells. Antigen contact signals the dendritic cell to leave the tissue and to reach a local lymph node via its lymphatics. En route the dendritic cell responds to signals produced by 'homeostatic' chemokines. Once arrived at the lymphoid destination, it gets embedded in T-cell-rich compartments and starts to present the freshly acquired antigen mainly to naive T cells. It is important to note that only dendritic cells are able to activate naive T cells, whereas memory T cells can also respond to nonprofessional antigen-presenting cells. Thus, dendritic cells are sentinels distributed throughout the body. They sense and present foreign structures, but also take up and display dying cells or their debris from surrounding tissue. While, in most cases, such self presentations communicate tolerogenic signals to self-reactive T cells, there may be pathological conditions under which they activate autoreactive T cells and start the autoimmune disease process.

Dendritic cells are the progeny of bone marrow-derived progenitors. For lineage-specific differentiation, these precursors require stimulation by cytokines, including granulocyte-macrophage colony-stimulating factor (GM-CSF), IL-4 and, for maturation, TNF-α. There are at least two sublineages of dendritic cells. Besides the classic variety, plasmacytoid cells were identified as an alternative lineage. These were already known to pathologists, and described in inflamed lymph nodes as 'T cells with plasmacytoid features' (Vollenweider and Lennert 1983). Plasmacytoid cells were discovered for immunology as a cell type with dendritic morphology, exhibiting some, but not all, T-cell markers (Grouard et al 1997). The cells gained particular attention as a major source of type I IFNs (M. Cella et al 1999; Siegal et al 1999).

It appears that classic dendritic cells and plasmacytoid cells have complementary functions. They differentiate from distinct progenitor cells – dendritic cells from the monocytic lineage and plasmacytoid cells from lymphoid cells. Each has distinct Toll-like receptor profiles for microbial determinants, and they possess somewhat different cytokine repertoires (Shortman and Liu 2002). Possibly, either cell is able to determine the Th1/Th2 lineage decision during the initial phase of a T-cell response (Rissoan et al 1999).

In short, dendritic cells are pivotal elements in the immune system. As professional antigen-presenting cells they contribute to the establishment of central self-tolerance in the thymic medulla. And they recognize foreign (microbial) antigens in the peripheral tissues, by linking innate to adaptive immune responses.

Antigen-presenting B cells

B cells express surface MHC class I and II antigens, along with a number of costimulatory determinants, and thus qualify for antigen presentation to T cells. B cells are special antigen-presenting cells. First, with their antigen-specific membrane immunoglobulin receptors, B cells are able to bind and focus specific protein antigens present even at low concentration. The immunoglobulin-bound antigen is engulfed by the lymphocyte and processed to become presentable in the MHC class I or II context (Abbas et al 1996). Hence B cells are especially efficient antigen-presenting cells specialized to present diluted soluble antigens. Moreover, B cells display sets of cytokines and surface costimulatory molecules, which radically differ from their counterparts in dendritic cells. B cells are not only the objects of instruction by T cells but, conversely, also influence their partners' function and fate. The nature and molecular context of antigen presentation determines the character of a resulting T-cell response, including Th1/Th2 polarity. With such different cytokine and costimulatory molecule repertoires from dendritic cells, B lymphocytes drive antigen-recognizing CD4$^+$ T cells preferentially towards the Th2 lineage (Abbas et al 1996; Finkelman 1995).

B lymphocytes produce humoral immunoglobulin antibodies, but they are not autonomous and they require help from CD4$^+$ T cells in order to create an optimal immunoglobulin response. T cells contribute to the processes that result in formation of antibodies having the best antigen-binding fit and immunoglobulin isotype, and they control duration of the humoral response. Regulation of B-cell activity by T cells is the result of a T-cell–B-cell interaction that hinges around antigen presentation by B cells.

T-cell differentiation in the thymus: self recognition shaping the (auto)immune T-cell repertoire

Most T cells are formed and reach their maturity in the thymus, the central organ of the immune system. Immature progenitor cells, coming from the bone marrow, reach the thymus where they undergo rapid proliferation before leaving as immunocompetent T lymphocytes. The thymus is thus the site where T-cell receptor diversity and the differentiation of T-cell lineages are generated. Both result from sequential interactions between immature thymic T cells and the various cellular milieus formed by the thymic stroma.

Intrathymic T-cell differentiation is a complex process requiring profound developmental change involving induction of genes within single cells as well as radical selection processes on a population basis. The primitive bone marrow-derived progenitor cells reach the thymus via the bloodstream. They first settle in cortical areas located just beneath the thymic capsule. During differentiation, the maturing T-cell progenitors move through different compartments towards the thymic medulla, which they reach mostly as competent but naive T cells (Van Ewijk 1991).

The thymus is composed of material that develops from several different sources. Until recently, it was assumed that, at least in the mouse, cortical epithelia are progeny of the third ectodermal cleft, whereas the medullary epithelium derives from the third endodermal pouch (Cordier and Haumont 1980). Now, this dichotomy appears too simple. Instead of being derived from one epithelial sheet, thymic medullary epithelium seems to be a mosaic of multiple and diverse epithelial islets, each derived from distinct progenitors invading the thymus in early embryonic development (Rodewald et al 2001). As will be discussed later, such a diversified origin of medullary cells would have profound implications for the shaping of autoimmune T-cell receptor repertoires. In addition to epithelial cells, stem cells immigrating from bone marrow differentiate into macrophages, dendritic cells (which act in the periphery as professional antigen-presenting cells) and lymphocytes (Owen and Jenkinson 1984).

Thymic microenvironments are strictly determined by local stromal cells but, in turn, their composition and character are controlled by local T lymphocytes. For example, mice with severe combined immunodeficiency, and those treated with ciclosporin A, have no differentiated thymic medulla. However, reconstitution with intact T cells regenerates the intact medullary milieu (Shores *et al* 1991). The relevant signals seem to be communicated through lymphotoxin receptors (Boehm *et al* 2003). This is not unique for the thymus. Induction of a specialized lymphoid tissue microenvironment by immigrating lymphocytes is also seen in peripheral immune organs. Here, activated B lymphocytes form the germinal centres with their typical follicular interdigitating cells, presumably by secreting proinflammatory cytokines such as lymphotoxin-α (Le Hir *et al* 1996). In general, however, it is the composition of stromal cells that determines actual function of the local microenvironment in T-cell differentiation. There must be particular sets of cell signalling molecules that fit best and encourage suitably differentiated T-cell maturation over a critical period.

The influences from membrane signals, along with soluble mediators, that characterize the individual thymic microenvironments and induce the next step of differentiation are finally being deciphered. Genetic studies of the athymic nude mutations in rat and mouse identify a particular transcription factor, *Whn*, as central in controlling differentiation of embryonic thymus epithelium right after the invasion of lymphoid progenitor cells. It regulates development of cortical, subcortical and medullary epithelia. Inactivation by mutation causes thymus aplasia, and in addition deficient hair growth (Nehls *et al* 1996). Other genes involved in creating the early thymic stromal environment are provided by the homeobox gene family, which act in early stages of endoderm/mesenchyme interactions (*Hoxa3*) and on the interaction between lymphocyte precursors and epithelium (*Pax9*: Manley 2000).

Clearly, epithelia must be acting in concert with bone marrow-derived stromal cells, such as thymic dendritic cells and macrophages. At least in the case of epithelium, regional diversity has been demonstrated using sets of monoclonal antibodies (Van Ewijk *et al* 1994). In any case, it is clear that the intact architecture of the thymus is absolutely essential for correct development and function of the immune system. Disruption of thymic structure, following infection or graft versus host attacks, leads to profound deficits in normal T-cell production. This has two equally undesirable consequences – compromised reactivity against microbial pathogens and autoimmune disease.

Gene expression during T-cell maturation

The developmental steps of T-cell differentiation have been defined by examining membrane markers and receptor-gene expression in thymic T-cell subsets during fetal development, after regeneration, and in transgenic animals. Obviously, productive rearrangement of the genes encoding T-cell receptor

α and β chains is the first key event. Moreover, the progression of T-cell receptor expression is closely related to induction and surface expression of the ancillary molecules CD4 and CD8 on differentiating T lymphocytes.

There is consensus that T-cell progenitors migrating from the bone marrow to the thymus have neither rearranged T-cell receptors nor CD4 or CD8 on their membranes. At this stage, the T-cell receptor genes are still located in germline formation at individual loci on the chromosome. The T-cell receptor β-chain genes are rearranged first. They appear on the cell membrane together with a primitive surrogate α chain. This signals several differentiation steps – induction of both CD4 and CD8, and subsequent rearrangement of the α-chain genes. The CD4$^+$ and CD8$^+$ T-cell receptor-expressing thymocytes are now ready to undergo selection events that result in the intact, functional T-cell repertoire composed of CD4$^+$ and CD8$^+$ single positive lymphocytes (Robey *et al* 1994).

Formation of the T-cell receptor repertoire: positive and negative selection events

The mature T-cell repertoire is generated in a sequence of intense interactions between the T-cell receptor of developing thymocytes and self-peptide-laden MHC products expressed on thymic stroma cells. It occurs in two separate global selection rounds. First, all thymocyte progenitors are pushed into proliferation by positive selection. At this stage they seem to generate a random spectrum of T-cell receptors. Some bind variously to self antigen with high or low affinity, whereas others do not bind anything present in the thymus. Most of these young T cells are doomed to die by programmed cell death. Only those that bind MHC products with low affinity are rescued and encouraged to expand. Non-binding T cells fail to receive a survival signal and die from neglect. Conversely, high-affinity binders receive a positive death signal. The nature of selecting MHC structures is not fully known. It appears, however, that, due to the low-affinity nature of positive selection, one particular complex of cortical MHC and peptide may select a broad range of (weakly) cross-reacting receptors.

The positively selected T-cell population now contains, *inter alia*, clones with receptors able to recognize self antigens in the periphery. Potentially, they could cause autoimmune disease (von Boehmer 1992). In a second, negative selection round, most truly self-reactive T-cell clones are eliminated. Negative selection takes place largely in the thymic medulla, as a result of interactions with medullary epithelium cells and bone marrow-derived dendritic cells. Interestingly, contact points between the differentiating T cells and selecting thymus epithelia are structured to form an immune synapse, reminiscent of that formed between mature T lymphocytes and antigen-presenting cells in the peripheral immune system (Bousso *et al* 2002; Hailman *et al* 2002; Richie *et al* 2002).

Very recent work supports an ancient hypothesis that the thymic medulla contains progenitor cells capable of producing and displaying a large diversity of antigenic structures specific for specialized tissues (J.R. Mackay and Goldstein 1967; Wekerle and Ketelsen 1977). Indeed, a large spectrum of putative tissue-specific antigens has been identified in the thymic medulla (Derbinski *et al* 2001). Transgenic mice expressing any one gene of interest under the control of a tissue-specific promoter express that gene not only in the target tissue but also in the thymus (Hanahan 1999). Most intriguingly, medullary expression of autoantigen seems to be controlled by epigenetic factors, in particular an autoimmune regulator, the *AIRE* (autoimmune regulator) gene, inactivation of which, either by spontaneous mutation or in transgenic mice, lowers the level of medullary autoantigen expression (Derbinski *et al* 2005). Such mutants suffer a multitude of autoimmune responses, through defective deletion of autoimmune T cells in the thymic medulla (Anderson *et al* 2002).

We cannot deny that T-cell differentiation in the thymus is an extremely complex event. It requires the sequential expression of genes within the differentiating cell. Positive and negative selection ultimately results in a T-cell population efficient in its reactions against foreign antigen and tolerant to self. The individual differentiation steps occur in specialized stromal microenvironments through which differentiating T cells pass until they enter the peripheral blood circulation. As we shall see later, mechanisms governing generation of the efficient immune repertoire, while safeguarding immunological self-tolerance, are not completely failsafe. Numerous organ-specific autoreactive T cells slip through negative selection in the intact thymus, and even fewer are held back in a pathologically altered thymus. These forbidden T cells are not only found in every healthy immune system but actually make up a substantial component of the entire population.

T-cell polarization: the Th1/Th2 dichotomy

We have mentioned that mature T lymphocytes can be considered in two major classes dependent on their expression of CD4 or CD8, two accessory molecules binding to MHC class II and I, respectively. Cytotoxic killer cells are characterized by the CD8 molecule, while helper T cells (required for full B-cell function and delayed-type hypersensitivity) express the CD4 molecule (Janeway 1992). However, the diversity of the T-cell population now goes further. Thus, the CD4+ T-helper lineage is composed of subsets producing different profiles of cytokines upon activation. In the classic study, a major part of the CD4+ cells was characterized by preferential secretion of IFN-γ and IL-2 (Mosmann and Coffman 1989). These T helper (Th) 1 cells were distinguished from another set of CD4+ T cells secreting IL-4 and IL-5, designated Th2 cells. Then, there are CD4+ T cells producing both IFN-γ and IL-4 (Th0 cells).

The Th1/Th2 dichotomy, firmly established for mouse lymphocytes, was also later outlined in principle for human T cells (Romagnani 1994). Although now considered rather too simple, the functional division of helper T lymphocytes into the Th1 and Th2 groups, and their corresponding cytokine release profiles, is still retained (Abbas *et al* 1996). Both cell populations also display distinct sets of functional marker structures on their surface (especially chemokine receptors) that can be used as differential markers (Figure 11.5: Sallusto *et al* 1998). The Th1 and Th2 pathways are to some extent symmetrical, balancing the development and suppression of cell subpopulations controlling the immune response. Depending on effector function, the Th1-associated cytokines are IFN-γ, TNF-α and IL-2 with an autocrine effect of IL-2. Conversely, Th-2 cells deploy IL-3, IL-4, IL-5, IL-10 and IL-13 with an autocrine loop mediated by IL-4.

To reach its lineage fate, the naive T lymphocyte has to pass several checkpoints on its way to maturation as an effector cell.

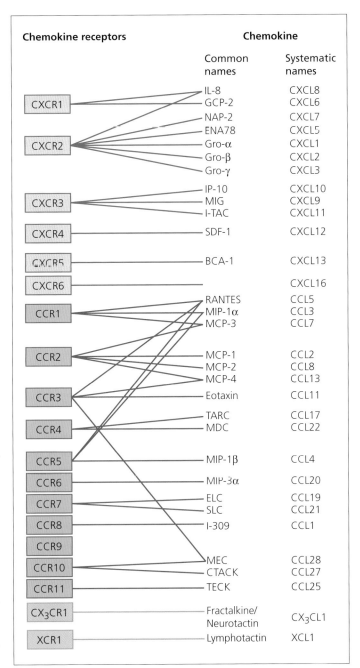

Figure 11.5 Scheme showing the main chemokine receptors and their respective chemokine ligands. Adapted from Proudfoot (2002).

Decisions are taken at different sites and times during differentiation. While the CD4 versus CD8 lineage choice is made in the thymus, the Th1/Th2 decision is made within the peripheral immune system, following first contact with specific antigen (Figure 11.6). The circumstances that govern first contact of naive T cells with antigen – the mode of presentation – dictate the prospective cytokine pattern.

The quantity and quality of cytokines secreted by a particular antigen-presenting cell, and the spectrum of costimulatory molecules displayed on its membrane, together determine whether a Th1 or a Th2 response is generated upon antigen recognition. Thus, IL-12 secreted preferentially by dendritic cells or

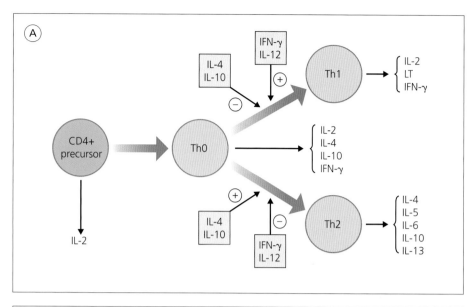

Figure 11.6 (A) Scheme to show the dichotomous development of T-helper (Th) subpopulations from CD4⁺ T cells, and their respective cytokine profiles. T cells expressing the α/β T-cell receptor (α/β⁺ T cells) constitute >95% of the T cells in blood. The rare γ/δ⁺ T cells are slightly enriched in certain multiple sclerosis lesions. The α/β⁺ T cells can be subdivided into CD4⁺ and CD8⁺ cells, and the latter can be divided into Th1 and Th2 cells. (B) Differentiation of Th1 and Th2 cells. CD4⁺ T precursor cells mature into Th0 cells. Under the positive or negative influence of various cytokines, Th0 cells differentiate into Th1 or Th2 cells. Note that the scheme is an oversimplification. In reality, cells are generally less polarized in their cytokine spectrum than are murine Th cells. Bold arrows indicate differentiation pathways; thin arrows indicate positive or negative regulatory influences or cytokine secretion. Adapted from Hohlfeld (1997).

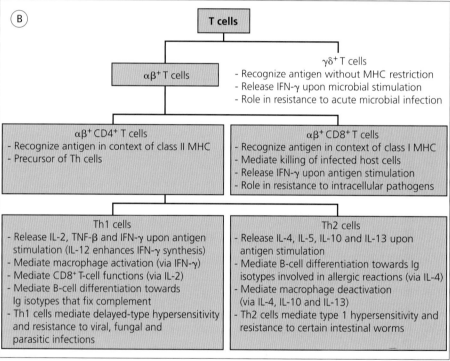

macrophages, induces production of IFN-γ in antigen-reactive CD4⁺ T cells, and at the same time suppresses IL-4 secretion. Under these conditions, Th1 differentiation would be expected. Conversely, antigen presentation by B cells tilts differentiation in the Th2 direction (Constant and Bottomly 1997). The cytokine pattern of an emerging CD4⁺ T-cell response is, however, not only imprinted by the instructing antigen-presenting cell but, in addition, depends strongly on the set of molecules recognized by the T-cell receptor and costimulatory molecules. The binding of B7-1 or B7-2 to T-cell CD28 structures may result in highly distinct cytokine responses, which can be reversed by soluble inhibitors (Reiser and Stadecker 1996), whereas binding to CTLA-4 has the opposite effect (Egen *et al*

2002). Furthermore, the antigenic peptide may itself determine distinct Th1/Th2 responses. Variation of peptide length or sequence of a given antigen affects the extent to which T cells are activated and, implicitly, their consequent cytokine secretion pattern (Kersh *et al* 1998).

Another, more indirect factor affecting this process is the microenvironment that surrounds antigen presentation. The composition of surrounding cells co-determines whether a naive CD4⁺ T cell assumes the Th1 or Th2 profile. The bystander cells – macrophages, mast cells, dendritic cells and a recently recognized natural killer NK1 T cell – shape ongoing T-cell responses both by surface structures and secreted cytokines (Coffman and von der Weid 1997).

At this point, innate immune reactivity comes into play. Recognition of microbial structures via Toll-like receptors activates cytokine responses in a number of cells, predominantly macrophages and dendritic cells, and thus influences activities of the maturing CD4$^+$ T cell. Activation of these cells by bacterial DNA set free during infection, and acting on Toll-like receptor-9 receptors, creates a milieu favouring Th1 induction. This mechanism explains the immunogenic effect of microbial adjuvants, such as Freund's complete adjuvant, which contains bacterial components that drive the Th1 orientation (H. Wagner 2001).

T-cell memory and homeostasis

The adaptive immune system is created to identify specific antigen, respond with maximal efficiency and remember the encounter. Repeated exposure triggers much faster and stronger responses than the initial reaction. Here, our metaphor linking the immunological and neural synapse is again appropriate: immunological and cognitive memory are functions that depend on altered structure driven by experience (Huntley *et al* 2002). The anamnestic immune response is determined by generation and persistence of specially differentiated, long-lived and antigen-specific memory T cells. Immune memory is explained by Macfarlane Burnet's clonal selection theory in purely quantitative terms. The concept rests on the expansion of specific immune cell clones in response to antigen stimulation, and their persistence in the repertoire. More specific immune cells produce a vigorous memory response. It is now known that in addition to numerical clonal expansion, immune memory requires the differentiation of a particular set of antigen-specific memory T cells, which respond to antigen more vigorously and efficiently than their naive, antigen-inexperienced counterparts.

Primary contact of naive T lymphocytes triggers massive cell division, which usually proceeds to elimination of the target antigen. Thereafter, the overwhelming majority of all the new lymphocytes are quickly eliminated by programmed cell death. Only a small subset, the memory T cells, survive this attrition – sometimes for life (Jenkins *et al* 2001). Memory T cells and their naive progenitors are clearly distinct. Following antigen-induced differentiation, they assume a particular profile of surface markers, including elevated levels of cell adhesion molecules (such as CD44), sets of cytokine and chemokine receptors, and isoforms of the leucocyte common antigen CD45 (Dutton *et al* 1998). Although there is marked functional plasticity, CD4$^+$ memory T cells seem to keep their Th1/Th2 lineage phenotype once this is acquired following initial antigen contact.

Most memory cells are migratory. In contrast to their naive counterparts, which travel from the thymus to peripheral immune organs and wait in expectation of specific antigen, a large set of memory T cells (termed effector memory cells by some investigators) indefatigably roam through the various organs in pursuit of their antigen. They go through blood and lymphatic vessels, and are attracted to putative antigen-presenting cells by chemotactic factors that are often induced by mechanisms of natural immune reactivity (Sprent and Surh 2002). A second type of memory cell, central memory cells, persist in lymphoid tissues where they wait for the eventual arrival of their antigen. The two types of memory cell are distinguishable by particular sets of surface markers, among these the chemokine receptor

CCR-7 (Sallusto *et al* 1999) and by the intensity of their response to antigen. Both have a long life expectancy although survival is not part of their birthright and must be earned. It appears that memory T cells receive signals from neighbouring cells, especially in immunologically rich environments, that trigger survival responses and allow cells to escape programmed cell death. The signals that encourage T-cell survival are provided by cells forming the local microenvironment. Cytokines (IL-7 or IL-15), cell adhesion molecules and even MHC determinants presenting random (unspecific) peptides may each participate in homeostasis (Seddon and Zamoyska 2003). It appears that, as for antigen-dependent T-cell activation, antigen-independent homeostatic stimuli are derived from synapse-like intercellular contacts (Revy *et al* 2001). The signals instruct local T cells not to proliferate in an uncontrolled way, but to survive without mitosis. The composition of signals controlling long-term persistence of naive and memory T cells is not known in detail. Most probably, they include positive signals that ensure clonal persistence and self-renewal, or negative messages that prevent precocious cell activation. Examples of gene products involved in negative regulation of T cells are cytotoxic T lymphocyte antigen-4 (CTLA-4) members of the suppressor of cytokine signalling (SOCS) gene family and lung Krüppel-like factor (LKLF), each of which work at different levels of suppressive gene regulation.

CTLA-4 is expressed on the surfaces of activated T cells. It is a receptor for costimulatory molecules of the B7 family. In contrast to the alternative B7 receptor, CD28, CTLA-4 does not activate antigen-recognizing T cells. Instead, it suppresses cell activation. Blockade of CTLA-4 by recombinant inhibitor proteins or antagonist monoclonal antibodies leads to exuberant T-cell responses against foreign and self antigens (Karandikar *et al* 1996; Perrin *et al* 1996). Transgenic knockout mice lacking *CTLA4* develop spontaneous organ infiltrations – presumably of an autoimmune nature – and die before adulthood (Tivol *et al* 1995). CTLA-4 limits T-cell activation at several levels: during primary or secondary antigen presentation and homeostatic regulation, acting both directly via interactions between T lymphocytes and antigen-presenting cells, or indirectly through CD4$^+$CD25$^+$ regulatory T cells (Sakaguchi 2000; Salomon and Bluestone 2001).

SOCS is a negative feedback inhibitor that acts on the signalling pathway triggered by cytokines. It interferes directly with activation of intracellular signalling molecules (jak/STAT families) through cytokine receptors. As a classic feedback inhibitor, it is induced by many proinflammatory cytokines, and reacts by suppressing the same cytokines (Alexander 2002). The pivotal regulatory role of SOCS in immune regulation is convincingly demonstrated by knockout mice, which, reminiscent of *CTLA4* mutants, die early in life with exuberant inflammatory disease (Marine *et al* 1999).

Finally, LKLF exemplifies suppressive regulation acting at the transcriptional level. The molecule derives its bizarre name from a *Drosophila* gene, which shares structural similarities with *LKLF* in their zinc-finger segment. LKLF is expressed in memory cells, apparently keeping them in a homeostatically acceptable resting state. Following antigen presentation and activation, LKLF is transiently lost from the T cell only to reappear with acquisition of the new memory state (Di Santo 2001).

B LYMPHOCYTES

B lymphocytes are agents of the humoral immune response. They determine the production of soluble antibodies (immunoglobulins), which bind antigenic structures and prepare these for elimination, using either the lytic complement cascade or the activation of phagocytes. B lymphocytes are centrally involved in immune responses against bacteria. In fact, many traditional vaccination strategies focus on B-cell production of protective antimicrobial antibodies. However, there is also a dark side to B cells. They play pivotal roles in pathological processes such as allergies, and they mediate certain autoimmune diseases.

B lymphocytes recognize antigen via receptors formed by membrane-bound immunoglobulins. They are clonally diverse – each clone recognizing one particular antigenic structure via a single immunoglobulin type. Unlike T cells and the thymus, mammalian B lymphocytes do not develop within one specialized central immune organ. Instead, they differentiate in particular milieus within the bone marrow from primitive precursors. Having reached immunocompetence, these naive B cells leave the cradle and settle in special compartments within the peripheral immune organs. The B-cell lineage develops from pluripotential stem cells – the origin of all bone marrow haemopoietic cells. But like T cells, the differentiating B lymphocyte interacts with local stroma cells, which offer microenvironments permissive for distinct steps in differentiation leading to rearrangement of the immunoglobulin V regions and assembly of intact immunoglobulin on the surface membrane of naive cells (at least for IgM and IgD).

A completely new phase of B-cell differentiation is triggered by first contact with antigen. After this encounter, the courtship with T cells leads to dichotomous differentiation pathways – relatively long-lived memory B cells and short-lived immunoglobulin-producing plasma cells. Fundamental changes take place within germinal centres of peripheral immune organs. Here, naive B cells encounter specific antigen presented by follicular dendritic cells (not to be confused with the professional antigen-presenting cells that interact with T cells) – the enigmatic stroma cell of germinal centres. In addition, some T-helper cells are present in these areas to provide a microenvironment facilitating maturation of the B-cell response by inducing somatic hypermutation of immunoglobulin complementarity-determining regions and isotype switching.

Experimental work indicates that B lymphocytes have diverse and complex roles in the pathogenesis of autoimmune disease. In addition to antibody production, they have ancillary functions in presenting autoantigen to T cells. B cells express costimulatory molecules (B7-1 and B7-2) on their cell membrane and are thus able effectively to activate resting specific T lymphocytes. By presenting antigen, B cells direct the responding T cell towards the Th2 pattern of cytokine secretion (Lenschow *et al* 1996). Having recognized their antigen on B cells, T cells are prone preferentially to secrete IL-4, IL-5 and IL-10 – the cytokines that, incidentally, are required for T-cell help for antibody-producing B lymphocytes.

Immunoglobulins

Immunoglobulins play several pivotal roles in B-cell immune responses. First, inserted in the surface membrane, they act as receptors, binding specific antigen and transmitting activation signals that initiate the immune response. In secreted, soluble form, they act as antibodies, binding and earmarking antigen for destruction by macrophages or proteases (via complement), thus exerting effector functions of the immune response. In both situations, immunoglobulins use the variable (V) segments, which specifically bind antigens having complementary structures. The immunoglobulin V region and corresponding antigenic epitope fit together no less tightly than the proverbial key and its lock. The immunoglobulin V region is formed in the course of B-cell differentiation by a complex series of diversification events. The steps in naive B-cell development include recombination of germline genes, addition of non-germline (N) encoded elements, and somatic mutation to improve further the fit (affinity) of immunoglobulin after encounter with the actual antigen.

Typical monomeric immunoglobulin is composed of two light and two heavy chains interconnected by disulphide bonds. A monomeric immunoglobulin possesses two identical antigen-binding sites, each formed by the V regions of adjacent light and heavy chains (see also Chapter 3). The immunoglobulin V regions are thus the structural basis for antibody diversity. Immunoglobulin V regions are composed of framework segments with genetically conserved sequences and interspersed hypervariable regions (sequences characteristic for each individual specific immunoglobulin). They combine to form the molecular surface of an antigen-binding site. As for T-cell receptors, structural similarity between these hypervariable immunoglobulins is reflected by their denomination as complementarity-determining regions. Structural genes for the immunoglobulin V region fall into three sets: variable (V), diversity (D) and joining (J) segments clustered on the chromosome as linearly arranged gene segments. Each group contains a large number of individual genes and the human heavy chain has literally hundreds of V, dozens of D and several J genes (Rajewsky 1996).

Early mechanisms of B-cell immunoglobulin diversification

Mature, antigen-binding immunoglobulins are formed in a complex process. As a first step, single members of each set are selected during gene transcription from the diverse gene cluster joined at random (Figure 11.7). This recombination of individual germline genes is brought about by a sequence of events directed by special enzymes known as recombinases (RAG proteins) expressed both in B and T cells, but only in the narrow time windows of lymphoid differentiation. Random recombination of preformed gene elements alone potentially offers many thousands of possible V regions but, in reality, antibody diversity is much higher. In stark contrast to T-cell receptors, which remain unchanged throughout the life of a T cell, immunoglobulins undergo somatic modifications, which improve antigen affinity, and switch to the ideal isoform. For example, imprecise joining of genes further increases variety of the B-cell repertoire. Furthermore, additional nucleotides (P and N region, neither encoded in the germline) are added. Nucleotides are added by terminal deoxynucleotidyl transferase (TdT). Like recombinases, this is only expressed transiently during B- and T-cell development. Interestingly, N-addition, especially prominent in the mature immune system, is almost lacking in neonates (Rajewsky 1996).

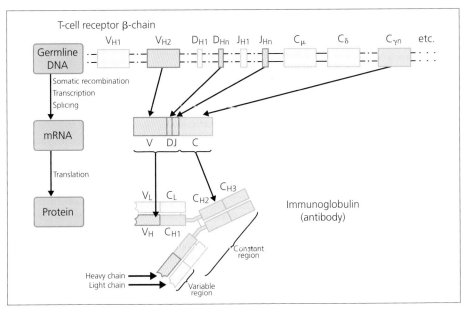

Figure 11.7 Rearrangement of germline genes in the formation of the immunoglobulin heavy chain. DNA encoding the variable region of the heavy chain contains variable (V_H), diversity (D_H) and joining (J_H) functional gene segments. The constant region genes code for the different immunoglobulin isotypes (e.g. $C\mu$ for IgM, $C\delta$ for IgD, etc.). A complete heavy chain V region gene is assembled by somatic recombination events that first join the D and J segments, and then join the V gene segment to the combined DJ sequence. The heavy chain C region sequences are spliced to the variable domain sequences during processing of the heavy chain gene RNA transcript. The mRNA coding for the two types of immunoglobulin light chain (κ and λ) is constructed by similar mechanisms (not shown). Adapted from Hohlfeld (1997).

Nothing lasts forever and freshly formed B-cell immunoglobulin receptors are no exception. A second round of B-cell receptor formation often takes place in the bone marrow. In a penultimate stage of B-cell maturation, certain immunoglobulin may happen to bind antigen, presumably expressed on unidentified bone marrow stroma, vetoing further B-cell production of its preferred receptor and rebooting the immunoglobulin recombination machinery. A new and distinct immunoglobulin chain is then formed providing the B cell with an amended, and more acceptable, antigen specificity – a process termed receptor revision or editing (Nemazee 2000), which presumably acts to avoid the formation of pathogenic autoantibodies.

Affinity maturation and immunoglobulin class switches

At this point in ontogeny, generation of the immunoglobulin repertoire is independent of exogenous antigen. Once activated, further changes affect immunoglobulin-binding sites on the B cell. During a primary reaction, the originally formed hypervariable complementarity-determining region sequences are further modified and diversified by somatic mutation. These improve the binding fit of antibodies (immunoglobulin affinity) through the ongoing immune response. Affinity maturation of immunoglobulin takes place in the germinal centres of secondary immune organs and involves complex intercellular responses between the differentiating B cell, helper T cells and dendritic cells (MacLennan 1994). Apparently, the selecting antigen is presented by follicular dendritic cells, which signal B cells with the best-fitting immunoglobulin receptors to amplify and persist, whilst those less fortunate die from neglect (Kelsoe 1996).

Immunoglobulins come in five different classes – IgD, IgM, IgG, IgA and IgE. These are defined by constant (C) regions of the heavy chain. Each B-cell clone is identified by its antigen specificity (V region) whilst still able to undergo a change in immunoglobulin class thereby grafting the same V regions to different heavy chain isotypes. Switches are not random but follow exact rules – IgM to IgA or IgG, but never in the reverse direction. This sequence follows the location of isotype structural genes on chromosome 12. Switch events are controlled by the interaction of B cells and helper T cells. Cytokines secreted by the T lymphocytes seem to provide the signals required to select individual isotypes. Thus, IL-4 favours production and secretion of IgE and IgG1, whilst IgG2a is preferentially induced by IFN-γ and IgA by TGF-β. Although the molecular mechanisms of affinity maturation and class switching are not yet fully characterized, there is good evidence that the activation-induced cytidine deaminase (AID) functions in both processes (Muramatsu and Honjo 2001).

AUTOIMMUNITY AND SELF-TOLERANCE IN THE CENTRAL NERVOUS SYSTEM

As emphasized before, the immune system is programmed to search out and remove suspicious organisms. This function is life saving, but at the same time carries a deadly risk. Immune cells with receptors for healthy tissues have the potential to divert immune responses against self, and thereby cause organ-specific disease. Immune cell clones with such a self-destructive potential should clearly be forbidden. Self-reactive, forbidden clones should be eliminated from the immune system early in development, ideally during embryonic life, as proposed by Burnet (Burnet 1959): no self-recognition, no autoimmune disease.

Burnet was partly right. Physical elimination of T-cell clones with receptors recognizing self antigen in the thymus was shown in pioneering experiments (von Boehmer *et al* 1989). This work was based on the construction of transgenic mice with a highly simplified, autoimmune-prone immune repertoire. The mice expressed a rearranged T-cell receptor transgene encoding a receptor for the male-specific H-Y autoantigen. In its absence (e.g. in females), most emerging T cells used the transgenic receptor. However, in the presence of autoantigen (as in male mice), recognition of H-Y peptides in the context of MHC class I protein led to thymic elimination of autoreactive T cells.

Clonal elimination is not absolute and, thus, additional ways of securing global self-tolerance must exist. In some cases, potentially autoreactive T lymphocytes that have escaped censure acquire profound nonreactivity against self antigen – a state of anergy. This concept stems from studies of transgenic mouse models, in which an experimental transgenic autoantigen is expressed at high level in a particular peripheral tissue, but only weakly in the thymus. In some (but not all) cases, anergy of self-reactive T cells is matched by downregulation of the self-reactive T-cell receptor (Arnold *et al* 1993).

The most intriguing, enigmatic and, for clinical immunology, important feature of tolerance, however, is the persistence of fully reactive, self-recognizing T-cell clones in the healthy immune repertoire. Under normal conditions, these remain harmless, but self-reactive T cells may escape control and become autoaggressive. One explanation offered for innocuous persistence of self-reactive T cells in the immune repertoire is clonal ignorance. This describes the situation in which a particular tissue remains secluded from blood and lymph circulation by a dense barrier. Therefore, whilst the immune repertoire contains T cells with receptors for this tissue, they are barred from entry and exert no effect until an accidental breach of the shielding barrier provides the portal for a less than friendly autoimmune encounter. As it turns out, this was always a naive concept, and truly secluded autoantigens are rare, if they exist at all. Few, if any of these antigens are 'tissue specific', and most are found outside the organ in question, and represented in the more distributed immune system.

Spectacular examples of autoimmune lymphocyte clones in the intact immune repertoire are T cells recognizing the brain myelin component, myelin basic protein. First isolated from lymph nodes of healthy rodents, these T cells unfolded a lethal autoaggressive potential when transferred in an activated state into healthy animals of the same strain (Schlüsener and Wekerle 1985). Later, myelin basic protein specific T-cell lines were also isolated from the peripheral blood of patients with multiple sclerosis and healthy volunteers (Pette *et al* 1990a). At first, inaccessibility of central nervous system target autoantigen was held responsible for the persistence of autoimmune T cells in the absence of obvious pathological consequences. Myelin basic protein and other brain autoantigens are, however, quite commonly produced outside the central nervous system and within the immune system, where they are readily accessible (K. Kojima *et al* 1997; Pribyl *et al* 1993; Zelenika *et al* 1993). Clonal ignorance cannot explain self-tolerance against central nervous system autoantigens. There must also be regulatory mechanisms, positive or negative, that normally hold autoimmune disease in check.

Now, we introduce the nature of autoreactive T cells and regulatory pathways that keep them from igniting the autoimmune process. We portray experimental autoimmune encephalomyelitis as proving phenomenally instructive as a model for certain aspects of multiple sclerosis and one that also offers essential insights into the cellular organization of immunological self-tolerance and immune reactivity within the immune system. We proceed by examining individual features of autoimmune reactivity targeted against the central nervous system, revealed by experimental autoimmune encephalomyelitis, and verify their contribution to the pathogenesis of multiple sclerosis.

Experimental autoimmune encephalomyelitis: a model of multiple sclerosis and more

Organ-specific autoimmune diseases are caused by autoimmune T cells that attack the body's own tissues. Thus, T cells that recognize brain structures can assault brain tissues, while T cells with receptors for pancreatic islet cells may cause immune diabetes. Autoreactive T cells are the pathogens of autoimmune disease, much like microbes qualify as pathogens in infectious diseases. The identification of autoimmune T cells consequently follows the rules established by Robert Koch in his search for pathogenic bacteria. A pathogen, autoimmune or microbial, must satisfy Koch's postulates: it must be regularly present in a particular tissue lesion; it must be isolated from the lesion and be propagated in pure culture; and, when transferred back into a healthy tissue, the pathogen must create tissue changes similar to the original lesion. Koch's postulates were first successfully applied to myelin autoreactive T cells, the pathogens of experimental autoimmune encephalomyelitis – often dubbed 'the' model of multiple sclerosis. The disorder has been invaluable in revealing the basic rules of organ-specific autoimmune reactions, and beyond that, the organization of immune reactivity in the central nervous system.

The classic experimental autoimmune encephalomyelitis models

Neurological complications observed at the turn of the century in the context of rabies vaccination, first suggested that autoimmunity targeted against nervous tissue elements can induce brain inflammation (Remlinger 1928). This concept was formally proven in experimental animals by the intentional induction of inflammatory demyelinating lesions after active immunization with brain tissue (Rivers *et al* 1933). Experimental autoimmune encephalomyelitis later became one of the most intensively studied experimental systems in autoimmune research, profoundly shaping our understanding of basic T-cell immunology and the pathogenesis of autoimmune inflammation. Experimental autoimmune encephalomyelitis can be induced in virtually all mammalian species, including humans. In the human, acute inflammatory demyelinating disease was reported after subcutaneous injection of brain tissue in the course of vaccinations (Uchimura and Shiraki 1957) and following unconventional cell therapy (Seitelberger *et al* 1958). The disease induced by sensitization with whole central nervous system tissue extracts in adjuvant has a complex pathogenesis and involves both cell-mediated and humoral immune mechanisms. It can usefully be considered as having several basic components (Lassmann 1983).

T lymphocytes, reactive against central nervous system proteins, are responsible for the induction of disease. Autoimmune-mediated inflammation of the brain can be transferred to naive recipients by T lymphocytes from sensitized donors (Paterson 1960) and even by monospecific T-lymphocyte lines and clones (Ben-Nun *et al* 1981b). Experimental autoimmune encephalomyelitis induced by T-cell lines is, in most models, an acute monophasic disease characterized pathologically by intensive inflammation (Figure 11.8). The disease develops in a very

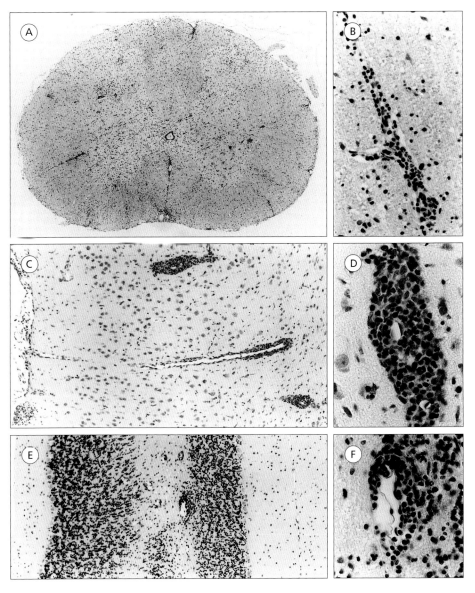

Figure 11.8 Inflammatory reaction in the central nervous system induced by T lymphocytes directed against different antigens. (A) Spinal cord inflammation in experimental autoimmune encephalomyelitis induced by transfer of an MBP-reactive T-lymphocyte line; ×30. (B) Perivascular inflammation with spread of leucocytes into the central nervous system parenchyma; ×400. (C) Inflammatory reaction in the cerebral cortex after transfer of an S-100-reactive T-cell line; ×100. (D) Prominent perivascular inflammatory reaction with little infiltration of leucocytes into the parenchyma; ×500. (E) Inflammation in the cerebellar white matter after transfer of a myelin oligodendrocyte glycoprotein-reactive T-cell line; ×100. (F) Inflammatory cells of cerebellar white matter are mostly located in the perivascular space; sections are stained with haematoxylin/eosin; ×500.

characteristic pattern, typically starting in lower parts of the spinal cord and progressing finally to reach the base of the brain. This is true for the development of inflammatory lesions, and reflected by the (motor) neurological deficits, which start with paralysis of tail muscles routinely spreading to affect hind and front limbs and, in severe cases, manifesting as brainstem disorders.

Demyelination and associated tissue damage are minimal or absent in most monophasic models. Nevertheless, in some animal strains, chronic progressive or relapsing disease variants may develop after a single transfer of encephalitogenic T cells (Mokhtarian *et al* 1984). In this situation, the inflammation may be accompanied by some demyelination and nonspecific tissue damage. Even in these models, and in contrast to the lesions of multiple sclerosis, inflammation is dominant and the sparse demyelination mainly restricted to the perivascular central nervous system parenchyma. These are the pathological features of acute disseminated leucoencephalomyelitis (ADEM; see Chapter 12).

In contrast to these purely T-cell mediated models of experimental autoimmune encephalomyelitis, sensitization with whole central nervous system tissue may result in prolonged chronic progressive or relapsing disease, in which the pathological appearances are inflammation, widespread primary demyelination and gliosis (Figures 11.9 and 11.10) (Raine *et al* 1974b; S.H. Stone and Lerner 1965). These models approximate more closely the pathology of multiple sclerosis, but are difficult to induce reproducibly. Their fickle nature depends upon many different factors, including the mode of sensitization and genetic background of the animal (Lassmann 1983). However, it is well established that chronic demyelinating experimental autoimmune encephalomyelitis models can nevertheless be induced in many different animal species and strains.

In addition to T-cell mediated inflammation, autoantibodies against myelin components seem to play a major role in the pathogenesis of chronic demyelinating variants of experimental autoimmune encephalomyelitis. Very similar disease and pathology can be induced when intravenous injection of anti-

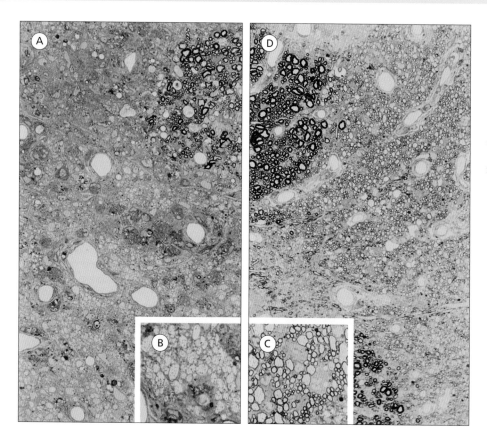

Figure 11.9 Demyelination and remyelination in chronic experimental autoimmune encephalomyelitis. (A) Early demyelinated plaque with complete demyelination; ×300. (B) Some macrophages contain myelin degradation products; ×900. (C) Late, partly remyelinated lesion; the axons are surrounded by thin myelin sheaths; ×900. (D) Toluidine blue-stained plastic section; ×300.

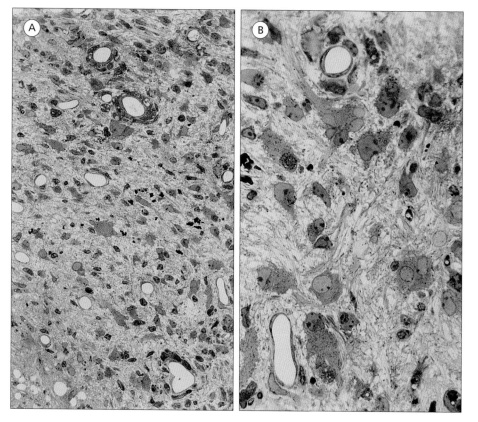

Figure 11.10 Astroglia reaction in demyelinated lesions in chronic experimental autoimmune encephalomyelitis. (A) Large hypertrophied astrocytes, some with multiple nuclei; ×300. (B) Occasional degradation products in the astrocyte cytoplasm; toluidine blue-stained plastic section; ×1000.

myelin antibodies is timed to coincide with the onset of the inflammatory reaction induced by transfer of encephalitogenic T lymphocytes (Linington *et al* 1988; Schlüsener *et al* 1987). Furthermore, in most models of chronic experimental autoimmune encephalomyelitis associated with widespread primary demyelination, significant serum titres of demyelinating antibodies can be detected (Linington and Lassmann 1987). Large confluent areas of demyelination develop, especially in DA and BN guinea pigs that had been immunized against recombinant myelin oligodendrocyte (MOG) protein, a minor protein component of myelin located on the surface of myelin-forming oligodendrocytes and myelin sheaths (Raine *et al* 1974b).

Experimental autoimmune encephalomyelitis in transgenic mice

Historically, most experimental autoimmune encephalomyelitis models used the Lewis rat or mouse strains PL/J (or B10PL for myelin basic protein-induced experimental autoimmune encephalomyelitis) and SJL/J (for proteolipid protein-induced experimental autoimmune encephalomyelitis), respectively. Many transgenic mice were generated and bred on the background of 129/J or C57BL strains. Unfortunately, neither was susceptible to the induction of experimental autoimmune encephalomyelitis. Thus, attempts to use available transgenic mice for experimental autoimmune encephalomyelitis research resorted to breeding the transgene onto a susceptible background – a time-consuming, expensive and bothersome procedure. Relief came when the group of Avi Ben-Nun identified the p35–55 peptide of myelin oligodendrocyte protein as a reliable and efficient encephalitogenic antigen in the C57BL mouse (Mendel *et al* 1995). Experimental autoimmune encephalomyelitis driven by the p35–55 epitope of myelin oligodendrocyte glycoprotein is now the most popular transgenic mouse system for modelling neuroimmunological disease (Owens *et al* 2001).

Spontaneous models of experimental autoimmune encephalomyelitis

These models are all induced by immunization of healthy animals with components of central nervous system protein. Spontaneously occurring experimental autoimmune encephalomyelitis has been observed only in transgenic mice that express genes encoding the myelin-specific T-cell receptor from an encephalitogenic T-cell clone. The first report was of a transgenic mouse in which most T cells used a myelin basic protein-specific T-cell receptor. Up to 40% of such transgenic mice developed spontaneous experimental autoimmune encephalomyelitis during the first 8 months of life. However, spontaneous experimental autoimmune encephalomyelitis emerged only in animals that were kept under conventional ('dirty') conditions. Animals of the same strain raised in a clean unit did not fall ill spontaneously (Goverman *et al* 1993).

High frequencies of spontaneous experimental autoimmune encephalomyelitis were observed in transgenic mice that had a comparable myelin basic protein-specific T-cell receptor, but lacked intact *RAG* genes. Since *RAG* genes are indispensable for generation of diverse T- and B-cell repertoires, these double transgenics possessed a monoclonal immune repertoire, comprising CD4$^+$ T cells with the transgenic anti-myelin basic protein

receptor. Practically all of these mice developed experimental autoimmune encephalomyelitis within 12 months of age (Lafaille *et al* 1994). As will be discussed later, a deficit of regulatory T cells appeared to be the pivotal event in determining the high frequency of autoimmune disease (Furtado *et al* 2001). It is worth mentioning that spontaneous experimental autoimmune encephalomyelitis is not limited to transgenic models of myelin basic protein-driven experimental autoimmune encephalomyelitis. Similar disease and in equivalent proportions was noted in transgenic mice with proteolipid protein-specific receptors (Waldner *et al* 2000). Optic neuritis developed in transgenics with myelin oligodendrocyte glycoprotein-specific T-cell receptors (Bettelli *et al* 2003).

Central nervous system-specific T cells as pathogenic agents of experimental autoimmune encephalomyelitis

Paterson (1960) provided formal proof that experimental autoimmune encephalomyelitis is an autoimmune disease mediated by cells and not humoral antibodies. At a time when immunologists were unaware of the distinction between T and B lymphocytes, he transferred experimental autoimmune encephalomyelitis from actively immunized rats to untreated recipients using large numbers of primed lymphocytes. The transferred cells were clearly organ specific and autoimmune, because they attacked the host brain tissue and ignored all others including the peripheral nervous system. Remarkably, these pathogenic lymphocytes came from donor rats that had been perfectly normal before immunization with myelin basic protein. Many questions immediately arose. Had the autoimmune encephalitogenic lymphocytes been formed *de novo* as a consequence of autoimmunization? Were they forbidden clones in the Burnetian sense? Or, alternatively, were encephalitogenic lymphocytes the progeny of precursors, pre-existing in the healthy rodent immune system but previously causing no harm because their target tissue, the brain, was inaccessible and shielded by the tight endothelial blood–brain barrier? We now know that none of these hypotheses provides a full explanation. Instead, healthy vertebrate immune systems contain ample numbers of potentially autoaggressive lymphocyte clones (T cells as well as B cells) that, once activated, readily access and attack their target tissues (see above).

General characteristics of encephalitogenic T cells

Most isolated encephalitogenic T-cell lines share essential characteristics. First, they are all members of the CD4$^+$ subset of Th cells and, as such, recognize target autoantigen in the molecular context of MHC class II proteins (Ben-Nun and Cohen 1982). Only very recently have CD8$^+$ killer T cells been described (Huseby *et al* 2001; D. Sun *et al* 2001). Secondly (and by definition), encephalitogenic T cells are principally able to transfer experimental autoimmune encephalomyelitis to naive syngeneic recipient animals. It is, however, crucial to note that activation is required to mediate disease by myelin-specific T cells. The same cells are harmless in the resting state. Interestingly, although encephalitogenic T cells qualify as CD4$^+$ T helper cells, many have a remarkable cytotoxic potential. In the Lewis rat, for example, myelin basic protein-specific encephalitogenic T-cell lines readily lyse all target cells that present the target encephalitogenic peptide in a recognizable MHC class II context. In sharp contrast, T-cell lines with nonencephalitogenic specificity (targeting ovalbumin or mycobacterial antigens) are not cytotoxic (D. Sun and Wekerle 1986). This behaviour is seen also in experimental autoimmune encephalomyelitis-inducing, myelin basic protein-specific T cells from SJL/J mice (Fallis and McFarlin 1989), and in human T-cell lines with the same specificity (J. Burns *et al* 1991; Martin *et al* 1990). Cytotoxic behaviour of encephalitogenic T cells correlates closely with their cytokine profile. Myelin basic protein-specific T cells transferring experimental autoimmune encephalomyelitis secrete IFN-γ and IL-2, but not IL-4 and thus qualify as members of the Th1 subset (Ando *et al* 1989). More precisely, these cells seem to belong to a subset of Th1 lymphocytes which is shaped by the cytokine IL-23 (Langrish *et al* 2005). Most, if not all encephalitogenic T-cell lines show these properties. Interestingly, the encephalitogenic potential is lost when CD4$^+$ T cells are manipulated to change from a Th1 to Th2-like cytokine pattern *in vivo* or *in vitro* (Racke *et al* 1994). Th1 bias is characteristic for adult myelin basic protein-specific T cells. In contrast, exposure of neonatal cells to the target autoantigen seems preferentially to induce Th2-like cells, and these are associated with lifelong resistance to experimental autoimmune encephalomyelitis (Forsthuber *et al* 1996).

However, it would be rash to conclude that Th2-like myelin-specific T cells are nonencephalitogenic, or even protective, under all circumstances. In fact, myelin basic protein-specific transgenic T cells can be re-educated *in vitro* to assume the Th2 phenotype. They mediate a vigorous central nervous system inflammatory disease when transferred into immunodeficient *RAG* knockout mice. Such lesional infiltrates are, however, dominated by polymorphonuclear leucocytes and thus thoroughly differ from classic Th1-dependent lesions (Lafaille *et al* 1997). Indeed, an 'anaphylactic' response was also observed in regular mice after challenge during recuperation from a preceding episode of experimental autoimmune encephalomyelitis. The allergic response was explained as pathological exaggeration of the physiological Th2-biased disposition prevailing during recovery from experimental autoimmune encephalomyelitis (Pedotti *et al* 2001).

Potentially pathogenic T-cell clones in the healthy immune repertoire

The fact that encephalitogenic T-cell lines can be isolated from autoimmunized rodents is in itself rather stunning. Ultimately, it indicates the presence of potentially pathogenic autoimmune T-cell clones in the regular immune repertoire. After all, it is safe to assume that, before immunization, the donor animal had enjoyed perfect health and possessed a normal immune system. Since, in striking contrast to B-cell immunoglobulin receptors, T-cell receptors are not somatically mutated at any stage of activation or proliferation (Ikuta *et al* 1985), encephalitogenic T lines must have been derived from clonal progenitors that pre-existed, without doing harm, in the donor's normal immune system. In fact, central nervous system-specific autoimmune T-cell clones have been demonstrated even more directly in healthy immune repertoires. Encephalitogenic T cells were first isolated from completely naive, nonimmunized Lewis rats. Their

myelin basic protein-specific T cells shared all functional and structural properties with conventional T-cell lines extracted from preimmunized animals. They were CD4$^+$, recognized the same peptide epitopes presented in an identical MHC class II antigen context, and used similar T-cell receptors. Most importantly, myelin basic protein-reactive T cells from naive rats roll out the same encephalitogenic potential as T cells derived from presensitized animals (Schlüsener and Wekerle 1985).

The existence of potentially autoaggressive T-cell clones in healthy immune systems is a general phenomenon, not restricted to myelin-specific T cells or Lewis rats. T-cell lines recognizing a virtually unlimited range of organ-specific autoantigens – including synovial, thyroid, retinal and pancreatic determinants (Cohen and Miller 1994) – have been raised in rodents by many laboratories. Encephalitogenic, myelin basic protein-specific T-cell lines were established from naive monkeys (Genain *et al* 1994; Meinl *et al* 1997) and similar T cells abound in the immune system of healthy human donors (see below). The relative number of myelin basic protein autoreactive T cells in immune compartments of naive rats is not known. There is, however, evidence that their concentration in the thymus is considerably higher than in peripheral immune organs (Lannes-Vieira *et al* 1995). One could argue that the frequency of myelin basic protein-specific T cells in the peripheral immune repertoire is insufficient to mount a spontaneous lifelong autoimmune attack. This, however, would not be the case in transgenic mice with myelin basic protein-specific TCR transgenes. The immune repertoires of these mice comprise >70% myelin basic protein-specific T cells and yet, kept under clean conditions, very few of these animals ever develop spontaneous experimental autoimmune encephalomyelitis (Goverman *et al* 1993). We argue later that regulatory control mechanisms seem to guarantee the nonreactivity of these potentially autoreactive T cells.

Thymic generation of the myelin autoreactive T-cell repertoire

It has been known for a long time that experimental autoimmune encephalomyelitis can be actively induced only in animals with an intact thymus. Thymectomized or congenitally athymic rodents fail to develop disease upon encephalitogenic immunization (Ortiz-Ortiz and Weigle 1976), although they are fully susceptible to experimental autoimmune encephalomyelitis transferred by activated myelin basic protein-specific CD4$^+$ helper T lymphocytes (Hinrichs and Humphres 1983). We have noted that the thymus affects susceptibility to autoimmune diseases (including experimental autoimmune encephalomyelitis) by controlling the development of mature immunocompetent T cells and eliminating many autoreactive T cells from the repertoire. Traditional theories explain tolerance by physical deletion of self-reactive lymphocytes from the immune repertoire – best guaranteed by the absence of a potentially autoreactive T-cell clone. Thereafter, the induction of autoimmune disease would depend on complex mechanisms, including pathological mutation of forbidden clones (Burnet 1959), or *de novo* exposure of sequestered autoantigens.

There is little doubt that deletion of self-reactive T-cell clones is a developmental feature of the immune repertoire. In transgenic mice with a self-reactive T-cell receptor, most T cells are removed during intrathymic development upon contact with the relevant autoantigen (von Boehmer *et al* 1989). More recent work has qualified that position. Self, presented in the context of MHC, plays a role in the positive selection of T-cell clones responding with low avidity. Conversely, the same peptide–MHC antigen product seems to select against T-cell clones with high avidity antigen receptors (Jameson *et al* 1995). Why then would brain-specific T-cell clones escape negative selection? The obvious explanation is clonal ignorance. It might be assumed that encephalitogenic proteins are localized exclusively within the central nervous system parenchyma, an immune privileged location secluded from the periphery by the intact blood–brain barrier (Wekerle *et al* 1986). In that situation, brain autoantigen would fail to reach the thymus and negative selection would not occur. Reality is, however, more complicated. Surprisingly, many encephalitogenic proteins are identified in thymic compartments. The first examples were unusual isoforms of myelin basic protein ('golli-protein'), a component of myelin appearing during postnatal development and in the thymus before birth as mRNA (Grima *et al* 1992; Pribyl *et al* 1993) and protein (Mathisen *et al* 1993). Myelin basic protein is by no means the only encephalitogen expressed in the thymus. Proteolipid protein has also been observed (Pribyl *et al* 1996), apparently within thymic macrophages. Furthermore, the calcium-binding S100b protein of astrocytes, the target autoantigen of an astrocyte directed experimental autoimmune encephalomyelitis model (Kojima *et al* 1994), is also expressed within the healthy adult thymus, where it directly coexists with S100b-specific encephalitogenic T-cell clones (Kojima *et al* 1997). Thus, the mere presence of autoantigen in the thymus by no means rules out the generation of autoimmune T-cell clones and their emigration to the periphery.

Encephalitogenic T cells must slip through a gap in the thymic negative-selection meshwork. While it is not clear how the cells manoeuvre their escape, there is evidence in favour of active central nervous system autoantigen-directed negative selection within the thymus. In the SJL mouse, the thymus mainly produces only the short isoform of proteolipid protein, DM-20, and not full-length protein. Most T cells recognizing DM-20 epitopes are retained in the thymus, whereas T cells specific for epitopes located on the extra sequences of full-length proteolipid protein, not covered by DM-20, reach the peripheral immune repertoire in substantial numbers (A.C. Anderson *et al* 2000; L. Klein *et al* 2000). Evidence from mice that lack particular myelin proteins due to natural mutation or transgenic inactivation complements these data. PLPI knockout mice lacking the entire proteolipid protein gene, and thus not expressing any protein variant in the central nervous system and thymus, display a much broader myelin protein-specific T-cell repertoire than wild-type animals (L. Klein *et al* 2000). Similar observations are available in myelin oligodendrocyte glycoprotein knockout (Delarasse *et al* 2003) and *shiverer* mutant mice, deficient in myelin basic protein (Targoni and Lehmann 1998). Both murine variants possess higher numbers and broader repertoires of myelin oligodendrocyte glycoprotein or myelin basic protein-specific T-cell clones.

The thymus should not, however, be viewed simply as a filter holding back (many) autoimmune T-cell clones. It plays an additional role in shaping the autoimmune T-cell receptor repertoire. Myelin basic protein-specific T cells in the Lewis rat use a very particular set of T-cell receptors. Instead of utilizing a broad set of available V genes, most cells are restricted to the Vβ8.2 gene along with a narrow spectrum of J chain genes. Unusually, most receptors have an exceptionally short MHC/peptide-binding segment (CDR3). The formation of this biased T-cell receptor repertoire depends on an intact, natural thymus. The chimeric thymus, composed experimentally of lymphocytes and dendritic cells from Lewis rats but epithelium from another animal, produces myelin basic protein-specific T cells that are fully functional but do not show the Vβ8.2 bias, and their complementarity-determining region 3 sequences are of conventional lengths (Wekerle *et al* 1996).

What could be the role of self-reactive T cells in the healthy immune system? Is their presence just the reflection of a porous regulatory mechanism? Or, could autoreactive T lymphocytes exert a positive homeostatic function, as postulated in the concept of the immunological homunculus (I.R. Cohen 1992)? The evidence supports a positive function for naturally self-reactive T cells – especially in tissue regeneration. Through their self-reactive receptors, lymphocytes are able to identify specific tissues, especially those undergoing degenerative or inflammatory changes, and provide molecules – such as neurotrophins – that mediate repair (Kerschensteiner *et al* 2003). Such beneficial autoimmunity has been proposed as a treatment (Schwartz and Kipnis 2001). These are evidently properties of autoreactive CD4$^+$ T lymphocytes, but it is not yet known whether cytotoxic CD8$^+$ T cells also participate in tissue regeneration.

Myelin-specific T-cell clones in the human immune repertoire

The existence of myelin-specific T-cell clones in the healthy immune repertoire is by no means a curiosity peculiar to rodent immune repertoires. The human immune system shows even higher proportions of myelin basic protein-specific T-cell lines (Burns *et al* 1983; Ota *et al* 1990; Pette *et al* 1990a). The data indicate that, with few exceptions, all are CD4$^+$ helper T lymphocytes recognizing autoantigenic epitopes with molecular restriction by DR products of the class II MHC, often of the DR2 haplotype (DRB1*1501 and DRB5*0101: Martin *et al* 1990; Ota *et al* 1990; Pette *et al* 1990b) . However, it should be noted that, in principle, every haplotype may act as an antigen-restricting element. In addition to DR, myelin basic protein presentation is described in the context of DQ and DP (Martin *et al* 1992a).

The cytokine patterns secreted by myelin basic protein-specific human T cells correspond to the Th1 subset of CD4$^+$ T cells. Upon antigen-dependent activation, these cells release large amounts of IL-2, IFN-γ and TNF-α (Voskuhl *et al* 1993). The Th1-like nature of human myelin basic protein-specific T cells has been confirmed by immunospot assays determining the cytokine release pattern of individually plated T lymphocytes (T. Olsson *et al* 1990b). An analysis of myelin basic protein-reactive T cells in the context of multiple sclerosis shows differences between cases and controls. These T cells have higher IFN-γ and IL-4 production, but do not polarize towards a distinct Th1 or Th2 profile, and clones produce IL-2, IL-4, TNF-α, IFN-γ and IL-10 but not IL-6 (Hermans *et al* 1997). As in the Lewis rat, many if not all human myelin basic protein-specific CD4$^+$ T-helper lymphocytes are in fact efficient cytotoxic killer cells. They destroy any antigen-presenting cell displaying myelin basic protein peptides in the appropriate MHC context (Martin *et al* 1990; J.R. Richert *et al* 1989; J. Zhang *et al* 1992).

The human T-cell repertoire contains not only clones reactive against myelin basic protein, but virtually all central nervous system autoantigens tested. Several groups have described healthy donor-derived T-cell lines specific for myelin oligodendrocyte glycoprotein (Lindert *et al* 1999), 2',3'-cyclic nucleotide 3'-phosphodiesterase (CNPase: Rösener *et al* 1997) and proteolipid protein (Markovic-Plese *et al* 1995; Ohashi *et al* 1995).

Autoantigen recognition by central nervous system-specific T cells

The isolation of central nervous system autoantigen-specific T cells from human donors has raised enormous hopes for a better understanding of the autoimmune pathogenesis and, implicitly, for the design of new, specific and efficient immune therapies. The study of such T cells should help elucidate the precise mechanisms of autoantigen recognition, the first critical step leading to the development of the inflammatory lesion. Then, therapies interfering with this recognition could be developed and used to curb ongoing plaque formation in the initial stage.

The dynamics of T-cell recognition: epitope and determinant spreading in experimental autoimmune encephalomyelitis

Comparison of myelin basic protein-specific T-cell lines isolated from primed or naive Lewis rats reveals that the overwhelming majority recognize the sequence p68–86 in the context of the RT1.A^l MHC class II product (Vandenbark *et al* 1985). Indeed, this is the fragment found to possess the strongest encephalitogenic potential in earlier active immunization experiments (Kibler *et al* 1977). A second, minor epitope at position p85–99 is presented in the Lewis rat in the context of an alternative MHC class II product, RT1.D^l. Immunization with intact myelin basic protein very rarely activates T cells specific for p85–99, but these can readily be selected after priming with this peptide. p85–99, is thus defined as a cryptic epitope (Mor and Cohen 1995).

To a greater or lesser extent, epitope dominance in encephalitogenic T-cell responses is seen in many experimental systems. There is considerable epitope dominance in experimental autoimmune encephalomyelitis induced by myelin basic protein in PL/J mice (and other strains exhibiting H-2^u). Most myelin basic protein-specific T cells from PL/J mice recognize the acetylated form of p1–11, with a minority responding to an epitope on p35–47 (Zamvil and Steinman 1990). The important encephalitogenic response of C57BL mice against myelin oligodendrocyte glycoprotein seems to be dominated by sequence 35–55, positioned on the extracellular portion of the molecule (Mendel *et al* 1995). The myelin basic protein epitope spectrum is, however, considerably broader in the SJL/J mouse, with multiple determinants nested in the central and N-terminal portions of the protein. Furthermore, in most rodents tested, the T-cell response against the second classic encephalitogenic myelin protein – proteolipid lipoprotein – is dissipated amongst several epitopes (Greer *et al* 1996), as is the response to myelin oligodendrocyte glycoprotein (Amor *et al* 1994).

The epitope response pattern in encephalitogenic T-cell responses is remarkably dynamic. In a landmark paper, Lehmann *et al* (1993) concluded that Ac1-11 is dominant only during the early active phase of experimental autoimmune encephalomyelitis in PL/J mice immunized against myelin basic protein. After remission and with the onset of chronic disease, additional but normally cryptic epitopes seem to be newly recognized by freshly recruited T cells – a phenomenon now known as determinant spreading and reported in the Lewis rat by some (Mor and Cohen 1993) but not all (Y. Matsumoto and Abo 1994) investigators. Although similar observations have been made in diabetes mellitus (D.L. Kaufman *et al* 1993; Tisch *et al* 1993), the universality of this phenomenon in autoimmune reactions remains to be established. What can be said is that similar broadening of epitope recognition is not seen in response to foreign antigens (Gammon *et al* 1990).

There is no ultimate explanation for intramolecular determinant spreading, and its relevance for the dynamics of relapse and remission is still debated. As we discuss below, it is possible that the first wave of encephalitogenic T cells, specific for the initially dominant epitope, enter the central nervous system parenchyma and are there eliminated by apoptosis. As a replacement, T cells recognizing minor or cryptic determinants then expand and dominate the demonstrable repertoire (J. Bauer *et al* 1995). Other hypotheses should also be considered. In fact, several reports highlight the late appearance of T cells reacting against proteolipid protein-induced chronic relapsing models of experimental autoimmune encephalomyelitis (L.L. Perry *et al* 1991). This *trans*-molecular determinant spreading is best explained by *de novo* immunization of T-cell populations as a consequence of local inflammatory responses. In this situation, primary encephalitogenic T cells could invade the central nervous system and trigger an inflammatory autoimmune attack, creating a proinflammatory milieu in which local debris is taken up by antigen-presenting cells (microglia, immigrant macrophages or dendritic cells) and offered to T cells already responsive to additional autoantigens (Vanderlugt and Miller 2002). In models of chronic relapsing experimental autoimmune encephalomyelitis, relapses can be stopped by treatments that block costimulatory receptors. Blindfolding B7-1 structures by blocking antibodies abrogates relapses and stops epitope spreading (S.D. Miller *et al* 1995b). Activation of B7-1 has the opposite effect (Vanderlugt *et al* 1997). It will be important for understanding relapses in multiple sclerosis to learn whether a causal relationship exists between epitope spreading and new episodes.

Human T-cell reactivity against brain autoantigens

The brain proteins known to provoke experimental autoimmune encephalomyelitis responses in animals have been examined for their immunogenicity to immune cells harvested from patients with multiple sclerosis. Myelin basic protein was the first brain autoantigen to be investigated. This putative autoantigen owes its candidature (and hence its devoted popularity amongst neuroimmunologists) to several properties. It is a small protein (main isoform about 18.5 kDa) positioned on the inner surface of the myelin membrane (see Chapter 10) but quantitatively a major component of the myelin membrane (30–40% dry weight). Due to its basic charge and solubility in water, it is easy to isolate to purity – in contrast to most other myelin proteins, which are either highly lipophilic or only minor components of myelin. Early attempts to study myelin basic protein reactivity in samples from patients with multiple sclerosis relied on simple proliferation or cytokine release tests confronting peripheral blood lymphocytes from patients or healthy control donors with purified antigen *in vitro*. The results of primary response assays were, however, often ambiguous or hardly reproducible despite the best efforts of competent investigators. It is now clear that simple bulk proliferation assays are not sufficiently sensitive to detect subtle differences in the myelin-specific repertoire of patients with multiple sclerosis. Detailed study of the disease-specific immune reactivity to brain determinants requires a technology allowing a large number of autoantigen-specific T-cell lines to be isolated from each patient. This has become possible with the development of the split-well cloning system, in which a primary limiting dilution approach allows the selection of mono- or oligoclonal T-cell lines from freshly isolated peripheral blood lymphocytes (Figure 11.11: Pette *et al* 1990a; 1990b). The principle is simple. Peripheral blood mononuclear cells are distributed into multiple microcultures containing decremental cell numbers. Addition of the putative autoantigen results in the activation and proliferation of individual autoreactive T cells contained within each well. At limiting (low) cell dilutions, some but not all parallel cultures respond by cell division. Initially, selectively presented antigen drives proliferation, but later this is sustained by cytokines such as IL-2. Microcultures containing a proliferating lymphocyte colony are selected and transferred in equal parts (split) to two culture wells. Autoantigen is added only to one split well. Colonies that require the presence of autoantigen for their further proliferation are, by definition, selected and propagated as autoantigen-specific T-cell lines. Often, but not always, this response takes its origin in the multiplication of one autoantigen-responsive T cell contained within the originally seeded lymphocyte population. In this case, the resulting cell line is truly monoclonal.

In terms of their membrane phenotype and cytokine secretion pattern, human peripheral blood-derived myelin basic protein-specific T lymphocytes closely resemble their rodent counter-parts. However, they differ strikingly in their interactions with target autoantigen. Epitope recognition pattern and T-cell receptor repertoire usage are much more complex in human than rodent T-cell responses. Whilst the myelin basic protein response in the Lewis rat focuses on a narrow segment of the molecule, the variety of epitopes recognized by human T cells is remarkably broad. The large body of data can be summarized: each individual human immune system contains T cells recognizing many epitopes distributed along the entire myelin basic protein molecule; any given MHC class II product (e.g. the DR2 molecule) can bind and present a variety of peptides (Wucherpfennig *et al* 1994a). Conversely, most peptides actually bind to different DR molecules and can therefore be presented in varied contexts (Martin *et al* 1991; Valli *et al* 1993); lastly, the central segment p87–106 and the C-terminal sequence p144–163 show relative immunodominance, recruiting more specific T-cell lines than most other segments (Martin *et al* 1992b; Ota *et al* 1990; Pette *et al* 1990b).

The epitope pattern characteristically found in the majority of human blood donors (with or without multiple sclerosis) showing reactivity to myelin basic protein is broad but not completely random. In a study of monozygotic twins, for example, disease concordant pairs showed remarkably uniform epitope recognition patterns, whilst there was more discrepancy between discordant twins (Utz *et al* 1993). Perhaps even more striking, and much in contrast to the majority of human anti-myelin T-cell repertoires, there is a small number of patients with multiple sclerosis who display an anti-myelin basic protein T-cell response focused against a narrow, dominant peptide segment reminiscent of the Lewis rat. Meinl *et al* (1993) describe a set of patients whose T lymphocytes (represented by panels of CD4[+] T-cell lines) almost exclusively recognize epitope(s) nested within one narrow myelin basic protein sequence – in one case with stability over 7 years. Similar patterns have been described in other patients using T-cell cloning (Lovett-Racke *et al* 1997; Salvetti *et al* 1993; Wucherpfennig *et al* 1994a), and polymerase chain reaction-based spectratype analyses (Goebels *et al* 2000; Muraro *et al* 2003; Musette *et al* 1996). The nature of these unusual human T-cell responses is obscure. They certainly do not result from isolated proliferation *in vivo* of one single T-cell clone, as indicated by T-cell receptor sequence analyses. However, some unrecognized antigen-driven oligoclonal proliferation event is not entirely excluded.

In multiple sclerosis, reactivity to the other mass protein of myelin, proteolipid protein, was first demonstrated using the immunospot assay. Olsson *et al* (1990b) reported a relative increase of reactivity to this and myelin basic protein, showing the presence of IFN-γ-secreting T cells both in peripheral blood and cerebrospinal fluid from patients with multiple sclerosis. Greer *et al* (1997) reported that immunodominant reactivity of peripheral blood mononuclear cells to proteolipid protein in patients with relapsing or progressive multiple sclerosis is confined to two overlapping peptides (PLP$_{184–199}$ and PLP$_{190–209}$) – these responses increase with disease duration and disability. At present, the number of antigen-specific T cells remains far lower than the availability of myelin basic protein-reactive T-cell lines, thereby limiting the opportunity to evaluate epitope dominance and T-cell receptor utilization. However, thus far, there is no evidence for unusual characteristics in proteolipid protein-specific human T-cell repertoires. And, most importantly, none

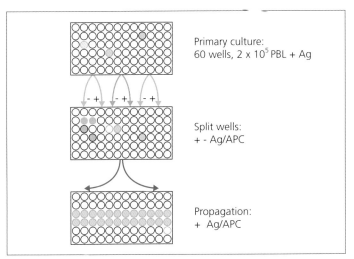

Figure 11.11 Establishment of autoantigen-specific oligoclonal T-cell lines (clonoids) by primary limiting dilution (split-well method). Ag = antigen; APC = antigen-presenting cell.

Primary culture:
60 wells, 2 x 10^5 PBL + Ag

Split wells:
+ - Ag/APC

Propagation:
+ Ag/APC

of the reported features is specific for multiple sclerosis. All this is reminiscent of investigations into myelin basic protein-specific T cells. Proteolipid protein-specific T cells mainly secrete the Th1 cytokine profile (Correale *et al* 1995a). Those harvested from patients with multiple sclerosis seem to express IL-2 receptors (J. Zhang *et al* 1994), have a broad spectrum of epitope recognition (Markovic-Plese *et al* 1995; Ohashi *et al* 1995), and offer no evidence for highly dominant T-cell receptor V gene usage (Kondo *et al* 1996).

A particularly intriguing candidate autoantigen in multiple sclerosis is myelin oligodendrocyte glycoprotein, first identified independently by Linington *et al* (1984) and Lebar *et al* (1986) as a minor myelin component exclusively located within the central nervous system. Two properties make it a particularly interesting molecule. First, the gene for myelin oligodendrocyte glycoprotein maps to the MHC (Pham-Dinh *et al* 1993). Secondly, it is an unusual member of the immunoglobulin super-gene family with a long extracellular domain that can readily be accessed by humoral mediators of immunity (Kroepfl *et al* 1996). Myelin oligodendrocyte glycoprotein-specific humoral antibodies thus can readily bind myelin membranes, and in cooperation with complement components and/or Fc-receptor bearing phagocytes, propagate large areas of demyelination (Linington *et al* 1988; Schlüsener *et al* 1987). In addition, myelin oligodendrocyte glycoprotein possesses highly autoimmunogenic T- and B-cell epitopes. In rodents, immunization with myelin oligodendrocyte glycoprotein peptides or recombinant protein causes activation of encephalitogenic T and B cells, mediating a disease that, in its similarity to multiple sclerosis, is strikingly distinct from myelin basic protein-induced experimental autoimmune encephalomyelitis (Johns *et al* 1995; Kerlero de Rosbo *et al* 1995).

The few reports on human myelin oligodendrocyte glycoprotein-specific T cells have raised considerable interest. In contrast to other brain autoantigens, their reactivity in patients with multiple sclerosis has been shown by primary proliferation responses *in vitro*. In one study using native myelin oligodendrocyte glycoprotein, proliferation responses were consistently stronger in T cells from patients with multiple sclerosis than from matched healthy donors (Kerlero de Rosbo *et al* 1993). While the original testing was done using native, brain-derived myelin oligodendrocyte glycoprotein, these findings were repeated using recombinant material (Kerlero de Rosbo *et al* 1997). Similar findings come from immunospot studies detecting cytokine release from myelin oligodendrocyte glycoprotein-specific T lymphocytes and specific autoantibodies from B cells. In both cases, the frequencies of positive lymphocytes were enhanced in peripheral blood mononuclear lymphocytes and cerebrospinal fluid from patients with multiple sclerosis (J. Sun *et al* 1991b). Definitive investigation of myelin oligodendrocyte glycoprotein-reactive immune cells appears hopeful but awaits confirmation by larger collections of cell lines and experiments.

Is there any evidence for epitope spreading in human T cells, as in rodent models of myelin autoimmunity? In principle, owing to the generally unfocused human anti-myelin response patterns, it is technically difficult to identify true epitope spreading over time. In some patients, however, epitope recognition is subject to marked changes. The number of epitopes recognized may increase but, in other cases, the range contracts (Goebels *et al* 2000; Mazza *et al* 2002; Tuohy *et al* 1998) and

epitope dynamics are often unconnected to the clinical course of multiple sclerosis (Ristori *et al* 2000). This may come as no surprise since, to date, the pathogenic target autoantigen in patients is itself unidentified. Thus, no clear linkage exists between epitope patterns and clinical courses in multiple sclerosis.

Myelin-specific T-cell receptors

Isolation of encephalitogenic T-lymphocyte lines from immune organs or central nervous system infiltrates of autoimmune rats using the protocol developed by Ben-Nun *et al* (1981a) paved the way for studies of the myelin autoimmune T-cell receptor repertoire. The initial descriptions were tantalizing. Myelin basic protein T cells both in Lewis rats and PL/J (or B10PL) mice used, almost uniformly, the Vβ8.2 gene along with a very narrow spectrum of Vα genes, and peculiar short complementarity-determining region 3 sequences. In particular, the preferential usage of Vβ8.2 by encephalitogenic T cells in diverse animals led to a 'V region disease hypothesis', which predicted selective use of particular T-cell receptor V genes in autoimmune disease (Heber-Katz and Acha-Orbea 1989). It later turned out that dominance of individual Vβ genes is the exception rather than the rule. In particular, the gene repertoire required to form functional T-cell receptors on human myelin basic protein-specific T lymphocytes is very broad and does not duplicate at all the unique arrangements of the Lewis rat. This may look unfortunate to creative therapists, because lack of T-cell receptor restriction undermines vaccination strategies directed at T-cell receptors or blocking of responses using peptides and small molecules (see Chapter 18).

The myelin-specific T-cell receptor repertoire in experimental autoimmune encephalomyelitis

The first studies of T-cell receptors used for recognition of central nervous system autoantigens were carried out using myelin basic protein-specific encephalitogenic T-cell clones isolated from Lewis rats. These indicated that anti-central nervous system autoimmune responses were characterized by their monotonous character and restriction to a minority of receptor subtypes. Thus, the Lewis rat T-cell response against myelin basic protein utilizes a strikingly simplified repertoire of structural genes. The earliest studies of myelin basic protein-specific T-cell receptors noted an almost complete utilization of Vβ8.2 genes, often combined with a limited set of Jβ elements (Burns *et al* 1989; Chluba *et al* 1989), and paired with an equally restricted repertoire of Vα genes. Most myelin basic protein T-cell receptors have complementarity-determining region 3 sequences – the receptor segments primarily dictating peptide specificity – encoded by unusually short base sequences (Kääb *et al* 1998; G. Kim *et al* 1998; X-M. Zhang and Heber-Katz 1992). Furthermore, myelin basic protein-specific complementarity-determining region 3 sequences are dominated by the Asp-Ser sequence, and they have a deficit of N-region inserts (Gold *et al* 1991; X-M. Zhang and Heber-Katz 1992). All these peculiarities are seen not only in T-cell lines isolated from myelin basic protein-primed rats but also in lines cloned out from naive Lewis rat thymus (Lannes-Vieira *et al* 1995). Short, N-insert-deficient complementarity-determining region 3 sequences are typical of immature T-cell responses (Bogue *et al* 1991). Strongly biased use of Vβ8.2 genes for myelin basic protein-specific T-cell receptors is also the rule in PL/J and B10.LP mice, both having the H-2ᵘ haplotype (Acha-Orbea *et al* 1988; Urban *et al* 1988).

The dominant use of Vβ8.2 and biased occurrence of one simple complementarity-determining region sequence motif in the encephalitogenic T-cell response raised high expectations for immunospecific therapy of brain autoimmunity. But, disappointingly, this seems to be an exception and not the rule. Even in the Lewis rat, Vβ8.2 dominance changes over time. It is strict in early phases of the encephalitogenic response but has a tendency to dissipate over time (Offner *et al* 1993). Furthermore, this bias seems restricted to T-cell responses against the dominant epitope p68–84 and not minor encephalitogenic determinants (Offner *et al* 1992; D. Sun *et al* 1992), or truncated versions of the dominant peptide where loss of a few key amino acids completely alters the Vβ8.2 focus (D. Sun *et al* 1995). Encephalitogenic T-cell responses have been analysed in many species and with many brain components as target autoantigens. Most data indicate diversity for T-cell receptor repertoires other than those directed at myelin basic protein. This applies especially to proteolipid protein (Kuchroo *et al* 1992) and myelin oligodendrocyte glycoprotein (Mendel *et al* 1996).

Autoantigen-reactive T-cell receptors in the human repertoire

Initial studies based on a limited number of myelin basic protein-specific T-cell lines suggested that preferential T-cell receptor gene usage is not uncommon, at least within the repertoire of an individual patient (Ben-Nun *et al* 1991; Kotzin *et al* 1991; Wucherpfennig *et al* 1990). Careful scrutiny of the accumulated data, however, does not show much conformity in T-cell receptor gene dominance or clonal expansion amongst patients with multiple sclerosis (Figure 11.12: Hafler *et al* 1996). Overall, there is no generally applicable and multiple sclerosis-associated T-cell receptor-α/β gene usage (comparable to Vβ8.2 in the Lewis rat or PL/J mouse). Furthermore, this repertoire is not fixed, as indicated by studies of bone-marrow transplant recipients (Muraro *et al* 2005). Whilst some studies indicate enhanced usage of certain Vβ genes (Vβ5.2 and Vβ6.1 in one study of T-cell lines: Kotzin *et al* 1991) in polymerase chain reaction material amplified from the lesions of multiple sclerosis (Oksenberg *et al* 1993), similar genes are not strikingly dominant in other series (Hafler *et al* 1996). Broad usage of the V gene repertoire has also been noted in T-cell line aggregates sorted for recognition of individual peptide epitopes and/or class II restricting elements (such as DR2 related molecules; Hafler *et al* 1996; Meinl *et al* 1993). In a few individuals, several independently isolated T-cell lines use the same receptor – based on identical complementarity-determining region 3 sequences – indicating clonal expansion that appears stable over years (Meinl *et al* 1993; Wucherpfennig *et al* 1994b).

Are the few putatively expanded T-cell clones related to the pathogenesis of multiple sclerosis? How might they change during clinical relapse? Would they expand further or, conversely, be eliminated? Would their elimination by therapeutic manipulation (T-cell receptor peptide therapies) demonstrably affect the clinical course of multiple sclerosis? These questions all remain to be answered, but the available results do not seem sufficiently coherent to advance strong guidelines for T cell-specific therapies. Antigen specificity of the T-cell receptor is mediated by the hypervariable complementarity-determining region 3 segment, which contacts antigenic peptide embedded within the central groove of the MHC product (Y. Li *et al* 2000; 2001; K.J. Smith *et al* 1998). The complementarity-determining region 3 sequence thus strongly determines peptide specificity of a T lymphocyte. Are there complementarity-determining region 3 sequence motifs related to recognition of myelin basic protein fragments? There is indirect evidence for structural sequence-specific constraints. One example is provided by two T-cell lines isolated from different individuals (one with multiple sclerosis and one healthy), each displaying the same unusual fine specificity. Both lines recognized the myelin basic protein peptide (p139–153) when presented either in the context of DR2 (DRB1*1501) or DR1 (DRB1*0101) using β chains identical at the protein, though not at the mRNA, level (Giegerich *et al* 1992). Obviously, it is tempting to relate the fine specificity of these cell lines to their T-cell receptor β-chain sequence and, more specifically, to the identical complementarity-determining region 3 sequence region.

Unfortunately, the search for sequence motifs predicting myelin basic protein epitope specificity is not yet conclusive. In one intriguing study, a T-cell receptor sequence (Vβ5.2-LRGA) amplified from post-mortem brain tissue had been previously found in a myelin basic protein-specific T-cell line from a different individual with multiple sclerosis (Oksenberg *et al* 1993). However, this identity may be an exceptional phenomenon. Most myelin-related motifs were identified by their similarity to complementarity-determining region 3 sequences from Lewis rat T cells, which recognize myelin basic protein peptides embedded in rat, not human, MHC class II proteins. Interestingly, myelin-related sequence motifs were noted in a panel of T cells selected from the blood of patients with multiple sclerosis for somatic mutation in the *hprt* (hypoxanthine guanine phosphoribosyltransferase) gene, a marker of extensive prior cell proliferation (see below; Allegretta *et al* 1990; Lodge *et al* 1995). This would indeed possibly relate myelin basic protein reactivity of CD4⁺ T cells to ongoing clonal expansion. On the other hand, at least two of the putative myelin basic protein-related complementarity-determining region 3 motifs (LRG, LGG) were also seen in a study of T cell receptors from peripheral blood-isolated CD8⁺ T lymphocytes of patients with multiple sclerosis (Monteiro *et al* 1996). Several studies have been performed of T-cell receptor repertoires selected in response to antigens other than myelin basic protein. In the case of anti-proteolipid protein, one study observed a broad V gene utilization (Correale *et al* 1995b), whereas a more restricted, epitope-related pattern was noted in another ethnically distinct population (Kondo *et al* 1996). Also the myelin basic protein-specific T-cell repertoire seems to use a broad spectrum of T-cell receptor V genes (Lindert *et al* 1999; Van der Aa *et al* 2003).

Over the past few years, new molecular approaches have evolved that are poised to illuminate the immune pathogenesis of multiple sclerosis. 'Humanized' transgenic mice have been constructed, with transgene inserts encoding key elements of the human myelin basic protein-specific T-cell recognition machinery – the two paired T-cell receptor chains, the peptide-presenting MHC class II protein (DR2), and the human coreceptor molecule

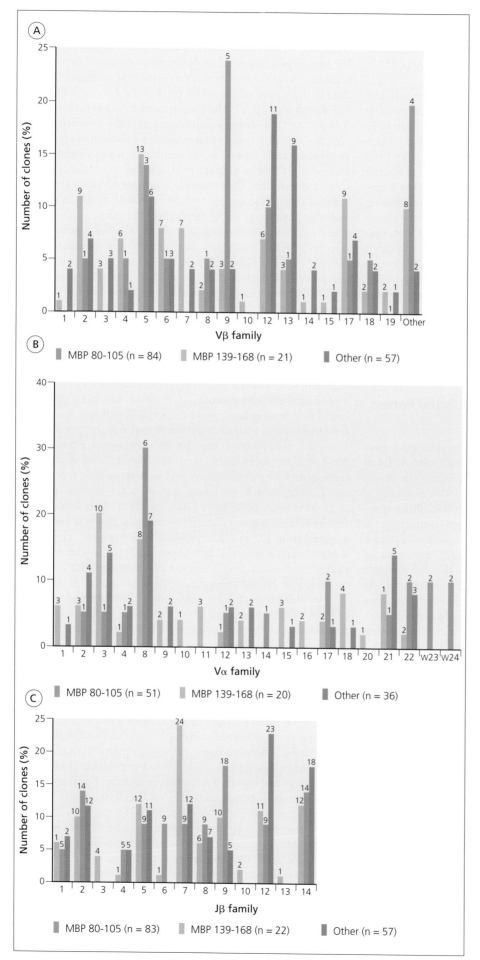

Figure 11.12 T-cell receptor genes used by human myelin basic protein-specific T-cell lines. (A) Analysis of Vβ family usage in human T-cell clones reactive to various myelin basic protein epitopes. Human myelin basic protein-reactive clones were grouped according to antigen fine specificity into three general categories: '80–105' includes clones reactive to 80–99, 80–105, 84–102, and 86–105; '139–168' includes clones reactive to 139–153, 143–168 and 152–162; 'other' includes clones reactive to all other epitopes. The number of clones in each category is indicated. (B) Analysis of Vα family usage in human T-cell clones reactive to various myelin basic protein epitopes. (C) Analysis of Jβ family usage in human T-cell clones reactive to various myelin basic protein epitopes. All three results show that there are no significant differences between groups. Adapted from Hafler *et al* (1996). © 1996, with permission from Elsevier.

CD4 (Madsen *et al* 1999). The behavioural properties of these triple transgene mice mimic transgenic mice with a murine anti-myelin basic protein T-cell receptor. About 5% of otherwise normal mice expressing this T-cell receptor develop spontaneous experimental autoimmune encephalomyelitis. In contrast, virtually all T-cell receptor transgenic mice bred on an immunodeficient, *RAG* knockout background become spontaneously unwell. Presumably, these lack the regulatory cells that prevent most autoreactive T cells from mounting autoimmune injury in wild-type animals.

'Spectratyping' – a polymerase chain reaction-based technique – allows the identification of individual T-cell clone expansions within immune populations, and permits the fate of such clones to be followed in individual patients over time. The method makes use of the highly variable lengths of MHC/peptide-recognizing T-cell receptor-αβ complementarity-determining region 3 regions, selecting individual sequences, depicting the relevant transcripts as individual peaks within the overall spectrum, and mapping these sequentially (Pannetier *et al* 1995). Musette *et al* (1996) first applied spectratyping to the study of myelin basic protein-specific T lymphocytes in patients with multiple sclerosis. They found complementarity-determining region 3 sequences suggestive of myelin basic protein specificity, and T cells bearing such receptors were expanded in some patients but not in matched controls. Spectratyping also documented the unusual longevity of myelin basic protein-specific T cells in patients with multiple sclerosis for up to seven years (Goebels *et al* 2000). Expanded cells were present both in peripheral blood and cerebrospinal fluid (Matsumoto *et al* 2003).

Very recently, a new tool became available to analyse T-cell function in fixed tissue preparations. 'Laser microdissection' allows the excision of single T cells from the lesions of multiple sclerosis. DNA segments and mRNA encoding both T-cell receptor chains of such individual cells can be amplified by combining complex elaborations of the polymerase chain reaction. The receptor genes can then be introduced into cell lines or even transgenic mice, thus making them accessible to study of their specificity and function. This approach literally permits the restoring to life of dead cells. To date, this has not only been restricted to the T-cell receptor β chain (Babbe *et al* 2000), but to the isolation of complete paired T-cell receptors of CD8 T cells infiltrating human multiple sclerosis brain tissue (Dornmair *et al* 2003).

Cytokine patterns of encephalitogenic T cells

Soon after their first description, encephalitogenic T lymphocytes sprung something of a surprise. Although clearly members of the CD4[+] helper T-cell subset, myelin basic protein-specific T-cell lines were shown to behave like CD8[+] cytotoxic killer lymphocytes. Encephalitogenic T cells effectively destroyed any cell presenting relevant myelin basic protein epitope in a recognizable fashion. Presentation was antigen dose-dependent, and restricted by the MHC class II product, RT1.B[1] (D. Sun and Wekerle 1986). This finding collided with the ruling dogma, but was seen with great regularity in most models of experimental autoimmune encephalomyelitis. Now, it is clear that classic encephalitogenic T cells are not only cytotoxic but also respond to activation by secreting IL-2 and IFN-γ (the Th1 response: Ando *et al* 1989).

It appears that the Th1-like cytokine pattern of encephalitogenic T cells is not merely associated with their pathogenic potential but may actually help generate the lesions (Table 11.2). Many current therapies for T-cell autoimmune disease are thus aimed at redirecting the Th1 cytokine production of autoreactive T cells to a Th2 profile. This can be achieved by changing the conditions of immune stimulation, presenting peptide variants rather than whole protein (Nicholson *et al* 1995), blocking costimulatory molecules (Khoury *et al* 1995), or changing modes of autoantigen administration through oral tolerance induction (Benson *et al* 2000; Y. Chen *et al* 1994). The nature of antigenic peptide presented by a suitable MHC protein determines polarity of the Th1 or Th2 immune response. This applies particularly to myelin protein fragments and potentially encephalitogenic T cells – a relationship that offers real therapeutic opportunities. Indeed, in experimental autoimmune encephalomyelitis models, sequence variants of encephalitogenic peptides have been successfully used to divert a pathogenic Th1 response to a protective Th2 orientation. Careful study of peptide interactions with MHC class II and the T-cell receptor surface, in experimental autoimmune encephalomyelitis induced by immunization against proteolipid protein peptide 139–151 in SJL mice, led to the discovery of an altered peptide ligand that is not only unable to induce experimental autoimmune encephalomyelitis but actively protects from experimental autoimmune encephalomyelitis induction. The altered peptide ligand acts by activating proteolipid protein-specific T cells to produce Th2, instead of Th1, cytokines (Nicholson *et al* 1995). A number of studies have confirmed the protective effects of altered peptides, including natural ligands (Ruiz *et al* 1999).

Needless to say, altered peptide ligand approaches have been translated into therapies for multiple sclerosis (see Chapter 18). Thus, a phase II trial of peptide 83–93, an analogue of myelin basic protein, showed positive effects in some patients (L. Kappos *et al* 2000), whereas other patients experienced exacerbations or hypersensitivity responses (Bielekova *et al* 2000). Clearly the best-known therapy based on altered peptide ligand peptide logic is glatiramer acetate or Copaxone, which behaves like a myelin basic protein altered peptide ligand, activating Th2 cells that may neutralize the activity of pathogenic myelin-specific Th1 lymphocytes (Duda *et al* 2000; Gran *et al* 2000b; Neuhaus *et al* 2000).

Other therapies aiming to drive Th1 to Th2 immune diversion include oral tolerization strategies (Bitar and Whitacre 1988; Higgins and Weiner 1988; Weiner 2000; Weiner *et al* 1993b). Oral application of myelin basic protein protects rats from subsequent attempts to induce experimental autoimmune encephalomyelitis. The mechanisms underlying oral tolerance induction include (in theory) deletion, anergy, regulation and activation of autoimmune T cells that secrete anti-inflammatory cytokines (IL-4, IL-10 and TGF-β) and therefore suppress the autoaggressive potential of Th1 effector T cells.

Maintenance and breakage of T-cell self-tolerance

It is difficult to understand in detail how the ability of autoreactive T cells to cause autoimmune disease is held in check so reliably. A number of distinct factors must cooperate normally to guarantee immunological health, and, conversely, more

Table 11.2 **Mediators associated with experimental autoimmune encephalomyelitis**

| Cytokines | Nature of association[a] | | Disease modulated by antibody or inhibitors (reference)* | |
	Active disease/ relapse (reference*)	Remission/ suppression (reference*)		
IL-1	+	*1	–	Yes	*22
IL-2	+	2,3	–	NR[b]	
IL-3	+	4	–	NR	
IL-4	–	+	–		
IL-6	+	1	–	NR	
IL-10	–	+	*1,5		
IL-12	+	5	–	Yes	12
IL-13	–	+	13		
IL-18	+	6	–	Yes	14
IFN-γ	+	1,3	+[c]	Yes[d]	3,15
TNF-α	+	1,5,7	–	Yes	16
LT-α	+	8	–	Yes	8
TGF-β	–	+	17,18		
IFN-α	?	+	19 (directly inhibited EAE)		
Chemokines[d]					
MCP-1	+	9	–	Yes	20,21
MIP-1α	+	9,10	–	Yes	10,20,21
MIP-1β	+	9	–	NR	
RANTES	+	9	–	No	20,21
IP-10	+	9	–	Yes	20
C10	+	11	–	NR	
MIP-2	–	–	10,20		
TCA-3	+[e]	9			

a References cited are as far as possible those that identified the mediators in question in the CNS, at or near sites of pathology, or reviews that summarize those data.

b NR: No reports.

c The viewpoint that IFN-γ suppresses experimental allergic encephalomyelitis is not consistent with recent data, but was a logical interpretation of antibody and knockout experiments in their time.

d The literature on this topic is broad, so only a few reviews have been cited.

e Association in this case was on the basis of expression by encephalitogenic T cells.

References: 1 = Okuda et al (1995); 2 = Litzenburger et al (1998); 3 = Owens et al (1994); 4 = Campbell et al (1998); 5 = Issazadeh et al (1995); 6 = Jander and Stoll (1998); 8 = Hjelstrom et al (1998); 9 = Stalder et al (1998); 10 = Karpus (1995); 11 = Bruce et al (1996); 12 = Leonard et al (1995); 13 = Cash et al (1994); 14 = Wildbaum et al (1998); 15 = Popko et al (1997); 16 = Selmaj and Raine (1995); 17 = Johns and Sriram (1993); 18 = Racke et al (1991); 19 = Billian et al (1988); 20 = Ransohoff (1999); 21 = Youssef et al (1998); 22 = Martin and Near (1995).

Reproduced from T. Owens et al (2001).

than one trigger is required for the development of a clinical autoimmune reaction. One essential prerequisite is activation of autoimmune T cells. Studies of experimental autoimmune encephalomyelitis proved that myelin basic protein-specific T cells only mediate autoimmune central nervous system inflammation after fresh activation. Resting cells neither reach nor attack their target tissue. However, lack of activation is probably not the only mechanism maintaining tolerance. There is additional, indirect evidence for active control through positive regulatory intercellular signals. For example, in rodent experimental autoimmune encephalomyelitis removal of CD8[+] T cells from mice by monoclonal antibody depletion (H. Jiang *et al* 1992) increases the incidence of spontaneous relapse, but does not interfere with recovery from the initial disease episode. Likewise, in transgenic mice lacking CD8[+] T cells, relapses in experimental autoimmune encephalomyelitis are more frequent than in control mice (Koh *et al* 1992). Also, relapses can be prompted by discontinuing immunosuppression previously achieved with ciclosporin A, which may result in an imbalance of immune regulatory circuits (Polman *et al* 1988). Formal demonstration of central nervous system-specific suppressor T-cell circuits has not been reported. Finally, spontaneous experimental autoimmune encephalomyelitis is rare in transgenic mice with myelin-specific T-cell receptors but otherwise intact immune systems; however, it happens regularly in mice having an immunodeficient genetic background.

We have to consider several mechanisms that could lead to autoimmune reactions. First, pathological mutation might lead to the appearance of forbidden lymphocyte clones in the immune repertoire. This is an improbable mechanism for T cells not using somatic mutation to shape their antigen receptors. A second possibility is the sudden gain of access to previously sequestered antigen. This can also be relegated to unimportant since most putatively sequestered antigens, including those encased within the central nervous system, turn out to be quite accessible. Accidental exposure, for example following central nervous system trauma, does not often result in autoimmune responses. More probable mechanisms revolve around activation, or derepression of self-reactive T cells. For example, microbial 'superantigens' have been shown semispecifically to activate relapses of experimental autoimmune encephalomyelitis (Brocke *et al* 1993; Schiffenbauer *et al* 1993). Next is antigenic mimicry of microbial structures sharing structural motifs with encephalitogenic proteins, thus engaging and activating the T-cell receptor. Fujinami and Oldstone (1985) showed that hepatitis virus polymerase shares the *aa* sequence with myelin basic protein and immunization with virus peptide caused experimental autoimmune encephalomyelitis in some rabbits. Finally, local microenvironments can be intensely stimulatory, using their cytokine content rather than specific cognate interactions to activate autoimmune T cells (Segal *et al* 1997).

Molecular mimicry

George Snell, the pioneer of MHC research and winner of the 1980 Nobel Prize for Physiology or Medicine, coined the concept of molecular mimicry. He reasoned that certain (viral) agents persist because they produce antigenic structures indistinguishable from self determinants and are thus invisible to immune cells. But what would happen if microbial antigen that mimicked self, activated potentially autoreactive immune cells? This scenario has long preoccupied immunologists. Originally, the search concentrated on contiguous peptide sequences shared between microbial and brain proteins (Jahnke *et al* 1985). Indeed, in their classic and often quoted study, Fujinami and Oldstone (1985) identified a peptide of hepatitis B virus polymerase sharing a contiguous sequence of six amino acids with myelin basic protein p69–75. Immunization of seven (outbred) rabbits against the viral peptide resulted in measurable anti-myelin basic protein antibody titres. Some animals had lymphocyte responses both to virus and myelin, and perivascular central nervous system infiltrates were observed at autopsy.

With improved understanding of antigen processing and presentation, it became clear that molecular mimicry at the T-cell level does not depend strictly and exclusively on the segregated identity of these two individual proteins. First, much rests on intracellular processing of (auto)antigenic proteins by the antigen-presenting cell. Intracellular proteases determine which particular peptides are excised from the parent protein and, among these, only those preferentially binding MHC products are selected for actual presentation on the membrane (Früh and Yang 1999; Geuze 1998; Villadangos and Ploegh 2000).

Sharing of MHC-binding motifs, and of structural profiles recognized by the T-cell receptor, is the basis for cross-reactivity. Thus, one investigation of synthetic peptide variants found that among the encephalitogenic peptides for PL/J mice (Ac1–11) only four amino acid positions are crucial for activation of encephalitogenic T cells, and with only two in continuity (Gautam *et al* 1994). Obviously, a multitude of microbial peptides could in theory fulfil these loose criteria but, as shown by other work, few qualify for a cross-stimulating mimicry reaction (Wucherpfennig 2001). Thus, mere structural resemblance is not sufficient for a peptide to qualify as a molecular agonist in central nervous system autoimmunity. Ideally, for this to be established, evidence that a given peptide will initiate experimental autoimmune encephalomyelitis (Gautam *et al* 1998), cross-prime an animal but fail directly to induce (Carrizosa *et al* 1998), or even protect against (Ruiz *et al* 1999), experimental autoimmune encephalomyelitis induction is required from direct testing in experimental models.

Two intriguing potential examples of molecular mimicry are mentioned here but also discussed in Chapters 2 and 5. Lang *et al* (2002) examined a cloned T-cell receptor previously considered simply to cross-recognize myelin basic protein (p85–99) and Epstein–Barr virus polymerase (p627–641) presented by the same human class II protein, DR2. However, the cross-reactive T-cell receptor turned out to recognize the two distinct peptides presented in separate molecular contexts – although each formed part of the DR2 haplotype – but nevertheless forming an antigenic surface complex that this T-cell receptor could not distinguish. Preliminary evidence from serology and cerebrospinal fluid suggested more often exposure to *Chlamydia pneumoniae* in people with multiple sclerosis compared with controls (Sriram *et al* 1999; S. Yao *et al* 2001), but this antibacterial response has been attributed to nonspecific polyclonal B-cell activation (Derfuss *et al* 2001; Gieffers *et al* 2001). Yet, *Chlamydia pneumoniae* does seem to affect anti-myelin autoimmune responses in rodent experimental autoimmune encephalomyelitis models. In the Lewis rat, immunization against a chlamydial peptide, which shares seven amino acid positions with a dominant myelin basic protein epitope, resulted in severe experimental autoimmune encephalomyelitis, suggesting a molecular mimicry response. Further, injection of living *Chlamydia pneumoniae* (but not other chlamydial organisms) into an autoimmunized mouse worsened the developing experimental autoimmune encephalomyelitis (Du *et al* 2002). And a crystallographic study of myelin-associated glycoprotein established structural similarity with a chlamydial protein of unknown function (Breithaupt *et al* 2003).

Finally, it should be pointed out that molecular mimicry is not limited to microbial antigens and autoantigens. In an intriguing set of studies, mimicry between a myelin autoantigen and nutritional milk component was found in the DA rat. Myelin-associated glycoprotein-specific encephalitogenic T cells recognized a peptide derived from butyrophilin, a component of cow's milk. Further immunization of these rats with butyrophilin led to mild experimental autoimmune encephalomyelitis, establishing symmetrical cross-reactivity between myelin and milk proteins (Stefferl *et al* 2000). Bovine butyrophilin, a member of a family of proteins that interestingly includes B7 costimulatory molecules (Tazi-Ahnini *et al* 1997), shares 50% sequence homology with the mouse myelin-associated glycoprotein extracellular domain (Gardinier *et al* 1992). One gene cluster for butyrophilin is located very close to MHC class I and class II regions in human and mouse (Stammers *et al* 2000). Whilst the concept of mimicry between myelin-associated glycoprotein and butyrophilin remains unproven, an increased frequency of butyrophilin-binding antibodies is described in patients with multiple sclerosis (De March *et al* 2003).

Microbial superantigens

Microbial products have evolved a second, semispecific means of activating autoreactive T cells. Microbial superantigen can activate central nervous system reactive T lymphocytes and thus initiate experimental autoimmune encephalomyelitis without structurally mimicking encephalitogenic peptide epitopes. Like specific peptide antigens, microbial superantigens activate T cells via the T-cell receptor and associated signal transduction pathways, and they also only activate T cells when complexed with MHC class II products. However, in contrast to antigenic peptides, the superantigens do not react with the hypervariable complementarity-determining region 3 portion of the receptor (which mediates peptide specificity) but bind to relatively constant determinants typical for $V\beta$ segments of the receptor (Herman *et al* 1991). Superantigens thus do not activate T cells in a clonally specific fashion but activate larger subsets of T-cell clones – those populations carrying the same relevant $V\beta$ determinant.

Activation of encephalitogenic T cells by bacterial superantigen was first shown in culture through triggering of Lewis rat myelin basic protein-specific $V\beta8.2$ T cells by the staphylococcal enterotoxin E, which also binds $V\beta8.2$ (Rott *et al* 1992) or enterotoxin D (Matsumoto and Fujiwara 1993). *In vivo*, the superantigen paradigm was validated by treatment of myelin basic protein-primed mice with staphylococcal enterotoxin B, another classic bacterial superantigen activating murine T-cell receptor containing $V\beta8.2$ determinants. Mice, recovered from experimental autoimmune encephalomyelitis mediated by $V\beta8.2^+$ T cells, were then exposed to staphylococcal enterotoxin B and underwent a new relapse. Similar treatment of unprimed mice did not trigger experimental autoimmune encephalomyelitis (Brocke *et al* 1993; Schiffenbauer *et al* 1993). Dormant, potentially encephalitogenic T cells must have been reactivated by the semispecific bacterial proteins. But, as discussed in Chapter 12, additional effects presumably contribute to the encephalitogenic activity of superantigens. By activating large populations of T cells, substantial doses of proinflammatory cytokines are released (Miethke *et al* 1992), which may activate cerebral endothelial cells and thus contribute to enhanced formation of brain infiltrates. Human endogenous retroviruses have been isolated from central nervous system tissues of people with multiple sclerosis (Perron *et al* 1997: see Chapter 2). Under certain conditions, these may produce superantigens, which in turn could activate autoimmune T lymphocytes (Sutkowski *et al* 2001). Their specific role in multiple sclerosis is disputed and awaits definitive validation (Brahic and Bureau 1997).

Bystander activation in inflammatory milieus: the link to innate immunity

Models of chronic virus infection exist that do not seem to involve the recruitment and activation of myelin-specific encephalitogenic T cells in response to molecular mimicry and superantigen responses. Coronavirus infection of Lewis rat brain, for example, may take a subacute course with round cell infiltration of central white matter (Watanabe *et al* 1983). Myelin basic protein (but not coronavirus virus)-specific $CD4^+$ T-cell lines isolated from infected donor rats mediate comparable disease. Mechanisms underlying the apparent activation of encephalitogenic T cells in the course of a slow virus infection of the brain remain to be elucidated. In another demyelinating central nervous system disease model, Theiler virus-induced encephalomyelitis, a chronic autoimmune response follows an acute phase of inflammation. While virus-specific T cells control the initial phase, the inflammatory response is subsequently driven by myelin-specific T cells (S.D. Miller *et al* 1995a). Release of brain autoantigen in concert with locally produced proinflammatory cytokines may be the key factor in virus-associated autoimmune encephalitis (Vanderlugt and Miller 2002).

The discovery of links between innate and adaptive immunity add a new component to our understanding of the role played by local tissue milieus in development and course of autoimmune disease. By activating mechanisms of innate immunity, microbial infections may create a local environment that is particularly supportive of T-cell activation (Bachmann and Kopf 2001). We have already described activation of innate immune mechanisms by the binding of microbial structures to Toll-like and other pattern receptors. Activation of dendritic cells by bacterial lipopolysaccharide, double-stranded RNA, CpG DNA or heat-shock proteins binding to Toll-like receptor induces costimulatory antigens in dendritic cells, and triggers secretion of proinflammatory cytokines including IL-12 (Reis e Sousa 2001). Alternatively, recent investigations suggest that the triggering of innate immune responses by engagement of Toll-like receptor may result in the neutralization of $CD4^+CD25^+$ regulatory T cells (Treg cells). The process apparently does not act via costimulatory structures and antigen presentation, but involves signalling through soluble IL-6. Functional inactivation of the regulatory T cells allows suppressed autoimmune T cells to become activated (Pasare and Medzhitov 2003). Radically different is the result of signalling via Toll-like receptor expressed on the Treg cells themselves where, rather than being blocked, the suppressive activity is enhanced (Caramalho *et al* 2003).

Taken together, the present evidence suggests that innate antibacterial immune responses promote the development of autoimmunity by creating a proinflammatory milieu, which strongly enhances the presentation of foreign or self antigen to T cells, or even facilitates 'bystander' activation of local T cells independent of antigen.

T cells carrying two sets of receptors

Both T and B lymphocytes normally only use genes from one of the two available alleles to code their antigen receptor, a phenomenon termed allelic exclusion (Nemazee 2000). This rule is firm but not unfailing. Violation of allelic exclusion, the expression of two types of receptor, was first described for T-cell receptor α chains in human (Padovan *et al* 1993) and transgenic mouse T cells (Heath and Miller 1993). Later, double expression of β chains was also reported (Balomenos *et al* 1995; Davodeau *et al* 1995; Padovan *et al* 1995). The theoretical implications of double T-cell receptor expression for the initiation of autoimmune disease are considerable. This might give rise to T-cell clones coexpressing self- and non-self-reactive T-cell receptors. Immunogenic ligation of non-self T-cell receptor by the appropriate foreign (microbial) antigen would activate the T cell and, at the same time, animate its autoimmune potential – defined and executed by the second autoreactive receptor. This mode of autoimmune activation is no doubt intellectually attractive, but so far unproven in clinical practice. The available experimental data are also not strongly supportive. Studies of double transgenic mice with two distinct T-cell receptor transgenes did identify a minor population of T cells with two T-cell receptors, one recognizing self and the other foreign antigen. In these dual receptor-expressing T cells, binding of a foreign ligand resulted in silencing of the cell, instead of activating its pathogenic potential (Dittel *et al* 1999; Fossati *et al* 1999). Activation of the autoimmune potential by recognition of microbial antigen remains to be demonstrated.

B-cell tolerance and autoimmunity

Thanks to B-cell tolerance, the production of pathogenic autoantibodies is prevented or suppressed, although our body fluids contain plenty of immunoglobulin binding harmlessly to self structures. Much knowledge of B-cell self-tolerance comes from transgenic mouse models. These animals have B cells, most of which use the transgenic autoantibodies as surface receptors. Autoreactive immunoglobulin production is restricted to the B lymphocyte subclass B-1. In normal animals, this population commonly makes polyreactive autoantibodies that are not autoaggressive. Release of pathogenic autoantibodies is triggered by microbial activation (Murakami and Honjo 1995). In classic B cells, however, self-tolerance is obligatory. It is effected by several mechanisms, and these are not necessarily mutually exclusive. Depending on the concentration of soluble self antigen, autoreactive B lymphocytes may either be physically eliminated from the immune repertoire by apoptosis or silenced to a state of profound nonreactivity or anergy (Goodnow 1992). Other B cells respond to the encounter of self antigen with replacement of their original, self-reactive immunoglobulin receptor by a newly arranged, non-self-reactive immunoglobulin chain – a mechanism termed immunoglobulin 'editing' (Radic and Zouali 1996). Receptor editing occurs in a late stage of B-cell maturation (Chen *et al* 1995b; Melamed and Nemazee 1997; Pelanda *et al* 1997), and may involve either the immunoglobulin H (C. Chen *et al* 1995a) or L chain (Brard *et al* 1999; Casellas *et al* 2001; H. Li *et al* 2001). Autoimmune prone strains, such as MRL-lpr/lpr mice, seem to have an editing machinery insufficient to delete autoimmune B-cell clones, and even allow their functional maturation by somatic mutation (Brard *et al* 1999; Pelanda *et al* 1997).

Autoimmune B lymphocytes in experimental autoimmune encephalomyelitis

So far, it has become clear that autoimmune T cells, especially CD4 T cells, are the pathogenic effectors in experimental autoimmune encephalomyelitis. They determine the location, activity and functional character of the central nervous system lesion. But this by no means excludes B cells from central nervous system autoimmune diseases. On the contrary, we shall see that B cells have essential functions in several stages of the unfolding experimental autoimmune encephalomyelitis lesion. Central nervous system autoantigen-specific B cells may help activate T lymphocytes as professional antigen-presenting cells, able to concentrate autoantigen due to their immunoglobulin surface receptors. Further, with their particular set of secreted cytokines, they are able to push antigen-recognizing CD4 T cells into particular functional pathways, usually along the Th2 pathway. Finally, binding of B-cell secreted anti-myelin autoantibodies to exposed surface structures of the myelin sheath or the myelin-forming oligodendrocyte is definitely one paramount mechanism of autoimmune demyelination.

Anti-myelin autoantibodies

Early studies on experimental autoimmune encephalomyelitis revealed that sera from affected animals may demyelinate organotypic central nervous system tissue cultures (Bornstein and Appel 1961). A similar demyelinating effect was later observed *in vivo* after injection of such sera into the central nervous system parenchyma or cerebrospinal fluid (Lassmann *et al* 1981b). The demyelinating factor turned out to be immunoglobulin – both IgG and IgM – and demyelination was mediated either via complement activation alone or in combination with activated macrophages. These observations suggest that antibodies against myelin can, at least in part, be responsible for demyelination in models of acute and chronic experimental autoimmune encephalomyelitis. This is further substantiated by studies of chronic experimental autoimmune encephalomyelitis, which show good correlation between the antibody response and amount of demyelination (Linington and Lassmann 1987).

Characterization of the fine specificity of demyelinating sera from experimental autoimmune encephalomyelitis animals first suggested that antibodies against certain glycolipids, such as galactocerebroside, are responsible for the demyelinating effect (Dubois-Dalcq *et al* 1970). However, the correlation between anti-glycolipid antibody titres and demyelinating activity of respective sera is generally poor. Much better correlation is found with antibody titres against myelin oligodendrocyte glycoprotein (Linington and Lassmann 1987). To date, no other myelin protein has been identified that serves as a target of demyelinating antibodies. The pathogenic role of demyelinating antibodies *in vivo* has formally been proven by the intravenous transfer of anti-myelin oligodendrocyte glycoprotein antibodies to animals in whom T-cell-mediated experimental autoimmune

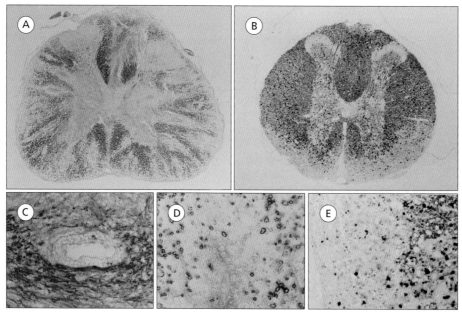

Figure 11.13 Demyelination in T-cell-mediated experimental autoimmune encephalomyelitis is augmented by the presence of demyelinating anti-myelin basic protein antibodies. (A) Injection of anti-myelin oligodendrocyte glycoprotein antibodies 3 days after transfer of myelin basic protein-reactive T cells; perivenous inflammation is associated with extensive perivascular loss of myelin; Klüver/PAS myelin stain; ×50. (B) Repeated cotransfer of myelin basic protein-reactive T cells and anti-myelin oligodendrocyte glycoprotein antibodies leads to confluent demyelinated plaques with loss of oligodendrocytes; myelin is stained by immunocytochemistry for proteolipid protein (blue) and oligodendrocytes by *in situ* hybridization for proteolipid protein mRNA (black cells); ×50. (C) Transfer of T lymphocytes in the absence of anti-myelin oligodendrocyte glycoprotein antibodies leads to perivenous inflammation without demyelination; Klüver/PAS myelin stain; ×300. (D) Extensive perivenous demyelination after cotransfer of myelin basic protein-reactive T cells and anti-myelin oligodendrocyte glycoprotein antibodies; Klüver/PAS myelin stain; ×500. (E) Higher magnification (×250) of the plaque in (B) with demyelination and oligodendrocyte loss; double staining for proteolipid protein immunocytochemistry and *in situ* hybridization.

encephalomyelitis had already been induced (Figure 11.13: Linington *et al* 1988; Schlüsener *et al* 1987). In this disease paradigm, the encephalitogenic T cells are required to prime the central nervous system parenchyma and open the blood–brain barrier to allow myelin oligodendrocyte glycoprotein-reactive monoclonal antibodies to enter the central nervous system. The antibodies cause demyelination, probably with the help of accessory macrophages and/or complement (Linington *et al* 1989; Piddlesden *et al* 1993). Rat experimental autoimmune encephalomyelitis mediated by double transfer of encephalitogenic T cells plus myelin-specific autoantibodies is certainly quite an artificial model of autoimmunity in the central nervous system. However, very similar inflammatory and demyelinating lesions have been created by very simple immunization with recombinant or myelin-derived myelin oligodendrocyte glycoprotein in adjuvant in rats (Johns *et al* 1995; Storch *et al* 1998b; Figures 11.14 and 11.15), mice (Amor *et al* 1994) and primates (Genain *et al* 1996). However, not all anti-myelin oligodendrocyte glycoprotein autoantibodies are demyelinating: only those recognizing a conformational epitope on myelin oligodendrocyte glycoprotein, but not linear peptide epitopes, are able to cause demyelination *in vivo* (Brehm *et al* 1999; von Büdingen *et al* 2002). At least in the mouse, production of anti-conformational autoantibodies seems to be controlled genetically by loci close to the MHC (Bourquin *et al* 2003).

Transgenic models of central nervous system-specific B cells

Transgenic mice with T-cell receptors for encephalitogenic autoantigen have provided models for understanding myelin self-recognition and autoimmunity. The same can be expected from transgenic mice with myelin autoimmune B lymphocytes (Litzenburger *et al* 1998). In contrast to T-cell receptor transgenics, these were gene replacement ('knock-in') mutant mice. Instead of randomly inserting the transgene into germline DNA, the germline J(H) locus was excised and replaced by the rearranged immunoglobulin H chain V gene of a pathogenic myelin oligodendrocyte glycoprotein-specific monoclonal antibody. It should be noted that expression of the transgenic H chain, in the absence of the paired transgenic L chain, was sufficient to produce a large proportion of myelin oligodendrocyte glycoprotein-binding B cells (>30% of all B cells in the repertoire) and high titres of myelin oligodendrocyte glycoprotein-binding serum immunoglobulins. Further, due to correct insertion of the H chain transgene, all essential features of immunoglobulin affinity maturation and isotype switching were recapitulated in transgenic B cells.

Study of the anti-myelin oligodendrocyte glycoprotein H chain knock-in mouse showed that the mere presence of myelin autoreactive B cells does not cause spontaneous experimental

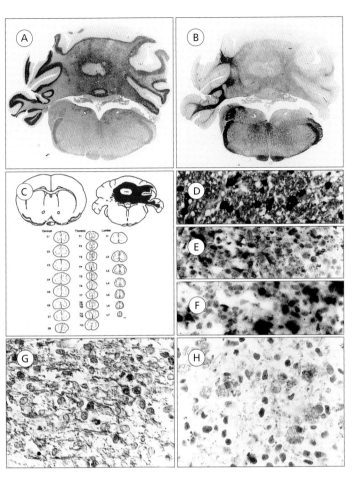

Figure 11.14 Patterns of demyelination in chronic experimental autoimmune encephalomyelitis in a DA rat induced by active sensitization with myelin oligodendrocyte glycoprotein. (A) Large inflammatory demyelinating lesion affecting most of the cerebellar white matter (hypercellular lesion); haematoxylin/eosin; ×10. (B) Extensive loss of myelin; Klüver/PAS myelin stain; ×10. (C) Topography of demyelinated lesions in the central nervous system of this DA rat; only two lesions are found – one in the cerebellar white matter, the other in the optic nerve; ×500. (D) Patterns of oligodendrocyte loss in demyelinating cerebellar lesion; periplaque white matter with normal density of oligodendrocytes; ×500. (E) Actively demyelinating area with granular myelin degradation products in macrophages (red granules) and nearly complete loss of proteolipid protein mRNA-reactive oligodendrocytes; ×500. (F) Inactive centre of the lesion with demyelination and a large number of proteolipid protein mRNA-positive oligodendrocytes, possibly recruited from the pool of progenitor cells; immunocytochemistry for proteolipid protein (red) and *in situ* hybridization for proteolipid protein mRNA (black cells); ×500. (G) Deposition of complement C9 in the demyelinating lesion; fibrillar staining of myelinated fibres at the actively demyelinating edge of the lesion; ×500. (H) Granular C9-reactive degradation products in macrophages; immunocytochemistry for C9; ×500.

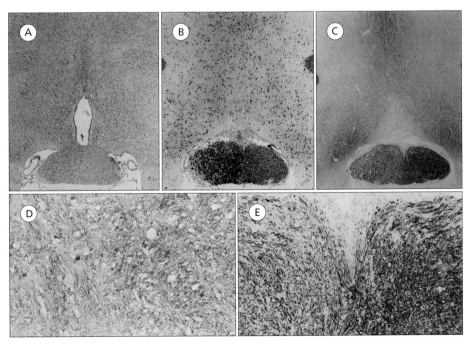

Figure 11.15 Remyelinating 'shadow plaque' in the optic chiasm of the same animal shown in Figure 11.13. (A) Increased cell density in the lesion occupying the left side of the optic chiasm; haematoxylin & eosin; ×45. (B) Reduced density of myelin but increased numbers of oligodendrocytes in the lesion; immunocytochemistry for proteolipid protein (red) and *in situ* hybridization for proteolipid protein mRNA (black cells); ×45. (C) Reduced axonal density in the affected portion of the optic chiasm; Bielschowsky silver impregnation for axons; ×45. (D) Reduced density of myelin in the affected portion of the optic chiasm (left half of the micrograph); Klüver/PAS myelin stain; ×300. (E) Higher magnification of (C) showing the reduced axonal density; Bielschowsky silver impregnation for axons; ×300.

autoimmune encephalomyelitis or demyelination. However, the same transgenic B cells and their autoantibody products became highly pathogenic in cooperation with transferred encephalitogenic T cells (Litzenburger *et al* 1998). The autoreactive B cells persisted throughout life in the transgenic mouse, and in high numbers. In contrast, B-cell differentiation was blocked in the bone marrow at a late pre-B-cell stage in double transgenic mice expressing both the myelin oligodendrocyte glycoprotein-reactive H and L chain. B cells underwent receptor editing, with replacement of the transgenic L chain by an endogenous L chain freshly created by renewed rearrangement (Litzenburger *et al* 2000). Clearly, it will be instructive to investigate transgenic mice with a myelin oligodendrocyte glycoprotein-biased immune repertoire, both at the T- and B-cell levels.

Autoimmune B cells in multiple sclerosis

In human multiple sclerosis an active participation of B cells in the immune pathogenesis has been postulated for many years. In fact, as will be detailed later, abnormal oligoclonal immunoglobulins in the cerebrospinal fluid (CSF), a fluid that normally contains no demonstrable immunoglobulins at all, is a diagnostic hallmark of multiple sclerosis. The antigen specificity of these immunoglobulins is completely obscure to date; curiously they do not bind any of the myelin candidate autoantigens. Remarkably, however, there is increasing evidence of specific antibody binding within particular types of multiple sclerosis plaques, and it appears plausible but remains yet unproven that such locally bound antibodies are indeed autoimmune and contribute to local myelin destruction.

Anti-myelin autoantibodies

Despite good evidence implicating B lymphocytes in the pathogenesis of multiple sclerosis, their precise role remains to be clarified. It has been known for many years that most, if not all, patients have abnormal oligoclonal immunoglobulin bands, reflecting intrathecal synthesis, in the cerebrospinal fluid. Although not specific, their detection is used as one laboratory criterion supporting the clinical diagnosis of multiple sclerosis. The specificity of the oligoclonal antibodies in cerebrospinal fluid remained enigmatic for many years, and attempts to identify myelin or other central nervous system structures as target antigens met with limited success (Cortese *et al* 1996). This uncomfortable situation may be changing. Several groups have described autoantibodies against myelin oligodendrocyte glycoprotein in the serum and cerebrospinal fluid of patients with multiple sclerosis (Lindert *et al* 1999; Reindl *et al* 1999; Xiao *et al* 1991). Others dispute this clarification (Karni *et al* 1999). When tested for the structural characteristics of binding epitopes, most myelin oligodendrocyte glycoprotein-reactive immunoglobulins were found to bind linear, rather than conformational epitopes (Haase *et al* 2001) – making the point that only autoantibodies directed against conformational determinants have a pathogenic demyelinating potential (see above: Brehm *et al* 1999; von Büdingen *et al* 2001). Nevertheless, a recent study correlated serum and cerebrospinal fluid myelin oligodendrocyte glycoprotein antibodies with disease severity (T. Berger *et al* 2003). An active role for anti-myelin associated glycoprotein autoantibodies in the pathogenesis of multiple

sclerosis is further supported by morphological analysis. Certain lesion types are characterized by myelin debris decorated with activated complement (Storch *et al* 1998a), possibly involving a humoral anti-myelin associated glycoprotein reaction (Genain *et al* 1999).

B cells in the central nervous system of patients with multiple sclerosis

The inflammatory infiltrates of active lesions commonly contain a relatively minor B lymphocyte or plasma cell infiltrate within a majority of T cells and macrophages (see Chapter 12). The B cells are often within plaque areas, rather than in the peripheral zones (Esiri 1980). It is tempting to assume that plaque-infiltrating B cells participate in inflammatory demyelination, perhaps by secreting anti-myelin oligodendrocyte glycoprotein autoantibodies. However, such a pathogenic function has not been demonstrated to date, perhaps for technical reasons. Early attempts to characterize B cells in tissue from individuals with multiple sclerosis used Elispot methods and B cells harvested from cerebrospinal fluid (Storch *et al* 1998a). This approach led to the identification of B cells specific for a range of myelin autoantigens, and semiquantification in various compartments at different stages of the disease (Archelos *et al* 2000). But cellular mechanisms underlying the antibody responses remained obscure.

Molecular approaches, especially those using polymerase chain reaction techniques, now seem poised to help out. The screening of cDNA libraries established from B cells infiltrating tissue favours an antigen-driven immune response. Comparison of antibody H chains documented extensive somatic mutagenesis. Individual sequence could be sorted as pedigrees probably derived from a few progenitor B cells (Owens *et al* 1998). A very similar observation was made using B cells or short lived plasmablasts (Cepok *et al* 2005a) from the cerebrospinal fluid of patients with multiple sclerosis. Expansion of a few individual B-cell clones, with strong somatic mutations, was again observed (Y. Qin *et al* 1998). These original reports were confirmed by more recent studies using immunoglobulin spectratyping (Baranzini *et al* 1999), and methods of single-cell gene cloning (A.M. Ritchie *et al* 2004).

REGULATION OF CENTRAL NERVOUS SYSTEM AUTOIMMUNE RESPONSES

We have stressed that the immune system achieves its well-dosaged reactivity against foreign structures by tight intercellular regulation. No individual immune cell, be it a T or a B lymphocyte, acts autonomously, but is subject to a chain of control exerted by neighbouring cells, which can be lymphocytes, macrophages, dendritic cells or components of the surrounding stroma. The principle of cell-to-cell regulation governs especially immunological self-tolerance. A failure of regulation may result in autoimmunity. Investigations into experimental autoimmune encephalomyelitis have revealed how failed immune regulation may cause or support autoimmune reactivity against the central nervous system, and studies of multiple sclerosis patients now confirm such failure in the pathogenesis of human disease. It now appears that an important part of the regulation is effected by check-and-balance interactions between two competing T-cell subsets, the Th1 and Th2 cells. This has been discussed above. In addition, however, there are specialized regulatory T cells that keep effector cells in check. These limit an ongoing immune response to its necessary duration, and help prevent activation of self-reactive T cells to warrant self-tolerance.

Chronic relapsing experimental autoimmune encephalomyelitis: a failure of regulation?

Although the mechanisms that control inflammation in acute monophasic experimental autoimmune encephalomyelitis are tolerably well understood, much less is known about pathogenic factors that operate in the induction of chronic disease or individual relapses. Most animal species and strains are resistant to re-induction of experimental autoimmune encephalomyelitis after a disease episode that follows active sensitization. However, certain mouse strains (SJL/J or Biozzi mice) are more exuberant and react with new inflammatory episodes after each fresh antigenic challenge (Kozlowski *et al* 1987). In these mice, a spontaneously developing chronic relapsing disease can be induced by single transfer of myelin-reactive T lymphocytes (Mokhtarian *et al* 1984; Zamvil *et al* 1985). Furthermore, in contrast to most animals with monophasic disease, in this situation the encephalitogenic reaction shifts from the originally transferred T cells towards an immune response directed against other cryptic determinants of myelin basic protein or even proteolipid protein (A.H. Cross *et al* 1993; Lehmann *et al* 1992). This indicates that liberation of antigen at the site of brain inflammation and/or its transport to local lymphatic tissue may in some animal species result in antigenic drift and uncontrolled autoimmunity. The reason for this lack of immune regulation in certain animal species is unknown. Suggestions include increased persistence of autoimmune effector cells in the central nervous system and immune system (Fritz *et al* 1998), participation of γδ-T-cell receptor cells (Rajan *et al* 1996) and increased expression of variant *golli* myelin basic protein in immune organs (MacKenzie-Graham *et al* 1997).

By active sensitization, chronic experimental autoimmune encephalomyelitis can be induced in a large variety of different animal species. In these models, chronic persistence of local antigen, made available from initial sensitization or repeated challenge, is critical for maintaining chronicity (Rivers *et al* 1933; Tabira *et al* 1984). By comparison with the transfer models described above, even less is known about the immunoregulatory events that lead to chronicity and relapse after active sensitization. Although no overt differences between active and inactive phases of the disease are noted in delayed-type skin responses against myelin basic protein (Tabira *et al* 1983), in one study increased antigen-specific suppression of T-cell activation was found during disease remission (Lyman *et al* 1981). In terms of the central nervous system lesions, there is little difference in the composition of inflammatory infiltrates between acute and chronic experimental autoimmune encephalomyelitis, or even between relapses and remissions (Figures 11.8, 11.16 and 11.17). Whether changes in local cytokine patterns *per se* can explain disease activity or remission in chronic experimental autoimmune encephalomyelitis models, such as described for acute experimental autoimmune encephalomyelitis (Kennedy *et al* 1992), remains to be determined.

Also relevant to the induction of chronic experimental autoimmune encephalomyelitis is the ability of animals to mount a humoral autoimmune response. In mice with identical MHC backgrounds, differences in the incidence of chronic experimental autoimmune encephalomyelitis can be traced to their production of high-affinity antibodies (Devey *et al* 1990). As discussed below, autoantibodies against antigens exposed on the surface of myelin sheaths play an important role in the induction of demyelination in chronic experimental autoimmune encephalomyelitis models (Linington and Lassmann 1987; Linington *et al* 1988). Furthermore, subclinical encephalitis induced by suboptimal numbers of encephalitogenic T lymphocytes can become clinically manifest in the presence of such autoantibodies (Lassmann *et al* 1988).

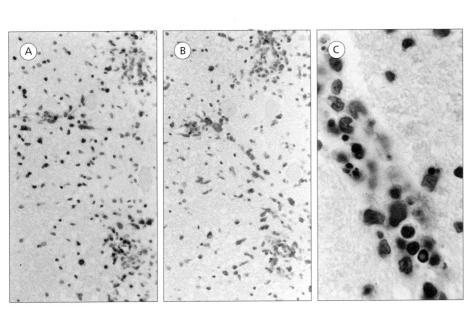

Figure 11.16 Composition of inflammatory infiltrates in T-cell-mediated experimental autoimmune encephalomyelitis. (A) Perivascular inflammation and tissue infiltration with T cells; immunocytochemistry with W3/13; ×200. (B) Large numbers of inflammatory cells express a lysosomal macrophage marker; immunostaining with ED1; ×200. (C) Many inflammatory cells (mainly T lymphocytes) show the typical alterations of apoptosis (nuclear condensation, margination of chromatin and nuclear fragmentation); haematoxylin & eosin stain; ×1000.

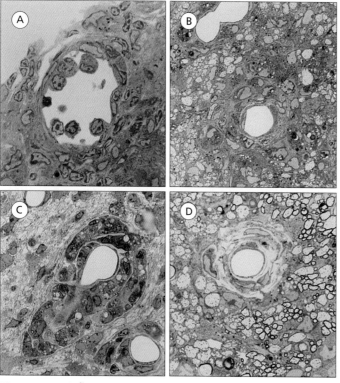

Figure 11.17 Inflammatory reaction in chronic demyelinating experimental autoimmune encephalomyelitis. (A) Leucocytes bind to the luminal surface of venules and migrate through the vessel wall; toluidine blue; ×1000. (B) Macrophages with myelin debris are located in the central nervous system parenchyma and perivascular space in actively demyelinating lesions; toluidine blue; ×1000. (C) Inactive lesion macrophages are mainly located in the perivascular Virchow–Robin space; toluidine blue; ×1000. (D) Inactive, remyelinating lesions show pronounced perivascular fibrosis of parenchymal vessels; toluidine blue; ×1000.

Regulatory CD8 T lymphocytes

Classic MHC class I restricted CD8$^+$ T cells are commonly equated with cytotoxic killer lymphocytes, which act as effectors in the context of tumour rejection, autoimmune inflammation and viral infection. Indeed, such cells may play an important role in mediating demyelination, axonal injury and global tissue destruction in the lesions of multiple sclerosis (see Chapter 12). Less clear is whether there is another type of CD8$^+$ T cell, with regulatory functions, bringing to a close otherwise ongoing cellular (auto)immune responses. The regulatory function of CD8$^+$ T cells has been revealed in two models of mouse experimental autoimmune encephalomyelitis where, in the absence of functional CD8$^+$ T cells, immunization against myelin basic protein enhances the encephalitogenic response. This has been shown, for example, after ablation of CD8$^+$ T cells by *in vivo* infusion of monoclonal antibodies directed against CD8. Mice depleted of CD8$^+$ T cells show more severe relapses, but their recovery from the individual attack is unimpaired (H. Jiang *et al* 1992). Furthermore, transgenic mice lacking CD8$^+$ T cells due to disruption of the CD8 gene also suffer increased severity of relapses, although the disease course

in general seems milder (D-R. Koh *et al* 1992). Recent work indicates that suppressive CD8$^+$ T cells are specific for peptide epitopes from T-cell receptors of CD4$^+$ effector T cells that dominate the encephalitogenic immune response (H. Jiang *et al* 2001), and recognize these epitopes in the unusual context of Qa antigens – atypical class I-related MHC products (class Ib) (Rodgers and Cook 2005). They thus can be defined as idiotype-specific regulatory cells.

The first reports of putative CD8$^+$ regulatory T cells were based on histological evidence. In the Lewis rat model of experimental autoimmune encephalomyelitis, CD8$^+$ T-cell infiltrates in the spinal cord persisted beyond clinical recovery, indicating a suppressive function for these lymphocytes (Hickey and Gonatas 1984). However, later work showed that depletion of CD8$^+$ T cells from the immune system altered neither the severity nor course of experimental autoimmune encephalomyelitis in the same strain (Sedgwick 1988). Regulatory CD8$^+$ T cells were first isolated from the spleens of Lewis rats that had previously received transfers of syngeneic encephalitic CD4$^+$ T-cell lines. Their transfer efficiently protected naive rats against the induction of experimental autoimmune encephalomyelitis by the relevant CD4$^+$ line (Lider *et al* 1988; D. Sun *et al* 1988). The cells are exquisitely specific for the inducing T-cell line and do not cross-react with or affect actively induced experimental autoimmune encephalomyelitis. They neutralize encephalitogenic target T cells *in vivo*, and specifically lyse these *in vitro* (D. Sun *et al* 1988).

Another CD8$^+$ T cell with potential regulatory function is described in studies of oral tolerization against myelin basic protein. Low-dose oral administration of antigen leads to the activation of CD8$^+$ T cells that suppress activation of encephalitogenic CD4$^+$ T lymphocytes in the host immune system (Lider *et al* 1989) by secreting anti-inflammatory TGF-β (A. Miller *et al* 1992). Thus far, activation of these T cells depends on pharmacological manipulations, and a physiological role remains to be defined. In a much quoted paper, Reinherz *et al* (1980) reported a dramatic loss of CD8$^+$ T lymphocytes from peripheral blood in patients with multiple sclerosis. In active disease, CD8$^+$ T cells (determined by cytofluorometry) were reduced to 5% of peripheral T cells compared with normal values of around 20%. Intriguingly, patients in remission showed much less pronounced changes. The interpretation seemed obvious. According to the prevailing view, active disease in multiple sclerosis was associated with, and possibly due to, the loss of CD8$^+$ suppressor T lymphocytes. Indeed, loss of negative immune regulation was corroborated in studies using functional suppressor assays. For example, Antel *et al* (1979), using a mitogen-driven T-cell suppressor assay, showed loss of suppressor activity during phases of active disease with restoration to normal levels during remission. Considered in their day to be pivotal results, they triggered a plethora of CD8/suppressor T-cell analyses using ever more elaborate (and expensive) panels of monoclonal antibodies as these became available. These accumulated data now seem to indicate much weaker disease-related effects than were initially claimed (Antel *et al* 1985), and this also holds true for the evidence of an inverse correlation between CD4$^+$/CD8$^+$ ratios and functional suppressor assays (P.J. Hughes *et al* 1988). Whilst it would be easy to conclude that this was a blind alley in multiple sclerosis research, active participation of regulatory CD8$^+$ T cells in the pathogenesis is by no means ruled out, and the functional significance of the markers used to define lymphocyte phenotypes has since systematically been refined. As suggested by the lessons from experimental autoimmune encephalomyelitis (see above), CD8$^+$ T cells have been observed after vaccination with attenuated myelin basic protein-specific CD4$^+$ T cells (J. Zhang *et al* 1995). They may participate both in immune regulation and cellular autoimmune attack. This topic should move forward with the ability to isolate CD8$^+$ T lymphocytes specific for myelin basic protein and proteolipid protein peptide determinants in the context of MHC class I molecules from the blood of patients with multiple sclerosis (Biddison *et al* 1997; Tsuchida *et al* 1995). New methods, such as recombinant MHC class I proteins complexed with (auto)antigenic peptides, now allow identification of specific CD8$^+$ T cells in blood and tissues. These approaches, together with single cell polymerase chain reaction techniques (Dornmair *et al* 2003), ought to improve our understanding of multiple sclerosis-related CD8$^+$ T cells, be they regulatory or effector cells (Appay and Rowland-Jones 2002; Skinner and Haase 2002).

Gamma/delta (γδ) T cells

In addition to the majority of T lymphocytes, which use classic antigen receptors of the αβ class, the immune system also harbours T cells with γδ receptors. Both populations are clonally diverse with antigen receptors composed of various gene segments linked by mechanisms of somatic recombination, sharing essential structural features of antigen-binding protein. However, the function(s) of γδ T cells are still largely obscure. They are by no means a homogeneous cell population and contain numerous subpopulations with diverse antigen recognition properties, cytokine spectra and tissue localizations. Curiously, while only few γδ T cells reside in peripheral lymph organs, they preferentially settle within epithelia, especially in the gut. Most γδ T cells lack CD4 and CD8, but some express one or the other of these markers (Hayday 2000).

The antigens recognized by γδ T cells are unusual and also diverse. Different subsets using distinct patterns of γδ receptors recognize small non-peptidic molecules (most prominently phosphorylated antigens from mycobacteria) without the need for a particular antigen-presenting molecule, heat-shock proteins, or more conventional peptides bound to variant MHC class Ib proteins (Allison and Garboczi 2002). This and additional evidence suggests that γδ T cells participate in antimicrobial immune responses, but other functions, such as regulation of immune responses, have also been proposed. Evidence for γδ T cells participating in autoimmune responses, as in the generation of experimental autoimmune encephalomyelitis lesions, remains indirect. The course of experimental autoimmune encephalomyelitis has been related to increased frequencies of γδ T cells in central nervous system infiltrates. Disease activity correlates with their state of activation, especially in chronic relapsing experimental autoimmune encephalomyelitis models. Relatively high frequencies (>10% of total T cells) were noted in active stages, whereas the concentration of γδ T cells was very low during remission. Depletion of γδ T cells by monoclonal antibody treatment increased experimental autoimmune encephalomyelitis susceptibility and severity, establishing the functional relevance of these cells (Rajan *et al* 1996).

γδ T cells may have an accessory role in experimental autoimmune encephalomyelitis but, unlike their αβ T-cell receptor-bearing counterparts, do not seem to be active mediators of disease. Transgenic mice lacking functional αβ T cells have unimpaired γδ T-cell receptor repertoires (Elliott *et al* 1996) but are completely resistant to active induction of experimental autoimmune encephalomyelitis. Conversely, transgenic mice lacking T-cell receptor γδ cells are no less susceptible to T-cell-transferred experimental autoimmune encephalomyelitis than their wild-type counterparts (Clark and Lingenheld 1998). Possibly γδ T cells regulate cytokine/chemokine production required for recruiting effector T cells into the central nervous system (Rajan *et al* 1999). It should also be mentioned that γδ T cells have been implicated only in selective models of experimental autoimmune encephalomyelitis, but seem to have no role in others. For example, their depletion in Lewis rats has no demonstrable effect on the induction of experimental autoimmune encephalomyelitis (Matsumoto *et al* 1998).

As in experimental autoimmune encephalomyelitis, most neuroimmunological studies of autoreactive T lymphocytes in multiple sclerosis have focused on T cells with αβ receptors, the agents of conventional cellular immune responses. There are, however, good reasons not to neglect γδ receptor T cells in the human disease. Selmaj *et al* (1991a) first observed notable proportions of γδ cells in the lesions of multiple sclerosis. These infiltrates commonly co-localize with enhanced expression of heat-shock proteins – a point of interest since these protein determinants are specifically recognized by some, but by no means all, γδ T cells (Chien *et al* 1996). What is the role of γδ T cells in multiple sclerosis? Are they, as we assume to be the case for their myelin-specific T-cell receptor αβ colleagues, primarily involved in the pathogenesis of individual lesions? Do they attack local brain cells? Or could they have a beneficial role, participating in the attempt to limit or restore the autoimmune injury?

To resolve these questions, and confirm or refute the pathogenic significance of γδ T-cell accumulation in multiple sclerosis lesions, and the reactivity of peripheral blood to heat-shock proteins, antigen-specific γδ T-cell lines are needed to facilitate the direct study of their T-cell receptor gene usage, antigen recognition, cytokine repertoire and cytotoxic potential (Pon and Freedman 2003). These reagents have proved more difficult to generate than T-cell receptor αβ-expressing cell lines. To obtain insights into the gene repertoire used by γδ T-cell receptor cells in selecting and responding to antigen, several groups have isolated this subpopulation from blood or cerebrospinal fluid of patients with multiple sclerosis (Nick *et al* 1995; Shimonkevitz *et al* 1993; Stinissen *et al* 1995). It should be noted that these γδ T-cell receptor cell lines were established using nonspecific polyclonal proliferation stimuli (such as anti-CD3 monoclonals or plant mitogens) rather than specific antigen. A set of short-term lines isolated from the cerebrospinal fluid of patients with early active multiple sclerosis contained an increased proportion of Vδ1- and Vδ2-bearing T cells. In this collection, some T-cell lines used identical receptor sequences (including complementarity-determining region 3 segments) and there was evidence for limited clonal expansion (Shimonkevitz *et al* 1993). Biased utilization of Vδ1 was also noted in short-term lines isolated from cerebrospinal fluid in patients with multiple sclerosis compared with peripheral blood (Nick *et al* 1995). An analysis combining immunocytochemistry and polymerase chain reaction also identified Vδ1- and Vδ2-bearing T cells in acute plaques with possible expansion of some individual clones (Wucherpfennig *et al* 1992b), while dominant usage of Vδ2 was described in another report (Battistini *et al* 1995).

Thus, there seems to be some bias in the Vδ gene repertoire used by brain-associated T cells in patients with multiple sclerosis. The significance of this is unclear, especially considering the limited gene usage typically seen in several physiological γδ T-cell receptor cell compartments, and the age-dependent shifts observed in responsiveness (Bluestone *et al* 1995). Unfortunately, the target epitopes of T-cell lines derived from patients with multiple sclerosis remain largely unknown – with the possible exception of some γδ cells that recognize brain membrane determinants produced, amongst others, by glioma cells (Nick *et al* 1995), and Vδ2 T cells isolated from peripheral blood and cerebrospinal fluid, which react with heat-shock protein 70 (Stinissen *et al* 1995). The key issue of whether the infiltrates of γδ receptor-expressing T cells attack myelin-forming cells in patients with multiple sclerosis, as suggested by the *in vitro* experiments (M.S. Freedman *et al* 1991), or actually limit the autoimmune process, remains unanswered.

T cells reactive against glycolipids (NK1 T cells)

With identification of the natural killer (NK1) T-cell subset, a newly identified and promising regulatory cell type arrived on the immunological stage. NK1 T cells share essential properties with natural killer cells and with classic T lymphocytes. Like T cells, some NK1 T cells express CD4, others CD8, while a third group expresses neither (Godfrey *et al* 2000). Besides NK receptors, they use regular T-cell receptors, mostly αβ but also the γδ type. The T-cell receptor collection used by NK1 T cells is highly simplified and differs from conventional repertoires. In humans, practically all NK1 T cells use the Vα24 chain, often together with a paired Vβ11 chain. The murine correlates are receptors composed of Vα14 mostly with Vβ8.2 chains (Godfrey *et al* 2000). However, unlike T lymphocytes, NK1 T cells display markers of the natural killer cell lineage on their membrane.

These monomorphic receptors recognize unusual target antigens. Observations using transgenic mice indicate that NK1 T cell development and function require β2-microglobulin (a component of MHC class I and class Ib molecules, but not the TAP peptide transporters; see Chapter 3: Vicari and Zlotnik 1996). Rather, it turns out that instead of responding to peptide bound to conventional MHC class I or II proteins, NK1 T-cell receptors bind Ib variants of the CD1 series. These present glycolipids but not peptides. Even more remarkable, the most powerful antigen recognized by NK1 T cells is an 'exotic' small glycolipid, α-galactosylceramide, the product of a marine sponge. No corresponding antigen has yet been found in vertebrates (Hong *et al* 1999).

Whereas there are several CD1 subtypes in humans (CD1a–e), the mouse has only CD1d. Like classic MHC class I proteins, they are composed of one heavy chain that bears the antigen-binding site, and the monomorphic β1-microglobulin. Crystallography shows an antigen-binding groove conformed so as to bind glycolipid antigen rather than short peptides.

Interestingly, like MHC class II antigens, CD1 seems to use the invariant (ii) chain for full structural maturation, membrane expression and antigen presentation to NK1 T cells (Moody and Porcelli 2001). Some NK1 T cells mature within the thymus (Schulz *et al* 1996), others in the periphery. Thymic NK1 T cells seem to differentiate following local interaction with CD1 antigens.

A possible connection of NK1 T cells with autoimmunity was first observed in nonobese diabetic (NOD) mice, which spontaneously develop autoimmune diabetes mellitus. They show a deficit of NK1 T cells, which is most notable in the thymus (Gombert *et al* 1996). The involvement of NK1 T cells was shown more formally in transgenic mice. Animals that express the Vα14 transgene of NK1 T cells, and thus possess increased numbers of these cells, are protected from disease (LeHuen *et al* 1998). Consequently, CD1 knockout mice completely lack NK1 T cells and are more susceptible to autoimmune diabetes (B. Wang *et al* 2001). In support of these findings, activation of endogenous NK1 T cells by their ligand α-galactosylceramide suppresses diabetes development in non-NOD mice (Hong *et al* 2001). The mechanism of NK1 T-cell-mediated protection is not yet clear. There is evidence that these cells act on autoimmune effector T cells, suppressing production of proinflammatory cytokines but without deletion of cells (Beaudoin *et al* 2002).

NK1 T cells play an indisputable role in different models of experimental autoimmune encephalomyelitis. NOD mice that overexpress NK1 T cells and are free from diabetes, are also resistant to the induction of experimental autoimmune encephalomyelitis (Mars *et al* 2002). Transfer of NK1 T cell populations decreases experimental autoimmune encephalomyelitis induction in transgenic mice (Fritz and Zhao 2001). Further, several groups have shown that activation of NK1 T cells by α-galactosylceramide (A.K. Singh *et al* 2001) or agonistic synthetic derivatives (Miyamoto *et al* 2001) protects mice from subsequent attempts to induce experimental autoimmune encephalomyelitis. It should, however, be noted that protection depends much on the treatment protocol. Altered regimens may even result in paradoxical exacerbation of disease (Jahng *et al* 2001). A comparable role for NK1 T cells in multiple sclerosis remains to be demonstrated but may be expected considering one study that showed a deficit of these cells in central nervous system plaque infiltrates, which could indicate an insufficient immune regulation (Illés *et al* 2000).

CD4+CD25+ regulatory T cells (Treg)

One hallmark of the adaptive immune response is regulation of its intensity and temporal course. The start of an immune response is marked by immune cell activation and expansion of the immune clones involved but, at the conclusion of this mission, activated cells either die by programmed cell death or are downregulated to the resting state. Either way, the population contracts. One mechanism contributing substantially to the termination of immune responses relies on suppressor T cells. They respond to antigen recognition by silencing, not activating, immune effector mechanisms. This concept enjoyed extreme popularity two decades back, but was then all but abandoned by most immunologists. Remarkably, specific programmed counterregulatory T cells were later resurrected, now wearing the new colours of T regulatory (Treg) cells (Bach 2003).

Tregs were discovered in mice that had been thymectomized shortly after birth. While growing to adulthood, these partly immunodeficient animals commonly develop spontaneous immune cell infiltrates in particular tissues, such as stomach, thyroid, pancreatic islets, adrenals or reproductive organs (Sakaguchi and Sakaguchi 2000). Interestingly, central or peripheral nervous tissues are missing from the list. The selection of affected organs within one particular strain of rodents is surprisingly stable. It is controlled by genetic factors that remain to be identified. Similar changes are seen in animals recovering from transient immunosuppression (ciclosporin), or after transfer of T cells into T cell-deficient animals. The key observation was that thyroiditis could be prevented by the transfer of spleen or thymus cells from normal syngeneic mice (A. Kojima *et al* 1976). Later, Sakaguchi and Sakaguchi (2000) showed that the protective anti-autoimmune cells are members of the CD4$^+$ subset of T lymphocytes. Tregs represent a particular set of T cells characterized by the expression of CD25 (the IL-2 receptor α chain) along with CD4 (Sakaguchi *et al* 1995).

The mechanisms used by Tregs for suppression of the ongoing immune response are not yet fully characterized. One is downregulation of effector T cells via the CTLA-4 molecule. CTLA-4 expression on Tregs is constitutive and, with CD4 and CD25, is a characteristic marker of this cell type (Sakaguchi 2000). The functional phenotype of Tregs is under the control of a transcriptional regulator of the Forkhead gene family, FoxP3. Mutant or transgenic mice lacking functional *FoxP3* develop an autoimmune syndrome, characterized by general immune hyper-reactivity and immune cell infiltration of diverse tissues. The syndrome, which also occurs in a few humans with mutant *FoxP3*, is typically associated with a deficit of CD25$^+$CD4$^+$ Treg cells (Wildin *et al* 2003). Conversely, *FoxP3* is specifically expressed in Treg cells. Introduction of the gene into regular CD4$^+$ T cells transforms them into specialized Tregs. These are not rare cells. They constitute around 10% of all immune competent CD4$^+$ T cells in the thymus and peripheral immune organs (Sakaguchi 2000). The way in which Tregs silence autoimmune effector T cells and participate in general immune responses is not well understood. First, the T-cell receptor specificity of Tregs remains to be established. The indirect evidence suggests that Tregs, possessing the relevant antigen specificity, are efficient regulators of organ-specific autoimmune responses. Thus, old results from neonatally thymectomized mice suggested that regulatory cells from male donors suppress autoimmunity in male (Taguchi and Nishizuka 1981; 1987) better than female gonads with corresponding inverse differential regulatory activities of female T cells (Taguchi and Nishizuka 1980). More recent work has established that tolerogenic treatment of T-cell receptor transgenic mice (using oral administration of autoantigen) involves expansion of antigen-specific Tregs, which downregulate effector or helper cells of identical antigen specificity (X. Zhang *et al* 2001).

Tregs depend on IL-2 for survival. Mice that lack either IL-2 or IL-2 receptor (including its α chain, CD25) develop spontaneous autoimmune disease, affecting especially the gastrointestinal tract (Sadlack *et al* 1993; Strober and Ehrhardt 1993). It appears that classic immunoregulatory cytokines such as IL-4, IL-10 or TGF-β do not play a pivotal role in Treg-mediated suppression (Bach 2003). Instead, direct cell-to-cell contacts, possibly involving the downregulatory molecule CTLA-4, are

involved (Salomon and Bluestone 2001). Recent work has shown that the regulatory function of Tregs is linked directly and indirectly to elements of the innate immune system. Activation of dendritic cells by ligation of Toll-like receptor seems to neutralize the suppressive potential of Tregs, presumably acting via soluble mediators that include IL-6 (Pasare and Medzhitov 2003). Tregs also express and use Toll-like receptors on their own membrane, and their activation has opposite results. Lipopolysaccharide activation of Tregs is reported further to enhance their suppressive action on other immune cells (Caramalho *et al* 2003).

Treg cells occur in several spontaneous and induced animal models of autoimmune disease. In addition to their effect in partly immune-deprived animals (neonatal thymectomy), Tregs protect against spontaneous and antigen-induced models of autoimmunity. Spontaneous autoimmune diabetes mellitus, which commonly develops in (female) NOD mice within the first 4 months of life, seems to coincide with a decline of CD4$^+$CD25$^+$ Treg cells. Their transfer from prediabetic NOD mice has a beneficial effect on the onset of diabetes in recipients of the same strain. The self-protective effect of Treg-like lymphocytes in anti-myelin autoimmunity was first demonstrated in monoclonal transgenic mice expressing a myelin basic protein-specific T-cell receptor on all T cells. The receptor came from an antigen-specific encephalitogenic T-cell clone isolated from a myelin basic protein-immunized wild-type mouse. (If a transgenic receptor is expressed in otherwise regular mice, the majority, but not all, T cells express the transgene, while the rest use receptors from the internal receptor gene repertoire: see Figure 11.17.) Most such transgenic mice with myelin basic protein-specific receptors rarely develop spontaneous experimental autoimmune encephalomyelitis (Lafaille *et al* 1994). This is in contrast to strictly monoclonal mice, which have the same receptor transgene but with a defective recombination machinery that prevents production of endogenous T- and B-cell receptors. Practically all of these monoclonal myelin basic protein-reactive mice eventually develop experimental autoimmune encephalomyelitis. This spontaneous autoimmune disease is prevented by transfer of Treg cells, most prominently those expressing both CD4 and CD25 (Furtado *et al* 2001). Unfortunately, as with other models of autoimmunity, the receptor specificity of the self-protective Tregs remains undefined.

Regulatory defects in multiple sclerosis

There are excellent reasons for immunologists to search for defective immune regulation in the pathogenesis of multiple sclerosis. One example is the undisputed presence of brain-specific autoreactive T cells in the healthy immune repertoire. Even though these must be activated in order to trigger autoimmune disease in the central nervous system, mere lack of activation seems too paltry a basis for lifelong self-tolerance. One would expect safeguards from active regulatory mechanisms to keep the potential autoimmune time bombs unexploded. Their identification in experimental autoimmune encephalomyelitis encourages the belief that similar regulatory mechanisms would directly lead to new and specific therapeutic approaches in human disease. We have discussed above early attempts to identify CD8$^+$ T lymphocytes as suppressor cells responsible for maintaining immunological self-tolerance. We noted that simple

T-cell subset enumeration or functional suppressor assays did not illuminate the matter, although an ever increasing number of publications seems to indicate a defect of regulatory cells (for example, Viglietta *et al* 2004). We omitted discussion of T-cell regulation via recognition of T-cell receptors (or their components). The concept of T–T-cell interactions as regulatory events in brain autoimmunity takes its origin from an observation made by Cohen and colleagues, namely that myelin basic protein-specific T lymphocytes not only act as pathogenic agents mediating the transfer of experimental autoimmune encephalomyelitis, but are themselves the targets for counter-regulatory cellular responses in the host immune system. Rats receiving myelin basic protein-specific T cells inactivated by irradiation not only fail to develop experimental autoimmune encephalomyelitis but also are protected against subsequent attempts to induce disease – the first example of vaccination against a T-cell-mediated organ-specific autoimmune disease (Ben-Nun *et al* 1981b). We referred to later experiments indicating that the vaccinating autoimmune T cells activate counter-regulatory T lymphocytes – mainly of the CD8$^+$ population – which then anticipate and destroy the activated encephalitogenic clones. Some indirect evidence suggests that the vaccination effect is directed against determinants of the brain-specific T-cell receptor (Lider *et al* 1988). A second, and unambiguously T-cell receptor-directed vaccination strategy was successfully used later by immunizing rats against peptide analogues to receptors typically used by encephalitogenic T cells (Howell *et al* 1989; Vandenbark *et al* 1989). Obviously, it is now known that profound differences exist between rodent and primate immune systems. But is there evidence for T-cell receptor-directed idiotypic T–T-cell interactions in the human immune system? T cells recognize receptor fragments of other T cells, but the relevance of these interactions for the pathogenesis and treatment of multiple sclerosis remains to be established.

T-cell receptor-specific human T-cell lines were first described by Saruhan-Direskeneli *et al* (1993), who used synthetic peptides representing sequences of the complementarity-determining region 3 and V regions of a known myelin basic protein-specific T-cell receptor β chain to select anti-idiotypic T-cell receptor-specific cells. Myelin basic protein-specific T cells were obtained from peripheral blood of the same (healthy) donor. A small panel of antigen- and receptor-specific T cells, all CD4$^+$ and restricted by DR2 products, proved strongly cytotoxic against antigen-presenting target cells. Importantly, all lines recognized specifically the relevant T-cell receptor-derived peptides when offered by antigen-presenting cells, but none of the anti-T-cell receptor lines showed any demonstrable interaction with the myelin basic protein-specific T cells. Following contemporary logic, the anti-T-cell receptor-specific T cells were recognizing cryptic T-cell receptor epitopes (Saruhan-Direskeneli *et al* 1993). More recently, complementarity-determining region 3 peptide-specific anti-idiotype reactive T cells were confronted *in vitro* with full-length recombinant T-cell receptor V chains. Some, but not all, of the peptide-specific T cells co-recognized their epitope when derived from the intact protein (Zipp *et al* 1998). While the anti-T-cell receptor-specific T cells were of the CD4 class, other investigators have isolated comparable anti-T-cell receptor-reactive T cells using shorter peptides. CD8$^+$ T cells were obtained that killed T cells with the suitable complementarity-determining region 3 and T-cell receptor sequence (Zang *et al* 2003b).

Two clinical studies support T-cell receptor-directed immune regulation controlling the T-cell response to myelin basic protein. We describe the preliminary therapeutic effects in Chapter 18, but here rehearse implications for understanding the immunology of multiple sclerosis. J. Zhang *et al* (1993) first directly applied Irun Cohen's T-cell vaccination scheme to multiple sclerosis. They isolated myelin basic protein-specific T cells from the peripheral blood of patients with multiple sclerosis, expanded these as lines, and transferred the T cells back to the original donors after irradiation. The autovaccinated patients underwent remarkable changes in their immune repertoire. For periods of several years, all myelin basic protein-reactive T cells were lost from the peripheral blood. During the same periods, CD8$^+$ T cells capable of specifically destroying the immunizing T cells developed in a clonotypic fashion (J. Zhang *et al* 1995). It is tempting to speculate, but premature to conclude, that elimination of myelin autoreactive T cells indeed affects the autoimmune pathogenesis of multiple sclerosis. An alternative strategy relied on vaccination of patients with synthetic peptides representing V region sequences from human myelin basic protein-specific T-cell receptors. This approach was based on the assumption of dominant usage of one particular Vβ gene (Vβ8.2) by human T cells recognizing myelin basic protein in the context of DR2 (DRB1·1501: Vandenbark *et al* 1996a). Such a biased repertoire was noted in some groups of patients (Chou *et al* 1994; Kotzin *et al* 1991; Oksenberg *et al* 1993), but not others (Afshar *et al* 1998; Hafler *et al* 1996), somewhat limiting general applicability of the therapy.

Vaccination of patients with multiple sclerosis using T-cell receptor peptide resulted in a partial loss of myelin basic protein-reactive T cells in patients who appeared to respond by entering disease remission. The effect of T-cell receptor peptide vaccination was attributed to the activation of Th2-like T cells suppressing pathogenic brain-reactive T cells in a bystander fashion (Vandenbark *et al* 2001). Unfortunately, like many other immunotherapeutic strategies, T-cell receptor-targeted vaccination has not yet yielded a satisfactory therapeutic success (Hohlfeld and Wiendl 2001). Taken together, the present data are compatible with idiotypic regulation of myelin-specific T cells, but the active role of Tregs in the pathogenesis of multiple sclerosis – plausible as a hypothesis – remains unproven.

IMMUNE REACTIVITY IN THE CENTRAL NERVOUS SYSTEM

Traditionally, the tissues of the nervous system have been considered exempt from immunological surveillance and devoid of immune reactivity. Barker and Billingham (1977) coined the term 'immune privilege' to describe this status. The concept carries with it the implication that immune surveillance, which protects most other tissues, does not extend to the nervous system. It follows that immunosurveillant lymphocytes, patrolling elsewhere in the organism, are excluded from brain and nerves. In its strict original version, the notion of immune privilege in the nervous system stood on somewhat shaky foundations. The brain parenchyma was considered to be totally secluded from the systemic circulation by a tight endothelial blood–brain barrier, excluding all recirculating immune cells. The central nervous system was thought to lack any lymphatic drainage, since fully differentiated lymphatic vessels, which permit transport of antigenic material from a primary site of infection into the local lymph node, were not found. In contrast to most other tissues, the healthy brain parenchyma was considered not to express MHC products, the essential prerequisite for antigen presentation to T lymphocytes. And, finally, professional antigen-presenting cells were thought not to be present in the normal brain. It is now clear that most of these assumptions, although not actually wrong, were somewhat exaggerated. It turns out that the central nervous system is far from absolutely immune privileged, although its behaviour differs from the classic pattern of immune reactivity seen in most other organs. Immune surveillance is restricted to a small set of activated lymphocytes, and antigen presentation can be induced in a number of brain cells by proinflammatory stimuli, such as IFN-γ (Wekerle *et al* 1986).

Lymphocyte traffic into the central nervous system

We have mentioned that the central nervous system tissues are secluded by a specialized endothelial blood–brain barrier that tightly seals the parenchyma from the bloodstream. The central nervous system endothelium differs indeed from endothelia lining the blood vessels in other organs, because it is lined by tight junctions that bar plasma molecules and circulating cells from entry. A few molecules that are required to feed the tissue, such as glucose or lipids, are taken up by transport systems on the luminal side and transferred in a controlled fashion into the tissue. For blood cells, such transportation is unknown. Yet, there must be some cellular traffic between blood and central nervous system. It is known that bone marrow-dependent progenitor cells slowly replace at least those microglial cells positioned close to the microvessels. Furthermore, there must be conditions that allow certain immune and inflammatory cells to enter the central nervous system. Without such mechanisms, the inflammatory lesions of multiple sclerosis would not occur (Sospedra and Martin 2005).

Migration of T cells into the central nervous system

Passage through the blood–brain barrier has been shown by metastasizing tumour cells (Subramaniam *et al* 2003), bone marrow-derived stem cells (Priller *et al* 2001), and – of significance in the present context – lymphocytes, provided that they are in a state of high activation (Wekerle *et al* 1986). Within the first few hours after transfer, a few highly activated T cells cross the resting blood–brain barrier and migrate into the central nervous system parenchyma. Assuming that brain antigen is not recognized, this T-cell infiltration is transient and lasts only a few hours. However, when the T-cell population is directed against a central nervous system antigen, the cells persist within the brain tissue (Hickey *et al* 1991; Wekerle *et al* 1986). After approximately 2–3 days, a sudden new influx of inflammatory cells occurs, which results in clinical disease associated with histological evidence for meningoencephalitis (Figures 11.8 and 11.16).

It is probable that the entry of activated lymphocytes through the initially resting blood–brain barrier is governed by the combination of chemotactic cytokines and special patterns of cell adhesion molecules displayed on the inner surface of brain microvascular endothelial cells. Prevailing wisdom distinguishes three steps in the attachment of lymphocytes to endothelial surfaces (Springer 1994). First, mutual contacts are made through selectins on one cell and glycoproteins on the other (L-selectins bind to GlyCAM, and P-selectin to the sLe^x glycoprotein). Although this selectin-mediated adhesion is relatively weak, selectin-bound lymphocytes roll along the endothelial surface directed by the streaming blood. In the second phase, the lymphocyte becomes activated either by selectin-glycoprotein binding or stimuli provided by chemokines. Additional cell adhesion molecules, including members of the integrin and immunoglobulin superfamilies, are quickly induced to form stronger bonds, tethering the T cell firmly to the endothelial membrane (Figure 11.17: von Andrian and Mackay 2000). Using proteases and glycosidases, in a third phase, the migrant T cells then puncture the blood–brain barrier and pass directly into the central nervous system parenchyma, presumably attracted by gradients of locally produced chemotactic factors (Butcher and Picker 1996; Kunkel and Butcher 2002).

There are observations suggesting that the general rules of leucocyte recirculation are not competely represented in the passage of activated lymphocytes across resting cerebral endothelial cells. One study combined fluorochrome labelling of activated T lymphocytes with *in vivo* microcinematography. It showed that, in contrast to regular lymphocyte penetration through blood vessel walls, activated T cells did not roll along the lining of cerebral vessels but directly adhered to the endothelium (Vajkoczy *et al* 2001). Initial adhesion involved binding of the VLA-4 integrin to vascular cell adhesion molecule 1 (VCAM-1), which seems to be constitutively expressed on resting cerebral endothelia, in contrast to most other endothelial cells. Importantly, interaction between VLA-4 and VCAM-1 leads to the enhanced production and T-lymphocyte secretion of gelatinases – enzymes that help the lymphocyte to break up the perivascular basal lamina and allow entry to the surrounding tissue (Hartung and Kieseier 2000).

VLA-4 was previously identified as a target of antibody-mediated immunotherapy (J.L. Baron *et al* 1993; Yednock *et al* 1992). Now, there is evidence that anti-VLA-4 antibodies act in a dual fashion. Initially they reduce the number of effector T cells entering the central nervous system in the early phase. Later, they block the influx of additional, nonspecific inflammatory cells (Brocke *et al* 1999). However, therapy using anti-VLA-4 blockade should be used with caution (see Chapter 18; Hohlfels and Wekerle 2005; Steinman 2005). Although it blocks entry of effector and accessory cells into the central nervous system when given early in a response, exposure at later time points may paradoxically cause exacerbation of chronic disease (Theien *et al* 2001). This has to be remembered in planning therapeutic trials, which, to date, have produced favourable clinical results (see Chapter 18: D.H. Miller *et al* 2003a; Tubridy *et al* 1999).

Cell migration through the primed blood–brain barrier: the second wave of immigration

Activation of the endothelial blood–brain barrier is central to the initiation of clinical experimental autoimmune encephalomyelitis. In T cell-transferred experimental autoimmune encephalomyelitis in the Lewis rat, mass invasion of the central nervous system by mononuclear cells coincides with acute onset of neurological defects. At this time, brain endothelia show notable changes. They become permeable, allowing influx of plasma macromolecules, and thus promote the formation of oedema (Butter *et al* 1991; Juhler *et al* 1984; Koh *et al* 1993). At the same time, the expression of MHC class I determinants and several cell adhesion molecules increases (Cannella *et al* 1991). The activated blood–brain barrier allows passage of mononuclear cells, including naive T cells, which are otherwise excluded by the resting unactivated blood–brain barrier (Krakowski and Owens 2000). Thus, activation of the blood–brain barrier endothelium is an essential prerequisite for formation of the pathogenic infiltrate in experimental autoimmune encephalomyelitis.

It remains unresolved where exactly in the central nervous system (and peripheral immune system) effector T cells are located, as the inflammatory infiltrate is assembled in the brain parenchyma, and how they influence the central nervous system tissue. The application of novel biological fluorochrome markers should help. Our position is that early effector T cells enter the central nervous system parenchyma, release proinflammatory cytokines and chemokines, and prime the local tissue. Accordingly, they are supposed to activate cerebral endothelia to express an inflammatory phenotype, and induce immune molecules in glia cells required for successful presentation of local autoantigens (Cross *et al* 1991; Wekerle *et al* 1986). The proportion and distribution of antigen-specific T-cell blasts in the lesions remain controversial. It was generally believed that antigen-specific cells in the lesion were rather sparse, representing only a few percent of the total T-cell population (A.H. Cross *et al* 1990; Fallis *et al* 1987; Stohl and Gonatas 1978), although others report a much higher proportion (Körner *et al* 1997; Matsumoto and Fujiwara 1988; Skundric *et al* 1994; Zeine and Owens 1992). We have used transgenic markers (J. Bauer *et al* 1998) and retroviral engineering (Flügel *et al* 1999) to trace transferred encephalitogenic T lymphocytes in the inflammatory infiltrates. As previously described, the small number of T cells arriving in the initial wave after transfer are all derived from the transferred antigen-specific pool. At the onset of clinical disease, 3 days after transfer, a massive influx of the transferred antigen-specific T cells is seen in the nervous system, and these constitute >90% of all CD4 T cells in the fresh infiltrate. As shown by recent two-photon imaging, the T cells rapidly cruise through the central nervous system parenchyma, apparently in search of the specific autoantigen (Kawakami *et al* 2005). This initial phase, however, is transient, and the antigen-specific T cells are gradually replaced in the lesions by secondarily recruited, host-derived T lymphocytes (Flügel *et al* 2001a).

One may assume that the activated blood–brain barrier surface *per se* is insufficient to attract inflammatory cells to the developing lesion. Soluble signals emanating from chemokines, perhaps produced by perivascular dendritic cells (Greeter *et al* 2005), should also play a vital role. In fact, an ever growing list of chemokines attracting T cells and monocytic cells has been demonstrated in the early phase of experimental autoimmune encephalomyelitis (Ransohoff *et al* 2003). Among the many chemokines making an appearance in the developing experimental autoimmune encephalomyelitis lesion, macrophage inflammatory protein MIP-1α seems especially important since

its neutralization by antibody stops disease (Karpus *et al* 1995). The chemokine attracts T cells and macrophages, but also participates in orchestrating the entire chemokine symphony. In general, chemokines such as MIP-1α, macrophage chemotactic protein MCP-1, RANTES and interferon induced protein IP-10 determine an inflammatory milieu, which controls the number and composition of inflammatory infiltrates in experimental autoimmune encephalomyelitis (Ransohoff 1999). It should be noted that chemokines contributing to the central nervous system infiltrate include not only those induced in response to inflammatory stimuli, but also molecules produced under homeostatic conditions. CCL21 (secondary lymphoid organ chemokine, SLC) and CCL19 (EBI-1 ligand chemokine, ELC), for example, chemokines that govern ordered migration of immune cells into and through lymphoid tissues, appear in chronic relapsing experimental autoimmune encephalomyelitis, although with different distributions from those characterizing the acute phases (Columba-Cabezas *et al* 2003).

Clearance of central nervous system inflammation

Experimental autoimmune encephalomyelitis in the Lewis rat (and other strains) is self-limiting and follows a monophasic course. Clinically, neurological signs develop, reach a peak, and thereafter resolve, often fully. The histological infiltrates usually, but not invariably, run a parallel course (Källen and Nilsson 1986; Levine and Sowinski 1980). Typically, the lesions of experimental autoimmune encephalomyelitis in the Lewis rat vanish within 2–3 weeks of disease onset. Clearance of inflammation in the central nervous system and recovery from an episode of experimental autoimmune encephalomyelitis are controlled by systemic immune regulatory mechanisms, as well as by events taking place within the nervous tissue. The severity of clinical disease and the time course of brain inflammation reflect the genetically determined ability of animals to mount a vigorous corticosteroid response (D. Mason 1991). In addition, adrenalectomy, or the blockade of glucocorticoid receptors, augments experimental autoimmune encephalomyelitis. Recovery from experimental autoimmune encephalomyelitis is also associated with changes in cytokine pattern within the circulation and local brain environment. In particular, cytokines associated with the suppression of T-cell reactivity (TGF-β and IL-10) are increased within the central nervous system lesions themselves (M.K. Kennedy *et al* 1992; Khoury *et al* 1992; Racke *et al* 1992). These cytokines have also been shown to suppress experimental autoimmune encephalomyelitis when systemically administered during the course of the disease (Racke *et al* 1991; 1994). Other data, however, indicate that local dysregulated expression of TGF-β may also augment inflammation (Wyss-Coray *et al* 1997).

How do inflammatory cells leave the central nervous system? Is this via blood vessels or other pathways? Alternatively, do they die and undergo local degradation? So far there is no convincing evidence for emigration of intraparenchymal T cells via a vascular route or cerebrospinal fluid (Wekerle 1993). Instead, several groups have found that antigen-activated T cells arriving in brain tissue undergo apoptosis at very high rates. Recovery from experimental autoimmune encephalomyelitis is associated with extensive apoptotic destruction of T and B lymphocytes in inflammatory brain lesions (Figure 11.16: Pender *et al* 1991; A.T. White *et al* 2000). In the late stages of T cell-transferred

EAE, up to 50% of the local T-cell population may synchronously be destroyed by this mechanism (Schmied *et al* 1993). To illustrate the significance of this high percentage it has to be understood that execution of the full apoptosis programme *in vitro* lasts for approximately 3 hours. A 50% apoptosis rate, observed within a given tissue section, suggests that about three times the number of cells present in the lesion are destroyed by programmed cell death within 24 hours. This clearance process is therefore so effective that an acute inflammatory lesion in the central nervous system can only be maintained by a continuous supply of new inflammatory T cells from the circulation.

T-cell apoptosis mainly affects the cell population that infiltrates the brain parenchyma, leaving inflammatory cells in the perivascular space and meninges unaffected (J. Bauer *et al* 1998). In experimental autoimmune encephalomyelitis induced by sensitization with myelin basic protein, most apoptotic T cells in the parenchyma carry the Vβ8.2 T-cell receptor, at least during the early phases of brain inflammation (Tabi *et al* 1994). Since this is also the receptor subtype of the transferred encephalitogenic T-cell fraction, it was originally suggested that the pool of autoreactive T cells dies selectively in the central nervous system by activation-induced cell death (Pender 1999). However, by transferring prelabelled T cells in the induction of experimental autoimmune encephalomyelitis, autoantigen-specific as well as irrelevant, it is clear that secondarily recruited T cells are also destroyed in the central nervous system lesions by apoptosis (J. Bauer *et al* 1998). Several different immunological mechanisms may be responsible for the induction of this T-cell apoptosis in inflammatory brain lesions. Programmed cell death of lymphocytes can be induced by the glucocorticoid response associated with recovery from experimental autoimmune encephalomyelitis. Indeed, myelin basic protein-specific T cells can synchronously be driven to apoptotic death when glucocorticoids are added *in vitro* at a late stage after T-cell activation (D.P. Gold *et al* 1991). Furthermore, high-dose corticosteroids significantly increase the rate of T-lymphocyte apoptosis in the lesions of experimental autoimmune encephalomyelitis (McCombe *et al* 1996; J. Schmidt *et al* 2000) and neuritis (Zettl *et al* 1995). Corticosteroids induce apoptosis not only in the Vβ8.2 positive, putative autoreactive T cells, but also in other T lymphocytes and microglia (McCombe *et al* 1996; Nguyen *et al* 1997).

Another possible mechanism of apoptosis induction in T cells lies in the action of TGF-β. The expression of this cytokine is massively upregulated in the recovery stage of experimental autoimmune encephalomyelitis, and TGF-β has been noted to have a potent suppressive effect on experimental autoimmune encephalomyelitis. *In vitro*, T cells can be driven into apoptosis by exposure to TGF-β (Weller *et al* 1994). On the other hand, it is known that apoptotic T cells themselves release substantial amounts of TGF-β (W. Chen *et al* 2001), making it difficult to determine whether enhanced cytokine levels are a cause or consequence of local apoptosis. In fact, the evidence suggests that neither the steroid response nor cytokines alone are responsible. Adrenalectomy does not prevent T-cell death in the brain lesions of experimental autoimmune encephalomyelitis, although it massively potentiates disease and mortality (T. Smith *et al* 1996). In addition, T-cell apoptosis in experimental autoimmune encephalomyelitis lesions is mainly found in the brain parenchyma and – at least in the early stages of the inflammatory process – predominantly involves the antigen-specific T-cell population. Thus, antigen-specific mechanisms may also play a central role in the induction of T-cell apoptosis in experimental autoimmune encephalomyelitis.

Antigen-specific induction of T-cell apoptosis could result from unbalanced signal transduction mediated by local nonprofessional antigen-presenting cells such as microglia or astrocytes. In line with this interpretation, apoptosis of antigen-specific T cells *in vitro* is readily induced by astrocytes (R. Gold *et al* 1996) and freshly isolated microglia (Ford *et al* 1996). Furthermore, the rate of T-cell apoptosis in the lesions *in vivo* is massively increased following treatment of animals with the respective soluble antigenic peptide (Ishigami *et al* 1998; Weishaupt *et al* 1997). On the other hand, it is unlikely that antigen presentation by local nonprofessional presenting cells alone is responsible for the induction of T-cell apoptosis, since its rate in brain lesions is identical when experimental autoimmune encephalomyelitis is induced in bone marrow chimeras or fully competent Lewis rats. In the former, antigen presentation on local tissue elements such as astrocytes or microglia cannot take place because of MHC antigen mismatch (J. Bauer *et al* 1998).

Since T-cell destruction by apoptosis is not restricted to the transferred antigen-specific cell population – being prominent in inflammatory lesions of the central (Schmied *et al* 1993) and peripheral nervous systems (Zettl *et al* 1994) but virtually absent in inflammatory lesions elsewhere (Schmied *et al* 1993; Schneider *et al* 1996) – should we conclude that the nervous systems have special mechanisms that control inflammation through effective destruction and elimination of T cells? One possible mechanism is by the Fas/Fas-L pathway. Activation of Fas through its specific ligand triggers an intracellular cell death pathway that can drive cells into apoptosis (Nagata and Goldstein 1995). In the central nervous system, Fas is widely expressed during inflammation, whereas Fas-ligand complex is mainly present on invading leucocytes, microglia (Dowling *et al* 1996; D'Souza *et al* 1996b) and possibly on astrocytes (Bechmann *et al* 2002; Kohji and Matsumoto 2000). When the Fas/Fas-L interaction is blocked, either pharmacologically or through genetic deletion of one binding partner, the rate of T-cell apoptosis is reduced in various *in vitro* and *in vivo* models (Bechmann *et al* 2002; Ciusani *et al* 2001; Flügel *et al* 2000). But in one other study, deletion of Fas or Fas-L had no effect on T-cell apoptosis in experimental autoimmune encephalomyelitis lesions, whereas, in the absence of tumour necrosis factor-receptor 1 (TNF-R1) signalling, T-cell apoptosis was reduced by 50% (Bachmann *et al* 1999). Taken together, there is good evidence that the network of microglia and astrocyte processes expressing Fas-L or TNF-α represents a hostile environment for activated Fas- or TNF-receptor-positive lymphocytes that enter the central nervous system from the circulation or become activated locally. Apoptosis of T cells in inflammatory brain lesions is further augmented by IFN-γ. In the absence of IFN-γ production in the central nervous system, T-cell apoptosis is massively reduced in experimental autoimmune encephalomyelitis lesions, and the clearance of CD4+ T lymphocytes from the central nervous system is disturbed (Chu *et al* 2000). Conversely, overproduction of IFN-γ in the central nervous system results in increased rates of lymphocyte apoptosis in animals with experimental autoimmune encephalomyelitis, reflected by reduced disease severity and earlier recovery (Furlan *et al* 2001). This may in part explain the unexpected effect of manipulating IFN-γ in the context of experimental autoimmune encephalomyelitis.

Whatever mechanisms are responsible for the induction of T-cell apoptosis in inflammatory brain lesions, dead cells are taken up locally by macrophages, microglia and (less effectively) astrocytes (Magnus *et al* 2002; Nguyen and Pender 1998). Uptake and digestion of apoptotic T cells by microglia leads to downregulation of their activation state (Magnus *et al* 2001).

The mechanisms described above may account for the removal of T cells from autoimmune lesions of the nervous system and consequently for downregulation of the inflammatory process. They do not, however, elucidate how secondarily recruited effector cells leave the lesion. Although in rare instances apoptotic macrophages and microglia are found in experimental autoimmune encephalomyelitis lesions (Nguyen *et al* 1994; White *et al* 1998), their low number does not offer a satisfactory explanation for effector cell clearance (T. Smith *et al* 1996). Macrophages containing tissue debris tend to accumulate in the perivascular space (Figure 11.17), from where they are able to reach the cerebrospinal fluid, suggesting that there is lymphatic drainage of the central nervous system (Cserr *et al* 1992; Weller *et al* 1996). Particulate substances injected into the central nervous system can be traced along the perivascular space into the leptomeninges (Weller *et al* 1992). From there, the material can further be transported along cranial and spinal nerve roots to reach the epidural space through channel systems in the arachnoid membranes of root pockets (Zenker *et al* 1994) and large brain vessels, as well as through the lamina cribrosa (Weller *et al* 1992). Consistent with the possible existence of lymphatic drainage of the central nervous system is the observation that in chronic experimental autoimmune encephalomyelitis in primates, myelin-reactive material ingested in macrophages or dendritic cells can be found in the deep cervical lymph nodes (De Vos *et al* 2002).

These data suggest that, in the normal brain and conditions of acute inflammation, T and B lymphocytes are effectively and rapidly cleared from the central nervous system by programmed cell death, while macrophages and microglia cells persist in the lesions for much longer. These cells may also be slowly removed by apoptosis. Alternatively, they have the capacity to migrate out of the central nervous system and reach regional lymph nodes. Apoptosis of T lymphocytes has been observed in similar quantity in the lesions of acute disseminated leucoencephalitis (Bauer *et al* 1999), suggesting that the basic mechanisms of T-cell clearance from inflammatory central nervous system lesions are similar between rodents and humans. However, in the lesions of multiple sclerosis, the rate of T-cell apoptosis is very low (Ozawa *et al* 1994). This may reflect the chronic course of the disease, in which a synchronous and simultaneous apoptosis of lymphocytes cannot be expected. In line with this interpretation is the low apoptosis rate of lymphocytes in chronic models of *Toxoplasma* encephalitis (Schlüter *et al* 2002). Alternatively it has been suggested that a genetically determined failure of activation-induced apoptosis of autoreactive T cells may underlie the chronic disease in multiple sclerosis (Pender 1998).

Regulation of major histocompatibility antigen expression in the brain

While it is clear that the healthy central nervous system displays very little MHC class I or class II antigen, it is equally apparent

that many, if not all, brain cells can be induced under suitable conditions to express these molecules. And from *in vitro* studies, we know that there is a clear hierarchy of MHC inducibility – microglia, astrocytes, endothelia, oligodendrocytes and then neurons (Wekerle 1994). MHC determinants are also induced *in vivo* under a variety of pathological conditions. Ectopic MHC expression is commonly noted in inflammatory responses, virus infections, tumour, development, and degenerative disorders. Whilst proinflammatory cytokines, such as IFN-γ, have a predominant role in MHC induction during inflammation of the central nervous system, mechanisms that result in the gene expression associated with noninflammatory neurodegenerative processes are less clear. Recent observations indicate that neurons have a crucial role in regulating MHC expression in the central nervous system. Electrically active neurons strongly suppress MHC expression on surrounding glia cells (H. Neumann *et al* 1996). However, neuronal degeneration following axotomy results in efficient induction of MHC class I components *in vivo* (Finsen *et al* 1993; Lindå *et al* 1998). Thus, paralysis of neuronal activity leads to the prompt inducibility of MHC determinants on all central nervous system cell classes. It is open to debate whether this negative signalling is mediated by diffusible neurotransmitters (glutamate, vasoactive intestinal peptide or catecholamines), or is the effect of electrical activity (H. Neumann *et al* 1996). Class I expression in the central nervous system is not an experimental curiosity, but is the hallmark of (human) neurodegenerative disorders. Alzheimer's disease (Tooyama *et al* 1990), Parkinson's disease (McGeer *et al* 1988), amyotrophic lateral sclerosis (Kawamata *et al* 1992) and brain trauma (Kaur *et al* 1995) are all associated with upregulation of MHC proteins, especially on microglia cells.

A particularly intriguing finding is the inducibility of MHC class I antigens on neurons. Traditionally, these were considered as the only cell types absolutely devoid of MHC antigens. Indeed, even high doses of IFN-γ, one of the strongest inducers of MHC, fail to induce class I molecules in electrically active neurons. However, after paralysis with sodium channel blockers, the same neurons become fully inducible (H. Neumann *et al* 1995; 1997). Some MHC class I expression appears during neuronal development (Huh *et al* 2000).

Neuronal MHC class I proteins are fully functional. They can present viral peptides to virus-specific class I restricted cytotoxic T cells. Recognition triggers cytolytic mechanisms, which start by disrupting axonal processes (Medana *et al* 2001b) and, with some delay, end up killing the entire neuron (Medana *et al* 2001a).

The central nervous system is therefore a conditionally privileged organ; it is accessible to immune surveillance and accessory inflammatory machinery; but this is well controlled so as not to threaten neurons, which are especially vulnerable and cannot be regenerated.

T-cell interaction with local glia

Once through the blood–brain barrier, activated T cells find themselves in contact with local glia (and neuronal) cells. By secretion of proinflammatory cytokines (IFN-γ, TNF-α and others), glia are induced to synthesize and express MHC products (Male *et al* 1987; Traugott and Lebon 1988c; Vass and Lassmann 1990), cell-adhesion molecules (Cannella *et al* 1991; Male *et al*

1994) and costimulatory molecules (Issazadeh *et al* 1998; Soos *et al* 1999; Williams *et al* 1994) needed to process and present self and foreign protein antigens to patrolling T cells. However, not all glia cells are equally responsive to the activating signals communicated by T lymphoblasts, and not all central nervous system cells are equally efficient antigen presenters. Perivascular cells and microglia, which scan the central nervous system tissue with fast moving processes (Davalos *et al* 2005; Nimmerjahn *et al* 2005), are undoubtedly the fastest and most proficient cytokine responders, whereas astrocytes and ependymal cells require more intense signals to become immunologically activated (Vass and Lassmann 1990).

The onset of overt brain inflammation is associated with a variety of immunopathological changes in the local tissue. First, different cytokines are produced locally in a time-dependent manner (Issazadeh *et al* 1995a; 1995b). The first cytokine to be expressed in the inflammatory lesion is IL-12 followed after a few hours by IFN-γ and TNF-α. Parallel with the expression of these cytokines, extensive upregulation of adhesion molecules and histocompatibility antigens takes place. In particular, endothelial cells of cerebral vessels express a variety of adhesion molecules – selectins, intercellular adhesion molecules (ICAMs), VCAMs and others – and endothelial cells acquire an activated phenotype (Cannella *et al* 1991; Lossinsky *et al* 1989; Wilcox *et al* 1990). These endothelial changes apparently are instrumental for the secondary recruitment of inflammatory cells (T cells and monocytes/macrophages) into the established lesions (Figure 11.17). Histocompatibility antigens are primarily expressed on meningeal and perivascular monocytes (Hickey and Kimura 1988; Matsumoto and Fujiwara 1987). In addition, a less pronounced expression of class I antigen is found on endothelial cells and, with more severe proinflammatory stimuli, on all other neuroectodermal elements in the lesions (Vass and Lassmann 1990). Class II MHC antigen expression in established lesions is more restricted and rarely found on elements other than leucocytes and resident microglia (Vass *et al* 1986). However, in rare instances, some expression is seen on cerebral endothelial cells, astrocytes and ependymal cells (Deckert-Schlüter *et al* 1994; Hickey *et al* 1985; Steiniger and Van der Meide 1988; Vass and Lassmann 1990). Although much emphasis has been placed on the possible role of class II MHC antigen expression and antigen presentation by neuroectodermal cells, studies in bone marrow chimeras clearly show that the expression of MHC antigens on local resident cells of the central nervous system, including astrocytes, ependymal cells, endothelial cells and resident microglia, is not required for the development of experimental autoimmune encephalomyelitis (Hickey and Kimura 1988; Lassmann *et al* 1993; Y. Matsumoto and Fujiwara 1988). In these animals, a model system is created in which experimental autoimmune encephalomyelitis is induced in a host environment where only meningeal and perivascular monocytes and haematogenous macrophages carry the specific MHC haplotype recognized by the transferred encephalitogenic T lymphocytes (Hickey *et al* 1992). Results obtained in this model indicate that induction, maintenance and downregulation of brain inflammation do not require antigen presentation on resident tissue elements. It has, however, yet to be determined whether local antigen presentation modifies experimental autoimmune encephalomyelitis, for example in the chronic models.

Is autoimmunity beneficial?

Traditionally, and throughout this text so far, autoimmunity has been treated as an unwanted upheaval of the immune system working against the organism – an illicit and pathological aberration. Consequently, early theories of immunity invoked emotive terms such as 'horror autotoxicus' (Ehrlich and Morgenroth 1901) to describe the catastrophic effects of immune reactions directed against self. Immune cells driving such responses were assigned the status of 'forbidden clones', having no place in health and therefore ripe for removal from the immune repertoire (Burnet 1959).

A dramatic revision of this thinking began with the discovery of organ-specific T-cell clones as normal components of the healthy immune system (Schlüsener and Wekerle 1985). Clearly, such T cells have receptors for antigenic structures on the body's own tissues and, yet, in most individuals they appear harmless throughout life. How then should we view these self-recognizing T-cell populations; can they be badged as flawed products of a sloppily evolved immune system? Irun Cohen formulated a theory that assigned a positive and physiological function to immunological self-reactivity. Briefly, his concept of the 'immunological homunculus' postulates that throughout the body, all major antigenic structures are reflected by complementary self-reactive T-cell clones in the immune system (Cohen 1992). These self-reactive T cells would be beneficial in more than one way. First, as proposed by Cohen, by activating a regulatory network, they would hold down exuberant, potentially pathogenic immune responses. More recently, tissue-specific T-cell activation occurring in response to trauma in the central nervous system was suggested to represent a mechanism of attempted tissue regeneration (Schwartz *et al* 1999). Indeed, a detailed series of experimental studies from Michal Schwartz and her group provides impressive evidence in support of this concept. Transfer of central nervous system autoreactive T-cell lines improves regeneration of severed central nervous system tissues in the optic nerve, spinal cord and retina (Schwartz and Kipnis 2001). In a key experiment, activated T cells were infused into Lewis rats after a unilateral optic nerve crush trauma. Myelin basic protein autoreactive, but not ovalbumin specific, T cells protected local axons from degeneration, as reflected by a threefold higher survival rate of relevant retinal ganglion cells (Moalem *et al* 1999). Active immunization against myelin basic protein or transfer of myelin basic protein-specific activated T cells, protected rats from degeneration of spinal cord motor neurons after contusion (Hauben *et al* 2000a) or ventral root avulsion (Hammarberg *et al* 2000). Intriguingly, neuroprotection derives not only from classically autoreactive T cells, specific to 'true' autoantigens such as myelin basic protein, but also from T cells responding to altered peptide ligands. Vaccination with a partially agonist myelin basic protein ligand protected spinal cord motor neurons from crush-induced degeneration (Hauben *et al* 2001). Similar therapeutic effects were obtained by vaccination with copolymer-1 (Kipnis *et al* 2000), which probably acts as a super-altered peptide ligand variant of myelin basic protein (see Chapter 18).

Therapeutic vaccination in neurodegeneration is an intriguing concept that is not yet fully understood or free from debate (Popovich and Jones 2003). Several properties of the central nervous system-directed autoimmune response act in favour of the approach. First, autoimmune T cells accumulate preferentially in central nervous system areas with ongoing degeneration, a behaviour that helps to target the therapy. This has been known ever since S. Levine and Hoenig (1968) showed in rat experimental autoimmune encephalomyelitis that immune cells strongly invade brain areas exposed to thermal injury but not the unlesioned tissue. Selective T-cell infiltration is also noted in central nervous system areas affected by peripheral nerve axotomy. Clipping of a facial nerve, for example, leads to retrograde degeneration of the facial nucleus embedded in the brainstem. In unilaterally axotomized rats, myelin-specific T cells infiltrate the lesioned facial nucleus, but avoid the contralateral intact side (Flügel *et al* 2000; Maehlen *et al* 1989). T-cell migration targeted to degenerative tissues has also been noted in the optic nerve (Hickey 1991; Konno *et al* 1990).

The signals that lure T cells into degenerative lesions are poorly understood. Endothelial cells of the local blood–brain barrier may be activated following neuronal injury, expressing profiles of cell adhesion molecules that favour inflammatory cell entry (Andjelkovic and Pachter 1998). No less important for degenerative lesions are the membrane profiles that support immune responses assumed by glial cells. Facial nerve axotomy leads to production and expression of MHC antigens, costimulatory structures, cell adhesion molecules and soluble mediators that all promote presentation of local (auto)antigen to T cells (Raivich *et al* 1999). The central nervous system milieu becomes immune friendly, allowing efficient processing of central nervous system autoantigen from cellular debris and its presentation to invading autoimmune T cells – as in antigen spreading following central nervous system infection (Vanderlugt and Miller 2002).

How might autoimmune T cells protect neurons from death and promote cell regeneration? It is notable that activated T cells produce and secrete a plethora of soluble mediators, cytotoxic as well as proregenerative. For example, T cells release neurotrophic factors including nerve growth factor (Ehrhard *et al* 1993) and brain-derived nerve growth factor (Kerschensteiner *et al* 1999), neurotrophin-3 (Besser and Wank 1999), and glia cell-derived neutrotrophic factor (GDNF) (Kerschensteiner *et al* 2003). Local deposition of neurotrophins could reduce cytotoxic inflammation, as has been found using nerve growth factor-engineered T-cell lines (Kramer *et al* 1995), and at the same time encourage survival and regeneration of central nervous system cells (Hammarberg *et al* 2000; Moalem *et al* 2000). In addition, proinflammatory mediators, like TNF-α, are known to play a dual role in the central nervous system. At high concentrations, TNF-α clearly damages central nervous system cells *in vivo* (Probert *et al* 1995), while *in vitro* (Nicholas *et al* 2002) it plays a role in tissue protection (see Chapter 10). In explant cultures, TNF-α protects hippocampus cells against the toxic effect of β-APP (Barger *et al* 1995) and glutamate (Cheng *et al* 1994). TNF-α also protects neurons *in vivo* from traumatic damage (Sullivan *et al* 1999).

To conclude, the concept of beneficial autoimmunity in the central nervous system and its application to therapy of central nervous system degeneration are fascinating. At present, the most formidable hurdle preventing practical application is the encephalitogenic potential of autoreactive T cells. Research must find ways to tune down the autoaggressive power of central nervous system reactive cells, while preserving or even amplifying the beneficial capacity of these cells. Newly emerging techniques of genetic engineering may realize that goal (T.N.M. Schumacher 2003).

PATHOGENESIS OF DEMYELINATION AND TISSUE DAMAGE

A variety of different mechanisms have been defined *in vitro* that lead, directly or indirectly through an effect on oligodendrocytes, to the destruction of myelin sheaths. These can loosely be considered as having immunological or neurobiological bases. We refer readers to Chapter 10 for additional discussion, especially of the latter category, but reiterate the point that the division is to some extent artificial, the evidence indicating complexity and interplay with, for example, an altered growth factor environment in the nervous system influencing the outcome of superimposed inflammatory injury. That said, the immunological mechanisms described here include both antigen-specific and nonspecific immune processes targeted against several components of the axon-glial unit. T-cell cytotoxicity is mediated either by αβ (D'Souza *et al* 1995) or γδ T lymphocytes (M.S. Freedman *et al* 1991), as well as antibody-mediated immune reactions targeting antigens expressed at the surface of myelin or oligodendrocytes (Linington *et al* 1988). Although it is easy to define such mechanisms *in vitro*, their role in the complex *in vivo* situation is more difficult to characterize.

Inflammation and tissue injury induced by Th1 and Th2 cells

MHC class II-restricted T lymphocytes, polarized to the production of classic proinflammatory cytokines such as IFN-γ and TNF-α (Th1), enter the central nervous system compartment in the process of immune surveillance and, encountering specific antigen, become reactivated and start an inflammatory process. These Th1 cells can themselves be cytotoxic and kill targets in the process of antigen presentation (D. Sun and Wekerle 1986). This direct cytotoxicity, however, appears to be limited *in vivo*, due to the low or absent MHC class II expression on glia cells within the lesions (Vass and Lassmann 1990). Th1 cells produce high amounts of proinflammatory cytokines, which attract haematogenous macrophages and activate the local microglia population.

Experimental models, induced by the transfer of autoreactive Th1 cells, are characterized in general by intense inflammation with rather limited tissue injury (Ben-Nun *et al* 1981a). An exception to this general rule is Th1-mediated brain inflammation in mice. In this species, a chronic disease with quite extensive demyelination and tissue destruction is induced even after a single transfer of myelin basic protein-reactive encephalitogenic Th1 cells (Mokhtarian *et al* 1984). Clinical disease and tissue damage in Th1-mediated encephalitis correlates with the extent of macrophage, but not T-cell infiltration (T. Berger *et al* 1997).

Class II-restricted T cells, polarized to the production of IL-4, IL-5 and IL-10, were initially regarded as having a role in downregulation of brain inflammation (during recovery from experimental autoimmune encephalomyelitis: Issazadeh *et al* 1995a; 1995b). Under favourable conditions, Th2 cells can themselves induce brain inflammation (Lafaille *et al* 1997). However, brain lesions in this model are fundamentally different compared with those induced by Th1 cells. They are characterized by massive nonselective tissue damage, associated with dense tissue infiltration by granulocytes, including basophils (Lafaille *et al* 1997). Although this model is rather artificial, requiring profound immunosuppression of the recipients, it shows that central nervous system-specific Th2 cells have, in principle, a pathogenic potential. Indirect evidence suggests that this may be the case in experimental autoimmune encephalomyelitis induced with myelin oligodendrocyte glycoprotein, where sensitization procedures that preferentially stimulate a Th2 response influence severity of disease and the extent of tissue damage (Genain *et al* 1996; Stefferl *et al* 1999). In these conditions, autoantibodies play a major role in the pathogenesis of lesions (Stefferl *et al* 1999). Infiltration of eosinophilic granulocytes (Storch *et al* 1998b) and the particular profile of antibody isotypes, indicate a Th2-driven immune response (Tsunoda *et al* 2000). Although such a spectrum of changes is rare in classic multiple sclerosis, it is found in the pathology of Devic's type of neuromyelitis optica (Lucchinetti *et al* 2002). As with Th1 cells, the damage induced by Th2 cells is most probably mediated by activated effector cells rather than the T cells themselves.

Tissue destruction through class I MHC-restricted cytotoxic T cells

There is recent evidence pointing to CD8[+] cytotoxic T cells as effectors in the lesions of multiple sclerosis (Friese and Fugger 2005). Cell destruction through cytotoxic T cells can be mediated through either the release of cytotoxic granules (mainly perforin and granzyme B) or the activation of cell death receptors on the target cells, such as Fas or other receptors of the TNF receptor family. All central nervous system neuroectodermal cells can be induced to express MHC class I molecules and are lysed by cytotoxic class I MHC-restricted T cells *in vitro* (H. Neumann *et al* 2002). Although cell death generally ensues through the induction of apoptosis, specific attack by CD8[+] T cells may exclusively affect the axon, leaving the rest of the neuron intact (Medana *et al* 2001b). The pathway of cell destruction mediated by cytotoxic granules or death ligands depends on the activation state of T cells as well as properties of the target cells. Thus under comparable *in vitro* conditions, in contrast to astrocytes, neurons may be protected against granule-mediated cytotoxicity, whilst still sensitive to lysis mediated through the activation of death receptors (Medana *et al* 2000). Transgenic models, in which virus antigens are selectively expressed in different central nervous system cells, show that class I MHC-restricted T cells can reach and destroy their targets *in vivo* (Cabarrocas *et al* 2003; C.F. Evans *et al* 1996; Oldstone and Southern 1993). In addition, new models of brain inflammation have been developed, induced by passive transfer of autoreactive class I MHC-restricted T cells (Huseby *et al* 2001; D. Sun *et al* 2001). Polarization to Tc1 cells (production of IFN-γ) and activation prior to transfer was required to induce brain inflammation and disease (Cabarrocas *et al* 2003; Huseby *et al* 2001; D. Sun *et al* 2001).

Brain inflammation induced by cytotoxic CD8[+] T cells differs in several essential aspects from that mediated by class II MHC-restricted cells. In the situation of mild inflammation associated with exquisitely selective destruction of antigen-containing target cells (and in the absence of any bystander damage of other tissue elements), inflammation is reflected by T-cell infiltration and microglial activation, with limited recruitment of haematogenous macrophages (Cabarrocas *et al* 2003). When the inflammatory reaction is more vigorous, tissue injury is induced, which in many respects resembles that seen in hypoxic brain damage (Huseby *et al* 2001). This may be due to liberation of antigen within the lesions and its diffusion to brain vessels. There, it may possibly be directly recognized by cytotoxic T cells at the luminal surface of endothelial cells, leading to vasculitis and thrombotic vessel occlusion. Alternatively, cytotoxic T cells may damage the nervous tissue by a nonspecific bystander mechanism. It has recently been shown that, after brain infection with JHM virus (mouse hepatitis virus strain JHM) in immunodeficient animals, the transfer of activated CD8[+] but not CD4[+] T cells directed against an irrelevant epitope of a completely unrelated virus may induce focal demyelination. Perhaps, these activated nonspecific cytotoxic T cells are recruited to sites of brain infection and induce tissue damage through activation of the local microglia population (Haring *et al* 2002; Haring and Perlman 2003).

The importance of class I MHC-restricted cytotoxic T cells in mediating clinical disease and tissue damage in the central nervous system is highlighted in the model of Theiler's virus-induced demyelinating encephalomyelitis. Studies on the genetic susceptibility to this disease (Altintas *et al* 1993; Rodriguez *et al* 1986) and disease induction in β2-microglobulin-deficient mice (Rivera-Quinones *et al* 1998) show that the clinical and pathological phenotypes depend on a class I MHC-restricted T-cell response. Disease can also be blocked by treatment with anti-CD8 antibodies (Rodriguez and Sriram 1988). Specific deletion of a virus peptide-specific class I-restricted T-cell response preserves motor function in infected animals (K.P. Johnson *et al* 2001). Cytotoxic T cells appear also to play a major role in the pathogenesis of demyelination and tissue damage in multiple sclerosis (H. Neumann *et al* 2002; see Chapter 12). CD8[+] cells dominate the T-cell infiltrates in all lesions, and clonal expansion within the central nervous system and cerebrospinal fluid mainly reflects this subset. Furthermore, a large proportion of CD8[+] T cells in actively demyelinating lesions express granzyme B. They are seen in close contact with injured oligodendrocytes and axons.

Antibody-mediated demyelination and tissue injury

We have illustrated the ways in which antibody plays a major role in the induction of demyelination and tissue injury in the central nervous system. This is particularly evident in models of chronic experimental autoimmune encephalomyelitis in rats, guinea pigs and primates, where a good correlation exists between the antibody response and amount of demyelination (Linington and Lassmann 1987; Stefferl *et al* 1999). The requirement for antibody to induce demyelination is epitope expression on the surface of myelin or oligodendrocytes. So far, only very few myelin antigens fulfil this criterion. More prominent are glycolipids (Dubois-Dalcq *et al* 1970) and myelin oligodendrocyte glycoprotein (Linington and Lassmann 1987). When demyelinating antibodies are injected intravenously into animals with experimental autoimmune encephalomyelitis, induced by encephalitogenic T cells at the point when T-cell-mediated inflammation becomes apparent in the central nervous system, they massively augment clinical disease and induce widespread demyelinating lesions restricted to the central nervous system (Linington *et al* 1988; Schlüsener *et al* 1987). Furthermore, size and shape of the demyelinating lesions depend upon the balance between encephalitogenic T lymphocytes and demyelinating antibodies (Lassmann *et al* 1988). A high T-cell response together with low antibody titres leads to inflammatory infiltrates ubiquitously distributed throughout the central nervous system, and associated with a small rim of perivascular demyelination. This pattern is similar to that found in acute disseminated encephalomyelitis. In contrast, a mild T-cell-mediated encephalomyelitis together with a pronounced demyelinating antibody response results in the occurrence of few focal plaques with extensive, confluent demyelination. This pattern more closely resembles that found in acute or chronic multiple sclerosis. Furthermore, when such cotransfers of encephalitogenic T cells and demyelinating antibodies are repeated several times, persistent demyelinating lesions with extensive gliosis and impaired remyelination are found, in most respects resembling those found in patients with multiple sclerosis (Figure 11.13: Linington *et al* 1992). In this situation, encephalitogenic T cells are required to prime the central nervous system parenchyma and open the blood–brain barrier to allow the entry of myelin oligodendrocyte glycoprotein monoclonal antibodies. Demyelination is due to antibody assisted by accessory macrophages and/or complement (Linington *et al* 1989; Piddlesden *et al* 1993). Depletion of macrophages strongly reduces the demyelinating effect of cotransferred anti-myelin-associated glycoprotein antibody (Huitinga *et al* 1995), while intrathecal injection of macrophage-activating IFN-γ amplifies antibody-dependent demyelination (Vass *et al* 1992). Depletion of complement ameliorates the demyelination (Piddlesden *et al* 1991; 1994). A similar disease is induced by direct sensitization of susceptible animals with myelin oligodendrocyte glycoprotein (Figures 11.13 and 11.15). Antibody converts monophasic and nondemyelinating experimental autoimmune encephalomyelitis in the Lewis rats immunized with myelin basic protein to a chronic relapsing variant characterized by large-scale demyelination (Johns *et al* 1995). Similar disease is inducible by myelin oligodendrocyte glycoprotein in some mouse strains (Amor *et al* 1994; Mendel *et al* 1995) and, as it now turns out, primates (Genain *et al* 1996). Thus, to date, myelin oligodendrocyte glycoprotein is the only myelin component that elicits B- and T-cell autoimmune responses that combine to establish histological changes reproducing many features typical of the lesions seen in multiple sclerosis (Storch *et al* 1998a).

An issue of major clinical and diagnostic relevance is therefore which myelin oligodendrocyte glycoprotein antibodies can induce demyelination. Myelin oligodendrocyte glycoprotein is a small folded glycoprotein that lies deeply embedded in the oligodendrocyte cell membrane (Kroepfl *et al* 1996). Thus, only a very small domain of the myelin oligodendrocyte glycoprotein molecule is exposed on the cell surface. Most antibodies binding peptide sequences of myelin oligodendrocyte glycoprotein or denatured protein in an ELISA or Western blot do not recognize intact antigen on the cell surface (Brehm *et al* 1999).

Direct evidence for a role of anti-myelin oligodendrocyte glycoprotein antibodies in the pathogenesis of demyelination has recently been described in primates with experimental autoimmune encephalomyelitis and in a subset of multiple sclerosis patients (Genain *et al* 1999). Here, the authors used labelled myelin-associated glycoprotein in glutaraldehyde-fixed and plastic-embedded tissue to detect antibody within actively demyelinating lesions, and found binding to damaged myelin. However, in support of this interpretation, O'Connor *et al* (2005) recently eluted anti-myelin oligodendrocyte glycoprotein immunoglobulin from the lesions of multiple sclerosis. This was interpreted as direct evidence for opsonization of degenerate myelin by anti-myelin-associated glycoprotein antibodies. That leaves unanswered the question of why labelled myelin-associated glycoprotein sticks selectively to damaged myelin sheaths, but not the more abundant supply in B lymphocytes and plasma cells. Furthermore, the studies were performed with labelled peptides – epitopes not recognized by demyelinating antibodies in intact oligodendrocytes or myelin. Amplification of tissue damage by antibodies within inflammatory brain lesions may not be restricted to demyelination and oligodendrocyte injury. In the search for other antibodies capable of damaging the axon-glial unit, circulating antibodies against AN-2 (an antigen expressed on oligodendrocyte progenitor cells) have been detected in patients with multiple sclerosis (Niehaus *et al* 2000). Clearly, such antibodies have the potential to eliminate progenitor cells from the lesions of multiple sclerosis in those lesions where shortage of progenitors contributes to the failure of remyelination.

Antigen-independent tissue injury by toxic macrophage products

Macrophages and activated microglia play an important role in the induction of tissue damage in the central nervous system. They are highly activated within acute and chronic inflammatory lesions. In most experimental autoimmune encephalomyelitis models, the extent of tissue damage correlates with macrophage infiltration (T. Berger *et al* 1997). In general, macrophage depletion ameliorates clinical disease and tissue damage (Huitinga *et al* 1990). Macrophages destroy tissue through the action of secreted toxic products in an antigen-independent and non-selective manner. Nevertheless, damage to different cellular components of the nervous system by macrophage toxins follows a hierarchical pattern. Myelin and oligodendrocytes are most susceptible followed by neurons and axons. In contrast, astrocytes and microglia are relatively resistant. Thus, a classic delayed-type hypersensitivity reaction, in which tissue injury is mainly mediated by activated macrophages and microglia, is reflected by a pseudoselective pattern of tissue damage showing primary demyelination with a variable extent of axonal and neuronal injury (Matyszak *et al* 1997; T.A. Newman *et al* 2001). It follows that selective primary demyelination associated with an inflammatory central nervous system lesion does not necessarily reflect a specific immune reaction against myelin antigens.

Proteases

Macrophages and microglia cells can induce tissue damage through a variety of different toxic molecules, including proteases, complement components, cytotoxic cytokines, reactive oxygen and nitrogen intermediates, and even excitotoxins. Proteases play a major role in the pathogenesis of inflammatory lesions in the central nervous system (Cuzner and Opdenakker 1999). This is best exemplified by the beneficial effects of protease inhibitors in the treatment of experimental autoimmune encephalomyelitis (Brosnan *et al* 1980; Clements *et al* 1997; Gijbels *et al* 1994) or other conditions of T-cell-mediated brain inflammation (Matyszak and Perry 1996c; T.A. Newman *et al* 2001). Proteases are produced by macrophages and microglia (Clements *et al* 1997; Teesalu *et al* 2001) and by astrocytes (Teesalu *et al* 2001). In general, they are secreted as inactive precursors requiring cleavage in order to become biologically active. Activity is strictly controlled, for example by tissue inhibitors of metalloproteases (TIMPs).

Proteases serve different functions in inflammation of the central nervous system. They are instrumental in the migration of inflammatory cells through vascular barriers and extracellular space by dissolving intercellular junctions or the extracellular matrix. It follows that inhibition of proteases has a direct anti-inflammatory effect. The decrease of enhancing MRI lesions in patients with multiple sclerosis treated with IFN-β may in part be due to inhibition of matrix metalloproteases (Leppert *et al* 1996). By cleaving proteins already released into the extracellular space, proteases increase the amount of peptides available for antigen presentation and therefore augment the immune reaction (Fabry *et al* 1994; Opdenakker and Van Damme 1994). In addition, proteases are directly involved in the induction of tissue damage, such as demyelination and axonal injury (Anthony *et al* 1998; Matyszak and Perry 1996c; T.A. Newman *et al* 2001).

Complement

There is good agreement that components of the complement system enter the brain under conditions of blood–brain barrier damage. Complement is also produced locally in pathological conditions by resident central nervous system cells (Morgan *et al* 1997). Deposition of complement components, including the lytic C9 neoantigen, characterizes a subset of multiple sclerosis patients (D.A.S. Compston *et al* 1989; Lucchinetti *et al* 2000; Prineas *et al* 2001; Storch *et al* 1998a). In general, experimental autoimmune encephalomyelitis induced in complement-deficient animals shows attenuated disease severity by comparison with wild-type controls (Mead *et al* 2002; Nataf *et al* 2000; G.T. Tran *et al* 2002). Complement may influence tissue injury in several ways. The induction of antibody-mediated demyelination is largely mediated through complement activation. Thus, demyelination and the subsequent axonal injury are effectively blocked in myelin oligodendrocyte glycoprotein-associated experimental autoimmune encephalomyelitis, induced in complement-deficient mice (Mead *et al* 2002). However, there are also effects of complement other than those attributable to the effect of antibody. The proinflammatory effects of leucotactic fragments, released in the course of complement activation, may explain why complement inhibition or deficiency not only blocks demyelination, but can also ameliorate inflammation in models of autoimmune encephalomyelitis – even in the absence of pathogenic antibodies (Nataf *et al* 2000; Piddlesden *et al* 1991; G.T. Tran *et al* 2002). In addition, complement may be activated in the central nervous system by components of myelin in the absence of antibody following the interaction of

myelin oligodendrocyte glycoprotein and C1q (T.G. Johns and Bernard 1997). Activated complement can lyse rat oligodendrocytes *in vitro* without anti-myelin antibodies (Piddlesden and Morgan 1993). Oligodendrocytes are more sensitive to this effect than other central nervous system cells (Benn *et al* 2001). Human oligodendrocytes, however, are less susceptible to complement-mediated damage since they express at least some cell surface complement inhibitory proteins (Scolding *et al* 1998a; Zajicek and Compston 1995). Complement also plays a role in the phagocytosis of myelin fragments through an interaction with the complement receptor 3 on microglia (Reichert and Rotshenker 2003).

Tumour necrosis factor α

TNF-α has pleotropic functions. It is expressed within the active lesions both of experimental autoimmune encephalomyelitis and multiple sclerosis (Issazadeh *et al* 1995a; Selmaj *et al* 1991b), produced by activated microglia and astrocytes (Frei *et al* 1987; Lieberman *et al* 1989). TNF-α exerts systemic immunoregulatory functions, but may act locally within lesions to act as a proinflammatory cytokine directly destroying oligodendrocytes (Probert *et al* 2000; Selmaj and Raine 1988). In transgenic animals overexpressing TNF-α under central nervous system-specific promoters, the pathology of lesions depends on the cellular source and amount of TNF-α produced. With low expression levels, no spontaneous disease occurs, but inflammation and demyelination are augmented in pre-existing experimental autoimmune encephalomyelitis (Taupin *et al* 1997). High levels in immature oligodendrocytes lead to spontaneous primary demyelination, while the expression in astrocytes is associated with very severe inflammation, demyelinating lesions and profound axonal injury (Akassoglou *et al* 1998). These effects are all mediated by signalling through the TNF-R1 pathway. Large vessel vasculitis with thrombosis and brain infarction induced in TNF-α transgenic animals, results in signalling exclusively through the TNF-R2 pathway (Akassoglou *et al* 2003).

These results in transgenic animals clearly highlight the pathogenic potential of TNF-α in the central nervous system and suggest that therapeutic blockade of this cytokine may have a beneficial effect in multiple sclerosis. Many studies have dealt with the effect of TNF-α blockade in experimental autoimmune encephalomyelitis either through pharmacological intervention or gene deletion. Although a beneficial effect has often been found, the results remain diverse and not easy to formulate (Willenborg *et al* 1995). Our synthesis is that, without TNF-α or TNF-R1, the extent of tissue injury is ameliorated, but with a variable effect on inflammation. That said, in some studies inflammation is augmented (Eugster *et al* 1999) and clearance of T-cell infiltration by apoptosis decreased (R. Bachmann *et al* 1999). Furthermore, major variations are found in the effects of TNF-R1 deletion on experimental autoimmune encephalomyelitis depending on mouse strain (Kassiotis *et al* 1999; Körner *et al* 1997; J. Liu *et al* 1998). Thus, TNF-α appears to be an important cytotoxic cytokine within inflammatory brain lesions, and blockade of its action may be beneficial. Conversely, the same molecule appears instrumental in immune regulation, involving the elimination of pathogenic T cells by apoptosis. Blockade of this function may augment inflammation and promote clinical disease (Probert *et al* 2000). Finally, TNF-α may also promote the survival and proliferation of oligodendrocyte progenitor cells, potentially contributing to remyelination (Arnett *et al* 2001).

Reactive oxygen and nitrogen intermediates

Reactive oxygen and nitrogen species, both produced by activated macrophages and microglia in their defence against pathogenic microorganisms, are highly cytotoxic molecules that can induce cell membrane damage and apoptosis. They can act synergistically through the formation of more toxic molecules such as peroxynitrite. Within the central nervous system they mediate a variety of toxic effects, and these can be highly relevant for the pathogenesis of demyelination and axonal injury (K.J. Smith and Lassmann 2002; K.J. Smith *et al* 1999; Willenborg *et al* 1999). Both sets of molecules are cytotoxic for oligodendrocytes and, as with most other macrophage toxins, selectively expose the myelin/oligodendrocyte complex (Y.S. Kim and Kim 1991; Merrill *et al* 1993; Noble *et al* 1994). However, as discussed in Chapter 13, nitric oxide may induce conduction block and degeneration when axons are electrically active (Kapoor *et al* 1999; K.J. Smith *et al* 2001a) due to modification of ion channels (Bielefeldt *et al* 1999) and impaired mitochondrial function (Bolanos *et al* 1997).

These observations identify reactive oxygen and nitrogen species as attractive candidates for therapeutic intervention in inflammatory demyelinating disease. Perhaps we should have expected that pharmacological blockade of nitric oxide production, or genetic deletion of inducible nitric oxide synthase, would yield the variety of conflicting results in experimental autoimmune encephalomyelitis – in many instances, aggravating, not settling the disease process (K.J. Smith and Lassmann 2002; Willenborg *et al* 1999). The explanation for this paradox lies in the additional roles of nitric oxide in regulating the inflammatory process. Nitric oxide inhibits T-cell activation (Albina and Henry 1991), downregulates endothelial adhesion molecule expression (Kubes *et al* 1991) and induces T-lymphocyte apoptosis (Okuda *et al* 1997; Zettl *et al* 1997). It is not surprising that inhibition of these activities augments the inflammatory process and exaggerates clinical manifestations of the disease.

Excitotoxins

Several studies suggest that excitotoxins contribute to tissue damage in inflammatory demyelinating lesions. First, the NMDA (*N*-methyl-D-aspartate) receptor inhibitor memantine was shown to inhibit experimental autoimmune encephalomyelitis (Wallstrom *et al* 1996). Later, blockade of AMPA/kainate receptors was shown to modify clinical disease and reduce demyelination as well as axonal and neuronal injury in animals with experimental autoimmune encephalomyelitis (Pitt *et al* 2000; T. Smith *et al* 2000). Excitotoxins are released from neurons as a consequence of brain damage. Microglia also represent a potent source of glutamate and the neurotoxin quinolinic acid (Espey *et al* 1997; Heyes *et al* 1996; Lehrmann *et al* 2001). Glutamate homeostasis is also implicated in the lesions of multiple sclerosis, as reflected by increased glutaminase expression in macrophages or microglia and reduced expression of gluta-

mate dehydrogenase in oligodendrocytes (Werner *et al* 2001). Finally, downregulation of glutamate transporters, as seen in the lesions of experimental autoimmune encephalomyelitis, may also increase the extracellular concentration of excitotoxins (Ohgoh *et al* 2002). Oligodendrocytes are highly susceptible to damage mediated by excitotoxins *in vitro* and *in vivo* (Cammer 2002; Matute *et al* 2001). Excitotoxic mechanisms are implicated in inflammatory demyelinating lesions targeting neurons in grey matter (T. Smith *et al* 2000).

Taken together, the immune system evidently packages a large repertoire of mechanisms for eliminating pathogens. However, the same molecules are also able to attack the body's own tissue in the context of autoimmunity. Since many of these mechanisms act in parallel, it follows that therapeutic blockade of one component may inadvertently affect another, yielding a mixed package of responses. In addition, several mechanisms instrumental in mediating tissue injury – for instance TNF-α or nitric oxide – are simultaneously used by the immune system in immune regulation, seeing off inflammatory cells once their task is fulfilled. In this context, the net effect of therapeutic blockade is often to exaggerate inflammation and the expression of disease – an inherently difficult problem to overcome in the treatment of immune-mediated diseases. But (as we discuss in Chapter 12) it remains possible that, in a disease like multiple sclerosis, one or other mechanism is dominant – generally or in particular groups – and so can be selectively targeted for disease-modifying effects.

PERIPHERAL BLOOD BIOMARKERS FOR MULTIPLE SCLEROSIS AND DISEASE ACTIVITY

Clinical and experimental investigations into multiple sclerosis and its experimental models provide an avalanche of data, in particular with regard to immune aspects of the disease. Clinicians and patients can be forgiven for expecting that much of this information can be applied to the diagnosis of human disease and in the assessment of treatment efficacy. But, sadly, this is not the case. In fact, many neurologists have been disappointed by the halting progress in this field. Up to now, there are only very few immunological biomarkers that are accepted as reliable and practicable parameters for determining the nature and state of activity of a given patient's affliction, or that follow the influence of any one drug on the disease process and its activity. At present, we use certain biomarkers to complement and confirm clinical, imaging or other findings, but there is no immunological test that convincingly diagnoses multiple sclerosis.

Biomarkers are needed to illuminate different aspects of the disease and its mechanisms. Apart from the initial diagnosis, they are required to monitor the course, potentially to help classify particular subsets of the disease and, ideally, to select optimal treatment and determine its efficacy over time. The current status of biomarkers for diagnosis and management of multiple sclerosis patients has been admirably summarized in a critical and comprehensive review by Bielekova and Martin (2004). The main results of this survey are shown in Table 11.3.

text continued on page 546

Table 11.3 Biomarkers for diagnosis and management of multiple sclerosis

Evaluated biomarkers according to categories	Biomarkers with potential for further development	Biological rationale	Correlation with disease activity	Correlation with disability progression	Correlation with treatment effect	Notes[a]
Biomarkers reflecting alteration of the immune system						Unlikely candidates for surrogate end points; may prove useful in studying disease heterogeneity and in developing of new therapies
(a) Cytokines and their receptors						The most extensively studied biomarkers in multiple sclerosis
IL-1, IL-2, IL-6, IL-10, IL-12, IL-18, TNF-α, LT-α/β, TGF-β, CD25	IL-6 (+ soluble interleukin sIL-6R and soluble glycoprotein sgp130)	+++[b]	++/–	+	+/+	Candidate cytokine system linking innate immune system with both arms of adaptive immune responses (T and B cells)
	IL-10	++	++/–	+	+/+	Candidate immunoregulatory cytokine
	IL-12 (p70)/IL-23	+++	++	++	+/+/+	Suggested as biomarker that can differentiate between relapsing-remitting and secondary progressive stages of multiple sclerosis
(b) Chemokines and their receptors						Biomarkers that may aid in studying disease heterogeneity and on proof of principle in therapy trials
CCR5, CXCR3, CXCL10, CCR2/CCL2	CCR5	++		nd[c]	+/–	Suggested as a candidate biomarker of Th1 T cells
	CXCR3/CXCL10	++	++	nd	–	Marker of activated T cells
(c) Antibodies						The least systematically studied category with some interesting novel markers; e.g. diagnostic relevance of antibody in neuromyelitis optica. These biomarkers need systematic development and standardization of techniques
CSF IgG index, κ light chains, oligoclonal bands, anti-MBP Ab, anti-MOG Ab	Anti-MBP and anti-MOG Ab	+++	nd	nd	nd	Suggested as a possible diagnostic tool for predicting the development of definite multiple sclerosis after first clinical symptom (clinically isolated demyelinating syndrome)
(d) Complement-related biomarkers						Biomarkers needed for assessment of disease heterogeneity (based on pathological classification of multiple sclerosis lesions) and for development of novel therapies

table continued on following page

Table 11.3 **Biomarkers for diagnosis and management of multiple sclerosis, cont'd**

Evaluated biomarkers according to categories	Biomarkers with potential for further development	Biological rationale	Correlation with disease activity	Correlation with disability progression	Correlation with treatment effect	Notes[a]
C3, C4, activated neo-C9. Regulators of complement activation (CD35, CD59)	Activated neo-C9	++	+	+	nd	Biomarker reflecting formation of membrane-attack complex (MAC) that is expected to contribute to demyelination at least in a subgroup of multiple sclerosis patients
(e) Adhesion molecules						It is unlikely that these biomarkers would become more useful than MRI-based markers of blood–brain barrier dysfunction
E-selectin, L-selectin, ICAM-1, VCAM-1, CD31, surface expression of LFA-1 and VLA-4						
(f) Biomarkers reflective of antigen processing and presentation						Very important category, little explored; needs further development for multiple sclerosis
CD40/CD40L, CD80, CD86, heat-shock proteins (hsp)	CD40/CD40L	++	+	nd	+	Suggested as candidate biomarker that can differentiate between relapsing–remitting and secondary progressive stages of multiple sclerosis
	hsp	+	nd	nd	nd	Dysregulation in the heat-shock protein system is the most prominent and consistent result of gene expression studies in multiple sclerosis and other autoimmune diseases
(g) Other activation markers						Markers reflecting activation of the innate immune system would contribute to studies of disease heterogeneity and aid in selection and screening of prospective novel immunomodulatory agents
CD26, CD30, CD71, perforin, OX-40 (CD134), osteopontin, macrophage-related proteins MRP-8 and MRP-16, neopterin, amyloid A protein, somatostatin	Neopterin	++	++	nd	+/–	

Table 11.3 Biomarkers for diagnosis and management of multiple sclerosis, cont'd

Evaluated biomarkers according to categories	Biomarkers with potential for further development	Biological rationale	Correlation with disease activity	Correlation with disability progression	Correlation with treatment effect	Notes[a]
(h) Cell-cycle and apoptosis-related biomarkers						Very important category of biomarkers because they may reflect both defects in regulation of immune cells as well as proapoptotic properties of central nervous system components
Fas (CD95) and Fas-L, FLIP, Bcl-2, TRAIL	FLIP	++	+	+	+	Anti-apoptotic protein overexpressed in multiple sclerosis
	TRAIL	+/?	nd	nd	+	Suggested as biomarker reflecting clinical response to IFN-β therapy in multiple sclerosis
(i) Biomarkers reflective of immune-mediated neuroprotection						Potentially very interesting biomarkers that need to be developed further; would contribute to disease heterogeneity studies and to development of process-specific therapies
BDNF expression						
(j) Changes in cellular subpopulations						Markers studied predominantly in the past; many should be reassessed by new, more precise techniques
NK cells, Vα24$^+$ NKT cells, CD4$^+$/CD25^{bright} and IL-10-producing immunoregulatory T cells, CSF cells, CD45RA$^-$/RO$^+$/CD4$^+$ (memory) T cells	CD4$^+$/CD25^{bright} T cells and IL-10-producing regulatory T cells, regulatory NK cells and NKT cells	+++	+	nd	+/nd	These cellular subpopulations were shown to have important immunoregulatory roles in animal models and other human autoimmune disorders and they merit careful evaluation in multiple sclerosis
(k) Functional assays for immunological reactivity						Although potentially very interesting, these assays are very tedious and therefore are likely to remain restricted to early phases of drug development and to proof-of-principle clinical trials
Proliferation assays (Ag-specific and polyclonal), cytokine-secretion assays, cytotoxic assays						

table continued on following page

543

Table 11.3 **Biomarkers for diagnosis and management of multiple sclerosis, cont'd**

Evaluated biomarkers according to categories	Biomarkers with potential for further development	Biological rationale	Correlation with disease activity	Correlation with disability progression	Correlation with treatment effect	Notes[a]
Biomarkers of blood–brain barrier disruption						It is unlikely that these biomarkers would become more useful than MRI-based markers of blood–brain barrier dysfunction
MMPs and their inhibitors (TIMP), platelet-activating factor, thrombomodulin						
Biomarkers of demyelination						Would greatly enhance the understanding of MRI/pathological correlations and have a potential for partial surrogacy
MBP and MBP-like material, proteolytic enzymes, endogenous pentapeptide QYNAD, gliotoxin	QYNAD – endogenous peptide with Na-channel blocking properties	++	nd	nd	nd	QYNAD is an endogenous substance in cerebrospinal fluid that probably originates from proteolytic cleavage during inflammation; deserves further evaluation
Biomarkers of oxidative stress and excitotoxicity						Very important biomarkers from the standpoint of disease heterogeneity and potentially for development of novel therapies; need to be developed further
NO and its stable metabolites (nitrite NO_2^- and nitrate NO_3^-), uric acid, isoprostane, marker for hypoxia-like tissue damage in multiple sclerosis	NO (+ NO_2^- and NO_3^-)	++	+/–	–/nd	nd	May help in disease heterogeneity studies
	Uric acid	++	++	+	+/–	Strong natural peroxynitrate scavenger
	Isoprostane	++	nd	+	+	Interesting candidate marker that merits further studies
	Marker for hypoxia-like tissue damage in multiple sclerosis	+	nd	nd	nd	Described in pivotal study as an endogenous epitope that is cross-recognized by monoclonal antibody against canine distemper virus and may become a diagnostic tool to identify specific multiple sclerosis subtype

Table 11.3 **Biomarkers for diagnosis and management of multiple sclerosis, cont'd**

Evaluated biomarkers according to categories	Biomarkers with potential for further development	Biological rationale	Correlation with disease activity	Correlation with disability progression	Correlation with treatment effect	Notes[a]
Biomarkers of axonal/ neuronal damage						Most likely category of biomarkers with surrogate potential in multiple sclerosis
Cytoskeletal proteins (actin, tubulin and neurofilaments), tau protein	Neurofilaments: light subunit (NF-L)	+++	+	+	nd	Might be the most likely candidate for surrogacy; its development warrants further efforts
	Tau protein	++	++	nd	nd	Also potentially very useful biomarker that needs further development
Biomarkers of gliosis						May be useful for disease heterogeneity studies but with unpredictable surrogacy potential
GFAP, S-100 proteins						
Biomarkers of remyelination and repair						Much-needed biomarkers that would guide development of repair-promoting strategies in multiple sclerosis and aid in disease heterogeneity studies
NCAM, CNTF, microtubule-associated protein-2 exon 13 (MAP-2 + -13), protein 14-3-3, CPK-BB, peptidylglycine α-amidating monooxygenase (PAM), neural-specific enolase (NSE)	NCAM – neural cell adhesion molecule	+	+	nd	nd	Very sparse data on both biomarkers. However, because these are so far the only potential candidates, their evaluation warrants further effort
	CNTF – ciliary neurotrophic factor	++	nd	nd	nd	

a Brief opinion of the authors about the potential use of the biomarkers and the need for further developments.

b We attempted to grade the strength of supportive evidence for each characteristic of the biomarker as low (+), medium (++) and high (+++). In treatment effects +/– implies positive correlation with one type of therapy and negative with another.

c No reliable data.

Ab = antibody; Ag = antigen; CNTF = ciliary neurotrophic factor; CSF = cerebrospinal fluid; FLIP = Fas-associated death domain-like interleukin-1β-converting enzyme inhibitory protein; GFAP = glial fibrillary acidic protein; hsp = heat-shock protein; ICAM-1 = intracellular adhesion molecule-1; IFN = interferon; Ig = immunoglobulin; IL = interleukin; LP = lumbar puncture; LT-α/β = lymphotoxin α/β; MAC = membrane-attack complex; MBP = myelin basic protein; MOG = myelin oligodendrocyte glycoprotein; MMP = matrix metalloproteinase; NCAM = neural cell adhesion molecule; NF-L = neurofilament light subunit; NK cells = natural killer cells; NKT cells = NK-like T cells; NSE = neuron-specific enolase; OCB = oligoclonal bands; PAM = peptidylglycine α-amidating monooxygenase; TGF-β = transforming growth factor β; TIMP = tissue inhibitor of matrix metalloproteinases; TNF-α = tumour necrosis factor α; VCAM-1 = vascular cell adhesion molecule 1.
BDNF = brain derived neurotrophic factor
CPK-BB = creatine phosphokinase-BB
LFA = lymphocyte function antigen
TRAIL = tumour necrosis factor related apoptosis-inducing ligand
VLA = very late appearing antigen

Simplified summary of reviewed biomarkers in multiple sclerosis taken from Bielekova and Martin (2004).

Markers for the diagnosis of multiple sclerosis

Multiple sclerosis presents a stunning variety of clinical symptoms, and histological lesion patterns, a complexity that often mimics other conditions of the central nervous system. Therefore a doubtfree diagnosis in an early stage of the disease is particularly difficult. Definite multiple sclerosis is often diagnosed only after repeated bouts, that is, only after some time following disease onset. Then, diagnosis is mainly based on a combination of clinical features with imaging, and cerebrospinal fluid abnormalities (oligoclonal immunoglobulin bands). The latter changes can be counted among immunological biomarkers, but they are not specific for multiple sclerosis. Additional supportive immune biomarkers are badly needed for the initial diagnosis but, to date, there is no such test that could be used on a routine basis.

Markers for disease diversity (pathogenesis)

As has been emphasized repeatedly, multiple sclerosis can evolve in distinct patterns and these variations in the clinical course may, in turn, reflect distinct pathogenic processes. Making these distinctions would assume additional importance if it were to be shown that the various disease subtypes require different therapeutic approaches. However, classification of lesion subtypes in multiple sclerosis has mainly emerged from morphological studies of post-mortem tissue samples with rather few available biopsies during the lifetime of the patient who, we hypothesize, might benefit from knowledge of their specific pathological features. For obvious ethical reasons, such biopsy material can be accessed only in very rare cases. Pieces of the central nervous system cannot be taken merely to confirm suspected multiple sclerosis, but the procedure may be justified to exclude other disorders, such as tumours.

Hence there is an urgent need for easily accessible biomarkers. As an obvious candidate, autoantibodies could serve as markers for the putative subtype mediated by humoral immunity. As described in Chapter 16, a subset of patients responds to plasma exchange, perhaps through the removal of circulating autoantibodies.

Lennon *et al* (2004) recently reported a possible immune biomarker for neuromyelitis optica (Devic's disease). A tight correlation was demonstrated between an IgG antibody binding to mouse brain sections, identified as acquaporin-4 (Lennon *et al* 2005), and the diagnosis of neuromyelitis optica. Time will tell whether this finding becomes of generalized use for diagnosis of this particular subset, and whether similar strategies will help to identify other categories of patients with multiple sclerosis.

Markers for the disease course

Especially in the relapsing–remitting phase, it would be of practical value to gain insight into the degree, distribution and consequences of the pathogenic inflammatory mechanisms. Is there a smouldering process that may evolve into overt clinical disease or is the force driving inflammation all but extinguished? Specific information would be invaluable for tailoring optimal treatment schemes according to the patient's current needs. Furthermore, relapse might be predicted and intercepted before the clinical manifestations erupted. Numerous activity-related blood and cerebrospinal fluid markers have been proposed and investigated, in particular those that relate to an ongoing inflammatory process (see box below).

Methods for detecting potential biomarkers

Soluble molecules (released into body fluids)
- ELISA (enzyme-linked immunosorbent assay)
- Western blotting (electrophoresis-separated proteins identified by specific antibody binding)

Cellular markers
- FACS cytofluorometry (membrane markers, soluble factors)
- Elispot (cytokine released by individual cells, bound to surfaces and identified by specific antibodies)

Molecular markers
- TPCR-related gene amplification

More hopeful are studies that use anti-myelin autoantibodies as a potential biomarker. Recently, Villar *et al* (2005) identified lipid-binding IgM antibodies in the oligoclonal cerebrospinal fluid bands, which (in their trial) predicted a particularly severe clinical course. T. Berger *et al* (2003) measured anti-myelin oligodendrocyte glycoprotein autoantibodies in a series of freshly diagnosed cases with possible/probable multiple sclerosis. High antibody titres were associated with a more severe disease course compared to cases with low titres or no antibody responses. Another study correlated the level of autoantibody titres against native glycosylated myelin oligodendrocyte glycoprotein with disease activity (Gaertner *et al* 2004). Both studies are intriguing, but it should be noted that the findings have not been repeated in other patient populations studied with similar technology (Lampasona *et al* 2004; Lim *et al* 2005). Without more information, we are unable to reconcile whether technical or other factors are responsible for the discrepancies.

Markers of therapeutic response

As a rule, drug treatments have diverse effects – some good, others not; they all require monitoring. Most obvious is the intended therapeutic effect, which ideally would be matched by clinical improvement. For this purpose, biomarkers are selected to resemble those used to follow the natural history of the disease. In addition, for most treatments, especially in the case of immunosuppressive or disease-modifying therapies, adverse effects must be recognized and, where necessary, quantified. Finally, biomarkers inform directly on the successful introduction and function of biological agents. The classic example is the MxA protein ('myxovirus resistance protein A'), the product of a gene induced by type I interferons. MxA-detecting immune assays are now commonly used as a sensitive parameter for bioavailability of therapeutic interferons (von Wussow *et al* 1990).

Biomarkers: assays and accessibility

To be useful, biomarkers should be clinically informative, correlated with a clinical outcome, easily measurable, and routinely accessible. On a more theoretical level, the biomarker might either relate to a mechanism that directly contributes to development and course of the disease, or serve as a marker of mechanisms that protect from or reduce the disease process.

The choice of suitable methods to monitor biological structures is not the limiting factor: a large repertoire of modern assays exists that is capable of measuring molecular and cellular components of body structures (Table 11.3). These allow the fast and reliable identification and quantification of soluble proteins circulating in body fluids, or of structures located on the surface of tissues or single cells.

A real problem in the context of multiple sclerosis is accessibility of biologically meaningful samples. Unfortunately, the most informative sample, namely the pathological lesion itself, is inaccessible, although the cerebrospinal fluid (see below) provides indirect access to markers of the disease process. But, even cerebrospinal fluid sampling at lumbar puncture requires a clear indication and cannot be repeated at the whim of the investigator. Cerebrospinal fluid originates from the interstitial fluid that drains tissues in the central nervous system. Therefore it contains some, but by no means all, soluble molecules interchanged between the brain parenchyma and cerebrospinal fluid-filled spaces (Teunissen *et al* 2005). Many details of its composition remain enigmatic. Thus, the character of cerebrospinal fluid antibodies, which form the characteristic oligoclonal bands, remains a matter of debate. Some investigators relate these proteins to processes that are considered relevant to the development of lesions in the central nervous system; other commentators, by contrast, maintain that the pathogenic autoantibodies are retained in the affected tissue, and only irrelevant antibodies are shed into the accessible cerebrospinal fluid. The same is true for the immune cells that are found in this compartment, and for their soluble products such as cytokines.

Other body fluids – such as blood, urine and saliva – are freely accessible to monitoring, but remote from the local pathogenic process. These fluids may display changes reflecting local processes powerful enough to spill over into the systemic circulation where, however, they may be overshadowed by unrelated events happening outside the central nervous system. Further, at least in theory, there may be systemic changes that have a direct impact on activity of the disease process in multiple sclerosis. Examples include concomitant infections with their multiple possibilities to act on pathogenic autoaggressive T cells (reviewed in this chapter). Such procedures have not, however, become part of routine clinical practice.

Markers that have been proposed and studied

Table 11.3 summarizes a large number of biomarkers, compiled by Bielekova and Martin (2004). The list contains:

- markers of immune activity – cytokines, chemokines, soluble membrane structures, proteases, peripheral immune cells, autoantigen reactivity, T-cell receptor profile, myelin autoantibodies, transcriptomics, Th1/Th2 profiles
- markers of neuronal damage (S100, neuronal filaments, etc.) and myelin damage (soluble myelin proteins)
- indicators of increased permeability through the blood–brain barrier in the form of blood-derived proteins.

Monitoring of these markers has been proposed for diagnosis, disease course (state of activity), therapeutic efficiency and, to a modest degree, subtype identification.

In addition, markers for drug bioavailability and drug-induced adverse effects are of importance. In the case of IFN-β, the interferon-induced MxA protein, which indicates the presence of biologically active interferon in the patient's system, and (conversely) the detection of interferon neutralizing antibodies (a response that can interfere with therapeutic efficiency) have entered clinical practice. In the case of treatment with glatiramer acetate, several groups recommend ELISPOT assays, which document cytokine conversion of T cells from Th1 to Th2 profiles.

Whilst there is perfect agreement that the identification of immunological biomarkers would be of enormous help for diagnosis, classification, and monitoring of natural course and therapeutic efficiency, only very few such markers are used widely in clinical practice. One example is the detection of oligoclonal immunoglobulin in the cerebrospinal fluid, a time-honoured assay. Other tests, based on the detection of specific antibodies in the central nervous system, have raised much interest but have yet to stand the test of time.

MARKERS OF MULTIPLE SCLEROSIS AND DISEASE ACTIVITY IN CEREBROSPINAL FLUID

The central nervous system is encased in strong layers of bone and connective tissue. These barriers protect the brain from traumatic injury but also make it inaccessible to the investigator. This inconvenience has impeded research into multiple sclerosis and other neurological diseases, but two windows permit some insight into the process of brain inflammation. One is the eye, which is commonly affected and where ophthalmoscopy can directly illuminate pathological processes (see Chapter 13: W.I. McDonald 1986). The other is cerebrospinal fluid, routinely sampled by lumbar puncture. It provides information that supplements clinical evidence for the diagnosis (see Chapter 7), whilst also offering clues to the pathogenesis. Typically, in patients with multiple sclerosis, cerebrospinal fluid contains abnormal levels of immunoglobulins distributed as oligoclonal bands, and inflammatory cells, which are mainly CD4$^+$ T lymphocytes and macrophages/monocytes. Immunoglobulins and T cells are both implicated in the autoimmune pathogenesis of multiple sclerosis. Although their direct roles and relative contributions remain to be determined, at the very least each contains signatures of the disease process and its activity.

However, the cerebrospinal fluid only partially reflects events taking place within central nervous system lesions. In immunological terms, the meningeal and subarachnoid compartment is different from the brain parenchyma (Matyszak and Perry 1996b; Schnell *et al* 1999). Furthermore, due to the narrow extracellular space, diffusion of immunological mediators is restricted, and thus cerebrospinal fluid does not necessarily mirror the composition of extracellular fluid in the parenchyma, especially when lesions are buried deep in the parenchyma. Pathogenic leucocytes, antibodies and inflammatory mediators are preferentially trapped within lesions, while those not directly involved in lesion pathogenesis may remain in the perivascular and meningeal compartments (Flügel *et al* 2000).

For these reasons, effective spillover of inflammatory components into the cerebrospinal fluid will only take place in the presence of multiple lesions or when they touch the meningeal or ventricular surface, and when massive oedema and widening of the extracellular space facilitate diffusion to the extracellular space. This is obviously not the case in many patients with multiple sclerosis, and direct correlation between cerebrospinal fluid alterations and lesional pathology is frequently disappointing. Thus, interpretation of cerebrospinal fluid changes in multiple sclerosis requires consideration of the basic physiology of its production and turnover.

Physiology of cerebrospinal fluid

The brain and spinal cord are bathed in cerebrospinal fluid. This reservoir fills the inner ventricles and outer subarachnoid space, including its cisterns. This compartment is sealed from the dural and epidural space by a tight layer of arachnoid membrane and separated, in turn, from the systemic circulation by the blood–brain barrier. There is communication with the extracellular space of the brain and spinal cord, although diffusion is limited by the narrow extracellular space in central nervous system tissue and by cellular layers of the ependyma and glia limitans (J.C. Lee 1972; see also Chapter 10).

Production, turnover and resorption

The molecular composition of cerebrospinal fluid and its sites of production, physiological turnover and resorption are reviewed in detail by Bradbury (1979) and Fishman (1992). Whereas its ionic composition is consistent with a plasma ultrafiltrate, the low protein content is explained by a stringent blood–brain barrier for nonpolar high molecular weight solutes (Felgenhauer 1974). The choroid plexus is the major source of cerebrospinal fluid. About 10% is of local extracellular origin, draining primarily into the perivascular (Virchow–Robin) spaces (Cserr 1984). From there, diffusion occurs into the subarachnoid compartment. In periventricular white matter, the brain extracellular fluid accumulates along fibre tracts and then passes through the ependymal lining of the ventricular walls (Weller et al 1992). It has to be remembered, however, that cerebrospinal fluid proteins are not exclusively derived from the choroid plexus and the brain extracellular space. A variety of proteins (enzymes, transport proteins, growth factors and cytokines) can be directly synthesized by leptomeningeal cells (Ohe et al 1996) and by leucocytes present in all central nervous system compartments (Renno et al 1994; Waage et al 1989).

Under pathological conditions, exchange between the brain extracellular space and cerebrospinal fluid appears much more pronounced, largely for two reasons. First, in conditions of acute pathology, the extracellular space is enlarged by vasogenic oedema, which facilitates the bulk flow of fluid into this compartment (J.C. Lee 1972). Secondly, as a result of tissue damage and scar formation, the perivascular spaces are enlarged, due to perivascular fibrosis (see Chapter 12). This may lead to the formation of connective tissue channels similar to lymphatic capillaries in other tissues (Prineas 1979). Since the central nervous system extracellular space is in continuity with the cerebrospinal fluid, alterations of the extracellular milieu in the

brain and spinal cord are, in principle, reflected in the composition of the fluid. There are, however, important limitations. Due to the narrow extracellular space in the nervous tissue, diffusion of molecules and migration of cells are somewhat limited (Cserr et al 1992) – the rate at which molecules move depending on radius (in a hydrated form) and charge. In general, diffusion is most rapid for small anionic or uncharged molecules. Large or cationic material moves more slowly. For example, after intrathecal injection, neutral protein tracers freely disperse in the extracellular space, whereas cationic molecules, such as myelin basic protein, largely remain trapped in the meningeal compartment (Vass et al 1984). In addition, molecules liberated in the central nervous system extracellular space may be removed by local uptake in macrophages (Broadwell and Salcman 1981) and also in neurons and glia. The uptake of different serum proteins into local macrophages in the lesions of multiple sclerosis lesions is well documented (see Chapter 12). Even more specific and effective uptake occurs with autoantibodies that are involved in the pathogenesis. These may be absorbed from cerebrospinal fluid through complexing with respective target brain antigens. For example, demyelinating activity is generally lower using cerebrospinal fluid than corresponding serum samples from patients with multiple sclerosis (S.U. Kim et al 1970). It is to be expected that antibody directed against any surface component of normal or pathological central nervous system tissue will largely be removed from the cerebrospinal fluid. Conversely, antibody directed against intracellular antigens, or targets not present in the central nervous system, will persist and may be enriched in the cerebrospinal fluid. In other words, the antigen specificity of cerebrospinal fluid antibodies shows a spectrum reflecting bystander reactions, not necessarily of relevance to the pathogenesis. One method for detecting antibodies that may directly be involved in tissue damage is to define antigen specificity by analysing antibodies secreted in vitro by B lymphocytes harvested from cerebrospinal fluid (J. Sun et al 1991a; 1991b) rather than by direct determination of antibody titres (Xiao et al 1991).

Taken together, the evidence suggests that – with respect to proteins and small molecular weight solutes (and acknowledging major inherent limitations) – cerebrospinal fluid offers a useful diagnostic window allowing the indirect study of pathological events taking place in the central nervous system.

Source and turnover of cells

As in the central nervous system parenchyma, a small number of mononuclear cells (0.3–6.2/µL) are normally present in the cerebrospinal fluid. These mainly consist of lymphocytes (86%) and monocytes/macrophages (12%) (Sörnäs and Östlund 1972). In a concise review, Oehmichen et al (1982) concluded that the normal turnover of cells in cerebrospinal fluid is below the limits of detection by transfer of labelled leucocytes, with a low rate of cell division, in vivo and in vitro, and a small number of cells undergoing necrosis – together indicating extremely low turnover under normal conditions and mainly resulting from proliferation and death of cells already present. In addition, the influx of haematogenous cells into the cerebrospinal fluid compartment in the context of inflammation is also supplemented by up to 25% local cell proliferation.

This traditional view now requires modification in the light of more recent experimental data. Activated T lymphocytes can pass through the normal blood–brain and cerebrospinal fluid barriers suggesting that, following peripheral immune activation, T cells selectively enter the cerebrospinal fluid compartment. In terms of numbers, five- to tenfold more lymphocytes express activation markers, such as IL-2 receptors and MHC class II antigens, in cerebrospinal fluid compared with peripheral blood. But the percentage of activated T lymphocytes in cerebrospinal fluid does not differ between patients with inflammatory and noninflammatory neurological diseases (Hafler *et al* 1985b; Noronha *et al* 1980; Tournier-Lasserve *et al* 1987). Since it is unlikely that lymphocytes are locally activated in the central nervous system compartment in noninflammatory diseases of the nervous system, these data suggest that lymphocytes enter the cerebrospinal fluid already activated, but are rapidly removed whilst continuing to express late activation markers. Kivisäkk *et al* (2003) used a large panel of antibodies against chemokine receptors and adhesion molecules, postulating that the normal cerebrospinal fluid mainly contains activated central memory T cells, which enter through the choroid plexus and the meninges in a P-selectin dependent manner. Conversely, the entry and turnover of monocytes may be much slower. It takes several months for donor-derived cells to repopulate the meninges in radiation bone marrow chimeras (Hickey and Kimura 1988; Hickey *et al* 1992). Slow turnover of cerebrospinal fluid monocytes is further supported by the observation that phenotypically they show a lower degree of activation than those in the peripheral circulation, and no differences in activation of monocytes are found in patients with inflammatory compared with noninflammatory neurological diseases (Salmaggi and Sandberg-Wollheim 1993). Little is known about the migratory properties and turnover in the cerebrospinal fluid of other inflammatory cells, such as B lymphocytes or natural killer cells. Granulocytes are extremely rare in normal cerebrospinal fluid, despite the local availability of lipopolysaccharide, cytokines and chemokines that trigger a granulocyte-dominated inflammatory reaction in the meningeal space and cerebrospinal fluid compartments (Andersson *et al* 1992; Bell *et al* 1996; Quagliarello and Scheld 1992). By comparison with the brain parenchyma, meningeal vessels appear more permeable both to proteins (Westergaard and Brightman 1973) and leucocytes (Perry *et al* 1995). This principle is clearly exemplified by T-cell-mediated brain inflammation in experimental autoimmune encephalomyelitis, in the many variants of which there is a dominance of meningeal over brain inflammation when the disease is induced by low numbers of encephalitogenic T cells (T. Berger *et al* 1997; Perry *et al* 1995). Furthermore, the dynamics and extent of brain inflammation are much more vigorous when foreign antigen or lipopolysaccharide is injected into cerebrospinal fluid compared with inoculation of the brain parenchyma (Matyszak and Perry 1996b; Perry *et al* 1995). This is also reflected by the presence of cells within the meninges and choroid plexus, which express dendritic cell antigens (Matyszak and Perry 1996c; McMenamin 1999; Pashenkov *et al* 2003b) and may be the origin of dendritic cells identified in cerebrospinal fluid (Pashenkov *et al* 2001).

In pathological conditions of the nervous system, leucocytes found in cerebrospinal fluid are derived not only from inflamed meningeal vessels but also as a result of cell migration from central nervous system lesions into the subarachnoid space or ventricles. It was noted in the earliest pathological studies on multiple sclerosis that debris containing macrophages in the spinal plaques of multiple sclerosis can pass directly into the superficial glia limitans to enter the spinal meninges and subarachnoid space (Marburg 1906). A similar exchange of inflammatory cells through the ependymal lining of the ventricles has been found in periventricular lesions of chronic experimental autoimmune encephalomyelitis (Lassmann *et al* 1981c). In addition, cellular drainage of deep white matter lesions can occur through the distended perivascular Virchow–Robin spaces (Prineas 1979). An additional barrier of leptomeningeal cells seals the perivascular from the subarachnoid space. Thus, although this barrier is permeable to fluid, solutes and the active migration of activated leucocytes, erythrocytes do not readily disperse into the Virchow–Robin space following subarachnoid haemorrhage (Hutchins and Weller 1986).

Lymphatic drainage

Labelled cells, erythrocytes or particulate material, injected into the cerebrospinal fluid, can reach regional lymph nodes (Oehmichen *et al* 1979; Weller *et al* 1992). Furthermore, haemosiderin-containing macrophages are found in peritracheal cervical lymph nodes in patients with subarachnoid haemorrhage (Oehmichen *et al* 1982). Antigen injected into the brain or cerebrospinal fluid may elicit specific immune reactions, predominantly in regional lymph nodes (Cserr *et al* 1992). de Vos *et al* (2002) described the appearance of macrophages with myelin degradation products in the cervical lymph nodes of animals with experimental autoimmune encephalomyelitis. These findings indicate active drainage of cells and antigens from the central nervous system to the lymphatic system. Several anatomical pathways have been identified. They include arachnoid channels in the cribriform plate (Weller *et al* 1992), tracking along cranial nerve roots (Bradbury and Cserr 1985), and additional pathways exiting through spinal root pockets (Zenker *et al* 1994). There are, however, several aspects that suggest much more complex drainage mechanisms. First, tracers injected on one side of the brain usually drain to ipsilateral lymph nodes (Yamada *et al* 1991). This argues against a diffuse drainage mechanism through the cerebrospinal fluid, and rather suggests the existence of more specialized lymphatic-like channels within the leptomeninges. These have recently been defined in periarteriolar meningeal sheaths (Preston *et al* 2003). The continuous leptomeningeal cell layer also inhibits diffusion of particulate material and nonactivated cells, even without sealing by continuous tight junction ridges. No detailed anatomical mapping of adhesion molecule expression, needed to enable the passage of activated cells, in meninges of the normal and diseased central nervous system is available. Meningeal cells from some mouse strains constitutively express P-selectin, and these show enhanced T-cell immune surveillance by comparison with animals lacking P-selectin expression in the meningeal compartment (Carrithers *et al* 2002). Finally, in contrast to the brain parenchyma proper, leucocyte apoptosis, as a mechanism for clearing inflammatory cells, rarely occurs in the meningeal space (J. Bauer *et al* 1998).

Multiple sclerosis-related cellular changes in cerebrospinal fluid

An increase in inflammatory cells in the cerebrospinal fluid is characteristic of multiple sclerosis. The total count may be 5–50 cells/mm^3 in acute disease, of which the majority are T lymphocytes. Many express late activation markers, such as CD26 (formerly referred to as Ta1; Hafler et al 1985b). Cell adhesion molecules that are potentially involved in interaction with cerebrovascular endothelium (e.g. VLAs and other integrins) are also expressed on lymphocytes present in cerebrospinal fluid (Svenningsson et al 1993). On the basis of their chemokine receptor profile, these represent activated memory T cells of the CD4$^+$ and CD8$^+$ subset (Giunti et al 2003; Kivisäkk et al 2003). We interpret this lymphocyte marker profile on the basis that activated T cells are selectively recruited from the periphery to the central nervous system, and thus to the cerebrospinal fluid. It is worth considering that these lymphocyte populations, accumulating in the cerebrospinal fluid, include activated T cells effecting physiological immune surveillance of the central nervous system (Wekerle et al 1986). This interpretation is consistent with the finding that (notwithstanding differences in absolute count) a predominance of activated T cells is found in samples from individuals who are healthy as well as those with neurological disease (Hedlund et al 1989; Vrethem et al 1998). It has, however, to be emphasized that the preferential recruitment of activated memory T cells into the cerebrospinal fluid is more pronounced in normal controls than in patients with inflammatory brain disease, in whom there is apparently also a secondary recruitment of leucocytes more closely reflecting cell populations in the circulation (Kleine et al 1999). Thus the appearance of nonactivated naive T cells in the cerebrospinal fluid is associated with active inflammation or disease activity (Kraus et al 2000b). As in the brain parenchyma of patients with multiple sclerosis, it is the CD8$^+$ T cell population in cerebrospinal fluid that undergoes preferential oligoclonal expansion (Jacobsen et al 2002).

B cells represent a small fraction of lymphocytes present in cerebrospinal fluid (Sandberg-Wollheim 1983). Whilst little information is available on their state of activation, a considerable number of B cells expressing cell surface CD5 is described in multiple sclerosis, although the functional status of these CD5$^+$ cells is undefined (Mix et al 1990). They may be members of the primordial B-1 population (containing a large proportion of B cells producing polyreactive natural autoantibodies and giving rise to B-cell lymphomas: Kantor and Herzenberg 1993) or regular activated B lymphocytes (R.A. Miller and Gralow 1984; Werner et al 1989).

In a systematic study of cerebrospinal fluid cytology during the evolution of multiple sclerosis, Cepok et al (2001) described inter-individual heterogeneity of cerebrospinal fluid cytological profiles, independent of stage and activity of the disease. While all patients showed a dominance of T lymphocytes in the cerebrospinal fluid, others showed a predominance of B cells or monocytes. Patients with high B-cell counts and intrathecal IgG production followed a more rapidly progressive course than those in whom monocytes were mainly found (Cepok et al 2001). These findings raise the possibility that high B-cell responses carry a worse prognosis. It is claimed that early conversion to definite multiple sclerosis is associated with the presence of anti-myelin antibodies at presentation with a first demyelinating episode (T. Berger et al 2003). These differences in clinical behaviour are also consistent with the evidence from pathological analyses for disease heterogeneity (see Chapter 12).

Immune function of cerebrospinal fluid lymphocytes

If immunosurveillant T cells do accumulate in the healthy central nervous system, one would expect a similar (or even increased) accumulation in cerebrospinal fluid in patients with multiple sclerosis at times of disease activity. The immunological properties of lymphocytes recovered from cerebrospinal fluid have therefore been intensively scrutinized. This work relies on several methodological approaches, including establishment of lymphocyte lines and characterization of products secreted by single lymphocytes using immunospot and in situ hybridization assays. Primary limiting dilution experiments using polyclonal mitogen (PHA) as the proliferating stimulus yield clonal T-cell lines, but none of these responds to known myelin autoantigens (Hafler et al 1985a). This result, superficially disappointing, presumably reflects a relatively low frequency of brain-specific T cells within the general T-cell repertoire contained in cerebrospinal fluid. In fact, application of more refined techniques, primarily selecting for autoantigen specificity, has led to the isolation of myelin-specific T-cell lines. In particular, the split well technique (Figure 11.11: Pette et al 1990b) helped to establish panels of myelin basic protein-reactive T-cell lines from the cerebrospinal fluid of patients with multiple sclerosis. The enrichment of autoreactive T cells within the overall population is estimated to be about tenfold higher than in peripheral blood. Many of the cells recognize a myelin basic protein epitope dominant response, both from patients with multiple sclerosis and healthy controls, involving the centrally located p84–102 and the C-terminal p143–168 fragments (Zhang et al 1994). γδ T cells, the lymphocytes implicated in lesions of multiple sclerosis that are seen to regenerate, have been isolated by several groups. Vδ1, often in conjunction with Vγ1 usage, was noted in one study of cerebrospinal fluid-derived T-cell lines from patients with multiple sclerosis. Some showed reactivity against human glioma determinants (Nick et al 1995). Another study demonstrated reactivity of γδ T cell receptor cell lines from patients with multiple sclerosis to heat-shock protein 70 (but not heat-shock protein 65; Stinissen et al 1995).

A second approach, pioneered by the groups of Tomas Olsson and Hans Link, for studying the functional repertoire contained within the cerebrospinal lymphocyte pool, relies on single-cell assays for secreted protein products (immunoglobulins or cytokines) and immunologically relevant mRNA. T lymphocytes isolated from peripheral blood or cerebrospinal fluid of patients with multiple sclerosis are exposed in vitro to putative autoantigens to allow specific activation of autoreactive lymphocytes. Cultured cells are then tested for release of activation-dependent cytokines by direct immunostaining. This extremely sensitive immunospot approach has demonstrated remarkably large proportions of myelin basic protein-specific T cells in peripheral blood, and even higher frequencies in the cerebrospinal fluid of patients with multiple sclerosis (Olsson et al 1990a). Enrichment of autoreactive T cells in cerebrospinal fluid was also found for other putative myelin autoantigens, such as proteolipid protein (J. Sun *et al* 1991a), myelin associated glycoprotein (Söderström *et al* 1994b) and myelin oligodendrocyte glycoprotein (Sun *et al* 1991b). The particular T-cell response profile is seen early in the course of the disease in the individual patient, and seems stable over time (Söderström *et al* 1994b). Although it is not surprising that myelin basic protein-reactive T cells are also enriched in optic neuritis (because of its close relationship to multiple sclerosis; Söderström *et al* 1994b), an unexpected elevation of such cells was documented in cerebrospinal fluid from patients with purely cerebrovascular diseases (W-Z. Wang *et al* 1992). Whilst these observations rely on the determination of secreted IFN-γ, the prototypic marker for Th1 cells, comparable analyses have more recently been extended to other cytokines such as IL-4, IL-10 and TGF-β (Söderström *et al* 1995) through the use of *in situ* hybridization. Preliminary data indicate a relative prevalence of IL-4 or TGF-β transcribing T cells in mild relapsing–remitting multiple sclerosis, with a reduction in clinically more severe cases (Link *et al* 1994).

Are cerebrospinal fluid lymphocytes involved in the pathogenesis of multiple sclerosis?

Close proximity of cerebrospinal fluid to the brain parenchyma, and the relative increase of myelin-specific autoreactive T lymphocytes within the mononuclear cell population in both compartments, might reasonably suggest that these T cells are autoaggressive immune cells. However, this is by no means proven. In fact, research using experimental models of myelin-specific autoimmune diseases (see above) shows that most, if not all, pathogenic T lymphocytes infiltrating the central nervous system die locally by apoptosis. Recirculation from the central nervous system to the periphery via the cerebrospinal fluid is assumed but not proven. Indeed, the origin of these cerebrospinal fluid cells is ambiguous. In experimental autoimmune encephalomyelitis, studies using cellular markers indicate that pathogenic T cells accumulate at high frequency in the parenchymal infiltrates, with many fewer cells in the perivascular and meningeal infiltrates. As in all inflammatory areas, post-activated T lymphocytes are additionally attracted to these locations in an antigen-independent manner. Thus, the enrichment of myelin-specific T cells in cerebrospinal fluid, both in multiple sclerosis and experimental autoimmune encephalomyelitis, may reflect their post-activated state rather than their recent participation in the demyelinating process.

Intrathecal immunoglobulin synthesis and oligoclonal bands

The central nervous system parenchyma is clearly not a physiological site for B-cell responses and antibody production, but individual B cells evidently can cross the blood–brain barrier, survive in the central nervous system and produce substantial amounts of immunoglobulin (Hickey 2001). Indeed B lymphocytes are readily demonstrable in a number of neuropathological contexts – such as viral encephalitides and lymphomas. In multiple sclerosis, small but consistent numbers of B lymphocytes at different stages of differentiation are present in inflammatory round cell infiltrates (see Chapter 12), as well as in the cerebrospinal fluid. B-lymphocyte infiltrations are also seen, although in variable degrees, in other pathological conditions,

Cellular basis of intrathecal immunoglobulin synthesis

Although the direct evidence is patchy, it seems likely that recirculating B lymphocytes share essential features with their T-cell counterparts (Hickey 2001). In the resting nonactivated stage, B lymphocytes are excluded by the specialized blood–brain barrier endothelium. However, after antigen-driven activation, B lymphoblasts cross into the central nervous system. In immuno-compromised individuals, most primary intracerebral lymphomas are Epstein–Barr virus (EBV)-transformed B-cell lymphomas (Morgello 1995). When transferred to immunodeficient mice, these lymphomas grow well after injection via the intracerebral but not the intravenous route (Bashir *et al* 1991; Nakamine *et al* 1991). This suggests that the brain parenchyma is not completely hostile to (xenogeneic) B cells and that specific contact-dependent interaction between recirculating B cells and the cerebral endothelium is required for correct lymphocyte migration through the blood–brain barrier. In xenogeneic (mouse/human) combination, this necessary fit of cell adhesion molecules is not reproduced. Rather, EBV-transformed B cells express a number of lymphocyte activation markers – most prominently MHC class II, costimulatory factors (B7-1 and -2) and cell-adhesion molecules, including LFA-1, LFA-3 and the ICAM family (Clark and Lane 1991). Although not clearly defined, a particular profile of surface adhesion molecules along with activation-dependent membrane proteases and chemokines must work together, selectively to allow activated B lymphocytes access to the brain parenchyma across the blood–brain barrier (Ambrosini *et al* 2003; Columba-Cabezas *et al* 2003).

The central nervous system lacks all stroma cells – such as follicular dendritic cells (which shape the germinal centres of secondary lymphoid follicles), and the fibroblast-like sinus cells that support B-lymphocyte formation in the bone marrow that normally make up the microenvironment of B-cell tissues (Weissman 1993). But even in the absence of these specialized lymphoid cells, there is no shortage of available cytokines in the central nervous system for survival and differentiation of antibody-forming B lymphocytes. While helper T cell-dependent cytokine signals are delivered by T-lymphocyte inflammatory infiltrates (e.g. IL-3, IL-4 and IFN-γ), local brain cells produce an impressive range of cytokines involved in B-cell biology. These include the proinflammatory mediators IL-1, TNF-α and IL-6; the chemokines MIP-1 and MIP-2; the B cell survival factor BAFF (Krumbholz *et al* 2005) and other cytokines of the epidermal, fibroblast and TGF families (Hopkins and Rothwell 1995). Each affects different aspects of B-cell function. Thus, for example, IL-6 was originally described as a B-cell growth factor (BGF-2) before its pleiotropic functions became evident. IL-6 is readily induced in brain microglia but also as part of the neuronal response to endotoxin, trauma, ischaemia and other insults. Besides acting on local brain cells, it has the capacity to maintain differentiation and activation of brain-infiltrating B cells up to the terminal plasma cell stage. IL-4, IFN-γ and TGF-β, and the chemokines MCP-1 and -2, influence immunoglobulin isotype switching and B-cell entry into the central nervous system.

Significance of intrathecal immunoglobulin for disease pathogenesis

In health, human cerebrospinal fluid contains little immunoglobulin or other plasma proteins. The appearance of immunoglobulin signifies pathological changes, reflecting either increased permeability of the blood–brain barrier or B cell-related immune processes active within the brain parenchyma (E.J. Thompson 1995). This is especially characteristic of samples taken from individuals with multiple sclerosis, which typically show immunglobulin distributed in oligoclonal patterns (see Chapter 7). Although not specific for multiple sclerosis, oligoclonal immunoglobulin bands have become a standard in providing laboratory support for the diagnosis of multiple sclerosis. Immunoglobulin permeating into the cerebrospinal fluid through a leaky endothelial barrier can be distinguished from that released by active plasma cells positioned within the brain or meningeal infiltrates by comparing the ratios of immunoglobulin and albumin concentrations in cerebrospinal fluid and plasma (the IgG index; see Chapter 7). Since albumin must reach the central nervous system from sources in the liver through the blood circulation, the albumin ratio can be considered as a pure permeability marker. Various formulas have been proposed for denoting the origin of immunoglobulins present in cerebrospinal fluid (Blenow et al 1994).

The elevated IgG index and presence of oligoclonal bands are general features of chronic brain inflammation and have achieved paraclinical diagnostic usefulness in multiple sclerosis (Fishman 1992; see also Chapter 7). It is the rare patient with multiple sclerosis who does not demonstrate oligoclonal bands and, in longitudinal studies, their absence may only be transient (Zeman et al 1996). However, the proportion lacking oligoclonal bands in the cerebrospinal fluid may be greater in cases with late-onset disease or chronic progressive disease variants (Pirttila and Nurmikko 1995) – perhaps reflecting contamination of these series with patients having other diagnoses. But, as discussed in Chapters 5, 7 and 8, the presence of oligoclonal bands is clearly low in other demyelinating disorders of the central nervous system, especially the optico-spinal form in Oriental peoples and in neuromyelitis optica (Fukazawa et al 1993; Wingerchuk et al 1999). Decoding the antigen specificity of oligoclonal IgG in multiple sclerosis has proved frustrating, and attempts to date have not illuminated our understanding of lesion pathogenesis. A large number of studies have focused on the occurrence of specific autoantibodies and found reactivity against myelin or oligodendrocyte proteins, glycolipids, axonal antigens, endothelial components and stress proteins (Archelos et al 2000; Ilyas et al 2003). Whether these antibodies are pathogenic is still unresolved.

Although brain specificity of oligoclonally distributed immunoglobulins has not regularly been shown, immunospot assays measuring myelin-specific immunoglobulin secretion by B lymphocytes harvested from cerebrospinal fluid in patients with multiple sclerosis show enhanced production of antibodies against a number of myelin proteins (M. Lu et al 1996). The groups of Hans Link and Tomas Olsson have used the immunospot assay to identify single B cells secreting brain-specific autoantibodies. Their results indicate that samples from patients with multiple sclerosis contain elevated numbers of myelin basic protein-specific B lymphocytes, but these do not change substantially with the clinical course (Link et al 1990; Olsson et al 1990a). As with T cells, the autoreactive B lymphocyte patterns are remarkably stable over time and do not parallel the clinical course (Link et al 1990). The B-cell response to myelin basic protein is directed against sequence p70–89. Reactions against proteolipid protein and myelin-associated glycoprotein have also been demonstrated (Baig et al 1991; Sellebjerg et al 1994). The antibody response against myelin-associated glycoprotein in the cerebrospinal fluid of patients with multiple sclerosis deserves special comment. These antibodies initiate myelin destruction in the presence of complement or macrophage-activating cytokines when injected into the cerebrospinal fluid of experimental animals (Vass et al 1992). Intrathecal production of anti-myelin-associated glycoprotein antibodies in patients with multiple sclerosis could therefore be directly involved in the pathogenesis of demyelination. By simple ELISA screening, anti-myelin-associated glycoprotein antibodies were detected only in a small number of patients with multiple sclerosis (Xiao et al 1991), perhaps because such antibodies are absorbed from cerebrospinal fluid by the excess antigen in brain tissue. With more sensitive techniques, such antibodies were found in the majority of individuals with multiple sclerosis but also in those with other inflammatory neurological diseases (Markovich et al 2003; Padberg et al 2001; Reindl et al 1999). For example, B lymphocytes secreting anti-myelin basic protein were present at high frequency in 8/10 patients with multiple sclerosis (J. Sun et al 1991b), and intrathecal synthesis of anti-myelin oligodendrocyte glycoprotein antibodies in multiple sclerosis is also reflected by an increased anti-myelin oligodendrocyte glycoprotein Ig index in cerebrospinal fluid (Reindl et al 1999). These data indicate that antibodies with demyelinating potential are produced intrathecally in patients with multiple sclerosis. However, anti-myelin oligodendrocyte glycoprotein antibodies, recognizing an epitope expressed on the surface of myelin and oligodendrocytes and therefore able to induce demyelination, may represent a small fraction of only the anti-myelin basic protein reactivity detected by ELISA or Western blot. Thus, the majority of such antibodies, present in cerebrospinal fluid, may not be directly involved in the demyelinating process (Haase et al 2001).

Using a broad-based new system of phage library screening for antigen specificity, no stereotyped pattern of intrathecal antibody production has been disclosed (Cortese et al 1996; 2001). For example, oligoclonal IgG in patients with multiple sclerosis contains reactivities against a variety of different virus antigens. But the patterns of antigen specificity are inconsistent and the virus-specific antibodies do not have the high affinity expected in the presence of specific antigen (Luxton et al 1995; Sindic et al 1994). More recent attempts to characterize oligoclonal bands include screening pooled cerebrospinal fluid from patients with multiple sclerosis against a murine oligodendrocyte precursor cell line-derived phage protein expression library. Five of seven positive clones, from amongst a pool of 1×10^6, contained an identical seven amino acid Alu repeat sequence spanning the B-cell epitope that reacted with 24/54 (44%) samples from patients with clinically definite multiple sclerosis, compared with <18% in patients with a variety of other neurological diseases. These differences were not seen when screening for reactivity to heat-shock protein (>50% in both groups), although antibody titres to both antigens were higher in the patients with multiple sclerosis (Archelos *et al* 1998). Finally, a recent study using expression arrays, identified Epstein–Barr virus proteins as common targets (Cepok *et al* 2005b). Taken together, it is likely that antibody responses in the cerebrospinal fluid of patients with multiple sclerosis, and contained in the oligoclonal response, represent a bystander reaction rather than direct markers of immune response driving the disease.

Soluble immune mediators in cerebrospinal fluid

Since multiple sclerosis is a chronic inflammatory disease of the nervous system, one would expect the cerebrospinal fluid to contain a variety of soluble immune mediators, such as cytokines, adhesion molecules and toxic effector molecules. By summarizing the data from a large number of studies on this topic, several general conclusions can be reached. First, a similar range and concentration of soluble immune mediators occur in the cerebrospinal fluid from patients with multiple sclerosis as in other chronic T-cell-mediated inflammatory diseases of the central nervous system and, to date, no disease-specific patterns have been revealed. Secondly, in general, the concentration of immune mediator proteins in cerebrospinal fluid correlates with the cellular reaction, indicating that inflammatory cells are their major source. Thirdly, cytokine patterns, as well as the appearance of antigens associated with inflammation in cerebrospinal fluid, may be useful in determining immunological activity of the disease process. Last, although not backed by much evidence, the patterns of toxic immune effector molecules in cerebrospinal fluid may help to identify mechanisms of tissue injury in these lesions.

Cytokines

Although early studies on cytokine patterns in cerebrospinal fluid from patients with multiple sclerosis were hampered by technical problems, improved assay sensitivity now makes it possible to detect practically all cytokines and chemokines (Navikas and Link 1996). There is a growing consensus that proinflammatory cytokines characterize cerebrospinal fluid during active stages of the disease, whereas anti-inflammatory mediators dominate the profile in remission (Rieckmann *et al* 1995). TNF-α appears to be particularly important during disease activity (Chofflon *et al* 1992; Hauser *et al* 1990; Maimone *et al* 1991b; Sharief and Thompson 1992; Spuler *et al* 1996; Tsukada *et al* 1991); levels correlate not only with clinical disease activity but also with measures of blood–brain barrier damage acting as a surrogate for acute inflammation (Sharief and Thompson 1992). This cytokine may be important not only for propagation of brain inflammation but also for playing a direct role in the destruction of myelin and oligodendrocytes. In addition, other cytokines that are important in regulation of T-cell-mediated inflammation, such as IL-2 (Gallo *et al* 1991; Sharief and Thompson 1993), IL-1 (Rovaris *et al* 1996), IL-10 (Navikas *et al* 1995), IL-15 (Kivisäkk *et al* 1998b), IL-18 (Losy and Niezgoda 2001) and lymphotoxin (Navikas *et al* 1996a), have been found. To this list can be added IL-4, IL-6 and Il-10

as indicators of intrathecal B-cell stimulation and antibody production (Nakashima *et al* 2000; Navikas *et al* 1996b; Perez *et al* 1995). But, again we should emphasize that the presence of proinflammatory cytokines in the cerebrospinal fluid is by no means specific for multiple sclerosis (Navikas and Link 1996).

Soluble adhesion molecules

Migration of inflammatory cells through the blood–brain barrier depends on the interaction between adhesion molecules on leucocytes and endothelial cells. Adhesion molecules in general are expressed on the surface of cells upon activation, but they may subsequently be shed and secreted. These soluble forms are not only reliable markers for cell activation in immunological processes, but they also function competitively to inhibit cell contact and migration. It is thus not surprising that practically all adhesion molecules, implicated in cell traffic through the blood–brain barrier, have been identified in soluble form in the cerebrospinal fluid (Dore Duffy *et al* 1995; S.J. Lee and Benveniste 1999; Mossner *et al* 1996; Sharief *et al* 1993; Tsukada *et al* 1993; 1995) and their concentrations differ with relapsing or progressive forms of the disease (Elovaara *et al* 2000). Serum levels of soluble ICAM-1 but not VCAM-1 correlate to some degree with MRI findings in relapsing–remitting and secondary progressive multiple sclerosis, and thus may offer an additional surrogate marker for disease progression (Giovannoni *et al* 1997). Soluble adhesion molecules are shed by leucocytes and resident meningeal cells (Jander *et al* 1993; Trojano *et al* 1996). Their concentration therefore correlates with pleocytosis (Sharief *et al* 1993) and is reduced after steroid treatment (Elovaara *et al* 2000). But, as with cytokines, the presence of soluble adhesion molecules in cerebrospinal fluid is not specific for multiple sclerosis (Rieckmann *et al* 1993; Mossner *et al* 1996).

Chemokines and chemokine receptors

Chemokines and their receptors are instrumental in the migration of inflammatory cells from the circulation to the central nervous system. Their patterns of expression within multiple sclerosis lesions reflect the composition of inflammatory infiltrates as well as activity and stage of the lesions (see Chapter 12). Although few members of the large family of chemokines and their receptors have so far been analysed in the cerebrospinal fluid of patients with multiple sclerosis, several general conclusions can already be reached. Overall, the patterns reflect the spectrum of inflammatory cells preferentially recruited into the central nervous system under normal and inflammatory conditions. Some apparently serve as useful markers for ongoing inflammatory activity. Furthermore, the patterns of chemokine and chemokine receptor expression in cerebrospinal fluid reflect those present within parenchymal lesions.

The cerebrospinal fluid from patients with multiple sclerosis contains elevated levels of CXCL 10 (previously called IFN-γ inducible protein 10; IP-10), and one of its receptors (CXCR 3) is expressed on the majority of lymphocytes present in cerebrospinal fluid (Narikawa *et al* 2004; T.L. Sorensen *et al* 1999). CXCR 3 is present on both T and B cells (T.L. Sorensen *et al* 1999; 2002b), and more detailed mapping of chemokine receptor expression in relation to other leucocyte markers shows that the population of activated memory cells is preferentially recruited (Giunti *et al* 2003; Kivisäkk *et al* 2003). This pattern of expression further suggests a bias in the recruitment of T cells polarized as Th1 and Tc1 cells (Giunti *et al* 2003; Misu *et al* 2001). Both are highly enriched in the active lesions of multiple sclerosis, but the same cell types also dominate the cerebrospinal fluid leucocyte population in controls (Kivisäkk *et al* 2002; 2003). These studies suggest that local production of IFN-γ in the central nervous system compartment induces the production of CXCL 10, which is then responsible for the dominant recruitment of Th1/Tc1 polarized T cells.

CCL2 (formerly monocyte chemoattractant protein 1; MCP-1) is present at increased concentration in cerebrospinal fluid from patients with multiple sclerosis and neuromyelitis optica compared with controls, and correlates inversely with disease activity (Franciotta *et al* 2001; Mahad *et al* 2002; Narikawa *et al* 2004; Scarpini *et al* 2002; T.L. Sorensen *et al* 1999). However, RANTES (regulated on activation, normal T cell expressed and secreted) is elevated in active lesions and may serve as a ligand for CCR 5 on T cells and monocytes (T.L. Sorensen *et al* 1999). Additional signals for cell recruitment are provided by the interaction of fractalkine (CX₃CL1) and its receptor (Kastenbauer *et al* 2003) and from CCL 17, CCL 19 and CCL 12 (Narikawa *et al* 2004; Pashenkov *et al* 2003a). The latter may play a role in retention and recruitment of dendritic cells in the cerebrospinal fluid (Pashenkov *et al* 2003b).

Although these studies define the major cell populations recruited into the cerebrospinal fluid of patients with multiple sclerosis, it remains to be determined whether the cerebrospinal fluid reflects the subtleties of chemokine and chemokine receptor expression within lesions (see Chapter 12), and whether their subtypes are mirrored by characteristic chemokine patterns in the cerebrospinal fluid.

Markers of inflammation and effector molecules

Macrophages are the dominant cells in actively demyelinating multiple sclerosis lesions. Thus, despite relatively low numbers in cerebrospinal fluid, their products can be liberated in lesions and are then readily detected. As a rather nonspecific marker of macrophage activation, cerebrospinal fluid neopterin levels are elevated in patients with multiple sclerosis – in particular during active stages of the disease (Fredrikson *et al* 1987; Ott *et al* 1993; Shaw *et al* 1995). Neopterin is released by cytokine-stimulated cells of the macrophage-monocyte lineage and may appear not only in cerebrospinal fluid but also in urine. Serial measurement shows urinary neopterin/creatinine ratios of 187, 187 and 218 in patients with relapsing–remitting and primary or secondary progressive multiple sclerosis, respectively, compared with 134 in controls. More days showed elevated ratios amongst patients than controls, and there were sustained elevations following relapses and identified infections (Giovannoni *et al* 1997). Elevated levels of β2-microglobulin (Bjerrum *et al* 1988; Us *et al* 1989) and the soluble alpha-chain of class I are also found in cerebrospinal fluid (Fainardi *et al* 2002).

Activated macrophages produce a variety of other toxic effector molecules that may be directly involved in the formation of multiple sclerosis lesions. Protease activity, which can be attributed to different specific proteases (Akenami *et al* 1996; Gijbels *et al* 1992; Liuzzi *et al* 2002) and their inhibitors, is increased in cerebrospinal fluid from patients with multiple sclerosis (Banik 1992; Price and Cuzner 1979; Richards and Cuzner 1978). As with cytokines and adhesion molecules, the concentration of proteases correlates with pleocytosis (Gijbels *et al* 1992) and is also elevated in other inflammatory neurological diseases (Akenami *et al* 1996). Treatment with corticosteroids may reduce matrix metalloproteinase and increase proteinase inhibitor activity in the cerebrospinal fluid (Rosenberg *et al* 1996). Prostaglandins and leucotrienes have been identified in cerebrospinal fluid from patients with multiple sclerosis (Dore-Duffy *et al* 1991; Neu *et al* 1992).

Studies of cerebrospinal fluid provide evidence for complement activation in multiple sclerosis. Complement is implicated both as an amplifier of the inflammatory process and mediator of demyelination. The concentrations of C2 (Delasnerie-Laupretre *et al* 1981), C4 (Jans *et al* 1984) and C9 (D.A.S. Compston *et al* 1986; Halawa *et al* 1989; Morgan *et al* 1984) are decreased, whereas soluble C5-9 complexes can be detected (Mollnes *et al* 1987; Sanders *et al* 1986). These observations indicate intrathecal complement activation. Others have not reproduced the alterations in late complement component concentrations comparing samples from multiple sclerosis patients with controls (M. Rodriguez *et al* 1990) and, at best, there is a wide concentration range for cerebrospinal fluid C5-9 between patients (Sanders *et al* 1986). One interpretation is that such measurements identify a subgroup of patients with an antibody-dependent complement-mediated pathway of myelin destruction (see Chapter 12). The situation, however, appears more complex, and complement activation in the cerebrospinal fluid may merely reflect local interaction with soluble immune complexes (Jans *et al* 1984; Rudick *et al* 1985). In addition, lack of complement inhibitory proteins in the cerebrospinal fluid may by itself lead to complement activation when the blood–brain barrier is damaged. In line with this observation, a similar activation of terminal complement complexes has been found in patients with subarachnoid haemorrhage as that reported in multiple sclerosis (Lindsberg *et al* 1996). Nevertheless, activation of terminal complement complexes correlates significantly with neurological disability, suggesting that patients with severe and destructive lesions have higher complement activation in the cerebrospinal fluid (Sellebjerg *et al* 1998a).

The potential role of reactive oxygen intermediates in the pathogenesis of demyelination and axonal pathology in multiple sclerosis is reflected by the appearance of lipid peroxidation products (Calabrese *et al* 1998; Hunter *et al* 1985) and increased levels of isoprostane in the cerebrospinal fluid (Greco *et al* 1999). Even more intriguing is the observation of increased nitric oxide-producing cells (Xiao *et al* 1996). A component of the cerebrospinal fluid of patients with multiple sclerosis, apparently unrelated to proinflammatory cytokines (Köller *et al* 1996), has been reported to block sodium channel activity (Chapter 13: Brinkmeier *et al* 1993; 1996). Later, a large number of studies looked for nitrite and nitrate as footprints of nitric oxide production in the cerebrospinal fluid of patients with multiple sclerosis. Both are elevated, especially in patients with active disease (Brundin *et al* 1999; Danilov *et al* 2003; Giovannoni 1998; Sveningsson *et al* 1999; Yamashita *et al* 1997), their concentrations correlating with the extent of blood–brain barrier damage (Acar *et al* 2003; Giovannoni *et al* 1998). Clinically, high nitrite and nitrate levels are associated with prolonged relapse duration and a more pronounced response to treatment with corticosteroids (Sellebjerg *et al* 2002). Other nitrosylation-induced metabolites, as well as nitric oxide synthase activity, are enhanced in the cerebrospinal fluid of patients with multiple sclerosis (Calabrese *et al* 2002). In cooperation with reactive oxgen species, nitric oxide induces mitochondrial dysfunction leading to hypoxia-like tissue injury (see Chapter 12; K.J. Smith and Lassmann 2002). Recently a new marker (D-110) has been identified, which selectively labels hypoxic tissue. The D-110 protein is liberated into the cerebrospinal fluid and detected by ELISA or Western blot. It is increased in a subset of patients with multiple sclerosis, and pre-liminary evidence correlating tissue biopsy with cerebrospinal fluid measurement indicates that it may indeed identify the subset of patients with hypoxia-like tissue damage (Lassmann *et al* 2003).

Finally, the cerebrospinal fluid of patients with multiple sclerosis possesses neurotoxic or gliotoxic activity. A factor, toxic for glia cells both *in vitro* and *in vivo*, has been identified. This is a small protein encoded by endogenous retrovirus sequence (Benjelloun *et al* 2002; Menard *et al* 1997) and found mainly in patients with active disease (Pierig *et al* 2002). It is present in urine and reported to show 91% sensitivity and 97% specificity for multiple sclerosis (Malcus-Vocanson *et al* 1998). Although as yet unidentified, a further factor is described in the cere-brospinal fluid of patients with multiple sclerosis that is able to induce neuronal apoptosis *in vitro* in a caspase-dependent manner (Cid *et al* 2002; 2003). This factor is mainly enriched in samples from patients with active disease and its activity seems to correlate with the destructiveness of lesions, as visualized by MRI (Cid *et al* 2002).

Markers of central nervous system damage

Damage to central nervous system tissue liberates intracellular proteins, which may diffuse through extracellular space into the cerebrospinal fluid compartment. These proteins offer an opportunity for monitoring acute tissue destruction in the course of multiple sclerosis. The first myelin protein analysed for this purpose was CNPase, since this is fairly specific for myelin and its enzyme activity provides a simple detection system. Activity was increased in active stages of multiple scle-rosis (Banik *et al* 1979; Eickhoff and Heipertz 1979) but not during remission (Banik *et al* 1979). However, a more reliable marker for demyclination is myelin basic protein (Cohen *et al* 1978). This parallels the increase in CNPase (Suda *et al* 1984). The validity of myelin basic protein as a marker of myelin destruction is supported by several investigations, although, not unexpectedly, it has become clear that its presence in cere-brospinal and other body fluids is not disease specific but also occurs in other conditions resulting in white matter destruction (Mukherjee *et al* 1985; Whitaker *et al* 1980). The detection of myelin basic protein in urine has not been adopted as a routine assay for assessing disease activity in multiple sclerosis.

Increased levels of myelin basic protein are present in cere-brospinal fluid during rather a short window of lesional activity (Gupta 1987; Lamers *et al* 1998; Sellebjerg *et al* 1998a;

Thompson *et al* 1985). Detailed epitope mapping of myelin basic protein molecules in cerebrospinal fluid reveals that not all portions of the molecule are detected, and neoepitopes of degraded myelin basic protein, not recognized in the intact molecule, may appear (Whitaker 1998; Whitaker *et al* 1986). Whereas the liberation of myelin basic protein appears restricted to the stage of active demyelination, S-100 protein also remains elevated in the cerebrospinal fluid during remission (Massaro *et al* 1985). In contrast, glial fibrillary acidic protein, which is also released into the cerebrospinal fluid in patients with multiple sclerosis, correlates more closely with the extent of disability than with lesion activity (Rosengren *et al* 1995), and neural cell adhesion molecule (NCAM) peaks at the time of recovery, possibly indicating synaptic remodelling (Massaro *et al* 1987). Furthermore, release of neurofilament protein into the cerebrospinal fluid in multiple sclerosis (Lycke *et al* 1998; Semra *et al* 2002) and optic neuritis (E.T. Lim *et al* 2004) may reflect axonal damage in lesions. In addition, antibodies against neurofilament protein were found to correlate with disease pro-gression and brain atrophy (Eikelenboom *et al* 2003; Silber *et al* 2002). For diagnostic purposes a combined analysis of different structural central nervous system components (myelin basic protein, S-100 and neuron-specific enolase) in the cerebrospinal fluid may be useful (Lamers *et al* 1995). Levels of the cytoskeleton protein tau and 14.3.3 in cerebrospinal fluid may reflect neuronal and axonal damage in the active lesions of multiple sclerosis (Bartosik-Psujek and Archelos 2004; Martinez-Yelamos *et al* 2001; Sussmuth *et al* 2001), although this has not been reproduced in another study (Jiminez-Jiminez *et al* 2002). A recent study describes the presence of Nogo-A antibodies in the cerebrospinal fluid (Reindl *et al* 2003). Antibody titres against this antigen were particularly high during the early stage of the disease, in patients with a relapsing disease course. They may be induced in the course of myelin and oligo-dendrocyte destruction within active lesions. It is not clear whether such Nogo-A antibodies are functionally active and may in part counteract the regeneration blockade mediated by Nogo.

Conclusion

With the introduction of MRI, the impact of cerebrospinal fluid analysis for the diagnosis of multiple sclerosis has declined, although, as we argue in Chapter 7, these laboratory investiga-tions provide qualitatively different yet complementary infor-mation. In many institutions the view now prevails that lumbar puncture is no longer necessary in patients with multiple scle-rosis. We hope that this attitude will change since, as we discuss here and in Chapter 12, the pathways involved in inflammation, demyelination and axonal destruction are diverse and require definition in each patient if treatment is to be individualized to suit people with specifically different pathological substrates. These classifications require an integrated approach combining clinical, neuroradiological and immunological analyses. In this respect, the analysis of cerebrospinal fluid offers a unique opportunity to define autoimmune responses in the central nervous system and to identify immunological pathways of myelin and axonal destruction.

The pathology of multiple sclerosis

12

Hans Lassmann and Hartmut Wekerle

INTRODUCTION

Multiple sclerosis has long been recognized as a disease of the central nervous system in which an inflammatory process is associated with focal destruction of myelin sheaths (Charcot 1868a; 1868b). Thus, the essential brain lesion in multiple sclerosis is the demyelinated plaque, which may occur at any place within the central nervous system where myelin sheaths are present. Demyelination is accompanied by astrocytosis and the formation of scars, reflected in the name multiple sclerosis, and signifying the occurrence of the many sclerotic plaques that are widely distributed throughout the brain and spinal cord.

Early descriptions of the macroscopic pathology of multiple sclerosis appeared in the first half of the 19th century (see Chapter 1: Carswell 1838; Cruveilhier c.1841), documenting multiple discoloured spots with induration of tissue in white matter and, in particular, within the spinal cord. The first histological investigations were published by Eduard Rindfleisch (1863), who made several remarkable observations. He noted that plaques were orientated around a central blood vessel, which revealed an increased density of intramural small round cells. This was interpreted by Rindfleisch as evidence for a chronic inflammatory process. Furthermore, he described loss of myelin sheaths in the lesions showing that axons, devoid of myelin, can be traced for a considerable distance into the plaques. This process was associated with increased density of 'connective tissue' in the form of scarring. Soon after, a systematic clinical and neuropathological survey of the disease was provided by Charcot. In particular, his fundamental neuropathological study defined in detail the demyelinating process that leads to the formation of plaques with glial scar formation (Charcot 1868b).

With time, and the steady accumulation of detailed pathological studies, it became clear that the classical clinicopathological pattern of multiple sclerosis represents only one of many closely related entities, summarized under the designation 'inflammatory demyelinating diseases' (Adams and Kubik 1952). Although, both from the perspective of clinical expression and pathological features, the separate inflammatory demyelinating diseases are quite diverse, continuous transitions from one to another strongly suggest that each has a close pathogenetic relationship (Krücke 1976).

In general, inflammatory demyelinating diseases affect both the peripheral nervous system and central nervous system, taking either an acute monophasic or a chronic (relapsing) course (Alvord 1985). For reasons that are not fully understood, disease of the central nervous system is typically chronic, in the sense that new episodes or steady deterioration are the rule, whereas inflammatory demyelination of peripheral nerves is more usually monophasic and with full recovery. The major differences between acute and chronic inflammatory demyelinating diseases of the central nervous system and peripheral nervous system lie in the extent of demyelination and the capacity for sustained remyelination. For example, in acute disseminated encephalomyelitis, massive inflammation is associated with only minor demyelination in the vicinity of the inflammatory infiltrates, whereas large confluent plaques of demyelination are the hallmark of a chronic disease, such as multiple sclerosis. Remyelination is patchy and of uncertain functional significance in relapsing–remitting multiple sclerosis, but routine, and the basis for functional recovery, in inflammatory demyelinating disorders of the peripheral nervous system. As discussed below, all inflammatory demyelinating diseases appear primarily to depend upon a T-cell mediated inflammatory reaction, but their clinical course and pathology may be modified by additional immune reactions.

PATHOLOGICAL CLASSIFICATION OF DEMYELINATING DISEASES

Before giving a detailed description of the pathology of multiple sclerosis, we start with a basic description and definition of individual inflammatory demyelinating diseases affecting the central nervous system.

Chronic multiple sclerosis

Chronic multiple sclerosis is the most frequent inflammatory demyelinating disease, affecting about 1:1000 individuals in the Western world (see Chapter 2). From the clinical perspective, it usually follows a relapsing course, at least in the early years, but may later transform into secondary progressive disease. In a minority of patients, the disease is progressive from onset. We make this point here because there are indications that there may be important differences in the pathology of primary progressive and relapsing or secondary progressive forms of multiple sclerosis (see below).

The neuropathologist usually only has access to tissue from individuals who have suffered from multiple sclerosis for many years. The pathology of such late chronic cases is characterized

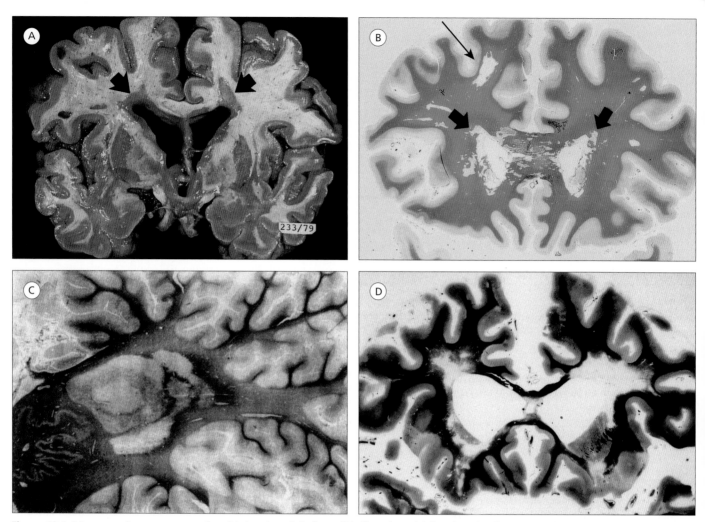

Figure 12.1 Macroscopic appearance of multiple sclerosis lesions. (A) Chronic multiple sclerosis of 23 years' duration; section through the fresh brain shows symmetrical demyelinated plaques in the periventricular white matter (arrows); ×0.5. (B) Acute multiple sclerosis of 7 months' duration; section through frontal brain shows multiple small, partly confluent demyelinated lesions in the periventricular area (thick arrows) and deep white matter (thin arrow). Myelin stain ×0.5. (C) Acute multiple sclerosis of 4.5 months' duration; concentric plaque in the cerebellar white matter; immunocytochemistry for myelin oligodendrocyte glycoprotein (MOG); ×2. (D) Myelin stain of chronic multiple sclerosis with long duration and severe clinical disability; in addition to multiple plaques, especially in the periventricular areas, there is severe atrophy of the white and grey matter; ×0.5.

by the presence of multiple demyelinated plaques in white and grey matter (Figure 12.1A). Demyelination in the chronic stage may still be accompanied by inflammation. In this situation, in addition to old sclerotic plaques, active lesions with ongoing myelin destruction may be present.

Sufficient data have only recently become available allowing conclusions to be reached on what happens during the first or second bout of typical chronic multiple sclerosis. Such early lesions can only be studied in tissue samples from patients who die from unrelated events during these early stages, or in diagnostic brain biopsies. The latter occasionally become available in neuropathological centres routinely performing stereotactic biopsy procedures for brain tumour diagnosis (Brück et al 1994; Kepes 1993; S. Poser et al 1992; Rodriguez and Scheithauer 1994). The pathological features of such early lesions in multiple sclerosis are similar to those in the chronic stage of the disease, although there are differences – in particular regarding the incidence of active demyelinating lesions, intensity of the inflammatory process, and the extent to which there is endoge-

nous remyelination and repair (Lucchinetti et al 1996; 1999; 2000; Ozawa et al 1994).

Acute multiple sclerosis

Acute multiple sclerosis was recognized as a subtype of the disease by Otto Marburg (1906). Clinically, it is characterized by rapid progression and an exceptionally severe course. Acute multiple sclerosis usually leads to death within a very few years from onset due to the severe neurological debilitation. Although at first glance the pathological alterations are very similar to those found in chronic multiple sclerosis, there are several profound differences. In general, the lesions are much more destructive. Many small lesions are typically seen throughout the brain and spinal cord, and these may form large confluent focal plaques (Figure 12.1B). In other cases, widespread demyelination is present throughout the white matter and resembles the lesions of diffuse sclerosis. Another important difference is that in many cases of acute multiple sclerosis, inflammatory demyelination is not restricted to the central nervous system but also affects peripheral nerves (Marburg 1906; Lassmann *et al* 1981a).

Concentric sclerosis of Balo

In 1928, Joseph Balo described a peculiar lesion in Hungarian patients with rapidly progressive multiple sclerosis. These have subsequently been seen in all cohorts, and are particularly prominent in patients from the Philippines (Kuroiwa 1985). The essential features are large demyelinated plaques that show peculiar alternating rims of myelin preservation and loss, giving lesions the macroscopic or microscopic structure of onion bulbs (Figure 12.1C; and see below). The formation of this impressive type of plaque has raised many pathogenetic speculations but its cause is still debated.

Neuromyelitis optica (Devic's disease)

The characteristic feature of the Devic subform of multiple sclerosis is dominant involvement of the spinal cord and the (anterior) visual pathway (Devic 1894). Due to the strategic location of the demyelinating lesions, and their failure to remyelinate, it is generally associated with very severe clinical manifestations attributable to involvement of the visual system and spinal cord. The disease is commonest in Oriental people (see Chapters 5 and 6).

Diffuse sclerosis (Schilder's disease)

Diffuse sclerosis was first described by Paul Schilder in 1912. The pathology was characterized by primary demyelination that, unlike chronic multiple sclerosis, was not restricted to focal plaques but affected large parts of the periventricular white matter. However, active demyelination was associated with chronic inflammation and, in this respect, did not differ from the pattern seen in multiple sclerosis. Some cases of diffuse sclerosis were later found to be examples of metabolic defects, such as adrenoleucodystrophy (Igarashi *et al* 1976). Diffuse lesions may, however, also be present in otherwise typical cases of the Marburg form of acute multiple sclerosis. In this instance they occur, in contrast to those in adrenoleucodystrophy, side by side with classical small 'multiple sclerosis-like' demyelinated plaques. Many have abandoned the concept of Schilder's disease and the disorder is not considered elsewhere in this book.

Acute disseminated encephalomyelitis and acute haemorrhagic leucoencephalomyelitis

Acute monophasic variants of inflammatory demyelinating diseases can, in rare instances, develop spontaneously, but more frequently they are associated with preceding vaccinations or infections (Alvord 1985). Between 6 days and 3–4 weeks after infection or vaccination, a rapidly progressive neurological disease appears, which can be fatal but more usually recovers without further disease activity. The pathology is characterized by inflammation and, in the case of acute disseminated encephalomyelitis, some perivascular demyelination (R.D. Adams and Kubik 1952). In the more severe variant, acute haemorrhagic leucoencephalomyelitis (Hurst 1941), the inflammatory reaction is associated with perivascular haemorrhages and severe brain oedema. Of those who survive the acute phase of the disease, some are disabled, but often little or no permanent neurological deficit is encountered and the brain lesions resolve with varying degrees of perivascular scar formation. A special form of acute disseminated leucoencephalitis is acute transverse myelitis due to one or several focal and very destructive inflammatory lesions in the spinal cord. Similar to acute disseminated leucoencephalitis, transverse myelitis may follow infection or vaccination.

Inflammatory demyelinating diseases of the peripheral nervous system

A similar disease process to that affecting the central nervous system in patients with multiple sclerosis may also involve peripheral nerves. The most frequent disease variant in the peripheral nervous system is the acute Guillain–Barré syndrome (Guillain *et al* 1916) in which acute monophasic inflammatory reaction in peripheral nerves and roots leads to destruction of myelin and, in very severe cases, also of axons. This disease may also take a chronic course, manifesting as chronic inflammatory demyelinating polyneuropathy (CIDP; Albers and Kelly 1989).

At first glance, it is surprising that we should choose to discuss such diverse conditions under the heading of inflammatory demyelinating diseases. However, there is good evidence that these disorders share common pathogenetic pathways. Transitional forms between the different diseases are observed (Fränkel and Jakob 1913; Pette 1928; Siemerling and Raecke 1914), which may cause problems in the diagnostic classification of brain biopsies (Kepes 1993). For example, the discrimination between acute disseminated leucoencephalitis and acute multiple sclerosis can be very difficult and may require the disease course to be monitored over several years before any final conclusion is reached. At one extreme, combined forms of acute haemorrhagic leucoencephalomyelitis and acute multiple sclerosis have been described (Krücke 1976). Conversely, the pathology of acute and chronic multiple sclerosis can be surprisingly similar. In addition, the combination of acute multiple sclerosis with acute or chronic inflammatory demyelinating polyneuropathy is occasionally seen in clinical practice (see Chapter 6), but this rare phenotype belies the fact that, from the neuropathology perspective, the combination is more the rule than the exception (Marburg 1906). Perhaps the most convincing argument for a common pathogenetic background to all these diseases comes from studies in experimental models of allergic encephalomyelitis (EAE) and neuritis (see Chapter 11). In these models, the whole spectrum of human inflammatory demyelinating diseases of the central nervous system and peripheral nervous system can be reproduced by different methods of autoimmunization (Lassmann 1983).

THE DEMYELINATED PLAQUE

The most characteristic pathological feature of multiple sclerosis is the demyelinated plaque with preserved axons set in a matrix of astrocyte scar formation distributed throughout the central nervous system, and showing a predilection for the optic nerves, periventricular white matter and corpus callosum, cerebellum and cervical cord (Fog 1950; Lumsden 1970; Oppenheimer 1978; G. Steiner 1931).

The basic lesion

In chronic multiple sclerosis, the plaque consists of a sharply demarcated lesion, which may have a diameter ranging from <1 mm to several centimetres (Figure 12.1). In general, plaques are centred on one or several medium-sized vessels (Rindfleisch 1863) and have a tendency to accumulate near the periventricular (G. Steiner 1931) or outer surfaces of the brain and spinal cord (Oppenheimer 1978). The lesions are normally round to oval but frequently show finger-like extensions in the periphery (Dawson 1916) that follow the path of a small or medium-sized vessel. By gross inspection of the unfixed brain, the plaques appear as grey discoloured areas with firm tissue texture. Microscopically, myelin sheaths are completely lost in the plaques. Axons are spared and embedded in dense astroglial scar tissue.

The demyelinating process is associated with persistent inflammation throughout the central nervous system (Babinski 1885b). Inflammatory infiltrates are located around small or medium-sized veins and may – especially in cases with ongoing disease activity – diffusely infiltrate the parenchyma of the central nervous system. Inflammatory infiltrates mainly consist of lymphocytes and macrophages. The inflammatory process in the nervous system is not restricted to the demyelinated plaques but also affects the so-called normal white and grey matter. It is present in the meninges that overlie the surface of the central nervous system tissue (Marburg 1906) and inflammation can sometimes even be found in areas devoid of myelin, such as the retina (Shaw et al 1987).

Definition of lesional activity

Actively demyelinating and inactive lesions may be encountered both in acute and chronic multiple sclerosis. Macroscopically, active plaques have a pink discoloration and their tissue texture is soft. Microscopically, they reveal demyelination with little astroglial scar formation. In addition, the lesions are infiltrated by numerous inflammatory cells (in particular macrophages) that contain myelin and tissue debris in their cytoplasm (Figure 12.2A,B).

A precise definition of lesional activity in multiple sclerosis is of major importance for biochemical and immunological studies of the pathogenesis. However, the morphological criteria for lesional activity in multiple sclerosis have been controversial and some of the essential features proposed in the literature are misleading. Active plaques are frequently defined by the presence of cholesterol esters and neutral lipids in macrophages. These are easily stained by lipophilic dyes, such as oil red O or Sudan II (sudanophilic stage of myelin degradation: Newcombe and Cuzner 1993; Newcombe et al 1991; V. Sanders et al 1993). Although the latter is a very convenient marker for macroscopic identification of the lesions in fresh or formaldehyde-fixed brain tissue, it is important to remember that this sudanophilic stage of myelin degradation may persist for several months after the actual destruction of myelin sheaths (Davie et al 1994; Lumsden 1970). It follows that lesional activity defined by the presence of sudanophilic lipids may have little relevance for immunological or biochemical studies.

The major criterion for definition of lesion activity in magnetic resonance imaging (MRI) investigations is gadolinium-DTPA leakage, taken to denote blood–brain barrier leakage (R.I. Grossman et al 1986; D.H. Miller et al 1988b). However, by comparison with imaging studies in multiple sclerosis, biopsy or autopsy material studied using neuropathological or immunocytochemical techniques shows variable degrees of blood–brain barrier leakage both in actively demyelinating as well as quiescent demyelinated plaques (Broman 1964; Tavolato 1975). In active plaques, the differences are quantitative in nature. Thus, from the pathological perspective, although representing an extremely useful research method for the evaluation of potential therapies aimed at modifying disease activity, the sharp distinction between active and inactive lesions based on gadolinium-DTPA MRI may in part reflect low sensitivity of these imaging techniques for detecting blood–brain barrier dysfunction. It is possible to demonstrate leakage of gadolinium-DTPA in a variety of acute and chronic lesions in which enhancement is not visible using standard imaging methods (Barnes et al 1991; Filippi et al 1995b; Silver et al 1997). Contrast enhancement occurs in the periplaque white matter, the rim of active myelin breakdown and the inactive plaque centre. Active demyelination, however, is matched by a small zone of decreased contrast in T_2-weighted images, located between the high-contrast areas of the periplaque oedema and the demyelinated plaque centre (Brück et al 1997).

In the pathology of demyelinating lesions, activity can be defined either by the inflammatory reaction (Figure 12.3) or by identifying early stages of demyelination. Criteria used to define inflammatory activity are diffuse infiltration of the vessel walls and central nervous system parenchyma by inflammatory cells (Hallervorden 1940), the increased expression of histocompatibility antigens (V. Sanders et al 1993; Traugott et al 1983a) or adhesion molecules (Raine et al 1990b; Sobel et al 1990), and the activation state of lymphocytes and macrophages within lesions (Brück et al 1995; Esiri and Reading 1987; H. Li et al 1993; Ozawa et al 1994).

A precise definition for lesional activity of demyelinated plaques can be achieved by studying the antigenic profile of myelin degradation products within macrophages in the lesions (Figure 12.2B,C: Hallpike et al 1970b; Lassmann 1983; H. Li et al 1993; Lumsden 1970; Seitelberger 1960). Detailed studies of demyelination using experimental material and human tissue have clarified the time sequence of myelin degradation in macrophages (Brück et al 1995; Lassmann and Wisniewski 1979c). Minor myelin proteins, such as myelin oligodendrocyte glycoprotein or myelin associated glycoprotein, are rapidly degraded within macrophages and their immunoreactivity disappears within 1–2 days after phagocytosis. Conversely, major myelin proteins, such as myelin basic protein or proteolipid protein, can be detected in macrophages for 6–10 days. In later stages, the macrophages contain sudanophilic lipids that may persist in the lesions for even longer (Lumsden 1970). The characterization of myelin degradation products in macrophages is the best and most precise method for the evaluation of lesional activity in multiple sclerosis. We should point out that when these stringent criteria are used, the incidence of active lesions in multiple sclerosis brains is low, especially in classical cases sampled at the chronic stage. Thus, when brain bank material is used for biochemical or immunological studies of multiple sclerosis pathogenesis, it is advisable to survey in detail the criteria used for describing the activity of individual lesions. An alternative method of evaluating tissue has been developed by Gay et al (1997). These

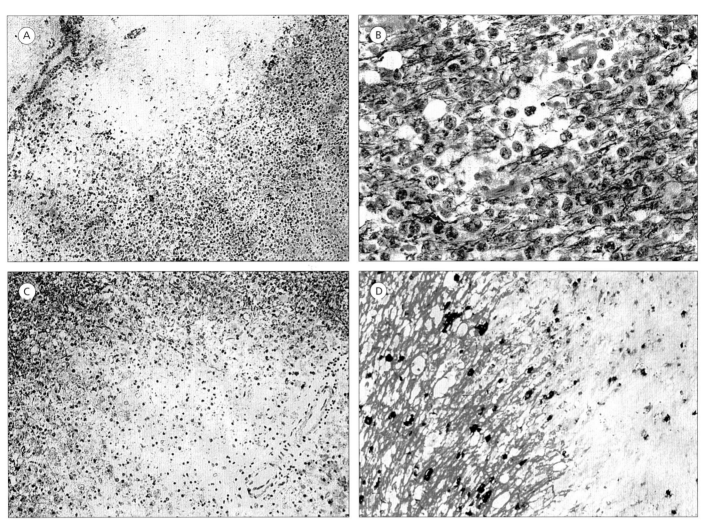

Figure 12.2 Lesional activity in multiple sclerosis. (A) Acute multiple sclerosis plaque; immunocytochemistry shows numerous macrophages stained with macrophage activation marker MRP14; ×80. (B) Acute multiple sclerosis, luxol fast blue myelin stain: very early lesion infiltrated by numerous macrophages containing luxol fast blue-positive degradation products; in between are preserved myelinated fibres; ×500. (C) Chronic multiple sclerosis, luxol fast blue myelin stain showing radially expanding lesion; numerous macrophages with luxol fast blue-positive myelin degradation products in the demyelinated area; ×80. (D) Chronic multiple sclerosis: *in situ* hybridization for proteolipid protein mRNA (black) and immunocytochemistry for proteolipid protein (red). Edge of a radially expanding lesion showing destruction of proteolipid protein-positive myelin sheaths (red) and proteolipid protein taken up by macrophages (small red granules). Oligodendrocytes with proteolipid protein mRNA (black cells) are reduced at the plaque margin. ×300.

authors suggest adopting a multifactorial cluster analysis, which includes parameters of clinical history, different aspects of inflammation and microglial activation, demyelination, and deposition of immunoglobulins and complement. Unfortunately the necessary clinical information is not always available, but the approach may help to identify stages of lesions that precede the structural dissolution of myelin sheaths.

When discussing lesion activity in multiple sclerosis, one aspect (generally ignored) that needs to be considered is whether active inflammation in multiple sclerosis necessarily leads to demyelination. In the pathology of active multiple sclerosis, vessels sometimes can be found with severe inflammatory infiltration of their walls and massive leakage of serum proteins but in the absence of active myelin destruction. Although such lesions may still represent a very early stage in the inflammatory process, followed later by demyelination, it remains entirely possible that not all inflammatory lesions evolve in this way. If this is the case,

separate criteria for inflammatory and demyelinating lesional activity are needed for studies on disease pathogenesis.

Lesion types

The characterization of lesions based on detailed histological features has provided neuropathologists with an extensive series of snapshots from which to reassemble a more dynamic concept of the pathogenesis, separating those lesion types that appear part of an evolving continuum from other appearances that may depend on an altogether different cascade of events.

Actively demyelinating lesions

The essential criteria for identification of actively demyelinating lesions are the presence of myelin sheaths in the process of dissolution and degradation products of myelin within macrophages

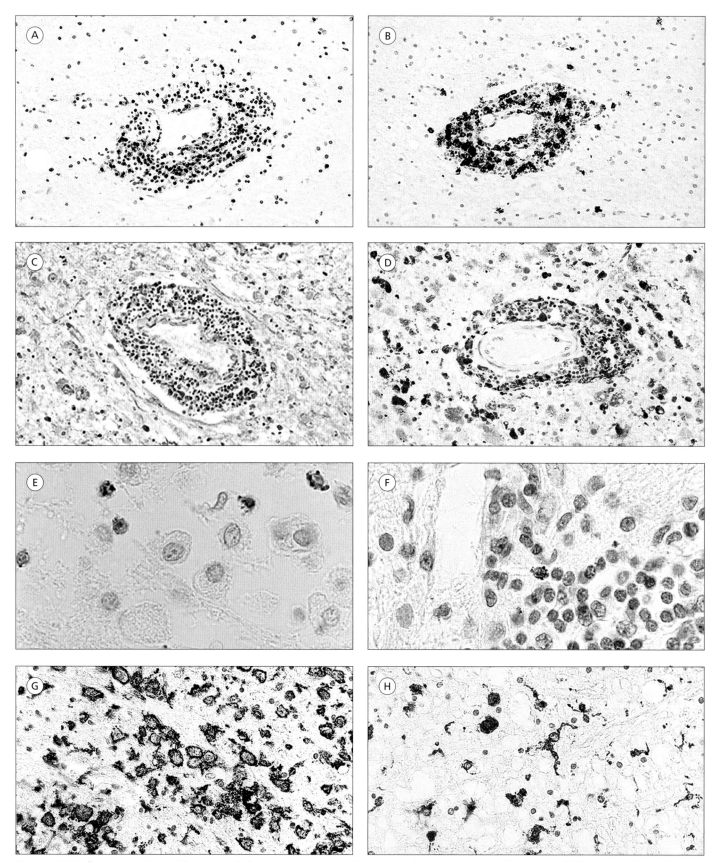

Figure 12.3 Inflammation in multiple sclerosis lesions. Acute multiple sclerosis. (A) Perivascular inflammatory infiltrates with CD3+ T cells. (B) CD8+ T cells. (C) IgG-containing plasma cells. (D) CD68+ macrophages; ×100. (E) Acute multiple sclerosis with granzyme B-reactive cytotoxic T cells in the lesion parenchyma. (F) A perivascular cuff; ×600. (G) Primary progressive multiple sclerosis lesion with CD68+ macrophages in an active plaque. (H) CD68+ microglia in the normal-appearing white matter; ×300.

that have infiltrated the tissue (Brück *et al* 1995; Gay *et al* 1997). Two different types of active lesions can be distinguished: the acute plaque and the chronic active lesions. In the acute plaque, the whole lesion is demyelinated simultaneously. Thus, in all plaque areas, myelin is at the same stage of dissolution or degradation. In contrast, chronic active plaques are characterized by a zone of ongoing demyelinating activity at the edge of the lesion, surrounding the already demyelinated centre of the plaque.

The identification of active plaques is straightforward at early stages of the disease, in particular in cases of acute or relapsing–remitting multiple sclerosis. There chronic active lesions are reflected by a dense infiltrate of macrophages, containing abundant early myelin degradation products. But the detection of active lesions is more difficult in late stages of multiple sclerosis and in patients with chronic progressive disease. In these cases, a slow-burning demyelinating process, perhaps only involving a few fibres at any one time, may take place at the borders of plaques (Prineas *et al* 2001). In such a situation, it is difficult to decide whether this is due to an ongoing immunological process or secondary fibre degeneration (Wallerian degeneration) due to transected axons in the centre of inactive plaques.

Inactive demyelinated lesions

The hallmark of chronic inactive lesions is the absence of ongoing destruction of myelin sheaths. This does not, however, imply that in all such lesions inflammation has already been totally cleared or that macrophages are no longer involved in further digestion of the myelin debris (Brück *et al* 1995). Macrophages may persist in central nervous system lesions for a considerable time, indicating that the complete process of dissolution and degradation of myelin remnants may be quite slow. Thus, for example, in Wallerian degeneration macrophages with sudanophilic myelin degradation products may persist for >6 months (Lumsden 1970), and in the plaques of multiple sclerosis, free lipids can be detected by magnetic resonance spectroscopy for several months after initiation of the lesion (Davie *et al* 1994). Thus, in the early stages, inactive plaques may still be hypercellular and diffusely infiltrated by lymphocytes and macrophages. At this stage macrophages may still contain abundant late myelin degradation products, and the dense astrocytic scar is not yet formed. In old 'burnt out' plaques, only few lymphocytes and macrophages are left at perivascular sites. The tissue texture appears hypocellular, due to profound loss of myelin and oligodendrocytes, and also of microglia. In these lesions, the remaining demyelinated axons are embedded in a dense astrocytic glial scar tissue.

These classical active and inactive plaques represent the vast majority of all lesions within a typical example of multiple sclerosis. However, additional lesions, rare in classical multiple sclerosis but more prominent in atypical disease variants, may occur.

The destructive lesion

Destructive lesions are responsible for very severe and rapidly progressive acute and chronic multiple sclerosis (Sugano *et al* 1992; Youl *et al* 1991a). Demyelination is accompanied by extensive additional tissue destruction, also affecting astrocytes and axons. In extreme situations, this may give rise to cystic brain lesions that can obscure the correct diagnosis, especially in brain biopsies. Furthermore, nonspecific tissue destruction in the plaques may result in pronounced atrophy of the grey and white matter in chronic multiple sclerosis (Figure 12.1D).

Shadow plaques

Shadow plaques were first depicted in a systematic study of acute multiple sclerosis by Marburg (1906), who noted incomplete demyelination in some lesions (see Chapter 1). Schlesinger (1909) later introduced the term *Markschattenherde* (translated as shadow plaque) to describe these lesions (see Figure 12.8A). In Schlesinger's original description, this term was applied to plaque-like lesions in the central nervous system, in which a reduced density of myelinated fibres was associated with unusually thin myelin sheaths. In later descriptions, this term was used for all lesions that revealed a decreased density of staining in sections stained for myelin. We consider that the term shadow plaque should only be used to describe the original type of lesion. Immunocytochemical and ultrastructural data strongly suggest that such lesions are areas of complete remyelination in previously demyelinated plaques (Lassmann 1983; Prineas 1985).

Besides remyelinated shadow plaques, areas of reduced myelin density within the central nervous system may also have other pathological substrates. In the early stages of active demyelination, some myelin sheaths may already have been destroyed while others are still preserved, accounting for reduced myelin staining as that seen in shadow plaques. In this situation, the decreased density of myelin is associated with extensive infiltration of the lesions by macrophages containing myelin in the earliest stages of degradation. In other lesions, a decrease in density of myelinated axons can be found in association with pronounced axonal loss. The surviving myelinated fibres have a similar myelin thickness and structure to that of surrounding white matter. In general, these lesions reflect secondary tract degeneration.

Balo's concentric sclerosis

The Balo plaque is a peculiar lesion characterized by concentric alternating layers of myelinated and demyelinated areas (Figure 12.1C) found in some cases of acute or rapidly progressive multiple sclerosis. Sometimes the rings can be detected by MRI (Revel *et al* 1993). This appearance was first illustrated and classified by Balo (1928) as a subform of multiple sclerosis. However, small concentric lesions can also be found in otherwise classical cases of acute or subacute multiple sclerosis (Courville 1970; Hallervorden and Spatz 1933; Marburg 1906). According to recent MRI and neuropathological studies, they may even represent a transient stage in the demyelinating process (Revel *et al* 1993; D.-L. Yao *et al* 1994). Neither the genetic background nor any one environmental factor has yet been implicated in the pathogenesis of this peculiar lesion.

In completely demyelinated areas, the concentric plaques of Balo are characterized by profound oligodendrocyte loss in addition to demyelination, and they show a considerable reduction in axonal profiles. In contrast, axon density is higher in the myelinated areas and many oligodendrocytes are present, although their total number is reduced compared with normal white matter (D.-L. Yao *et al* 1994). There is ambiguity concerning the nature of concentric bands of myelin – the view being expressed that these are either areas of preserved myelin (D.-L. Yao *et al* 1994) or bands of remyelination (G.R. Moore *et al* 1985). Our position, in agreement with previous studies (Courville 1970), is that the basic mechanism operating within these lesions is hypoxia-like tissue injury, the concentric bands of myelin resulting from hypoxic preconditioning of the tissue (Stadelmann *et al* 2005).

The 'preactive' lesion

The existence of preactive lesions has been postulated on the basis of studies correlating MRI appearances and tissue pathology. These observations depend largely on evidence from a single patient who died in the active stage of multiple sclerosis (De Groot *et al* 2001). There were many areas of MRI abnormality that – on the basis of pathological features – can be subsumed under one of the categories described above. Some areas of MRI abnormalities, however, revealed only inflammation, some blood–brain barrier damage and oedema, and a reduction in myelin density. It was suggested that these lesions represent stages of plaque development that precede the overt dissolution of myelin sheaths. Applying their scheme of multifactorial cluster analysis, Gay *et al* (1997) had previously reached similar conclusions. They also postulated the existence of an ultra-early stage in development of the lesion in multiple sclerosis characterized by a moderate degree of inflammation, microglia and complement activation, some reduction of myelin density, and few myelinated fibres in the initial stages of dissolution. It seems likely that such an initial stage of lesion formation does exist. It is, however, highly unlikely that all brain lesions characterized by T_2-weighted MRI abnormalities in which histological analysis reveals myelin pallor and some diffuse inflammation and oedema are preactive plaques. Most importantly, although such abnormalities are relatively frequent in brain tissue from multiple sclerosis, more or less identical changes occur in other inflammatory brain diseases and in conditions not followed by the development of demyelinated plaques. In addition, areas of Wallerian tract degeneration and remyelinated shadow plaques may show pathological features very similar to those characterized as the hallmarks of preactive multiple sclerosis plaques. Thus, the identification of a preactive lesion in multiple sclerosis requires more than MRI signal abnormality and inflammation, oedema and myelin pallor expressed as a T_2-weighted MRI signal abnormality. Identification of the earliest stages of demyelination still requires evidence for active myelin destruction and/or oligodendrocyte damage with myelin debris in macrophages.

IMMUNOPATHOLOGY OF INFLAMMATION

Having weighed the evidence, we conclude that the conduit through which all players involved in the pathogenesis of lesions in multiple sclerosis must pass is the process of inflammation. This is pivotal and the motor that drives forward the disease process. Our own view is that despite the lack of evidence implicating one or more specific candidate autoantigens or microbial triggers, that process is sustained by autoimmunity (see Chapter 11). It follows that special attention must be given to the description of cells making up the inflammatory infiltrates, the molecules on which their passage into the brain parenchyma depends, and the factors that determine their effector mechanisms and regulation.

Inflammation can be driven by an immune-mediated process or may occur as a secondary consequence of tissue injury. Immune-mediated inflammation is mediated by cells of the adaptive immune system such as T and B lymphocytes, and is thus reflected by their presence within lesions. In addition, cytokines produced by the lymphocytes stimulate effector cells such as macrophages and microglia to express and produce molecules involved in propagation and regulation of the immune response or in the induction of tissue injury. Reactive inflammation, which occurs as a response to tissue injury, is mainly reflected by activation of cells involved in innate immunity, which in the central nervous system consist mainly of macrophages, microglia and possibly dendritic cells. Activation antigens expressed under these conditions are mainly those involved in phagocytosis and antigen presentation. Recruitment of lymphocytes in such lesions is sparse or absent. It has, however, to be noted that this simple distinction between immune-driven and reactive inflammation is far from absolute and a broad overlap exists between these two conditions.

Inflammation and disease activity

Chronic persistent inflammation in the central nervous system is one of the most characteristic pathological features of multiple sclerosis. Inflammation is not restricted to the areas of demyelination but also affects large parts of the so-called normal white and grey matter and, to a lesser extent, the meninges. The density of inflammatory infiltrates in general is higher within demyelinated plaques compared with the surrounding white matter. Whether inflammation is a primary event in the evolution of demyelination and plaque formation or, conversely, merely a reaction to tissue injury resulting from alternative non-inflammatory mechanisms has been disputed for many years. Our position is that the various arguments favour the primary role of the inflammatory process, although the question has not been formally settled to the satisfaction of every commentator.

Inflammation, signified by T and B lymphocyte infiltrates, is regularly present during ongoing disease activity. Very exceptionally has active demyelination been described in the absence of inflammation (Guseo and Jellinger 1975). In such instances, lack of inflammation was defined by the absence of perivascular infiltrates. However, these sparse accounts based on morphology did not make use of immunocytochemical markers for the identification of inflammatory cells, and recent data show that diffuse parenchymal infiltration by T cells can occur in the absence of overt perivascular infiltrates (see below). In addition, those cases showing very little or no perivascular inflammatory infiltrates had all been treated with immunosuppressants. Using serial MRI, new clinical exacerbations are usually associated with focal blood–brain barrier damage (R.I. Grossman *et al* 1988; D.H. Miller *et al* 1988b). Confirmation that this is associated with brain inflammation is provided by biopsy or autopsy studies (Estes *et al* 1990; Katz *et al* 1993; Nesbit *et al* 1991).

As discussed below, the inflammatory reaction in active multiple sclerosis lesions is associated with local upregulation of immunoregulatory molecules such as histocompatibility antigens, adhesion molecules, cytokines or chemokines. By analogy with the immunopathology of experimental models of demyelination (see Chapter 11), these findings strongly endorse our interpretation that an immunologically driven inflammatory response – at least in the majority of patients with multiple sclerosis – is the primary pathogenetic event. This view is further supported by serial brain biopsies performed in a single patient with the Marburg type of acute multiple sclerosis. Whilst the first biopsy showed a purely inflammatory disease of the white matter, a second biopsy of the same lesion performed 76 days later revealed large confluent demyelinated lesions (Bitsch *et al* 1999).

The primary nature of inflammation in the plaques of multiple sclerosis has recently been challenged in a study describing the pathological features of a brainstem lesion in a 13-year-old patient with chronic relapsing multiple sclerosis dying a few hours after onset of brainstem symptoms. In this lesion a decrease in myelin staining intensity and massive oligodendrocyte apoptosis were described, occurring in the absence of inflammation (Barnett and Prineas 2004). From these observations it was concluded that oligodendrocyte injury is the primary event in plaque formation, followed by a secondary inflammatory reaction. Although this study is based on a very careful neuropathological description, there may be alternative explanations for this finding. A role of inflammation in these lesions cannot altogether be excluded, since some perivascular inflammatory infiltrates were present and a detailed analysis of lymphocyte subsets within the lesions was not performed. In addition, the patient was treated with high-dose corticosteroids, which may downregulate the inflammatory response. Alternatively, as will be discussed below, very similar lesions with oligodendrocyte apoptosis can be found regularly in a subset of multiple sclerosis patients in the presence of inflammation (pattern III: Lucchinetti *et al* 2000). However, an identical pattern of myelin and oligodendrocyte pathology is also found in acute white matter ischaemia or hypoxia in the absence of an inflammatory response (Aboul Enein *et al* 2003). Fulminating brain diseases are frequently complicated by brainstem hypoxia, occurring either as a result of herniation damage or due to systemic preterminal complications. To us, these seem not to have been excluded in the study of Barnett and Prineas (2004).

Cellular composition of inflammatory infiltrates

As noted in the earliest studies of multiple sclerosis pathology, inflammatory infiltrates are mainly composed of mononuclear cells (Figure 12.3). In active multiple sclerosis lesions, inflammatory cells are present in the perivascular space and also dispersed throughout the central nervous system parenchyma. This holds true for lymphocytes as well as macrophages (Prineas and Wright 1978). However, B lymphocytes and plasma cells are more concentrated in the perivascular space and meninges, while parenchymal infiltration is relatively rare.

T lymphocytes

The vast majority of infiltrating lymphocytes are T cells (Nyland *et al* 1982; Traugott *et al* 1983a; 1983b). Immunocytochemical attempts to differentiate lymphocyte subsets in multiple sclerosis lesions have proved controversial. All investigators agree that both CD4$^+$ (helper) and CD8$^+$ (suppressor/cytotoxic) T lymphocytes are present in the lesions but some claim that the dominant cell population present in the active plaque is the CD8 cell (Booss *et al* 1983; Gay *et al* 1997; Hayashi *et al* 1988) and others that it is the CD4 T lymphocyte (Traugott *et al* 1983a; 1983b). The most recent studies on this topic (Babbe *et al* 2000; Gay *et al* 1997) show that T-cell infiltrates within the perivascular inflammatory infiltrates are composed of equal numbers of CD4$^+$ and CD8$^+$ cells. In contrast, the tissue infiltrates are invariably dominated by CD8$^+$ T cells, irrespective of clinical disease type (acute or chronic multiple sclerosis), or activity of the lesions. Analysing the T-cell receptor of single cells within lesions by single cell polymerase chain reaction showed that, on average, 65% of CD8$^+$ but only 25% of CD4$^+$ cells were clonally expanded (Babbe *et al* 2000), indicating that these cells may have recognized specific antigen within the lesions. In acute multiple sclerosis a high proportion of CD8$^+$ T cells also express granzyme B, indicating their activation as cytotoxic effector cells (Figure 12.3). The T-cell infiltrates in lesions are associated with expression of class I MHC molecules on infiltrating leucocytes, but also on astrocytes, oligodendrocytes and axons (Höftberger *et al* 2004). Furthermore, using confocal laser microscopy, the attachment of granzyme B-positive T cells on oligodendrocytes and axons in actively demyelinating lesions is frequently encountered. Taken together, these data suggest that activated cytotoxic class I MHC-restricted T cells play a major role in the propagation of inflammation and the induction of tissue injury in multiple sclerosis (Neumann *et al* 2002).

Cytotoxic class I MHC-restricted T cells are, however, not the only immune cells present in lesions. Clonal expansion of CD4 lymphocytes (Babbe *et al* 2000) suggests that these cells are also driven by the recognition of specific antigen. Furthermore, B lymphocytes and plasma cells accumulate and undergo clonal expansion in the perivascular and meningeal tissues in the chronic lesions of multiple sclerosis (G.P. Owens *et al* 2001). This suggests that inflammation in multiple sclerosis is driven both by class I and class II restricted T cells. In addition, there appears to be a significantly lower incidence of CD45R (putative suppressor/inducer) cells in active compared with inactive multiple sclerosis lesions or other inflammatory diseases of the nervous system (Hayashi *et al* 1988; Sobel *et al* 1988), indicating dysregulation of the immune response within the plaques.

Experimental and clinical immunological studies reveal that particular T-cell receptor subtypes may be of fundamental importance in T-cell mediated autoimmunity (for review see Lassmann and Vass 1995; Wekerle *et al* 1994). T cells carry a dimeric receptor composed either of αβ or alternatively γδ chains (see Chapters 3 and 11). αβ T cells generally dominate in the mature immune system and characterize the vast majority of T lymphocytes in blood, lymph nodes and spleen. These cells are mainly responsible for specific immune functions involved in the elimination of pathogens. The γδ T lymphocyte is mostly found in the lymphatic system of the gut and other mucosal tissues. The majority are responsive to highly conserved epitopes of cellular proteins, such as heat-shock proteins, that are homologous throughout a wide spectrum ranging from bacteria to mammalian cells. By these relatively nonspecific mechanisms, γδ T cells in humans are involved in early defence against bacteria and other cellular pathogens (Kaufmann 1990).

In addition to these principal differences in T-cell receptor chain usage of different T-cell populations, recent studies suggest that, even within a given αβ or γδ T-cell population, specific subtypes of T lymphocytes may be selected in the induction of autoimmunity. Thus, most autoreactive T lymphocyte lines directed against myelin basic protein that are able to transfer autoimmune inflammation after intravenous transfer in mice and rats, express the T-cell receptor chain Vβ8.2 (Wekerle *et al* 1994). These data suggest that T-cell autoimmunity may be restricted to a small population of very specific T-cell receptor subtypes – an observation that, although as yet unproven, has nevertheless stimulated novel therapeutic approaches.

For reasons discussed above, several studies have focused on the characterization of T-cell receptors in multiple sclerosis lesions. The vast majority found in multiple sclerosis plaques carry (as expected) the αβ T-cell receptor. Some results suggest clonal expansion of certain γδ T-cell subsets in multiple sclerosis plaques (Oksenberg *et al* 1993), but this has not been confirmed by others (Birnbaum and van Ness 1992; Wucherpfennig *et al* 1992a). In addition to αβ T cells, a variable number of γδ T lymphocytes can also be found in the lesions of multiple sclerosis (Selmaj *et al* 1991a; Wucherpfennig *et al* 1992b). Because γδ T cells are capable of specifically lysing oligodendrocytes *in vitro* (M.S. Freedman *et al* 1991), their presence may be of significance in the pathogenesis of lesions in multiple sclerosis.

B lymphocytes

Besides T lymphocytes, a variable but low number of B cells are found within plaques (Prineas and Wright 1978; Figure 12.3). The number of antibody-producing cells is, in general, very low in the lesions of acute multiple sclerosis or those that arise during early bouts in the chronic phase of the disease. However, their absolute and relative numbers are much higher in the typical case of chronic multiple sclerosis (Ozawa *et al* 1994). As with all other inflammatory cells, B lymphocytes are more evident in active than inactive lesions (Esiri 1977). Relatively little is known about the antigen specificity of B lymphocytes and plasma cells in multiple sclerosis lesions. Clonal expansion of B-cell populations in the lesions is suggested by the antibody spectrum characterized in cerebrospinal fluid or the tissue itself, and some data suggest that this process may be driven by specific antigen(s) (Gilden *et al* 2001). A multiple sclerosis-specific pattern of antibody reactivity has so far not been identified, even using random screening with peptide libraries (Archelos *et al* 1998; 2000; Cortese *et al* 1998; 2001; Gilden *et al* 2001; Jolivet Reynaud *et al* 1999). However, in a single unconfirmed study, many of these B lymphocytes and plasma cells were found to produce antibodies against myelin basic protein (Gerritse *et al* 1994).

Macrophages and microglia

The vast majority of haematogenous cells within multiple sclerosis plaques are monocytes and macrophages (Adams and Poston 1990; Adams *et al* 1989; Babinski 1885b; Newcombe and Cuzner 1994; Traugott *et al* 1983a; 1983b). These cells are dispersed throughout the whole lesion and are especially prominent in actively demyelinating plaques (Figure 12.2). In fact, the

presence of early myelin degradation products in macrophages is at present the most reliable marker for ongoing demyelinating activity (Brück *et al* 1994). In addition, there is extensive uptake of low-density lipoproteins in macrophages and microglia within active lesions, which is probably important for the metabolism of lipids liberated in the course of active myelin destruction (Newcombe and Cuzner 1994). Besides these myelin degradation products, the expression of activation antigens in macrophages and microglia is a good marker for actively demyelinating plaques (Brück *et al* 1995; Ozawa *et al* 1994; Ulvestad *et al* 1994). Although the majority of macrophages within multiple sclerosis plaques are thought to come from blood-borne monocytes, resident microglia may be even more important in lesion development. Ramified activated microglia that express histocompatibility antigens, adhesion molecules or markers of activated peripheral macrophages are present mainly in the white or grey matter that surrounds actively demyelinating as well as inactive lesions. Detailed quantitative analysis of the inflammatory response in lesions at different stages of development reveals that microglial activation and demyelination precede recruitment of the vast majority of haematogenous cells into the lesions (Gay *et al* 1997). Furthermore, the profiles of CCR1 and CCR5 chemokine receptor expression in the lesions of multiple sclerosis suggest that, in the earliest stages, ramified microglia mediate demyelination, digest debris and are then transformed into macrophage-like cells. Conversely, haematogenous macrophages make a small contribution to lesion formation (Trebst *et al* 2001). Irrespective of their primary origin, macrophages and microglia in multiple sclerosis lesions express a variety of molecules required for propagation and regulation of the inflammatory response, and for the induction of tissue injury. These include costimulatory molecules (Gerritse *et al* 1996; Windhagen *et al* 1995), MHC antigens (Esiri and Reading 1987), Toll-like receptors (Bsibsi *et al* 2002), macrophage colony-stimulating factor (K. Werner *et al* 2003), adhesion molecules (Peterson *et al* 2002), annexin 1 (Probst-Cousin *et al* 2002), Fc receptors (Ulvestad *et al* 1994), inducible nitric oxide synthase (J.S. Liu *et al* 2001), proteases (Anthony *et al* 1997; Cossins *et al* 1997; Hallpike *et al* 1970a; Maeda and Sobel 1996), different ion channels (Craner *et al* 2005) as well as many different cytokines (Woodroofe and Cuzner 1993) and cytokine receptors (Bonetti and Raine 1997; Hulshof *et al* 2002; Ramanathan *et al* 2001). Furthermore, MRI studies indicate the presence of free radicals in macrophages at the edge of expanding demyelinating lesions (Powell *et al* 1992). Besides these cell types characteristic of multiple sclerosis, some lesions may be infiltrated by mast cells (Olsson 1974; Toms *et al* 1990), granulocytes (Lucchinetti *et al* 2002) or cells expressing dendritic cell markers (Plumb *et al* 2003). Granulocytes and, in particular, eosinophils are mainly present in lesions with profound antibody and complement deposition and this is particularly evident in the lesions of Devic's disease (Lucchinetti *et al* 2002).

Inflammation-induced reaction of local tissue components in demyelinating plaques

A distinction can be made between those molecular signals and mediators of tissue injury and repair that are expressed constitutively in the central nervous system and others that result from inflammation and other inaugural components of the disease process. In turn, their identification and characterization may illuminate important aspects of the pathogenesis.

Major histocompatibility complex antigens

A very characteristic feature of inflammatory lesions in the brain and other organs is the expression on local tissue components of histocompatibility antigens and adhesion molecules. T lymphocytes do not recognize soluble molecules or peptides but react to antigen, presented in the context of major histocompatibility complex (MHC) molecules on the surface of antigen-presenting cells. Thus, the distribution of MHC antigens within tissue pinpoints the possible sites where T lymphocytes are able to recognize specific antigen in propagation of the inflammatory reaction. There is now good agreement that the vast majority of cells in the central nervous system that express class II MHC antigens are resident microglia and haematogenous macrophages (Boyle and McGeer 1990; Cuzner *et al* 1988; Esiri and Reading 1987; Traugott *et al* 1983a). In addition, some immunoreactivity has been described on astrocytes and endothelial cells (S.C. Lee *et al* 1990; Ransohoff and Estes 1991; Sobel and Ames 1988; Traugott and Lebon 1988a), although this has not been reproduced by others (Bo *et al* 1994). The situation is different for class I MHC molecules. *In vitro*, their expression can be induced on virtually all cell types upon appropriate immunological stimulation (Neumann *et al* 2002). *In vivo*, class I antigens can be detected in the normal central nervous system on endothelial cells and a subpopulation of microglia. Their expression is variable in different inflammatory conditions. For example, abundant expression on neurons is seen in paraneoplastic encephalitis or Rasmussen's encephalitis (Bien *et al* 2002). We have found MHC class I mainly in active lesions of acute and, to a lesser extent, chronic multiple sclerosis diffusely expressed (as in normal brain) not only on infiltrating inflammatory cells but also endothelial cells, microglia, oligodendrocytes, astrocytes and axons (Höfteberger *et al* 2004). Thus, it seems that all cellular elements of the central nervous system have the potential to present antigen to class I MHC restricted T cells thereby exposing themselves to potential antigen-specific T-cell mediated cytotoxicity.

Antigen-specific activation of T lymphocytes requires the additional interaction of costimulatory molecules. In their absence, the interaction of T lymphocytes with antigen-presenting cells may lead to anergy and restriction of the inflammatory response rather than proliferation. In the lesions of multiple sclerosis, macrophages express CD40 and B7-2, while CD40 ligand and B7-1 are mainly present on lymphocytes (Gerritse *et al* 1996; Windhagen *et al* 1995). If the expression of these costimulatory molecules is instrumental in perpetuation of the inflammatory response, they may offer themselves as potential targets for immunosuppressive treatment.

Adhesion molecules

Because T lymphocytes can pass the intact blood–brain barrier in a non-antigen-specific manner (Hickey *et al* 1991; Wekerle *et al* 1986), the role of adhesion molecules that guide the traffic of leucocytes through body compartments and steer inflammatory cells to lesions has been much studied (Shimizu *et al* 1992). In normal brain vasculature, adhesion molecules are expressed only on endothelial cells at very low levels (Lassmann *et al* 1991b; Male *et al* 1990). Thus, selected leucocyte subsets, in particular activated T lymphocytes, appear to bind these adhesion molecules and attach to the endothelial surface before migrating across the blood–brain barrier. When an inflammatory focus is initiated, adhesion molecules on cerebral endothelial cells and local cellular constituents are upregulated and may then function as adhesion partners for a large variety of secondary effector cells (Cannella and Raine 1995).

Migration of inflammatory cells through the endothelial barrier involves a variety of different consecutive steps (Shimizu *et al* 1992). Initially, an interaction of selectins with carbohydrate moieties induces a loose interaction of leucocytes with endothelia, involving a slow rolling motion of inflammatory cells along the luminal surface of endothelial cells. Next, the interaction between adhesion molecules of the immunoglobulin supergene family with integrins results in firm binding of the inflammatory cells at the luminal surface of endothelial cells. This adhesion, together with the expression of proteolytic enzymes on the surface of inflammatory cells, allows the latter to pass either between or through channels of the endothelial cells and reach the perivascular space (Engelhardt and Wolburg 2004). However, in brain vessels, which are sealed by the blood–brain barrier, the transendothelial route appears to be preferred, while paracellular migration, associated with opening of tight junctions, is an unusual portal of entry (Engelhardt and Wolburg 2004; Raine *et al* 1990; Wisniewski and Lossinsky 1991).

Only some active adhesion partners have been identified in the lesions of multiple sclerosis (Cannella and Raine 1995). For example, E-selectin (Washington *et al* 1994), intercellular adhesion molecule 1 (ICAM-1; Sobel *et al* 1990; Tsukada *et al* 1994), vascular cell adhesion molecule 1 (VCAM-1; Dore-Duffy *et al* 1993) and unclassified vascular addressins (Raine *et al* 1990) are expressed on endothelial cells in active plaques. That said, Peterson *et al* (2002) found VCAM on activated microglia cells in close contact with oligodendrocytes rather than endothelial cells. Despite this controversy, blockade of the interaction between VCAM and its specific ligand through an antibody against α4 integrin effectively ameliorates the inflammatory reaction in the active stage of multiple sclerosis (Tubridy *et al* 1999). Other molecules that have been suggested to be involved in recruitment and activation of inflammatory cells are CD97 and its binding partner CD55. They are expressed on endothelial cells and leucocytes in the lesions of multiple sclerosis, but their functional role is so far undetermined (Visser *et al* 2002). In addition, other molecules involved in cell–cell interactions, such as fibronectin (Sobel and Mitchell 1989), urokinase, plasmin activator receptor and activated complement components, have been identified on vessels in active multiple sclerosis plaques (see below: D.A.S. Compston *et al* 1989; Washington *et al* 1994), resulting in major changes in the composition of the extracellular matrix in the lesions of multiple sclerosis in comparison with normal brain (Sobel 2001).

Chemokines

In addition to adhesion molecules, a set of newly discovered chemokines appears to be of major importance in the recruitment of inflammatory cells to brain lesions (Luster *et al* 1998).

Chemokines are small peptides liberated by inflammatory cells as well as by local parenchymal cells in response to inflammatory stimuli. Delivered into the extracellular space, they are able either directly, or by modifying the expression and affinity of adhesion molecules, to attract effector cells (in particular, monocytes, macrophages or granulocytes). These then follow the concentration gradient of secreted chemokines (Luster et al 1998). Indeed, abundant mRNA for chemokines has been detected in the lesions of multiple sclerosis (Schlüsener and Meyermann 1993). The more detailed analysis of chemokines and their receptors provides some interesting clues to the pathogenesis of inflammation in multiple sclerosis. The dominant T-cell population recruited into lesions is CD3/CCR5/CXCR3 positive and this profile apparently reflects a population of activated memory T cells (Goldberg et al 2001; J. Simpson et al 2000a; Sorensen et al 1999; 2002), whereas macrophages, recruited into the lesions from the circulation, are mainly CCR1/CCR5 positive (Sorensen et al 1999; Trebst et al 2000). A variety of different chemokines, which may interact with these receptors, has been described in the plaques of multiple sclerosis, the most important being MCP-1, MIP-1a, RANTES and IP-10 (Balashov et al 1999; McManus et al 1998; J.E. Simpson et al 1998; 2000b; for review see D.Huang et al 2000). Besides macrophages and microglia cells, astrocytes are an important source of chemokines in the central nervous system (McManus et al 1998).

Taken together, these data suggest that chemokines are key molecules in the process of recruiting inflammatory cells into the lesions of multiple sclerosis. Their blockade by small molecules could become a very attractive target for anti-inflammatory therapies. In addition, differences in the spectrum of chemokines expressed in lesions may reflect variation in the immunological mechanisms of inflammation and account for the detailed composition of inflammatory infiltrates between groups of patients. As an example, the high prevalence of granulocytes and eosinophils in active lesions of Devic's type of neuromyelitis optica is associated with a chemokine receptor expression, which is typical for Th2 mediated inflammatory responses (Lucchinetti et al 2002).

Local expression of stress proteins

Stress proteins comprise a variety of polypeptides that are synthesized by cells in response to injury. They have diverse functions, including the regulation of gene expression, intracellular traffic and delivery of proteins, and the degradation of denatured or damaged protein molecules. Inflammation is one mechanism that can be responsible for local upregulation of stress proteins (D'Souza et al 1994).

Since they are essential for cell survival during metabolic stress, it is not surprising that stress proteins are highly conserved in evolution and present in nearly identical forms from bacteria to mammals. The immune system has utilized this high degree of conservation for a nonspecific but effective defence mechanism (Cohen and Young 1991; Kaufmann 1990). γδ T lymphocytes use recognition of these highly conserved stress proteins to destroy microorganisms that have invaded the organism. However, immune responses directed against stress proteins may become dysregulated and augment inflammation through autoimmune mechanisms. It has been proposed that

this sequence operates in the lesions of multiple sclerosis (Freedman et al 1991; Selmaj et al 1991d). γδ T lymphocytes, enriched in some active multiple sclerosis lesions, apparently by local clonal expansion (Wucherpfennig et al 1992b), lyse oligodendrocytes through heat-shock proteins 65 and 70 (Freedman et al 1991; Selmaj et al 1992). Another stress protein implicated in the pathogenesis of multiple sclerosis is αβ-crystallin, which appears to be the dominantly recognized autoantigen in a subgroup of patients with multiple sclerosis (Van Noort et al 1995). Although astrocytes express this protein within active and inactive lesions, its expression in oligodendrocytes is restricted to areas of ongoing demyelination (Bajramovic et al 1997).

In general, the patterns and intensity of expression appear to depend upon the type of stress protein as well as severity and stage of the inflammatory reaction. Whilst stress proteins are ubiquitously found in different cellular elements, they are not expressed to a major degree in normal tissues of the central nervous system. However, pronounced upregulation is typical of the inflammatory lesions in multiple sclerosis. Here, the pattern is of selective heat-shock protein 65 and αβ-crystallin upregulation in oligodendrocytes (Selmaj et al 1992; Van Noort et al 1995). Conversely, other molecules such as heat-shock proteins 27, 70 and 90 (Hans Lassmann, unpublished observation) or c-fos (J.S. Yu et al 1991) are mainly present in astrocytes and inflammatory cells. Their pattern of expression and possible release into the extracellular space are consistent with the hypothesis that stress proteins are recognized by specific T-cell mediated autoimmune reactions (Van Noort et al 1995). Although final proof for the involvement of such a mechanism in multiple sclerosis is still lacking, autoimmunity against these antigens could augment inflammation in established lesions and, by this mechanism, amplify the inflammatory process and its consequences. However, the upregulation of heat-shock proteins 65 and 70 in oligodendrocytes at the edge of active lesions may protect these cells against further damage in an expanding active lesion. This seems to be a major controlling mechanism in the formation of concentric demyelinating lesions in Balo's concentric sclerosis.

Cytokines in multiple sclerosis lesions

Immune-mediated inflammation, such as that present in multiple sclerosis, is influenced by a large battery of different cytokines (T. Olsson 1994). These are produced either by inflammatory cells or local tissue components. They mediate communication between inflammatory cells and local tissue constituents. Some are proinflammatory, activating certain components of the immune system and thereby propagating immune reactions and inflammation. For example, elevated levels of TNF-α in the cerebrospinal fluid of patients with multiple sclerosis correlate with disease activity and blood–brain barrier damage (Sharief and Thompson 1992). On the other hand, interleukin 4 (IL-4) and IL-10 may suppress delayed-type hypersensitivity reactions and downregulate T-cell mediated inflammation or macrophage activation (M.K. Kennedy et al 1992; Weinberg et al 1993). A similar action may also be induced by the more general immunosuppressive effect of transforming growth factor β (TGF-β; Johns et al 1991; Racke et al 1992). Furthermore, in addition to the induction of nonspecific tissue damage, molecules such as lymphotoxin (TNF-β: Selmaj et al 1991b), TNF-α (Selmaj and Raine 1988) and perforin

(Scolding *et al* 1990) may be directly involved in the destruction of oligodendrocytes and myelin. Conversely, cytokines – for example, insulin-like growth factor I (IGF-I) – may be essential for oligodendroglia survival and remyelination (Komoly *et al* 1992; see Chapter 9). Cytokine-like immunoreactivity has been detected in various cell types of the central nervous system. In particular, immunocytochemical analysis of inflammatory cells, astrocytes and microglia has demonstrated IL-1, IL-2, lymphotoxin, TNF-α, interferons (IFNs), IL-6 (Cannella and Raine 1995; Hofman *et al* 1989; Merrill 1992; Selmaj *et al* 1991a; Traugott and Lebon 1988b; 1988c) and IL-10, IL-12 and IL-18 (Canella and Raine 2004). In our view, immunocytochemical studies on these topics are difficult to interpret. Apart from technical problems relating to antibody specificity and avidity with possible central nervous system peptide cross-reactivity, no conclusions can be drawn about whether the cytokines are synthesized locally or taken up secondarily at the site of immunoreactivity. Polymerase chain reaction amplification reveals the presence of IL-1 in all active multiple sclerosis lesions, whereas mRNAs for IL-2, IL-4 or IL-10 are found in a minority of lesions (Schlüsener and Meyermann 1993; Wucherpfennig *et al* 1992a). Gene microarray analysis of multiple sclerosis lesions shows increased transcripts of genes encoding for IL-6, IL-13, IL-17, TNF-α and IFN-γ (Lock *et al* 2002; Mycko *et al* 2003; Tajouri *et al* 2003; Whitney *et al* 1999). Although there appears generally to be rather low expression of cytokine mRNAs, this may not be the case for chemokines such as IL-8 and MCP-1 (Schlüsener and Meyermann 1993). *In situ* hybridization studies reveal mRNAs for a variety of cytokines, including IL-1, IL-2, IL-4, IL-6 and IL-10, IFN-γ, TNF-α and TGF-β1 and -β2 (Bitsch *et al* 2000b; Werner *et al* 2002; Woodroofe and Cuzner 1993).

In summary, these studies describe the presence of many different cytokines and the expression of various cytokine receptors in the lesions of multiple sclerosis, apparently reflecting the chronic immunologically driven inflammatory process. Similar findings have been observed in other inflammatory neurological diseases (Canella and Raine 2004) and, so far, no pattern of cytokine expression specific for multiple sclerosis has been proposed. Cytokines seem to be more prominent in actively demyelinating compared with inactive lesions or 'normal' white matter, but a clear-cut differential pattern of expression, which allows different lesion stages to be distinguished, is not yet apparent.

Antibodies and complement components

As already mentioned, active lesions in multiple sclerosis are associated with pronounced damage to the blood–brain barrier, potentially allowing serum components such as antibodies or complement to enter the nervous system. In addition, B lymphocytes accumulate and may persist at the sites of active inflammation (Guseo and Jellinger 1975; Prineas and Wright 1978). These cells produce antibodies locally as reflected by the increased immunoglobulin index and oligoclonal bands in cerebrospinal fluid. IgG is mainly produced in the lesions of multiple sclerosis. Although some IgA- and IgM-producing plasma cells are also detected in lesions, they make a small contribution (Auff and Budka 1980; Bernheimer *et al* 1983; Esiri 1977; Mussini *et al* 1977). The number of B lymphocytes and plasma cells is variable and depends on stage of the disease and the

activity of lesions (Prineas and Wright 1978). During lesional activity, the high number of infiltrating leucocytes includes an increased number of B lymphocytes compared with inactive lesions (Esiri 1977). However, there is also a major difference in the extent of B cell and plasma cell infiltration in lesions formed during initial bouts compared with those arising after several years of disease duration. In the former, infiltrates are mainly composed of T lymphocytes and macrophages, and only a minority (around 0.5–1%) of inflammatory cells actually produce immunoglobulins. Conversely, during late phases of the disease, the ratio of B to T lymphocytes is about 1:7 (Ozawa *et al* 1994). These stage-dependent changes in the composition of inflammatory infiltrates are also reflected in cerebrospinal fluid. Whereas in chronic multiple sclerosis, an elevated IgG index and oligoclonal pattern of immunoglobulins is typical, similar changes may be absent during the first or second bout of the disease. In active lesions, T cells and macrophages infiltrate the brain parenchyma, whereas B lymphocytes and plasma cells tend to remain in the perivascular space and meninges (Esiri *et al* 1989).

Immunoglobulin deposition, concentrated at sites of active myelin destruction and located either on activated macrophages or dressing the surface of myelin sheaths that are in the process of being destroyed, characterizes actively demyelinating plaques (Prineas 1985). Complement components are deposited in actively demyelinating lesions, mainly at the vessel walls (D.A.S. Compston *et al* 1989). In a subset of patients with multiple sclerosis, deposition of complement components, including the C9 neoantigen (a reliable marker for the lytic membrane attack complex), is present at the active edge of demyelinating plaques. In addition to lysosomal myelin degradation products in macrophages, C9 neoantigen is detected on disintegrating myelin sheaths (Lucchinetti *et al* 2000; Storch *et al* 1998a). Using biotinylated myelin oligodendrocyte glycoprotein as a probe, deposition of anti-myelin oligodendrocyte glycoprotein antibodies on disintegrating myelin has been described in lesions of acute multiple sclerosis (Genain *et al* 1999). Although complement appears mostly to enter through the damaged blood–brain barrier, additional local synthesis by macrophages and microglia is suggested. Complement inhibitory proteins are also present in multiple sclerosis lesions. For example, SP40 immunoreactivity is found in reactive astrocytes (E. Wu *et al* 1993). There is, however, no spatial relationship between the deposition of complement and the inhibitory proteins to suggest a functional role for the latter (Storch *et al* 1998a).

Blood–brain barrier alterations

Widespread blood–brain barrier damage has been demonstrated in multiple sclerosis lesions using post-mortem tracer studies (Broman 1964). Immunocytochemical studies on the distribution of serum proteins within lesions (Kwon and Prineas 1994; Tavolato 1975) indicate that the blood–brain barrier in plaques is impaired compared with the normal white and grey matter of patients with multiple sclerosis and controls. These pathological findings were not immediately consistent with some of the early MRI studies showing gadolinium-DTPA leakage restricted to active multiple sclerosis lesions (Kermode *et al* 1990; McLean *et al* 1993). As pointed out above, however, low levels of gadolinium-DTPA leakage can be detected in chronic lesions (Barnes *et al* 1991). And in experimental autoimmune encephalomyelitis, gadolinium-DTPA is transported in such vessels in an energy-dependent manner (C.P. Hawkins *et al* 1990a; 1990b).

Infiltration of the vessel walls by inflammatory cells shows that the most intense leakage of the blood–brain barrier is in lesions with active inflammation (Gay and Esiri 1991), although intense perivascular deposition of serum proteins sometimes can also be noted around vessels that are devoid of inflammation. Whether such alterations are restricted to the vicinity of inflamed vessels is unresolved. Inflammatory infiltration of the vessel walls with perivascular accumulation of leucocytes and deposition of serum proteins is not necessarily associated with demyelination. The proposal that lesions with sparse inflammatory infiltration of the surrounding tissue and no myelin-containing macrophages represent early stages in the process of lesion formation is not fully convincing because, in experimental models of inflammatory demyelination, these features are rarely present beyond the first few hours of tissue injury. It is therefore likely that active inflammation in multiple sclerosis does not invariably result in myelin destruction. Indeed, studies of experimental autoimmune encephalomyelitis and other experimental models of inflammatory demyelination suggest that, in addition to the primary T-cell response that induces inflammation, additional immunological mechanisms are required for the establishment of demyelination (Lassmann *et al* 1988; Linington *et al* 1988).

Ultrastructural studies show increased endothelial pinocytotic vesicles, possibly reflecting enhanced permeability of the blood–brain barrier. The ultrastructure of endothelial tight junction systems has been considered normal (W.J. Brown 1978), but more detailed immunocytochemical analysis of occludin and ZO-1 proteins revealed focal discontinuities of tight junction ridges (Plumb *et al* 2002). Besides endothelial alterations, pathological changes of astrocytic foot processes are encountered (Rafalowska *et al* 1992), which may represent a footprint for the passage of inflammatory cells through the blood–brain barrier.

Vascular pathology

It is clear from the earliest histological descriptions of multiple sclerosis pathology that blood vessels play a central role in this disease. Thus, it is not surprising that interest in the pathogenesis of multiple sclerosis has often focused on possible essential vascular mechanisms (Courville 1968; Putnam 1935). These ideas eventually emerged as the concept of vasculomyelinopathy, in which a primary vascular lesion leads to myelin destruction (C.M. Poser 1987b). Vessels in active lesions may show features of vasculitis. Here, inflammation of the vessel wall is reflected by diffuse mononuclear cell infiltration, perivascular accumulation of leucocytes, leakage of serum proteins, upregulation of adhesion molecules on endothelial cells and some deposition of complement components on the luminal surface of the vessel wall. However, this accumulation of immune cells and mediators does not lead to vascular necrosis, intraluminal deposition of immune complexes and complement, or granuloma formation. Thus, it is different from the changes found in most other types of cerebral vasculitis (M.M. Brown and Swash 1989) and closely reflects the type of inflammation found in experimental models of delayed-type hypersensitivity reactions.

In rare instances, more pronounced acute vascular changes can be encountered. These consist of intraluminal platelet aggregation and thrombosis resulting in complete thrombotic occlusion of small inflamed veins and venules (Putnam 1935; Wakefield *et al* 1994). These alterations, however, are restricted to cases with extraordinarily severe inflammatory reactions. Such severe blood vessel changes may even result in blood extravasation, later marked by perivascular iron deposition within the affected tissue (Craelius *et al* 1982). That damage of cerebral endothelial cells occurs in a subset of patients with multiple sclerosis is further suggested by the presence of endothelial microparticles in plasma during active stages of the disease (Minagar *et al* 2001).

Vascular fibrosis is present in most cases of longstanding duration (Prineas and Wright 1978). Using ultrastructural criteria, many of the connective tissue channels that form in areas of vascular fibrosis show anatomical characteristics similar to those of lymphatics (Prineas 1979). Vascular fibrosis is not specific to the pathology of multiple sclerosis, but represents an alteration found in all types of chronic brain inflammation (Spielmeyer 1922). The degree of vascular fibrosis is most pronounced in the periventricular white matter and in lesions close to the pial surface of the spinal cord. Because inflammatory infiltrates are partly cleared through the cerebrospinal fluid (Cserr *et al* 1992; Weller *et al* 1992), vascular fibrosis may indeed facilitate the removal of inflammatory cells from chronically inflamed brain lesions.

Finally, inactive multiple sclerosis lesions contain a much higher density of vascular profiles compared with normal white matter. This is not only due to shrinkage and atrophy of the tissue, which by itself will result in a relative increase of vessel density, but reflects profound angiogenesis during the active phase of plaque formation (Ludwin *et al* 2001). In turn, this may result from local induction of vascular endothelial growth factor (VEGF) within active lesions (Proescholdt *et al* 2003).

Leucocyte destruction in multiple sclerosis lesions: a mechanism for clearance of inflammatory infiltrates

Experimentally, the majority of T lymphocytes invading the brain parenchyma do not leave the central nervous system during the clearance of inflammation but are destroyed *in situ* by programmed cell death (Pender *et al* 1991; Schmied *et al* 1993). Similarly, T cells with nuclear changes typical of apoptosis are found in active multiple sclerosis plaques, being most numerous in lesions from cases of acute or subacute multiple sclerosis (Figure 10.4: Ozawa *et al* 1994). However, the percentage of apoptotic T cells within multiple sclerosis lesions is much lower than that found in monophasic models of acute experimental autoimmune encephalomyelitis. This is not surprising because synchronous self-destruction of T cells cannot be expected in chronic inflammation, nor is it present in chronic models of experimental autoimmune encephalomyelitis. However, in acute disseminated leucoencephalomyelitis, very high numbers of apoptotic T lymphocytes are found within inflammatory infiltrates, comparable both in absolute and relative numbers to those found in acute experimental autoimmune encephalomyelitis (J. Bauer *et al* 1999).

We have only identified a single case – with primary progressive multiple sclerosis and receiving high-dose corticosteroid treatment despite the absence of relapses – where complete and

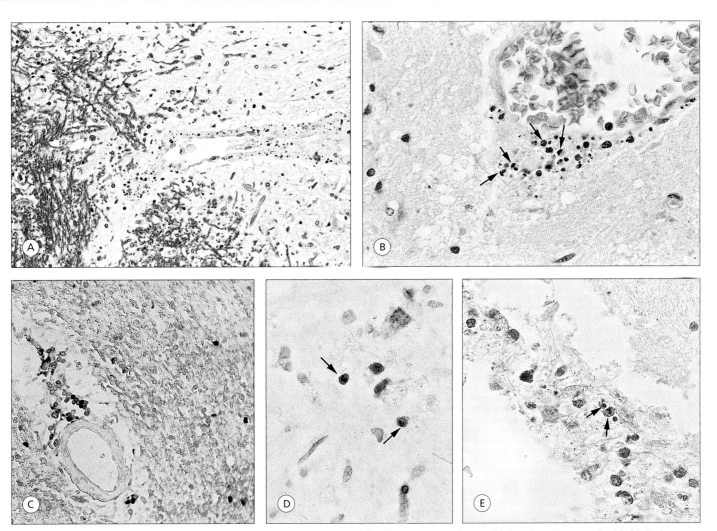

Figure 12.4 Apoptosis of T lymphocytes in multiple sclerosis lesions. (A) Primary progressive multiple sclerosis treated with high-dose steroids: immunocytochemistry for proteolipid protein. Most cells in the perivascular infiltrate at the lesional border and some in the central nervous system parenchyma (arrows) show apoptosis. ×100. (B) Typical appearances of apoptosis in perivascular inflammatory cells (arrows); ×300. (C) Chronic relapsing multiple sclerosis: *in situ* tailing for DNA fragmentation and immunocytochemistry with anti-CD3 (T lymphocytes). DNA fragmentation (black nuclei) in cells in the perivascular infiltrate and parenchyma. ×100. (D) Acute multiple sclerosis: immunocytochemistry with anti-CD3. Apoptotic cells identified by nuclear condensation (arrows) are labelled with a T-cell marker. ×300. (E) Primary progressive multiple sclerosis: immunocytochemistry with anti-CD3; perivascular infiltrate with numerous T cells (brown), some of which show nuclear condensation of apoptosis (arrows); ×300.

synchronous apoptosis of T lymphocytes was present both in the perivascular space and parenchyma (Figure 12.4). Because apoptosis of autoreactive T cells may be induced by steroids (Zettl *et al* 1995), our observation in this particular patient may reflect an effect of therapy.

Inflammatory cells in the lesions of multiple sclerosis express neurotrophins

Basic immunological studies tell us that inflammatory cells may also produce trophic cytokines, known to be essential in wound repair. Activated, and to a lesser extent resting, T and B cells and macrophages all produce neurotrophins, which stimulate neuronal survival *in vitro* (Kerschensteiner *et al* 1999; Moalem *et al* 2000). Neurotrophin expression is more pronounced in inflammatory cells within lesions than on adjacent neurons and glia.

Neurotrophins may downregulate MHC expression in inflammatory lesions and thereby be involved both in downregulation of brain inflammation and the provision of immune privilege for the central nervous system (Flügel *et al* 2001b). Neurotrophins produced by activated leucocytes seem also to exert neuroprotective functions – at least in the context of brain trauma or ischaemia.

Brain-derived neurotrophic factor (BDNF) is highly expressed in lymphocytes and macrophages in actively demyelinating lesions. Receptors for this ligand are found on different cell types in the vicinity of lesions (Stadelmann *et al* 2002; Valdo *et al* 2003). Neurotrophins may be needed for remyelination, because myelin formation and repair require the local presence of macrophages (Kotter *et al* 2001). In addition, increased expression of nerve growth factor as well as its receptor, trkA, have been found in optic nerve lesions (Micera *et al* 1999).

Brain inflammation in multiple sclerosis: a summary

The following sequence is suggested as a summary of findings on the immunopathology of multiple sclerosis. The driving force for the inflammatory reaction appears to be a T-cell mediated immune reaction. The composition of leucocyte subsets is in accordance with the pattern of a delayed-type hypersensitivity reaction. Different subpopulations of T helper cells have been identified according to their cytokine profiles and functional properties (for review, see Clerici and Shearer 1993; Mosmann and Coffman 1989). Th1 cells predominantly secrete IFN-γ, IL-2 and TNF-α. Their major property is the recruitment and activation of macrophages at sites of inflammation. In contrast, Th2 cells mainly secrete IL-4 and IL-10 and their major task is to promote B-lymphocyte differentiation and antibody production. They can inhibit the Th1 reaction through the production of IL-10. In addition to these T helper subsets, the subpopulation of CD8+ T lymphocytes may either be cytotoxic or mediate suppression of cellular immune reactions. Class I MHC-restricted T cells undergo a polarization into T cytotoxic (Tc1 and Tc2) cells similar to that described for CD4+ T lymphocytes.

The initial event in the induction of inflammation in multiple sclerosis appears to be infiltration of the nervous system by Th1 cells and CD8+ Tc1 cells, the latter dominating the T-cell infiltrates in active as well as inactive lesions. By producing their cytokine cocktail, mainly IFN-γ and TNF-α, local central nervous system elements become immunologically activated. Resident microglia express histocompatibility antigens and thereby facilitate antigen recognition by T lymphocytes in the brain. Upregulation of adhesion molecules at the blood–brain barrier together with local chemokine production adds to the recruitment of inflammatory cells (predominantly other T cells, B cells and macrophages). The antigen recognized by these Th1 and Tc1 cells in multiple sclerosis brains is not known. Autoantigens as well as foreign (virus) antigens are possible candidates. Secondary effector cells are recruited into the nascent inflammatory focus and the blood–brain barrier is compromised. This results in protein leakage into the nervous system, registered by the increased gadolinium uptake in MRI studies of active lesions. In addition, resident microglia become activated and differentiate into phagocytic effector cells. A range of effector cells including macrophages/microglia and T lymphocytes, together with humoral factors, including antibodies and/or complement components, are involved in the destruction of myelin sheaths.

Downregulation of the inflammatory process coinciding with remission may take place through various mechanisms. It has been shown in experimental models of allergic or virus-induced inflammatory disease of the nervous system, and for a low proportion of cells in the lesions of multiple sclerosis, that T lymphocytes are effectively removed from the brain parenchyma through apoptosis. That said, the significance of programmed T-lymphocyte death for the clearance of inflammation in multiple sclerosis remains to be determined. Other factors that do appear to be involved in the downregulation of brain inflammation in multiple sclerosis are the cytokines IL-10 and TGF-β, and neurotrophins. In models of experimental autoimmune encephalomyelitis, the primary encephalitogenic Th1 reaction may switch to a Th2 reaction coinciding with recovery and increased pro-

duction of IL-4 and IL-10 (Issazadeh et al 1995a; 1995b). Both cytokines have been shown to inhibit the delayed-type hypersensitivity reactions induced by Th1 cells (Fiorentino et al 1989). Although the exact time course of cytokine expression in the lesions of multiple sclerosis is not yet known, the prominent IL-10 expression in some cases suggests that similar mechanisms may be operating. TGF-β, a cytokine with prominent immunosuppressive activity, has been detected in local tissue components, especially astrocytes, during the recovery from inflammation. Because intravenous administration of TGF-β may block or suppress experimental autoimmune encephalomyelitis (Johns et al 1991), its local production in lesions suggests a prominent role in downregulation of the inflammatory response. Systemic endocrine responses, such as glucocorticoid release, may additionally be involved in downregulation of disease activity. In experimental autoimmune encephalomyelitis, the peak systemic corticosteroid response coincides with the phase of resolving inflammation (see Chapter 13) and the susceptibility of different animal strains to experimental autoimmune encephalomyelitis partly depends upon their ability to mount a corticosteroid response in the course of immune activation. In patients with multiple sclerosis, high-dose corticosteroids stabilize blood–brain barrier dysfunction and, possibly by this mechanism, improve clinical signs and shorten the duration of relapses (Burnham et al 1991; D.H. Miller et al 1992b). In addition, steroid therapy may have a direct effect on T-cell apoptosis within lesions. But a neuroprotective role for inflammation has been shown in several models of brain disease (Moalem et al 1999; 2000), and inflammatory cells are an important source for neurotrophin production in the lesions of multiple sclerosis (see Chapter 10: Kerschensteiner et al 1999; Stadelmann et al 2002).

DEMYELINATION AND OLIGODENDROGLIAL DAMAGE

The demyelinated plaque is the pathological hallmark of multiple sclerosis. In its classical form, this is a sharply demarcated lesion with complete loss of myelin sheaths and demyelinated axons embedded in a dense matrix of glial scar tissue. In general, there is a sharp transition between the demyelinated plaque and adjacent normal white matter. Yet, in chronic lesions, a small rim of thinly myelinated fibres, typical of remyelination, is frequently encountered at the lesional border. The demyelinating process is primary and segmental (Figure 12.5). Thus, at the edge of the lesions, myelin sheaths terminate at the node of Ranvier, the naked axon traversing the lesion boundary.

Immunological mechanisms of demyelination

The myelin sheath is a complex structure formed through spiral ensheathment of the axon by the oligodendrocyte plasma membrane (Bunge et al 1962). A single oligodendrocyte can form multiple segments, yet the number of myelin sheaths provided by a single cell depends upon axon and myelin thickness (see Chapter 10; A. Peters and Proskauer 1969). Biochemically, myelin sheaths are composed of lipids and protein. Major central nervous system myelin proteins are myelin basic protein and proteolipid protein. Both apparently have important func-

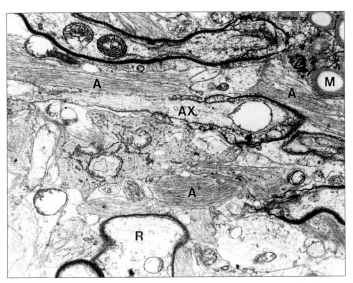

Figure 12.5 Chronic multiple sclerosis: electron micrograph of inactive plaque; dense astroglial scar tissue. Segmental myelin loss in a nerve fibre: A = astrocyte; AX = axon of the demyelinated fibre; M = macrophage; R = myelinated fibre with thin myelin sheath, suggestive of remyelination. ×10 000.

tions in the stabilization of complex lipid layers. Minor myelin proteins – myelin associated glycoprotein, myelin oligodendrocyte glycoprotein and 2′,3′-cyclic nucleotide 3′-phosphodiesterase (CNPase) – may play a role in the axon–myelin interaction or as surface receptors of oligodendrocytes (Morell 1984; Quarles 1989).

In principle, all myelin proteins are potential target antigens for T-cell mediated encephalitogenic reactions. To be recognized by CD4 lymphocytes, these antigens must be released into the extracellular space and processed by antigen-presenting cells – principally perivascular macrophages or microglia but possibly also astrocytes. This type of T-cell mediated immune reaction appears responsible for the induction of inflammation although, alone, it is not capable of destroying the myelin sheaths (Wekerle et al 1986). The *in vitro* data indicate that myelin sheaths can be damaged by several immunological mechanisms. Oligodendrocytes have a limited capacity to express histocompatibility antigens and present antigen (S.C. Lee and Raine 1989; Lisak et al 1983; Mauerhoff et al 1988), although they express class I MHC molecules in the inflammatory background of active multiple sclerosis lesions (Höfteberger et al 2004). Thus, they may become a direct target for antigen-specific T-cell mediated cytotoxicity. In addition, myelin sheaths are particularly sensitive to cell-surface or soluble immunotoxins produced by lymphocytes or macrophages, such as TNF-α (Selmaj and Raine 1988; Zajicek et al 1992), lymphotoxin (Selmaj et al 1991b), complement (Scolding et al 1989b) and perforin (Scolding et al 1990). Alternatively, T lymphocytes can themselves destroy oligodendrocytes and myelin without the need for MHC-restricted antigen recognition (D'Souza et al 1996b; M.S. Freedman et al 1991).

T-cell mediated cytotoxicity may be accomplished either through the release of cytotoxic granules or the activation of membrane-bound death receptors. The first pathway involves the liberation of perforin and granzymes from cytotoxic T cells.

These are attached to target cells by the 'immunological synapse'. Indeed, close contact of CD8 cells with a polar orientation of cytotoxic granules towards the surface of oligodendrocytes and axons can be found in the actively demyelinating lesions of multiple sclerosis (Neumann et al 2002). Cell destruction through death receptors involves the interaction of TNF-like receptors with their specific ligands. For example, activation of the Fas antigen by Fas ligand can trigger an intracellular death domain and induce apoptotic death of target cells. Fas expression has been described mainly on oligodendrocytes in chronic active lesions, whereas Fas ligand is expressed reciprocally on reactive microglia (Brosnan and Raine 1996; D'Souza et al 1996b). In another study, widespread expression of Fas was described on all central nervous system cells whereas Fas ligand was mainly identified on oligodendrocytes and astrocytes (Dowling et al 1996). In addition, Fas-positive oligodendrocytes were taken up by reactive macrophages/microglia. No satisfactory explanation for these ambiguous results is apparent. Furthermore, the prominent expression of Fas and other members of the TNF receptor family on oligodendrocytes in multiple sclerosis lesions is not necessarily associated with apoptotic oligodendrocyte death (Bonetti and Raine 1997). Such resistance to apoptotic cell death may be due to activation of the NF-κB and c-jun transcription factors in oligodendrocytes within the lesions of multiple sclerosis (Bonetti et al 1999).

Demyelination may also follow the specific recognition and opsonization of myelin sheaths by antibodies present on the extracellular surface of myelin or oligodendrocytes (Bornstein and Appel 1961; Lassmann et al 1981b; Linington et al 1988). Thus far, however, only a few myelin antigens are known to be exposed at the extracellular surface, potentially serving as targets for antibody-mediated demyelination. Apart from myelin lipids such as galactocerebroside (Dubois-Dalcq et al 1970), myelin oligodendrocyte glycoprotein appears to be an important target antigen for antibody-mediated demyelination (Linington and Lassmann 1987; Linington et al 1988). In other patients, circulating antibodies against oligodendrocyte progenitor cells and surface antigens of neurons have been detected (Lily et al 2004; Niehaus et al 2000). Furthermore, high-affinity anti-DNA antibodies, which have been rescued from the intrathecal antibody response of patients with multiple sclerosis, were found to bind the surface of neuronal cells and oligodendrocytes (Williamson et al 2001). Destruction of antibody-opsonized myelin is mediated either by complement (Linington et al 1989; Piddlesden et al 1993a) or activated macrophages (Brosnan et al 1977; Scolding and Compston 1991) through interaction with their Fc receptors (Ulvestad et al 1994).

Apart from specific immunological processes, tissue may also be destroyed nonspecifically in inflammatory lesions by toxic molecules of activated effector cells, such as macrophages or microglia. Macrophages produce a spectrum of molecules that are lethal to cells and invading microorganisms or dissolve the extracellular matrix. Those that have been identified in actively demyelinating multiple sclerosis lesions include proteolytic (Anthony et al 1998; Cuzner and Opdenakker 1999; Cuzner et al 1996; R.L.P. Lindberg et al 2001; Scarisbrick et al 2002; Vos et al 2003) and lipolytic enzymes, reactive oxygen and nitrogen species (J.S. Liu et al 2001; K.J. Smith and Lassmann 2002; K.J. Smith et al 1999), complement components, cytotoxic cytokines (Probert et al 2000) and excitotoxins liberated in the lesions due to an altered glutamate homeostasis in neurons and glia (S.A. Lipton 1998; P. Werner et al 2001). These exert their toxic action nonselectively on all cellular components of the inflamed tissue. Certain cells and structures are, however, more vulnerable than others. Myelin sheaths and oligodendrocytes are particularly sensitive, and are destroyed by most of these toxins at concentrations far below those needed to injure other cells. Thus, macrophage-mediated inflammatory tissue damage in the central nervous system is always reflected by a pseudoselectivity of tissue injury – demyelination and oligodendrocyte loss being most pronounced, followed by some degree of axonal injury associated with nearly complete preservation of astrocytes and microglia cells. A key question for understanding the immunopathogenesis of multiple sclerosis lesions is therefore to identify the extent to which these mechanisms of demyelination are reflected in the various patterns of myelin and oligodendrocyte destruction in this disease.

Structural patterns of myelin destruction

There has been no shortage of speculation on mechanisms of myelin destruction, from the earliest descriptions of the demyelinating process in multiple sclerosis. In a very artistic image, Babinski (1885b; see Chapter 1, Figure 1.28) illustrated the interaction of debris containing cells with the demyelinating fibre and concluded that myelin destruction is accomplished by invading white blood cells. Conversely, Marburg (1906) described a primary lysis of myelin followed by the infiltration of phagocytic cells, and postulated a pathogenetic role for humoral myelinotoxic factors. A new dimension to this discussion was added by the application of electron microscopy to the study of multiple sclerosis. Several different patterns of myelin damage have since been described. Receptor-mediated phagocytosis of myelin (pinocytosis vermiformis) was first described by Prineas et al (1984). It is characterized by the interaction of 'coated pits and vesicles' on macrophages containing elongated myelin-containing channels. It is suggested that macrophages react with opsonized myelin (Moore and Raine 1988; Prineas 1985) through Fc and complement receptors, which are upregulated on the cell surface of macrophages in active lesions (Ulvestad et al 1994). Myelin, bound to the macrophage surface, is then internalized into the cell through vesicles or tubular channels. This view receives support from the finding of IgG deposition at the sites of macrophage–myelin interactions (Prineas and Graham 1981).

Myelin stripping, a prominent feature in animals with experimental autoimmune encephalomyelitis, appears relatively rare in multiple sclerosis and is restricted to very severe lesions with extensive inflammatory infiltration (Lassmann 1983). In this pattern, lymphocytes and macrophages, or their cell processes, invade myelin sheaths and are then found between myelin lamellae or the myelin sheath and axon. Disorganization or vesicular dissolution of myelin is present in the vicinity of these inflammatory cells. Vesicular disruption of myelin sheaths consists of partial or complete vesicular transformation of the myelin sheath. It has mainly been found in cases of acute multiple sclerosis, characterized by very severe and destructive lesions (Guo and Gao 1983; Lassmann 1983; S.C. Lee et al 1990) and, to a lesser extent, in active chronic multiple sclerosis (J. Kirk 1979; Lumsden 1970). These features characterize

experimental models of demyelination in which the lesions are mediated by antibody and complement (Lassmann et al 1988). Although it is clear from experimental studies that this pattern of demyelination is a real phenomenon in vivo, studies on human tissue suggest that the process is augmented by post-mortem autolysis (Prineas 1985). However, because vesicular disruption is not a prominent feature of autolysis in normal post-mortem brain, it may – besides being a direct reflection of complement-mediated lysis – also indicate increased susceptibility of predamaged myelin to autolysis after death.

Dying back oligodendrogliopathy is characterized by pathological alterations in the most distal parts of the oligodendrocyte cell process. It was first described in a model of toxic oligodendrogliopathy and demyelination (Ludwin and Johnson 1981) and more recently has been reported as a typical feature of brain biopsies taken during early bouts of multiple sclerosis (M. Rodriguez and Scheithauer 1994; M. Rodriguez et al 1993b). Dying back oligodendrogliopathy is particularly frequent in models of virus-induced demyelination (M. Rodriguez 1992). Furthermore, similar alterations have been found in myelin associated glycoprotein-deficient mice (Lassmann et al 1997). Because the expression of some myelin proteins and their mRNAs in oligodendrocytes is dramatically downregulated in experimental models of virus infection or severe inflammation as well as in some multiple sclerosis cases (Itoyama et al 1980; Jordan et al 1989; Rodriguez et al 1994a), the changes of dying back oligodendrogliopathy may reflect impairment of oligodendrocyte metabolism in multiple sclerosis lesions. In line with this interpretation, a closely similar pattern of distal oligodendrogliopathy typically reflects early myelin damage in conditions of energy failure, such as hypoxia or ischaemia of the white matter (Aboul Enein et al 2003).

Most ultrastructural studies aim to define the unique and characteristic pattern of demyelination that pinpoints a ubiquitous mechanism of myelin destruction. It now appears likely that this concept is misleading. The original ultrastructural findings were based on very small numbers of cases and lesions. More recent observations show that multiple immunological pathways can potentially destroy myelin. Therapeutic inhibition of one mechanism is often compensated by another. Similarly, across the spectrum of patients with multiple sclerosis, disparate pathogenetic factors may prevail and result in diverse ultrastructural patterns of demyelination. This multiplicative concept of demyelinating pathways is further supported by the analysis of oligodendrocytes in lesions.

Fate of oligodendrocytes in multiple sclerosis lesions

Neuropathological studies on demyelinated plaques in multiple sclerosis have often claimed the complete absence of oligodendrocytes. But this view has been challenged. Using histochemical techniques, Ibrahim and Adams (1963; 1965) and Friede (1961) described the abundance of oligodendrocytes within early plaques, suggesting their numbers are actually increased compared with surrounding periplaque white matter. This analysis was confirmed by Raine et al (1981) in an ultrastructural study of a single lesion. In a more detailed quantitative study of another case, Prineas et al (1984) found a partial reduction in oligodendrocytes within an actively demyelinating mul-

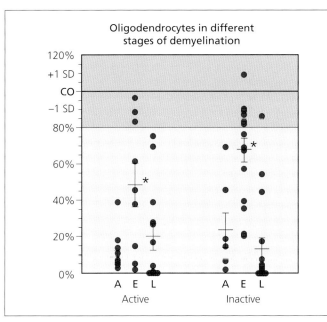

Oligodendrocytes in different stages of demyelination

Figure 12.6 Percentage of oligodendrocytes in the centre of demyelinated lesions in different forms and stages of multiple sclerosis lesions. A = acute multiple sclerosis; E = early multiple sclerosis; L = late multiple sclerosis; 'active' = actively demyelinating lesions; 'inactive' = demyelinated plaques without recent demyelinating activity. During the early bouts of multiple sclerosis, there are significantly higher numbers of oligodendrocytes in the plaques than in the destructive lesions of acute multiple sclerosis, and in the demyelinating plaques that develop late in the course of the disease. There is pronounced variation in the oligodendrocyte density between lesions of different patients. The differences in oligodendrocyte loss are apparently not due to stage of the demyelinating process (active vs. inactive). CO = control.

tiple sclerosis lesion. There now appears to be good agreement that oligodendrocytes are largely absent in the lesions of typical chronic multiple sclerosis when several years' disease duration have taken their toll. However, in early bouts of the disease a high or even normal density of oligodendrocytes can be found (Figure 12.6: Brück *et al* 1994; Lassmann 1983; Ozawa *et al* 1994; Prineas *et al* 1984; 1989; 1993a; Raine *et al* 1981; D.-L. Yao *et al* 1994) and remyelination is pronounced in these lesions (Lassmann 1983; Prineas *et al* 1993b). There are, however, different interpretations for these findings. Prineas (1985) suggested that oligodendrocytes are effectively destroyed within active lesions. Early in the course of multiple sclerosis, these may rapidly be replaced by new oligodendrocytes, recruited from the pool of progenitor cells. The final number of oligodendrocytes in a given lesion is then dependent upon the availability of oligodendrocyte progenitors. Another view is expressed by Raine *et al* (1981) and Selmaj *et al* (1991a; 1992), who described very high numbers of oligodendrocytes, identified by immunohistochemical and ultrastructural criteria, in active lesions and a reduction in older lesions. Their interpretation is that oligodendrocytes survive the primary attack only to be destroyed in the later phases of plaque formation, possibly through additional immune-mediated mechanisms. Finally, we have postulated that the degree of oligodendrocyte pathology may differ between the early and late stages of multiple scle-

rosis, as well as between patients (Lassmann 1983). At first sight, these fundamentally divergent interpretations of quite similar neuropathological observations appear surprising. But we feel that they can be reconciled.

As already confessed, assigning a mechanistic interpretation for neuropathological appearances requires animation of these static observations. In multiple sclerosis lesions, this can be achieved by correlating oligodendrocyte numbers with stages of myelin degradation products in macrophages. Until recently, quantitative studies on oligodendrocytes in multiple sclerosis plaques have not managed a sufficient sample size of lesions representing different stages of the disease. Patterns of oligodendrocyte death in active lesions were not systematically studied. Furthermore, the unambiguous identification of oligodendrocytes has met with pronounced difficulties. Ultrastructural confirmation, although based on relatively safe criteria is – by nature of the poor availability of suitable material and the tedious process of investigation – inevitably restricted to very few examples (Prineas 1985). Previously, immunocytochemical markers used in multiple sclerosis plaques were directed against myelin antigens expressed on oligodendrocytes only at the peak of myelination or remyelination (Prineas 1985; Prineas *et al* 1984; 1989). Thus, indirect criteria for oligodendrocyte recognition were introduced – such as cells with typical oligodendrocyte structure that have not labelled with leucocyte markers (Prineas *et al* 1993a), or round cells that are larger than leucocytes (D.-L. Yao *et al* 1994).

New markers have subsequently become available allowing positive identification of oligodendrocytes in lesions of routinely fixed and processed autopsy tissue (Brück *et al* 1994; Lucchinetti *et al* 1996; Ozawa *et al* 1994). They include mRNAs for myelin proteins, especially myelin oligodendrocyte glycoprotein, CNPase and proteolipid protein (Figures 12.2 and 12.8). The expression of mRNA for proteolipid protein is a very early marker of oligodendrocyte differentiation, seen on cells of the oligodendrocyte lineage during myelination and maintenance of myelin. It is, however, not present in surviving oligodendrocytes that have lost their myelin sheaths. Furthermore, myelin protein mRNA expression may be reduced when oligodendrocytes are exposed to immunological attack (Shirazi *et al* 1993) or virus infection (Jordan *et al* 1989; Rodriguez *et al* 1994a). In contrast, myelin oligodendrocyte glycoprotein is not expressed on the surface of myelin sheaths and oligodendrocytes until late in myelination. It persists during myelin maintenance and is detectable on oligodendrocytes that have survived demyelination following Wallerian (axonal) degeneration (Ludwin 1990). Thus, myelin oligodendrocyte glycoprotein appears to be a good marker for terminally differentiated oligodendrocytes both in myelinated and demyelinated tissue. CNPase is abundant in oligodendrocytes actively engaged in myelination, but still present at lower amounts in mature oligodendrocytes. These cell markers for oligodendrocytes can be combined with methods for the identification of dying cells dependent on DNA fragmentation (Figure 12.7: R. Gold *et al* 1994).

To date, rather few studies have used a sufficient number of well-characterized cases and adopted stringent criteria for the categorization of lesions from each, with quantification of oligodendrocyte numbers. Lucchinetti *et al* (1999) analysed the density of oligodendrocytes within >300 lesions from 119 patients with multiple sclerosis. In the primary analysis, a profound

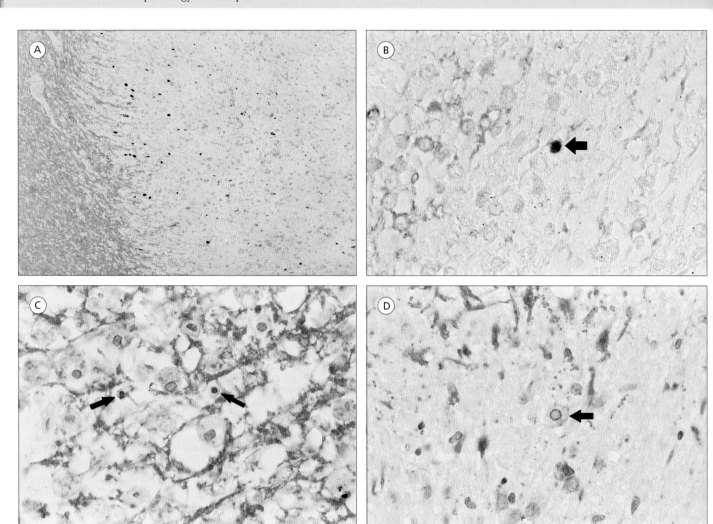

Figure 12.7 Oligodendrocyte death in multiple sclerosis lesions. (A) Chronic multiple sclerosis: detection of DNA fragmentation by *in situ* tailing (black); immunocytochemistry with anti-myelin oligodendrocyte glycoprotein antibody (red); radially expanding lesion; numerous cells with DNA fragmentation at the lesional border; ×50. (B) Dying oligodendrocyte identified by immunoreactivity against myelin oligodendrocyte glycoprotein (red); DNA fragmentation is visualized by *in situ* tailing (black; arrow); ×500. (C) Acute multiple sclerosis: immunocytochemistry with anti-myelin oligodendrocyte glycoprotein antibody. Actively demyelinating lesion with numerous macrophages that contain myelin oligodendrocyte glycoprotein-immunoreactive myelin debris. Two oligodendrocytes are identified by their surface immunoreactivity for myelin oligodendrocyte glycoprotein with condensed nuclei, typical for apoptosis (arrows). ×350. (D) Chronic multiple sclerosis: immunocytochemistry with anti-myelin oligodendrocyte glycoprotein antibody. In an actively demyelinating lesion, the oligodendrocyte is identified by myelin oligodendrocyte glycoprotein immunoreactivity, with swollen cytoplasm and nucleus suggestive of cell necrosis (arrow). ×350.

variation of oligodendrocyte density was found within plaques (Figure 12.6). Cells were virtually absent in some lesions and cases, whereas in others, relative numbers within the tissue were even higher than in the adjacent normal white matter. The most pronounced differences related to the histological stage of demyelinating activity and inter-individual variations. Although there appears to be profound heterogeneity of oligodendrocyte damage between patients (Lucchinetti *et al* 1999), lesions of a single individual exactly matched for state of activity showed very similar oligodendrocyte densities. Together, these data suggest that, not unexpectedly, oligodendrocyte survival undergoes dynamic changes with the evolution of activity and onset of remyelination.

More detailed analysis of the quantitative data on oligodendrocytes reveals, first, that in all cases there is a loss of oligodendrocytes in actively demyelinating lesions – the extent of

which varies from trivial to near complete. Secondly, the recruitment of oligodendrocytes into the lesions varies between the highly effective, leading to a plethora of oligodendrocytes in inactive or remyelinating lesions, to apparent inhibition of recruitment leaving persistently demyelinated plaques, devoid of oligodendrocytes and with no demonstrable remyelination. On the basis of these observations, different patterns of oligodendrocyte pathology can be defined, which at least in part reflect different clinical manifestations of the disease (Lucchinetti *et al* 1999).

As a general rule, the recruitment of new oligodendrocytes is more efficient in the early stages of relapsing–remitting multiple sclerosis. Thus, in acute multiple sclerosis, rapid and extensive remyelination is seen in about two-thirds of cases despite the fulminant and destructive disease process still taking place in fresh lesions. In the remainder, very few new oligodendrocytes appear in inactive lesions and remyelination is low or absent (Lucchinetti *et al* 1999). These patterns of oligodendrocyte reaction correlate with different immunopathological patterns of demyelination (Lucchinetti *et al* 2000). The pattern is fundamentally different after several years' disease duration and in patients with chronic progressive disease. Here, oligodendrocyte numbers within the plaques are in general very low (Mews *et al* 1998). Although a minority of cases in the late chronic stage of multiple sclerosis – while still in the relapsing–remitting stage of the disease – show partial or even extensive oligodendrocyte preservation and rapid remyelination similar to that found during the early stages (Figures 12.6 and 12.8), destruction of oligodendrocytes in the active phase of demyelination is then not followed by significant recruitment of progenitor cells.

Source of new oligodendrocytes in the lesions of multiple sclerosis

Two different types of oligodendrocytes can be seen within the early demyelinating plaques of multiple sclerosis (Lucchinetti *et al* 1999; Wolswijk 2000). The first are small round cells, which express myelin oligodendrocyte glycoprotein in high density on their surface and with low cytoplasmic levels of CNPase but virtually devoid of mRNA for any of the myelin proteins. These cells most probably are oligodendrocytes that survived the demyelinating episode but lost their peripheral cell processes and myelin sheaths. The other population consists of large reactive cells with very intense production of myelin protein mRNA and high cytoplasmic density of CNPase. Myelin oligodendrocyte glycoprotein expression is absent or low. These cells are believed to be derived from the pool of oligodendrocyte progenitors. At later stages of lesion development, the small myelin oligodendrocyte glycoprotein-positive cells are gradually lost and replaced by others with high expression of myelin protein mRNAs, engaged in remyelination.

The fate of surviving myelin oligodendrocyte glycoprotein-positive oligodendrocytes is so far not clear. Most experimental data suggest that new remyelinating oligodendrocytes exclusively come from the pool of undifferentiated progenitor cells and their further differentiation into remyelinating oligodendrocytes requires proliferation (Keirstead and Blakemore 1999). If that also applies to human inflammatory demyelinating lesions, oligodendrocytes that survive the demyelinating attack should be useless and gradually disappear from the lesions by programmed cell death. Indeed, in some lesions, myelin oligodendrocyte glycoprotein-positive oligodendrocytes are partly preserved in areas of active demyelination but gradually lost from more inactive lesions in the absence of newly recruited remyelinating oligodendrocytes (Lucchinetti *et al* 1999; Wolswijk 2000). However, this does not exclude the possibility that the specific growth factor environment in the vicinity of lesions may drive terminally differentiated oligodendrocytes back into an undifferentiated stage thereby maintaining a pool of potential remyelinating cells.

Because proliferation is evidently a prerequisite for oligodendrocyte precursors to differentiate into remyelinating cells, the issue of which cells proliferate in the lesions of multiple sclerosis is of interest. Using immunocytochemical identification of the proliferation markers Ki67 or proliferating cell nuclear antigen (PCNA), dividing cells are frequently encountered in actively demyelinating lesions. Within expanding plaques, these proliferating cells are mainly located at the active lesional border. By double labelling experiments, the majority of proliferating cells are identified either as T cells or macrophages and very few glial fibrillary acidic protein (GFAP) astrocytes are labelled. Oligodendrocytes, distinguished by binding antibodies against CNPase or myelin oligodendrocyte glycoprotein, are rare in the proliferating cell fraction. These data suggest that proliferation of myelinating or mature oligodendrocytes does not contribute significantly to the number of oligodendrocytes in these lesions. Yet, recruitment of new oligodendrocytes from a pool of dividing undifferentiated progenitor cells that still have proliferating capacity may be a significant event in lesion repair. In keeping with this interpretation a significant fraction of proliferating cells in the lesions of multiple sclerosis express the platelet-derived growth factor A receptor – a marker of oligodendrocyte progenitors (Maeda *et al* 2001; Solansky *et al* 2001).

Oligodendrocyte progenitors have recently been visualized in multiple sclerosis lesions using specific markers for this cell population (Maeda *et al* 2001; Wolswijk 2002). The expression of developmentally regulated proteins and chemokine receptors in oligodendrocytes within the lesions of multiple sclerosis may control their recruitment and differentiation. (A. Liu *et al* 2005; Omari *et al* 2005). These studies clearly show that their presence and density correlate with the capacity of lesions to recruit new oligodendrocytes and start the remyelinating programme (Wolswijk 2002). Although the absence of remyelination is in part determined by the availability of progenitor cells, remyelination may also be blocked despite the presence of large numbers of oligodendrocyte progenitors (A. Chang *et al* 2002). This observation suggests that, in some patients and lesions, the differentiation of progenitor cells into remyelinating oligodendrocytes may be disturbed either by inadequate axonal signals or inhibitory factors that actively suppress oligodendrocyte differentiation and remyelination (Charles *et al* 2002a; John *et al* 2002).

Can these seemingly divergent findings regarding oligodendrocytes in multiple sclerosis lesions be reconciled? All the data suggest that oligodendrocytes are destroyed in actively demyelinating lesions, although to an extent that varies between different patients. The terminally differentiated oligodendrocytes, which have survived the demyelinating insult, seem to be slowly removed from lesions by apoptotic cell death. Although it is not yet completely clear whether terminally differentiated oligodendrocytes can dedifferentiate in the specific inflammatory environment, the major source of remyelinating oligodendrocytes depends on recruitment of progenitors, and the extent of lesion repair largely depends on their availability and functional properties. Remyelination and repair are features of the early disease stages in acute and relapsing–remitting patients, but poor thereafter and especially in patients with progressive disease.

Heterogeneity of multiple sclerosis lesions: individual differences in structural and immunological pathology of actively demyelinating plaques

As discussed above, recent studies have shown profound inter-individual differences in the patterns of myelin destruction and oligodendrocyte pathology. Conversely, when multiple lesions in

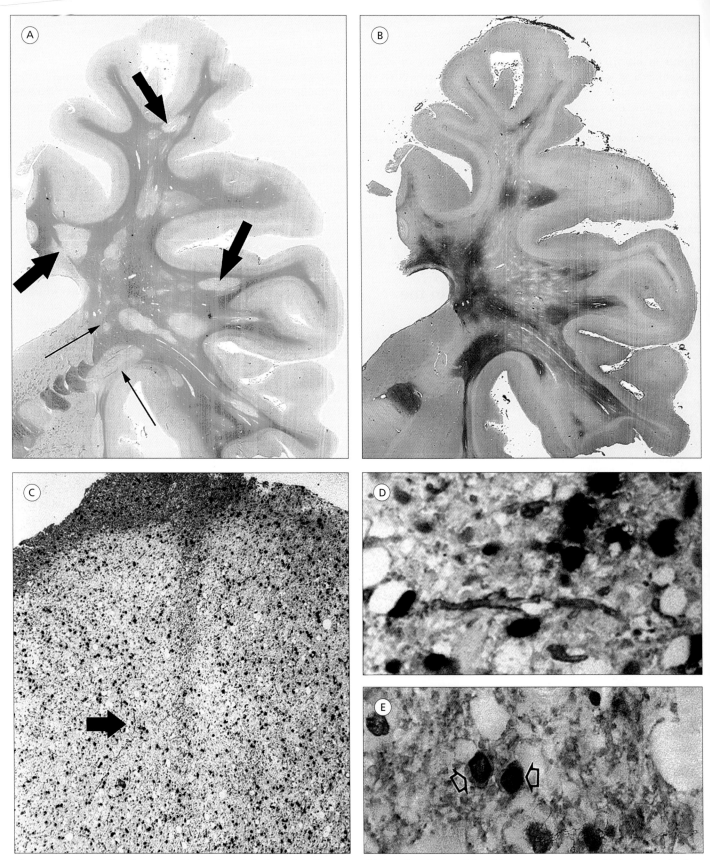

Figure 12.8 Remyelination in multiple sclerosis lesions. (A) Chronic multiple sclerosis: luxol fast blue myelin stain; multiple lesions in the white matter; some lesions are completely demyelinated (thick arrows), whereas others are shadow plaques (thin arrows); ×1. (B) Tissue adjacent to the section shown in (A) stained with Holzer stain for gliosis; the completely demyelinated plaques from (A) show very little gliosis and, thus, represent fresh active lesions; the shadow plaques reveal extensive fibrillary gliosis and are therefore old repaired lesions; ×1. (C) Brain biopsy obtained during the first bout of chronic multiple sclerosis: *in situ* hybridization for proteolipid protein mRNA (black) and immunocytochemistry for proteolipid protein (red); large plaque with numerous oligodendrocytes in the lesion; the arrow marks the position shown in high magnification in (D); ×40. (D) Oligodendrocyte with proteolipid protein mRNA (black) connected to remyelinated sheath with proteolipid protein immunoreactivity (red); ×500. (E) Same lesion as in (C) and (D): immunocytochemistry with anti-proteolipid protein antibody; immunoreactivity for proteolipid protein is not only located in myelin sheaths but also in the cytoplasm of remyelinating oligdendrocytes (open arrows); ×800.

the brain autopsy of a single patient were compared in detail, based on an exact and stringent classification of lesional activity, the patterns of demyelination and oligodendrocyte injury were highly homogeneous (Lucchinetti *et al* 1999; 2000). These data suggest that mechanisms of demyelination and oligodendrocyte damage are similar in any one patient at a given stage of disease development, but differ between patients or, perhaps, in the same patient at different stages of the disease (acute or early relapsing versus late chronic and/or progressive disease).

By analysing in detail the immunopathological nature of the inflammatory response, the structural patterns of myelin and oligodendrocyte injury as well as the topography and cellular reaction within lesions, four different patterns of demyelination have been defined in patients with multiple sclerosis (Lucchinetti *et al* 2000). In immunological terms, these can be measured against one basic pattern – inflammation, some demyelination and tissue destruction – that characterizes all multiple sclerosis patients and every lesion (pattern I). But our position is that this core pattern is sometimes modified by additional factors, including antibodies, hypoxia or a genetically determined increase in susceptibility of the target tissue.

Basic general pattern of all lesions in multiple sclerosis (pattern I)

The inflammatory reaction is always dominated by T lymphocytes and macrophages. Whereas different T cells are present in the lesions, class I MHC restricted T cells invariably outnumber other T-cell populations, irrespective of the stage of the lesion. This T-cell dominated inflammatory process is associated with activation of local microglia cells and, to a lesser extent, the recruitment of haematogenous macrophages. Such activated microglia and macrophages may form clusters of increased cell density, associated with the generation of focal demyelinated plaques. They may, however, also be diffusely dispersed in the normal-appearing white matter, associated with diffuse myelin and axonal injury. Activated macrophages and microglia are found in close contact with demyelinating nerve fibres and disintegrating axons. They take up and digest the tissue (myelin) debris. Thus all these features suggest that, through their toxic secretory products, activated macrophages and microglia are instrumental in the induction of tissue damage. Indeed, activated proteolytic and lipolytic enzymes (Cuzner *et al* 1996), molecules involved in oxidative and nitrative damage (Broholm *et al* 2004; K.E. Hill *et al* 2004; J.S. Liu *et al* 2001), cytotoxic cytokines (Cannella and Raine 1995; Hofman *et al* 1989; Merrill 1992; Selmaj *et al* 1991b) and excitotoxins (Lipton 1998) can be produced by macrophages and have been detected in the lesions of multiple sclerosis and other conditions.

Besides macrophage/microglia-mediated tissue damage, there is additional evidence for direct T-cell mediated toxicity within these lesions. Massive class I MHC expression is found on oligodendrocytes, astrocytes, axons and neurons in active lesions of acute and chronic multiple sclerosis (Höfteberger *et al* 2004), and CD8[+] T cells can be found in very close association with oligodendrocytes and axons in the lesions (Neumann *et al* 2002) – their cytotoxic, granzyme B reactive granules being arranged in a polarized fashion towards the contact area with oligodendrocytes or axons. This closely mimics the formation of an immunological synapse between the cytotoxic T cell and its target, as shown convincingly *in vitro*. Some oligodendrocytes within the lesions show all the classical features of apoptosis, including nuclear condensation and fragmentation.

This immunological pattern of tissue injury is associated with the formation of confluent demyelinated lesions and relative axonal sparing. Oligodendrocytes are partly lost in the active stages of demyelination, yet a high frequency of surviving myelin oligodendrocyte glycoprotein-positive oligodendrocytes is typical for this lesion type. In addition, reappearance of new oligodendrocytes is frequent and remyelination extensive, in particular at the early stage of the disease (acute or relapsing multiple sclerosis). Later, in patients with chronic progressive disease, a similar pattern of tissue injury is present leading to very slow progression of myelin destruction with reduced numbers of activated phagocytes containing myelin degradation products. Interestingly, the loss of oligodendrocytes in such lesions is extensive and remyelination sparse (Prineas *et al* 2001). These data indicate that the inflammatory mediators of T cells and macrophages, involved in demyelination and tissue injury, differ between the early relapsing and later progressive stages of the disease.

Augmentation of demyelination by specific antibodies (pattern II)

A large proportion of patients with multiple sclerosis show – in addition to the basic features of active lesions described above – deposition of immunoglobulins (Prineas 1985; Prineas and Graham 1981) and activated complement in the areas of active myelin destruction (Lucchinetti *et al* 2000; Storch *et al* 1998c). All components of the complement system are present in these lesions, whereas complement inhibitory proteins are sparse (Storch *et al* 1998a; 1998b; 1998c). Complement C9 neoantigen, a conformational epitope of the ninth complement component only exposed with formation of the lytic membrane attack complex, is deposited on myelin sheaths, the surface of oligodendrocytes and within myelin degradation products in macrophages (Schwab and McGeer 2002; Storch *et al* 1998a; 1998b; 1998c). Complement activation correlates strictly with the demyelinating activity of these lesions, being present only during the earliest stages of myelin destruction (Figure 12.9). Antibody-mediated demyelination is also associated with significantly higher numbers of B lymphocytes and plasma cells within the plaques. Antibody-mediated demyelinated plaques in multiple sclerosis are sharply demarcated (Figure 12.9) and centred on an inflamed vein or venule. Extensive primary demyelination is frequently associated with profound nonselective tissue damage and destruction, and a high degree of oedema and axonal loss. Recruitment of new oligodendrocytes and remyelination is extensive.

The most extreme variant of antibody-mediated demyelination and tissue destruction is seen with Devic's type of neuromyelitis optica (Lucchinetti *et al* 2002). In these patients, complement activation is extensive not only at sites of active demyelination but also within the walls of small and medium-sized parenchymal vessels. In contrast to typical forms of multiple sclerosis, the lesions of neuromyelitis optica show profound infiltration with granulocytes, especially eosinophils. In more chronic lesions, vascular sprouting and perivascular fibrosis are extensive. These findings suggest that antibodies dominate

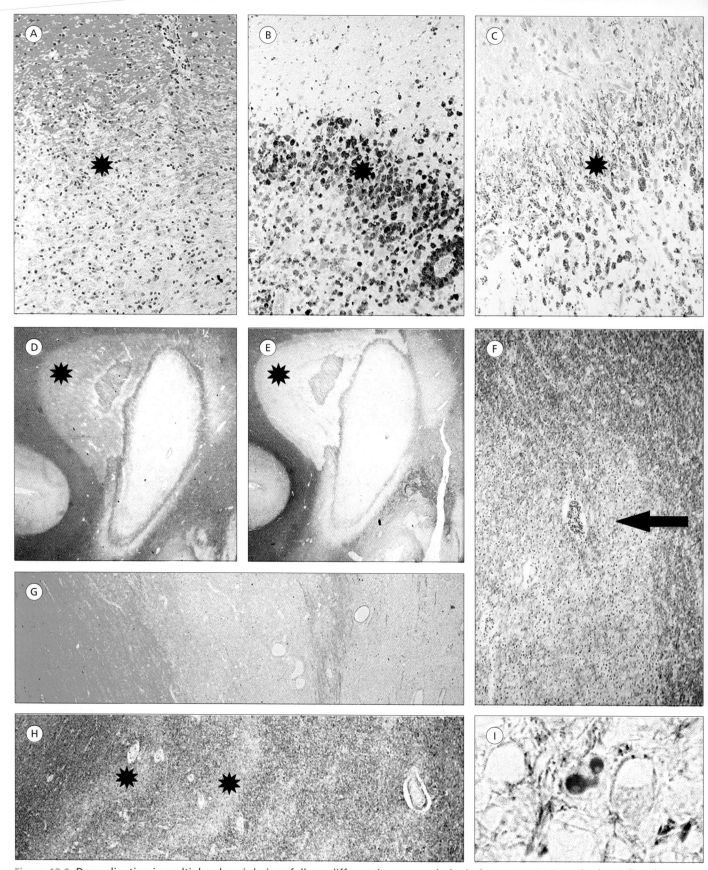

Figure 12.9 Demyelination in multiple sclerosis lesions follows different immunopathological patterns. A–C, antibody-mediated demyelination (pattern II). (A) The lesion is sharply demarcated and the zone of active myelin destruction (*) infiltrated by macrophages containing myelin degradation products (luxol fast blue; ×100). (B) The macrophages at the lesion edge express CD68; ×100. (C) Myelin sheaths at the lesion edge and myelin degradation products within macrophages are immunoreactive for C9 neoantigen; ×200. D–I, demyelination following a pattern of hypoxia-like tissue injury (pattern III). (D,E) The area of active demyelination (*) still contains myelin oligodendrocyte glycoprotein (D) but has completely lost myelin-associated glycoprotein immunoreactivity; ×2. (F) The lesion edge (*) is ill defined and contains a broad zone of partial demyelination. In the surrounding of inflamed vessels the myelin sheaths are better preserved than in the depth of the lesion (arrow); ×100. (G, H) The edge of the lesion shows profound reduction of myelin density in Luxol fast blue staining (G) and alternating rims of demyelinated (*) and myelinated tissue, when stained for myelin oligodendrocyte glycoprotein (H; G and H: ×30). (I) Numerous oligodendrocytes show the morphological changes of apoptosis (nuclear condensation and fragmentation); ×1000.

the immune reaction in neuromyelitis optica, directed against myelin and/or antigens present in the walls of cerebral vessels. This view is supported by the recent identification of a 'Devic's disease-specific' antibody response directed against a so-far-unknown determinant in perivascular and subpial astrocytic foot processes (Lennon *et al* 2004). In addition, the pattern of brain inflammation more closely resembles experimental models of brain inflammation induced by Th2 rather than Th1 polarized T cells (Lucchinetti *et al* 2002).

Augmentation of demyelination and tissue damage by hypoxia-like tissue injury (pattern III)

A proportion of patients present with a pattern of acute demyelination that has histological appearances fundamentally different from those described above or seen in experimental immune-mediated models of inflammatory demyelination (Lucchinetti *et al* 2000). The hallmark of these lesions is a profound and selective loss of myelin-associated glycoprotein and CNPase, early in the development of demyelination, with preservation of other myelin antigens such as myelin basic protein, proteolipid protein and myelin oligodendrocyte glycoprotein (Figure 12.9). These changes in myelin protein expression are associated with pathological alterations in the most distal processes of oligodendrocytes – the paranodal and peri-axonal oligodendrocyte loops – followed later by apoptotic death of oligodendrocytes (Figure 12.9). This pattern of demyelination can be described as a distal or dying back oligodendrogliopathy. Although previously recognized (Itoyama *et al* 1980) in multiple sclerosis and virus-induced white matter inflammation (Itoyama *et al* 1981), it only recently became clear that such a distal oligodendrogliopathy is indicative of hypoxic/ischaemic white matter damage (Aboul Enein *et al* 2003). The existence of hypoxic tissue injury in inflammatory brain lesions could have several explanations. Massive oedema or inflammation within the vessel walls might impair the microcirculation within actively demyelinating lesions, reducing oxygen tension and disturbing energy metabolism within the tissue. Alternatively, reactive oxygen and nitrogen species may impair mitochondrial function, resulting in hypoxia-like tissue damage (Bolanos *et al* 1997; Aboul-Enein and Lassmann 2005). Indeed, some data suggest changes in mitochondrial enzymes, which occur in parallel to oxidative tissue damage in chronic active multiple sclerosis lesions (F. Lu *et al* 2000). Reduced expression of genes encoding mitochondrial proteins has also recently been observed in a gene array study comparing cerebral cortex from multiple sclerosis patients and controls (McDonough *et al* 2003). Whether such alterations are more pronounced in lesions showing the hypoxia-like tissue injury pattern remains to be determined.

Pattern III lesions differ in several other important respects from those designated as pattern I and II plaques. Although the global extent of inflammation, reflected in the number of T and B cells and macrophages/microglia cells is similar, the lesions contain fewer foamy macrophages. Furthermore, the activation state of microglia seems less pronounced and different from that seen in pattern II lesions. The expression pattern of chemokine receptors more closely reflects that characterizing ischaemic stroke than other types of lesion seen in multiple sclerosis (Mahad *et al* 2004). Finally, the distribution of pattern III lesions is different from other plaques. Their edges are ill-defined and

the lesions not necessarily centred on small vessels. When inflamed, these small vessels are often surrounded by small rims of intact myelin (Figure 12.9). This also is a characteristic feature of hypoxia, where myelin surrounding small vessels is generally better preserved than within the rest of the lesion (Aboul-Enein *et al* 2003).

The most severe and dramatic manifestation of pattern III lesions in multiple sclerosis is Balo's concentric sclerosis. The active lesions invariably show a rim of hypoxia-like tissue injury at the border with surrounding white matter. There is conspicuous oligodendrocyte expression of stress proteins, especially heat-shock proteins 70 and 65 and hypoxia-inducible factor 1α (Hif-1α) within the distal concentric rims and in a small zone outside the active lesions, consistent with the hypothesis that hypoxia at the lesion edge induces their expression rendering the rim of tissue more resistant to the next wave of hypoxic injury, finally resulting in the expansion of lesions with alternating layers of demyelination and myelin preservation. In short, the findings suggest that concentric rings in Balo lesions are due to hypoxic preconditioning at the edge of rapidly expanding plaques (Stadelmann *et al* 2005).

Augmentation of demyelination and tissue damage due to a genetically determined increased susceptibility of the brain tissue for immune-mediated injury (pattern IV)

Pattern IV lesions were initially defined as actively demyelinating plaques showing unusually severe, often lethal, damage to oligodendrocytes in a small rim of periplaque white matter, adjacent to the zone of active myelin destruction. Such lesions were thus interpreted as examples of primary oligodendrocyte damage with secondary demyelination (and possibly also inflammation: Lucchinetti *et al* 1996; 2000). This is not a common type of lesion in multiple sclerosis (<2% in our series). One mechanistic interpretation comes from studies on inflammatory demyelination in patients or experimental animals with a deficiency of ciliary neurotrophic factor. Patients with multiple sclerosis, who have a genetic polymorphism conferring a functional deficit in ciliary neurotrophic factor, appear to have a more aggressive disease with earlier age at disease onset (Giess *et al* 2002). When autoimmune encephalomyelitis is induced in ciliary neurotrophic factor-deficient mice, clinical disease, demyelination and oligodendrocyte death are more severe than in wild-type littermates (Linker *et al* 2002). *In vitro*, ciliary neurotrophic factor protects oligodendrocytes against apoptosis, induced by TNF-α (D'Souza *et al* 1996a). These data suggest that a genetic deletion or polymorphism alters the susceptibility of central nervous system tissue to immune-mediated damage. Several genes have been identified that may change the outcome of inflammatory demyelinating diseases, including apolipoprotein E (apoE4: Fazekas *et al* 2000; and see Chapter 3), mitochondrial DNA (Mojon *et al* 1999b), or the spinocerebellar ataxia gene 2 (Chataway *et al* 1999a). Another possible candidate gene, associated with severe oligodendrocyte damage, is that coding for p53 (Wosik *et al* 2003).

The relation between mitochondrial gene defects and multiple sclerosis deserves separate attention. As described in Chapter 3, mitochondrial mutations typical for Leber's optic atrophy may manifest as bilateral optic neuropathy and multifocal demyelinating lesions in other brain areas (Harding *et al* 1992). Given the number of such cases described in the literature and the low incidence of isolated Leber's optic atrophy, it is unlikely that the simultaneous presence of both types of lesion in the same patient is a mere coincidence. Furthermore, considering mitochondrial injury, induced by oxygen or nitrogen radicals, as a possible mechanism of tissue destruction in multiple sclerosis, it is not unlikely that a genetic defect of mitochondria may synergistically augment mitochondrial dysfunction and subsequent tissue damage. Only recently has the neuropathology of such a case been extensively characterized (Kovacs *et al* 2005). Besides symmetrical inflammatory demyelinating lesions in both optic nerves, multiple plaques in different stages of demyelinating activity were found. Active lesions revealed massive inducible nitric oxide synthase (iNOS) expression in macrophages and microglia and upregulation of manganese superoxide dismutase. Such a pattern of tissue damage is consistent with oxidative injury.

Although genetic mechanisms accounting for lesion heterogeneity in the pathology of multiple sclerosis remain entirely speculative, we can predict that a systematic analysis of genes determining susceptibility and the clinical course will further refine the definition of pathological features representing extremes of the clinical phenotype, including those that show disproportionate demyelination or axonal and neuronal degeneration.

Differences in the patterns of demyelination between acute, relapsing and progressive multiple sclerosis

The four patterns of demyelination described above are observed in the fresh white matter lesions in patients at the early stage of the disease. Overall, pattern III lesions are most frequently encountered in patients with acute multiple sclerosis, whereas patterns I and II have their highest frequency in early chronic stages of the disease. To date, pattern IV lesions appear rarely and only in a subset of patients with a rapidly progressive disease course. These patterns of demyelination cannot explain the slow progression of disease in patients suffering from classical primary or secondary progressive disease. In these patients, there is apparently a very slowly progressive demyelination at the edges of pre-existing plaques (Prineas *et al* 2001), chronic axonal injury and destruction within the plaques (Kornek *et al* 2000), a diffuse inflammatory process with slow-burning myelin and axonal injury in the normal white matter, and profound demyelination in the cortex.

Demyelination in multiple sclerosis plaques: a summary

The mechanisms contributing to tissue injury in multiple sclerosis are complex and heterogeneous between different patients and stages of the disease. There seem to be two essentially different pathogenetic events – the rapid formation of actively demyelinated well-circumscribed plaques and, as will be described in detail in the section dealing with the pathology of progressive multiple sclerosis, a slower and more diffuse process of inflammation, demyelination and axonal injury (Peletier *et al* 2003). Although these processes may overlap, each characterizes a fundamentally different stage of the disease. Although the formation of new white matter plaques is the dominant feature of acute and relapsing–remitting multiple sclerosis, the slow pro-

gressive tissue injury underlies disease chronicity in primary and secondary progressive multiple sclerosis. Inflammation, dominated by T lymphocytes and macrophages, is the driving force behind both lesion types. Especially in fresh white matter plaques of acute or relapsing multiple sclerosis, new inflammatory cells enter the central nervous system through small parenchymal vessels. The inflammatory foci are characterized by acute blood–brain barrier damage, tissue oedema, demyelination and a variable degree of acute axonal injury. Conversely, in the progressive stage of multiple sclerosis, the inflammatory reaction is apparent within the central nervous system but contained and compartmentalized. Rather few new lesions are therefore formed and most of the cumulative damage occurs by expansion of pre-existing plaques as well as diffuse damage to the normal white matter and cortex.

Besides these stage-dependent features of the evolving disease process in any one individual, there is additional inter-individual heterogeneity in the immunological mechanisms responsible for demyelination and tissue injury as well as in structural aspects of the lesions, such as the extent of remyelination (Lassmann *et al* 2001). Our position is that genetic background modulates the basic pattern of inflammatory demyelination and tissue damage, mediated mainly through cytotoxic T lymphocytes and activated macrophages. As a result, inflammation leads to focal demyelinated plaques (pattern I), amplification by pathogenic antibodies together with complement and activated macrophages (pattern II), hypoxia-like tissue injury (pattern III), or susceptibility of selected sites for immune-mediated demyelination and axonal injury (pattern IV). These different patterns of demyelination segregate clinically into distinct disease entities in the most severe forms of the disease, explaining the characteristic pathological features of neuromyelitis optica and Balo's concentric sclerosis. In the more classical forms of multiple sclerosis, lesions differ in the patterns and extent of myelin destruction, oligodendrocyte and axonal damage, as well as in their geography and gross appearance. Self-evidently, serum and cerebrospinal fluid biomarkers are needed to identify these subgroups and classify patients with multiple sclerosis according to the dominant immunological pathways responsible for the plaque formation.

REMYELINATION

It is a matter of great significance to people with multiple sclerosis that the lesions may undergo spontaneous remyelination, and that – in the experimental context – this restores function. News of this simple fact, gathered in the laboratory, has reached the clinic and provides hope that there is a path back from tissue injury. Now, the pressure is on to improve upon these endogenous processes and capture their principles as a treatment (see Chapter 19).

Central remyelination

Although the morphological changes had been depicted by Babinski (1885b; see Chapter 1), Otto Marburg first realized that remyelination is a feature of acute multiple sclerosis (Marburg 1906). His interpretation of the very thin myelin sheaths, detected by osmic acid impregnation in many plaques, depended on the comparison with changes already described in regenerating peripheral nerves (Stransky 1903). Marburg first suggested that these changes may reflect some degree of remyelination. It later became clear that remyelination of nerve fibres, defined by the appearance of uniformly thin and short internodes and by aberrant myelination around nonaxonal cell processes, is a frequent finding at the edge zones of inactive plaques (Perier and Gregoire 1965; Prineas and Connell 1979; Suzuki *et al* 1969; see Chapter 1). In chronic multiple sclerosis lesions, these signs of remyelination are generally restricted to a small zone around demyelinated plaques (Figure 12.10). As a result, many commentators have proposed that remyelination is defective in multiple sclerosis and should be stimulated either by the application of trophic factors or implantation of new oligodendrocytes into the lesions (see Chapters 10 and 13). But evidence emerging in recent years suggests that, at least in the early stages of multiple sclerosis, rapid and extensive remyelination may be the rule rather than the exception (Lassmann 1983; Prineas 1985; Prineas *et al* 1984; 1993a; 1993b; Raine and Wu 1993). This conclusion is, however, difficult to reconcile with the electrophysiological evidence for a one-way path from normal to demyelinated axons. However, whilst delays in the visual evoked potential usually persist following optic neuritis, except in childhood, there may be a slow crawl back towards normal latency if the period of observation is extended from months to years (see Chapter 13).

The abundance of shadow plaques is apparent from studies of acute and early multiple sclerosis. Described in detail by Schlesinger (1909), these sharply demarcated areas of myelin pallor and gliosis (Figure 12.8) very frequently are found in the early stages of multiple sclerosis and other acute demyelinating disorders. Although shadow plaques were at one time regarded as areas of incomplete demyelination (Schlesinger 1909), we now know that these represent remyelination of previously fully fledged plaques (Lassmann 1983; Prineas 1985). This view is further substantiated by more recent detailed ultrastructural and immunocytochemical studies (Brück *et al* 1994; Ozawa *et al* 1994; Prineas *et al* 1989; 1993a; 1993b).

Together, these studies clarify several aspects of remyelination in multiple sclerosis. By identifying all essential ultrastructural criteria for remyelination in the thinly myelinated fibres of shadow plaques (Prineas 1985; Prineas *et al* 1989), clear evidence is provided that complete remyelination of lesions can occur. Correlating the presence of remyelinating fibres with stages of myelin degradation products in macrophages (Brück *et al* 1994; Lassmann 1983) or with clinical course of the disease (Prineas *et al* 1989; 1993a), suggests that remyelination may be a very early event in the evolution of plaques. Remyelination is a dominant feature in cases of early or acute multiple sclerosis (Brück *et al* 1994), whereas it is limited in classical chronic multiple sclerosis (Ozawa *et al* 1994). But remyelinated lesions can again become targets for new waves of demyelination (Prineas *et al* 1993b).

Two cellular events may account for the rapid and complete remyelination in early multiple sclerosis. First, oligodendrocytes or their progenitor cells appear to be preserved to a much larger extent in lesions formed during the first years of multiple sclerosis than in those arising later in the course (Brück *et al* 1994; Ozawa *et al* 1994). Thus, in early multiple sclerosis lesions, more oligodendrocytes are available for myelin repair (Figure 12.8). Secondly, in experimental studies, repeated demyelinations and remyelinations induced by cuprizone toxicity are deleterious with respect to lesion repair (see Chapter 10). Whereas progenitor cells are available to differentiate into mature oligodendrocytes and start remyelination after a single episode of demyelination and oligodendrocyte destruction, repeated cycles may exhaust this reserve of progenitor cells, culminating in persistent demyelination (Ludwin 1980). Although such a mechanism has for long been accepted as a major reason for remyelination failure in chronic demyelinating diseases, it has to be acknowledged that a recent study failed to reproduce these results in a different model of toxic demyelination (Penderis *et al* 2003a). It is currently unresolved whether this discrepancy can be explained by differential vulnerability of oligodendrocyte progenitor cells to separate toxic insults. However, in a model of relapsing inflammatory demyelinating disease, repeated demyelinating episodes also reduced the capacity for repair (Linington *et al* 1992).

Schwann cell remyelination

Besides remyelination by oligodendrocytes, multiple sclerosis lesions may also partly be repaired by Schwann cells (Feigin and Ogata 1971; Ghatak *et al* 1973; Ogata and Feigin 1975). Schwann cell remyelination is mainly found in the spinal cord (J.M. Andrews 1972; Feigin and Popov 1966), apparently due to inward migration from the meninges and/or peripheral roots. Although Schwann cell engagement of naked axons is, in general, restricted to a few nerve fibres, some cases show extensive peripheral remyelination. This is particularly the case in severe spinal forms of multiple sclerosis, mainly described in Oriental people (Itoyama *et al* 1983; 1985). Apparently, the major obstacle confronting Schwann cells aiming to reach the central

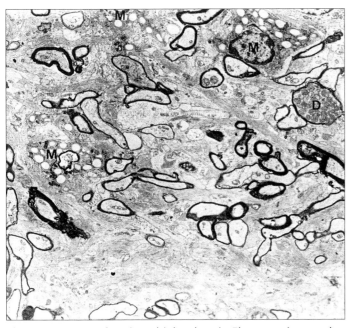

Figure 12.10 Late chronic multiple sclerosis. Electron micrograph of inactive demyelinated plaque with abundance of thinly myelinated nerve fibres, suggesting remyelination. M = macrophage; D = dystrophic axon; ×8000.

nervous system parenchyma and remyelinate naked axons is the astrocytic environment (Blakemore 1976; Itoyama *et al* 1985). Thus, as in models of chronic experimental autoimmune encephalomyelitis (Lassmann *et al* 1980), Schwann cell remyelination is (paradoxically) most evident in cases with severe destructive demyelinating lesions characterized by extensive loss of astrocytes (Itoyama *et al* 1985; Yamamoto *et al* 1991).

Why do some lesions in multiple sclerosis remyelinate and others not?

As described above, the extent of remyelination in multiple sclerosis ranges from complete in the majority of plaques to virtually absent throughout the entire brain. Many explanations for this diversity have been offered, and most likely all of them may play a role in different situations (Chari and Blakemore 2002b; Franklin 2002; D.J. Miller *et al* 1996).

In principle, the extent of remyelination depends on the presence and functional state of myelinating oligodendrocytes, and the availability of surviving axons for remyelination. The extent of oligodendrocyte destruction and recruitment of progenitor cells within the lesions of multiple sclerosis is highly variable and partly determined by the pathogenic mechanism of demyelination in a given case (Lucchinetti *et al* 1999). Many different macrophage toxins can induce demyelination, and their toxic effects on either mature oligodendrocytes or progenitor cells differ. Some macrophage toxins, cytokines and growth factors have trophic effects on progenitor cells but induce apoptosis in mature oligodendrocytes (Arnett *et al* 2001; Muir and Compston 1996). Conversely, reactive oxygen species differentially damage immature compared with mature oligodendrocytes (Almazan *et al* 2000). Similar differential selectivity has been described for serum antibodies in patients with multiple sclerosis. Whereas anti-myelin oligodendrocyte glycoprotein antibodies mainly lyse terminally differentiated oligodendrocytes (Linington *et al* 1988), those that target the proteoglycan AN-2 may preferentially eliminate progenitor cells (Niehaus *et al* 2000). Finally, rather than inducing demyelination, certain low-affinity antibodies against oligodendrocyte surface molecules may stimulate remyelination (Mitsunaga *et al* 2002).

Thus, remyelination will be poor when the pool of oligodendrocyte progenitor cells is depleted, either through repeated focal demyelination or through specific immune mechanisms – although impoverished remyelination cannot always be explained by the loss of progenitor cells (A. Chang *et al* 2002). Rather, recent data suggest that in some progenitor cells the differentiation programme is arrested by astrocyte-derived cytokines (John *et al* 2002), although the proposed pathway of Notch1/Jagged1 signalling is not a limiting factor for remyelination in experimental demyelinated lesions (Stidworthy *et al* 2004). The problem may, however, also reside in the properties of axons within plaques. Self-evidently, massive axonal destruction will limit the opportunity for remyelination and functional repair. In some plaques, demyelinated but surviving axons re-express polysialylated neuronal cell adhesion molecule (PSA-NCAM), an axonal molecule that actively suppresses myelination (Charles *et al* 2002a).

Activated macrophages produce cytokines and trophic factors that stimulate myelination *in vitro* (Diemel *et al* 1998) and promote remyelination *in vivo* (Kotter *et al* 2001). Thus, it is likely that activity of the inflammatory reaction influences remyelina-

tion – negatively by inducing more demyelination and damage of oligodendrocytes or their progenitor cells, and positively by producing neurotrophic factors.

These data identify several potential explanations for the absence of remyelination. These will differ between patients and lesions depending on the mechanisms of tissue damage, activity of the disease process and properties both of the remyelinating cells and axons. Against this background, it seems naive to believe that single strategies to stimulate remyelination, such as this or that growth factor, or a shot of stem cells, will be a panacea for repair and remyelination in such a biologically complex situation.

AXONAL PATHOLOGY

The status of demyelination as a defining feature of the pathology in multiple sclerosis implies, as first emphasized by Marburg (1906), that axons are relatively preserved. But it is now accepted that – to an extent varying between individual patients – acute axonal pathology is seen in active demyelinating lesions, and axonal density is reduced in most chronic multiple sclerosis plaques (Ferguson *et al* 1997; Trapp *et al* 1998). Evidence for active destruction of axons is generally more pronounced in acute multiple sclerosis and in actively demyelinating lesions, but sometimes may be extensive even in chronic plaques (Figure 12.11; Barnes *et al* 1991). That said, given the much longer time course over which axons are able to degenerate, axonal attrition may accumulate more in the chronic than acute phases of plaque formation. When large numbers of multiple sclerosis plaques are analysed, axonal density ranges from nearly normal to a loss of around 80% of all axonal profiles, with an average of 67–70% in established inactive lesions (Mews *et al* 1998). This wide range of axonal loss applies equally to different patients with multiple sclerosis, and to the totality of plaques within the same individual.

Although in certain cases the loss may be unambiguously devastating (Figure 12.11), axonal density within given lesions allows only a rough estimate of axonal loss. The density of axons is influenced by diverse factors, most obviously genuine destruction; but tissue oedema and atrophy, and infiltration by inflammatory cells, may spuriously alter the apparent density of axons per unit area, thus masking the true extent of axon loss in areas of demyelination. In general, assessments of axonal density tend to overestimate the extent of axonal destruction. To overcome this problem detailed quantitative studies on the number of axons in defined tract systems have been performed (Bjartmar *et al* 2000; 2001). These studies confirmed results obtained by simple determination of axonal density, showing also an average loss of axonal profiles in established lesions by 60–70%. In addition, loss of axons was not restricted to demyelinated plaques themselves, but also found in more remote tract systems (Bjartmar *et al* 2001; Ganter *et al* 1999; Lovas *et al* 2000), and spinal cord atrophy was found to be similar in areas with demyelinated plaques in comparison with areas devoid of lesions (Evangelou *et al* 2005). These data strongly suggest that secondary Wallerian degeneration is an important feature of multiple sclerosis pathology. Such tract degeneration has directly been demonstrated in the corpus callosum, where its extent correlates with the degree of axonal damage in adjacent plaques within the hemispheric white matter (Evangelou *et al* 2000a).

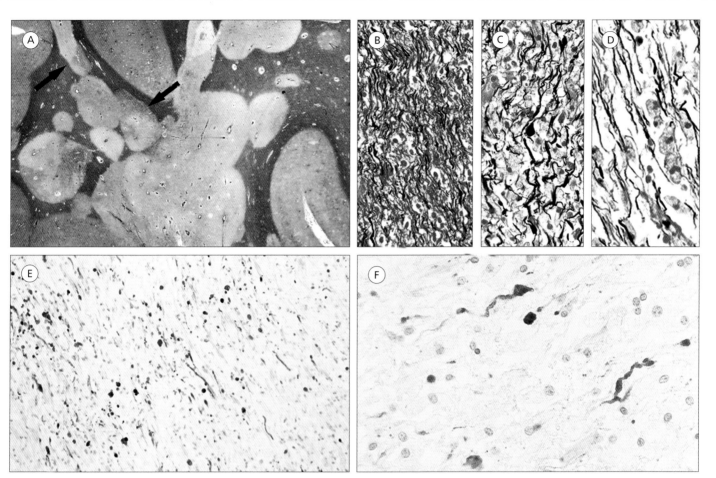

Figure 12.11 Axonal pathology in multiple sclerosis lesion. (A) Multiple demyelinated plaques with variable axonal density in the white matter of a patient with longstanding chronic multiple sclerosis. The areas marked with arrows represent new demyelinated areas in previously existing plaques. These lesions show reduced axonal density compared with the rest of the pre-existing lesion. Bielschowsky silver impregnation for axons; ×2. (B–D) Axonal density in the normal-appearing white matter (B) and in two different plaques of the same patient (C and D); axonal density differs between demyelinated plaques; Bielschowsky silver impregnation; ×400. (E) Expression of β-amyloid precursor protein in dystrophic axons from an actively demyelinating lesion, indicating acute axonal injury; ×300. (F) As in (E); ×600.

Acute axonal injury is particularly apparent in actively demyelinating lesions formed in the very severe cases of acute multiple sclerosis (Marburg 1906) and in active plaques of patients with chronic multiple sclerosis (Bitsch *et al* 2000b; Trapp *et al* 1998). The damage consists of axon interruption and swelling with formation of spheroids and regenerative sprouts (Figure 12.12; Dahl *et al* 1989). In some of the acute multiple sclerosis cases, these changes affect the vast majority of axons in the lesions. Although axonal injury is much less pronounced in the actively demyelinating lesions of chronic multiple sclerosis than in acute plaques (Bitsch *et al* 2000b), it is nonetheless a consistent feature found in every demyelinating lesion (Figure 12.13).

Focal accumulation of amyloid precursor protein is a particularly valuable marker for acute axonal injury. This protein moves by fast axonal transport and accumulates at sites where traffic is blocked, either as a result of axonal transection or from disturbed axonal metabolism. Being easily accessible for quantification, the intra-axonal accumulation of amyloid precursor protein closely reflects acute axonal injury in a given lesion. Using this technique, it was shown that large numbers of

axons are damaged during and shortly after the process of acute demyelination (Ferguson *et al* 1997; Kornek *et al* 2000). Thus, as often suggested (Kornek and Lassmann 1999), this implies that the active inflammatory process, apparently responsible for demyelination, also affects axons – especially those that have lost their myelin sheaths acutely. In addition, a slow-burning axonal injury affects completely demyelinated plaques in which inflammation is quiescent (Kornek *et al* 2000). Although the incidence of axonal injury in such lesions is <1% of that seen in active plaques, this rate may eventually prove functionally significant, because chronic lesions can smoulder for several years. Acute axonal injury in the plaques of multiple sclerosis has also been studied in relation to disease duration (Kuhlmann *et al* 2002b). The most extensive axonal injury was found in patients with a disease duration of <1 year, and the incidence of axonal injury decreased with disease duration, despite the presence of actively demyelinating lesions. From this study, it was concluded that axonal injury is most extensive at early stages of the disease and decreases over time. This interpretation may, however, be misleading. Patients with a disease duration of

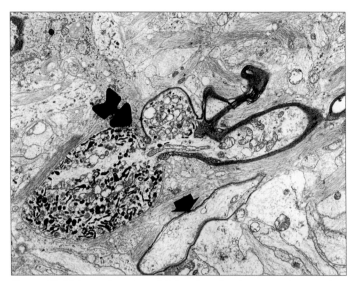

Figure 12.12 Late chronic multiple sclerosis: electron micrograph of inactive demyelinated plaque with extensive astrocytic scar formation. Dystrophic axon, loaded with axonal organelles; large arrow indicates the node of Ranvier; small arrow shows a thinly myelinated fibre, suggestive of remyelination. ×20 000.

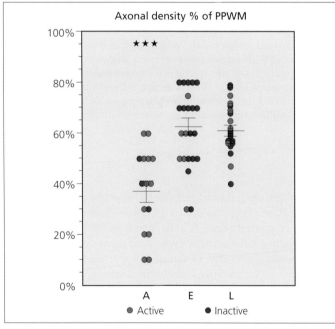

Figure 12.13 Axonal density in multiple sclerosis lesions. The number of axons in plaques was determined in ten microscopic fields at different sites and compared with the number of axons similarly determined in the periplaque white matter (PPWM). The values are given as a percentage of the axon density in plaques relative to that in the periplaque white matter. A = acute multiple sclerosis; E = early chronic multiple sclerosis (first or second bout of the disease); L = late chronic multiple sclerosis (several years' disease duration). There is a significantly higher reduction of axonal density in lesions of acute multiple sclerosis compared with other groups; the reduction of axonal density is, however, highly variable, ranging from <20 to >80%.

<1 year were either those who died with acute multiple sclerosis or underwent biopsy for diagnostic purposes. This is obviously a sample heavily biased towards disease severity. Our view is that the extent of axonal injury reflects severity of the disease process rather than the stage or duration of disease. Acute axonal injury and loss are not restricted to demyelinated plaques but are also present – although at much lower incidence – in the periplaque and normal-appearing white matter (Evangelou *et al* 2000a; 2000b; B. Ferguson *et al* 1997; Kornek *et al* 2000), perhaps due in part to Wallerian degeneration. Furthermore, diffuse axonal injury in normal-appearing white matter is seen in primary progressive multiple sclerosis (see below).

Acute axonal injury may either lead to complete transection or reversible structural and functional alterations of axons. Complete transection is reflected by the appearance of axonal end bulbs or spheroids (Trapp *et al* 1998). Reversible damage generally leads to enlargement of the axon calibre and/or focal axonal swellings. Overall, small-calibre axons and neurons appear to be selectively affected in the lesions of multiple sclerosis (Evangelou *et al* 2001). At least in actively demyelinating lesions, inflammatory cells and their toxic mediators appear to be directly responsible for the induction of axonal injury. Dystrophic axons in active plaques are in close contact with activated macrophages and microglia cells (B. Ferguson *et al* 1997; Fraenkel and Jacob 1913; Trapp *et al* 1998). The degree of axonal injury, both in active (B. Ferguson *et al* 1997) and inactive lesions (Kornek *et al* 2000) correlates significantly with the extent of tissue infiltration by activated macrophages or microglia cells. There is a weaker correlation between cytotoxic class I MHC restricted T-cell infiltration and axonal damage (Bitsch *et al* 2000b). Experimental data show that axons can be destroyed by the products of activated phagocytes (Anthony *et al* 1998) as well as directly by cytotoxic T cells (Neumann *et al* 2002). Oxygen and nitric oxide radicals (K.J. Smith and Lassmann 2003) or proteolytic enzymes (Anthony *et al* 1998) seem to be the most important macrophage toxins involved in axonal injury. In addition fibrin and its cleavage products, which are chronically deposited in the plaques of multiple sclerosis (Gveric *et al* 2001; 2003), may trigger axonal and neuronal degeneration (Akassoglou *et al* 2004). Following this initial immune-mediated injury, further axonal dissolution appears to involve the influx of Ca^{2+} ions, activation of intra-axonal proteases, ubiquitination of axonal proteins (Giordana *et al* 2003; Kornek *et al* 2001) and, finally, dissolution of the axonal cytoskeleton. The resulting impairment of axonal transport is reflected by the focal accumulation of proteins, such as amyloid precursor protein (B. Ferguson *et al* 1997), sodium channels (Nav1.2 and Nav1.6) and the Na^+/Ca^{2+} exchanger (Craner *et al* 2004a; 2004b), metabotropic glutamate receptors (Geurts *et al* 2003) or voltage-gated calcium channels (Kornek *et al* 2001). Aberrant expression of ion channels and the Na^+/Ca^{2+} exchanger at sites of axonal damage may further amplify Ca^{2+} influx and, thereby, augment and sustain axonal damage.

In addition to acute axonal injury and transection, other axonal alterations have also been described in the lesions of multiple sclerosis. Thus, axons entering areas of demyelination at the plaque edge generally show changes in diameter when passing the last node of Ranvier. It had already been noted by Marburg (1906) that, particularly in active plaques, axons are thicker than in the normal surrounding white matter. This observation was further substantiated by electron microscopic studies providing clear quantitative evidence for axon thickening and increase of axonal filaments (Shintaku *et al* 1988). Conversely, axonal atrophy with a decreased axon diameter is a typical feature of the chronically demyelinated plaque. Over and above these structural changes, demyelinated axons may change the composition of their axolemmal surface molecules, evidently with profound functional consequences. Unlike the contribution of PSA-NCAM re-expression to impaired remyelination (Charles *et al* 2002a), redistribution of sodium channels extending from the previous node of Ranvier to the entire demyelinated segment (Craner *et al* 2004a; Moll *et al* 1991) may restore electrophysiological conduction and functional recovery. In addition, however, abnormal patterns of sodium channel expression in demyelinated axons and their cell bodies, as described in multiple sclerosis and autoimmune encephalomyelitis, may result in more subtle functional disturbances of neurons (Black *et al* 2000; Craner *et al* 2003a).

Axonal loss in multiple sclerosis is a very important pathological feature because it is an irreversible change that sooner or later leads to severe neurological deficit (see Chapter 13; M.A. Lee *et al* 2000). Indeed, recent MRI observations suggest that brain and spinal cord atrophy and axonal loss (determined by magnetic resonance spectroscopy or magnetization transfer ratios) correlate better with clinical deficit than the total number and size of demyelinated plaques (Davie *et al* 1996; Losseff *et al* 1996b). In this respect, it is important to note that the degree of axonal loss is more uniform in a single individual than in the lesions of different patients. It follows that evaluating the degree of axonal damage by magnetic resonance may serve as an important prognostic marker (Bjartmar *et al* 2003; Medana and Esiri 2003).

GREY MATTER PATHOLOGY AND CORTICAL PLAQUES

Although multiple sclerosis lesions are most obvious in white matter, the grey matter is also severely affected (Figure 12.14) both by classical demyelinated plaques and by global neuronal loss and atrophy, due to retrograde degeneration following axonal destruction in the neighbouring white matter. Demyelinated plaques may be present in all grey matter areas of the central nervous system (Brownell and Hughes 1962; Lumsden 1970; Sander 1898). As in white matter plaques, myelin remains the principal target, resulting in areas of demyelination with relative axonal and neuronal sparing and some remyelination. Despite these similarities, lesions in the white matter and cerebral cortical grey matter lesions differ in many respects.

Three types of cortical lesions can be distinguished (Bo *et al* 2003b; T. Kidd *et al* 1999; Peterson *et al* 2001):

* intracortical perivascular lesions
* cortico-subcortical compound lesions affecting grey and white matter
* surface-oriented bandlike cortical lesions.

The first two develop, as in white matter, around small veins and venules. In contrast, the third type – by far the most common

cortical lesion – is characterized by demyelination of the outer 3–5 layers of the cortex, resulting in bandlike demyelinated lesions spanning several millimetres or centimetres of the cortical surface (Peterson *et al* 2001). They are related to inflammatory infiltrates in the meninges and are particularly prominent in areas where access to the cerebrospinal fluid circulation is restricted. Thus, predilection sites for such lesions are the cortical sulci, the cingulate, temporal and insular cortex, and the cerebellar cortex. Factors produced in the meninges that diffuse into the brain parenchyma seem instrumental in the development of these lesions.

Microscopically, cortical lesions are fundamentally different from those seen in the white matter (Peterson *et al* 2001). Intensity of the inflammatory reaction is much less and this is particularly impressive when cortico-subcortical compound lesions are analysed. Clear separation between the heavily inflamed white matter portion and the weakly inflamed grey matter component is obvious. In addition, perivascular inflammatory cuffs are rare or absent in cortical plaques and blood–brain barrier damage is negligible, even when the lesions are in the stage of active demyelination. Moreover, a quantitative study of T- and B-cell infiltrates showed no significant differences between the normal cortices of control patients and multiple sclerosis patients nor between demyelinated or non-demyelinated cortex in multiple sclerosis (Bo *et al* 2003a). Finally, the cortical pathological process is much more selective than in white matter. Although there is some acute axonal and neuronal injury during the active stage of demyelination (Peterson *et al* 2001), this is much less pronounced than in white matter. Again, this is most convincingly seen in demyelinated plaques that straddle the grey and white matter. Thus, cortical plaques are lesions with limited inflammation and blood–brain barrier damage, minimal oedema and very sparse tissue loss due to the low amount of myelin and restricted axonal and neuronal injury. It is not surprising that direct MRI visualization of cortical plaques is difficult and at best incomplete (Boggild *et al* 1996; Bozzali *et al* 2002).

Little is known about immunological mechanisms responsible for the formation of cortical demyelinated plaques. Their orientation towards the meningeal surface of the cortex, the association with meningeal inflammation, and the near complete absence of inflammatory infiltrates argue for the diffusion of a soluble factor responsible for selective destruction of myelin. In some active cortical lesions, myelin sheaths are dressed with antibodies and activated complement (C9 neoantigen), but this is the exception, not the rule (Brink *et al* 2005). A general feature of cortical plaques in all patients with multiple sclerosis is the massive activation of cortical microglia (Bo *et al* 2003b), associated with very high expression levels of inducible nitric oxide synthase (iNOS: Figure 12.14).

Besides demyelination, the cerebral cortex of patients with multiple sclerosis may also be affected by tissue loss and atrophy, particularly at sites of severe focal or diffuse white matter injury. The classical literature established that neurons in such lesions may show signs of retrograde reaction, such as central chromatolysis. Unlike the demyelinating component (Geurts *et al* 2005), cortical atrophy can be readily detected and quantitated by MRI (Bozzali *et al* 2002). These analyses show that cortical atrophy may occur early and to some extent predicts the clinical course and the development of cognitive problems.

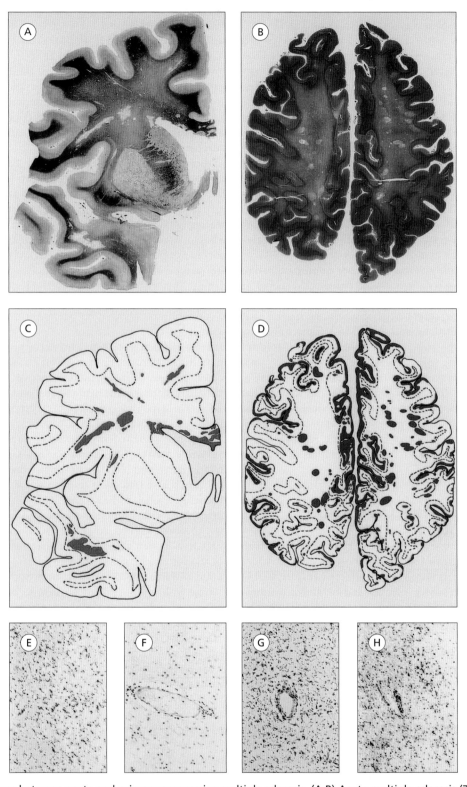

Figure 12.14 Differences between acute and primary progressive multiple sclerosis. (A,B) Acute multiple sclerosis (7 months' disease duration); multiple partly confluent plaques of demyelination in the white matter (green lesions in B). (C,D) Primary progressive multiple sclerosis with multiple small plaques in the white matter (green lesions in D) and massive diffuse white matter injury (light myelin staining in C); in addition there is extensive demyelination in the cerebral cortex (red lesions in D). A,C: Klüver myelin stain, ×0.3; B,D: graphical lesion map. (E, F) Normal-appearing white matter in acute multiple sclerosis with expression of HLA-D in microglia (E) but no expression of iNOS (F); ×50. (G, H) Normal-appearing white matter in primary progressive multiple sclerosis with massive expression of HLA-D (G) and iNOS (H) in microglia; ×50.

ASTROGLIAL REACTION

As the name makes clear, scar formation is a major aspect of the pathology in multiple sclerosis. Thus, in the majority of inactive plaques in chronic disease, the demyelinated axons are embedded in a dense, fibrillary network of astrocytic processes (Figure 12.8) containing increased amounts of glial fibrillary acidic protein (GFAP) and sometimes so-called Rosenthal fibres (Herndon *et al* 1970; Ogasawara 1965). But in other chronic multiple sclerosis plaques, the tissue texture may be quite loose, the extracellular space wide, astrocytes and their processes reduced in density, and naked axons may traverse the extracellular space (Barnes *et al* 1991). Such lesions are especially frequent in the spinal cord where an ingrowth of Schwann cells may result in peripheral remyelination (Feigin and Ogata 1971; Itoyama *et al* 1985). In actively demyelinating and subacute lesions, the astrocytic reaction is different. Large, bizarre, sometimes multinucleated astrocytes with high immunoreactivity for glial fibrillary acidic protein are present. These highly reactive astrocytes sometimes contain cell debris or myelin degradation products (Marburg 1906; Lassmann 1983; S.C. Lee *et al* 1990), may also express histocompatibility antigens (S.C. Lee *et al* 1990), and often contain abundant lysosomal enzymes (I.V. Allen *et al* 1979a). Alternatively, large reactive astrocytes are found with their cell body completely engulfing apparently intact oligodendrocytes (Ghatak 1992; Prineas *et al* 1990; Wu and Raine 1992). This pattern has primarily been taken to indicate phagocytosis of oligodendrocytes by reactive astrocytes. Ultrastructural studies suggest alternatively that these oligodendrocytes are surrounded but not taken up by astrocytes and that specific cell contacts are present between the membranes of each cell type. This interaction between astrocytes and oligodendrocytes is not specific for multiple sclerosis but can be found in a variety of other conditions where myelin is destroyed (Ghatak 1992). What remains uncertain is whether this relationship is protective or harmful for oligodendrocytes.

Apart from the reactive change that culminates in formation of a glial scar within the demyelinated plaque, astrocytes may also be destroyed through the immunological process. Although this is a rare phenomenon, restricted to the very severe lesions of acute and subacute multiple sclerosis, it may have important consequences. In such lesions, generally demarcated from the adjacent white matter by a dense glial scar, the number of astrocytes is much reduced compared with surrounding white matter. During lesional activity, some astrocytes show nuclear DNA fragmentation indicating active destruction of the cells (Ozawa *et al* 1994). More chronic lesions of this type show extensive reduction of parenchymal elements including myelin, oligodendrocytes, astrocytes and axons leading to a pronounced increase in width of the extracellular space. The most obvious explanation for such lesions is that they result from severe inflammatory tissue injury, indicative of severe but nonspecific tissue damage by immune mediators. Indeed, most of these lesions are associated with extremely severe inflammation with dense infiltration of highly activated macrophages. It has been shown *in vitro* that astrocytes may become a target for T lymphocytes during the process of antigen presentation (Sun and Wekerle 1986), suggesting that their destruction in the course of T-cell mediated inflammation may also be a specific immunological event.

In addition to glial scar formation within plaques, changes in astrocytes may also be found in the normal periplaque white matter of patients with multiple sclerosis. This led to the suggestion that a primary defect of astrocytic metabolism is responsible for lesion formation (see Chapter 1: Müller 1904). Reactive hypertrophy of astrocytes is frequent and generally associated with increased expression of lysosomal enzymes (I.V. Allen *et al* 1981). The cause of this diffuse astrocyte reaction in multiple sclerosis is unknown. Several mechanisms have been proposed, such as secondary Wallerian (axonal) degeneration, persistence of reactive astrocytes in remyelinated lesions (Lassmann 1983), or a general astrocyte activation due to the presence of soluble inflammatory mediators in the brain extracellular space. The latter explanation is most likely because a variety of cytokines, particularly TNF-α and other mediators, may stimulate the proliferation and glial fibrillary acidic protein expression of astrocytes *in vitro* (Fontana *et al* 1980; Selmaj *et al* 1990).

ABNORMALITIES IN THE 'NORMAL' WHITE MATTER OF PATIENTS WITH MULTIPLE SCLEROSIS

The advent of magnetic resonance imaging and spectroscopy has directed attention to diffuse abnormalities within the so-called 'normal' white matter of multiple sclerosis patients. These changes consist of diffuse signal alterations, identified using various imaging protocols, such as magnetization transfer ratio and diffuse reduction of *N*-acetyl aspartate peaks in MR spectroscopy. These alterations are generally associated with a progressive loss of brain volume (see Chapter 7). Such changes may already be apparent early in the relapsing–remitting stage of the disease, but become most prominent in patients with primary and secondary progressive multiple sclerosis.

To date, pathological studies have paid little attention to these diffuse alterations in the 'normal' white matter. Axonal loss in the late stage of chronic multiple sclerosis may be reflected by pronounced atrophy of the white matter and dilatation of the cerebral ventricles (Figure 12.1D) associated with secondary degeneration in the long ascending and descending tracts of the brainstem and spinal cord (Bjartmar *et al* 2001; Ganter *et al* 1999; Lovas *et al* 2000). Thus, diffuse abnormalities in the 'normal' white matter have long been considered a secondary consequence of axonal injury and loss occurring within the plaques, and have been designated the 'encephalopathy' of multiple sclerosis (Jellinger 1969). Not surprisingly, these diffuse brain alterations are the main morphological substrate of dementia in this clinical context (Fontaine *et al* 1994). On a microscopic basis, these changes are reflected by mild inflammation, some microglia activation, astrocytic scarring, increased expression of proteolytic enzymes within astrocytes and microglia, together with some microscopic foci of demyelination (I.V. Allen *et al* 1979; 1981; 2001; McKeown *et al* 1978).

Although the presence of secondary 'Wallerian' degeneration in the normal white matter of patients with multiple sclerosis, arising from axonal loss in plaques, is undisputed, recent MRI studies describe profound alterations in the 'normal' white matter in patients either with early multiple sclerosis or with primary progressive disease, in whom focal lesion load is small and cannot account for the extent of diffuse changes (Bozzali *et al* 2002; Filippi *et al* 2003). We therefore readdressed this question by comparing in detail the pathology of 'normal' white matter in patients with acute or relapsing multiple sclerosis and that found in the progressive stage of the disease. We found a diffuse inflammatory process, reflected by perivascular inflammatory infiltrates and parenchymal inflammatory infiltration in the patients with progressive but not acute and relapsing disease, which was globally distributed throughout the entire brain and showed no relation to the number, distribution, activity or destructiveness of focal white matter lesions. This diffuse inflammatory process was associated with profound and global activation of microglia, and the formation of small microglial nodules. Activated microglia expressed CD68, a marker for phagocytic activity, MHC class II antigen and iNOS. Primary demyelination was rare or absent within the 'normal' white matter, but many axonal spheroids and terminal axonal swellings were scattered throughout the tissue (Kutzelnigg *et al* 2005).

These data suggest that, in the brain of patients with multiple sclerosis, two independent and essentially different pathological processes develop in parallel. One is the formation of focal inflammatory demyelinating plaques; evidently, this depends upon the infiltration of tissue by new waves of inflammatory cells, derived from the peripheral circulation. Axonal destruction within the plaques may in part lead to degeneration of axons in white matter tracts, distant to the site of focal injury. In addition, however, there is a second pathological process, reflected by a gradual accumulation of inflammatory cells with diffuse and global axonal injury occurring in the absence of primary demyelination within the entire white matter. Focal white matter lesions are the hallmark of acute and relapsing multiple sclerosis, whereas the diffuse damage of 'normal' white matter is particularly prominent in the progressive stage of the disease.

DISTRIBUTION OF LESIONS IN THE NERVOUS SYSTEM

Plaques may appear randomly within the central nervous system, although certain locations in the brain and spinal cord are preferentially affected (Fog 1950; Ikuta and Zimmerman 1976; Lassmann 1983; Lumsden 1970; G. Steiner 1931).

Demyelination

In patients with chronic multiple sclerosis, there are two major sites of predilection within the forebrain hemispheres: the periventricular white matter and the cortico-subcortical white matter (Lumsden 1970; G. Steiner 1931). Other sites commonly affected are the optic nerves and chiasm, midbrain, pons and cerebellar white matter – in particular the cerebellar peduncles (Field 1979) – and medulla. There is a loose correlation between lesion load and clinical dysfunction, especially when patients with chronic relapsing and secondary progressive multiple sclerosis are compared (Gonzalez *et al* 1994). Although the largest lesions and the highest lesion volume are generally present in the periventricular white matter of the forebrain, lesion load – based on numbers of lesions per tissue weight – appears highest in the brainstem, especially the pons and medulla, in cases with very severe clinical disease (Lumsden 1970). This may, however, be a sampling error because such

cases generally show severe and atypical clinical disease and, thus, are likely to be over-represented in autopsy series. Similarly, lesions in the spinal cord may appear at any location (Fog 1950). However, when large numbers of lesions are analysed, demyelinated plaques cluster in the cervical spinal cord. In these areas, the majority of lesions are located in the lateral column and have a triangular or fanlike shape with the tip of the triangle pointing towards the centre of the cord (Oppenheimer 1978).

The topography of brain lesions within the central nervous system changes with disease chronicity and especially in relation to disease course. In patients with acute multiple sclerosis (Marburg type) and during the early stages of relapsing–remitting disease, demyelinated plaques are predominantly present in the deep white matter but also in grey matter of brainstem nuclei, whereas cortical lesions or plaques touching the inner or outer surface of the brain are rare. In contrast, patients with late chronic multiple sclerosis who have reached the progressive phase have a majority of lesions oriented towards the ventricular or meningeal surface of the central nervous system and, thus, show a very high frequency in the cerebral and cerebellar cortex. Chronic persistent inflammation in the ventricles and meningeal spaces appears to be a driving force for the gradual development and enlargement of demyelinated lesions in primary and secondary progressive multiple sclerosis (see below). The topography of lesions may also have a direct effect on disease severity and progression. Active lesions in the hypothalamus may lead to downregulation of mRNA for corticotropin-releasing hormone, thus reducing corticosteroid secretion. This pathological feature is associated with an unfavourable disease course (Huitinga *et al* 2004).

Vascular pathology

Whereas demyelination in multiple sclerosis is typically focal and restricted to sharply demarcated areas, inflammation is much more widespread. In particular, perivascular inflammatory infiltrates are not only present within demyelinated plaques but also abundant in the normal white matter. In addition, meningeal inflammation is regularly encountered. This widespread inflammation may be associated with extensive MRI abnormalities in brain areas that do not contain demyelinated plaques (Newcombe *et al* 1991).

Peripheral nerve involvement

Pathological changes are often observed in the peripheral nervous system of patients with multiple sclerosis (Pollock *et al* 1977). The commonest alterations in the peripheral nerves are secondary changes due to very severe lesions in the spinal cord, those resulting from pressure damage of peripheral nerves in immobilized patients, and the consequences of metabolic disturbance and malnutrition (Hasson *et al* 1958). Thus, a moderate degree of axonal damage with secondary Wallerian (axonal) degeneration can be found in a large proportion of cases. Small series of cases have documented primary inflammatory demyelinating lesions in the peripheral nervous system of patients with multiple sclerosis (P.K. Thomas *et al* 1987) but primary inflammation and demyelination are rare in chronic multiple sclerosis (C.M. Poser 1987a). In a systematic survey of peripheral nerve involvement, Jellinger (1969) found only 1 of 70 cases with peripheral nerve lesions suggestive of a demyelinating disease. In this case, no active inflammation or demyelination was found and the peripheral nerve pathology consisted of abundant onion bulb-like lesions, suggesting repeated demyelination and remyelination. The relation of the lesion to the ongoing inflammatory demyelinating disease process in the central nervous system was not established, nor was it possible to exclude coincidental association with a genetic demyelinating polyneuropathy. But, noting that such lesions are infrequent in classical chronic multiple sclerosis, the spectrum of alterations in acute cases includes inflammation (Lassmann *et al* 1981a; Ninfo *et al* 1967; Pette 1928), primary demyelination (Dinkler 1904; Lassmann *et al* 1981a; Marburg 1906; Pollock *et al* 1977), plaquelike distribution of demyelinating lesions (Lassmann *et al* 1981a; Van Gehuchten 1966) and remyelination with the formation of onion bulb-like lesions (Dinkler 1904; Jellinger 1969; Pollock *et al* 1977; Schob 1923). Thus, in acute multiple sclerosis, these are almost invariable features when adequate sampling is performed, arising by the same pathogenic process that attacks the central nervous system. Inflammatory demyelinating lesions are randomly distributed throughout peripheral nerves, although the highest incidence of lesions is found in cranial and spinal roots.

Ocular involvement

Involvement of the eye in patients with multiple sclerosis is an interesting aspect of the disease because no (or very few) myelin sheaths are normally present. Inflammation affecting the retina, uveal tract and iris has been reported in patients with multiple sclerosis, but in the absence of myelin sheaths these lesions only show inflammation. The association of periphlebitis retinae with multiple sclerosis is still a matter of debate (see Chapter 6). Estimates for the incidence range from 10 to 45% (Annunziata *et al* 1988; Engell *et al* 1984; Lightman *et al* 1987; Rucker 1972). However, considering the transient nature of retinal inflammation in this disease, the actual incidence may be higher. On the other hand, it has to be considered that periphlebitis retinae is not specific for multiple sclerosis and may occur in infectious diseases, such as tuberculosis or sarcoidosis. Close similarities between the composition of inflammatory infiltrates in the retina and other brain regions in patients with multiple sclerosis suggest a common pathogenic background. Histological examination in a few cases reveals perivenous cuffing with lymphocytes, monocytes and plasma cells infiltrating the retina (P.J. Shaw *et al* 1987). As expected, chronic lesions are characterized by less cellular infiltration but more extensive perivascular scar tissue characterized by dense deposition of connective tissue.

Inflammation has also been observed in the uveal tract of patients with multiple sclerosis (Boskovich *et al* 1993). The incidence of these alterations ranges from 5 to 27% (Bammer *et al* 1965; Berger and Leopold 1968; Lightman *et al* 1987; Tschabitscher 1958). Iridocyclitis has been described at a similar frequency. Although, in general, the appearance of uveitis and iridocyclitis in multiple sclerosis are regarded as events unrelated to the primary pathogenesis, recent experimental evidence suggests an alternative explanation. In experimental autoimmune encephalomyelitis induced by T lymphocytes reactive against S100 protein (K. Kojima *et al* 1994), inflammatory lesions are not confined to the nervous system but also occur in the retina (periphlebitis retinae), uvea or iris.

Pathogenetic factors determining lesion topography

Clinical and experimental evidence indicates that many different factors are responsible for the precipitation of lesions at a given site in the brain of patients with multiple sclerosis. As noted in the earliest clinicopathological correlations (J. Dawson 1916; Rindfleisch 1863; Siemerling and Raecke 1914), multiple sclerosis plaques tend to develop around one or more centrally located venules or veins. For these reasons, brain and spinal cord areas with high densities of postcapillary venules and veins are more likely to contain plaques than others (Fog 1950). The brain regions with high densities of postcapillary venules are the periventricular white matter, cortical/subcortical border zone of the forebrain and white matter tracts of the spinal cord.

In addition, the close topographical relation of multiple sclerosis plaques to outer and inner surfaces of the brain and spinal cord suggested to other investigators that factors present in the cerebrospinal fluid might play some additional role in the precipitation of lesions (H. Pette 1928; G. Steiner 1931). Whereas adjacent small perivenous lesions in deep periventricular white matter sometimes fuse and appear secondarily to reach the ventricular surface (Adams *et al* 1987), in other cases periventricular lesions are primarily related to the ventricular surface. A possible explanation for this difference may lie in the relative contribution made by T-cell and antibody-mediated immune reactions to the pathogenesis of lesions at different sites in the central nervous system.

The principal orientation of lesions towards veins and brain surface areas does not account for the fact that they are focal and involve selected parts of the nervous system. Nor does it explain why, in patients with neuromyelitis optica, white matter lesions accumulate only in the spinal cord and optic system, whereas in chronic multiple sclerosis they preferentially affect the forebrain. Thus, there have to be additional precipitating factors determining the distribution of lesion formation. The topography of plaques in the spinal cord has led others to suggest that minor traumatic events may play a role (Oppenheimer 1978). We do not subscribe to this view. The argument goes that the precipitation of lesions in the lateral cervical spinal cord coincides with areas of highest tearing and shearing forces during head and neck movements. Focal traumatic events induce upregulation of histocompatibility antigens and, thus, locally precipitate inflammation in a state of latent autoimmunity (Hickey *et al* 1991). Trauma clearly does not precipitate the autoimmune reaction itself. We defer to the epidemiological evidence in failing to provide any direct evidence in support of this hypothesis and consider that, however deserving an unfortunate victim of multiple sclerosis may be for financial support, the scientific position cannot be jettisoned for the convenience of plaintiffs seeking compensation for their ailment through offices of the law (see Chapter 3).

An additional factor determining lesion topography in multiple sclerosis may be the antigen, recognized by T cells, responsible for induction of the inflammatory reaction. Certain patients develop a dominant form of disease in the spinal cord, whereas in others the majority of lesions are located in the periventricular white matter of the forebrain. By systematically studying lesion topography in experimental autoimmune encephalomyelitis induced by T-lymphocyte lines directed against different brain antigens, we found that antigen specificity of the pathogenic T cell profoundly influences the topography of lesions (T. Berger *et al* 1997). For example, T-lymphocyte lines that recognize antigens present in compact myelin (myelin basic protein or proteolipid protein) induce a disease that predominantly affects areas having very thick myelin sheaths, such as the spinal cord or brainstem. Conversely, those directed against myelin oligodendrocyte glycoprotein and myelin-associated glycoprotein, antigens present in equal amounts in thick or thin myelin sheaths, predominantly precipitate lesions in areas with many thin myelin sheaths, such as the periventricular or cerebellar white matter. Alternatively, autoimmunity against S100 protein leads to inflammation, more pronounced in the grey than white matter and also resulting in inflammation of the retina and uveal tract – areas devoid of myelin sheaths (K. Kojima *et al* 1994). For these reasons, it seems logical to propose that the topography of lesions in multiple sclerosis may reflect variations in the autoimmune spectrum recognized by autoreactive T lymphocytes. In line with this hypothesis, different forms of multiple sclerosis have been found to be associated with humoral immune responses against myelin basic protein or proteolipid protein (K.G. Warren *et al* 1994).

IS THERE EVIDENCE FOR AN INFECTIOUS AGENT IN THE LESIONS OF MULTIPLE SCLEROSIS?

There are a substantial number of claims for the presence of infectious agents in the brain lesions of multiple sclerosis (see Chapter 2; Carp *et al* 1972; Gudnardottir *et al* 1964; Perron *et al* 1992; Pertschuk *et al* 1976; G. Steiner 1931; Ter Meulen *et al* 1972; for review, see R.T. Johnson 1994). The spectrum of possible viral candidates is broad, ranging from paramyxovirus, herpes virus and retrovirus to prions. None of these virus isolations has been consistently reproduced in subsequent investigations, nor has it yet been possible to transmit the disease to experimental animals using defined pathogens. Nevertheless, this failure of Koch's postulates does not exclude the possibility that infections play a role either in the induction of disease, by triggering autoimmune reactions, or through direct invasion of the central nervous system. Thus, the search for possible infectious agents continues as part of epidemiological studies and by screening brain tissue from affected individuals (for reviews see: Ascherio and Munch 2000; Gilden 2002; Marrie and Wolfson 2001; I. Steiner *et al* 2001; Swanborg *et al* 2003). Here, we focus on attempts to detect infectious agents within the brain tissue of patients with multiple sclerosis.

With the introduction of electron microscopy in multiple sclerosis research, it became possible to search for viral structures within lesions. Indeed, in the early studies, nuclear and cytoplasmic inclusions attributed to paramyxovirus infections were reported (Dubois-Dalcq *et al* 1973; J. Kirk and Hutchinson 1978; Narang and Field 1973; Raine *et al* 1974a; I. Watanabe and Okazaki 1973). Most of these structures have subsequently been identified either as polymorphic myelin degradation products (Prineas 1975) or altered nuclear chromatin of activated cells,

accentuated during tissue autolysis (I. Allen 1991). Thus, ultrastructural studies provide little evidence for a direct role of virus infections in the pathogenesis of multiple sclerosis lesions.

It is possible that a chronic, persistent, nonreproductive virus infection recognized by the immune system as a target antigen for the inflammatory response remains to be detected, either by virus isolation or ultrastructural search for virus particles. In line with this hypothesis, the pathology of certain experimental models of virus-induced inflammatory demyelinating diseases closely resembles that of chronic autoimmune encephalitis or even multiple sclerosis itself (M. Rodriguez 1992). Indeed, the presence of virus-specific genomic material has been found in a proportion of multiple sclerosis cases by *in situ* hybridization (Cosby *et al* 1989; A.T. Haase *et al* 1981; R.S. Murray *et al* 1992).

Currently, three different infectious agents are the focus of interest: human herpes virus 6 (HHV 6), an endogenous retrovirus, and *Chlamydia pneumoniae* (see also Chapter 2). HHV 6 was first isolated from and detected by immunocytochemistry in the brain tissue of patients with multiple sclerosis but not controls (Chaloner *et al* 1995). Immunocytochemistry showed a peculiar granular staining pattern in the cytoplasm of oligodendrocytes and in neurons. Our own experience, using the same antibodies and immunocytochemical staining techniques, revealed that most of the reactivity seen in multiple sclerosis is due to nonspecific antibody binding to lipofuscin. Several investigators later used the polymerase chain reaction amplification and *in situ* staining of brain material and cerebrospinal fluid from patients with multiple sclerosis, but these have not settled the matter – not least because the presence of viral DNA is not disease specific (Blumberg *et al* 2000; Swanborg *et al* 2003). The situation with chlamydia is similar to HHV 6. Here too, initial claims for disease-specific infection in multiple sclerosis have not been substantiated and the jury remains out (Swanborg *et al* 2003). Endogenous retroviruses and their possible association with multiple sclerosis require more detailed consideration.

A replication competent retrovirus was first isolated from the meninges of an affected patient (Perron *et al* 1992). Later, many different endogenous retrovirus sequences were found by PCR in the brains of patients with a variety of different diseases. Overall, these studies are in agreement that in patients with multiple sclerosis – but probably also those with other inflammatory central nervous system diseases – these endogenous retrovirus sequences are expressed in significantly higher amounts than in noninflammatory controls (Perron *et al* 2005). Increased expression correlates with the degree of macrophage/microglia activation (Johnston *et al* 2001). Thus, the expression of endogenous retrovirus sequences, incorporated in every human genome, may be upregulated by proinflammatory cytokines. These antigens then become targets for specific cellular and humoral immune reactions, thus behaving as autoantigens (Christensen *et al* 2003; M. Clerici *et al* 1999; Jolivet-Reynaud *et al* 1999; Trabattoni *et al* 2000). Furthermore, some products of endogenous retrovirus sequences may act as superantigens (Perron *et al* 2001) inducing T-cell mediated brain damage in experimental models (Firouzi *et al* 2003). Although these effects are evidently not specific for multiple sclerosis, they could represent one additional factor potentiating central nervous system tissue damage. Focal immune stimulation within multiple sclerosis plaques may also be stimulated by bacterial products. Recently bacterial peptidoglycans have been identified in the lesions of multiple sclerosis trapped within cells having macrophage or dendritic cell characteristics, and expressing various proinflammatory cytokines and costimulatory molecules (I.A. Schrijver *et al* 2001). Such peptidoglycans are components of Gram-positive bacteria with potent proinflammatory properties. But it is not clear how these bacterial components reach the brain and whether they are footprints of systemic sepsis. Being present within the lesions, they may, however, promote the local inflammatory response by stimulating innate immunity.

In summary, despite the epidemiological clues, there is no secure evidence for an infectious aetiology in multiple sclerosis. But absence of evidence is not evidence of absence. Current technology does make it possible to conclude whether or not different agents are capable of reprogramming the immune system towards central nervous system autoimmunity through molecular mimicry in multiple sclerosis. A persistent noncytopathic infection by one or several pathogens may be present in the central nervous system of patients with multiple sclerosis, and recognized by the immune system as autoantigen, especially following rechallenge in the periphery by the same or a related infectious agent.

DYNAMIC EVOLUTION OF MULTIPLE SCLEROSIS PATHOLOGY

There is a wide spectrum of structural abnormalities in the inflammatory demyelinating lesions of patients with multiple sclerosis. In principle, this variation may be due to changes that take place during evolution of the lesions or of the disease itself. Alternatively, it may reflect disease subtypes or variant pathogenic mechanisms, operating in different patients. Attempts have been made to clarify the relative contribution of each aspect, and to establish a dynamic analysis of the pathogenesis of lesion formation and repair. For this purpose, evidence from highly informative biopsies and autopsies at different stages of the disease, together with serial MRI studies, have proved informative.

Dynamics of lesion formation

There is good agreement that tissue injury in multiple sclerosis lesions starts with inflammation, associated with leakage of the blood–brain barrier (Gonzalez-Scarano *et al* 1987; R.I. Grossman *et al* 1986; 1988; Kermode *et al* 1990; McDonald and Barnes 1989; D.H. Miller *et al* 1988b). The evidence comes from serial MRI studies showing that early gadolinium-DTPA leakage precedes structural change in T_2-weighted scans (J.O. Harris *et al* 1991; Kermode *et al* 1990). Biopsy samples taken from such lesions invariably show brain inflammation, although the extent and stage of demyelination are variable (Brück *et al* 1994; Estes *et al* 1990; Nesbit *et al* 1991). In particular, in a detailed study correlating post-mortem imaging with neuropathology (Newcombe *et al* 1991), extensive MRI abnormalities were found in the presence of very few and small demyelinated plaques. In addition, two sequential biopsies in the same patient initially showed an inflammatory process, which a few months later had developed into an inflammatory demyelinating plaque (Bitsch *et al* 1999). These observations suggest that whereas, at least in chronic relapsing and secondary progressive multiple sclerosis, demyelinating lesions are initiated by inflammation and blood–brain barrier damage, inflammation does not invariably lead to demyelination.

Recent observations challenge this concept. In some new lesions, gadolinium-DTPA leakage is sparse and follows the appearance of signal abnormalities in T_2-weighted images. In addition, neuropathological studies suggest that, at least in a subset of patients with multiple sclerosis, the sentinel plaques are characterized by demyelination, microglia activation and complement deposition, followed by substantial leucocyte infiltration of the tissue (De Groot *et al* 2001; Gay *et al* 1997). However, even in such lesions, inflammation is present at most initial stages of lesion formation (Gay *et al* 1997). Our position is that, initially, all lesions are driven by inflammation but with different subsequent pathways of evolution. In some, the process starts with massive inflammation followed by demyelination and tissue injury. These lesions are characterized on MRI by early gadolinium-DTPA leakage, followed by T_2-weighted signal abnormalities and pathological patterns I and II, described above. In other individuals, plaques initially start with a milder inflammatory response, microglia activation, demyelination and hypoxia-like tissue injury followed later by massive influx of inflammatory cells. These lesions appear as focal areas of enhancement on MRI; only at later stages do they show rather mild and spotty enhancement. The pathological correlate is hypoxia-like tissue injury (pattern III). Nothing is known so far on the MRI correlates of pattern IV lesions.

New imaging techniques (mainly fluid-attenuated inversion recovery sequences (FLAIR) and diffusion weighted images) show that, in yet other cases, signal abnormalities anticipate the formation of classical plaques by several weeks or months. Some observers have interpreted this observation as an indication that there is a primary phase of tissue degeneration with secondary inflammation, blood–brain barrier leakage and demyelination. Much the same issues arise in considering the pathology of primary progressive multiple sclerosis, where serial MRI reveals surprisingly small numbers of T_2-weighted lesions and very few areas of enhancement (A.J. Thompson *et al* 1991). This is, however, associated with more diffuse damage of the normal-appearing white and grey matter than can reasonably be explained on the basis of damage emanating from focal plaques (Peletier *et al* 2003; Rocca *et al* 2003c). This observation forms the basis for proposing that the pathogenesis of multiple sclerosis includes a degenerative component independent of inflammation, extending beyond the classical focal demyelinated plaque. But pathological analysis does not support this notion. In primary progressive multiple sclerosis, although the intensity is reduced compared with other forms of multiple sclerosis, inflammation is present in all cases and at all stages (Brück *et al* 2003; Revesz *et al* 1994). Furthermore, despite rigorous searching, pathologists working over the last 100 years have found no evidence for this putative neurodegenerative process occurring in the absence of inflammation and reactive changes affecting microglia. Our position is that the formation of new lesions and propagation of chronic central nervous system damage in multiple sclerosis are driven by the inflammatory process.

It is therefore important to consider for how long the lesions in chronic relapsing multiple sclerosis stay active with respect to inflammation, blood–brain barrier damage and demyelination. Serial MRI generally reveals increased blood–brain barrier permeability within single lesions for several weeks or longer (Kermode *et al* 1990; D.H. Miller *et al* 1992). High-dose corticosteroid treatment decreases gadolinium enhancement within the lesions and this correlates with clinical recovery (Barkhof *et al* 1992; Burnham *et al* 1991; D.H. Miller *et al* 1992). However, gadolinium-DTPA leakage may reappear within a few days of discontinuing steroid treatment. Taken together, these data suggest that individual episodes of inflammatory activity in relapsing–remitting multiple sclerosis may be brief in some patients but, in others, can persist for many weeks.

Dynamics of demyelination and remyelination

Once initiated, the destruction of myelin appears to be a very rapid process. In experimental systems, immune-mediated destruction of myelin is accomplished within a few hours (Lassmann *et al* 1988; Linington *et al* 1988). Although no data are available from patients with multiple sclerosis, there is no reason to believe that the dynamics of myelin destruction are different. Remyelination may also be a very rapid process. In experimental models, remyelination starts within a few days of myelin sheath destruction and can be completed within one week (Linington *et al* 1988). This is not dependent on the fate of oligodendrocytes during the demyelinating episode because the extent and speed of remyelination mainly depend upon the recruitment of glial progenitors and this is rapid, even with complete destruction of mature oligodendrocytes in the core lesion (Linington *et al* 1992; Ludwin 1980).

Although the evidence is indirect, the same dynamics of remyelination apply to the lesions of multiple sclerosis. Extensive remyelination of axons is seen in close apposition to macrophages containing myelin degradation products in cases of acute multiple sclerosis and those with early bouts of chronic disease (Brück *et al* 1994; Lassmann 1983; Ozawa *et al* 1994; Prineas *et al* 1993a). Thus, the rapid recovery of patients with multiple sclerosis from early bouts of the disease may not only be due to clearance of inflammation and oedema, and to plasticity in association with redistribution of sodium channels (see Chapter 13) but also to remyelination and lesion repair. This analysis is further supported by correlative studies of MRI and neuropathology, showing that the normalization of T_1 signal intensity in fresh black holes is associated with the clearance of oedema and with remyelination (Bitsch *et al* 2001). However, plaques that arise late in disease evolution generally show more persistent demyelination (Ozawa *et al* 1994).

Dynamic changes during disease evolution

There are two pathological aspects that change during the long-term evolution of multiple sclerosis. The first relates to axonal loss and brain atrophy, and the second to oligodendrocyte depletion and remyelination. Brain atrophy is a characteristic feature of the neuropathology in patients who have longstanding and severe disease. It apparently reflects the progressive destruction and loss of axons during active phases of plaque formation. This leads to secondary Wallerian (axonal) degeneration of white matter tracts and eventually to neuronal loss and atrophy of grey matter. In addition, diffuse inflammatory myelin and axonal damage in the normal-appearing white matter, characteristic features of progressive multiple sclerosis, contribute to the accumulation of atrophy. The final result of these injuries is summarized under the designation of multiple scle-

rosis encephalopathy (see above; Jellinger 1969; Seitelberger 1973).

The extent of axonal destruction in multiple sclerosis lesions differs between patients but is consistent across different plaques in the same individual. Losseff *et al* (1996a) have shown that an increase in cerebral atrophy (as measured by MRI) occurred in 16/29 patients over as short a time as 18 months. Axon loss and secondary brain atrophy are more reliable markers of disability in multiple sclerosis than the total number or collective lesion load (E. Fisher *et al* 2000). Axonal and neuronal loss, resulting in brain atrophy, start early in the course of the disease. Thus, significant acute axonal injury occurs in every new plaque formed at onset or during the course of the disease (B. Ferguson *et al* 1997; Kornek *et al* 2000; Trapp *et al* 1998). It has been suggested that lesions that develop early are more aggressive than those formed later (Bitsch *et al* 2000b). This observation may, however, incorporate a sampling error because autopsies or biopsies at early stages of multiple sclerosis generally come from patients with exceptionally severe disease course. Due to the high reserve capacity of the central nervous system, axonal loss only leads to permanent clinical deficit at later stages, and when a critical threshold of nerve fibre degeneration is surpassed (Bjartmar *et al* 2003).

Whereas the increase in brain atrophy during multiple sclerosis disease evolution merely reflects the accumulated burden of axonal and neuronal loss, differences in the degree of oligodendrocyte damage seen at different stages of the disease may indeed reflect a dynamic evolution in the pathogenesis. Overall, chronic multiple sclerosis appears to start as a disease of myelin, in which oligodendrocytes are often preserved. Only in more severe cases are they destroyed early together with other tissue elements. But with further evolution of the disease process, the destructive force increasingly focuses on the myelin–oligodendrocyte complex, resulting finally in persistent demyelinated lesions, devoid of oligodendrocytes and without significant remyelination. Both the dense fibrillary gliosis within the plaques and the depletion of oligodendrocyte progenitors contribute to this lack of repair. Over and above these factors, a profound change in the immunopathogenesis must occur to explain the substantial variation in oligodendrocyte destruction that characterizes active demyelination in lesions arising early and late in the disease process. In experimental models, antigen and epitope spreading lead to broadening of the immune response during the evolution of chronic experimental autoimmune encephalomyelitis (Lehmann *et al* 1992). Similar mechanisms may operate in multiple sclerosis as new cellular reactions (possibly directed against stress proteins: Van Noort *et al* 1995) and humoral immune responses (induction of antibodies against myelin or oligodendrocyte progenitor cells: Niehaus *et al* 2000; J. Sun *et al* 1991) are recruited. Thus, it is not surprising that patients with chronic multiple sclerosis mount a very broad autoimmune response against a multitude of different central nervous system antigens (Olsson 1992).

DIFFERENCES BETWEEN ACUTE, RELAPSING AND PROGRESSIVE MULTIPLE SCLEROSIS

Due to the paucity of available biopsy and autopsy material, pathological studies in multiple sclerosis mainly concentrate on the two prototypic stages of the disease. Most autopsy material comes from patients with the late stage of chronic (and mostly secondary progressive) disease. Many of these cases are burnt out, with very little evidence for ongoing demyelination or tissue damage. Thus, studies on immunologically active phases of the disease mainly depend on patients with fulminant acute multiple sclerosis or with aggressive relapsing disease. Most of our knowledge derives from these cases. The lessons are that acute and early relapsing multiple sclerosis is mainly a white matter disease, characterized by the formation of new foci of perivenous inflammation, resulting in dispersion of the inflammatory infiltrates into the surrounding tissue and leading to primary demyelination with some associated axonal injury and loss. In these stages of the disease, inflammation and tissue injury are mainly concentrated in the plaques, while the white and grey matter outside the plaque remains more or less normal.

In brain autopsies sampled at much later stages of the disease – the burnt-out cases – there is persistent inflammation and numerous inactive demyelinated and sclerotic plaques. This is associated with global damage to the brain, reflected by microglia activation, diffuse white and grey matter atrophy and astrocyte scarring (I.V. Allen *et al* 2001). This diffuse damage, epitomized by the multiple sclerosis encephalopathy, is generally regarded by neuropathologists as a secondary consequence of tissue damage in the demyelinated plaques. But to us, this simplistic view seems to be incorrect for several reasons.

Although there is clear evidence that diffuse white matter injury can be the result of secondary Wallerian degeneration in multiple sclerosis (Evangelou *et al* 2000a), there are also cases in which the lesion load is so small that the extensive brain atrophy cannot be explained on the basis of secondary damage in plaques (Bozzali *et al* 2002). This is particularly evident in cases with primary progressive multiple sclerosis. Brain atrophy (reflected by loss of brain volume) occurs very early, at a stage where the diffuse volume loss cannot reasonably be attributed to focal demyelination in plaques (Filippi *et al* 2003; Lassmann 2003b). Furthermore, the neuropathology has to account for the fact that clinical progression in primary or secondary progressive multiple sclerosis generally occurs on the background of minimal MRI-defined disease activity.

For these reasons, the pathology of primary progressive multiple sclerosis is especially illuminating. Do we find a pathological process in primary progression that is different from that responsible for the development of classical plaques in acute and relapsing multiple sclerosis? To address this question, a subset of patients with a typical clinical and pathological profile has to be studied selectively. The informative cohort has primary progressive disease without relapses and remissions, leading to significant permanent neurological deficit after several years. The cerebrospinal fluid alterations are typical for multiple sclerosis, with positive oligoclonal bands. MRI shows a low lesion load but with additional diffuse abnormalities of the normal-appearing white matter.

At first sight, the pathology in these cases shows the expected changes – a chronic inflammatory process with associated multiple plaques of demyelination. Axonal injury and loss are variable and similar to other cases of multiple sclerosis, any differences being quantitative rather than qualitative. Inflammation in the plaques is significantly less pronounced. Their number and size are smaller with less axonal injury (Brück *et al* 2003; Revesz *et al*

1994). Thus, neither specific features of the plaques nor their location to strategic sites of the central nervous system can account for the clinical phenotype of primary progressive multiple sclerosis. Rather, this seems to have its explanation in the involvement of the normal-appearing white matter and patterns of demyelination in the cerebral cortex (Figure 12.14).

The normal-appearing white matter in progressive multiple sclerosis shows a diffuse inflammatory process throughout the whole brain, mainly due to perivascular accumulation and diffuse tissue infiltration by class I MHC-restricted T cells. This is matched by profound activation of the whole microglia population associated with widely distributed injury and destruction of single nerve fibres. These pathological features appear as diffuse myelin pallor and reactive gliosis throughout the whole hemispheric white matter. Cortical atrophy on MRI correlates with profound grey matter involvement in primary progressive multiple sclerosis extending outside the regions of abnormal white matter. Extensive large bandlike demyelinated plaques affecting the outer three to five layers may be seen in up to 50% of the cortex. Microglia are highly activated and apparently the major cell type involved in the process of myelin destruction and tissue injury because these cortical plaques show very little lymphocyte infiltration, even during the stage of active demyelination. But, significantly, these are always orientated towards foci of persistent inflammation in the overlying meninges.

Thus far, the immunological mechanisms responsible for diffuse injury in the grey and white matter lesions of primary progressive multiple sclerosis are not characterized. The evidence suggests a role for soluble factors produced by meningeal inflammatory cells acting on microglia, with cytotoxic T cells making an additional contribution in the white matter. The most striking feature is the ubiquitous expression of iNOS in microglia, unlike acute and relapsing multiple sclerosis in which the detection of iNOS is moderate and confined to the edges of active plaques. This is also reflected by biochemical evidence for nitrosative damage in the normal appearing white matter (Bizzozero *et al* 2005). A possible role of nitric oxide and oxygen radical induced mitochondrial injury in the pathogenesis of diffuse white matter injury in progressive multiple sclerosis is also suggested by the marked upregulation of genes involved in (hypoxic) tissue preconditioning (Graumann *et al* 2003). That said, more detailed analysis reveals that similar patterns are observed in secondary progressive multiple sclerosis, albeit in the context of many classical demyelinating plaques.

All these observations suggest that the classical demyelinated plaques are initiated by new foci of vascular inflammation, associated with blood–brain barrier damage, dispersion of inflammatory cells into the parenchyma and the induction of tissue damage through cytotoxic T cells, activated macrophages/ microglia and specific antibodies. Conversely, in progressive multiple sclerosis, the inflammatory reaction is already established and chronically active within the central nervous system such that new vascular inflammatory foci with blood–brain barrier damage are rare. The compartmentalized inflammation is mainly present in the meninges and the perivascular Virchow–Robin spaces and may form local, and hence ectopic, B-cell follicles with germinal centres (Serafini *et al* 2004). These local inflammatory cells produce factors that, directly or indirectly through microglia activation, lead to slow-burning chronic enlargement of existing demyelinated plaques (Prineas *et al* 2001), diffuse axonal injury within the plaques (Kornek *et al* 2000), nerve fibre degeneration in the normal-appearing white matter, and massive demyelination and atrophy of the cerebral cortex.

The vascular inflammatory process of acute and relapsing multiple sclerosis is evidently a more accessible target for anti-inflammatory treatment (see Chapter 16) unlike the compartmentalized inflammatory process in progressive multiple sclerosis. We recently had an opportunity to study the brain autopsy of a patient with primary progressive multiple sclerosis, dying 4 weeks after autologous bone marrow transplantation. As expected, classical perivascular inflammatory infiltrates were sparse or absent. However, despite the intense immunosuppressive therapy, diffuse inflammation of the white matter by cytotoxic T cells and massive microglia activation were no different from untreated cases – as were the slow-burning enlargement of some demyelinated plaques and diffuse nerve fibre injury in the normal-appearing white matter.

MOLECULAR APPROACHES TO THE STUDY OF THE MULTIPLE SCLEROSIS LESION: PROFILING OF TRANSCRIPTOME AND PROTEOME

In contrast to other human inflammatory diseases affecting skin, muscle, gut or liver, the pathological lesions in multiple sclerosis are sacrosanct and often inaccessible. Brain biopsies are taken only in exceptional circumstances. As a result, fresh tissue samples are generally not available for research purposes and exploration of the pathogenesis in intact tissue depends much on the use of experimental models, which allow reasonable extrapolation to the human disease, and the morphological study of autopsy material.

Immunocytochemistry and *in situ* hybridization

The application of immunocytochemistry to studies on multiple sclerosis tissue, which started in the late 1970s, has to a large extent broadened our understanding of the inflammatory nature of the disease and of the mechanisms of tissue injury and repair. With the availability of new and better antibodies and the adaptation of *in situ* hybridization techniques for human archival biopsy and autopsy material, these techniques are major tools for research in studies aimed to clarify the nature and pathogenesis of the lesions in multiple sclerosis. But there are limitations relating to sensitivity and specificity, in particular when these techniques are applied to archival autopsy material. In addition, the methods are in essence qualitative and very limited in providing information on quantitative differences in the expression patterns of different proteins or their respective mRNAs.

The common view amongst immunologists and molecular biologists is that analysis of unfixed fresh-frozen tissue material is most suitable for detecting antigens or mRNAs in tissue sections. There are, however, major limitations with this approach in its application to neuropathology of human disease. First and most obvious is the apparent problem of access to well-preserved frozen material from human autopsies and biopsies. Reasonable preservation of frozen tissue can only be achieved in small tissue

blocks and when special care is taken in snap freezing the material. This is a major obstacle in multiple sclerosis where, even in a single plaque, the stages of demyelinating activity or the structural patterns of tissue injury may show regional differences. Furthermore, even under the best conditions of tissue preservation, structural integrity of the tissue in frozen material is at best suboptimal, creating problems with precise classification of lesions and the unambiguous identification of immunoreactive cells. Finally, nonspecific binding of antibodies is not uncommon in tissue sections of fresh-frozen material. For all these reasons it is not surprising that many results have proved difficult to reproduce.

The situation is different when formaldehyde-fixed and paraffin-embedded materials are used. Such material is abundantly available in the archives of neuropathological laboratories and the preservation of tissue is limited only by the pre-mortem condition of the patient and the post-mortem autolysis time, factors that also limit the use of frozen material. Immunocytochemistry and *in situ* hybridization can be performed on large tissue sections, including hemispheric or double hemispheric brain sections. Obviously, some antigens are denatured by the fixation and embedding procedure, but many of these can be restored by recently developed methods of antigen retrieval; or specific staining can be achieved by selecting antibodies that recognize epitopes not affected by denaturation of the respective protein. A major limiting factor for the use of embedded material is the time to formaldehyde fixation. Satisfactory results can be achieved when material is used that has been embedded within one week of formaldehyde fixation, and when staining conditions are optimized by selecting suitable antibodies and defining for each individual antibody the most suitable method of antigen retrieval. Short formaldehyde fixation and a standardized embedding protocol are also instrumental in preservation of mRNA and DNA in archival tissue material. If done properly, *in situ* hybridization as well as DNA and RNA extraction can be achieved satisfactorily.

Immunocytochemistry and *in situ* hybridization on human brain tissue have proved successful but nonetheless largely descriptive and limited to elucidating static features of the evolving disease processes and associated interactions between individual cellular elements. However, developments in molecular genetics seem poised to break down these barriers. Using available post-mortem material, it is now possible to establish global profiles of gene expression in tissue, and at the single cell level. Even more intriguing, the 'dead' material can be called back to life and various expression systems used to ascertain the functions of these genes.

Microarrays: scanning the transcriptome

Microarrays exploit knowledge of the identification of genes accumulated through sequencing of genomes. The principle of microarray technology is simple. Minute samples of available genes – as complementary DNA (cDNA) or oligonucleotides – are printed on glass or plastic surfaces to form a delicate filigree. Contemporary arrays print tens of thousands of individual spots on a single glass, plastic or silicon grid. For gene profiling, mRNA is extracted from a tissue or cell sample, and reverse transcribed to cDNA. These molecules are fluorochrome labelled and layered over the chips to allow each individual cDNA to search for and bind its best fitting spot on the microarray. After washing, the loaded microarray is screened in a fluorescence scanner to determine the relative number of red, green or yellow bound fluorescent cDNA probes. Localization of an individual spot identifies the gene in question. Everything is done robotically using automated high throughput photosensor technology.

One strategy for relating gene expression to function involves direct comparison of gene profiles between samples that represent a difference of interest. This might be affected versus normal tissue, or plaques from different stages of the disease process and locations. cDNA preparations from each source are then labelled with two distinct fluorochromes, adjusted to similar concentrations, mixed and layered on a microchip. The ratio between fluorescent colours reflects differential binding and thus indicates increased, decreased or unchanged transcription of a particular gene. Thus stated, gene profiling by microchip arrays seems powerful, easy and plausible. But there are considerable limitations. One is the information technology resource needed to store and analyse the information in order to sort individual signals from noise and integrate findings into coherent gene clusters. Once a gene of potential interest has been spotted, its relevance must be examined by more conventional biological testing in the postgenomic phase. Any new and unexpected gene requires additional experimental approaches to confirm its significance. These may range from verification of the candidate gene in informative samples using real-time polymerase chain reaction, *in situ* hybridization or immunocytochemistry, to cell culture, transfection of the gene and the construction of transgenic mice.

Microdissection of single cells

Many investigators settle for establishing gene profiles in tissue samples. This approach, however, is limited by complexity of the sampled material. Even in health, most tissues comprise a multitude of cell components differing in lineage, activation state and age. Pathologically changed tissues are still more complex. In a tissue lesion, gene expression in autochthonous cells will be affected by degeneration and compensatory activation. In addition, exogenous infiltration from blood-borne inflammatory cells is to be expected. It is rarely possible to relate changed transcriptional patterns to individual cell components. Laser capture microdissection of single cells from a stained microscopic tissue slide offers one potential solution. The excised single cell sample is catapulted into a vial, to be further processed using reverse transcription and polymerase chain reaction methods. Single cell microdissection produces highly specific results, but the amount of mRNA/cDNA obtained is minute and usually insufficient to be combined with microarray analyses. Large numbers of individual cells can be excised and collected in the expectation that they exist in a similar functional state. Alternatively, mRNA of single cells can be amplified in order to obtain sufficient amounts of cDNA, keeping constant the quantitative proportion of individual mRNAs between the original cell extract and amplified material. Each strategy has met with success. In one report, a thousand small or large neurons were isolated from fixed and stained rat dorsal root ganglion slices by laser microdissection. The samples were pooled and subjected to microarray profiling (Luo *et al* 1999). Elsewhere, the preamplification approach was applied to char-

acterize neurons and their progenitors in the developing murine olfactory system (Tietjen *et al* 2003), and to distinguish different neurons from the rat hippocampus (Kamme *et al* 2003).

The quality of extracted mRNA is a factor limiting microdissection of human material. Especially in human post-mortem material, mRNA is often degraded to a degree that excludes polymerase chain reaction amplification and scanning of the transcriptome. Even so, this material can be used to study the more stable nuclear DNA. This allows the study of genes that undergo somatic recombination and/or mutation, as in T and B lymphocytes. Single cell microdissection followed by polymerase chain reaction amplification has been used to identify T-cell receptors in autoimmune infiltrates of the lesions in multiple sclerosis. Here, and in polymyositis, the T-cell receptors of single CD8 T cells infiltrating brain and muscle, respectively, were amplified, used to characterize the individual immune repertoire, and followed over time using complementarity-determining region 3 spectratyping (Babbe *et al* 2000; Hofbauer *et al* 2003).

What has microarray analysis contributed thus far to the study of multiple sclerosis? Using a microarray of 9000 cDNA probes, Whitney *et al* (1999) compared gene expression profiles between a plaque and normal white matter. As expected from morphological experience, a considerable number of genes were enhanced in multiple sclerosis, many of potential relevance to inflammation (Duffy chemokine receptor, interferon regulatory factor-2 (IRF-2), and TNF-R p75). More recent reports addressing differential gene expression sharpened the focus. The core of floridly active lesions displayed dynamic transcription of proinflammatory cytokine genes and related members of their activation cascade whereas silent plaques displayed a heterogeneous set of gene expressions, including IL-17, TGF-β and structures involved in scar formation (Lock *et al* 2002; Mycko *et al* 2004).

Several recent studies have examined the therapeutic effect of IFN-β on peripheral blood immune cells from patients with multiple sclerosis. Searching for effects on the Th1 phenotype of CD4 T cells, Wandinger *et al* (2001) described upregulation of Th1 cytokines (IL-12 β chain) and functional surface markers (chemokine receptor CCR5). Upregulation of Th1-related genes was also noted in a Japanese study (Koike *et al* 2003). Gene profiles have been used to compare responses to therapy and magnetic resonance imaging lesions. Differences between blood cells from responders and nonresponders to IFN-β were reported but the correlation between *in vitro* and *ex vivo* patterns remained ambiguous, with conspicuous differences between individual patients (Stürzebecher *et al* 2003). A longitudinal study of changes in peripheral blood cells in response to IFN-β treatment showed increased expression of genes involved in antiviral responses and in interferon signalling as well as in lymphocyte activation (Weinstock-Guttman *et al* 1997). To what extent these changes are related to the therapeutic effect in patients with multiple sclerosis is so far unclear.

Functional expression studies

The identification of potentially interesting genes in pathological tissue is a means, not an end in itself, providing a basis for further functional studies. This is certainly true for global transcriptome profiling by microarrays, and for polymerase chain reaction analyses of single cells in histological slides. One instructive example is given by the detection of osteopontin as a component in the inflammatory tissue in autoimmune disease of the central nervous system. Osteopontin did not start life as an immune molecule. It was discovered as a glycoprotein involved in bone (re-)modelling (Oldberg *et al* 1986), and only later found in freshly activated T lymphocytes (Patarca *et al* 1989). But in a recent microarray study of lesions in multiple sclerosis, osteopontin emerged as a strongly upregulated gene, and its potential relevance held up in histological analyses derived from these studies (Chabas *et al* 2001; Tajouri *et al* 2005; Sinclair *et al* 2005). Increased osteopontin levels were found in the plasma of patients with relapsing–remitting but not those with progressive multiple sclerosis (Vogt *et al* 2003). More telling, osteopontin-deficient knockout mice proved resistant to active induction of experimental autoimmune encephalomyelitis, possibly by preferential activation of protective Th2 T cells (Chabas *et al* 2001).

Applying the strategy of resurrecting gene functions from post-mortem samples, paired T-cell receptor (TCR) α and β chains have been cloned from one CD8 T cell in a patient with acute polymyositis. The 'donor' T cell qualified as a putative autoimmune effector cell, because it infiltrated a muscle fibre. Furthermore, the receptor was part of an expanded T-cell clone (Dornmair *et al* 2003). Paired TCR genes can now readily be used in functional studies – introduced to a cellular read-out system by transfection, in order to screen for potential target autoantigens, and eventually used to provide ultimate proof of T cell pathogenicity through the creation of TCR transgenic mice.

Probing the universe of proteins: proteomics

The investigation of transcriptomes gets one step closer to the issue of functional relevance for gene expression profiles in a cell or given tissue. However, not every transcription event leads to equally efficient protein synthesis. For many questions, including post-translational protein modification, direct information on the protein composition of cells is preferable. Recent progress in protein isolation and sequence determination brings closer this aim. A typical approach is to identify the proteome of a small tissue sample starting with the isolation of protein from the sample, and separation into single protein components by two-dimensional gel electrophoresis. Present technology allows resolution to roughly one thousand single spots, in patterns that are highly reproducible. Stability of the pattern formation, identified by computer-assisted imaging, is a key issue since it is the basis for declaring newly appearing or disappearing spots between samples. The next and decisive step is elution of protein from identified gel spots and matrix-assisted laser desorption/ionization (MALDI) mass spectroscopy. Minute amounts of homogeneous protein are sufficient for sequencing using modern hardware. Mass spectroscopy identifies protein sequences of lengths that allow determination of the protein by screening suitable databases.

Strategies for informative proteomics present no fewer challenges than for transcriptome profiling. Since quality and definition of the starting material are of crucial importance, combining protein scanning with single cell or even subcellular technologies remains a methodological challenge likely to be tackled by microdissection (Craven *et al* 2002; Gillespie *et al*

2002) and the use of subcellular structures (Théry *et al* 2002). At first, changes of gene expression during cellular development and differentiation, often paired with transcriptome analyses using cDNA or oligonucleotide microarrays, were used to validate the applications of this technology (Zucchi *et al* 2001). After some delay, proteomics has entered research in multiple sclerosis. A recent study used protein (not gene) microarrays in an effort to identify central nervous system structures that could be used for self-tolerizing immunotherapies. The strategy was to use myelin proteome arrays to identify autoantibodies appearing in SJL mice after immunization with diverse myelin components. The microchips were produced – following the principles of cDNA arrays – by depositing peptide and proteins on 'sticky' slides, and probing for binding of putative autoantibodies in experimental sera. This study shows that the evolution of chronic autoimmune encephalomyelitis is associated with an extensive intra- and intermolecular epitope spreading of autoreactive B-cell responses. The study further provided information on autoantigen profiles, which are applicable to the development of DNA vaccines designed to suppress autoimmune neuroinflammation (W.H. Robinson *et al* 2003).

ASSOCIATION OF MULTIPLE SCLEROSIS WITH OTHER DISEASES

From the pathological perspective, the association of multiple sclerosis with other diseases, especially those involving altered immune regulation, might identify factors that precipitate inflammatory demyelinating lesions in the nervous system, or reveal unexpected aspects of the aetiology and pathogenesis. No significant associations with putative autoimmune diseases have been identified with probands (see Chapter 6 for more detailed discussion), neoplasms (Currie and Urich 1974; K.L. Ho and Wolfe 1981) or other systemic diseases (for review, see Reder and Arnason 1985). There is, however, a decreased prevalence of IgE-mediated allergic diseases in patients with multiple sclerosis, suggesting some immunological deviation towards a predominant use of Th1-mediated immune responses (Oro *et al* 1996). In addition, some systemic factors are implicated in the precipitation of relapses in multiple sclerosis. Epidemiological studies support the role of infections, but not vaccinations, as triggers for disease activity (see Chapter 4). Taken with the evidence that systemic administration of IFN-γ may also induce relapses of the disease (Panitch *et al* 1987a; 1987b), generalized stimulation of the immune system appears to be an important factor in disease reactivation in patients with multiple sclerosis. Rarely, and in defined episodes presumably related to the inoculum, a disease that resembles multiple sclerosis can occasionally be induced by specific vaccinations. When they occur, the brain lesions that accompany vaccinations are generally characterized by inflammation and perivenous demyelination (acute postvaccinal or postinfectious leucoencephalomyelitis). Large demyelinated plaques are not normally present. However, widespread demyelination may be encountered when the vaccine contains central nervous system tissue and is applied serially over a period of several months. In these cases, the brain pathology is indistinguishable from the Marburg type of acute multiple sclerosis (Seitelberger 1967; Uchimura and Shiraki 1957).

The association of demyelinated plaques with other brain lesions is surprisingly low (I.V. Allen *et al* 1978; Jellinger 1969; Lumsden 1970). This may partly be due to the relatively low average age of patients with multiple sclerosis coming to autopsy. Additional stroke lesions or vascular malformations are occasionally revealed (Jellinger 1969). Although such lesions may sometimes colocalize with a demyelinated plaque, such a direct association is surprisingly rare. This indicates that blood–brain barrier damage at a given site of the central nervous system is not sufficient to precipitate demyelination in patients with multiple sclerosis – placing additional obstacles in the way of hypotheses that seek to establish a mechanistic link between trauma and multiple sclerosis. Another theory for the pathogenesis of multiple sclerosis, advanced in recent decades, is a possible disturbance of the neuroendocrine axis, resulting in dysregulation of the general immune response (for review, see T. Smith and Cuzner 1994). Indeed, some abnormalities in the immune system of patients with multiple sclerosis are suggestive. They include hints of a global defect in immune suppression (Reder and Arnason 1985), changes in β-adrenergic receptors on the lymphocytes of patients with multiple sclerosis (Zoukos *et al* 1994), and global changes in the corticosteroid responses. Reder *et al* (1994) reported that adrenal weight in patients with multiple sclerosis is on average 36% higher than controls. In addition, immunocytochemistry for hypothalamic corticotropin-releasing factor (CRF) has revealed a significant increase in immunoreactive neurons in patients with multiple sclerosis (Purba *et al* 1995). Both studies indicate that the neuroendocrine axis in patients with multiple sclerosis is overactivated, resulting in a perturbation of immune regulation. Alternatively, neuroendocrine abnormalities may be a secondary phenomenon due to defective glucocorticoid feedback regulation, as also described in patients with multiple sclerosis (Reder *et al* 1994).

CONCLUSION

Taken together, the pathology of multiple sclerosis consists of two essentially different features – the focal demyelinated plaque and the diffuse global brain injury. Both types of pathology occur on the background of an inflammatory response, dominated by T cells and activated macrophages or microglia.

Focal plaques are characterized by primary demyelination and astrocytic scarring. Although axons are partly preserved, their destruction and loss is present in variable extent in all lesions and seems to be an important correlate of permanent functional deficit in the patients. Focal plaques are heterogeneous between patients with respect to the dominant mechanisms of tissue injury as well as structural aspects, such as the extent of remyelination and axonal damage. New focal inflammatory demyelinating lesions may occur at any stage of the disease, but are most prominent in patients with acute or relapsing disease.

Diffuse brain injury seems to develop even during the relapsing phase of the disease, but is particularly prominent in patients with primary and secondary progressive multiple sclerosis. Global brain damage is mainly reflected by diffuse injury of the 'normal' white matter and by widespread subpial demyelination in the cerebral and cerebellar cortex. Diffuse white matter injury mainly affects axons in the absence of primary demyelination and is associated with global brain inflammation and microglia activation. It seems to develop through a slowly progressive accumulation of inflammatory cells behind an unimpaired or repaired blood–brain barrier.

The pathological features of these lesions suggest that new focal inflammatory demyelinating lesions may be well accessible for peripheral immunomodulatory or immunosuppressive therapies, since they form on the background of new waves of inflammation, entering the central nervous system at onset. In contrast, it seems unlikely that the compartmentalized inflammation, which accumulates behind an intact blood–brain barrier and is associated with global and diffuse brain injury particularly in the progressive stage of the disease, can be targeted with current anti-inflammatory treatments.

The pathophysiology of multiple sclerosis

13

Kenneth Smith, Ian McDonald, David Miller and Hans Lassmann

INTRODUCTION

Although the disease process in multiple sclerosis appears to be directed mainly against glial cells, the clinical features arise primarily from the electrophysiological consequences for axons. The effects can be profound, ranging from complete conduction block, to axonal hyperexcitability and the spontaneous generation of spurious, ectopic impulses. These particular changes are believed to result in the production of both 'negative' and 'positive' symptoms and signs – that is, the loss and gain of inappropriate function, respectively. While the conduction block can arise from factors such as demyelination, hyperexcitability is likely to represent a maladaptive response to demyelination, probably involving the expression of an inappropriate balance of ion channels across the segment of demyelinated membrane.

In previous years, attention focused on the conduction deficits arising directly from demyelination but, although these are still considered important in the pathophysiology of multiple sclerosis, our understanding has now widened to appreciate the additional contribution made by inflammatory mediators *per se*, axonal degeneration, and synaptic dysfunction resulting from cortical lesions. Thus a modern formulation recognizes that demyelination, inflammation, axonal degeneration and cortical lesions can result directly in major functional deficits, such as blindness, paralysis and numbness, as well as a range of more subtle deficits. This chapter summarizes our current understanding of how these factors affect neurons and axons, and how the resulting physiological changes result in the symptoms experienced by patients. As befits its longer research history, our understanding of how demyelination contributes to conduction deficits far surpasses current knowledge on the roles of inflammation and cortical lesions.

Diversity of symptoms and the disease course

Patients with multiple sclerosis can exhibit a surprising variety of symptoms and signs. One may be blind and another paralysed, numb, tingling or in pain. The explanation for this variety is mainly anatomical, arising from the distribution of lesions in different patients so that a range of separate pathways are disturbed and a variety of symptoms expressed, but it is also partly explained by the variety of conduction properties of affected axons.

Variability exists not only between patients, but also in the same individual at different times, as lesions affect new pathways and the clinical course changes. Early in the disease, a patient may have an episode resulting in paraplegia that may appear to recover completely within only a few weeks and remain stable thereafter for many years. Eventually, however, remissions may be incomplete, or absent, so that disability begins to accumulate and the disease enters a more progressive course. When they occur, remissions are believed to arise from a range of mechanisms including restoration of conduction due to the resolution of inflammation, axolemmal plasticity restoring conduction to the persistently demyelinated axon, adaptive synaptic changes, and repair by remyelination. However, over time these compensatory processes prove less effective and another factor gains dominance, namely axonal degeneration. In fact it is now clear that axons start to degenerate from very early in the disease, but the loss has to accumulate before becoming clinically apparent, due to inherent redundancy of the nervous system. Once the capacity of this protective reserve has been exceeded, additional degeneration results in a progressive deficit.

Do the lesions of multiple sclerosis cause the neurological deficit?

It may at first seem obvious that the lesions are themselves responsible for causing the neurological deficit in multiple sclerosis but, in fact, the correlation between lesions and deficit is not so close as might intuitively be expected. The explanation has several parts. It is certainly true that there can be an excellent correlation between the appearance of new lesions and the onset of a corresponding clinical deficit. This is well illustrated in pathways that are anatomically circumscribed, such as the optic nerve, and can be monitored using magnetic resonance imaging (MRI) techniques. Indeed, MRI has been particularly valuable in shaping our current understanding of the disease process (see below). MRI scanning of the optic nerves in a large cohort has shown that gadolinium enhancing lesions are present in the symptomatic nerve in almost all patients with acute optic neuritis (101/107, 94%: Kupersmith *et al* 2002). In a study of ten patients with optic neuritis, Youl *et al* (1991b) found that visual deficits were always initially associated with the presence of an enhancing lesion in the ipsilateral optic nerve (see below). In addition to poor vision, impaired conduction along the affected nerve fibres was also indicated by a reduction in amplitude of the visual evoked potential. Additional evidence that lesions can directly cause neurological deficits has been provided by the correlation of imaging abnormalities in the cervical dorsal root entry zone with the acute useless hand syndrome (D.H. Miller *et al* 1987a), and those in the medial longitudinal fasciculus associated with acute internuclear ophthalmoplegia (Ormerod *et al* 1987). Such observations provide convincing evidence that the lesions probably caused the functional deficits.

However, there may also be little difference in MRI appearance between patients with longstanding benign disease, and those with severe deficits. Thus although it is safe to say that, where a functional deficit exists, there will almost certainly also be a causal lesion, identifiable by MRI or autopsy, the reverse is not necessarily true. Indeed, it is common for patients to have lesions, perhaps many, but no discernible deficits. In these situations, the disparity between lesion load and severity of the clinical deficits can be explained by a combination of physiological recovery mechanisms and the location of lesions in clinically 'silent' areas of the brain. For example, many lesions occur in the periventricular white matter, producing deficits that often yield no symptoms or signs and, at best, are difficult to detect by either the patient or the physician, unless the lesions are very large. From such observations has emerged the clinical concept of the 'eloquent' and, conversely, the 'silent' or 'reticent' lesion. The high prevalence of silent lesions can explain why serial MRI examinations have revealed that patients may have ≥30 new inflammatory lesions in a single monosymptomatic episode (Figure 13.1; Isaac *et al* 1988; A.J. Thompson *et al* 1991; Willoughby *et al* 1989). The frequency of relapses therefore greatly underestimates the number of new lesions, and clinical episodes simply represent the (apparently) chance location of disease activity in a clinically eloquent pathway.

Apart from lesions in silent areas, there are also examples of demyelination affecting tracts from which clinical manifestations would ordinarily be expected but which, paradoxically, caused little or no neurological deficit during life (Gilbert and Sadler 1983; R.P. Mackay and Hirano 1967; Namerow 1972; Namerow and Thompson 1969; O'Riordan *et al* 1998a; Phadke and Best 1983; Ulrich and Groebke-Lorenz 1983). In the visual system, for example, vision has been found to be transmitted over an optic nerve that is completely demyelinated over a length of 1.2 cm (Ulrich and Groebke-Lorenz 1983). The presence of such lesions poses a problem because it is difficult to believe that large lesions can form suddenly in eloquent pathways and yet produce no symptoms at onset. It follows that they may grow gradually. In this case, those axons that were demyelinated first might regain the ability to conduct (see below) before other axons were demyelinated. In this way, the number of blocked axons could remain below the threshold necessary for a clinical deficit to become apparent.

It is not clear whether this reasoning might provide a plausible explanation for the observations of Rivera-Quinones *et al* (1998). These investigators report the absence of neurological deficit in major histocompatibility complex (MHC) class I-deficient mice with Theiler's murine encephalomyelitis, despite the presence of substantial demyelinating lesions in the spinal cord (Figure 13.2). The lesions would normally have been expected to cause significant deficits, as indeed occurred in mice with similar lesions that expressed class I molecules. Lesions in the Theiler's model tend to form more slowly than is typical for rodent

models of experimental autoimmune encephalomyelitis. It is therefore possible that the number of nonfunctioning axons present at any one time had always remained below the level required to detect the deficit, especially when difficulties of the murine neurological examination are taken into account. The findings are all the more intriguing when the electrophysiological findings are considered. Given the extent of demyelination it is surprising that the authors did not find a conduction delay in the class I-deficient mice, although more sophisticated tests for detecting an electrophysiological deficit (such as the refractory period of transmission) were not performed. The absence of neurological deficits specifically in class I-deficient mice focuses attention on the role of CD8$^+$ T cells (see below).

In summary, although it is clear that the lesions of multiple sclerosis can, and often do, directly cause symptoms, this is not always the case even when the lesions are large and located in pathways that are normally clinically eloquent. In these latter lesions, function must be restored, or retained, by the mechanisms described later in this chapter.

METHODS FOR EXPLORING THE PATHOPHYSIOLOGY OF MULTIPLE SCLEROSIS

It is not possible to predict with any certainty the conduction properties of pathological axons based on their morphological appearance, but a range of electrophysiological techniques are available that can examine axonal function. Here, we describe the increasing detail of information that can be gained by methods that, usually, depend upon increasing disturbance of tissue structure and function.

Electrophysiological techniques

A superficial indication of axonal function can be gained from intact preparations, be they human or animal, by simple observation and neurological examination. Paralysis, blindness and numbness, for example, demonstrate loss of function, and loosely imply loss of axonal function, but axonal damage is, of course, not the only possible explanation. A more direct assessment of function can be obtained by examination of evoked potentials.

Evoked potentials

Evoked potentials are typically obtained by repeatedly presenting a stimulus and then averaging the evoked changes in electrical potential recorded from the activated part of the nervous system. The stimulus employed is simply one that is appropriate for the pathway to be studied. Thus, to record a visual evoked potential a light flash can repeatedly be shone into the eyes, although superior results are often obtained with a higher contrast stimulus, such as that obtained by a reversing chequerboard, namely a stimulus composed of many black and white squares, continuously illuminated but repeatedly and suddenly reversed in colour. Recording electrodes are applied to the scalp, typically near the visual cortex, although with sufficient averaging a signal of some sort can be recorded from almost any location on the body (even away from the head). Averaging is a very powerful way of discerning the usually small-

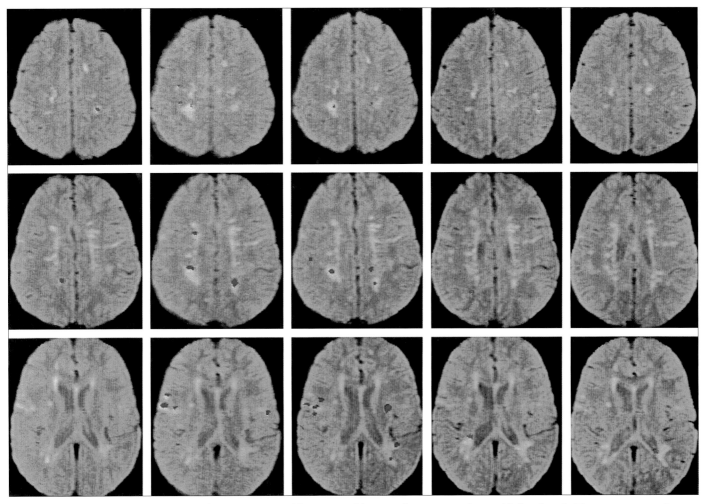

Figure 13.1 Serial enhanced MRI scans from a 25-year-old woman with secondary progressive multiple sclerosis. The scans were taken approximately every 4 weeks, and are presented in five columns. Areas of enhancement are superimposed in red on the unenhanced scans; enhancement typically persists for a particular lesion for approximately 1 month. New lesions are frequent and during the 6-month study period this patient developed 97 new lesions, but only suffered two clinical relapses.

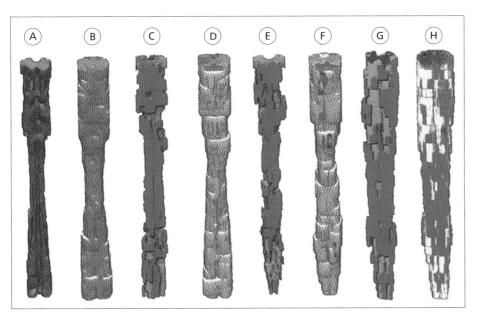

Figure 13.2 Three-dimensional reconstruction of demyelinated lesions from mice chronically infected with the Theiler's murine encephalomyelitis virus model of demyelination. Non-mutant mice (A and B) show no demyelination, but class I-deficient (C and D), SJL/J (E and F) and class II-deficient (G and H) mice show similar demyelination. The class I-deficient mice were functionally normal. Green = grey matter; white = white matter; red = demyelinated lesions. From Rivera-Quinones *et al* (1998) with permission.

amplitude (microvolts) evoked signals that may be totally hidden in electrically noisy records. A computer is used to sum the electrical signals that are linked to the stimulus, and the electrical noise is progressively eliminated because it is not time-locked and so tends to average to zero over time. The sensitivity of the technique can lead to unintended artefacts: it is possible to obtain a spurious 'visual' evoked potential in a patient lacking eyes if the change in visual stimulus is accompanied by an audible mechanical click (in reality, an auditory evoked potential).

True auditory evoked potentials can be obtained in response to deliberate click stimuli applied by headphones, and somatosensory evoked potentials by, for example, electrical stimulation of selected peripheral nerves (such as the median or posterior tibial, depending on clinical need), or mechanical tapping of the fingernails. In the latter cases, recordings can be made over the somatosensory cortex, or earlier along the conduction pathway by recording over the spinal cord. The pattern of evoked waveforms is reasonably uniform between different normal individuals, allowing the discrimination of changes in the waveform in response to disease. If the pathway examined is affected by the lesions of multiple sclerosis, the major components of the waveform can be delayed or diminished (or may be absent), and these changes are typically interpreted as indicating conduction slowing due to demyelination, and conduction failure due to demyelination and/or axonal degeneration, respectively. Whether such straightforward interpretations are routinely correct is questionable, but they have important diagnostic value nonetheless.

The first evoked potentials to be examined employed sensory pathways, as described above, but it is also possible to examine motor evoked potentials. These can be derived from magnetic stimulation of motor pathways, with recording from the musculature. The study of motor evoked potentials tends to be of more limited value in multiple sclerosis because abnormalities in the records are usually only found when abnormalities can also be detected by clinical examination.

Evoked potentials provide only an indirect indication of axonal function, because abnormal records can result from different kinds of pathology. In recent years, a much more direct and detailed assessment of axonal function has arisen from the study of stimulus-response characteristics and threshold electrotonus (M.C. Kiernan *et al* 2001). However, at present these techniques cannot be applied to the study of axons within the central nervous system, and so they are of limited value with regard to the study of multiple sclerosis.

Chronic implantation

More detailed recordings can be obtained by chronically implanting stimulating and/or recording electrodes on parts of the nervous system (Felts *et al* 1992; K.J. Smith *et al* 1979). Recordings are usually made during intermittent periods of general anaesthesia. An advantage of chronically implanted preparations is that the records obtained can be highly reproducible over months so that small alterations are reliably monitored and interpreted. It is therefore possible serially to examine the changing conduction properties of pathological axons as they pass through different stages, such as demyelination and remyelination. This ability can substantially reduce the number of investigations required, but the benefit is offset by the inherent increase in technical complexity.

Acute terminal examination

Still more detailed recordings can be made in preparations under terminal general anaesthesia, with the nervous system exposed and covered with warmed mineral oil to avoid drying. This is the traditional approach employed by physiologists. It has the important advantage (compared with the other detailed methods below) of examining the nervous system under physiological conditions, and with an intact vascular supply (W.I. McDonald and Sears 1970; K.J. Smith and McDonald 1982). This is especially important when examining pathological tissue, because the acquisition of such tissue is extremely sensitive to any variation in the environment, including abnormally low, or high, oxygenation. As soon as tissue is removed and placed *in vitro* there are many compromises that have to be made, not least the fact that the bathing fluid will be artificial and its composition is, at best, only ever an approximation to the true environment. Indeed, in our experience conduction in demyelinated axons, particularly in the central nervous system, is often so insecure that it promptly fails if exposed to any environment that is in any way suboptimal. It therefore frequently occurs that axons able to conduct *in vivo* may fail to do so if removed and placed *in vitro*.

Acute terminal preparations allow stimulating and recording electrodes to be placed precisely on the tissues of interest, so that limitations over stimulus spread and volume recording are diminished. This advantage has contributed to the fact that examinations in terminal preparations have been crucial in revealing nearly all the pathophysiological properties of demyelinated axons.

Excised tissues

The most detailed examinations of axons tend to employ excised tissues studied *in vitro*. The main disadvantage of *in vitro* approaches has been mentioned above, but sometimes the benefits of being able to control the external environment can outweigh the fact that the environment is no longer physiological. For example, an extracellular fluid that lacks any large molecules like proteins is a clear advantage when using patch-clamp examinations, since otherwise the molecules can coat the patch electrode thereby preventing the very high resistance electrical seal onto the cell membrane that is an essential component of the standard technique (see below). Another undoubted advantage of the *in vitro* approach for microelectrode work is that pulsatile and breathing movements are eliminated, although it is nonetheless possible to achieve prolonged micropipette impalements of individual axons *in vivo* (Kapoor *et al* 1993).

Voltage-sensitive dyes have been used to monitor impulse conduction in axons (Shrager and Rubinstein 1990), but these techniques are sophisticated and require specialized equipment, including very low light microphotography.

Sharp and patch micropipettes

It is possible to measure the internal potential of cells by impaling them with a glass micropipette, drawn to a very fine (submicron) point from small-diameter glass tubing. The micropipette is filled with an electrically conducting solution, typically having high potassium ion concentration. The pipette is held in a very stable micromanipulator and advanced, perhaps using a stabbing motion, into the cell to be studied. Axons can be impaled in this way (Kapoor *et al* 1997), but their small diameter makes it difficult to 'hold' a penetration over a prolonged period. Demyelinated axons can be impaled with difficulty: the stability and electrical sealing provided by a myelin sheath at the site of impalement are an advantage. It is possible to label the cell or axon from which recordings are made by iontophoresing a marker into it before withdrawing the micropipette (Felts *et al* 1997).

The use of 'sharp' micropipettes in this way is the traditional method for making intracellular recordings, but the advent of low-resistance patch techniques (using relatively blunt micropipettes) has opened new possibilities, including the use of patch voltage clamp (Scholz *et al* 1993). Patch micropipettes have a comparatively wide aperture (around 1 μm), which is polished smooth using heat. The intention is not to penetrate the cell, but rather to stick the tip of the pipette to the cell membrane: the smooth glass bonds to the membrane, giving a very high resistance seal (giga-ohm seal, or gigaseal). Recordings can be made using a number of configurations, and in patch voltage clamp the patch electrode is used for both voltage clamping and current measurement.

Initially the patch arrangement is cell attached, and this allows measurements to be made of the currents flowing through ion channels in the patch of membrane on the end of the pipette, while the channels are influenced by cellular processes, such as second messengers. If the cell membrane across the pipette tip is broken, the pipette makes electrical connection with the inside of the cell, permitting whole-cell voltage clamp. This configuration allows the current flowing through all the ion channels in the cell membrane to be measured. Alternatively the pipette can be pulled from the cell, in which case the patch of membrane can remain attached to the end of the pipette. In this 'inside out' configuration, it is possible to study the currents flowing through the ion channels in the patch, with full control over the composition of the fluid bathing the formerly internal surface of the membrane. If suction is applied in the cell-attached configuration to break the membrane patch, and then the pipette is simply pulled from the cell, the torn membrane can reseal to form a patch, permitting 'outside out' recordings. Unfortunately, patch clamp techniques are not easily applied to demyelinated axons because their small diameter and elongated shape compromise adequate space clamping.

Nodal voltage clamp

The nature of the currents flowing across myelinated and (usually acutely) demyelinated axon membranes has been studied using voltage clamp techniques. These methods are sophisticated and, as with patch electrodes, it is not possible to provide a detailed account. However, gap methods (air-, sucrose-, grease- or Vaseline-gaps) provided early information and revealed the surprising finding that repolarization of the action potential in mammalian myelinated axons is not directly achieved by potassium efflux from voltage-gated potassium channels, as had been assumed (see below). In the Vaseline-gap method an individual living nerve fibre is teased from a nerve over a distance of a few millimetres, cut free and positioned across an apparatus composed of different fluid filled compartments. A node is manoeuvred into the appropriate compartment and these are then largely electrically isolated from each other by a method such as piping Vaseline seals (grease-gaps) between

them, over the nerve fibre. The two compartments containing the cut ends of the fibre are usually filled with a fluid similar in ion composition to axoplasm. Effectively the only electrical connection between the compartments is now via the inside of the axon and across the nodal membrane. The apparatus allows the voltage across the nodal membrane to be controlled at will and set, or clamped, at different potentials. If voltage-gated ion channels in the axolemma open in response to imposed changes in the transmembrane potential, ions will flow through the open channels, across the membrane, according to the driving force obtained from their electrochemical gradient. Because the transmembrane potential is clamped, the current carried by the ions is exactly balanced by an opposing current provided by the apparatus, and it is this current that is plotted as the voltage-clamp record. The nodal voltage is stepped in successive records through a range of different values, and so over a short time a family of different records is obtained. During plotting, these are typically superimposed, providing the familiar (if initially baffling) illustrations characteristic of such investigations. It is realistic to study only peripheral nerve fibres in this way, because central nerve fibres lack the connective tissue support (collagen matrix) required to give tensile strength to the nerve fibre during the dissection and manoeuvring steps.

Insights to the pathophysiology of multiple sclerosis from MRI

As mentioned in Chapters 7 and 18, respectively, magnetic resonance imaging (MRI) and spectroscopy measures have provided important advances for the diagnosis of multiple sclerosis and for monitoring potential new disease modifying treatments. In addition, MR measures provide a sensitive and direct way of monitoring the evolving pathology noninvasively during life. In so doing, new insights into the pathophysiology have emerged. MRI mainly provides a correlate of morphological events that can be predicted to have defined histopathological substrates. At present, it lacks cellular and molecular resolution but it is expected that molecular imaging will increasingly play a role in the evaluation of disease processes, to some extent obviating the need for tissue inspection. However, additional information is already provided on chemical and adaptive processes through magnetic resonance spectroscopy (MRS) and functional MRI (fMRI) respectively. Within these limitations, MRI has allowed a more extensive survey of the disease at all stages, especially early in the course when access to neuropathological tissue tends to be limited. In a sense, the information on pathophysiology derived from MRI falls somewhere between the direct neuropathological or neurophysiological evidence, and the information provided by clinical observation. Throughout, we review insights for the pathophysiology of multiple sclerosis derived from the main MR techniques deployed at different stages of the disease (Table 13.1). From this, a framework of the evolving pathology and pathophysiology is constructed, which in turn helps to understand key aspects of the clinical course of the disease – relapse, remission and progression.

T_2-weighted lesions

The standard way of depicting focal lesions in the brain and spinal cord is by T_2-weighted images (Figure 13.3A). These

Table 13.1 **Magnetic resonance imaging methods used to study multiple sclerosis and their proposed pathophysiological correlates**

MRI technique	Pathophysiological correlate
T_2-weighted lesions	Focal white matter lesions – pathologically nonspecific
Gadolinium enhancing lesions	Blood–brain barrier breakdown, perivascular inflammation, macrophage infiltrates
T_1-weighted hypointense lesions (persistent)	Greater extent of axonal loss than T_1 isointense lesions

Tissue volume loss (atrophy):
   Whole brain
   Brain regions (e.g. white/grey matter)
   Spinal cord
   Optic nerves
	Axonal loss (main cause), demyelination, anti-inflammatory treatment and (?) gliotic retraction

MR spectroscopy metabolites:
   N-acetyl aspartate
   Myo-inositol
   Choline-containing compounds
   Creatine/phosphocreatine
   Glutamate/glutamine
   Lipid resonances
	Neuroaxonal dysfunction or loss
	 Glial proliferation, inflammation
	 Membrane turnover
	 Cellular activity
	 ?Neuronal activity/neurotoxicity
	 Active demyelination

Magnetization transfer ratio	Demyelination in lesions; subtle pathology in normal-appearing white and grey matter

Diffusion tensor imaging
   Mean diffusivity
   Fractional anisotropy
	
	 Size of extracellular space
	 White matter tract integrity

T_1 relaxation	Sensitive to pathology in normal-appearing white and grey matter
T_2 relaxation	Demyelination (short T_2), expanded extracellular space (long T_2)
Functional MRI	Cortical adaptive responses to underlying pathology
Perfusion MRI	Neuronal loss (decreased grey matter perfusion) Inflammation (increased white matter perfusion)

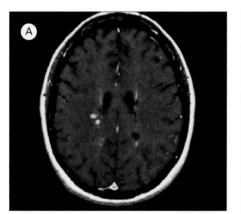
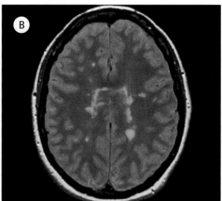
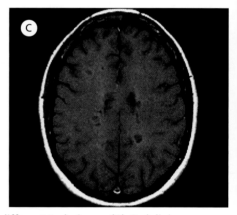

Figure 13.3 MRI scans illustrating the appearance of lesion types in multiple sclerosis using different techniques. (A) Gadolinium-enhanced T_1-weighted. (B) T_2-weighted. (C) Unenhanced T_1-weighted images. Panels (B) and (C) reproduce Figures 7.16A and B for the convenience of the reader.

images readily identify focal white matter areas that have an increase in the density and/or mobility of water protons, as occurs in regions of inflammation or demyelination. Many, but not all, T_2-weighted lesions correspond pathologically with foci of demyelination (Ormerod *et al* 1987). Some lesions visible by T_2 examination are not apparent on macroscopic examination of post-mortem brain slices. These often lack demyelination but show more subtle signs of activity, with clusters of microglial cells, perivascular lymphocytes and oedema. It has been suggested that these lesions represent reactive lesions (De Groot *et al* 2001). It can be concluded, however, that T_2-weighted lesions *per se* are pathologically nonspecific.

Gadolinium enhancing lesions

Gadolinium-containing chelates are used as intravenous contrast agents to show areas of the central nervous system in which there is a breakdown of the blood–brain barrier. The accumulation of gadolinium leads to enhanced T_1 relaxation, and increased signal, on T_1-weighted images (Figure 13.3A). In multiple sclerosis, gadolinium enhancement is a consistent feature of new lesions in bout onset (relapsing–remitting and secondary progressive) disease (Cotton *et al* 2003; H.M. Lai *et al* 1996; D.H. Miller *et al* 1988b; A.J. Thompson *et al* 1991). Several studies correlating post-mortem or biopsy data of enhancing lesions have shown consistent evidence for inflammatory activity, most notably macrophage infiltrates with active myelin breakdown, and also the presence of perivascular inflammatory cuffs including lymphocytes (Brück *et al* 1997; Katz *et al* 1993).

T_1 hypointense lesions

About 20–30% of T_2 lesions are hypointense on T_1-weighted images (these are sometimes called 'black holes': Figure 13.3C). Such lesions are often seen transiently during the gadolinium enhancing phase when new lesions appear (van Waesberghe *et al* 1998). About 50% of such lesions remain persistently hypointense after many months or years. These have a greater extent of axonal loss when compared with T_1 isointense lesions (van Walderveen *et al* 1998).

Tissue volume loss (atrophy)

Progressive regional or global loss of brain tissue is a predictable feature of primary neurodegenerative diseases, of which Alzheimer's disease is the most characteristic. Atrophy of the brain and spinal cord is also commonly observed in multiple sclerosis. It reflects several processes. First and foremost is neuroaxonal loss, which is likely in most instances to account for the majority of tissue loss because neurons and axons are the largest bulk element in the central nervous system (D.H. Miller *et al* 2002). Other causes of tissue loss are demyelination *per se*, reduction in brain water and inflammation; and possibly retraction effects from gliosis (in theory, however, gliosis could also increase tissue volume). Brain atrophy can be measured globally or regionally in white matter, grey matter or in terms of ventricular size. Spinal cord and optic nerve atrophy can also be quantified.

MR spectroscopy

Whereas MRI depicts water protons, MR spectroscopy investigates other proton-containing metabolites, typically present in much smaller, millimolar, concentrations. This means that reliable measurement requires relatively large volumes of tissue to be studied in order to achieve sufficient signals from these metabolites. The typical spatial resolution for spectroscopy at the standard 1.5 tesla field strength used on clinical scanners is 1–4 cm^3 (1000–4000 mm^3), which contrasts with a resolution of $1 \times 1 \times 3$ mm (3 mm^3) for two-dimensional and $1 \times 1 \times 1$ mm (1 mm^3) for three-dimensional MR images of water protons. Single slice, multi-voxel spectroscopic imaging can, however, be used to investigate normal-appearing grey and white matter in the cerebral hemispheres (Figure 13.4).

The main peak seen on MR spectroscopy is N-acetyl aspartate, an amino acid that in the adult central nervous system is contained almost exclusively in neurons and axons (M.L. Simmons *et al* 1991). It is also found in oligodendrocyte precursor cells (Urenjak *et al* 1993) but, being present at low concentration, their contribution to the overall signal is probably negligible. An *in vitro* study reporting the presence of N-acetyl aspartate in mature rat oligodendrocytes under stringent laboratory conditions (Bhakoo and Pearce 2000) is unlikely to be of much relevance to the study of human brain *in vivo*.

The peak due to choline-containing compounds (Cho) reflects several molecules and is sensitive to an altered turnover of cell membranes, as, for example, would be expected with inflammation or demyelination (R.E. Brenner *et al* 1993). The creatine/phosphocreatine peak (Cr) is probably related to the concentration and metabolic activity of cells within the region being studied. Glial cells produce *myo*-inositol (Brand *et al* 1993), which is detected in the normal white matter using short echo time MR spectroscopy. An increase probably reflects changes in the number and/or activity of glial or inflammatory cells. Both glutamate and glutamine produce spectral peaks, although at 1.5 tesla it is normally only possible to measure their combined concentration (known conventionally as Glx). This ambiguity makes it difficult to interpret increases and decreases of Glx, both of which have been reported in multiple sclerosis. Mobile lipid peaks at 0.9 and 1.3 parts per million in the proton MR spectrum are detected in acute multiple sclerosis lesions, in which situation they probably indicate active breakdown of myelin (Davie *et al* 1994). However, it is more feasible selectively to measure the resonance from glutamate on higher field (3 Tesla) scanners. A recent study of multiple sclerosis used a single voxel TE-averaged PRESS technique and reported an increase in the concentration of glutamate in both gadolinium-enhancing lesions and normal-appearing white matter (Srinivasan *et al* 2005).

Magnetization transfer ratio (MTR)

Magnetization transfer imaging involves the application of an additional radio frequency pulse to saturate the protons bound to macromolecules. Because these 'bound' protons are in exchange with the 'free' or non-bound proton pool from which conventional MR images are obtained, their saturation alters the image such that it provides a quantifiable measure of the extent of the bound proton pool (Figure 13.5A; Dousset *et al* 1992). It is thought by some that myelin is mainly responsible for the magnetization transfer effect in normal white matter. MTR correlates not only with myelin content in the lesions of multiple sclerosis (Mottershead *et al* 2003) but also with axonal density both in the lesions and normal-appearing white matter (van Waesberghe *et al* 1999). Recent work in postmortem multiple sclerosis tissue using multiple regression analysis to compare the relative contributions from myelin content and axonal density indicated that the former has a more direct influence on the measured MTR (Schmierer *et al* 2004). MTR is a robust and stable quantitative measure and, using histogram analysis (Figure 13.5B), has proved sensitive enough to detect subtle abnormalities in the normal-appearing tissues in multiple sclerosis (Table 13.2). These small changes in MTR could reflect inflammation, mild disruption of myelin, or axonal loss.

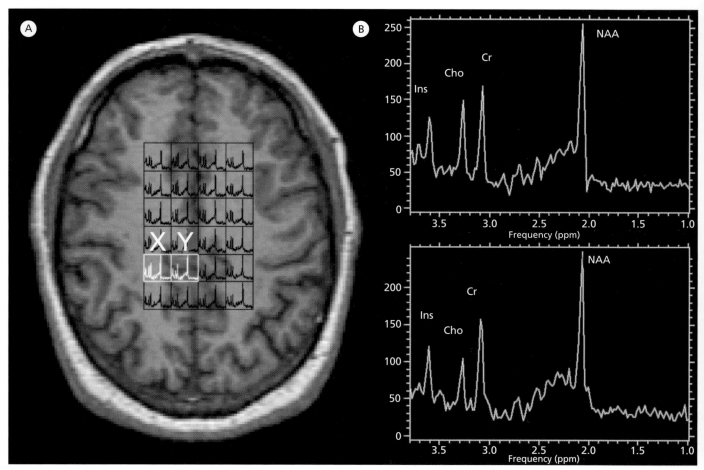

Figure 13.4 ¹H-MR spectra from normal-appearing grey and white matter. (A) Normal-appearing white matter voxel. (B) A cortical grey matter voxel (X is the top panel; Y is the lower panel). From Chard *et al* (2002a). © 2002, reprinted with permission of John Wiley & Sons.

Diffusion tensor imaging

Using additional gradient pulses, it is possible to generate MR images that are sensitive to the diffusion properties of water protons. The mean diffusivity can be measured and it is sensitive in detecting pathological change in lesions and normal-appearing tissues (Cercignani *et al* 2001b; Ciccarelli *et al* 2001), although it is probably less sensitive in the latter region when compared with MTR. Increased diffusion implies a decrease in structural barriers and an increase in extracellular spaces, as occurs in acute inflammation or chronic lesions with demyelination and axonal loss. Fractional anisotropy is a measure of directionally preponderant diffusion. This is observed in white matter tracts because there is greater diffusion *along* versus *across* directions in which the axons are travelling. This fractional anisotropy is highest in coherently organized tracts such as the corpus callosum, optic radiation and corticospinal pathways. Fractional anisotropy thus provides an indication of structural integrity in white matter tracts. The anisotropy properties can be used further to define major tracts by the application of tracking algorithms (Figure 13.6). Preliminary work has revealed abnormalities of the volume and anisotropy of the optic radiation in patients with isolated optic neuritis, suggesting possible transsynaptic degeneration (Ciccarelli *et al* 2005).

T_1 relaxation time

T_1 (longitudinal) relaxation time is a fundamental nuclear magnetic resonance (NMR) property that reflects the exchange of magnetization between protons and their environment once the initial excitatory radio frequency pulse has stopped. An increase in T_1 is expected when the density and mobility of water protons are increased, and it is seen both in the lesions of multiple sclerosis and the normal-appearing white and grey matter, even in early relapsing–remitting disease (Griffin *et al* 2002b; Laule *et al* 2004). It is sensitive to pathology but unlikely to be pathologically specific, although a correlation with axonal density has been reported in multiple sclerosis (Van Waesberghe *et al* 1999).

T_2 relaxation time

T_2 (transverse) relaxation time is also a fundamental NMR property sensitive to the interaction between neighbouring water protons that have been excited by the initial radio frequency pulse. If multiple spin echo pulses with short inter-echo times are used, the process of T_2 relaxation can be mapped in detail. In normal white matter, prominent peaks are observed at short (<50 ms), intermediate (50–150 ms) and long (>150 ms)

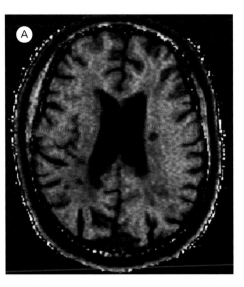

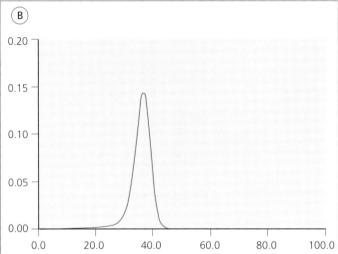

Figure 13.5 Magnetization transfer MRI of normal-appearing brain tissue. (A) Brain magnetization transfer image and histogram from normal-appearing brain tissue. (B) The magnetization transfer histogram for normal-appearing brain tissue. From Traboulsee *et al* (2003) with permission.

echo times. These three peaks are conventionally attributed to myelin-associated water (short T_2), extracellular water (intermediate T_2) and cerebrospinal fluid (long T_2; MacKay *et al* 1994). In multiple sclerosis white matter lesions, the short T_2 component has been reported to be absent and this has been proposed as indicating demyelination. A post-mortem study of two cases revealed loss of the short T_2 component in areas with demyelination (G.R. Moore *et al* 2000).

Functional MRI

This modality has been widely applied over the last decade to investigate normal and abnormal brain function. The core steps of an fMRI study are, first, to stimulate neuronal activity in a particular brain region (the stimulus may be motor, visual, sensory, cognitive or auditory). The increase in neuronal activity is closely followed by the haemodynamic response that increases regional blood flow in response to the increased metabolic needs of the tissue. This alteration in blood flow results in a decreased local concentration of deoxyhaemoglobin and, because deoxyhaemoglobin is paramagnetic, the change in regional signal can be detected on the MR image. Second, after a combination of repeated on–off experiments (to generate sufficient signal-to-noise ratio) and spatial mapping (using statistical parametric mapping), it is possible to locate the altered cerebral blood oxygenation (and, by implication, neuronal activation) in response to the original stimulus. In pathological states, including multiple sclerosis, fMRI has been used to investigate alterations in cortical activation from those seen in healthy individuals (Cifelli and Matthews 2002). Such changes may reflect adaptive mechanisms of functional benefit to the patient, although this remains to be definitively proven. A genuine adaptive response may be due to the release of existing pathways that are normally inhibited, or structural (hardwire) changes resulting from new synaptic connections.

Perfusion studies

It is possible to measure cerebral perfusion in multiple sclerosis either by performing rapid scanning following the injection of a

Table 13.2 **Magnetization transfer ratios in patients with relapsing–remitting and secondary progressive multiple sclerosis**			
	Control (63)	**Relapsing–remitting multiple sclerosis (70)**	**Secondary progressive multiple sclerosis (25)**
Mean MTR	34.4 + 0.5	33.2 + 0.9[a]	32.6 + 1.3[a]
% Decrease		− 3.0%	− 4.9%
Peak height	10.4 ± 0.8	10.1 ± 0.8	9.3 ± 1.1[a]
Peak location	37.0 ± 0.6	36.1 ± 0.8[a]	36.0 ± 0.7[a]
25th Percentile	31.8 ± 0.6	30.7 ± 1.2[a]	29.7 ± 1.6[a]
50th Percentile	35.1 ± 0.5	34.3 ± 0.8[a]	33.7 ± 1.2[a]
75th Percentile	37.5 ± 0.5	36.8 ± 0.7[a]	36.5 ± 1.1[a]

a $p < 0.001$ for comparisons between patients with relapsing–remitting or secondary progressive multiple sclerosis and controls. From Traboulsee et al (2003) with permission.

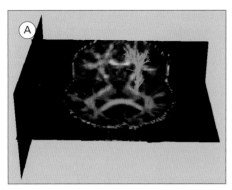

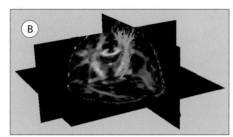

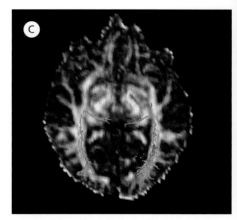

Figure 13.6 Diffusion tractography. (A, B) Pyrimidal tract. (C) Optic radiation. Green tracking lines indicating the optic radiations and pyramidal tracts are superimposed on fractional anisotropy images, which show high signal in the major white matter tracts.

bolus of intravenous contrast agent, or using the selective magnetization of flowing protons to generate perfusion images. The latter approach (arterial spin tagging) is less invasive but yields lower signal-to-noise ratio images.

RELAPSING–REMITTING MULTIPLE SCLEROSIS: LOSS OF FUNCTION

Patients with relapsing–remitting multiple sclerosis typically exhibit periodic episodes where new functional deficits arise spontaneously over days or a few weeks, and then resolve over the ensuing weeks or months. Although MRI can often detect the new area of disease activity, it is not effective in monitoring the loss or restoration of function within that lesion, as illustrated in Figure 13.7 showing two images of a patient taken one month apart. The images are indistinguishable (other than changes in background contrast) and yet the first was captured when the patient was paraplegic and incontinent, whereas normal function had been restored (save for an extensor plantar response) by the time of the second study. The nonspecificity of MRI in this respect is because the changes responsible for deficits, and the restoration of function, occur at the molecular level in the membranes of individual axons. Indeed, it is not possible to predict the function of axons even from their appearance under the electron microscope.

The main cause of relapse is the failure of axonal conduction at the site of a lesion – as predicted by Charcot (1868b). In fact, it is not surprising that function is lost so frequently in inflammatory demyelinating lesions, because several mechanisms are operating, each of which may contribute to conduction block. The evidence that conduction does fail in patients is inevitably more indirect than can be achieved in experimental preparations in the laboratory, but there is support from the study of evoked potentials. Figure 13.8 shows recordings from a child with bilateral optic neuritis. At the time of the first recording, vision was reduced to counting fingers using either eye. There was no detectable cortical evoked response from the left eye and only a small delayed response from the right. By the time of the second recording, only six days later, visual acuity had substantially recovered and was accompanied by the return of fairly well-formed evoked responses, albeit with delayed latency. Given

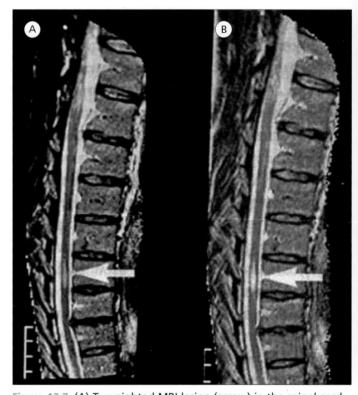

Figure 13.7 (A) T$_2$-weighted MRI lesion (arrow) in the spinal cord taken when the patient had severe paraparesis. (B) One month later when there had been virtually complete resolution of symptoms. From Prineas and McDonald (1997) with permission.

that there were lesions in the optic nerves, and vision was restored within days coinciding with return of the evoked potential, by far the most likely explanation is that the visual deficit arose from temporary block of conduction in the optic nerve axons. This interpretation is strongly supported by the study of experimental lesions (see below).

The role of demyelination

Conduction block is the predominant electrophysiological feature when experimental demyelinating lesions are examined in

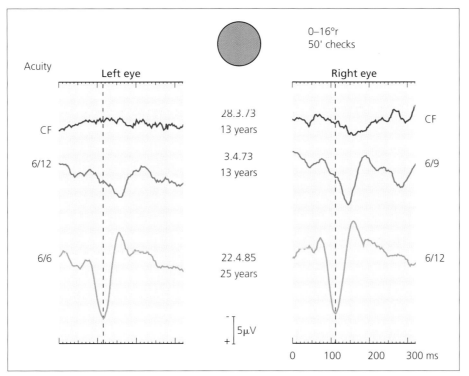

Figure 13.8 Visual evoked potentials to pattern reversal recorded from a girl aged 13 years at presentation, 3 days, 9 days and 12 years after onset of an attack of acute bilateral optic neuritis. Kindly provided by Drs Martin Halliday and Anthony Kriss. Adapted from McDonald (1986) with permission from Elsevier.

the laboratory. The pathology most clearly responsible for conduction block is segmental demyelination resulting in the loss of whole internodes of myelin. Such studies have revealed that conduction fails specifically at the site of the lesion, whereas morphologically unaffected portions of the axon on either side of the lesion continue to conduct normally (W.I. McDonald 1963). As with so many electrophysiological observations in demyelinated axons, this finding was first made in demyelinated peripheral fibres (Denny-Brown and Brenner 1944; W.I. McDonald 1963) and later confirmed in central axons as the requirement for more challenging techniques was fulfilled (W.I. McDonald and Sears 1969; 1970) (Figure 13.9). At first, central experimental lesions were induced by the direct intraspinal injection of diphtheria toxin, which resulted in a complex mixture of partial and segmental demyelination, remyelination and axonal degeneration. Recent studies have employed lesions exhibiting more homogeneous pathological features, such as those that result from the local injection of lysolecithin – lysophosphatidylcholine (LPC) (Blakemore *et al* 1977; Bostock *et al* 1980; Bowe *et al* 1987; K.J. Smith and Hall 1980; K.J. Smith and McDonald 1980; 1982; K.J. Smith *et al* 1979; 1981; 1982; Targ and Kocsis 1985; 1986) or ethidium bromide (Felts *et al* 1997; Honmou *et al* 1996; Kapoor *et al* 1997; Redford *et al* 1997; K.J. Smith *et al* 1994; 1997; 2000a).

The main determinants of whether conduction in a demyelinated axon is blocked are the time elapsed since demyelination occurred, the size of the lesion, and the extent of myelin loss along the internode. The duration of demyelination matters because loss of myelin triggers a series of adaptive axonal responses. Perhaps the most important is the appearance along

the demyelinated membrane of a revised population of ion channels, which can result in the restoration of conduction (see below). Lesion size is important because axons seem to repair centripetally within the lesion, and so long lengths of demyelination are repaired more slowly. Thus the probability of functional recovery tends to relate inversely to lesion size. A practical consequence of this is that conduction is sequentially restored to axons with progressively longer segments of demyelination. Thus, as the lesion repairs, progressively later components are added to the compound action potential and this can give the misleading impression that conduction is deteriorating over time. Also, as the length of a demyelinated segment increases, so does the statistical chance of including any portion of the axon that may have particularly insecure conduction. It follows that the possibility of conduction block also increases with length of the lesion. With regard to myelin loss, complete loss of a single internode of myelin is more than sufficient to block conduction, but partial myelin thinning anywhere along the internode can also cause conduction failure. In practice, myelin loss involving the paranodal region and resulting in widened nodes is much more potent in blocking conduction than a comparable loss distributed along the internode (see below).

Mathematical models suggest that conduction could occur in fresh, cleanly demyelinated axons, particularly if they are of small diameter (Bostock 1994). However, our practical experience in experimentally demyelinated axons in the spinal cord, spinal roots and sciatic nerve is that conduction is invariably blocked if the demyelination is segmental (involving loss of the whole internode), and conduction remains blocked for several days thereafter (McDonald and Sears 1970; K.J. Smith *et al* 1979;

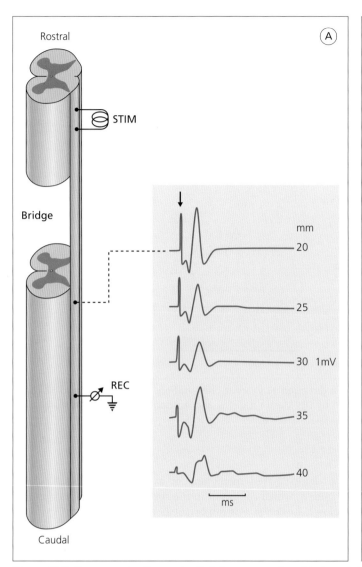

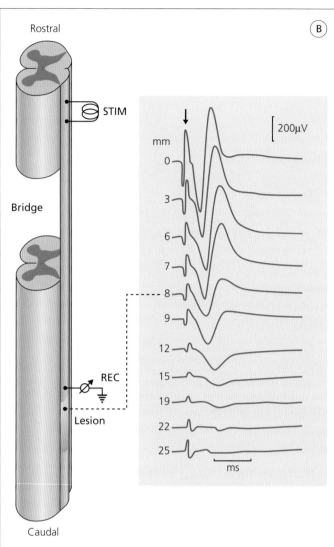

Figure 13.9 Compound action potentials from normal and lesioned dorsal column fibres in the cat. (A) The records were made at the distances indicated (mm) caudal to the stimulating electrodes after conduction through a dorsal column 'bridge'. Note the change in gain at 35 and 40 mm. Positivity at the active electrode gives a downward deflection. (B) Conduction distances measured from the first recording site. Note the abrupt transition in the form of the compound action potential with differential reduction in the amplitude of the negative component, indicating focal conduction block, between 7 and 8 mm (at the site of the lesion). STIM = stimulate; REC = record. The arrow indicates the location of the stimulus artefact. Adapted from W.I. McDonald and Sears (1970).

1981). This seemingly mandatory period of conduction failure is probably related to the initial paucity of sodium channels in the freshly exposed internodal axolemma (Waxman and Ritchie 1993). Compared with the nodal membrane, the axolemma beneath the myelin sheath has a much lower density of the sodium channels needed for conduction, and this may simply be insufficient for the support of conduction (Waxman 1989; Waxman and Ritchie 1993; see also Utzschneider *et al* 1993); the freshly demyelinated axolemma may be both inexcitable, as well as nonexcited (for more detailed reviews see Bostock 1984; Hille 1992; K.J. Smith 1994; Waxman and Brill 1978; Waxman and Foster 1980).

The effect of nodal widening

Apart from the obvious loss of whole myelin internodes (segmental demyelination), a recent confocal examination has

shown that some nodes are inappropriately wide in the lesions of multiple sclerosis due to paranodal demyelination, or retraction of the paranodes (Wolswijk and Balesar 2003). A similar phenomenon occurs in some forms of postinfectious polyneuritis (J.W. Griffin *et al* 1996; J.L. Lu *et al* 2000), and we have produced the phenomenon experimentally by the intraneural injection of tumour necrosis factor α (TNF-α) (Redford *et al* 1995). As in the human disease (Gilliatt 1982; J.L. Lu *et al* 2000), our own unpublished studies and other people's experimental work (Sumner *et al* 1982) suggest that nodal widening is sufficient to block conduction, in keeping with predictions made using computer models (Bostock 1993; 1994; Chiu and Ritchie 1981; Koles and Rasminsky 1972; Stephanova and Chobanova 1997).

The sensitivity of conduction to increases in the area of membrane exposed at the node, whether caused by myelin retraction or segmental demyelination, has several causes. Perhaps easiest to understand is the fact that the loss of the myelin reduces the

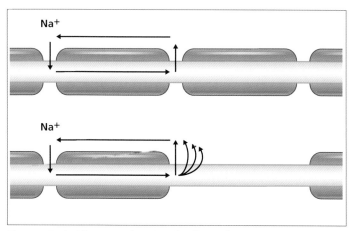

Figure 13.10 Diagrams showing the flow of local action currents along a normal fibre (upper illustration) and one that has lost an internode of myelin (lower). The myelin normally helps to limit the flow of action current to the minute portion of excitable axolemma at the node of Ranvier but, in the absence of myelin, the current becomes dispersed over a much larger area of axon membrane.

constraints on local current generated by the driving node (the last intact node before the demyelinated region) to act just at the localized (former) nodal membrane, but rather to become dissipated over a much larger area (Figure 13.10). This is one consideration contributing to a reduction in the safety factor for conduction (see below). A less intuitive, but perhaps more important, cause derives from the fact that cell membranes have substantial electrical capacitance, and this must be discharged if the node is to be depolarized. The capacitance of a membrane is proportional to its area, and so demyelination dramatically increases the capacitance of the affected (hemi)node, thereby increasing the amount of local current required to depolarize the membrane to its firing threshold. This effect further reduces the safety factor. More detailed accounts, of varying complexity, are provided by Waxman and Brill (1978), Bostock (1984), Hille (1992) and K.J. Smith (1994).

Loss of nodal sodium channels

Sodium channels are reported to be lost from the nodes of Ranvier in experimental autoimmune neuritis (Novakovic *et al* 1998), which presumably renders the nodes inexcitable and results in conduction block. The timing of this loss correlates with the appearance of clinical signs but the mechanism is unknown. Possible explanations include molecular mimicry between the immunogen and sodium channels, complement-mediated injury (Hafer-Macko *et al* 1996) and internalization of the channels (Dargent *et al* 1994). Whether similar events occur in multiple sclerosis is not known.

Safety factor for conduction of the nerve impulse

The safety factor is a useful concept for understanding conduction deficits in multiple sclerosis. It can be defined as the 'current available to depolarize the axolemma, divided by the current necessary to do so' (W.A.H. Rushton 1937). Normal myelinated axons have a safety factor of around 3–5, namely the

action potential at an individual node generates approximately 3–5 times more current than is actually required to fire the next node along the axon (Tasaki 1953). In demyelinated axons, the safety factor is reduced to around unity (K.J. Smith 1994). Self-evidently, this is a critical level because it places the success of conduction in many demyelinated axons on the cusp of success or failure. If conditions favour a safety factor >1.0, conduction will be successful but, conversely, adverse conditions reduce the safety factor below unity and conduction promptly fails. Where many axons in an individual lesion have safety factors near unity (as is often the case), it follows that small changes in the environment of axons have pronounced effects on the expression of symptoms. Temperature is one variable that strongly affects the safety factor, and it can have dramatic effects on the expression of symptoms (see below). Disruption of the blood–brain barrier (Abbott 2002; Petty and Lo 2002) will also markedly affect the microenvironment of axons, and thereby influence the conduction properties of fibres traversing an individual lesion.

The role of glial dysfunction

Thus far, we have discussed the consequences of demyelination only from the standpoint of structural loss of the myelin sheath, but dysfunction of glial cells is likely to play an important role in influencing the conduction properties of axons. Astrocytes play a crucial role in maintaining homeostasis of the extracellular milieu in the central nervous system, without which normal function is severely compromised. Astrocytes are clearly abnormal in the lesions of multiple sclerosis, and this may result in an improperly regulated ionic milieu for the demyelinated axons. This problem is compounded by deficits in the integrity of the blood–brain barrier. Furthermore, axons that are threatened by an inflammatory environment are likely to be especially dependent on an optimal combination of growth factors and other forms of trophic support provided by glial cells (see Chapter 10). Astrocytes also play an important role in the organization of ion channels along the axonal membrane. Aggregations of sodium channels (identified by patches of subaxolemmal density along demyelinated central axons) often make intimate contact with astrocytic processes (Blakemore and Smith 1983; Rosenbluth *et al* 1985), and oligodendrocytes are important in the appearance of node-like sodium channel accumulations in developing optic nerve axons (Figure 13.11; Kaplan *et al* 1997; Rasband *et al* 1999a; 1999b). Schwann cells play a comparable role in the peripheral nervous system (J.D. England *et al* 1996; Novakovic *et al* 1996; Rasband *et al* 1998). Finally, the paranodal loops of myelin are normally in intimate contact with the axolemma, and this interaction will undoubtedly be important not only in maintaining precise channel organization, but also in guiding the flow of local current to ensure secure impulse conduction. There is evidence that these intimate contacts can be disrupted at nodes near the borders of the lesions in multiple sclerosis (see Chapter 12; Wolswijk and Balesar 2003), and this can be expected to have adverse effects on axonal function.

The role of inflammation

Our understanding of the mechanisms responsible for loss of function during the individual episode has been substantially

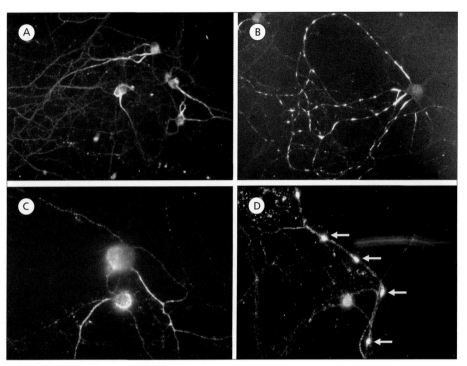

Figure 13.11 (A,C) Immunohistochemical micrographs showing the clustering of sodium channels along nonmyelinated, developing axons from rat central nervous system retinal ganglion cells in culture. (B,D) In the presence of oligodendrocyte conditioned medium the diffuse labelling changes to show the clustering of sodium channels. Adapted from M.R. Kaplan *et al* (1997) and kindly provided by Ben Barres and colleagues.

reassessed over the last decade, with the appreciation that inflammation can play an important – and perhaps the dominant – part in causing transient neurological deficits. Thus, whereas loss of function was once attributed almost entirely to demyelination, it now appears that some relapses (especially those that are brief) depend entirely on inflammatory mediators *per se*. This change in perspective was stimulated in large part by the MRI study of optic neuritis (Youl *et al* 1991b), and from surprising observations resulting from the evaluation of novel immunotherapy using the humanized monoclonal antibody, Campath-1H (Moreau *et al* 1996). This new appreciation was further supported by inferences from a biopsy study concluding that 'inflammation alone may be sufficient to cause significant clinical deficits without demyelination' (Bitsch *et al* 1999). These findings in multiple sclerosis are mirrored by experimental observations (see Chapter 11).

Oedema

Oedema and its dispersal are often invoked as an explanation for functional loss and recovery in multiple sclerosis, and some authors have interpreted observations obtained in experimental autoimmune encephalomyelitis as supporting this mechanism (Kerlero de Rosbo *et al* 1985; R.D. Simmons *et al* 1982). It should be noted, however, that almost nothing is known about the effects on conduction of increased extracellular fluid, or of the changes in ionic composition that may result from oedema and myelin breakdown. In view of the extensive oedema that can be asymptomatic in other disorders such as cerebral tumour and sagittal sinus thrombosis, we consider it unlikely that oedema plays a significant role, except perhaps through pressure effects in regions of tight constriction such as the optic nerve in the scleral and optic canals (D.H. Miller *et al* 1988).

The role of T cells and their soluble mediators

Infiltration of the lesions in multiple sclerosis by CD4$^+$ and CD8$^+$ T cells (see Chapter 12; Booss *et al* 1983; Gay *et al* 1997) may be directly responsible for impairing axonal conduction. However, the evidence is circumstantial because it is difficult, both in the experimental and clinical context, to disentangle any contribution to the conduction deficits arising directly from T cells from those attributable either to structural changes (such as demyelination) or other cells (particularly macrophages) recruited to the lesion.

Yarom and colleagues (1983) provided seemingly decisive evidence that T cells could impair axonal conduction by showing that activated T cells reactive for myelin basic protein block conduction in almost half the axons of isolated optic nerves within 40 minutes of exposure. Conduction block was reversed on removing the cells unless the period of incubation was >2 hours. T cells directed against a non-optic nerve antigen had no effect on conduction. The anti-myelin basic protein T cells had no effect on conduction along allogeneic optic nerves, or syngeneic peripheral nerves. These observations strongly suggest that an immunologically specific interaction between T cells and axons led to conduction block. However, after an interval of 20 years, it has recently been reported that the findings could not be reproduced using a similar protocol. The addition of T cells to syngeneic optic nerve did not depress axonal conduction, even though the same T cells were capable of inducing lethal experimental autoimmune encephalomyelitis *in vivo* (Devaux *et al* 2003b). This latter study suggested that other cells or factors present in intact animals, but not replicated *in vitro*, effect conduction block. Interestingly, it has recently been reported that activated human γδ T cells (but not αβ T cells) obtained from the blood or cerebrospinal fluid of patients with multiple sclerosis can block conduction in excised rat optic nerves (Freedman *et al* 2004). The conduction block was detected after 6 hours, and was substantial (>90% reduction) after 19 hours, appearing to occur in conjunction with axon and myelin pathology.

Using an *in vivo* approach, CD8⁺ T cells have been implicated in the production of neurological deficits in mice infected with Theiler's murine encephalomyelitis virus (Rivera-Quinones *et al* 1998) through a perforin-mediated mechanism (P.D. Murray *et al* 1998). Perforin, produced by cytotoxic CD8⁺ T cells, forms pores in target cell membranes, and permeated cells are killed by loss of ionic and osmotic homeostasis. Recent two-photon confocal microscopy has revealed that T cells cause calcium oscillations within neurons and calcium-dependent degeneration. Both events are prevented by blocking perforin and glutamate receptors (Nitsch *et al* 2004). Perforin-deficient mice infected with Theiler's virus exhibit minimal neurological deficits compared with normal mice, despite showing similar magnitudes of demyelination. It remains to be shown whether perforin mechanisms are implicated in other experimental models of multiple sclerosis. We describe the role of major histocompatibility complex antigen expression and neuronal function in Chapter 11.

The role of nitric oxide (NO)

The enzyme inducible nitric oxide synthase (iNOS) can be abundant especially in the acute inflammatory lesions of multiple sclerosis. This form of the enzyme produces nitric oxide continuously, and at high concentration (Alderton *et al* 2001). Accordingly, there is much evidence that nitric oxide can be present at high concentration within the lesions of multiple scle-

rosis (see Chapter 12; K.J. Smith and Lassmann 2002), and even within the normal-appearing white matter (Bizzozero *et al* 2005). It is therefore noteworthy that nitric oxide has been found to act like a local anaesthetic in reversibly blocking axonal conduction (Kapoor *et al* 1999; Redford *et al* 1997; Shrager *et al* 1998), and demyelinated axons are especially vulnerable (Figure 13.12; Redford *et al* 1997). Thus, at low concentrations of nitric oxide, demyelinated axons would be selectively affected, providing a plausible explanation for the transient exacerbation of previously expressed clinical features observed upon the administration of Campath-1H (see above, and Chapters 10 and 18). Given that nitric oxide is prominent in many lesions, it seems reasonable to suspect that nitric oxide contributes to neurological deficits arising during the normal course of multiple sclerosis. Thus, an unusual observation made in the setting of experimental therapy may have illuminated a general mechanism of tissue dysfunction in multiple sclerosis.

Experimentally, axonal conduction block can be imposed within minutes of nitric oxide exposure, maintained for hours in its presence, and relieved within minutes of its removal. Following block, the axons continue to conduct normally for at least 10 hours, and presumably permanently (Kapoor *et al* 1999; Redford *et al* 1997; Shrager *et al* 1998). There are several possible mechanisms underlying this reversible conduction block, each of which is theoretically sufficient to block conduction. Which mechanism is dominant remains to be elucidated (for review see Santiago *et al* 1998; K.J. Smith and Lassmann 2002; K.J. Smith *et al* 1999).

Perhaps the most obvious potential NO-mediated mechanism is impaired function of the sodium channels upon which conduction depends (Figures 13.13 and 13.48) (Ahern *et al* 2000; Bielefeldt *et al* 1999; Ding *et al* 1998; Duvall *et al* 1998;

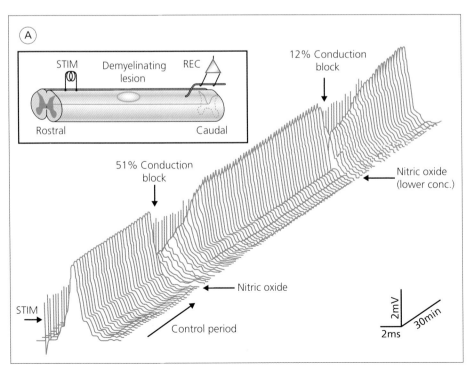

Figure 13.12 Reversible block of conduction in central demyelinated axons mediated by the injection of nitric oxide into the lesion, which was located within the rat dorsal columns (see inset: STIM = stimulate; REC = record). The records are plotted with three-dimensional perspective, with the earliest records shown at the front. Records were made every 2 minutes and show about 5 hours of recording time. All the axons contributing to the compound action potentials were known to be affected by the demyelinating lesion as determined from other electrophysiological data, and confirmed upon histological examination. Conduction along the axons was stable until exposed to nitric oxide released by the nitric oxide donor spermine NONOate, when conduction in approximately half the axons was promptly blocked. The block was gradually released over the ensuing half hour as the rate of nitric oxide release diminished, and the donor diffused away. A second injection of a lower concentration of donor reinstated the block, in a smaller number of axons. Adapted from Redford *et al* (1997).

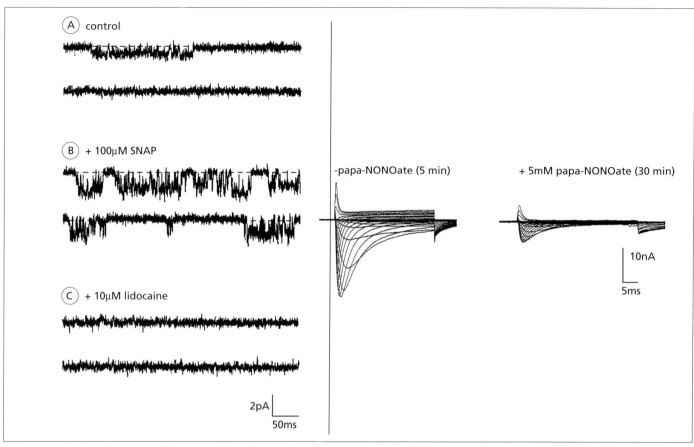

Figure 13.13 Records showing different effects of nitric oxide on sodium channels (see also Figure 13.48). Patch clamp records from an excised inside-out patch from a rat hippocampal neuron showing currents resulting from the openings of individual sodium channels. (A) Under control conditions channel openings are few so that the persistent sodium current experienced by the whole cell would be very small, but after 5 minutes in the presence of the nitric oxide donor *S*-nitroso-*N*-acetyl-DL-penicillamine (SNAP), the channel openings were much increased. In the presence of the donor the whole cell would experience a much enhanced persistent inward sodium current. (B) Families of voltage clamp records showing slow sodium currents in a neuron that only expressed such currents. On the left and right are shown records before and after exposure to nitric oxide released by the nitric oxide donor papa-NONOate. Exposure to nitric oxide reduces the magnitude of the sodium currents. (C) The openings were completely blocked after 4–5 minutes of exposure to the sodium channel blocking agent lidocaine despite the presence of SNAP, indicating that the currents are the result of sodium channel activity. Adapted from Hammarstrom and Gage (1999). © 1999 with permission of Blackwell Publishing Ltd, and Renganathan *et al* (2002b).

Hammarstrom and Gage 1999; Z. Li *et al* 1998; Renganathan *et al* 2000; 2002a; Sawada *et al* 1995). Some of these effects are observed with endogenous nitric oxide production (Q-S. Liu *et al* 1997; Z. Li *et al* 1998; Renganathan *et al* 2000). They may be mediated by chemical reactions between nitric oxide (or related reactive nitrogen species such as nitrosothiols: Hogg 2002) and targets on the sodium channel, including channel thiols (Ahern *et al* 2000; Becchetti *et al* 1999; Z. Li *et al* 1998; Renganathan *et al* 2002b; Shrager 1977). The sodium channel may also be modified by the action of cyclic guanosine 3′,5′-monophosphate (cGMP), production of which is stimulated by nitric oxide-mediated activation of guanylate cyclase (Sawada *et al* 1995).

Nitric oxide and related molecules can also affect axons through effects on potassium channels (Ahern *et al* 1999; Bari *et al* 1996; Bolotina *et al* 1994; C-H. Chen *et al* 1998; Erdemli and Krnjevic 1995; Furukawa *et al* 1996; Moreno *et al* 1995) and calcium channels (Kurenny *et al* 1994; Snider *et al* 2000; Zsombok *et al* 2000). L-type calcium channels are normally present on myelinated axons (A.M. Brown *et al* 2001; Ouardouz *et al* 2003), whereas N-type calcium channels become expressed

on demyelinated axons (Kornek *et al* 2001). Thus, several paths exist by which nitric oxide might interact with ion channels and impair axonal function, or affect the function of calcium channels at axon terminals, thereby perturbing synaptic transmission.

In addition to these effects on ion channels, nitric oxide might block conduction by depolarizing axons (Figure 13.14; Garthwaite *et al* 1999; 2002), either acting though cGMP-mediated effects (Bains and Ferguson 1997) or, perhaps, by direct effects on the electrogenic Na^+/K^+ ATPase sodium pump (Guzman *et al* 1995; Sato *et al* 1995). Nitric oxide can also impair mitochondrial metabolism (Bolanos *et al* 1994; 1997; G.C. Brown 1999; G.C. Brown *et al* 1995), reducing the supply of ATP, perhaps below the level required to maintain those ion gradients upon which conduction depends.

Nitric oxide may also contribute to conduction deficits in multiple sclerosis by modifying many biological properties of glial cells (Chao *et al* 1995; S.C. Lee *et al* 1995; Merrill and Benveniste 1996; Ridet *et al* 1997), and it is easy to imagine that a disturbance of the metabolic functions of glia, particularly those that regulate ionic activity and neurotransmitter avail-

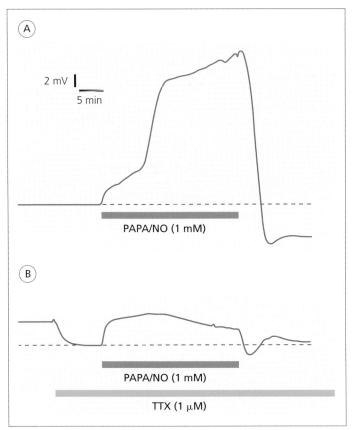

Figure 13.14 Depolarization of optic nerve produced by nitric oxide. (A) The nitric oxide donor PAPA NONOate (blue bar) caused a small rapid depolarization that was followed by a larger, delayed depolarization that reversed rapidly on washout. (B) Application of the sodium channel blocking agent tetrodotoxin (TTX) (green bar) caused a small hyperpolarization and abolished the delayed depolarization, but not the early depolarization caused by the nitric oxide donor. Adapted from Garthwaite *et al* (2002). © 2002, with permission from Elsevier.

delicately balanced processes would be completely overwhelmed by a continued presence of the higher concentrations of nitric oxide expected at sites of inflammation Given the complex chemistry of NO, especially in the context of inflammation, it is not yet possible to predict with certainty which of its reactions and effects primarily determine events occurring within the lesions of multiple sclerosis. The role of reactive oxygen and nitrogen species in demyelinating disease has been reviewed in more detail by Santiago *et al* (1998), K.J. Smith *et al* (1999) and K.J. Smith and Lassmann (2002).

It would seem at first glance that a therapy could be based on the inhibition of nitric oxide production by the iNOS enzyme. However, apart from the difficulty of selectively inhibiting iNOS using the currently available pharmacological agents, the goal may itself be misplaced. Nitric oxide exerts complex functions in health, including immunosuppressive activities, so that inhibition of nitric oxide could adversely affect those components of the disease driven by autoimmunity. The dual action of nitric oxide may explain the unpredictable consequences of its inhibition in the context of experimental autoimmune encephalomyelitis (see reviews in Singh *et al* 2000; Willenborg *et al* 1999; and also more recent publications of A.H. Cross *et al* 2000; D.C. Hooper *et al* 2000; Pozza *et al* 2000; Shin *et al* 2000; Spitsin *et al* 2000). Frustratingly, despite >40 studies examining the role of nitric oxide and its related compounds in experimental autoimmune encephalomyelitis, no consensus has emerged. With regard to a potential therapy, it is also worth pointing out that, although it appears plausible and altogether likely that nitric oxide does play an important role in the alteration of neurological function in multiple sclerosis, so far the evidence remains circumstantial.

Finally, it is worthwhile noting that interferon-β (IFN-β) inhibits iNOS expression in astrocytes (Guthikonda *et al* 1998; Hua *et al* 1998; V.C. Stewart *et al* 1997; 1998), which are arguably the main source of nitric oxide in the lesions of multiple sclerosis (Z. Liu *et al* 2001; Oleszak *et al* 1998). Moreover, IFN-β also inhibits the production of reactive oxygen species by monocytes from patients with relapsing–remitting multiple sclerosis (Lucas *et al* 1998). Thus, despite our reservations based on theory and observations in the experimental context, iNOS inhibition may be an unintended component of the treatment provided by some of the currently licensed therapies.

Circulating factors that block conduction

It has long been suspected that extracellular factors present in the lesions of multiple sclerosis may impair neurophysiological function. Indeed, it was discussed at some length in an earlier edition of this book (Lumsden 1972). Common sense seems to dictate that such factors probably exist, and supporting observations of various kinds, spanning 40 years, have been offered but without a consensus emerging on the identity of such factors. Many of the claims have not been reproducible. More recently, some potential candidates in the inflammatory soup have been identified.

The literature on putative 'neuroelectric blocking factors' present in the serum of patients with multiple sclerosis is both tantalizing – because, if such factors exist, it may be possible to modulate their production for therapeutic gain – and yet confusing, because the findings based on different models lack

ability, could impair the electrophysiological properties of axons, especially if their function was already compromised by demyelination. In addition, disruption of the normal cellular contacts between axons and macroglia would be expected to impair normal axonal function in axons, as, for example, astrocyte processes are integral components of many central nodes of Ranvier (Sims *et al* 1991). These processes might be damaged or retracted in response to nitric oxide exposure.

Nitric oxide can also be expected to affect neuronal function in the grey matter, as inflammatory lesions may occur in this compartment. It can cause both the excitation and inhibition of spontaneous activity in spinal neurons (Pehl and Schmid 1997; S.L. Smith and Otis 2003), and also interfere with synaptic transmission. Depending on the location of lesions, the latter effect may not only impair function in motor and sensory pathways but also contribute to cognitive deficits (Jeffrey *et al* 2000). In the normal nervous system low concentrations of nitric oxide are produced locally in short bursts to modulate synaptic function and contribute to synaptic plasticity (Baranano *et al* 2001; Bon and Garthwaite 2003; Holscher 1997; Kiss and Vizi 2001). It is easy to envisage how these coherence and appear contradictory. The story began in 1965 with a small study that included few controls (Bornstein and Crain 1965) showing that sera obtained from patients with multiple sclerosis during acute exacerbation, or from animals with experimental autoimmune encephalomyelitis, blocked reflex activity in cultured central nervous system tissue within minutes of exposure. The effect was considered to be complement dependent, and it was usually found to be prompt and reversible. These findings triggered a number of further investigations. Some were confirmatory (Cerf and Carels 1966) whereas others questioned the data, claiming that the findings were nonspecific – although this does not, of course, diminish their potential role in multiple sclerosis (Seil et al 1975). The blocking activity was typically found in the serum, diminished by plasma exchange, and some evidence favoured a role for IgG (Schauf and Davis 1981), whereas other evidence suggested that factors other than antibodies were primarily responsible (Seil et al 1976).

Although the terminology can superficially suggest that the factors block axonal conduction, the sera were in fact screened for their effects on synaptic transmission, and even those that had potent neuroelectric blocking effects were found not to affect conduction in demyelinated axons (Schauf and Davis 1981). Furthermore, the activity is not necessarily present in the cerebrospinal fluid, even in patients with potent blocking activity in serum (Schauf and Davis 1981). Superficially, these observations argue against the factors playing an important role in the pathophysiology of multiple sclerosis. However, even if the effects are true and confined to disruption of synaptic activity, serum factors could access grey matter through breakdown of the blood–brain barrier, and so they may contribute to the pathophysiology of multiple sclerosis. As matters stand, there remains a potential role for neuroelectric blocking factors in multiple sclerosis, but there is as yet no widely reproducible evidence (Koller et al 1997; K.J. Smith 1994).

The possibility that nitric oxide contributes to serum neuroelectric blocking effects is worth consideration. Although any free nitric oxide present in clinical samples would have far too short a half life to contribute an effect on conduction when tested later in vitro, some nitrosothiols (formed by the interaction of nitric oxide with protein and other thiols) can preserve the biological activity of nitric oxide, acting in a similar way as nitric oxide donors (Stamler et al 1992). As with the putative neuroelectric blocking factors, such activity would be more apparent in serum than cerebrospinal fluid, due to the greater abundance of thiol-containing proteins. The classic neuroelectric blocking factors are putatively present in the serum, but a recent study has reported that the cerebrospinal fluid from some patients with multiple sclerosis can induce a reversible conduction block in isolated rat optic nerve (Centonze et al 2005). Thus the fluid (diluted one-third in control medium) from 7 of 15 patients reversibly reduced the amplitude of the compound action potential by 9–41% within 30–50 minutes of exposure. The mechanism remains unclear, but the authors discuss the potential role of QYNAD.

QYNAD (endocaine)

A pentapeptide with the amino acid sequence QYNAD (Gln-Tyr-Asn-Ala-Asp) has been found specifically in the cerebrospinal fluid of patients with multiple sclerosis and the Guillain–Barré syndrome. At endogenous concentrations, QYNAD is reported to have local anaesthetic-like effects on sodium channels (Aulkemeyer et al 2000; Brinkmeier et al 2000; Meuth et al 2003; Padmashri et al 2004), hence the name endocaine, and to cause conduction block in sciatic nerve axons (F. Weber et al 2002). However, careful studies in several laboratories have failed to reproduce the findings (Cummins et al 2003; Quasthoff et al 2003). Our own unpublished observations show that the compound can impair conduction in demyelinated central axons, but only at much higher concentrations than previously described. Whether this short peptide can nonetheless exist in forms offering different biological activities, thereby explaining the contradictory literature, remains unanswered.

Antibodies

It is possible that antibodies contribute directly to the impairment of conduction in multiple sclerosis, perhaps by binding to ion channels or their associated molecules (for discussion, see Ariga et al 2001; Waxman 1995). Although no antibodies have so far been shown to affect axonal conduction in multiple sclerosis, clear effects of antibodies on the electrophysiological properties of central nervous system neurons have recently been demonstrated in HTLV-1 myeloneuropathy (Figure 13.15; Levin et al 2002). Furthermore, anti-ganglioside antibodies are present in some individuals with multiple sclerosis (Acarin et al 1996; Sadatipour et al 1998), especially those with prominent axonal damage, and some (although not all) studies have found that such antibodies can impair axonal conduction in peripheral axons (reviewed in K.J. Smith and Hall 2001; Willison and Yuki 2002). Antibodies could also, of course, act indirectly in a very wide variety of ways, most obviously by causing demyelination through immunological mechanisms, or by disturbing the composition of the extracellular milieu by influencing integrity of the blood–brain barrier, perhaps mimicking the activity of anti-ganglioside GM1 antibodies acting at the blood–nerve barrier (Kanda et al 2000).

Cytokines

Active lesions in multiple sclerosis are notable for intensity of the inflammatory response, and a number of studies have accordingly described the prominence of cytokines within the cerebrospinal fluid, including interleukin 1β (IL-1β) (Hauser et al 1990; Tsukada et al 1991), IL-2 (Gallo et al 1988, 1991), IL-6 (Maimone et al 1991b; Weller et al 1991) and TNF-α (Franciotta et al 1989; Hauser et al 1990; Sharief and Hentges 1991; Tsukada et al 1991; for review see Koller et al 1997; Rothwell et al 1996). IL-1 and TNF-α are also detected within lesions (Cannella and Raine 1995; Hofman et al 1989; Wucherpfennig et al 1992a). These cytokines may well result in neurological deficits because several are known to affect the electrophysiological properties of neurons and axons, directly and by inducing vascular changes (Brosnan et al 1989). As potent inducers of iNOS, TNF-α and IFN-γ may indirectly affect axonal function by the production of NO, but these cytokines can also directly influence voltage-gated ion channels (Brinkmeier et al 1993; Kaspar et al 1994; McLarnon et al 1993; Mimura et al 1994; Plata-Salaman and ffrench-Mullen 1992;

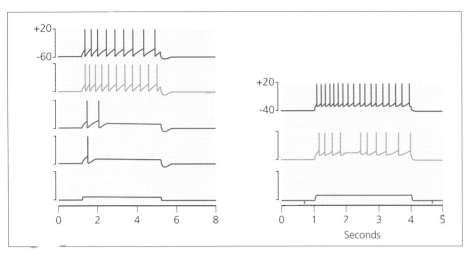

Figure 13.15 Patch clamp recording from a rat neuron in a brain slice showing the reduction in neuronal firing upon the extracellular infusion of increasing physiological concentrations of IgG from patients with human T lymphotropic virus type 1-associated myelopathy (HAM)/tropical spastic paraparesis (TSP). Recordings were made in current clamp mode and show the train of action potentials evoked in response to a depolarizing plateau stimulus in the presence of normal cerebrospinal fluid (red) and 5, 10, 15, and 20 µg/mL HAM/TSP IgG (green, blue, purple, brown, respectively).

Visentin and Levi 1997). For example, IL-1β inhibits the calcium current in hippocampal neurons (Plata-Salaman and ffrench-Mullen 1992), and IL-2 inhibits neuronal calcium currents (Plata-Salaman and ffrench-Mullen 1993; P. Song *et al* 2002) and muscle sodium channels (Kaspar *et al* 1994). TNF-α inhibits sodium currents, at least in *Aplysia* neurons (Sawada *et al* 1991).

In the context of grey matter lesions, several studies have found effects of cytokines such as IL-1β and IL-6 on synaptic transmission (Kelles *et al* 2000; S. Wang *et al* 2000). Direct effects on axonal conduction have proved more difficult to demonstrate (Dugandzija-Novakovic and Shrager 1995; E.J. Redford *et al* 1995; Uncini *et al* 1999), but a systematic study of cytokines on axons, particularly those that are demyelinated, may now be warranted given the availability of a wide range of cytokines for experimental study in a variety of laboratory species.

Cytokines and other factors associated with inflammation may, of course, also exert indirect effects on neurons by influencing glial cells (Köller *et al* 1993; 1996; 1997; 1998). In line with their role as immunocompetent cells, inflammatory mediators predictably have pronounced effects on astrocytes and microglia. In turn, astrocytes can signal directly to neurons via a number of routes including, at least in culture, gap junctions (Nedergaard 1994).

Prostaglandins

It is possible that prostaglandins may play a role in modulating the electrophysiological properties of demyelinated axons. Prostaglandin E₂, in particular, has been found to affect the tetrodotoxin-resistant sodium current (J.D. England *et al* 1996; M.S. Gold *et al* 2002) and the potassium current (A.R. Evans *et al* 1999) of neurons, resulting in increased excitability (S. England *et al* 1996) mediated by intracellular pathways (A.R. Evans *et al* 1999; M.S. Gold *et al* 2002). Arachidonic acid (which is metabolized to prostaglandins) also inhibits potassium currents, resulting in broadening of the action potential (Keros and McBain 1997). Together, these observations raise the possibility that prostaglandins may well affect conduction in multiple sclerosis.

Neurological deficits and experimental autoimmune encephalomyelitis

The various forms of experimental autoimmune encephalomyelitis model different aspects of multiple sclerosis, with varying degrees of accuracy. The animals typically exhibit inflammatory demyelinating lesions within the central nervous system, and show neurological deficits that mirror the more florid features of multiple sclerosis, such as weakness and paralysis. However, thus far, the study of experimental autoimmune encephalomyelitis has not been particularly helpful in identifying specific factors that underlie the disruption of neurological function because the pathological processes in this disease often combine several factors simultaneously. Furthermore, animals with experimental autoimmune encephalomyelitis tend spontaneously to make a relatively complete recovery, preventing the analysis of factors associated with remission from those that cause chronic deficits. With regard to mechanisms underlying loss of function, the evidence suggests that inflammation and demyelination each make an independent contribution to the clinical deficit. Thus, severe neurological deficit is found not only in models of chronic experimental autoimmune encephalomyelitis characterized by extensive demyelination, but also in the acute forms induced by Th1 polarized T cells, which show massive inflammation but very little demyelination or tissue injury. Unfortunately, it is difficult to segregate and identify each and every factor responsible for the neurological deficit. For example, in passive T-cell-dependent experimental autoimmune encephalomyelitis it is difficult to prove that inflammation *per se* is responsible for the clinical deficit because, although there may be no demyelinated plaques, animals with severe neurological deficit exhibit some structural damage of nerve fibres around the inflammatory infiltrates, and these are abundantly distributed throughout the neuraxis. Thus, even small penumbral deficits around the T-cell infiltrates may constitute quite significant myelin and axonal damage when the central nervous system is considered as a whole. Of course, a long axon only needs conduction to be blocked at one, possibly discrete, location somewhere along its length for that fibre to be rendered functionally useless. Electrophysiological studies, needed to clarify the roles of different pathologies, have so far been performed in only very few experimental autoimmune encephalomyelitis models.

In general the correlation between inflammation within the central nervous system and the expression of a neurological deficit is good (Alvord and Kies 1959). However, even in the early studies of experimental autoimmune encephalomyelitis, discrepancies emerged between the severity of neurological deficits and the degree of inflammation in clinically important regions, such as the spinal cord. In particular, profound inflammation can persist in animals when they are nonetheless undergoing significant recovery of function after an individual attack. Furthermore, severe neurological deficits, and even death, can occur in acute experimental autoimmune encephalomyelitis despite the presence of only mild inflammation. In these animals, the deficits correlate with marked vascular congestions, small haemorrhages and massive oedema (Alvord and Kies 1959; S. Levine and Wenk 1965). This pathological picture is similar to that found in acute haemorrhagic leucoencephalomyelitis (see Chapter 12; Hurst 1941). A role for inflammation is, however, suggested by some chronic models of experimental autoimmune encephalomyelitis. For example, the severity of the neurological deficit is often more pronounced during the inaugural (mainly inflammatory) phase of chronic disease than during the later stages, characterized by large confluent demyelinated plaques (Lassmann and Wisniewski 1979a; 1979b). One chronic relapsing model of experimental autoimmune encephalomyelitis (Lorentzen et al 1995) has been described as exhibiting prominent central nervous system inflammation, but no demyelination, at the first occurrence of the neurological deficit (Tanuma et al 2000). Prominent demyelination becomes apparent with the second phase. This model appears to indicate that, at first, inflammation can cause significant neurological deficits. However, our own unpublished examination of this model has revealed that active demyelination is in fact present in the spinal cord during the first attack, although whether it is sufficient to explain the entire neurological deficit is uncertain.

Although animals with substantial neurological deficits show corresponding electrophysiological abnormalities, mainly the conduction block that is typically attributed to demyelination, electrophysiological studies performed to date have not clearly illuminated the specific contribution of this histological feature (Chalk et al 1994; Deguchi et al 1992; Heininger et al 1989; Kojima et al 1994; Stanley and Pender 1991; Vass et al 1992). Some earlier reports of myelin basic protein-induced experimental autoimmune encephalomyelitis in the rat emphasized the presence of neurological deficit despite relative lack of demyelination. However, Pender and colleagues found that demyelination was in fact quite prominent in these rats, arguing that the earlier studies had overlooked this aspect of the pathology because it was concentrated in the spinal roots rather than the cord (Chalk et al 1994; 1995; Pender 1988a; 1988b; Pender and Sears 1984; Stanley and Pender 1991). These root lesions were associated with prominent conduction block. Additional evidence favouring a predominant role for demyelination underlying the neurological deficits was provided by the observation that clinical remission was associated with the recovery of conduction in both the central and peripheral nervous system, but recovery correlated better with the restoration of conduction in the periphery, where demyelination was located (Chalk et al 1995; Pender 1989). These studies

highlight the need to investigate the pathology of experimental autoimmune encephalomyelitis throughout the entire neuraxis if the neurological deficit is to be accurately explained. That said, root lesions cannot account for the neurological deficits observed in all experimental autoimmune encephalomyelitis models. For example, the transfer of T cells targeting myelin oligodendrocyte glycoprotein in DA rats causes a severe neurological deficit, but myelin oligodendrocyte glycoprotein is not expressed in the peripheral nervous system and T-cell mediated inflammation driven by myelin oligodendrocyte glycoprotein-reactive T cells does not affect the spinal roots (T. Berger et al 1997).

The role of inflammation in causing conduction deficits has partly been obscured by lack of precision in interpretation of the word 'inflammation'. Rather, it is helpful to focus on the contribution of specific cellular populations involved in the inflammatory response. Thus, a recent systematic comparison of experimental autoimmune encephalomyelitis induced by a variety of antigen-specific T-cell lines in different rat strains showed that it is the antigen-specific reactivation of T cells within the central nervous system that determines their ability to cause neurological deficits, more than the amount of T-cell infiltration (Kawakami et al 2004). In animals with lymphocyte infiltrates but no symptoms, the intrathecal injection of soluble antigen effectively provokes the reactivation of T cells, resulting in the local production of proinflammatory cytokines and chemokines. T-cell reactivation is effective, and necessary, in recruiting large numbers of activated ED1$^+$ macrophages into the central nervous system. These observations augment the previously reported close association between the severity of the neurological deficit in experimental autoimmune encephalomyelitis and the extent of macrophage activation and infiltration into the lesions (see Figure 13.16; T. Berger et al 1997), and other studies that have highlighted the crucial role of macrophages in the expression of a neurological deficit in experimental autoimmune encephalomyelitis (Brosnan et al 1981; Huitinga et al 1990; Martiney et al 1998; Tran et al 1998).

These data suggest that inflammation of the central nervous system is able to provoke a neurological deficit in the absence of demyelination, provided that the driving T cells are locally activated in an antigen-specific manner. It is the subsequent recruitment of activated macrophages that seems to trigger the neurological deficit, either by impairing axonal conduction (see below) or, in severe conditions, through structural damage of axons in the absence of primary demyelination. It may be of interest in this context that our unpublished observations show, in addition to the macrophage infiltration initiated by reactivated T cells (Kawakami et al 2004), some associated perivascular acute axonal injury, occurring in the absence of primary segmental demyelination.

However, to emphasize the complexity of experimental autoimmune encephalomyelitis as a system for the examination of neurological deficits, Kojima and colleagues (1994) have described a model with no neurological deficit despite the presence of prominent (largely T-cell) inflammation within the central nervous system. This deploys passive transfer of T cells specific for the S100β molecule found primarily (at least within the central nervous system) in astrocytes. Production of the neurological deficit in this model requires the administration of appropriate antibodies in order to provoke demyelination.

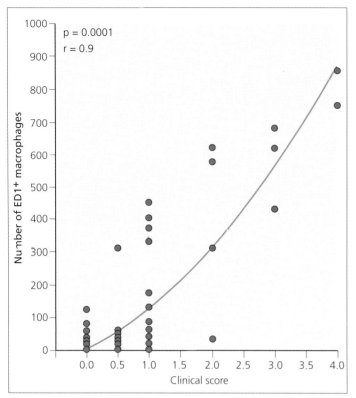

Figure 13.16 Graph showing the positive relationship between the number of macrophages within the central nervous system and the expression of neurological deficit in animals with experimental autoimmune encephalomyelitis. Adapted from T. Berger *et al* (1997).

Neurological deficits and multiple sclerosis

Perhaps the clearest, and certainly most striking, evidence that inflammation can cause clinical deficits in multiple sclerosis came from experimental therapy involving the administration of Campath-1H, directed against the CD52 antigen expressed by lymphocytes and monocytes (see Chapter 18; Moreau *et al* 1996). In the original study, within only a few hours of antibody administration and the onset of lymphocyte depletion, patients experienced a rehearsal of deficits expressed earlier in the course of their disease, but from which they were in remission. The effect was transient, and recovery generally completed within 24 hours. As old symptoms were resurrected rather than new ones appearing, the observations suggested that something to do with the therapy caused conduction to be temporarily blocked in axons previously damaged by the disease process (see Figure 18.48). The exacerbations were sufficiently brief that structural changes, such as demyelination with repair by remyelination, seemed unlikely (these processes take weeks), implying a physical or chemical mechanism. Temporary conduction block mediated by body warming (Uhthoff's phenomenon, see below) was a possible explanation, but that was excluded by manipulation of body temperature. However, Campath-1H did cause a surge in the circulating concentration of cytokines, particularly TNF-α, IFN-γ and IL-6 (Moreau *et al* 1996; Wing *et al* 1996), although subsequent observations suggested that the prime candidate (TNF-α) was not the culprit (Coles *et al* 1999a). The cytokine surge peaked at 2–4 hours, approximately correlating with onset of the clinical exacerbation. Pretreating the patients with intravenous methylprednisolone prevented both the cytokine surge and expression of the symptoms.

It appeared that one or more of the cytokines might be blocking conduction in damaged axons, but an electrophysiological examination of conduction along experimentally demyelinated axons did not find any cytokines (including TNF-α, IFN-γ and IL-6) that acutely blocked conduction (Redford *et al* 1997). However, this study did reveal a different candidate for the blocking effect, namely nitric oxide. Significantly, its production is markedly enhanced by the presence of TNF-α and IFN-γ, which act synergistically to promote formation of the inducible form of nitric oxide synthase (iNOS) in inflammatory cells and microglia (Goureau *et al* 1997).

Synaptic dysfunction: grey matter lesions and cognitive decline

It has long been known that lesions can occur within the grey matter. In fact, these are rather common (see Chapter 12) and may explain the reduction in cognitive function seen in multiple sclerosis (Camp *et al* 1999; Demaree *et al* 1999; DeSousa *et al* 2002; Foong *et al* 1999; Jeffrey *et al* 2000). Involvement of white matter is probably also relevant because cognitive impairment correlates with the volume of MRI lesions in periventricular white matter (Franklin *et al* 1988; S.M. Rao *et al* 1989a; Ron *et al* 1991).

The mechanisms involved remain unclear, but several factors associated with inflammation can disturb synaptic transmission in normal tissue, including IL-1 (L.G. Miller and Fahey 1994), IL-2 (H.J. Park *et al* 1995), TNF-α (Tancredi *et al* 1992), IFN (D'Arcangelo *et al* 1991) and, especially, nitric oxide (Fossier *et al* 1999; Holscher 1997; Kara and Friedlander 1998; Kilbinger 1996; S. Wang *et al* 2000). Furthermore, it is easy to imagine that the physical disturbance associated with oedema in the cortex as distinct from white matter, together with any dysregulation of the composition of the extracellular fluid due to impairment of the blood–brain barrier or glial dysfunction, could disrupt the delicately balanced processes of normal synaptic function.

If synaptic depression does contribute to the neurological deficit, it might help to explain why 4-aminopyridine provides a modestly effective therapy for certain symptoms (Bever Jr *et al* 1994; Davis *et al* 1990; R.E. Jones *et al* 1983; Polman *et al* 1994a; 1994b; Stefoski *et al* 1987; van Diemen *et al* 1992). 4-Aminopyridine blocks potassium channels and it might act clinically either by restoring conduction to blocked axons – prolonging the duration of the action potential as originally demonstrated experimentally using high concentrations of the agent (Figure 13.17; Bostock *et al* 1981; Sherratt *et al* 1980; Targ and Kocsis 1985; 1986) – or by potentiating synaptic transmission, as suggested more recently (Figure 13.18; Felts and Smith 1994; K.J. Smith *et al* 2000).

Glutamate is produced by activated microglia and leucocytes within the brain (Piani *et al* 1991) and its concentration is raised in the inflammatory lesions of multiple sclerosis. Indeed, glutamate concentrations may be further amplified by the inhibitory

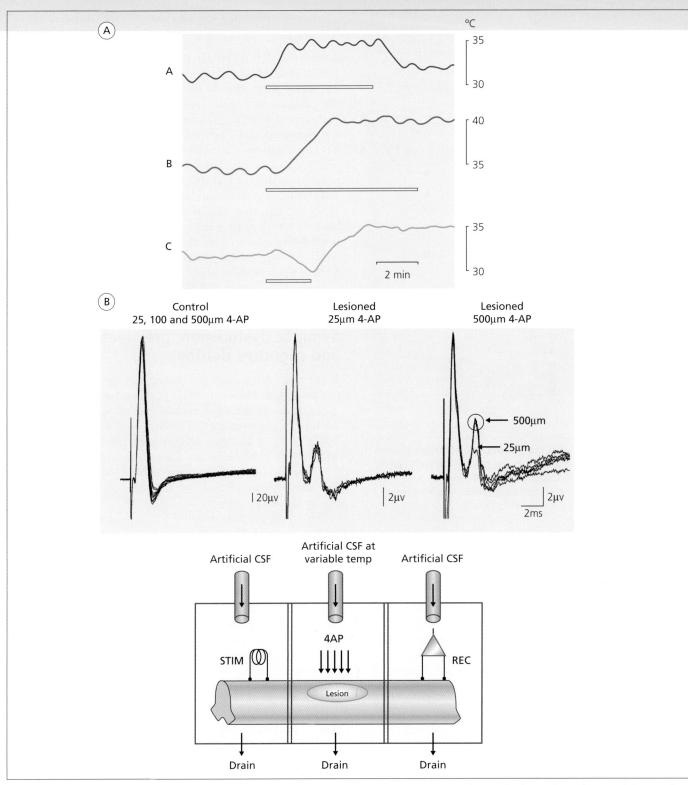

Figure 13.17 Data showing the beneficial effect of potassium channel blocking agents on conduction in demyelinated axons. (A) Records showing an increase in the security of conduction of individual demyelinated axons following administration (indicated by bars) of the potassium channel blocking agents (A) tetraethylammonium ions (TEA), or (B and C) 4-aminopyridine at 1 mM or 5 mM concentrations respectively. The drugs increase the temperature at which conduction becomes blocked, by several degrees centigrade. Adapted from Bostock et al (1981). (B) Three families of superimposed compound action potentials recorded from excised control rat dorsal columns (left group), or similar tissue in which a focal experimental demyelinating lesion had been induced 21 days previously by the intraspinal injection of ethidium bromide (centre and right groups). The inset illustrates the recording arrangement. The records were obtained at 5-minute intervals before and after the solution in the central lane was changed from control artificial cerebrospinal fluid to identical fluid containing the concentrations of 4-aminopyridine indicated: each was applied for 20 minutes. The control records show that 4-aminopyridine has almost no effect on conduction in normal central axons. The 'lesioned' records show two peaks to the compound action potentials; the first peak results from conduction in axons spared by the lesion, while the second shows delayed conduction in axons that are almost certainly demyelinated. The lesioned records are divided into two groups for clarity. The central panel shows one record obtained before the addition of 25 μM 4-aminopyridine, and then three records obtained following 4-aminopyridine exposure: 25 μM 4-aminopyridine has little or no effect on conduction in either the normal, or the demyelinated axons. The right panel shows five superimposed records, comprising one obtained in 25 μM 4-aminopyridine (the latest record from the central panel), and four in 500 μM 4-aminopyridine. Exposure to 500 μM 4-aminopyridine results in an increase in the number of demyelinated axons conducting successfully through the lesion. The records result from the same two pieces of tissue as those illustrated in Figure 13.35. STIM = stimulate; REC = record. Adapted from K.J. Smith et al (2000).

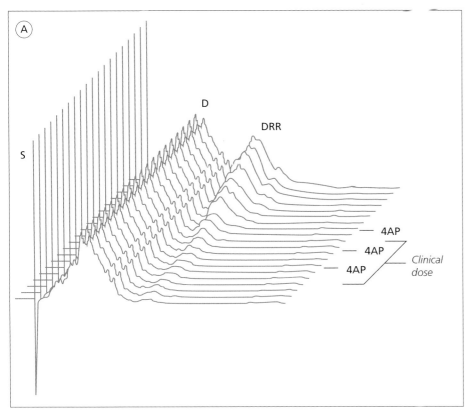

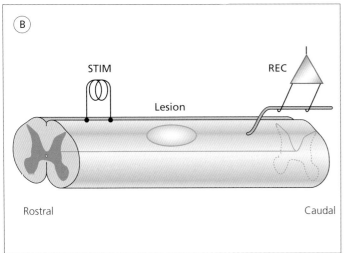

Figure 13.18 Superimposed records of compound action potentials made from the ipsilateral L5 dorsal root of an anaesthetized rat following supramaximal stimulation of the dorsal columns rostral to a central demyelinating lesion induced by the intraspinal injection of ethidium bromide 33 days previously. The recording arrangement is illustrated in the inset. The records are shown in three-dimensional perspective, with the earliest records displayed towards the front. Two peaks to the compound action potential can be discerned. The first peak (labelled D) represents direct conduction in dorsal column axons; almost all the axons contributing to this peak were known to be affected by the demyelinating lesion (data not shown). The second peak (DRR) shows activity resulting from the dorsal root reflex, namely action potentials resulting from synaptic activity within the dorsal horns. Before the administration of 4-aminopyridine the DRR makes very little contribution to the waveform, but the amplitude of the reflex activity increases many fold in response to the intravenous administration of the drug, which was injected in small, equal aliquots at 10 minute intervals; the first two administrations resulted in a similar dose to that administered to patients. Although the 4-aminopyridine dramatically enhanced the DRR, it had very little, if any, effect on the success of conduction along the lesioned dorsal column axons, even though the lesion contained many axons that were just on the verge of conducting, and to which conduction could be restored by small decreases in temperature. S shows the position of the stimulus artefact. STIM = stimulate; REC = record. Adapted from K.J. Smith *et al* (2000).

action of proinflammatory cytokines (IL-1β and TNF-α) on glutamate uptake by astrocytes (Hu *et al* 2000). It is reasonable to propose that raised concentrations of this neurotransmitter may impair synaptic transmission, and it is therefore particularly noteworthy that blockade of NMDA/AMPA/kainate receptors can ameliorate experimental autoimmune encephalomyelitis (Pitt *et al* 2000; T. Smith *et al* 2000b; Wallstrom *et al* 1996; Werner *et al* 2000). Although this effect may primarily be mediated by the protection of oligodendrocytes and neurons from glutamate-mediated toxicity, an additional effect on synaptic transmission remains a possibility.

In view of the potent effects of nitric oxide on such fundamental neuronal properties as ion channel function and membrane polarization, it is not surprising that nitric oxide also has strong effects on synaptic transmission, which may not only compromise transmission in motor and sensory pathways, but also help to explain the loss of cognitive function in multiple sclerosis (Jeffrey *et al* 2000). Indeed, some synaptic effects of nitric oxide occur at relatively low concentrations as part of normal physiological function (reviewed in Baranano *et al* 2001; Holscher 1997; Kara and Friedlander 1998). However, in the lesions of multiple sclerosis, pathological concentrations of nitric oxide, probably sufficient to disrupt synapses, can be anticipated because lesions expressing iNOS are common within the grey matter (Kidd *et al* 1999a; Peterson *et al* 2001). These high nitric oxide concentrations may simply swamp the normal, delicately balanced physiological synaptic processes. Furthermore, each of the several different forms of nitric oxide can directly affect NMDA and AMPA receptors (Choi and Lipton 2000). Indeed, a vicious cycle has been hypothesized involving sodium channels, glutamate release, NMDA receptors and local nitric oxide production, which can act synergistically to cause degeneration (Strijbos *et al* 1996).

Contributions from abnormalities of peripheral axons and muscle

It is an assumption that the functional deficits in patients with multiple sclerosis necessarily result exclusively from pathophysiological events confined to the central nervous system. As discussed in Chapter 12, peripheral nerves are occasionally involved in patients with multiple sclerosis, but it is difficult to dissect their contribution to neurological deficits because peripheral nerve damage usually occurs at late stages of the disease, when pronounced irreversible deficits of central origin are already established. In this setting, many peripheral nerve lesions and their functional consequences can reasonably be attributed to secondary complications, such as pressure palsies in immobilized patients, or metabolic disturbances and malnutrition. However, primary inflammatory demyelination of the peripheral nervous system is sometimes present in patients with acute fulminant (Marburg type) multiple sclerosis, providing a better opportunity to assess its contribution to the functional deficit.

High-dose corticosteroid therapy can reportedly reduce the excitability of denervated muscle fibres (Rich *et al* 1998). Although such therapy is routinely used to shorten the duration of acute relapses in multiple sclerosis, there is no evidence that it compromises function by a direct effect on peripheral nerve and muscle.

MRI of the acutely symptomatic lesion: optic neuritis

The most suitable location for studying the evolution of acutely symptomatic lesions in the central nervous system in multiple sclerosis is the optic nerve. This site offers several advantages:

- Optic neuritis is a frequent manifestation of multiple sclerosis, being the presenting feature in 25% of patients and occurring at some stage of the illness in about 75%.
- The clinical course can be monitored using sensitive neuro-ophthalmological measures such as Logmar visual acuity, Humphrey fields and Pelli–Robson colour vision assessment.
- Conduction through the symptomatic lesion can be evaluated with the visual evoked potential.
- The symptomatic lesion can be directly imaged and followed using structural MRI focused on the anterior visual pathway.
- The cortical response can be followed using fMRI to study the primary visual cortex and other cortical areas.

Furthermore, because optic neuritis is usually unilateral, it is possible to compare MRI findings in the affected and unaffected nerve. In 80–90% of instances there is a good clinical recovery. The study of optic neuritis should therefore help in understanding the mechanisms of relapse and recovery that operate in acutely symptomatic inflammatory/demyelinating lesions.

Conventional T_1- and T_2-weighted MRI have proved insensitive in detecting the lesions of optic neuritis, due to the problem of high signal from surrounding orbital fat with an associated chemical shift artefact. This problem was first overcome by using a STIR (short T_1 inversion recovery) sequence that suppresses the fat signal allowing the depiction of intrinsic nerve lesions in most cases (D.H. Miller *et al* 1986b). In a study of ten patients with acute optic neuritis, STIR imaging was undertaken on two occasions before and after the administration of gadolinium. The first scan was obtained within two weeks of symptom onset and the second one month later (Youl *et al* 1991b). Initially, all 11 symptomatic nerves displayed gadolinium enhancement, indicating the presence of acute inflammation. The VEP amplitude was markedly reduced at this time and vision was usually impaired. One month later, when visual recovery had occurred in most patients, only 2/11 nerves continued to show gadolinium enhancement and the VEP amplitude had increased. However, VEP latency was prolonged, indicating the presence of persistent demyelination (Figure 13.19). The investigators concluded that acute inflammation and conduction block were present at the time of initial visual loss, and that both recovered with the resolution of the inflammation, despite the persistence of demyelination as indicated by a prolonged VEP latency. The study provides evidence that resolution of inflammation *per se* is a mechanism for functional recovery.

Recently, Hickman *et al* (2004a; 2004b; 2004c) have related the dynamics of early MRI, and the clinical and electrophysiological features to final visual outcome in a serial study over 1 year. At presentation, within four weeks of onset, 27/28 symptomatic nerves displayed gadolinium enhancement (see Figure 7.27). Enhancement lasted a mean of 61 days. Improved prognosis at one year was associated with having a short acute optic

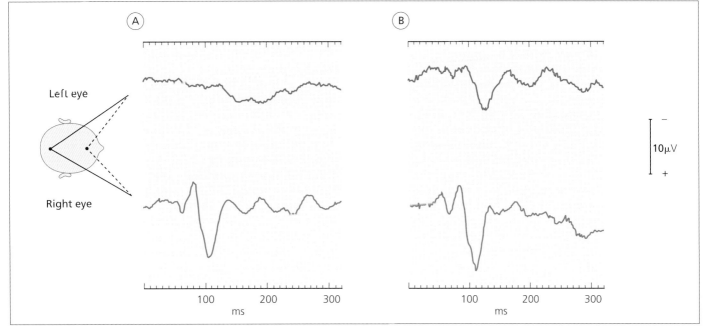

Figure 13.19 Visual evoked potentials obtained from a patient with left optic neuritis. (A) The left eye shows an acute attack with conduction block and slow conduction. (B) One month later the amplitude has partly recovered, with slow conduction.

nerve lesion on gadolinium enhanced MRI, a higher amplitude VEP during recovery, and a steep gradient of initial improvement in vision. There was no relationship between the duration of enhancement and visual outcome. While the extent of inflammation along the nerve may have some prognostic value, this did not emerge as a powerful predictor of outcome in this study. The STIR sequence has been used to investigate the effect of high-dose intravenous methylprednisolone on the structural outcome of symptomatic lesions. In a randomized, placebo-controlled trial involving 66 patients scanned immediately pretreatment and six months later, there was no effect of treatment on the final length of the optic nerve lesion (Kapoor *et al* 1998) nor on the development of optic nerve atrophy (Hickman *et al* 2003), which was observed in both treatment arms.

One limitation of the STIR sequence arises from cerebrospinal fluid in the optic nerve sheath. This produces high signal so that it is difficult to quantify the size of the nerve itself. However, a short echo time fat suppressed fast FLAIR sequence (sTEfFLAIR) has been developed that suppresses the signal from both orbital fat and optic nerve sheath cerebrospinal fluid. Using this sequence it is possible to measure the cross-sectional area of the optic nerve from coronal images. Such studies have revealed that in acute optic neuritis, swelling of the affected nerve is usually present. There was a mean increase in cross-sectional area of 20.1% (Figure 13.20) compared with the contralateral unaffected nerve at first presentation a median of 13 days from symptom onset in a recent prospective study (Hickman *et al* 2004b). The swelling resolves in a few weeks to months, and with follow-up after one year or longer, a decrease in optic nerve area of 10–15% has been reported (see Figure 7.29B; Hickman *et al* 2001). In a prospective serial study, the decrease in area was 11.7% compared with the clinically unaffected nerve after one year (Hickman *et al* 2004b). The subsidence of swelling

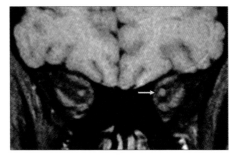

Figure 13.20 MRI of acute left optic neuritis. A sTEfFLAIR scan shows swelling of the left optic nerve (arrowed).

during the early weeks reflects resolution of oedema and inflammation and coincides with cessation of gadolinium enhancement. There is also some evidence that atrophy may continue for several years (Hickman *et al* 2002a). Continued loss of nerve tissue may reflect a slower time course for clearing the products of Wallerian degeneration in the central nervous system. Alternatively, it may indicate continuing axonal loss occurring in persistently demyelinated, and hence more vulnerable, axons.

The presence of optic nerve atrophy probably indicates both demyelination and axonal loss, and is more severe in patients with poor visual recovery (Inglese *et al* 2002b). However, some atrophy is seen despite good clinical recovery (Hickman *et al* 2001). This dissociation may have several explanations, some of which can be inferred from recent structural and fMRI studies. We have described above that conduction can be restored to demyelinated axons by the insertion of sodium channels along the axonal membrane. This process would not alter the size of the optic nerve. Also, repair by remyelination will make conduction more secure but it does not follow that the diameter of the nerve will be restored because the new myelin is thinner than normal. In addition, optic nerve MTR has been correlated inversely with VEP latency in patients following an attack of optic neuritis (Thorpe *et al* 1995) suggesting that, at least in part, MTR provides an assessment of myelination in the optic nerve. A recently completed serial study reported MTR changes in the optic nerve over one year from presentation with acute optic neuritis (Hickman *et al* 2004c). MTR decreased to a minimum at 240 days after which it appeared to rise, although the increase was not significantly different from the nadir value. The authors suggested that the gradual fall in MTR over six or more months might reflect the gradual clearance of myelin debris, and that remyelination may have influenced subsequent MTR changes: that there was a significant time linked association between MTR and VEP latency further suggests that MTR provides an indication of myelination. Shortening of the VEP latency over a 2-year period of follow-up from presentation with acute optic neuritis has been interpreted as indicating evidence for delayed remyelination after optic neuritis (Brusa *et al* 2001). Cortical reorganization may also allow recovery or maintenance of function even if there is irreversible damage, including axonal loss in the symptomatic optic nerve.

An interesting feature of the acute relapse in multiple sclerosis is the occasional concurrence of symptoms attributable to dysfunction at several, sometimes widely separated, sites: for example, trigeminal sensory loss occurring with acute optic neuritis. The explanation probably lies in the observation that it is common to find enhancement on MRI not only in the several areas implicated by clinical symptoms but also at several other locations (R.I. Grossman *et al* 1986; Kappos *et al* 1999). The implication is that relapse is driven by a systemic factor distributed simultaneously to several sites throughout the nervous system. An obvious candidate is the infiltration of inflammatory cells.

MRI and the clinical course of clinically isolated syndromes and early relapsing–remitting multiple sclerosis

Much work has been devoted to describing the MRI findings, both in cross-sectional and longitudinal studies, at all stages of the clinical course of multiple sclerosis. The following represents a summary of the key findings that have emerged. The earlier and clinically milder stages of multiple sclerosis (noting that this discussion refers only to patients with clinically isolated syndromes who go on to develop multiple sclerosis) are characterized on MRI by multifocal white matter lesions in the cerebrum, posterior fossa and spinal cord. There are, however, very large variations between individuals in the number and location of lesions. On average, serial scanning reveals 5–10 new T_2 lesions for every clinical relapse (Barkhof *et al* 1991; A.J. Thompson *et al* 1992). New lesions occur 4–10 times more often in the brain than the spinal cord (Silver *et al* 2001; Thorpe *et al* 1996a).

When frequent (monthly or weekly) scanning has been performed, it becomes evident that new lesions almost invariably start by displaying gadolinium enhancement (Cotton *et al* 2003; J.O. Harris *et al* 1991; H.M. Lai *et al* 1996). Enhancement may even precede the appearance of a T_2 abnormality by a few days (H.J. Barratt *et al* 1988; Kermode *et al* 1990). Such observations have understandably led to the hypothesis that breakdown

of the blood–brain barrier is the first event in the pathogenesis of a new lesion in multiple sclerosis.

The phase of gadolinium enhancement lasts on average 2–6 weeks, but with some variation between lesions. Most form a small homogeneous region of enhancement before partially resolving, although persistent T_2 abnormality is the rule. Larger lesions sometimes evolve from homogeneous regions showing ring enhancement, which probably reflects the active advancing edge of acute inflammation. Enhancing lesions may also display prominent lipid peaks on proton MR spectroscopy-indicated concurrent demyelination (Davie *et al* 1994).

New enhancing lesions are more likely to be symptomatic when they occur at clinically eloquent sites such as the spinal cord or optic nerves. Enhancing brain lesions are seen more often during relapse than periods of remission (R.I. Grossman *et al* 1986). Many acute enhancing lesions are hypointense on the non-contrast T_1-weighted image, although follow-up of these lesions shows that only about 50% show persistent hypointensity (van Waesberghe *et al* 1998). When it persists, this feature indicates a greater degree of axonal loss than is seen in T_1 isointense lesions (van Walderveen *et al* 1999a; 1999b). Not unexpectedly, enhancing lesions occur less often in patients with relapsing–remitting disease of long duration and low disability (Kidd *et al* 1994; A.J. Thompson *et al* 1992), so-called benign multiple sclerosis.

There is a consistent and quite robust relationship between new and enhancing lesions and the occurrence of relapse (Kappos *et al* 1999), especially in early disease. Indeed, new lesions appearing within 3–12 months of a clinically isolated syndrome are associated with a high probability of having a further clinical relapse within 3 years (Dalton *et al* 2002a; Tintore *et al* 2003). In contrast, little or no relationship has emerged between T_2 or gadolinium enhancing lesions and disability accumulation (Kappos *et al* 1999). This discrepancy may partly reflect the short-term nature of these studies with corresponding small changes in disability. Thus, there is much interest in the long-term relationship of early MRI findings to future disability. Two recent follow-up studies from onset with a clinically isolated syndrome have shown that the location and volume of T_2 lesions at presentation predicts disability as measured on the EDSS after 8.7 years (Minneboo *et al* 2004) and 14 years (Brex *et al* 2002). But the lack of a strong relationship between imaging at presentation and outcome suggests that pathological features other than the visible lesions determine the long-term clinical course.

It has become clear from a number of studies that both the normal-appearing white and grey matter are abnormal in the early stages of relapsing–remitting multiple sclerosis and patients with clinically isolated syndromes (Iannucci *et al* 2000b; Traboulsee *et al* 2002). Other studies have shown that the abnormalities within the normal-appearing white matter may precede the development of focal inflammatory (gadolinium enhancing) lesions by several months or longer. Abnormalities reported to precede lesions or to occur in very early disease include lipid peaks in white matter (Narayana *et al* 1998), decreased MTR and *N*-acetyl aspartate and increased T_1 relaxation time in both white and grey matter (Chard *et al* 2002a; 2002b; De Stefano *et al* 2003; Filippi *et al* 1998a; 1999a; Griffin *et al* 2002a), and increased diffusion (Werring *et al* 2000a), and *myo*-inositol (Fernando *et al* 2004) in white matter. Serial studies have shown progressive grey matter atrophy and ventricular enlargement in the early years following a clinically isolated syndrome (Dalton *et al* 2004a) and in early relapsing–remitting multiple sclerosis (Chard *et al* 2004). A progressive decline in the MTR of both normal-appearing white and grey matter has been observed over 2 years in early relapsing–remitting multiple sclerosis (Davies *et al* 2005). The intrinsic abnormalities in normal-appearing tissues, including atrophy, are related only modestly to lesion load, and may therefore reflect an early and diffuse process with associated neuroaxonal damage that is potentially independent of lesion formation. In the main, these abnormalities are quite mild and thus it is not surprising that they have not led to overt clinical impairment. Follow-up is required to determine if they predict any aspect of the future clinical course or disability.

Superficially, such findings challenge the hypothesis that the first event in focal white matter lesion formation is breakdown of the blood–brain barrier with subsequent trafficking of inflammatory cells into the brain. However, the existence of low grade leakage and distributed microglial activation has been demonstrated by histological examination of normal-appearing white matter, indicating that the visual detection of gadolinium enhancement has limited sensitivity.

RELAPSING–REMITTING MULTIPLE SCLEROSIS: RECOVERY OF FUNCTION AND REMISSION

One remarkable feature of multiple sclerosis is the ability of patients to make an apparently complete recovery from relapses, including those characterized by severe neurological deficits. Such complete remissions occur most commonly early in the disease course. Three main mechanisms can be identified, whose relative importance probably varies between different patients and lesions, and within a single patient at different stages of the disease. First is the relief of conduction block or synaptic dysfunction that may have been imposed on structurally normal tissue by, for example, inflammatory mediators. The second mechanism involves plastic changes, perhaps involving alterations in functional cortical organization, so that surviving neuronal networks take over functions lost as a result of the disease process. Lastly, is the restoration of function to axons in which conduction has previously been blocked, either through adaptive changes or in association with repair by remyelination.

Recovery through the resolution of inflammation

We have argued above that inflammation can result directly in neurological deficits, and it is therefore reasonable to conclude that the resolution of inflammation may contribute to remission. Certainly function improves as inflammation wanes in animals with experimental autoimmune encephalomyelitis (Chalk *et al* 1995). More specifically, if nitric oxide is involved in causing the deficit associated with inflammation, it is worth mentioning the striking extent and rapidity with which conduction is restored upon removing nitric oxide in experimental systems (see below, and the left plot in Figure 13.21; Redford *et al* 1997; K.J. Smith *et al* 2001a). Although less easily studied in the clinical context, the studies to which we have already

referred correlating symptom onset and recovery with the gadolinium DTPA-enhancing phase of optic nerve MRI lesions, and the associated increase in amplitude of the visual evoked potential, can also be interpreted as indicating the direct and reversible effect of inflammatory mediators on the conduction properties of myelinated axons in the central nervous system. The transient neurological manifestations associated with cytokine release in the context of treatment with Campath-1H also provide indirect evidence that the removal of inflammatory mediators restores conduction and leads to symptom recovery (see above).

Restoration of function by adaptive changes and plasticity

The possibility that conduction may occur in demyelinated axons was first predicted on the basis of clinical observations, namely the presence of large but silent demyelinating lesions in pathways where symptoms would have been expected (Ghatak *et al* 1974; Gilbert and Sadler 1983; Mackay and Hirano 1967; Namerow 1972; O'Riordan *et al* 1998a; Phadke and Best 1983; Ulrich and Groebke-Lorenz 1983; Wisniewski *et al* 1976). Despite the characterization of experimental lesions, definitive proof of conduction in central demyelinated axons awaited a study in which the properties of single axons, identified as passing through lesions, were determined. These informative axons were labelled and reconstructed in three dimensions at the electron microscope level (Figure 13.22; Felts *et al* 1997). It is now clear that although conduction is initially blocked by segmental demyelination, it can be restored within 2–3 weeks of demyelination in the central nervous system, even when several internodes are affected, and in the absence of remyelination (Felts *et al* 1997). The restoration of conduction can occur even more promptly in the peripheral nervous system (Bostock and Sears 1976; 1978; K.J. Smith *et al* 1982), where recovery can be seen within 6 days of demyelination (K.J. Smith *et al* 1982). Whether conduction in central demyelinated axons occurs by continuous or microsaltatory conduction (Bostock and Sears 1976; K.J. Smith *et al* 1982) is not known. It is reasonable to accept that it is the restoration of conduction that reverses the neurological deficit (Chalk *et al* 1995).

Although conduction can occur in demyelinated axons, conduction block may persist. Whether conduction does occur depends on a number of factors. Conduction is favoured by a small axon diameter (Bostock 1994; Bostock and Sears 1978; Waxman 1989), a short internode preceding the demyelinated segment (Bostock 1994; Shrager and Rubinstein 1990; Waxman and Brill 1978), a short lesion (see above), the absence of inflammation (see above), and cool body temperature (see below). The first two factors characterize axons in the optic nerves and pyramidal tracts, and this may help to explain the potential for recovery with lesions of these pathways. However, conduction can occur in demyelinated axons as large as 5.5 μm in diameter (Felts *et al* 1997), and so it is likely that almost all central demyelinated axons should be capable of conduction, at least under ideal conditions (which may often not prevail within lesions). Because remyelinated internodes are short, it also follows that remyelination might be expected to promote successful conduction, even if the repair is restricted (as is often the case) to the margins of each lesion. The presence of a short internode

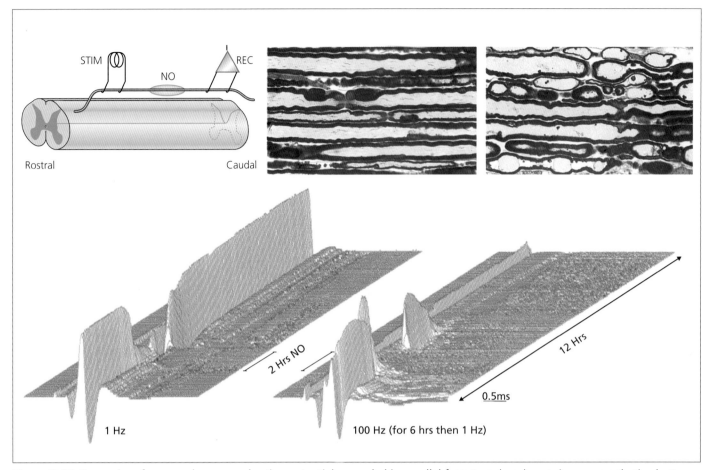

Figure 13.21 Two series of averaged compound action potentials recorded in parallel from two dorsal roots in an anaesthetized rat, using the arrangement indicated (see inset). The data are shown in three-dimensional perspective, with the earliest records at the front, and with a 2 minute interval between adjacent records: each plot therefore shows approximately 12 hours of recorded data. The left plot shows records obtained at continuous 1-Hz stimulation. The records were stable for the first 2.5 hours, but conduction block was imposed on nearly all the axons by a 2 hour exposure to nitric oxide. This block was released upon removal of nitric oxide, and the axons continued to conduct for the remaining 7.5 hours of the experiment. In contrast, the right plot shows the effect of the same exposure to nitric oxide, but in axons stimulated continuously at 100 Hz for the first 6 hours of recording. The nitric oxide again causes a prompt block of conduction, but now washing results in the recovery of conduction in only some axons, and the recovery is transient. The combination of nitric oxide exposure and sustained impulse activity results in persistent conduction block; this persisted despite reduction of the stimulus frequency to only 1 Hz for the last 6 hours of the experiment. Histological examination of the roots at the end of the experiment revealed that whereas the root stimulated at only 1 Hz during the period of nitric oxide exposure was quite normal in appearance, all the axons exposed to nitric oxide in conjunction with stimulation at 100 Hz had undergone degeneration. STIM = stimulate; REC = record. Adapted from K.J. Smith *et al* (2001).

facilitates the driving node to fulfil its role of depolarizing the demyelinated axolemma, because this reduces dissipation of the available action current (through resistive loss and discharge of internodal capacitance) before reaching its target. A short internode may thus be able to compensate for other factors that may not be optimal for conduction in a particular axon (Shrager and Rubinstein 1990). Conduction is also favoured by the mere presence of some residual glial wrapping (Shrager and Rubinstein 1990), especially the presence of glial contacts. These can be associated with axolemmal specializations suggestive of increased excitability, such as the presence of an electron dense axolemmal undercoating similar to that observed at nodes of Ranvier and believed to represent a high density of sodium channels (see below; Black *et al* 1991; Blakemore and Smith 1983; Rosenbluth and Blakemore 1984; Rosenbluth *et al* 1985).

Changes in the distribution and expression of ion channels

It is often assumed that action potentials can simply jump across a single demyelinated internode but this is far from the case. Detailed electrophysiological observations in peripheral demyelinated axons (which are likely to reflect the properties of central demyelinated axons) have revealed that, if conduction is successful, the action potential crawls along the demyelinated axolemma, either in a purely continuous manner (Bostock and Sears 1976; 1978), or by microsaltation between new node-like foci, termed phi-nodes, that form along the demyelinated axolemma every 100–400 μm (mean 255 μm) (K.J. Smith *et al* 1982). As the internodal axolemma normally sheltered beneath the myelin sheath has a low sodium channel density, the

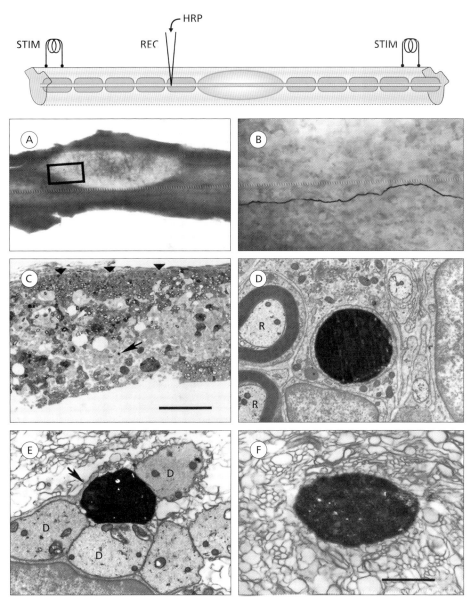

Figure 13.22 Conduction properties of single demyelinated central axons with their ultrastructural appearance. A single axon is impaled with a recording micropipette (diagram) and the conduction properties of the axon along its normal and demyelinated portions determined. The axon is then labelled by iontophoresing horseradish peroxidase before the micropipette is withdrawn. After a delay to allow horseradish peroxidase to pass along the axon into the lesion, the tissue is fixed for microscopic examination, and longitudinal vibratome sections taken. (A) The lesion is apparent as a translucent area. The horseradish peroxidase is developed to reveal the labelled axon. (B) At the region marked in A, can be seen the only axon in the tissue for which the conduction properties are known. The vibratome section is embedded in resin to allow serial, semi-thin sections to be obtained, now in the transverse plane, in which the labelled axon can be distinguished (C, arrow). Selected semi-thin sections are trimmed and re-embedded for ultrathin sectioning and examination (without additional EM stain) at the ultrastructural level (D, E and F), where the electron dense label is clearly distinguishable. In this way the same axon can be examined ultrastructurally at different locations across many millimetres of its length. In the example illustrated, the axon was demyelinated and it passed from a region where it was ensheathed by a Schwann cell (D, two adjacent axons are remyelinated [R]), through a region where it lay alongside other demyelinated axons and was in contact with a glial process along part of its circumference (E, arrow), to a region where it was unensheathed by cellular processes, but located in a foam of vesicular myelin debris (F). From Felts *et al* (1997) with permission.

restoration of conduction has long been believed to depend on reorganization of, at least, the sodium channel population. In recent years our understanding of this process has been substantially augmented by immunohistochemical and molecular analyses. It is now possible, for example in immunolabelled axons, to see the exquisite precision with which different types of channel are arranged, and in some cases strictly segregated, at nodes of Ranvier (Figure 13.23; Arroyo and Scherer 2000; Caldwell *et al* 2000; Kazarinova-Noyes and Shrager 2002; Peles and Salzer 2000; Rasband and Shrager 2000). Previously, this precision could only be inferred from electrophysiological and freeze-fracture studies. Indeed, there are probably few structures in mammalian biology as finely honed by evolution as the node of Ranvier, which has been elaborated to permit rapid and reliable transmission of the nerve impulse. It is easy to appreciate that disruption of this tightly ordered pattern in demyeli-

nated axons will contribute to the conduction abnormalities arising directly from the myelin loss, and the most recent studies have started to reveal that not only are existing channels disrupted, but new types are inserted in the axonal membrane.

Although detailed description of the molecular changes accompanying demyelination and remyelination is beyond the scope of this chapter, it is clear that the organization of sodium and potassium channels at nodes is intimately dependent upon the maintenance of ordered paranodal myelin (Arroyo *et al* 1999; Baba *et al* 1999; Dupree *et al* 1999; J.D. England *et al* 1990; 1996a; Novakovic *et al* 1998; Rasband *et al* 1998; 1999b; J.R. Schwarz *et al* 1991; H. Wang *et al* 1995). It follows that demyelination will cause conduction deficits not only by the removal of the myelin, but also through the consequent disruption of ion channels. Indeed, the timing of changes in ion channel distribution correlates directly with the loss of function.

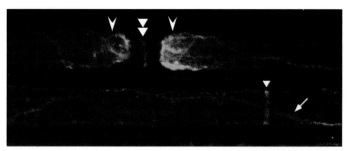

Figure 13.23 Fluorescent micrograph of a node along a rat sciatic nerve fibre showing the immunohistochemical labelling of sodium (red) and potassium (Kv1.2; green) channels. The sodium channels are restricted to the nodal gap (double arrowheads), whereas the potassium channels are segregated to the juxtaparanodal region (arrowheads) and apposed to a Schmidt–Lanterman incisure (arrowhead). From Arroyo and Scherer (2000). © 2000, with permission of Springer-Verlag GmbH.

Sodium channels

Research in peripheral axons has advanced more rapidly than in the central nervous system, and most of our knowledge regarding channel organization is derived from demyelinating peripheral nervous system lesions produced by either focal injection of lysolecithin or the induction of experimental allergic neuritis. Demyelination results in loss of the highly organized focal ring of sodium channels normally present at normal nodes of Ranvier. This is replaced by a more diffuse pattern correlating with loss of function (Novakovic et al 1998; J.R. Schwarz et al 1991). As described above, there is good evidence from animal studies that the distribution of sodium channels changes in response to demyelination.

Following the onset of demyelination there is a highly significant increase in the number of sodium channels within peripheral nerves experimentally demyelinated with adriamycin (J.D. England et al 1991). Furthermore, nodelike clusters of sodium channel immunoreactivity can be identified along entirely naked central axons demyelinated with ethidium bromide (Felts et al 1998), although it is not clear whether these are new or the remnants of old nodes. The precise role of glial cells in the organization of ion channels at new nodes formed during remyelination is still being elucidated, although it is already clear that glial cells play a crucial role. Whether the role of Schwann cells in the peripheral nervous system exactly mimics that of oligodendrocytes remains unclear but, in the peripheral nervous system, new clusters of sodium channels develop only in association with the edges of remyelinating Schwann cells, which seem to control the distribution and mobility of channels (Ching et al 1999; J.D. England et al 1996a; Kazarinova-Noyes and Shrager 2002). Sodium channel clustering at the supposed sites of new nodes during development of the peripheral nervous system appears to be dependent on contact with Schwann cells (Ching et al 1999; Custer et al 2003), and there is evidence that oligodendrocytes play a similar role in the central nervous system, at least during development (Rasband et al 1999a). Contact between oligodendrocytes and axons is not required for sodium channel clustering during development, at least in vitro (Figure 13.11; Alessandri-Haber et al 1999; M.R. Kaplan et al

1997; 2001), although it is not yet clear whether these clusters are at the later sites of nodes of Ranvier.

Apart from changes in the distribution of existing channels, it has recently become clear that demyelination can also result in the expression of novel channel subtypes in the demyelinated axolemma. At least ten genes encode sodium channels in mammals (Caldwell et al 2000). Thus expression of the sensory neuron-specific Nav1.8 sodium channel, not normally expressed within the brain, appears on cerebellar Purkinje cells in patients and animals with multiple sclerosis and experimental autoimmune encephalomyelitis, respectively (Black et al 2000), together with its accessory molecule annexin II (Craner et al 2003a). Demyelination in the *taiep* rat is also associated with expression of the Nav1.8/SNS/PN3 sodium channel mRNA and protein in cerebellar Purkinje cells (Black et al 1999b), and with changes in expression of the β1 and β2 sodium channel subunits in dorsal horn neurons (Blackburn-Munro and Fleetwood-Walker 1999). The β subunits of sodium channels affect their biophysical properties, influencing the bulk electrophysiological and conduction properties of the axolemma in which they are present. Interestingly, it has now been found that the type of sodium channel expressed at nodes of Ranvier can change in optic nerve axons in response to experimental autoimmune encephalomyelitis (Craner et al 2003b; 2004a). In normal tissue, there is a marked predominance of sodium channel Nav1.6$^+$ nodes over Nav1.2 but, in experimental autoimmune encephalomyelitis, the balance shifts in favour of Nav1.2. Also, axons that appear to be demyelinated show diffuse Nav1.2 labelling. These findings suggest that demyelinated axons may adapt so that they resemble immature axons, at least with regard to the expression of sodium channel subtypes.

Observations derived from the lesions of multiple sclerosis have until recently been limited. Increased binding of saxitoxin, a sodium channel blocking agent, was demonstrated immuno-histochemically (Moll et al 1991), but at that time the spatial resolution was insufficient to distinguish axonal from glial binding. Most recently, a change in both the distribution and type of sodium channels has been reported along denuded axons within the plaques of multiple sclerosis. In particular, whereas the Nav1.6 subtype of sodium channel is confined to the nodes of Ranvier in normal axons, both Nav1.6, together with Nav1.2, are expressed along extensive regions of demyelinated axons within acute plaques (Craner et al 2004b). It thus seems that the changes in sodium channel distribution found in animal models are representative of the lesions in multiple sclerosis.

It remains uncertain whether changes in the distribution of sodium channels are linked to the association of channels with other axolemmal or extracellular proteins. There is evidence from knockout mice that the localization of sodium channels at nodes is strongly influenced by the L1 cell adhesion molecule family members, neurofascin and neural cell adhesion molecule and by 480/270 kD ankyrin$_G$, which may bind directly to sodium channels in a ternary complex (V. Bennett and Lambert 1999; Lambert et al 1997). The channels also have associations with molecules such as tenascin-R in the extracellular matrix (P. Weber et al 1999). As well as the effect on their distribution, these different interactions may have important influences on channel excitability.

Inflammation resulting from the subcutaneous injection of Freund's adjuvant has been shown to result in a marked increase in immunoreactivity for sodium channels in primary sensory neurons (H.J. Gould *et al* 1998). Indeed, inflammation within the central nervous system significantly alters the expression of genes encoding ion channels (Carmody *et al* 2002), and these changes are compounded by post-transcriptional changes due to phosphorylation and nitrosation (see above). Similar changes will occur in potassium channels. These findings have led to the interesting suggestion that multiple sclerosis has some characteristics of an acquired channelopathy (Waxman 2005; Waxman *et al* 2000), with the attendant possibility of novel therapies based on subtype-specific channel modulation (Waxman 2002).

It seems likely that the changes in expression of sodium channels in multiple sclerosis will be accompanied by detectable alterations in the function of neurons and their axons, and although detailed biophysical observations are lacking, this expectation is supported by several observations. Thus, *in vitro*, the biolistically (to describe the situation in which a cDNA is gunned into the cell, transcribed and then the protein product is expressed) induced expression of Nav1.8 in Purkinje cells at levels similar to those normally expressed in dorsal root ganglion cells results in altered electrophysiological properties, including an increase in amplitude and duration of action potentials, and the production of sustained pacemaker-like impulse trains in response to depolarization (Figure 13.24; Renganathan *et al* 2003; Saab *et al* 2004). Such changes may well contribute to cerebellar dysfunction in multiple sclerosis (Waxman 2005). There is also evidence from the peripheral nervous system that pathological changes mimicking those seen in multiple sclerosis have functional consequences. Thus, chronic constriction injury of the sciatic nerve results in inflammation, demyelination and axonal degeneration, and these events are associated with changes in the β subunits associated with sodium channels (Shah *et al* 2000), and in the sodium currents expected to result in hyperexcitability (Kral *et al* 1999). Furthermore, it is known that the channel expression of dorsal root ganglion neurons alters in response to injury, and is accompanied by changes in the electrophysiological properties of the neurons and their axons (Black *et al* 1999a; Cummins *et al* 2000; Dib-Hajj *et al* 1999; Nonaka *et al* 2000; Sleeper *et al* 2000). It seems reasonable to suppose that such fundamental changes in the electrophysiological properties of neurons and axons will contribute to the signs and symptoms of multiple sclerosis, especially with respect to hyperexcitability and positive symptoms (see below).

These observations show that inflammation and demyelination can alter the ion channel repertoire of cell bodies and axons, and it seems that these changes may well be superimposed on inherent differences between axons. For example, there is evidence that motor axons in different nerves can have subtly different electrophysiological properties, perhaps indicating differences in the properties and/or distribution of their ion channels. It also seems that the electrophysiological properties of individual myelinated axons may vary along their length (differing, e.g., at the knee compared with the ankle: Kuwabara *et al* 2000). Clearly, if the channel changes resulting from disease processes are superimposed on inherently different patterns of axonal ion channel expression, the resulting spectrum of electrophysiological consequences may be considerable, contributing to the complex neurological manifestations of inflammatory demyelinating disease.

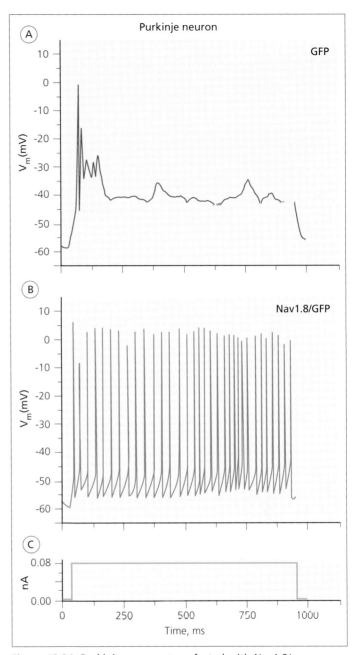

Figure 13.24 Purkinje neurons transfected with Nav1.8/green fluorescent protein (GFP) show sustained repetitive firing on injection of depolarizing current. (A) Control Purkinje neuron transfected with GFP (a marker for transfected cells) produces a conglomerate action potential consisting of five spikes. (B) Purkinje neurons also expressing Nav1.8 produce action potentials of larger amplitude and sustained, pacemaker-like activity in response to the stimulus indicated in C. Adapted from Renganathan *et al* (2003). © 2003, with permission from Elsevier.

Potassium channels

As demyelination has such dramatic effects on sodium channel distribution and expression, it is not surprising that the potassium channel population is also affected. Traditionally, it was anticipated that fast potassium channels would be present in abundance at the mammalian nodal axolemma, as in the larger

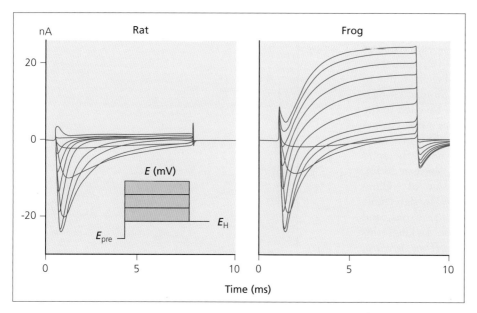

Figure 13.25 Membrane currents recorded from rat and frog nodes of Ranvier under voltage clamp conditions (protocol indicated). The mammalian node exhibits only a small outward potassium current, whereas these currents are large in the frog. The inward sodium currents (predominantly downward deflections) are almost the same in both species. Adapted from Roper and Schwarz (1989). © 1989, with permission of Blackwell Publishing Ltd.

but not smaller (Smith and Schauf 1981c) amphibian myelinated fibres (Smith and Schauf 1981c). Unexpectedly, this was not confirmed by voltage clamp studies in the early 1980s (Brismar 1981a; 1981b; Brismar and Frankenhaeuser 1981; Chiu and Ritchie 1980; Smith and Schauf 1981a; 1981b). These revealed that the nodes of Ranvier on mammalian peripheral axons had much less potassium current than the amphibian nodes with which they were compared (Figure 13.25). However, although the mammalian axons initially seemed to lack large numbers of nodal potassium channels, they had abundant potassium channels of the fast Kv1.1 and 1.2 subtypes in the juxtaparanodal axolemma (Arroyo and Scherer 2000; Rasband and Trimmer 2001; Scherer and Arroyo 2002), and these channels were exposed by demyelination (Brismar 1981a; 1981b; Chiu and Ritchie 1980; Ritchie et al 1981; Schauf and Smith 1981; Smith and Schauf 1981c). Later, voltage clamp studies (Corrette et al 1991; Roper and Schwarz 1989; Safronov et al 1993) revealed that two or three types of potassium current are present in the region of mammalian peripheral nodes, with channels responsible for the fast current located in the juxtaparanodal membrane, and channels underlying the slow current at the nodal axolemma. Recent immunohistochemical studies have revealed that a subset of larger axons in the spinal cord possess Kv3.1 potassium channels at the nodal axolemma (Devaux et al 2003a), whereas the KCNQ2 potassium channel is present at this site in both central and peripheral axons (Devaux et al 2004). Rather few peripheral mammalian axons have nodes positive for Kv3.1. As with sodium channels, it appears that the ordered distribution of different potassium channel subtypes at the node of Ranvier (at least with respect to the Kv1.1 and 1.2 channels) is strongly dependent on the presence of intact paranodal axo-glial interactions. If these are disrupted in mutant mice, the channels become much more widely distributed along the axon (Boyle et al 2001; Dupree et al 1999; H. Wang et al 1995). Kv1.1 and Kv1.2 channels initially become dispersed along the axon, and are then no longer detectable in peripheral axons experimentally demyelinated by the injection of lysolecithin. They remain undetectable even during the early stages of remyelination, but reappear in the

nodal gap at 14 days postinjection. The distribution becomes more ordered as remyelination continues, again emphasizing an important role for myelinating cells in channel organization (Rasband et al 1998; J.V. Wu et al 1993). As expected, the altered potassium channel distribution is accompanied by abnormalities in axonal pharmacology and function (Rasband et al 1998), as also occur in Kv1.1 knockouts, which have hyperexcitable axons (Zhou et al 1999). Axonal injury also affects potassium channel expression, in that axotomy of dorsal root ganglion cells reduces neuronal immunoreactivity for several types of potassium channel (Ishikawa et al 1999).

It is clear that potassium channels can profoundly change the behaviour of nonexcitable cells, over and above their effects on axons. Kir4.1 channels (inward rectifying potassium channels) appear not to be synthesized by neurons or astrocytes, but are present on myelinating oligodendrocytes (Neusch et al 2001). Kir4.1 knockout mice show a marked motor impairment due, it seems, to hypomyelination in the spinal cord, severe spongiform vacuolation and axonal degeneration. This knockout indicates that myelin abnormalities can result from ion channel mutations, adding to the complexity of gene changes that could contribute to polygenic demyelinating diseases (Neusch et al 2001).

Calcium channels

Apart from the L-type calcium channels that appear to be functional in normal central axons (Brown et al 2001), immunohistochemical examination of axons demyelinated by multiple sclerosis or experimental autoimmune encephalomyelitis has also revealed the presence of N-type calcium channels (see Chapter 12; Kornek et al 2001). Whether these are functional is not yet clear.

Chloride channels

In addition to the cation channels discussed above, lysolecithin-mediated demyelination uncovers at least three types of anion channel, at least in peripheral *Xenopus* axons (J.V. Wu and Shrager 1994), including outwardly rectifying, inwardly rectifying and maxi-chloride channels. It seems likely that similar channels are present in mammalian central axons but these have not yet been characterized in physiological or pathological situations.

The role of astrocytes in restoring conduction

Gliosis is usually considered to be a deleterious response in multiple sclerosis. However, the close apposition of glial membranes to demyelinated axons should theoretically aid conduction by affecting the passive cable properties of the axons (Shrager and Rubinstein 1990). Furthermore, astrocytic processes make intimate contacts with demyelinated axons specifically at sites that exhibit a node-like undercoating (Black *et al* 1991; Blakemore and Smith 1983; Rosenbluth and Blakemore 1984; Rosenbluth *et al* 1985). The belief that this undercoating indicates the presence of sodium channels at high density is supported by freeze-fracture studies (Rosenbluth *et al* 1985), encouraging the belief that glial ensheathment helps to re-establish the apparatus necessary for restoration of conduction to demyelinated axons. However, immunocytochemical evidence has revealed the presence of node-like aggregations of sodium channels along demyelinated axons in the absence of any nearby glial contacts (Felts *et al* 1998), indicating that these contacts are not essential for excitability. Confirmation that this interpretation is correct is provided by an ultrastructural three-dimensional study (Felts *et al* 1997), which established that demyelinated axons are able to conduct even when at least 88% of their surface area is entirely devoid of glial contacts across several internodes. It follows that the paucity of glial processes in the lesions of multiple sclerosis having a greatly expanded extracellular space, completely demyelinated axons and few glial processes (Barnes *et al* 1991) need not preclude the possibility of axonal conduction. These axons should be capable of conduction, even if local circumstances may hold this in abeyance. As probes become available it will be interesting to see how many different types of ion channels, pumps and exchangers (Waxman and Ritchie 1993) owe their positioning along axons, at least in part, to the locations of glial processes and vice versa.

In addition to their effects on the locations of ion channels along axons, astrocytes also regulate the composition of the extracellular fluid, particularly the concentrations of potassium ions and neurotransmitters (Largo *et al* 1996), and provide trophic support for axons. Astrocytes also contribute to regulation of the cerebral microcirculation (Anderson and Nedergaard 2003). These roles might be performed just as well by astrocytes organized into a gliotic 'scar' as under normal conditions. In contrast with the traditional view that gliosis is an unfavourable development, it is worth considering that it may actually be beneficial for axonal function.

Cortical plasticity

Intuitively, it seems likely that the loss of function resulting from axonal degeneration in multiple sclerosis will also be partially compensated by the same types of cortical changes that provide a degree of recovery from traumatic or vascular damage to the central nervous system (R. Chen *et al* 2002). There is now good evidence from functional MRI studies that such cortical plasticity does, indeed, play a role in the recovery of symp-

toms due to multiple sclerosis (Pantano *et al* 2002; H. Reddy *et al* 2002; Rocca *et al* 2002a; Spitzer 1999; Toosy *et al* 2005; Werring *et al* 2000b). For example, compared with controls, patients with multiple sclerosis have been found to activate a larger area of cortex during vision or whilst accomplishing motor tasks. Abnormal activation patterns are seen in patients after a single clinical attack (Rocca *et al* 2003a), and in those with no disability (Rocca *et al* 2002a) or few MRI lesions (Rocca *et al* 2003a; Filippi *et al* 2004b). Thus, an fMRI study of seven patients several years after each had presented with a single isolated episode of optic neuritis, showed activation of multiple extrastriate areas of cortex (Toosy *et al* 2002; Werring *et al* 2000b; see Figure 7.22). Motor tasks have usually involved the upper limb and movements such as flexion-extension or repetitive finger tapping. Whereas in normal individuals fMRI activation is largely confined to the contralateral primary motor cortex, in patients with multiple sclerosis it is also seen in other cortical regions including the ipsilateral primary motor cortex, supplementary motor areas, and more distributed regions (Figure 13.26; M. Lee *et al* 2000; Pantano *et al* 2002; H. Reddy *et al* 2002). It has been observed that the area of activation is related to lesion load (Rocca *et al* 2002a) and the extent of abnormality in the normal-appearing tissues as measured using indices of diffusion (Rocca *et al* 2003c) or axonal damage (H. Reddy *et al* 2000). In a recent study, some of the processes underlying plasticity have been observed in response to an experimental inflammatory lesion affecting the rat corticospinal tract (Kerschensteiner *et al* 2004). Remodelling was found at multiple levels, including sprouting of local interneurons around the lesion, sprouting of corticospinal tract axons in a detour to their target area, and terminal sprouting of spared corticospinal axons. New neurons were also recruited to the cortical motor pool. It seems likely that similar mechanisms may play a role in multiple sclerosis. It is possible that the nature of the adaptive change may change with disease severity and with time since disease onset.

Remyelination

Remyelination is a feature of multiple sclerosis (see Chapters 10 and 12; Prineas and Connell 1979; Prineas *et al* 1987; 1993b). Although it seems logical to imagine that morphological repair will result in improved conduction and the restoration of function, this cannot be assumed. In common with remyelination seen in experimental lesions, the new internodes are both thinner and shorter than normal (Gledhill and McDonald 1977; Gledhill *et al* 1973; B.M. Harrison *et al* 1972). These features will raise the internodal capacitance and reduce internodal resistance, both acting to impair conduction. Although the short internodal length will tend to compensate, this also means that new nodes are formed at sites on the axolemma previously covered by myelin, lacking the specializations characteristic of normal nodes, including the dense accumulation of the sodium channels essential for impulse formation. However, despite these limitations, serial studies of conduction in a single group of central axons undergoing demyelination and remyelination have demonstrated restoration of fast and secure conduction, probably in all remyelinated axons (Figure 13.27; K.J. Smith *et al* 1979; 1981). Indeed, conduction has been documented in axons ensheathed with new myelin composed of only five lamellae (Felts *et al* 1997). At least in thicker sheaths, not only is the

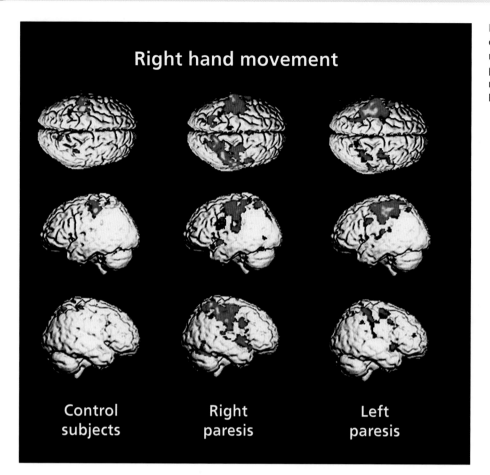

Right hand movement

Control subjects | Right paresis | Left paresis

Figure 13.26 Statistical maps showing cortical activation during right hand movement in controls and patients with previous right or left hemiparesis due to multiple sclerosis (see also Figure 7.22). From Pantano *et al* (2002) with permission.

velocity almost fully restored and the refractory period for transmission returned to within normal limits, but remyelinated axons can also conduct trains of impulses faithfully at high frequency (K.J. Smith *et al* 1979; 1981). Accordingly, remyelination has been associated with the restoration of behavioural function (Jeffery and Blakemore 1997) and it is reasonable to conclude that, where it occurs in multiple sclerosis, remyelination will contribute to the remission of clinical deficits resulting from demyelination. This view is supported by the observation that latency of the visual evoked potential progressively shortens during the two years following an attack of optic neuritis, particularly during the 3–6 months when remyelination might be expected to occur (Figure 13.28; Brusa *et al* 2001). The changes in visual evoked potential are accompanied by improvements in contrast sensitivity and sensitivity of the central visual field. Latency of the evoked potential may eventually be restored to normal following optic neuritis, especially in children (Figure 13.29; Kriss *et al* 1988). This is less predictable in adults, and the age-related differences may reflect the extent of remyelination, or greater likelihood of recurrent episodes of inflammatory demyelination in the adult optic nerve.

Remyelination restores conduction irrespective of whether it is achieved primarily by oligodendrocytes (K.J. Smith *et al* 1979; 1981), endogenous Schwann cells (Felts and Smith 1992), transplanted normal or frozen human Schwann cells (Honmou *et al* 1996; Kohama *et al* 2001), olfactory ensheathing cells (Imaizumi *et al* 1998; 2000; Utzschneider *et al* 1994), human neural precursor cells (Akiyama *et al* 2001), or bone marrow

cells (Akiyama *et al* 2002). Although not proven beyond doubt, it seems safe to assume that each new node of Ranvier formed by remyelination will be excitable, and actually excited during conduction, as occurs in peripheral remyelinated axons (K.J. Smith *et al* 1982). Certainly, the new nodes have aggregations of sodium channels, at least in experimental preparations of peripheral axons (Dugandzija-Novakovic *et al* 1995) and central axons (Felts *et al* 1998).

It is understandable that the promotion of remyelination is a major research goal in multiple sclerosis, especially because repair may not only improve conduction, but also perhaps provide protection from degeneration (see Chapter 10). Furthermore, where remyelination is dependent on Schwann cells or other non-oligodendrocyte cells, the new myelin might be less vulnerable to antigen-specific inflammatory demyelination. As discussed in Chapters 10 and 19, attempts to promote remyelination are being pursued using immunological (Asakura and Rodriguez 1998; Warrington *et al* 2000) and biological strategies (Baron-Van *et al* 1997; Blakemore 2000; Blakemore and Franklin 2000; Blakemore *et al* 2000).

PHYSIOLOGICAL EXPLANATIONS FOR CLINICAL SYMPTOMS IN MULTIPLE SCLEROSIS

Although conduction can eventually be restored to demyelinated axons, it remains markedly slower than normal, and also

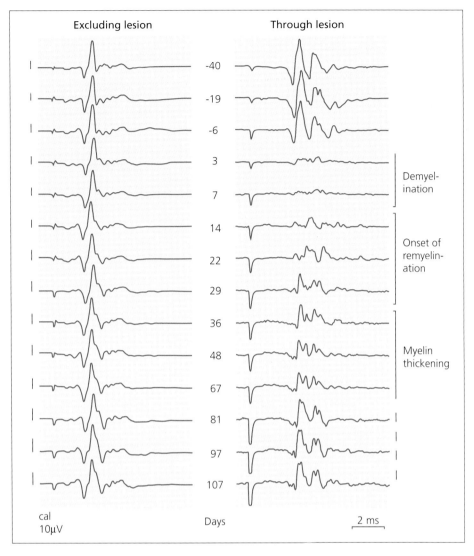

Figure 13.27 Series of records obtained over a 5 month period showing changes in conduction occurring through a central demyelinating lesion located in the dorsal columns. Records obtained excluding the lesion from the conduction pathway (left) were quite stable throughout, as were those obtained including the site of the lesion, but before the lesion was induced (right, top three records). After the lesion was induced (by the intraspinal injection of lysolecithin at day 0) conduction was blocked during the period of demyelination, but progressively restored during the period of repair by remyelination. Remyelination also restored the ability of the axons to conduct closely spaced impulses (not shown). Adapted from Smith *et al* (1979) Reproduced with permission from Nature Publishing Group (www.nature.com/nature).

insecure, failing especially at higher firing frequencies. These deficiencies result in a range of conduction abnormalities and functional deficits, some of which can seem bizarre.

Conduction slowing

A reduced conduction velocity in segmentally demyelinated axons is invariable, and often so prominent that it is erroneously considered diagnostic for demyelination. Detailed axonal recordings reveal that the slowing occurs specifically at the site of demyelination, with the myelinated portions on either side of a focal lesion appearing to conduct normally, in both peripheral axons (Kaeser 1962; Kaeser and Lambert 1962; W.I. McDonald 1961; 1962; 1963; Rasminsky and Sears 1972) and central axons (J.I. Hall 1967; W.I. McDonald 1983; W.I. McDonald and Sears 1970). In peripheral axons, a sophisticated recording technique has revealed that even in a large-diameter (normally fast) axon, conduction along the demyelinated portion occurs at only around 0.5–2.5 m/s (Bostock and Sears 1976; 1978; K.J. Smith *et al* 1982). Under these circumstances, even a short segment of demyelination results in a prominent increase in latency. In peripheral demyelinating disease, this can be measured

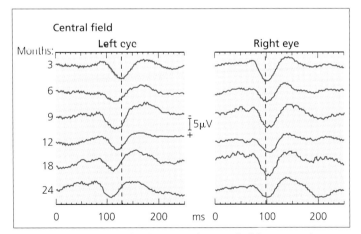

Figure 13.28 Visual evoked potentials recorded from a patient with unilateral optic neuritis after different periods (indicated). Records from the affected eye (left) show an initial delay, but this improves to within normal limits over time, during which remyelination is supposed to have occurred. The latency of the response from the right eye does not change appreciably. Adapted from Brusa *et al* (2001).

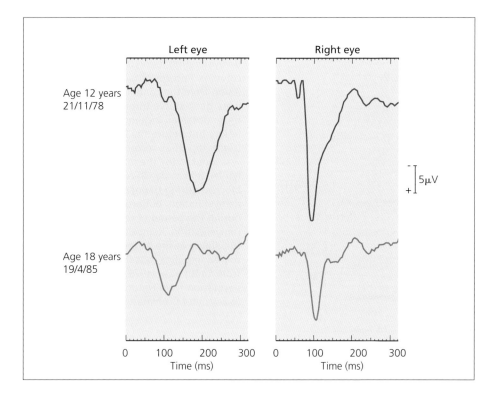

Figure 13.29 Visual evoked potentials recorded from a young patient with unilateral optic neuritis affecting the left eye (upper records), and at follow-up (lower records). Note the delayed and broadened 'P100' wave (downward deflection) from the left eye upon initial recording. The latency, but not the amplitude, had returned to normal upon re-examination 6 years later. Adapted from Kriss *et al* (1988). Reproduced with permission from the BMJ Publishing Group.

directly, as it can in animals with experimental demyelinating lesions. However, increased latency in central nervous system axons in patients can usually only be inferred from the delay in evoked potentials, although it has more recently become possible to measure the central motor conduction delay (D. Kidd *et al* 1998; Schmierer *et al* 2002).

The first evidence of delayed central conduction in humans was through the use of visual evoked potentials in optic neuritis (Halliday *et al* 1972), although delays had earlier been observed in the cortical responses to peripheral nerve stimulation (J.B. Baker *et al* 1968; Halliday and Wakefield 1963; Namerow 1968b). Delays in the visual evoked potential are usually substantial at around +30–35 ms, or even up to 100 ms (see below; Halliday *et al* 1972; 1973a; 1973b; Shahrokhi *et al* 1978). Although often well preserved, even in the presence of reduced amplitude, the shape of the waveform may also change and measures of latency then become subjective. Whether all of the delay is due to slow axonal conduction is doubtful, and slow retinal (B.A. Milner *et al* 1974) and cortical (J.H. Cook and Arden 1977) transmission may also contribute. Because the number of active axons influences the latency of the evoked potential, both persistent conduction block and axonal degeneration may also play a role in determining latency. However, these uncertainties do not detract from the pragmatic value of evoked potentials in clinical practice. Delays in these potentials have proven to be valuable laboratory adjuncts to clinical assessment in diagnosis (see Chapter 7), in exploring the visual pathways (Halliday *et al* 1972; 1973b), somatosensory pathways (Desmedt and Noel 1973; D.G. Small *et al* 1978; Trojaborg and Petersen 1979) and brainstem auditory pathways (Chiappa *et al* 1980; Eisen and Odusote 1980; Hume and Waxman 1988; K. Robinson and Rudge 1977). Delays in the motor response

evoked by electrical (Merton and Morton 1980; Merton *et al* 1982; Mills and Murray 1985) or magnetic (Barker *et al* 1985; 1986; Hess *et al* 1986) stimulation of the cortex have subsequently been observed.

The delays in evoked potentials usually cause few symptoms. Patients with gross abnormalities of the visual evoked potential may have normal visual acuity (Halliday *et al* 1972; 1973b; Hume and Waxman 1988). The absence of neurological deficit generally reflects the relative insensitivity of most parts of the nervous system to the precise timing of impulses (Brindley 1970). However, where precise timing is important, the delays may have interesting consequences. Difference in the arrival time of visual information to each hemisphere can result in the Pulfrich phenomenon (Pulfrich 1922), in which normal individuals perceive a pendulum to swing in an ellipse instead of a straight line if a neutral density filter is placed in front of one eye, thereby slowing the visual signal from that eye. In patients with unilateral optic neuritis, delay in impulse transmission through the lesion may produce the Pulfrich phenomenon without the aid of a neutral density filter (Frisen *et al* 1973; D. Rushton 1975). Interestingly, this effect may be compensated by placing a neutral density filter over the good eye (Alan Bird, personal communication). It is likely that this class of abnormality underlies the difficulty that some patients experience in judging velocity and anticipating the future position of moving objects, such as whilst playing tennis or negotiating moving traffic, following an attack of optic neuritis. A person with multiple sclerosis reported to one of us (KJS) that oncoming traffic disturbingly appeared to veer in a curve towards him. Conduction delays can also have subtle effects on auditory function, particularly where precise inter-aural time discrimination is crucial (R.A. Levine *et al* 1994).

Conduction of pairs of impulses

Focal slowing of conduction at the site of demyelination is one of the factors that limits the minimum interval between successive impulses, if these are to be transmitted faithfully through the lesion. In their early study, W.I. McDonald and Sears (1970) coined the phrase 'refractory period for transmission' to describe this deficit, defining this as the maximum interval between two conducted impulses such that the second fails to be conducted successfully through the lesion. In normal axons, the refractory period of transmission is equal in value (although not in concept) to the absolute refractory period, but in demyelinated axons it is longer, sometimes considerably so, than the absolute refractory period of the same axon measured across its myelinated portion. Indeed, in proven segmentally demyelinated central axons, Felts *et al* (1997) found prolongations from 0.5–1.4 ms in the normal portion to 1.0–6.0 ms across the demyelinated region, with one axon having a refractory period of transmission of 27 ms.

If demyelinated axons have long refractory periods of transmission and reduced ability to conduct closely spaced impulses, it can at first seem surprising that these deficits may not also be obvious in axons having no myelin (amyelinated), where the absolute refractory periods may be short (Utzschneider *et al* 1993). The explanation lies in the fact that the major cause of prolongation in the refractory period for transmission along demyelinated axons is the low safety factor for conduction imposed by the need to depolarize the beginning of the demyelinated segment to its firing threshold by action currents generated an internodal distance away. This need does not arise in axons that are free of myelin along their length and, in common with unmyelinated axons, amyelinated axons have a relatively high security for conduction.

Some relatively new approaches have been added to the electrophysiological examination in humans of normal and demyelinated axons using threshold tracking techniques (reviewed in Bostock *et al* 1998; Burke *et al* 2001). These allow the excitability of nerve fibres to be assessed, providing infor-mation about membrane properties of axons at the site of stimulation. Changes in membrane potential caused by activation of ion channels and electrogenic ion pumps can be assessed, but unfortunately the methods are not directly applicable to central axons and, hence, to the evaluation of conduction in axons affected by multiple sclerosis. However, the methods have been applied to the study of peripheral axons affected by Guillain–Barré syndrome, where prolongation of refractory period of transmission was observed in some forms of the disease (Kuwabara *et al* 2002).

Conduction of trains of impulses

Prolongation of the refractory period of transmission inevitably limits the maximum transmissible frequency of demyelinated axons. It also underestimates the magnitude of the deficit because the refractoriness accumulates with repeated activation. Thus, the refractory period of transmission between the second and third impulses of a train is longer than between the first and second, and tends progressively to increase for subsequent impulses. The problem arises from the fact that the second impulse of a train conducts across the demyelinated region in the relative refractory period of the first, and so it conducts even more slowly than its predecessor, and so on. The maximum transmissible frequency therefore decreases progressively (to well within the physiological range) as the number of action potentials in the train increases. Indeed, alternation of response to suprathreshold stimuli at frequencies as low as 1 Hz can be seen in experimentally induced and naturally occurring peripheral demyelinating lesions (W.I. McDonald 1982; R. Gilliatt *et al*, unpublished observations). This feature was recognized in the earliest studies (W.I. McDonald and Sears 1970), where one axon was able to conduct impulses along its normal portion at up to 1000 Hz whereas conduction through the lesion was reduced to only 410 Hz, and this frequency was only maintained for three transmissions before alternate impulses failed resulting in an output frequency of 205 Hz (Figure 13.30). Failure to transmit impulses at physiological frequencies offers a ready

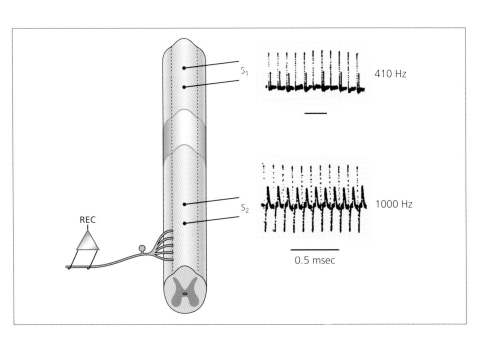

Figure 13.30 Records of activity in a single unit in a dorsal root filament teased from an intercostal nerve caudal to a demyelinating lesion (yellow shaded region). The lesion was earlier induced in the dorsal columns by the intraspinal injection of diphtheria toxin. The stimulus artefacts appear as dotted lines, and the action potentials as solid lines. Stimulation at S_1 includes the lesion in the conduction pathway, whereas the lesion is excluded by stimulation at S_2. Although the axon can conduct faithfully at 1000 Hz excluding the lesion, it only conducts three impulses through the lesion at 410 Hz before alternate impulses are blocked. REC = record. Adapted from W.I. McDonald and Sears (1970).

410 Hz

1000 Hz

0.5 msec

explanation for many symptoms in multiple sclerosis, including impaired sensory and motor function, as indicated experimentally (Kaji *et al* 1988).

More recent studies have revealed several additional problems that are now known to arise with repeated activation. Thus, other than the failure of alternate impulses in a train, repeated activation of demyelinated axons can result in intermittent periods of complete conduction block, interspersed with periods when conduction through the lesion occurs faithfully (Figure 13.31D). The cause of this activity-dependent conduction block was initially suspected to be progressive membrane depolarization due to the intracellular accumulation of sodium ions, but some elegant experiments revealed just the opposite. Rather, conduction is blocked due to membrane hyperpolarization in response to potentiated activity of the electrogenic Na$^+$/K$^+$ ATPase (sodium pump) caused by the raised intracellular sodium (Bostock and Grafe 1985). The hyperpolarization is easily induced, even at natural levels of impulse activity, and is particularly prominent in motor axons (Vagg *et al* 1998). Strikingly, the hyperpolarization can chop a train of impulses into intermittent bursts separated by completely silent periods

of, in our experience, around 0.2–2.0 s (Felts *et al* 1995). The hyperpolarization can be seen by the shift in baseline membrane potential of the intra-axonal record shown in Figure 13.31D. It seems that the hyperpolarization is sufficient to block conduction in demyelinated axons, due to their inherently low safety factor. Examination of patients with chronic inflammatory demyelinating polyradiculoneuropathy (Cappelen-Smith *et al* 2000) or multifocal motor neuropathy (Cappelen-Smith *et al* 2000; Kaji *et al* 2000) has provided good evidence that activity-dependent hyperpolarization can lead to conduction block and cause motor fatigue in humans. Apart from these effects, it remains possible that the intracellular accumulation of sodium ions (Rasminsky and Sears 1972) or of extracellular potassium ions (Brismar 1981b) may add to the conduction impairments exhibited by some demyelinated axons.

The phenomenon of intermittent conduction has now been demonstrated in human peripheral axons affected by various pathologies (Burke *et al* 1998; Cappelen-Smith *et al* 2000; Kaji *et al* 2000; Petajan and White 2000). Correspondingly, drugs that inhibit Na$^+$/K$^+$ ATPase have been reported to improve conduction in both central (Kaji and Sumner 1989a) and peripheral

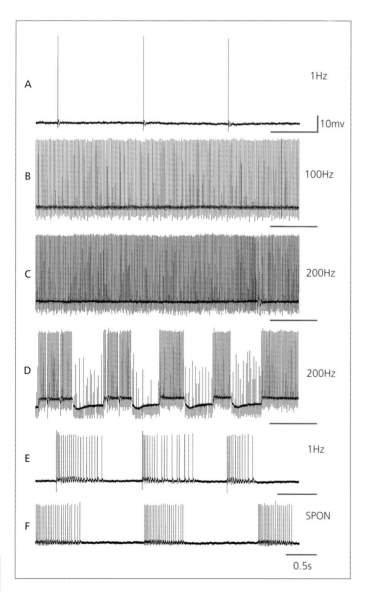

Figure 13.31 Several portions from a long, intra-axonal record (resting potential –60 mV) obtained from a central axon at or near a site of demyelination induced by the injection of ethidium bromide into the dorsal column 14 days previously. The refractory period of transmission was prolonged from 0.77 ms in the unaffected portion of the axon, to 1.32 ms through the lesion. The record illustrates several electrophysiological properties of demyelinated axons. (A) Initially the axon propagated a single action potential through the lesion in response to each supramaximal electrical stimulus presented distal to the lesion at 1 Hz (the stimulus artefacts are not distinguishable). (B) The axon was also initially able faithfully to propagate action potentials in response to 10 s of stimulation at 100 Hz and (C) at 200 Hz. (D) After about ten seconds of such stimulation, the axon entered intermittent periods of complete conduction block (the irregular spikes during these periods represent stimulus artefacts occasionally captured by the analogue-to-digital converter). The periods of conduction block were separated by periods when the axon conducted action potentials in response to approximately 75% of the stimuli, indicating that the lesioned portion of the axon accumulated refractoriness upon repeated activation causing it to filter its input of impulses at 200 Hz into an output of only about 150 Hz. Note that in these intra-axonal records, it is clear that conduction block coincides exactly with periods of membrane hyperpolarization. This finding is consistent with conduction block mediated by activity of the electrogenic Na$^+$/K$^+$ ATPase (see text). (E) After a total of 30 s of stimulation at 200 Hz, the axon responded to individual stimuli presented at 1 Hz, with bursts of impulses rather than single impulses, as in A. (F) Furthermore, in the absence of any electrical stimulation, the axon generated spontaneous bursts of impulses approximately every 2–3 s. Prior to the stimulation at 100 or 200 Hz, this axon was found to generate records similar to those in (E) and (F), but with briefer bursts, following only 2 s of stimulation at 50 Hz: such an impulse load is well within the normal physiological range. Adapted from Felts *et al* (1995).

(Kaji and Sumner 1989b; Shrager 1993) demyelinated axons, and some benefit occurred upon drug administration in 3/7 patients with multiple sclerosis (Kaji *et al* 1990).

Interestingly, intermittent conduction failure can appear after just one second of stimulation at 500 Hz (W.I. McDonald and Sears 1970), or within 10–30 seconds of stimulation at frequencies well within the physiological range (100–200 Hz: unpublished observations) These deficits may therefore underlie the reduced flicker fusion frequency seen in some patients (Titcombe and Willison 1961) and the failure of visual and somatosensory evoked potentials to follow rapidly presented stimuli (Milner *et al* 1974). It is easy to appreciate that the periodic switching on and off of impulse transmission will markedly impair normal sensation and motor activity.

The progressive conduction deficits upon repeated activation described above provide a plausible explanation for the fading or blurring of vision upon prolonged fixation of gaze (W.I. McDonald 1998; Waxman 1981) reported by some patients, or the progressive weakness experienced by some patients after walking only a short distance (W.I. McDonald 1975). A period of rest allows homeostasis of sodium ions and the restoration of function.

Although demyelinated axons typically conduct less securely with repeated activation, an interesting exception has been reported in demyelinated peripheral axons in *Xenopus* (Shrager 1993). In this example, action potentials presented at low frequency did not make it through the lesion, whereas at higher frequencies the second and subsequent action potentials were sometimes transmitted. It seems that if action potentials travel in the supernormal period following a preceding impulse (when conduction velocity and amplitude of the second action potential are enhanced), their enhanced safety factor can result in successful conduction. By varying the timing of impulses within a train entering a lesion, it is therefore possible to derive various output patterns (Figure 13.32). These patterns doubtless contribute to the everyday experiences of people with multiple sclerosis.

Over and above the well-established differences that exist between axons subserving different modalities, such as sensory and motor functions (Bostock and Rothwell 1997; Mogyoros *et al* 2000), there is growing evidence that regional differences exist for fibres responsible for a single modality. For example, motor axons in the median nerves exhibit more prominent slow potassium conductances than peroneal motor axons (Kuwabara *et al* 2001). These properties may differentially predispose populations of axons to disease processes, and determine their responses.

Uhthoff's phenomenon

Many patients with multiple sclerosis exhibit a worsening of symptoms with a rise in body temperature – an effect known as Uhthoff's phenomenon, after the German neuro-ophthalmologist Wilhelm Uhthoff (1890) (Selhorst and Saul 1995). In fact, Uhthoff's original description was restricted to the worsening of vision upon exercise, and the role of temperature was missed, even though one of his patients reported that she experienced the same deterioration of vision when standing in front of a hot stove. Interest in Uhthoff's phenomenon was resurrected after the First World War when induced pyrexia became a fashionable

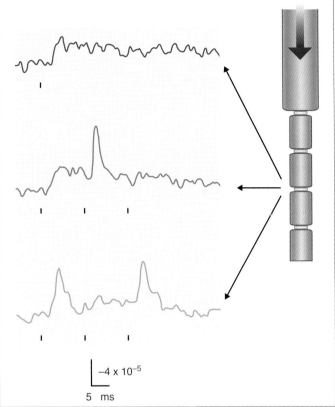

Figure 13.32 Optical records from a node of Ranvier (indicated in the sketch) forming on an axon in the sciatic nerve of *Xenopus*; the nerve had been demyelinated with lysolecithin 20 days previously. The records show how the frequency at which impulses are delivered to a damaged region can affect the pattern of transmission (records are averaged, n = 64). Top record: there appears to be total conduction block when impulses are delivered at 10 Hz. Middle record: only the middle impulse is conducted when a burst of three impulses is delivered at 10 ms intervals. Bottom record: only the first and third impulses are conducted when a burst of three impulses is delivered at 3.3 Hz. Adapted from Shrager (1993). © 1993, with permission from Elsevier.

therapy for multiple sclerosis (see Chapter 1), and many authors reported benefits even though it was appreciated that warming could result in neurological deterioration, and even death. Indeed, the worsening was sufficiently robust and reproducible that the phenomenon later underpinned the diagnostic 'hot bath test' (Guthrie 1951; Malhotra and Goren 1981). This procedure was shown to be associated with clinical deterioration in >80% of patients, and 60% seemingly developed new signs. In fact, the Uhthoff phenomenon can be provoked by a hot shower (Waxman and Geschwind 1983), sunbathing (Avis and Pryse-Phillips 1995; J.R. Berger and Sheremata 1985; Harbison *et al* 1989), use of a hair dryer (Brickner 1950), exercise (van Diemen *et al* 1992) as slight as ascending stairs (Edmund and Fog 1955), or even by the normal circadian change in body temperature (D.G. Baker 2002; F.A. Davis *et al* 1973; Namerow 1968a; Romani *et al* 2000). For example, a pilot with multiple sclerosis experienced blurred vision each afternoon (changing from an acuity of 20/30 in the morning to 20/50 by the afternoon), associated with corresponding changes in the pattern visual evoked potential (Figure 13.33; Scherokman *et al* 1985).

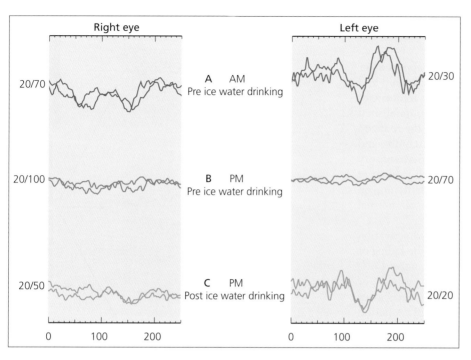

Figure 13.33 Visual evoked potentials recorded from a patient who showed a version of Uhthoff's phenomenon, namely an improvement in vision upon body cooling. In this patient, the improvement in vision showed a circadian rhythm and was correlated with improvements in the evoked potential, and a measure of the temperature of the tympanic membrane. The records suggest that the conduction block normally experienced in the afternoon was reversed upon drinking cold water. Adapted from Scherokman *et al* (1985). © 1985, reprinted with permission of John Wiley & Sons.

The exacerbations due to warming occur very promptly. In extreme instances, support to prevent drowning in a hot bath has been described (Guthrie 1951). Deaths due to scalding and hyperthermia have been reported from immersion in hot water and sunbathing, respectively (Harbison *et al* 1989; Waxman and Geschwind 1983) indicating that patients can be overcome by weakness so rapidly that they are unable to summon help (Avis and Pryse-Phillips 1995). Cooling can not only reverse the deficits caused by warming, but also prove inherently beneficial (Schwid *et al* 2003). Thus an improvement in clinical function is often reported by patients following a cold bath, or even after drinking cold water. The pilot referred to above found that several minutes after drinking iced water his normally blurred vision was improved sufficiently to read newsprint for 30–40 minutes. This improvement was accompanied by an increase in amplitude of the pattern evoked response (Figure 13.33). On a different day, a similar improvement in acuity was accompanied by reduction in temperature of the tympanic membrane of 0.25°C. In another case, improvements in vision and amplitude of the visual evoked potential were documented over time after drinking iced water (Figure 13.34; Hopper *et al* 1972; W.I. McDonald 1986). These effects of temperature are typically reversible, although persistent deficits are reported (J.R. Berger and Sheremata 1983; 1985; F.A. Davis 1985). (A website regarding the effects of temperature, organized by educated patients and without the contents necessarily having been professionally scrutinized, has been established at *http://www.mscooling.org/index.html*.)

The clinical observations suggest that warming and cooling can cause transient block and restoration of conduction, respectively, and these effects are easily reproduced in experimentally demyelinated axons both in central axons (Figure 13.35; K.J. Smith *et al* 2000) and peripheral axons (Bostock *et al* 1981; F.A. Davis and Jacobson 1971; F.A. Davis *et al* 1975; Pencek *et al* 1980; Pender and Sears 1984; Rasminsky 1973; Sears and Bostock 1981; Sears *et al* 1978).

Evidence for conduction failure in patients has been provided by Persson and Sachs (1981), who showed that impairment of visual acuity induced by exercise is accompanied by a reduction in amplitude of the visual evoked potential without a change in latency, indicating that conduction block has developed. Recovery of acuity was accompanied by restored amplitude of the evoked potential. An earlier study showed a prominent (40%) reduction in flicker fusion frequency upon exposure to heat, even though the patient underwent only a 0.2°C rise in temperature (Figure 13.36; Namerow 1972).

Because heating one arm caused weak muscles in other limbs, an effect that could be prevented by applying a tourniquet to the arm, Uhthoff's phenomenon was first attributed to humoral effects or to a reflex reduction in cerebral blood flow (Guthrie 1951). However, this hypothesis was challenged when a large quantity of blood, sampled at a time when heat-induced visual loss was at its maximum, failed to induce the same symptoms after transfusion back into the cooled patient once normal vision had been restored. It is now believed, on the basis of experimental studies, that the exacerbations upon warming are primarily due to shortened duration of the action potential at the node just before the demyelinated region, namely the node responsible for driving the current to depolarize the demyelinated axolemma to its firing threshold (Paintal 1966). Duration of the action potential changes because the temperature coefficient for sodium inactivation is larger than that for activation (F.A. Davis and Schauf 1981). We have described above how demyelinated axons have a reduced safety factor for conduction, such that many hover between conduction block and successful transmission of the nerve impulse. In this situation, the minute shortening in duration of the action current can be the deciding factor in causing conduction failure.

Although the generally accepted view is that temperature-mediated conduction block arises from effects on duration of the action potential, a different mechanism is suggested by a

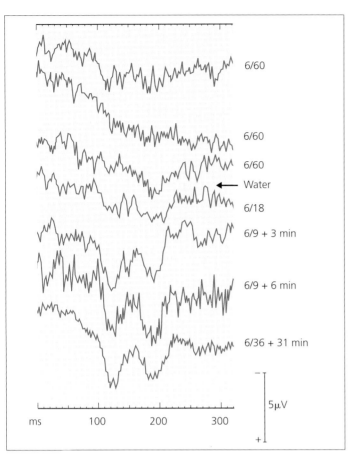

6/60

6/60

6/60

Water ⟵

6/18

6/9 + 3 min

6/9 + 6 min

6/36 + 31 min

5μV

ms   100   200   300

Figure 13.34 Pattern reversal visual evoked potentials from a patient with multiple sclerosis. Visual acuities are given at the end of each trace. There is no consistent response in the top three traces, but then the patient drank a litre of ice-cold water over the course of 7 minutes (arrow). Subsequent records show the appearance of a delayed visual evoked potential, which persisted for approximately one hour. Note the difference in time course of the changes in the evoked potentials and the visual acuity. Kindly provided by Drs Anthony Kriss and Bryan Lecky. Adapted from W.I. McDonald (1986).

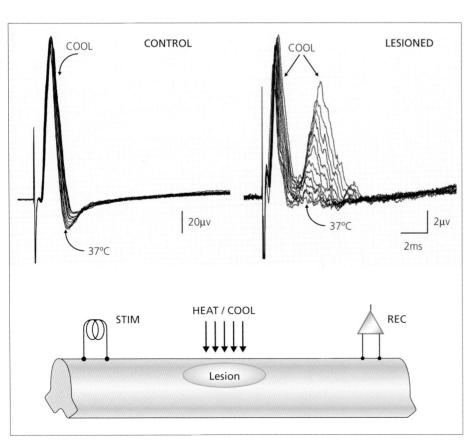

Figure 13.35 Two families of superimposed records obtained from excised dorsal columns examined *in vitro*. The records on the left are from a naive animal, whereas those on the right are from tissue in which an experimental demyelinating lesion had been induced 21 days previously. (A) The temperature of the tissue in the central recording lane (containing the lesion, where present) was raised from 25 to 37°C in 1°C intervals. (B) The temperature changes had little effect on conduction along the normal central axons, but caused prominent changes in the lesioned tissue. When cooled, the compound action potential from the lesioned tissue was composed of two peaks. The early peak occurred with a latency similar to that of control tissue, whereas the second was delayed and comprised of axons with a prolonged refractory period of transmission (data not shown) indicating that the axons were affected by the demyelinating lesion. The axons comprising the second peak were markedly temperature sensitive, such that very few were able to conduct at normal body temperature. Other records from the same tissues are illustrated in Figure 13.17B. Adapted from K.J. Smith (1994). Reproduced with permission from Nature Publishing Group (www.nature.com/nature).

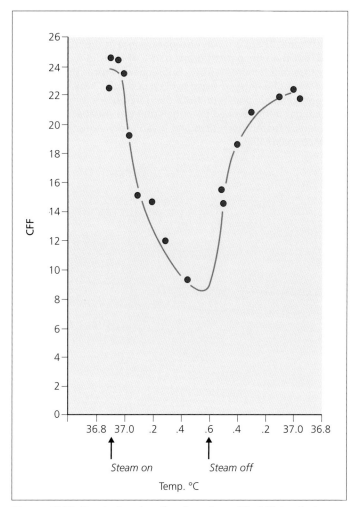

Figure 13.36 Graph showing the changing critical flicker fusion frequency (the ability to discriminate flashes presented in rapid succession) of a patient with multiple sclerosis who had a history of optic neuritis and residual visual impairment. When the patient was exposed to heat, the flashes had to be presented further apart if they were still to be discriminated. Adapted from Namerow (1972). © 1972, with permission from Elsevier.

study that examined the consequences, both on body temperature and leucocyte nitric oxide production, of wearing a cooling garment (Beenakker *et al* 2001). Cooling did not reduce core temperature as measured from the tympanic membrane but did decrease mean leucocyte nitric oxide production by 41%, when this was assessed from blood samples taken 3 hours later. The authors argue that if core temperature was unchanged, the traditional explanation involving prolongation of action potential duration cannot be offered for supposed improvement in the success of axonal conduction. Thus, although temperature has profound effects on axonal conduction in demyelinated axons, these effects may not account for the measured improvement in function associated with wearing a cooling garment. Rather, the authors attribute the beneficial effects of cooling to the reduction in nitric oxide production, as nitric oxide can promote conduction block, especially in demyelinated axons (Redford *et al* 1997). The reduction in nitric oxide production has been attributed to elevated plasma norepinephrine (noradrenaline) caused by cooling the sympathetic nervous system, which in turn leads

to reduced release of proinflammatory cytokines by mononuclear cells and lowered NOS activity in leucocytes (Beenakker *et al* 2001). These effects may offer a partial explanation for the decreased sense of fatigue reported by patients during a month of daily cooling (Schwid *et al* 2003).

If these effects are confirmed, it seems to us that cooling may be beneficial for two reasons. First, in circumstances where core cooling is reliably achieved, it will restore conduction in demyelinated axons. This is a very robust observation in the laboratory, where our unpublished observations show that conduction can be blocked and restored many times per minute if the temperature of the lesion is rapidly modulated. Secondly, cooling may have prolonged beneficial effects arising from the modulation of nitric oxide production. This latter mechanism would explain why patients can experience a sustained benefit from wearing a cooling garment for 45–60 minutes, two to three times each day (Beenakker *et al* 2001; Schwid *et al* 2003).

It is a curious fact that Uhthoff's phenomenon is rarely encountered in demyelinating peripheral neuropathy. Why this should be is unclear. One of us (KJS) has formed the casual impression that whereas conduction in all demyelinated axons is very insecure when first restored, peripheral axons achieve a higher security than central fibres over time. In patients, any such benefit will be augmented by the fact that the temperature of peripheral nerves is often substantially cooler than central nerve fibres. This difference will tend to persist even in a hot patient due to evaporative cooling of the periphery, although it is acknowledged that this argument would not apply if lesions were present in the intrathecal portions of spinal roots. Another consideration is that peripheral axons are more likely to be repaired by remyelination than their central counterparts, and remyelinated axons do not exhibit the conduction changes responsible for Uhthoff's phenomenon. Curiously, some patients with peripheral neuropathy report a negative Uhthoff's finding, such that their symptoms increase with body cooling. We suspect that this finding is due to the markedly different magnitude of temperature change that can occur in peripheral compared with central nervous system axons. On a cold day, temperature of the extremities may reduce to the point where other factors come into play, including the depression of metabolic activity and compromise in blood supply due to vasoconstriction.

The beneficial effects of cooling (Figure 13.35) have encouraged the view that a useful symptomatic therapy for multiple sclerosis may result from drugs that, at normal body temperature, mimic the effects of body cooling by prolonging duration of the action potential (Davis and Schauf 1981; Sears and Bostock 1981; Waxman 1992; Waxman *et al* 1994b). This can be achieved by potassium channel blockade using 4-aminopyridine or by delaying sodium channel inactivation with scorpion venom or pyrethroids. Both strategies can be shown to restore conduction in the laboratory (Bostock *et al* 1978; 1981; Bowe *et al* 1987; Lees 1998; Sherratt *et al* 1980; Targ and Kocsis 1985). As discussed in Chapter 17, 4-aminopyridine is an effective symptomatic therapy in multiple sclerosis (reviewed in Bever 1994; Schwid *et al* 1997b), although whether its efficacy depends on prolonging action potentials at the driving node, or effects on the demyelinated axolemma remains uncertain. Indeed, it is not even clear that 4-aminopyridine acts at the site of the lesion (K.J. Smith *et al* 2000). Laboratory examination has revealed that the drug has no discernible influence on the success of conduction through central demyelinating lesions at therapeutic concentrations (which are orders of magnitude below the concentrations applied directly to demyelinated axons in the initial experimental studies), but it strongly potentiates synaptic transmission (K.J. Smith *et al* 2000). However, if 4-aminopyridine does not restore conduction, what underlies its beneficial effects? It seems possible that, in pathways where conduction in many axons fails due to demyelination or degeneration, potentiating the synaptic efficacy of surviving axons may help to compensate for conduction failure. Whatever its mechanism of action, the adoption of 4-aminopyridine as a therapy has been limited, largely because most patients find its modest advantages are offset by the inherent risk of convulsions (Bever *et al* 1994; Blight *et al* 1991). It is even less surprising that scorpion toxin has also failed to achieve clinical use, although inadvertent 'field trials' in desert regions have apparently resulted in some favourable chance consequences (Breland and Currier 1983).

Fatigue

An excessive sense of fatigue affects the great majority of patients with multiple sclerosis (see Chapter 6; Krupp *et al* 1988) and up to 40% claim this to be their dominant complaint (T.J. Murray 1985). However, despite its importance, fatigue is poorly understood, and progress hampered both by the ambiguity of definition and subjective nature of the deficit (reviewed in Comi *et al* 2002; Rosenberg and Shafor 2005). It is helpful to distinguish motor fatigue from mental exhaustion. Motor fatigue is the better understood, but not necessarily what patients mean when they complain of fatigue. Mental fatigue is the overwhelming sense of tiredness or exhaustion, the need to rest, or the feeling that tasks take too much energy to complete or even contemplate (Freal *et al* 1984).

Motor fatigue can be relatively easily measured (Djaldetti *et al* 1996) and in patients it can result in an unusually rapid decline in tension upon tetanic stimulation. This effect has been attributed to biochemical changes within muscles (C.L. Rice *et al* 1992), and perhaps also to a failure of excitation-contraction coupling (Kent-Braun *et al* 1994). The muscle fibre population of chronically inactive muscles may also switch towards a fatiguable phenotype (Lenman *et al* 1989). Apart from changes associated with the muscles themselves, there is evidence that the motor drive can be compromised such that, in one study, patients rarely achieved >60% activation (C.L. Rice *et al* 1992; Sheean *et al* 1997). In keeping with this finding, voluntary activation of muscles may be suboptimal in patients, so that force can be augmented by artificial stimulation of the motor cortex or motor nerves (Gandevia *et al* 1996).

The role played by frequency-dependent conduction block described in experimentally demyelinated axons remains uncertain (Sheean *et al* 1997). It is difficult to conceive that such block will not reduce motor output, but several studies have emphasized the importance of changes upstream of the motor cortex (Colombo *et al* 2000; Gandevia *et al* 1996; Leocani *et al* 2001; Sheean *et al* 1997), perhaps associated with functional deafferentation of the cortex. Certainly there is ample anatomical substrate for such a deficit, given that cortical lesions can be extensive in multiple sclerosis (see Chapter 12). Cortical deficits are also implicated by the observation that patients with multiple sclerosis show cognitive fatigue, namely a decline in

verbal memory and conceptual planning tasks during testing sessions, in contrast to control subjects who show an improvement in these measures (Krupp and Elkins 2000). Furthermore, the experience of fatigue in patients is associated with a slowing of reaction times on memory tasks (Sandroni *et al* 1992). A role for demyelination in the pathogenesis of fatigue is indicated by the fact that up to 90% of patients consider their fatigue to be worse in warmer environmental conditions, or after vigorous exercise (see also discussion of Uhthoff's phenomenon; Freal *et al* 1984). Accordingly, a daily cooling regimen using a temperature-controlled garment has been reported to improve fatigue (Flensner and Lindencrona 2002; Schwid *et al* 2003; A.T. White *et al* 2000).

The amount of exercise-induced fatigue in patients does not correlate with the level of fatigue experienced in daily life, suggesting that other factors contribute to the symptom (Sheean *et al* 1997). Whatever their nature – and a role for factors associated with inflammation, such as cytokines, has been proposed (Rosse 1989) and denied (Giovannoni *et al* 2001; Iriarte and De Castro 2002; Rudick and Barna 1990) – it seems likely that factors other than the conduction properties of axons, operating upstream from the primary motor pathways, contribute to the symptom (Sheean *et al* 1997). Fatigue appears unrelated to global impairment, or depression (Krupp *et al* 1988), although it can correlate with mood (H.L. Ford *et al* 1998). Fatigue has also been linked to dysfunction of the premotor, limbic, basal ganglia or hypothalamic areas, together with disturbance of the neuroendocrine axis leading to low arousal (Krupp 2003; Gottschalk *et al* 2005). There is a significant association between fatigue, as assessed by interview, and the burden of MRI lesions (Colombo *et al* 2000). Fatigue also correlates with axonal dysfunction or loss, as assessed by a reduction in *N*-acetyl aspartate levels (Tartaglia *et al* 2004).

Another factor that may contribute to fatigue is the fact that patients with multiple sclerosis need to activate much more of the cortex than normal to accomplish even simple motor tasks, or to see (Pantano *et al* 2002; Reddy *et al* 2002; Rocca *et al* 2002a; Spitzer 1999; Werring *et al* 2000b). If more brain energy is required to achieve even simple daily functions, with the consequent implications for cerebral metabolism, it would be surprising if this feature of the disease did not contribute to the sense of fatigue in patients.

Hyperexcitability and positive symptoms

We have described how demyelination initially results in the loss of axonal conduction due, in part, to low excitability of the newly exposed and demyelinated axolemma. We have explained how this membrane can regain excitability over time so that conduction is restored. However, in some axons these alterations lead to hyperexcitability and these axons may become spontaneously active. This results in a variety of positive symptoms such as tingling paraesthesiae, trigeminal neuralgia, pain, triggered and movement-induced sensations, myokymia and the paroxysmal manifestations of multiple sclerosis (see Chapter 6). Other positive phenomena suggest that populations of axons can fire *en masse* in relatively synchronous discharges, as might arise from ephaptic interactions between axons.

Hyperexcitability results in the generation of trains of impulses that arise ectopically, and conduct away from the demyelinated site in both directions (M. Baker and Bostock 1992; K.J. Smith and McDonald 1980; 1982). Both central (K.J. Smith and McDonald 1980; 1982) and peripheral (M. Baker and Bostock 1992; C.M. Bowe *et al* 1987; Burchiel 1980; Calvin *et al* 1982; Nordin *et al* 1984) demyelinated axons are affected in this way, together with amyelinated axons (Huizar *et al* 1975; Rasminsky 1978; 1987). Sensory demyelinated axons are more prone to developing hyperexcitability than their motor counterparts, perhaps because of the greater expression of persistent sodium currents (Bostock and Rothwell 1997; Mogyoros *et al* 2000). The excitability probably explains the greater incidence in multiple sclerosis of positive sensory than motor phenomena, although manifestations such as facial myokymia and paroxysmal dystonia do occur (Andermann *et al* 1961; Y. Chen and Devor 1998; Hjorth and Willison 1973; L. Jacobs *et al* 1994; Kapoor *et al* 1992; Sedano *et al* 2000; Uncini *et al* 1999; Waubant *et al* 2001). Hyperexcitability is likely to be based, in part, on an atypical expression of ion channels, perhaps augmented by the influence of nitric oxide on axonal sodium channels (Hammarstrom and Gage 1999).

Both continuous (at 10–50 Hz) and bursting spontaneous ectopic discharges have been described (Figure 13.37). The individual bursts often show a similar pattern in individual axons, but with interaxonal variation in duration (from 0.1 to

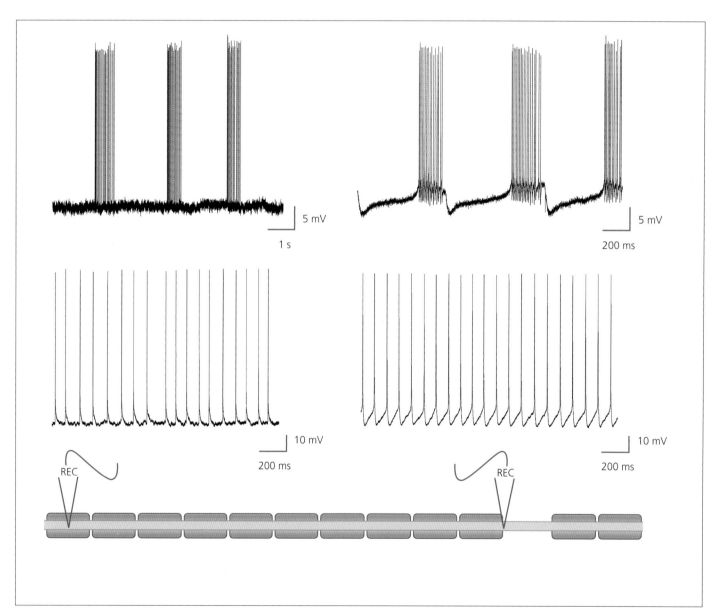

Figure 13.37 Four intra-axonal records obtained from four different demyelinated central axons. The records on the left were obtained with the recording micropipette positioned at a site slightly remote from the demyelinating lesion, while those on the right were obtained at, or near, the lesion. All the records show ongoing activity, evoked in the absence of any intentional stimulus, although the lower records were obtained in the presence of the potassium channel blocking agent 4-aminopyridine; similar records could be obtained in the absence of the drug. Two types of activity are apparent, namely a bursting discharge (upper records) and a more even discharge (lower records). The changes in membrane potential associated with the generation of the impulses can be observed in the records obtained at or near the site of demyelination. REC = record. Adapted from Felts *et al* (1995) and Kapoor *et al* (1997).

5 s) and separation (0.1–100 s). Individual axons appear consistent in firing either as a continuous or bursting discharge, but both types may coexist in different axons within a single lesion. The discharges are protracted, and one of us (KJS) has monitored a continuous discharge in one central demyelinated axon for more than 10 hours, during which the frequency of firing was stable throughout.

In sensory axons, impulses travelling antidromically (i.e. centrifugally towards the periphery) probably do so without much consequence, but it seems reasonable to propose that those propagating in an orthodromic direction and generated concurrently in hundreds of different spontaneously active axons are likely to be perceived as a tingling sensation referred to the body part normally innervated by those axons. This intuitive view has received convincing support from recordings in patients with multiple sclerosis (see below; Nordin *et al* 1984). It seems likely that the formation of ectopic action potentials in axons subserving the sensation of itch can explain the occurrence of paroxysmal itching in patients with multiple sclerosis (Osterman 1976). Similar discharges, perhaps arising from lesions in the thalamus and basal ganglia, may be responsible for the uncommon occurrence of phonic tics (spontaneous throat clearing sounds: Lana-Peixoto *et al* 2002).

The mechanisms underlying these spontaneous activities have been probed using a number of techniques, including intra-axonal recordings and pharmacological manipulations (for review see M.D. Baker 2000; Mogyoros *et al* 2000; K.J. Smith and McDonald 1999; K.J. Smith *et al* 1997). Continuous discharges have been related to the appearance of a slow, persistent inward sodium current appearing at demyelinated membranes (Cummins and Waxman 1997; Honmou *et al* 1994; Kapoor *et al* 1997; Rizzo *et al* 1996; Stys *et al* 1993). The bursting discharges can arise from an atypical, inward potassium current due to the accumulation of potassium ions in an extracellular compartment surrounding demyelinated axons (Felts *et al* 1995; Kapoor *et al* 1993; see also Burke 1993; W. Young *et al* 1989). However, it is not possible rigidly to assign different types of discharges to particular mechanisms. Our unpublished observations show that each type can sometimes arise from either sodium or potassium currents.

The therapeutic efficacy of sodium channel blocking agents such as carbamazepine, lamotrigine, lidocaine and mexiletine indicates that sodium currents contribute to the generation of paraesthesiae and pain in patients with multiple sclerosis (Cianchetti *et al* 1999; Leandri *et al* 2000; Petersen *et al* 1986; Sakurai and Kanazawa 1999; Schwarz and Grigat 1989). Direct evidence for periaxonal potassium accumulation is understandably lacking, but impaired potassium homeostasis seems likely in chronic 'open' lesions (Barnes *et al* 1991), meaning lesions with a large extracellular space, axonal loss and a paucity of astrocytes, the cells primarily responsible for potassium regulation. Furthermore, bursting discharges can be provoked in central demyelinated axons by just a few seconds of impulse conduction at physiological frequencies (2 s at 50 Hz: see Figure 13.37), consistent with the hypothesis that such activity is sufficient to load periaxonal compartment(s) with potassium ions.

Positive symptoms are enhanced by hyperventilation in multiple sclerosis (F.A. Davis *et al* 1970) and in animals with experimental demyelinating lesions (Burchiel 1981), and this manoeuvre tends generally to enhance neuronal excitability

(Mogyoros *et al* 2000). Mechanisms responsible for the increase in excitability are unclear. The classical view, which invokes hypocalcaemia, has been questioned. A more recent interpretation is that the increase in excitability depends primarily on extracellular H^+, perhaps in addition to Ca^{2+} ions (Baker and Bostock 1999; Mogyoros *et al* 1997), which may either affect gating, by changing axolemmal surface charge, or impede ion fluxes through the channels (Hille 1992). The late or persistent sodium current is particularly sensitive to changes in pH, including shifts within the physiological range (Baker and Bostock 1999). Hyperventilation raises pH and, in turn, increases the late current. Its magnitude potently affects the excitability of axons and so it is likely that the effects of hyperventilation on axons are mediated by changes in pH. These also affect the unitary conductance of sodium channels (Baker and Bostock 1999), with conductance diminishing after acidification. The contribution made by atypical ion channels inserted along the demyelinated membrane, perhaps with post-translational changes, to the generation of ectopic activity is described above.

Triggered sensations

It is not uncommon in experimental demyelinated axons to find that a spontaneous burst of ectopic activity is provoked by the conduction of a single impulse through the lesion (Bowe *et al* 1987; Burchiel 1980; Calvin *et al* 1982; Felts *et al* 1995; Huizar *et al* 1975; see also Bostock 1994; Calvin *et al* 1977; Howe *et al* 1976). Interestingly, axons can sometimes be conditioned to exhibit such triggered activity by prior stimulation at high frequency (Figure 13.31E) consistent with a mechanism involving potassium loading of the periaxonal space (see above; Kapoor *et al* 1993). It seems likely that such triggered bursts may underlie the positive phenomena sometimes reported by patients, such as when localized light touch evokes pain referred to the same receptive field.

Readers with a penchant for self-experimentation may like to know that one of us (KJS) believes these triggered bursts can be induced in the normal nervous system, if sensory axons are repeatedly stimulated at high frequency, such as by holding a vibrating object (we favour the handle of a hedge trimmer) for an hour or more. If, following such an experience, the hands are clapped together, there is not only a sharp sensation as contact is made, but also an immediately ensuing sense of vibration, as if placing the hands on a vibrating cymbal. Some patients with multiple sclerosis can experience such sensations without clipping hedges. A similar sensation can be triggered in the feet from prolonged standing on a vibrating surface, such as the floor of a small boat above the engine. These sensations are consistent with the interpretation that a long train of sustained, naturally evoked impulses results in loading of the periaxonal space beneath the internodal myelin with potassium ions. This arrangement results in axons being poised on the threshold of generating a spontaneous burst of ectopic impulses at multiple points along their length. Passage along the axons of impulses generated by clapping the hands triggers release of the ectopic bursts, as previously described (Felts *et al* 1995; Kapoor *et al* 1993). More stoic experimenters have achieved continuous tingling sensations within only 10–20 minutes of applying tetanic electrical stimulation to the sensory nerves (Kiernan *et al* 1997).

Impulse reflection

Sometimes an action potential entering the demyelinated portion along an axon triggers the formation of a daughter impulse that travels back along the axon in the opposite direction (Howe *et al* 1976). Such impulse reflections arise because the prolonged duration of the action potential as it crosses the demyelinated axolemma re-excites the node immediately before the demyelinated stretch once the node has recovered from its absolute refractory period. It can be imagined that a pair of such sites along an axon could set up a reverberating condition whereby action potentials shuttle back and forth between the lesions, generating a train of impulses emerging at each site.

Mechanosensitivity

At about the same time that demyelinated axons become spontaneously active they are also likely to become unusually mechanosensitive. Here, demyelinated portions of the axon acquire properties similar to those of mechanoreceptors, such that distortion of the lesion evokes a phasic and/or tonic burst of activity (Figure 13.38; K.J. Smith and McDonald 1980; 1982). Demyelinated axons can become exquisitely mechanosensitive such that even the relatively small deformations of the central nervous system resulting from normal body movement can stimulate sensations resulting from the ectopic generation of impulses. In patients with demyelinating lesions affecting sensory axons in the cervical posterior columns, mechanosensitivity provokes electric shock or tingling sensations (Lhermitte's symptom), which radiate down the limbs and body upon bending the neck (Kanchandani and Howe 1982; J. Lhermitte *et al* 1924). The perception of tingling evoked by neck movement is associated with a burst of activity in cutaneous nerve fascicles, presumably representing impulses conducted antidromically following their ectopic generation in a cervical lesion (Figure 13.39; Nordin *et al* 1984). Similarly, in patients with optic neuritis, axonal mechanosensitivity leads to the perception of flashes of light, or phosphenes, provoked by movements that distort the optic nerve (Davis *et al* 1976).

The mechanisms responsible are not understood in detail, but similarity of the discharges with those arising from primary sensory mechanoreceptors (phasic and/or tonic discharges upon sustained deformation) suggests that the demyelinated axolemma acquires properties similar to those present at normal mechanoreceptor endings.

Ephaptic activity

Certain clinical phenomena (such as tonic spasms, see Chapter 6) imply that axons affected by demyelinating lesions can fire *en masse* in relatively synchronous discharges (Kapoor *et al* 1992; B. Matthews 1998; W.B. Mathews 1975; W.B. Mathews 1998). Ephaptic interactions (Holt and Koch 1999; see also Shinder *et al* 1998) between adjacent axons are sometimes invoked as a mechanism (ephaptic interactions are electrical interactions that occur at sites other than synapses). Although other explanations are possible, some complicated paroxysmal phenomena are best explained by postulating the lateral spread of excitability across different, but anatomically adjacent, spinal or brainstem tracts (Kapoor *et al* 1992). A particularly interesting

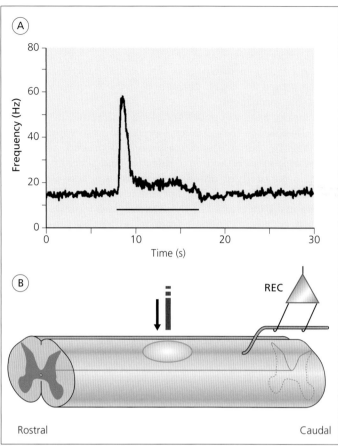

Figure 13.38 Graph showing mechanosensitivity of a central demyelinated axon isolated in a teased dorsal root filament caudal to a demyelinating lesion (yellow) induced in the spinal dorsal columns by the injection of lysolecithin. The unit is spontaneously active, generating a train of impulses at approximately 18 Hz that arise at the lesion. The unit is mechanosensitive and responds to a sustained 10 second 0.75-mm deformation of the lesion by a phasic burst of activity, followed by a slower, more tonic discharge. The activity was unaffected by similar deformations applied to the dorsal columns at sites remote from the lesion. REC = record. Adapted from K.J. Smith and McDonald (1980). Reproduced with permission from Nature Publishing Group (www.nature.com/nature).

example concerned a patient, later diagnosed with multiple sclerosis, who experienced the intense pain of trigeminal neuralgia on the right side triggered by auditory stimuli such as the ringing of a telephone (Hartmann *et al* 1999; see also Devor *et al* 2002). The experience of pain was confined to the duration of the telephone ring. MRI showed a lesion in the pons that involved the right lateral lemniscus and the trigeminal pathway. It seems likely that the auditory impulses ephaptically excited activity in trigeminal axons.

Ephaptic interactions have been difficult to demonstrate in experimental preparations, but one particularly well-documented example involved just two axons, one normal and one amyelinated in the dystrophic mutant mouse (Rasminsky 1978; 1980). Impulses in the amyelinated axon ephaptically excited daughter impulses in the normal axon that travelled in both directions away from the site of ephapse (Figure 13.40). In this example, ephapsis occurred in peripheral, rather than central, nervous tissue (spinal roots) but, in general, ephaptic transmission is expected to be rare in the peripheral nervous system. This is because peripheral axons, even demyelinated ones, are normally prevented from intimate contact by intervening Schwann cell processes and the basal lamina. In the experimental case cited above, cross-talk between axons was possible due to the unusual pathology present in the dystrophic mouse. In the lesions of multiple sclerosis, demyelinated axons can be in direct contact thereby increasing the likelihood of ephaptic activity.

Despite the paucity of proven examples, it is plausible to believe that ephaptic transmission involving demyelinated axons might be quite common. It is easy to imagine circumstances where a hyperexcitable, but quiescent, axon may be poised just on the verge of firing such that it would be triggered by action currents generated in a neighbouring axon. This simple idea can easily be extended to populations of hyperexcitable axons. In this context it is interesting that, albeit rarely, massed synchronous firing can sometimes be recorded from the spinal roots of experimental demyelinating lesions of the dorsal columns (K.J. Smith *et al* 1997). It seems likely that the phenomenon arises from self cross-excitation of a large population of axons or neurons, but whether this occurs within the lesion, or in the dorsal horn, is currently uncertain. If mass synchronous firing occurs in the grey matter, it may release mechanisms similar to those involved in epilepsy, which occurs more frequently in people with multiple sclerosis than in the general population (see Chapter 6; Eriksson *et al* 2002; Ghezzi *et al* 1990; Sokic *et al* 2001). We have never observed any activity suggestive of mass ephaptic interactions in experimental preparations with experimental demyelinating lesions of the dorsal columns in awake animals. The slow spread of ephaptic excitation has been proposed as the mechanism underlying paroxysmal manifestations of multiple sclerosis, such as painful tonic seizures and episodic dysarthria (see Chapter 6; Matthews 1975). Ephaptic transmission may well contribute to brief paroxysms (lasting <1 min), but longer durations (lasting, say, 15–30 min) are more likely to be caused, or augmented, by local transient changes in ion composition perhaps resulting from glial cell dysfunction (Largo *et al* 1996).

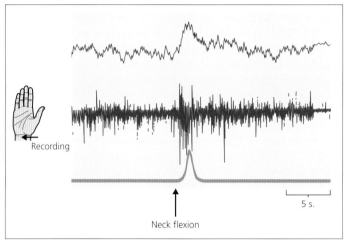

Figure 13.39 Recording from a skin fascicle in the right median nerve (see diagram) of a patient with multiple sclerosis and a six-month history of Lhermitte's symptom. On neck flexion (vertical arrow) the patient experienced a nonpainful paraesthesia ('electric feeling') in all the fingers of her hands, indicated by the peak in the lower grip force record. The middle record shows the evoked multiunit burst of activity, which coincides with the paraesthesiae, and the upper record shows the integrated neurogram (time constant 0.5 s). Adapted from Nordin *et al* (1984). © 1984, with permission from the International Association for the Study of Pain.

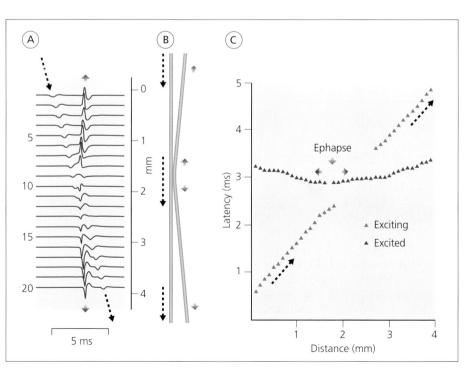

Figure 13.40 Plots showing ephaptic transmission between two nerve fibres in the ventral root of a dystrophic mouse. (A) Ladder plot showing external longitudinal currents recorded at intervals of 200 μm from proximal (top) to distal. The directions of travel of the exciting and excited action potentials are indicated by the dashed and red arrows, respectively. (B) Diagram showing the site of ephaptic interaction. The fibre to the left is the exciting one, and it initiates an ectopic impulse in the right fibre, which propagates away from the ephapse in both directions. (C) Graph showing the latency of the exciting and excited action potentials. The slow conduction velocity of the exciting impulse (travelling from bottom left to top right) indicates that the exciting axon is not myelinated. Adapted from Rasminsky (1980). © 1980, with permission of Blackwell Publishing Ltd.

Pain

Pain is often described by patients with multiple sclerosis (Ehde *et al* 2003; Shibasaki *et al* 1981) but its origins are not well understood. The varieties are discussed in Chapter 6. It may have ischaemic or mechanical explanations in spasticity and after prolonged immobilization. Pain in optic neuritis can be due to meningeal stretch and experienced when the nerve is mechanically distorted upon eye movement (Fazzone *et al* 2003). Electrophysiological properties may cause pain in Lhermitte's symptom and paroxysmal events such as trigeminal neuralgia. Here, we confine our discussion to neuropathic pain. Although spontaneous and triggered discharges in demyelinated nociceptive axons are a likely mechanism (especially in view of the study noted above: Hartmann *et al* 1999), we are not aware that this possibility has been emphasized in the literature. Nonetheless, there is good evidence that demyelination at the dorsal root entry zone is responsible for intractable trigeminal neuralgia in patients with multiple sclerosis. Thus, ultrastructural examination of six biopsies found that, in all samples, the central nervous system component of the trigeminal nerve showed demyelination. Interestingly, the denuded axons lay juxtaposed with no intervening glial processes (Love *et al* 2001). A role for sodium channels in initiating the pain is indicated by the efficacy of partial sodium channel blockade as therapy in multiple sclerosis, for example using carbamazepine (Cianchetti *et al* 1999; Leandri *et al* 2000; Petersen *et al* 1986).

There is also evidence that TNF-α is involved in the generation of neuropathic pain (Sorkin and Doom 2000). Applying low concentrations (0.001–0.01 ng/mL) to normal peripheral nerve can induce ectopic discharges in nociceptive (Aδ and C) axons (Figure 13.41; Sorkin *et al* 1997), and enhance the responses of wide dynamic range neurons to noxious stimulation (Onda *et al* 2002). Furthermore, antibodies to TNF-α or to the tumour necrosis factor-receptor 1 (TNF-R1) reduce thermal hyperalgesia and mechanical allodynia in the chronic constriction injury model of peripheral demyelination and inflammation (Sommer *et al* 1998). TNF-α is present in the inflammatory lesions of multiple sclerosis (Carrieri *et al* 1998). It is therefore possible that its presence within the central nervous system may provoke pain, especially when exposed to demyelinated nociceptive central axons. The electrophysiological consequences of TNF-α exposure may, as expected, be dependent on the site of exposure, because intrathecal administration of TNF-α (or IL-1α) has been reported to promote analgesia (Bianchi *et al* 1992). A concentration effect may also be important because higher concentrations of TNF-α reduce firing in nociceptors (Sorkin *et al* 1997). TNF-α may exert some of its effects by inducing IL-1β and nerve growth factor (Woolf *et al* 1997).

As well as the action of specific cytokines on normal nerve, it has also been reported that neuropathic pain can be generated by the demyelination resulting from experimental application of lysolecithin to the saphenous nerve (Wallace *et al* 2003). This interesting finding had not previously been suspected from several earlier studies by other groups of a similar lesion induced in the sciatic nerve. A change in the expression of sodium channel subtypes (involving Nav1.8 and Nav1.3) has been implicated (Wallace *et al* 2003).

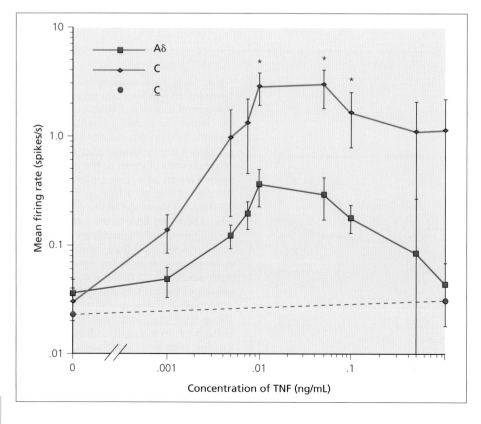

Figure 13.41 Graph showing the effect on firing rate of individual small myelinated (Aδ) and unmyelinated (C) axons of administering the proinflammatory cytokine TNF-α to the rat sciatic nerve. Adapted from Sorkin *et al* (1997). © 1997, with permission from Elsevier.

PERMANENT LOSS OF FUNCTION IN THE CONTEXT OF DISEASE PROGRESSION

We described earlier how complete recovery of function often follows relapses early in the course of multiple sclerosis, even when these are clinically severe. However, recovery is not always complete and tends to diminish with time. Furthermore, by definition, the deficit increases systematically in primary and secondary progressive multiple sclerosis. Several mechanisms probably contribute to the failure of recovery and disease progression.

Persistent conduction block

We have described how conduction can be restored to persistently demyelinated axons through the reorganization of ion channels along the demyelinated axolemma, and argued that, when present, this contributes to remission. However, we emphasize that even when conduction is restored, it is much less secure than normal such that the safety factor for conduction is near unity. It follows that this form of conduction is perilously close to failure, and likely to fail with repetitive activity. This is partly because, in some demyelinated axons, conduction only occurs when local conditions (such as temperature and extracellular ion concentration) are optimal. In other axons, the safety factor is so low that conduction is effectively permanently blocked. Contributory factors could include a long internode preceding the demyelinated stretch, or an internode with partial-thickness demyelination spread along its length. The composition of the extracellular fluid may also be disadvantageous, due perhaps to a paucity of glial cells buffering the local ionic environment. In some patients and lesions it seems likely that persistent conduction failure is the norm, perhaps due to genetic characteristics that might, for example, favour a less advantageous balance of ion channel subtypes or distribution, or an inadequate glial response. Differences may also exist in the potential for repair of individual axons, throughout the course, or at particular times (Black and Waxman 1996). Figure 13.35 shows an example of conduction through a lesion that contains many demyelinated axons capable of conduction, but virtually none of them transmits nerve impulses at normal body temperature. Although the demyelinated membrane is excitable and has all the equipment necessary for conduction, and is indeed excitable when cooled, these axons would persistently fail to conduct in patients as they would be maintained at 37°C.

It is worth noting that persistent conduction block characterizes the lesion in multifocal motor neuropathy (Lewis *et al* 1982), where block can persist for years despite axonal continuity. The physiological mechanisms underlying this block are not known, but the use of threshold tracking techniques has revealed that axons within the nerves are hyperpolarized distal to the site of block, perhaps linked to a depolarization within the lesion itself that may directly block conduction (Kiernan *et al* 2002). An immunological contribution is indicated by the fact that conduction block is associated with the presence of circulating antiganglioside antibodies; 80% of patients improve with intravenous immunoglobulin (IVIg) therapy, and some patients respond to IFN-β (Nobile-Orazio *et al* 2002). Although the detailed mechanisms responsible for these changes in membrane polarization are not yet clear, it is reasonable to consider that similar mechanisms block conduction in some lesions due to multiple sclerosis, contributing to persistent functional deficits.

Axonal degeneration

Axonal degeneration in multiple sclerosis has been discovered and forgotten repeatedly over the past 140 years. It is gratifying to those who have for years been emphasizing its importance to find that axonal loss is now central to much clinical, pathological, pathophysiological and therapeutic discussion about multiple sclerosis. Rather than reiterate this history (see Chapter 1), here we consider how axon degeneration relates to the symptomatology and course of multiple sclerosis. In brief, axonal loss is now considered to be a main cause, perhaps 'the' main cause, of irrecoverable deficit and progression.

The mechanisms responsible are partly discussed in Chapters 10 and 12, but it is clear that at least two patterns of degeneration occur. Axons degenerate in large numbers in acute, inflammatory demyelinating lesions where the magnitude of the damage is proportional to the intensity of inflammation (B. Ferguson *et al* 1997; Trapp *et al* 1998), but there is also a slow-burning axonal degeneration in chronic inactive demyelinated plaques (Kornek *et al* 2000). Furthermore, axons may also be lost secondary to neuronal apoptosis in cortical lesions (Peterson *et al* 2001), although it is not clear how much this contributes to global axonal loss in the white matter. A role for nitric oxide is proposed as contributing to the acute inflammatory mechanisms. Loss of trophic support from growth factors for neurons and axons normally produced by cells of the oligodendrocyte lineage is implicated in the putatively inactive axonal and cortical lesions. In fact, as we argue in Chapter 10, separating the inflammatory and neurobiological components is somewhat artificial and there is evidence, at least *in vitro*, for growth factors conditioning the response to injury by inflammatory mediators (Wilkins and Compston 2005).

The fact that axonal degeneration leads to a loss of conduction is obvious, and has been known for >150 years (Gunther 1843; Waller 1850), so it is easy to accept that MRI evidence for atrophy of the spinal cord shows a graded correlation with disability as measured on the Kurtzke EDSS (Figure 13.42; Losseff *et al* 1996b). Cerebral atrophy also correlates with worsening disability (see Figure 7.18; Kalkers *et al* 2001; Losseff *et al* 1996a; Miller *et al* 2002). Notably, slits in the retinal nerve fibre layer due to axonal loss are readily visible in multiple sclerosis (Frisén and Hoyt 1974) and one of us (WIMcD) has seen this appearance after a single attack of optic neuritis. These slits correspond to arcuate field defects, providing a convincing demonstration that an absolute loss of function corresponds with specific axonal loss (Figure 13.43).

Further evidence for axonal loss is provided by magnetic resonance spectroscopy The ^1H spectrum from the brain of healthy individuals is dominated by a peak due to *N*-acetyl aspartate, an abundant amino acid that is virtually confined in the adult to neurons (including axons), where it is mainly located in mitochondria. That a reduction in *N*-acetyl aspartate is associated with neuronal loss is shown by its inverse correlation with cerebral infarction (Gideon *et al* 1992) and (of more interest in the present context) cerebellar atrophy in dominantly inherited cerebellar atrophy, in which axon loss is known to be the mechanism of atrophy (Davie *et al* 1995). In patients with multiple sclerosis manifesting severe ataxia, there is a similar persistent reduction in *N*-acetyl aspartate, in association with a measured reduction in cerebellar volume (Figure 13.44), whereas the *N*-acetyl aspartate and cerebellar volume are normal in non-ataxic patients. Longitudinal study of a single patient showing a strong correlation between the *N*-acetyl aspartate:creatine ratio and clinical disability indicates that axonal loss or dysfunction contributes to functional impairment in multiple sclerosis (De Stefano *et al* 1997). Reduced *N*-acetyl aspartate in the normal-appearing white matter is well established to correlate with disability (Davie *et al* 1997; Fu *et al* 1998; Sarchielli *et al* 1999). This is already detectable early in relapsing–remitting multiple sclerosis (Chard *et al* 2002a), although not obviously present when patients first present with a clinically isolated syndrome such as optic neuritis (Fernando *et al* 2004). Although whole brain *N*-acetyl aspartate is reduced in clinically isolated syndrome patients, this technque is methodologically more difficult

than standard spectroscopic approaches that use smaller voxels and the finding should be interpreted with caution (Filippi *et al* 2003). Nevertheless, the overall evidence from studies of *N*-acetyl aspartate indicates that neuroaxonal loss or damage occurs in lesions and normal-appearing tissues from very early stages of the disease. However, it should be remembered that reduction in *N*-acetyl aspartate may, in some instances, be reversible, reflecting transient metabolic dysfunction of axons rather than their irreversible loss. This has been clearly demonstrated within evolving inflammatory white matter lesions (Davie *et al* 1994), and has also been reported in a small group of patients after treatment with IFN-β (Narayanan *et al* 2001).

Taken together, the evidence shows a correspondence between irrecoverable deficit, atrophy and axonal loss in the central nervous system, which is graded in degree and progresses over the course of a year or so. Although the evidence is gathered from a variety of sources, none in itself definitive, it is reasonable to conclude that axonal loss is an important mechanism contributing to irrecoverable disability in multiple sclerosis.

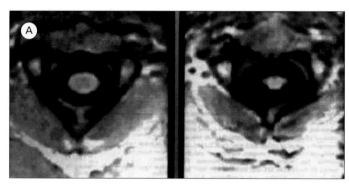

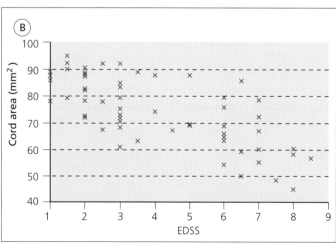

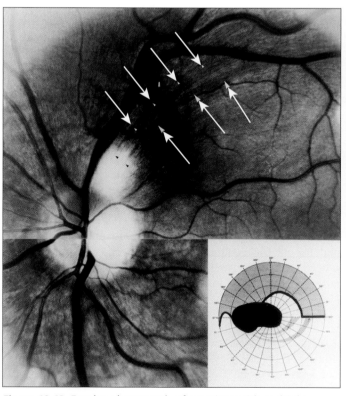

Figure 13.42 MRI scans and graph showing atrophy of the upper cervical spinal cord, and its relationship to disability in multiple sclerosis. (A) The scans compare the normal cord size in a patient without disability (benign multiple sclerosis; EDSS = 1; left), with marked cord atrophy in a patient with secondary progressive multiple sclerosis and severe disability (EDSS = 8; right). (B) The scatter graph shows the correlation between C2 cord area and EDSS (r = 0.7). From Losseff *et al* (1996b) with permission. (This image is also shown in Figure 7.19).

Figure 13.43 Fundus photograph of a patient with multiple sclerosis. There are myelinated nerve fibres at the upper temporal margin of the disc. Arrowheads indicate slits in the retinal nerve fibre layer, some of which can be traced down into the myelinated region. The lower part of the figure illustrates arcuate scotomata, which correspond in position to the location of the slits in the retinal nerve fibre layer. From Sharpe and Sanders (1975). Reproduced with permission from the BMJ Publishing Group.

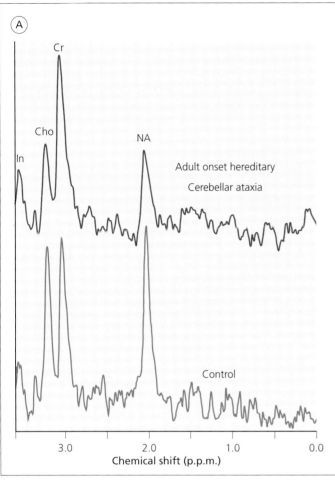

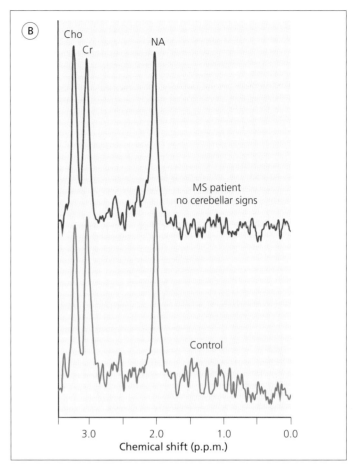

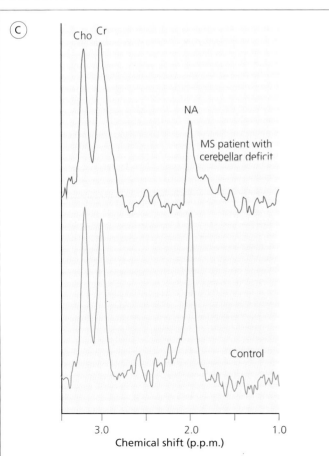

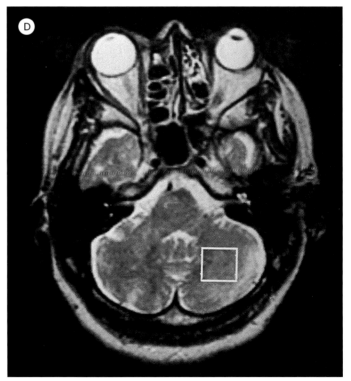

Figure 13.44 Magnetic resonance spectra. (A) Patient with autosomal dominant cerebellar ataxia (above) and a healthy control (below). (B) Patient with multiple sclerosis but no cerebellar deficit (above) and a healthy control (below). (C) Patient with a severe cerebellar deficit due to multiple sclerosis (above) and a healthy control (below). (D) Proton density scan showing a volume of interest localized to the cerebellar white matter (box) in a patient with severe ataxia due to multiple sclerosis. From Davie *et al* (1994) with permission.

A different MRI approach to investigating axonal loss is the correlation between progression of disability and an increase in T_1 hypointensity in T_1-weighted images, which correlates at post mortem with axonal loss in the brain (Truyen *et al* 1996; Van Walderveen *et al* 1998). However, T_1 hypointense lesions are almost never seen in the spinal cord, despite the presence of extensive axonal loss (Bjartmar *et al* 2000; Lovas *et al* 2000; Mottershead *et al* 2003). Atrophy would seem a more reliable measure of axonal loss in the cord. Nor is hypointensity of brain lesions specific for axonal loss. Some acutely hypointense lesions resolve with follow-up, perhaps reflecting resolution of oedema and the impact of remyelination (Barkhof *et al* 2003a; Bitsch *et al* 2001). Another issue with respect to T_1 hypointense lesions is that they provide no indication of axonal loss occurring in normal-appearing white and grey matter. Overall, atrophy measures can be considered the most robust approach for *in vivo* assessment of axonal loss in multiple sclerosis.

Cortical lesions and neuronal loss in grey matter

Much less is known about the contribution made to disability in multiple sclerosis by neuronal loss. As discussed in Chapter 7, magnetic resonance studies of atrophy and *N*-acetyl aspartate have indicated the presence of neuroaxonal loss in cortical and deep grey matter, not only (as expected) in advanced secondary progressive disease (Cifelli and Matthews 2002), but also in early

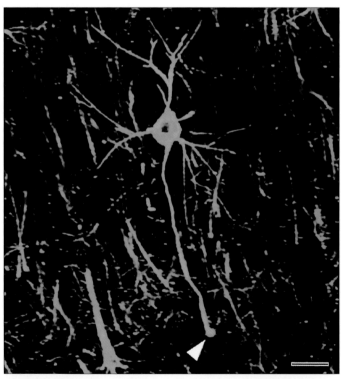

Figure 13.45 Confocal image of a neuron from a cortical lesion in multiple sclerosis. The axon has been truncated and now ends in a terminal swelling (arrowhead). Scale bar = 90 μm. From Peterson *et al* (2001). © 2001, reprinted with permission of John Wiley & Sons.

relapse onset disease (Chard *et al* 2002a; Dalton *et al* 2004a; De Stefano *et al* 2003). This implies that grey matter neuroaxonal pathology is an important factor in the overall disease course. Just as permanent loss of function will typically follow axonal transection, so too it results from cortical neuronal loss, synaptic stripping and severance of dendrites (Figure 13.45; Peterson *et al* 2001). Clearly, a paucity of synaptic complexity will prevent the subtle balancing of multiple inputs upon which sophisticated behaviours are based. Wherever the fundamental substrate of electrical activity is lost, a deficit (detectable or not) must ensue.

Nitric oxide and axonal degeneration

Several studies have concluded that the magnitude of axonal degeneration in the lesions of multiple sclerosis is related to intensity of the inflammatory response (B. Ferguson *et al* 1997; Trapp *et al* 1998), suggesting that factor(s) associated with inflammation are responsible. Many potential mechanisms may be operating in the inflammatory milieu, and they may differ between lesions or at different stages of the disease. Degeneration may also be the consequence of several small insults, individually innocuous but lethal to the axon if acting in unison. However, although complicated, the goal of characterizing mechanisms responsible for degeneration is not hopeless, and several are already identified. Here, we focus on the potential role of nitric oxide. Study of the pathology in multiple sclerosis suggests that cells capable of iNOS expression, such as macrophages and astrocytes, are intimately involved (see Chapter 12; K.J. Smith and Lassmann 2002). Clearly, cells that become activated and iNOS positive will also be producing a host of other inflammatory factors that may be deleterious for axons, but there is evidence that nitric oxide may be particularly toxic, especially if it occurs in association with impulse activity.

That nitric oxide is inherently toxic to axons is shown by their selective sensitivity when peripheral (Kapoor *et al* 2000; 2003) or central (Garthwaite *et al* 2002) nerve tissue is incubated with nitric oxide donors *in vitro*. Axons degenerate upon exposure to nitric oxide at lower concentrations, and after shorter durations of exposure, than do Schwann cells, oligodendrocytes and astrocytes. Interestingly, this sensitivity to nitric oxide is markedly exacerbated if the axons are electrically active (Figure 13.46; Smith *et al* 2001a), and this vulnerability is clearly expressed at physiological frequencies of impulse conduction. Thus, Figure 13.21 shows the degeneration of 100% of axons exposed to nitric oxide and sustained impulse activity at 100 Hz, and Figure 13.47 shows that 100 Hz is below the average firing frequency of primary afferent fibres from the cat gastrocnemius during the normal stepping cycle of limb movement (Prochazka and Gorassini 1998). As both nitric oxide exposure and electrical activity will occur within the lesions of multiple sclerosis, it follows that this combination of events could contribute to axonal degeneration. The characterization of their biochemical mechanisms may identify rational protective therapies.

The mechanisms responsible for degeneration appear to involve the intracellular accumulation of sodium ions. Certainly there are several reasons to believe that demyelinated axons will be inherently vulnerable to such accumulation, and this vulner-

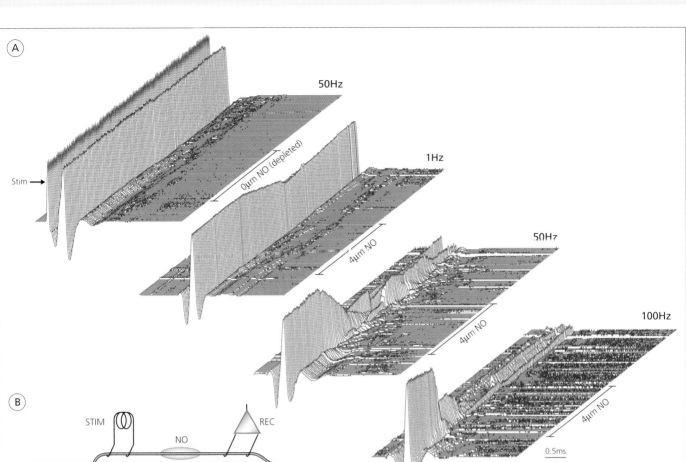

Figure 13.46 Four series of averaged compound action potentials recorded in parallel from four separate dorsal roots using the arrangement indicated (see inset), in an anaesthetized rat. The data are illustrated in the same way as in Figure 13.21, but here each plot shows approximately 5 hours of recorded data. The first plot shows control data obtained in response to continuous supramaximal stimulation of the root at 50 Hz. The stimulus artefact (indicated) can easily be distinguished from the compound action potential, which remains constant in configuration and amplitude throughout the recording period. During a 2 hour period (indicated) the culture medium in a 7 mm long bath surrounding the middle portion of the root was exchanged for one containing the nitric oxide donor DETA NONOate, but the donor applied to this root alone had been depleted of its nitric oxide content. The second plot, also a control, shows the effect at 1 Hz stimulation of a medium liberating nitric oxide at 4 μM concentration; the nitric oxide has little effect on conduction when the axons are conducting at low frequency. However, the same nitric oxide concentration causes persistent conduction block – shown in other experiments (see Figure 13.21) to be due to axonal degeneration – if the axons are conducting impulses at either 50 or 100 Hz. STIM = stimulate; REC = record. Adapted from K.J. Smith *et al* (2001a). © 2001, reproduced with permission of John Wiley & Sons.

ability will be enhanced at sites where axons are exposed to nitric oxide. We have described above that demyelinated axons acquire sodium channels along the axolemma formerly covered by myelin. This adaptation is normally regarded as beneficial because of the opportunity for restoration of conduction and relief of the neurological deficit. However, although such conduction is very welcome from a clinical standpoint, the impulses cross the demyelinated segment using a continuous or micro-saltatory mode of conduction (Bostock and Sears 1976; K.J. Smith *et al* 1982), and this exposes the axons to a very much greater sodium load per impulse than is normal. The newly acquired sodium channels can also include subtypes that are atypical for myelinated axons (Craner *et al* 2003b), raising the possibility that they could contribute unduly to sodium loading. Secondly, sodium entry into the axon may be multiplied many times if the axon becomes hyperexcitable and spontaneously active. We have already made the point that demyelinated axons affected in this way can generate continuous trains of ectopic impulses at frequencies of up to 50 Hz (Baker and Bostock 1992; Kapoor *et al* 1997; Rizzo *et al* 1996; K.J. Smith and

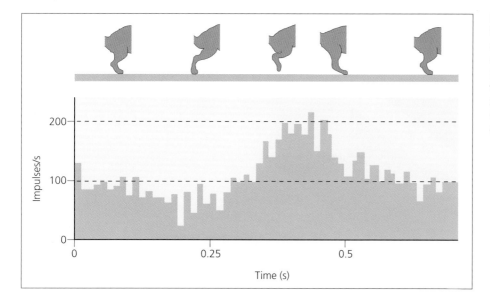

Figure 13.47 Graph showing the mean firing rate of a spindle secondary afferent arising from the cat hamstring muscle during the normal stepping cycle (indicated). The average firing rate for this nerve fibre during normal activity is >100 Hz. Adapted from Prochazka and Gorassini (1998). © 1998, with permission of Blackwell Publishing Ltd.

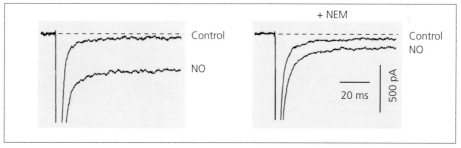

Figure 13.48 Records showing the effect of nitric oxide (released by flash photolysis of sodium nitroprusside) on the persistent sodium current recorded from myocytes. The augmentation of the persistent current was reversed by the sulfhydryl alkylating agent *N*-ethylmaleimide (NEM). Adapted from Ahern *et al* (2000). Reproduced with permission from The American Society for Biochemistry and Molecular Biology.

McDonald 1980; 1982). This activity, which occurs in addition to the normal physiological impulse traffic, can add very substantially to the impulse (and hence sodium) load. A continuous train of impulses at 50 Hz amounts to 180 000 additional impulses per hour! This is an impressive achievement for axons that are already undergoing pathological changes. Although it seems that axons can sustain such activity indefinitely under ideal circumstances (K.J. Smith and McDonald 1982), whether this poses an intolerable burden on those additionally exposed to insults, especially nitric oxide, is another matter. This free radical (nitric oxide) is produced in high concentrations within the inflammatory lesions of multiple sclerosis due to prominent expression of the inducible form of nitric oxide synthase (iNOS) (Bagasra *et al* 1995; Cross *et al* 1998; Hooper *et al* 1997; Oleszak *et al* 1998).

Exposure of axons to nitric oxide may well be doubly damaging, because it can be expected both to exacerbate the magnitude of sodium loading and simultaneously deprive the axon of its ability to restore sodium homeostasis. On the first point, there is indirect evidence (M.D. Baker 2000; M.D. Baker and Bostock

1992; Kapoor *et al* 1997; Rizzo *et al* 1996; K.J. Smith *et al* 1997) that demyelinated axolemma acquires properties resulting in a persistent sodium current, arising from continuous drift of sodium ions into the axon. This type of current may be dramatically enhanced in the presence of nitric oxide (Figure 13.48 and see also Figure 13.13A; Ahern *et al* 2000; Hammarstrom and Gage 1999) or hypoxia (Hammarstrom and Gage 1998) there is evidence that hypoxia-like conditions exist within the inflammatory lesions of multiple sclerosis (see Chapter 12; Aboul-Enein and Lassmann 2005; Aboul-Enein *et al* 2003), perhaps due to a direct modification of the sodium channels resulting in a much increased probability that individual channels will open spontaneously. The load of sodium ions will have to be removed from the axon if sodium homeostasis is to be maintained, and this requires energy in the form of ATP to supply the Na^+/K^+ ATPase (sodium pump). Increased energy demand may well explain the increased numbers of mitochondria that appear along demyelinated portions of axoplasm (Mutsaers and Carroll 1998), but there are reasons to believe that the energy supply may nonetheless be compromised. This problem arises from another property of nitric oxide, namely that it is a potent inhibitor of mitochondrial metabolism (Bolanos *et al* 1997; Brorson *et al* 1999; G.C. Brown 1999; Duchen 2000; Heales *et al* 1997). Whether such inhibition occurs at sites of inflammation is not clear. However, mitochondrial inhibition occurs at low (nanomolar) nitric oxide concentrations, and lactic acidosis has also been noted in experimental autoimmune encephalomyelitis during the onset of clinical signs (R.D. Simmons *et al* 1982). This indicates that, under these circumstances, the mitochondria are not working sufficiently to supply the energy needs, triggering the switch to anaerobic respiration. It therefore seems reasonable to propose that axons exposed to nitric oxide may lack sufficient ATP to maintain function of the sodium pump. As the opening of sodium channels is not itself dependent on ATP (and so will continue unabated, adding to the sodium load), it is clear that axons exposed to nitric oxide may experience a significant rise in internal sodium ion concentration. This rise may be particularly severe in spontaneously active, demyelinated axons. The rise in internal sodium may be exacerbated even further, in all axons, by the fact that nitric oxide can also directly impair the function of the sodium pump itself (Guzman *et al* 1995; Sato *et al* 1995). Although sodium ions are not particularly toxic, a high internal sodium concentration can cause the axolemmal sodium/calcium ion exchanger to operate in reverse, as has been demonstrated in a laboratory model of anoxic injury (Stys and LoPachin 1997; Stys *et al* 1991; Waxman *et al* 1994a). Reverse operation of the exchanger will result in a potentially catastrophic rise in intra-axonal calcium, especially when this occurs in an axon already metabolically compromised and so deprived of its normal mechanisms for sequestering or extruding calcium. A significant rise in intra-axonal calcium can be expected to activate calcium-dependent degradative enzymes and initiate Wallerian type degeneration (for review see Bechtold and Smith 2005).

There is recent evidence to support the belief that the above mechanism may play an important role in axonal damage in both experimental autoimmune encephalomyelitis and multiple sclerosis. Our preliminary findings (KJS) indicate that axons can be protected from degeneration in chronic relapsing experimental autoimmune encephalomyelitis by selective blockade of the reverse mode of action of the sodium/calcium exchanger, clearly implicating this molecule in the pathogenesis of axonal damage. Furthermore, there is also recent immunohistochemical evidence that the sodium/calcium exchanger co-localizes with regions of axonal damage in both experimental autoimmune encephalomyelitis (Craner *et al* 2004a) and acute multiple sclerosis lesions (Craner *et al* 2004b).

An interesting recent finding suggests that the rise in internal calcium could be augmented, or achieved, by depolarization-driven opening of axolemmal calcium channels and the release of internal calcium stores via activation of ryanodine receptors (Ouardouz *et al* 2003). The discovery of this mechanism may prove to be an important advance for research into the consequences of brain ischaemia, but it is not yet clear that conditions within the lesions of multiple sclerosis are sufficiently severe for this mechanism to be initiated. Whether the combination of nitric oxide exposure and impulse activity contributes to axonal degeneration in multiple sclerosis remains uncertain. In support

of this possibility, it is notable that small diameter axons are particularly vulnerable to this combination of events (K.J. Smith *et al* 2001a), and small axons degenerate selectively in multiple sclerosis (Evangelou *et al* 2001; Ganter *et al* 1999).

The mechanism of degeneration involving reverse operation of the sodium/calcium exchanger may have particular relevance for the inflammatory lesions of relapsing–remitting multiple sclerosis where iNOS expression is particularly prominent and axons degenerate in large numbers. However, it may also be relevant to the slow-burning degeneration of progressive multiple sclerosis (Kornek *et al* 2000). In such types of the illness, although intense active inflammation is less common, axonal degeneration occurs on a background of residual chronic inflammation (Prineas and Wright 1978) and many microglial cells are intensely iNOS positive. Thus, chronic exposure of axons to nitric oxide may be responsible for slow-burning degeneration, with individual axons succumbing if they happen over time to be located near iNOS-positive microglia, and to fire for sustained periods at high frequency.

If nitric oxide exposure does encourage the sodium loading of energy-deficient axons, resulting in their degeneration via reverse operation of the sodium/calcium exchanger, is it possible to protect axons pharmacologically and so provide a degree of neuroprotection? Theoretically, axonal protection could be achieved by inhibition of the sodium/calcium exchanger, the enzymatic activity of iNOS, or the axolemmal sodium channels. With regard to the exchanger, axonal protection from nitric oxide-mediated axonal degeneration has been demonstrated *in vitro* with bepridil, which inhibits the exchanger (Kapoor *et al* 2003). It remains to be shown whether blocking this exchanger would constitute an acceptable chronic therapy in clinical practice. Research into the inhibition of iNOS has been hampered by the lack of highly specific, nontoxic drugs that penetrate the blood–brain barrier, but nonetheless a number of studies have examined the efficacy of available iNOS inhibitors in models of experimental autoimmune encephalomyelitis (Cross *et al* 2000; D.C. Hooper *et al* 2000; Pozza *et al* 2000; Shin *et al* 2000; V.K. Singh *et al* 2000; Spitsin *et al* 2000; Willenborg *et al* 1999). No consistent picture has emerged. Some combinations of model, drug and timing of administration have shown such therapy to be highly beneficial, but other cocktails have resulted in exacerbation of the disease. In part the problem reflects the 'Janus faces' of nitric oxide, both at the level of individual cells (Bishop *et al* 2005) and at the level of the intact organism, where the agent can be damaging to tissues but also protective in autoimmune disease via immunosuppression (K.J. Smith and Lassmann 2002). Given the very variable consequences of iNOS inhibition in animal models, currently it seems premature to explore this therapy in patients

However, this latter concern may not apply to the partial blockade of sodium channels. Several sodium channel blocking agents have been examined in a range of different models. Lidocaine, flecainide (Kapoor *et al* 2000) and tetrodotoxin (Garthwaite *et al* 2002) protect axons from degeneration mediated by incubation of nervous tissue with nitric oxide, and lidocaine and flecainide are effective in protecting axons from degeneration following combined exposure to nitric oxide and impulse activity (Figure 13.49; Kapoor *et al* 2003; K.J. Smith

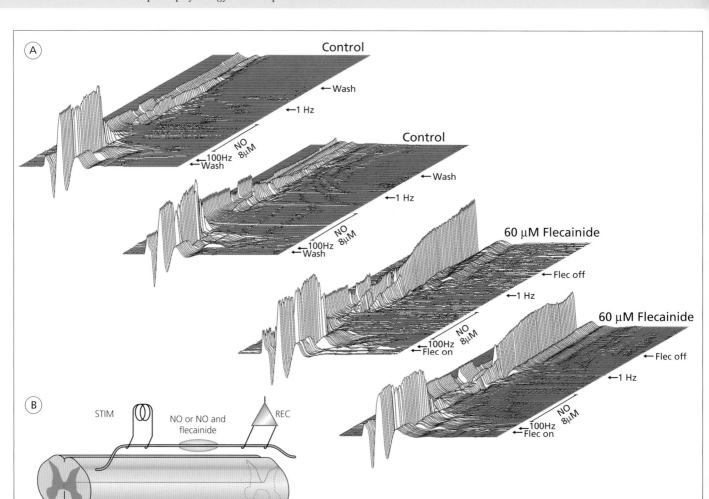

Figure 13.49 Four series of recordings made in parallel from four dorsal roots in an anaesthetized rat (see description for Figure 13.46). In the upper two plots the combination of impulse activity and nitric oxide exposure, as will occur in the lesions of multiple sclerosis, results in persistent conduction block in almost all of the axons due to axonal degeneration (see Figure 13.21). However, in the adjacent roots almost all the axons survive, despite experiencing exactly the same protocol. In these roots the sodium channel blocking agent flecainide was included with the nitric oxide donor, although in a sufficiently low dose that conduction persisted despite the presence of the drug. The inclusion of flecainide protected the axons from degeneration. STIM = stimulate; REC= record. Adapted from Kapoor *et al* (2003). © 2003, reproduced with permission of John Wiley & Sons.

et al 2001b). Perhaps more closely relevant to a potential therapy for multiple sclerosis, flecainide and phenytoin have been found to protect axons from degeneration in models of relapsing–remitting (Figure 13.50; Bechtold *et al* 2004a) and progressive experimental autoimmune encephalomyelitis (Lo *et al* 2002; 2003), respectively. Subsequently, lamotrigine has also been shown to be effective in relapsing–remitting experimental autoimmune encephalomyelitis (Bechtold *et al* 2004b), and flecainide in experimental autoimmune neuritis (Bechtold *et al* 2005). In experimental autoimmune encephalomyelitis, daily administration of flecainide significantly reduced peak severity of both acute and persistent neurological deficits. The number of functioning axons in the dorsal columns was also increased at the end of the trial, together with the number of surviving axons in the same pathway. These beneficial effects were observed irrespective of whether drug administration commenced prior to immunization, or was delayed until after the onset of neurological deficits (Bechtold *et al* 2004a). At the time of writing, these findings regarding axonal protection have encouraged proposals to examine sodium channel blocking agents, especially lamotrigine and phenytoin, as potential therapeutic agents in clinical trials of patients with multiple sclerosis.

Glutamate and axonal degeneration

Extracellular glutamate concentrations are raised in the inflammatory lesions of multiple sclerosis, due both to local gluta-

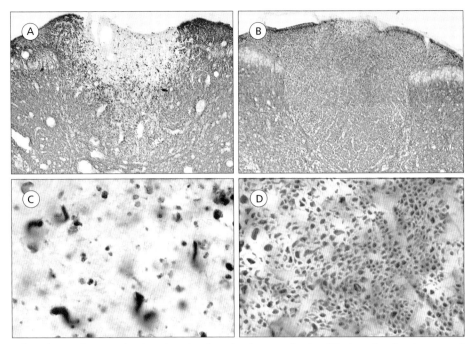

Figure 13.50 Representative photomicrographs showing the dorsal columns of rats with chronic relapsing experimental autoimmune encephalomyelitis treated with daily administration of vehicle (A and C, higher power) or the sodium channel blocking agent flecainide (B and D, higher power). The axons have been labelled immunohistochemically for neurofilaments. (C) Whereas many axons degenerate in vehicle-treated control animals (pale area in the medial dorsal columns), (D) most are protected by flecainide administration. Modified from Bechtold *et al* (2004a). © 2004, reproduced with permission of John Wiley & Sons.

mate release by activated microglia and leucocytes (Piani *et al* 1991), and to cytokine-impaired glutamate uptake by astrocytes (Hu *et al* 2000). Apart from these mechanisms, there is evidence that large quantities of glutamate may be released by the reverse operation of sodium-dependent glutamate transport, if sodium and potassium gradients are run down (S. Li and Stys 2001; S. Li *et al* 1999; 2000). We describe above that energy insufficiency at sites of inflammation may lead to diminished ion gradients, due to nitric oxide-mediated mitochondrial inhibition and consequent lack of sufficient ATP to supply the sodium pump. A high extracellular glutamate concentration would be expected to activate AMPA receptors and thereby result in injury due to raised intracellular calcium. The beneficial effects of blocking NMDA/AMPA/kainate receptors in experimental autoimmune encephalomyelitis (Pitt *et al* 2000; T. Smith *et al* 2000b; Wallstrom *et al* 1996; Werner *et al* 2000) and the efficacy of riluzole (Gilgun-Sherki *et al* 2003) provide evidence that these mechanisms play an important role in axonal and perhaps oligodendrocyte degeneration.

MRI in primary and secondary progressive multiple sclerosis

A paradoxical finding in early studies of primary progressive multiple sclerosis was that although patients were more disabled and had a poorer prognosis, fewer MRI lesions were visible when compared with a cohort having benign relapsing–remitting

disease (A.J. Thompson *et al* 1990b). New T$_2$ lesions in primary progressive disease are also less likely to exhibit gadolinium enhancement (A.J. Thompson *et al* 1991), suggesting that they are less inflammatory in nature, a finding confirmed by pathological examination (Revesz *et al* 1994). The small lesion load and lower frequency of inflammatory lesions partly explains why patients with primary progressive disease rarely experience relapses. What therefore is the explanation for their progressive disability? Several factors are probably relevant.

There is evidence for significant and progressive spinal cord atrophy (Ingle *et al* 2003; Losseff *et al* 1996b). Most patients with primary progressive disease present with myelopathy. It follows that progressive axonal loss also occurs preferentially in the spinal cord, leading to atrophy and clinical disability, but progressive cerebral atrophy is also seen (Ingle *et al* 2003), implying more generalized neuroaxonal loss. The normal-appearing white and grey matter also shows intrinsic abnormalities in primary progressive multiple sclerosis. These include increased diffusion and decreased MTR in both tissue compartments (Dehmeshki *et al* 2003; Rovaris *et al* 2001b; 2002a) and decreased *N*-acetyl aspartate in white matter (Leary *et al* 1999). The inferences from MRI are that the pathology in primary progressive multiple sclerosis exhibits less in the way of multifocal inflammatory white matter lesions, but rather more in the way of diffuse abnormalities that include neuroaxonal loss – often, but not exclusively, in the spinal cord.

Patients with secondary progressive multiple sclerosis have more T_2 and gadolinium enhancing lesions than those with primary progressive multiple sclerosis (A.J. Thompson *et al* 1991). The frequency of such lesions is related to whether or not there are concurrent relapses (Molyneux *et al* 2001; Tubridy *et al* 1998b). Patients with relapsing secondary progressive multiple sclerosis have an even higher prevalence of gadolinium enhancing lesions and, in conventional radiological terms, appear similar to patients with active relapsing–remitting disease. On the other hand, nonrelapsing patients have fewer lesions and in this respect resemble primary progressive multiple sclerosis. It seems clear that, in general, inflammatory white matter MRI lesions located in clinically eloquent pathways are related to relapses but not to clinical progression.

Clear differences emerge when patients with relapsing–remitting and secondary progressive multiple sclerosis are compared with respect to atrophy or abnormalities of the normal-appearing tissues. In the spinal cord, there is often marked atrophy in secondary progressive multiple sclerosis (Losseff *et al* 1996b), whereas it is mild or even absent in relapsing–remitting disease. Progressive brain atrophy is also seen in secondary progressive multiple sclerosis, and the atrophy is largely independent of lesion load and activity (Losseff *et al* 1996a; Molyneux *et al* 2000). There are greater abnormalities of MTR (Filippi *et al* 1999; Kalkers *et al* 2002b; Traboulsee *et al* 2003) and diffusion (Bozzali *et al* 2002) in the normal-appearing tissues in secondary progressive disease. In addition, the reduction in *N*-acetyl aspartate in the normal-appearing white matter is more marked in those with progressive disability (Davie *et al* 1995; Fu *et al* 1998; Sarchielli *et al* 1999), indicating the presence of more severe and diffuse axonal loss.

Extensive neuronal loss affecting deep grey matter structures is seen in progressive forms of multiple sclerosis. When a group of 14 patients with secondary progressive multiple sclerosis were compared with healthy controls, thalamic volume was reduced by 17% and thalamic *N*-acetyl aspartate by 19% (Cifelli and Matthews 2002; Cifelli *et al* 2002). The combined decrease of volume and *N*-acetyl aspartate suggested a 30% decrease in the effective thalamic neuronal density. A parallel *in vitro* study of ten patients who died in the secondary progressive stage of the disease reported a 21% reduction of thalamic volume and a 22% decrease in the density of thalamic neurons compared with ten controls, giving an overall decrease in total neuronal number of 35%.

Perfusion MRI using arterial spin tagging has reported a substantial decrease in deep grey matter perfusion in 12 patients with primary progressive multiple sclerosis, most notably in the caudate nucleus and thalamus (see Figure 7.24; Rashid *et al* 2004). Decreased grey matter perfusion was also observed in 14 individuals with secondary progressive disease. No such reduction was observed in 21 patients with relapsing–remitting multiple sclerosis. In fact, this subgroup exhibited an increase in white matter perfusion attributed to inflammation. A plausible explanation for the finding of decreased deep grey matter perfusion in progressive multiple sclerosis is loss or dysfunction of neurons in that region, with a consequent decrease in metabolic activity and, hence, perfusion.

Studies of cortical plasticity using fMRI have revealed complex abnormal patterns of activation in primary progressive (Filippi *et al* 2002b; Rocca *et al* 2002b) and secondary progressive (Rocca *et al* 2003a) multiple sclerosis. That said, a consistent pattern that characterizes disease subtypes has not emerged. This is perhaps not surprising when one considers the variable and heterogeneous pathology that affects different individuals, the potential for cortical networks and adaptive mechanisms to be interrupted in a largely unpredictable manner, and the apparently minimal nature of the initial pathological process that can on occasions lead to widespread alterations in the fMRI response. fMRI is undoubtedly a powerful tool for investigating the response of the brain to structural diseases of the brain, but thus far it has been difficult to evaluate the significance of the changes observed in multiple sclerosis at least in part because of the complex underlying pathology.

CONCLUSION

The plethora of neurological deficits experienced by patients with multiple sclerosis can be traced both to the diverse location of lesions and the consequences for affected nerve fibres. All parts of the central nervous system may be involved, and the pathophysiological effects on nerve fibres range from inexcitability to hyperexcitability, and from functional repair to permanent structural loss due to degeneration. However, the presence of a lesion does not necessarily equate with the awareness of symptoms, even when the lesion is in a clinically eloquent pathway. The central nervous system has a substantial functional reserve capacity, so that 50% or more of axons may be lost without clinical deficits becoming manifest. However, that said, lesions often do cause symptoms because many demyelinated axons fail to conduct effectively, and all demyelinated axons probably pass through an initial period – lasting at least a week or two – in which they cannot conduct through the lesion at all. Provided that many axons are not synchronously affected, this enforced period of conduction block may remain subclinical. However, the pathophysiology of demyelination is not limited to the success or failure of conduction, because axons can also become hyperexcitable, generating trains and bursts of spurious, ectopic impulses. These activities contribute to various 'positive' phenomena, including tingling sensations and, perhaps, pain.

Deficits also result from two other cardinal pathological features of the lesion in multiple sclerosis, namely axonal degeneration and inflammation. It is easy to understand that axonal degeneration can cause neurological deficits, perhaps permanent ones, but the role of inflammation has only been recognized more recently, and its direct contribution is perhaps not yet proven beyond all doubt. However, if factors associated with inflammation are capable of impairing conduction, any list of potential culprits is likely to include nitric oxide in a prominent position. Nonetheless, it is not yet clear whether it is inflammation *per se* that may be responsible for conduction deficits, because inflammation might almost inevitably result in some subtle degree of myelin pathology, short of denuding axons, especially at the paranodes. Even partial myelin damage, if it occurs at this site, may have significant effects on conduction. Thus, whether it is myelin damage or inflammatory mediators, or indeed anything at all, that affects axonal conduction at a site of pure inflammation, is currently unknown.

Although any current discussion of the pathophysiology of multiple sclerosis is likely to centre on axons and white matter, this should not be construed as implying that we believe all other structures to be functioning normally. On the contrary, already there is clear evidence for grey matter pathology, and almost certainly this contributes to neurological deficits. Writing in 2005, it remains a matter of speculation as to which other components of the central nervous system, and mechanisms of injury, may yet be implicated in the pathophysiology of multiple sclerosis.

The pathogenesis of multiple sclerosis: a pandect

14

Hans Lassmann, Kenneth Smith, Hartmut Wekerle and Alastair Compston

For many years, the central concept underlying ideas on the pathogenesis of multiple sclerosis has been that the cascade of inflammatory events culminating in demyelination depends on the peripheral activation of autoreactive T lymphocytes. According to this analysis, activated T cells express adhesion molecules and chemokine receptors on their surface and upregulate complementary molecules within the central nervous system tissue and on the luminal surface of blood vessels, allowing them to cross the blood–brain barrier by diapedesis and then disperse into the brain parenchyma. Within the central nervous system, these T cells re-encounter specific antigen and set up an inflammatory process that resembles delayed-type hypersensitivity. As a result, axon–glial arrangements are disturbed, saltatory conduction breaks down and the symptoms of multiple sclerosis follow. This could be considered the standard 'immunocentric' position representing 1990s dogma. Recent studies, however, indicate that the pathogenesis is much more complex. Some of these data suggest a primary neurodegenerative process independent from immune-mediated inflammation. We argue that, just as genes and environment interact in the aetiology of multiple sclerosis, so too the inflammatory and degenerative components are inter-related and should not be regarded as fully independent events.

In addition to effects on the myelin sheath, axons and neurons are also affected. Functional deficits may be caused not only by the loss of myelin and consequent failure of saltatory conduction, but also through the direct effects of inflammatory mediators on axonal impulse conduction, and by the destruction of axons. The cascade of damage does not stop with disordered function. Perturbation of the complex normal interaction between axons and myelin sheaths not only influences the clinical deficit but may also compromise remyelination and repair. An important concept, and one that currently excites much debate, is that the complex anatomical and physiological environment of the central nervous system is disturbed in multiple sclerosis patients by two processes: the formation of focal demyelinated plaques and a global and diffuse injury of the entire nervous system. Thus, especially in patients with chronic progressive disease, multiple sclerosis is not simply a focal white matter condition but one that is also characterized by widespread neurodegeneration. The fact that these components of tissue injury may, in part, develop independently from each other, and proceed at different rates, has led some commentators to conclude that the neurodegenerative component has nothing to do with inflammation – and may even be the primary defect in the pathogenesis. Because this debate is not settled to everyone's satisfaction, our pandect on the pathogenesis of multiple sclerosis addresses the following questions.

- What is the neurobiological and pathological basis of the disease?
- What is responsible for the functional deficits?
- What is the relation between inflammation and neurodegeneration?
- What is the role of autoimmunity?
- What are the implications of complexity and disease heterogeneity?

CORE FEATURES IN THE NEUROPATHOLOGY OF MULTIPLE SCLEROSIS

The bulk of the central nervous system is made up of systems each containing neurons and their parallel bundles of axons, coated with the compacted myelin membranes of mature oligodendrocytes. The axons synapse with the processes of neurons placed next in line. Together, these axon–glial units, supported in a network of astrocytes and blood vessels, and diffused with microglia, make up the cellular architecture of the central nervous system through which electrical sophistication in the form of saltatory conduction of the nerve impulse is achieved. The rules and regulations of how these elements develop are only now being defined, but the principles are clear. Stem cells deploy intrinsic genetic programmes for proliferation, migration from germinal centres, and differentiation into fate-defined progeny in response to growth factors. Precursor cells must express the receptors for these growth-promoting factors and, in turn, activate signal transduction pathways that lead to gene expression and protein production. The concept of a busy phase of development followed by fixed structure is outdated. Now, not only is there clear evidence for adaptation and plasticity both at the neuronal–axonal level and in terms of cortical receptor zones – expanding and switching in the face of impoverished afferent activity – but also there seems to be a considerable capacity for replacement of cells through the differentiation of adult neural stem cell precursors. Patients expect this new neurobiology to be harnessed in their interests; and clinical scientists are not reticent in claiming that this might soon be done.

As defined more than a hundred years ago, the core features of the pathology in focal multiple sclerosis lesions consist of inflammation, primary demyelination with relative sparing of axons, and reactive astrocytosis leading to glial scar formation. The blood–brain barrier is selectively permeable in health to allow access of cells and molecules – probably in both directions. Transport across the barrier is continuously changing. For example, any part of the central nervous system that is actively working requires nutrients. These needs are met by an alteration in the calibre of blood vessels, and a change in their permeability providing increased blood flow and allowing a surge in extraction of oxygen and glucose. Under these circumstances, opening of the barrier is physiological. However, permeability of the blood–brain barrier may alter, selectively or generally, and allow the entry of cells or substances having the potential to inflict injury on one constituent or another of the central nervous system. Thus, increased permeability of the blood–brain barrier may contribute to disease processes. Lymphocytes normally traffic to the central nervous system as part of physiological immune surveillance. This increases significantly with immune activation. Migration operates through specific transport mechanisms involving sophisticated recognition signals between receptors and ligands on circulating immune cells and brain endothelia. It is specificity, rather than the fact of passage, that determines subsequent events culminating in inflammatory demyelination and axonal injury of affected pathways. Only specific transport mechanisms can account for the focal inflammation in acute lesions of multiple sclerosis. Being smaller than lymphocytes, erythrocytes (red blood cells) would also accumulate if a nonspecific mechanism (such as trauma) was operating. This does not happen.

According to the analysis of multiple sclerosis as a focal inflammatory disease of the central nervous system, infiltrating T cells activate microglia and set up a proinflammatory loop which provides an infiltrate rich in activated T cells and microglia. At all stages of the disease process in multiple sclerosis, the inflammatory reaction in the central nervous system is dominated by T lymphocytes and activated phagocytes, being mainly derived from the pool of activated microglia. All T-cell subsets are present in the lesions, although class I major histocompatibility complex-restricted CD8-positive cells dominate, and show preferential clonal expansion. The vast majority of these cells are cytotoxic T cells with a Tc1 cytokine polarization. They seem to be the major stimulus for microglial activation, although it is likely that class II major histocompatibility complex-restricted T cells of both T helper types 1 and 2 polarity also contribute to the propagation of inflammation and tissue damage. On this analysis, demyelination is mediated either directly by the cytotoxic T cell or – in a bystander reaction – through toxic products of activated microglia and macrophages. The reason for selective demyelination with relative axonal preservation may reside in antigen specificity of the immune reaction, selecting one or more components of the myelin sheath or oligodendrocyte cell body. Alternatively – and probably in parallel – specificity is also introduced by differential vulnerability for macrophage toxins of myelin and oligodendrocytes by comparison with other cellular elements of the central nervous system (see Chapter 10). Our position is that – to a greater or lesser degree – this core process of T-cell- and macrophage-mediated demyelination and tissue injury is present in all patients with multiple sclerosis and at all stages of the disease, irrespective of whether the illness is relapsing or has advanced to the progressive phase.

That said, when new white matter lesions are formed in acute or relapsing multiple sclerosis, the basic pattern of tissue injury may become modified by additional immunological mechanisms, resulting in interindividual disease heterogeneity (Figure 14.1). In some patients, antibody-mediated immune reactions against myelin, oligodendrocytes and their progenitors amplify the demyelinating reaction and/or impair the recruitment of new oligodendrocytes and remyelination. In others, hypoxia-like injury is a major force in the propagation of tissue injury. Hypoxia-like damage may, in different patients, result either from inflammation-induced vascular damage or macrophage toxins that impair mitochondrial function. Finally, in other patients, a genetic defect or polymorphism may change susceptibility of the target tissue (switching from myelin to oligodendrocytes or axons) to immune-mediated injury. These distinct mechanisms of tissue damage account for differences in the extent of demyelination, oligodendrocyte injury, remyelination and axonal damage seen across the spectrum of multiple sclerosis and its atypical or related forms – Devic's and Balo's diseases.

These features account for the formation of the focal white matter lesions that dominate the pathological picture in acute and relapsing stages of multiple sclerosis. However, in patients with primary and secondary progressive disease, the formation of new white matter plaques is rather rare and the pre-existing lesions grow slowly by radial expansion. In addition, there is a diffuse injury of the whole 'normal' white matter, reflected by a slowly progressive diffuse axonal injury in the absence of primary demyelination. The cortex, too, is severely affected in the progressive stage of the disease, showing large areas of demyelination associated with a variable amount of axonal and neuronal degeneration.

The cellular pathology of the progressive stage is more uniform. Here, the perivascular inflammatory infiltrates contain T and B lymphocytes, plasma cells and some macrophages – albeit in lower numbers compared to those in active plaques of acute and relapsing multiple sclerosis. It is mainly activated microglia that accumulate at sites of ongoing demyelination and tissue damage. It seems that diffuse and continuous damage in the central nervous system, the pathological hallmark of progressive multiple sclerosis, is mediated by microglia which, in contrast to classical neurodegenerative diseases, are permanently driven by inflammatory mediators produced in the lymphocyte infiltrates.

Thus, multiple sclerosis has two pathological components. The first is formation of focal white matter plaques. This occurs mainly during the acute and relapsing phase of the disease and is driven by a focal inflammatory response. The second is diffuse injury, which affects the central nervous system more globally. This component of the pathology is particularly pronounced in the progressive stage of multiple sclerosis but, according to the evidence from magnetic resonance imaging (MRI), it may gradually develop in parallel with the formation of white matter plaques already established during the relapsing phase of the disease. It is important to note here that the diffuse central nervous system damage in progressive multiple sclerosis is invariably associated with brain inflammation, although the intensity of the inflammatory response is less severe compared

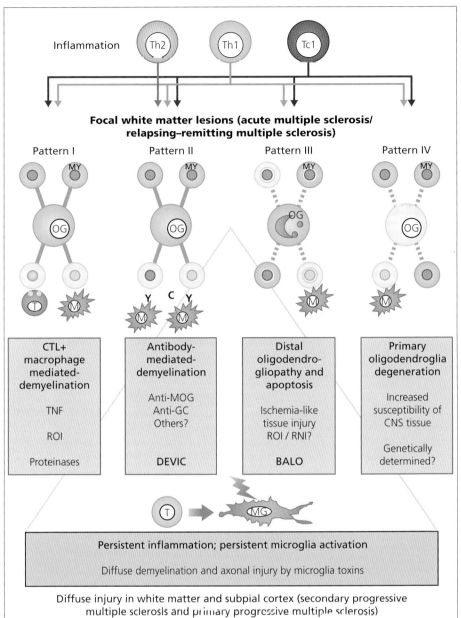

Figure 14.1 The lesions occur on the background of a T-cell-mediated inflammatory reaction. Cytotoxic CD8+ cells (Tc-1 cells) dominate the lesions, although there seems to be an additional contribution of T helper type 1 and type 2 polarized CD4+ cells. In acute and relapsing multiple sclerosis, focal white matter lesions are formed by new waves of inflammatory cells entering the central nervous system from the circulation. Depending upon the genetic background of the patients different immunological mechanisms are involved in demyelination and tissue injury, reflected by distinct immunopathological patterns of demyelination. In parallel, inflammation becomes trapped within the central nervous system compartment, resulting in a chronic persistent inflammatory activation, cytokine production and subsequent microglia activation. Activated microglia cells induce a chronic progressive diffuse injury of the grey and white matter. This process is associated with disease progression in primary and secondary progressive multiple sclerosis: OG = oligodendrocytes; ROI = reactive oxygen intermediates; RNI = reactive nitrogen intermediates; T = T cells; M = macrophages; MG = microglia; MY = myelin; TNF-α = tumour necrosis factor-α; MOG = myelin oligodendrocyte glycoprotein; GC = galactocerebroside.

to that seen in fresh white matter plaques. Whether this inflammatory response is driving the neurodegenerative process or is a secondary consequence of neurodegeneration remains part of the current debate. But should the two be separated even for the purposes of discussion? Our position is that the extent to which tissue survives inflammatory injury is modulated by its underlying condition. We argue that, initially, the inflammatory process must be relatively intense to inflict tissue damage whereas, later, injury may occur in response to a degree of inflammatory injury from which protection would be anticipated under more favourable conditions. This concept has two implications. First, in the setting of focal inflammation, such a safeguard would limit bystander damage to myelin and oligodendrocytes whilst allowing cell-contact-dependent mechanisms of injury and phagocytosis of irreversibly damaged tissue at the centre of the developing lesion to operate appropriately after microglial activation. Second, although the amount of inflammation may wane

as the disease progresses, the residual immunological activity continues to exert a significant effect on cumulative tissue injury since it is now occurring in an environment much compromised by prior injury and hence more vulnerable. Thus, tissue injury continues to accumulate across the spectrum of the disease, albeit with an altered dynamic, and in the face of changing contributions from the inflammatory and degenerative components (Figure 14.2).

THE PATHOPHYSIOLOGY OF FUNCTIONAL DEFICITS AND RECOVERY

The seemingly straightforward sequence of events associated with a relapse, namely the onset of a deficit followed by a gradual and perhaps incomplete recovery, can in reality arise from a complex interplay of different pathophysiological perturbations.

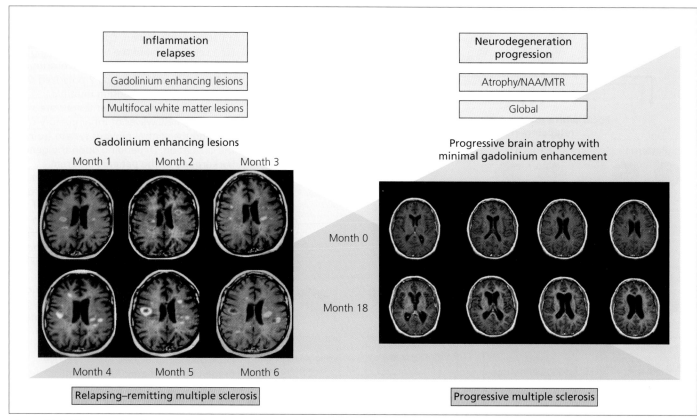

Figure 14.2 Diagram showing the dual pathogenic model of multiple sclerosis. This model proposes an early phase dominated by multifocal inflammation and relapses, and a later phase dominated by progressive neuroaxonal loss and increasing disability. NAA/MTR = N-acetyl aspartate/magnetization transfer ratio. Adapted from D.H. Miller (2004b). © 2004, with permission from the American Society for Experimental Neurotherapeutics.

Function will most likely be primarily compromised by loss of axonal activity, probably in a white matter tract, but possibly also in the grey matter. The loss of axonal function will result in a neurological deficit appropriate for the pathway affected. Initially, it is explained by inflammation and the action of inflammatory mediators on cells or axons. Although it is not yet clear whether inflammation alone is sufficient to block conduction in morphologically normal axons, there is evidence that inflammation does arrest conduction in axons damaged by previous lesions (that is, demyelinated and perhaps remyelinated axons). Attention has focused so far on a mechanism involving nitric oxide, but it seems likely that other inflammatory factors will be discovered, perhaps acting in combination. It seems certain that any conduction block caused by inflammation will often merge seamlessly into that caused by demyelination. Whereas inflammation may or may not affect conduction depending on its intensity and nature, demyelination will affect conduction if whole internodes of myelin are lost, or if more limited demyelination is focused at the paranodes.

Apart from axonal conduction block, it is likely that deficits may also result from synaptic disturbances, as a result of inflammatory and/or demyelinating lesions in the grey matter. For example, cortical lesions can be extensive and it is safe to assume that they will impair normal function, either through the action of cytokines on synaptic transmission, or by the intervening presence of inflammatory cells physically distorting delicate synaptic interactions.

Just as the loss of function has several causes, so too the restoration of function during remissions also has a number of component parts. If inflammation does not result in structural changes, such as demyelination, its resolution will allow the reappearance of successful conduction and the resolution of symptoms. Where demyelination does occur, it inherently imposes a number of electrophysiological limitations on axons; but even when multiple internodes of myelin are lost, conduction block can be reversed after as little as 2 or 3 weeks (based on observations in experimental lesions) by molecular changes in the demyelinated axolemma, especially the appearance of internodal sodium channels. However, even when the necessary molecular changes occur, it is not inevitable that conduction will be restored. It seems that, in some demyelinating lesions, virtually no axons are functional, at least at physiological temperatures. In this situation, neurological deficits are likely to persist. Genetic influences doubtless play a role, but purely structural factors also contribute, such as length of the internode preceding the demyelinated stretch. Although some demyelinated axons fail to regain function, other, particularly sensory, axons can become hyperexcitable, generating trains of spurious, ectopic impulses at the site of the lesion. Bursts of ectopic impulses can also be released at lesions by the passage of a conducted impulse. Trains of ectopic impulses may be generated continuously for hours, and probably days, at a time. In sensory axons, this can be expected to result in tingling sensations. There is convincing evidence that excitation can sometimes also traverse lesions, from one axon to its neighbours, resulting in paroxysmal phenomena appropriate for the pathway affected.

Chemical composition of the extracellular fluid, particularly the concentration of potassium ions, is likely to be important in determining whether conduction is restored to demyelinated axons, and this composition will be affected by the balance and dysfunction of glial cells, and the integrity of the blood–brain barrier. When demyelinated axons successfully regain the ability to conduct, they contribute to the restoration of function, but conduction in such axons is insecure, sometimes resulting in a range of peculiar phenomena. One example is the loss of axonal function upon body warming (Uhthoff's phenomenon), and this results in unpredictable experiences for patients as lesioned parts of the central nervous system may effectively 'turn off' with the rise in body temperature. Demyelinated axons also fail reliably to conduct trains of impulses, exhibiting either the 'drop out' of individual impulses at the lesion site, or intermittent periods of complete conduction failure. It is easy to imagine that these deficits will result in the scrambling of sensory information, and weakness in motor performance.

Remissions can perhaps most reliably occur as a result of the structural repair of demyelinated lesions by remyelination, as Joseph Babinski saw but did not perceive (Chapter 1). Remyelination restores secure conduction, and there is every reason to believe that remyelinated shadow plaques are responsible only for minimal neurological deficits – assuming that most axons survived the initial insult – or none at all. Quite apart from changes in the lesions themselves, remissions are also explained in part by adaptive and plastic changes dependent upon cortical reorganization.

Remissions may however be incomplete, especially where many axons undergo degeneration as a consequence of the inflammation. It is easy to appreciate that function will be lost when axons degenerate, but rather more difficult to understand why they degenerate. There is no shortage of potential mechanisms that have been advanced, but knowing which ones operate significantly in multiple sclerosis is more of a challenge. One possibility is that they succumb to the deleterious effects of sustained impulse activity when this is combined with exposure to nitric oxide, as will occur when axons conduct the physiological impulse traffic at sites where they are affected by inflammation. Another possibility is that demyelinated axons suffer from a loss of trophic support normally provided by cells of the oligodendrocyte lineage, perhaps accentuated by chronic low-grade inflammation. It seems likely that in many cases axons will succumb to a combination of deleterious events, any one or several of which might be survived if they occurred individually.

THE RELATION BETWEEN INFLAMMATION AND NEURODEGENERATION IN MULTIPLE SCLEROSIS

From the standpoint of neuropathology, there is little doubt that multiple sclerosis in all its manifestations is a chronic inflammatory disease of the central nervous system. This statement needs to be made since the notion that inflammation is invariably the engine driving tissue destruction has been challenged. If the pathological evidence is not considered convincing, additional evidence is provided by the beneficial effects of immunomodulatory and immunosuppressive treatments in acute and relapsing stages of the disease. Nevertheless, several arguments are offered to support the concept of a primary neurodegenerative component in the disease process. In our judgement, they are not fully convincing.

Is there evidence that neurodegeneration precedes inflammation in the formation of focal demyelinated plaques?

Serial MRI studies show that gadolinium enhancement, in most instances, precedes the appearance of T_2 lesions. However, some recent studies have emphasized subtle focal changes in magnetization transfer ratio in areas that subsequently mature into enhancing focal plaques. These studies suggest that focal alterations may occur in the affected tissue before onset of the inflammatory response. The concept of primary neurodegeneration in multiple sclerosis has gathered momentum from a recent neuropathological study reporting a fresh brainstem lesion in a 14-year-old patient with chronic relapsing multiple sclerosis, who died within a few hours of developing a massive new clinical exacerbation, having presented acutely with brainstem symptoms (M.H. Barnett and Prineas 2004). In this particular lesion, some areas showed damage of the myelin sheaths and apoptotic cell death of oligodendrocytes, occurring on the background of microglial activation but without detectable T-cell infiltration. In other, putatively more advanced, stages of the same lesion, loss of myelin was associated with classical lymphocyte- and macrophage-dominated inflammation. Based on this observation, the authors conclude that degeneration of oligodendrocytes precedes inflammation in the evolution of demyelination. The same appearances have been described as pattern III (hypoxia-like tissue injury) lesions (Lucchinetti *et al* 2000). It appears that in some patients with multiple sclerosis, the inflammatory response is initially mild but is followed by massive additional T-cell recruitment, after tissue injury is already established (F.W. Gay *et al* 1997). With the apparent exception of the single case reported by M.H. Barnett and Prineas (2004), T cells are invariably present even at the earliest stages of plaque formation. Their failure to detect a cellular infiltrate in the areas already showing oligodendrocyte damage in that instance might have several explanations. A detailed study of different subsets of inflammatory cells, including, most importantly, CD8$^+$ class I major histocompatibility complex-restricted T lymphocytes, was not performed. The patient was treated with high-dose corticosteroids. The pattern of demyelination in this case resembled hypoxia-like tissue injury. In our opinion, brainstem hypoxia as a secondary complication of fulminating multiple sclerosis, contributing to the development of this particular lesion, was not excluded. Thus, considering all available evidence, our position is that – to date – no convincing evidence has been presented showing that demyelination and tissue injury occur in the earliest stages of plaque formation in multiple sclerosis in the absence of inflammation.

Is the course of neurodegeneration in the progressive phase of multiple sclerosis independent of inflammation?

Evidence that the progress of neurodegeneration is not directly dependent on inflammation includes the observation that tissue remote from areas of macroscopic inflammation can be radiologically abnormal (Filippi *et al* 2003). Serial MRI mainly associates gadolinium enhancement with the stage of acute and relapsing–remitting multiple sclerosis but this may be trivial or even absent in patients with steady progression that is attributable to secondary or primary progressive disease in whom axonal loss and disability continue to accumulate. Diffuse changes in so-called normal-appearing white matter, together with slowly progressive atrophy of the white and grey matter, are observed early in the disease. In addition, systematic studies of anti-inflammatory or immunomodulatory treatments indicate that, despite reducing the relapse frequency, these have little effect on disease progression or the accumulation of chronic permanent neurological deficit. Postulating the existence of a neurodegenerative component in the pathogenesis of multiple sclerosis, independent of inflammation, is therefore attractive.

Pathology offers two different explanations for diffuse brain injury, which is particularly prominent in patients with progressive multiple sclerosis. Although primary demyelination with axonal preservation is a characteristic hallmark of multiple sclerosis lesions, the preservation of axons is far from complete. Cut axons are seen in acute inflammatory plaques and they degenerate further over the ensuing months, possibly through loss of the survival effects normally provided by oligodendrocytes and myelin. Axonal destruction in plaques inevitably leads to distal Wallerian degeneration, affecting brain structures, far away from the actual lesion, thus in part explaining diffuse white matter abnormalities. As a result of the high functional reserve capacity of the central nervous system permanent clinical deficit will only ensue when a critical threshold of axonal loss is reached. Thereafter, even minor additional axonal injury, either as the result of a slowly progressive axonal loss in pre-existing plaques or of age-related neurodegenerative events, will produce progressive functional deficit. Under these conditions, progressive brain damage is clearly a secondary consequence of the pathology driven by inflammation within the plaques, but deploying anti-inflammatory therapeutic strategies at this late stage is unlikely to have a beneficial effect.

However, diffuse brain injury cannot be completely explained by this mechanism. In patients with primary progressive multiple sclerosis extensive diffuse damage of the 'normal' white matter may occur in the presence of only very few and small focal plaques. Similarly, diffuse white matter injury may already be present in patients with few focal lesions, and at early stages of relapsing multiple sclerosis. Given these findings, the degeneration can be attributed to mechanisms independent from those driving focal demyelinated lesions. However, as discussed above, pathological studies show that diffuse white matter injury occurs on the background of persistent and global inflammation. Why does this inflammatory process escape detection by MRI?

MRI studies are relatively insensitive to tracer leakage resulting from breakdown of the blood–brain barrier in association with inflammation. Although, when it is present, gadolinium enhancement offers a reliable marker for acute blood–brain barrier disturbance, failure to detect such leakage by no means excludes the presence of brain inflammation. It is well known from neuropathological studies that blood–brain barrier leakage in the brain of patients with multiple sclerosis is much more widespread than the evidence from gadolinium enhancement would suggest. Furthermore, the quality of this diffuse inflammation in progressive multiple sclerosis is different from that present in active focal lesions. The persistence of a compartmentalized inflammatory response in the central nervous system, which is trapped behind a normal or repaired blood–brain barrier, appears to be a driving force for diffuse damage of the white and grey matter, seen typically but not exclusively in patients with primary and secondary progressive multiple sclerosis. Neuropathological analysis of tissue illustrating the progressive phase of multiple sclerosis following intense immunosuppression – as for instance in the course of autologous bone marrow transplantation – indicates that such therapies may have surprisingly little effect on this compartmentalized immune reaction in the central nervous system. The lack of therapeutic success in the progressive stage of multiple sclerosis may therefore reflect lack of efficacy rather than a pathogenesis that has nothing to do with inflammation.

Adrenoleukodystrophy is a metabolic disease, caused by a gene defect in a peroxisomal ABC transporter and leading to the accumulation of very long chain fatty acids in various tissues including the central nervous system. It may present as a fulminating inflammatory demyelinating disease of the central nervous system, leading to severe disability and death within a few months or years (Ito *et al* 2001; Moser 1995). However, many patients, with the same gene defect do not develop inflammatory brain disease. Instead they suffer at later time points in life from a slowly progressive neurodegenerating disease – adrenomyeloneuropathy (Powers *et al* 2000). Thus, adrenoleukodystrophy also exemplifies a progressive degenerative disease, modified (and amplified) in some patients by an inflammatory process. Whether the inflammatory component is driven by additional modifying genes or an exogenous trigger is unknown.

THE ROLE OF AUTOIMMUNITY IN MULTIPLE SCLEROSIS

The plaque in multiple sclerosis has many faces, but inflammation seems to be the common denominator of most, if not all, florid and active lesions. Inflammatory responses can be triggered by a broad range of events, which include microbial infection or endogenous cell degeneration. In the case of the multiple sclerosis plaque, another process seems to underlie inflammation: an autoimmune attack against myelin or other structures of the central nervous system parenchyma.

The lines of evidence favouring an autoimmune pathogenesis are manifold but indirect. Inflammatory responses very similar to the active inflammatory lesions of multiple sclerosis can be induced experimentally (in rodents and nonhuman primates) by immunization against components of myelin. Myelin-specific T cells cloned from affected animals mediate central nervous system inflammation when transferred to healthy hosts. Furthermore, many investigators have found evidence for autoimmune reactions in patients with multiple sclerosis. Most importantly, therapies targeting putative autoimmune T cells have been successful, especially in patients with early active multiple sclerosis.

How can the immune system attack the body's own tissues? Obviously, the immune system has evolved to protect the organism from life-threatening processes such as microbial infection and tumour growth. Protection is achieved by combining two complementary strategies, innate and adaptive immune responses. Innate responses act immediately on microbial intruders, but their discrimination between the pathogenic agents and the surrounding self tissue is blunt, and their efficiency is leaky. The adaptive immune response is much more sophisticated. It has the capability to focus exclusively on the one pathogenic structure that acutely threatens the organism, while exquisitely it spares the body's own cells. The agents of the adaptive immune response are lymphocytes – T and B cells. With specific sensors on their surface, antigen receptors, lymphocytes can identify any foreign structure, and mount an appropriate response. Each lymphocyte family (clone) has one particular receptor for one particular antigen structure. Since the immune system holds millions of different lymphocyte clones, the diversity of antigen receptors is almost infinite. Each foreign structure finds a complementary receptor preformed in the immune repertoire, and binding of the antigen to this specific receptor triggers an immune response with the aim of destroying and eliminating the antigen.

But how does the immune system spare all the cells and proteins of its own organism? Why, for example, is a piece of skin accepted, when grafted from one part of the same body to another, but rejected when transplanted to another individual? The answer is because the immune system tolerates self tissues. Tolerance to self is learned, whilst diverse immune repertoires are being generated in the thymus (T cells) and the bone marrow (B cells). During maturation, most lymphocytes with self-specific receptors are eliminated in the thymus or bone marrow as soon as they encounter their specific self-antigen.

Self-tolerance by deletion is, however, not absolutely fail-safe. Quite a number of autoreactive lymphocytes, including those specific for brain autoantigens, sneak through the self-tolerizing checkpoints and settle in the healthy peripheral immune repertoire. In most people, lymphocytes with autoimmune potential are innocuous throughout life. They remain in a state of rest, first, because they do not encounter the specific autoantigen under particularly stimulating circumstances; and, second, because they are held in check by counter-regulatory suppressor T cells. However, these lymphocytes can unfold their autoimmune potential when accidentally activated, often in connection with microbial infections. Only upon such activation, does a self-reactive lymphocyte become autoaggressive. It should be noted that a large spectrum of microbes, especially viruses and bacteria, may activate autoimmune lymphocytes under particular, permissive conditions. The autoimmune receptors of lymphocytes may erroneously bind a microbial antigen, which structurally resembles the myelin autoantigen. Alternatively, microbial 'superantigens' – proteins which activate groups of T-cell receptors in an antigen-independent fashion – may preferentially stimulate autoimmune T cells. Most important, however, are mechanisms that amplify the local microenvironment. Responses of the innate immune system against microbial components (microbial oligonucleotides and membrane products, such as endotoxin or polysaccharides) may create a milieu of local inflammation that indirectly results in the activation of resting autoimmune T cells. Under these conditions, antigen-presenting cells may become increasingly efficient, and the suppressor T cells lose their counter-regulatory power. It should be noted that all these microbial mechanisms can be triggered by nonspecific infections, in the absence of a particular 'multiple sclerosis' agent.

How do activated autoimmune lymphocytes attack the central nervous system tissue? Briefly, they use the immune apparatus which is so efficient in neutralizing and eliminating exogenous agents, or newly arising tumours. Activated T cells can act on neural cells, directly or indirectly, by recruiting ancillary macrophages or microglial cells. They secrete inflammatory cytokines, such as tumour necrosis factor-α, which impede neural or glial function, or, in the case of $CD8^+$ cytotoxic killer T cells, attach to central nervous system cells and destroy them via the release of perforin. Other inflammatory mediators, cytokines and chemokines, attract macrophages and activate these to produce an additional set of inflammatory mediators, leading to the lysis and phagocytosis of the incriminated organisms.

Viewing the immune system as it reacts against foreign and even self structures may look pretty frightening. Indeed, the immune system and its connected inflammatory responses constitute a formidable fighting machinery, primarily evolved to keep the body free of microbial and other menaces. However, inflammation has its beneficial side. Inflammatory responses, be they controlled by autoimmune reactions or antigen independent, are critically required for tissue regeneration. Skin wounds, for example, are inflamed irrespective of bacterial superinfection, and the inflammation accelerates wound healing. It is known that inflammatory and immune cells produce and deposit mediators, such as neurotrophic factors, in the central nervous system that protect neuronal cells from exogenous injury and help them to function and survive. This makes it difficult to assess the actual character of an inflammatory infiltrate within the brain parenchyma. Inflammatory infiltrates in multiple sclerosis may be detrimental, by inducing tissue damage, but simultaneously may stimulate remyelination and repair.

COMPLEXITY AND HETEROGENEITY IN MULTIPLE SCLEROSIS

Everyone working in any area of multiple sclerosis research is confronted by the profound variability of the disease. Clinically the manifestations are unpredictable, as is the course and response to treatment. The pathophysiology is complex. Major differences are seen between patients in the structural features of lesions, and in the evidence for defined immunological mechanisms responsible for tissue injury. These complexities correlate with various different factors, such as the age and gender of the patients, the stage and severity of the disease, the genetic background of the patients, and (as seems likely) exposure to environmental factors.

A question that needs to be defined carefully is whether this reflects complexity or heterogeneity. By complexity, we mean the situation in which the same root cause subsequently evolves through different pathways to produce phenocopies – defined at the pathological, clinical and radiological levels. By heterogeneity, we infer a situation in which specifically different aetiological conditions (susceptibility genes and environmental triggers) determine altogether different disease mechanisms that nonetheless converge on a single set of clinical and radiological features fitting within the spectrum of one disorder.

Pathology reveals disease complexity on several different levels. As discussed above, the pathological substrate of focal white matter lesions, which mainly occur in acute and relapsing multiple sclerosis, is fundamentally different from that of diffuse white matter injury and the cortical lesions, predominantly encountered in patients with progressive disease. In essence, focal white matter lesions seem to be formed by new waves of inflammation, which result in immune-mediated damage of myelin and oligodendrocytes, and to a lesser extent of axons. In contrast, the global brain injury in progressive multiple sclerosis appears to be driven by a compartmentalized inflammatory reaction in the whole brain and meninges, resulting in gradual expansion of pre-existing plaques, diffuse axonal injury in the 'normal' white matter and extensive cortical demyelination. It seems obvious that essentially different therapeutic strategies will be necessary to treat these different conditions. Thus it is likely that a therapy that mainly inhibits the migration of inflammatory cells through the blood–brain barrier will be effective in relapsing multiple sclerosis, but may show little effect in the progressive stage.

There are, however, also major differences between patients with multiple sclerosis in the structural aspects of lesions. In particular, the extent of oligodendrocyte injury, the loss of oligodendrocyte progenitor cells, and the degree of remyelination are profoundly different. Thus, in some patients nearly all plaques within the central nervous system are remyelinated shadow plaques. In others, remyelination is sparse or completely absent. Interestingly, the degree of remyelination bears little relationship to the stage (early or late) and severity of the disease, or disease type (relapsing versus progressive).

Furthermore, differences reflecting complexity have recently been shown in the immunopathological mechanisms of demyelination and tissue injury of active plaques. Some patients reveal a pattern consistent with T-cell- and macrophage-mediated tissue damage whereas, in others, antibodies and complement or hypoxia-like tissue injury may play an (additional) role. Finally, some lesions show exceptionally severe oligodendrocyte injury or axonal damage. What could be the reasons for these profound interindividual differences?

In most patients, the disease begins with a relapsing–remitting course. After several years, this converts into the progressive phase. We favour the interpretation that the pathology of (secondary) progressive disease is induced by a gradual and continuous accumulation of inflammatory cells in the central nervous system compartment, while plaques in relapsing multiple sclerosis are precipitated by massive focal influx of inflammatory cells. Both processes may develop in parallel, explaining detectable diffuse white matter injury even at early stages of the disease. Age, however, may profoundly accelerate the pathology of progressive multiple sclerosis. Since the damage of cortex and 'normal' white matter in secondary progressive multiple sclerosis is mainly associated with microglial activation and the expression of nitric oxide synthase in these cells, age-related augmentation of oxidative brain damage could accelerate the development of disease progression.

However, the complexity goes further. We have described in detail the four patterns of pathology seen across the spectrum of cases with multiple sclerosis. Here, we favour the interpretation that true heterogeneity in structural aspects of plaques and in the immunopathological mechanisms of demyelination does exist as a result of differences in the genetic background of the patients. Of course, in the absence of identified susceptibility genes in multiple sclerosis these arguments remain hypothetical. It is not in dispute that genetic factors are involved in regulating susceptibility to multiple sclerosis but evidence for effects on the clinical course are much less secure. Perhaps valuable lessons can be gained from experimental studies. Here, the genetic background of animals determines whether T-cell-mediated or antibody-mediated tissue injury dominates in experimental autoimmune encephalomyelitis, and how systemic effector cells are recruited, and local effector cells activated. In addition, gene polymorphisms and mutations can change the susceptibility of the target tissue for immune-mediated attack. From these studies it can be predicted that differences in the genetic background of the patients will also have major effects on structural and immunological features of the lesions.

Thus, our view is that multiple sclerosis is both complex and heterogeneous – using these terms as defined above. It will be a major challenge in the future to identify the genes that are responsible for disease heterogeneity in multiple sclerosis, and thereby stratifying the patients for more specific therapeutic interventions. For all these reasons, it is logical to improve the characterization of the immunopathology in each patient, perhaps using neuroimaging techniques, and to use this information in designing individual therapeutic strategies that are appropriate for every subgroup and stage of the disease – designer immunotherapy based on a personalized tissue read-out. We consider the implications of an improved understanding of the pathogenesis in Chapter 19.

Section Five

THE TREATMENT OF MULTIPLE SCLEROSIS

Chapter 15 Care of the person with multiple sclerosis
David Miller, John Noseworthy and Alastair Compston

Chapter 16 Treatment of the acute relapse
John Noseworthy, Christian Confavreux and Alastair Compston

Chapter 17 The treatment of symptoms in multiple sclerosis and the role of rehabilitation
John Noseworthy, David Miller and Alastair Compston

Chapter 18 Disease-modifying treatments in multiple sclerosis
John Noseworthy, David Miller and Alastair Compston

Chapter 19 The person with multiple sclerosis: a prospectus
Alastair Compston, David Miller and John Noseworthy

Care of the person with multiple sclerosis

15

David Miller, John Noseworthy and Alastair Compston

It is self-evident that many detailed and specific aspects related to the management of people with multiple sclerosis need to be addressed by neurologists and other health care professionals to provide the best available treatment for affected individuals. The protean clinical manifestations and their social implications, the variable and uncertain course of the illness, and the evidence needing to be digested from a plethora of clinical trials all combine to challenge health care professionals as they advise and implement treatment strategies. People with multiple sclerosis are also becoming better informed about the nature of their disorder and the therapeutic options, in part through information saturation arising from the internet era. There is little doubt that a good deal can be done to ameliorate disease symptoms and, together with the assumption that the course of the disease can now be modified, expectation has – in recent years – tended to replace the traditional sense of therapeutic nihilism with one of unbridled optimism. The burgeoning knowledge of underlying pathogenic mechanisms and the increasing range of potential pharmacotherapies sustain the belief that, before long, there will be progress in developing disease-modifying treatments that are more effective than those currently available. In short, the present climate for managing multiple sclerosis is well informed, complex and hopeful. The task that lies ahead is simply to realize this potential and complete the saga of disease treatment and prevention in multiple sclerosis.

While the specific aspects of symptomatic and disease-modifying treatments are dealt with in Chapters 16, 17 and 18, it is also necessary to consider care of the person with multiple sclerosis as a whole. It is readily understood that actual treatment interventions are fundamentally influenced by individual patient choice. The experience of having multiple sclerosis can have a major impact on lifestyle, employment, recreational activities, family life, independence and driving – to name but a few aspects of daily living. Self-evidently, the impact of a given cluster of symptoms will vary enormously depending on individual circumstances. Effects on immediate carers and the extended family of the person with multiple sclerosis are also profound. This chapter addresses these more 'holistic' issues. First, we provide some general guidelines for the provision of care that it is hoped will help to meet direct needs of the person with multiple sclerosis. There follows a more detailed consideration of issues relevant to the care of people with multiple sclerosis, stratified according to level of disability and stage of disease. This approach is adopted because, although there is

much individual variation in perception and coping with the illness, issues requiring attention inevitably increase in frequency as the affected person matures through the early and middle stages of multiple sclerosis, when disability starts to accumulate, through to the later stages, by which time participation becomes impossible and dependence on others is increasingly apparent. That is not to say that our categorizations preclude particular issues emerging earlier or, alternatively, continuing to dominate the reality of having multiple sclerosis, in many individuals throughout the course of their illness. Again, there are no rules or set patterns, and the style of management needs to be sensitive to the particular needs of each affected person whatever their circumstances or clinical status. We conclude with a brief discussion of a guideline for the care of people with multiple sclerosis recently published in the United Kingdom that offers a generic menu of clinical management and care.

GENERAL APPROACH TO THE CARE OF PEOPLE WITH MULTIPLE SCLEROSIS

The principles of how best to interact with the person newly diagnosed with multiple sclerosis or fearing that this may be the explanation for recent neurological symptoms are summarized in Table 15.1.

Provide a timely service during the diagnostic phase

The presentation with neurological symptoms and impairments due to multiple sclerosis, the nature of which is not immediately apparent, is a time of considerable anxiety requiring sensitive, competent and experienced professional management. People in whom multiple sclerosis is suspected should be referred and seen in a timely manner by a specialist in neurology. If the neurologist wants to perform further diagnostic investigations, these should be arranged and the patient should be re-assessed promptly. We recommend that this diagnostic process is completed over a maximum interval of 1 month, although whether this is achievable will vary across different countries and depend on local arrangements for the provision of health services.

Give adequate time for clinic appointments

Most contact between people with multiple sclerosis and their neurologist will be in a hospital outpatient clinic. It is important

Table 15.1 General approach to the care of people with multiple sclerosis

- Provide a timely service during the diagnostic phase
- Give adequate time for clinic appointments
- Provide an accessible and rapidly responsive service to deal with acute problems as they arise
- Provide a convenient service for patients
- Keep up to date with current practice and literature
- Recognize the need for and provide a multidisciplinary service
- Be vigilant for serious physical or psychiatric problems
- Keep in mind the implications of the disease for the patient's carer and family
- Remember that people with multiple sclerosis develop other medical problems

to recognize that, for several reasons, considerable time is needed to provide adequate care – at and beyond the phase of diagnosis – in this environment. Initially, many different sets of symptoms may need to be described and evaluated requiring a careful history, supported by neurological examination to clarify the specific problems and decide on their management. Later, there often needs to be a detailed discussion of treatment options including informed decisions on the use of disease-modifying treatments. Throughout, the management plan should be seen as a joint process agreed between the patient and neurologist (Leary *et al* 2005). It follows that these conversations cannot be hurried and sufficient time must be allocated to ensure that people are well informed in contributing to this process.

Provide an accessible and rapidly responsive service to deal with acute problems as they arise

People with multiple sclerosis often develop acute problems, directly (relapses) or indirectly (for example, urinary tract infections) related to the disease, that require prompt access to the appropriate medical care (Leary *et al* 2005). All clinic-based multiple sclerosis teams should ensure that a rapidly responsive system is in place.

Provide a convenient service for patients

Attendance at a specialist centre can be difficult for patients with neurological disability and, where possible, provision of local or community services may be preferable – but balance is needed. The expertise of a dedicated multiple sclerosis service is of overriding importance even if not at the most convenient location.

Keep up to date with current practice and literature

It behoves all clinicians to keep up to date in their field of special interest and expertise. Patients are entitled to expect nothing less and are themselves increasingly well informed, in part as a result of the much readier access to medical information made possible through the internet. Electronic access to relevant medical and scientific literature can also be extremely valuable to clinicians in maintaining their knowledge base as part of continuing medical education. It will be possible for many to access most of the relevant literature through electronic media, often using the institutional subscription of their employer. However diligent the neurologist, patients will frequently bring to their attention novel websites offering informed and more maverick advice to which the listener should be sympathetically receptive but nonetheless sensible in offering advice.

Recognize the need for and provide a multidisciplinary service

Because there is a complex range of dysfunctions that can affect the daily activities and participation of the person with multiple sclerosis, optimal care includes input from professionals with multiple skills appropriate for the stage reached by each affected individual. Amongst these are neurology, neuroradiology, psychiatry, ophthalmology, physiotherapy, occupational therapy, speech therapy, uroneurology, nursing care, psychology and social work. Specialist multiple sclerosis nurses have become increasingly vital and valued members of the professional team, providing a first line of contact and advice for patients whatever the nature of the problem. They are rightly seen as available, accessible, informed and sympathetic – traits that the neurologist does not always match – and provide regular follow-up as well as coordinating referral to other health care professionals.

Be vigilant for serious physical or psychiatric problems

Although uncommon, it should be remembered that multiple sclerosis is sometimes acutely life threatening in the context of respiratory compromise as a result of lower brainstem or upper cervical cord lesions, or from mass effect and coning as a result of large acutely inflamed cerebral hemisphere lesions. Prompt admission and appropriate care in an intensive treatment unit may be required in such circumstances. Depression is common and the suicide rate is higher in multiple sclerosis patients than in the general population. Neurologists should be alert to the clinical features of serious depression because these can usually be effectively treated.

Keep in mind the implications of the disease for the patient's carer and family

There has been recognition in recent years that the disease has a major impact on carers and the families of people with multiple sclerosis. The physician should always remember the implications of diagnosing multiple sclerosis for a spouse, partner, child or any other family member or carer (L.P. McKeown *et al* 2004). There is an increasing literature addressing the value of peer support groups for people with multiple sclerosis. In fact, one recent study demonstrated that participation in a peer support group does not invariably improve quality of life and emphasized the need to validate that peer support is actually beneficial (see Uccelli *et al* 2004). There is evidence that care givers may become depressed in response to the reality of multiple sclerosis, and may need treatment, even when the affected person improves as a result of interventions targeted at the disease. In turn, these effects on carers have reciprocal implications for disability and health status in the patients (Pozzilli *et al* 2004).

People with multiple sclerosis develop other medical problems

As for any individual, the person with multiple sclerosis may develop other important but unrelated disorders. If the manifestations are neurological, they may inadvertently be attributed to multiple sclerosis. All experienced neurologists will have encountered cases of multiple sclerosis coexisting with another central nervous system disorder. Thus, the astute clinician is not only alert to the possibility of an alternative diagnosis when neurological manifestations occur that are atypical for demyelination but also to comorbidity arising from double diagnoses.

THE EARLY STAGES OF MULTIPLE SCLEROSIS: MINIMAL DISABILITY

The neurologist seeing for the first time a young person, on the threshold of adult life with all the bright enthusiasms of youth, describing a cluster of neurological symptoms that immediately suggest the likelihood of multiple sclerosis may experience an inner sinking of the spirits – seeing ahead the possibilities of a lifestyle compromised by neurological impairments. However, equally, that neurologist knows that – for a proportion of these incident cases – many years or decades of near normal neurological life may lie ahead. Any sense of pessimism in anticipation of events should therefore be suppressed, and management oriented around cautious optimism without jettisoning reality. These issues make the management of multiple sclerosis a specialist trade.

Diagnosis and prognosis counselling

Until the relatively recent past, clinicians did not hurry to pursue a definite diagnosis at presentation with early symptoms suggestive of multiple sclerosis because the potential benefit for patients was considered limited. Further diagnostic investigations were sometimes deferred in the hope of limiting psychological distress to the patients. A diagnosis of multiple sclerosis *per se* was believed by some clinicians to reduce quality of life, even in the absence of physical disability. This is now rightly considered to be an antiquated style, although discretion may yet be needed, even in the age of transparency.

When to communicate the diagnosis

There is more to be gained than lost by early and informed disclosure of the diagnosis once the probability or certainty of multiple sclerosis is established in the mind of the attending neurologist. Timing is important. Some clinicians prefer to wait until there is sufficient clinical or laboratory evidence to rule out misdiagnosis on the grounds that telling people that they have multiple sclerosis when they do not is bound to cause distress (and indeed has landed several doctors, including a few neurologists, in the law courts). We have already referred to the issue of suicide in response to learning the diagnosis (see Chapter 6). However, over-caution and avoidance of discussion have proved much more damaging. There are many more patients who harbour bitterness over the delay in learning the true nature of their illness than those who wish they had not been told so soon, or at all. Patients are better informed than ever with increasing access to medical information. Many patients now quickly learn that remitting neurological symptoms may suggest multiple sclerosis and most will quickly connect the once intentionally imprecise description of 'inflammation of the myelin sheath' with multiple sclerosis. Patients increasingly appreciate and anticipate frank discussions about their diagnosis and prognosis. The previous paternalistic approach of reassuring patients that 'perhaps they have experienced a virus-induced disorder that may not return' is – categorically – no longer acceptable. On the contrary, there is a clear move to discuss the possibility of multiple sclerosis even at an early stage when the diagnosis remains provisional – such as following a first and anatomically isolated clinical episode.

The need to acknowledge the possibility of multiple sclerosis early in the clinical course stems at least in part from the fact that laboratory results, in particular magnetic resonance imaging (MRI) findings, can now be used to make a definitive diagnosis before there is sufficient clinical evidence for dissemination in space and time. An international panel developed the most recently revised criteria for the diagnosis of multiple sclerosis (W.I. McDonald *et al* 2001). These use imaging features as a surrogate for the second clinical episode, sufficient to fulfil the criteria of dissemination in space and time, in patients with clinically isolated syndromes. However, if the neurologist plans to perform MRI in such a patient, it would be evasive not to admit that one purpose of the investigation – in addition to excluding alternative diagnoses – is to confirm that the symptoms are probably the result of multiple sclerosis. As we discuss in Chapter 7, these criteria are set to be revised, in particular with respect to the status of imaging abnormalities.

Given the move towards discussing and making an earlier diagnosis, it is reassuring that there is considerable evidence from the more contemporary literature to suggest that, in the main, patients prefer to know the name of their illness at an early stage, and they perceive benefits from early disclosure. Indeed, to those whose experience of medicine is confined to the last few decades, anything other than full and frank discussion as soon as the clinical situation has been formulated must seem alien. Heesen *et al* (2003) assessed the current status of diagnostic and therapeutic information relating to multiple sclerosis from the perspective of both patients and neurologists. They concluded that, in contrast to beliefs held by some physicians, patients prefer having information about a possible diagnosis, even if this is not yet confirmed. This is in line with an earlier study (Strasser-Fuchs *et al* 1997), in which patients reported a high rate of anxiety, depressed mood, uncertainty and concern in advance of learning the diagnosis of multiple sclerosis. Receiving the diagnosis caused a further slight increase of these negative sentiments, offset by more positive feelings such as a sense of determination to fight the disease and relief that ambiguity was now resolved. Only three out of 50 (7%) of these patients would have preferred discussion to have been deferred, although opinions regarding the optimal timing of full diagnostic information were variable.

Mushlin *et al* (1994) also attempted to determine the perceived value of diagnostic information to patients with suspected multiple sclerosis. Most considered themselves to be advantaged through having received diagnostic information, but subgroups of patients differed in their responses. Whereas individuals in whom no definitive diagnosis emerged tended to be more anxious, those to whom a definitive diagnosis could be communicated expressed favourable feelings about the diagnostic work-up even though they often faced the prospect of coping with a chronic disease. Removal from diagnostic uncertainty was accompanied by a sense of improved well-being. Taken together, these observations suggest that, because they bring forward the point of diagnosis, the most recently revised criteria for multiple sclerosis (W.I. McDonald *et al* 2001) bring the added dividend of reducing uncertainty for the individual. These applications are endorsed by the evidence, discussed in Chapter 7, that the new criteria, and their planned revisions, based on imaging, show high specificity and accuracy for the diagnosis of multiple sclerosis using traditional clinical criteria. The multiple benefits of applying the new criteria at the time of first clinical presentation are summarized by Miller *et al* (2005).

Communicating the diagnosis

Making the diagnosis of multiple sclerosis often requires more than one consultation. If at the first assessment the clinical picture suggests the diagnosis but the evidence is inconclusive, it is likely that further investigations will be ordered and the patient reviewed later. It is important that investigations are expedited and the patient seen promptly after the completion of these investigations because the period of waiting for diagnostic clarification is bound to promote anxiety. We recommend that patients should not have to wait more than 1 month for investigations such as MRI and should be followed up within 2 weeks of investigations being completed.

It is appropriate to communicate the diagnosis face-to-face at a clinic appointment, with ample time set aside to provide further information and deal with the many questions that will arise both from the patient and any companion. It is highly inadvisable to transmit the diagnosis, deliberately or inadvertently, through communication with a third party or by telephone, letter or email. Given the increase in public awareness of medicine in general and multiple sclerosis in particular, formal delivery of the diagnosis rarely comes as a surprise to patients with tell-tale symptoms. The fact that the possibility of multiple sclerosis will probably already have been mentioned at an earlier visit, either by the patient or the neurologist, makes the process of confirmation more straightforward. However, there will be occasions when the diagnosis does come as a thunderbolt. For these reasons, it is sensible to deliver the news carefully in a few sentences which move from confirmation that the symptoms are significant; that they indicate an illness affecting the central nervous system; that they suggest a tendency for patches of inflammation (with suitable metaphors to explain this term) in the brain or spinal cord; that a high proportion of people in whom this pattern develops turn out to have the illness known as multiple sclerosis; and that this appears to be the diagnosis for this patient. Clearly style matters, and although many neurologists will have developed their own preferred method for initiating and conducting these interviews, without much formal education, training in communication skills is now rightly seen as an important aspect of good doctoring. Fallowfield and Jenkins (2004) offer an analysis and provide generic advice but without specific reference to disclosing potentially distressing neurological diagnoses. Dealing with the specific issue of communicating the diagnosis of multiple sclerosis, J. Johnson (2003) perceived

a much greater degree of distress, feelings of abandonment and isolation than might be appreciated from the neurological perspective and urged for communication always to be linked to the provision of sources of information, advice and ongoing practical support as individuals adjust to the naming of the illness.

At the first consultation where discussion of the diagnosis takes place, it is usually possible to convey the picture of an illness which, despite public perceptions and hard-hitting advertising campaigns (see Figure 1.11) designed to raise awareness and generate charitable donations, is not necessarily severe. It is convenient to describe the three phases of relapse with recovery, relapse with persistent symptoms (which may not be noticeable to others) and progression, and it is appropriate to err on the side of optimism at this stage.

There is a basic human need to know why a thing has happened and most patients enquire about causation. Explaining the interplay between genetic susceptibility and environmental triggers conveniently introduces the topic of risk to others in the family, especially children, and, in turn, this allows the subject of pregnancy and multiple sclerosis to be introduced. Mentioning current ideas on the aetiology also allows the point to be made that multiple sclerosis is not infectious. Some remarks on self-help usually follow and it should be emphasized that changes in domestic activities or professional aspirations are inappropriate, merely in anticipation of problems that may never arise. Clearly, for a proportion of patients, subsequent events may dictate revision of this optimism.

Finally, it is worth summarizing the available treatments, distinguishing those designed to deal with acute episodes from remedies for persistent symptoms and the use of drugs that may modify the longer-term course of the illness. Many patients cope well with existing symptoms but are concerned that they might be losing an opportunity, or compromising their future, through ignorance. Important issues surrounding the early use of disease-modifying treatments need to be discussed (see section below). We point out that, in our view, patients who, for whatever reason, remain untreated are not missing out on anything which is known to be safe, effective and readily available. This aspect of the conversation can be concluded by mentioning the enormous research effort and available resources aimed at solving the problem, and expected to pay dividends for the individual patient before too long. Further questions may arise but the consultation with the neurologist at which the diagnosis is divulged can usually be completed in 30–45 minutes. This is time well spent and a worthwhile investment early in the management of the individual patient.

Once the diagnosis has been declared, it is very important to maintain close support from the multiple sclerosis care team during the immediate post-diagnostic phase, when patients will often experience a good deal of anxiety and identify a number of questions for which they would like answers. On subsequent occasions, it may be necessary to go over aspects of the illness, its natural history and treatments that were not fully appreciated or dealt with at the initial consultation. Multiple sclerosis nurses can provide very valuable and readily accessible support during this period (J. Johnson 2003; B. Porter and Keenan 2003). A seamless provision of care during the diagnostic phase sets the framework for a healthy continuing relationship between the person with multiple sclerosis and their health care team.

Sources of information and support

Newly diagnosed patients can receive support and information from a variety of sources. Many National Multiple Sclerosis Societies offer an extensive welfare service, including (in some countries) a telephone helpline, along with a compendium of relevant literature, presented in a manner that is easily understood. Multiple sclerosis clinic services must recognize that newly diagnosed patients require much ongoing support, and with repeated and easy access when needed. Some of us have found it useful to establish workshops for people who are newly diagnosed. These provide an informal setting in which patients can meet others in a similar situation and ask questions of professional carers who attend the meetings.

The internet provides much excellent information for patients on authoritative websites such as the United States National Multiple Sclerosis Society (*www.nmss.org*), the Multiple Sclerosis Society of Great Britain and Northern Ireland (*www.mssociety.org.uk*), and Multiple Sclerosis International Federation (*www.msif.org*) to name but three. However, a 'Google' search for multiple sclerosis will also reveal many other links to information, not all of it reliable. Newly diagnosed patients should be warned to treat with scepticism the many unwarranted and unverified claims that can be read on the internet and in the lay press, and which so often reflect interests and approaches that are nonscientific, emotive and sometimes driven by the desire for unscrupulous commercial gain.

Pregnancy counselling

Because multiple sclerosis is most prevalent amongst females in the reproductive age group, it is often necessary to discuss in detail the relevant facts concerning pregnancy and multiple sclerosis (see also Chapter 4). The discussion should include the effects of pregnancy on relapse rate (decreased during pregnancy and increased during the postpartum phase), the lack of any recognized effect of pregnancy on the long-term course of multiple sclerosis, and the slightly increased but nonetheless low risk for multiple sclerosis in offspring. It is worth emphasizing that, if the disease does develop in a child, this is not likely to happen for a few decades, by which time there is the possibility of fully effective treatments having been developed.

In patients with a recent diagnosis and minimal symptomatology, it is nevertheless appropriate to hint at the possibility that significant disabilities may develop during the next 10–20 years, the period during which parental care is most needed. One should be careful not to discourage women who are keen to have a family, and in this circumstance it probably makes sense for them have children at a time when any effects of the disease are still minimal. When the disease is mild, obstetric complications are no different from those for pregnancy in healthy women. If there is moderate or severe disability, obstetric management may be affected with the need to shorten labour because of fatigue or to perform an elective Caesarean section if there is severe lower limb spasticity and adductor spasm. Multiple sclerosis is not a contraindication to performing epidural anaesthesia or conventional breast-feeding.

Family life and child care

Given the uncertain prognosis that it implies, the diagnosis of multiple sclerosis can be expected to cause anxiety for the patient's spouse or partner. It is therefore appropriate to involve both patient and partner in discussion of the diagnosis and prognosis. Sometimes the person diagnosed may wish to discuss the illness and ask questions of the neurologist whilst accompanied by a parent, sibling, or older child. These conversations are likely to include assessment of recurrence risks for members of the family.

Even in the early stages, there may be symptomatic problems for patients, such as fatigue or intermittent periods of disability because of relapses, which disrupt normal family life and the carrying out of parental tasks. Additional support from other extended family members or close friends may be helpful. Additional child-care support may be possible through social or community services during periods of transient incapacity attributable to relapses.

Principles of relapse management

For the 80% of affected individuals who present with relapsing–remitting disease, a major issue during the early years is the management of individual episodes. It is prudent to anticipate these events and discuss the appropriate strategy prospectively with patients. This discussion should take place at the time of, or soon after, diagnosis. Some explanation of the pathophysiological mechanisms thought to underlie both relapse and remission is helpful. It should be emphasized that the natural history is usually, but not invariably, for full recovery at least from the initial series of relapses. Patients should be informed that most episodes recover spontaneously and without the need for specific therapy. They should be made aware that a short course of high-dose corticosteroids (usually intravenous methylprednisolone for 3–5 days) will shorten the duration of dysfunction, and is appropriately used when the symptoms are sufficiently troublesome or disabling. However, it should also be emphasized that there is no treatment known to alter the final outcome of an individual episode.

An important point is that the system for providing intravenous steroids should be available at short notice so that treatment is given promptly when indicated. Since the effect of treatment is to abbreviate the episode, much of the benefit will be lost if there is a long delay before corticosteroid administration. In one of our services, we have established a relapse clinic that operates each week. Patients who have presented with a relapse during the previous week are treated with intravenous methylprednisolone, 1 g daily for three consecutive days. Some clinics will provide a home service for intravenous treatment, when there is an appropriately qualified domiciliary professional who can supervise and administer the infusion. It should be remembered that, although generally well tolerated, occasional serious adverse effects from intravenous methylprednisolone may be seen (see Chapter 16). Caution should also be taken to avoid too frequent repeated administration, given the risk of cumulative adverse effects related to total duration or amount of exposure – notably osteoporosis. A short course of oral prednisolone (typically starting at 60 mg/day and reducing to zero over 3 weeks) or higher dose oral methylprednisolone (for 3–5 days) may be a more practical therapy if access to intravenous methylprednisolone is difficult, although the evidence for efficacy is less convincing.

Continuity of care

Multiple sclerosis is an unpredictable disease at the individual level, and the issues, symptoms and disabilities that arise are complex and varied. From the earliest stages, patients deserve access to a service that provides care in a timely and consistent manner. Having a key contact person (sometimes called the key worker) in the multidisciplinary care team may be helpful. In many services, nurses provide the primary link between the patient and available care services. With regard to neurological follow-up, it is always preferable if people see the same neurologist, who comes to understand both the person and their disease. Although this may be difficult to achieve in practice, it is a familiar experience to hear patients complain that they have had to see a different doctor at each of their follow-up visits to the neurology clinic. The multidisciplinary, hospital or medical centre-based, multiple sclerosis clinic – as occurs in some large centres, particularly in North America – has proved to be an efficient and popular system for providing care; it also provides an excellent template for conducting epidemiologically sound research (Confavreux and Paty 1995).

Discussion of disease-modifying therapies

A major change in practice over recent years has been the introduction of licensed disease-modifying treatments – interferon-β and glatiramer acetate – often started early in the course of relapsing–remitting multiple sclerosis. The (as yet unproven) rationale for this strategy is to prevent or delay the pathological process that later culminates in disability. Although due in part to the sincere belief of many neurologists in the results of randomized trials, the recent enthusiasm for early treatment has been managed and sustained by commercial marketing. Crucially, it is not known whether the existing disease-modifying treatments are effective in the long-term and it is also the case that early treatment of large numbers of patients will undoubtedly include a sizeable group in whom a favourable long-term course will occur as part of the natural history.

Given that the issues surrounding use and timing of disease-modifying treatments are complex, a good deal of time must be set aside to ensure that these are adequately discussed with patients, especially since increasingly well-informed patients are requesting advice about the choice and timing of medication using one or more of the currently available agents. These discussions should begin from the time of diagnosis. People should be given information on the results from randomized trials on relapse rate and the development of disability, the uncertainties regarding long-term treatment (beyond 2 years), the effects on MRI, the methods of treatment administration, and the adverse effects. Deciding who to treat and when will depend partly on local prescribing guidelines and drug availability, each of which varies from country to country.

Assuming that a patient is eligible according to local guidelines, we support a shared decision-making model in which the neurologist reviews the treatment options (including no treatment) coupled with a clear review of what is known, and unknown, about the short- and long-term expectations of medications and the disease itself. It is naturally the case that patients bring immutable aspects of their personality and expectations for health to this decision. Some express considerable uncertainty and will look to their neurologist for guidance as to whether a disease-modifying treatment should be started and, if so, which one. Others will want to do 'all they can' to improve long-term health prospects and will opt to start treatment with one of the disease-modifying agents at an early stage. Some in this category will want the neurologist to advise on which agent should be chosen. Others will have their own views based on factors such as the frequency and route of administration, or perceived differences in efficacy and adverse effects profile. Other patients will weigh up the merits and demerits and opt not to begin disease-modifying treatment early in the disease course. Here, the neurologist needs to keep in touch so that the period in which an individual remains a candidate for treatment – both from the perspective of health care policy and the underlying pathogenesis – does not pass that person by.

In those with early relapsing–remitting disease, there is often no right or wrong answer in deciding when and who to treat. It is easier to be dogmatic in those with nonrelapsing, progressive forms of multiple sclerosis. Some of us have found evidence-based treatment guidelines – such as those developed in 2001 by the Association of British Neurologists (*www.theabn.org*) – useful in identifying relapsing patients for whom treatment is most appropriate. As further evidence emerges, especially that related to the long-term effects of existing treatments, and as new therapies are identified, it seems inevitable that current practices will continue to evolve and new treatment guidelines will be developed.

Diet and alternative treatments

At one time, hypotheses for the pathogenesis of multiple sclerosis found their expression in clinical trials of altered diet (Bates *et al* 1978; Dworkin *et al* 1984; Millar *et al* 1973; Paty *et al* 1978), hyperbaric oxygen (B.H. Fischer *et al* 1983; C.M. Wiles *et al* 1986) and other so-called alternative therapies. Kleijnen and Knipschild (1995) analysed 14 trials of hyperbaric oxygen and concluded that in seven of the eight they judged to be competent, oxygen at 1.75–2.0 atmospheres pressure in daily sessions for several weeks or longer had no effect in patients with chronic progressive or chronic stable multiple sclerosis. Nevertheless, some centres remain active and attendees perceive themselves to benefit from regular hyperbaric immersions. Dworkin *et al* (1984) summarized the results of three double-blind trials of linoleic acid involving 87 patients (treated for 2.5 years) and 85 controls and concluded that treated patients with minimal or no disability at entry had a smaller increase in disability, and reduced severity and duration of relapse (considering all levels of disability and length of illness at entry). We are not so sanguine about these putative remedies and do not review them in detail. Although worthy in their time, they represent steps towards an improved understanding of the basis for treatment in multiple sclerosis and have not secured a lasting place in therapy. We are relaxed about endorsing the adoption of these diets as self-help measures for individual patients – despite the absence of evidence for a therapeutic effect – because they are not inconvenient and, in the main, they are healthy. However, we are surprised that linoleic acid is being promoted as an evidence-based disease-modifying treatment in a recent national guideline published in the United Kingdom (see below).

THE MIDDLE STAGES OF DISEASE: MODERATE DISABILITY

For most people with multiple sclerosis, the illness brings a prolonged period during which moderate and persistent disabilities impact significantly on the extent of activity and participation in daily life. The disease-related symptoms are multiple and complex: ongoing expert care and advice are required from many health care professionals, including neurologists with experience of the disease, in their management.

Employment issues

As physical and/or cognitive impairments emerge, it may be difficult for people to maintain employment. The loss of earning potential can have serious financial implications for patients and their families, leading to loss of self-esteem and social difficulties. Understandably, many patients want to maintain employment at all costs. Neurologists may be able to assist by writing to the employer, explaining the medical problems and proposing adaptations to the workplace designed to accommodate that patient's disability, thus making it possible to continue the job. In other instances, a compromise may be appropriate, whereby there is an agreement with the employer to work part time. In some individuals, flexible working hours concentrated during the morning, if that is the time when an affected individual is least fatigued, may be helpful. For some jobs, such as those involving extensive use of computers or the internet, it may be possible for the patient to work from home, at least for a part of the week. Other individuals accept the impracticalities and strain of struggling to continue at work, and they seek early retirement on medical grounds. In such circumstances, mechanisms for continued financial support should be explored. These might involve state or government benefits, work-related pension schemes, or personal health insurance policies held by the patient. The neurologist will often be called on to write medical reports explaining the consequences of the illness and supporting the need for the patient to stop working.

Driving

Specific locomotor impairments such as ataxia, weakness, spasticity, visual loss, and – if marked – sensory loss can all cause difficulty with, or even preclude, driving. Spasticity of the lower limbs may significantly impede the rapid and precise foot controls needed for braking and acceleration, with the potential for disastrous consequences. In some cases it may be possible to continue driving by using hand controls, because upper limb function is often preserved in the context of severe lower limb spasticity.

Whilst driving regulations, and procedures for their enforcement, will vary between countries, the neurologist is frequently asked to give an opinion on the safety of the person with multiple sclerosis continuing to drive. This is likely to become an issue of major importance to patients for whom driving is a necessary part of their employment. However, despite these practical considerations, driving is a privilege, not a constitutional right, and it may reasonably be denied on health grounds even against the patient's expressed wishes. It may be difficult to judge from the neurological examination alone how safe someone will be when driving a vehicle. In forming an opinion and giving advice, there should be a consideration of the interests of the patient, on the one hand, balanced against the risks to the affected person and third parties. An independent driving assessment by an appropriate authority can be performed in some countries. This usually involves a simulated assessment of driving performance and may be very helpful in deciding how best to proceed. In the United Kingdom, the final responsibility for determining fitness to drive rests not with neurologists but with a governmental agency – the Driving Vehicle Licensing Authority.

Sporting and recreational activities

In general, people with multiple sclerosis should be encouraged to continue with normal daily activities, both work and domestic, as far as the limitations imposed by their illness allow. For most people in the early stage, leisure activities will not be affected. However, restrictions will inevitably occur with advancing disability. Issues of safety may arise even for those activities that remain accessible and a source of pleasure – such as swimming in deep water. But that said, maintaining a regular fitness programme through sports and recreational activities, or through regular exercises advised by a neurophysiotherapist, and within the constraints imposed by the disease, makes good sense.

Symptomatic therapies

The stage of moderate disability is one where symptomatic treatments are frequently used and bring most advantage to affected individuals (see Chapter 17). Both pharmacological and physical therapies will be used, sometimes together. The most tractable symptoms to manage are bladder and sexual dysfunction, neuropathic or mechanical pain syndromes, spasticity and fatigue. Often, less can be achieved to help ataxia, weakness, visual loss and cognitive impairments. Regular follow-up with a neurologist and other health care professionals will help to ensure continuity of care and adjustment of symptomatic treatments optimized to changing needs.

Physical therapies and rehabilitation

Many still regard physical therapies and rehabilitation as routine responsibilities of the physician caring for a patient. However, the specialty of neurological rehabilitation has defined a more precise role in managing both physical manifestations of multiple sclerosis and their impact on the affected individual as a person with domestic, social and professional aspirations. It is important that affected individuals benefit from all that is available for the chronic young sick. Multidisciplinary care provided within the framework of a comprehensive rehabilitation service can help to achieve this aim. The limitations provided directly by available disease-modifying or symptomatic pharmacological treatments are often apparent, and the need to help more severely affected individuals to deal with disability and handicap is all too evident in everyday neurological practice. There are prospects for neurological rehabilitation itself to progress from the present emphasis on coping or optimizing function within the constraints of disease pathology to one in which nervous systems are re-educated, realizing the full potential for new therapies, through plasticity and restoration of structure and function – an era of biological rehabilitation.

The process of rehabilitation may not be relevant for many patients for many years, if at all. To some extent the need to consider secondary consequences of physical impairment, including contractures, urinary tract infection, osteoporosis (arising from immobility and repeated use of corticosteroids, as well as individual risk factors), and decubitus ulceration, represents failure of the more pharmacologically orientated approaches. These complications are best prevented by awareness and anticipation because, in the severely affected individual, they usually develop quickly yet take months to resolve. Maximizing activity and participation by attention to social, vocational, marital, sexual and psychological aspects of the illness are more important to most patients than drug treatment. In situations where the natural history has led to loss of mobility despite attempts at disease modification, it may be appropriate to advise the use of mechanical walking aids (foot-raising splints, walking sticks or crutches), despite the negative perceptions of dependency that some people associate with such appendages. A wheelchair may be self-propelled, electric or lightweight and can be adapted for access to and from a vehicle. In the home, it may be necessary to provide rails, transfer boards, ramps, hoists and lifts (elevators), to widen doorways and build facilities for drive-in bathing at ground floor level. Maintaining communication and outside interests for the person who is no longer able to come and go as they please can lessen frustration and boredom and home-based information technology, requiring reasonable vision but minimal hand control, can provide a welcome link with other people.

People with multiple sclerosis are aware that physiotherapy is one way to maximize the usefulness of their remaining functions and, although it is rarely necessary to provide continuous or prolonged access, the contribution of physiotherapy may be more important than rest or medication in restoring function after a temporary reduction in mobility arising from coincidental infection or recent relapse. Patients with chronic progressive multiple sclerosis, on the verge of losing their independence from impaired mobility, may be kept ambulant for a while through the use of physiotherapy, sometimes undertaken intensively during a programmed in-patient admission to a rehabilitation service lasting for several weeks. Hand function may also be amenable to physical therapy and there will be opportunities for improving quality of life through attention to speech, swallowing and the provision of low visual aids, amongst other devices.

The specialist in rehabilitation is especially alert to the possibility of depression in patients with multiple sclerosis. At diagnosis, the problems are those of facing an uncertain future. Later, the possibility of impending disability has to be confronted. Eventually, for some patients, there may be complete loss of independence. Counselling and sympathy seem to make as much sense as pharmacology but drug treatment is sometimes needed. However, antidepressants may have consequences, beneficial and adverse, for physical aspects of the disease, including bladder control. The combination of fatigue and low mood inevitably leads to poor self-esteem and tends to promote social isolation and inertia. This may aggravate physical aspects of the disease. Tackling and ameliorating both fatigue and depression are important steps towards successful outcome during a period of rehabilitation.

Managing cognitive dysfunction

Cognitive dysfunction is common and is frequently a significant problem for the person with multiple sclerosis. It can be readily overlooked in patients during a cursory neurological assessment that focuses primarily on physical aspects of the illness. It may manifest as poor coping with aspects of daily living, work and family or other responsibilities without much evidence of physical impairments to account for the apparent difficulties. Some patients report problems with memory or the organization of daily activities. Others may complain of fatigue – a common and disabling symptom in its own right. In some patients, it may be difficult to distinguish between cognitive impairment and depression. Indeed, the two commonly coexist. If cognitive impairment is suspected, formal neuropsychological assessment will help to confirm whether it is present and also to quantify its nature and severity. Where cognitive impairment is demonstrated, patients may be helped by advice on daily planning, limiting the number of tasks tackled, establishing routines and keeping written lists of what needs to be accomplished.

The role of formal cognitive therapy is unproven and no drug treatments are shown to enhance cognition, although the recent demonstration that a central-acting choline esterase inhibitor can modify the functional MRI response to a cognitive paradigm (Parry *et al* 2003) suggests the potential for pharmacotherapy favourably to influence cognitive performance. A course of antidepressant medication may be warranted if it is thought possible that cognitive performance is impaired by coexistent depression.

Disease-modifying therapy

Patients with moderate disability and frequent relapses may be eligible for existing disease-modifying treatments. Most neurologists would agree that affected individuals who are accumulating disability as a result of severe relapses with incomplete recovery are especially eligible for one of the licensed treatments. Some neurologists would opt for interferon-β rather than glatiramer acetate in patients with frequent new or gadolinium enhancing MRI lesions, given the evidence for a greater anti-inflammatory effect on MRI. In patients with clinically very active disease, more powerful forms of immunosuppression are also likely to be considered (see Chapter 18).

When moderate disability is the result of slow progression – either from onset (primary progressive) or after a relapsing–remitting phase (secondary progression) – the licensed disease-modifying treatments, and indeed more powerful immunosuppression, appear to be ineffective. Some neurologists will not use any disease-modifying treatments in this situation. Others – despite the lack of evidence (and perhaps in part as a result of pressure from patients to 'do something') – will use a variety of unproven treatments, usually exploiting an immunosuppressive or immunomodulatory mechanism. This group of patients represents an especially large area of need for therapeutic progress. Participation in well-designed, well-controlled clinical trials of promising new therapies may enable patients to feel that something is being done to address their particular needs. Participation in clinical trials also often brings more frequent contact with the clinical services, which can be helpful in its own right. The use of agents with a putative neuroprotective mechanism is currently seen as a rational and promising strategy for tackling the progressive phase of multiple sclerosis.

Involvement with lay support groups

As the disease evolves, many patients and their carers find much benefit from involvement with lay support groups. Most countries have a National Multiple Sclerosis Society that offers a range of services to patients including information and welfare support. Some Societies are also a major source of research funds. In many countries, there will be local chapters or branches with which people can become involved, both to receive and provide support. Some people with multiple sclerosis, or their carers, derive considerable satisfaction from contributing to the organization, funding and development of their lay society. The Multiple Sclerosis International Federation provides a global framework for communication between the national societies and people with the disease (*www.msif.org*) and it is now also committed to research funding (see Chapter 18).

THE LATER STAGES OF DISEASE: SEVERE DISABILITY

For a significant number of individuals, the fears and frustrations of having multiple sclerosis do, in due course, come to pass. Whilst the balance of responsibilities may shift, and new members of the team providing comprehensive care now become more relevant, the treating neurologist still has a role to play in helping the individual patient face the daily practicalities of living with significant disabilities but nevertheless retaining participation and personal dignity consistent with advanced multiple sclerosis.

The caring physician

Dedicated neurologists have always tried to give practical help to the large number of patients with multiple sclerosis for whom they have responsibility, throughout the illness. They use the range of medications described in Chapters 16–18, adjusting thresholds to reflect the aim of improving quality of life, even in situations where there is no prospect of a cure. Neurologists advise on adaptation of the local environment for affected individuals depending on the level of disability and the impact this has on activities of daily living. Whenever possible, they negotiate the necessary financial resources available from social security or insurance schemes for domestic alterations, loss of mobility and earning potential and financial repercussions on carers, which are often the consequence of having multiple sclerosis. Physicians ensure access to physical, occupational and speech therapists, and to psychologists and social workers. They encourage patients to contact lay groups (the Multiple Sclerosis Societies) and other self-help organizations. These activities are traditionally the pastoral aspects of good doctoring and they merge imperceptibly with prescribing and the provision of accurate information on all aspects of the disease to those with a vested interest.

Symptomatic treatments and multidisciplinary care

Inevitably, as there are still only limited strategies available for disease modification, many of the patients with multiple sclerosis that a neurologist meets eventually develop severe physical and cognitive disabilities so that the role of pharmacology diminishes and the need for pragmatic measures increases with time. As these more severe manifestations develop, the requirements for provision of care become more complex, necessitating increased input from multidisciplinary and specialized teams. Now, in place of drug treatment, interventions for spasticity may include intrathecal baclofen or intrathecal phenol only available through a highly experienced service. Severe dysphagia may require percutaneous endoscopic gastrostomy, and this again should be performed in specialized centres with the close involvement of speech therapists. An active preventive programme to reduce the chances of bed sores should always be instituted in disabled patients. When decubitus ulceration does occur, management may require the use of a specialized bed and mattress, regular dressing and sometimes more aggressive surgical intervention.

Family and carer issues

The burden on family and carers is greatest when the person with multiple sclerosis has become severely disabled. The stresses and strains that are imposed on interpersonal relationships are large and it is not surprising that marriages and partnerships may break up. On many occasions, however, the commitment of the spouse, partner and other carers is sustained and profound. Professional carers need to be sensitive to these pressures and, correspondingly, to nurture loyalty and dedication to the task, providing additional support as and where possible. Periods of respite residential care enable others to take much needed holidays and thereby sustain a stable existence in the community for the affected person.

The effect is considerable on children who have a parent with multiple sclerosis. The impact of the disease on family life may restrict opportunities for a normally balanced and active childhood. Children may receive less emotional and physical support than normal and have inner anxieties about what will happen to the affected parent – or, indeed, to themselves. A study of 87 offspring from 52 families where one parent had multiple sclerosis showed that daughters cope better than sons, irrespective of which parent is affected (Steck *et al* 2001). Healthy mothers and daughters coped better with the increasing disability of a male proband.

Community support and residential care

It is often impractical for severely disabled patients to attend hospital clinics, and provision of care within the community is then more appropriate. Good liaison between hospital and community services is essential to ensure that a responsive and efficient system of care is still provided for the patient. Whereas care may have predominantly been provided in a hospital setting during the early diagnostic phase or the stage of moderate disability, the general practitioner may become more involved at this stage. Residential care may be necessary when it is no longer feasible for carers or other support services to maintain and manage the patient's needs in their own home. However, the decision on where care is best provided will depend on the nature of the available support services, and the views of all concerned in this significant decision. In many situations, the increasing difficulties and escalating demands present no obstacle to continued domestic care of a loved one for the remainder of their life.

Palliative care

When multiple sclerosis reaches a point of very severe disability, it may be appropriate to involve a palliative care service in the management. Such services are especially equipped to meet the needs of people who have severe and irreversible diseases and skilfully to provide symptomatic care that is optimized to relieve distress and maintain quality of life as far as is possible. In the United Kingdom, the Multiple Sclerosis Society has recently funded a post of palliative care clinician, and in due course the outcome of this initiative will be audited to learn more of the value of such a service for people with severe multiple sclerosis.

GUIDELINES FOR THE MANAGEMENT AND INVESTIGATION OF MULTIPLE SCLEROSIS

A number of guidelines or reviews have been developed to inform and guide those working in the health care or research fields. Such individuals are involved in providing care for people with multiple sclerosis or in trying to discover more about its cause and cure, respectively. Two recent issues on this theme have come from the National Institutes of Health in the United States and the National Institute for Health and Clinical Excellence in England and Wales (NICE). The former document is more focused on a review of scientific and medical knowledge, and points the way towards important areas for future research (see *www.ninds.nih.gov/health_and_medical/pubs/multiple_sclerosis.htm*). The latter is focused on care for people with multiple sclerosis (see *www.nice.org.uk* clinical guideline in multiple sclerosis, 2003).

Some studies have investigated the costs of the disease (Amato *et al* 2002; Anon 1998; D.T. Grima *et al* 2000; N. Murphy *et al* 1996) and some guidelines have considered the cost effectiveness of interventions, most notably the expensive disease-modifying treatments (see *www.nice.org.uk* technology appraisal of beta interferon and glatiramer acetate, 2002). This approach has been motivated by a desire to allocate resources most efficiently in a health care environment where there are limitations on what can be afforded. Such efforts have inevitably evoked a great deal of controversy and have also resulted in widely differing estimates of cost effectiveness. To be reliable, these estimates require not only an accurate estimation of the progression of the disease but also a detailed understanding of health economics; this topic is beyond the scope of the present discussion, which deals with the care of individual patients. Before doing so, there are, however, some general points worth making about the cost of the disease:

- In countries where multiple sclerosis is common, it is a major cost for the health care system.
- The disease results in both direct and indirect costs. Examples of the former are pharmacological and other treatments, and hospitalization; the latter includes loss of employment earnings for the patients and their carer.
- The costs of the disease increase sharply with increasing disability.

Patient-centred guidelines may be treatment-specific or symptom-specific or they may apply to the disease as a whole. They can be useful to health care professionals and patients in providing information and setting a uniform standard for delivery of appropriate health care. Because of its contemporary and comprehensive nature, the NICE guideline is discussed in some more detail, although we recognize that there will be other suitable guidelines that usefully address the management of either specific issues or the disease as a whole.

NICE guidelines for the management of the person with multiple sclerosis

The NICE guidelines for the management of multiple sclerosis in primary and secondary care in the United Kingdom were issued in November 2003. Their recommendations hold for not more than 6 years. The immediate context is the needs of adults at all ages available through the National Health Service. Evidence that formed the basis for the expressed views is categorized. The need for further research in prospective epidemiological studies of morbidity is identified. The prognostic role of investigations at baseline; improved measurement of impairment and participation; health economics studies of morbidity; hospital versus domestic management of relapses using oral or intravenous corticosteroids and rehabilitation interventions; and comparison of interferon-β, glatiramer acetate, linoleic acid and azathioprine in terms of benefit, costs, adverse effects and duration of exposure are all evaluated.

The NICE guidelines will probably be seen as pastoral and sensitive to the needs and perspective of the person with multiple sclerosis. They undoubtedly contain much valuable information, albeit presented in documents that somewhat overwhelm in their length and breadth. As is eloquently elaborated in the guidelines, it is essential to provide a seamless, timely and multiskilled service in order to meet all of the complex needs of people with multiple sclerosis, from the early diagnostic phase through to the late stage of severe disability. The guidelines are substantially focused on rehabilitation and the comprehensive approach to management, and a considerable increase in National Health Service resources and personnel will be required to meet many of the service delivery goals that have been laid down.

The guidelines are somewhat rigid on the algorithm for managing the sensitive stage of diagnosis. On the one hand, they emphasize the need to discuss the possibility of multiple sclerosis at the earliest opportunity, whilst at the same time downplaying the use of laboratory investigations – in particular MRI – to establish (in conjunction with the clinical picture) an early diagnosis. Taken at face value, this could lead to many people having to live with the possibility that they might have multiple sclerosis without benefiting from the investigations needed to ensure that the diagnosis is made in a timely manner. The guidelines are eccentric in the faith held in certain medications (linoleic acid and alternative therapies) and in the limited attention that is paid to licensed and unlicensed disease-modifying therapies (although in defence of the latter approach, it is accepted that the benefits of existing disease-modifying treatments are modest). They are pragmatic but not sufficiently versed in clinical neurology with respect to some symptomatic treatments. Through their advocacy of treatments for most situations, the guidelines remove flexibility and may lead to overprescribing in contexts where patient and clinician may prefer a waiting game or interventions other than pharmacology. Notwithstanding such caveats and inconsistencies – perhaps inevitable in a document that is very large (the full version runs to 213 pages) and written by committee with much consultation – there is a great deal of information and advice that should make the guidelines a valuable resource for neurologists and other health care professionals who provide care to people with multiple sclerosis.

CONCLUSION

The care of people with multiple sclerosis is a process that starts at the time of diagnosis and continues throughout the duration of the illness, although the needs and timing of care will vary much from one individual to the next. Optimal delivery of care requires the continuous availability of a skilled multidisciplinary service that is accessible and responsive, providing the range of medical and paramedical skills that may be called upon by people with multiple sclerosis. Neurologists play a major role – especially in diagnosis, and the use of disease-modifying and symptomatic treatment – but should always work closely with a broadly based group of fellow professionals who make up the expert team. Good care of people with multiple sclerosis mandates a ready awareness of the impact of the disease on carers; it should also allow the patient to participate – according to their wishes and abilities – in management decisions.

16

Treatment of the acute relapse

John Noseworthy, Christian Confavreux and Alastair Compston

THE FEATURES OF ACTIVE MULTIPLE SCLEROSIS

Multiple sclerosis is the classical relapsing–remitting and potentially disabling neurological disease of young adults. Few medical disorders demonstrate such variability in their clinical expression; few are so frightening for the affected individual; and few are so prone to misunderstanding of the clinical course. Affected individuals are subject to change in clinical features with time of day and environment – relating to circadian changes in body temperature and stress – menstrual cycle, and intercurrent infections. These expressions of reduced safety factor for conduction of the nerve impulse (see Chapter 13) are of interest to the clinical scientist and alarm the patient but do not necessarily signify disease activity. Conversely, clinical relapses are the expression of complex changes in the disease process. Synonyms for relapse include exacerbations, attacks, bouts, flare-ups and episodes. There is widespread awareness that function may suddenly worsen in people with multiple sclerosis, and that full recovery is by no means certain in this setting. Indeed, this tendency for unpredictable clinical worsening contributes to the cruel reputation of multiple sclerosis. Until a patient has experienced meaningful recovery from a relapse, few will share their physician's confidence that significant recovery can be expected, even from a disabling episode. Early in the disease course (the clinically isolated syndrome and initial episodes of relapsing–remitting multiple sclerosis), episodes take an enormous toll on the affected person's emotional state – and many affected individuals are naturally fearful of irreversible disability. Each relapse reminds the patient that multiple sclerosis is unpredictable and generally recurs despite a positive attitude to the disease, good diet, regular exercise, self-help measures and whatever treatment plan the neurologist suggests. The relapse brings stark reminders that the person with multiple sclerosis cannot fully control the future. Most patients eventually learn this lesson although, for some, the knowledge is slow in coming and achieved at great emotional cost. Since it often brings into focus the hopes and fears of the newly diagnosed individual, management of the acute episode has a special significance for disease management. Happily, not only is the natural history usually for useful recovery but much can be done to ameliorate the symptoms and signs through drug treatment.

New episodes do not only occur during the relapsing–remitting phase of multiple sclerosis. At one extreme, the development of a *bona fide* new event in a patient previously experiencing a clinically isolated syndrome clarifies the diagnosis of multiple sclerosis. At least for a while, many patients who have entered the secondary progressive stage continue to experience relapses ('secondary progressive multiple sclerosis with ongoing relapses') and a small percentage of people with primary progressive multiple sclerosis experience episodes at some point during the course of their disease. The term 'progressive relapsing multiple sclerosis' is sometimes applied to such cases (for more detailed discussion, see Chapter 4). Recent population-based studies suggest that these occasional relapses have no impact on outcome in primary progressive patients, providing little justification for expanding the classification (Kremenchutzky *et al* 1999; Weinshenker *et al* 2000). Apart from the tendency for better spontaneous recovery from the individual episode and, hence, less accumulation of fixed disability after clinically isolated syndromes and the early phase of relapsing–remitting multiple sclerosis, the nature of relapse is indistinguishable across the subtypes of people with multiple sclerosis. Our preferred position is therefore to stick with the simple descriptors: clinically isolated syndromes, relapsing–remitting multiple sclerosis, and primary and secondary multiple sclerosis. Here, we retain those terms but recognize that others may prefer also to identify relapsing progressive and transitional forms of multiple sclerosis.

Definition of relapse

Relapses have been variously defined, both by lay societies and investigators designing clinical trials (Table 16.1). Inherent in all these definitions is the concept that symptoms and signs suggesting a relapse represent the clinical manifestations of new or ongoing disease activity within the central nervous system. Episodes are especially likely to be recognized, and separated from the everyday experience of multiple sclerosis for that individual, when function is disturbed in clinically eloquent pathways such as the optic nerve, medial longitudinal fasciculus, medial lemniscus or corticospinal tract. Symptoms typically evolve over hours or days although some are by their nature more explosive and fully recognized within moments of onset. That said, the features typically mature subacutely over days or weeks. Clinical findings often include several manifestations of white matter disease during the course of a single acute attack. This clinical evolution may indicate the growth of a single symptomatic lesion as inflammation spreads through juxtaposed tracts and structures

Table 16.1 **Definition of relapse used in a sample of phase I and II randomized trials and prospective studies conducted since 1993**

Clinical trial	Duration of symptoms	Objective evidence of relapse	Comments
INFβ-1b (The IFNB Multiple Sclerosis Study Group 1993)	≥24 hours	Not required	
Glatiramer acetate (Johnson et al 1995)	≥48 hours	Increase of ≥0.5 EDSS points or 1 point on ≥2 functional systems (FS) scores, or ≥2 points on one functional system score	Bowel/bladder or cognitive functional system scores alone could not be used to indicate objective worsening
INFβ-1a (Jacobs et al 1996)	≥48 hours	Increase of ≥0.5 EDSS points or ≥ 1.0 worsening on pyramidal, cerebellar, brainstem or visual functional system score	
PRISMS (PRISMS Study Group 1998)	≥24 hours	Not required	Relapse severity measured by Scripps neurological rating scale
CHAMPS (Jacobs et al 2000)	≥48 hours	Increase of ≥1.5 EDSS points	
ETOMS (Comi et al 2001a)	≥24 hours	Worsening in EDSS or FS (excluding bladder/bowel and cognitive change)	
SPECTRIMS (SPECTRIMS Study Group 2001)	≥24 hours	Not required	Relapse severity measured by Scripps neurological rating scale
MIMS (Hartung et al 2002)	≥48 hours	FS worsening ≥2.0 or ≥1.0 of either pyramidal, cerebellar, brainstem or visual scores	Relapse data contributed to 2/5 components of the primary outcome measure
EVIDENCE (Panitch et al 2002)	≥24 hours	Abnormality on examination corresponding to the symptoms of the relapse	
SPECTRIMS (SPECTRIMS Study Group 2001)	≥48 hours	'Objective relapse': Increase of ≥1.0 EDSS point, 1 point on two functional systems scores, or ≥2 points on one functional system score	'Total relapses' in trial analysis included non-objective relapses
Berger (Berger et al 2003)	≥48 hours	Not required	

(such as the sensory symptoms of a dorsal spinal cord lesion). Alternatively, clinical worsening may reflect an increase in the number of discrete lesions as, for example, occurs with multifocal involvement of the spinal cord and optic nerve during a single episode. Definitions vary with respect to the minimum period of involvement constituting a new relapse but most require at least 24 hours of worsening at a time when the patient is otherwise free from intercurrent illness (typically an infection producing fever). For us, this is an interval over which spontaneous fluctuations in symptoms that do not necessarily constitute a biologically significant new episode may occur, making for some difficulty in the definition and enumeration of new episodes. We prefer a longer period of change – say, two or three days at a minimum – but acknowledge the pragmatic need for tighter limits in clinical trials.

The mechanisms and natural history of relapse

We have already made the point that, early in the disease course, it may be difficult for patients to differentiate minor fluctua-tions in baseline from those portending a clinical relapse. Many patients recognize that they feel best early in the day, becoming more symptomatic by the middle afternoon and early evening in association with the normal diurnal increase in body tempera-ture. Others volunteer that they are at their best late in the evening when core temperature is at its nadir. Personal stress, nonrestorative sleep, menses and intercurrent infections (espe-cially those accompanied by fever) characteristically worsen existing symptoms or rehearse previously experienced features. Patients should be instructed on these important points. Febrile illnesses should be identified, diagnosed and treated appropriately. In so doing, transient clinical worsening associated with fever ('pseudorelapse') will often remit within days. However, viral illnesses may also trigger genuine relapses of multiple sclerosis, and prolonged clinical worsening despite resolution of the infection suggests disease activity that may require treatment. Unsatisfactory sleep patterns may improve with appropriate guidance. Personal stress should be identified and addressed in so far as this is possible. Patients with coexisting psychiatric disease or psychological problems may declare symptoms that blur with the genuine manifestations of multiple sclerosis (conversion disorder, malingering and somatization) thus presenting a considerable challenge of interpretation for the neurologist. In all these situations, errors in diagnosis may lead to inappropriate therapy or prolonged morbidity. It is usually not necessary to suggest hormonal therapy for menses-related clinical worsening. Failure to recognize the importance of minor clinical fluctuations and pseudorelapses may result in the excessive use of corticosteroids with predictable and nontrivial adverse effects. Additionally, the mistaken belief that multiple sclerosis is still clinically active despite the recent use of conventional therapies may lead to the use of potentially hazardous and, in the context, inappropriate immunosuppressive therapies (see Chapter 18).

We describe the relationship between environmental events and disease activity in Chapters 2 and 4, and here merely summarize the several situations that may trigger a relapse. Taken together, the evidence for an association is strongest for the postpartum period, modest for a role of infection, minor or nonexistent for trauma, surgery and stress, and absent for vaccinations (Confavreux *et al* 1998a; Confavreux *et al* 2001; Goodin *et al* 1999; Mohr *et al* 2000).

Relapse severity depends on a number of mechanistic factors. The likelihood that a relapse will be detected clinically increases with the location, number and size of lesions. Presumably, this reflects accumulated damage from previous attacks taking up the slack on the complex interplay of compensatory mechanisms, including resolution of inflammation and recovery from conduction block, neuronal and cortical plasticity, and remyelination (see Chapter 13). The involvement of clinically eloquent pathways typically evokes symptoms and signs in most patients. Conversely, individual subcortical, callosal and periventricular lesions usually go unnoticed. In clinical trials, relapse severity is typically measured by the degree of change from baseline disability [using, for example, the Kurtzke Expanded Disability Status Scale (EDSS) and Scripps Neurological Rating Scale]. As noted in published trials (Milligan *et al* 1987; O'Connor *et al* 2004), more than half of episodes improve within 4 weeks, and up to two-thirds within 6–8 weeks. With the lessening of symptoms and return towards better health, patients regain confidence that recovery is possible. This positive experience helps the affected person to cope emotionally with future attacks so that, with time, many patients with relapsing–remitting multiple sclerosis adjust to what can be expected from both mild and more severe episodes. We discuss in Chapter 13, the evidence mainly derived from studies using functional magnetic resonance imaging (MRI), that the cortical receptor zone subserving specific functions may increase following an episode of isolated demyelination or established multiple sclerosis, presumably to maximize capture of the impoverished signals reaching that part of the cortex. Plasticity also operates at the neuronal level, restoring various forms of conduction through axons where the normal myelinated arrangements and saltatory conduction are perturbed. There is limited literature on how much failure to recover from each relapse contributes to long-term disability. Lublin *et al* (2003) reported that 42% of patients enrolled in placebo groups from clinical trials still have ≥ 0.5 EDSS change 2 months after a clinical relapse. Evaluation of a subset of patients seen an average of 113 days post-relapse, showed a similar proportion with unresolved findings, suggesting that relapses contribute to medium-term dysfunction if not prolonged and sometimes unremitting disability.

The role of magnetic resonance imaging in treatment decisions

The advent of MRI has demonstrated unequivocally that multiple sclerosis is frequently active without this being expressed as new clinical manifestations. Serial MRI studies estimate that as few as 10% of new biological episodes are expressed clinically. Even quite large lesions may be silent. The key issue is whether these asymptomatic, short-lived changes in MRI signal (new, recurrent or enlarged lesions, and areas with gadolinium enhancement) carry the same immediate or future prognostic significance as an episode that does produce symptoms. MRI also endorses the clinical formulation that, despite restricted symptoms and signs, many relapses are multifocal. Others reactivate previously affected anatomical sites and so tend to rehearse old and familiar manifestations of the disease.

In many countries, well-resourced practices are increasingly performing MRI with gadolinium to clarify the likelihood that a patient is undergoing a clinical relapse when this cannot be determined with certainty from the clinical presentation. This may be particularly informative in the context of apparent failure of response to disease-modifying therapies; where a change in treatment plan is under discussion; or in clarifying that nonorganic features are influencing current clinical status. Our impression (but this is not supported by published data) is that MRI studies do not invariably demonstrate worsening (new, larger, recurrent or enhancing lesions) during obvious clinical relapses. Increasingly, patients in remission expect – and neurologists are requesting – MRI to clarify whether the disease is active as the basis for providing guidance on prognosis, and to assist with therapeutic decisions. In the absence of a secure evidence base, at present we discourage this practice despite the previously noted superior sensitivity of MRI compared with clinical evaluation alone. Intuitively, it seems likely that MRI inactivity is preferable to activity, but this has not been demonstrated prospectively. In short, there is considerable dissociation between clinical and MRI activity. Some patients remain clinically stable despite extensive lesion loads on MRI, whereas others progress and accumulate disability without any apparent change in the number, size or location of lesions. The situation more commonly arises of practitioners debating how best to advise a patient on the meaning of MRI worsening in the setting of apparent clinical stability. In the absence of studies that guide the practitioner in making an informed therapeutic decision, the approach has to be empirical. In the current climate of partially effective therapies, and with only limited evidence for subclinical MRI activity, one approach is reassurance and continuation of the current active or expectant treatment plan. Some patients find it comforting that neurologists are familiar with this dichotomy and prefer to treat the patient, not the MRI scan. Others remain anxious that their illness is not in full remission and request a change in treatment, or early re-evaluation of the MRI study to update their disease activity status. Increasingly, practitioners also are persuaded by evidence for MRI activity alone to start treatment or modify the dose and frequency of existing medication. Few neurologists would advocate the use of corticosteroids in an asymptomatic patient. Some are occasionally sympathetic to the request for repeated courses in patients with fixed disabilities, seeking to maintain a precarious hold on valuable functions, who feel that a top-up may provide cover for an impending downward lurch in function or for a forthcoming social call on their vulnerable abilities. These are individual matters of judgment that the experienced neurologist will be prepared to take and defend even in the absence of evidence backing up their decisions.

THE TREATMENT OF RELAPSES

Whenever possible, we instruct patients to rest until their symptoms improve, reasoning that this is an important part of the treatment plan for any acute inflammatory illness. If practical and not counterproductive (for example in situations where the affected person does not have a satisfactory insurance plan such that stopping work reduces income or threatens job security), we suggest avoiding strenuous physical or mental effort and stressful circumstances. Until recently there has been little evidence to support this practical advice – best articulated as good medical practice in the 19th century before pharmacology made any discernable impact on the management of disease (J. Hilton 1876). However, K.J. Smith *et al* (2001a) have now shown that sustained impulse activity in the setting of acute inflammation may lead to irreversible axonal injury through a mechanism that involves nitric oxide, energy failure and exposure to excitotoxic mechanisms (see Chapter 13). Perhaps this experimental evidence accounts for the anecdotal experience, familiar to many neurologists, of the patient who fails to recover from a particularly memorable period of extended physical activity either during an apparent period of remission or, more especially, in the midst of a relapse.

When no treatment was available, patients with exacerbations due to multiple sclerosis were encouraged that the natural history of the acute attack is spontaneous and complete recovery. Time remains the most predictable factor in recovery from the acute episode (Figure 16.1) but there is also a useful role for drug treatments in abbreviating the attack (Figure 16.2).

Corticotropin

Corticotropin given as pulsed intramuscular treatment was first shown to shorten the duration of acute events but with no effect on the degree of recovery and with no influence on the long-term course of the disease. For many years, corticotropin remained the preferred treatment for exacerbations of multiple sclerosis. Undoubtedly many patients were spared periods of morbidity but, in the face of significant adverse effects (including weight gain, acneiform skin eruptions, mild hypertension and glycosuria), physicians and their patients often took the view that treatment was not appropriate for each and every exacerbation. Once the evidence for an effect, albeit modest, of corticotropin was in place, no new trials were conducted, even though some neurologists preferred to use orally active corticosteroids. Whilst this approach avoided the need for daily medical supervision, usually involving hospital admission, the adverse effects of treating an acute attack were not reduced since these relate more to the duration of corticosteroid therapy than dose or mode of administration.

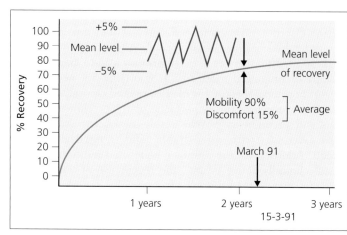

Figure 16.1 **Natural history of recovery from relapse depicted by one introspective academic patient with multiple sclerosis.**

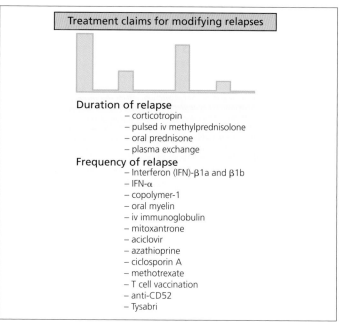

Figure 16.2 **Drug treatments which alter the duration and frequency of relapse in multiple sclerosis.**

H. Miller *et al* (1961b) treated 22 patients within 14 days of an acute exacerbation due to multiple sclerosis with a decremental regimen of corticotropin (initially 60 units by intramuscular injection twice daily) over 3 weeks, and reported an improvement compared to 18 matched, placebo-treated controls. The United States Cooperative Study (Rose *et al* 1970) included 103 patients treated within 8 weeks of new symptoms with a tapering dose of corticotropin (initially 40 units by intramuscular injection twice daily), and confirmed the increased rate of improvement compared with 94 placebo-treated controls. However, improvement was not sustained beyond the first 2 weeks after completion of treatment (Figure 16.3). Corticotropin is now rarely, if ever, used in the care of patients with multiple sclerosis, partly because of the unpredictable rise in serum cortisol and the inconvenience of intramuscular administration. Instead, glucocorticoids administered orally or by the

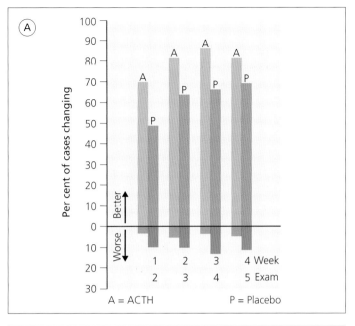

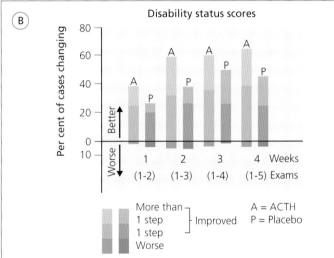

Figure 16.3 Corticosteroids in multiple sclerosis. (A) Estimate of overall condition at each weekly examination versus pretreatment examination according to treatment. A = ACTH (corticotropin) versus P = placebo for those judged better or worse in the interval. Figures are cumulative frequency percentages. (B) Disability status score changes by week of study in 103 cases on ACTH versus 94 on placebo. Adapted from Rose *et al* (1970). © 1970, reproduced with permission from Lippincott Williams & Wilkins (lww.com).

intravenous route achieve levels up to ten-fold higher than those resulting from stimulated release of endogenous hormones by corticotropin (R. Gold *et al* 2001).

Methylprednisolone

The next advance in the treatment of acute episodes due to multiple sclerosis was the introduction of much shorter courses of high-dose intravenous methylprednisolone. Subsequently, this route of administration has not been shown to be more effective than the use of intramuscular corticotropin or oral corticosteroids (prednisone and high-dose methylprednisolone), but recognition that the shorter course is not inferior has had a

major impact on clinical practice. Acute exacerbations can now effectively be treated in 3 days, without the need for hospital admission, and with a conspicuously lower adverse effects profile. The cost of methylprednisolone is offset by the rapidity with which clinical improvement may occur. Patients, physicians and hospital administrators have all felt the impact of this change in approach to treatment and, as a result, a much higher proportion of acute attacks is now managed pharmacologically than was formerly the case. There is also an emerging biological rationale for abbreviating the duration of exposure to inflammatory mediators during an acute episode (see Chapters 10 and 13).

Following the initial report of clinical improvement in five of seven patients with acute demyelination given methylprednisolone (Dowling *et al* 1980), several small studies were carried out using either historical controls (Goas *et al* 1983) or none at all (Buckley *et al* 1982; P.K. Newman *et al* 1982; T. Smith *et al* 1986). On the basis of these promising results from open studies, a number of controlled trials were completed and reported in the mid-1980s. Using a complicated design, Durelli *et al* (1986) showed an improvement in rate but not degree of recovery in 13 treated patients compared with ten controls. However, as the latter were then given methylprednisolone openly, and both groups subsequently received oral prednisolone for 120 days, no controlled assessment of results was possible after the initial 15 day treatment. Milligan *et al* (1987) carried out a randomized controlled trial of high-dose pulsed methylprednisolone in 50 patients with multiple sclerosis. Twenty-two were in acute relapse and 20 had chronic progressive disease. All patients were assessed at entry using the EDSS and were then randomized within each group to receive 0.5 g methylprednisolone by slow intravenous infusion daily for 5 days. Nineteen of the 26 methylprednisolone-treated patients showed decreased disability score at 4 weeks. Seven were unchanged and, of these, six had secondary progressive multiple sclerosis (Figure 16.4). In the control group, seven of the 24 cases showed a decrease in disability and ten were unchanged. One patient did not complete the study. Eight of 13 patients treated during an acute relapse had improved 1 week after starting methylprednisolone and in four of eight cases the decrease in disability ranged from 2.5 to 4.5 points on the EDSS. This initial rapid response was followed by a further clinical improvement in seven of eight cases so that, at 4 weeks, ten of 13 patients showed a useful decrease in disability score. Two control patients improved, four were unchanged and two had deteriorated by the end of the trial as a result of new relapses. Six of 13 actively treated patients with progressive multiple sclerosis showed a reduction in disability score which was more than 1 point on the EDSS at 4 weeks. All six showed improved pyramidal function largely as a result of a decrease in spasticity. Two of six patients also showed improved sensory function after treatment with methylprednisolone but scores in other functional systems were unchanged. Controls were unaffected by placebo treatment and two relapsed during the trial. Subsequently, Oliveri *et al* (1998) demonstrated that 2.0 g of methylprednisolone given by daily intravenous injection may be more effective than the conventional daily dose of 0.5–1.0 g dose in reducing MRI evidence of disease activity. Because spontaneous recovery is the rule, the beneficial effect of corticosteroids used to treat acute symptomatic relapses is only measurable over weeks, using magnetic resonance surrogates of

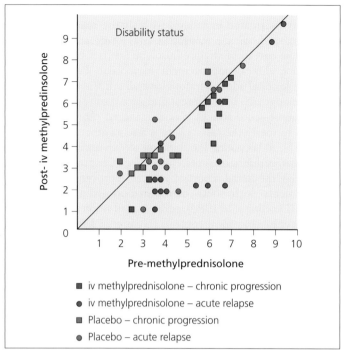

Figure 16.4 Clinical disability scores before and 4 weeks after treatment with methylprednisolone in 50 patients with multiple sclerosis. Patients in whom disability scores did not change appear on, or adjacent to, the diagonal line. A decreased disability score after treatment is indicated by a point below, and an increased disability score by a point above this line. Analysis of covariance revealed a significant effect in favour of methylprednisolone treatment ($t = -3.85$; $p < 0.001$). Adapted from Milligan *et al* (1987) with permission from the BMJ Publishing Group.

disease activity (Barkhof *et al* 1994), except perhaps when given together with another disease-modifying agent (Gasperini *et al* 1998).

Bethoux *et al* (2001) studied the timing of recovery following methylprednisolone treatment in patients with acute relapses of multiple sclerosis. Improvements in subjective health status (quality of life) occurred later than effects on impairment and disability, suggesting a complementary role for subsequent rehabilitative measures in this setting. The Multiple Sclerosis Functional Composite (MSFC) was shown by T. Patzold *et al* (2002) to be more sensitive than the EDSS in measuring improvement at days 5 and 20 following corticosteroid treatment for an acute relapse (26/27 improved on the MSFC and 7/27 on the EDSS at day 20).

The effects of methylprednisolone do not last for more than a few months. The original placebo-controlled trial of methylprednisolone (Milligan *et al* 1987) sought to determine whether there are long-term implications for patients with multiple sclerosis from a single course of treatment. Forty-eight of 50 participants were reviewed between 13 and 35 months (mean 23± months) later under open conditions (and in some cases after additional treatment with methylprednisolone). Four had improved, eight were unchanged and 12 of 48 had worsened in the methylprednisolone-treated group at late follow-up compared with six, eight and ten patients, respectively, in the placebo group, providing (as expected) no evidence for a long-term effect on disability.

These studies show that pulsed therapy with high-dose methylprednisolone is effective in patients with multiple sclerosis in relapse. The initial rapid improvement, usually noticeable by the third dose, is followed by further recovery at 4 weeks in the majority of responsive patients. Treatment shortens the duration of hospital admission and can be given on an outpatient or community basis. Nos *et al* (2004) showed that, amongst the 44% of 54 improving episodes, severity of the attack at the time of treatment predicted change in the EDSS at 1 month. But this may be an artefact of the greater numerical potential for change in those with higher scores rather than a real difference in the biological response to corticosteroids. The role of methylprednisolone in patients with progressive multiple sclerosis is less certain but there appears to be a specific effect on the reduction of spasticity (Milligan *et al* 1987).

In 2003, an international shortage of methylprednisolone triggered a change in practice patterns. At that time, the American Society of Health System Pharmacists provided helpful background information on comparative pharmacology and equivalent dosing, suggesting alternative corticosteroid regimens for common indications on their website: *http://www.ashp.org/shortage/methyl-prednisolone.cfm*. In response to this shortage, one approach was to substitute dexamethasone 35 mg, also given by intravenous infusion daily, for 1 g methylprednisolone taking into consideration the comparative pharmacology and five- to six-fold superior anti-inflammatory properties of dexamethasone. The crisis has passed but the options for alternative regimens remain valid.

The use of corticosteroids should not be at the expense of general management for the acute episode. There is increasing evidence that a multidisciplinary approach to the rehabilitation of patients with multiple sclerosis may optimize functional recovery and symptom control (see Chapter 17). Craig and colleagues (2003) randomized patients seen during an acute relapse to receive either standard in-patient care or multidisciplinary team assessment by a specialist multiple sclerosis care team. This included staff to provide health promotion advice, treatment by physical and occupational therapists and orthoptists, advice to family members to assist in stretching exercises, speech therapy, and bladder management – in addition to standard treatment with 3 days of intravenous methylprednisolone (1 g daily). Mean length of stay in the care facility was not significantly prolonged by this additional intervention (3.5 days for the treated patients versus 4.8 days for the control group). The addition of multidisciplinary team assessment and treatment improved functional recovery at 3 months, as measured by the Guy's Neurological Disability Scale and the Amended Motor Club Assessment, compared to standard nursing care alone. Gains were seen primarily in motor function. The patients and evaluators were not blinded to the treatment assignment. After correcting for the confounding effects of interval since treatment with corticosteroids, and re-admission, C. Liu *et al* (2003) showed more improvement on the EDSS, Barthel Index and Functional Impairment Measure, and on subjective indices of improvement in patients involved in an active programme of rehabilitation during the acute episode.

Taken together, we adopt rather a low threshold for the use of corticosteroids, given as short intravenous courses of methylprednisolone 1 g daily for 3 days, but with some increase in duration and reduction in dose depending on the build of the patient and the clinical circumstances, in managing the acute episode. Rarely, we follow an intravenous course with oral prednisone and use oral corticosteroids alone when attendance at hospital is impractical. We aim to combine rest, corticosteroid administration and rehabilitation strategies to assist in the care of patients during the acute and recovery periods of each relapse and thus have a significant effect on neurological function. But, as we point out on theoretical grounds in Chapters 10 and 19, there is an argument for *ultra* early use of corticosteroids on the basis that axons may well slip beyond the period of reversible injury after no more than 12–24 hours' exposure to inflammatory mediators. It seems to us that, if corticosteroids are to be prescribed, the sooner they are administered the better. The next sensible trial in this area might usefully compare measures of axonal injury in individuals treated with corticosteroids stratified for interval from onset of symptoms to uptake of treatment.

High-dose oral corticosteroids

In many centres, high-dose intravenous methylprednisolone is the preferred treatment for relapses due to multiple sclerosis. Convenient outpatient protocols have been developed to enhance efficiency and improve convenience for patients. Although the considerable institutional and personnel costs associated with this approach are reduced or eliminated by adopting oral therapy, until recently, the efficacy and safety of high-dose oral corticosteroids had not been much studied. The unconfirmed, yet troubling, finding from the Optic Neuritis Treatment Trial (ONTT: see below) that high-dose oral prednisone may increase short-term relapse rate in the 6–24 months after treatment, together with the expectation of unacceptable gastrointestinal effects, may have held back formal evaluation of this pragmatic therapy.

Two recent studies now suggest that high-dose oral methylprednisolone may be effective in treating acute relapses. Sellebjerg *et al* (1998b) randomized 51 patients with relapsing–remitting multiple sclerosis in the midst of a recent episode (less than 1 month duration) either to placebo or oral methylprednisolone 0.5 g daily for 5 days followed by a tapering course over 10 days. The patients were well matched for disease duration, disability at onset (mean EDSS 4.5 and 4.0 in the methylprednisolone and placebo groups, respectively) and relapse duration. The methylprednisolone group improved to a greater degree by all measures [Scripps Neurological Rating Scale (NRS), visual analogue scale (Millar *et al* 1967), EDSS and patient rating scale] at both 3 and 8 weeks. At 12 months, methylprednisolone-treated patients had a mean EDSS improvement of 0.75 compared with 0.5 points for the placebo patients. A greater percentage had improved by ≥ 1.0 EDSS point (50% compared with 22%). Although there were no serious complications from treatment, insomnia (65% vs. 8% placebo) and gastrointestinal (38% vs. 8%) side effects were more frequent in the methylprednisolone group. The success of blinding was not reported but probably was compromised such that the perceived benefits of treatment may have been exaggerated in individuals noticing adverse effects of methylprednisolone. Given concerns raised by the ONTT, the authors evaluated patients for post-treatment relapse rate but no increase was observed.

Metz *et al* (1999) evaluated the effect of high-dose oral and intravenous corticosteroids on gastric permeability to address concerns that oral administration may preferentially damage gastric mucosa. In this small but unique study, 21 patients with multiple sclerosis who were to receive pulsed corticosteroids chose either to receive five doses of oral prednisone [1.25 g (25 × 50 mg tablets in two divided doses)] or 1 g methylprednisolone intravenously on alternate days. Both groups then received an 18 day oral tapering dose of oral prednisone. Gastric permeability was evaluated at baseline and at the end of the high-dose protocol (day 10) by a sucrose excretion method. Of the 17 patients completing the study, 12 were treated with oral prednisone and five were given intravenous methylprednisolone. Both treatments were well tolerated although insomnia and mood change were slightly more troublesome in the methylprednisolone group. There was a similar frequency and degree of disrupted gastric permeability in both groups, but this was judged to be mild and acceptable. The authors concluded that short-term, high-dose oral prednisone is safe in patients with multiple sclerosis having no prior history of gastrointestinal disorder, renal disease, diabetes and concomitant nonsteroidal anti-inflammatory drug use (exclusion criteria in this study).

Comparing routes of administration

Initially, open comparisons between different methods of administering corticosteroids did suggest that short intravenous courses of methylprednisolone are more effective than prolonged treatment with corticotropin. In the interests of improved efficacy, and putting aside the inconvenience and discomfort, intrathecal administration has been used in an attempt to achieve higher doses of corticosteroids within the central nervous system but this was associated with a high prevalence of adverse effects, attributed to the vehicle in which the steroids were delivered. Heun *et al* (1992) reported the open use of intrathecal triamcinolone (n=22) and intravenous methylprednisolone followed by a tapered dose of oral corticosteroids (n=24). Patients were assigned in sequence to the alternate regimens. At 3 weeks, 13 of the 22 receiving intrathecal treatment had improved by >0.5 EDSS points (mean score changed from 4.2 to 3.7) compared with ten of the 24 in the intravenous/oral group (mean score changed from 5.4 to 5.0; these patients were self-evidently more severely affected at the onset of the study). A corresponding improvement of >1 EDSS point was achieved in seven and five individuals in the two treatment groups, respectively. No functional system seemed to benefit selectively from intrathecal therapy. The only comparable study reported that intrathecal methylprednisolone appeared no better than oral prednisone in patients with (unclassified) forms of multiple sclerosis (Mazzarello *et al* 1983). We do not recommend the use of intrathecal methylprednisolone under any circumstances.

The recent literature does not fully resolve the issue of whether different regimens confer special advantages and hence whether choice can be entirely determined by convenience. Abbruzzese *et al* (1983) failed to show a significant difference between patients randomized to receive treatment with either corticotropin or bolus 6-methylprednisolone in a study involving 60 patients. Intravenous methylprednisolone (1 g daily for 7 days) was compared by M.P. Barnes *et al* (1985) with intramuscular corticotropin administered once weekly at doses of 80, 60, 40 and 20 units. There was a significant increase in rate of recovery in 25 patients receiving methylprednisolone but with no effect on final outcome. In an attempt to reduce the dose of methylprednisolone below that likely to produce adverse effects but without eliminating the therapeutic effects, P.K. Newman and Saunders (1989) compared, in an open design, a single infusion of 1 g and a 5 day course of 5 g in total of methylprednisolone and found the lower dose to be inferior in terms of effect on the EDSS. In an important study, A.J. Thompson *et al* (1989) compared methylprednisolone (3 g over 3 days) and corticotropin (a decremental regimen starting at 80 units by intramuscular injection over 14 days) in 61 patients not yet spontaneously improving within 4 weeks of an acute relapse (51 had relapsing–remitting disease and 10 were in the secondary progressive phase). Both treatment groups improved (there were no placebo controls) but with an equivalent rate and degree of recovery. There was no difference in the response of relapsing–remitting and secondary progressive cases within groups.

Alam *et al* (1993) randomized 35 patients with acute relapse to treatment either with oral methylprednisolone (500 mg for 5 days) and intravenous placebo (n=20) or intravenous methylprednisolone (500 mg for 5 days) with oral placebo (n=15). There were no differences in EDSS at 5 and 28 days (mean score changed from 4.8 to 3.5 in those receiving intravenous treatment compared with a change from 4.8 to 3.7 in the oral group). Sixteen of 20 patients receiving active intravenous treatment reported improvement compared with ten of the 15 patients in the oral methylprednisolone group. Since no increase in adverse effects was seen in patients taking high-dose oral corticosteroids, the authors recommended this as the preferred regimen. La Mantia *et al* (1994) compared oral dexamethasone with low and high doses of oral methylprednisolone over 1 year in 31 patients. Low-dose methylprednisolone was inferior to the other treatments in the short term and seemed to be associated with early clinical reactivation, either at the original or a new clinical site. Overall, the treatment most closely associated with early reduction of the EDSS and clinical inactivity over the 1 year period of observation was high-dose methylprednisolone.

In an increasingly cost aware medical culture, the expense of hospital admission for intravenous methylprednisolone (estimated in the United Kingdom at £500 or $825) prompted a further randomized and masked comparison of oral prednisolone (a decremental dose of 48 mg – which is equivalent to 60 mg prednisone – down to 12 mg of methylprednisolone daily over 3 weeks, costing £2.80 or $4.60) and intravenous methylprednisone (1 g daily for 3 days by slow infusion in dextrose). No difference in response, judged by a variety of outcome measures, was seen at 4, 12 and 24 weeks between groups, and the treatment protocols were equally uncomplicated. However, there was a surprising overall lack of improvement in both groups from the relapse determining entry into the trial (D. Barnes *et al* 1997). Perhaps either the dose or duration of therapy was not sufficient to achieve full benefit. Many patients were significantly disabled at entry and therefore perhaps less likely to recover. In an editorial discussion of this trial, Barkhof and Polman (1997) suggest that the study required confirmation (perhaps with MRI as the outcome) and warned against sliding into the habit of chronic oral corticosteroid use given the relative ease of administration. Later, the authors stuck by their preference for using oral prednisone to manage acute relapses of multiple sclerosis in the outpatient setting (Barnes *et al* 1997). Sharrack *et al* (2000) followed this cohort of patients for 2 years after treatment to determine whether route of administration affected subsequent relapse rate but no differences were seen.

Tremlett *et al* (1998) surveyed 212 United Kingdom neurologists to ascertain their prescribing habits. Most used corticosteroids at some time in their management of patients with multiple sclerosis. There was a strong preference (74%) for 3 days of intravenous methylprednisolone in the setting of an acute relapse. Little consensus was obtained on the indications for, or preferred regimen and dose of, oral corticosteroids either given alone or as a tapering course following intravenous methylprednisolone (50% of neurologists never prescribed concomitant intravenous and oral corticosteroids). Subsequently D.M. Miller *et al* (2000) performed a meta-analysis of published trials using corticosteroids in acute relapses of multiple sclerosis. They found no difference in EDSS improvement between high-dose and low-dose methylprednisolone regimens. Consequently, there is reason to believe that oral and intravenous high-dose methylprednisolone are equally effective. In practice, we continue to use the conventional intravenous route but cannot claim that it is superior to oral administration.

OTHER APPROACHES TO THE TREATMENT OF ACUTE RELAPSE

Approximately 50% of patients fail to recover satisfactorily from severe attacks despite the use of corticosteroids. Until recently, there were few therapeutic options in this setting but the issue arises of whether alternative or additional therapy might rescue the affected individual from otherwise poor recovery.

Plasma exchange

The Mayo Clinic experience with plasma exchange in the management of six patients with multiple sclerosis who failed to improve after corticosteroid administration for the treatment of devastating acute relapses was published by M. Rodriguez *et al* (1993a). These patients either had severe acute motor deficits (paraplegia, quadriplegia), aphasia or ventilator dependence. All demonstrated unequivocal improvement, often within days of starting plasma exchange. Five enjoyed excellent recovery, and improvement appeared to persist for months thereafter.

This uncontrolled study was followed by a National Institutes of Health funded, randomized, double-blind, and sham-plasma exchange controlled study of patients (two of whom were aphasic) who had not responded to high-dose corticosteroids in the setting of a catastrophic relapse thought to be – on the basis of demyelinating disease – multiple sclerosis, transverse myelitis, neuromyelitis optica or acute disseminated encephalomyelitis (Weinshenker *et al* 1999b). Because the entry criteria were unusually stringent, 165 individuals were screened to identify 31 potentially eligible patients. Patients needed to agree to a protracted period of observation for at least 2 weeks after high-dose corticosteroids to determine nonresponsiveness. After randomization, plasma exchange or sham-exchange was carried out on alternate days for 14 days (seven exchanges). Apparent nonresponders crossed over to the alternative (true or sham) form of exchange.

Eventually, 21 patients were randomized and the results were convincing despite this limited sample size. Five of 11 patients treated with active plasma exchange demonstrated moderate or marked improvement (primary outcome) within days of treatment compared with only one of the 11 patients treated initially with sham-plasma exchange. Similarly, moderate or marked improvement was seen when plasma exchange was administered to three of eight patients failing sham treatment. Conversely, none of the patients who failed plasma exchange improved after subsequently receiving sham-exchange. Overall, eight of the 19 patients improved following plasma exchange (42%), compared with only one of 17 following sham treatment (6%).

Plasma exchange was associated with anaemia in most patients and this association was similar in both groups (sham and true exchange). Anaemia was mild in most patients but was severe (at least one value <8.0 g/dL) in four. A central line was needed to complete the treatments in 13, and this was accomplished without incident. Two patients died during the initial sham-exchange treatment programme and never received plasma exchange. One developed fatal increased intracranial pressure. The other died from pulmonary embolism complicating heparin-induced thrombocytopenia. Four responders suffered repeated relapses within 4 months of completing the protocol.

To date, others have not attempted to confirm this result. To launch a second study of this magnitude would be demanding on effort and resources. The patients were terribly disabled, travelled hundreds of miles to the study centre because of the relatively uncommon nature of their illness, and then complied heroically with the protocol. Keegan *et al* (2002) reported a retrospective review of the entire Mayo Clinic experience (1984–2000) with plasma exchange in the setting of severe demyelination (relapsing–remitting multiple sclerosis, 40%; other variants, 60%). Of 59 consecutively treated patients, 44% demonstrated at least moderate improvement comparable to that originally reported by Weinshenker *et al* (1999b). Responders usually demonstrated a benefit early in the treatment programme. Male gender and preserved reflexes at onset of treatment predicted a better response. Subsequently, in a retrospective and uncontrolled observational series, Keegan *et al* (2005) reported that patients in whom brain biopsy showed antibody and complement deposition (pattern II) were more likely to experience moderate to substantial functional improvement from episodes of demyelination refractory to corticosteroids than cases with the type 1 and type III histological patterns described in Chapters 12 and 14. Others report the same benefits from plasma exchange but without prior selection based on histology (Bennetto *et al* 2004).

Monoclonal antibody therapy of acute relapses

Lublin *et al* (1999) provided a preliminary report on their experience comparing the efficacy and safety of the humanized anti-CD11/CD18 monoclonal antibody Hu23F2G in 169 patients treated in the setting of an acute relapse. The CD11/18 complex consists of glycoprotein dimers made up of a common β-chain and individual α-chains (CD11a/18 or CD11b/18 and CD11c/18). CD11a/18 is a receptor for C3bi, a complement component: CD11b/18 is lymphocyte function activator; CD11c/18 is a lectin-like glycoprotein involved in cell adhesion. CD11 is found on lymphocytes, granulocytes, monocytes and macrophages; CD11b is present on myeloid and natural killer cells; and CD11c is expressed on myeloid cells. Patients were randomized to receive either three daily 1 g doses of methylprednisolone, Hu23F2G (1 or 2 mg/kg), or placebo within 1 week from the onset of an acute relapse. The monoclonal antibody performed no better than placebo with respect to clinical (day 0 and 90) or MRI (day 0 and 5) outcomes, whereas corticosteroid-treated patients did improve more rapidly. O'Connor *et al* (2004) have reported their experience with natalizumab (Tysabri), a humanized anti-α4 integrin monoclonal antibody. In this trial, 180 ambulatory patients were randomized within 2–4 days from the onset of an acute relapse to receive a single intravenous dose of either 1 mg/kg or 3 mg/kg of the active drug or placebo. Clinical and MRI studies were performed regularly for 14 weeks (MRI scans at baseline, and at weeks 1, 3 and 14). Sixty-seven per cent of patients (all groups) had improved clinically by 8 weeks. There was no difference in clinical improvement between the treated and placebo groups. Overall, patients improved by about 1.2 EDSS points at week 4 and by 1.6 EDSS points by week 8. MRI studies showed fewer gadolinium enhancing lesions in antibody-treated patients at weeks 1 and 3 than in the placebo group. In summary, the study failed to demonstrate clinical benefit from a single dose of this agent despite its known effect on blocking central nervous system traffic of activated T cells. Considerable recovery occurred promptly in placebo-treated patients. These two studies remind us how difficult it is to demonstrate benefit with putative therapeutic manoeuvres in the setting of an acute attack due to multiple sclerosis.

Intravenous immunoglobulins

Until recently, there has been no definitive study of intravenous immunoglobulins in the setting of acute relapse. There continue to be anecdotal reports of isolated impressive responses in patients who are otherwise corticosteroid unresponsive. This raises the possibility that there may be a subgroup of patients responsive to intravenous immunoglobulin, analogous to those with neuromyelitis optica (see above) who benefit from plasma exchange. The reported benefit of plasma exchange (Weinshenker *et al* 1999b) suggests that a proper trial may be warranted considering that these two treatment approaches are equally effective in the context of acute inflammatory demyelinating polyradiculoneuropathy (Bril *et al* 1996; Kleyweg *et al* 1998; van der Meche and Schmitz 1992; Plasma Exchange/Sandoglobulin Guillain–Barré Syndrome Trial Group 1997). Nos *et al* (1996) reported that intravenous immunoglobulin did not reverse the blood–brain barrier defect identified by MRI in a study of six patients randomized to 5 consecutive days of treatment with either high-dose intravenous methylprednisolone (1 g, followed by oral prednisone) or intravenous methylprednisolone (400 mg/kg) during an acute attack. Visser *et al* (2004) randomized 19 consecutive patients to receive either intravenous methylprednisolone (500 mg daily for 5 days) and intravenous immunoglobulin (0.4 g/kg for 5 days) or intravenous methylprednisolone with placebo in the setting of an acute relapse. No difference was seen in the two groups. Sorensen *et al* (2004) randomized 76 patients with multiple sclerosis seen in the setting of acute relapse (optic neuritis or motor relapse) to receive a single intravenous dose of either intravenous immunoglobulin

(1g/kg) or placebo prior to a 3 day course of intravenous methyl-prednisolone (1 g daily for three doses) to determine if this approach improved outcome. However, no benefit was seen at 12 weeks in the primary outcome measure (Z score of the targeted deficit).

TREATMENT OF ACUTE OPTIC NEURITIS

The same general principles apply to the management of acute demyelination affecting the optic nerve as other central nervous system demyelinating syndromes. Until recently, except in patients with severely compromised vision in the other eye, most episodes of optic neuritis were allowed to recover sponta-neously. This situation altered with the publication in 1992 of a randomized controlled trial of corticosteroids in the treatment of acute optic neuritis which proved influential, especially amongst ophthalmologists (R.W. Beck et al 1992; R.W. Beck and the Optic Neuritis Study Group 1992).

The prognosis for spontaneous recovery of vision in optic neuritis was first assessed by Bradley and Whitty (1968) who showed that 75% improved to 6/9 (20/30) vision by 6 months. Much the same visual prognosis was described by Earl and Martin (1967). Attempts to demonstrate a therapeutic effect of corticosteroids in optic neuritis began with Rawson et al (1966) who showed quicker recovery, but no difference in visual function at one year, in 50 patients entered into a double-blind placebo-controlled randomized trial of intramuscular corticotropin (see also Rawson and Liversedge 1969). This modest thera-peutic effect was not confirmed by Bowden et al (1974) who studied 54 patients with optic neuritis. However, in reporting their final evaluation of corticotropin in multiple sclerosis, Rose et al (1970) mentioned 41 examples of acute optic neuritis and confirmed more rapid improvement in the 22 patients receiving active treatment compared with 19 in the placebo group. Arguing that the local optic nerve dose of corticosteroid achieved with oral therapy might be insufficient, E.S. Gould et al (1977) assessed retro-orbital triamcinolone against controls, using a single-blind design, and again found faster improvement in the group receiving corticosteroids. The study design made it difficult to draw comparisons with more conventional forms of corticosteroid administration used at the time.

Spoor and Rockwell (1988) treated 12 patients presenting consecutively with acute (idiopathic) optic neuritis using high-dose intravenous methylprednisolone (between 1 and 4 g daily for 3–7 days, either with abrupt cessation or gradual withdrawal). Recovery to near normal visual acuity was reported in eight of the patients, some of whom had shown progressive visual loss over several weeks, and a further two showed useful improve-ment. The authors considered this to demonstrate a beneficial effect of corticosteroids but the study was uncontrolled. The frequency and range of complications was as expected following the use of high-dose methylprednisolone.

In the Optic Neuritis Treatment Trial (R.W. Beck et al 1992), patients were recruited within 8 days of a first attack of acute optic neuritis (even though demyelination may previously have occurred in the other eye or at other sites). Treatment was with intravenous methylprednisolone 1 g for 3 days followed by oral prednisone (1 mg/kg/day for 11 days), oral prednisone alone for 14 days, or placebo preparations. Blinding was maintained only

in patients receiving oral therapies. The visual field, colour vision and contrast sensitivity improved to normal faster in the group receiving intravenous methylprednisolone than in the placebo-treated patients but the effect on degree of visual recovery was less marked. There was no difference between groups in the number of patients with acuities of 6/12 (20/50) or worse at 6 months. The effects of treatment were most marked within the first 15 days and in those most severely affected at entry. Conversely, oral prednisolone had no effect compared with placebo for any index of visual function.

It is important to point out that this high profile publication in the *New England Journal of Medicine* was later qualified in somewhat more understated publications (R.W. Beck 1995; R.W. Beck et al 1993a). At 1 year, visual acuity [documented in 409/457 (89%) participants] had reached 20/40 (6/12) or better in 126/133 (95%) of the placebo group compared with 129/137 (94%) and 126/139 (91%) in the methylprednisolone and prednisolone groups, respectively (R.W. Beck et al 1993a). This lack of a long-term benefit was seen irrespective of severity at entry. There were no differences in the results at 1 year for contrast sensitivity, visual fields or colour vision.

Subsequently, a treatment trial in optic neuritis attempted to stratify patients for high and low risk of poor visual recovery. Previous MRI studies had shown that long lesions and those located within the intracanalicular portion of the optic nerve carry a relatively poor visual prognosis (Figure 16.5: D.H. Miller et al 1988c). Kapoor et al (1998) performed MRI of the optic nerve in the acute phase of optic neuritis, and randomized 66 patients to treatment with methylprednisolone or placebo within high-risk (long lesions and those involving the intra-canalicular portion of the nerve) and low-risk groups. Patients who presented early were more likely to have normal scans or short lesions which often lengthened over time. The clinical detection of papilloedema did not correlate with optic nerve swelling on MRI or the presence of an intracanalicular or ante-rior lesion. Swollen nerves tended to have long lesions. The use of methylprednisolone did not affect visual outcome or maximum lesion length. In those who recovered fully, normal visual acuity may have been achieved a little quicker in the treated group. Serial imaging showed that lesions tended to shorten with time but this was uninfluenced by treatment and only one lesion dis-appeared altogether at follow-up. Poor visual recovery correlated with the development of optic nerve atrophy. Stratification for lesion length or site did not identify a methylprednisolone respon-sive subgroup, although patients with short lesions receiving active treatment had less prolongation in visual evoked potential at 6 months and, as expected, there was a trend for longer lesions to carry a worse prognosis irrespective of treatment.

The possibility of a difference in the frequency of subsequent episodes of demyelination between groups featured in a follow-up analysis of the Optic Neuritis Treatment Trial. This attracted much attention but also caused some confusion. In their initial paper, R.W. Beck et al (1992) reported that the percentage of patients having a further episode of optic neuritis in the 6–24 months after treatment was higher following oral pred-nisone [42/156 (27%)] than either intravenous methylpred-nisolone [20/151 (13%)] or placebo [24/150 (15%)]. Between 1 and 4 years, recurrent optic neuritis occurred in 30/133 (22%) placebo patients compared with 28/137 (20%) and 52/139 (37%) in the methylprednisolone and prednisone groups,

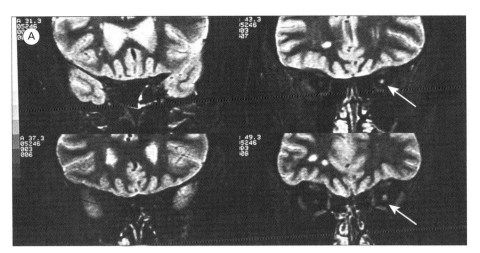

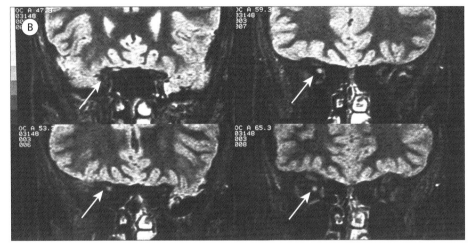

Figure 16.5 Magnetic resonance STIR sequences showing lesions in the right optic nerve. (A) Good prognosis; the lesion does not extend posteriorly into the canal; white matter lesions are also seen in the frontal lobes. (B) Poor prognosis; the optic nerve abnormality is seen in all four slices including the canal. Kindly provided by Professor David Miller and Dr Raj Kapoor.

respectively, providing a relative risk for recurrent disease of 1.83 (95% CI 1.1–2.3) associated with the use of oral prednisone during the presenting episode (R.W. Beck 1995).

R.W. Beck *et al* (1992) also suggested that, in contrast to previous reports (Herishanu *et al* 1989), treatment of acute optic neuritis with methylprednisolone was protective with respect to the subsequent rate of conversion to multiple sclerosis. This question was subsequently addressed by follow up at 2 years of patients as part of the Longitudinal Optic Neuritis Study (R.W. Beck *et al* 1993b). This cohort was restricted to those without clinical evidence of multiple sclerosis at presentation and included 389/457 of the original participants. Clinically definite multiple sclerosis was considered to have developed in ten of the 134 (7%) patients in the intravenous methylprednsiolone group, compared with 19 of 129 (15%) and 21 of 126 (17%) placebo-treated and oral prednisone-treated patients, respectively (Figure 16.6). An additional 6%, 9% and 9% in each group, respectively, were classified at follow-up as having probable demyelinating disease; and 13%, 30% and 16%, respectively, had experienced further attacks of optic neuritis in one or other eye. The apparent effect of methylprednisolone in reducing the conversion rate to multiple sclerosis was mainly confined to patients with abnormal cerebral MRI at presentation. Few patients from any group who were clinically and radiologically normal developed widespread demyelination. On the face of it, these results suggest that intravenous methylprednisolone fol-

lowed by oral prednisone protects individuals with a high risk of multiple sclerosis (abnormal MRI at presentation: D.H. Miller *et al* 1988a) from clinical expression of further demyelination, whereas oral prednisone alone is not effective and may even increase the risk (at least for recurrent optic neuritis).

Given the initial forceful recommendations (R.W. Beck and the Optic Neuritis Study Group 1992), it was inevitable that re-evaluation of the role of oral prednisone in acute episodes of multiple sclerosis, based on an unexpected result in patients with optic neuritis, would draw a good deal of fire in the correspondence columns of journals. Although the investigators excluded chance as the explanation for their observations, no rational explanation was offered and many observers were not convinced that this or any other study provided reliable evidence that the use of corticosteroids in patients with monophasic demyelination at a single clinical site alters the proportion or conversion rate for those who later develop multiple sclerosis. This study was not initially designed to include long-term follow-up. More patients were lost to follow-up than converted to definite multiple sclerosis. It therefore came as no surprise when R.W. Beck (1995) subsequently presented additional results on the conversion rate to multiple sclerosis in those recruited to the Optic Neuritis Treatment Trial who had no evidence of widespread demyelination at entry. Now, there was no effect of treatment (beneficial or adverse) on the proportions developing clinically definite multiple sclerosis (17% in the intravenous

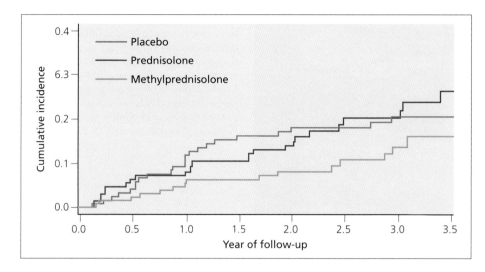

Figure 16.6 Kaplan–Meier curves showing the cumulative incidence of definite multiple sclerosis according to treatment group (p = 0.09 and p = 0.12 by the Wilcoxon test for the comparison of curves for the three groups evaluated together for the first 2 years and the entire follow-up period, respectively). The 2 year cumulative incidence of definite multiple sclerosis was lower in the intravenous methylprednisolone group than the placebo group (p = 0.03) but the value in the prednisone group did not differ significantly from that in the placebo group (p = 0.54). Adapted from R.W. Beck *et al* (1993b). © 1993, with the permission of the Massachusetts Medical Society.

methylprednisolone group compared with 21% in the placebo group at 3 years, and 25% and 27% at 4 years, respectively).

Sellebjerg *et al* (1999) compared high-dose oral methylprednisolone (500 mg daily for 5 days, tapered over 10 days) with placebo in a randomized trial of 60 patients with acute optic neuritis. They demonstrated benefit at weeks 1 and 3 (but not at week 8) and concluded that this route of administration was safe and effective. To date, there has not been a head-to-head comparison of oral versus intravenous methylprednisolone in acute optic neuritis. Consequently, the preferred route of administration (and, for some practitioners, the decision to treat) remains a matter of personal preference for the physician who is prescribing treatment in this setting. In order to determine whether intravenous immunoglobulin might hasten recovery in acute optic neuritis, Roed *et al* (2005) randomized 68 patients within the first 4 weeks of onset of visual symptoms to receive five doses of either intravenous immunoglobulin (0.4 g/kg) or placebo over a period of 60 days. The investigators detected no benefit from this acute treatment in either the primary outcome measure (contrast sensitivity) or in physiological measures of optic nerve function.

MANAGEMENT OF OTHER ISOLATED SYNDROMES AND ACUTE DISSEMINATED ENCEPHALOMYELITIS

Although rare by comparison with the requirement for neurologists to manage and treat individuals with clinically isolated episodes of demyelination or established multiple sclerosis in relapse, it is advisable to have a strategy for dealing with rarer forms of isolated and multifocal demyelination, and to know what may be achieved over and above the natural history of these disorders.

Transverse myelitis and isolated brainstem syndromes

As noted in Chapter 8, a wide differential diagnosis must be considered in the patient with either complete or incomplete transverse myelitis (Cordonnier *et al* 2003; Harzheim *et al* 2004; Scotti and Gerevini 2001; Scott *et al* 1998; Transverse

Myelitis Consortium Working Group 2002), isolated brainstem syndromes or a relapse in the setting of neuromyelitis optica (Devic's disease: Wingerchuk *et al* 1999). It is essential to evaluate the patient carefully for metabolic, traumatic, infectious, vascular and neoplastic or paraneoplastic disorders, some of which potentially have specific and effective remedies. There are no definitive, phase III trials that provide a solid evidence basis for treatment decisions. As noted in the discussion on management of relapses due to multiple sclerosis, we recommend a short course of corticosteroids to hasten recovery in the setting of a significant spinal cord attack. Appropriate steps should be taken to reduce the risk of deep vein thrombosis if a period of immobility is anticipated. Subcutaneous heparin (5000 units by subcutaneous injection twice daily), perhaps supplemented by the use of pneumatic compression stockings and early mobilization, reduces the risk of this important complication. We have used the same plasma exchange protocol (seven exchanges performed on alternate days) for paraplegic patients who have not responded to high-dose corticosteroids. The results appear to us to be comparable to those expected in multiple sclerosis – approximately a 40% chance of moderate improvement.

Acute disseminated encephalomyelitis: Marburg and Balo's variants of multiple sclerosis

It may be difficult to distinguish acute disseminated encephalomyelitis from patients presenting with the first attack of cerebral multiple sclerosis. As outlined in Chapter 12, there are important differences in the underlying pathology (innumerable inconspicuous or small sites of perivenous inflammation and demyelination in acute disseminated encephalomyelitis compared with macroscopic lesions in multiple sclerosis, and massive zones of demyelination with necrosis in the Marburg variant) and risk of recurrence in these two conditions.

As with transverse myelitis, there are no pivotal trials to guide management decisions. The treatment of acute disseminated encephalomyelitis and the Marburg variant of multiple sclerosis is similar to that which we advise for a severe relapse in multiple sclerosis – corticosteroids followed by plasma exchange in nonresponders (Hindley *et al* 1993; Kanter *et al* 1995; Keegan *et al*

2002; Miyazawa *et al* 2001; Pasternak *et al* 1980; M. Rodriguez *et al* 1993a; Weinshenker *et al* 1999b). There are a number of reports claiming that acute disseminated encephalomyelitis may respond to intravenous immunoglobulin (Finsterer *et al* 1998; J.S. Hahn *et al* 1996; Kleinman and Brunquell *et al* 1995; Marchioni *et al* 2002; Pittock *et al* 2001; Pradhan *et al* 1999; Sahlas *et al* 2000) and one report that cyclophosphamide may be of benefit (S. Schwarz *et al* 2001).

Occasionally, patients with acute disseminated encephalomyelitis and cerebral forms of multiple sclerosis develop a life-threatening increase in intracranial pressure from massive swelling of the inflamed brain (diffuse swelling in acute disseminated encephalomyelitis and focal cerebral herniation in the Marburg variant). Acute disseminated encephalomyelitis is potentially a fully reversible condition even in the context of coma arising from cerebral swelling. As such, we recommend that patients with impaired consciousness should be treated in an intensive care setting by physicians experienced in the management of impending cerebral herniation. Treatment measures may include (in addition to high-dose corticosteroids) elevating the head of the bed, blood pressure control, avoidance of hypotonic intravenous solutions, fluid restriction, respiratory support with hyperventilation (to a target pCO_2 of 28–32 mmHg), intravenous mannitol (20% solution as 1–1.5 g/kg by rapid infusion) and (rarely) phenobarbitol coma or induced hypothermia (Takata *et al* 1999). The patient with Marburg variant may require craniotomy as a life-saving measure in the setting of medically refractory, focal cerebral swelling from a single massive area of necrotizing demyelination. Little is known about the management of Balo's concentric sclerosis and we can offer no general guidance based on anecdotal experience.

ADVERSE EFFECTS

The many adverse effects of corticosteroids are well known. These include insomnia, mood change, mania, depression, acute confusion, dyspepsia, a metallic taste (with intravenous administration), hyperglycaemia and acneiform eruptions. Chronic administration is now rarely used in the care of patients with multiple sclerosis and consequently the adverse effects seen with prolonged administration (Cushingoid facies, bruising, thinning of the skin and poor wound healing) are rarely a problem. Repeated short courses of corticosteroids, however, may increase the development, or worsening, of existing osteoporosis with fractures.

Milligan *et al* (1987) reported slight reddening of the face, transient ankle oedema and a metallic taste in the mouth during infusion of methylprednisolone. These were also commented on by P.R. Lyons *et al* (1988), who retrospectively reviewed the adverse effects of 350 methylprednisolone treatments given to 240 patients (mostly a single course but up to seven in some instances) over approximately a 10-year period covering the introduction of methylprednisolone (given as 5 g over 5 days followed by a decremental course of oral prednisolone starting at 60 mg daily, for 10 days). Most patients had acute exacerbations but some were in the chronic progressive phase. Complications attributable to methylprednisolone included urinary tract infections (two cases), candidiasis (two cases), epileptic attacks (three cases; single seizures only), glycosuria (12 cases; one of whom subsequently became diabetic), upper abdominal discomfort (five cases; one of whom was shown to have duodenitis), mood

alteration (six cases; four with euphoria and two with depression), ankle oedema (two cases), transient hypertension (one case), acne (three cases), deep vein thrombosis (one case) and skin excoriation (two cases). Chrousos *et al* (1993) summarized the experience of adverse effects in patients participating in the Optic Neuritis Treatment Trial (see below). The frequency of minor alterations in sleep pattern, facial flushing and gastrointestinal disturbance was significantly higher in patients receiving corticosteroids, as was transient weight gain. One example each of acute severe depression and pancreatitis amongst the 151 patients randomized to intravenous methylprednisolone appeared related to treatment.

Minden *et al* (1988) had previously reported that nine of 50 patients receiving corticosteroids became manic or hypomanic early in the course of treatment. The risk seemed to be higher with corticotropin and, as expected, was influenced by a prior personal or family history of psychiatric disease or alcoholism. Symptoms did not always recur with repeated therapy. Acute and near fatal anaphylaxis has been described (Beaudouin *et al* 1992; van den Berg *et al* 1997; D.L. Patterson *et al* 1995; Pryse-Phillips *et al* 1984). Clear (1999) reported an anaphylactoid reaction to methylprednisolone, in a patient with multiple sclerosis who had previously tolerated corticosteroids, after starting interferon-β (IFN-β1b). The putative mechanism was increased production of interleukin-2, thereby triggering an allergic response.

Not all of these associated conditions can necessarily be attributed to the use of methylprednisolone and most investigators have found this to be surprisingly free from complications despite the theoretical risks. Acute effects on joints – aseptic necrosis – are not reported. It has not proved easy to assess the long-term risk of osteoporosis attributable to the use of corticosteroids since a study of this kind would need to control for the effects of chronic immobility and other confounding factors. Troiano *et al* (1992) retrospectively assessed 103 patients treated with corticosteroids (using different methods of administration) and reported fractures (hips, pelvis, ribs and vertebrae) in 3% of patients per year over 7 years at-risk. The frequency seemed to increase after 5 years but was not related to cumulative dose. Schwid *et al* (1996) reported that, although bone density in 30 ambulatory patients with multiple sclerosis was less than normative data, absolute values were not affected by a single course of high-dose methylprednisolone. Their retrospective analysis suggested that the level of activity (ambulation) is more important than repeated brief courses of corticosteroids in determining risk of osteoporosis. Ardissone *et al* (2002) demonstrated that laboratory markers of increased bone resorption and reduced new bone formation associated with intravenous methylprednisolone administration were reversed within a few weeks of treatment. Tuzun *et al* (2003) assessed bone mineral density of the lumbar spine and hip, together with biochemical markers of bone metabolism. They showed a direct correlation between disease duration and an inverse relationship between functional status in women and bone density, but no correlation with exposure to corticosteroids. More recently, Weinstock-Guttman *et al* (2004) reported on the risk of bone loss in men with multiple sclerosis and found that amongst 40 moderately disabled men with relapsing–remitting (17%) or primary (25%) and secondary (58%) progressive multiple sclerosis, 40% had osteoporosis and 80% showed reduction in bone mass below normative age-related values. Eight of 38 patients had experienced a bone fracture. Risk factors related more to disability and body mass index than to prior exposure to intravenous corticosteroids but against that evidence is the finding that some female patients with spasticity may have indices indicating stronger bone (based on quantitative speed of ultrasound in the tibia) perhaps as a result of spasticity (Achiron *et al* 2004a). Zorzon *et al* (2005) conclude that high-dose intravenous methylprednisolone does not contribute significantly to the development of osteopenia and osteoporosis when used repeatedly in the treatment of patients with multiple sclerosis. In their study of 43 patients treated electively with pulsed corticosteroids (n = 25) or for relapse (n = 18) compared with 61 healthy age- and sex-matched controls, they note that patients with limited mobility are at risk of bone loss and recommend monitoring bone mineral density when corticosteroids are used repeatedly in the management of this disease.

Hoogstraten *et al* (1987) compared bedrest with and without corticotropin retrospectively in 55 patients suffering 99 relapses due to multiple sclerosis. Bedrest alone emerged as a treatment in terms of outcome, but there are arguments in favour of also abbreviating an attack with drug treatment – not least to reduce the complications of immobility. Subsequently, Hoogstraten and Minderhoud (1990) compared bedrest for 3 weeks (with vitamin B complex) and a course of intramuscular corticotropin (lasting 3 months) in 29 patients with acute episodes assessed at 6 and 12 months. There was selective improvement in some functional systems over the first few weeks (but not at 6 months) in the group receiving steroids, but these patients also showed more adverse effects and a higher frequency of further relapse during the period of observation (12 per 161 patient-months compared with six per 163 patient-months in the bedrest group). We generally encourage patients to rest as much as possible until they recover from a relapse. This is not always possible, of course, for individuals in employment who are the key (or sole) source of income for a family.

In 1997 it was found that high-dose methylprednisolone improved event-related potentials, suggesting enhanced ability to process auditory stimuli (S.R. Filipovic *et al* 1997). Conversely, Oliveri *et al* (1998) reported that treatment with intravenous methylprednisolone is associated with worsening of explicit memory in patients with multiple sclerosis treated during an acute episode. Cognitive function recovered within 2 months. It was shown by M. Kaufman (1997) that high doses of corticosteroids (methylprednisolone and dexamethasone) could significantly prolong prothrombin times in patients taking warfarin in conjunction with other medications. Pulsed treatment with methylprednisolone can also rarely trigger atrial fibrillation (Fujimoto *et al* 1990; McLuckie and Savage 1993; Moretti *et al* 2000; N. Ueda *et al* 1988). Hawley (2000) reported a case of fatal hyperammonaemic coma in a patient treated with high-dose corticosteroids for suspected multiple sclerosis. Although the aetiology of this metabolic coma was unproven, unsuspected urea cycle enzyme defects and other causes of reduced hepatic glutamine synthetase activity (including concomitant medications, infection or inflammation) perhaps worsened by the catabolic state induced by corticosteroid administration may have been responsible (Berry *et al* 2000). These need to be identified and corrected quickly in the setting of metabolic encephalopathy accompanying the use of corticosteroids in multiple sclerosis.

MODE OF ACTION OF CORTICOSTEROIDS

Methylprednisolone rapidly enters the central nervous system, the concentration reaching a peak in cerebrospinal fluid at 6 hours and falling to undetectable levels 48 hours after a bolus infusion of 1.5 g (Defer *et al* 1995). Many effects of corticosteroids on immunological, biological, physiological and imaging features of demyelinating disease have been demonstrated acting at multiple molecular, cellular and systems levels in the central nervous system. Genomic mechanisms are triggered by binding of steroids to the cytosol steroid receptor, and function at low concentrations of circulating steroids (R. Gold *et al* 2001). At higher concentrations, however, additional mechanisms of action come into play including effects on the resolution of oedema, permeability of the blood–brain barrier, ion channel activity and the systemic and intrathecal immunological interactions that underlie the inflammatory process. Much of the more recent evidence derives from brain imaging. It is not really possible currently to determine the precise mechanism(s) of action that are primarily responsible for the beneficial effects of corticosteroids in the patient with multiple sclerosis. Corticosteroid-induced improvement of blood–brain barrier permeability is most apparent in serial MRI studies (see below). It is tempting to assume that rapid symptomatic improvement relates, at least in part, to the anti-inflammatory effects of corticosteroids somehow optimizing axonal function (see Chapter 13). Effects on the immune response are less predictable (see below) and, therefore, perhaps less likely to mediate symptom improvement in the setting of a relapse.

Troiano *et al* (1984) showed that contrast enhancement in lesions demonstrated by computerized tomography is eliminated within a matter of hours following treatment with methylprednisolone. Kesselring *et al* (1989) carried out quantitative MRI in 50 patients before and after treatment with methylprednisolone to show that abnormal signals attributable to increased water content are reduced in the cortex and normal-appearing white matter, consistent with an effect on oedema of the central nervous system. However, new lesions develop and alterations occur in pre-existing abnormalities, indicating that the effect of methylprednisolone is temporary without an effect on disease activity. Methylprednisolone also temporarily eliminates gadolinium enhancement, confirming the effect on permeability of the blood–brain barrier. Barkhof *et al* (1991) studied the effect on gadolinium enhancement of administering 21 courses of methylprednisolone (1 g for 10 days). Ninety-eight lesions were detected in 12 patients before treatment, of which 93 were also visible without gadolinium. Of these, 78 were no longer enhancing (but were still visible) after the courses of corticosteroids at which stage six new areas of enhancement had appeared. Barkhof *et al* (1992) described clinical improvement in 15 of 20 patients receiving a single pulse of intravenous methylprednisolone associated with a 76% reduction in gadolinium enhancing lesions (seen on 16/20 scans). There was also a change in cerebrospinal fluid myelin basic protein. These correlations led the authors to conclude that methylprednisolone influences clinical activity by reducing inflammation and demyelination. An effect of corticosteroids on the permeability of the blood–brain barrier was also described by Burnham *et al* (1991). D.H. Miller *et al* (1992c) emphasized the important point, to be expected on the basis of the transient clinical efficacy of methylprednisolone, that the reduction in permeability of the blood–brain barrier demonstrated by a change in gadolinium enhancement, following a course of intravenous corticosteroids, is itself of short duration. Scanning ten patients within 6 weeks of an acute relapse showed that 81 of 85 (96%) lesions enhancing at presentation (day 1) displayed absent or reduced enhancement on day 3. However, most lesions (33 of 43 that were inactive on day 3 and 27 of those which showed reduced enhancement) had reactivated after 1 week (although they still showed less enhancement than before treatment) and remained so at 1 month (Figure 16.7).

The mechanism underlying this alteration in blood–brain barrier permeability was studied by Rosenberg *et al* (1996) who correlated changes in gadolinium enhancement on MRI with reduced production of a tissue inhibitor to metalloproteinase, arguing that this would alter the availability of gelatinase B and so inhibit brain inflammation by an effect on cell migration across cerebral endothelia. High-dose intravenous methylpred-

nisolone increased the levels of tissue inhibitors of metalloproteinase and reduced levels of gelatinase B and urokinase type plasminogen activator in seven patients with multiple sclerosis treated for an acute relapse. The authors hypothesized that steroids may enhance recovery from acute relapses by reversing the effect of metalloproteinase and other proteolytic enzymes on blood–brain barrier permeability. In a related study, Brundula *et al* (2002) reported that minocycline inhibited matrix metalloproteinase-9 production, reduced T-cell trafficking *in vitro* in a transmigration model, and delayed clinical disease onset in myelin oligodendrocyte glycoprotein-induced experimental autoimmune encephalomyelitis. Against the background of reduced circulating baseline levels of tissue inhibitor to metalloproteinase-1 and metalloproteinase-2, and elevated concentrations of metalloproteinase-9, Mirowska *et al* (2004) reported a transient increase in metalloproteinase-9 attributed to activation of granulocytes and monocytes, but no other effects of methylprednisolone.

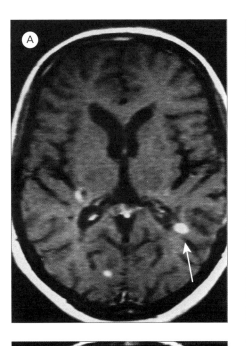
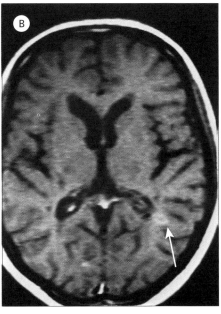
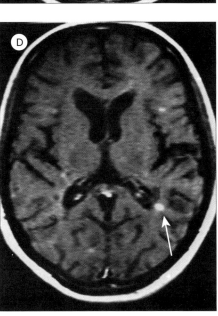

Figure 16.7 Effect of treatment with methylprednisolone on gadolinium enhancement in a demyelinating lesion. (A) Before treatment there is a prominent, round enhancing lesion in the right parietal white matter (arrow). (B) After 1 day of methylprednisolone, the lesion shows much reduced enhancement (arrow). (C) There is no enhancement after 3 days. (D) At 1 week, the lesion re-enhances although to a lesser degree than prior to treatment (arrow). Although image (D) is at a slightly different level than images (A)–(C), there was no enhancement on slices adjacent to (D). From D.H. Miller *et al* (1992c). © 1992, with permission of Lippincott Williams & Wilkins (lww.com).

Hoogervorst *et al* (2002) showed that brief courses of corticosteroids do not affect MRI measures of brain volume, whereas more prolonged courses (5 days of intravenous methylprednisolone followed by a tapering course of oral corticosteroids for 4 weeks) are associated with moderate but transient reductions in brain volume. However, A.B. Rao *et al* (2002) reported that brief courses of intravenous methylprednisolone (3 or 5 days without a prednisone taper) may be followed by reductions in brain fraction volume and contrast enhancing lesions that persist for as long as 3 months in patients receiving IFN-β1b by subcutaneous injection three times weekly. The duration of reduction in enhanced MRI abnormalities achieved with methylprednisolone may be extended by concurrent use of IFN-β1a (Gasperini *et al* 1998). In a longitudinal MRI study, N.D. Richert *et al* (2001) also showed that methylprednisolone and IFN-β1b each facilitate recovery of magnetization transfer in the lesions of individuals with relapsing–remitting multiple sclerosis.

Treatment with methylprednisolone does not rapidly or persistently alter immune responsiveness in patients with multiple sclerosis. In the original placebo-controlled clinical evaluation of methylprednisolone, the effect of treatment was to lower the cerebrospinal fluid cell count and immunoglobulin G index (D.A.S. Compston *et al* 1987). Earlier studies had demonstrated that methylprednisolone reduces intrathecal immunoglobulin G synthesis, but not qualitative immunoglobulin G abnormalities in cerebrospinal fluid (Durelli *et al* 1986; Trotter and Garvey 1980; K.G. Warren *et al* 1986), and the production of anti-myelin antibodies (Wajgt *et al* 1983; K.G. Warren *et al* 1986). Subsequently, P.F. Kirk and Compston (1990) characterized the effect of methylprednisolone on the function of circulating T and B lymphocytes. B-cell activity was enhanced in patients with multiple sclerosis compared with controls. Both groups showed a modest *in vitro* increase in mitogen-stimulated immunoglobulin G synthesis with low doses of methylprednisolone, but with inhibition at higher doses. These findings indicate increased B-cell activity in patients, perhaps as a result of impaired activity of T regulatory cells. Wandinger *et al* (1998) reported that treatment with 3 days of intravenous methylprednisolone reduced concentrations of interleukin-1 and other cytokines without changing baseline immunoglobulin levels in 18 patients with multiple sclerosis who were evaluated during an acute relapse. It was reported by T. Yoshida *et al* (1999) that pulsed methylprednisolone may suppress neutrophil production of superoxide, possibly by an effect on macrophages. Sellebjerg *et al* (2000b) studied immune parameters in 50 patients treated with 15 days of high-dose oral methylprednisolone (5 days at 500 mg, then tapered and discontinued over the next 10 days) for acute attacks of multiple sclerosis or optic neuritis. They observed that treatment was followed by reductions in immunoglobulin G synthesis and myelin basic protein levels in cerebrospinal fluid and serum immunoglobulin G levels without changes in cerebrospinal fluid leucocyte counts, matrix metalloproteinase-9 (gelatinase-B) levels or CD4 T cells in blood and cerebrospinal fluid. They postulated that corticosteroids reduce T-cell activation and immunoglobulin synthesis and increase levels of transforming growth factor-β1 in cerebrospinal fluid.

Gallo *et al* (1994) reported on changes in T-lymphocyte phenotype and function in patients with multiple sclerosis receiving methylprednisolone but there were no consistent effects. Patients showed a slight increase in activation markers, and a

reduction in natural killer cells and interleukin-2 production. In an analysis of peripheral blood, Crockard *et al* (1995) correlated lymphocyte subpopulations and mitogen-induced cytokine production with treatment. There was a reduction in the proportion of most subpopulations (total T cells, helper–inducer CD4 cells, naive and memory CD8 cells but not γδ T cells or B lymphocytes) and cytokine production (interleukin-2 and IFN-β) within 24 hours of the first infusion with rebound and subsequent return to normal. Human leucocyte antigen (HLA)-DR expression was transiently reduced on B cells and monocytes. In a subsequent study, Crockard *et al* (1996) showed that the known effect of methylprednisolone in downregulating HLA-DR expression was reduced in patients receiving IFN-β. Using samples from participants in the double-blind, multicentre, controlled trial comparing oral (48 mg methylprednisolone daily for 1 week then tapered to 24 mg for 1 week and then 12 mg for a final week) with intravenous methylprednisolone (1000 mg daily for 3 days; D. Barnes *et al* 1997), Pitzalis *et al* (1997) studied immunological phenotypes and showed a comparable reduction in circulating levels of tumour necrosis factor-α and the CD11a/CD18 marker but no effect on the majority of adhesion molecules or lymphocyte subpopulations.

The *in vitro* effect of methylprednisolone on mediators of inflammation (prostaglandin E2, leukotriene B4 and thromboxane B2 synthesis by adherent monocytes) was examined by P.F. Kirk *et al* (1994) in peripheral blood from 15 patients with multiple sclerosis and 18 normal controls. Eicosanoid release by monocytes was reduced in the samples from patients with multiple sclerosis compared with controls and there was a further dose-dependent inhibitory effect *in vitro* of methylprednisolone on the production of prostaglandin E2 and thromboxane B2 but not leukotriene B4 in patients with multiple sclerosis following intravenous treatment with methylprednisolone compared with pretreatment samples. These results suggest that methylprednisolone inhibits monocyte–macrophage function but indicate that the effect may not be specific for patients with multiple sclerosis.

Studies on cell and soluble adhesion molecule expression suggest that methylprednisolone influences integrin biology. In summary, high-dose methylprednisolone may transiently reverse the putative changes in levels of adhesion molecules accompanying activity in multiple sclerosis. Droogan *et al* (1998) studied 15 patients with multiple sclerosis receiving intravenous methylprednisolone (500 mg daily for 5 days) in the context of acute relapse. Prior to treatment, T-cell and monocyte adhesion molecule expression was similar between patients with multiple sclerosis and controls. Methylprednisolone affected monocyte expression but not T-cell adhesion molecule expression. Specifically, consistent changes following methylprednisolone administration were early monocyte expression of very late antigen-4 (VLA-4; reduced levels at 4 and 24 hours after methylprednisolone), L-selectin (increased at 24 hours) and Mac-1 (decreased at 6 hours). Soluble levels of E-selectin were decreased at 6 and 24 hours after treatment. However these effects were transient with all levels returning to baseline values by day 7. Adhesion molecule changes may alter monocyte traffic across the blood–brain barrier for the first few days after exposure to corticosteroids. Elovaara *et al* (1998) showed differences in adhesion molecule levels in 23 patients with multiple sclerosis, studied during relapse, compared to controls. They reported higher lymphocyte levels of

VLA-4 and lymphocyte function activator-1 (LFA-1) in patients with multiple sclerosis than controls prior to and following treatment with corticosteroids – particularly for those with larger T_2 lesion loads on MRI. Corticosteroids reduced levels of adhesion molecules [VLA-4, LFA-1 and intracellular adhesion moelcule-1 (ICAM-1)] both on peripheral blood lymphocytes and monocytes and in cerebrospinal fluid leucocytes at day 5 after treatment. Kraus *et al* (2000a) reported lower cerebrospinal fluid CD3$^+$ T-cell expression of ICAM-3 in 25 patients with multiple sclerosis who were studied during relapse than in eight patients in remission. Treatment with high-dose methylprednisolone was followed by an increase in cerebrospinal fluid ICAM-3 levels at day 10, suggesting a possible marker for the anti-inflammatory effect of corticosteroids in the treatment of relapse. Luján *et al* (1998) reported that intravenous methylprednisolone reduced the percentage of HLA-DR$^+$ CD3$^+$ peripheral blood lymphocytes and the population of these cells expressing VLA-4 but did not affect the expression of CD3, CD4, DR, or LFA-1 in their series of 17 patients studied during relapse. Using an *in vitro* model of the blood–brain barrier, Gelati *et al* (2002) showed that methylprednisolone administration reduces monocyte migration *in vitro*.

Keles *et al* (2001) found that levels of nitric oxide in serum and cerebrospinal fluid were generally elevated during relapse, in 20 patients with multiple sclerosis and 20 controls, but were reduced following administration of intravenous methylprednisolone, suggesting another potential mechanism of action for corticosteroids in the treatment of multiple sclerosis. They reported that elevated levels of malondialdehyde (indicating active lipid peroxidation) in cerebrospinal fluid and serum in association with acute relapse are lowered by corticosteroid administration although the mechanism of action in this setting is not yet known (Keles *et al* 2001). Martínez-Cáceres *et al* (2002) noted that changes in lymphocyte populations (immediate reduction in CD4$^+$ and relative increase in CD4$^+$ and CD45R0$^+$), IFN-γ production, chemokine expression and other immunological functions are no longer apparent 6 months after a short course of intravenous methylprednisolone thus confirming, as expected, that many steroid-related changes in immune function are transient.

Leussink *et al* (2001) studied the effect of intravenous methylprednisolone (0.5 or 1 g) on T-cell apoptosis in 66 patients with multiple sclerosis and 16 individuals with other neurological disorders. Blood samples taken immediately before and after treatment demonstrated that unstimulated peripheral blood lymphocytes exposed to corticosteroids *in vivo* undergo apoptosis *in vitro*. This effect is particularly prominent for CD4$^+$ T cells. Bcl-2 expression in T cells is unaffected. Additionally, these authors demonstrated that T-cell receptor stimulated peripheral blood lymphocytes isolated after treatment produce less interleukin-2, IFN-β and tumour necrosis factor-α compared with cells isolated before treatment. They propose that corticosteroids both accelerate the physiological elimination of inflammatory cells by apoptotic mechanisms and downregulate T helper type 1 cytokine production by activated T cells, thereby reducing local central nervous system inflammatory

injury in multiple sclerosis. Zipp *et al* (2000b) demonstrated that corticosteroids work through caspase-mediated mechanisms to induce apoptosis in T-cell lines. However, corticosteroids also protect T cells from CD95-dependent apoptosis, including activation-induced cell death. The suggestion is that by preventing apoptosis of cells committed to ongoing pathogenic immune responses in multiple sclerosis, corticosteroids only provide a transient therapeutic effect. A recently updated systematic review of the use of corticosteroids or corticotrophin for the management of acute relapses in multiple sclerosis (Filippini *et al* 2005) again confirmed that the limited data available support the conclusion that these agents enhance short-term recovery, with no evidence to inform the issue of whether there is any long-term benefit.

PRACTICE GUIDELINES

Clinically significant relapses improve more quickly following prompt treatment with corticosteroids. This basic approach is widely used by neurologists both for relapses of multiple sclerosis and isolated episodes of demyelination. It seems intuitive that enhancing the speed and degree of recovery from relapse will benefit patients. However, there remains a critical need for careful, properly controlled, long-term studies to evaluate whether reducing the duration of each relapse improves the eventual prognosis in multiple sclerosis. It also remains to be established whether other treatments are superior to the use of corticosteroids.

The Therapeutics and Technology Assessment subcommittee of the American Academy of Neurology (Goodin *et al* 2002) recently published practice guidelines for disease-modifying agents in multiple sclerosis. Evidence from Class I and II studies that corticosteroids shorten the time to recovery led the committee to recommend that corticosteroids should be considered for the treatment of acute attacks (Type A recommendation). The committee found insufficient data to favour a specific dose, route or type of corticosteroid and concluded that there was currently no convincing evidence for a prolonged treatment benefit. The committee advised that it is possible that plasma exchange may be of benefit in the management of severe episodes of demyelination based on the single, small, class I study (Type C recommendation).

The treatment of people with multiple sclerosis occupies a rapidly changing landscape. Increasingly, we are guided by the principles of evidence-based medicine. With improved trial design and proper validation of available biomarkers (providing convincing evidence that short-term changes do indeed predict long-term disability), we anticipate that practice guidelines will be increasingly helpful in directing our treatment decisions. For now, however, we recommend that physicians continue carefully to review the design, conduct and analysis of each published trial. In so doing, they should weigh new evidence in the context of what has been published to date, and then proceed to guide their patients in every treatment decision from an informed and compassionate perspective.

The treatment of symptoms in multiple sclerosis and the role of rehabilitation

17

John Noseworthy, David Miller and Alastair Compston

THE GENERAL PRINCIPLES OF SYMPTOMATIC TREATMENT IN MULTIPLE SCLEROSIS

Several manifestations of multiple sclerosis that cause persistent disability can usefully be improved by symptomatic therapies (Table 17.1). It is a rare conversation with any affected individual, other than those free from symptoms, that does not identify one feature or another that might be amenable to drug treatment or other approaches to management. Whether these options are taken up is a different matter and the choice of intervention is much influenced by the severity of the problem, personal inclination, morbidity attributable to multiple sclerosis, and the impact of that treatment on the overall functional status of the individual. It follows that treatments that are worth considering in people with moderately advanced and severe multiple sclerosis would not be instituted at earlier stages in the illness (Figure 17.1). Thus, by way of example, early manifestations of the unstable bladder might be managed by an anticholinergic; later clean intermittent self-catheterization becomes useful and appropriate; and, in the context of immobility with dribbling incontinence, the preferred management might be suprapubic catheterization. Equally, measures needed to control spasticity in the absence of useful mobility differ markedly from those considered in patients with equivalent degrees of increased muscle tone who are still ambulant and depend on stiffness to maintain the upright posture and independent movement. High on the list of symptoms amenable to pharmacological intervention are the unstable bladder, spasticity, paroxysmal manifestations and dysaesthesiae. Some impact can be made on sexual dysfunction in the male, bowel dysfunction, and fatigue.

As is the case in management of any chronic illness, we suggest concentrating efforts on no more than a few symptomatic issues during any given visit. We advise spending enough time adequately to review the symptoms and general principles of their treatment but rarely advise starting more than one medication at any single visit (with obvious exceptions, such as the need to prescribe antibiotics or antidepressants in the context of urinary tract infection and depression, respectively). The symptoms complicating multiple sclerosis tend to fluctuate and recur, and the time course is long, providing ample opportunity to design and conduct a variety of treatment plans. Some symptoms are notoriously refractory to treatment (ataxia, tremor, chronic pain, fatigue that does not respond readily to medication, altered sleep habits, and impaired cognitive function). For these symptoms, it is helpful for the patient to appreciate the challenge that satisfactory management presents so as to maintain confidence if, as is probable, these manifestations of multiple sclerosis subsequently prove refractory to drug treatment and other interventions (Krupp and Rizvi 2002). Other symptoms and signs including focal cortical manifestations (aphasia, limb apraxia and visual agnosia) or extrapyramidal disorders (chorea, athetosis, tics, ballism and parkinsonism) are important in that their presence usually may suggest comorbidity or even an alternative diagnosis.

DISTURBANCES OF AUTONOMIC FUNCTION

The high prevalence of involvement of autonomic fibres in the spinal cord, especially in the secondary progressive stage of multiple sclerosis, means that alterations in the control of bladder, bowel and sexual function are commonplace and almost invariable in the person with multiple sclerosis beyond the first few years of the illness. It is usual for there to be a hierarchy of involvement: impotence then bladder symptoms and constipation developing in that order in males; and urinary urgency, with or without incontinence, dominating the clinical picture in females, whereas constipation and disturbances of sexual function are complained of less often in women. In both sexes, the other features of autonomic dysfunction that we describe are less prevalent manifestations of multiple sclerosis.

Bladder function

Impaired bladder control affects up to 80% of patients with all forms of multiple sclerosis at some stage during the course of the illness (H. Miller *et al* 1965). Bladder problems generally predate those affecting the bowel. The impact varies from a slight nuisance to significant interference with social and professional aspects of daily living, and potentially life-threatening complications resulting from impaired renal function (Betts *et al* 1993). The normal mechanisms of bladder filling and emptying are described in Chapter 6. The more usual complaint is failure to store urine, causing bladder irritability manifesting as frequency, urgency, urge incontinence, nocturia and nocturnal enuresis. Although apparently normal, asymptomatic incomplete bladder

text continued on page 708

Table 17.1 Medications used in managing the symptoms of multiple sclerosis. The reader is advised to use this table as a guide only since the adverse effect profiles for these agents may change with time. Ref: Micromedex ® Healthcare Series

Indication	Agent	Dose	Contra-indications	Precautions	Adverse events	Pregnancy category; breast feeding	Comments
Erectile dysfunction	Alprostadil	Urethral suppository 125–1000 µg Intracavernosal injection initial dose under medical supervision 1.25 µg (1.25–30 µg not more than three times weekly)	Anatomical deformity of penis, penile implant, Peyronie's disease, priapism	Anticoagulants and vasoactive agents	Priapism, bradycardia, fever, hypotension and pain in penis, testes	C; unknown	Seek treatment for erections lasting longer than 4 hours. Review every 3 months if using intracavernosal injections
	Sildenafil citrate	25–100 mg (usually 50 mg) orally 1 hour before sexual activity not more than once daily; with elderly patients and hepatic or renal disease, P450 3A4 inhibitors and HIV agents: reduce to 25 mg	Nitrates (risk of hypotension)	Anatomical penile deformities, bleeding disorders, ischaemic heart disease, multi-drug hypertension, retinal abnormalities, and hepatic and renal impairment	Flushing, dizziness, headache, diarrhoea, dyspepsia, visual change and nasal congestion; rare myocardial infarction and priapism	B; unknown	Not approved for use in women; studies in progress
	Vardenafil	10–20 mg orally; reduce dose to 5–10 mg in elderly patients	Nitrates (risk of hypotension)	Similar to sildenafil	Similar to sildenafil	Not stated	Not approved for use in women; studies in progress
Fatigue	Amantadine HCl	100 mg orally qd or bd (rarely tds); last dose at midday; reduce to 100 mg qd or less in presence of renal impairment		Hepatic disease, eczema, heart failure, oedema, hypotension, seizures and glaucoma	Livedo reticularis, nausea, headache, insomnia, dizziness, nightmares, confusion, oedema and orthostatic hypotension	C; unsafe	Discontinue after 4 weeks if no benefit; rare neuroleptic malignant syndrome
	Modafinil	100 mg orally qd or bd in morning and at midday		Cardiovascular disease, hypertension and oral contraceptives	Agitation, dizziness, headache, insomnia, diarrhoea, arrhythmia and hypertension	C; unknown	May reduce effectiveness of contraceptive agents
Spasticity	Baclofen	5 mg orally tds; may increase to 80 mg/day (in three or four daily doses)		Dose reduction in elderly and renal insufficiency; avoid rapid dose reductions; seizures, autonomic failure and lactation; severe psychiatric disease and stroke patients	Constipation, nausea, paraesthesia, headache, hepatic dysfunction and somnolence	C; safe	Abuse or rapid withdrawal may cause confusion, agitation, seizures, coma, cardiovascular instability and hypothermia. In oral overdose use activated charcoal and gastric lavage
	Baclofen intrathecal pump	Test dose: 50 µg in 1 mL intrathecal over at least 1 minute; increase daily by 25 µg increments for 4–8 hour benefit; for titration, consult references	Test dose: failure to respond to 100 µg/2 mL test dose				

Table 17.1 Medications used in managing the symptoms of multiple sclerosis. The reader is advised to use this table as a guide only since the adverse effect profiles for these agents may change with time. Ref: Micromedex ® Healthcare Series, cont'd

Indication	Agent	Dose	Contra-indications	Precautions	Adverse events	Pregnancy category; breast feeding	Comments
	Tizanidine HCl	Initial dose 4 mg orally; increase by 2–4 mg over 4 weeks using tds or qds schedule (maximum: 36 mg/day)		Oral contraceptives, heart failure, cardiac arrhythmia, hepatic or renal disease, hypertension and hypotension	Abnormal hepatic function tests, asthenia, dry mouth, hypotension, somnolence, dizziness; uncommon cardiac and haematological abnormalities, syncope, phlebitis, hepatitis, gastrointestinal bleeding	C; unknown	May reduce effectiveness of oral contraceptive agents
	Clonazepam	0.5–2 mg orally for nocturnal spasticity	Glaucoma and severe hepatic disease	Renal, hepatic and respiratory insufficiency; acute intermittent porphyria	Dizziness, behavioural change, drowsiness	D; unknown	Multiple drug interactions; avoid rapid discontinuation in patients receiving long-term treatment
	Dantrolene sodium	25 mg orally once daily; gradual increase to maximum 100 mg orally qds	Active hepatic disease	Myocardial or respiratory disease	Constipation, diarrhoea, dizziness, drowsiness, headache, fatigue, diplopia, hepatic toxicity, pleuropericarditis	C; unknown	Monitor hepatic function studies. Multiple drug interactions
	Botulinum toxin type A	30–245 units by intramuscular injection divided amongst muscles	Infection at injection site	Neuromuscular junction disorders and use of aminoglycosides	Oedema and erythema at injection site, and weakness; rare anaphylaxis	C; unknown	Repeated dosing needed approximately every 12 weeks
Neurogenic bladder	Oxybutynin chloride	5 mg orally bd or tds (maximum 5 mg qds) or 10 mg XL (delayed release) qds.	Gastric and urinary retention, glaucoma and myasthenia gravis	Autonomic neuropathy, arrhythmia, heart failure, angina, bladder neck obstruction, and hepatic and renal disease	Constipation, dry mouth, decreased sweating, dizziness	B; Unknown	
	Tolterodine tartrate	1–2 mg orally bd 2–4 mg CER (extended release) orally qds	Gastric and urinary retention and glaucoma	Hepatic and renal disease	Constipation, blurred vision, dry mouth, headache	C; unsafe	Multiple drug interactions
	Terazosin HCl	Initial dose: 1 mg orally; increase to 1–10 mg orally qd (maximum 20 mg)	Dose reduction in presence of hepatic disease	Other antihypertensives and orthostatic hypotension	Hypotension, oedema, dizziness, syncope; rare priapism, blood dyscrasias	C; unknown	Drug interactions with antihypertensives and midodrine

table continued on following page

Table 17.1 Medications used in managing the symptoms of multiple sclerosis. The reader is advised to use this table as a guide only since the adverse effect profiles for these agents may change with time. Ref: Micromedex ® Healthcare Series, cont'd

Indication	Agent	Dose	Contra-indications	Precautions	Adverse events	Pregnancy category; breast feeding	Comments
	Propantheline bromide	15–30 mg orally qds; increase weekly to maximum of 90 mg qds (often used with self-catheterization)	Glaucoma, gastrointestinal or bladder obstruction and myasthenia gravis	Heart, hepatic and renal disease, autonomic neuropathy and arrhythmias; multiple drug interactions	Constipation, dry mouth, decreased sweating, confusion	C; unknown	Multiple drug interactions
	Prazosin HCl	0.5–2.0 mg orally bd or qds	Reduce dose in elderly, and patients with hepatic disease or those using antihypertensives	First dose hypotension, syncope, palpitations and tachycardia	Hypotension, angina, palpitations and asthenia	C; unknown	
	Phenoxy-benzamine HCl	10 mg orally bd or qds	Reduce dose with antihypertensives, and renal impairment	Ischaemic heart disease, cardiac failure, hypertension and renal impairment	Hypotension, fatigue, tachycardia, dizziness, dry mouth, nausea, ejaculatory failure and seizures	C; unknown	
	Desmopressin acetate; DDAVP	Initial dose: 0.2–0.6 mg orally as necessary. Initial dose: 20 µg intranasal hs; (one 10 µg spray to each nostril; 10–40 µg hs)	Type IIB von Willebrand's disease	In the presence of factor VIII antibodies, reduce fluid intake, especially in the elderly, with hypertension and electrolyte abnormalities	Flushing, headache, nausea; hyper- or hypotension, hyponatraemia, palpitations and thrombotic events	B; safe	Monitor for water intoxication
Constipation	Senna	One tablet (364 mg) orally (maximum two tablets daily); also available as rectal suppository and syrup or oral tea	Inflammatory bowel disease and bowel obstruction		Abdominal pain, nausea, cramps, electrolyte disturbance and melanotic staining of bowel wall	C; safe	
	Psyllium	Granules: 1–2 teaspoons orally. Liquid: 2–4 mL orally tds or qds. Seed husks: 3 g orally tds or qds Seed: 5–10 g orally tds or qds	Oesophageal narrowing and bowel obstruction or impaction		Bloating	Unknown; unknown	Drug interaction with antidiabetic agents, carbamazepine and lithium
	Lactulose	15–45 mL orally tds or qds (20 g/30 mL)		Diabetes	Bloating, cramping and diarrhoea; rare hypernatraemia	B; unknown	

Table 17.1 Medications used in managing the symptoms of multiple sclerosis. The reader is advised to use this table as a guide only since the adverse effect profiles for these agents may change with time. Ref: Micromedex ® Healthcare Series, cont'd

Indication	Agent	Dose	Contra-indications	Precautions	Adverse events	Pregnancy category; breast feeding	Comments
Pain and paroxysmal syndromes	Carbamazepine	Initial dose: 100 mg orally bd, increase by 200 mg daily in two doses; or initial dose, 200 mg extended release tablets orally qds, increase by 200 mg/day in two doses, as needed	Active hepatic disease, MAO inhibitors and previous blood dyscrasia	Breast feeding, elderly patients, glaucoma, renal and hepatic dysfunction, pregnancy	Dizziness, nausea, confusion, blurred vision, nystagmus, ataxia, hypertension, hypotension, allergic skin rashes, SIADH, blood dyscrasia, arrhythmias, heart failure, hepatitis and hypocalcaemia	D; safe	Do not stop abruptly; monitor baseline, periodic urinalysis and renal and hepatic function; maintain carbamazepine blood levels below toxic range. Multiple drug interactions
	Phenytoin	300 mg orally qds; use scored 50 mg tablet and 100 mg capsule to adjust dose	Cardiac arrhythmia and heart block	Alcohol abuse, diabetes, hepatic and renal dysfunction, porphyria and pregnancy	Dizziness, ataxia, nystagmus, gingival hyperplasia, confusion, skin rash, osteomalacia and renal and hepatic toxicity	D; safe	Do not stop abruptly; monitor baseline, urinalysis, blood count and hepatic function; maintain phenytoin blood levels below toxic range. Multiple drug interactions
	Gabapentin	Initial dose: 300 mg orally tds; increase to 1800 mg/day in three doses as necessary (maximum 2400–3600 mg/day)		Renal insufficiency	Dizziness, confusion, ataxia, somnolence, fatigue, personality change, myalgia	C; unknown	Multiple drug interactions
	Divalproex sodium	250 mg orally bd (maximum 1000 mg/day), or 500 mg ER (extended release) orally qds; may increase in 1 week to 1000 mg orally qds	Hepatic dysfunction	Pancreatitis; lower dose for elderly	Asthenia, abdominal pain, anorexia, weight gain or loss, alopecia, rash, tremor, constipation, visual changes; hepatic failure, pancreatitis, thrombocytopenia	D; safe	Full blood count, amylase and hepatic function tests at regular intervals first 6 months. Multiple drug interactions
	Diazepam	2–10 mg orally tds or qds	Lower doses for elderly, in hepatic dysfunction and glaucoma	Avoid abrupt withdrawal or concomitant use of other psychotropic drugs, in hepatic or respiratory insufficiency, the elderly, and pregnant or with alcohol use	Drowsiness, fatigue, hypotension and respiratory depression	D; controversial	Multiple drug interactions; dependency

table continued on following page

Table 17.1 Medications used in managing the symptoms of multiple sclerosis. The reader is advised to use this table as a guide only since the adverse effect profiles for these agents may change with time. Ref: Micromedex ® Healthcare Series, cont'd

Indication	Agent	Dose	Contra-indications	Precautions	Adverse events	Pregnancy category; breast feeding	Comments
	Amitriptyline HCl	10–25 mg orally; may increase weekly by 10–25 mg (maximum 150–200 mg/day)	Immediate post-myocardial infarction, cisapride and MAO inhibitor use	Cardiovascular disorder, concomitant ECT, the elderly (lower dose), glaucoma, and with hepatic dysfunction, hyperthyroidism, urinary retention, epilepsy, pregnancy, bipolar disorder or schizophrenia	Blurred vision, nausea, drowsiness, fatigue, headache, dry mouth, weight gain, constipation, bloating, syncope, blood dyscrasias and arrhythmias	C; controversial	ECG if cardiac disease. Monitor complete blood count and hepatic function periodically. Multiple drug interactions
	Nortriptyline HCl	Initial dose: 10 mg orally daily; increase by 10 mg/day every 3–5 days as necessary	Immediate post-myocardial infarction and MAO inhibitor use	Lower dose for elderly, hepatic dysfunction; cardiovascular disorder; concomitant use of reserpine, glaucoma, epilepsy, hyperthyroidism, urinary retention and schizophrenia	Blurred vision, drowsiness, fatigue, headache, dry mouth, weight gain, constipation, bloating, syncope, blood dyscrasias, rashes, arrhythmias, hepatic dysfunction and seizures	D; controversial	ECG in cardiac disease; monitor blood count and hepatic function periodically. Multiple drug interactions
	Topiramate	25–50 mg orally; increase by 25–50 mg/day at weekly intervals; usual dose 200 mg orally bd (maximum 1600 mg/day)		Cognitive disorders, glaucoma, hepatic or renal dysfunction and urolithiasis	Asthenia, paraesthesia, tremor, ataxia, confusion, inattention, breast pain (women), dysmenorrhoea, visual change, glaucoma, nausea; rare blood dyscrasia, hepatitis and pancreatitis	C; unknown	Multiple drug interactions; withdraw gradually
	Lamotrigine	Initial dose: 25 mg orally daily for 2 weeks, then increase every 2 weeks to 50–100 mg orally daily in two divided doses		Risk of severe rash if given with valproic acid; rapid dose escalation leading to excessive dose	Ataxia, blurred vision, dizziness, headache, nausea, rash; erythema multiforme (Stevens-Johnson syndrome), toxic epidermal necrolysis, blood dyscrasias, angioedema and liver failure	C; unknown	Multiple drug interactions
	Misoprostol	200 µg orally qds or 300 µg orally bd	Pregnancy	Elderly, children, and those with renal impairment or vascular disease	Abdominal pain, diarrhea, nausea; rare arrhythmias and anaemia	X; unsafe	Multiple drug interactions

qd = once a day; bd = twice daily; tds = three times daily; qds = four times daily; hs = at bedtime; HCl = hydrochloride; MAO = monoamine oxidase; SIADH = syndrome of inappropriate antidiuretic hormone production; ECT = electroconvulsive therapy.
Food and Drug Administration (USA) Use-in-Pregnancy ratings:

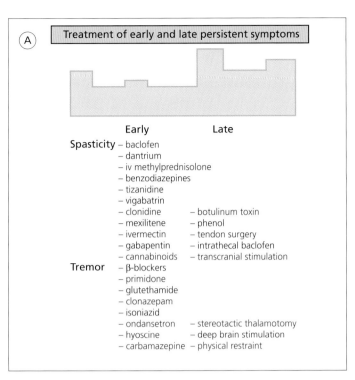

A

Treatment of early and late persistent symptoms

	Early	Late
Spasticity	– baclofen	
	– dantrium	
	– iv methylprednisolone	
	– benzodiazepines	
	– tizanidine	
	– vigabatrin	
	– clonidine	– botulinum toxin
	– mexilitene	– phenol
	– ivermectin	– tendon surgery
	– gabapentin	– intrathecal baclofen
	– cannabinoids	– transcranial stimulation
Tremor	– β-blockers	
	– primidone	
	– glutethamide	
	– clonazepam	
	– isoniazid	
	– ondansetron	– stereotactic thalamotomy
	– hyoscine	– deep brain stimulation
	– carbamazepine	– physical restraint

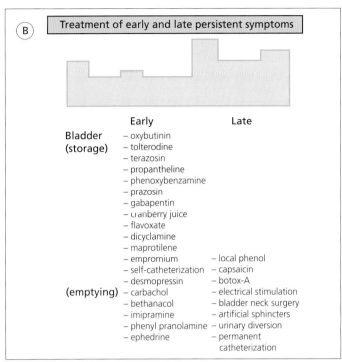

B

Treatment of early and late persistent symptoms

	Early	Late
Bladder (storage)	– oxybutinin	
	– tolterodine	
	– terazosin	
	– propantheline	
	– phenoxybenzamine	
	– prazosin	
	– gabapentin	
	– cranberry juice	
	– flavoxate	
	– dicyclamine	
	– maprotilene	
	– empromium	– local phenol
	– self-catheterization	– capsaicin
	– desmopressin	– botox-A
(emptying)	– carbachol	– electrical stimulation
	– bethanacol	– bladder neck surgery
	– imipramine	– artificial sphincters
	– phenyl pranolamine	– urinary diversion
	– ephedrine	– permanent catheterization

Figure 17.1 Drug treatment and the management of persistent symptoms in patients with multiple sclerosis; interventions are listed in groups which are appropriate for the overall level of disability and handicap.

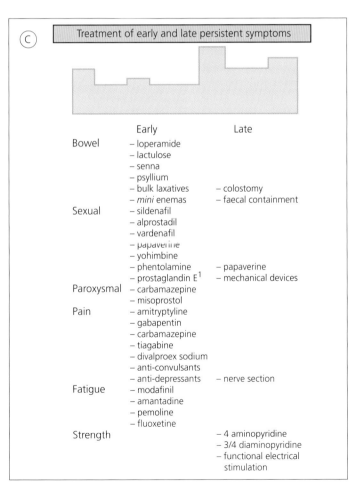

C

Treatment of early and late persistent symptoms

	Early	Late
Bowel	– loperamide	
	– lactulose	
	– senna	
	– psyllium	
	– bulk laxatives	– colostomy
	– *mini* enemas	– faecal containment
Sexual	– sildenafil	
	– alprostadil	
	– vardenafil	
	– papaverine	
	– yohimbine	
	– phentolamine	– papaverine
	– prostaglandin E[1]	– mechanical devices
Paroxysmal	– carbamazepine	
	– misoprostol	
Pain	– amitryptyline	
	– gabapentin	
	– carbamazepine	
	– tiagabine	
	– divalproex sodium	
	– anti-convulsants	
	– anti-depressants	– nerve section
Fatigue	– modafinil	
	– amantadine	
	– pemoline	
	– fluoxetine	
Strength		– 4 aminopyridine
		– 3/4 diaminopyridine
		– functional electrical stimulation

emptying is actually rather common in these patients. Inability to empty may be the dominant symptom and, in many patients, bladder detrusor and sphincter function become uncoupled as a result of spinal cord disease, leading to a combination of urgency and hesitancy (bladder sphincter dyssynergia). Urodynamic evaluation is necessary to determine the aetiology of the symptoms (making the distinctions between detrusor hyper- or hypo-reflexia, alone or in combination with bladder neck dyssynergia), to guide treatment, and to assess its outcome. We refer the interested reader to a comprehensive review of the evaluation and management of bladder dysfunction in multiple sclerosis by K.L. Andrews and Husmann (1997).

Some patients train themselves to achieve bladder emptying by light suprapubic tapping, abdominal pressure (Credé manoeuvre) or perineal stimulation, and straining. We advise patients to time voiding for approximately every 3 hours during the day. It is now possible using ultrasound techniques to measure residual urine noninvasively. For the patient with chronic impairment of bladder emptying, the effectiveness of each technique can be assessed. Most patients learn to tolerate occasional small volume incontinence. Special pads and under garments are helpful for those with more frequent leakage. In a recent report, Prasad et al (2003) compared the relative effectiveness of bladder emptying using abdominal pressure, a percutaneous bladder stimulator (Queen Square Bladder Stimulator; Malem Medical) and no treatment in 28 patients with voiding dysfunction. Both active methods of assisting bladder emptying were superior to no treatment. The percutaneous vibrating device was marginally preferable to manual pressure. Other self-help measures include the use of cranberry juice: the suggestion is that this acts by inhibiting the adhesion of infecting bacteria to the uroepithelium, or by acidification and antiseptic effects on the urine. Meta-analysis of studies, not specifically involving people with multiple sclerosis (Jepson et al 2004), suggests that cranberry juice is preventive (relative risk 0.62: 95% CI 0.4–0.97) and reduces the risk of recurrent urinary tract infections (0.61: 95% CI 0.4–0.91). Cranberry juice is safe, inexpensive and marketed with a pleasant taste, mainly because of added sweeteners.

We generally advise patients troubled with nocturia to reduce their late afternoon and evening intake of fluids, especially alcohol and caffeine-containing drinks. Most will notice less nocturia if they imbibe not more than 1800 mL of liquid per day and drink little after 16.00 hr. A urinal or bedroom commode is appropriate for some patients.

Symptoms that result from bladder instability respond well to medication (those most commonly used are shown in Table 17.1). To improve filling, drugs that inhibit the detrusor include oxybutynin, tolterodine and propantheline. Treatments that inhibit the urethral sphincter include phenoxybenzamine, diazepam, baclofen and dantrium (so that the treatment of spasticity, see below, may decrease bladder emptying). Where the problem is impaired emptying, drugs that stimulate the detrusor are carbachol and bethanecol. Those that stimulate opening of the urethral sphincter include ephedrine, phenylpropanolamine and imipramine. In practice, anticholinergics are the mainstay of treatment because they are effective and because failure to store urine is the common problem (Fowler et al 1992a). They cause dry mouth, constipation and visual disturbance and may require dose adjustment and acceptance by the patient in the presence of these adverse effects.

When patients present with recent symptoms of bladder urgency, hesitancy or nocturia, we generally perform urinalysis and Gram stain (culturing the urine if these suggest infection) and measure postvoiding residual volume by ultrasound. If this is < 100 mL, the best first step is to reduce fluids after midafternoon, prescribe pelvic floor exercises (Vahtera et al 1997) and initiate occasional use of anticholinergics to control symptoms. Oxybutynin chloride (2.3–5.0 mg orally, one to three times daily), propantheline bromide (7.5–15 mg orally, one to four times daily) and tolterodine (2–4 mg orally once or twice daily) are often helpful. Some patients prefer the delayed release preparations taken at bedtime if their symptoms are primarily nocturnal (oxybutynin SR, 15 mg; tolterodine SR, 4 mg). Patients must be apprised of the risk of urinary retention. We usually recommend consultation with a urologist or uroneurologist if these simple measures fail to control symptoms, or patients experience repeated urinary tract infections. When residual urine volumes (before or after starting anticholinergics) regularly exceed 100 mL, we suggest clean intermittent self-catheterization. This is quickly taught and easily adopted by motivated patients with adequate vision and arm function, or by a partner. It can be performed discreetly at work or in the home using a rigid or low friction catheter and ensures complete bladder emptying with immeasurable advantages to social confidence and sleep. It is particularly useful in patients who are socially disabled by bladder symptoms but not otherwise significantly impaired. The frequency is dictated by symptoms and may be necessary every 3–4 hours (more often, as needed, to achieve a volume of 400 mL per intervention), whereas others only need to empty their bladder fully on retiring. Kornhuber and Schutz (1990) make the important point that a short period of intermittent self-catheterization combined with bladder retraining can achieve a useful and lasting reduction in residual bladder volume, even in individuals with severe motor and cognitive disabilities. In some patients, the combination of an anticholinergic and intermittent self-catheterization provides effective control and deals with the detrusor hyper-reflexia and incomplete bladder emptying that often coexist. In more intractable cases, permanent use of a catheter (see below) is preferable to constant dribbling incontinence, which leads to skin excoriation and aggravates other manifestations of spinal cord disease.

A simple means for reducing the volume of urine in the bladder, and hence the desire to micturate, is to recommend intranasal or oral desmopressin spray, especially at night. A double-blind crossover design was used by P. Hilton et al (1983) to assess 1-desamino, 8-[D] arginine vasopressin (DDAVP; 20 µg intranasally) in 16 women with multiple sclerosis. Nine of 16 felt better and there was reduction in night-time voiding rate from 2.5 to 2.0 in treated patients compared with 1.3 in controls. Valiquette et al (1992) assessed eight patients (given 10 µg intranasally at bedtime with fluid restriction). Some also used anticholinergics and intermittent self-catheterization over 1 week. Five were judged to be completely better and two were somewhat improved. Various dose-related adverse effects were reported. Valiquette et al (1996) later reported in a double-blind, placebo-controlled, crossover trial of 17 patients with multiple sclerosis, that DDAVP reduced the number of nights with nocturia, and voidings per night, whereas the number of uninterrupted sleep hours increased. Four patients withdrew because of hyponatraemia (serum sodium nadirs reached

126–133 mEq/L). A double-blind, placebo-controlled, crossover trial of intranasal DDAVP was performed by S. Fredrikson (1996) in 26 patients. DDAVP in a daily dose of 20 mg reduced the number of voidings during the 6 hours after treatment and was preferred to placebo by two-thirds of the patients. The magnitude of this benefit, however, seemed modest (mean number of voidings reduced from 3.1 to 2.6; $p < 0.05$). Hoverd and Fowler (1998) reported almost identical outcomes in their trial of 22 patients with multiple sclerosis using a similar trial design. Oral DDAVP (0.2 mg, titrating up as needed to 0.6 mg) or intranasal DDAVP (10–40 µg) at bedtime may be helpful for short-term or occasional use. Tubridy et al (1999) reported apparently equal (oral vs. nasal) effectiveness in one of their patients who reported taking DDAVP orally (100 µg) although we have little experience with this route of administration. Headache, nausea, rhinitis, nasal excoriation and epistaxis are reported occasionally. Water intoxication, hypertension and oedema are rare but potentially serious complications of DDAVP use. These are best prevented by occasional use of medication, fluid restriction and avoiding this agent in patients with severe cardiovascular disease and hypertension. Bosma et al (2005) conclude from meta-analysis of the published literature that desmopressin has an important role in the symptomatic treatment of bladder dysfunction in multiple sclerosis. This treatment reduced the number of voids and the 6 hour post-treatment urine volume.

Where failure to empty the bladder occurs in isolation, the cholinergic drugs that enhance detrusor contraction, such as carbachol and bethanecol, can be used but these are often less satisfactory than intermittent catheterization. This class of medications should be avoided in patients at risk for obstructive uropathy (such as those with prostatic hypertrophy).

Fowler et al (1992b; 1994) developed a method for reducing detrusor contractions in patients with multiple sclerosis using local injection with capsaicin for 30 minutes to inhibit unmyelinated C-fibre-dependent afferent activity. Despite early deterioration, four of eight patients with bladder hyper-reflexia reported improved bladder control (also using intermittent self-catheterization) within a few weeks. There was objective evidence for increased bladder capacity, fewer hyper-reflexic contractions and a fall in detrusor pressure. The effect may last up to 6 months and can be repeated. Others have applied intravesicular oxybutynin *via* intermittent self-catheterization using a 5 mg tablet dissolved in sterile water or commercially available liquid oxybutynin. Weese et al (1993) found that nine of 42 patients who attempted this protocol encountered practical difficulties, but that 18 of 33 (six with multiple sclerosis) who managed to retain the solution were able to reduce mean usage of protective pads from 3.7/day to 1.2/day, and nine of the 18 who reported improvement had complete resolution of symptoms. Other approaches currently under investigation include the use of synthetic cannabinoids (given orally or as a sublingual spray: C.M. Brady et al 2004) and intravesicular botulinum toxin. Six patients with multiple sclerosis were included in a study of 59 individuals with an unstable bladder whose usual practice of intermittent catheterization was supplemented by a single injection into the detrusor of botulinum toxin (BTX-A 200 or 300 units), or placebo; BTX-A (at either dose) was associated with subjective and objective measures of improvement in all patients for ≥ 24 weeks, and there were no

adverse effects (Schurch et al 2005). C.P. Smith et al (2005) reviewed their institutional experience of treating 110 patients with an unstable bladder or lower urinary tract disorders using bladder or urethral BTX-A (100 or 200 units); 67% improved, including the patients with multiple sclerosis, of whom two noticed an increase in stress incontinence and one other had an increase in residual volume. Although their role remains to be determined in trials dedicated to patients with multiple sclerosis, we sense a growing enthusiasm for the use of intravesicular Botox amongst uroneurologists and their patients (Claire Fowler, personal communication).

Attempts have been made to influence bladder emptying through afferent electrical stimulation of S3 nerve root fibres. Rudd Bosch and Groen (1996) selected six multiple sclerosis patients with stable disability showing detrusor hyper-reflexia and a bladder capacity of > 150 mL. Four patients underwent chronic S3 nerve root stimulation for between 24 and 39 months. There was a reduction in the mean number of episodes of incontinence from 4/day to 0.3/day, and two patients became completely dry. Urodynamic results were less clear cut but showed some favourable responses in three of the four women. The reversible nature of this procedure and its apparently low complication rate would appear to offer some advantages over other local measures for dealing with sphincter dyssynergia. It is nevertheless an invasive treatment with very limited anecdotal experience to support its use. This approach has rarely been utilized in our practice.

Bladder infections can usually be satisfactorily managed with short courses of antibiotics. In the past, physicians often prescribed low-dose maintenance, 'prophylactic' antibiotic therapy but this is likely to encourage the emergence of resistant bacterial strains. Although this approach still persists, and some patients find the perception that recurrent infection can be prevented in this way reassuring, the practice is not sound from the bacteriological perspective and we no longer recommend the use of prophylactic antibiotics. Repeated infections promote the development of bladder stones and urinary tract obstruction with a consequent deterioration in renal function. In all patients with a neurogenic bladder, preservation of upper urinary tract function is essential to avoid renal failure. Screening for upper urinary tract abnormalities should be considered in patients with recurrent urinary tract infections or known prior pyelonephritis, kidney stones or elevated serum creatinine levels. Sliwa et al (1996) showed that ultrasound examination of the upper urinary tract may detect asymptomatic upper tract pathology in up to one-fifth of patients with multiple sclerosis having urinary tract symptoms regardless of neurological impairment. Findings included renal stones, calyceal dilatation and cortical atrophy. They recommend the inclusion of regular upper urinary tract ultrasound screening in the long-term management of patients with bladder symptoms and in asymptomatic, moderately disabled patients with multiple sclerosis. It is nevertheless reassuring that renal failure, complicating the neurogenic effects of multiple sclerosis on the lower urinary tract, is a very uncommon event.

Paraplegic and quadriplegic patients with a poorly controlled neurogenic bladder and bowel dysfunction may develop significant problems with perineal health, including unacceptable pelvic hygiene, urethral erosions, bladder neck dilatation, urethrocutaneous fistulae, bladder stones and recurrent infection It is essential that the perineum be dry to avoid skin excoriation and decubitus ulcers. These are slow to heal and can cause life-threatening sepsis (see below). Condom catheters may be useful in men with refractory incontinence and no outlet obstruction, often as a temporary measure because chronic use can lead to urethral diverticulae proximal to the attachment site of the condom, and leaking around the condom. Chronic indwelling catheters are complicated by sepsis, stone formation, urethral stricture, squamous metaplasia of the bladder (J.M. Kaufman et al 1977) and fistula formation between the urethra and the skin.

Once the decision has been taken to manage the bladder by permanent drainage, it is generally preferable to implant a suprapubic catheter with closure of the lower urinary tract, rather than rely on urethral catheterization. Alternative approaches can be considered in this setting to avoid the long-term complications resulting from a chronic indwelling bladder catheter. These measures include urinary diversion through an ileal conduit, insertion of an artificial mechanical sphincter (F.B. Scott et al 1973) or electrical stimulation of the spinal nerve roots in an attempt to synchronize sphincter contraction and relaxation. Desmond and Shuttleworth (1977) reported on 12 patients with multiple sclerosis in whom an ileal conduit was created. Inevitably, the majority were severely disabled and currently managed by indwelling catheterization or were tolerating incontinence. Nine of 12 had not been helped by previous surgical procedures. Although there were several perioperative complications (especially in patients with decubitus ulceration), and two patients associated the procedure with a permanent increase in physical disability, bladder symptoms were judged to have improved in 11 of the 12 patients and these benefits outweighed the perceived disadvantages. This remains a treatment option in patients with severe incontinence and may be preferable to the use of an indwelling catheter. Malone et al (1985) retrospectively assessed 13 women who underwent urinary diversion by ileal conduit for incontinence. The seven with multiple sclerosis had more operative complications than other patients (one died 4 months after surgery from decubitus ulceration, and another experienced a significant increase in disability) but bladder function was improved thereafter and 67% of patients had resumed social activities that previously had been impossible. In a recent report, Chartier-Kastler et al (2002) reported on a group of 33 consecutive neurologically impaired patients, unable to perform clean intermittent self-catheterization, in whom urinary diversion with cutaneous drainage was initiated for management of the neurogenic bladder. They found that ileocystostomy, alone or in combination with either cystectomy or cutaneous urinary diversion, was effective and relatively free from important complications in this patient group. Cannabinoids (cannabis extract or Δ^9-tetrahydrocannabinol vs. placebo; p = 0.149) were not found to benefit bladder function in a recent large trial (Zajicek et al 2003). But the continued enthusiasm of patients is borne out by further open label studies. Extracts containing delta-9-tetrahydrocannabinol (THC) and cannabidiol (2.5 mg of each per spray) were evaluated by C.M. Brady et al (2004) for 8 weeks followed by THC only (2.5 mg THC per spray) for a further 8 weeks before entering a long-term extension phase. All aspects of bladder function improved in 15 of the 21 treated patients available for assessment whether or not they had indwelling catheters.

Bowel dysfunction

Bowel dysfunction is common in Western society and a significant symptom in patients with multiple sclerosis. Abnormal bowel habit is not easily defined but up to two-thirds of patients with multiple sclerosis admit to constipation. Faecal incontinence is reported by up to 50% although fortunately it is less often a recurring complaint (Chia et al 1995; Hinds et al 1990). Factors increasing the frequency of constipation include delayed transit time (Glick et al 1982; J. Weber et al 1990), immobility, fluid restriction, and use of medications prescribed to control other symptoms complicating the disease, especially anticholinergics to enhance bladder instability. Intussusception can occur in patients with chronic constipation and a history of chronic straining at stool (Gill et al 1994). Surgery may be helpful in these cases. Faecal incontinence may be associated with reduced awareness of rectal fullness (Nordenbo et al 1996).

The principle of managing constipation is dietary alteration and the use of bulk laxatives, avoiding agents that act directly on the bowel wall. Reflex emptying of the bowel at socially convenient times and places should be encouraged. It is important to enhance mobility and facilitate timely visits in response to the sensation of a full rectum. In practice it is helpful to have these principles of patient education reinforced by staff experienced in bowel care for spinal cord injury patients. In such settings, patients and their partners can be taught the fundamental principles of dietary management (roughage and liquids), bulk laxatives (psyllium fibre, lactulose 10 mL orally per day, polyethylene glycol: Attar et al 1999), retraining to optimize reflex bowel emptying, and the use of stool softeners and fibre supplements (see Table 17.1).

In severe constipation, the use of glycerol suppositories can be helpful. We recommend that enemas be avoided except in the setting of impaction as these may lead to adverse effects on sacral reflexes from excessive distention of the rectum. Small volume enemas comprising 50–100 mg of docusate sodium work well, produce little mucus and can be administered no more than once daily to patients with refractory constipation and incontinence to enhance their feeling of control over this disabling problem. When this approach fails, bisacodyl and senna may be used occasionally to stimulate bowel emptying. In severe cases, digital stimulation of the anal ring or local application of a vibrating device may be needed to initiate rectal emptying (P. Dasgupta et al 1997). In severe constipation, the use of glycerol suppositories can be helpful and we have anecdotal experience suggesting that anticholinesterases may provide symptomatic benefit in patients with refractory constipation. Loperamide or oxybutynin may be useful where the predominant complaint is urge faecal incontinence. Bowel incontinence in the absence of constipation may indicate a cause other than multiple sclerosis and should trigger further investigation (Fowler 1997). When these simple measures do not control the symptoms of constipation, we generally request evaluation by a gastroenterologist to exclude coexisting conditions (Hirshsprung's disease, diverticulosis or obstruction) and to determine additional treatment options. Despite these strategies, for some patients inability to empty their bowels according to expectation or former habit remains a major concern and a cause of significant morbidity. Some will seek surgical measures including colostomy – and may find compliant surgeons – but our threshold for recommending such interventions is very high.

Sexual dysfunction

Sexual dysfunction is common in multiple sclerosis (Fowler *et al* 1999; Ghezzi 1999) – decidedly more so than in age-matched controls or patients afflicted by other chronic medical illnesses (Zorzon *et al* 1999). Multiple sclerosis may compromise sexual function in a number of ways. To a variable degree fatigue, depression, poor self-esteem, weakness, ataxia, spasticity (axial, leg and pelvic muscles), pain and sensory loss, neurogenic bladder and bowel symptoms, decubitus ulcers and the need for catheters each reduce libido, performance and satisfaction from sexuality. Despite mutual understanding, the symptom may contribute to marital discord. Counselling may temporarily mollify feelings of guilt and inadequacy but practical measures are also needed. The physiological basis for sexual dysfunction can be assessed using pudendal and posterior tibial nerve evoked potentials, and one or other is abnormal in 80% of patients (Betts *et al* 1994). The contribution of psychological factors should be considered in males with multiple sclerosis and erectile dysfunction but in most cases, even when erections are still occurring, the problem is the result of spinal demyelination. In a prospective survey, Stenager *et al* (1996) demonstrated that the reporting of sexual dysfunction increased in both genders on repeated inquiry after a disease duration of 5 years.

Many patients with multiple sclerosis and their partners either request help or anticipate guidance from their physicians for support in managing sexual dysfunction. Whenever possible, couples must be encouraged to express their needs and fears openly. Everyone must feel comfortable discussing these issues for progress to be made. Successful management is much enhanced by a trusting and supportive relationship. The physician must be sensitive to the needs of the patient and partner, scheduling adequate time to address their concerns. After the initial interview, it may be helpful to have both partners present for subsequent discussions. Involvement of a sexual dysfunction specialist is appropriate but not always possible or necessary.

Much can be done practically to optimize sexual satisfaction (Chandler 1999; Fowler *et al* 1999; Ghezzi 1999; Hulter and Lundberg 1995). Sexual performance is easier when privacy is secure and attention is given to personal hygiene. In severely disabled patients this may require preparation of the perineum, bladder emptying, catheter removal (or, for some disabled women, taping the catheter to the anterior abdominal wall). When fatigue is a major factor, partners should consider timing sexual intercourse to follow sleep or for the early morning when men may experience spontaneous erections. Antispasticity drugs, a stretching programme and a warm bath may temporarily relax spastic muscles. Patients should determine their preferred sexual position to reduce fatigue and spasms, and improve the prospects of orgasm.

Medications that may contribute to sexual dysfunction should be identified and either reduced or substituted by other agents whenever possible. For both genders, these include antihypertensives, antidepressants, antispasticity agents, anticonvulsants and neuroleptics. In the past, manoeuvres for strengthening and sustaining erections included topical application of vasodilator creams such as aminophylline (Gomaa *et al* 1996). Prostaglandin E (alprostadil) may enhance erectile function in men within 15–30 minutes when given either as an intra-urethral pellet or by injection into the corpora cavernosa (Porst 1997). Yohimbine, an α-adrenergic agonist, may enhance ejaculation and orgasm in men (5–10 mg orally) taken 1 hour before intercourse (G.S. Brindley 1994). The previous practice of using self-administered cavernous injection of papaverine (Strachan and Pryor 1987) carried obvious social disincentives, and could not necessarily reliably be timed to start and finish with successful intercourse. Semi-rigid prostheses are available and vacuum-pump-induced tumescence can be achieved. Electroejaculation techniques are available to achieve fertility in impotent males who wish to have children (G.S. Brindley *et al* 1982).

In recent years, these mechanical approaches have largely been replaced by the use of sildenafil, a phosphodiesterase type 5 inhibitor that prolongs the effect of cGMP (I. Goldstein *et al* 1998; Fowler *et al* 1999) administered as 50 mg orally. Nitric oxide release from the vasa nervorum of arterioles within the corpora cavernosa induces smooth muscle relaxation mediated by cyclic guanosine monophosphate (cGMP) leading to vascular engorgement and penile erection. A second cGMP phosphodiesterase inhibitor, vardenafil, is now licensed in the United States. These agents are undoubtedly the treatments of first choice in males with erectile dysfunction, if not contraindicated by associated ischaemic heart disease. Fowler *et al* (2004) reported that sildenafil is extremely effective for the management of erectile dysfunction in a randomized, double-blind, placebo-controlled study of 217 men with multiple sclerosis. Treatment was well tolerated with no unanticipated toxicities. The authors note that the patients in this study were only moderately disabled (mean EDSS 4.0) and relatively young (mean age 45–47 years) but, since this class of agents affects the peripheral neurovasculature, they suggest that sildenafil may also benefit more disabled patients.

Sexual dysfunction in women is less easy to manage. Common concerns include reduced libido and difficulty reaching orgasm. Concerns about incontinence, adductor spasticity, reduced perineal sensation and vaginal dryness are common. There is much to be gained from dealing with associated bladder symptoms and spasticity. The evidence suggests that bladder dysfunction directly compromises sexual activity in women with multiple sclerosis despite normal libido although, paradoxically, urge incontinence may enhance orgasm (Borello-France *et al* 2004) presumably through loss of descending spinal inhibition. Vaginal dryness may respond to estrogen creams. Water-soluble lubricants are often helpful. Scattered reports that sildenafil may enhance female sexual response are emerging (S.A. Kaplan *et al* 1999; Sipski *et al* 2000) but there is no definitive evidence for benefit in women with multiple sclerosis. Clitoral (and occasional penile) hypersensitivity may either require medications to reduce local pain and tenderness (analgesics, tricyclic antidepressants and anticonvulsants) or local cooling with a cloth-wrapped ice pack. We are told that, in this situation, some women advocate the use of a bag of frozen vegetables. Anecdotal reports suggest that in some patients reduced clitoral sensitivity may be enhanced by sildenafil or (as in all women) by manual stimulation and the use of a mechanical vibrator. However, a recently published randomized, double-blinded, placebo-controlled crossover study by R. DasGupta and colleagues (2004) in 19 female patients with multiple sclerosis suggests that the beneficial effects of sildenafil for women are minimal and may be restricted to enhanced vaginal lubrication and sensation without benefit in the orgasm response.

Cardiovascular and temperature dysregulation

With the exception of neurogenic bowel, bladder and sexual dysfunction, autonomic dysfunction rarely complicates the care of patients with multiple sclerosis. Most centres are not equipped to measure autonomic function (Linden *et al* 1997; Meh and Denislic 1998) and interpretation of autonomic testing, especially sympathetic skin responses, is challenging (Linden 1998a). Indeed, McDougall and McLeod (2003) report that there is at best a limited correlation between symptoms of autonomic dysfunction and abnormalities found by autonomic testing. In their recent large series, up to one-fifth of patients with multiple sclerosis were found to have abnormalities on two or more tests of sudomotor and cardiovascular autonomic function with abnormalities predominantly affecting the more disabled and those with secondary progressive disease. Orthostatic hypotension was uncommon (3%). Patients with multiple sclerosis sometimes volunteer subjective changes in temperature and sweating on the trunk or extremities. In such cases there is rarely clinical confirmation or a pressing need to consider treatment options.

Multiple sclerosis is not routinely considered to represent a significant cause of cardiac dysfunction. Recent investigations, however, suggest that autonomic dysfunction, possibly from extensive spinal cord damage, in patients with multiple sclerosis may lead to disorders of ventricular repolarization (for example, QT interval prolongation; Drouin *et al* 1998; De Sèze *et al* 2000b). It might be appropriate, therefore, to perform a baseline electrocardiogram before prescribing medications that can prolong the QT interval (including tricyclic antidepressants, anti-epileptic and anti-arrhythmic agents). One study by Olindo *et al* (2002) reported that patients with multiple sclerosis have reduced right and left ventricular ejection fractions as measured by radionuclide angiocardiography compared with age-matched controls. The authors speculate that this could be on the basis of unrecognized autonomic involvement attributable to multiple sclerosis but further studies are needed. That said, the experience gathered from systematic cardiac ultrasound echography before initiating treatment with mitoxantrone to patients with aggressive multiple sclerosis (see Chapter 18) rarely uncovers unanticipated cardiac disease.

Loss of central regulation of temperature control may occur in patients with lesions in the hypothalamus. These individuals can have unrecognized, sometimes profound, hypothermia and coma especially in the setting of intercurrent illnesses, particularly sepsis. Rare patients, again with presumed lesions in the hypothalamus, may develop profound disorders of temperature regulation rendering them essentially poikilothermic. We have not seen patients with central dysregulation of satiety, diabetes insipidus or inappropriate antidiuretic hormone secretion although the latter has been described (Apple *et al* 1978).

MOBILITY AND GAIT DISTURBANCE

Reduced mobility is the most obvious disabling manifestation of multiple sclerosis. It may result from weakness, impaired co-ordination, spasticity, fatigue, dizziness or loss of proprioception – alone or in combination – and affecting the upper limbs, legs or axial musculature. A multidisciplinary approach to management is essential. Experts in rehabilitation are often best placed to provide gait training and appropriate aids for patients with multiple sclerosis (De Souza and Ashburn 1996; Frzovic *et al* 2000; Lord *et al* 1998a; 1998b; Rodgers *et al* 1999). Many with moderate distal leg weakness and spasticity will benefit from an ankle–foot orthosis. With time, needs change and repeated gait evaluation is often helpful. Eventually, walking sticks, canes, crutches, walking frames, wheelchairs and motorized scooters may be required. The physician plays a crucial role in helping patients to accept the need for these aids – balancing the emotional cost of sensing that a threshold has been crossed, and disability declared, against the advantages of safer mobility or an extended range of activities. For many, the stigma of using a wheelchair outside the home is readily offset by the advantage of re-establishing a more normal range of mobility allowing active participation, minimizing the risk of personal injury and preventing social isolation. For others, the price in terms of appearance and self-esteem remains high. These individuals prefer to remain ambulant without support, however slow and difficult walking may have become. Neither is right or wrong and the experienced physician will support individuals preferring either option.

Weakness

The experimental work of Bostock and Sears (1978) demonstrated that it is possible to overcome conduction block in demyelinated axons pharmacologically or by alterations in ion concentration (systemically and within the central nervous system). Clinical examples of temperature sensitivity for some symptoms in a proportion of patients, and anecdotes relating to symptomatic improvement after scorpion bites (Breland and Currier 1983), subsequently led to the evaluation of aminopyridines as symptomatic treatments in multiple sclerosis. Aminopyridines block potassium channels on the axolemma of demyelinated axons and so act to stabilize the disruption of conduction that arises from simultaneous opening of sodium and potassium channels (see Chapter 13). Although aminopyridines were first used in patients with impaired vision due to multiple sclerosis (R.E. Jones *et al* 1983), their main application has since been to improve muscle strength. In this context, the initial reports were concerned with establishing safety (which remains an issue in view of their epileptogenicity), dose and the role of prolonged administration (Stefoski *et al* 1987).

Clinical improvement was reported in nine of 13 temperature-sensitive male patients receiving 10–25 mg 4-aminopyridine as a single oral dose (F.A. Davis *et al* 1990). Motor function was selectively improved although objective changes in visual psychophysics were also observed. Onset was within 1 hour and lasted between 4 and 7 hours. Stefoski *et al* (1991) gave 4-aminopyridine (7.5–52.5 mg daily in divided oral doses for up to 5 days) to 17 temperature-sensitive patients under placebo-controlled and single-blind conditions. Patients received 86 doses over 47 days and 13 of 17 reported improvement lasting 7–10 hours on 30 of 47 (64%) occasions. By comparison, 3 of 9 controls improved with 4 of 11 (36%) doses. Although several systems were assessed, the main influence was on motor function. The adverse effects were paraesthesiae, dizziness and nausea. After a preliminary evaluation of 3,4-aminopyridine, Bever and colleagues aimed for a compromise between efficacy and toxicity in their dose-ranging double-blind, randomized, placebo-controlled crossover (placebo, low-dose and high-dose arms) trial involving eight patients with temperature-sensitive motor and visual symptoms (Bever *et al* 1990; 1994). Although clinical and laboratory effects were observed, the high dose produced unacceptable adverse effects (convulsions and confusion).

Van Dieman *et al* (1992) also used a crossover design in 70 patients treated for 12 weeks each with 4-aminopyridine or placebo. Improvement during treatment of > 1 Expanded Disability Status Scale (EDSS) point was observed in 10 of 61 (16%) patients and subjective changes were reported by 18 of 61 (29%), especially those with temperature sensitivity, a long clinical history or onset of the chronic progressive phase. One patient improved whilst receiving placebo medication but the effect of 4-aminopyridine was not influenced by the sequence in which therapy was given. Subsequently, van Dieman *et al* (1993) described the neurophysiological effects of a single intravenous dose of 4-aminopyridine (3–7.5 mg/hour for several hours). Concentrating on the visual system, they reported a reduction in latency and an increase in amplitude of the visual evoked response (curiously, this was much more marked – and only statistically significant – in the left eye) and increased velocity of saccadic eye movements. Duration of treatment, physiological effects and clinical usefulness of these rather trivial alterations in latencies and amplitude were not discussed. The same group (Polman *et al* 1994b) described improvements in ambulation, fatigue and cognition in 13, 13 and four of 31 patients, respectively, on long-term 4-aminopyridine (up to 0.5 mg/kg/day; self-selected on the basis of a favourable response). In a double-blind, placebo-controlled, crossover trial in patients with stable motor deficits producing EDSS scores of 6–7.5, 4-aminopyridine improved timed walking and was preferred by seven of the eight participants, but did not achieve a statistically significant effect on most indices of motor performance (Schwid *et al* 1997b). Together, these studies leave no doubt that the use of 4-aminopyridine is limited by adverse effects. Apart from the risk of convulsions and confusion, doses which have a clinical effect are associated with dizziness (50%), paraesthesiae (25%), abdominal pain (10%) and ataxia (10%).

However, nothing else has emerged as a more reliable means of improving muscle strength in people with multiple sclerosis. On the theoretical grounds that (experimentally) digitalis reverses conduction block in demyelinated nerve fibres, Kaji *et al* (1990) reported clinical and evoked potential effects (at the appropriate site) in three of seven temperature-sensitive patients treated with intravenous digitalis (0.02 mg/kg). One patient showed clinical and physiological responses which were topographically dissociated, and three were unaffected. In the Theiler's virus animal model of multiple sclerosis, immunoglobulin administration promotes abundant remyelination (Asakura *et al* 1996; M. Rodriguez and Lennon 1990; M. Rodriguez and Miller 1994; M. Rodriguez *et al* 1996). This observation inspired one of us (J.N.) to evaluate the potential for intravenous immunoglobulin to reverse long-standing weakness attributable to multiple sclerosis. In a double-blinded, placebo-controlled trial of 67 patients, however, repeated infusions of intravenous immunoglobulin (0.4 g/kg administered 11 times over a 12 week period) did not lead to a measured improvement in muscle strength (Noseworthy *et al* 2000b).

Spasticity

Spasticity is a common symptom, interfering with mobility and causing muscle spasms, pain and disturbed sleep. Patients may notice diurnal variability in their levels of spasticity and some are aware of cold intolerance (Chiara *et al* 1998). Spasticity may worsen in the setting of an intercurrent illness (especially urinary tract infection or decubitus ulceration), with use of the interferons (especially in patients disabled by progressive multiple sclerosis), and with bladder and bowel retention or fatigue. In ambulant patients, treatment is aimed at reducing muscle tone but this may be at the expense of increased weakness so that, despite dose titration, there is no net improvement in function. Patients with weak legs who rely on increased tone to maintain standing and walking should be warned that antispasticity medications may transiently reduce extensor muscle tone to the degree that they may fall (see below). This consideration is less relevant in nonambulant patients where the priority may be to ease nursing and increase comfort irrespective of an effect on mobility. The pharmacological treatment of spasticity is therefore dependent on clinical context, and management often involves both physical measures and drug therapy.

Spasticity can be reduced by local treatments that interfere with spinal reflexes or by systemic medication (Table 17.1). Pharmacology remains the first-line treatment for the majority of patients but physiotherapy has a complementary role by optimizing the balance of activity in agonists and antagonists. Medication carries certain disadvantages and none of the available drugs are both fully effective and entirely free from adverse effects. When increased muscle tone causes pain and other distressing symptoms, and voluntary movement is no longer possible, destructive procedures that interrupt the spinal reflex arc (surgically or chemically) can be considered. These are not appropriate for patients who retain some use of their limbs. Corticosteroids (given as pulsed high-dose intravenous methylprednisolone) reduce spasticity in patients with secondary progressive multiple sclerosis but the effect is of short duration and decreases with subsequent treatments (Milligan *et al* 1987).

Despite their limitations and adverse effects profiles, benzodiazepines, baclofen and dantrolene sodium have proved to be the mainstay of treatment for spasticity alone or in combination for many years (R.R. Young and Delwade 1981a; 1981b), with the more recent addition of tizanidine. Baclofen remains the most widely used antispastic agent in multiple sclerosis. It is thought to act by stimulating γ-aminobutyric acid B (GABA$_B$) receptors. Since GABA is the main inhibitory neurotransmitter active in the spinal cord, the effect is to suppress both monosynaptic and polysynaptic transmission through effects both on presynaptic calcium release and postsynaptic potassium conductance, reducing spasticity and improving motor function or comfort (Cartlidge *et al* 1974; Feldman *et al* 1978; R.F. Jones *et al* 1970; Sawa and Paty 1979). Achieving the most effective dose may be limited by the development of adverse effects, including drowsiness, unsteadiness and nausea. A direct action on muscle contraction inevitably introduces weakness that may eliminate its overall usefulness. Others suggest that weakness associated with the use of baclofen is perceived rather than real. It was noted by C.R. Smith *et al* (1991) that 15–20% of patients exceed the recommended dose of baclofen without adverse effect and many settle for a dose of > 80 mg/day. M.B. Smith *et al* (1992) measured torque production in 30 patients using a complicated crossover design with placebo, and reported no weakness during the 1 week periods on baclofen, suggesting that 'weakness' may be used by patients to describe the sensation of reduced muscle tone. Baclofen use is further complicated by an appreciable incidence of impaired liver function (1%) that can occasionally be life threatening (0.1%; Ladd *et al* 1974; R.T. Schmidt *et al* 1976). In practice, however, we have not experienced significant liver injury from the use of baclofen and do not routinely monitor liver function tests when it is used. As noted in the summary table, sudden withdrawal of baclofen may be complicated by encephalopathy and seizures. Accordingly, when the decision to discontinue medication is taken, baclofen should be tapered gradually over a period of weeks.

Dantrolene sodium has a direct effect on skeletal muscle and acts by uncoupling excitation–contraction mechanisms in individual fibres. It is occasionally associated with serious hepatic toxicity. This agent is perhaps more widely used in France than in North America or the United Kingdom. When dantrolene sodium is prescribed, we recommend baseline and monthly evaluations of liver function because of the known hepatotoxicity, particularly when high doses (at least 300 mg/day) are used. Benzodiazepines (diazepam, clonazepam and tetrazepam) reduce spasticity by activating $GABA_A$ receptors throughout the central nervous system, thereby increasing presynaptic spinal inhibition and reducing the activity of brainstem neurons that influence spinal interneurons. Their use is often limited by increased muscle weakness, drowsiness and altered sleep patterns, ataxia and mental confusion. Diazepam (which also is presumed to enhance GABA transmission in the spinal cord) is probably less effective than baclofen and has a more complicated profile in terms of drowsiness and habituation at clinically effective doses (or so it is perceived). It is considered a second-line medication in the treatment of spasticity.

Tizanidine is an imidazoline derivative that is not available in all European countries. It has several sites of action (Coward 1994; J. Davies 1982). Tizanidine is thought to affect conduction in descending noradrenergic pathways of the spinal cord via a stimulatory effect on central $\alpha 2$ receptors leading to pre- and postsynaptic modulation of release and response to excitatory amino acids, respectively. Since tizanidine differs from other medications used to treat spasticity, and there is a need for drugs that selectively interfere with muscle tone without reducing strength in the affected muscles, it may have a particular role in the management of ambulant patients with spasticity.

Lapierre *et al* (1987) assessed the use of tizanidine for 8 weeks in a double-blind placebo-controlled trial involving 66 patients and reported a clinically useful reduction in stretch reflexes, ankle clonus and cumulative limb tone. Muscle strength did not deteriorate. A double-blind, placebo-controlled trial coordinated in the United States used an incremental dose of tizanidine (titrated to a maximum of 36 mg/day) and reported a significantly greater reduction in self-reported muscle spasms and clonus than with placebo but no objective reduction in muscle tone using the Ashworth scale. Minor adverse effects were common and occasionally limited the dose or tolerability of treatment (C.R. Smith *et al* 1994). Tizanidine was also evaluated in a prospective, double-blind, randomized and placebo-controlled trial in 187 patients with multiple sclerosis (United Kingdom Tizanidine Trial Group 1994). Taken orally for 9 weeks, and preceded by a titration phase over 3 weeks starting at 2 mg daily, tizanidine achieved a significant reduction in spastic muscle tone compared with placebo. The effective dose range was around 16 mg daily in divided doses and this resulted in a 20% mean

reduction in muscle tone. Approximately 75% of patients, with all degrees of spasticity, reported subjective improvement without an increase in muscle weakness but there was no improvement in activities of daily living dependent upon movement. Tizanidine achieved its maximum effect on spasticity within 1 week of starting treatment and the benefit was maintained for at least 1 week after discontinuation of therapy. Various adverse events were recorded by patients taking tizanidine but these rarely limited drug usage. No clear preference emerged from comparative studies but tizanidine appears neither less effective nor more toxic than baclofen (Bass *et al* 1988; Eyssette *et al* 1988; Lataste *et al* 1994; Rinne 1980; R. Stein *et al* 1987), although it tends to induce less muscle weakness (Hoogstraten *et al* 1988).

Other drugs have been tested in patients with multiple sclerosis and comparable clinical contexts. These include progabide (Rudick *et al* 1987; now withdrawn because of hepatic toxicity), vigabatrin, clonidine (Nance *et al* 1989), threonine (S.L. Hauser *et al* 1992), mexiliteme (Jimi and Wakayama 1993) and ivermectin (Costa and Diazgranados 1994). Different sites of action can be exploited by combining drug use on the same or different occasions. In an open label study, Solaro *et al* (2000) reported that of 24 patients with multiple sclerosis and painful nocturnal flexor or extensor spasms, 20 responded favourably within 5 days to a low dose (300–600 mg orally) of the GABA agonist, gabapentin, at bedtime. In a double-blind, placebo-controlled crossover study, N.C. Cutter *et al* (2000) reported that gabapentin was superior to placebo in controlling symptoms of spasticity (including spasm frequency and severity, interference with function and painful spasms) in 21 patients with multiple sclerosis followed for 2 weeks at doses of 900 mg orally three times daily.

In general, we advise a combined approach of physiotherapy with a daily stretching programme and oral medication for ambulant patients with troublesome spasms, disabling spasticity in the setting of relatively preserved strength or nocturnal spasms, and spasticity interfering with sleep. We generally avoid antispasticity medications in the setting of borderline leg strength. Most patients will tolerate a gradually increasing dose of either baclofen or tizanidine. These agents may also be used in combination, with a reduced dosage of each. Patients with troublesome nocturnal spasms may benefit from a warm bath, a gentle stretching programme, and a single dose of baclofen, tizanidine or clonazepam at bedtime.

The word has got around amongst patients with multiple sclerosis that symptoms improve with the use of cannabis. Many take this substance through inhalation or ingestion of illicit material, or using nabilone. Some feel subjectively better and report a specific benefit on bladder symptoms. Others find that cannabis reduces spasticity. Forty-three per cent of patients with multiple sclerosis responding to a recent survey indicated that they had used cannabinoids (although for medicinal purposes in only a minority) and many reported improved control of anxiety, chronic pain and spasticity (S.A. Page *et al* 2003). Recent studies have extended the potential role of cannabinoids to immune-mediated and viral experimental animal models of multiple sclerosis (Arevalo-Martin *et al* 2003; Croxford and Miller 2003). Treatment-induced, pro-inflammatory changes in cytokine expression have been demonstrated in patients with multiple sclerosis (Killestein 2003). Recent reviews summarize the pharmacology and biology of this agent (D. Baker and Pryce 2003; Iversen 2003; P.F. Smith 2002).

Petro and Ellenberger (1981) first showed a reduction in spasticity through the use of cannabis using a composite score and this was matched by reduced electromyographic activity. Consroe *et al* (1997) reported that cannabis reduced pain, spasticity, tremor and paroxysmal symptoms in nearly all patients studied. Killestein *et al* (2002a) performed a randomized, double-blind, placebo-controlled, two-fold crossover study of oral Δ^9-tetrahydrocannabinol (THC) and *Cannabis sativa* plant extract in 16 patients with severe spasticity. There was no evidence for improved spasticity (Ashworth score), disability (EDSS) or fatigue with active treatment. Deterioration was seen in the brainstem functional status score and Multiple Sclerosis Functional Status (MSFC). Using a visual analogue scale, patients indicated deterioration in the 'subject's global impression' while on active treatment. Zajicek *et al* (2003) published a much advertised trial in the United Kingdom. Six hundred and fifty-seven patients were randomized either to receive oral cannabis extract, Δ^9-THC, or matching placebos during a 15 week blinded period. The primary outcome (Ashworth scale score) did not confirm an objective effect on spasticity. Patients randomized to the active agent reported subjective improvements in pain, sleep and spasticity and there was a minor improvement (a few seconds) in the median time to walk 10 m, although improvement was also seen in placebo-treated patients. Blinding is difficult in studies of cannabinoids and, in this regard, the study failed. The authors remind us that a recent Cochrane report failed to find sufficient evidence on which to recommend treatment guidelines for the evaluation of spasticity (Shakespeare *et al* 2003). They also noted the inconsistent literature on whether tizanidine reduces spasticity using the Ashworth scale (United Kingdom Tizanidine Trial Group 1994; C.R. Smith *et al* 1994) with no evidence that tizanidine improves walking times, pain relief or sleep. An accompanying editorial (Metz and Page 2003) suggested that cannabinoids are similar in potency to other, more accepted, agents but should be reserved for patients failing standard treatment. The situation remains confused. Vaney *et al* (2004) did not observe an effect on spasticity using an intention to treat analysis although spasm frequency and mobility were improved in individuals who actually received $\geq 90\%$ of the intended dose. Conversely, in a double-blind randomized and placebo-controlled study involving 160 patients, Wade *et al* (2004) reported improvement in a visual analogue scale score for each patient's most troublesome symptom using oromucosal sprays of matched placebo, or whole plant extracts containing equal amounts of Δ^9-THC and cannabidiol; the effect was most apparent for spasticity. Despite the lack of objective evidence, 36% of 220 patients with multiple sclerosis have tried cannabis and 14% are regular users – 3% meeting criteria for drug dependence (A.J. Clark *et al* 2004). We do not advise our patients to take cannabis. Nor do we censure its medicinal use although cannabis remains an illegal substance in many countries.

A modification of the pharmacological approach has been to use intrathecal drugs (Ochs *et al* 1989) and local injection of botulinum toxin to relieve spasticity (Borodic *et al* 1992; Das and Park 1989; O'Brien 2002). In the context of multiple sclerosis, these are usually only appropriate for patients with advanced disease, and drug treatment is to be preferred.

Injected locally, purified botulinum-A exotoxin produces a dose-related weakness by interfering with the release of acetylcholine for several months, or longer. Snow *et al* (1990) assessed the role of botulinum toxin in reducing adductor tone in ten chair- or bed-bound patients with multiple sclerosis in whom spasticity had not adequately been controlled with oral medications. After 6 weeks, treatment had a statistically significant and clinically useful effect on spasticity but not on spasms compared with placebo. There were no drug-related adverse effects. Borg-Stein *et al* (1993) reported an improvement in adductor spasm, restoring assisted ambulation or transfer, and reducing more distal flexor spasm after local injection of botulinum toxin at multiple sites. Hyman *et al* (2000) randomized 74 patients with adductor spasticity to one of three botulinum toxin doses (500, 1000 and 1500 units) or placebo. They noted an important reduction in the frequency of spasms, muscle tone and measures of perineal hygiene (assessed using a six-point scale describing the degree of independence with perineal cleaning and catheter care) at 4 weeks and recommended that the 500–1000-unit dose range was optimal for patients requiring bilateral injections (weakness was more common at higher doses). A potential major advantage of regional neuromuscular blockade with botulinum toxin is the opportunity selectively to reduce muscle tone in one group of muscles whilst leaving others (for example, the leg extensors needed for standing) intact.

Selective chemical denervation with botulinum toxin may improve symptoms in the occasional patient with intractable spasticity or dystonia involving a limited number of muscle groups in one or two limbs. This approach is costly and the results are usually short lived (lasting ≤ 3 months). Very high doses of botulinum toxin are needed for large muscle groups (hip adductors), making this approach impractical.

Intrathecal baclofen delivered by an implantable pump may help in the management of painful spasms and medically refractory adductor tone in paraplegic patients (Coffey *et al* 1993; Penn and Kroin 1985; Penn *et al* 1989). The effect of treatment is optimized by using a single daily dose of around 0.4 mg. Intrathecal baclofen can be used continuously to help patients with multiple sclerosis for up to 3–4 years. There is some evidence that the prolonged use of intrathecal baclofen produces a lasting reduction in muscle tone even after discontinuation of therapy. Ochs *et al* (1989) included 12 patients with multiple sclerosis in their series of 28 nonambulant individuals with severe spasticity treated by continuous infusion of intrathecal baclofen for up to 2 years. Quality of life was much improved in those who were nonambulant because of a reduction in muscle tone and spasms. Weakness (and difficulty in titrating the dose) posed problems (not insuperable) for patients with useful function in the legs. Complications related more to local aspects of the apparatus than to the drug itself (including infection). Patients may experience drowsiness and two in this series became comatose (apparently as a result of concomitant medication). This is an expensive approach to treatment and requires special expertise to insert and manage the pump. Dressnandt and Conrad (1996) studied 27 patients (not all with multiple sclerosis) with severe spasticity affecting at least two limbs, given continuous infusion at T10 for 60 months (mean dose 189 µg/mL/day). Seven were able to stop treatment, ten reduced their dose, and the remaining ten needed the same or a larger dose to maintain the beneficial effect on muscle tone. In their prospective series,

Azouvi *et al* (1996) reported that intrathecal baclofen remained effective throughout 36 months of follow-up in reducing tone and improving function in severely disabled patients with multiple sclerosis. Dose escalation was often needed after 6 months. Symptoms were less well controlled in patients with severe upper limb spasticity. The authors cautioned about the risk of baclofen overdose and the occasional technical problems with pump function. In their series of 99 patients with multiple sclerosis treated with intrathecal baclofen, Schuele *et al* (2005) reported an increased risk of seizures compared with standard antispasticity treatment measures (7% of those receiving intrathecal baclofen had seizures compared with 1% of a matched control group of equally disabled patients; three individuals with multiple sclerosis developed status epilepticus). We rarely use intrathecal bacofen in ambulatory patients. In the occasional patient with severe, intractable spasticity, who remains mobile, the likelihood that this approach may be effective can be assessed by administering a test dose. However, this may prove to be misleading because the test dose may exceed that delivered by the pump.

Intrathecal phenol (or alcohol) may also be useful in patients with severe lower limb spasticity (Jarrett *et al* 2002). In cases that are refractory to drug therapy, there is a role for surgical interruption of the reflex pathways or tenotomy. These chemical, neurosurgical (anterior and posterior rhizotomy, myotomy, selective neurotomy and destruction at the dorsal root entry zone) and orthopaedic procedures should be considered irreversible and only considered in situations where all use in the legs has already been lost. Motor point blocks using phenol are inexpensive and long lasting (up to 1 year) but should not be used in sites where there is a risk of damaging sensory nerves (for example, finger flexors; see review by Stolp-Smith *et al* 1997). A further recent modification to the pharmacological approach has been to use magnetic stimulation to relieve spasticity. In a double-blind and placebo-controlled trial, Nielsen *et al* (1996) showed over 7 days that (in addition to a placebo effect) magnetization reduced objective measures of spasticity, although the optimum protocol for its routine use remains to be determined. There is an important risk of contractures and decubitus ulcers in immobile patients. Clearly these are best prevented by careful and repeated education of the patient and caregivers.

Taken together, the needs of the patient with spasticity change as the illness unfolds. Shakespeare *et al* (2005) reported a systematic review of oral antispasticity drugs in the management of multiple sclerosis. They conclude that the published studies are insufficiently convincing to provide guidelines for treatment of this important and sometimes disabling symptom. We recommend stretching and strengthening exercises for all patients. These may need to be done passively by a caregiver in the severely disabled patient. The appropriate use of antispasticity medications will reduce the frequency and severity of spasms in most patients and may improve the sensation of stiffness in those with symptomatic spasticity but preserved strength. However, only rarely will these medications completely improve stiffness and dexterity, and they may cause troublesome loss of antigravity power in paretic patients.

Pressure ulcers

Patients with multiple sclerosis who are either bed-bound or confined to a wheelchair are at risk of skin breakdown, cellulitis,

pressure (decubitus) ulcers and osteomyelitis (see reviews by Ditunno and Formal 1994; P.Y. Takahashi *et al* 2004). The principal causes of ulcers are excessive pressure, friction, shear forces and moisture (Figure 17.2). The risk is increased in the elderly and in those with poor nutrition, altered mental status, chronic immobility and diabetes – especially, in the setting of incomplete control of continence. The risk of ulcer formation can be predicted by the Braden score (Table 17.2: C. Fife *et al* 2001).

Decubitus ulcers are most often seen over bony prominences (the sacrum, ischium, hip, heels, elbows and base of skull) and are best prevented and treated by attention to several key principles. These include mobilization, repositioning, pressure management devices, and keeping the skin clean and dry. Pressure and shearing forces cause injury in part by interference with blood supply; wheelchair cushions will not prevent ulcer formation in patients who do not shift their weight at least every 15 minutes (Cuddigan *et al* 1998). Chronic immobilized patients must be turned regularly (at least every 1–2 hours). The skin over sites at risk must be kept dry through control of continence and perspiration in skin-folds, and inspected regularly to watch for impending breakdown. Lotions to moisturize dry skin and, as needed, transparent adhesive film dressings that reduce surface tension help to minimize friction and shear skin injury. Patients who are confused, inattentive or unable to shift their position will benefit from proper seating and mattresses including pressure relieving devices (low air loss or air–fluid mattresses). Attention to nutrition and hydration enhance wound healing. Debilitated patients may require protein supplementation (for example, 1.0–1.5 g/kg/day).

Early identification of infection is important through awareness of redness and warmth at the edge of the ulcer, purulent discharge and foul odour. Antibiotics should cover both streptococcal and staphylococcal organisms; Gram-negative and anaerobic organisms may also require treatment. The depth of the ulcer may be difficult to judge. In this respect, magnetic resonance imaging (MRI) may help in formulating a treatment plan. Necrotic skin should be excised and the formation of granulation tissue should be encouraged by keeping the wounds moist either using saline gauze dressings, changed at least three times

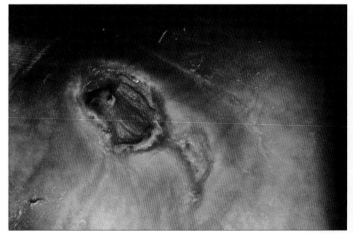

Figure 17.2 Decubitus ulceration resulting from pressure on damp perineal skin in a patient with multiple sclerosis.

Table 17.2 Braden score for characterizing risk of pressure ulcer

Sensory perception Ability to respond meaningfully to pressure-related discomfort	1. Completely limited	2. Very limited	3. Slightly limited	4. No impairment
Moisture Degree to which skin is exposed to moisture	1. Constantly moist	2. Very moist	3. Occasionally moist	4. Rarely moist
Activity Degree of physical activity	1. Bedfast	2. Chairfast	3. Walks occasionally	4. Walks frequently
Mobility Ability to change and control body position	1. Completely immobile: cannot make even slight changes in body or extremity position	2. Very limited: makes occasional slight changes in body or extremity position	3. Slightly limited: makes frequent though slight changes in body or extremity position independently	4. No limitation
Nutrition Usual food intake pattern	1. Very poor: never eats a complete meal (< two-thirds of meal)	2. Probably inadequate: usually eats about half a meal	3. Adequate: usually eats over half a meal or is on tube feeding or total parenteral nutrition (TPN) regimen	4. Excellent: eats most of every meal
Friction and shear	1. Problem: requires moderate to maximum assistance in moving. Slides frequently	2. Potential problem: moves feebly or requires assistance. Some sliding	3. No apparent problem: moves in bed or chair independently	

daily, or occlusive dressings (gels, colloids, biomembranes or polymer films). In severe cases, wide excision and covering the ulcer with a mucocutaneous flap may be needed for closure. In many tertiary centres, multidisciplinary wound-care teams comprised of physicians and nurses with expertise in dermatology, rehabilitation, infectious disease and plastic surgery assist in treating this complication of chronic immobility.

FATIGUE

Fatigue, occurring in the apparent absence of physical symptoms, may handicap patients with multiple sclerosis who otherwise have no physical impairments or disabilities by nevertheless severely limiting their ability to participate. Up to 75% of patients are affected (Edgley *et al* 1991; Fisk *et al* 1994; Krupp *et al* 1988). Physicians and caregivers might anticipate that other symptoms (weakness, sphincter disturbances, pain or paraesthesia) would be of greater concern but many patients rate fatigue as the number one problem in multiple sclerosis. This is a poorly understood feature not explained by increased cytokine production, the release of any other putative biological marker of disease activity, or altered metabolic activities in muscle. Spouses and family members are often not aware that this symptom is a *bona fide* manifestation of the disease, and attention to this issue by the neurologist may relieve tension and foster support at home. Fatigue may, of course, signal an intercurrent medical condition (infection or depression) and these secondary causes should be recognized and treated accordingly.

Fatigue may improve usefully following attention to coexistent depression but people with multiple sclerosis are sensitive and rightly resistant to the formulation that this is often an affective disturbance. Lack of a mechanistic explanation does not alter the status of fatigue as a physical manifestation of multiple sclerosis. In line with the interpretation of fatigue as a physical symptom, Sheean *et al* (1997) correlated subjective improvement in fatigue with electrophysiological measures of enhanced motor performance.

Patients typically describe a diurnal, circadian pattern with most prominent fatigue after the middle of the day. Typically, symptoms peak in the mid- to late afternoon. Patients may develop a second wind later in the evening. Occasional individuals will even delay chores or schedule other activities (such as reading for pleasure) until late at night to take advantage of the effects of their lower core body temperature at that time on levels of energy and neurological function. Activity, heat, stress and concomitant medical illness (infection, anaemia, depression and hypothyroidism) may each aggravate the severity of fatigue (Krupp and Pollina 1996). Patients discriminate fatigue attributable to multiple sclerosis from normal weariness and describe an unpleasant lack of ability to complete desired tasks. They use terms like 'dish-ragged' and 'unplugged' to characterize the symptom. The severity of fatigue may vary and fluctuate during the course of the illness. Fatigue is invisible, difficult to measure and, consequently, rarely evokes intuitive understanding and compassion from employers and others unaware of its troublesome nature.

The treatment of fatigue in multiple sclerosis is partly pragmatic and focused on education of the patient, family and employer to evoke understanding and maximize flexibility in home life and work schedules. All possible steps must be taken to optimize sleep. These include a thorough sleep history and treatment of nocturia, spasticity, restless legs syndrome, sleep apnoea, pain, and other causes of insomnia. Strategically timed daytime napping is often helpful. The physician can support the patient's need to rest in the middle of the working day by explanation to employers. Patients should be encouraged to enter a graded exercise programme to optimize fitness.

Using a crossover design, the Canadian MS Research Group (1987) treated patients with amantadine hydrochloride (100 mg orally twice daily) and noted marked or moderate improvement in 47% compared with 1% of controls. R.A. Cohen and Fisher (1989) used subjective measures in a similar design to assess 22 patients receiving amantadine (ten with progressive and 12 with relapsing multiple sclerosis). They reported improvement in some aspects of fatigue (energy level, sense of well-being, perceived attention and memory, or problem-solving capacity) in 15. There was a conspicuous dissociation between the effect on motivational and motor aspects of fatigue. Weinshenker et al (1992) reported a comparable clinical effect from pemoline, also in a crossover trial, but found this to be poorly tolerated. These agents were compared by Krupp et al (1995) and amantadine emerged as the more promising therapeutic agent. Pemoline is no longer used for this indication following release of a precaution about hepatic toxicity from the United States Food and Drug Administration.

There have been reports that the potassium-channel blocker, 4-aminopyridine, may be more effective than 3,4-aminopyridine (Polman et al 1994a) in treating fatigue. As noted above, reported side effects include light headedness, abdominal pain, confusion and seizures (Bever 1994). Further work is in progress with a slow-release preparation. Rossini et al (2001) could not, however, confirm that 4-aminopyridine is superior to placebo in a double-blinded trial using the Fatigue Severity Scale scores. Taken together, the aminopyridines have not been widely used for this therapeutic indication.

Recent reports suggest a role for modafinil, introduced primarily for the treatment of narcolepsy, at an oral dose of 200 mg daily (Rammohan et al 2002). Side effects, including headache, nausea and a sense of nervousness, occur in a minority of patients. Stankoff et al (2005) randomized 115 patients with multiple sclerosis to receive either oral modafinil (200 mg/day initial dose, increased as tolerated to 400 mg/day) or placebo in a double-blind study. Patients in both groups reported that their level of fatigue improved as measured by the Modified Fatigue Impact Scale at 5 weeks but there was no difference in apparent efficacy between placebo and modafinil-treated subjects. This parallel group study questions the value of modafinil in the treatment of fatigue in multiple sclerosis. As noted in the accompanying editorial (Schwid and Murray 2005), the previous cross-over study of modafinil (Rammohan et al 2002) may have underestimated the placebo effect and, thereby, incurred a type-one error. There have been repeated anecdotal reports that the selective serotonin reuptake inhibitors relieve fatigue in multiple sclerosis but this has not been demonstrated in adequate clinical trials nor has it been our clinical experience that these are helpful. Wingerchuk et al (1998; 2005) reported that

1300 mg/day of aspirin may have a role in the management of fatigue due to multiple sclerosis. In this randomized, double-blind, placebo-controlled, cross-over study, 30 patients were randomized to active drug or placebo and later crossed over to the second arm. Their analysis suggested a benefit of aspirin as measured by the Modified Fatigue Impact Scale scores and patient preference. A definitive, controlled, blinded, parallel group confirmatory trial is needed. The MS Council for Clinical Practice Guidelines has published a comprehensive algorithm to assist the physician in the evaluation and management of this common and vexing symptom (Fatigue Guidelines Development Panel of the Multiple Sclerosis Council for Clinical Practice Guidelines 1998). A recent randomized, three-arm study suggested that participation in either yoga or an exercise class for a 6 month period reduced the severity of fatigue compared with a waiting list control group (Oken et al 2004). In planning an exercise programme for patients with multiple sclerosis, it is important to note that it has been recently shown that there is a correlation between exercise capacity and level of disability (EDSS) even in mildly disabled patients (Romberg et al 2004).

When medication is needed for fatigue, we generally begin with amantadine 100 mg orally in the late morning, increasing to one tablet twice (or rarely three times) daily, and instructing the patient to take their last dose before mid-afternoon. Patients are told that up to 60% may notice a moderate degree of improvement (representing no more than a change of one grade in severity) and that those who do benefit are likely to notice improvement within 4 weeks. We generally discontinue this drug if there has been no response after 1 month. Those who respond can take amantadine indefinitely. If tachyphylaxis develops, a drug holiday for 1 month may restore benefit. It seems likely that modafinil will increasingly be used for this indication but evidence for efficacy is needed rather than high expectations sustained by anecdotal experience.

DISTURBANCES OF BRAINSTEM FUNCTION

The primary role of many brainstem structures in coordinating the precision and success of movement, the concentration of nuclei, and the high density of axonal traffic through the brainstem leave many functions dependent on the integrity of these pathways. It follows that several symptoms requiring treatment will develop when these pathways are affected by the disease process in multiple sclerosis.

Ataxia and tremor

Tremor in multiple sclerosis is typically most noticeable during goal-directed actions and at the terminal stages of movement. Axial and limb posture may also be contaminated in isolation or, more commonly, in combination with intention tremor. The most disabling disturbance is wide-amplitude proximal upper limb and head tremor, more or less completely interfering with all skilled movement. This has as its basis disruption of connections between the dendate nuclei and contralateral thalamus in the superior cerebellar peduncle or red nucleus. Although tremor may occur, and subsequently recover, in the context of an acute exacerbation, once established, it is more typical for this disability to persist. Irreversible axial and appendicular ataxia and tremor may ruin motor function in otherwise mildly disabled patients, but more commonly this complicates the later phases of long-standing, advanced multiple sclerosis. The development of persistent upper limb tremor is therefore usually an ominous sign and one that proves tough to manage.

Even in the absence of the Uthoff phenomenon, the amplitude of upper limb tremor may reduce with cooling, proportionate to the degree of temperature lowering and without loss of strength, but the effect is short lived (Feys *et al* 2005). Loss of coordination as a result of tremor can also be managed by partial physical restraint using weights of around 4 kg (Aisen *et al* 1993). A pilot study of 26 patients with multiple sclerosis evaluated neuromuscular rehabilitation methods with and without Johnstone Pressure Splints. The splints were developed with the premise that pressure from the splints might stimulate cutaneous nerve endings and thereby enhance proprioception. This study demonstrated some minor, usually poorly sustained, benefits in individuals with axial and appendicular ataxia (Armutlu *et al* 2001).

The mainstay of pharmacological treatment is to use β-blockers, of which the most predictable are propranolol, metoprolol, nadolol and sotalol. Primidone probably acts through metabolism to barbiturate and the parent drug can be used itself. Clonazepam and carbamazepine may help but, paradoxically, toxicity will increase unsteadiness and intention tremor. Isoniazid has been assessed in a placebo-controlled crossover design involving six patients with superior cerebellar peduncular tremor (Bozek *et al* 1987; Hallett *et al* 1985) with some claims for success. Ondansetron (a 5-hydroxytryptamine-3 antagonist, given as 8 mg orally) was evaluated in a small pilot study (G.P.A. Rice *et al* 1995) and has its devotees. Recent anecdotal reports suggest that oral gabapentin (300–600 mg orally three times daily up to a maximum of 3.6 g daily) may be useful in this setting but efficacy has not been substantiated in adequate clinical trials. Cannabinoids (5–15 mg of THC orally) were reported to improve tremor but not ataxia in two patients, and five others experienced no change in symptoms or signs (D.B. Clifford 1983). This led H.S. Greenberg *et al* (1994) to measure postural control in ten patients with multiple sclerosis who had moderately severe spastic paraparesis and ten controls matched for physiognomy. A single reefer had no discernible effect on the objective neurological examination and postural control deteriorated in both groups.

Stereotactic neurosurgical procedures creating a lesion in the ventrolateral nucleus of the thalamus can be used to achieve one useful (contralateral) arm in patients who are no longer able to manage basic aspects of daily living. Speech deficits are frequent when the procedure is bilateral and, despite stability at rest and during movement, patients often choose not to use the limb. Thus, tremor is replaced by bradykinesis. However, with improved stereotactic techniques, we anticipate that functional neurosurgery may be used more readily in the management of incoordination resulting from the lesions of multiple sclerosis. There is, of course, the inherent risk in using invasive procedures of this type that early gains may be reversed by later disease progression.

Thalamic electrostimulation within the ventrolateral nucleus just above the intercommissural line, in front of the anterior commissure and lateral to the wall of the third ventricle, produces results comparable to those achieved with destructive procedures (J.P. Nguyen and Degos 1993). The device can be used intermittently. Whittle *et al* (1998) have drawn attention to the practical difficulties and unpredictable results. Of 17 patients considered for thalamic stimulation, in only five of the eight who proceeded to stereotactic exploration could a target be identified for implantation of a thalamic stimulator, although one other subject appeared to benefit from the stereotactic procedure alone. Frequent adjustments to the stimulator were subsequently needed to suppress the movement disorders, and these patients required support from a dedicated rehabilitation team postoperatively.

Recent reports from several groups confirm that clinical benefits from unilateral thalamotomy and thalamic stimulation in multiple sclerosis are modest and transient compared with those seen in Parkinson's disease and essential tremor (Alusi *et al* 2001a; 2001b; Schuurman *et al* 2000). These procedures may be more effective at reducing tremor than at reducing ataxia (J. Matsumoto *et al* 2001). Given the unsatisfactory therapeutic options, it follows that despite best medical attention, ataxia and ataxic tremor remain enormously challenging to patients and their caregivers.

Other movement disorders

Hyperkinetic and hypokinetic movement disorders are rarely seen as manifestations of multiple sclerosis (see Chapter 6; C.C. Mao *et al* 1988). Indeed, chorea, athetosis, tics, ballism (Riley and Lang 1988), spasmodic torticollis (Plant *et al* 1989) and parkinsonism usually suggest alternative diagnoses. Ruprecht *et al* (2002) recently reported a patient with multiple sclerosis and symptomatic hyperekplexia who was responsive to gabapentin. Roos *et al* (1991) and Rozza *et al* (1993) each reported single cases of paroxysmal kinesigenic choreoathetosis and kinesigenic dystonia. The nosology of these two cases is controversial in that each had movement-initiated transient motor phenomena. In fact, our reading of the literature suggests that many of these cases do not primarily have movement disorders but, rather, are examples of paroxysmal manifestations of multiple sclerosis and should therefore be treated as such. We share this interpretation (suggested by Honig 1992) of the case reported by Roos *et al* (1991) because there is no description of the patient's chorea. The patient described by Rozza *et al* (1993) also appears likely to have had typical paroxysmal tonic spasms provoked, as they often are, by movement or hyperventilation. The same interpretation can be placed, in our opinion, on the report of paroxysmal kinesigenic choreoathetosis by De Sèze *et al* (2000a). One case of 'alternating-side paroxysmal dystonia' (Lugaresi *et al* 1993) seems likely to be no more than paroxysmal tonic spasms that became bilateral. Coleman *et al* (1988) described two patients presenting with paroxysmal dystonic writer's cramp, suggesting that sustained dystonia may rarely be the first symptom of this disease. Kapoor *et al* (1992) described a case of propriospinal myoclonus possibly originating from cervical spinal cord involvement in multiple sclerosis but did not discuss treatment. There are isolated reports of patients developing parkinsonian features in the setting of suspected long-standing multiple sclerosis (Vieregge *et al* 1992). This suggests comorbidity rather than a direct relationship. The treatment of these rare cases needs to be evaluated individually and using medications appropriate for the shared condition.

Dizziness, vertigo, dysequilibrium and nystagmus

An inseparable part of the motor disabilities that characterize demyelination of brainstem cerebellar pathways is the disorganization of eye movements. Gaze-evoked nystagmus more often ranks as a sign than a symptom requiring treatment. The most common abnormality directly to produce symptoms of oscillopsia or visual instability is bilateral internuclear ophthalmoplegia. Ocular flutter and bobbing are no less disruptive. Starck *et al* (1997) compared scopolamine given by cutaneous patch for 3 days with oral memantine (a glutamate antagonist, given orally at doses of 15–60 mg daily for 7 days) in a small group of patients with acquired pendular nystagmus due to multiple sclerosis. Memantine was considered effective in all patients on the basis of eye movement recordings, whereas scopolamine improved nystagmus in only two of eight. Stabilizing eye movements reduced the symptom of dysequilibrium and improved visual acuity but had no effect on cerebellar function. Some patients continued to derive benefit from memantine and were able to tolerate the drug in the long term. This treatment for a distressing symptom seems an improvement on the essentially negative responses to L-dopa, baclofen, carbamazepine, tetrabenazine, prochlorperazine, primidone, or vigabatrin (Bandini *et al* 2001; Mossmann *et al* 1985), and the partial but unpredictable effects of alcohol, trihexiphenidyl, hyoscine, isoniazid or sodium valproate and clonazepam (Herishanu and Louzoun 1986; Leigh *et al* 1991; Mossmann *et al* 1985; Traccis *et al* 1990). The recent approval of memantine by the Food and Drug Administration (United States) will probably lead to further reports of its putative benefit in patients with multiple sclerosis. A number of recent studies have demonstrated that gabapentin is useful in the treatment of acquired pendular nystagmus due to multiple sclerosis (Averbuch-Heller *et al* 1995; 1997; Bandini *et al* 2001; Stahl *et al* 1996). Both oscillopsia and visual acuity improve in these cases. A patient with both acquired horizontal and vertical nystagmus was described by S. Jain *et al* (2002). Gabapentin improved the horizontal nystagmus and inferior oblique muscle recession thereafter reduced the remaining primary position vertical nystagmus (acuity improved to 6/9 from the pretreatment values of 6/24 and 6/60, respectively). Others have used local injections of botulinum toxin to relieve nystagmus (J. Lee *et al* 1988; Menon and Thaller 2002) and a recent report claimed benefit from both cannabis and ethanol in a single patient with multiple sclerosis (Schon *et al* 1999).

Unsteadiness arising from altered vestibular input may improve with the use of a vestibular sedative such as prochlorperazine or cinnarizine. Vertigo as a manifestation of brainstem disease involving the eighth nerve root entry zone or nuclei may be either a presenting symptom of multiple sclerosis, or may herald a relapse. However, as clearly shown by E.M. Frohman *et al* (2000), other causes of vertigo (particularly benign paroxysmal positional vertigo) must be considered. In their retrospective series, this explained over half the cases of vertigo whereas one-third were attributed to a relapse of multiple sclerosis. It is, of course, important to distinguish these aetiologies to plan appropriate treatment (especially, the particle repositioning manoeuvre of Epley). In their experience, vertigo related to multiple sclerosis usually improves spontaneously or with corticosteroids; one of their patients responded fully to clonazepam.

Swallowing, dysarthria and other manifestations

Although not a common manifestation of multiple sclerosis early in the course, altered bulbar function becomes increasingly obvious and contributes significantly to morbidity as disability increases, usually in the secondary progressive phase.

Dysphagia from disruption of the mechanisms of swallowing develops in many moderately and severely disabled patients with multiple sclerosis and may be potentially life threatening through aspiration or malnutrition (Abraham *et al* 1997; Calcagno *et al* 2002; Daley *et al* 1962; J.C. Hughes *et al* 1994; Thomas and Wiles 1999). As outlined in the recent study by De Pauw *et al* (2002), permanent dysphagia occurs in up to one-quarter of all patients with multiple sclerosis and increases in prevalence as disability advances. Up to two-thirds of the most disabled patients (EDSS > 7.5) and those with severe brainstem dysfunction (Calcagno *et al* 2002) are at risk of aspiration. The disturbance is more common in the oral phase and only rarely affects the pharyngeal component of swallowing. Mildly disabled patients generally have dysphagia for liquids but more disabled patients may have problems also with solids. Patients and their families should be questioned about coughing and choking episodes during meals or previous episodes of pneumonia to identify those that merit study. We recommend a formal swallowing evaluation with video imaging to determine the site and severity of the disorder as videofluoroscopy has been shown to be a sensitive diagnostic study for this complication of multiple sclerosis (Wiesner *et al* 2002). Reminding patients to eat small quantities of food slowly, to chew adequately and avoid talking whilst swallowing may often be sufficient. 'Chin tucking' during swallowing significantly reduces the risk of aspiration. Patients with significant dysphagia for liquids may benefit from the use of thickening agents during meals although this approach is contraindicated in patients with pharyngeal dysfunction. Anecdotally, we have occasionally found that anticholinesterases, used as in the treatment of bulbar weakness due to myasthenia gravis, may improve swallowing in advanced multiple sclerosis but the benefit is transient and may be offset by increased secretions.

Dysarthria, particularly ataxic or mixed spastic–ataxic dysarthria, is a common finding in disabled patients with multiple sclerosis. Speech therapy may be helpful in teaching precision during articulation. In severe examples, communication devices including spelling boards and computer-assisted communication programs may be of value (see below).

Pulmonary complications

There are several situations in which patients with multiple sclerosis and other demyelinating disorders (especially neuromyelitis optica) face significant pulmonary complications (see review by J.L. Carter and Noseworthy 1994). This is most common in the nonambulatory patient with advanced disease. This potentially life-threatening complication should be remembered in the management of the quadriparetic patient. Extensive cervical spinal cord involvement may lead to respiratory muscle weakness from unilateral or bilateral diaphragmatic paralysis (Table 17.3). Patients with neuromuscular respiratory failure may report orthopnoea, a reduced cough and inability to

Table 17.3 Patterns of respiratory involvement with multiple sclerosis

Abnormality	Anatomic localization	Clinical findings at bedside
Paralysis of voluntary respiration	Bilateral corticospinal tracts, brainstem, or upper cervical cord	Unable voluntarily to increase tidal volume or hold breath, automatic respirations intact
Paralysis of automatic respiration	Dorsomedial medulla, nucleus ambiguus, and medial lemnisci	Apnoea during drowsiness, normal voluntary control of respiration while awake
Diaphragmatic paralysis (unilateral or bilateral)	Upper cervical cord (C1–C4 level)	Paradoxic movements of chest wall and abdomen, use of accessory muscles, orthopnoea
Apneustic breathing preserved	Lower brainstem	Inspiratory apneusis, voluntary control between episodes
Paroxysmal hyperventilation	Lower brainstem	Apnoeic pauses after hyperventilation with or without bulbar 'tonic spasms'
Obstructive sleep apnoea	Tegmentum of medulla	Snoring, sleep apnoea, with or without hiccups
Neurogenic pulmonary oedema	Medulla in region of nucleus tractus solitarius and floor of fourth ventricle	Pulmonary oedema without signs of heart failure

Adapted with permission from Carter and Noseworthy (1994).

clear their secretions. On examination, these patients are often unable to increase their tidal volume, to hold their breath, or to count aloud beyond 15 with a single breath. They may demonstrate paradoxical breathing with the use of accessory muscles of respiration. This complication may ultimately be followed by pneumonia, respiratory failure and death. Rarely, however, respiratory muscle weakness heralds a cervical cord relapse and prompt treatment with corticosteroids (or plasma exchange in steroid failures) can prove life saving. In either setting, pulmonary function tests will confirm neuromuscular weakness. Appropriate diagnostic studies and care by physicians skilled in managing respiratory failure are needed. There is recent evidence that respiratory muscle training may be beneficial in the setting of chronic respiratory muscle weakness attributable to multiple sclerosis (Gosselink *et al* 2000).

Much less commonly, acute lesions in the brainstem cause central nervous system disorders of respiration (such as apneustic breathing and central nervous system hyperventilation; Table 17.3). The most dramatic of these complications is neurogenic pulmonary oedema. Acute neurogenic pulmonary oedema is a rare early manifestation of multiple sclerosis (Barnett and Prineas 2004; Crawley *et al* 2001; Gentiloni *et al* 1992; Melin *et al* 1996). The causative lesion is usually in the medulla and affects the nucleus tractus solitarius (Darragh and Simon 1985; R.P. Simon *et al* 1991). Patients present with the clinical picture of acute pulmonary oedema (severe dyspnoea, bloody sputum, diaphoresis, tachycardia and circulatory collapse) and may die within minutes if untreated. This rare disorder must be recognized at once to initiate immediate, potentially life-saving ventilatory support and high-dose corticosteroids.

PERTURBATIONS OF NERVE CONDUCTION

We describe in Chapter 13 the pathophysiology of symptom production and recovery in multiple sclerosis. Amongst these alterations in normal properties of the nerve impulse are a variety of symptoms that arise from perturbations of saltatory conduction. Because they depend on alterations in the passage of ions across the cell membrane, that are increasingly well characterized and amenable to pharmacological manipulation, many can be satisfactorily treated.

Paroxysmal manifestations

The paroxysmal manifestations of multiple sclerosis, resulting from spontaneous discharge in partially demyelinated axons or ephaptic transmission between neighbouring nerve fibres (see Chapters 6 and 13), are amongst the most satisfactory symptoms to treat. Frequently greeted with frank bewilderment or incorrectly attributed to emotional issues, transient ischaemic attacks, epilepsy, or new episodes of demyelination, these characteristic manifestations are amongst the most poorly recognized features of multiple sclerosis, even by competent neurologists, and yet they are so treatable. Understandably, the patient is frustrated or discouraged having experienced many weeks of very frequent episodes without a proper diagnosis. In most patients, a low dose of carbamazepine, valproate or other anticonvulsants that increase membrane stability, will quickly bring these attacks under control to the immediate satisfaction of everyone involved. Generally dubbed 'tonic brainstem paroxysmal attacks', the anatomical basis for these symptoms may be more distributed within the central nervous system. Waubant *et al* (2001) demonstrated convincing evidence from a single patient with multiple sclerosis that a lesion in the posterior internal capsule and adjacent lenticular nucleus may be followed by contralateral paroxysmal, acetazolamide-responsive, dystonia. Zenzola *et al* (2001) reported MRI evidence that a lesion in the thalamus may cause contralateral painful tonic spasms ('paroxysmal dystonia'). Paroxysmal attacks frequently occur relatively early in the course of the illness when disability is limited (Tüzün *et al* 2001).

We generally start with a small dose of carbamazepine (100 or 200 mg orally twice or three times per day) and increase weekly, as needed. Most patients will notice a dramatic response at a dose lower than conventionally needed to control epileptic seizures. Once these episodes are abolished, we usually recommend that the patient continues on medication for about 2–3 months before gradually reducing the dose, then stopping if possible. Some patients will subsequently experience recurrence of these symptoms later in the illness and will quickly call for help. We tell our patients to anticipate a rapid reduction in the frequency of these paroxysms. If the response to treatment is delayed or incomplete, we first advance slowly to the maximum tolerated dose before switching to an alternative anticonvulsant. Rare patients require two anticonvulsants. Solaro *et al* (1998) reported that gabapentin in doses of 600–1200 mg/day is usually effective in the management of paroxysmal symptoms in multiple sclerosis. Recently, Solaro and Tanganelli (2004) reported that four of seven individuals with previously refractory painful tonic spasms benefited within 4 weeks from a gradually increasing dose of tiagabine (starting at 5 mg orally per day, increasing as needed to a maximum of 30 mg/day) when more conventional agents had previously failed.

Pain

Nonparoxysmal pain is more complex, less completely understood and generally more refractory to treatment than paroxysmal pain in patients with multiple sclerosis. It is not a trivial or uncommon problem. Two papers, published in the 1980s, highlighted the problem of pain in the context of multiple sclerosis (Clifford and Trotter 1984; Moulin *et al* 1988). These two large surveys highlighted that between 28 and 55% of patients may suffer from significant acute or chronic pain syndromes at some stage during their illness.

In a recent postal survey from Denmark, Svendsen *et al* (2003) reported that patients with multiple sclerosis are more likely than those with other disorders to report severe pain, require analgesics or acknowledge that pain interferes with their quality of life. Although the frequency of pain may not differ significantly between these two populations of patients, the impact appears greater in multiple sclerosis. Ehde *et al* (2003) found that >40% of those responding to a survey reported a significant and moderately severe pain disorder in the preceding 3 months. One-quarter reported chronic pain of a severe degree interfering with daily life. Advanced disability (EDSS >6.5) and depression increased the risk both of the likelihood that pain would be reported and that it would interfere with daily activities. Although there is inherent bias in a self-reporting survey of this nature, the report indicates that pain may be an important component of life with multiple sclerosis.

Each of these studies reminds us of the need to ask about pain in patients with multiple sclerosis and then to seek an accurate diagnosis to guide therapy. Acute, chronic and recurrent back and extremity pain may be persistent, cramping, lancinating or burning in nature. Pain may be restricted to one limb, the face or a combination of sites. Pain can be unilateral or bilateral, mild or severe. Pain may accompany very specific syndromes (such as the acute discomfort triggered by eye movements in optic neuritis; Lhermitte's symptom; painful tonic spasms; painful flexor spasms; painful band-like tightness involving the trunk or an extremity). It is rather common for patients to describe troublesome pain disorders that evolve gradually and are seemingly independent of an acute relapse. Patients with long-standing sensory loss may experience disagreeable paraesthesiae or burning

in the extremities. These symptoms are often constant or primarily noticed during periods of rest or inactivity. Others will describe lightning-like lancinations that are often restricted to one body site.

Additionally, the physician must be vigilant for common and often treatable pain syndromes that may be seen in any disabled population, including shoulder and trochanteric bursitis, epicondylitis, cervical and lumbar spondylosis, spinal stenosis, entrapment neuropathies, overuse injuries, and other ligamentous and arthritic conditions. Severely disabled patients often notice trunk and low back discomfort in association with prolonged sessions in one posture. As discussed above, spasticity may be complicated by painful spasms involving either trunk or limb extensor and flexor muscles. We have seen acute radicular symptoms both in the setting of acute multiple sclerosis relapses (presumably the demyelinating plaque involves the root entry or exit zone) and as a result of conditions other than multiple sclerosis such as disc herniation.

Optimal patient management requires accurate diagnosis and involvement of the patient and caregivers in the treatment plan. Diagnostic procedures (especially imaging) are often informative when there are underlying structural causes for the pain disorder. Empirical treatment may be useful for patients suffering from focal bursitis (including corticosteroid injections, local application of ice, and avoidance of local trauma to the site).

The same approaches apply to the management of chronic pain in multiple sclerosis as in any other medical context. The physician must carefully evaluate the symptom complex, the patient's premorbid personality, the social situation, comorbidity (depression, insomnia or diabetic neuropathy) and willingness to participate in a comprehensive pain management strategy. Typically each of these variables needs attention. Difficult or threatening home situations must be identified and addressed. Insomnia and mood disorders must be treated appropriately. Mechanical stressors (improperly fitting or inadequate orthoses, a poorly fitted wheelchair, abnormalities of posture and seating hygiene, amongst other issues) must be corrected.

Nonsteroidal anti-inflammatory medications and physical therapy may have a role in many pain disorders. Spasticity should be addressed (see above), and paroxysmal disorders should be recognized and treated appropriately. Decubitus ulcers have to be managed systematically and successfully. In refractory cases, consultation with a comprehensive, multidisciplinary pain management team may be helpful. The role of antidepressants is complex and often requires tact in explaining that the mechanism of action is primarily an effect on neurochemical properties of pain pathways in the central nervous system and not because pain in multiple sclerosis is invariably a symptom of depression. That said, all these sensations are coped with less well in the context of impaired mood. In our opinion, tricyclic antidepressants (especially amitriptyline) are superior to the selective serotonin reuptake inhibitors for the management of chronic, burning, dysaesthetic extremity pain, and when taken at bedtime may help insomnia.

Dysaesthetic pain syndromes are difficult to treat but gabapentin is widely used for many pain disorders; it is generally well tolerated and the dose range is vast (300–3600 mg/day). Anecdotal evidence (Samkoff *et al* 1997) and an open uncontrolled study involving 25 patients support the general belief that gabapentin has a role in the management of painful syndromes associated with multiple sclerosis, although adverse effects can limit the perceived benefits in these clinical contexts (Houtchens *et al* 1997). Table 17.1 lists commonly used medications employed in the management of pain disorders in multiple sclerosis.

Trigeminal neuralgia

The most discrete pain syndrome occurring as a symptom of multiple sclerosis is trigeminal neuralgia but focal, tic-like lancinating pain may involve other sites in the head, neck, trunk and extremities in patients with multiple sclerosis. The mainstay of treatment is the use of anticonvulsants – carbamazepine and valproate in conventional doses. Trigeminal neuralgia also responds to the prostaglandin E1 agonist misoprostol in an oral dose of 300 mg twice daily, presumably by an effect on cytokines which mediate painful inflammation of trigeminal nerve roots (Reder and Arnason 1995; DMKG Study Group 2003). Following an earlier report that lamotrigine may be effective in treating trigeminal neuralgia (Lunardi *et al* 1997), Leandri *et al* (2000) reported that all but one of 18 patients with multiple sclerosis who failed carbamazepine reported either complete or nearly complete pain relief with lamotrigine at a dose of between 75 and 100 mg orally per day, although one patient had to discontinue treatment because of a rash. Glossopharyngeal neuralgia is much less common in multiple sclerosis than trigeminal neuralgia but may also respond to carbamazepine (Minagar and Sheremata 2000).

Microvascular decompression has rarely been used in patients with multiple sclerosis given the general sense that the neuralgia is likely to be lesion-related and not the result of vessel ectasia (see Figure 6.18). However, Broggi *et al* (2000) reported that five of ten patients with multiple sclerosis in a series of 250 with trigeminal neuralgia treated with microvascular decompression achieved excellent results. Recurrence risk for their series was 15% during a mean follow-up of 38 months. At present there is not sufficient information on which to advise patients with multiple sclerosis of recurrence after microvascular decompression and it seems reasonable to prefer other surgical procedures given their superior outcomes in medically refractory cases. Kanpolat *et al* (2000) reported on 17 patients with multiple sclerosis treated with percutaneous controlled radiofrequency rhizotomy from a large series (1672 patients). The majority (82%) had complete relief with one or repeated multiple rhizotomies (< 20% required repeated procedures) and 17% received partial benefit but required adjunctive medical management. Berk *et al* (2003) reported similar response rates in 13 patients, with a 50% recurrence risk at 52 months. No serious adverse effects were reported in either series, and few patients seemed to mind the facial numbness introduced by this procedure. The results of gamma-knife neurosurgery, reporting on a dose of 70–90 Gy to a single 4-mm isocentre at the trigeminal nerve root entry zone, have also now been evaluated. Brisman and Mooij (2000) reported that patients with multiple sclerosis are less likely to achieve excellent pain relief at 6 and 12 months using a maximum dose of 75 Gy (multiple sclerosis: five of 21 improved at 6 months and two of 15 improved at 12 months; others, 47 of 105 improved at 6 months and 28 of 41 improved at 12 months). Excellent results were reported by E. Huang *et al* (2002) for all seven patients treated using a dose of 80–90 Gy (latency 1 day to 8 months; one recurrence at 24 months). Rogers *et al* (2002)

reported an 80% response rate in 15 patients with multiple sclerosis (with peak effect seen after a mean latency of 56 days). Delayed facial numbness may follow this procedure.

Rasche *et al* (2004) reported a case of refractory trigeminal neuralgia that responded to microvascular decompression of the superior cerebellar artery. In this case, repeated radiofrequency rhizotomies had failed to control the patient's symptoms. Preoperative MRI demonstrated the site of trigeminal nerve compression. The patient remained free of pain on no medications at 14 months. McNatt *et al* (2005) reported that gamma knife radiosurgery provided benefit to 61% of 49 patients with previously medically intractable trigeminal neuralgia due to multiple sclerosis. Fifty per cent of responders were pain free off medications but a total of 23% suffered a recurrence of pain after a mean interval of 9.6 months. Forty-seven per cent reported mild to moderate facial numbness or dysesthesias following treatment. Considering the theoretical potential for long-term sequelae and the known morbidity from radiation therapy in multiple sclerosis, we feel that further experience is needed before recommending radiosurgery in this setting. Pickett *et al* (2005) reported that percutaneous retrogasserian glycerol rhizotomy resulted in complete (78%) or partial (13%) pain control in their series of 53 patients with trigeminal neuralgia due to multiple sclerosis. However, 59% experienced a recurrence (at a mean interval of 17 months), and one-half of re-treated patients had recurrent symptoms within a further year. It seems that radiosurgery and percutaneous rhizotomy are effective for many patients with refractory trigeminal neuralgia but both seem to be associated with a high and relatively early risk of recurrence. Alternative measures that may prove necessary include cutaneous electrical stimulation of the dorsal spinal cord, transcutaneous nerve stimulation (TENS), regional sympathetic blockade or destruction of nerve fibres using alcohol or phenol and differential nerve root section.

Heat sensitivity and Uhthoff's phenomenon

As discussed earlier, many patients are sensitive to changes in ambient temperature. It is important to understand this phenomenon, both to anticipate and control the transient symptomatic worsening that follows and to recognize that such changes are not heralding a relapse. In general we recommend avoiding exposure to excessively hot climates (air conditioning); adequate hydration with cool liquids, soaking the shirt or headband, or blanketing the head and shoulders with light, wet towels during planned exercise; and the use of tepid baths and antipyretics in the setting of febrile illnesses. Profoundly heat-sensitive patients with previous paraparesis should avoid using hot baths and spas unaccompanied, because a severe Uhthoff's reaction could (theoretically) place them at risk of drowning – although we are not aware of any such accidents. Cooling vests are marketed for patients with multiple sclerosis but the simple measures described above usually suffice.

Seizure disorders

Seizures are not especially common in patients with multiple sclerosis. Although several reports suggest an increased incidence of seizures (Ghezzi *et al* 1990; Kinnunen and Wikström 1986; Olafsson *et al* 1999), this was not confirmed in a recent population-based study (Nyquist *et al* 2002). Our experience is that most patients with multiple sclerosis complicated by seizures can readily be controlled with a single anticonvulsant. This experience is substantiated by the evidence that only 11% of patients with seizures had medically refractory epilepsy (Nyquist *et al* 2001). Although there are reports of death from status epilepticus occurring in patients with multiple sclerosis (R.S. Allison 1950), refractory seizures are uncommon. It has been our experience that the rare patient who experiences a first seizure in the setting of a relapse consistent with a lesion in the cerebral hemispheres (usually frontal or temporal lobe origin) may not require long-term anticonvulsant medications.

COGNITIVE FUNCTION

As outlined in Chapter 6, patients with multiple sclerosis may develop important problems with cognitive function, particularly memory, abstracting ability, attention, executive functioning and processing speed, whereas speech and recognition memory, and implicit learning are often spared (Beatty and Monson 1996; Brassington and Marsh 1998; M. Grossman *et al* 1995; Lincoln *et al* 2002; Litvan *et al* 1988; Rao *et al* 1989a; 1989b; 1993). Minor abnormalities can often be noted on cognitive testing in apparently asymptomatic patients. The prevalence of important cognitive dysfunction increases with disease duration and is seen more often in patients with progressive disease. Patients, family members and employers may notice problems with multitasking. Deficits often progress with time (Amato *et al* 2001).

We urge patients who hold responsible jobs to undergo formal psychometric testing when concerns arise about cognition, so as to reduce the consequences of poor judgment and decision-making. Similarly, we instruct patients and their families to be aware that cognitive dysfunction may impact on important personal domestic and professional decisions.

The treatment of cognitive dysfunction in multiple sclerosis is limited. Acute worsening of cognitive function may accompany a relapse and respond to corticosteroids. Patients with cerebral multiple sclerosis are prone to reversible worsening in the setting of disturbances in metabolic function (including electrolyte imbalance, sepsis and drug side effects). However, chronic, irreversible cognitive dysfunction must currently be managed by educating the patient and caregivers – much as for other dementing illnesses. There need to be safeguards that limit the chance of personal injury from cooking, smoking or domestic hot water (we advise turning down the water temperature to avoid accidental scalding injuries) and important financial decisions should be made with input from others. It is sometimes also necessary to reduce the executive independence of the patient in the work place, in order to reduce the impact of poor decision-making. Patients may benefit from consultation with a multidisciplinary team that has expertise in managing disorders of memory. Aids may be useful (especially a personal hand-held computer). Preliminary evidence suggests that computer-assisted retraining may benefit patients with impairments in attention (Plohmann *et al* 1998).

In a small randomized, placebo-controlled trial involving 45 patients, Geisler *et al* (1996) demonstrated that amantadine and pemoline do not improve cognitive functioning in multiple sclerosis. Clearly there is the hope that early treatment with dis-

ease-modifying agents may delay or reduce the complication, but this remains unproven. Weinstein *et al* (1999) recently reported that 248 individuals with relapsing–remitting multiple sclerosis treated with glatiramer acetate remained cognitively unchanged over a 2 year period. Fischer *et al* (2000) reported that patients randomized to receive weekly intramuscular injections of interferon-β1a for 104 weeks did better than patients receiving placebo on the Comprehensive NP Battery, particularly within the domains of information processing and learning and memory. Clearly longer follow-up of many more patients is needed for a definitive statement to be made.

Jønsson *et al* (1993) reported a randomized controlled trial designed to determine whether specific cognitive treatment (including direct training, compensatory strategies and psychotherapy) is superior to a control strategy (deliberately diffuse mental stimulation). After a mean of 46 days of treatment, important differences in measures of depression and visuospatial memory favoured the directed strategy. More recently, Lincoln *et al* (2002) reported the results of a single-blind, randomized trial to determine whether knowledge of the results of cognitive testing, or this information together with a treatment programme tailored to the patient's deficits, would result in better outcomes at 4 and 8 months. The results did not favour intervention; in general, the control group (no knowledge of the results of testing, and no intervention) did no worse than individuals exposed to the bespoke intervention. This disappointing result of cognitive assessment and rehabilitation may reflect a number of trial design deficiencies (acknowledged by the authors) but overall suggests that much work needs to be done to provide meaningful help for this important complication of the disease. Krupp *et al* (2004) reported that oral donepezil hydrochloride (10 mg orally daily for 24 weeks) may provide some improvement based on the findings of their randomized, double-blind, placebo-controlled study of 69 patients with memory complaints associated with multiple sclerosis. As noted in an accompanying editorial (Doraiswamy and Rao 2004), this study will likely be followed by others addressing this important and occasionally disabling symptom. A larger study is planned to confirm these promising findings.

Competency and 'the vulnerable adult'

The neurologist may be asked to judge the ability of a chronically disabled patient with multiple sclerosis to understand both the issues that they face in making important life decisions (such as competency) and the nature of their acts (capacity; see review by David 2004). This situation arises most commonly in the patient with cognitive impairment from cerebral involvement in multiple sclerosis. In this setting, we recommend neuropsychological testing and, often, a psychiatric consultation to assist in providing advice.

Demented and chronically disabled patients are 'vulnerable adults' and, as such, are at risk of emotional, physical and sexual abuse by others. The physician should remain vigilant for behaviours and physical signs that may indicate abuse or neglect. The clues include change to a more passive demeanour, the presence of a dominant (controlling) partner or caregiver at all visits, non-compliance with appointments, evidence of 'accidental injuries' (burns, laceration or bruising), vague 'somatic' complaints, the development of a chronic pain disorder, drug-seeking behaviour or substance abuse, pseudoseizures, a suicide attempt and presentation with a conversion reaction, or other apparently 'functional' manifestations. In this setting, considerable care is needed to confirm that abuse or neglect are taking place. Once confirmed, the physician is responsible for initiating appropriate steps to protect the patient (see review by Massey 2003).

Psychiatric abnormalities

Psychiatric illness complicates multiple sclerosis in many patients and may contribute to morbidity and risk of suicide (Caine and Schwid 2002; Feinstein 2002; Patten *et al* 2002; Ron and Feinstein 1992; Sadovnick *et al* 1991b). As discussed in Chapter 6, the full range of psychiatric illness is seen in this chronic illness but anxiety and mood disorders predominate. Major depression has been shown in a recent population-based study to be increased in affected individuals (odds ratio 2.3) compared with persons without multiple sclerosis (Patten *et al* 2003). As discussed earlier, patients with multiple sclerosis are at risk of suicide (Sadovnick *et al* 1991b), especially young patients with mild or moderate disability. The effect on quality of life cannot be overstated in this chronic and unpredictable disease. Patients face an uncertain future. Many volunteer that the relative absence of readily apparent outward, physical evidence of illness coupled with the high prevalence of (sometimes disabling) fatigue compounds their fear. With progressive physical disability, social isolation becomes an important issue for many. There is some evidence that bipolar disorder may be associated with multiple sclerosis (Joffe *et al* 1987; Schiffer *et al* 1986). Brief episodes of psychosis may occur as manifestations of multiple sclerosis (Davison and Bagley 1969; Feinstein and Ron 1990). Corticosteroids may provoke anxiety, acute confusional states, depression, mania and psychosis. Although the literature remains ambiguous on whether interferons provoke or worsen depression (Borràs *et al* 1999; European Study Group on Interferon β-1b in Secondary Progressive MS 1998; L.D. Jacobs *et al* 1996; Klapper 1994; Patten and Metz and Group SS 2002; PRISMS Study Group 1998), recent evidence suggests that response to antidepressant medication is unaltered by interferon therapy (Feinstein 2002). Early diagnosis of psychiatric comorbidity is essential to reduce the burden of these disorders. There is no reason to conclude that patients with multiple sclerosis respond differently to standard psychiatric treatment strategies than any other individuals.

VISUAL LOSS

Pain on eye movement commonly accompanies acute optic neuritis. This generally resolves quickly following treatment with corticosteroids, or (perhaps) more slowly in untreated patients. An occasional patient will complain of recurrent or chronic eye pain. These individuals should consult an ophthalmologist for other more treatable causes but, in our experience, nothing is usually discovered. In the absence of clinical evidence for active optic neuritis, we generally recommend a trial either of non-steroidal anti-inflammatory medication or gabapentin. The results are often disappointing. Anecdotal reports suggest that a short course of oral corticosteroids may be helpful. Clearly, prolonged or repeated courses should be avoided in the management of this uncommon symptom.

Visual symptoms often persist after optic neuritis, manifesting as reduced colour intensity, loss of edge definition and depth perception, and after images in patients not necessarily noticing significant loss of acuity. Currently little can be done for these patients.

Patients with acute diplopia in the setting of a relapse are more comfortable using a cloth eye patch until they recover. With time, even in the setting of unresolved internuclear ophthalmoplegia, diplopia generally clears completely – presumably as a result of cortical extinction of the ghost image. Prism lenses are often a great help in this setting (either temporary or ground into glasses providing the deviation is < 40 prism dioptres). Much less commonly, botulinum toxin injection into extra-ocular muscles may temporarily restore muscle imbalance or reduce the amplitude of persisting nystagmus for the occasional patient with persistent diplopia.

In the United States, persons must have vision of at least 20/40 in at least one eye to hold a driving licence but laws (especially those governing visual field requirements) vary extensively between countries and even across regions (i.e. states). In the United Kingdom, patients are required to declare multiple sclerosis to the licensing authorities who, on the advice of the treating physician, may require confirmation that a vehicle number plate can be read at 20 m – which acts as an indicator of adequate acuity. Impairment of colour vision may reduce driving safety in the setting of flashing traffic signals. Clearly in evaluating whether the person with multiple sclerosis is safe to operate a motor vehicle, other issues must be considered. These include assessment of additional complex cognitive (attention, visuo-spatial processing, executive function, memory and learning) and sensorimotor impairments (proprioception, coordination, spasticity and speed, strength and accuracy of movement) that place the patient or other road users at risk (M. Rizzo and Kellison 2004).

As noted previously, extreme bilateral, persistent visual loss from irreversible optic neuritis is uncommon in multiple sclerosis (more often seen in neuromyelitis optica). Rare patients will experience persistent hemianopia or cortical blindness. For patients rendered nearly blind from long-standing optic neuritis, referral to a low-vision specialist is in order. These ophthalmologists and optometrists are able to offer appropriate assistance, often working together with other health care professionals (social workers, occupational therapists and visual rehabilitation workers). Low-vision rehabilitation utilizes low-vision aids, illumination and training to maximize participation in independent living. These aids include magnifiers, telescopes, electronic devices, and large-text reading material, as well as nonoptical devices such as playing cards, books on tape and compact discs, software for computers, reading stands and lamps. Rehabilitation services for the blind may assist with devices and training in the home (operator assistance for phone calls), to assist in the activities of daily living and to reduce personal risk (for example, from cooking and house fires). The rehabilitation of patients with hemianopia or full cortical visual loss (again, uncommon and more likely to be on the basis of another diagnosis) is more difficult. The use of prismatic corrections and training to maximize visual function can be effective. The results of 'blindsight' training using forced choice techniques and performance feedback to facilitate saccades toward or pursuit of objects into the blind field is controversial and beyond the scope of this text

(Pambakian and Kennard 1997; J.A. Sharpe 2003; Zihl and Werth 1984).

REHABILITATION IN MULTIPLE SCLEROSIS

In many communities, the availability of specialty services offered by rehabilitation facilities for people with multiple sclerosis is sparse and access throughout the course of their illness is intermittent. Within the last decade there has been an increasing effort to improve and validate the benefits of these services as part of the strategy for optimizing treatment methods used to control symptoms accompanying the disorder. It follows that this is a changing landscape with much yet to be done. In this era of rising medical costs and increasing governmental scrutiny of health care delivery, it is appropriate that the principles of evidence-based research be applied to the delivery of rehabilitation services. The preliminary work is promising and a number of treatment approaches are now validated. Against this background, we anticipate increasing investment in validated programmes designed to provide these services for people with multiple sclerosis.

The Disability Committee of the Royal College of Physicians (1991) defined rehabilitation as 'an active process of change by which a person who has become disabled acquires and uses the knowledge and skills necessary for optimal physical, psychological and social functioning'. This definition underscores the principles of empowerment inherent in rehabilitation. The patient and their family must actively engage in effecting change in attitudes and activities so as to promote an optimal quality of life. Multiple sclerosis affects physical, psychological and social functions. A multidisciplinary rehabilitation facility provides resources to deal with many of these needs. The changing clinical challenges and social threats accompanying a lifetime with multiple sclerosis make it necessary for patients and their physicians to understand the dynamic role of rehabilitation services during the course of the illness. The temporary challenge presented by an acute relapse differs substantially from that of chronic or recurring symptoms (for example, the neurogenic bladder and altered bowel function, fatigue or spasticity) and from the steady loss of ambulation that may accompany the progressive phase of multiple sclerosis. As such, treating physicians should regularly re-evaluate their patients' needs for rehabilitation services. The interested reader is referred to a number of recent reviews that provide useful insights into the benefits of a comprehensive, multidisciplinary, individualized, carefully coordinated rehabilitation programme for patients with multiple sclerosis (Freeman and Thompson 2003; Gibson and Frank 2002; Kraft 1998; LaBan et al 1998; Reitberg et al 2005; A.J. Thompson 1998; 2002b). At some time during the illness, most patients will require the expertise of one or more members of such a team including those with skills in nursing, physical and occupational therapy, psychiatry and psychology, sexual counselling, speech and language, nutrition, wound care, continence (including urology, physical medicine and rehabilitation physicians, therapists and nurses), orthotics, wheelchair needs, evaluation of motor vehicle operation (including assessment for hand controls), social work, and employment advice. Assembling such a team may seem daunting but, without these inputs, the person with multiple sclerosis may be at a disadvantage. Increasingly such teams are focusing on goal setting and evaluation of out-

comes both for the individual patient and the new treatment programmes themselves. Within this context, it is essential that a health care provider, knowledgeable about the needs of people with multiple sclerosis and wise to resources available in the community, offers continuous care. The added value of rehabilitation in the management of acute relapse is discussed in Chapter 16.

Increasingly, clinical research is utilizing more sensitive outcome measures to determine the value of innovative treatments. As outlined in our discussion on the use of MRI technology to study the course of multiple sclerosis (see Chapters 7 and 13), recent functional MRI (fMRI) and positron emission tomography (PET) studies have provided insights into possible mechanisms of recovery (including cortical activation and brain reorganization) in multiple sclerosis (Hillary et al 2003; Pantano et al 2002; Reddy et al 2002; Staffen et al 2002). It seems likely that these and other sensitive physiological and imaging outcome measures will increasingly be used to validate rehabilitation strategies. Functional MRI has recently been used to show an alteration in the cortical response when subjects with multiple sclerosis receive a cholinergic pharmacotherapeutic intervention during cognitive testing (A.M. Parry et al 2003).

Delivery of out-patient rehabilitation services

There are now several studies demonstrating the utility of out-patient rehabilitation services. Di Fabio et al (1998) compared the frequency of symptom control and functional status in a group of 46 disabled patients with multiple sclerosis (EDSS 5.0–8.0) studied whilst on the waiting list for an out-patient rehabilitation programme (compared with 26 controls) and during and at 1 year after enrolment (n = 20). Extended out-patient rehabilitation (5 hours of services on 1 day per week for 1 year) reduced symptom frequency and fatigue levels but had no effect on functional status. Pozzilli et al (2002) randomized a group of 201 patients with multiple sclerosis to receive 1 year of either home-based or hospital care (control group). Home-based care included an individualized needs assessment by a multidisciplinary team that included two neurologists, a urologist, a rehabilitation physician, a physical therapist, a nurse, a social worker and a care coordinator. These patients then had access to nursing care, physiotherapists, psychologists, home intravenous medication administration, and educational and social services. The control group continued to receive care from their physicians with access to hospital, as needed. The authors concluded that home care is slightly more cost-effective than conventional management. Home-based care achieved important gains in measures of general health, pain, role–emotion, and social functioning on the Short Form General Health Survey (SF-36). The functional status was equivalent with both systems of care delivery. Patti et al (2002) studied 111 patients with multiple sclerosis randomized either to an intense out-patient rehabilitation programme (6 days per week for 6 weeks) or waiting list with instruction in a home exercise programme. They conclude that this out-patient rehabilitation programme improved practically every measured quality of life index as well as mood (Beck Depression Index) and social functioning (Social Experience Check-list). Romberg et al (2004) reported that a 6 month graded exercise programme enhanced walking speed, leg strength and arm endurance and dexterity when studied in a randomized, controlled study of 114 mild or moderately disabled patients (EDSS 1.0–5.5). A recently completed systematic review of the literature on exercise therapy by Rietberg *et al* (2005) provides support for its use in the management of multiple sclerosis in remission. Conversely, based on systematic review, Steultjens *et al* (2004) conclude that published studies on the role of occupational therapy in the management of multiple sclerosis are inconclusive.

Delivery of in-patient rehabilitation services

Early studies of inpatient rehabilitation services in multiple sclerosis suggested a variety of benefits to patient care but few were randomized or adequately controlled (Aisen *et al* 1996; Carey *et al* 1988; Feigenson *et al* 1981; Francabandera *et al* 1988; Greenspun *et al* 1987; Kidd and Thompson 1997; Reding and LaRocca 1987). Petajan *et al* (1996) assessed the role of aerobic training on several somewhat ephemeral aspects of daily living in 54 patients randomized to exercise or non-exercise in three 40 minute training sessions each week. Apart from getting fitter, the patients who exercised were happier, less angry, less fatigued, and more active domestically and in recreation. In short, life was better. In the first controlled study of in-patient rehabilitation, Freeman *et al* (1997) randomized 66 patients with progressive multiple sclerosis either to a waiting list or to early in-patient treatment. The in-patient programme addressed the individual needs of each patient using a multidisciplinary approach to create a package structured to improve quality of life. Services included those provided by the primary care physician, psychiatry, psychology, urology, speech and language therapists, nursing, and occupational and physical therapy. Measures of impairment (EDSS and FS) did not differ between groups at the end of 6 weeks. However, treated patients demonstrated improved disability (the motor domain of the Functional Independence Measure and other subscales) and handicap measures (London Handicap Scale). The authors followed 50 of these patients at 3 monthly intervals for 1 year (Freeman *et al* 1999). The early benefits were maintained for several months (disability and handicap were stable for the first 6 months; emotional status for 7 months; and several quality of life measures were stable for up to 10 months) despite evidence for clear clinical neurological worsening in the majority of patients (median EDSS changed from 6.8 at baseline to 8.0 at 1 year). The authors stressed the need to maintain continuous care of patients with progressive multiple sclerosis so as to optimize treatment needs after an initial in-patient rehabilitation programme. In a randomized, crossover trial of 40 patients with multiple sclerosis, Wiles *et al* (2001) reported benefits in the Rivermead Mobility Index both for in-patient and home physiotherapy programmes.

In terms of the preferred location, Wiles *et al* (2001) investigated the effect of both hospital and home-based physiotherapy in 40 patients with chronic multiple sclerosis using a randomized crossover trial design with an 8 week period of physiotherapy or no treatment. Compared to no treatment, they found that physiotherapy in either location was associated with improved mobility, sense of well-being and mood, but the benefits may last for only a few weeks. Improvement was also reported by C. Liu *et al* (2003) in a number of clinical and patient-based outcome measures following a period of in-patient neurorehabilitation in a cohort of 90 patients with relapsing–remitting multiple sclerosis. The benefit was most apparent in those with incomplete recovery from relapses who had accumulated moderate to severe disability, and was independent of the timing of corticosteroid treatment. This is also a subgroup of patients in whom there is at least some prospect of stabilizing the underlying relapse-related activity of the disease using one of the existing disease-modifying treatments. Thus, the introduction of drug treatment in parallel with neurorehabilitation offers a better chance for the rehabilitation intervention to result in sustained benefits to the patient.

Delivery of rehabilitation using community services

The perception is that people with multiple sclerosis are heavy consumers of community facilities. Clearly, patients with advanced progressive multiple sclerosis require access to these resources but many are infrequent users of community or rehabilitation services. Conversely, other patients have important needs that are never adequately recognized or addressed. As demonstrated by Stolp-Smith (1998) in a population-based study of a resource-rich community (Olmsted County, Minnesota served by the Mayo Clinic), > 80% of patients with multiple sclerosis never utilize home health services and 90% were currently not tapping these resources. Many admitted to low compliance with equipment they had acquired whereas others had unmet needs. The authors demonstrated a clear relationship between disease severity, unemployment status and utilization of services but could not correlate service use with disease duration, age of onset or educational achievements. Williams and Bowie (1993) reported that severely disabled patients were more likely to receive appropriate community and other services if a multidisciplinary team rather than a single provider coordinated their care. Freeman and Thompson (2000) recently reported findings from a survey of 150 patients with multiple sclerosis. The majority received no community services (including 39% with moderate and 12% with severe disability). As such, there appeared to be important discrepancies in access to community services for this population.

Adaptive and assistive devices

A wide array of adaptive devices is now available to help manage the disabilities of multiple sclerosis (Stolp-Smith *et al* 1997). An incomplete list would include transfer devices (sliding boards, transfer slings, and floor-based or ceiling-mounted transfer devices), hygiene aids [toothbrushes and hairdryers, bidets, microcomputerized toilet seats (Washlet SIII)], environmental control units, voice-dial speaker phones, and power-assisted hospital beds) and communication aids (computer-based onscreen keyboards, word prediction programs and voice recognition software). Occupational therapists are usually best suited to advise on home modifications including ramps, bathroom remodelling (seats, toilet modifications, shower stalls and lifts). Neurologists caring for disabled patients with multiple sclerosis need to familiarize themselves with the expertise of rehabilitation facilities in their region and access these and other evolving technologies on behalf of their patients.

CONCLUSION

The management of symptoms in multiple sclerosis is more than the prescribing of drugs. The principles of providing comprehensive care to the patient with multiple sclerosis are similar to those guiding the care of any patient with chronic illness. The physician must earn the trust of the patient and family and help them to understand the complex problems that multiple sclerosis may bring to their lives. The physician must remain vigilant to the needs of each patient and pay particular attention not only to their mental and physical health but also to the stability of the home environment and financial security. The physician must be familiar with the support services available in the community and recruit these, as needed. The physician must remain current with the literature and be comfortable prescribing symptomatic treatments. The therapeutic armamentarium continues to grow at a rapid pace, making it increasingly possible to ameliorate the symptoms of this life-long condition.

Disease-modifying treatments in multiple sclerosis

John Noseworthy, David Miller and Alastair Compston

THE AIMS OF DISEASE-MODIFYING TREATMENT

There have been many developments since we last reviewed the role of disease-modifying treatments in multiple sclerosis. Collectively, these represent progress but fall well short of a solution to the problem. Results of the pivotal interferon and glatiramer acetate trials led to approval of these treatments by licensing bodies throughout the world. For the first time, patients with multiple sclerosis had a treatment. This was welcome and fuelled further efforts to improve on the evidence for efficacy and indications for the timing, dose and duration of therapy. Increasingly sensitive diagnostic criteria, bolstered by serial magnetic resonance imaging (MRI) studies (W.I. McDonald *et al* 2001), now allow more rapid diagnosis and hence – in our current climate – earlier exposure to treatment. However, further work is needed on many strategic issues and points of detail:

- Will early treatment make a difference?
- Can sensitive clinical and MRI measures detect early favourable trends that predict long-term benefit?
- Might the trials be made even shorter?
- How early in any study should a monitoring committee conclude with certainty that a trial is positive and recommend early termination with generalized access to the therapy?

It is axiomatic that doctors want to make their patients better. Patients want to lead normal lives unencumbered by any physical, psychological or life-style baggage related to multiple sclerosis. As clinical scientists, we need to structure that pastoral position around concepts of the pathogenesis and strategies for what realistically can be achieved. Patients with multiple sclerosis need treatment before the onset of fixed disability. Throughout, we have argued that the clinical manifestations of multiple sclerosis can be attributed to perivascular inflammation and the tissue injury with which it is inextricably linked. Since we last reviewed the subject in 1998, the diversity of mechanisms that injure nerve fibres throughout the illness and the contribution these processes make to the clinical course have been intensively studied. Concepts have been updated and revised. Thus, whilst we remain of the view that inflammation is pivotal to the destruction in parallel of axons and oligodendroglia, the inflammatory process also triggers biological processes that increasingly contribute to tissue destruction. What position should the prescribing physician take on how and when to treat the person with multiple sclerosis? Our stance is pragmatic but informed by the neurobiology and neuroimmunology, and by the evidence from clinical trials.

We structure this discussion around the formulation that, typically, the early clinical course of multiple sclerosis is marked by relapses from which symptomatic recovery is usually complete. Inflammation drives the process. Subsequent episodes may affect the same or different myelinated pathways. Before long, clinical deficits, which correlate with abnormalities in saltatory conduction of the nerve impulse, accumulate. These reflect loss of functional reserve in the adaptive capacity of the nervous system to make best use of surviving electrical activity, and the impoverished but detectable signals that reach the cortex or distant parts of major pathways. Then, inflammation wanes (without necessarily ceasing) and the relative contribution of cumulative axonal damage, amplified by loss of trophic support, makes an impact (Figure 18.1). Initially, the clinical course is intermittent in 80% of affected individuals but a high proportion do later enter the secondary progressive phase in which impairment, loss of ability, and impact on health-related quality of life are each affected. For these patients, disability is established in 40% by 10 years, in 60% by 15 years and in 80% (that is 50% of all patients) by 25 years. It is the onset of secondary progression that gives multiple sclerosis the frightening reputation it has amongst affected individuals. Progression is the main factor distinguishing mild from severe forms of multiple sclerosis. In 20% of patients, the disease progresses slowly from onset, most typically with predominant spinal involvement, and this form of multiple sclerosis is even more predictably disabling. The analysis that fully reversible deficits mainly result from inflammtion, oedema and the physiological action of cytokines whereas persistent symptoms and signs can be attributed to demyelination and the initial wave of axonal damage with failure of recovery mechanisms, and that chronic progression is attributable to cumulative axon degeneration, has obvious implications for treatment.

Immunological therapies are most likely to be effective in the inflammatory (relapsing–remitting and relapsing–persistent) phases. Conversely, it will be more difficult to influence progression with immunotherapy. Any treatment that reduces the accumulation of disability, and inhibits or delays time to onset of the progressive phase, is most likely to have a clinically useful disease-modifying effect whether or not that treatment also

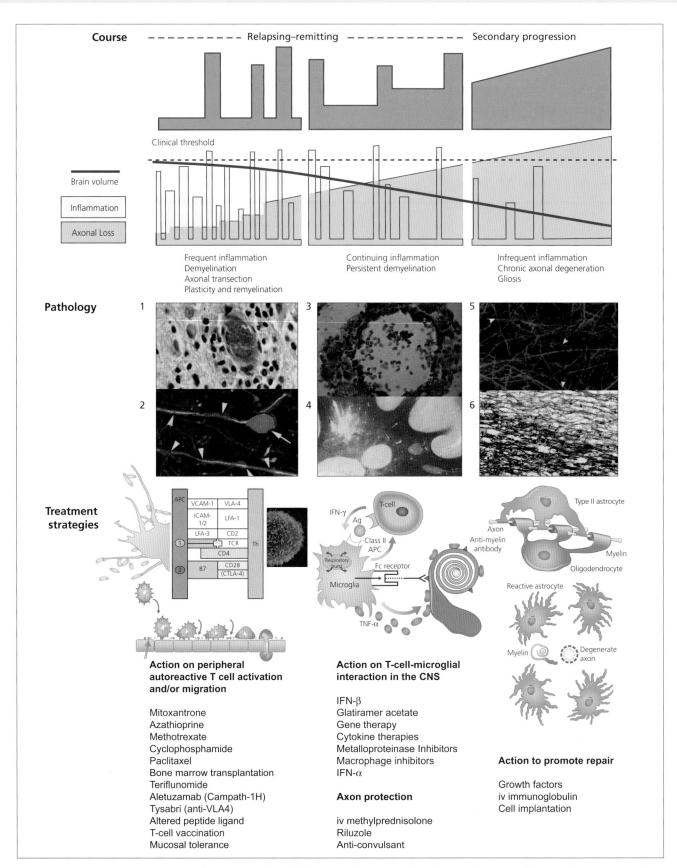

Figure 18.1 The course, pathogenesis and treatment of multiple sclerosis. *Course*: the clinical phases of relapse with recovery, relapse with persistent deficits and progression depend mainly on the effect of inflammation, demyelination and axon degeneration, respectively. Disease activity is often presymptomatic and, later, not invariably expressed clinically. As inflammation wanes, brain volume reduces with accumulated axonal loss. *Pathology*: perivascular inflammation (panel 1) causes acute axonal transection (panel 2), and microglia-mediated removal of myelin (panel 3) with persistent demyelination despite some remyelination (panel 4); chronic lesions show further axonal loss (panel 5) and gliosis (panel 6). The scheme does not depict primary progressive multiple sclerosis in which there is significant axonal degeneration with or without a preceding inflammatory phase. *Treatment strategies*: target the phase of T-cell activation in the periphery or cell migration; interactions between the activated T cell and microglia in the central nervous system; and axon protection and remyelination. Adapted from Compston and Coles (2003). © 2003, with permission from Elsevier.

affects the number of new episodes or lesions detected by brain imaging. Therefore, it makes sense to deploy strategies for treatment that address this evolution of events – choosing those interventions that preferentially tackle (or, preferably, anticipate) the individual components so as to be maximially effective. Although much contemporary research in multiple sclerosis is appropriately directed at identifying disease-modifying treatments, many patients already make clear that merely aspiring to shape the future course of the disease is not sufficient. They want to get better. If repair is a matter of restoring structure and function, it follows that dealing with the rewriting of neurological history requires treatments that enhance plasticity and reconstruct the myelinated axon in its network of connectivity. Thus, repair involves applying the lessons of neurobiology to the problems of multiple sclerosis. It remains possible that enhanced remyelination will occur in an immunologically stable environment. The experimental evidence already hints at this possibility (see Chapter 10). Remyelination may protect injured axons from further damage resulting from loss of trophic support. Conversely, optimizing their growth factor environment may reduce the extent to which axons, already insulted, are affected by further exposure to inflammatory mediators. Conversely, it is logical to assume that sophisticated repair strategies will have a low dividend for success without first having available a treatment that reliably stabilizes the disease process. Just as the dichotomy of genes versus environment is a somewhat sterile aetiological debate, so too separating inflammatory and biological mechanisms of injury to the axon–glial unit is somewhat strained.

But to go back a step, in Chapter 1 we reviewed the development of ideas concerning disease-modifying treatments in multiple sclerosis. The era prior to 1980, summarized by W.I. McDonald (1983), was empirical and largely uncluttered by serious concern about disease mechanisms. This period of intellectual freedom concerning the nature of multiple sclerosis provided ample opportunity for wild, and at times frivolous, approaches to treatment, some of which (rightly) gave the disease the bad therapeutic name from which it has not yet fully recovered. An important development in the treatment of multiple sclerosis in the 1980s was the acceptance that therapeutic claims must adopt orthodox clinical trial methodology based on blinding (single or double), use of controls (preferably placebo but sometimes receiving best existing medical practice), matching groups at entry for potentially confounding variables, setting primary outcome measures at the outset of the study and not trawling for the best result on completion, and considering power calculations during the planning stage. Working groups were convened to issue guidelines (see, for example, J.R. Brown *et al* 1979; Weiss and Dambrosia 1983). The impact of papers laboriously listing trial design tactics encouraged journal editors and referees to flex their methodological muscles – factors which undoubtedly led therapists to conform and resulted in the steady demise of therapeutic generalizations based on anecdote. The rubric 'double-blind, randomized and placebo-controlled' became commonplace. Since progress in identifying useful treatments was disappointingly slow, through no fault of those who designed the studies, separate trials of many agents proliferated and none could be regarded as definitive. Patients violated protocols and left studies for open label treatments, making it necessary to sort those who completed studies from 'intention to treat' cohorts. Commentators struggled to put

their thoughts in order by cataloguing published material and seeking a best position on disparate data. Faced with too few studies involving sufficient numbers of patients from which to draw firm conclusions, the meta-analysis emerged as a device for 'seeing the wood for the trees'. Considered by some as scientific sophistry, this analytical procedure exposed the criticism of mixing chalk with cheese and creating statistical noise, not least because outcome measures in multiple sclerosis are an integral of up to three independent clinical features – acute events, persistent deficits, and progression – which contribute to impairment, loss of ability, autonomy and participation (formerly referred to as impairment, disability and handicap).

Later, came the interim analysis – often used to stop trials either on the grounds of futility or issues of patient safety. Recent examples include studies of intravenous immunoglobulin designed to measure clinical recovery in multiple sclerosis and optic neuritis; trials of altered peptide ligands; the story of agents that have an impact on tumour necrosis factor-α (TNF-α); the glatiramer acetate study in primary progressive multiple sclerosis; and the use of oral glatiramer acetate (see below for more detailed discussion). However, the interim analysis has also recently been used increasingly to stop trials early on the basis of perceived efficacy, thereby allowing active treatment to be made immediately available for all patients without the disadvantaged controls waiting for completion of the protocol. We have seen this happen repeatedly, dating from the first wave of pivotal trials in relapsing–remitting multiple sclerosis [the North American IFNβ-1a trial (Avonex)] and, subsequently, with trials in possible (CHAMPS) and secondary progressive multiple sclerosis (the European trial, SPECTRIMS) – all discussed below. More recently, trials have been reported and widely accepted as valid with as little as 6 months follow-up (for example, EVIDENCE). The lesson from the failed Mayo Clinic Canadian Sulfasalazine Trial that early benefit may wane with further blinded follow-up seems often to have been forgotten (Noseworthy *et al* 1998; Rudge 1999). Hence, we now have to provide wise counsel to a generation of patients, some treated immediately after an inaugural clinical episode (clinically isolated syndromes), others when the illness has been established for only a few years (early relapsing–remitting multiple sclerosis), and many long into the illness with advanced secondary progressive disease – despite the lack of convincing evidence for protracted benefit – aiming to steer a course between managing their expectations and not shirking our responsibilities as clinical scientists.

The concentration of clinical research on the evaluation of therapies that target the immune response in multiple sclerosis itself represents something of an advance, displacing hypotheses for the pathogenesis finding their expression in less rational clinical trials. We hope that those who contributed to these studies will accept our decision to concentrate on contemporary immunotherapy and applied neurobiology. Of course, we accept that some (or indeed many) of the agents which we have selected for detailed discussion may in time join those which we have placed on the well-stacked shelves of therapeutic history in multiple sclerosis.

By the late 1980s, Noseworthy *et al* (1989b) were able to tabulate a large number of potential therapies which experienced investigators considered to be promising options for treatment. Many are still being evaluated but some degree of consensus on the basis for treatment in multiple sclerosis has emerged in recent years. At first, physicians were cautious when considering the use of immunotherapy for multiple sclerosis even though many of the available medications had been used successfully in other inflammatory and autoimmune diseases. This caution was appropriate since a significant proportion of affected individuals remain free from disability despite having intermittent symptoms over several decades, and it is not possible to segregate individuals destined to have benign forms of multiple sclerosis early in the course. In our opinion, however, the focus on treating secondary progressive multiple sclerosis held up progress for a generation. Since the late 1990s, that lesson has been clear. Wait until late and the contribution of anti-inflammatory therapy is so small as to not be cost effective. For many affected individuals, this is a formula for disappointment leading to cynicism that, despite intense research, no useful progress is being made in understanding the disease. It seems clear that, in the context of disease progression, the focus should now be on neuroprotective and biologically motivated approaches – alone or in combination with immunotherapy. Treat early and the dividend may be greater but still the dilemma remains. Drugs that are partially effective may not sufficiently stabilize the disease processes whereas the more actively anti-inflammatories are likely to carry nontrivial adverse-effect profiles. As we wrote in the early 1990s, the comprehensive management of multiple sclerosis is about both limiting and repairing the damage.

Progress has been made in improving outcome measures in the assessment of treatments for multiple sclerosis. Totting up the number of acute events requires them to be reliably defined, but patients will understandably assign significance to transient alterations in symptoms, perhaps having explanations other than disease activity. Conversely, motivation and the hope of a therapeutic effect will lead others to ignore clinical changes even though these are biologically meaningful. Periods of disease activity measured by high relapse rates tend to oscillate and, overall, slow with time so that a reduction in relapse rate *per se* is not necessarily impressive unless the placebo group has behaved less well and in keeping with the known natural history of the disease. The problems are even greater for the assessment of disability. There have probably been more critiques of the Expanded Disability Status Scale of Kurtzke (EDSS) (Kurtzke 1983a) and related clinical outcome measures than clinical trials in multiple sclerosis. The problems are well known. The EDSS mixes activity with disability and ignores participation. It is excessively weighted towards the motor system. It is ordinal not linear. Patients tend to cluster in the lower and higher echelons and it is insensitive in the middle range. However, it survives and despite much squabbling has yet to be replaced by a better, fully validated and universally accepted system. In this context, we welcome the deliberations of a panel convened by the United States National Multiple Sclerosis Society to make recommendations for a comprehensive clinical outcome system applied universally to treatment trials in multiple sclerosis, so allowing more meaningful comparisons between studies of the same or different agents (Rudick *et al* 1996a). The original guidelines were subsequently updated with special emphasis on the need for advisory/steering (to comment on the rationale, design, protocol, accrual and ownership of the data) and safety committees (to monitor operational aspects of trials), and the involvement of a group to supervise publication (Lublin *et al*

1997). The panel derived the Multiple Sclerosis Functional Composite scale (MSFC; G.R. Cutter *et al* 1999; Rudick *et al* 1996a; 1997) specifically to resolve these matters. The MSFC integrates scores on a timed 25 foot (7.5 m) walk (T25FW), Nine-Hole Peg Test (9HPT) of upper limb function, and Paced Auditory Serial Addition Test (PASAT). Values are reported as a Z-score, derived from comparison with an index population from the National Multiple Sclerosis Society Task Force dataset (G.R. Cutter *et al* 1999). The scale awaits validation as an accepted outcome for clinical trials and the MSFC has yet to be embraced by practising and academic neurologists. In large part, this is because, using this metric, most do not understand what is meant by changes in the Z-score, whereas few have difficulty with a single or multiple step change in the EDSS.

The introduction of novel scales has been trivial by comparison with the introduction of surrogate MRI markers as indices of therapeutic efficacy. The apparently favourable impact of approved but, in the event, partially effective treatments on relapse rates and MRI appearance solidified the sense that trials could increasingly use surrogate markers to detect a treatment effect. Clearly, reduction in the initial frequency of relapse and MRI activity may genuinely predict prolonged benefit but this requires evidence and has yet to be demonstrated. Such a study design aims to push new and existing therapies over a very high hurdle, requiring huge investments of time and money. Only recently have investigator-led studies adopted this long-term view but attention to effects that last and shape the neurological future is in the interests of patients and should be seen as motivated by the highest principles of clinical science, with a real dividend for improvement from the investment of hope in treatment. Worried by the sustained use of imperfect instruments for assessing outcome, investigators have created and partially validated increasingly sensitive measures of disability (such as the MSFC) and shown that these may detect treatment differences between treated patients with secondary progressive multiple sclerosis and controls, when standard measures (the Kurtzke EDSS) do not. Is the problem that our measures of disease progression are too insensitive to recognize a favourable response to treatment? Rather, it seems increasingly likely that existing treatments are insufficiently effective, or are deployed too late, completely to inhibit advancing disability.

The essential yet daunting task of confirming that these sensitive measures matter clinically in the long term – and are thereby predictive of a meaningful long-term benefit – has yet to be established. Here, a difference in agenda exists between physicians and the pharmaceutical industry, spawning secondary tensions between doctor and patient. The clinical scientist has a responsibility to proselytize secure knowledge even if this is gathered slowly and is disappointing in its scope. Sponsors need an early return on investment. In the context of multiple sclerosis, *Big Pharma* can be caricatured as having avoided engaging investigators in a dialogue about the importance of establishing long-term disability benefits. In turn, licensing agencies have not required that industry, assisted by teams of clinical investigators, demonstrate continued benefit for these expensive drugs as the necessary qualification for a drug licence. We have seen a proliferation of extension trials designed to demonstrate continued benefit. However, as discussed below, most are degraded by bias resulting from the recurring reality that failing patients drop out at the completion of the proper trial. Conversely, responders are better motivated to participate in the extension limb of the study. Although re-randomized, loss of the original 'treatment failures' introduces selective sampling that subsequently haunts the trial, thereby reducing confidence that any long-term benefit claims are real. The push to earlier treatment, and acceptance by patients and physicians of the need for prolonged use of the currently available drugs (even in the face of obvious ongoing disease activity dressed up around 'perhaps the treatments are helping a bit'), is bolstered by several factors. Sponsors of the approved agents have failed to press for clinical and laboratory biomarkers that characterize responder status. As a result, far more patients are being treated than might be appropriate given the partial benefits noted in the literature.

These recent changes in the attitudes of specialists in multiple sclerosis should not be seen as mulish obstruction to the pharmaceutical agenda. Investigators and sponsors share the sense of urgency in wanting to provide patients with effective drugs as soon as possible. More than $1 billion is spent annually on these agents, in the United States alone, with no funds invested to confirm sustained benefit. This hope that treatment with existing agents will provide an extended benefit, especially for patients treated early, remains just that – an unconfirmed, elusive concept without proof for patients and physicians. Meanwhile, little (if any) progress is being seen in creating a robust strategy to validate this goal. If we appear critical, it is in the spirit of prioritizing real not virtual progress. Our attitude is in the interests of people with multiple sclerosis and the advancement of clinical science, with personal reputation and commerce well down the motivation stakes.

THE PRINCIPLES OF EVIDENCE-BASED PRESCRIBING IN MULTIPLE SCLEROSIS

As discussed in the preceding section, over the last decade clinical investigators have become increasingly familiar with the principles of clinical trial design and have adopted these structures in the evaluation of putative new treatments. Thus, practice has shifted from the extrapolation of anecdotal experience to a more evidence-based stance on prescribing (Sackett *et al* 2000). The concepts of levels of evidence and grades of recommendation are slowly becoming part of the clinical trials lexicon. The neurological community is increasingly demanding that published reports of clinical trials clearly state how each trial was conducted and wishes to know how the data were analysed and by whom. Prior to 1994 it was common to see trials that were neither randomized, blinded, nor adequately controlled. Patients with different disease courses (relapsing–remitting, and primary or secondary progressive) were often included in the same study; this latter concern is still rarely addressed. At that time, trials rarely performed an intention to treat analysis, often accounted incompletely for drop-outs, and rarely assessed the adequacy of efforts to blind patients and evaluators. Outcome measures were usually not validated (regrettably, this is still largely the case). Nor were the sensitivity and specificity of these measures provided in the reports. Sample size estimates and power calculations were often not stated, leaving open the possibility of type 2 ('false-negative') errors resulting from an underpowered sample size. Many authors did not state the pre-determined primary outcome measure and post-hoc analyses

were often not identified as such. Authors rarely corrected for multiple statistical comparisons (the Bonferroni correction).

With time, the clinical trials community in multiple sclerosis has become increasingly sophisticated about these essentials of trial design and conduct. Most of the design flaws already listed are now appropriately filtered during design of the protocol, and policed by the peer review process before a report is published. However, some problems remain. As emphasized repeatedly throughout this chapter, clinical trials in multiple sclerosis are rarely of sufficient duration to determine whether the intervention affects eventual outcome in terms of disability but there are many seemingly insurmountable obstacles that block the path to longer trials. These include the lack of 'equipoise' for selecting both the active treatment(s) and the control group, since many investigators have strong opinions about which treatments they consider to be superior. There is reticence by both the sponsor and patients to commit to long trials. To date, every treatment has proved incompletely effective and this regrettable truism results in an inevitable but variable degree of 'treatment failure' for most participants – most patients experiencing clinical or MRI evidence for worsening. Naturally, the disappointed patients who detect clinical worsening remain anxious to try another form of treatment and many options are now available. Whitaker (1993), on behalf of the Advisory Committee on Clinical Trials of New Agents in Multiple Sclerosis of the National Multiple Sclerosis Society (NMSS), argued against named patient prescribing (compassionate use of investigational drugs) since this bypasses or otherwise compromises the double-blind, randomized and placebo-controlled trial. His views are no less relevant today when patients have been given high expectations of drug treatment and efficacy has been proselytized through a combination of altruism and exploitation. Many doctor–patient relationships have been strained by these helter-skelter events. Agreement on trial design and protocol management and policing of methodology in treatment trials continues into the new millennium. With increasing duration, drop-outs accumulate and blinding of the patient and evaluator become increasingly difficult. Similarly, as discussed later in this chapter, extension trials are flawed by the late loss of protection from the initial randomization step that is so essential to reduce bias by balancing unknowable prognostic variables across each study group. Most reports of positive trials do not discuss the 'numbers needed to treat' analysis (see below), although independent editorials and correspondents frequently raise this matter; there remains a pressing need to establish that MRI measures can serve as reliable predictive biomarkers of disease course.

It is regrettable to acknowledge that few investigators participating in industry-sponsored trials yet have full access to raw data or the process of analysis. This continues to be a vexing problem in multiple sclerosis research despite requirement by major clinical journals for authors to confirm that an opportunity was provided to participate both in the collection of results and their analysis (Davidoff *et al* 2001). The academic community is gradually accepting the importance of so-called integrity policies that mandate full disclosure of competing interests with sponsors but greater transparency on this issue is still needed (Noseworthy *et al* 2003). The strong stance taken recently by major biomedical journals to require that trials be fully registered, if they are to be accepted for publication, may provide much needed clarity within the clinical trials arena (De Angelis *et al* 2005).

With the proliferation of partially effective, disease-modifying treatments, fewer untreated patients are available to participate in clinical trials. In 1998, a small group of investigators decided to create a research centre independent of commercial influence and with the goal of hastening the search for therapeutic advances (Noseworthy *et al* 2003). The Sylvia Lawry Centre for Multiple Sclerosis Research at the Technical University of Munich (named in honour of the founder of the National Multiple Sclerosis Society of the United States and the International Multiple Sclerosis Society – see Chapter 1 – and directed by Albrecht Neiss and Martin Daumer) has amassed an impressive repository of data from natural history and completed clinical trials. In 2004, it had access to 43 data sets involving 14 700 cases and representing 62 000 patient years of follow-up. These data were primarily orientated towards controls since pharmaceutical sponsors had yet to donate information on individuals receiving study medications. Efforts are already under way to use this resource as the basis for understanding the contribution of demographic variables and laboratory measures (primarily MRI data) in identifying characteristic of the short- and long-term clinical course. The aim is to apply this knowledge in predicting the long-term course early in what is, for most affected individuals, almost invariably a chronic illness. Several countries (Denmark, Canada and Spain amongst others) have developed national registries to monitor the use of expensive therapies. Such databases will increasingly provide insights on long-term treatment efficacy with these drugs.

THE ROLE OF MAGNETIC RESONANCE IMAGING IN CLINICAL TRIALS

Over the last decade, the application of a range of MRI outcome measures has become a standard means of assessing therapeutic efficacy in the context of controlled clinical trials. The potential to monitor both natural history and treatment interventions was quickly recognized when MRI was introduced into clinical practice in the 1980s. As a direct and sensitive surrogate measure of the evolving disease process, it promised outcome measures that were simultaneously more objective and efficient than the cumbersome clinical markers on which clinical trials exclusively depended at that time. In the first clinical trial of interferon-β (IFN-β), culminating in a drug licence, the unequivocal evidence that new lesions could be prevented was seen as strong supporting evidence to accompany the principal clinical effect of a reduction in relapse rate (Paty *et al* 1993).

Individual magnetic resonance imaging lesions

The sensitivity of counting new MRI lesions in treatment monitoring has been amply confirmed. In relapsing–remitting or relapsing secondary progressive multiple sclerosis, serial monthly brain MRI reveals about ten new gadolinium enhancing or new T_2 lesions for every clinical relapse. It can thus be anticipated that the number of subjects and length of follow-up is reduced when using MRI lesions as the primary outcome measure (D.H. Miller *et al* 1991). Significant reduction in the number of new

MRI lesions can be demonstrated in a matter of months using a relatively small number of patients and, as a result, MRI has been proposed – and is widely accepted – as the primary outcome measure in exploratory trials of potential new disease-modifying agents in relapsing multiple sclerosis (D.H. Miller *et al* 1996). This approach is biologically plausible when the treatment is intended to suppress inflammation, since gadolinium-DTPA (gadopentetate dimeglumine) enhancing lesions identify areas of active inflammation. Monthly T_2-weighted and gadolinium-DTPA enhanced (0.1 mmol/kg of a gadolinium chelate) brain MRI are usually performed in phase I/II studies. In relapsing–remitting multiple sclerosis, a parallel groups design with placebo requires about 40 patients per arm to show a 60% reduction in new enhancing lesions over 6 months (McFarland *et al* 1992; Sormani *et al* 1999; Tubridy *et al* 1998a). A single run-in scan at 1 month reduces the sample size by about 30% (Tubridy *et al* 1998a). Slightly larger numbers are needed in secondary progressive multiple sclerosis. Crossover designs are more powerful, because there is less intra- than inter-patient variability in MRI activity. A single crossover design with 6 months run-in followed by 6 months of treatment requires between 10 and 12 patients to show a 60% reduction in activity (McFarland *et al* 1992). Double crossover designs are even better, but there needs to be a wash-out period between the two phases. Both crossover designs are compromised by regression to the mean. If a safe and cheap drug shows only a moderate reduction in activity (c.50%) in a small crossover study, this might be sufficient evidence to justify going straight to a phase III trial using a clinical end point. However, if the drug has more side effects or is expensive, a parallel group design with the larger sample sizes (such as 2 groups of 40 individuals treated for 6 months) should first be undertaken to gain more certainty about the MRI effect. An important limitation of studies with this size and duration is that they will not detect infrequent, severe or delayed side effects. It is therefore still considered necessary for the definitive (phase III) trial to be longer, to involve larger cohorts and to have a primary clinical end point.

A major limitation in the interpretation of gadolinium enhancing or T_2 lesions as outcome measures in trials is that these do not strongly predict or correlate with the long-term clinical course. Although concordance of the treatment effect on MRI lesions and relapses has been observed with most (but not all) agents that have been investigated in placebo-controlled trials (Table 18.1), the magnitude of reduction on MRI has not reliably predicted the extent of any decrease in relapse rate. For example, IFN-β and glatiramer acetate both reduce relapse rate by about 30% but, whereas IFN-β reduces the new MRI lesion rate by 50–70%, glatiramer acetate is associated with only 30% reduction. More importantly, the extent of T_2 and gadolinium-DTPA enhancing lesions has consistently demonstrated little or no relationship with concurrent or future disability (Kappos *et al* 1999). This lack of a relationship may partly be the result of limited follow-up – most published studies have lasted no more than a few years and may not have allowed sufficient time for substantial changes in disability to be revealed. Two recently published cohorts of patients presenting with clinically isolated syndromes have been followed for 8.7 and 14 years, respectively. One study of 42 patients showed that infratentorial lesions at presentation are associated with greater disability after 8.7 years (Minneboo *et al* 2004). In the second, the number and

Table 18.1: Treatment effects on active MRI lesions and relapses reported in parallel groups, placebo-controlled multiple sclerosis treatment trials

Therapy	Sub-group	Treatment duration	Patient number	MRI effect %	Relapse effect %	Reference
Beta interferon 1b SC	RR	4 years	372	−60 to 75	−33	IFNB Study Group (1995)
Beta interferon 1a IM	RR	2 years	301	−50	−31	Jacobs et al (1996)
Beta interferon 1a SC	RR	2 years	560	−75	−27 to 33	PRISMS Study Group (1998)
Beta interferon 1b SC	SP	3 years	718	−65	−31	D.H. Miller et al (1999)
Beta interferon 1a IM	CIS	2 years	383	N/A	−44	Jacobs et al (2000)
Beta interferon 1a SC	CIS	2 years	308	−33	−23	Comi et al (2001)
Beta interferon 1a SC	SP	3 years	618	−73	−30	SPECTRIMS Study Group (2001)
Beta interferon 1a IM	SP	2 years	436	−46	−33	J.A. Cohen et al (2002)
Alpha interferon	RR	6 months	20	−95	None[a]	Durelli et al (1994)
Linomide	RR	6 months	31	−70	None[a]	Andersen et al (1996)
Linomide	SP	6 months	30	−55	None[a]	Karussis et al (1996)
Anti-CD4 antibody	RR/SP	6 months	71	None	−41	van Oosten et al (1996)
Mitoxantrone	RR/SP	6 months	42	−90	−77	Edan et al (1997)
Lenercept	RR	6 months	168	+30 to 60	+50 to 68	Lenercept MS Study Group (1999)
Tysabri	RR/SP	2 months	72	−50	None[a]	Tubridy et al (1999)
Cladribine	SP/PP	1 year	159	−80	None	G.P. Rice et al (2000)
Glatiramer acetate	RR	9 months	239	−29	−33	Comi et al (2001)
Mitoxantrone	RR/SP	2 years	194	−85	−60	Hartung et al (2002)
Oral beta interferon	RR	6 months	173	None	None	Polman et al (2003)
Tysabri	RR/SP	6 months	213	−90	−50	D.H. Miller et al (2003)

a Study too small to reliably evaluate relapses.
RR = relapsing–remitting; SP = secondary progressive; CIS = clinically isolated syndrome; PP = primary progressive.
− = decrease in activity rate treatment versus placebo.
+ = increase in activity rate treatment versus placebo.
SC = subcutaneous; IM = intramuscular.
N/A = not possible to assess because of patient censoring on developing clinically definite multiple sclerosis.

volume of T_2 lesions in 71 patients at presentation correlated modestly with EDSS after 14 years (Brex et al 2002). The increase in T_2 volume during the first 5 years correlated somewhat more strongly with disability at year 14 (r = 0.61), suggesting that early accumulation of an increased lesion load does partially relate to long-term outcome. These studies are, however, quite small and the strength of the relationship between lesions and disability remains modest, suggesting that it is not sufficient to rely on MRI lesions *per se* (or their modification by treatment) to predict long-term disability (or its prevention by treatment).

The poor predictive value for disability of T_2 and gadolinium-DTPA enhancing lesions is that they are neither specific nor sensitive to axonal loss – the major pathological substrate for irreversible disability in multiple sclerosis. These markers do not reflect axonal attrition within lesions, or the loss that occurs more widely in normal-appearing white and grey matter. As a result, increasing attention has been placed on surrogate MR measures of axonal loss to study disease progression in multiple sclerosis and its modification by treatment.

It has been suggested that axonal loss in MRI lesions may be inferred by the presence of T_1 hypointensity. Such lesions (col-loquially described as T_1 black holes) account for 20–30% of all T_2 visible lesions and have been found in post-mortem studies to indicate a greater extent of axonal loss than lesions that remain T_1 hypointense (van Walderveen et al 1998b). However, the use of T_1 hypointense lesions as a surrogate marker for axonal loss has important limitations. First, not all such lesions are irreversible – acute enhancing lesions frequently display transient hypointensity, and their resolution with follow-up may simply imply that reversible mechanisms such as oedema contribute significantly to the appearance. Secondly, T_1 hypointensity is a subjective assessment that is less reproducible than T_2 lesion identification and is highly dependent on MR sequence parameters. Thirdly, T_1 hypointense lesions are almost never seen in the spinal cord, yet axonal loss in this location is crucially related to locomotor disability. Fourthly, being a subset of visible lesions, assessment of T_1 hypointensity provides no indication of the axonal loss occurring in normal-appearing tissues.

It has been useful in placebo-controlled clinical trials to follow the evolution of acute inflammatory gadolinium enhancing lesions through to areas of persistent T_1 hypointensity. The frequency of such an evolution is reduced in patients treated with glatiramer acetate compared to the placebo group (Filippi et al

2001a) and Tysabri (Dalton *et al* 2004a) but not IFN-β (Brex *et al* 2001b). This outcome could be considered as the MR equivalent of an incomplete recovery from relapses. However, given the abundant evidence for neuronal and axonal loss in the white matter and grey matter beyond MR visible lesions, attention is being focused on global MR measures as a more plausible surrogate marker of irreversible and progressive disability.

Global magnetic resonance measures of neuronal and axonal loss: atrophy

Tissue loss (atrophy) is the most widely used measure of neuroaxonal loss in treatment trials. Axons contribute 45% to white matter volume, followed by myelin (25%) and other tissue elements (glial and vascular tissues and water: D.H. Miller *et al* 2002). Neuronal cell bodies and axons constitute the bulk of grey matter volume although myelin is also present, albeit to a lesser extent than in white matter. Atrophy of white or grey matter in multiple sclerosis in large part reflects axonal and neuronal loss. In a study of the spinal cord of five people with multiple sclerosis, marked atrophy and axonal loss were both observed (Bjartmar *et al* 2000). However, neuroaxonal loss is not the only cause of atrophy. Loss of myelin, variations in glial bulk, inflammation and tissue water content also affect global or regional volume measures in multiple sclerosis. Pertinent to treatment trials, it should be noted that anti-inflammatory therapies (such as high-dose corticosteroids or IFN-β) reduce brain volume without axonal loss having occurred. We recommend that a period of 3 months should elapse after receiving such therapy before inferring that atrophy is measuring axonal loss.

The optimal technique for detecting atrophy should be reproducible, sensitive to change, accurate and pragmatic. The two distinct methodological aspects involved in measuring tissue volumes are data acquisition and data analysis. The ability to reduce partial volume errors with high resolution scans means that 3-D acquisitions are attractive, although 2-D sequences (Molyneux *et al* 2000) have also been used successfully to derive cerebral volume measures. Segmentation of the brain is necessary for whole brain atrophy measurements, and suppression of cerebrospinal fluid helps to generate a sharp distinction in signal between cerebral and extracerebral matter. The most widely used 3-D sequence is a T_1-weighted gradient echo. Specific study of white or grey matter requires good contrast at the cortical boundaries and interfaces both with cerebrospinal fluid and the individual lesions. It is aided by multiple contrast acquisitions (e.g. T_1, T_2 and proton density).

Manual outlining provides the simplest approach to measuring changes in volume and is useful in small structures or regions such as the third ventricle, where significant atrophy occurs in multiple sclerosis. Disadvantages of manual segmentation include operator bias, long analysis time and poor reproducibility when compared with automated techniques. Semi-automated methods improve speed and reproducibility. Regional segmentation algorithms are used to outline lesions, spinal cord, optic nerves and ventricles. Many automated methods exist for segmentation (and thus volume measurement) of the whole brain. Both single contrast (Chard *et al* 2002c) and multispectral data (Ge *et al* 2000) are utilized for whole brain segmentation. Usually, the difference in signal intensity between brain parenchyma and cerebrospinal fluid on a single contrast acquisi-

tion is enough to drive the segmentation process. Segmentation of grey and white matter may also be accomplished with either single contrast or multispectral data, although additional sophistication is required to separate the two tissue types. Methods include Statistical Parametric Mapping (SPM) based segmentation (Ashburner and Friston 2000) and the fuzzy C-means algorithm (Pham and Prince 2000). Masking of lesions is necessary to avoid misclassification.

Estimates of absolute volume at separate time points are not necessarily needed. Evidence for atrophy may be obtained by looking for differences between serial scans (S. Smith *et al* 2001). Nonlinear registration of such scans produces deformation fields that yield information concerning regional and global atrophy, and rigid body registration can be used to track displacement of the brain surface during atrophy (Freeborough and Fox 1997; 1998). Normalizing to head size reduces intersubject variations in brain volume. Relative volumes also remove variability due to scanner instability. The scalp, and the total intracranial capacity (determined by the sum of the volumes of grey matter, white matter and cerebrospinal fluid, or the sum of the brain and ventricular and sulcal cerebrospinal fluid) have all been used to adjust brain volumes for normalization. Atrophy is seen in both the brain and spinal cord in secondary and primary progressive multiple sclerosis. It is most marked in secondary progressive disease and correlates with disability (Kalkers *et al* 2001; Lin *et al* 2003; Losseff *et al* 1996b). In primary progressive multiple sclerosis, significant atrophy of brain and cord over 1 year was evident in a large cohort of primary progressive patients drawn from six European centres (Stevenson *et al* 2000). Change in cerebral volume over this period correlated only weakly with change in T_1 and T_2 brain load. More recently, progressive cerebral and cervical cord atrophy has been observed over a 5 year follow-up in a cohort of 41 primary progressive patients with multiple sclerosis (Ingle *et al* 2003). The rates of atrophy appeared relatively constant within individual patients but varied between subjects.

Atrophy, however, is not confined to advanced stages of the disease. Brain atrophy is also seen in established relapsing–remitting multiple sclerosis within 3 years of the onset of symptoms (Chard *et al* 2002a). Both white and grey matter atrophy are observed (Chard *et al* 2002a; de Stefano *et al* 2003). Even early follow-up of patients with clinically isolated syndromes has shown that significant brain atrophy emerges over 1–3 years in those subjects who later develop multiple sclerosis. This is most clearly seen in the grey matter and also as progressive ventricular enlargement (Dalton *et al* 2002b; 2004a). The apparent absence of progressive white matter tissue loss at this early stage of disease may reflect bulk tissue compensation by inflammation or gliosis (Fernando *et al* 2004). Possibly, grey matter atrophy will be a more sensitive measure of neuroaxonal loss because inflammation is less evident in this location (Bo *et al* 2003b; Petersen *et al* 2001). Atrophy of about 10–15% has also been observed in the optic nerve following a single attack of optic neuritis (Hickman *et al* 2001). We discuss later the evidence for atrophy as an outcome in the context of specific clinical trials.

From these data emerge a crucial lesson for the pathogenesis of multiple sclerosis and the timing of its treatment. The point is made repeatedly throughout this and other chapters. Despite effective suppression of inflammatory MRI lesions, treatments may not slow the rate of ongoing cerebral atrophy (Coles *et al*

1999a; Filippi *et al* 2000a; 2000b; Molyneux *et al* 2000) or have only a modest effect (Filippi *et al* 2004b). While differences in tissue loss from baseline can be detected in multiple sclerosis within 12 months, little work has been done to determine the optimal sample sizes and length of study required to demonstrate significant slowing of progressive atrophy as a result of therapeutic intervention. This is a priority area for further research, which should include consideration of the stage of disease, type of data acquisition, method of image analysis, region of the central nervous system being studied, frequency of scanning, and other potential confounding factors such as age or concomitant atrophy due to reduction of oedema.

Magnetic resonance spectroscopy: *N*-acetyl aspartate (NAA)

The main peak in the proton MR spectrum from human adult brain is *N*-acetyl aspartate (NAA), an amino acid contained almost exclusively in neurons and axons. A reduction in NAA provides evidence for axonal dysfunction or loss, and has been consistently reported in lesions and normal-appearing white matter in multiple sclerosis (Fu *et al* 1998). A greater reduction of normal-appearing white matter NAA is observed in secondary and primary progressive than relapsing–remitting multiple sclerosis, and disability has been correlated with reduced NAA in both cerebral (Sarchielli *et al* 1999) and cerebellar (Davie *et al* 1995) tissue. Decreased NAA (by 7%) has also been observed in cortical grey matter in early relapsing–remitting multiple sclerosis, suggesting that early neuronal cell body damage is occurring (Chard *et al* 2002b). It is reduced by c. 20% in thalamic grey matter in secondary progressive multiple sclerosis and, in a post-mortem study, the decrease in NAA (accompanied by atrophy) was associated with reduced numbers of neurons (Cifelli *et al* 2002).

Two approaches have been used to measure NAA: an absolute measure of concentration using an external standard reference of known concentration; and a ratio of NAA : Cr which assumes that Cr (creatine and phosphocreatine) remains stable in pathological situations. Although both approaches have produced robust evidence that NAA is reduced in the lesions and normal-appearing tissues, abnormalities of Cr may also occur. Therefore absolute measures are preferable. A methodological approach of recent interest is the quantification of whole brain NAA (Gonen *et al* 2000). This has been reported as low in patients with clinically isolated syndromes, implying extensive axonal damage even at this very early stage of disease (Filippi *et al* 2003). However, the resonance for whole brain NAA is broad and requires manual delineation for quantification – its analysis is potentially subject to bias and poor reproducibility. In contrast, the narrow NAA resonances from small voxels, obtained as a single region or as part of a spectroscopic imaging slice, can be automatically identified and quantified with a model that uses as reference a solution with a known concentration of NAA (Provencher 1993). Using such an approach, the normal-appearing white matter in patients with clinically isolated syndromes does not reveal a significant reduction of NAA (Fernando *et al* 2004). The time of onset and location of neuro-axonal damage should therefore be considered as uncertain.

A limitation of spectroscopy is the low signal to noise ratio and modest reproducibility of the measured metabolite concentrations. For this reason, it has been little used in multicentre therapeutic trials. Highlighting the problem, two small single-centre studies of patients treated with IFN-β have produced conflicting results. One study showed an increase in NAA, suggesting that therapy induced reversal of axonal dysfunction (Narayanan *et al* 2001). The other showed a decrease in NAA indicating that progressive axonal loss continues despite treatment (Parry *et al* 2003). Nevertheless, more vigorous efforts to investigate NAA as a surrogate outcome in trials of neuroprotection in multiple sclerosis are warranted, given that it provides specific information on axonal survival and function.

Diffusion tensor imaging

Diffusion tensor imaging offers potentially more specific access to the integrity of white matter tracts. Fractional anisotropy indicates the orientation of diffusion and is high along well-defined pathways such as the corpus callosum, pyramidal tracts and optic radiations. A reduction in such pathways is therefore a potential marker of axonal structural integrity. Algorithms have been developed for identifying individual white matter tracts. Diffusion tractography can be performed using several approaches (G.J. Parker *et al* 2002). Problems arise where pathways cross and there are sharp bends in the tract. However, tractography algorithms can quantify the size and fractional anisotropy of major pathways in the brain such as optic radiation and pyramidal tract (Ciccarelli *et al* 2000b; 2003a).

Other global measures

Many other quantitative MR measures have been applied to the study of multiple sclerosis. These include magnetization transfer ratio (MTR), T_1 relaxation time, and the apparent diffusion coefficient. Such measures are sensitive in depicting subtle abnormalities in normal-appearing white and grey matter, and convincing evidence has emerged that increasing abnormality in these tissues is associated with clinical progression (Filippi *et al* 1999a; Traboulsee *et al* 2003). However, these subtle MR changes do not denote specific pathological findings and could potentially represent the effects of inflammation, gliosis or axonal loss, each of which occurs in normal-appearing white matter (D.H. Miller *et al* 2003b). MTR may be valuable for monitoring clinically relevant disease progression in clinical trials. In a recent placebo-controlled study of IFN-β in secondary progressive disease, there was a significant increase in whole brain MTR abnormality in both the treated and placebo arms but no beneficial effect of treatment (Inglese *et al* 2003). This finding is consistent with lack of efficacy in the context of progressive disability. However, it is important to remember that progressive MTR abnormality may not be specific for neurodegeneration.

The process of neuronal and axonal degeneration is diffuse throughout the central nervous system and becomes more prominent with increasing disability and the progressive phase of multiple sclerosis. The two most specific MR methods for detecting neuroaxonal loss are atrophy and decreased NAA. For several reasons, atrophy has emerged as the preferred method for monitoring the neurodegenerative process in multiple sclerosis. Robust methods for detecting tissue loss are available. It is progressive from onset and increases with disability, correlates only modestly with inflammatory lesions, and thus provides additional information in therapeutic monitoring. Whereas a number of existing therapies have shown good suppression of inflammatory lesions, an effect on progressive atrophy has been less evident (for review, see D.H. Miller *et al* 2002). Although other MR markers of diffuse disease (such as MTR) are not specific for axonal loss, along with atrophy they provide sensitive measures of a diffuse, progressive underlying process that relates to clinical progression. MTR measurement in lesions may have a more specific role in therapeutic monitoring in that decreases and increases (which are larger than the subtle changes seen in normal-appearing tissues) may reflect demyelination and remyelination, respectively (Barkhof *et al* 2003; Schirmer *et al* 2004).

It is therefore recommended that atrophy should be measured in trials aiming to prevent disability at all stages of disease (clinically isolated syndromes, relapsing–remitting, primary and secondary progressive) and, where feasible, NAA should also be measured along with other techniques (such as MTR) to monitor progressive normal-appearing white and grey matter. It is nevertheless important to remember that the MR surrogates for neuroaxonal loss and diffuse disease have not yet unambiguously been shown to predict future disability and its prevention by treatment. Long-term follow-up studies of well-characterized cohorts, including those participating in controlled clinical trials, are needed to clarify this relationship. Meanwhile, definitive trials should continue to measure an appropriate clinical end point.

DRUGS THAT STIMULATE THE IMMUNE RESPONSE

In the past, attention was more or less equally divided between strategies designed to stimulate the immune system (initially, in the belief that immunological injury is sustained by persistent viral infection) or provide specific antiviral therapy, and those that suppress immunity. Now, it is clear that immune stimulants are either not effective or increase disease activity – perhaps as a result of increased expression of class II major histocompatibility complex (MHC) antigens on antigen-presenting cells. Some of these discarded treatments are briefly reviewed as part of the evidence that suppression of immunity and inflammation, not its stimulation, holds most promise for modifying the clinical course of multiple sclerosis.

Isoprinosine

Isoprinosine is a physicochemical complex of inosine and the para-acetamidobenzoic acid salt of *N,N*-dimethylamino-2-propranolol, that enhances B-lymphocyte activity, perhaps through an effect on T helper cells. It also increases macrophage phagocytosis, release of cytokines that induce macrophage proliferation, including immune interferon and interleukin-1 (IL-1) and IL-2, and augments the action of T-cell mitogens (Hadden and Speafico 1985). Pompidou *et al* (1986) compared the clinical and immunological effects of isoprinosine, chlorambucil and a placebo preparation in a small cohort of patients with multiple sclerosis over 2 years. Relapses occurred in all patients treated with chlorambucil or placebo but in only a minority of those receiving isoprinosine. Relapses did not differ in severity

between the three groups but the authors reported a reduction in disability associated with the use of isoprinosine. Immunological studies showed increased suppressor cell number and function in isoprinosine-treated cases, whereas cells with the T helper phenotype and delayed-type hypersensitivity were reduced in patients receiving chlorambucil.

Milligan and Compston (1994) used isoprinosine under double-blind, randomized and placebo-controlled conditions in 52 patients with relapsing–remitting or progressive multiple sclerosis. All patients initially received pulsed treatment with methylprednisolone. There was no significant effect of treatment on clinical disability or the accumulation of MRI abnormalities, after correction of results for multiple comparisons.

Linomide

Linomide is an immunomodulator that appears primarily to affect natural killer cells without inducing the release of IFN-γ. It also increases T-cell proliferative responses, the proportion of the CD45-Ra-positive subpopulation and IL-2 production. Its use in multiple sclerosis arose from the apparent ability of linomide to prevent and reverse the clinical and histological manifestations of experimental autoimmune encephalomyelitis (see Chapter 11). Karussis *et al* (1996) evaluated linomide (2.5 mg/day for 6–12 months) in 24 patients with secondary progressive multiple sclerosis who had deteriorated by >1 EDSS point in the previous 2 years, and showed either three regular or one enhancing MRI lesions on a single screening scan. There were no major adverse effects although minor events were reported in a high proportion of all participants. On this evidence, linomide appeared safe. An increase in disability (EDSS) at 6 months occurred in three of the 15 linomide-treated patients, and in six of the 15 placebo-treated patients; five and two of the 15 cases improved, respectively. Active lesions were present in 16% of linomide-treated patients and 33% of the placebo group at onset. Subsequently, 11 of 33 (33%) and 24 of 32 (75%) had active scans, with a difference in mean number of new enhancing lesions of 0.2 and 0.4 per scan, respectively.

Andersen *et al* (1996) reported a somewhat greater range and prevalence of adverse effects (one requiring drug withdrawal and another a reduction in dose) in 28 patients with relapsing multiple sclerosis randomized to oral linomide (2.5 mg/day for 6 months). MRI showed a lower rate of active T_2-weighted lesions in treated patients (1.4 compared with 4.2 in the placebo group; 0.8 and 2.6 for new lesions, respectively; constituting a 68% reduction in activity) and this effect seemed to increase with the duration of treatment. Three patients on linomide had four relapses and six of the placebo group had nine new episodes. Whilst the placebo group showed no change in disability, patients on linomide had a modest reduction in EDSS (−0.4). The numbers who improved, remained unchanged or deteriorated were ten, one and three in the treated group, respectively, compared with five, one and eight in the placebo-treated patients.

Enthusiasm for the use of linomide in multiple sclerosis collapsed with the decision to terminate early the North American and European phase III trials after enrolling >1380 patients with relapsing–remitting and secondary progressive multiple sclerosis because of serious cardiopulmonary and other adverse effects in the treated groups (Noseworthy *et al* 2000c; I.L. Tan *et al* 2000; Wolinsky *et al* 2000). Two linomide-treated patients died in the course of the trial from suspected cardio-pulmonary complications of linomide, but autopsies were not performed. An unacceptable number of patients treated with linomide developed pleuro-pericarditis (nine patients), chest pain, myocardial infarction (five patients), and possible pulmonary embolic disease as well as arthralgia, myalgia, bursitis and facial and peripheral oedema. These trials again emphasize that experimental treatments can place patients at risk of life-threatening adverse events. The importance of scrupulous surveillance by data-monitoring committees cannot be overstated. If there are safety concerns, immediate action may be needed to lessen risks to patients. Unless a preventable mechanism for these events becomes apparent, it looks as if linomide will join the ranks of drugs no longer to be used in patients with multiple sclerosis. However, Polman *et al* (2005) have recently studied the oral agent laquinimod (ABR-215062), a synthetic compound structurally related to roquinimex (linomide) in a randomized, double-blind, placebo-controlled trial of 209 patients with multiple sclerosis in three groups (laquinimod 0.1 mg or 0.3 mg, or placebo daily for 6 months). There were no serious adverse side effects (notably, no cardiopulmonary events or serositis; see above for linomide). High-dose laquinimod reduced the frequency of active MRI lesions significantly compared with placebo. These results, if confirmed in a larger controlled trial of sufficient duration and statistical power, suggest reasons for optimism in the search for oral agents that might one day simplify the management of relapsing–remitting multiple sclerosis.

Interferon-γ

The clinical trial of IFN-γ reported by Panitch *et al* (1987a, 1987b) proved extremely influential because it made patients worse and so told an important story (Figure 18.2). The logic for using IFN-γ was based on the hypothesis that multiple sclerosis is caused by persistent viral infection or an immunoregulatory defect that requires stimulation. If the study had shown clinical benefit in such a small group of patients, replication would have

been immediately demanded, but this result was readily accepted because, at the time of publication, knowledge of autoimmune processes had advanced to the stage where it could be predicted that disease activity would increase with promotion of class II MHC molecule expression. Panitch *et al* (1987a; 1987b) recruited 18 patients known retrospectively from case records to have had two or more relapses in the previous 2 years. All were in remission and ambulatory at the start of treatment. Follow-up was to be for 6–12 months after receiving three doses of IFN-γ (1, 30 and 1000 mg by intravenous injection) on eight occasions over 4 weeks. Within 1 month of treatment, seven of the patients had experienced a new relapse. Based on pretreatment rates, no more than two relapses were expected. Onset and severity were unrelated to the dose given. Recovery was complete and the relapse rate stabilized during follow-up at the former frequency with no overall change in disability. There was an increase in MHC class II-positive circulating lymphocytes. The implication of the study was that systemic IFN-γ had a rapid and causal effect on stimulating inflammatory processes within the central nervous system. In their discussion, the authors recommended others to assess treatments, including IFN-α and IFN-β, that specifically inhibit IFN-γ. Not surprisingly, this study is often cited as a clear example of clinical science in which lessons learned from the experience of treatment led to new concepts of disease mechanisms and, in turn, the development of more rational and effective therapies. Self-evidently, there are no subsequent studies on which to comment.

Interferon-α

The demonstration of a deficient interferon response in patients with multiple sclerosis stimulated the use of IFN-α at a time when the adverse effects of IFN-γ and the logic for using anti-inflammatory cytokines were not fully understood. Fog (1980) failed to show a beneficial effect on the disease course over 18 months in six patients with chronic progressive multiple sclerosis openly treated with intramuscular IFN-α. Next, Knobler *et al* (1984) reported fewer and shorter new episodes during IFN-α treatment in 24 patients with relapsing multiple sclerosis compared with retrospective assessment of relapse frequency over 2 years before starting the trial. Although the crossover design made for difficulties in judging the magnitude of this treatment effect, there was a reduction in relapse frequency with time in all participants. This was most apparent in patients receiving IFN-α after the placebo period. The reduction in relapse rate was maintained and improved in those patients showing a treatment effect over the initial 2 year period of observation in the subsequent 2 years, but the extent to which this could be attributed to treatment rather than to the natural history of the disease remained uncertain. Compared with the relapsing–remitting patients, those with relapsing progressive disease demonstrated evidence of mild to moderate symptom worsening during the prestudy period and they continued to have exacerbations during treatment (Figure 18.3). There was no effect on disability (Panitch 1987). Recombinant IFN-α, given by self-administered subcutaneous injection three times weekly for 1 year, was first used in a study of 98 patients with multiple sclerosis with at least two relapses during the previous 2 years. The results were not encouraging. All patients showed a reduction in relapse rate as part of the natural history of the

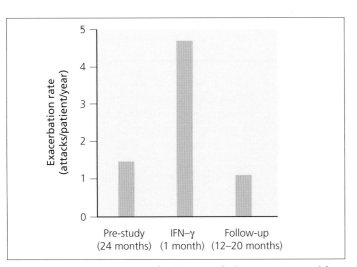

Figure 18.2 Increase in exacerbation rate during treatment with IFN-γ compared with pretreatment and follow-up periods. Adapted from Panitch *et al* (1987b). © 1987, with permission from Elsevier.

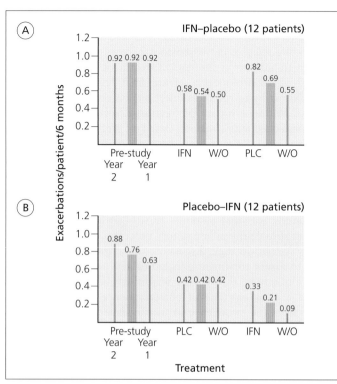

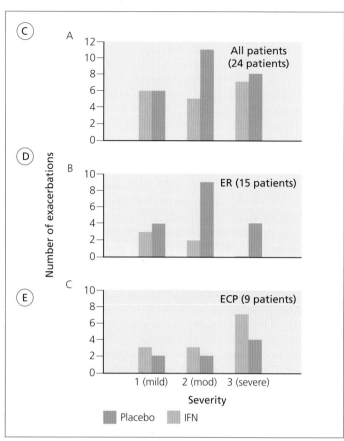

Figure 18.3 Treatment of multiple sclerosis with IFN-α. (A and B) Relationship between treatment sequence and response. The effect of interferon (IFN), placebo (PLC) and respective washout (W/O) periods on mean number of exacerbations/patient/6 month period are indicated by red and blue solid lines. The orange bars are average values for the flanking red and blue lines. Exacerbations occurring during prestudy year 2 or year 1 are also expressed per 6 month period. There is a greater reduction in exacerbation frequency associated with the PLC–IFN sequence than the IFN–PLC, which may reflect carryover effects of the crossover design or composition of the two groups. (C–E) Relationship between subgroup of multiple sclerosis patients, treatment and exacerbation severity. The latter was graded as mild (MLD), moderate (MOD) or severe, dependent on change in the Scripps (SNRS) score and duration of the exacerbation in days, during IFN and placebo treatment and respective washout periods. (C) IFN did not appreciably alter exacerbation severity when all 24 patients were compared. (D) However, the 15 exacerbating–remitting (ER) patients had no severe and fewer moderate exacerbations (p = 0.10) on IFN compared with placebo. (E) In contrast, the nine exacerbating chronic progressive (ECP) patients had more exacerbations of each grade during IFN treatment than during placebo treatment. Adapted from Knobler *et al* (1984). © 1984, reproduced with permission of Lippincott Williams & Wilkins (lww.com).

disease. However, more treated than placebo cases moved from the relapsing to the progressive phase of the disease and, unlike those on placebo preparations, treated cases experienced an increase in disability after discontinuing treatment (Camenga *et al* 1986).

It is perhaps surprising that, in the face of these results, Durelli *et al* (1994) repeated the study of IFN-α given by intramuscular injection on alternate days to patients with relapsing–remitting multiple sclerosis. Individuals on IFN-α showed a lower exacerbation rate (Figure 18.4), longer time to first relapse, and milder episodes less often requiring supplementary treatment with corticosteroids compared to the placebo group. However, disability was unaffected. Fatigue and other systemic adverse effects associated with the use of interferon were the main complications of treatment. There was an effect on disease activity measured by MRI. One of 12 patients on active treatment had a single enlarging lesion (which corresponded to a new clinical episode) whereas six of the eight controls had both new and enlarging lesions (27 of either type, equivalent to five for

each active scan). The treated group also showed some suppression in the systemic production of IFN-γ.

In a follow-up study, Durelli *et al* (1996) examined the resumption of clinical, MRI and immunological activity in patients who had to discontinue IFN-α (after 6 months of treatment) for administrative and financial reasons. In the four 6 month epochs preceding treatment, the numbers of patients remaining relapse free in the 12 patient cohort later randomized to IFN-α were two, one, four and three. The numbers without episodes in the group of eight patients randomized to placebo were two, zero, three and one, respectively. Against the background of these baseline estimates, two further relapses occurred during treatment with IFN-α compared with eight in the placebo group. In the 6 months after completion of the active treatment phase, there were three relapses in individuals who had received IFN-α compared with four in the placebo group. The numbers of patients remaining relapse free during and after the period of treatment with IFN-α were ten and nine, compared with two and four of the eight patients in the placebo

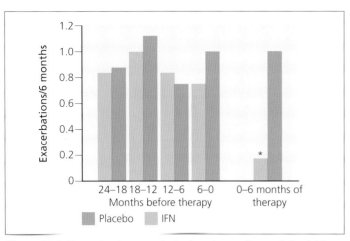

group. Taken together, these observations suggest a transient increase in the number of relapse-free patients during treatment with IFN-α.

The MRI results also suggested a transient reduction in disease activity which reversed on discontinuing treatment with IFN-α. There was one active lesion in the IFN-α patients during treatment and 14 after treatment, compared with 27 and 17 in the placebo group, repectively. Corresponding results for the number of active scans were one (during) and six (after) of the 12 IFN-α-treated patients, compared with six and six for the placebo group. There was no obvious effect on disability during treatment or apparent acceleration after discontinuing IFN-α. Durelli *et al* (1996) concluded that two of the 12 patients receiving IFN-α and seven of the eight placebo-treated patients had active disease during treatment, compared with six (IFN-α-treated) and six (placebo-treated) after completion of the active treatment phase. Immunological assessments showed that reduced IFN-γ and TNF-α levels, associated with the use of IFN-α for 6 months, also returned to baseline values on discontinuing treatment. Adverse effects attributed to the use of IFN-α were reversed within 1 or 2 months of treatment. This study adds to the evidence that clinical, radiological and immunological observations can directly be attributed to IFN-α, but are rapidly washed out on discontinuing treatment.

Myhr *et al* (1999b) randomized 97 patients with relapsing–remitting multiple sclerosis to receive either 4.5 or 9 million international units (MIU) of IFN-α2a or placebo, by subcutaneous injection three times weekly for 6 months. Relapses were not reduced although monthly MRI measures suggested a possible benefit during the period of treatment. The authors reported that neutralizing antibodies developed early in the group given low-dose IFN-α, and they speculated that this may have reduced the treatment effect. However, as discussed below, in most of the large-scale recent IFN-β trials, changes in clinical and MRI measures of disease activity correlating with antibody formation are generally difficult to detect unless a large number of patients are followed up for a protracted period.

Brod *et al* (2001) reported that oral IFN-α2a (10 000 or 30 000 units administered on alternate days for 9 months) was no better than placebo in suppressing MRI evidence of disease activity in a study of 30 patients with relapsing–remitting multiple sclerosis. However, despite some favourable results, we understand that IFN-α is not to be developed further for use in patients with multiple sclerosis.

Transfer factor

Although the biological properties of IFN-α were already characterized, patients with multiple sclerosis were also treated in the 1980s with transfer factor – a dialysable leucocyte extract thought to restore cell-mediated immunity and to have antiviral actions similar to IFN-α and IFN-β. The AUSTIMS Research Group (1989) compared these two biological reagents [IFN-α $(3 \times 10^6$ units); transfer factor (0.5 units) made from the leucocytes of cohabitees to maximize the prospect of achieving specificity against whatever agent might be causing multiple sclerosis] with placebo preparation(s) in 182 patients. There was no stratification for relapsing versus progressive disease. Clinical outcome was assessed using the EDSS. There was no difference in progression of disability between groups and no apparent effect of treatment on laboratory indices. In fact, the only clear result was that transfer factor was poorly tolerated and many individuals withdrew from the treated group. Soon after, van Haver *et al* (1986) treated 105 patients with multiple sclerosis (a mixed group with relapsing–remitting and secondary progressive disease) using transfer factor prepared from the leucocytes of random donors or family members. They also failed to demonstrate an effect on disability, activities of daily living or laboratory indices of demyelination. Treatment did not affect IFN-γ production.

Aciclovir

Although not strictly an immune modulator, we include discussion of the antiviral treatment, aciclovir, because (as with IFN-γ) it has been used on the basis that tissue injury in multiple sclerosis might result from persistent viral infection. Aciclovir (2.4 g orally for 2 years) has been evaluated in 60 patients with frequent relapses but very few persistent disabilities (C. Lycke *et al* 1996). There was a reduction in relapse frequency (from 1.7 to 1.0 in the aciclovir group and from 1.7 to 1.6 in placebo-treated patients; p = 0.08). Aciclovir did not affect the time to first and second exacerbations over the 2 years of the study. Despite the reduction in relapse rate, patients accumulated clinical deficits at an equivalent rate in both groups and there was no difference in disability on completion of the study. This dose of aciclovir achieved some reduction in herpes simplex virus-2 but not varicella zoster, Epstein–Barr virus or cytomegalovirus antibody titres. As expected, aciclovir was well tolerated with few adverse effects.

A second phase two, randomized, double-blinded, placebo-controlled study of anti-herpes therapy was reported by Bech *et al* (2002). They compared valaciclovir (1 g orally three times daily for 24 weeks) with placebo in 70 patients with relapsing–remitting multiple sclerosis. To be eligible, patients needed to have a history of two or more relapses in the previous 2 years yet still be ambulatory (EDSS 0–5.5). The primary outcome (number of new active MRI lesions over the 24 week course of the trial) was negative (valaciclovir: 11.9 ± 17.6 SD; placebo 14.5 ± 21.4 SD) and there were no differences in any of the clinical end points. A planned exploratory analysis detected that the valacilovir-treated patients who had at least one active MRI lesion during the pretreatment phase of the trial (4 weeks plus baseline MRI) had fewer new MRI lesions and were more likely to remain free of new MRI evidence for disease activity during the treatment period. An accompanying editorial encouraged further well-designed trials with antiviral agents while acknowledging that valaciclovir at conventional doses has no apparent role in the treatment of multiple sclerosis (Goodman and Miller 2002). Friedman *et al* (2005) reported that a placebo-controlled, randomized trial of valaciclovir (3000 mg/d) involving 58 patients with multiple sclerosis failed to demonstrate convincing clinical or MRI evidence for benefit although there were statistical trends in favour of some outcomes in the most severely affected patients.

Against this background, the further use of drugs that are known to stimulate one aspect or another of the immune response seems inappropriate and unlikely to satisfy scrutiny by ethical committees. Rather, the focus of therapeutic attention has turned to a range of strategies that have in common suppression of the immune response. It would take a very churlish observer to conclude that nothing has been learned and no patients helped from this approach (but such therapeutic nihilists exist). Equally, no informed critic could reasonably argue that the achievements to date are anything other than modest and represent no more than an indicator of the way forward. Perhaps, the crucial limitation has been the timing of treatment and the exposure of patients to drugs that are not fully appropriate for the stage reached in the illness by that particular patient. Now, we review in detail the various drugs that suppress one aspect or another of the immune response through a variety of mechanisms – some identified, others mysterious.

DRUGS THAT NONSPECIFICALLY SUPPRESS THE IMMUNE RESPONSE

Advances in understanding the nature of tissue injury in multiple sclerosis, and the lessons from attempts to stimulate the immune response and so purge the nervous system of persistent viral infection, prompted the use of drugs that suppress the immune response. This seemed logical even though most inflict prolonged punishment on the whole immune system for the misdemeanours of a small proportion of its constituent cells.

Azathioprine

Azathioprine, used for many years to treat individual patients with multiple sclerosis, was evaluated in clinical trials during the 1970s and 1980s (Mertin *et al* 1982; U. Patzold *et al* 1982; Rosen 1979; Swinburn and Liversedge 1973). The possibility that this reasonably well-tolerated nitroimidazole substituted form of 6-mercaptopurine might reduce progression of the disease in patients with moderately severe forms of multiple sclerosis prompted the (United Kingdom) Medical Research Council to sponsor a double-blind, placebo-controlled trial involving 354 unselected patients, on the advice of its working party on clinical trials (British and Dutch Multiple Sclerosis

Azathioprine Trial Group 1988b). There was slower deterioration and fewer relapses in patients treated with azathioprine but these differences were not statistically significant or considered clinically useful for the individual patient. Other work in progress at that time was subsequently reported including a trial in which small numbers of patients were treated with azathioprine, methylprednisolone or placebo preparations. The treatment groups each contained fewer than 30 patients (Ellison *et al* 1989). No significant differences emerged, although subgroup analysis showed that patients tolerating the combination of active treatments deteriorated less rapidly. The authors recommended that, because of the poor risk to benefit ratio, azathioprine should not be given alone or with corticosteroids to patients with progressive multiple sclerosis. After publishing a preliminary account, and including their data in the meta-analysis of azathioprine (see below), Milanese *et al* (1993) subsequently provided a final report on their study of 40 patients with relapsing or chronic progressive multiple sclerosis receiving 2 mg/kg/day for 3 years. There was a very high drop-out rate but the authors concluded, on an intention to treat analysis, that a treatment effect was demonstrated on relapse rate (90% remained relapse free on azathioprine vs. 60% of the placebo group) and the proportion of patients remaining clinically stable (62% vs. 18%).

Kappos *et al* (1990) reported on 37 matched pairs selected retrospectively from amongst 277 with clinically definite multiple sclerosis who had all been fully ambulant when treatment with azathioprine was started >10 years previously. Six treated patients were bedridden and four had died compared with 13 and eight, respectively, amongst untreated historical controls. The mean EDSS at 10 years was less in the azathioprine-treated group (4.9 vs. 6.0). There were similar numbers of patients in both groups who remained nearly normal (EDSS 0–2.5), reflecting again the important observation that a subgroup of untreated patients with multiple sclerosis remain with limited disability for prolonged periods. Goodkin *et al* (1991) also showed a lower relapse rate in 43 of 59 patients recruited to a study of azathioprine (3 mg/kg/day) compared with placebo in relapsing multiple sclerosis. Annual pretreatment, year 1 and year 2 rates in the azathioprine and control groups were 1.6, 0.7 and 0.3 and 1.5, 1.2 and 0.8, respectively. The numbers having a relapse in years one and two, for each group, were 16 and 7, and 17 and 11, respectively. The proportions showing progression in the EDSS and ambulation index in the treated group were 19% and 22% compared with 32% and 40%, respectively, in the placebo group. Not surprisingly, azathioprine does not prevent the onset of multiple sclerosis. Constantinescu *et al* (2000) described two patients developing multiple sclerosis after treatment for inflammatory bowel disease with azathioprine after 3.5 and 10 years, respectively.

Against this background of small studies suggestive of a treatment effect, Yudkin *et al* (1991) performed a meta-analysis of published trials. Ten were considered, of which seven were included. In five, the design was double-blind and placebo-controlled but not all had been analysed on an intention to treat basis. Of the 793 participants, 719 (91%) were followed for at least 1 year, 563 for 2 years and 459 for 3 years (with information available on 94% and 90%, respectively). Patients with relapsing–remitting and both primary and secondary progressive multiple sclerosis were included but evenly distributed between

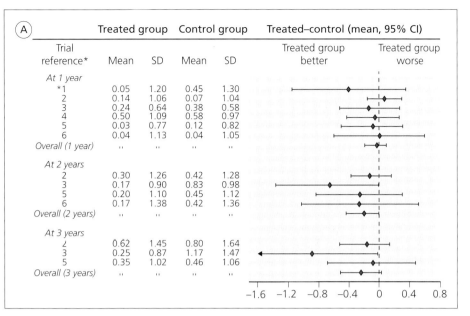

Figure 18.5 Meta-analysis of treatment trials using azathioprine in multiple sclerosis. (A) Changes in [E]DSS. (B) Probability of freedom from relapse. Adapted from Yudkin *et al* (1991). References: 1 = Mertin *et al* (1982); 2 = British and Dutch Multiple Sclerosis Azathioprine Trial Group (1988); 3 = Milanese *et al* (1988); 4 = Ghezzi et al (1989); 5 = Ellison *et al* (1989); 6 = Goodkin *et al* (1991); 7 = Swinburn and Liversedge (1973). © 1991, with permission from Elsevier.

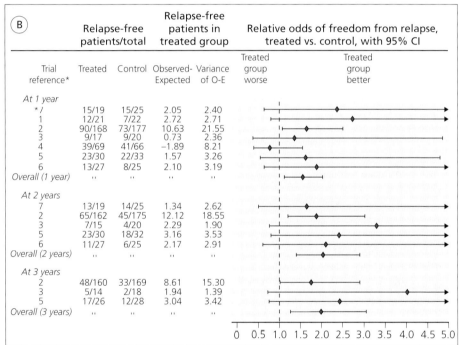

active and placebo treatment groups. The odds ratio for a treatment effect achieving a reduction in the EDSS attributable to azathioprine was −0.03 (95% CI −0.19, +0.12) but this had increased after 2 and 3 years to −0.22 (95% CI −0.43, +0.003; $p \leq 0.06$) and −0.24 (95% CI −0.51, +0.03; $p < 0.09$: Figure 18.5A). The probability of remaining free from relapse, attributable to azathioprine, at 1, 2 and 3 years was 1.5 (95% CI 1.1–2.0; $p < 0.01$), 2.0 (95% CI 1.4–2.9; $p < 0.001$) and 2.0 (95% CI 1.3–3.0; $p < 0.01$), respectively (Figure 18.5B).

Although the mode of action of azathioprine is well established, little is known concerning its effects on those aspects of immunity considered most relevant to multiple sclerosis. Salmaggi *et al* (1997) compared a range of immunological markers in individuals receiving up to 3 mg/kg azathioprine daily and untreated patients with multiple sclerosis. Therapy was characterized by

pan-neutropenia which disguised selective increases attributable to azathioprine in the proportion of lymphocytes coexpressing the CD3/4, CD3/56, CD3/16 and CD4/45Ra markers, with a corresponding reduction in natural killer cells (but not natural killer cell activity) and TNF-α production. There was no effect on immunoglobulin production despite the increase in CD4/45Ra cells. These findings do not obviously enhance our understanding of the immunopathogenesis of multiple sclerosis or provide an independent logic for reintroducing azathioprine as a disease-modifying treatment in multiple sclerosis.

Reduction in relapse rate with a delayed and modest effect on disability anticipates results subsequently obtained using the currently licensed therapies but the tone of discussion around these earlier treatments could not have been more different. The meta-analysis of azathioprine is a model of caution and understatement, emphasizing that the effects are modest, probably explained by interobserver variation, of doubtful value to the individual patient, quite possibly attributable to unblinding, and potentially posing serious long-term risks. Nevertheless, until the advent of IFN-β, many clinicians used azathioprine in patients with multiple sclerosis despite general concern over the long-term risks (Kinlen 1985). Reassuringly, Amato et al (1993) provided evidence against an increased rate of malignancy in patients with multiple sclerosis receiving azathioprine. Five of 207 patients taking 2 mg/kg daily for a mean of 4.2 years developed a malignancy compared with seven of 247 controls, giving prevalence rates of $3.6/10^3$ patients (95% CI 1.2–8.4) and $4.2/10^3$ patients (95% CI 1.7–8.7) and a relative risk (RR) of 0.8 (age adjusted) for cancer in the treated patients with multiple sclerosis. In a more detailed assessment, Confavreux et al (1996) showed in a case–control study that 14 of 23 patients with multiple sclerosis who developed one form or another of cancer had been treated with azathioprine for at least 1 month (RR = 1.7; 95% CI 0.6–4.6). There was a direct relationship between risk and duration of exposure (<5 years, RR = 1.3, 95% CI 0.4–4.0; 5–10 years, RR = 2.0, 95% CI 0.4–9.1; >10 years: RR = 4.4; 95% CI 0.9–20.9). Nevertheless, adverse effects appear to influence decisions over the use of azathioprine.

Most clinicians concluded, when these studies were published, that the clinical benefits of azathioprine fall short of satisfactory treatment for the individual patient, and as new immunosuppressants became available, they were evaluated in the hope that the new medicines would prove more effective. Nevertheless, azathioprine has not disappeared from the list of drugs used in multiple sclerosis. Some consider that prolonged oral azathioprine is no less effective than IFN-β and glatiramer acetate – since efficacy was not evaluated using MRI outcomes at the time opinions were being formed. Later, Massacesi et al (2000) reported that MRI measures of disease activity were reduced by treatment with azathioprine in 14 patients followed for 2 years. Meanwhile, Palace and Rothwell (1997) reviewed published data for the 2 year probabilities of freedom from relapse with each of the approved but partially effective agents including azathioprine and compared these projections with the observed outcomes of placebo-treated patients from these studies. The overall odds ratios for an effect on relapse rate demonstrated that oral azathioprine may indeed be comparable to the now more widely used parenteral agents (glatiramer acetate, 1.37; IFN-β1a, 1.68; IFN-β1b, 2.38; intravenous immunoglobulin, 2.01; and azathioprine 2.04) – and at a fraction of the cost (Clegg and Bryant 2001).

The recent trend has been to use azathioprine in combination with other therapies. Intravenous immunoglobulin was given in divided doses (total 2 g/kg) over 72 hours followed by monthly infusions of 0.2 g/kg for 3 years to 38 patients with relapsing–remitting multiple sclerosis who also received oral azathioprine (3 mg/kg/day: Kalanie and Tabatabai 1998). Combination therapy was well tolerated by the 34 patients completing this trial. After 3 years of monthly evaluations by an assessor blinded to details of the protocol, no patients developed clinical evidence of worsening (relapse rate or disease progression). These results are rather remarkable, and more favourable than expected from experience with natural history and clinical trial data sets. However, the study was uncontrolled and, to date, has not been replicated. Moreau et al (2001) reported that the combination

of azathioprine and IFN-β1a appears safe and well tolerated, at least for the 6 months of follow-up available at the time of abstract submission – but, to date, the study has not generated a full research publication. Recently, Lus et al (2004) reported their small prospective study of 23 patients treated with a combination of azathioprine and IFN-β1a (Rebif) followed for 2 years. For the purpose of data analysis, patients were considered in three groups: previously untreated individuals (n = 8) and patients previously treated with either azathioprine (n = 8), or IFN-β1a (n = 7). Combination therapy was safe and generally well tolerated. Relapse rates and MRI evidence of disease activity (T_2 lesions, contrast enhancements and T_1 hypodense lesions) were reduced in the prospective phase of the study compared with historical data. In a small study (n = 6), Markovic-Plese et al (2002) reported that the combination of azathioprine and IFN-β1b (Betaseron) provided synergistic effects on stabilization of the blood–brain barrier as determined by MRI studies.

Whilst alert to the changing landscape of treatment trends in multiple sclerosis, at present we do not routinely use azathioprine, pending evidence of superior efficacy and adequate safety from contemporary controlled trials but it remains an acceptable approach in patients who are unable to contemplate injected therapies. That said, Craner and Zajicek (2001) consider that, unlike those with myasthenia gravis or rheumatoid arthritis, the majority of patients with multiple sclerosis (55%) are unable to tolerate azathioprine. It has been recommended that levels of thiopurine methyltransferase should be measured in advance of a prescription, so as to avoid serious bone marrow toxicities (F.J. Thomas et al 2001; Weinshilboum and Sladek 1980).

Ciclosporin

Although not now routinely used in clinical practice or featuring in new trial protocols, we retain our earlier account of ciclosporin (formerly cyclosporine) for the lessons it provides in the evolution of ideas concerning the basis for treatment in multiple sclerosis. In a modest way, ciclosporin influences progression of multiple sclerosis, relapse rate and severity but only at doses that produce unacceptable adverse effects. Rudge et al (1989) showed no difference in the number of patients remaining relapse free between ciclosporin-treated and placebo-treated groups during a 2 year clinical trial. However, episodes were more frequent in the placebo group, and these were judged to be more severe and to have occurred earlier. More ciclosporin-treated patients than controls remained stable, in terms of the EDSS, over the first 6 months of the trial but this effect was not maintained thereafter. One difficulty that arose was the need to stratify the analysis to account for a centre effect. Selection of patients on the basis of clinical course and the dose of ciclosporin that was tolerated differed between the two participating centres. Critics therefore assume that, for many participants, the study was unblinded. They worry about the dependence on subgroup analysis and conclude that there is no clinical role for ciclosporin. We know of very few patients with multiple sclerosis in whom this immunosuppressant is still used. This trial taught the useful lesson that the course of multiple sclerosis is more likely to be altered by immunological treatments used at doses producing significant adverse effects that outweigh the modest clinical advantages. In a comparison with azathioprine, low-dose ciclosporin is shown to be less well tolerated and no more beneficial in terms of disease stabilization (Kappos *et al* 1988). Although the participants experienced very little deterioration during the trial, this study was not designed to show that either drug influenced the natural history of the disease.

Subsequently, in a placebo-controlled study of ciclosporin involving 547 patients with moderate to severe progressive multiple sclerosis (EDSS between 3 and 7 with a change in the year before entry of between 1 and 3 points) treated with a range of doses, some aspects of disability were significantly influenced. However, a substantial number of patients withdrew from the active treatment group because of adverse effects, notably nephrotoxicity and hypertension (Multiple Sclerosis Study Group 1990). Reduction in the mean increase in EDSS in treated patients compared with controls (0.39 ± 1.07 vs. 0.65 ± 1.08; mean $\pm$ SD) was associated with delay in time to use of a wheelchair but not to sustained progression, and there was no effect on activities of daily living. Ruutianen *et al* (1991) compared ciclosporin (7.5 mg/kg) with oral prednisolone (tapering from 0.8 mg/kg). Despite no immediate difference in outcome, greater improvement was reported in patients on corticosteroids at 3 months. There was no difference in the frequency of adverse effects.

Taken together, clinicians are not persuaded that ciclosporin represents a significant advance over the modest effects associated with the use of azathioprine. Long-term oral therapy with azathioprine appears better tolerated but not sufficiently useful (see above), whereas ciclosporin is considered more effective but unacceptably complicated in patients with multiple sclerosis.

Cyclophosphamide

The same problems have characterized the evaluation of treatment with cyclophosphamide. This immunosuppressant has been used on an open uncontrolled basis for many years, especially in continental Europe. Attention was drawn to its use with the publication of a study reporting that high-dose intravenous cylcophosphamide stabilizes the clinical course in patients with progressive multiple sclerosis when given with corticotropin by comparison with patients receiving corticotropin alone, or plasma exchange with corticotropin and low-dose oral cyclophosphamide (S.L. Hauser *et al* 1983). By present standards, this study was of short duration and underpowered, only involving between 18 and 20 patients in each arm. Summarizing the quantitative observations in an overall qualitative assessment, four of the 20 patients receiving corticotropin stabilized or improved at 1 year, compared with 16 of the 20 patients in the cyclophosphamide/ corticotropin group and nine of 18 patients in the plasma exchange. As a result of this trial, many patients received high-dose intravenous cyclophosphamide for several years, tolerating a variety of unpleasant short-term adverse effects in the hope of disease stabilization. Subsequent experience with dose ranging studies in which maintenance therapy was adjusted against indices of immune suppression (circulating CD4 counts) merely confirmed the potential toxicity of cyclophosphamide and led some to conclude that the drug is too toxic for routine use (L.W. Myers *et al* 1987). Nevertheless, an approach using repeated pulses of well-tolerated doses, given at monthly or longer intervals, was later evaluated in 14 patients using a partial crossover design. Those treated with cyclophosphamide were considered to have less frequent and shorter episodes than the placebo group and the trial sustained the belief that the beneficial effects of cyclophosphamide could be maximized and the adverse effects could be reduced using pulsed therapy (Killian *et al* 1988).

The Kaiser study (Likosky *et al* 1991) examined the efficacy of pulsed intensive immunosuppression with intravenous cyclophosphamide (c.500 mg/day until the leucocyte count reached $<4000/mm^3$) given in an outpatient setting under randomized single-blind conditions with folic acid as the comparator. At 1 year, 14 of 22 (64%) immunosuppressed patients were unchanged or stable compared to 14 of 20 (70%) taking folic acid. At 2 years, the figures were nine of 19 (47%) and nine of 17 (53%), respectively. There was no change in the rate of disability at 1 year between groups and each had worsened by approximately 0.5 EDSS points. However, at 2 years, patients on folic acid were accumulating disability at a faster rate than immunosuppressed patients (+0.4, 95% CI 0.4–1.2: the corresponding figure for the ambulation index was +0.8, 95% CI 0.5–2.2). Throughout, the authors nicely understate these results showing wide confidence intervals, in marked contrast to some other enthusiasts for the use of cyclophosphamide.

The definitive clinical trial of cyclophosphamide involved 168 patients (Canadian Co-operative Multiple Sclerosis Study Group 1991). Participants had progressive multiple sclerosis which had deteriorated by >1 EDSS point in the previous year. The proportions showing sustained deterioration of a further point (or more) were 35%, 32% and 29% in three groups – given intravenous cyclophosphamide with oral prednisolone, daily oral cyclophosphamide with alternate day prednisolone and weekly plasma exchange, or placebo preparations of all these treatments, respectively. There were no differences between groups in the proportions who improved, stabilized or worsened, nor in the final EDSS scores (Figure 18.6). Despite the necessarily complicated trial design, failure to demonstrate a difference in the overall outcome or interim assessments between groups was conclusive with respect to cyclophosphamide, not least because the study involved nearly three-fold more patients than earlier evaluations. However, perhaps the conclusion that 'immunosuppressive treatments do not stabilize or improve the clinical course in patients with multiple sclerosis' was overstated. Our position is that physician blinding prevented an erroneous conclusion being reached about the efficacy of intravenous cyclophosphamide in the Canadian study since Noseworthy *et al* (1994) point out that a treatment effect would have been reported (for the 6, 12 and 24 month epochs) had the analysis been based on the scores of neurologists who were unblinded during the trial and not (as was the case) the masked investigator. This analysis demonstrates, as well as any in the literature, the importance of evaluator blinding in the assessment of a putative treatment effect.

Although the Canadian study offered cyclophosphamide little future prospect as a treatment for multiple sclerosis, new studies have continued to appear. Weiner *et al* (1993a) extended their previous assessment of intravenous cyclophosphamide, modifying the induction regimen and adding so-called 'boosters' to maintain the effects. This required a comparison of four treatment groups but there was no difference in outcome between the two methods of induction. A higher proportion of patients who received further treatments with intravenous cyclophosphamide

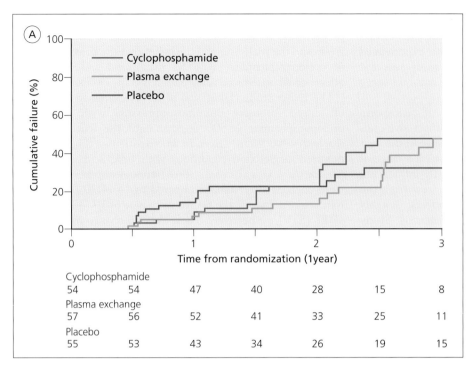

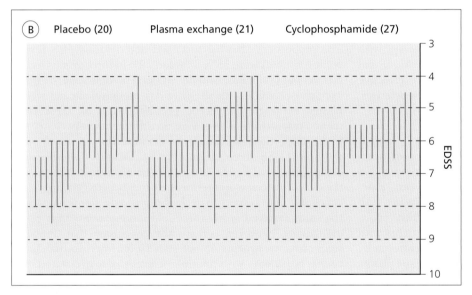

Figure 18.6 Canadian cyclophosphamide trial. (A) Time to treatment failure. (B) Extent of deterioration in EDSS. Every patient whose EDSS increased by >1 point (evaluating neurologist's assessment) at any one time during the trial is represented by a line connecting the EDSS at entry with the worst EDSS recorded during the trial. Numbers in parentheses are the numbers in each group who showed an increase of at least 1 EDSS point. Adapted from the Canadian Co-operative Multiple Sclerosis Study Group (1991). © 1991, with permission from Elsevier.

every 2 months for 2 years was clinically stable or improved at 24 and 30 (but not 6, 12 and 18) months and the time to treatment failure was prolonged in these two groups. Thirty-eight per cent responded clinically at 24 months in the two groups receiving boosters compared with 24% in the induction-only groups. Comparable figures at 30 months were 27% and 17%, respectively (Figure 18.7).

Weiner *et al* (1993a) emphasize that these clinical effects (which we consider to be modest and achieved at some price in terms of risk and potential adverse effects) are more likely to occur in young patients (aged <40 years) and not in individuals with primary progressive multiple sclerosis. In another report from this group, Gauthier *et al* (2003) reported a retrospective analysis of their experience using cyclophosphamide in 47 relapsing–remitting patients with multiple sclerosis considered unresponsive to glatiramer acetate and the various forms of

IFN-β. The combination of pulsed intravenous methylprednisolone and cyclophosphamide appeared to stabilize MRI and clinical measures of progression in up to 75% of cases.

There have been no recent, randomized, controlled trials using cyclophosphamide but several investigators have reported apparently positive clinical experience. Based on an open label series of 17 patients with advanced disability (EDSS 6.0–8.5), who had deteriorated by at least 1.5 EDSS points despite recent treatment with corticosteroids, Weinstock-Guttman *et al* (1997) consider that high-dose intravenous cyclophosphamide and methylprednisolone followed by IFN-β therapy may stabilize rapidly worsening multiple sclerosis. They administered intravenous cyclophosphamide 500 mg/m^2 and 1.0 g intravenous methylprednisolone daily for 5 days along with abundant intravenous fluids to reduce the risk of haemorrhagic cystitis. Patients were then given a tapering course of oral prednisone for 12 days.

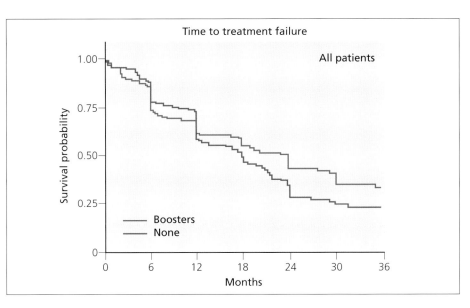

Time to treatment failure

Figure 18.7 Kaplan–Meier survival curves comparing time to treatment failure in patients receiving and not receiving bimonthly cyclophosphamide booster therapy. Percentages of individuals who were not treatment failures are plotted against time. No significant difference was found (p = 0.18) over the entire course of follow-up, but in examining booster effects starting at 1 year, a significant benefit (p = 0.03) was detected. Adapted from Weiner *et al* (1993a). © 1993, reproduced with permission of Lippincott Williams & Wilkins (lww.com).

Thereafter, 'maintenance immunotherapy' was continued at the discretion of the prescribing physician. This varied from repeated bimonthly treatments with intravenous cyclophosphamide and methylprednisolone, to weekly methotrexate or bimonthly intravenous methylprednisolone, and IFN-β1b. They reported that this complex immunological regimen was well tolerated (one patient had fever and two developed severe nausea and vomiting). Thirteen of 17 were either stable or improved at 1 year, and nine of 13 at 2 years. Although encouraging, collective experience has shown that nonrandomized, uncontrolled studies are often not validated by prospective studies using rigorous trial designs. In addition, the extreme variability of the 'maintenance immunotherapy' given to these patients leaves open too many freedoms in concluding what has and has not contributed to the complex equation of efficacy and clinical cost. Hohol *et al* (1999) reported their consecutive series of 95 patients with progressive forms of relapsing–remitting, secondary progressive and primary progressive multiple sclerosis. Each patient received 5 days of 1 g intravenous methylprednisolone followed on day 4 or 5 by a single course of intravenous cyclophosphamide (800 mg/m²). Thereafter, patients received repeated single courses of 1 g intravenous methylprednisolone and cyclophosphamide (monthly dose increasing as needed to induce a midmonth leukopenia of 1500–2000 cells/mm³). Patients were treated monthly for 1 year, every 6 weeks in year 2, and then every 8 weeks in year 3. This approach appeared most beneficial for patients with relatively recent onset secondary progressive multiple sclerosis (mean 2.1 years) whereas those with primary progressive disease responded less well. The authors reported that, at 2 years, 76% of the chronic progressive patients were stable or had improved using EDSS criteria. However, when using a combined outcome of either EDSS change or the examining physician's global impression of worsening, 54% of the patients with chronic progressive disease were judged to have deteriorated at 2 years. This experience is again unblinded and uncontrolled. Perhaps of equal importance, 70 of 95 patients discontinued the planned protocol prior to analysis, with approximately an equal number dropping out during each of the 3 years of follow-up. The authors conclude, as have many others, that the yield from treating secondary progressive multiple scle-

rosis using intensive immunosuppression diminishes with time. Gobbini *et al* (1999) administered high-dose pulse intravenous cyclophosphamide monthly for 6 months in a hospital setting to five patients with relapsing–remitting disease judged to have failed licensed therapies. Patients were adequately hydrated and underwent a 24 hour bladder irrigation protocol to reduce the likelihood of haemorrhagic cystitis. Cyclophosphamide was administered as 1 g/m² monthly with dose adjustments as needed to achieve a peripheral white blood cell count nadir of 1500–2000 cells/mm³ at 10 days. Ondansetron hydrochloride 10 mg by intravenous injection was used to reduce nausea and vomiting. Monthly MRI studies demonstrated that all patients had a reduced number of gadolinium enhancing lesions by month five and two patients demonstrated a reduced T₂ lesion load. Two others could not be evaluated because of inadequate MRI. One patient continued to demonstrate an increase in T₂ lesion load despite stabilization of contrast enhancing lesions. One patient developed alopecia, another developed herpes zoster and, in two patients, a seizure disorder was observed but attributed to advanced multiple sclerosis. The authors conclude that this approach may be useful in patients failing approved therapies.

Monthly pulses of intravenous cyclophosphamide were used by S. Khan *et al* (2001a) in 14 patients with 'rapidly deteriorating' relapsing–remitting multiple sclerosis. Each had worsened by at least 3.0 EDSS points in the preceding year despite at least 6 months of an approved immune-modulating parenteral therapy and at least two courses of intravenous methylprednisolone. They administered 1 g/m² cyclophosphamide by monthly intravenous infusion, adjusting the dose based on a target peripheral white blood cell nadir of 2000–2200 cells/mm³ at 14 days. Most patients were treated for 6 months and then started on one of the approved therapies. Dexamethasone (20 mg) and ondansetron (32 mg, each by intravenous injection) were administered, along with intravenous fluids to prevent haemorrhagic cystitis. All patients were thought to have stabilized or improved by 6 months and this apparent clinical benefit persisted for an additional year (assessed at 18 months, postinduction). Mild or moderate nausea and transient alopecia were reported but no participant experienced haemorrhagic cystitis or clinical relapses. Self-evidently, cyclophosphamide is a complicated drug to administer and the net contribution to the welfare of people with multiple sclerosis is hard to evaluate. For example, in a comparative study of patients receiving monthly infusions of methylprednisolone (n = 15), bimonthly intravenous cyclophosphamide with methylprednisolone (n = 32), methotrexate (n = 5) or IFN-β (n = 15), there was early and sustained selective increase in eosinophilia and raised levels of stimulated CD4 T-cell-secreted IL-4 and IL-10 with a reduction in production of IFN-γ in the cyclophosphamide group – representing both inhibition and enhancement of potentially immunopathogenic processes – not seen with the other putative therapeutic agents (D.R. Smith *et al* 1997). A recent Cochrane systematic review concluded that cyclophosphamide does not prevent worsening of the EDSS but appears favourably to influence the rate of EDSS change at 12–18 months (La Mantia *et al* 2002). Astonishingly, only four randomized trials from a total of 326 published reports were judged suitable for review because of limitations in trial design and conduct. These authors cautioned against the use of this agent because of the frequency of sepsis and amenorrhoea in treated patients.

We rarely, if ever, use cyclophosphamide in our clinical practice. It may be that this powerful immunosuppressive agent has a role in stabilizing patients with very active disease but our reading of the published reports suggests extreme caution. As in many trials where the first reported effect has not been confirmed, the treated group fared no better than patients receiving placebo but nonetheless participating in trials of chronic progressive multiple sclerosis. This calls to mind the remark of the late Dale McFarlin:

> *when I get multiple sclerosis, put me in a trial and make sure I get the placebo.*

Plasma exchange

Plasma exchange has been used in patients with multiple sclerosis in the hope of matching the uncomplicated benefits achieved in other inflammatory disorders. It has been evaluated both as a disease-modifying agent and in the management of refractory acute episodes (see Chapter 16). Although the mode of action in disorders where details of the immunopathogenesis remain to be fully characterized is obscure, plasma exchange presumably removes or indirectly restores to balance soluble mediators of immunity. The same general principle is thought to underlie the use of immune globulin (see below).

Khatri *et al* (1991) reviewed their experience of plasma exchange in 200 patients with progressive multiple sclerosis (based on a recent retrospective review of case records) also receiving cyclophosphamide, prednisolone and symptomatic treatments. Pooled human globulin was used to replace fluid after exchanges given weekly for 3 months with a subsequent weaning period, the duration of which depended on initial response. The results showed a reduction in EDSS at 1, 2 and 3 years by comparison with scores at entry, and the authors considered that >80% of patients had improved or stabilized by 3 years. Four potentially active treatments were used in the study. Patients were selected on the basis of ability to pay for therapy through insurance. There were no controls. It is therefore difficult to reach any conclusions from this evidence on whether plasma exchange has an independent effect, comple-

ments immunosuppressants or makes no contribution to the management of disease progression. Whereas the Canadian Cooperative Multiple Sclerosis Study Group (1991) concluded on the basis of their study that immunosuppressants (then available) were generally ineffective in multiple sclerosis, Khatri *et al* (1991) reached diametrically opposite conclusions using a comparable regimen of combined therapies.

Most reported studies use plasma exchange as an adjunct to other forms of immunological treatment. Thus, the clinical course has been shown to stabilize in patients with progressive disease treated with corticosteroids and cyclophosphamide, whether or not plasma exchange is also used (Khatri *et al* 1985). An earlier trial comparing plasma exchange in patients also receiving azathioprine showed that both groups deteriorated at a comparable rate (Tindall *et al* 1982). Confirming that the short-term consequences of relapse are reversed more rapidly in patients receiving plasma exchange in addition to intramuscular corticotropin and cyclophosphamide, Weiner *et al* (1989) were unable to demonstrate any long-term effects. The contribution made by plasma exchange in patients also receiving azathioprine was assessed in a crossover design by P.S. Sorensen *et al* (1996). Fourteen exchanges were given over 20 weeks in the active period. Plasmapheresis had no effect on disease activity as assessed by gadolinium enhanced MRI, although the total lesion load and central motor conduction times were reduced during the exchange period. A specific role for plasma exchange in the treatment of fulminant demyelination was reported by M. Rodriguez *et al* (1993a). This observation is substantiated by both a randomized, double-blinded trial (Weinshenker *et al* 1999b) and an uncontrolled, prospective series (Keegan *et al* 2002) of patients who failed to improve following a course of steroid treatment in the setting of acute inflammatory demyelination because of established multiple sclerosis, neuromyelitis optica or a first episode of demyelinating disease. Bringing together empirical observations treating fulminating episodes of demyelination with plasma exchange and histological observations made in the highly selected group of cases studied by brain biopsy, Keegan *et al* (2005) subsequently correlated the presence of antibody and complement deposition (type 2: see Chapter 12) with moderate to substantial functional improvement – responses that were not seen in patients with other histological features. It remains unclear at what point in the natural history of an episode with poor recovery, plasma exchange might be considered as one option for limiting the extent of persistent or long-term disability, thereby constituting a disease-modifying treatment (see Chapter 16).

Intravenous immunoglobulin

We refer elsewhere (see below, and Chapters 10 and 19) to the potential for remyelination from the use of intravenous immunoglobulin in experimental demyelination and the clinical setting. Intravenous immunoglobulins are widely used in the management of peripheral and central nervous system disorders (Wiles *et al* 2002). Intravenous immunoglobulin has been assessed in detail for a variety of indications in multiple sclerosis (Stangel and Hartung 2002), including attempts to alter the natural history of relapsing–remitting and secondary progressive disease, and to reverse established deficits by enhancing remyelination (Asakura 1996; Rodriguez and Lennon 1990; M. Rodriguez *et al*

1996). Immunoglobulins may stimulate remyelination in the Theiler's murine encephalomyelitis virus animal model. Other possible mechanisms of action include an effect on anti-idiotypes (Tenser *et al* 1993), interference with complement (M.M. Frank *et al* 1992) or Fc-receptor-mediated interactions between microglia and their opsonized targets (Jungi *et al* 1990), or a reduction in cytokine production (U.G. Anderson *et al* 1993). Whatever the mode of action, intravenous immunoglobulin appears to be safe and generally well tolerated.

Schuller and Govaerts (1983) first used immune globulin in multiple sclerosis, reporting that 11 of 31 patients with chronic progressive disease showed improvement. Nine were unchanged and the remaining 11 deteriorated. These results are rather reminiscent of the rule of thirds in multiple sclerosis treatment trials (one-third each better, same and worse). Achiron *et al* (1992b) later reported an open controlled trial using 0.4 g/kg intravenous immunoglobulin given for 5 days and then every 2 months for 1 year in ten patients and ten controls. Treatment was well tolerated. Relapse rate changed in the treated group from 3.7 ($\pm$ 1.2)/year to 1.0 ($\pm$ 0.7)/year, and from 3.3 ($\pm$ 1.4)/year to 3.0 ($\pm$ 1.6)/year in controls (which is rather high for unselected patients). At 12 months, the EDSS had changed from 4.5 to 4.2 in treated patients and from 3.5 to 3.7 in controls. Cook *et al* (1992) combined intravenous immunoglobulin (0.5–2 g/kg) with methylprednisolone given monthly to 14 patients with progressive multiple sclerosis. These were unusual in that 11 of the patients were considered to be corticosteroid dependent. During follow-up (mean duration 7.8 months) 11 patients experienced 17 relapses, many of which occurred within 1 month of treatment or coincided with attempts to taper the dose of corticosteroids. Tenser *et al* (1993) treated six patients with relapsing progressive multiple sclerosis for 2 days with 0.8 g/kg of intravenous immunoglobulin. Whilst we question the value of learning that two of them felt better, the main purpose of this study was to demonstrate immunological effects on immune function. van Engelen *et al* (1992) treated five patients with stable visual deficits, in the context of multiple sclerosis which had not previously responded to intravenous methylprednisolone, with 0.4 g/kg intravenous immunoglobulin for 5 days followed by a single dose twice monthly for 3 months. Vision started to improve within 12 months of treatment and was maintained for >1 year, but this did not correlate closely with psychophysical tests or imaging appearances.

Fazekas *et al* (1997) randomized a larger group (150 patients with relapsing multiple sclerosis having clinical evidence for moderate but neither trivial nor severe disability and without chronic progression) to a single monthly infusion of intravenous immunoglobulin (0.15–0.2 g/kg). This is a low dose. Exposure to other forms of immunosuppression up to 3 months (2 weeks for corticosteroids) previously was permitted, as was methylprednisolone in pulses of up to 10 g during intercurrent relapses. This design limits the confidence with which the otherwise impressive and statistically significant effects on disability (the primary outcome measure) and relapse activity can be assessed. In an intention to treat analysis, the proportions improving, worsening or unchanged in the treated group were 31%, 16% and 53% compared with 14%, 23% and 63% in placebo patients, respectively. However, the magnitude of change was small, being −0.2 EDSS points in treated patients and +0.1 in the placebo group (a difference of 0.3; p = 0.008). The effect on

relapse frequency shows the now familiar pattern. Treated patients had a reduction in baseline rate from 1.3 to 0.5 relapses during the first year (a reduction of 0.8 per year), which stabilized at 0.4 per annum in the second year compared with baseline, 1 year and 2 year rates of 1.4, 1.3 and 0.8 (reductions of 0.1 and 0.5, respectively) in the placebo group. Thus, the impact was all in the first year. Adverse effects were few and probably unrelated to medication. On closer inspection, however, a couple of additional points should be mentioned. Surprisingly, less reduction in relapse rate was seen in the placebo group than is usual in comparable trials. We wonder whether blinding was adequate. Failure of regression to the mean in the control group may have inflated the apparent treatment benefit. Investigators did not require a second confirmatory examination to determine that the apparent delay in EDSS progression was sustained at further examinations separated by 3, 6 or 12 months. The effect of intravenous immunoglobulin on MRI behaviour was not assessed in this study. However, in a small study, G.S. Francis *et al* (1997) demonstrated that intravenous immunoglobulin had no apparent effect on MRI behaviour in nine patients given induction and monthly booster doses. They continued to relapse, progress and accumulate T_2-weighted MRI lesions.

Achiron *et al* (1998) randomized 40 patients to induction and maintenance treatment with intravenous immunoglobulin (0.4 g/kg for 5 days with a single treatment every 2 months for 2 years) or placebo. Primary outcome measures related to relapse frequency, interval, time to next episode, and severity. These were patients with high pretreatment relapse rates and, unusually, the placebo cases showed fluctuations in relapse rate (1.5, 1.8 and 1.4 per year before and during each of the 3 years of the study, respectively), whereas treated patients showed a reduction (1.8, 0.7 and 0.4 per year, respectively; p = 0.0006, overall). Annual change in relapse rate across the 3 years of observation was −1.1 and −0.3 in patients receiving intravenous immunoglobulin compared with +0.2 and −0.4 in the placebo group. Thus, the effect on relapse rate depended entirely on the first year effect during which treated patients improved and the placebo group deteriorated (a difference in activity of 1.4 relapses/year). A greater proportion of treated patients (six of 20) than controls (none of 20) remained exacerbation free during the entire period of the study, and the time to first relapse was longer (233 compared with 82 days). There was no difference in mean EDSS scores between groups but a favourable distribution in the proportion within each group who worsened, improved or remained stable (14%, 24% and 63% in those receiving immunoglobulin compared with 17%, 11% and 72% in the placebo group, respectively) was observed. The protocol for MRI does not allow useful conclusions to be drawn. Twenty-six patients were treated by P.S. Sorensen *et al* (1998) in a crossover design with intravenous immunoglobulin 2 g/kg or placebo monthly each for 6 months. There were fewer new enhancing lesions on MRI (the primary end point; however, no benefit was seen in the number of new T_2 lesions) and a greater proportion of patients was relapse free (the secondary outcome) during periods of active therapy. Although promising, these smaller studies all failed to reproduce the original claim of Fazekas *et al* (1997). Consequently, intravenous immunoglobulin is not widely used as maintenance therapy to reduce relapse frequency in relapsing–remitting multiple sclerosis but, rather, is considered a second-line therapy (Rieckmann and Toyka 1999).

In a preliminary study involving 108 pregnancies, Achiron *et al* (2004b) investigated the specific issue of reducing the possibility of disease activity – manifesting as new relapses – in the puerperium by prophylactic use of intravenous immunoglobulin. Two treatment groups (intravenous immunoglobulin 0.4 g/kg/day for 5 consecutive days in week one after delivery with the same regimen at weeks six and twelve after delivery; or 0.4 g/kg/day for 5 consecutive days within 8 weeks of conception, and once every 6 weeks until 12 weeks postpartum) were compared with untreated mothers. No confounding factors were identified and there were no serious adverse events. The group treated during pregnancy showed fewer relapses during pregnancy (0.43, 0.15 and 0.0 annualized rates for each trimester compared with 0.72, 0.61 and 0.41 in controls); both treated groups had fewer episodes in the puerperium (0.28 and 0.58 annualized rates, respectively) compared with controls (1.33). This initial study suggests that further controlled trials of intravenous immunoglobulin in this clinical setting are needed.

A recently completed phase three study of intravenous immunoglobulin in secondary progressive multiple sclerosis involved 318 patients randomized to receive monthly infusions of either intravenous immunoglobulin 10% at a dose of 1 g/kg body weight (to a maximum of 80 g; eight vials) or the same volume of placebo with 0.1 g albumin per vial. Although there was a treatment advantage over the first year of the trial, this benefit was soon lost since treatment did not influence the proportion of patients classified as treatment failures (confirmed progression of EDSS of 1.0, or 0.5 for baseline EDSS of ≥ 6.0), or reduce MRI evidence of T_2 lesion accumulation. The trial was stopped after 27 months based on this interim analysis demonstrating futility (Hommes *et al* 2004). Of interest, however, was a reported beneficial effect on the development of brain atrophy (Lin *et al* 2002).

Following one clinical report that intravenous immunoglobulin might benefit patients with longstanding visual loss due to multiple sclerosis (van Engelen *et al* 1992), Noseworthy *et al* (2000b; 2001) conducted two randomized, double-blinded, placebo-controlled phase two trials to determine if intravenous immunoglobulin might restore function in the setting of persistent (visual) clinical deficits. In the first study, 67 patients with either relapsing–remitting (n = 19) or secondary progressive multiple sclerosis (n = 48), known to have a moderately severe fixed motor deficit (confirmed by isometric biomechanical muscle strength testing), were randomized to receive either 0.4 g/kg intravenous immunoglobulin daily for 5 days then every 2 weeks for 3 months (representing a total of 11 infusions) or placebo. Treatment failed to demonstrate an improvement in strength of the targeted muscle groups or benefits in any secondary outcome measures. In the second study, 55 patients with persistent visual loss from inflammatory optic neuritis were randomized to receive either 0.4 g/kg intravenous immunoglobulin daily for 5 days then monthly for 3 months (a total of eight infusions) or placebo. Treatment did not improve the primary visual outcomes (visual log acuity scores at 6 months) and the trial was again stopped on the futility principle. Stangel *et al* (2000a) were also unable to demonstrate that treatment with either placebo or intravenous immunoglobulin (0.4 g/kg/day for 5 days) separated by 6 weeks improved central conduction motor conduction velocity in ten patients with multiple sclerosis.

In summary, there is only limited evidence to support a role for intravenous immunoglobulin in patients with demyelinating disease of the central nervous system (other than those who have failed to respond to high-dose steroids or plasma exchange in the setting of a catastrophic relapse; see above and Chapter 16). Future randomized studies may change this recommendation.

Methotrexate

Despite being available for many years, methotrexate has only recently been evaluated in multiple sclerosis. The first study (J.W. Neumann and Ziegler 1972) alternated treatment with methotrexate (2.5 mg/day) and 6-mercaptopurine (75 mg/day) in 3-monthly cycles. There was no clinical effect but the study design was not ideal. Subsequently, Currier *et al* (1993) reported a reduction in relapse rate for patients in the relapsing–remitting phase treated with methotrexate but there was no effect on disability in patients with progressive multiple sclerosis. The role of methotrexate in this clinical situation was specifically assessed by D.E. Goodkin *et al* (1995). Sixty patients with secondary or primary progressive disease were randomized to treatment with a weekly oral dose of 7.5 mg methotrexate or placebo. Methotrexate was well tolerated and the relative absence of adverse effects allowed blinding to be maintained throughout the study. Overall, patients and independent observers were unimpressed by the results. Objective assessments, using a complex composite scale which independently assessed the EDSS, ambulation index, box and block and nine-hole peg tests (upper limb function), and new or enlarging MRI lesions, showed a statistically significant effect of methotrexate on function in the peg test but not the box and block method for assessing upper limb function or mobility.

Subsequently, D.E. Goodkin *et al* (1996) reported on changes in active MRI lesions and T_2-weighted total lesion load but, by comparison with other claims for an effect on surrogate markers of disease activity, methotrexate was relatively unimpressive. In correspondence, Olek *et al* (1996) indicated that weekly subcutaneous injections of a higher dose (20 mg) of methotrexate were generally well tolerated by 38 patients although one developed an injection site abscess and transient liver enzyme elevation was occasionally seen. The full report of this study appears not to have been published.

In a preliminary trial of 15 patients, Calabresi *et al* (2002b) showed that, when added to weekly IFN-β1a, methotrexate 20 mg orally, also in a single dose each week, seemed to reduce gadolinium enhancements and may have provided an additional protection against relapses. In a very small study, Rowe *et al* (2003) reported preliminary findings from adding high-dose intravenous methotrexate (2 g/m^2) every 2 months for 1 year in 15 patients with relapsing–remitting multiple sclerosis who had demonstrated neurological worsening during the preceding period on IFN-β1a weekly by intramuscular injection. Patients continued on weekly IFN-β1a tolerated combination therapy with evidence for stabilization of the clinical course as judged by the MSFC (see above), and with immunological markers suggesting an influence on disease mechanisms. We understand that a four-arm trial designed to determine whether methotrexate (20 mg orally per week) alone or in combination with methylprednisolone (1000 mg by intravenous infusion for 3 days every 2 months) provides a treatment advantage over weekly IFN-β1a in 900 patients with relapsing–remitting multiple sclerosis who have failed interferon alone is in progress. However, despite these ongoing studies, at present methotrexate joins cyclophosphamide and azathioprine as medications rarely, if ever, prescribed in our clinical practice.

Mitoxantrone

Mitoxantrone is an anthracenedione antineoplastic agent that intercalates with DNA and inhibits both DNA and RNA synthesis, suppressing T-cell and B-cell immunity. Mauch *et al* (1992) first treated 12 patients perceived to have rapid progression of disability with mitoxantrone (12 mg/m^2). All reported clinical stabilization and eight of them were considered to have improved at 1 year. The patients had 169 gadolinium-DTPA enhancing lesions at entry but only 10 were visible on completion of the study. Adverse effects were minimal. Mitoxantrone was next assessed in a small open study involving 13 patients with progressive multiple sclerosis (Noseworthy *et al* 1993). Participants received seven intravenous infusions over 3 weeks. Nine of the 13 patients had been observed over the previous 18 months and, in the remainder, historical evidence for rate of progression was available from case records. Initially, the clinical course appeared to stabilize and no changes in EDSS were seen for up to 12 months, but progression was apparent 6 months later. Although the authors considered progression to have occurred at a slower rate than expected from pretreatment observations in this cohort of patients, the changes were consistent with the natural history of multiple sclerosis previously seen in their placebo-controlled study of cyclophosphamide (see above). In eight of the 12 patients, there was evidence for continuing MRI activity during treatment with mitoxantrone.

In a subsequent study (Edan *et al* 1997), 42 patients with aggressive active clinical and radiological disease all receiving monthly injections of methylprednisolone were randomized to 6 months of treatment with intravenous mitoxantrone (20 mg/month) or no additional therapy. The baseline relapse rate was three per year in those who met the radiological guidelines for inclusion (there had to be gadolinium enhancing lesions) compared with 0.7 per year in patients who reported attacks in advance of selection but did not meet the radiological criteria for inclusion. Mitoxantrone was associated with a significantly higher frequency of conversion to disease inactivity as judged by gadolinium enhanced MRI activity. The mean number of enhancing lesions was reduced by about 90%, similar to that seen with other aggressive immunosuppressive regimens. Although both the number of participants and duration of follow-up prevented detailed assessment, there was an apparent beneficial effect of treatment on relapse rate and disability. The profile of adverse effects inhibited blinding, but no serious consequences of treatment were observed. In a 1 year study aimed at demonstrating whether mitoxantrone is cardiotoxic, De Castro *et al* (1995) showed a reduction in relapse rate in treated patients. There were no electrocardiographic or echocardiographic abnormalities. Millefiorini *et al* (1997) treated 27 patients monthly for 1 year with intravenous mitoxantrone (8 mg/m^2) or placebo. The differences in rate of accumulation of disability and number of relapses favoured a treatment effect. Nine of 24 placebo-treated patients deteriorated by up to 1 point on the EDSS compared with two of 27 patients given mitoxantrone. Five of 24 from the placebo group were free from exacerbations during the trial compared with 17 of the 27 patients given mito-

xantrone. This was reasonably well tolerated and, again, with no cardiac toxicity. However, MRI did not show a significant reduction in disease activity and, in this respect, the results provide less persuasive evidence for the therapeutic role of mitoxantrone than those reported by Edan *et al* (1997).

After a 4 year interval between the initial declaration of results in abstract form and full publication, Hartung *et al* (2002) reported on MIMS (Mitoxantrone in MS Study Group). In this double-blind, placebo-controlled, multicentre study (17 centres in four European countries: Germany, Belgium, Hungary and Poland), MIMS randomized 194 patients with either worsening relapsing–remitting (progressive relapsing) or secondary progressive multiple sclerosis to treatment either with placebo (3 mg methylene blue) or mitoxantrone (5 or 12 mg/m^2 intravenously every 12 weeks for 24 months). Inclusion criteria required that patients had deteriorated by up to 1.0 EDSS point in the 18 months prior to enrolment with a baseline EDSS of 3.0–6.0. Annual MRI scans were performed on a subset of 110 patients. The primary outcome measure was a composite score comprised of five clinical measures: change in EDSS at 2 years; change in ambulation index at 2 years; change in the baseline standardized neurological status at 2 years; number of relapses requiring corticosteroid treatment; and time to first relapse. Seventy-seven per cent completed 24 months of follow-up (71% completed 36 months in the study). Those who discontinued treatment were slightly more common in the control group. At 24 months, benefit was reported in all five components of the composite measure for both active treatment arms, with the overall greatest benefit noted between placebo and the group receiving mitoxantrone at a dose of 12 mg/m^2 (p < 0.0001: Figure 18.8). That said, the magnitude of the effect on EDSS was rather modest [essentially mild benefit vs. mild deterioration; mean EDSS change for high-dose mitoxantrone, –0.13 (SD 0.90) vs. +0.23 (SD 1.01) in the placebo group] as expected in a trial of relatively brief duration. Preliminary MRI analysis also indicated a treatment effect with fewer T$_2$-weighted lesions and fewer patients experiencing enhancing lesions at 2 years in the high-dose group (see below). Post hoc analysis was performed

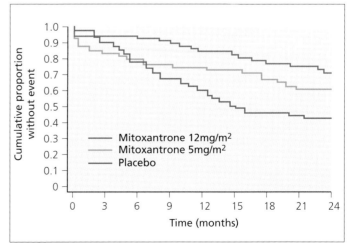

Figure 18.8 Treatment of progressive multiple sclerosis with mitoxantrone. Time to first relapse. Both doses of mitoxantrone delayed time to first recorded relapse by the treating physician. This individual was aware of the treatment assignment. Adapted from Hartung *et al* (2002). © 2002, with permission from Elsevier.

based on the 18-month pre-enrolment relapse history, to determine whether mitoxantrone was equally effective in patients with ongoing relapses and those progressing with superimposed relapses. This subgroup analysis was underpowered but showed a similar benefit in both groups of patients. However, there was a trend for EDSS progression in all relapse-free patients irrespective of treatment assignment, albeit to a lesser degree in those who received mitoxantrone. Indeed, the mean EDSS worsening at 2 years in previously relapse-free mitoxantrone recipients was virtually the same as that seen in the placebo-treated relapsing patients.

A few points merit additional comment. This study generated widespread use of mitoxantrone in patients failing to respond to the interferons and glatiramer acetate (K.K. Jain 2000). It contributed to the Food and Drug Administration (FDA; United States) approval of mitoxantrone for use in progressive multiple sclerosis even though a peer-reviewed manuscript was not published for a further 2 years. This delay remains unexplained. Additionally, the detailed MRI analysis is still not available. With respect to design and conduct of the study, an unblinded physician was used to determine relapse status. Success of the blinding procedure was not assessed. Nausea and mild alopecia were reported but tolerated. Secondary amenorrhoea lasting at least 1 year developed in 25% of women receiving high-dose mitoxantrone. No patients developed significant cardiomyopathy. Goodin *et al* (2003) recently highlighted an important concern that re-analysis by the sponsor (Immunex) with selective censoring of the treatment arms contributed to the reported treatment and its magnitude. Goodin *et al* (2003) point out that, at 3 years, the benefit in standardized neurological status persisted but the EDSS and ambulation index results did not. They question whether methylene blue may have been neurotoxic and thereby contributed to the clinical and MRI decline in control patients. They also emphasize that high-dose mitoxantrone did not affect the mean number of gadolinium enhancing lesions (p = 0.1). The apparent effect of low-dose mitoxantrone was not subjected to statistical analysis. High-dose mitoxantrone reduced T_2 number (p = 0.03) and the number of new contrast enhancing lesions (p = 0.02) but there was no apparent effect on T_2 lesion load.

Taken together, the limited evidence to date supports the conclusion that mitoxantrone reduces relapse frequency and MRI evidence for blood–brain barrier disruption in patients with very active multiple sclerosis. The benefit for patients with relapse-independent progression is less certain. The recently published report of the Therapeutics and Technology Assessment Subcommittee of the American Academy of Neurology (Goodin *et al* 2003) recommends caution in the use of this drug, and calls for confirmatory studies. We recommend this report as a balanced and comprehensive review of the evidence for efficacy and the range of toxicity associated with the use of mitoxantrone in multiple sclerosis. The magnitude of the expected treatment effect is perhaps best stated using the 'numbers needed to treat (NNT)' approach (Sackett *et al* 2000). From the MIMS results, one would need to treat 11 patients with secondary progressive multiple sclerosis for 2 years to prevent one person from worsening by 1.0 EDSS point.

Mitoxantrone is a toxic agent that must be administered with care to reduce the likelihood of marrow suppression, opportunistic infection and cardiomyopathy. Amenorrhoea is an important concern for many young women. The risk of cardiomyopathy is generally dose dependent and may be as great as 6% in cancer patients receiving up to 140 mg/m² (Dukart 1984; Mather 1987). In most trials involving patients with multiple sclerosis, and in our clinical practice, regular pretreatment echocardiograms can be used to screen for reduced left ventricular function. The MIMS investigators recommend measuring cardiac output at baseline and thereafter, once patients have received a total of 100 mg/m². In practice, we measure cardiac output before each infusion and discontinue mitoxantrone if there is evidence for a reduction. Irreversible cardiomyopathy requiring transplantation has been reported in patients with multiple sclerosis exposed to excessive doses of this agent. Pathological findings in such cases include noninflammatory myofilament rarefaction and degeneration, sarcoplasmic dilatation, and interstitial fibrosis (Gbadamosi 2003b). Goffette *et al* (2005) reported three cases of delayed cardiomyopathy (heart failure) beginning 24–80 months after the last dose of mitoxantrone (total cumulative dose 144 mg/m²) with no adequate explanation other than prior treatment with cyclophosphamide (two patients). This report reminds us of the need to use caution in the decision to use this agent and to be rigorous in maintaining close follow-up thereafter. Mitoxantrone is a topoisomerase II inhibitor and therefore may predispose to treatment-related leukaemia. There are now several reports possibly linking mitoxantrone to the development of acute leukaemia (Brassat 2002; Cattaneo 2003; Mogenet *et al* 2003; A.M. Vicari 1998). In a review of the literature, Ghalie *et al* (2002) estimated the risk of therapy-related acute leukaemia in patients with multiple sclerosis receiving mitoxantrone at 0.05–0.1%. This perceived rate may be on the low side; by 2004, there were currently five examples of acute leukaemia amongst a register of 2336 patients with multiple sclerosis receiving mitoxantrone, representing a cumulative incidence of 0.21% (Voltz *et al* 2004).

In the United States, Novantrone (mitoxantrone) is licensed by the FDA for

reducing neurologic disability and/or the frequency of clinical relapses in patients with secondary (chronic) progressive, progressive relapsing, or worsening relapsing-remitting multiple sclerosis (i.e. patients whose neurologic status is significantly abnormal between relapses). Novantrone is not indicated in treatment of patients with primary progressive multiple sclerosis.

In Europe, although unlicensed, mitoxantrone is not infrequently used to treat patients who are deteriorating along the lines described in the FDA licence. We use the drug sparingly, reserving mitoxantrone for patients who continue to suffer clinical and MRI evidence of active disease (frequent significant relapses and multiple contrast enhancements) despite treatment with interferons (or glatiramer acetate). In one of our centres (D.H.M.), it is required that there has been a deterioration of at least 2 EDSS points within 12 months, accompanied by evidence for active inflammatory disease based either on the occurrence of clinical relapses or the presence of gadolinium enhancing MRI lesions. We generally administer 12 mg/m² by intravenous infusion every 3 months for not more than eight cycles but hope for a stronger evidence base from ongoing trials resolving the issue of whether higher cumulative doses offer increased efficacy but without increasing the risk. We sometimes use the protocol of Edan *et al* (1997), namely mitoxantrone 20 mg monthly by intravenous injection for 6 months, in the small group of patients with particularly aggressive fulminant disease, in whom rapidly increasing disability has accumulated on the basis of frequent, severe relapses and many active inflammatory lesions on gadolinium enhanced MRI.

Cladribine

Cladribine specifically induces apoptotic death in resting and dividing lymphocytes but is otherwise relatively nontoxic. After assessing safety and obtaining a preliminary impression of efficacy, Sipe *et al* (1994) compared monthly pulses of cladribine given by an indwelling intravenous line with placebo in 51 patients with progresssive multiple sclerosis. The analysis was confined to 48 participants randomized initially to receive cladribine or placebo, completing the assessment at 1 year. Of the three remaining patients, one died from acute hepatic failure, one withdrew after suffering a hip fracture and one was lost to follow-up. Three other treated patients had significant episodes of infection and there was evidence for bone marrow suppression in another, but these all continued in the study. This was terminated on the basis of results at 1 year without embarking on the planned crossover phase. Placebo-treated patients deteriorated by approximately 1 EDSS point and by a comparable amount on a locally designed neurological rating scale (the Scripps scale), whereas those receiving cladribine remained stable or showed modest clinical improvement in pre-existing disabilities. The numbers of patients showing deterioration (by >1 EDSS point), improvement or stabilization were seven, one and 15 of the 23 patients in the placebo group compared with one, four and 19 of the 24 patients randomized to cladribine, respectively. Within pairs, a greater number showed no disease activity in serial MRI characteristics in the cladribine group compared with their placebo-treated partners (Figure 18.9A and B). There was some evidence for a difference in concentration, but not in the number, of oligoclonal bands in cladribine-treated patients compared with the placebo group. Since cladribine can now be given subcutaneously, the authors recommend its use at a lower dose than was evaluated in their trial of chronic progressive multiple sclerosis on the basis of efficacy and acceptable risks. Critics have argued that the original trial design was not strictly followed, and that the result was largely achieved through the atypical and severe course of the placebo group. However, in a preliminary communication, others have since endorsed the difference in natural history of progressive multiple sclerosis between patients receiving pulsed treatment with cladribine and placebo (Grieb *et al* 1994).

In a subsequent publication, Beutler *et al* (1996) extended the period of observation for the original study. Maintaining the blinded design, they crossed over the two randomized groups of patients, administering placebo to the original cladribine group and gave a reduced dose of cladribine to the patients who had first received placebo. A treatment effect was still claimed. The magnitude was reduced but toxicity was also less marked with the lower dose. The authors noted that cladribine can be given safely and with apparent equal efficacy by the subcutaneous route. Our position is that bone marrow toxicity (especially thrombocytopenia), herpetic infection in six patients and

reported protocol violations undermine the likelihood that the trial was sufficiently blinded to be convincing.

There are several more recent reports exploring the potential use of cladribine in multiple sclerosis. Romine *et al* (1999) claimed clinical benefit, measured as a reduction in the combined outcome of relapse severity and frequency, in a short (18 month) double-blind, placebo-controlled trial of cladribine (0.07 mg/kg subcutaneously daily for 5 days and repeated monthly for 6 months; total 2.1 mg/kg) given to 52 patients with relapsing–remitting disease. Relapse rate fell dramatically during the first 6 months of the trial, especially in the placebo group but, thereafter, treated patients continued to show fewer episodes. Cladribine-treated patients also had fewer gadolinium enhancing MRI lesions. In a phase three trial involving patients with progressive multiple sclerosis, Rice *et al* (2000) demonstrated that each of two doses of cladribine (0.07 mg/kg subcutaneously daily for 5 days each month repeated for either 2 or 6 months) reduced MRI evidence of disease activity in the subset of patients with secondary progressive disease. Unfortunately, this trial was limited to 1 year of follow-up and no clinical benefit was apparent in the primary outcome measures (EDSS and Scripps Neurologic Rating Scale). Both doses reduced the number and volumes of contrast enhancing lesions. The higher dose also reduced T_2 lesion load. Significantly, there was no effect on the progression of cerebral atrophy (Filippi *et al* 2000a; 2000b). We remain to be convinced that cladribine is useful, and do not recommend its use in the management of patients with multiple sclerosis.

Sulfasalazine

Noseworthy *et al* (1998) conducted a phase three trial designed to determine whether prolonged administration of sulfasalazine might reduce disease activity in patients with active multiple sclerosis. The trial was started before completion of the first definitive trial of IFN-β and at a time when there were no approved therapies for multiple sclerosis. Sulfasalazine is a well-tolerated oral agent for which a number of relatively mild immunosuppressive activities had previously been claimed together with moderate efficacy in other chronic immune-mediated disorders including rheumatoid arthritis and inflammatory bowel disease. Interim analysis suggested that treatment had been mildly effective early in the trial. Wisely, the data monitoring committee recommended that the study be continued to completion – and the early benefits disappeared so that, in the final analysis, there was no overall benefit (Figure 18.10). The decision to continue this trial without informing the investigators or sponsors of the early apparent benefit, and the subsequent recognition that early effects are often transient, provides an important lesson for the design and conduct of treatment trials in multiple sclerosis that has subsequently been well learned. Thus, sulfasalazine joins the list of agents that do not have a role in the treatment of multiple sclerosis.

Corticosteroids

Despite the unambiguous evidence that corticosteroids hasten clinical recovery in the setting of acute relapse (see Chapter 16), it has previously been held as axiomatic that they have no effect on the natural history of multiple sclerosis. But until recently,

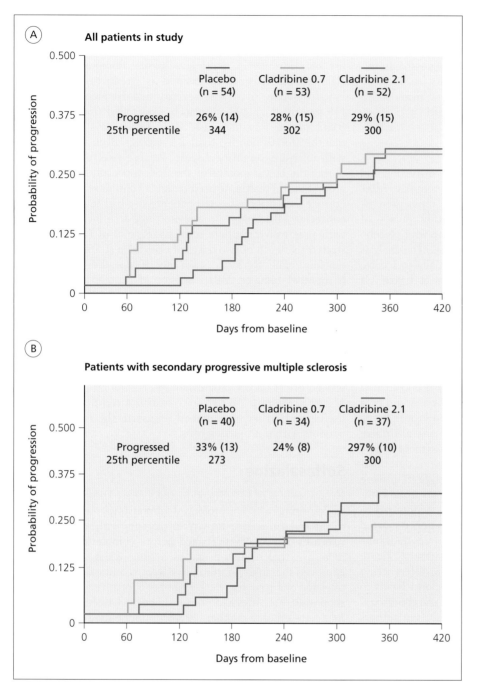

Figure 18.9 Treatment of multiple sclerosis with cladribine. Probability of disease progression (A) All patients; (B) Secondary progressive multiple sclerosis. This study was underpowered and of insufficient duration to determine whether cladribine would benefit patients with secondary progressive multiple sclerosis. Adapted from Rice *et al* (2000). © 2000, reproduced with permission of Lippincott Williams & Wilkins.

there had not been an adequate, long-range, properly controlled study to establish the validity of this axiom.

In a recent report, Zivadinov *et al* (2001a) randomized 88 ambulatory (baseline EDSS ≤ 5.5) patients with relapsing–remitting multiple sclerosis to receive either corticosteroids as needed to treat acute relapses, or on a predetermined schedule (every 4 months for 3 years and then every 6 months for 2 years). The regimen used methylprednisolone 1000 mg by intravenous infusion for 5 days followed by 4 days of oral prednisone (2 days each of 50 and 25 mg). To be eligible, patients needed to be at least 3 months removed from prior corticosteroid treatment and on no immune-modulating agents. Only the radiologist was blinded to study assignment. The results of this study were impressive. Only seven patients were lost to

follow-up. The primary (MRI) and secondary (disease progression as measured by EDSS) outcomes favoured the scheduled regimen. Patients randomized to regular courses of corticosteroids showed a benefit in terms of T_1 lesion volume and brain parenchymal volume. Although no significant differences were seen in T_2 volume, surprisingly there was a trend suggesting that T_2 volume increased more in the group receiving scheduled corticosteroids. Clinical measures also favoured the scheduled regimen. These included confirmed EDSS change (≥ 1.0 worsening for baseline EDSS ≤ 5.0; ≥ 0.5 points for EDSS ≥ 5.5 at baseline; and changes confirmed for at least 8 months in the first 2 years and at least 12 months in years four and five), proportion with EDSS worsening, proportion converting to secondary progressive multiple sclerosis, and mean EDSS change. There were no

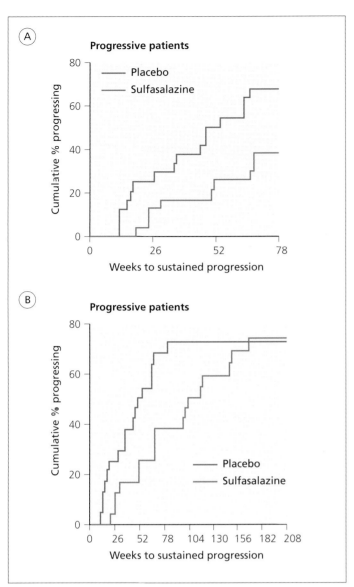

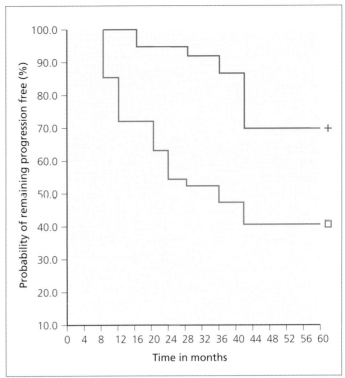

Figure 18.11 Treatment of relapsing–remitting multiple sclerosis with scheduled pulses of methylprednisolone (MP). Time survival curve to the onset of sustained EDSS score worsening. Log rank test p < 0.001. + = pulse MP; □ = control group. Adapted from Zivadinov *et al* (2001a). © 2001, reproduced with permission of Lippincott Williams & Wilkins (lww.com).

Figure 18.10 Treatment of active multiple sclerosis with sulfasalazine. (A) At the time of the interim analysis, there appeared to be an early treatment advantage for patients with progressive MS. (B) This later disappeared with prolonged follow-up. The data monitoring committee wisely did not terminate the trial early 'for apparent efficacy'. Adapted from Noseworthy *et al* (1998). © 1998, reproduced with permission of Lippincott Williams & Wilkins (lww.com).

differences in relapse rates, number, or time to relapse (Figure 18.11). Are these findings definitive? Regrettably not. Although certainly they are of great interest in that this is the longest trial to date (5 years) and corticosteroids are inexpensive and generally well tolerated; the putative effects on cerebral atrophy reported are, to date, unmatched so that the study needs to be repeated. The decision not to blind the evaluator was a major design flaw. This omission may have significantly biased the clinical assessments, lending a spurious credence to the reported result (Noseworthy *et al* 1994). That said, the MRI evaluations were blinded and seem robust, although cerebral atrophy measures have not been validated as definitive outcomes. Cerebral volumetric measures are clearly influenced in the short term by the use of corticos-

teroids, and artefacts arising from suppression of inflammation. If independently confirmed, the findings would suggest that regularly administered corticosteroids delay or prevent irreversible tissue injury. In turn, such a result would support the hypothesis that corticosteroids act to inhibit nitric oxide and excitotoxic mechanisms of neuronal and axon injury (see Chapter 10). We are not aware that a confirmatory trial is under way.

As we discuss in Chapter 4, new episodes cluster in women with relapsing–remitting multiple sclerosis during the puerperium. For this reason, De Séze *et al* (2004) treated 20 women who had recently completed a pregnancy prophylactically with methylprednisolone (1 g monthly for 6 months) and noted a lower relapse rate (0.8 ± 0.41) compared with 22 females observed expectantly a few years earlier (2 ± 0.66).

THE BETA INTERFERONS

The 1990s were dominated by the publication of large clinical trials evaluating the three brands of IFN-β and glatiramer acetate as disease-modifying drugs in multiple sclerosis, and the consequent managed introduction of these products into clinical practice. Interferons were first used in multiple sclerosis because of their antiviral activities. At first, no emphasis was placed on the type of interferon and each was assessed after administration by the systemic or intrathecal route. A series of pilot studies, mostly uncontrolled and involving small numbers of patients, was performed in the 1980s. These involved IFN-α (Camenga *et al* 1986; Knobler *et al* 1984), IFN-β given systemically

(Baumhefner *et al* 1987; M. Huber *et al* 1988; K.P. Johnson *et al* 1990; Ververken *et al* 1979) or by the intrathecal route (Confavreux *et al* 1986; Jacobs *et al* 1981; 1982; Milanese *et al* 1990), and IFN-β (Panitch *et al* 1987a; 1987b). The role of IFN-α and IFN-γ is discussed above. In general, many details of these inaugural studies are now more of historical interest than providing evidence for the clinician wishing to assess the role of IFN-β in the management of multiple sclerosis, since they have been updated and superseded by the pivotal clinical trials discussed below. However, the pioneering work of Larry Jacobs (1938–2001) should be mentioned.

Initially, Jacobs carried out an unblinded trial of intrathecal natural IFN-β in 20 patients (Jacobs *et al* 1981). There was an effect on relapse rate and this work was extended to a single-blind (sham lumbar puncture) study in which 69 patients also showed a reduction in annual relapse rate (0.8 in treated patients compared to 1.5 in controls; p < 0.001: Jacobs *et al* 1986b; 1987). There were practical problems associated with the use of intrathecal interferon and difficulties in obtaining natural IFN-β. Together with results suggesting an increase in disease activity in patients receiving natural interferon (Milanese *et al* 1990), no further progress was made until recombinant IFN-β was shown to be effective after parenteral administration. It was subsequently recognized that the immunological effects and physiological situations that characterize release of the naturally occurring interferons differ for IFN-α and IFN-β from IFN-γ. The results of clinical trials led to the conclusion that IFN-γ is contraindicated in multiple sclerosis and that IFN-α is not obviously effective, although its use has not altogether been abandoned (see above). However, IFN-β survived this filtration process, attracting increasing attention because of the accumulation of evidence for its partial efficacy together with vigorous marketing on a scale to which neurologists looking after people with multiple sclerosis had not previously been exposed. By comparison with azathioprine, for example, the processing of comparative clinical results attributable to IFN-β (see below) has been demonstrably less restrained.

In summary, the IFNB Multiple Sclerosis Study Group trial showed that patients receiving IFN-β1b (Betaseron 8 MIU by self-administered subcutaneous injection on alternate days) had a reduced relapse rate, although the effects on disability and disease progression did not reach conventional levels of statistical significance. Much was made of the reduction in MRI activity seen in the IFN-β1b (Betaseron) study and the extent to which this provided evidence for a disease-modifying effect. Subsequently, IFN-β1a (Avonex; 6 MIU intramuscularly on a weekly basis) was shown to reduce relapse rate and slow the rate of disability and the time to progression. The report on IFN-β1b (Betaseron) appeared in 1993, with an update in 1995. The study of IFN-β1a (Avonex) received much advance publicity but did not appear until January 1996. Sandwiched between these primary publications was a deluge of commentaries, vigorous marketing efforts by the pharmaceutical companies who stood to gain from the introduction of these products, and the jottings of several seriously ill-informed journalists. The immediate consequence was that, initially, neurologists were asked to prescribe IFN-β before it was licensed or widely available and often in settings where governments restricted its use. This complex situation subsequently evolved. Interferons became widely available for use in relapsing–remitting multiple sclerosis and, in some countries, for secondary progressive disease. Governmental efforts to ration their use still vary widely. Many countries and groups of opinion leaders have developed guidelines for prescribing these agents. Despite these efforts, however, there remains no evidence-based definition of 'responder' status or 'treatment failure'. Consequently, practitioners and patients struggle daily with decisions of when to start, change or stop the use of these agents.

The mechanisms of action

Most cells express receptors for type 1 interferons. IFN-α and IFN-β share and compete for the same site, transducing signals through protein tyrosine kinases, phosphorylation of signal transducers and activation of transcription factors (STAT1 and STAT2), formation of the IFN-stimulated gene factor 3 from the association of STAT1 and STAT2 with the p48 protein, and binding of this gene factor to promoter elements resulting in gene transcription (Karpusas 1998). IFN-γ uses a different receptor but stimulates some of the same intracellular signalling molecules. Collectively, the interferons show a variety of antiviral, antimicrobial, antitumour and immunological effects (for review, see Goodkin 1994; Weinstock-Guttman *et al* 1995; Yong 2002). If IFN-β has a role in modifying the long-term course of multiple sclerosis, it is almost certainly not through any effect on the response to viral infection, as originally suggested, and the recent logic for continued use in clinical practice rests on the results of laboratory studies that shift the emphasis on mode of action to immunological properties. T-cell-derived IFN-γ has mainly proinflammatory effects and this explains why it increases disease activity in multiple sclerosis.

The logic for using IFN-β is now based not only on the argument that IFN-β inhibits the actions of IFN-γ, but also from a wide variety of additional presumed mechanisms of action including inhibition of T-cell activation, modulation of cytokine production and reduction in T-cell migration. In this respect, IFN-β can be considered as an anti-inflammatory cytokine but it also enhances some components of the immune response. This literature is abundant and often conflicting. Research remains active and, as expected given the plethora of potential sites of activity, the story is self-evidently incomplete and not without its share of ambiguities on the specific immunological effects and their relevance for treated patients. Inevitably, individual commentators tend to focus on the mechanisms that address their preferred concepts for the pathogenesis of multiple sclerosis. We are not exempt from these accusations of parochialism. Table 18.2 provides contemporary references for recent work on the potential mechanisms of action of IFN-β, a subject comprehensively reviewed by J. Zhang *et al* (2002). Exposure of microglia to IFN-γ *in vitro* increases the expression of cell surface class II MHC antigen (Woodroofe *et al* 1989) and the constitutively expressed T helper type 1 (Th1) costimulatory molecule B7 (K.E. Williams *et al* 1994). This upregulation is inhibited by IFN-β in a dose-dependent manner. The effect is most pronounced when IFN-β is introduced *in vitro* prior to IFN-γ exposure but is still evident when IFN-β is added after exposure of microglia to IFN-γ. Since this inhibition is not associated with a decrease in class II mRNA within cells, the mechanism is considered to be post-transcriptional and, given that class II heavy chain accumulates within cells, presumably post-translational. Revel *et al* (1995) have shown that the molecular interactions of IFN-β and IFN-γ involve the STAT1 transcription

Table 18.2 Presumed mechanisms of action of the beta interferons

Inhibits T-cell costimulation and/or activiation processes

- Inhibits IFN-γ-induced expression of MHC class II molecules and other molecules required for T-cell activation (Arnason *et al* 1996)
- Modulates costimulatory molecules on dendritic and other cell types (Y.M. Huang *et al* 2001a; 2001b; 2001c; 2001d; Z. Liu *et al* 2001)
- Reduces precursor frequency of myelin-reactive T cells (Kozovska *et al* 1999; Zang *et al* 2000b)
- Treatment-induced reduction in costimulatory molecules (Shapiro *et al* 2003)
- Treatment-induced reduction in the number of antigen presenting dendritic cells (Bergh *et al* 2004)

Modulates anti-inflammatory and proinflammatory cytokines

- Increases IL-10 and IL-4 production/expression at protein and mRNA levels (Ozenci *et al* 2000; Rep *et al* 1996; Rudick *et al* 1996b; 1998b; Tuohy *et al* 2000)
- Decreases IL-12 production (Karp *et al* 2001; McRae *et al* 1998; Tuohy *et al* 2000)
- Decreases TNF-α and IFN-γ production (Kozovska *et al* 1999; Rep *et al* 1996; Zang *et al* 2000b)
- Suppresses Th1 cells and upregulates IL-10 production (Zang *et al* 2003)

Decreases aberrant T-cell migration

- Enhanced shedding of VCAM-1 from endothelium into soluble form (Calabresi *et al* 1997c)
- Decreases T-cell migration (Prat *et al* 1999)
- Reduced integrin gene expression (Muraro *et al* 2004)
- Inhibits expression of mRNA for MIP-1α, RANTES, and CCR5 (Zang *et al* 2000a; 2001)
- Reduces migration of T cells toward the chemokines RANTES and MIP-1 (Zang *et al* 2001)
- Decreases IL-2-stimulated secretion of MMP (Leppert *et al* 1996; Lou *et al* 1999)
- Treatment-induced reduced MMP-9 levels in PPMS (Yushchenko *et al* 2003)
- Treatment-induced enhanced TIMP-1 levels in RRMS (Karabudak *et al* 2004)
- Reduces secretion of TNF-α and IL-1 (Lou *et al* 1999)

MHC = major histocompatibility complex; IL = interleukin; mRNA = messenger ribonucleic acid; TNF = tumour necrosis factor; VCAM = vascular cell adhesion molecules; MIP = macrophage inflammatory proteins; RANTES = regulated on activation, normal T-cell expressed and secreted; CCR = chemokine receptor; MMP = matrix metalloproteinases; TIMP-1 = natural tissue inhibitors of MMPs. Adapted from Zhang et al *(2002) with permission.*

factor and they propose a model involving antagonistic and synergistic actions on different genes whose products relate to cell activation. The increased class II antigen expression on microglia enables these to function as antigen-presenting cells and the proliferation of primed T cells exposed to antigen and IFN-γ activated microglia is inhibited by IFN-β (G. Hall *et al* 1997a). It is well recognized that IFN-β has an antiproliferative effect on T (and other non-immune) cells, inhibiting markers of activation such as IL-2 receptor, transferrin receptor and CD2 (A. Noronha *et al* 1993). Others have shown that the release *in vitro* of IFN-γ by mononuclear cells is reduced in patients treated with IFN-β (Petereit *et al* 1997).

Antigen-specific and IL-2-stimulated proliferation of Th1 cells are inhibited by IFN-β but without reducing their secretion of IFN-γ, TNF-α or macrophage inflammatory protein-1α. In fact,

IFN-γ secretion is slightly increased, further demonstrating that the effects of IFN-β are complex and cannot simply be seen as suppression of IFN-γ-stimulated proinflammatory events (M. Pette *et al* 1997). In a comprehensive assessment, H. Jiang *et al* (1995) showed that IFN-β inhibits the ability of human antigen-presenting cells and B lymphocytes to induce T-cell proliferation. These inhibitions are associated with reduced expression of class II MHC antigens and adhesion molecules.

Taken together, these *in vitro* results suggest that IFN-β prevents the arrival of T cells and limits antigen presentation within the central nervous system, disengaging the amplification of local immune responses involving microglia and (antigen-specific) infiltrating T cells. IFN-γ also promotes the cytotoxic and phagocytic activities of microglia by increasing their respiratory burst and inducing the release of many mediators, but the interaction of IFN-γ and IFN-β on these properties is less straightforward. Rodent microglia exposed to IFN-γ increase the expression of Fc receptors and this effect is enhanced by IFN-β (G.C. Hall *et al* 1997b). IFN-β also directly stimulates the production of potentially harmful cytokines including TNF-α by microglia, further promoting their cytotoxic and phagocytic properties. TNF-α has a complementary effect on the ability of IFN-γ to increase class II antigen expression, demonstrating that intricate networks exist between pro- and anti-inflammatory cytokines. In samples obtained from patients before and during treatment, Brod *et al* (1996) showed that mitogen-induced production of cytokines (IFN-γ, IL-2, IL-6 and IL-10 but not IL-4 or TNF-α) is increased by IFN-β. Porrini *et al* (1995) took a slightly different position claiming that, *in vitro*, IFN-β induces the production of IL-10 and cytokines characterizing Th2 cells – a response not reproduced by IFN-γ. IL-10 released in response to IFN-β inhibits the production of TNF-α and IL-6 induced by IFN-γ and other macrophage activators. Others have since confirmed the antiproliferative effect of IFN-γ on human T cells *in vitro*, adding the observation that cooperation between T and B cells is also inhibited and emphasizing the anti-inflammatory consequences of the associated enhanced IL-10 production (Rep *et al* 1996; Rudick *et al* 1996b; see Chapter 11). IL-1 and IL-10 and transforming growth factor-β (TGF-β) tend to reduce class I antigen expression, providing evidence for a cascade of anti-inflammatory effects on antigen presentation in the central nervous system (Cowan *et al* 1991b; Racke *et al* 1991). IFN-β also inhibits antigen presentation of peripheral blood mononuclear cells through an effect on class II antigen expression (H. Jiang *et al* 1995). IFN-β inhibits IL-1-induced and IFN-α-induced production of nitric oxide (L.L. Hua *et al* 1998) and protects neurons from nitric oxide-mediated damage to mitochondrial complexes II/III and IV (Stewart *et al* 1998).

IFN-β and IFN-γ may therefore independently enhance the cytotoxic and phagocytic properties of microglia. At the very least, there does not appear to be complete reciprocal inhibition. Conversely, the antigen-presenting effects of IFN-γ-stimulated microglia are inhibited by IFN-β (G. Hall *et al* 1997a; 1997b). Given the part inhibitory and part complementary effects, it would be too simple to designate IFN-γ and IFN-β as entirely proinflammatory and anti-inflammatory cytokines, respectively.

The fact that IFN-β also inhibits class II expression on endothelial cells [in this situation, probably through a transcriptional mechanism (A. Miller *et al* 1996)] provides an additional potential mechanism of action through effects on cell migration across the blood–brain barrier (Huynh *et al* 1995). Further evidence is provided by the demonstration that the IL-2-induced secretion of metalloproteinases by T cells, which normally enhances their ability to adhere and migrate through endothelial barriers, is reduced by preincubation *in vitro* with IFN-β, probably by a direct effect on IL-2 receptors (Leppert *et al* 1996). Others have assessed changes in the endothelium and conclude that IFN-β, by reducing the secretion of matrix metalloproteinases, inhibits cell migration and limits the ability of T cells and natural killer cells to cleave fibronectin on the basement membrane of endothelial cells (Stuve *et al* 1996). These studies specifically implicate matrix metalloproteinase-9. Corsini *et al* (1997) showed a reduction in adherence between mononuclear cells from patients treated for at least 6 months with IFN-β on cultured brain endothelia derived from a patient with multiple sclerosis. This was associated with reduced expression of HLA-DR on endothelial but not mononuclear cells, and with no effect on other adhesion molecules. Related work shows also that IFN-β affects the migratory activity of mononuclear cells by inhibiting their production of matrix metalloproteinase-9 (Stuve *et al* 1997). Recently, two groups have studied the effects of interferons on matrix metalloproteinase-9 and a tissue inhibitor of metalloproteinase (TIMP-1). Yushchenko *et al* (2003) showed that treatment with IFN-β1b produced reduced levels of serum matrix metalloproteinase-9 in all but one of 19 patients with primary progressive multiple sclerosis; there were no consistent changes in TIMP-1 levels. Karabudak *et al* (2004) reported that IFN-β1a treatment induced transient increases in TIMP-1 levels compared with baseline (at 3 and 6 months but not at 1 year) in a study of 16 patients with relapsing–remitting multiple sclerosis. However, no consistent changes were detected in matrix metalloproteinase-9 levels. Again, the relevance of these findings remains uncertain.

In a study of 35 patients with relapsing–remitting multiple sclerosis and 12 with secondary progressive disease, Shapiro *et al* (2003) demonstrated that treatment with IFN-β1a (Rebif) may induce changes in the ratio of costimulatory molecules (for example, suppression of CD80 and induction of CD86) detected within the first year of treatment that favour a Th2 predominance. They raise the theoretical concern that these patients could be at risk of humoral mediated autoimmunity or allergic phenomena.

An effect of IFN-β on lymphocyte migration, and hence inflammation, is also provided by the demonstration of reduced very late antigen-4 (VLA-4) expression on monocytes (Soilu-Hanninen *et al* 1995) and lymphocytes from a small group of treated patients, but this finding could not be reproduced *in vitro* (Calabresi *et al* 1997a; Muraro *et al* 2000). The interferons may increase shedding of vascular cell adhesion molecule (VCAM) and intracellular adhesion molecule-1 (ICAM-1) from endothelial cells thereby increasing circulating levels of these adhesion molecules (Calabresi *et al* 1997c). IFN-β treatment could thereby block migration of activated T cells by reducing the concentration of endothelial membrane-bound adhesion molecules. Alternatively, once shed from the cell surface, these soluble adhesion molecules may block their respective receptors on activated peripheral blood mononuclear cells [for example, soluble ICAM-1 binding to lymphocyte function associated antigen (LFA) and Mac-1; and soluble VCAM binding to VLA-1]. In a recent study of 50 patients with relapsing–remitting multiple sclerosis treated with IFN-β1a and IFN-β1b, Muraro *et*

al (2004) reported that integrin gene expression of VLA-4 and LFA-1 is reduced in patients classified as 'IFN responders', raising the intriguing (but unconfirmed) suggestion that transcription of integrin genes may correlate with the treatment effect.

In summary, IFN-β probably exerts its effects through a variety of mechanisms. These include actions that reduce T-cell and monocyte activation and lymphocyte proliferation, decrease the proinflammatory cytokine bias that is thought to underlie some of the steps in tissue injury, reduce the IFN-γ upregulation of class II expression, diminish antigen presentation, and reduce T-cell migration through the blood–brain barrier. As discussed later, the putative mechanisms of action of glatiramer acetate differ from those for the interferons but with some interesting overlap and redundancy. These major differences raise a possible role for combination therapy.

The pivotal trials

The evidence that informed prescribing patterns, and led to product licences for the three brands of IFN-β, was derived from a series of pivotal studies incorporating randomized, double-blind and placebo-controlled designs carried out in the 1990s. IFN-β1b is produced by recombinant DNA technology using *Escherichia coli*. It differs from natural human and recombinant IFN-β1a (made in Chinese hamster ovary cells) in having 165 amino acids (lacking the methionine at position 1), a serine residue substituted for cysteine at position 17 to prevent incorrect disulphide bond formation, and no glycosylation of the asparagine residue at position 80. In the pivotal trials IFN-β1a (Avonex) was administered by weekly intramuscular injection (6 MIU), and IFN-β1a (Rebif; 22 or 44 μg thrice weekly) and IFN-β1b (Betaferon; 8 MIU), and as alternate day subcutaneous injections. These regimens were justified by the demonstration that serum levels of IFN-β1b peak between 8 and 24 hours and return to baseline by 48 hours (O.A. Khan *et al* 1996). There are no obvious differences between IFN-β1b and IFN-β1a in their biological activity or *in vivo* pharmacokinetics. Each is associated with the development of neutralizing antibodies. Here, we review the efficacies and adverse effects of these therapies, and the position that has emerged on the timing of treatment with respect to disease course. In turn, these inform the evidence base for the role of IFN-β in the management of multiple sclerosis at several stages of the illness. The sponsors of trials n multiple sclerosis have used an inconsistent and unhelpful format for designating doses of the interferons. To avoid controversy with regard to bio-equivalence, we refer to these studies using the doses as published. For reference, subcutaneous IFN-β1b has been tested in doses of 1.6 and 8 MIU (Betaseron) and 22 and 44 μg (Rebif). Intramuscular IFN-β1a (Avonex) has been tested predominately at 30 μg. On a mass basis, 6 MIU equates to 22 μg and 8 MIU to 44 μg.

IFN-β1b (Betaferon)

The pilot study of IFN-β1b was used to determine primary outcome measures for the definitive trial (K.P. Johnson *et al* 1990). Compared with seven controls, treatment in 24 patients using different doses of IFN-β1b showed a modest effect on relapse frequency. During treatment, patients receiving IFN-β1b had a relapse rate of 0.7 per year compared with 0.9 per year in the placebo group; and the probability of remaining relapse free at 3 years was 83% compared with an estimated pretreatment rate of 63%. There was no effect on disability. In fact, the treated group did marginally worse.

The phase three trial was conducted simultaneously in Canada and the United States (IFNB Multiple Sclerosis Study Group 1993). It involved 372 patients, each having two relapses in the previous 2 years and with pre-entry EDSS scores <5.5 (the mean was about 3.0; Table 18.3). Treated cases were younger and had slightly longer disease duration. Corticosteroids were used during the trial period by 35% and 50% of treated and placebo cases, respectively. Those who did not complete the study (19%) were considered to have remained stable from the point at which they dropped out. The study was not therefore analysed strictly on an intention to treat basis. The results were broadly similar in the Canadian and United States groups. Most commentators consider this to have been a single trial, although attempts were made to represent these as independent and hence confirmatory studies, respectively.

In patients receiving 8 MIU of IFN-β1b, both primary outcome measures – relapse rate and number of relapse-free patients – achieved statistically significant results (p = 0.0001 and p = 0.007, respectively). Of the secondary end points, reduction in relapse rate in those who continued to relapse (p = 0.001), increase in time to first relapse (p = 0.015) and second relapse (p = 0.007),

and reduction in the proportion of relapses judged to be moderate or severe (placebo vs. 8 MIU, p = 0.002) were also achieved.

The subsequent experience of these participants was later reported. The overall tone of the second publication (IFNB Multiple Sclerosis Study Group and the University of British Columbia MS/MRI Analysis Group 1995) was notably more sober than the initial paper. Participants had remained in the study for a median time of just under 4 years. Taking this entire period, the reduction in relapse rate associated with the use of IFN-β1b reported in 1993 was maintained at follow-up (8 MIU: 0.78 per year compared with 1.12 for the placebo group; p = 0.0006). The main effect of treatment was achieved in the first year. Although there was a reduction in relapse rate, both in treated patients and the placebo group, in each subsequent year, the cumulative reduction beyond year 1 was in fact greater as part of the untreated natural history (–0.63 between years 2 and 5 in placebo-treated patients compared with –0.39 in the treated group; Table 18.3 and Figure 18.12). However, this observation may be somewhat disingenuous since the baseline was lower at the start of year 1 in the treated group, therefore providing less room for manoeuvre in terms of further reduction in relapse rate by comparison with controls. Understandably, the authors emphasized these results as showing a continuing difference in exacerbation rates between treated and placebo groups, year on year, borrowing the substantial reduction in the first year for the subsequent cumulative reduction in

Table 18.3 **IFN-β1b: updated report of pivotal trials**	Placebo	1.5 MIU	8 MIU
Exacerbation rates			
Enrolled	123	125	124
Number entering year 5	56	52	58
Overall exacerbation rate	1.12[a]	0.96	0.78[a]
(baseline–year 5)	(1.02–1.23)	(0.87–1.06)	(0.70–0.88)
Year-on-year exacerbation rates			
Year 1	1.44	1.22	0.96
Year 2	1.18	1.04	0.85
Year 3	0.92	0.80	0.66
Year 4	0.88	0.68	0.67
Year 5	0.81	0.66	0.57
Reduction in exacerbation rate			
Baseline–year 1	–0.36	–0.48	–0.74
Year 2–5	–0.63	–0.56	–0.39
Disability			
Enrolled	123	125	124
Number entering year 5	56	52	58
No. with EDSS >1 point	56/122 (46%)	59/125 (47%)	43/122 (35%)[b]
Baseline EDSS <3	26/58 (45%)	30/59 (51%)	20/55 (36%)
Baseline EDSS >3	30/64 (47%)	29/66 (44%)	23/67 (34%)
Median time to progression (years)	4.18	3.49	4.79[c]
MRI: lesion load			
Enrolled	73	66	78
Number entering year 5	72	61	75
Baseline MRI (median)	1503	1086	1525
Completing year 1	+6.7	+5.7	–4.9
Completing year 4	+30.2[d]	+10.6	+3.6[d]
Increase: year 2–5	+23.5	+4.9	+8.7
a p = 0.0001; b p = 0.096; c p = 0.087; d p = 0.04.			

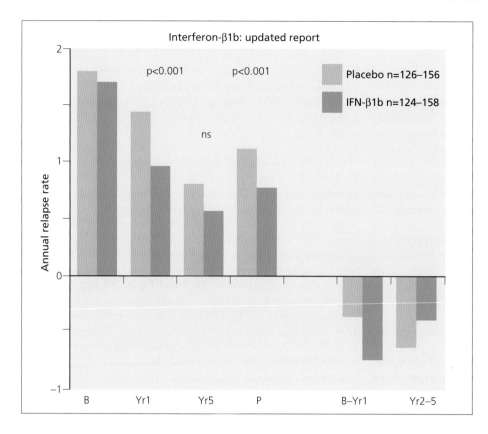

Figure 18.12 Annual relapse rates at baseline (B), baseline to year 1 (Yr1) and baseline to year 5 (Yr5) and in placebo-treated patients (P) in a trial of IFN-β1b; the rate of reduction is shown from baseline to end of year 1 (B-Yr1) and end of year 1 to end of year 5 (Yr2-5). Adapted from the IFNB Multiple Sclerosis Study Group (1993; 1995). © 1993, 1995, reproduced with permission of Lippincott Williams & Wilkins (lww. com).

relapse rate over the entire period. In this second report, once again IFN-β1b at a dose of 8 MIU reduced the proportion of patients judged to have a moderate or severe relapse compared with placebo (p = 0.012) although the data are not shown.

It has since been much debated whether a modest effect on relapse rate is useful for the majority of patients with multiple sclerosis. Relapses are distressing but usually self limiting, although they cause disability if recovery is poor. IFN-β1b may reduce relapse severity but the magnitude of this putative protection is somewhat unclear. In the IFN-β1b trial reports, 'moderate and severe' relapses are grouped together. The numbers of patients with each type of relapse, including those of 'unknown' severity, are not given. That said, it may be that, in protecting individuals from about one relapse every 3 years, IFN-β1b may be more likely to reduce a severe attack than a mild one. Relapses affecting the pyramidal and cerebellar systems are often relatively disabling, at least in the short term, and there were fewer of these in the treated patients. The effect on relapse rate reduced the need for hospitalization, and presumably also the impact on aspects of daily living, although this could not directly be assessed. Critics pointed out that the relapses were self reported and not universally confirmed by the attending neurologist. We understand that analysis only of those relapses that were physician confirmed was still highly significant and so take a charitable view on this design fault, accepting that there was no bias in the distribution of pseudo- and non-relapses in treated patients compared with the placebo group.

In many natural history studies, relapse frequency has not emerged as a factor which predicts disability. In recent studies from the Mayo Clinic (with a small cohort of patients followed closely for several decades), it has been difficult to confirm a close link between relapses and disability. No single demographic or disease variable (including relapse number in the first year) closely predicted prognosis (Pittock et al 2004a). In this series, as reported previously (Confavreux et al 2000), relapses did not influence further progression after reaching EDSS 3.0 (Pittock et al 2004b). In the large Canadian series, however, the number of relapses in the first 2 years, and time to the first relapse after presentation, did each correlate with eventual disability (Weinshenker et al 1991a; see also Chapter 4). This has encouraged people with multiple sclerosis that the reduction in relapse rate may have a dividend for an altered natural history of disease. It remains completely unknown, however, whether a reduction in relapse rate attributable to treatment (if this was shown to be long lasting by appropriately designed trials) shares the same good prognosis enjoyed by untreated patients experiencing a relatively relapse-free existence as part of their natural history.

Much has been made of the extent to which the MRI results influenced the overall impact of the IFN-β1b study. The IFNB Multiple Sclerosis Study Group studied a cohort of cases with serial assessments of lesion load (an indicator of the volume of affected brain), supplemented by measures of new and active lesions (Paty et al 1993). Comparable at entry, IFN-β1b-treated cases showed a reduction in lesion load within the first year (−4.9%) compared with the placebo group (+6.7%). These differences were maintained into the year 5 but, here too, the early effect attributed to IFN-β1b slipped marginally with time (Figure 18.13). Thus, both for the effect on relapse frequency and MRI lesion load, the experience of the first year proved crucial in this pivotal trial (Table 18.3).

In a subsequent study involving patients not recruited for the IFN-β1b (Betaseron) trial, L.A. Stone et al (1995) compared the contrast enhancing new lesion rate in the 7 months before and 6 months after introduction of IFN-β1b. A minimum pretreatment rate of 0.5 lesions/month was required for entry and

13 of the 14 participants showed a reduction in active lesions. This represented an average change from 3.1/month to 0.5/month (p = 0.002). The number was 230 before and 20 after starting treatment with IFN-β1b, a reduction of 90%. Many patients had been studied over a longer period (up to 50 months) and the new lesion rate changed from 2.7/month to 0.2/month. These patients had eight clinical episodes in the pretreatment period and four during treatment – a surprisingly high number given the MRI results. As an extension of this work, L.A. Stone *et al* (1997) prospectively studied 29 patients having

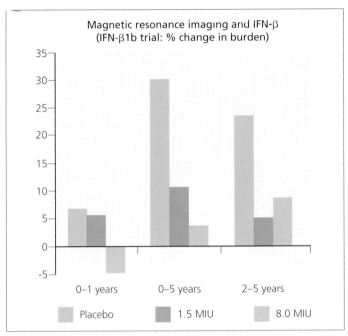

Figure 18.13 Annual change in MRI disease burden at baseline, baseline to year 1 and baseline to year 5 in patients receiving IFN-β1b; the rate of reduction is shown from baseline to end of year 1 and end of year 1 to end of year 5. Adapted from Paty *et al* (1993) and the IFNB Multiple Sclerosis Study Group (1993; 1995). © 1993; 1995, reproduced with permission of Lippincott Williams & Wilkins (lww.com).

>0.5 lesions/month during a 7 month qualification period. Eighty-six per cent of scans were active before and 33% were active during treatment with IFN-β1b. The median number of new lesions per patient per month dropped from 2.5 to 0.17 (p < 0.0001). Inevitably, there was variation between patients, prompting the authors to define a group of nonresponders but these did not have identifiable clinical or natural history characteristics.

A different marker of biological efficacy, measurement of urinary myelin basic protein-like material, was used for some participants in the IFN-β1b study (Whitaker *et al* 1995b). In so far as levels of this breakdown product represent a marker of disease progression and both number of lesions and total MRI lesion load, this result provided further surrogate evidence for efficacy. However, randomization bias prevented detailed analysis of the effect of IFN-β on urinary myelin basic protein.

There was no statistically significant effect of IFN-β1b on disability in these mildly affected patients participating in the North American study and that situation did not change with extension to 5 years (Figure 18.14). Thus, 43 of 122 (35%) treated patients showed a sustained (>6 months) deterioration of ≥ 1 EDSS points compared with 59 of 122 (46%) of the placebo group (p = 0.10). These results were uninfluenced by stratification for disability (baseline EDSS <3 and ≥ 3 at entry). It has been argued that restriction of the trial to include only stable, ambulant, relapsing–remitting patients did not give the study adequate power to assess this outcome. Thus, the results can be read as providing evidence for no effect on disability, or no evidence for an effect on disability. This difference in outcome may relate to the relative ease with which new episodes can be defined and the low stringency conditions used to assign relapses in this study, together with the insensitivity of scales routinely used to define disability. We have made the point repeatedly that inflammation and degeneration make different contributions to the pathological processes underlying relapse and progression. Saida *et al* (2005) randomized 205 patients from Japan with relapsing–remitting multiple sclerosis either to receive high-[250 μg (8 MIU)] or low-dose [50 μg (1.6 MIU)] IFN-β1b (Betaseron) three times weekly. As reported previously in the original North American trial, high doses of IFN-β1b were superior to low doses in reducing relapse rates and other measures of

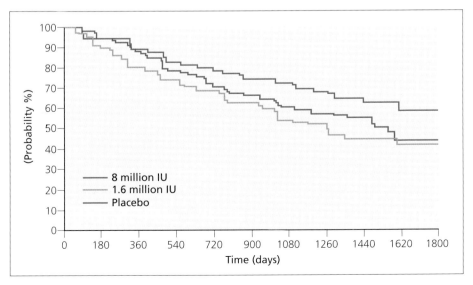

Figure 18.14: Kaplan–Meier curves showing, by treatment arm, the probability of avoiding progression of multiple sclerosis equal to at least 1 EDSS point. Adapted from the IFNB Multiple Sclerosis Study Group and the University of British Columbia MS/MRI Analysis Group (1995). © 1995, reproduced with permission of Lippincott Williams & Wilkins (lww.com).

disease activity. This suggests that, despite some differences in phenotype, IFN-β may be no less effective in Japanese populations than elsewhere.

IFN-β1a (Avonex)

The results of a study using IFN-β1a, with disability as the primary outcome measure, were first presented to a joint meeting of the American Neurological Association and Association of British Neurologists in October 1994 and immediately published in abstract form (Anon 1994). Despite widespread distribution of fly-sheets further advertising these results at scientific meetings and a description of the methodology (Jacobs *et al* 1995), no peer-reviewed publication of the results appeared until early 1996 (Jacobs *et al* 1996) by which time the procedure for granting a product licence in the United States and Europe was well advanced. In the trial, existing symptomatic treatments were not discontinued. Relapses were treated (at the discretion of physicians) with corticosteroids and immediate adverse effects of IFN-β1a were prophylactically managed with acetaminophen. Three hundred and one patients with clinically definite multiple sclerosis in the relapsing phase (some with persistent symptoms and signs), and with EDSS scores ranging from 1 to 3.5, were treated with placebo (n = 143 at entry; n = 87 for 2 years) or IFN-β1a (n = 158 and n = 85, respectively; Table 18.4). Each had two or more physician-documented relapses in the preceding 3 years but none in the previous 2 months, and the pretreatment exacerbation rate was >0.67 per year. Compliance with the trial protocol was good, with >99% of assessments completed. There were 23 early exits from the study but assessments continued in these patients. Sample size calculations allowed for 25% of patients to discontinue treatment but remain available for analysis on an intention to treat basis and with 10% lost to follow-up. The drop-out rate was <3%. The decision was taken to restrict recruitment to 288 patients (in fact, 301 had already been enrolled) and to stop the study a year earlier than planned. In retrospect, this was unwise because it has been assumed (wrongly according to the manufacturer) that premature termination of the study was taken with reference to interim efficacy analyses. Whatever the reason, this decision left the study significantly underpowered.

Treatment with IFN-β1a was shown to be associated with a slower rate of disability (defined in advance as deterioration by ≥ 1 point on the EDSS for ≥ 6 months; Table 18.4). The decision to stop the trial early left only 172 (IFN-β1a, n = 85; placebo, n = 87) participants observed for the intended duration of the study. Two years after the start, 22% of 158 patients who had received IFN-β1a were classified as treatment failures compared with 35% of the 143 placebo cases. At this point, two patients had not completed 6 months on the study; 14 (seven in each arm) had been involved for <1 year; 67 (IFN-β1a, n = 32; placebo, n = 35) had been studied for <18 months; and 134 (IFN-β1a, n = 56; placebo, n = 73) had been involved for <2 years (Figure 18.15). The numbers of treatment failures in those who completed 2 years were 18 of 85 (21%) in the IFN-β1a-treated group and 29 of 87 (33%) in the placebo group, respectively. Using the probability of sustained progression in the first year as an outcome also revealed the modest effect on disability (22% and 16% during year one, and 12% and 11%

Table 18.4 IFN-β1a (Avonex): pivotal trial

	Placebo	IFN-β1a
Number enrolled	143	158
Number completing year 1	136	151
Number completing year 2	87	85
Change in disability		
Sustained progression at year 1	22%	13%
Sustained progression at year 2 (all patients)[1]	35%	22%
Sustained progression at year 1	22%	13%
Sustained progression at year 2 (patients completing 2 years on study)	33%	21%
Change in EDSS at 2 years: −<1 point	12%	19%
Change in EDSS at 2 years: +<1 point	37%	24%[a]
Change in relapse frequency		
Relapse frequency at 2 years: <2	56%	68%
Relapse frequency at 2 years: >2	44%	32%
Change in relapse rate: all cases	−0.38	−0.53[b]
Change in relapse rate: at 2 years	−0.30	−0.59[c]
MRI		
Change in T$_2$ lesion volume: year 1	−3%	−13%[a]
Change in T$_2$ lesion volume: year 2	−7%	−13%
Number of Gd+ lesions: baseline	>174	>196
Mean number of Gd+ lesions: baseline	2.32	3.17
Number of Gd+ lesions: year 1	>124	>85
Mean number of Gd+ lesions: year 1	1.59	1.04[a]
Number of Gd+ lesions: year 2	>78	>49
Mean number of Gd+ lesions: year 2	1.65	0.80[d]

a p = 0.02; b p = 0.04; c p = 0.0002; d p = 0.05. Gd = gadolinium.

during year two, for placebo and treated patients, respectively; p = 0.02: Figure 18.16). These proportions did not differ between those who completed a second year in the study and those who did not.

Relapse rate (each exacerbation had to last >48 hours and be confirmed by a neurologist) was a secondary outcome measure. Overall, the reduction amongst treated patients was 18%. Fewer treated patients in the cohort who completed 2 years (12 of 85, 14%) had three or more exacerbations during the study than controls (28 of 87, 32%; p = 0.03). In the group studied for 2 years, annual exacerbation rates reduced from 1.2 to 0.61 per year (−0.59) in patients receiving IFN-β1a compared with a reduction from 1.2 to 0.90 per year (−0.30) in the placebo group (a 31% difference; p = 0.002). The reduction in the annual exacerbation rate per patient per year suggested less benefit for all randomized patients (0.82 for placebo compared with 0.67 for treated patients; p = 0.04) than for the subset who completed 104 weeks of follow-up (0.90 for placebo compared with 0.61 for treated patients; p = 0.002; Figure 18.17). In marked contradistinction to the IFN-β1b study, the change in relapse rate was not apparent until the second year of the study. The proportions free from any relapse at 2 years in the IFN-β1a and placebo-treated groups were 38% and 26%, respectively (p = 0.03), and there was no significant difference in time to first relapse between the groups (36 and 47 weeks, respectively; p = 0.34; Table 18.4). Partly in response to critical comments on the IFN-β1a study, the investigators subsequently re-analysed their results using more stringent outcome measures (Rudick

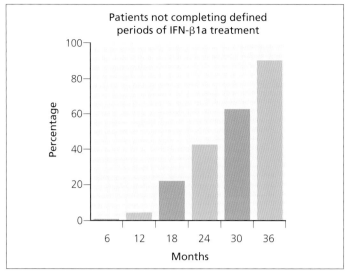

Figure 18.15 Percentage of patients not completing defined periods of treatment with IFN-β (Avonex). Data taken from Jacobs *et al* (1996). © 1996, reproduced with permission of John Wiley & Sons.

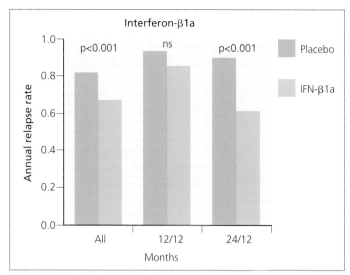

Figure 18.17 Annual relapse rates over the course of the study for all participants taking IFN-β1a (Avonex; All), and those completing year 1 (12/12) and year 2 (24/12). Adapted from Jacobs *et al* (1996). © 1996, reproduced with permission of John Wiley & Sons.

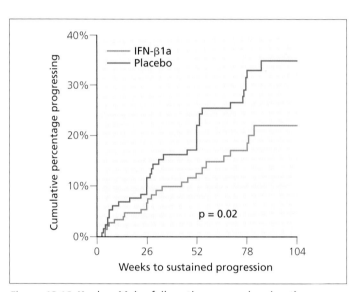

Figure 18.16 Kaplan–Meier failure time curve showing the cumulative percentage of patients taking IFN-β1a (Avonex) progressing according to number of weeks to beginning of sustained disability progression, compared with placebo-treated patients. Adapted from Jacobs *et al* (1996). © 1996, reproduced with permission of John Wiley & Sons.

et al 1997). Widening the gap between treated and placebo patients to >2 EDSS points or lengthening the duration of the >1 point difference to 1 year improved the benefits of IFN-β1a to 61% and 67% reductions, respectively, compared with the original estimate of 37% based on differences in the rates of accumulation of disability between groups. For those who did worsen, IFN-β1a failed to discriminate between functional systems. The authors concluded that IFN-β1a affects the magnitude but not the pattern of involvement in multiple sclerosis and that no factor other than randomization to the treatment arm could explain the outcome in this cohort of patients.

This trial also included surrogate markers of disease activity and lesion load. By year one, fewer IFN-β1a-treated patients had gadolinium enhancing lesions (30%) than in the placebo group (43%; p = 0.05) and there were also reductions in the number (p = 0.02) and volume (p = 0.02) of enhancing lesions. The assessment of T_2 lesion volumes, which featured strongly in the study of IFN-β1b, proved more difficult to resolve in the trial of IFN-β1a and the significant difference apparent at year one (−3% in IFN-β1a-treated patients compared with −13% in the placebo group; p = 0.02) was not maintained on completion of the second year (−7% and −13% respectively; p = 0.36; Table 18.4). The investigators subsequently updated these imaging results using a different method to measure T_2 lesion volume and reported a decrease in the number of new, enlarging, and new or enlarging T_2 lesions over 2 years. The increase in T_2 lesion volume was 628 mm^2 in patients receiving IFN-β1a compared with 1410 mm^2 in controls. In the subgroup with active lesions in advance of treatment, these differences were 1285 and 2980 mm^2, respectively, over the 2 years but with an increase in acquisition of new lesions in the treated group during the second year (J.H. Simon *et al* 1997). Pohl *et al* (2005) reported their experience treating 51 children and adolescents with relapsing–remitting multiple sclerosis using IFN-β1a once weekly. Although this was not a controlled trial, their report and the accompanying editorial (Banwell and Tremlett 2005) comparing pre- with post-treatment relapse rates suggested that children aged <16 years may benefit and tolerate IFN-β1a in this setting.

IFN-β1a (Rebif)

The effects of IFN-β1a (Rebif) were first assessed in 68 patients using MRI measures as outcome (Pozilli *et al* 1996). The average number of gadolinium-DTPA enhancing lesions decreased from three (SD 4.3) per month during the 6 months prior to treatment with 3 or 9 MIU subcutaneously three times weekly, to 1.3 (SD 2.2) lesions per month during the 6 months on treatment. The

OWIMS study (Once Weekly Interferon for MS Study Group 1999) demonstrated that even small doses of IFN-β1a (22 or 44 μg) administered once weekly influenced MRI evidence of disease activity. In this study, 293 relapsing–remitting patients randomized either to placebo or two doses of IFN-β1a were followed for 1 year. MRI features, combined unique lesions (showing either proton density/ T_2 or T_1 gadolinium activity) and lesion load, favoured the active treatment groups over placebo although clinical effects were not apparent at either dose. Resolving these issues of dose and frequency of administration has been the subject of several studies carried out since IFN-β1a and IFN-β1b were licensed (see below).

In the pivotal study of IFN-β1a (PRISMS; Prevention of Relapses and disability by Interferon-β1a Subcutaneously in Multiple Sclerosis 1998), 560 patients with relapsing–remitting multiple sclerosis with two or more episodes in the 2 years before (but not within 2 months of) treatment, and an EDSS score of 0–5, received IFN-β1a by subcutaneous injection (6 or 12 MIU) or a placebo preparation three times each week for 2 years. The primary outcome of this 2-year study was the relapse count over the course of the trial. Both doses were associated with a significant reduction in relapse rate compared with controls (1.82, 1.73 and 2.56 over 2 years, respectively; p < 0.0002), achieving about a 33% reduction (12 MIU compared with placebo) across the study period. The proportion of patients free from relapse during the 2 years of the study was 32% (12 MIU), 27% (6 MIU) and 16% (placebo) in the two treated groups and controls (p < 0.005 and p < 0.05, respectively). Both doses achieved a reduction in the severity of those relapses that did occur. Time to confirmed progression of >1 EDSS point increased in each group but, much as in the trials of IFN-β1b and other IFN-β1a preparations, this was less marked than the effect on relapse rate (p < 0.04: Figure 18.18). A novel composite score of integrated disability (amounting to the 'area under the EDSS curve over time') showed a 77% reduction in accumulated burden of disability during the study period. MRI was performed twice during the study and a subgroup underwent more frequent analyses. There was a reduction, by around 70% but higher in the more frequently studied cohort, in median number of active lesions per patient on each MRI scan in both treated groups compared with controls. Burden of disease increased by 11% in the control patients and decreased by 1% and 4% in the low-dose and high-dose groups, respectively (p < 0.0001).

The authors did not evaluate the success of blinding. As with other contemporary interferon studies, it is likely that patients were able correctly to guess whether they were receiving placebo or active therapy. Whether blinding was maintained for the evaluating physician was not reported. For reasons that remain unclear, the number of patients available for assessing the rate of nonprogression was only 76% of the study population at 1 year, and 70% at 18 months. Follow-up at the time of primary analysis was only 2 years. The authors reported 'confirmed worsening' at 3 months but did not present the data on 6 month and 12 month confirmed worsening. The analysis did not address the degree to which EDSS worsening attributable to relapse contributed to the data on sustained worsening.

An extension trial was started upon the completion of PRISMS. Patients originally receiving placebo were randomized to either low- or high-dose IFN-β1a. Those already receiving interferon continued on their original regimen of active drug (PRISMS Study Group 2001). Ninety per cent of the original 560 patients participated in the extension trial and almost 88% of this cohort completed the 2 year extension study.

The primary outcome in the extension study was relapse count per patient over the 4 years of the entire study. As such, the clinical behaviour (relapse count) in the first 2 years of the original study contributed substantially to the 4 year analysis of the extension. Not surprisingly, the extension trial demonstrated that IFN-β1a provides some protection (in terms of reduction in relapse rate) for those originally treated with placebo, although the trial was no longer blinded since patients and evaluators knew that all were receiving interferon therapy (Figure 18.19). Relapse rates over the 4 years of the study were 0.72 and 0.80 for the 12 MIU and 6 MIU groups, respectively, compared with 1.02 for the placebo patients who were randomized to 12 MIU at the time of the extension phase (p < 0.001 for both 'always interferon' groups compared with the group that started on placebo). There was a trend suggesting a marginal benefit for the higher dose of IFN-β1a (p = 0.07). Secondary analyses also showed a possible delay in time to confirmed progression for the high-dose group. MRI analyses supported a greater effect on lesion load for the high-dose group ('always 44 μg', 6.2% reduction; all other groups showed an increase in lesion load). Once again, the proportion of patients with neutralizing antibodies was higher in the low-dose group (23.8% vs. 12.5%) and, for the first time, the PRISMS investigators acknowledged that the presence of neutralizing antibodies reduced the clinical benefit on relapse rate (44 μg antibody-negative group, 0.50; 44 μg antibody-positive group, 0.81). In the analysis of this study, the authors did not correct statistically for multiple comparisons. The largest proportion of drop-outs was seen in the high-dose (44 μg) group (23%) – a finding that somewhat undermines confidence in these data. Analysis of the MRI results (Li and Paty 1999) confirmed the previously reported benefit on lesion load at 2 years (placebo, increase of 10.9%; 22 μg, decrease of 1.2%; 44 μg, decrease of 3.8%). Fifty per cent of placebo patients showed >10% increase in lesion load. Similarly, treatment reduced the frequency of active lesions (22 μg, 67% reduction; 44 μg, 78% reduction) and the proportion of patients with inactive scans (placebo, 8%; 22 μg, 19%; 44 μg, 31%). A subset of patients studied with more frequent MRI provided evidence that the treatment benefit could be identified as early as 2 months after starting interferon therapy. MRI atrophy was not evaluated.

As noted, the decision to include the 'relapse counts per patient' in the first 2 years of the original trial seems to have served the sponsor well in the extension phase, as did the accompanying editorial reporting that 'the placebo group never caught up' with the patients originally receiving interferon (Schwid and Bever 2001). This is hardly surprising. To catch up, the original placebo patients would either have had to be more responsive to the effects of interferon than those who were first randomized to the active agents, or the trial would have needed to be sufficiently sensitive to a loss of treatment effect in the third and fourth years of exposure. It is unlikely that the study was powered to demonstrate this effect. Lack of blinding in the extension study limits the conclusions that can be drawn from this phase of the trial considering the subjective nature of the primary outcome. The authors did not report on use of corticosteroids in the patients who changed treatments. Regrettably,

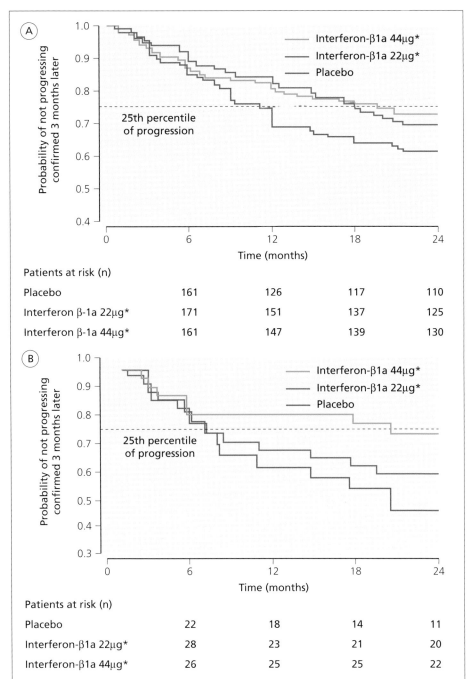

Figure 18.18 Treatment of relapsing–remitting multiple sclerosis with subcutaneous IFN-β1a (Rebif; PRISMS study). (A) Time to confirmed progression in disability in whole study group. (B) Patients with baseline EDSS >3.5. *p < 0.05 compared with placebo. Adapted from PRISMS Study Group (1998). © 1998, with permission from Elsevier.

this study demonstrates once again that multiple sclerosis disease activity continues despite treatment with interferons even at high dose.

Secondary progressive multiple sclerosis

Although there are many remaining questions surrounding the use of interferons in relapsing–remitting multiple sclerosis, there is at least a general belief that patients who choose to start therapy either with an interferon or glatiramer acetate (see below) can expect up to a 30% reduction in relapse rate over the initial 2 years on treatment. Treating physicians should indicate that there is no definite proof that treatment delays the development of persistent symptoms and signs. In secondary pro-

gressive multiple sclerosis, there is much less consensus on the short-term benefits of treatment. Although the interferons appear to reduce relapse frequency in the subset of individuals with secondary progressive disease who continue to experience attacks, it is hard to avoid the conclusion that clinical progression and MRI evidence of cerebral atrophy continue despite treatment. The published trials in secondary progressive multiple sclerosis are summarized in Table 18.5.

The European IFN-β1b study has been published in most detail (Kappos *et al* 1998; D.H. Miller *et al* 1999; Molyneux *et al* 2000). Thirty-two centres contributed 718 patients with secondary progressive multiple sclerosis (EDSS 3.0–6.5). Patients receiving active treatment demonstrated benefit for the primary outcome – time to worsening by 1.0 EDSS point confirmed at

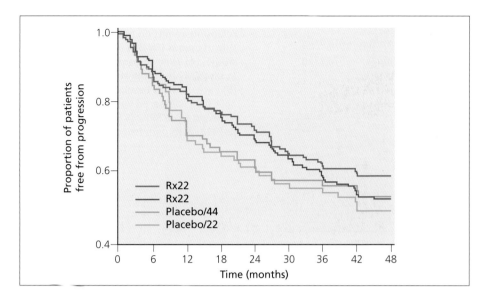

Figure 18.19 Treatment of relapsing–remitting multiple sclerosis with subcutaneous IFN-β1a (Rebif; PRISMS-4 extension study). Kaplan–Meier curves for time to confirmed progression in disability for years 1 through 4 (all patients). Proportions of patients are those free from progression. Adapted from the PRISMS Study Group (2001). © 2001, reproduced with permission of Lippincott Williams & Wilkins (lww.com).

Table 18.5 **Recent randomized trials in secondary progressive multiple sclerosis**

Trial (number enrolled; follow-up)	Treatment	Primary outcome	Secondary outcome	Comments
European IFN-β1b (718; 3 years)	8 MIU IFN-β1b by subcutaneous injection on alternate days vs. placebo	Time to EDSS worsening confirmed at 3 months (39% versus 50%; p = 0.0048). Probability of remaining progression-free noted by 1 year	Time to become wheelchair bound, hospitalizations, annual relapse rate, effect on MRI T$_2$ volume and activity. Time to 1.0 and 2.0 point EDSS change. Proportion with either relapses or progression	Year 3, increase of T$_2$ volumes in IFN-β-treated patients. Minor effect on preventing progressive cerebral atrophy
SPECTRIMS (618; 3 years)	22 μg or 44 μg IFN-β1a s.c. on alternate days vs. placebo	No effect on time to 3 month confirmed EDSS worsening (p = 0.88)	Treatment reduced relapse rate. Delayed progression in women at both doses. MRI effect seen on number of active lesions per patient per scan, combined unique activity and T$_2$ volume	Male placebo patients did unusually well. Patients with neutralizing antibodies showed no MRI effect
IMPACT (436; 2 years)	IFN-β1a s.c. 60 μg i.m. 1×/week vs. placebo	Benefit on MSFC noted in year 2	No effect on EDSS	MSFC not validated as disability measure
North American IFN-β1b (939; 3 years)	IFN-β-1b s.c. 8 MIU or 5 MIU/m^2 q2d vs. placebo	No effect on proportion with confirmed EDSS worsening	Positive effect on relapse rate, MRI activity and T$_2$ volume	No effect on EDSS
European mitoxantrone (188; 2 years)	5 or 12 mg/m^2 mitoxantrone every twelfth week vs. placebo (methylene blue)	Benefit on composite measure (EDSS, AI, SNS, time to first attack needing steroids, time to attack)	Number of patients with EDSS progression. Fewer new T$_2$ and Gd+ lesions	Outcome measure not validated, potential cardiotoxicity

GA = glatiramer acetate; Gd+ = gadolinium enhancing MRI lesions; IFN = interferon; EDSS = Expanded Disability Status Scale; MIU = million international units; AI = Ambulation index; SNS = Scripps Neurologic Scale; s.c. = subcutaneous; i.m. = intramuscular. Adapted from Noseworthy and Hartung (2003) with permission.

3 months (0.5 EDSS points, if baseline EDSS was 6.0 or greater; p = 0.0008). There was a 21.7% relative reduction in the proportion of patients reaching this outcome (placebo, 49.8%; IFN-β1b, 38.9%; p = 0.0048: Figure 18.20). This benefit was supported by an analysis of 6 month confirmed worsening, irrespective of whether patients lost to follow-up were counted as stable or worse (p = 0.0016). There was a difference in time to reach the primary end point between the two treatment arms of 9 months that first became apparent by survival analysis in the second year of treatment. A number of secondary outcomes also supported a treatment effect including time to unconfirmed wheelchair dependence (delayed by 9 months; and with a 32% reduction in the number of patients reaching this end point), progressive worsening without relapses, number of hospitalizations, annual

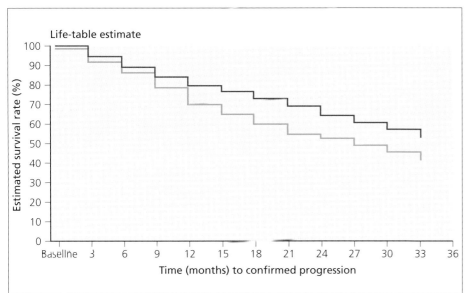

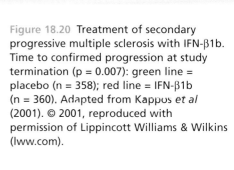

Figure 18.20 Treatment of secondary progressive multiple sclerosis with IFN-β1b. Time to confirmed progression at study termination (p = 0.007): green line = placebo (n = 358); red line = IFN-β1b (n = 360). Adapted from Kappos *et al* (2001). © 2001, reproduced with permission of Lippincott Williams & Wilkins (lww.com).

relapse rate, time to first relapse, proportion with moderate or severe relapses, and MRI T_2 volume (placebo, 8% increase; IFN-β1b, 5% reduction). An analysis of the 125 patients selected for frequent MRI studies (monthly scans between months 1 and 6 and 18 and 24) demonstrated fewer active scans early (65% reduction between months 1 and 6) and late in the study (78% reduction between months 18 and 24). The development of neutralizing antibodies in 27.8% of the IFN-β1b recipients reduced the benefit on relapse rate but not the disability findings (Polman *et al* 2003). Further analysis of the clinical findings reported a small number of patients lost to follow-up (48 of 358 placebo-treated patients; 40 of 360 patients given IFN-β1b). The proportion of patients with 3 month confirmed worsening of at least 2.0 EDSS points was reduced by 27% (p = 0.007). There was a 30% reduction in the proportion of patients either with fewer relapses or no progression (Kappos *et al* 2001). Subsequent analysis apparently confirmed that benefit from IFN-β1b was more likely in patients either with more than two pre-enrolment relapses or worsening of >1.0 EDSS points in the 24 months preceding randomization.

Two additional manuscripts detailed the MRI analysis of this large trial. It was reported by D.H. Miller *et al* (1999) that, at 3 years, there were persistent MRI lesion volume differences between the treatment arms (placebo, 16% increase; IFN-β1b, 2% decrease) although the MRI lesion volume increased for the first time in the IFN-β1b-treated cohort in the third year (p = 0.0001: Figures 18.21 and 18.22). Molyneux *et al* (2000), reporting on a subset of 95 patients in five centres that had MRI studies twice yearly during the 3 years of the study, found that atrophy continued in both treatment groups (placebo, 3.9%; IFN-β1b, 2.9% at 36 months). IFN-β1b treatment seemed to reduce the degree of atrophy developing in patients without evidence of contrast enhancing lesions at baseline (placebo, 5.1% loss of volume; IFN-β1b, 1.8%; p < 0.05: Figure 18.23). These atrophy studies, however, were underpowered because only 65 of 95 patients had the 3 year MRI scan.

The European study resulted in drug approval for the indication of secondary progressive multiple sclerosis in Europe although enthusiasm for its use varies widely amongst neurologists. The second large study of secondary progressive multiple

sclerosis failed to confirm an effect on disability (SPECTRIMS; Secondary Progressive Efficacy Clinical Trial of Recombinant Interferon-β1a in MS: SPECTRIMS Study Group 2001). Failure of the other trials in secondary progressive multiple sclerosis to demonstrate a convincing benefit has influenced the degree to which this drug is used sparingly in clinical practice.

SPECTRIMS involved 22 centres in North America, Europe and Australia and included 618 patients with secondary progressive multiple sclerosis (baseline EDSS 3.0–6.5) randomized either to receive three subcutaneous doses of placebo each week or IFN-β1a (22 µg or 44 µg). The study failed to demonstrate a significant impact on the primary outcome measure (3 month confirmed EDSS worsening at 3 years; p = 0.146) although an early benefit was apparent at 1 year (Figures 18.24 and 18.25). Secondary analyses revealed the unexpected finding that the primary outcome was positive in female patients for both doses of IFN-β1a compared with placebo (22 µg, p = 0.036; 44 µg, p = 0.006). This may, in part, relate to the observation that men treated with placebo did unusually well (better than women treated with placebo). Interferon-treated patients with pre-enrolment relapses demonstrated a delay in time to progression. Treatment significantly reduced relapse rates (p < 0.001). Subsequent MRI analysis of SPECTRIMS (D.K. Li *et al* 2001) demonstrated a treatment effect on MRI parameters. Specifically, mean number of T_2 active lesions per patient per scan was reduced (placebo, 0.67; 22 µg: 0.20, 44 µg: 0.17, p < 0.001) as were monthly combined unique MRI activity (T_1 and T_2; p < 0.001) and accumulation of lesion load (baseline vs. 3 years; placebo, 10% increase; 22 µg, 0.5% decrease; 44 µg, 1.3% decrease; p < 0.0001). An effect of IFN-β1a was seen particularly in patients who reported relapses in the 2 years preceding randomization. The presence of neutralizing antibodies completely abrogated the evidence from MRI for a treatment effect in this trial.

The North American trial of IFN-β1b in secondary progressive multiple sclerosis is currently only published in abstract format (Goodkin 2000; see Table 18.5). Nine hundred and thirty-nine patients with secondary progressive multiple sclerosis were randomized either to receive placebo or one of two subcutaneous doses (8 MIU or 5 MIU per m^2) of IFN-β1b on

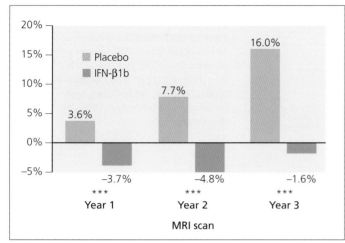

Figure 18.21 Treatment of secondary progressive multiple sclerosis with IFN-β1b. Annual MRI analysis. Percentage change in total lesion volume (TLV; mean) seen in the study cohort during years 1–3 compared with MRI scan at study entry. ***p < 0.0001 for difference between treatment groups. Adapted from D.H. Miller *et al* (1999). © 1999, reproduced with permission of John Wiley & Sons.

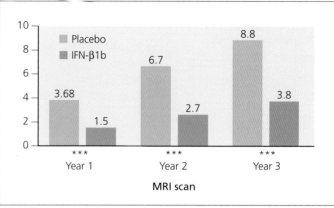

Figure 18.22 Treatment of secondary progressive multiple sclerosis with IFN-β1b. Annual MRI analysis. Cumulative number of active lesions (mean) seen in the study cohort during years 1–3 compared with MRI scan at study entry. ***p < 0.0001 for difference between treatment groups. Adapted from D.H. Miller *et al* (1999). © 1999, reproduced with permission of John Wiley & Sons.

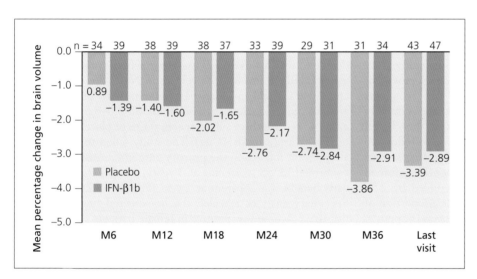

Figure 18.23 Treatment of secondary progressive multiple sclerosis with IFN-β1b. Percentage change in cerebral volume compared with baseline for all patients. M = month. Adapted from Molyneux *et al* (2000).

three occasions per week. The primary outcome (proportion of patients with confirmed EDSS progression at 3 years) was not reached although, as in SPECTRIMS, there were apparent treatment effects on relapse frequency and MRI measures (activity indices and T_2 lesion volume).

The final trial, of IFN-β1a in secondary progressive multiple sclerosis (IMPACT; International Multiple sclerosis secondary Progressive Avonex™ Controlled Trial; Cohen *et al* 2002) evaluated whether high dose (60 µg; compared with 30 µg used in relapsing–remitting multiple sclerosis) IFN-β1a given once weekly by intramuscular injection was more effective than placebo as measured by changes at 2 years in the MSFC. These investigators reported benefit using this 'more sensitive' but, as yet, incompletely validated outcome measure. Two components of the MSFC (the nine-hole peg test and the paced auditory serial addition task – PASAT) contributed to the positive findings in this trial (Figure 18.26). No benefit was seen in the timed gait or EDSS (secondary outcome). After reviewing these data, the FDA (United States) did not grant approval for once weekly IFN-β1a in secondary progressive multiple sclerosis.

Although much can be done to alleviate persisting symptoms (Chapter 17), the treatment of secondary progressive multiple sclerosis is largely unsolved. The classification of secondary progression is usually made retrospectively in a patient who, upon reflection, after a period of relapses with recovery appears to have worsened in recent months (years) either as a result of incomplete recovery from relapses or through a relapse-independent gradual decline in performance. In this context, the decision on whether or not to start (or continue) treatment is never easy and involves a careful discussion with the patient of expectations matched against the evidence available from published trials. The case for using IFN-β is perhaps most compelling for untreated patients who also report ongoing relapses. In this subset of patients, there is a good chance that treatment may reduce relapse frequency although the patient should be

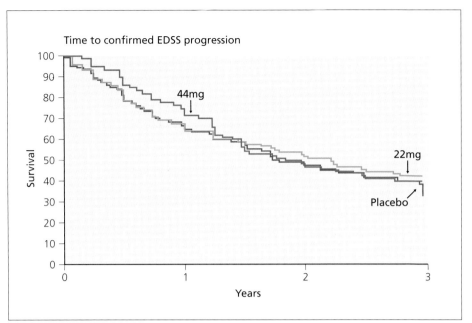

Figure 18.24 Treatment of secondary progressive multiple sclerosis with IFN-β1a subcutaneously three times weekly. Kaplan–Meier curves for time to confirmed EDSS progression for all patients. Adapted from SPECTRIMS Study Group (2001).

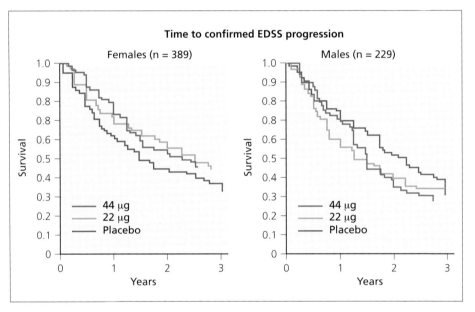

Figure 18.25 Treatment of secondary progressive multiple sclerosis with IFN-β1a subcutaneously three times weekly. Kaplan–Meier curves for time to confirmed EDSS progression for male and female patients. Adapted from SPECTRIMS Study Group (2001). © 2001, reproduced with permission of Lippincott Williams & Wilkins (lww.com).

advised that attack rate and progression do not necessarily correlate. The situation is no more promising for people with primary progressive multiple sclerosis.

Primary progressive multiple sclerosis

Trials initiated before the mid1990s frequently failed to distinguish the various chronic progressive disease subtypes and primary progressive patients were lumped with those who once experienced or continued to suffer clinical relapses. In the absence of biomarkers to help determine that a therapeutic intervention is providing early benefit, treatment trials in primary progressive multiple sclerosis have relied upon changes in disability to determine efficacy (Neuhaus and Hartung 2001). Leary *et al* (2003) reported that IFN-β1a (30 μg and 60 μg weekly by intramuscular injection) was well tolerated at the lower dose but neither provided convincing evidence of benefit in a 2 year randomized, placebo-controlled, double-blinded trial of 50 patients with primary progressive disease. The lower dose may have marginally reduced T_2 lesion load accumulation but, paradoxically, measures of progressive brain atrophy appeared worse in those randomized to 60 μg weekly. Possibly this group had a greater lesion load at entry and, with a significant anti-inflammatory effect, the higher dose resulted in a more obvious reduction in brain volume.

Montalban (2004) has recently reported the preliminary analysis of a randomized, placebo-controlled phase two trial of IFN-β1b in 73 patients with either primary progressive or transitional multiple sclerosis. This preliminary report suggests that the IFN-β-treated patients demonstrated moderate benefits in the MSFC and MRI parameters (T_1 and T_2 lesion volume) at 2 years. The full report is awaited.

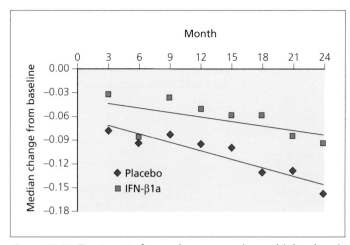

Figure 18.26 Treatment of secondary progressive multiple sclerosis with IFN-β1a by intramuscular injection once weekly. Median MS Functional Composite change from baseline every 3 months. The trend lines were determined by linear regression. Adapted from J.A. Cohen *et al* (2002). © 2002, reproduced with permission of Lippincott Williams & Wilkins (lww.com).

Clinically isolated syndromes

Syndromes that may represent the inaugural episode in the natural history of multiple sclerosis have been the focus of subsequent attention with respect to disease-modifying treatments. Three reasons for this shift in attention can be suggested. First, the relative failure of IFN-β to influence features of multiple sclerosis, other than relapse rate, identifies the need to treat patients before the onset of disability and disease progression. Secondly, disease mechanisms that are predicted to be less responsive to cytokine therapy than inflammation are thought to increase with disease duration (see Chapter 10). Not only is there evidence from several sources that immune-mediated axonal injury is seen early in cases of relapsing–remitting multiple sclerosis but it also follows that early intervention with an anti-inflammatory agent might inhibit the cascade of events that leads to disease progression and thereby improve the long-term outlook. However, it should be pointed out that, whilst convincing for cases severe enough to warrant tissue examination, the same logic may not apply to more entrepreneurial examples of clinically isolated syndromes or relapsing–remitting multiple sclerosis. Thirdly, and to adopt a more entrepreneurial stance, early use of drug treatments makes good marketing sense, and each of these studies has been sponsored by pharmaceutical companies poised to benefit from prescribing drift.

Two recent randomized, double-blinded and placebo-controlled trials have addressed the issue of whether treatment with IFN-β1a at the time of presentation protects from recurrent clinical disease activity (Table 18.6). Fifty centres from the United States and Canada participated in the first of these two studies (CHAMPS; Controlled High risk subjects Avonex™ Multiple sclerosis Prevention Study; Jacobs *et al* 2000). Three hundred and eighty-three patients were randomized to receive either IFN-β1a at 30 µg weekly by intramuscular injection (n = 193) or a matched placebo (n = 190) for the duration of follow-up. Prior to starting active or placebo treatment, all patients were treated with methylprednisolone 1 g daily by intravenous injection for 3 days followed by 14 days of oral

prednisone (1 mg/kg daily for 11 days then tapering in the final 4 days as follows – 20 mg on the first day, 10 mg on the second day, 0 mg on day three and 10 mg on the final day). Treatment commenced within 4 weeks from onset of the sentinel clinically isolated symptom. To be eligible, patients had to have two or more asymptomatic MR lesions on cranial imaging. Patients were assessed clinically at 4 weeks and every 6 months thereafter. The primary outcome measure was 'conversion to clinically definite multiple sclerosis (CDMS)' as defined by a further clinical relapse (Figure 18.27). When this occurred, patients were removed from the study and offered active treatment with IFN-β1a in an unblinded fashion. MRI studies were not performed at the time of putative conversion to multiple sclerosis. This high profile study was terminated early because of 'evidence for efficacy' in that fewer actively treated patients converted than controls (p = 0.002). At this point, 274 of the original 383 patients (71%) had completed 1 year of follow-up. We are struck by how quickly this study was brought to closure [of the 383 original subjects 210 (55%) were followed for 18 months; 131 (34%) were followed for 24 months; and only 61 (16%) were followed for 36 months]. Within months of publication, the United States FDA approved IFN-β1a for use in patients with clinically isolated syndromes deemed to be at high risk of developing multiple sclerosis.

The study bears further scrutiny. The trial was regrettably short, limiting the amount of available clinically relevant information. It is inconceivable that patients were blinded to the treatment received given the nearly universal occurrence of side effects from intramuscular administration of interferon. As such, patients receiving IFN-β1a would almost certainly have been aware that they were on active treatment, and vice versa. The possibility remains that incomplete blinding influenced the reporting of symptoms suggesting a first relapse. The primary outcome in this study was soft and merely required patients to identify symptoms suggesting a relapse. The conversion rate to clinically definite multiple sclerosis seems surprisingly rapid in CHAMPS (at 1 month: 18% in the placebo group vs. 9% of IFN-β1a-treated patients; and 26% compared with 12%, respectively, at 4 months). There have been many other examples where the placebo group did less well than expected thereby inflating the apparent treatment effect. The benefit of treatment in CHAMPS is less impressive if the patients who either converted or dropped out of the study and thereby could not benefit from treatment are considered together (44% of patients receiving IFN-β1a and 56% of the placebo group).

MRI data are presented as number of lesions rather than the proportion of patients showing MRI activity. The study design did not require MRI studies at the time of clinical conversion to multiple sclerosis. Furthermore, there are very few published clinical details and, as noted, no MRI data on two very important subsets of patients – the 46% of those enrolled who converted to clinically definite multiple sclerosis and the 15% who dropped out of the study. The absence of information beyond 18 months brings into question the durability of the effect on MRI features.

The relatively modest benefit of early treatment is perhaps seen more clearly in the observation from a subsequent paper that 50% of patients with clinically isolated syndromes treated with IFN-β1a demonstrated either clinical or MRI evidence of relapse while on treatment within the first 18 months of the study (R.W. Beck *et al* 2002: Figure 18.28). Additional analyses

Table 18.6 Recent randomized trials in clinically isolated syndromes			
Trial (number enrolled; follow-up)	**Treatment**	**Primary outcome**	**Comments**
CHAMPS (383; 71% 1 year, 34% 2 year, 16% 3 year)	Corticosteroids, then: IFN-β1a 30 μg by intramuscular injection weekly vs. placebo	Delayed conversion to clinically definite multiple sclerosis (p = 0.002)	Patient unblinding likely. 'Soft' outcome measures. Limited follow-up. MRI only on 'stable' patients. No MRI studies beyond 18 months. Limited clinical data published
ETOMS (309; 2 year)	IFN-β1a 22 μg by subcutaneous injection once weekly vs. placebo	Delayed conversion to clinically definite multiple sclerosis (45% versus 34%)	Patient unblinding likely. 'Soft' outcome measures. Limited follow-up. MRI only on 'stable' patients. Not all MRI studies available for analysis of volume change
IFN = interferon. Adapted from Noseworthy and Hartung (2003) with permission.			

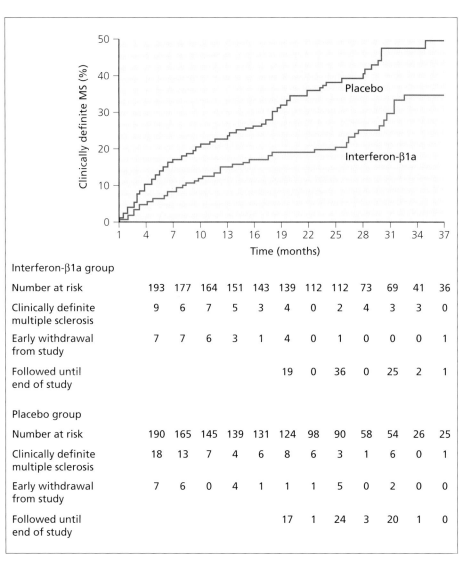

Figure 18.27 Treatment of patients with clinically isolated syndromes and abnormal cerebral MRI with once weekly intramuscular IFN-β1a (Avonex; CHAMPS Study). Kaplan–Meier estimates of the cumulative probability of the development of clinically definite multiple sclerosis according to treatment groups. Adapted from Jacobs *et al* (2000). © 2000, with permission of the Massachusetts Medical Society.

Interferon-β1a group

Number at risk	193	177	164	151	143	139	112	112	73	69	41	36
Clinically definite multiple sclerosis	9	6	7	5	3	4	0	2	4	3	3	0
Early withdrawal from study	7	7	6	3	1	4	0	1	0	0	0	1
Followed until end of study						19	0	36	0	25	2	1

Placebo group

Number at risk	190	165	145	139	131	124	98	90	58	54	26	25
Clinically definite multiple sclerosis	18	13	7	4	6	8	6	3	1	6	0	1
Early withdrawal from study	7	6	0	4	1	1	1	5	0	2	0	0
Followed until end of study						17	1	24	3	20	1	0

have reported that IFN-β1a provides only partial (and we would suggest limited) protection regardless of the specific syndrome (optic neuritis, brainstem/cerebellar or cerebral involvement) and that risk of conversion to clinically definite multiple sclerosis is slightly greater for individuals with optic neuritis (R.W. Beck *et al* 2002), for patients with two or more contrast enhancing MR lesions, and for those already fulfilling MRI criteria for multiple sclerosis in this clinical context (Barkhof *et al* 1997a; CHAMPS Study Group 2002).

In a trial of similar design, the ETOMS (Early Treatment Of Multiple Sclerosis; Comi *et al* 2001a) investigators from 57 centres in 14 European countries randomized 309 patients having

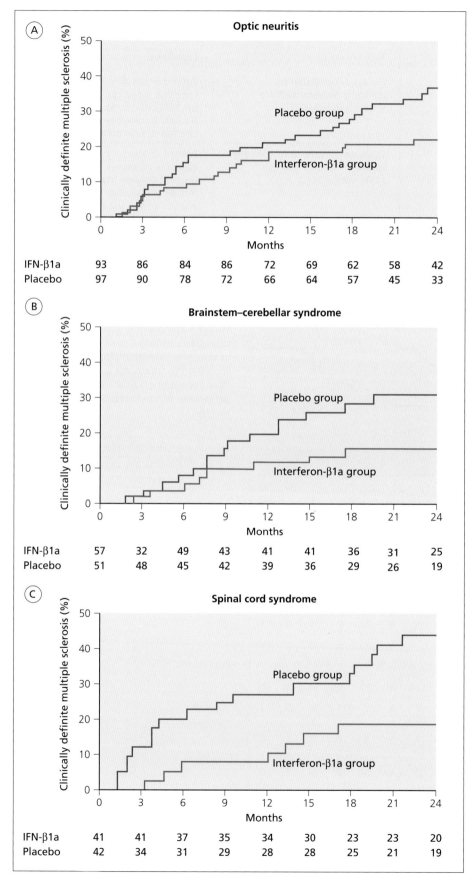

Figure 18.28 Treatment of patients with clinically isolated syndromes and abnormal cerebral MRI with once weekly intramuscular IFN-β1a (Avonex; CHAMPS Study). Cumulative probability of the development of clinically definite multiple sclerosis by treatment groups according to type of presenting event. (A) Optic neuritis; (B) Brainstem–cerebellar syndrome; (C) spinal cord syndrome. Adapted from Beck *et al* (2002). © 2002, reproduced with permission of John Wiley & Sons.

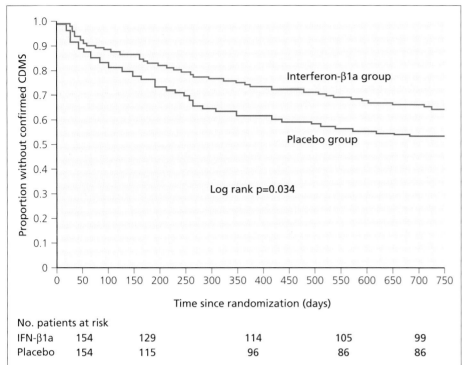

Figure 18.29 Treatment of patients with clinically isolated syndromes within the last 3 months and abnormal cerebral MRI with once weekly subcutaneous IFN-β1a (Rebif; ETOMS Study). Kaplan–Meier survival curve of probability of no conversion to clinically definite multiple sclerosis over 2 years. Adapted from Comi *et al* (2001a). © 2001, with permission from Elsevier.

clinically isolated syndromes within the previous 3 months if they had four or more MRI lesions, to receive either once weekly low dose (22 μg) IFN-β1a subcutaneously or a matched placebo. Patients were assessed clinically at 1 month and then every 6 months for 2 years, with annual MRI scans. Ninety per cent completed follow-up. At 2 years, the authors claimed a treatment advantage with 45% of placebo-treated patients converting to multiple sclerosis compared with 34% of those receiving IFN-β1a (Figure 18.29). As with CHAMPS, no attempt was made to determine the success of blinding in this trial. In a subsequent manuscript, Filippi *et al* (2004b) reported an apparent benefit on the development of brain atrophy at 24 months in the treated group (30% reduction in the observed decrease in brain volume; –1.18% IFN-β1a vs. –1.68% for the placebo group; p = 0.0031). It remains to be determined whether this very small weekly dose of interferon offers an important and potentially long-term benefit. Indeed, the degree of atrophy is so small in the untreated patient (<2% of normalized brain parenchymal volume) that it stretches the imagination to accept that a 30% reduction in this metric will be biologically meaningful in this chronic disease. Accordingly, in an accompanying editorial, D.H. Miller (2004a) offers optimism for genuine protection from irrreversible brain injury but cautions that it remains to be confirmed that this effect on brain atrophy will translate into delayed or reduced disability.

The same concerns arise with respect to the subjective primary outcome measure as in CHAMPS. The frequency with which the MRI studies of asymptomatic patients showed evidence of recurrent disease activity (MRI conversion) has not been published but there are differences between the trials. The patients in ETOMS had a high frequency (39%) of multifocal symptoms at onset (compared with 0% in CHAMPS). The

ETOMS patients, therefore, were at approximately a two-fold increased risk of converting to multiple sclerosis in a short time frame. Additionally, the longer interval between symptom onset and entry in the study (3 months vs. 1 month for CHAMPS) probably increased the conversion rate in ETOMS. Only 70% of participants in ETOMS received corticosteroids at the time of randomization compared with 100% in CHAMPS. Despite their limitations, these studies provide evidence that early treatment with IFN-β1a may have a partial, and at least short-term, benefit in delaying further episodes of demyelination either in patients at risk of multiple sclerosis or in those already established in the early stages of the illness. We emphasize again the obvious need to determine whether any of these therapies provides a treatment benefit that is sustained over a prolonged period and is clinically useful. In part, this reflects the lack of robust mechanisms for evaluating the long-term benefits of treatment but it is an enormously important question since there are theoretical benefits in strategies that arrest axonal injury before it has contributed to the progressive and presumably irreversible axonal degeneration that underlies the later stages of multiple sclerosis.

Using a whole brain ratio method, brain atrophy was assessed over 2 years in a placebo-controlled trial of IFN-β1a in relapsing–remitting disease (C.K. Jones *et al* 2001). Atrophy measures were available in 519 patients, 172 of whom were on placebo treatment. Significant brain atrophy was seen in the total cohort. Whole brain ratio at baseline correlated weakly with T_2 lesion load and decreased by 1.4% over 2 years but no difference in the rate of atrophy was seen between treatment arms. Cerebral atrophy has been evaluated in 52 relapsing–remitting patients for 6 months before and 24 months following treatment with IFN-β1a, and correlated with other MRI lesion and clinical parameters (Gasperini *et al* 2002). During the 2 years of treatment, there was a significant reduction of brain volume (mean −2.2%) that correlated weakly with the mean number of enhancing lesions on 6 monthly pretreatment scans. Over the 2 years, 26 patients exhibited significant atrophy and 26 did not. Of the former, 13 experienced an increase in disability whereas only three of the latter became more disabled. This confirms other studies showing a link between increasing atrophy and disability (Losseff *et al* 1996b; Paolillo *et al* 1999). In a 2 year placebo-controlled trial of IFN-β1a in relapsing–remitting multiple sclerosis, atrophy was measured from yearly scans using brain parenchymal fraction. The mean decrease was similar in both arms in year one, but smaller in the IFN-β1a arm in year two (Rudick *et al* 1999). The changes in brain parenchymal fraction during this 2 year period showed little or no correlation with lesion measures. There was c.1% loss of central cerebral volume per year in both the treated and placebo arms. Prolonged 8 year follow-up of the placebo cohort from this trial assessed the long-term relationship between earlier brain parenchymal fraction change and later disability (E. Fisher *et al* 2002). Comparison of quartiles based on change over the first 2 years revealed a greater likelihood of developing severe disability (EDSS ≥ 6 at follow-up) in patients with most atrophy during the initial 2 years.

Devic's disease (neuromyelitis optica)

As discussed in Chapter 16, the treatment of acute symptomatic neurological syndromes in patients with Devic's disease (neuromyelitis optica) is essentially the same as for multiple sclerosis in relapse. A significant proportion of these patients relapse and stepwise worsening may lead to severe and irreversible neurological disability, often with troublesome pain (Wingerchuk *et al* 1999; Wingerchuk and Weinshenker 2003). Some patients have a malignant course with early disability or shortened life expectancy.

There is limited published experience to guide treatment decisions. There are no proper, phase III randomized trials on which to make evidence-based decisions. Karussis *et al* (1998) have recommended that antiplatelet agents or anticoagulants be used to treat patients with Devic's disease if anti-phospholipid antibodies are present. Mandler *et al* (1998) published an uncontrolled series of seven patients, reporting that long-term oral prednisone and azathioprine may stabilize the course of neuromyelitis optica for a period of up to 18 months. Patients were initially treated with intravenous methylprednisolone (500 mg twice daily) for 5 days and then started on oral prednisolone (1 mg/kg). Prednisone was gradually tapered and then converted to an alternate day schedule, and continued for the full 18 months; on day 21, oral azathioprine was begun at 2 mg/kg. Clearly, confirmatory studies are needed. Anecdotal experience suggests that IFNs are not effective and, theoretically, glatiramer acetate might be contraindicated given the possibility that enhanced Th2 activity would be expected to worsen a humorally mediated disorder such as Devic's Disease (Duda *et al* 2000; Gold and Linington 2002). With recent publications describing antibody- and complement-dependent effector mechanisms of tissue injury (Lucchinetti *et al* 2002) and response to plasma exchange (Keegan *et al* 2002), it seems increasingly likely that immunosuppressive strategies focusing on reducing B-cell function should take preference in seeking

to build on immediate improvements (see Chapter 16) and stabilize the longer-term clinical course. Cree *et al* (2005) administered rituximab, a chimeric murine/human monoclonal antibody that binds to the CD20 antigen and depletes B cells, to eight patients with Devic's disease in an open label, pilot trial. Treatment was well tolerated and seemed to suppress relapses. The treated patients generally improved (seven of eight) but – as the authors acknowledge – in the absence of controls, recovery might have been spontaneous. Lennon *et al* (2004) identified a serum autoantibody that may contribute to diagnostic certainty in the evaluation of Devic's disease (see Chapter 7). This IgG antibody has now been shown to bind to the aquaporin-4 water channel suggesting that Devic's disease may be an autoimmune channel disorder (Lennon *et al* 2005). This bioassay should enhance efforts to describe the full clinical spectrum of neuromyelitis optica and hasten the discovery of key antigens involved in triggering the disease and maintaining disease activity.

Dose effects and comparison of different interferons

Placebo controls were uniformly used during the early period of clinical trials of interferons in multiple sclerosis. There were no 'head-to-head' studies comparing the relative efficacy of different drugs, doses and routes of delivery. This situation has subsequently changed (Table 18.7). Several direct comparisons of licensed and unlicensed products are available and more are under way. It is apparent, and in the main regrettable, that these studies are motivated primarily by competition for market share. Will they provide novel insights that lead to better treatment strategies?

The pivotal trials led to much speculation about the relative merits of subcutaneous injections of IFN-β1b three times weekly compared with the more convenient schedule of giving IFN-β1a by the intramuscular route once each week. The North American IFN-β1b trial showed that alternate day treatment reduced relapse rates by 28–33% in each of the first 3 years of use, and clearly demonstrated a dose effect. The pivotal IFN-β1a study did not report a reduction in relapse rate over the first year, and had a lesser effect in the second than already reported for IFN-β1b, yet it was granted approval by the FDA (United States) for its claim to reduce disease progression. Much like the pivotal North American IFN-β1b trial, PRISMS and SPECTRIMS indicated that a higher dose of interferon was perhaps more effective in reducing relapses than a lower dose when each was administered three times weekly. A study evaluating two doses (30 and 60 μg) of once weekly intramuscular IFN-β1a failed to support a dose effect except for MRI outcomes during the third year (Clanet *et al* 2002). Clanet *et al* (2004) extended the opportunity to these patients to remain on the same dose of IFN-β1a for up to 4 years (56% of the original cohort had completed 4 years of treatment at the time of publication). Again, clinical outcomes were similar between the two groups (30 μg or 60 μg weekly). The Once Weekly Interferon for Multiple Sclerosis Study (OWIMS 1999) showed that a higher dose of once weekly IFN-β1a influenced MRI features more than a lower dose, although neither had a convincing effect on clinical outcomes. Eighty-four percent of the OWIMS subjects agreed to remain on study for the duration of a 4 year extension trial. Freedman *et al* (2005b) reported that once

Table 18.7 Recent randomized trials in relapsing–remitting multiple sclerosis

Trial (number enrolled; follow-up)	Treatment	1° Outcome	Comments
North American GA Extension Study (208; up to 6 years)	Glatiramer acetate 20 mg subcutaneous daily daily injection	Annual relapse rate: reduction reported	Patients enrolled in extension trial had fewer relapses and disability worsening than non-participants. Historical control group contained progressive patients
European-Canadian GA (239; 9 months)	Glatiramer acetate 20 mg subcutaneous daily injection vs. placebo	Total number of Gd+ lesions (29% reduction, p = 0.003)	Delayed, partial benefit: first seen by 6 months and many new lesions in GA group; proportion of patients with Gd+, T_1 black hole lesion volumes not significant and T_2 volumes continue to increase. Short follow-up
PRISMS-4 (506; 90% of initial study; 2 + 2 years)	After 24 months, placebo patients randomized to 22 µg or 44 µg IFN-β1a by subcutaneous injection × 3/week	Relapse count over 4 years (p = 0.001)	Unusual primary outcome; no chance for placebo cases to catch up; largest drop-out in 44 µg group. No adjustment for multiple comparisons. Almost achieves a benefit on disability benefit but effect is modest
INCOMIN (188; 1 year)	IFN-β1a 30 µg by intramuscular injection × 1 per week vs. 9 MIU IFN-β1b by subcutaneous injection on alternate days	Months 6–12, IFN-β1b superior reduction in relapse rate, proportion relapse-free and EDSS	Only radiologist blinded
EVIDENCE (677; 6–12 months)	IFN-β1a 30 µg by intramuscular injection × 1 per week vs. 44 µg by subcutaneous injection × 3 per week	Proportion relapse free favours high dose (75% vs. 63%)	Efforts to blind the evaluators but not patients. Short duration hard to evaluate
Tysabri (213; 1 year)	Tysabri 3 or 6 mg/kg by intravenous injection × 1 per month vs. placebo once per month	Fewer Gd+ lesions (p < 0.0001)	Effect disappeared when treatment stopped. Safety concern when given with IFN-β1a

Gd+ = gadolinium enhancing MRI lesions; IFN = interferon; EDSS = Expanded Disability Status Scale; MIU = million international units; Tysabri = humanized monoclonal anti-α_4 integrin antibody. Adapted from Noseworthy and Hartung (2003) with permission.

weekly IFN-β1a retains a slightly positive MRI effect with no clinical benefit in patients with relapsing–remitting multiple sclerosis. The results of recent direct comparisons (INCOMIN and EVIDENCE, see below) have been used to strengthen the claim that, although less convenient, exposure to interferon three times weekly outperforms weekly administration, at least for the first 6–12 months of treatment.

The INCOMIN study (Independent Comparison of Interferon Trial) randomized 188 relapsing–remitting patients with multiple sclerosis from 15 centres in Italy either to once weekly intramuscular IFN-β1a or alternate day subcutaneous injections of 8 MIU IFN-β1b, under single-blind (evaluator) conditions (Durelli *et al* 2002). The primary outcome measures were the proportion of relapse-free patients, and no new MRI lesions at 2 years. Both primary outcomes favoured the alternate day dose of IFN-β1b, and the magnitude of the effect became more evident in the second year of study (Figure 18.30).

In the EVIDENCE (Evidence of Interferon Dose–response: European North American Comparative Efficacy) trial, investigators from 56 centres in Europe and North America completed a randomized study directly comparing once weekly intramus-

cular IFN-β1a with high-dose subcutaneous (44 µg) three times weekly IFN-β1a in 677 patients with relapsing–remitting multiple sclerosis each having a baseline EDSS of <5.5 (Panitch *et al* 2002). This study was powered to demonstrate a treatment difference within the first 6 months of follow-up. The patients were not blinded but evaluators of clinical and MRI outcomes were unaware of the treatment randomization. The primary outcome was the proportion of relapse-free patients at 6 months, although patients were also evaluated at 1 year. At both 6 and 12 months patients receiving three times weekly IFN-β1a were more likely to be relapse free and with a reduced number of active MRI lesions (Figure 18.31). Fewer patients in the once weekly group developed neutralizing antibody (2% vs. 25%) and injection site reactions or liver enzyme elevations were also less frequent. Long-term safety data at ≥64 weeks confirmed that adverse events were more frequent with the high-dose group and were mainly attributable to the frequency of injection site reactions and hepatic and haematological abnormalities. Objectively, most events were rated as mild, and more serious adverse effects were equally distributed between groups (Sandberg-Wollheim *et al* 2005).

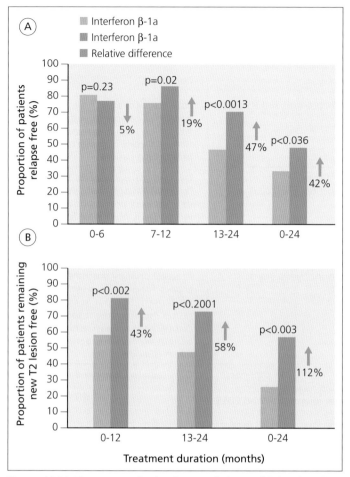

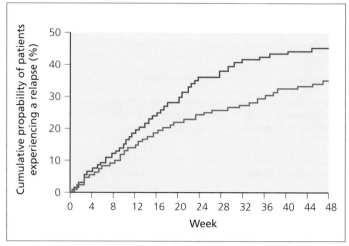

Figure 18.31 Treatment of relapsing–remitting multiple sclerosis either with three times weekly subcutaneous IFN-β1a (Rebif; blue line) or once weekly intramuscular IFN-β1a (Avonex; red line; EVIDENCE Study). Kaplan–Meier curves illustrating the cumulative probability of patients experiencing a first relapse during the study. Adapted from Panitch et al (2002).

Figure 18.30 Treatment of relapsing–remitting multiple sclerosis either with every other day subcutaneous IFN-β1b or once weekly intramuscular IFN-β1a (INCOMIN study). (A) Relative difference (proportion in IFN-β1b group minus proportion in IFN-β1a group divided by proportion in IFN-β1a group) between the proportion of patients free from relapses. (B) New proton density or T$_2$ MRI lesions in the treatment groups at different time points. Adapted from Durelli et al (2002). © 2002, with permission from Elsevier.

Proponents of once weekly interferon hold that the findings of these trials are suspect since in neither study were patients blinded to the treatment assignment. As has been the case with all trials performed to date, there is no mechanism in place adequately to define the long-term implications of these early efficacy claims, or the potential that neutralizing antibody formation will eventually compromise any treatment effect on disability. In 2004, more patients were receiving once weekly intramuscular IFN-β1a than other preparations – primarily because of convenience and more effective sponsor marketing, but also through physician preference given the lower incidence of neutralizing antibody formation and FDA approval for the putative reduction in disability.

The first systematic Cochrane review of interferons in relapsing–remitting multiple sclerosis appeared in 2003 (Filippini et al 2003a). The authors concluded that there was evidence only for a reduction in relapse frequency during the first year of treatment with no convincing benefit thereafter, and no effect on disability (Figures 18.32 and 18.33). As expected, this publication triggered considerable editorial discussion and correspondence

centred, in large part, on methods used to conduct the systematic review (such as handling of drop-outs, comparability of studies, lumping trials of IFN-α and IFN-β, and ignoring MRI effects; Filippini et al 2003b; 2003c; M. Freedman et al 2003; Goodin 2003; Kappos and Kesselring 2003; Paty et al 2003; Rudick et al 2003). As with mitoxantrone, independent calculation of the 'number needed to treat' measure from each of the published trials turns out to be somewhat discouraging (Figure 18.34). In the setting of patients presenting with a clinically isolated syndrome, seven must be treated to prevent one patient developing clinically definite multiple sclerosis at 3 years. In the setting of relapsing–remitting multiple sclerosis, nine have to receive interferon for 1 year to prevent a single relapse, and eight patients must be treated for 2 years to prevent one patient from worsening by a single EDSS point. Although these numbers needed to treat may actually be superior to those quoted for other chronic medical conditions (see Sackett et al 2000), the high cost of interferon therapies and the apparent enthusiasm for their widespread use justify some reflection on cost–benefit ratios and health care economics. In a recently published systematic review, Rice et al (2005) concluded that the IFNs provide modest reduction in relapse risk for up to 2 years but there is insufficient evidence to judge efficacy beyond this time point. As with every systematic review, much hinges on an estimate of the behaviour of those lost to follow-up. In this example, if – to take a worst case – IFN-treated drop-outs worsened, the statistical benefit of treatment would no longer be judged significant.

Adverse effects

In the pivotal trials, blinding was not thought to have been undermined by the local or systemic effects of subcutaneous IFN-β1b but was maintained less well in patients receiving intramuscular IFN-β1a (Avonex; 32% of patients were unblinded but the number of placebo cases correctly guessing the treatment code was not recorded). Now, several years on and with more

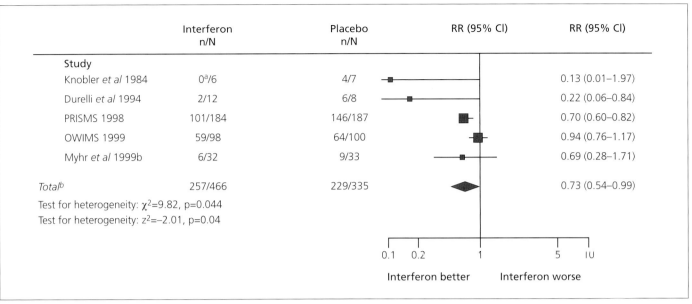

	Interferon n/N	Placebo n/N	RR (95% CI)	RR (95% CI)
Study				
Knobler *et al* 1984	0[a]/6	4/7		0.13 (0.01–1.97)
Durelli *et al* 1994	2/12	6/8		0.22 (0.06–0.84)
PRISMS 1998	101/184	146/187		0.70 (0.60–0.82)
OWIMS 1999	59/98	64/100		0.94 (0.76–1.17)
Myhr *et al* 1999b	6/32	9/33		0.69 (0.28–1.71)
Total[b]	257/466	229/335		0.73 (0.54–0.99)

Test for heterogeneity: $\chi^2=9.82$, p=0.044
Test for heterogeneity: $z^2=-2.01$, p=0.04

0.1   0.2   1   5   IU
Interferon better   Interferon worse

Figure 18.32 Meta-analysis of patients who had at least one exacerbation during the first year of treatment. n/N = number of patients who had exacerbations/number of patients randomized. To estimate relapse rate, 0.5 was added to each cell of the 2×2 table for the trials. a = no patients with exacerbations in the IFN group; b = random effects model. Adapted from Filippini *et al* (2003a).

experience of these agents, we doubt that patients can be adequately blinded to the side effects of interferons. The main adverse effects of IFN-β1b and IFN-β1a are local injection site reactions (Figure 18.35), flu-like symptoms and hyperthermia at onset, and depression. Fortunately, there is no significant drug hypersensitivity. Based on the evidence from clinical trials, contraindications to the use of IFN-β are pregnancy, epilepsy and depression. Post-marketing experience in the United States indicates that patients in whom fatigue and depression occur prior to starting IFN-β1b, especially those with secondary progressive disease, often abandon treatment because of adverse effects (Neilley *et al* 1996). Events may be delayed for up to 29 months and usually consist of injection site reactions (Gaines and Varrichio 1998). The long-term risks of IFN-β1b are unknown.

With time, most patients are better able to tolerate the adverse effects commonly associated with the use of IFN-β (Walther and Hohlfeld 1999). Injection site reactions are more frequent with subcutaneous than intramuscular administration. These may become intolerable leading to discontinuation of treatment. Careful attention to technique (avoiding intradermal injections, excessive sun exposure, overly cooled solutions and nonsterile technique) and local icing of the injection site may help. Necrosis at the injection site is more common in women, especially if the medication is not warmed to room temperature before injection. Intramuscular injections seldom cause tissue reactions but abscess formation, although rare, may lead to significant morbidity. Many patients are able to tolerate the transient flu-like symptoms that frequently occur for the first 4–12 hours after each injection by administering the dose in the evening along with an oral anti-inflammatory agent (acetominophen or ibuprofen: G.P. Rice *et al* 1999; Rio and Montalban 2000). Occasionally it may be necessary to reduce the dose of interferon and to co-administer oral prednisone for a few weeks to improve compliance (Rio *et al* 1998). Patients often develop transient elevations of liver function tests, neutropenia and, less

commonly, anaemia requiring dose reduction or a drug holiday.

We routinely measure liver function and a full blood count at baseline, after the first week and month of exposure and then every 3 months thereafter. Menstrual function may be affected, usually resulting in menorrhagia. The issue of depression remains controversial. We generally advise patients and family members that interferons may either expose or worsen underlying depression. They should remain alert to a change in mood that may require treatment. There are reports that spasticity may increase with interferons (Bramanti *et al* 1998; Frese *et al* 1999). Occasionally treated patients develop serological abnormalities suggesting the induction of autoimmunity, including antibodies to thyroid, nuclear and muscle antigens. There are several reports of treatment-induced thyroid dysfunction associated with the use of IFN-β in multiple sclerosis. The initial reported frequency varied from 0% to 34% (Colosimo *et al* 1997; Durelli *et al* 1998; 1999; Kivisakk *et al* 1998c; Monzani *et al* 1999; 2000; Rotondi *et al* 1998; Schwid *et al* 1997a). These trials involved small cohorts of patients treated for varying durations, and to us the overall estimated prevalence (23%) seems high based on personal experience, although that there is a genuine relationship is unambiguous (see below). A more recent study followed 106 patients receiving IFN-β for between 31 and 84 months (Caraccio *et al* 2005). Thyroid autoimmunity affected one-quarter of the patients. The majority were examples of hypothyroidism, half of which were transient. Hyperthyroidism occurred in one-fifth of the cases, and was always characterized by an initial hyperthyroid phase, followed by a plateau culminating in hypothyroidism. It also was often subclinical or transient. Clinical thyroid disease and the development of thyroid autoantibodies in isolation occurred most commonly in the first year after treatment. Females were preferentially affected, but thyroid disease was more persistent in males. The presence of thyroid specific antibodies at baseline (8.5%), the presence of subclinical hypothyroidism prior to

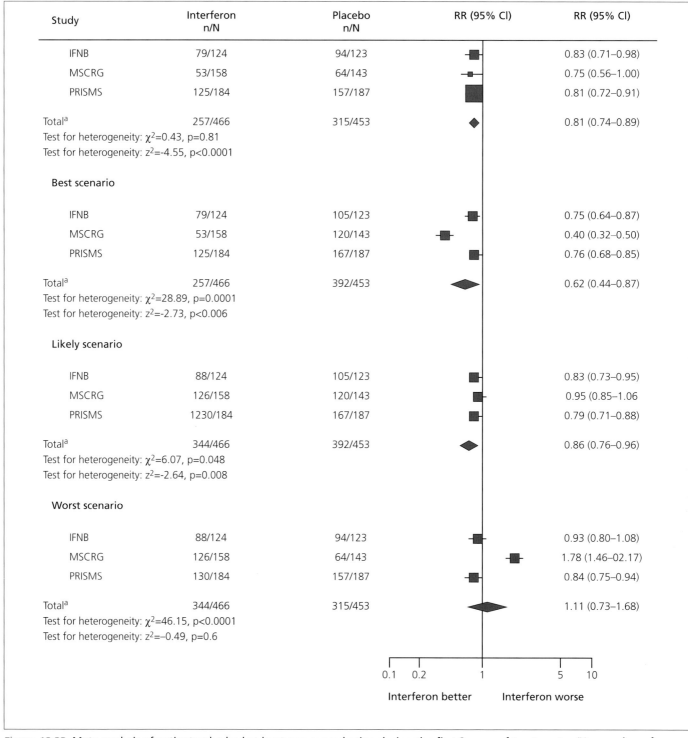

Study	Interferon n/N	Placebo n/N	RR (95% CI)	RR (95% CI)
IFNB	79/124	94/123		0.83 (0.71–0.98)
MSCRG	53/158	64/143		0.75 (0.56–1.00)
PRISMS	125/184	157/187		0.81 (0.72–0.91)
Total[a]	257/466	315/453		0.81 (0.74–0.89)

Test for heterogeneity: χ^2=0.43, p=0.81
Test for heterogeneity: z^2=-4.55, p<0.0001

Best scenario

IFNB	79/124	105/123		0.75 (0.64–0.87)
MSCRG	53/158	120/143		0.40 (0.32–0.50)
PRISMS	125/184	167/187		0.76 (0.68–0.85)
Total[a]	257/466	392/453		0.62 (0.44–0.87)

Test for heterogeneity: χ^2=28.89, p=0.0001
Test for heterogeneity: z^2=-2.73, p<0.006

Likely scenario

IFNB	88/124	105/123		0.83 (0.73–0.95)
MSCRG	126/158	120/143		0.95 (0.85–1.06
PRISMS	1230/184	167/187		0.79 (0.71–0.88)
Total[a]	344/466	392/453		0.86 (0.76–0.96)

Test for heterogeneity: χ^2=6.07, p=0.048
Test for heterogeneity: z^2=-2.64, p=0.008

Worst scenario

IFNB	88/124	94/123		0.93 (0.80–1.08)
MSCRG	126/158	64/143		1.78 (1.46–02.17)
PRISMS	130/184	157/187		0.84 (0.75–0.94)
Total[a]	344/466	315/453		1.11 (0.73–1.68)

Test for heterogeneity: χ^2=46.15, p<0.0001
Test for heterogeneity: z^2=–0.49, p=0.6

0.1   0.2   1   5   10

Interferon better   Interferon worse

Figure 18.33 Meta-analysis of patients who had at least one exacerbation during the first 2 years of treatment. n/N = number of patients who had exacerbations/number of patients randomized. a = random effects model. References: IFNB = IFNB Multiple Sclerosis Study Group (1993); MSCRG = Jacobs et al (1996); PRISMS = PRISMS Study Group (1998). Adapted from Filippini et al (2003a). © 2003, with permission from Elsevier.

starting treatment (2.3%: defined as raised thyroid stimulating hormone without abnormalities of serum thyroxine or tri-iodothyronine) or the development of thyroid-specific antibodies following treatment (23%) were the only predictive factors for the development of thyroid disease. There was no difference in frequency depending on exposure to IFN-β1a or IFN-β1b. There are isolated reports of treatment-related myasthenia gravis (Blake and Murphy 1997), systemic lupus erythe-matosus (Watts 2000), rheumatoid arthritis (Alsalameh et al 1998; Jabaily and Thompson 1997), inflammatory arthritis (Altintas et al 2002; Levesque 1999; Russo et al 2000), urticaria (D.L. Brown et al 2001), Raynaud's phenomenon (Cruz et al 2000; Linden 1998b), worsening of psoriasis (Kowalzick 1997; Webster et al 1996), acute hepatitis (Christopher et al 2005) liver failure (E.M. Yoshida et al 2001), a fatal capillary leak syndrome (in a patient with pre-existing acquired C1 inhibitor

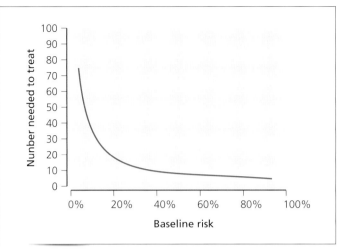

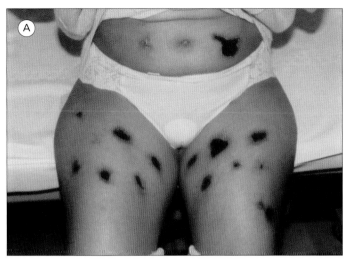

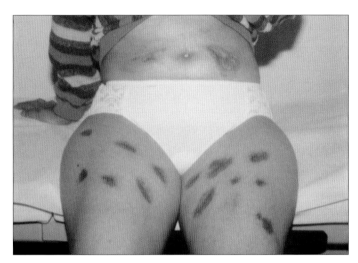

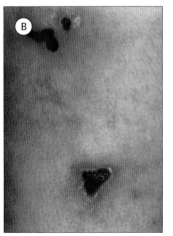

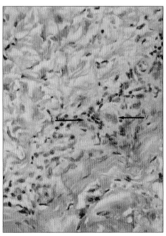

Figure 18.34 Number needed to prevent one patient having at least one exacerbation at 1 year in relation to baseline risks. Adapted from Filippini *et al* (2003a). © 2003, with permission from Elsevier.

deficiency; Niederwieser 2000; S. Schmidt *et al* 1999), intracerebral hemorrhage (Niederwieser *et al* 2001) and anaphylaxis (Clear 1999; Corona *et al* 1999). From amongst this catalogue, the one clear message is that patients with monoclonal gammopathy should not receive IFN-β as they may be at risk for developing a life-threatening capillary leak syndrome.

Neutralizing antibodies to interferons

It is now revealed that up to 45% of patients on 8 MIU IFN-β1b develop neutralizing activity. In the original series, this usually occurred in the first year (34 of 124) with fewer examples thereafter (7 of 124 in year 2, and only 2 of 124 in year 3; IFNB MS Study Group and the UBC MS/MRI analysis Group 1995). In the trial of IFN-β1a (Avonex; Jacobs *et al* 1996), persistent neutralizing anti-interferon activity was seen in 14% of treated individuals by one year and 23% at two years. This compared with 4% in the placebo group, but the positive tests always disappeared with repeat testing. The tendency for neutralizing antibodies to be present transiently has since been confirmed, an early response but at low titre having predictive value for subsequent reversion to seronegativity (Gneiss *et al* 2004) Subsequent experience confirms the significant antigenicity of IFN-β1b and shows cross-reactivity between neutralizing and binding antibodies to IFN-β1b, IFN-β1a and naturally occurring IFN-β. At first, the clinical significance of neutralizing antibody responses remained uncertain (Kivisäkk *et al* 1997). Antibodies are detected by a cytopathic effect on virus-infected cells. Preliminary enzyme-linked immunosorbent assay screening has since been introduced and the prevalence of antibodies in more recent cohorts of patients treated with IFN-β1a is lower than previously published or that seen with IFN-β1b. For IFN-β1b, the original primary and secondary outcome measures have been re-analysed, stratified for the presence of neutralizing antibodies and different epochs within the initial 3 year period of exposure for comparisons of relapse rate, MRI activity and disability. This has generated much uncertainty (and spin) about whether the drug would be even more effective were it not for antibody development or, conversely, is doomed to short-term efficacy (at best) by immunogenicity.

Figure 18.35 (A) Severe necrotizing lesions in a woman with multiple sclerosis undergoing treatment with IFN-β1b at onset (top panel) and on recovery (lower panel). (B) Macroscopic and microscopic appearance of an individual area of necrosis. From Albani and Albani (1997) with permission. © 1997, reproduced with permission of the BMJ Publishing Group.

In support of the first interpretation is the conclusion that patients who do not develop neutralizing activity have an even lower relapse rate than that reported for all IFN-β1b-treated patients. For the period 13–36 months, the attack rate was 1.06 per year in the placebo group compared with 1.08 per year in

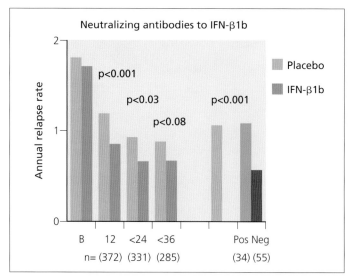

Figure 18.36 Annual relapse rates at baseline (B), and on completion of years 1 (12), 2 (<24) and 3 (<36) in patients taking IFN-β1b; the annual relapse rate is also shown in a subgroup of patients with (Pos) and without (Neg) neutralizing antibodies compared with a cohort of controls studied for the same period. Adapted from the IFNB Multiple Sclerosis Study Group (1993; 1995). © 1993, 1995, reproduced with permission of Lippincott Williams & Wilkins (lww.com).

the IFN-β1b-treated antibody-positive patients and 0.56 per year in those without neutralizing activity (Figure 18.36: IFNB MS Study Group and the UBC MS/MRI Analysis Group 1995). It follows that, at least in this series, the development of neutralizing activity is associated with a relapse rate which is greater than that reported for other treated patients. In fact, patients destined to develop neutralizing antibodies showed a higher relapse rate before neutralizing activity was detected. This increased further after the assay became persistently positive. For this reason, it has been proposed that patients who develop neutralizing antibodies may have a different profile of immune responsiveness which promotes both neutralizing activity and the disease process, culminating in the symptoms of multiple sclerosis. This formulation seems to us contrived.

In the early analyses of these trials, patients who developed neutralizing activity did not become more disabled than the remaining participants. In fact, the converse was true. This was seen as evidence that the development of neutralizing activity does not disadvantage patients in the longer term. However, taken with the increased relapse rate associated with neutralizing activity, this observation merely reflects the poor correlation between relapse and disability, and suggests that inactivity of IFN-β1b *in vivo* does not adversely affect the course of the disease – a conclusion prompting the response that IFN-β1b is therefore not a disease-modifying drug. The effects on MRI activity and total lesion load in patients developing antibodies parallel the observations relating to relapse rates.

To clarify these emerging issues, investigators using IFN-β1b in the pivotal study subsequently published a detailed report on the development of neutralizing antibodies (IFNB Multiple Sclerosis Study Group and the University of British Columbia MS/MRI Analysis Group 1996). They validated the cytopathic assay and confirmed that the original antibody results were not

false-positives; although with a change in cut-off point for a positive titration result the prevalence dropped to 35%. Antibodies mainly, but not exclusively, developed in the first year and this complication was not dose dependent. Relapse rates differed depending on the presence of antibodies, as originally reported (IFNB Multiple Sclerosis Study Group 1995). There was more disease activity on MRI in patients who developed antibodies on high (but not low) dose IFN-β1b than the antibody-negative group, but the cumulative number of enlarging lesions was still less than in the placebo group. There was no detrimental effect on disability progression and antibody-positive patients had less disability progression than those patients who remained antibody negative. No new adverse events correlated with the development of neutralizing activity. In fact, beyond 18 months, fewer events occurred than previously reported in studies using IFN-β1b. Individuals who developed antibodies were no more or less likely than others on active treatment to discontinue IFN-β1b.

In the trial of IFN-β1a (Rebif; PRISMS 1998), all the adverse effects were as reported for other brands of IFN-β but they were no more prevalent. Specifically, neutralizing antibodies to IFN-β1a developed in 18% of treated patients and 1% of controls. Although initially reassuring, the extension study (PRISMS-4) did show a detrimental effect on relapse rate in antibody-positive patients (44 μg group, antibody-negative relapse rate was 0.50 per year compared with 0.81 per year in antibody-positive patients). The formation of neutralizing antibodies reduced the protective effect on relapse recurrence in the European trial of secondary progressive multiple sclerosis but did not influence disability progression (Polman *et al* 2003). Neutralizing antibody formation was shown to inhibit the MRI benefit from treatment in the SPECTRIMS trial (SPECTRIMS Study Group 2001).

The neutralizing antibody story has continued to unfold. Although there is still no definitive study of adequate size and duration to provide a final statement on this complex issue, the suspicion that antibody formation reduces both the biologic effect of IFN-β and the clinical and MRI evidence for efficacy have since increased. In a study of 754 Danish patients, Ross *et al* (2000) found that neutralizing antibodies are more common in patients receiving IFN-β1b than IFN-β1a; in patients treated with subcutaneous compared with intramuscular injections, and in those receiving three times weekly injections; compared to once weekly administration. Bertolotto *et al* (2002) found similar results based on a cytopathic effect assay in a study of 125 patients. They reported that those receiving IFN-β1a (Rebif) three times weekly developed neutralizing antibodies with a frequency between that reported for the other preparations (18 month results for persistently positive: IFN-β1b, 31%; subcutaneous IFN-β1a three times weekly, 15%; and intramuscular IFN-β1a once weekly, 2%). Also reviewing the nationwide Danish prescribing experience, P.S. Sorenson *et al* (2003) reported similar findings in 541 IFN-β-treated patients followed for up to 5 years. Using three techniques of varying sensitivity (the findings were similar regardless of the assays used), they found that approximately one-third of IFN-β-treated patients developed neutralizing antibodies in the first year of treatment. This percentage stayed largely unchanged with prolonged follow-up. However, there was considerable variability between the different preparations. Factors leading to a greater risk of neutralizing antibody formation included exposure to IFN-β1b (compared with IFN-β1a), subcutaneous injection (compared with intramuscular; p = 0.022) and repeated dosing (three times weekly compared with once weekly; p = 0.0001). Antibody levels fell in the third year in some patients (p = 0.023), particularly those receiving IFN-β1b. The presence of neutralizing antibodies influenced the observed relapse rates in this study. Relapse rates were greatest during antibody-positive epochs (0.64–0.70 vs. 0.43–0.46; p < 0.03). They confirmed that antibody-positive patients relapse more often than those without antibodies (odds ratio during antibody positive periods: 1.51–1.58; p < 0.03) although this loss of protection is usually delayed. MRI data were not reported. These authors speculate that the reduction in prevalence of antibodies with time, and the associated fall in relapse rate may relate, in part, to changing avidity of the antibodies. Bellomi *et al* (2003) reported that the type of IFN-β exposure does not determine whether antibodies are lost with time.

The Danish series found no effect of antibody formation on disability progression as measured by the EDSS (P.S. Sorenson *et al* 2003). Approximately 50% of patients had deteriorated by 1.0 EDSS point (confirmed at 6 months) at the 42 month follow-up. Survival curves, stratified for the presence of neutralizing antibodies, seemed to separate thereafter, suggesting that antibody-negative patients accumulated disability more slowly after the 3 year follow-up, but the number of patients available for follow-up fell sharply after 3 years and this difference was not significant (p = 0.14). Taken together, the Danish investigators conclude that the development of antibodies does compromise the effect of IFN-β. They recommend that antibody status should be monitored in patients with active disease and suggest changing to another class of treatment (such as glatiramer acetate or mitoxantrone) in antibody-positive patients.

Oger *et al* (1997) reported that antibody formation correlated with high levels of immunoglobulin production in an *in vitro* immunoglobulin G secretion assay but others (Bellomi *et al* 2003; Rudick *et al* 1998a) were unable to identify markers that predict the development of antibodies. Lawrence *et al* (2003) developed a rapid, inexpensive radio-immunoprecipitation assay to measure binding antibodies to IFN-β. Using a cohort of 33 patients with relapsing–remitting multiple sclerosis, they reported that the assay is predictive both for the presence of neutralizing antibodies and reduced efficacy in preventing MRI outcomes. Gilli *et al* (2003) reported that neutralizing antibodies reverse the putative protective influence of IFN-β on reduction of matrix metalloproteinase-2 and -9 expression but do not influence endogenous levels of the tissue inhibitor (TIMP-1).

In a recent report, Petkau *et al* (2004) analysed the neutralizing antibody data collected during the pivotal North American IFN-β1b trial. They determined that neutralizing antibodies reduce the clinical benefit (relapse reduction) from both doses of IFN-β1b but the detrimental effect of these antibodies is more marked in those receiving the low dose (that is, relapse rates were higher by 28% for 1.6 MIU compared with 2% for 8 MIU: Figure 18.37A and B). They also reported that this reduction in efficacy reverses with restorations of antibody-negative status (60% who were once antibody-positive later had at least one antibody-negative value). Gilli *et al* (2003) reported that neutralizing antibodies developing during the course of treatment with each of the available interferons abrogated the effect of IFN-β on reducing matrix metalloproteinase-9 expression, suggesting a possible mechanism of action for these antibodies.

Against this background, the transactions of a conference devoted to antibody formation in multiple sclerosis have since appeared (Pachner 2003). Attendees reached consensus (>70% agreement) on many of the conclusions already discussed relating to antibody-mediated decrease in bioactivity. They called for more universal standards in the assays used to measure binding and neutralization, longitudinal data analyses to avoid the limitations of previously reported cross-sectional studies (Petkau 2003), and prospective efforts to identify strategies for reducing

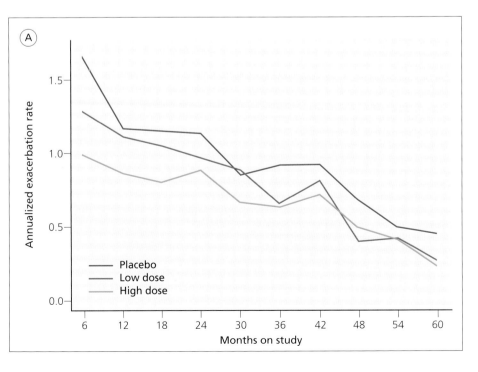

Figure 18.37 (A) Annualized exacerbation rates in the preceding 6 month periods (number of exacerbations beginning in preceding 6 month period/number of patient years on study in preceding 6 month period). Adapted from Petkau *et al* (2004). © 2004, reproduced with permission of Hodder Education.

illustration continued on following page

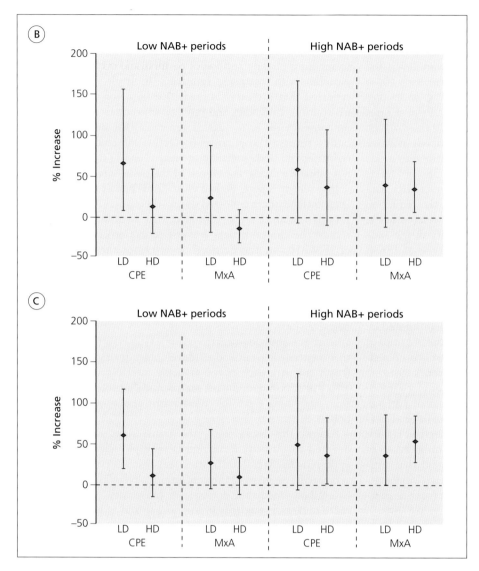

Figure 18.37, cont'd (B and C) Increase in exacerbation rate (and 95% CI) for eventually neutralizing antibody (NAB)+ subgroups in low NAB+ (confirmation required) and high NAB+ (no confirmation required) periods relative to NAB− periods: (B) 'Once positive, always positive' classification of NAB status. (C) 'All switches considered' classification of NAB status. LD = low dose; HD = high dose; CPE = cytopathic effect; MxA = myxovirus protein A. Adapted from Petkau et al (2004). © 2004, reproduced with permission of Hodder Education.

antibody formation in patients treated with IFN-β. Strategies for inhibiting the formation of antibodies so as to maintain the perceived efficacy of IFN-β1b include using higher doses, concurrent use of corticosteroids or other immunosuppressants, and switching brands – although the prevailing view is that antibodies to IFN-β1a and IFN-β1b cross-react. In 2005, there are still no proven strategies for reducing antibody formation. The interested reader is referred to a series of recent papers comprising the proceedings of an international consensus conference held in August 2002 (Bertolotto et al 2004; Billiau et al 2004; Deisenhammer et al 2004; Hartung and Munschauer 2004; Hartung et al 2004; Schellekens and Casadevall et al 2004; Vartanian et al 2004).

Malucchi et al (2004) recently reported on their non-randomized study of 78 patients treated with either subcutaneous IFN-β1b (Betaseron; n = 20), subcutaneous IFN-β1a (Rebif; n = 25) or IFN-β1b by intramuscular injection (Avonex; n = 33). Neutralizing antibody assays were performed every 3 months for up to 3 years. Their frequency was similar to previous reports in the literature (subcutaneous IFN-β1b, 35%; subcutaneous IFN-β1a, 20%; and intramuscular IFN-β1a, 3%).

Relapses were most consistently reduced in the patients without antibodies; patients 'persistently positive' demonstrated less relapse suppression and a greater likelihood of EDSS worsening during the course of the study. In another recent report, Frank et al (2004) reported that subcutaneous IFN-β1b reduced the number of contrast enhancing lesions and the cumulative white matter lesion load over a period of up to 3 years in 30 patients using a baseline versus treatment crossover design. The MRI effect was reduced in antibody-positive patients. The authors suggested that IFN-β1b by subcutaneous injection reduced the progression of cerebral atrophy but, from our review of this paper, the benefit is less certain given the small sample size.

Thus, the issue of whether neutralizing antibodies matter is not settled. On one side of the debate is the theory that IFN-β is biologically inactive in the presence of neutralizing antibodies and so should not be prescribed. Antibodies very clearly reduce biological activity and seemingly reverse any effect on frequency of relapse, reducing antibody-positive patients to nearly the same risk of relapse as untreated controls. Several recent studies support the concept that neutralizing antibodies decrease the therapeutic effects of the IFN-βs (G.S. Francis et al 2005;

Giovannoni and Goodman 2005; Kappos *et al* 2005; P.S. Sorensen *et al* 2005). The observation that disability continues regardless of antibody formation suggests that this group of drugs provides little in the way of long-term disease modification. Others present these findings and their implications for efficacy and safety in the best possible light; they argue that the development of neutralizing activity has led to the true efficacy of IFN-β1b being underestimated; that neutralizing activity is not associated with additional adverse effects; and that, at worst, it may only make the drug harmlessly inactive.

The licences for IFN-β

By 1996, approximately 35 000 patients in the United States were receiving Betaseron for ambulant, relapsing–remitting disease. The number of patients attending some centres who received a prescription was estimated at >50%. Presumably, there was some laxity in the policing of reimbursements by the insurance companies with a good deal of drift at the prescribing margins. The unofficial guidelines, drafted by neurologists involved in the clinical trials and with postmarketing experience, were orientated towards expanding the group eligible for a prescription and offered advice on managing difficulties which might arise, such as perceived lack of efficacy, without discontinuing treatment (Lublin *et al* 1996). In the first few months after a licence was granted for Avonex, the company claimed 15 000 prescriptions, with a proportion switching from IFN-β1b to IFN-β1a (Avonex), creating considerable confusion with respect to the carryover of clinical benefits, adverse effects and neutralizing antibodies. Because the clinical trials were published later and the granting of a licence was delayed, Rebif lagged in the United States market. In 2003, the approximate number of patients receiving these treatments in the United States (total 172 000 prescriptions) and Europe (94 000 prescriptions) respectively were: Avonex – 47% and 15% (94 500 total); Betaseron – 17% and 38% (65 500 total); Rebif – 10% and 31% (46 500 total); and Copaxone (see below) – 26% and 15% (59 500 total).

It did not take long for a debate to begin on the managed entry of the interferons in continental Europe and the United Kingdom, with jockeying for position on who should take the decision to prescribe and who pays (Walley and Barton 1995). In Europe, where Betaferon was granted a product licence in late 1995, Avonex in 1997 and Rebif in 1998, the professional analysis was much more measured than in the United States. The take-up of prescriptions was slower and in many countries this resulted from delay in establishing guidelines for clinical use, closely linked to decisions on funding. All forms of IFN-β and glatiramer acetate are currently provided in the United Kingdom through a Risk Sharing Scheme, organized by the Department of Health, in which patients on treatment will undergo annual EDSS evaluations for up to 10 years. From these long-term data, the price of the drug may in future be adjusted to meet an acceptable level of cost-effectiveness. Meanwhile, pressure from the neurological community and the commercial realization that the arguments with respect to efficacy and cost are not yet won has led to new trials, some already completed (see above). However, comparative studies with other immunosuppressive drugs, which the prescribing community would want to have available – such as the proposed ERAZMUS (EEC

concerted action) trial comparing IFN-β1a (Avonex) with azathioprine and placebo in 1200 patients with early relapsing–remitting or secondary progressive multiple sclerosis, taking time to EDSS 3 over 4 years as the primary outcome measure, are commercially unattractive and have never materialized.

Information distributed by the pharmaceutical companies which make or market Betaseron in the United States recommends that

Betaseron™ (interferon beta-1b) is indicated for the treatment of relapsing forms of multiple sclerosis to reduce the frequency of clinical exacerbations.

In the European Community, Betaferon is currently indicated [European Agency for the Evaluation of Medicinal Products (EMEA) European Public Assessment Report (EPAR), Revision 5, 12 June 2003]

for the treatment of patients with relapsing-remitting multiple sclerosis and two or more relapses in the last two years. Betaferon is also indicated for patients with secondary progressive with active disease evidenced by relapses.

In North America, Avonex

is indicated for the treatment of patients with relapsing forms of multiple sclerosis to slow the accumulation of physical disability and decrease the frequency of clinical exacerbations. Patients with multiple sclerosis in whom efficacy has been demonstrated include patients who have experienced a first clinical episode and have MRI features consistent with multiple sclerosis. Safety and efficacy in patients with chronic progressive multiple sclerosis have not been established.

Caution is advised in using Avonex in patients with a history of depression and in those with a prior history of epilepsy. Breastfeeding and Avonex-use should not be combined. In the European Community: Avonex is currently indicated (EMEA EPAR, revision 4, 24 February 2004)

for ambulatory patients with relapsing multiple sclerosis characterized by at least two recurrent attacks of neurologic dysfunction (relapses) over the preceding three year period without evidence of continuing progression between relapses. It slows the progression of disability and decreases the frequency of relapses over a two year period. Contraindications are known hypersensitivity to IFN-β or human albumin, pregnancy, breast feeding, severe depression or suicidal ideation, and poorly controlled epilepsy.

Avonex is also indicated for the treatment of patients who have experienced a single demyelinating event with an active inflammatory process if it is severe enough to warrant treatment with intravenous corticosteroids; if alternative diagnoses have been excluded; and if they are determined to be at high risk of developing clinically definite multiple sclerosis. The EMEA goes on to suggest that *a high risk patient is one who has ≥ 9 T2 lesions on a baseline MRI and at least one new T2 or gadolinium enhancing lesion on a follow up scan performed at least 3 months later. Treatment should be discontinued in patients who develop disease progression*

In the United States

Rebif™ (interferon beta-1a) is indicated for the treatment of patients with relapsing forms of multiple sclerosis to decrease the frequency of clinical exacerbations and delay the accumulation of physical disability. Efficacy of Rebif™ in chronic progressive multiple sclerosis has not been established.

In the European Community, Rebif is currently indicated (EMEA EPAR, revision 6, 4 December 2003)

for the treatment of patients with multiple sclerosis with two or more relapses within the last two years. Efficacy has not been demonstrated in patients with secondary progressive multiple sclerosis without ongoing relapse activity.

This licence is now updated to recommend 44 μg as the preferred dose.

In the climate which has emerged following the marketing of IFN-β, working in health care systems with competitive and limited resources, such as the United Kingdom, maintaining a balanced and responsible position, remains intermittently stressful but still of importance. Well-tried mechanisms for challenging decisions on prescribing, where medical and fiscal motives are easily confused, have already been exercised. It is somewhat ironic and, for some, frankly perplexing, that the introduction of a treatment that might have a disease-modifying effect in multiple sclerosis should have provoked so much apparent controversy. On one side of this debate are professional and lay enthusiasts who argue that this is the first useful drug treatment for a frightening and potentially disabling neurological disease affecting young adults. On the other, are those who have experienced previous short-lived therapeutic claims and, therefore, remain sceptical about the newly licensed therapies having more than a transitional role on the way to more effective remedies.

In the United Kingdom, all three interferon preparations are currently used according to the guidelines of the Association of British Neurologists (January 2001, see *www.theabn.org*) which require that there have been two or more clinically significant relapses in the previous 2 years in ambulant patients with relapsing–remitting multiple sclerosis and two disabling relapses as the main clinical feature of disease activity in ambulant patients with secondary progressive disease. The guidelines also suggest the following be considered as potential stopping criteria:

- the occurrence of two severe relapses within 12 months
- the development of secondary progression for >6 months
- the loss of ability to walk.

These somewhat rigorous stopping guidelines have not always proved feasible to apply in clinical practice (B.D. Dubois *et al* 2003). The EMEA reports provide a variety of recommendations for monitoring patients and deciding when treatment might be continued or discontinued. These reflect the uncer-

tainties that exist concerning the long-term effectiveness of all the interferons and the frequent difficulties in determining for individual patients whether or not treatment is providing benefit. The use of IFN-β is contraindicated in young people aged <16 years, although the experience of treating a group of Italian children or adolescents is that the reduction in relapse rate is no less than in adults (Ghezzi *et al* 2005). The pivotal trials were usually confined to the 16–55 year age groups, and no upper age limit is included in the summary of product characteristics.

There is a critical need for thorough and transparent analysis of all the prescribing experience with each of these partially effective drugs to characterize, if possible, what determines 'responder' vs. 'nonresponder' status. To date, these analyses have not been possible as the informative clinical trial data are largely unavailable to investigators, being held *in camera* by the sponsors. Given the importance for all parties of identifying clinical and biological markers of response, both to predict who will respond and to clarify the magnitude and duration of a positive response, none of the approved drugs has yet been subjected to such comprehensive analysis. Indeed, investigators have yet to create clinical and MRI guidelines that are either consensus driven or, preferably, biologically meaningful. It remains uncertain whether the 'partial response' so universally reported in contemporary trials relates to a partial response for many or a biologically meaningful response for only a minority of patients. Consequently, patients and their physicians are left to speculate as to when drugs should be started, changed or stopped. This ambiguity has prompted some experts to suggest that since one cannot predict who may respond, virtually all affected individuals should be considered for treatment at the time relapsing–remitting multiple sclerosis is diagnosed (Van den Noort 1998). However, disbelievers amongst the prescribing community argue that the drugs are sufficiently limited in effectiveness as to make their use purely optional and determined more by the desire of the patient and physician to 'do something' rather than realistic expectation of a brighter neurological future.

MOLECULES THAT INHIBIT T-CELL–PEPTIDE BINDING

The principle that immune responses can be manipulated by the use of peptides or other molecules that mimic closely the naturally occurring ligand for T-cell binding has shown that it is possible to promote clonal anergy. These strategies have therefore been applied to the treatment of multiple sclerosis.

Oral myelin

One approach that has already received preliminary clinical application (Weiner *et al* 1993b) is inhibition of the autoimmune processes with oral antigen. Thirty patients, having two or more relapses in the previous 2 years, were treated with 30 mg of oral bovine myelin or placebo for 1 year. Six of the 15 myelin-treated patients had major attacks compared with 12 of the 15 placebo patients. There was no effect on disability, although a rather contrived subgroup analysis claimed a selective effect in DR2(15)-negative males. The clinical observations could not be correlated with changes in the proportion or specificity of T-cell clones reactive to myelin basic protein, or its encephalitogenic peptides. In other contexts, oral feeding of antigen has been shown to favour the induction of T cells which secrete IL-4, TGF-β and IL-10 at low doses and to delete both Th1 and Th2 cells at higher doses (Y. Chen *et al* 1995). Although superficially attractive, the results of the pilot study always seemed to us overstated and few were surprised by the widely publicized news that the phase three trial of oral myelin (515 patients, 14 sites) showed no clinical effect. However, this negative study remains unpublished several years after the trial was stopped and seems destined never to be reported in full.

Altered peptide ligands

Antigen-specific immunotherapy was dealt a further tough blow in 2000 when two phase two trials of altered peptide ligand therapy designed to interfere with T-cell responses were terminated early because of concerns about patient safety. In the first, use of the altered peptide ligand (CGP77116) was associated with clinical relapses and systemic hypersensitivity reactions that persisted despite dose reduction (Bielekova *et al* 2000). The trial was terminated after only eight patients were enrolled. The finding that two-thirds of patients who had clinical relapses after starting therapy were shown to have developed high T-cell precursor frequencies to the ligand and myelin basic protein peptide 83–89 suggested that the intervention incited clinical relapses. In the second study, three doses of the altered peptide ligand NBI5788 (5, 20 or 50 mg weekly by subcutaneous injection) were compared with placebo administration. The trial was stopped when nine of the 142 patients experienced hypersensitivity reactions. Immunological studies suggested that treatment induced a Th2 profile of immune response (Kappos *et al* 2000). This study was of insufficient duration to detect a clinically meaningful response but MRI monitoring suggested a possible benefit using the lowest dose of altered peptide ligand. D.E. Goodkin *et al* (2000) demonstrated that various doses of a complex of HLA-specific DR2 solubilized with the myelin basic protein peptide 84–102 (AG284) were well tolerated but the trial was not powered for an efficacy analysis.

Copolymer-1 or glatiramer acetate (Copaxone)

Following the logic that immunological damage in multiple sclerosis is mediated by antigen-specific T cells, a synthetic peptide composed of L-alanine, L-glutamic acid, L-lysine and L-tyrosine was designed specifically to mimic the structure of myelin basic protein. Copolymer 1 [Cop-1, later renamed glatiramer acetate (Copaxone) by the sponsor upon approval of this agent for use in multiple sclerosis by the FDA in North America] was neither encephalitogenic nor toxic, and was shown to suppress experimental autoimmune encephalomyelitis (perhaps by inducing antigen-specific suppressor cells). It moved into clinical practice in the early 1980s (Abramsky *et al* 1977).

Clinical studies

Bornstein *et al* (1982) first reported in detail on the therapeutic use in 16 patients with multiple sclerosis. In a subsequent blinded and placebo-controlled study of patients having two or more relapses in the previous 2 years, and EDSS scores of <6 at entry, randomization to active or placebo preparations was within EDSS bands (Bornstein *et al* 1987). Participants received subcutaneous Cop-1 for up to 2 years. A neurologist assessed disease activity, and analysis was on an intention to treat basis. Taking absence of relapse during the trial as the primary end point, a greater proportion of individuals in matched pairs randomized to Cop-1 were relapse free on completion than placebo cases (ten of 22 compared with two of 22 in whom the placebo partner but not the Cop-1-treated individual was free from relapse, and ten of 22 pairs in whom the course was concordant within individual pairs; p = 0.039: Figure 18.38A). There were 62 exacerbations in 23 placebo-treated patients compared with 16 amongst 25 Cop-1-treated individuals. Although the placebo group showed a reduction in relapse rate during the trial as part of the natural history, or regression to the mean, the difference between groups was 4.9 in the first year and 3.3 in the second, favouring treatment with Cop-1. Overall 14 of 25 treated patients were free from relapse compared with six of 23 in the placebo group (p < 0.001). An apparent difference in the rate at which Cop-1- and placebo-treated patients deteriorated (five of 25 and 11 of 23, respectively), which was especially marked in less affected individuals (EDSS <2 at entry), was not statistically significant. There was, however, a delay in time to progression by one EDSS point amongst Cop-1-treated patients (Figure 18.38B). Local injection site reactions seriously undermined blinding in this study and 29 of 40 participants (in whom information was available) correctly guessed treatment assignments (the authors suggest that unblinding was also influenced by the response to treatment). Subsequently, Bornstein *et al* (1991) completed a study of 106 patients with secondary progressive multiple sclerosis who had documented evidence for an increase in disability over the preceding 6–18 months. Treatment had no effect on the proportion of patients showing sustained progression by a further one EDSS point. Apart from local skin reactions at the injection site, Cop-1 was well tolerated.

The result of the above study was presumably influential in the decision to design a phase three trial involving patients with relapsing–remitting multiple sclerosis and using relapse rate as the primary outcome. This involved 251 patients randomized to Cop-1 (20 mg by daily subcutaneous injection for 2 years; n = 125) or placebo (n = 126; K.P. Johnson *et al* 1995). The relapse rate over 2 years in treated patients was 1.2 ± 0.1 compared with 1.7 ± 0.1 in controls (a 29% reduction giving annual rates of 0.6 and 0.8, respectively; p < 0.007: Figure 18.39A). More Cop-1-treated patients were free from relapse, and treatment also favoured a delay in time to relapse. With respect to disability, the proportions of patients taking Cop-1 who were unchanged, improved or worse by 1 EDSS point were 54%, 25% and 21% compared with 56%, 15% and 29%, respectively, in the placebo group (Figure 18.39B). Results of the pivotal North American trial led the FDA to approve Cop-1 for the reduction of exacerbations in patients with relapsing–remitting multiple sclerosis. (As noted above, following FDA approval for licensure the company renamed the agent glatiramer acetate or Copaxone.) A United Kingdom licence for the same indication followed in 2000 and in the rest of the European Union in 2001 (*www.tevapharm/com/copaxone/*). In the United Kingdom, the

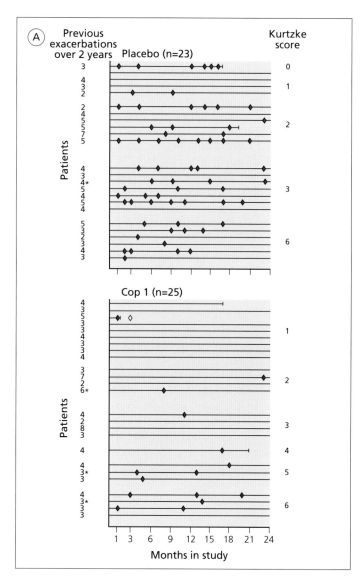

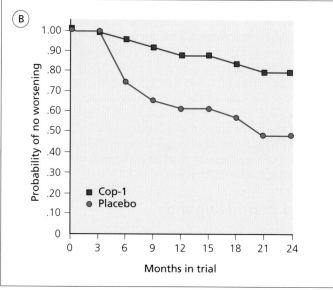

Figure 18.38 Treatment of multiple sclerosis with copolymer-1. (A) Exacerbations occurring during the 2 years of the trial; each line represents a patient and each diamond represents an exacerbation. Patients are grouped according to their EDSS on entry. The number of pretrial exacerbations is indicated to the left. Discontinuous lines represent patients who withdrew before completion. The open diamond indicates an exacerbation occurring after withdrawal which was included as a study event. Patients who were not included in the matched-pair analyses are indicated by an asterisk. (B) Survival curves representing the probability of no worsening from the baseline EDSS; worsening was determined when first observed but was counted only if it continued for 3 months. Adapted from Bornstein *et al* (1987). © 1987, reproduced with permission of the Massachusetts Medical Society.

Association of British Neurologists guidelines on eligibility criteria for glatiramer acetate are:

- ambulant patients with relapsing–remitting multiple sclerosis able to walk at least 100 m without support (EDSS ≤5.5)
- at least two clinically significant relapses in the last 2 years
- age ≥ 18 years.

The pivotal North American glatiramer acetate (or Copaxone, see above) study has been continued. In a blinded extension for up to 11 additional months, there was no loss of effect on relapse rate. Sustained disability was seen in 23% of patients receiving glatiramer acetate compared to 29% of controls (K.P. Johnson *et al* 1998). The European–Canadian glatiramer acetate MRI study was designed to evaluate the effect of treatment on MRI features of disease activity in relapsing–remitting multiple sclerosis (Comi *et al* 2001b). Two hundred and thirty-nine patients with relapsing–remitting multiple sclerosis from 29 centres in seven countries were randomized to receive daily subcutaneous injections of placebo or glatiramer acetate (20 mg). Monthly MRI studies were performed for 9 months.

This study demonstrated that treatment reduced the total number of gadolinium enhancing lesions (overall reduction, 29%; p = 0.003: Figure 18.40) although a large number of enhancing lesions were still seen in treated patients. This effect was first apparent after approximately 6 months of treatment (Figure 18.41). There was no difference, however, in the proportion of patients showing MRI contrast enhancements (although the specific data were not reported). Notably, only three treated patients remained free of contrast enhancing lesions during the 9 month study. T_2 volume continued to worsen in both groups but to a lesser degree in those receiving glatiramer acetate. The change in hypodense lesion volume was not significantly different between groups. Treatment also reduced the number of relapses but not for the first 6 months. A subsequent publication from this prospective study reported that treatment with glatiramer acetate reduced the proportion of the 1722 new contrast enhancing MRI lesions that developed into persisting hypodense T_1 'black holes', at 7 months (p = 0.004) and 8 months (p = 0.0002) after they were first detected in the 239 participants (Filippi *et al* 2001a) but not at the 6 month assessment (Filippi *et al* 2002c; N.D. Richert 2002). These reports suggest

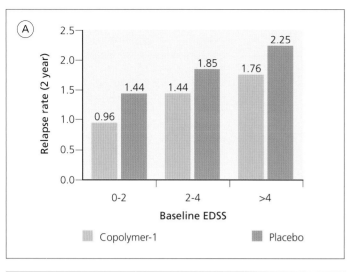

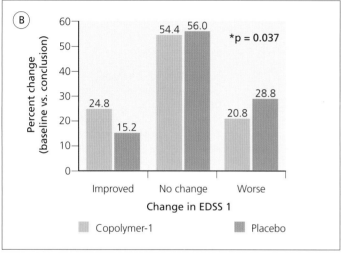

Figure 18.39 Treatment of multiple sclerosis with copolymer-1. (A) Changes in relapse rate observed over 2 years, by baseline EDSS. Numbers above each bar represent the mean 2 year relapse rate for each group. (B) Percentage of patients who improved, were unchanged, or were worse by ≥1 EDSS points between baseline and the last (24 month) measurement (repeated measures ANCOVA). Numbers above each bar represent the percentage of patients in the respective copolymer-1 or placebo group. Adapted from K.P. Johnson *et al* (1995). © 1995, reproduced with permission of Lippincott Williams & Wilkins (lww.com).

that glatiramer acetate has less immediate impact on MRI markers of inflammatory demyelination than IFN-β but may favourably affect the proportion of MRI lesions that develop significant axonal loss.

A 9 month, placebo-controlled trial of glatiramer acetate in 239 pateints with relapsing–remitting multiple sclerosis revealed a mean 0.7–0.8% reduction in central cerebral volume with no significant differences between the patient groups (Rovaris *et al* 2001c). The study showed a weak association between enhancing lesion numbers and atrophy. Rovaris *et al* (2002b) later designed a small, prospective study of glatiramer acetate on the formation of new T_2 lesions and (new and total) contrast-enhancing MRI lesions. This cohort of 20 patients with relapsing–remitting multiple sclerosis underwent monthly MRI

studies during both pretreatment and posttreatment periods of observation (two sessions of monthly scans beginning 5 months before and then restarting 90 days after treatment with daily subcutaneous injections of glatiramer acetate, 20 mg). Patients were given both a standard and triple dose of gadolinium separated by 12–24 hours. Using MRI measures of disease activity based on pretreatment behaviour, the authors concluded that treatment reduced both new T_2 and new and total gadolinium enhancing lesion formation. The benefit was detectable within 4 months of starting therapy. In addition, glatiramer acetate reduced the number of contrast enhancing lesions using all doses of contrast enhancing agent. These observations suggested that, in the context of multiple sclerosis, glatiramer acetate may reduce the number of inflammatory lesions in situations of both mild and severe blood–brain barrier disruption – although this conclusion is necessarily based on an indirect measure of blood–brain barrier integrity.

A large, phase III, randomized, double-blinded, placebo-controlled trial designed to determine whether either of two doses of daily oral glatiramer acetate (5 and 50 mg) were superior to placebo in reducing relapse rate (primary outcome), MRI activity (secondary outcome) or disability (tertiary and other end points) was terminated after an interim analysis at 14 months suggested little likelihood of a positive outcome. The results are not yet published.

The clinical relapse rates of 85 patients with relapsing–remitting multiple sclerosis who switched from IFN-β1a (6 MIU by intramuscular injection for 18–24 months) to glatiramer acetate (20 mg by subcutaneous injection daily) either for reasons of perceived lack of efficacy (62 patients) or persistent intolerance to treatment-related side effects (23 patients) were evaluated by O.A. Khan *et al* (2001b). After a further period of 18–24 months prospective follow-up, the authors concluded that glatiramer acetate administration reduces relapse rate in patients previously not fully responsive to IFN-β. The degree of reduction is no less than in patients who responded but switched because of drug intolerance.

Although this result invites the conclusion that glatiramer acetate can rescue patients who fail on treatment with IFN-β, no definitive studies comparing the relative efficacies of these drugs are available although several trials are in progress. A comparison was made by O.A. Khan *et al* (2001c) of clinical outcomes at 18 months in a group of 156 patients with relapsing–remitting multiple sclerosis followed prospectively. In this open label, non-randomized and unblinded study, patients were permitted to choose no treatment (n = 33) or standard doses of intramuscular IFN-β1a (Avonex; n = 40), subcutaneous IFN-β1b (Betaseron; n=41) or glatiramer acetate (n = 42). At 18 months, 122 patients remained in the study (18/34 drop-outs were from the 'no treatment' group). Annual relapse rates were significantly reduced only by glatiramer acetate (0.49; p = 0.001) and subcutaneous IFN-β1b (0.55; p = 0.001) but not by intramuscular IFN-β1a (0.81) compared with the 'no treatment' group (1.02). Similarly, the percentage of relapse-free patients was significant only for glatiramer acetate and subcutaneous IFN-β1b (33% for both; p = 0.05; intramuscular IFN-β1a, 12%; no treatment, 7%). Mean change in EDSS also favoured these two treatment groups (IFN-β1b: –0.25, p = 0.010; glatiramer acetate: –0.44, p = 0.003; IFN-β1a +0.19, p = 0.452 compared with untreated patients: +0.60).

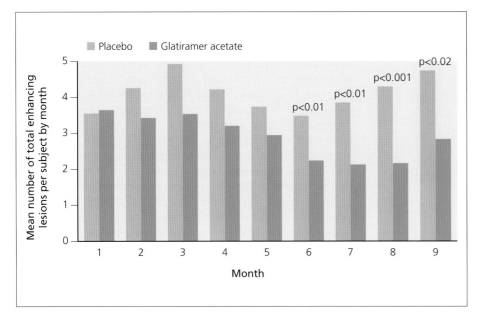

Figure 18.40 European/Canadian trial of glatiramer acetate in relapsing–remitting multiple sclerosis. Median number of total enhancing lesions per subject observed at each month on study using the last observation carried forward. Repeated measures analysis favoured a treatment effect for glatiramer acetate (p = 0.003). Adapted from Comi *et al* (2001b). © 2001, reproduced with permission of John Wiley & Sons.

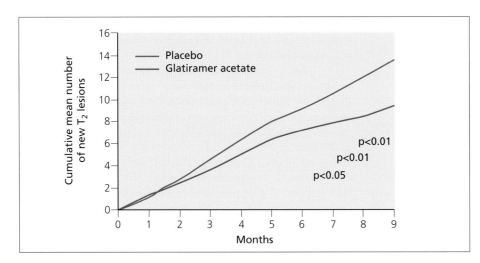

Figure 18.41 European/Canadian trial of glatiramer acetate in relapsing–remitting multiple sclerosis. Cumulative mean number of new lesions observed on the T_2-weighted images at each month on study. Statistically significant differences first emerged after 5 months on treatment. Adapted from Comi *et al* (2001b). © 2001, reproduced with permission of John Wiley & Sons.

The impact of this study is clearly reduced by the design, but nevertheless it provides some evidence that, in practice, glatiramer acetate may have similar efficacy to IFN-β1b, and both are superior to IFN-β1a. A large, National Institutes of Health funded, phase three trial comparing IFN-β1a by once weekly subcutaneous injection (Avonex) and glatiramer acetate (Copaxone) given either alone or in combination (four treatment arms) to patients with relapsing–remitting multiple sclerosis is in progress in the United States (Fred Lublin, personal communication) An open label prospective study of modest size is already reassuring with respect to safety issues (Lublin *et al* 2001; 2002). Clearly, these turf wars are not yet settled.

Munari *et al* (2004; 2004b) completed a systematic review of glatiramer acetate and concluded that there is no conclusive evidence that this agent alters relapse or progression rate in patients with multiple sclerosis. The interested reader is referred to correspondence rebutting and supporting the methodological assumptions that led to this conclusion (Caramanos and Arnold 2005; Comi *et al* 2005; deJong *et al* 2005; Munari and Filippini 2005).

PROMISE was a massive, randomized, double-blind, placebo-controlled phase three study involving 943 primary progressive patients randomized in a 2:1 ratio either to receive glatiramer acetate or placebo. It was recently terminated after an interim analysis suggested futility (Wolinsky *et al* 2004). There were no safety concerns and doubtless post-hoc analyses will add greatly to our understanding of the nuances of testing therapies in this disease category. PROMISE was not fulfilled.

Adverse effects

Glatiramer acetate is generally well tolerated. It is usually possible to initiate treatment at full strength (20 mg by subcutaneous daily injection) without dose titration. Although a daily subcutaneous injection is required, rarely do patients discontinue this drug because of intolerance. In the early reports (Bornstein *et al* 1982; 1987) and pivotal North American trial (K.P. Johnson *et al* 1995; 1998), there is comment on an unpredictable, sometimes frightening but transient and usually self-limiting systemic reaction (facial flushing, chest tightness, anxiety, palpitations and dyspnoea) lasting for around 30 minutes immediately after an injection. This is experienced by up to 15% of patients (but not recurring in 50%) with an estimated frequency of one episode per 840 injections (K.P. Johnson *et al* 1998). It is important to warn patients but, although alarming, it is seemingly an innocent adverse effect. Approximately two-thirds of patients notice pain at the injection site. Local irritation may occur in 2–3% (K.P. Johnson *et al* 2000) but skin breakdown is very rare (Johnson *et al* 1998). Focal atrophy of subcutaneous tissue at injection sites and adjacent lymphadenopathy may develop (Windhagen *et al* 2001). Glatiramer acetate is not associated with laboratory abnormalities and routine blood studies are not needed to monitor its safety. There are no important drug interactions.

Treated patients may develop antibodies to glatiramer acetate. However, unlike the situation with neutralizing antibodies to IFN-β, experimental and clinical evidence does not suggest that these anti glatiramer acetate antibodies reduce biological function (Teitelbaum *et al* 2003). This has been shown in assays that measure binding to MHC molecules, T-cell stimulation, interference of competition between glatiramer acetate and myelin basic protein peptide, cytokine production by glatiramer acetate-specific T-cell clones and *in vivo* inhibition of experimental autoimmune encephalomyelitis (Aharoni *et al* 1998; T. Brenner *et al* 2001; C. Farina *et al* 2002; Teitelbaum *et al* 1973; 1991; 2003).

Mechanism of action

As for IFN-β, the precise mechanism(s) whereby glatiramer acetate influences the course of multiple sclerosis continues to be discussed (Dhib-Jalbut 2002; Neuhaus *et al* 2001; Yong 2002). Table 18.8 and Figures 18.42 and 18.43 itemize many of the key findings and provide references to the supporting literature. As discussed earlier, interferon administration is generally followed within weeks by a striking reduction in MRI evidence of blood–brain barrier disruption. This effect is much less dramatic following the administration of glatiramer acetate although MRI activity reduces gradually over a period of several months (see above, Comi *et al* 2001b). This may be explained by the finding that glatiramer acetate does not significantly inhibit T-cell migration (Dufour *et al* 2000; Prat *et al* 1999).

Each drug influences T-cell function (especially CD4 cells) in ways that both overlap and are distinctive. Each agent blocks T-cell activation and promotes Th2 (IL-4, IL-5, IL-10, IL-13 and TGF-β) cytokine production. Unlike IFN-β, however, glatiramer acetate induces the production of regulatory T cells in the periphery. These glatiramer acetate reactive cells cross the blood–brain barrier, respond to central nervous system myelin antigens by secreting Th2 (M. Chen *et al* 2001; Y. Qin *et al* 2000) and Th3 cytokines (Aharoni *et al* 2003) that inhibit Th1 cells, thereby effecting so-called 'bystander suppression'. Glatiramer acetate-reactive cells may also induce anergy (Gran *et al* 2000b).

Recently, abundant evidence has accumulated that glatiramer acetate-specific cells secrete brain-derived growth factors (Aharoni *et al* 2003; Kappos and Duda 2002; Ziemssen *et al* 2002) raising the intriguing possibility that this agent may enhance repair at the site of the multiple sclerosis lesion by inducing a degree of localized 'neuroprotective autoimmunity'.

Table 18.8 Presumed mechanisms of action of glatiramer acetate (adapted from J. Zhang *et al* 2002 with permission)

Modulates T-cell activation and/or proliferation
  Competes for binding sites of MHC class II antigens (MBP, PLP, MOG: Ben-Nun *et al* 1996; Fridkis-Hareli *et al* 1994; Fridkis-Hareli and Strominger 1998; Racke *et al* 1992; Teitelbaum *et al* 1996; 2003)
  May modify dendritic cell costimulation processes (Hussien *et al* 2001) or act as weak/partial T-cell receptor agonist (Wiesemann *et al* 2001)
  Reduces proliferation of MBP-reactive T cells (Duda *et al* 2000; Karandikar *et al* 2002; Neuhaus *et al* 2000)
  Actives both Th1 and Th2 cells (Zang *et al* 2003)

Increases ratio of anti-inflammatory (Th2) to proinflammatory (Th1) cytokines
  Increases IL-10, IL-4, and IL-6 production (C. Farina *et al* 2001; Hussien *et al* 2001; Neuhaus *et al* 2001a) and decreases IL-12 production (Hussien *et al* 2001)
  Increases and then decreases IFN γ secretion with repeated antigen stimulation (Aharoni *et al* 1997)
  Upregulates CD8+ T-cell responses (Karandikar *et al* 2002)
  Induce regulatory Th2/3 cells that penetrate the central nervous system and express their anti-inflammatory cytokines and neurotrophic factors *in situ* in animal models of multiple sclerosis (Aharoni *et al* 2003)

Induces TNF-α and IFN-γ production (C. Farina *et al* 2001; Neuhaus *et al* 2000; Zang *et al* 2003)
Enhances production of brain-derived nerve growth factor (Ziemssen *et al* 2002)
Reduces monocyte (Weber *et al* 2004) and antigen-presenting cell function (S. Jung *et al* 2004; H.J. Kim *et al* 2004)

MHC = major histocompatibility complex; IL = interleukin; ; TNF = tumour necrosis factor; MBP = myelin basic protein; PLP = proteolipid protein; MOG = myelin oligodendrocyte glycoprotein; Th = T-helper cell.

The idea that inflammation may enhance remyelination has attracted great interest in the experimental literature (Kipnis *et al* 2000; M. Rodriguez and Lennon 1990; Schori *et al* 2001; Schwartz 2001; Schwartz *et al* 1999; Schwartz and Kipnis 2001) and is discussed more fully in Chapter 10. Recently, M.S. Weber *et al* (2004) have reported that glatiramer acetate blocks monocyte reactivity *in vitro* using cells from treated patients. Both S. Jung *et al* (2004) and H.J. Kim *et al* (2004) have shown that glatiramer acetate also reduces the function of antigen-presenting cells. Together, these studies demonstrate that the mechanisms of action of glatiramer acetate extend well beyond the lymphocyte population of immune cells.

An enzyme-linked immunoadsorbent spot (ELISPOT) assay was developed by C. Farina *et al* (2002) that may correlate 'responder' status to glatiramer acetate. They created three immunological criteria (reduced proliferative response to glatiramer acetate, *in vitro* activation of IFN-γ-producing cells, and activation of IL-4-producing cells) and found that 13 of 15 clinical responders (87%) met two or all three criteria, compared with 22% of patients who appeared to be failing treatment. If correct, this assay may ultimately find more widespread use and lead to the development of other *in vitro* measures to inform treatment decisions.

Antibodies to glatiramer acetate develop within 3 months and may later diminish (T. Brenner *et al* 2001; C. Farina *et al* 2002).

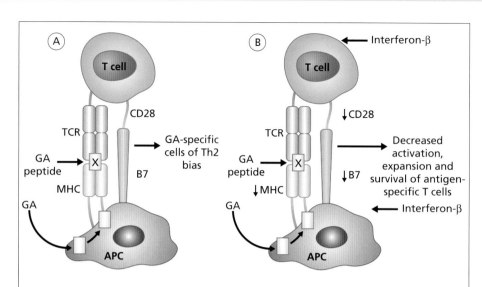

Figure 18.42 Mechanisms of action of glatiramer acetate (GA) and beta-interferons on antigen presentation. (A) The high affinity of GA for the MHC groove or the uptake of GA by an antigen-presenting cell leads to the presentation of GA as an antigen and the generation of GA-specific Th2-biased cells. (B) IFN-β acts on its receptor on T cells and antigen-presenting cells. This decreases the expression of molecules needed for antigen presentation. Together with a further activity of interferon on T-cell expansion and survival, this leads to the decreased generation of antigen-specific T cells. X refers to an antigen-siting in the MHC groove; TCR = T-cell receptor. Adapted from Yong (2002). © 2002, reproduced with permission of Lippincott Williams & Wilkins (lww.com).

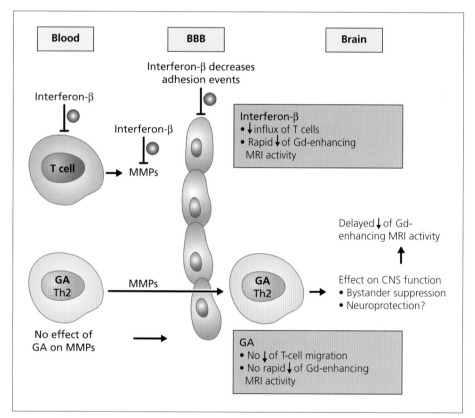

Figure 18.43 Effects of glatiramer acetate (GA) and IFN-β on the blood–brain barrier (BBB) and within the central nervous system. IFN-β reduces the production of matrix metalloproteinases (MMP) by T cells and diminishes the adhesion of T cells to endothelium. These two effects reduce the influx of T cells into the central nervous system. GA-specific Th2 cells traffic into the central nervous system to produce local bystander immune suppression and possibly exert neuroprotection. Gd = gadolinium. Adapted from Yong (2002). © 2002, reproduced with permission of Lippincott Williams & Wilkins (lww.com).

There is great interest in whether these antibodies reduce the clinical benefit of glatiramer acetate (see the discussion of the possible influence of neutralizing antibodies on clinical effects of the interferons). In a large series of *in vitro* and *in vivo* experiments, Teitelbaum *et al* (2003) reported that these antibodies do not seem to reduce activity. A subsequent study, however, reported that antibodies to glatiramer acetate reversed many of these putative activities, including the effect on T-cell proliferation and both pro- and anti-inflammatory cytokines (Salama *et al* 2003). More work is therefore needed to clarify these ambiguities.

Early work of great interest suggests that antibodies to glatiramer acetate induce remyelination in the Theiler's virus animal model of demyelinating disease (Ure and Rodriguez 2002). This finding parallels the observation that immunoglobulins directed against central nervous system antigens also induce abundant remyelination in this animal model (Bieber *et al* 2003; Ciric *et al* 2003; 2004; Mitsunaga *et al* 2002; M. Rodriguez and Lennon 1990) and raises the possibility that anti-glatiramer acetate antibodies may enhance repair of the lesion in multiple sclerosis.

In what ways might these two agents complement their mechanisms of action? Zang *et al* (2003a) showed that, when tested together *in vitro*, IFN-β1a and glatiramer acetate act to antagonize their respective modes of action. Specifically, IFN-β1a blocked glatiramer acetate-induced T-cell proliferation and the drug-specific pattern of cytokine production was lost. Glatiramer acetate induced both Th1 (TNF-α and IFN-γ) and Th2 (IL-4 and IL-10) cytokines. Conversely, IFN-β inhibited Th1 cytokine production. Together, IFN-β reduced the number of IFN-γ-producing cells compared to glatiramer acetate alone – suggesting another type of antagonism between these two agents. Firm conclusions on the practical and immunological aspects of combination therapy seem premature.

The licence for Copaxone

In the United States, information distributed by the pharmaceutical company that markets glatiramer acetate states that this agent is

> *recommended for reduction of the frequency of relapses in patients with relapsing remitting multiple sclerosis. It is contraindicated in patients with known hypersensitivity to glatiramer acetate or mannitol and is not recommended for use in pregnancy. The safety and efficacy of glatiramer acetate is unknown in nursing women, in those with impaired renal function, in patients <18 years old, and in the elderly.*

Copaxone was approved for marketing in the United Kingdom and launched in December 2000 with the same general indications. This first approval in a major European market led to extension throughout the European Union by the end of 2001 under the European Mutual Recognition Procedure with the United Kingdom acting as reference member state.

TREATMENTS THAT TARGET T CELLS

In view of the conditional benefits of immune suppression in the treatment of patients with multiple sclerosis, attention has turned to alternative means of interfering with the sequence of events that leads to tissue injury. The theoretical basis for designing therapies, the experimental evidence that they might work, such clinical evidence as there is for efficacy, and the reasons why theory does not always translate into clinical success were admirably reviewed by R. Hohlfeld (1997). These approaches include:

- the use of monoclonal antibodies that achieve much more precise immunological effects than nonspecific immunosuppressants
- reagents which block recognition between antigen-presenting cells and responder lymphocytes
- depletion of autoreactive lymphocyte populations by T-cell vaccination
- bone marrow transplantation.

The validity of these approaches has yet to be confirmed and most are conditional on whether the central hypothesis for the role of T cells in the pathogenesis of inflammatory demyelination is correct. Most of these therapies target circulating white blood cells, in particular lymphocytes, and so qualify as potential disease-modifying treatments in multiple sclerosis. We retain a brief discussion of the earlier studies as background to the current interest in this strategy.

Anti-lymphocyte globulin

The first trial, assessing treatments designed to target circulating lymphocytes and adopting a double-blind and placebo-controlled protocol, was reported in 1982. Inevitably it was underpowered. Forty-three patients with relapsing–remitting multiple sclerosis were randomized to treatment with anti-lymphocyte globulin, azathioprine and prednisolone in combination for 1 month, followed by azathioprine (3 mg/kg) alone for a further 14 months, or placebo preparations. The reduction in relapse rate from 1.0 to 0.7 in the treated group, time to first episode and accumulation of disability all favoured an effect of treatment but the magnitude of these results did not impress the investigators, who reported their findings as offering no more than an indication for continuing to evaluate immunosuppression in the context of multiple sclerosis (Mertin *et al* 1982).

Total lymphoid irradiation

Cook *et al* (1986) first compared total lymphoid irradiation given over 5 weeks with sham irradiation in a group of 45 patients with secondary progressive multiple sclerosis. They reported a beneficial effect on time to further sustained progression, especially over the first 12 months of the study. This clinical response was anticipated by a reduction in absolute lymphocyte count to <850/mm^3 and only these patients showed lower functional impairment scores for up to 4 years after the start of treatment. Wiles *et al* (1994) studied 27 patients (the plan was to study 56 but recruitment proved difficult) randomized to active or sham irradiation with 1980 cGy to the lymphoid system and spleen. There was no difference between groups in the clinical course over 2 years, other than a small improvement in bladder function. However, MRI activity was reduced. Three patients died – two, sham-treated, from respiratory complications of multiple sclerosis, and one, who received total lymphoid irradiation, from cardiac failure. Although these fatalities were not related to lymphoid irradiation, the treated group experienced more adverse effects than controls. Subsequently, Cook *et al* (1995) claimed that the concomitant use of corticosteroids further improved the effects of total lymphoid irradiation, and that this additional benefit correlated with the emergence of T cells having the CD$^+$/CD3$^-$ or CD8$^+$/CD3$^-$ phenotype. Mortality after total lymphoid irradiation was 1% compared with 14% in the sham-treated group. With EDSS scores at entry of >6.5, these were moderately severely affected patients at the outset.

Monoclonal antibodies

With developments in therapeutic immunology came the opportunity to design small molecules and monoclonal antibodies targeting one component only of the immune system, and leaving the rest intact. In theory, chimaerization and humanization reduce the immunogenicity of therapeutic antibodies and allow courses of reagents having prolonged effects to be given repeatedly (Winter and Milstein 1991). A single pulse of treatment can induce prolonged alteration in immunological behaviour long after the targeted immune population has been reconstituted (S. Qin *et al* 1993). Anti-CD6 (Hafler *et al* 1986), anti-CD2 (Hafler *et al* 1988), anti-CD3 (Weinshenker *et al* 1991b), anti-CD4 (Lindsey *et al* 1994a; 1994b; van Oosten *et al* 1997; Racadot *et al* 1993) and anti-CD52 (Moreau *et al* 1994; 1996) antibodies have all been administered to patients with multiple sclerosis. In some instances, anti-globulin responses and acute adverse effects limited the usefulness of these potential treatments and an additional problem has been modulation of the targeted lymphocyte antigen, allowing some cells to survive.

Anti-CD6

Using a murine antibody which recognizes the T12 antigen (CD6) present on most (post-thymic) T lymphocytes (but neither chimaeric nor humanized), together with corticosteroids, Hafler *et al* (1986) reported clinical stabilization in six of 12 patients with secondary progressive multiple sclerosis (severe enough to require the recent use of a wheelchair in two cases) at 6 months in an open uncontrolled study. This effect was maintained for a further 3 months in three of these responders. Human anti-mouse antibodies developed within 7 days in seven of nine patients in whom assays were performed. Recovery of circulating T12 cells was rapid and there was evidence *in vitro* for antigen modulation. Studies of cerebrospinal fluid did not suggest that antibody had entered the central nervous system.

Anti-CD3

Weinshenker *et al* (1991c) treated 16 patients, selected for recent rapid accumulation of disability or a high relapse rate, with 50 mg of an anti-CD3 monoclonal antibody (OKT3) over 10 days. Each received corticosteroids and non-steroidal anti-inflammatory drugs. One patient developed anaphylaxis within minutes of receiving the first dose of OKT3 and did not continue in the protocol. A variety of systemic symptoms occurred in all patients despite prophylactic measures (typical symptoms included hypotension, fever, nausea, vomiting, diarrhoea and skin rash). Six out of 16 deteriorated during the course of treatment but this alteration was transient in three. Two patients died from complications of severe multiple sclerosis between 9 and 12 months after enrolling in this trial. Overall, the authors were uncertain that the treatment provided any lasting benefit to this group of patients. At the 1 year follow-up examination, of the 15 patients who completed the treatment protocol, four had worsened by ≥ 1.0 EDSS points (including the two deaths), nine were unchanged (EDSS changed by ≤ 0.5 points) and two improved by ≥ 1.0 EDSS point. No conclusions could be reached in the three patients with relapses of whom one each improved, remained stable and deteriorated. A small number of serial MRI scans failed to show an effect on lesion load. Rapid but transient reductions in circulating lymphocytes and their subpopulations were observed. All patients developed high titres of human anti-mouse antibodies. The systemic manifestations of OKT3 administration are known to be cytokine mediated, to correlate with sequential release of circulating TNF-α and IFN-γ followed by IL-6, and to be suppressed with methylprednisolone (Pececs *et al* 1993). Each of the two patients

studied by Weinshenker *et al* (1991c) showed a transient surge in circulating TNF-α and IFN-γ on the first day of treatment. Therapy was complicated by oral candidiasis, and two patients were thought on clinical grounds to have aseptic meningitis. Whilst not promoting the continued use of murine monoclonals in multiple sclerosis, Weinshenker *et al* (1991c) advocated the development of more specific and less toxic reagents, manipulated to restrict their immunogenicity.

Anti-CD4

The first reported study using murine anti-CD4 monoclonal antibody therapy in multiple sclerosis (Racadot *et al* 1993) included 21 patients with disease progression or frequent relapse and showed no acute effects (good or bad). Clinical stabilization was claimed for 12 of 20 patients at 3 months and eight of the 20 at 6 months. No new relapses were documented. The reductions in circulating lymphocytes had returned to normal ranges within 90 days. A transient elevation was observed in circulating TNF-α, soluble TNF receptor and IL-6 but not IFN-γ, IL-1 or soluble CD8 and CD4 antigen. Unlike most other investigators, Racadot *et al* (1993) reported a detectable rise in cerebrospinal fluid TNF-α levels.

Lindsey *et al* (1994a) treated 29 patients in an open uncontrolled study with a chimaeric anti-CD4 antibody in doses ranging from 10 to 200 mg given as a single infusion, or over 3 days. The reduction in total circulating lymphocytes was partial and recovered within 6 months. The same pattern was observed for CD4 cells but without complete return to the normal range. Five patients developed anti-murine antibodies. Small improvements were noted in three of 26 patients undergoing clinical evaluation, but the majority remained unchanged (16 patients) or deteriorated (seven patients). Fourteen of 25 patients in whom serial scans were obtained had enhancing lesions on baseline MRI. One hundred enhancing lesions were seen on 91 scans obtained during follow-up, and 17 of 25 patients showed an increase in T$_2$-weighted lesions. The patients reported minor systemic symptoms and there was an increase in infections requiring treatment.

Most of these patients were subsequently considered for re-treatment on the basis that their CD4 count returned to >300 cells/mm^3 (Lindsey *et al* 1994b). Several were withdrawn or elected not to continue and one died suddenly after aspiration whilst eating. Twenty-one of the original cohort received up to three further treatments (a total of 36 courses were administered), responding with a drop in CD4 count on each occasion and sometimes showing prolonged lymphopenia. There seemed to be no increase in the development of anti-idiotype antibodies with this second exposure. One patient improved, three worsened, 16 remained unchanged and one was lost to follow-up. MRI activity was seen on ten of 16 scans before treatment and on 12 of 26 scans (from 16 patients) at follow-up (six of 17 in the subgroup with persistently low CD4 counts). Other than minor infections, some requiring treatment, and one episode of herpes zoster, there were few complications of repeated treatment. On the basis of these preliminary results, van Oosten *et al* (1997) randomized 71 patients, most with clinical and radiological evidence for disease activity, to treatment with chimaeric anti-CD4 or placebo under double-blind conditions.

Although circulating CD4 counts were reduced, both groups showed persistent radiological activity (at around 1.5 new lesions per patient per month) although the number of clinical exacerbations was lower, by 41%, in the treated than placebo group. A mild cytokine release syndrome was apparent in these patients leading to withdrawal from the study in a few instances. Serial immunological observations in a subgroup of participants showed, as expected, reduced numbers of CD4$^+$ naive memory cells (which persisted for 12 months after treatment) but there was no effect on serum levels or on mitogen-stimulated release of TNF-α (Llewellyn-Smith et al 1997). These blood markers did not correlate with MRI activity.

Natalizumab (anti-VLA4)

Lymphocytes and monocytes express α$_4$β$_1$ integrin on their cell surface. This glycoprotein binds the endothelial VCAM-1 and thereby mediates cell adhesion and transendothelial migration. Natalizumab (initially marketed as Antegren, Elan Pharmaceuticals and Biogen) is a humanized monoclonal antibody that blocks the α$_4$ integrin adhesion molecule and so reduces cell migration across the blood–brain barrier. Since serial gadolinium-DTPA enhanced MRI scans indicate breakdown of the blood–brain barrier as a consistent feature of new lesions (Kermode et al 1990), these properties suggested a potential therapeutic role during the active inflammatory stage of active multiple sclerosis. Data from the experimental autoimmune encephalomyelitis model of multiple sclerosis (Engelhardt et al 1998; van der Laan et al 2002) indicated that adhesion molecule inhibition might have therapeutic effects in inflammatory brain disease independent of the effect on cell migration. Natalizumab administration reduced new MRI activity in a placebo-controlled pilot study where two intravenous doses were given 1 month apart (Tubridy et al 1999; and see Schwid and Noseworthy 1999).

Against this background, D.H. Miller *et al* (2003a) reported a phase two randomized, double-blind, placebo-controlled study comparing two doses of natalizumab (3 and 6 mg/kg) administered intravenously once monthly for 6 months in 213 patients with relapsing–remitting multiple sclerosis. Both doses favourably influenced the primary end point (number of new MR lesions as determined by monthly scanning). Significantly fewer patients reported clinical relapses in the active treatment arms at 6 months (relapse-free: placebo, 62%; both active groups, 81%; p = 0.02: Figure 18.44). However, the apparent benefit of these treatments was not prolonged beyond the period of treatment. During the subsequent 6 months of follow-up, during which patients were untreated, those previously randomized both to the placebo and natalizumab groups, had essentially identical numbers of relapses and amounts of MRI activity. Treatment was well tolerated although there were a few allergic responses (including one episode of anaphylaxis causing bronchospasm and urticaria that responded quickly to emergency treatment with antihistamines), and perhaps a minor trend suggesting increased risk of infection (pharyngitis) in treated subjects. In a follow-up report, Dalton *et al* (2004b) demonstrated that gadolinium enhancing MRI lesions developing in the natalizumab-treated patients were less likely to develop into T$_1$ hypointense lesions (T$_1$ black holes) at 1 year than those present in the placebo patients. This report suggests that even a relatively limited period of treatment with this agent might have a degree of prolonged benefit on MRI behaviour. The clinical relevance of this finding remains to be determined.

These encouraging early findings led to further evaluation in two large phase III trials. Nine hundred and forty-two patients with relapsing–remitting multiple sclerosis, who had not received any other drug treatment for at least 6 months, were randomized to treatment with either natalizumab (300 mg) or placebo intravenously every 4 weeks for 28 months. A second placebo-controlled trial was designed to determine whether

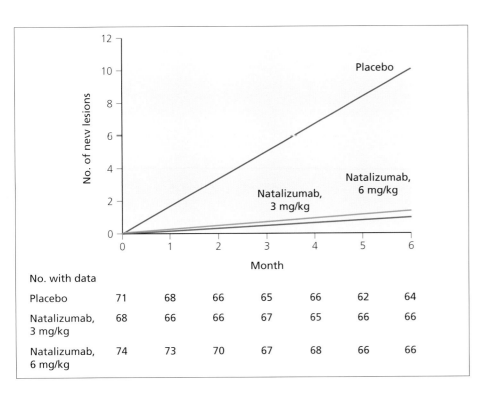

Figure 18.44 Treatment of relapsing–remitting multiple sclerosis with intravenous natalizumab (a humanized monoclonal antibody against anti-α$_4$ integrin) at 3 mg/kg (blue line) and 6 mg/kg (green line). Cumulative mean number of new gadolinium-enhancing lesions on MRI while on treatment. However, in the subsequent 6 months, upon discontinuing treatment, the patients originally treated with the active antibody had equal numbers of relapses and MRI markers of disease activity to those originally randomized to placebo. Adapted from D.H. Miller *et al* (2003a). © 2003, reproduced with permission of the Massachusetts Medical Society.

No. with data							
Placebo	71	68	66	65	66	62	64
Natalizumab, 3 mg/kg	68	66	66	67	65	66	66
Natalizumab, 6 mg/kg	74	73	70	67	68	66	66

prolonged administration of natalizumab provides additional benefit to weekly IFN-β1a in 1171 individuals who have already experienced at least one episode whilst on IFN-β1a. Preliminary data on safety, immunogenicity, pharmacokinetics and pharmacodynamics indicated that there were no unfavourable interactions between these therapeutic agents (Vollmer *et al* 2004a). In a similar but smaller trial, investigators randomized 110 patients treated with glatiramer acetate to monthly doses either of natalizumab or placebo for a period of 6 months.

Preliminary results of the first two studies described above, after patients had received treatment for a median duration of 13 months, led the Food and Drug Administration (*http://www.fda.gov/*) to license natalizumab (Tysabri) 300 mg by intravenous infusion every 4 weeks, late in 2004 for the 'reduction of clinical exacerbations in patients with relapsing forms of multiple sclerosis'. The advice on use in pregnancy is ambiguous ('only if clearly needed'); administration to individuals aged under 18 years is contraindicated; advice on the upper age limit is noncommittal. Although experience beyond 13 months was limited at that time, the only adverse effects of note were headache, arthralgia, infections and hypersensitivity reactions but these were infrequent and rarely limiting. In study 1, the annualized relapse rate was 0.25 in individuals receiving natalizumab compared to 0.74 in the placebo group; the percentages of patients remaining relapse free were 76% and 53%, respectively. In study 2, annualized relapse rate was 0.36 in patients receiving natalizumab compared to 0.78 (the same as placebo-treated cases from study 1) in those only being treated with IFN-β1a; the percentages of patients remaining relapse free were 67% and 46%, respectively – even less than the placebo rate for these individuals receiving IFN-β1a. As expected, the clinical results were matched by comparable reductions in disease activity using imaging surrogates. Again, there was no difference in the proportion or number of cases showing activity comparing the placebo group of study 1 and the IFN-β1a-only group of study 2 but this may reflect differences in the study populations. About 6% of patients developed a persistent antibody response to natalizumab that was associated with an apparent loss of clinical effectiveness. Clearly, these data do not provide support that IFN-β1a is effective in reducing clinical or MRI evidence of disease activity in patients who continue to report clinical relapses while receiving this agent.

The patients involved in the 2 year placebo-controlled trials are being followed in an extension study while on natalizumab; in order to obtain long-term data on effectiveness, tolerability and safety in addition to immunogenicity. The intention was to follow what happens to these patients in the 6–12 months after infusions cease, so as to determine whether this more prolonged antibody administration proves more durable against clinical and MRI indicators of disease activity than the results reported to date.

On 28th February 2005 the sponsors of Tysabri (Biogen Idec and Elan Pharmaceuticals) voluntarily removed this agent from clinical and research trial use because progressive multifocal leukoencephalopathy was reported in two patients treated with the combination of Tysabri and IFN-β1a (Avonex) for more than 2 years. A third case was soon reported in a patient treated with Tysabri for Crohn's disease (eight doses over a period of 18 months), again in the context of a randomized trial; the patient died from what initially was thought to have been a fatal glioma and later confirmed to be progressive multifocal leukoencephalopathy. This patient had been refractory to corticosteroids, azathioprine and other immunosuppressants – perhaps contributing to the risk of additional immunosuppression with this experimental agent. Two additional unconfirmed cases have been subsequently reported in the context of clinical trials for multiple sclerosis but, at the time of writing, the details are scarce. Tysabri-treated patients from these trials are now under close scrutiny to detect progressive multifocal leukoencephalopathy as early as possible and investigators are reviewing the available data to understand the mechanism(s) of presumed reactivation of the JC virus in this setting. As highlighted earlier, these events remind us of the potential risks inherent in clinical trials (Drazen 2005). It remains uncertain that this once-approved therapeutic agent will resurface for use in multiple sclerosis and other inflammatory disorders.

In late spring, 2006, an FDA advisory committee completed their review of all available clinical and laboratory data on the association of PML with exposure to natalizumab. Finding no additional cases, this committee recommended that natalizumab be made available as a monotherapy to adult relapsing-remitting patients (e.g., without concomitant corticosteroids, beta-interferon or other immunomodulating agents). The FDA has delayed its decision pending their review of a risk management plan that is being designed to both limit the likelihood of patients developing PML and to optimize early detection of future cases. A decison is expected in early summer, 2006.

Anti-Vβ5.2/5.3+ T cells

In a study designed to determine whether administration of the humanized monoclonal antibody ATM-027 (with specificity for Vβ5.2/5.3+ T cells) would reduce MRI measures of disease activity, Killestein *et al* (2002b) stratified relapsing–remitting patients by HLA-DR2 status to receive monthly intravenous infusions either of the antibody (n = 47) or placebo (n = 12). The dose was titrated to deplete the target T cells. Treatment successfully suppressed the Vβ5.2/5.3+ T-cell population and was well tolerated. There was a trend suggesting a reduction in MRI activity (lesion count, volume of enhancing lesions) but this result did not achieve the goal of the study.

Anti-CD52

Campath-1H may emerge as an important treatment for multiple sclerosis. From the clinical science perspective, its credentials are already established. Clinical observations provided the stimulus for basic research that has illuminated key aspects of the pathogenesis (Coles *et al* 1999a; Moreau *et al* 1996; Redford *et al* 1997; K.J. Smith *et al* 2001; Wilkins *et al* 2003). In turn, these are now being recycled into clinical practice and with provisionally encouraging results. Campath-1H is a humanized monoclonal antibody suitable for therapeutic use that targets the CD52 antigen present on all lymphocytes and a proportion of monocytes. As a result of its isotype, Campath-1H is exceptionally good at activating complement and mediating antibody-dependent cell-mediated cytotoxicity (M.Q. Xia *et al* 1993). CD52 does not lose its potential for lysis through modulation by antibody. Lymphopenia is rapid and prolonged following a pulse of treatment since the CD52 antigen is expressed in high density on the target cell membrane (Hale *et al* 1990). The median times to recovery of baseline counts for CD3, CD4, CD8 and total lymphocytes are 51, 61, 30 and 66 months, respectively. Conversely, B-cell numbers return more rapidly and tend to overshoot above baseline but rarely rise above the upper limit of the normal range. Although a single treatment does not elicit an anti-globulin response, this may not be the case if repeated courses of antibody are given. Campath-1H has been studied in three cohorts of patients with multiple sclerosis treated on an open label basis.

The change in MRI evidence for disease activity following treatment with Campath-1H established that a reduction in the availability of circulating lymphocytes is associated with a more or less complete cessation in new lesion formation and prompted the further evaluation of Campath-1H as a possible disease-modifying treatment (Moreau *et al* 1994). A second cohort of 36 patients with secondary progressive multiple sclerosis (duration of the progressive phase, 3.6 + 2.6 years; mean EDSS 5.8 ± 0.8; increase in disability in the year before treatment, ≥ 1 EDSS point; annual relapse rate, 0.7 per patient per year) confirmed that radiological evidence for disease activity was suppressed by >90% for at least 18 months (Coles *et al* 1999a; Paollilo *et al* 1999). Relapse rate, expected to decline as part of the natural history of multiple sclerosis in the secondary progressive phase, changed from 0.7 per patient per year before treatment to an annualized rate of 0.02 per patient per year at mean follow-up of 6.7 (SD ± 2.1) years. When 13 patients from this original cohort were re-examined 5.8 years (± 0.5) after their last scan (which was itself 18 months after Campath-1H), there was no evidence for an increase in proton density or T_1 lesion volume in the intervening period.

However, dissociation emerged between this suppression of inflammation and disease progression. Disability increased by +0.2 EDSS points per patient per year. Although this represents a statistically significant reduction in rate of progression compared to the year before treatment (p < 0.001), the toll of incremental progression over time has led to substantial accumulation of disability with no overall benefit from treatment (Figure 18.45). Disease progression was associated with brain atrophy. Patients who progressed from baseline at the first follow-up interval (18 months) showed reduced brain volume at the time of treatment with Campath-1H by comparison with patients showing initial stability of clinical progression. Those who progressed early had most inflammatory activity prior to treatment. Furthermore, despite continued suppression of cerebral inflammatory activity, this poor prognosis group with atrophy at the time of treatment and early disease progression demonstrated sustained reduction in brain volume and altered MR spectroscopy (*N*-methyl-aspartate) indicating progressive axonal loss. After 7.5 years, mean percentage change in cerebral volume was –0.48% (± 0.46) per year. The mean absolute change was –1.37 (± 1.28) mL/year (p = 0.002). Two patients in this group had measurable cerebral atrophy despite clinical stability. Early loss of brain volume was an indicator of sustained atrophy. The six of 13 patients who had already shown increased cerebral atrophy at 18 months after Campath-1H had a mean further loss of 2.13 mL per year (± 0.65), compared to only 0.7 (± 1.4) mL per year in those whose cerebral volume was stable for the initial 18 months after treatment (p = 0.042). The lesson is clear. Once the cascade of events leading to tissue injury is established, effective suppression of inflammation does not limit brain atrophy or protect from clinical progression.

Against this background, a third cohort consisted of 22 patients with active relapsing–remitting multiple sclerosis, a short clinical history and no disease progression (Coles *et al* 2005). As a group, they had experienced a total of 133 relapses over 60 patient-years of combined disease history before treatment, giving an annual relapse rate of 2.2 per patient. This rose to 2.94 per patient in the year before Campath-1H. The cohort included 17 drug naive patients and five who had already failed treatment with IFN-β. After treatment this cohort has had five investigator-confirmed episodes, giving a relapse rate of 0.14, and representing a 94% reduction in relapse rate (Figure 18.46). By comparison with many of the pretreatment episodes, all but one was clinically mild with full spontaneous recovery and leaving no stepwise increase in EDSS.

It is instructive to compare the accumulation of disability in the relapsing and progressive groups (Figure 18.47). In the year before treatment, the relapsing patients showed a mean annual increase of +2.2 EDSS points. Mean annualized changes over the periods 0–6, 6–12 and 12–24 months were –2.4, –0.6 and –0.4, respectively. This compares with –3.8, –0.6 and –0.2 in the relapsing–remitting cohort (excluding the more advanced group of patients who had failed previous treatment with IFN-β). Nine of 15 patients observed at 1 year had an improved EDSS. All but one of the others was stable, and the mean effect was an improvement by 1.2 points compared to baseline. This improvement was sustained in the nine patients observed at 24 months, whose mean EDSS was –1.3 points from baseline. One patient had a sustained deterioration from EDSS 6.0 to 6.5 within the first 3 months after Campath-1H, but no subsequent change in disability. This stabilization of disability stands in marked contrast to the group with secondary progressive multiple sclerosis.

Patients treated for multiple sclerosis with Campath-1H experience an acute cytokine release syndrome with severe but temporary rehearsal of previous clinical features - specific manifestations varying with previous clinical features (see Chapters 10 and 13; Figure 18.48; Moreau *et al* 1996). Pretreatment with corticosteroids abolishes or minimizes these neurological exacerbations. Infections that may represent adverse effects of Campath-1H are mild and relatively infrequent given the profound and prolonged depletion of lymphocytes. These include spirochaetal gingivitis (at 10 days), measles (at 11 days), herpes zoster (three instances; at 6 and 9 months, respectively), varicella zoster (at 2 years), recurrent aphthous mouth ulcers (from 6–9 months), pyogenic granuloma (at 22 months), and listeria meningitis after eating soft cheese at 2 weeks. One patient with secondary progressive multiple sclerosis (EDSS 8.5) died of sepsis 7 years after Campath-1H treatment.

The principal adverse effect of Campath-1H therapy in patients with multiple sclerosis is Graves' disease (Coles *et al* 1999b). One patient had experienced Graves' disease prior to Campath-1H treatment and, to date, 15 new cases have been observed after treatment in the remaining 57 patients (27%), with one additional case of autoimmune hypothyroidism. One patient in the relapsing–remitting group developed acute renal failure as a result of Goodpasture's syndrome, with no lung involvement. This occurred 10 months after treatment with Campath-1H and was associated with the development of high titre anti-glomerular basement membrane antibodies, which were not detectable in serum taken before Campath-1H treatment,

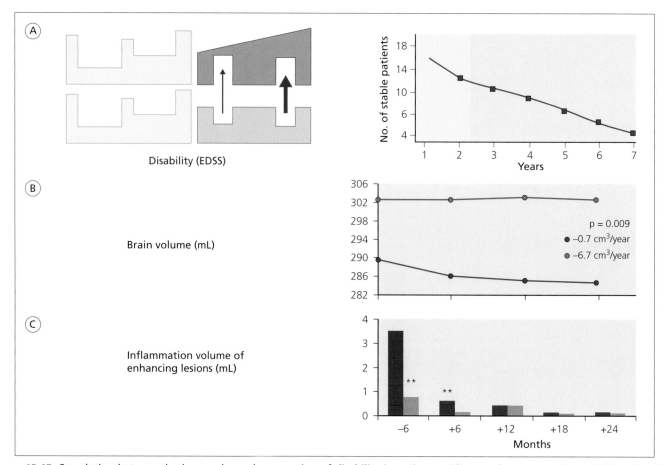

Figure 18.45 Correlation between brain atrophy and progression of disability in patients with secondary progressive multiple sclerosis showing substantial reduction in new lesions after treatment with Campath-1H. Adapted from Coles *et al* (1999a). © 1999, reproduced with permission of John Wiley & Sons.

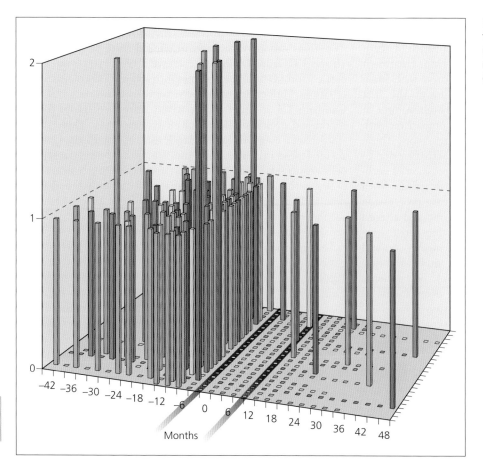

Figure 18.46 Reduction in new episodes following treatment with Campath-1H in patients with active relapsing–remitting multiple sclerosis. Adapted from Coles *et al* (2005).

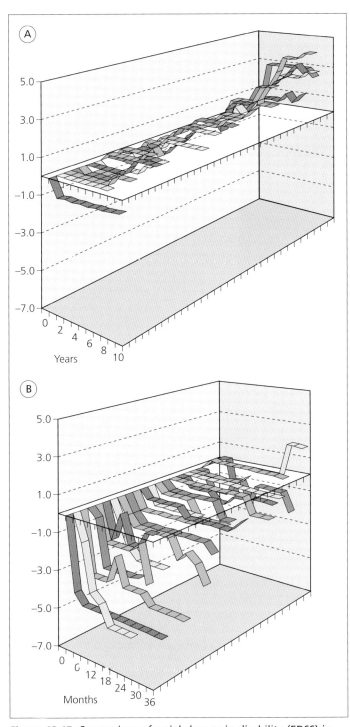

Figure 18.47 Comparison of serial change in disability (EDSS) in 36 patients with secondary progressive multiple sclerosis and 22 with early active relapsing–remitting disease. Adapted from Coles *et al* (2005).

nor 1 month before her illness. Systematic screening of sera from all other patients for autoantibodies against glomerular basement membrane, reticulin, gastric parietal cell, endomysial, anti-acetylcholine receptor and anti-voltage gated calcium channel have shown no abnormalities. One patient has developed positive anti-double-stranded DNA antibodies without any clinical evidence of systemic lupus erythematosus, impaired renal function, or arthritis. Another patient with a positive

family history of coeliac disease had elevated positive IgA and IgG anti-gliadin antibodies, without IgA tissue transglutaminase antibodies, in a single serum sample at 1 month after Campath-1H. These were undetectable in both the subsequent serum samples and those taken before treatment. Recruitment closed in April 2004 for a phase II multicentre randomized study comparing two doses of Campath-1H (60 mg and 120 mg over 5 days at baseline, repeated at 1 and 2 years) with IFN-β1a (Rebif; 22 μg three times weekly increasing at 1 month to 44 μg three times weekly by subcutaneous injection) in patients with early clinically active relapsing–remitting multiple sclerosis. The primary outcome is time to sustained disability as determined at 3 years. A press release issued by the sponsors in September 2005 reporting the first interim analysis indicates at least a 75% treatment effect on relapse rate, and >60% on sustained accumulation of disability, each at 1 year, compared with Rebif. These preliminary results appear to confirm the high efficacy of Campath-1H but, as before, the major adverse effect relates to autoimmunity with three cases of idiopathic thrombocytopaenic purpura, one of which proved fatal

Anti-CD25 (daclizumab)

There are few studies that systematically address the management of patients failing to respond adequately to approved therapies. In an uncontrolled series, Rose *et al* (2004) treated 19 patients, 17 of whom were not responding to other therapies, for between 5 and 25 months with daclizumab and claimed that all showed reduced MRI activity, compared with pre-treatment images, and 'sustained clinical improvement (10) or 'stability' (9). In a recent report, Bielekova *et al* (2004) administered a humanized monoclonal antibody (daclizumab) directed against the IL-2 receptor on activated T cells (IL-2Rα-chain; CD 25) to 11 patients with multiple sclerosis who appeared not to be responding to IFN-β1b treatment. All patients continued to receive IFN-β1b therapy during this study. 'Failure to respond' was defined as either one or more relapses or continued progression of ≥ 1.0 EDSS worsening over a period of 18 months on IFN-β1b treatment. Patients were selected for participation if they demonstrated ≥ 0.67 new MRI lesions per month during a 4-month period on IFN-β1b treatment. Treatment was given as 1.0 mg/kg per intravenous dose at baseline and week two, and then five additional infusions given at 4-weekly intervals. This agent was well tolerated although there were more infections and liver enzyme elevation over the period during which the antibody was given. There was a 78% reduction in new contrast enhancing lesions compared with baseline that began approximately 6–8 weeks after the first antibody infusion. One patient seemed to respond only to a higher dose (2 mg/kg per dose administered every 2 weeks). Secondary measures of benefit included a reduced relapse rate, better motor performance on the nine-hole peg test, improved scores on the Scripps Neurological Rating Scale, and reduced volume of contrast enhancing lesions. Further studies are planned.

T-cell vaccination

One therapeutic approach has been to eliminate antigen-specific autoreactive T cells by vaccination with X-irradiated cells primed against myelin basic protein. It was J. Zhang *et al* (1993)

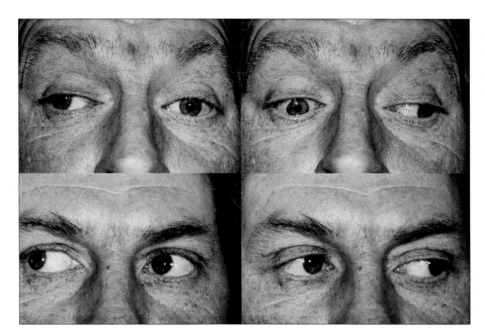

Figure 18.48 Recurrence of internuclear ophthalmoplegia with complete recovery developing in a patient during (top) and after (bottom) the first infusion of CAMPATH-1H. From Moreau *et al* (1996) with permission.

who first showed that inoculation of myelin basic protein reactive T cells induces responses that deplete circulating antigen-specific T cells, confirming that clonotypic interactions regulating autoreactive lymphocytes can be induced in humans by T-cell vaccination. Subsequently, in a small pilot study involving eight patients, five showed a reduction in relapses from a total of 16 to three in the 2 years before and after treatment, whereas controls showed no apparent reduction (12 and 10 before and after treatment). These clinical changes were accompanied by a difference in MRI lesion load of +8% and +39.5%, respectively. Clinical and MR indices of disease activity worsened in three patients in whom autoreactive T cells (showing different antigenic specificity) reappeared after vaccination (Medaer *et al* 1995).

Building on their earlier experience with experimental autoimmune encephalomyelitis (see Chapter 11) and clinical laboratory studies, Vandenbark *et al* (1996a) immunized 23 HLA-DRB1*1501-positive patients with T-cell receptor Vβ5.2 (residues 38–58 in two variations, with and without a tyrosine to threonine substitution at position 49), or placebo (n = 6) peptides on 14 occasions over 1 year. T-cell responses were more predictable and rapid with the substituted than natural peptide but were difficult to sustain in both groups. Several who were vaccinated continued to show T-cell reactivity on completion. However, there was a reduction in myelin basic protein reactivity which also correlated with altered disease progression. An unusually high number of patients with primary progressive multiple sclerosis was included (eight of 23 patients) and neither these nor the secondary progressive cases showed a clear clinical benefit (or deterioration) from the vaccination protocol (those who responded immunologically remained unchanged by comparison with all other participants, both placebo-treated and nonresponders; p = 0.02). Peptide-specific T-cell clones tended to show Th2 cytokine profiles (predominant production of IL-10) in contrast to the Th1 features of their myelin basic protein-specific T-cell clones.

Bone marrow and stem cell transplantation

Bone marrow transplantation following immune ablation has received much attention in recent years. More research is needed before it is clear whether this is a useful approach to treatment, and sufficiently safe to justify whatever clinical dividend emerges in due course. Currently patients either with advanced secondary progressive multiple sclerosis or refractory, aggressive relapsing–remitting disease are being assessed. If efficacy is established, the next step may be to assess whether patients who are at an earlier stage of the disease, but can genuinely be predicted to have a poor prognosis, should be selected for further trials. In the context of multiple sclerosis, the term stem cell transplantation is currently used primarily to refer either to bone marrow or peripheral blood autologous stem cell transplantation applied in the setting of immune system ablation. Experimental work with neural stem cells is moving quickly in model systems but is not yet applied to patients. The rationale for stem cell transplantation in all immune-mediated disorders is the premise that after near complete ablation of the host immune system (full ablation is not currently possible), the reconstituted immune system will be reprogrammed, resulting either in prolonged remission or amelioration of immune-mediated attack on the host. However, it remains to be established whether therapy depends more on the immunosuppressive induction with autologous stem cell rescue than these strategies for immune tolerance to autoantigens. Whatever the precise mechanisms, preliminary evidence in experimental animal model systems and multiple sclerosis is considered promising (Burt *et al* 1995; 1997).

Allogenic stem cell transplantation requires an HLA identical donor and, as such, has rarely been feasible for patients with multiple sclerosis. With advances in umbilical cord blood screening methods for bone marrow donors and cord blood banks, it will soon theoretically be possible to identify HLA compatible donors for haematopoietic stem cell transplantation (Laughlin *et al* 2001). Bone marrow harvesting requires a general anaesthetic, yields few T cells and is associated with a longer reconstitution time. Currently, most programmes therefore harvest autologuous stem cells from peripheral blood (as opposed to bone marrow) since this requires only a brief exposure to the risks of bone marrow suppression (Comi *et al* 2000; Tyndall and Koike 2002). Currently, peripheral blood stem cell harvesting is achieved using high-dose cyclophosphamide (2–4 g/m^2) either alone or with granulocyte colony-stimulating factor (G-CSF). G-CSF has been used without cyclophosphamide but may increase the likelihood of triggering an exacerbation of multiple sclerosis. This occurred in four of ten patients receiving G-CSF for peripheral blood stem cell harvesting (Openshaw *et al* 2000a). Three patients responded to methylprednisolone but one relapse proved fatal. These investigators reportedly now administer methylprednisolone together with recombinant G-CSF and do not use G-CSF after the patient is transplanted. There are several options for cytotoxic drug conditioning, including BEAM (*B*CNU, *E*toposide, cytosine *A*rabinoside, and *M*elphalan) alone or with anti-thymocyte globulin. Others use cyclophosphamide together with total body irradiation and a combination of busulfan and cyclophosphamide. The field has moved away from T-cell purging as there is no clear advantage and the risks of infection in the setting of T-cell depletion are high.

During the mobilization phase, patients may experience fever, seizures and infection. Allergic reactions to cyclophosphamide, G-CSF or the stem cells may occur during the intervention. Following transplantation, patients can experience allergic responses to anti-thymocyte globulin. Mucosal infections, prolonged fever, bleeding, neutropenia, thrombocytopenia, neurotoxicity and autoimmune thyroiditis (as with Campath-1H) are all encountered. Late complications, especially in T-cell-depleted grafts, include serious infections (such as aspergillosis), veno-occlusive liver disease, thrombotic thrombocytopenic pur-

Table 18.9 Published results with haematopoietic stem cell transplantation in multiple sclerosis

Investigator	Conditioning and immune ablation	Comments
Mancardi *et al* 2001 (ten patients; five Italian sites)	30–40 days following BEAM	Median follow-up only 18 months. Most stable. No Gd+ or new T$_2$ lesions. Atrophy (1 year) and oligoclonal bands continued at 2 years
Kozák *et al* 2002 (15 patients)	BEAM-ATG. 9/15 also received *ex vivo* T-cell depletion of graft	One death from progressive multiple sclerosis. Median follow-up 20 months with 11/15 stable or improved
Saiz *et al* 2004 (15 patients)	BCNU, high-dose cyclophosphamide, ATG and T-cell-depleted grafts	3 year median follow-up: 46% free of disease activity. No deaths. 4/14 continued to relapse (3 of these at multiple times). MRI no new lesions but atrophy continued
Openshaw *et al* 2000b (five patients)	Busulfan, cyclophosphamide and T-cell-depleted blood autografts	One died early post-transplant; histology showed macrophages but few T cells surrounding demyelinated plaques
Nash *et al* 2003 (26 patients; four United States sites)	Prednisone 1 mg/kg/day by mouth, TBI 2Gy × 4 doses, cyclophosphamide 60 mg/kg × 2 doses, horse ATG 15 mg/kg/ daily × 6 doses, GCSF 5 µg/kg/daily by intravenous injection	27% progressed by ≥ 1.0 EDSS at 3 years. Four new Gd+ lesions. Nine of 12 still had oligoclonal bands. One died with EBV-PTLD. Two relapses during mobilization, one proving fatal; 91% survival at 3 years
Burt *et al* 2003 (21 patients; three United States sites)	Cyclophosphamide 60 mg/kg iv, TBI with lung shield, 150 cGy bid on days −3, −2, −1	No transplantation-related deaths. Two died from progressive multiple sclerosis after 13–18 months. Eight of 12 at EDSS >6 worsened. All nine of nine at EDSS < 6 remained stable
Kimiskidis *et al* 2002 (35 patients)	Cyclophosphamide, G-CSF, BEAM, busulfan	G-CSF may have caused radiological deterioration. Subclinical MRI activity persisted in five patients. MRI atrophy progressed at 12 and 24 months. Two cases developed post-transplantation autoimmunity: thyroiditis (1) and refractory factor VIII-inhibitor (one with massive haemorrhage and death). Progression-free survival, 67% at 5 years
Fassas *et al* 2002 (85 patients; nine European sites and one United States site)	BEAM for 54/85 93% peripheral blood stem cell transplants (BMT 7%) 60% had *ex vivo* graft T-cell depletion	Median 16 months follow-up. 27% worsened in early post-transplant period. Seven of 85 (8.2%) died; two from progressive multiple sclerosis with high pretransplantation EDSS scores; five from toxic causes – four infections and one from heart failure. 3 year death rate was 10%; 20% progressed and 21% improved by ≥1.0 EDSS. MRI active after TPT in 8%. 74% progression-free survival at 36 months

BEAM = BCNU, etoposide, cytosine arabinoside, melphalan, rabbit ATG (anti-thymocyte globulin); TBI = total body irradiation; G-CSF = recombinant human granulocyte colony-stimulating factor; PTLD = post-transplantation lymphoproliferative disorder; EBMT Study = European Group for Blood and Marrow Transplantation Study.

pura, hypogonadism, cataract formation, and the development of malignancy related to the prolonged period of immunosuppression (Fassas *et al* 2000). Although autologous peripheral blood stem cell transplantation has a lower risk than allogenic transplantation, mortality rates are still reported to be in the 5% range or slightly higher. This relatively high risk of a fatal complication for an experimental therapy given in the context of a chronic, rarely life-threatening disorder places the burden on proof of superiority for those conducting this work.

The numbers of cases treated worldwide is ever increasing. In 2000, it was estimated that 74 patients with multiple sclerosis had been transplanted. This had risen to 109 by the third quarter of 2002, and approximately 200 people with multiple sclerosis had been transplanted by mid-2003. A position paper summarizing the opinion of selected European multiple sclerosis specialists has been published making recommendations for each step in this complex therapeutic programme (Comi *et al* 2000). The published results to date are summarized in Table 18.9. As noted, the numbers are small, the follow-up is modest and the evidence for clinical benefit is minimal to date. Several studies have shown MRI evidence for stability or apparent improvement, although serial MRI studies have shown that cerebral atrophy continues to progress after transplantation. Again, it is unclear to what extent the reduction in new MRI lesions relates to the transplant procedure rather than the profound degree of immunosuppression associated with induction.

In the trial reported by Nash *et al* (2003), death from post-transplantation lymphoproliferative disorder was attributed to a change from horse to rabbit anti-thymocyte globulin in the high-dose immunosuppressive therapy protocol. A second death was attributed to a relapse of multiple sclerosis during mobilization (another episode in a second patient during mobilization reversed within 6 months). Thirteen of the first 18 patients developed a fever and rash, sometimes associated with neurological worsening ('engraftment syndrome'). Burt *et al* (2003) reported two late multiple sclerosis-related deaths, and EDSS progression in eight of 12 patients with baseline EDSS scores of 6.0 or higher. They concluded that intense immunosuppression with total body irradiation and haematopoietic stem cell transplantation should not be offered to patients with advanced progressive multiple sclerosis. Conversely, in a retrospective review

of bone marrow transplantation, Fassas and Kimiskidis (2003) conclude that the early results are encouraging despite the morbidity and mortality experienced in their protocol. In a recent update of the series from Barcelona, Saiz *et al* (2004) reported on their experience of autologous stem cell transplantation after a course of high-dose chemotherapy. As outlined in the accompanying editorial (Freedman and Atkins 2004), at 3 years median follow-up, four of 14 patients continued to experience relapses (several each in three individuals) suggesting incomplete or ineffective suppression of disease activity although 46% were disease free. This protocol seemingly prevented the development of new contrast enhancing lesions and was followed by reductions in T_2 lesion load. In parallel, however, there was progressive brain atrophy. It remains to be determined whether the reduction in brain volume reflects true progressive atrophy or is fully explained by a reduction in active inflammation. The current status of autologous haematopoietic stem cell transplantation in multiple sclerosis is reviewed elsewhere (Blanco et *al* 2005; Burt *et al* 2005). Muraro *et al* (2005) recently reported that there is an important change in the immune profile of T cells 2 years after stem cell transplantation in patients with multiple sclerosis. Post-transplantation there are fewer memory T cells and a greater diversity of expressed T cell receptors, suggesting that delayed benefit may extend beyond that explained by lymphocyte depletion. The trials in progress will bring more insights but each is relatively small and insufficiently powered to prove definitive.

AGENTS INHIBITING MACROPHAGES AND THEIR MEDIATORS

Drugs that inhibit the function of macrophages (and microglia), or the release of their mediators, have been evaluated in multiple sclerosis although it is unclear whether these studies are primarily motivated by attempts to modify the course of the illness or merely to suppress symptoms.

Monoclonal antibodies targeted against TNF-α have been used in rheumatoid arthritis and appear to stabilize joint symptoms for several months. We have used very short pulses of humanized soluble TNF receptor for the specific purpose of suppressing the

	Placebo	Lenercept (mg)			
No. of patients	43	44 (10 mg)	40 (50 mg)	40 (100 mg)	p value
Patients with ≥1 exacerbation through week 24	15	21	28	27	0.003[a]
Patients with ≥1 exacerbation through week 48	22	26	32	32	0.007[b]
Exacerbations with onset ≤ week 24	22	28	37	33	
Duration (days) of these exacerbations	28.3	38.6	41.6	42.0	0.62[c]
Range (median)	28 (1–91)	31 (6–189)	31 (6–201)	25 (4–261)	
Annualized exacerbation rate	0.98	1.0	1.64	1.47	

Table 18.10 Number, duration and annual rate of exacerbations during the Lenercept multiple sclerosis trial

a Chi-square tests: global.
b Kruskal–Wallis test.
c Kaplan–Meier (KM) (means and medians are estimated from the KM curves).

cytokine release syndrome associated with the use of Campath-1H without apparent benefit or adverse effect (Coles *et al* 1999a). In a randomized, double-blind, placebo-controlled study of a recombinant soluble TNF-α receptor p55 immunoglobulin fusion protein (lenercept), Arnason *et al* (1999) demonstrated that this agent is associated with an increase in disease activity (earlier, more frequent and possibly more severe clinical relapses) than placebo (Table 18.10). The drug was poorly tolerated (headaches, nausea, abdominal pain; Schwid and Noseworthy 1999). A previous small study had also demonstrated an increase in MRI markers of disease activity in response to anti-TNF-α monoclonal antibody (van Oosten *et al* 1996b). In addition, 17 patients are reported to have developed signs and symptoms suggesting central nervous system demyelination after treatment with the anti-TNF-α agent etanercept, and two patients have had similar reactions to infliximab administration (Mohan *et al* 2001). As such, despite the theoretical arguments in favour of its use, anti-TNF-α strategies do not appear to have a therapeutic future in multiple sclerosis.

A few preliminary results are available on the use of macrophage inhibitors in multiple sclerosis but the choice (or availability) of agents is such that their therapeutic role remains largely unexplored. Deoxyspergualin suppresses the maturation of lymphocytes and also inhibits production of oxygen radicals by macrophages. It received attention amongst multiple sclerosis sufferers through publicity surrounding an individual case and on the basis of effects in experimental autoimmune encephalomyelitis (Schorlemmer and Seiler 1991). Deoxyspergualin was subsequently evaluated in a placebo-controlled study in which 2 or 6 mg/kg deoxyspergualin was given intravenously for 1 month as 5 day pulses (Kappos *et al* 1994). Preliminary results showed no effect on the pretreatment level of disease activity assessed by MRI but the clinical evaluation remains unpublished. Different doses of pentoxifylline were given to 14 patients by L.W. Myers *et al* (1998) to identify that which best suppressed TNF-α production in both a bioassay and enzyme-linked immunosorbent assay. These were sensitive assays since TNF-α was detected in the majority of cerebrospinal fluid samples before treatment. There was no immunological effect of treatment at any dose and almost all the patients deteriorated, objectively and subjectively. MRI abnormalities continued to accumulate. van Oosten *et al* (1996b) also were unable to demonstrate any effect of pentoxifylline (800–1200 mg daily for 4 weeks) on a range of Th1 and Th2 cytokine productions in 20 patients with multiple sclerosis. By contrast, Rieckmann *et al* (1996) showed *in vitro* and *in vivo* suppression by pentoxyfilline (1600 mg/day by oral administration) on TNF-α and IL-12 production, with corresponding stimulation of IL-10 and IL-4 in patients with relapsing–remitting multiple sclerosis.

Nineteen patients (nine with primary progressive and ten with secondary progressive disease) were treated by S.G. Lynch *et al* (1996) using the iron chelator desferroxamine by subcutaneous infusion for 14 days to enhance iron chelation and prevent hydroxyl radical formation. The study was open and uncontrolled and rather little can be learned from the claim that nine, six and three and three, five and six patients improved, were unchanged or worsened by >1 EDSS point at 6 and 12 months, respectively. The same reservations apply to an earlier study of 12 patients with more marked disabilities (EDSS 5.5–8) of whom seven, four and three improved, stabilized or worsened in the 3 months after treatment with desferroxamine (Norstrand and Craelius 1989).

RECENT MISCELLANEOUS TREATMENTS

The National Multiple Sclerosis Society (of the United States) keeps a checklist on trials in progress. The most recent version lists more than 150 current clinical trials (*http://www.nationalmssociety.org/Clinical%20Trials.asp*). Several are likely to be completed in the near future and new options for treatment or fresh insights into preferred strategies for the timing and choice of interventions may be provided. A few new faces are already on the street.

Statins

As outlined in recent editorials (D. Baker *et al* 2003; Neuhaus *et al* 2004), statin drugs are attracting interest in both the scientific and lay literature as potential treatments for multiple sclerosis, and for several reasons. Statins have a wide variety of immunoregulatory effects, are relatively inexpensive, generally well tolerated and available as oral agents. Lovastatin was shown to be partially effective in acute experimental autoimmune encephalomyelitis (Stanislaus *et al* 2001). Neuhaus *et al* (2002) demonstrated that simvastatin, mevastatin and lovastatin each had significant immunosuppressive activities in humans, including treatment-induced reduction in the proliferation of stimulated peripheral blood mononuclear cells, reduced adhesion molecule expression (CD54; ICAM-1), altered Th1/Th2 cytokine profile (paradoxically favouring a so-called 'proinflammatory profile'), reduced matrix metalloproteinase-9 levels and expression of B-cell and T-cell cytokine receptors. In further animal studies, Youssef *et al* (2002) showed that oral atorvastatin promoted a Th2 anti-inflammatory cytokine profile, reduced the expression of MHC class II and costimulatory molecules, and prevented the development of chronic experimental autoimmune encephalomyelitis. There are probably multiple mechanisms whereby statin drugs affect the immune response but inhibition of mevalonate with subsequent reduction in isoprenoids (and, hence, reduced post-translational isoprenylation of proteins) may be important (D. Baker *et al* 2003). In an open label trial of 30 patients with multiple sclerosis, Vollmer *et al* (2004b) reported an effect on contrast enhanced MRI indicators of disease activity (reduction in 44% by number and 40% by volume of contrast enhancing lesions) at months 4, 5 and 6 following the administration of simvastatin (80 mg orally per day) compared with pretreatment data. This small study did not demonstrate a reduction in relapse rate but patients were only followed for 6 months. Being unblinded, the study did not adequately address the possibility of regression to the mean. Exploratory immunological studies did not demonstrate an impressive *in vitro* effect. Much more work is clearly needed to raise the status of statins as a disease-modifying treatment in multiple sclerosis.

Estriol

Pregnancy provides an important, though transient, benefit for patients with relapsing–remitting multiple sclerosis (see Chapter 4). This example from nature has long provoked interest in estrogen therapy as a potential treatment option. Sicotte *et al* (2002) completed a small open label trial of daily high-dose oral estriol administration (8 mg/day – an amount designed to simulate pregnancy levels) in 12 women (six each with relapsing–remitting and secondary progressive multiple sclerosis). The relapsing–remitting cohort, but not those with secondary progressive multiple sclerosis, experienced a reduction in MRI evidence for disease activity (number and volume of gadolinium-DTPA enhancing lesions). This result was unexpected since the natural history of gadolinium enhancing lesions appears similar in both clinical subgroups and the response to other therapies such as IFN-β has been similar. Treated relapsing–remitting patients also demonstrated reduced immune function compared with pretreatment values (such as reduced delayed-type hypersensitivity to tetanus and serum levels of IFN-γ). MRI and immune functions returned to pretreatment levels when estriol was discontinued. The authors do not discuss safety issues other than to say that 'pregnancy levels' of estriol were associated with uterine bleeding requiring endometrial biopsy. They recommend that future trials consider combining estriol with progesterone to prevent uterine endometrial hyperplasia. Other safety issues known to be associated with high-dose estrogen therapy would need to be considered carefully in future trials (including effects on thromboembolic disease, migraine, breast cancer, endometrial hyperplasia and cancer, menstrual irregularity, gallbladder disease, cholestatic jaundice, pancreatitis and hypertension).

Minocycline

Based on its anti-inflammatory properties, acting through the inhibition of matrix metalloproteinases, and evidence for efficacy in experimental autoimmune encephalomyelitis (Popovic *et al* 2002), minocycline seems set for thorough evaluation as a treatment for multiple sclerosis. Metz *et al* (2004) treated 10 patients with relapsing–remitting disease, observed to have a mean number of episodes during the previous 2 years of 2.6 (range 2–4 over the 2 years) with minocycline (100 mg twice daily for 6 months); interim analysis of this uncontrolled series showed no change in the frequency of episodes but mean total

enhancing lesion number changed from 1.4 per scan before treatment to 0.2 lesions per scan whilst receiving minocycline, representing > 84% reduction; however, these data (before and after treatment) depended exclusively on the experience of only five patients.

POSTSCRIPT

We have reviewed much that has gone into recent efforts to develop more effective therapies for people with multiple sclerosis. Clearly progress has been made but more is needed. We are cautiously optimistic that the decade ahead will bring even more hopeful news for our patients and trust that progress will accelerate. We say this, fully aware of the vast investment in biomedical research worldwide and the tremendous collaborative spirit that is evident in the work already accomplished and currently under way. We are encouraged by the creativity of the scientific community and anticipate that continued productive collaboration across the research and biotechnology communities will pay further dividends. The currently available, licensed medications demonstrate favourable effects on relapse rates and on MRI indicators of (presumably inflammatory) disease activity. We do not yet know for certain that treatment delays clinical disability progression or the progression of brain and cord atrophy. We strongly suspect that the progression of clinical disability often developing as the years pass is largely attributable to gradual loss of axonal number and function. This assumption brings great hope that meaningful benefits will follow closely on our increased understanding of the factors that determine axonal loss. Until such time as the 'breakthrough' arrives, we must remain objective and humble about what is known and what is not. We must continue to ask the right scientific questions and demand useful answers even if these are hard to acquire. Patients have a right to be informed about the knowledge base and zones of ignorance in multiple sclerosis. They should understand fully the limits of our ability to control the course of their illness and be encouraged to participate actively in debating the merits and demerits of existing and new treatments.

The person with multiple sclerosis: a prospectus

19

Alastair Compston, David Miller and John Noseworthy

A PERSPECTIVE ON THE RECENT HISTORY OF THERAPEUTIC ENDEAVOUR IN MULTIPLE SCLEROSIS

In 2005, the person with multiple sclerosis faces an array of opinion and directives concerning treatment that must seem bewildering. Caught in the trap of history, with the problems identified but no answers delivered, public lobbying has raised the temperature of the health care agenda; chronic illness is a pawn in the political game; Biotech and Big Pharma sense a return on investment yet find themselves operating in an increasingly defensive climate; governmental legislation and guidelines define 'who' may receive 'what' – rationing by any other name; definitions for meaningful and clinically useful outcomes are adjusted so as to raise the status of selected 'medicines' to 'treatments'; hawks compete with doves in pronouncing on meta-analyses of treatment trials; fact merges with fiction – truth with hyperbole. In short, expectations are high; people with multiple sclerosis are confused or frankly disappointed; and the traditional working relationship between doctor and patient is periodically strained in attempting to negotiate the gap between what is promised and what can actually be delivered. The sense of disappointment for patients who see that medication will not immediately solve all their problems can be worse than the frustration of remaining untreated. There is a risk that overstating the results of trials inhibits decisions about the need for other competent research promising equal or better therapeutic options. The declaration that there are effective therapies has already established a gold standard against which all new treatments need to be assessed. This has profound implications for the design, size and expense of new studies.

A consolidated position for existing treatments, the disappearance of some others, and the assessment of new strategies based on more precise dissection of interactions between the immune system and structures of the central nervous system, all seem scheduled for the next few years. But when and how will the dividend of so much effort and sustained hope be realized? As investigators, we need to decide collectively that our mission is to discover treatment programmes that favourably influence long-term outcomes for this chronic illness, and raise the game from a focus on short-term objectives that sell drugs but do not necessarily provide lasting benefits to people with multiple sclerosis. There are, as yet, no mechanisms in place to accomplish this difficult goal. We expect that international cooperatives will help to demonstrate how clinical features, neuroimaging measures and biomarkers (each of which must be validated using appropriate long-term methodologies) contribute to the reliable recognition of meaningful outcomes, based on further analyses of the natural history datasets that are already available and increasingly well coordinated.

SETTING AN AGENDA: THE WINDOW OF THERAPEUTIC OPPORTUNITY

We approach prospects for managing the many problems of multiple sclerosis in the future from the same perspective as we laid out the present situation in Chapters 15–18: the treatment of acute episodes; reducing the impact of persistent manifestations through symptomatic treatments and rehabilitation; and modifying the course of the disease. But there are shifts in emphasis, nuances of interpretation: the expectation is that more will be achieved through theoretically motivated rather than purely empirical strategies. We anticipate that the trend will be towards tailoring treatments to disease types, in individuals or groups, and timing interventions to match the stage reached in the clinical course. Once, the key event in multiple sclerosis was assumed to be damage to the myelin oligodendrocyte unit resulting in breakdown of saltatory conduction. Now, the importance of acute and chronic axonal injury is emphasized – not for the first time. To us, it seems self-evident that anticipating and preventing damage to axons and glia will be easier to accomplish than restoring structure and function in the already damaged brain and spinal cord; but, as before, the challenge is both to limit and to repair the damage.

Management of the acute episode

In Chapters 10 and 13, we made the case that inflammatory mediators *per se* transiently interrupt function in myelinated or hypomyelinated nerve fibres; more prolonged exposure adds structural damage to axons and myelin, especially if the pathway is electrically active. It follows that, from the outset, the inflammatory process is as hazardous for axons as it is for myelin and oligodendrocytes. Whilst this is not a new formulation (see Chapter 1), 'demyelinating' disease might seem to be misnamed. At the molecular level, the main candidates for mediating acute

803

axonal injury are nitric oxide and excitotoxicity acting through damage to mitochondrial function, with altered ion exchange mechanisms leading to increased calcium entry (see Figure 10.19). In the experimental context, corticosteroids protect axons from the effects of media conditioned by activated microglia; direct inhibition of nitric oxide activity and the blocking of NMDA (*N*-methyl-D-aspartate) receptors have the same effect. Again, in experimental inflammatory conditions, membrane stabilizing agents (phenytoin, lamotrigine and flecainide) protect axons from excess sodium influx via the voltage-gated sodium channels that triggers reverse sodium–calcium exchange and excitotoxic injury (for review see Stys 2004; Waxman 2005). In the clinical setting, corticosteroids prevent the cytokine release syndrome associated with the use of some monoclonal antibodies (see Chapter 18) – itself attributed to the effects of nitric oxide. Although a single course of intravenous methylprednisolone administered a median of 8 days after symptom onset did not prevent the development of optic nerve atrophy in patients with acute optic neuritis (Hickman *et al* 2003), the rate of brain atrophy was reduced in patients with multiple sclerosis following repeated doses of oral methylprednisolone (Zidavinov *et al* 2001a); but this study was incompletely blinded and remains to be confirmed.

Taken together, these data have implications for management of the person with multiple sclerosis. First, there should be minimal delay in the interval between onset of symptoms and the start of treatment with corticosteroids for patients not at high risk of complications from pulse corticosteroid administration. If exposure of axons for $\geq$ 72 hours *in vitro* leads to irreversible axonal damage, it makes little sense to wait for several days before issuing a prescription in the clinic, although this hypothesis needs to be tested. We cannot exclude a series of type 2 errors in the current evaluation of corticosteroids, because most studies have achieved no more than a median interval of 7–10 days from onset to institution of treatment. Secondly, if many inflammatory events are not expressed clinically and occur more often than new episodes – and normal-appearing white and grey matter is, in reality, far from normal – a case could be made for a properly controlled trial to test whether repeated courses of corticosteroids, given electively and not timed merely to follow clinical episodes of proven MRI activity, provide long-term benefit to patients with active relapsing–remitting multiple sclerosis. Clearly, such an approach must be balanced against the reality of adverse effects, and before any change in practice is contemplated this would have to be evidence based. Despite the logistic difficulties, we would like to see an evaluation of ultra-early use of corticosteroids versus later administration in acute relapse, using neuroimaging and biomarkers of axonal injury as outcomes; and, until studies have been conducted having an interval from onset of the inflammatory process measured in hours, not days, we keep an open mind on the long-held view that the use of corticosteroids is limited to abbreviation of the acute episode with no effect on the accumulation of disability (see Chapter 1). For us, this debate is not settled by the optic neuritis treatment trial and its many analyses (see Chapter 16).

Because the chain of events mediating axonal degeneration in inflammatory conditions bears close similarity to those operating in hypoxic/ischaemic injury of the central nervous system, therapeutic strategies recently developed to prevent white matter damage in stroke may be effective for short- or long-term neuroprotection in patients with multiple sclerosis. Those who visit health stores, take vitamin (E) supplements and consume red wine *ad libitum* may justify their self-medicating around this formulation. Appropriate studies designed to test antioxidants in multiple sclerosis have been proposed (Gilgun-Sherki *et al* 2004). These, and plans for clinical trials of agents that block Na^+ channels or glutamate receptors, have a reasonable theoretical basis, and the results are awaited with interest. We expect a steady pipeline of new candidate agents from the drug discovery routes, and anticipate that the next generation will focus on axonal protection. For example, Pryce *et al* (2003) demonstrated the role of the cannabinoid system in mediating axonal loss in experimental autoimmune encephalomyelitis. Mice deficient in CB_1 cannabinoid receptors had more extensive axonal loss than controls; and administration of CB_1 agonists limited retinal neurodegeneration in an experimental uveitis model. Cannabinoids may act by blocking glutamate excitotoxicity although other mechanisms are implicated including antioxidation and interference with the cell death pathway. Cannabis, of course, remains illegal in many countries but we expect it to be evaluated under appropriate licence for this and other potential new indications. It will not be alone in attracting interest and the investment of hope from people with multiple sclerosis.

Symptomatic treatment and rehabilitation

On the question of relieving persistent symptoms, too few manifestations of multiple sclerosis are at present satisfactorily managed by existing therapies. The gaps are obvious: cognitive function, low vision, weakness, poor balance, tremor and fatigue, *inter alia*, are hardly ever helped by medication; even spasticity, bladder dysfunction and pain are often not relieved to the degree required by individual patients; only the paroxysmal manifestations of multiple sclerosis could be seen as more or less invariably treatable. Making pharmacological inroads into these deficits will involve drug development with generic indications for the individual products, because the potential market for particular symptoms in multiple sclerosis is small. That said, the needs of the affected individuals are real. Occasional surprises may identify new indications for existing therapies: effective treatments for pain – amytriptyline and carbamazepine/gabapentin – were first introduced as antidepressant and antiepileptic medications, respectively; botulinum toxin – used to treat focal spasticity – was first used to treat focal dystonias; sildenafil and the anticholinergics – used to treat erectile or bladder dysfunction, respectively – are also effective in a range of medical disorders in which similar symptoms occur. Increasingly, specialists in the management of unremitting pain are making strides that can be applied to people with multiple sclerosis including nonpharmacological measures involving medical disciplines other than pharmacology and neurology.

But perhaps the greatest potential for improving quality of life in the presence of disabling symptoms is to expand the ambitions and availability of rehabilitation so that the opportunities for combining pharmacological, immunobiological and physical therapy interventions with tactics for coping, reducing disability and improving participation are fully exploited. The agenda includes an understanding of activity and environmental input in driving neuroplasticity in healthy and injured brains; determining the role of brain-behaviour relationships and their application to attention, motivation, mood and goal setting in neurorehabilitation by adopting the principles of cognitive neuroscience; and using technologies that both explore and may themselves modulate brain function including, for example, transcranial magnetic and deep brain stimulation. Experimental work has already established that interventions must be 'taught to work' by behavioural techniques if the desired improvements in function are to follow the restoration of structure. These and many related matters are usefully summarized in a report with supporting evidence on restoring neurological function from the United Kingdom Academy of Medical Sciences (2004).

Disease-modifying treatments

The immediate aim of disease-modifying treatments is to inhibit disease activity, but the hope is that this will also limit the accumulation of disability and prevent the onset of disease progression. We began our discussion of these agents (Chapter 18) with an established view of the pathogenesis, having inflammation as the pivotal process from which all other aspects of tissue injury follow. We assumed that genetic predisposition and environmental triggers initiate an inflammatory process sustained through immunological mechanisms – a 'hit and run' scenario rather than persistent (viral) infection. For over a decade the emphasis of disease-modifying therapy has therefore focused more or less exclusively on immunological therapies. As we move from an entirely empirical to a more rational basis for treatment, consolidating the validity of this central inflammatory hypothesis becomes more crucial, but it has recently been challenged. Tissue remote from areas of macroscopic inflammation is abnormal; lesions sampled ultra-early in the course show loss of oligodendrocytes in the absence of inflammatory injury; and suppression of inflammation in chronic multiple sclerosis rarely does much to limit the accumulation of disability through sustained progression. Superficially, these observations question the central dogma of multiple sclerosis as a disorder in which the priority is for suppression of the inflammatory process.

But if inflammation does trigger a cascade of secondary consequences in multiple sclerosis, it follows that there is all the more reason to anticipate those events, and prevent the dominoes tumbling, by limiting the process before the onset of irreversible tissue injury. But how early is early? The establishment of a definite diagnosis – the prerequisite for any aggressive anti-inflammatory therapy – has, using traditional clinically based criteria, taken place after the disease has already caused tissue injury in the central nervous system, perhaps over several years. The development of new criteria (W.I. McDonald *et al* 2001) that use laboratory investigation – in particular neuroimaging findings – now enables earlier diagnosis in a substantial number of patients, even within 3 months of a first characteristic clinical episode. Such criteria will facilitate earlier disease-modifying treatment although, even at the first clinical manifestation, it is apparent from magnetic resonance imaging that, in many patients, the pathological process is already well established. We continue to debate whether the use of MRI criteria to confirm 'definite multiple sclerosis' after intervals as short as 12 weeks merit becoming the accepted standard.

Having reaffirmed the rationale for early anti-inflammatory treatment, it is logical to look more imaginatively at steps in the cascade of events leading to tissue injury at which a spanner might most effectively be placed in the immunological works. By analogy with success achieved in the drug management of some malignancies, there may be a place for induction of a clinical effect with a more intensive immunosuppressant followed by maintenance therapy using one or other of the licensed medications. Many drug combinations can be contemplated and, given the freedom to prescribe, their use seems inevitable, but we advocate caution in instituting polypharmacy. There is now a proliferation of 'head-to-head' trials comparing many established cocktails containing symptomatic treatments (theoretical and empirical), licensed treatments and immunosuppressive agents (usefully summarized, as at 2004, by Gonsette 2004). It is clear that many of these trials are significantly underpowered and others, we predict, will be terminated early because of apparent evidence of short-term efficacy, leaving open the question of whether there is a lasting therapeutic advantage from drug combinations with respect to disability or brain atrophy.

We have set out a sufficiently detailed account of the immunological synapse (Chapter 11), and the structure-function relationships of axons and glia (Chapters 10 and 13), for the reader to see that there is no shortage of candidate molecules or pivotal pathways at which new treatments might be targeted. The options have been rigorously catalogued, covering all the options (Hohlfeld 1997; Nepom 2002) or selected therapeutic targets (Opdenakker *et al* 2003). Suffice it to say that the zones where therapies are most likely to be deployed (and the category of medicine that will most probably be used) would include the following:

- depleting the systemic lymphocyte pool and inducing immune tolerance (monoclonal antibodies, immunosuppression, pheresis technology)
- increasing the regulation of T cells (cytokine-based therapies, immune tolerization)
- restricting the movement of activated T cells across endothelial barriers (monoclonal antibodies and small molecules, corticosteroids)
- preventing the diffusion of cells into the brain parenchyma (chemokine-based treatments)
- limiting antigen presentation and microglial activation (cytokine-based treatments, monoclonal antibodies)
- protecting intact myelinated axons from activated macrophages/microglia (macrophage inhibitors)
- inhibiting the establishment of immunological chronicity (anti-B cell and monoclonal antibodies)
- protecting intact axons from acute injury (anti-excitotoxic and membrane stabilizing agents)
- providing trophic support of persistently demyelinated axons (growth factors and remyelination strategies that might include pharmaceutical strategies for enhancing remyelination)
- promoting plasticity and axon regeneration (extracellular matrix molecules and manipulation of inhibitory environments).

PROSPECTS FOR THE TREATMENT OF PROGRESSIVE MULTIPLE SCLEROSIS

If axonal loss and inflammation are independent pathologies, then no single immunotherapy is likely to influence progression of disability; but if axons degenerate directly as a result of the inflammatory process, or indirectly through loss of trophic support normally provided by cells of the oligodendrocyte lineage, the dividend from early suppression of inflammation may be considerable; and if the naked axon is resistant to the inflammatory milieu but has poor survival properties, strategically timed interventions leading to enhanced remyelination may also be directly neuroprotective. In Chapter 10, we challenged the dogma that rigidly separates the immunological and neurobiological components of tissue injury in multiple sclerosis. Clearly the nervous system does much to limit and contain the inflammatory process. We emphasized that molecules traditionally considered part of the immunological repertoire nevertheless act on cell-based structures in the central nervous system. Conversely, neurotrophins provide autocrine protection from inflammatory mediators, and have their own short-range immunosuppressant properties. Here, therefore, are endogenous mechanisms for limiting the potential damage to viable but threatened neurons and myelinated axons in the vicinity of an inflammatory focus, sealing the area of damage and creating the sharply demarcated lesions that characterize the pathology of multiple sclerosis. Thus, it follows that a clever course has to be steered in limiting those aspects of the inflammatory response that contribute to tissue injury, without compromising benefits for tissue repair. Furthermore, combining anti-inflammatory and neuroprotective treatments may be a sensible strategy for disease-modifying therapy throughout the clinical course. Taking the evidence gathered from a variety of clinical and experimental sources, our position is:

- The areas of focal damage, constituting plaques, are driven by inflammation; it remains to be shown that diffuse injury of normal-appearing white matter has a cause other than inflammation resulting in microglial activation.
- Regions of the central nervous system or the brain and spinal cord as a whole may have an intrinsic vulnerability to damage – a neurodegenerative diathesis – resulting from genetic or environmental events but this vulnerability nevertheless needs to be exposed by inflammation: the pathogenesis is not primarily and independently neurodegenerative.
- The impact of inflammation is conditioned by the prior state of the inflamed tissue: previously damaged regions are further injured by a minimal amount of active inflammation; intact tissue has a higher threshold and resists this potentially pathological insult.
- At the extremes of this interplay, the early stage of the disease is entirely inflammatory whereas, in the end, axon degeneration through loss of trophic support may proceed in the absence of ongoing inflammation.

The therapeutic implications of this analysis for disease progression are self-evident (Figure 19.1). There is no evidence that any form of currently available treatment alters the natural history of primary progressive multiple sclerosis. We take an equally reserved position on the success from current strategies for altering the natural history of secondary progression, once transition from the relapsing–remitting phase is unambiguously established. As a result, individuals with progressive multiple sclerosis feel disenfranchised, and their needs not well served by the recent attention to other disease types. Discouraged by the spectacle of their slow decline, these patients regularly remind

neurologists that they are keen to participate in trials. Recent epidemiological evidence suggests that the clinical decline is similar in both primary and secondary cases once a moderate, fixed degree of disability has accumulated, suggesting that relapses do not significantly impact the rate of progression after this threshold has been crossed (see Chapter 4). Once a patient has entered the secondary progressive phase of multiple sclerosis, the emphasis shifts to neuroprotection – although, as set out above, we do not exclude a modest further contribution from the suppression of inflammation.

Aside from the measures we would like to see explored for acute axonal protection (see above), the mechanisms of chronic axonal attrition need separate consideration. If axons die from loss of trophic support and exquisite sensitivity to residual inflammation, it follows that replacing the missing trophic factors should be tried. But first, the trophic factors must be identified and catalogued. To date, we have IGF-I and glial cell line-derived neurotrophic factor (GDNF) on the list but others are bound to be added. Perhaps the characterization will never be complete or adequate, in which case the best dressing for threatened axons is myelin.

REMYELINATION AND AXON REGENERATION

Remyelination occupies a special role in ideas on the treatment of multiple sclerosis. To the affected person, it is an icon of hope – a holy grail – sustaining the vision of reversing chronic deficits and thereby rewriting the neurological natural history. For the clinical scientist, remyelination seems the neatest trick for protecting axons in the chronic stages, both through the direct provision of trophic support and in order to raise the threshold for further injury from residual inflammatory activity. In addition, if axonal outgrowth and connectivity could be ordered in the context of late chronic multiple sclerosis through one or other of the neurobiological strategies suggested from the identification of inhibitory molecules and growth support, it would be necessary to clothe these fragile processes with myelin in order to restore function. This analysis lifts the status of remyelination above that of a luxury – icing on the therapeutic cake – to one in which it plays an essential part in any coherent strategy for limiting and reversing the clinical deficits that invariably accumulate once recovery from the individual episode proves incomplete. The extent to which endogenous remyelination already contributes to clinical recovery, and the factors that determine the dynamics of this process, are discussed in Chapters 12 and 13. Failure of remyelination, and the reasons for this limitation from the experimental perspective, are set out in Chapter 10. So what are the prospects for making progress with this much discussed aim? It is convenient to list the issues:

- Will cessation of the inflammatory process allow sufficient repair and reversal of deficits or is assistance needed?
- Do remedies already exist that promote remyelination?
- Does suppression of the inflammatory process inhibit remyelination?
- Are some individuals good, and others bad, remyelinators; and if so, might this propensity change with time?
- Is the potential for enhancing endogenous remyelination real enough to make the concept of exogenous rescue unnecessary?

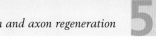
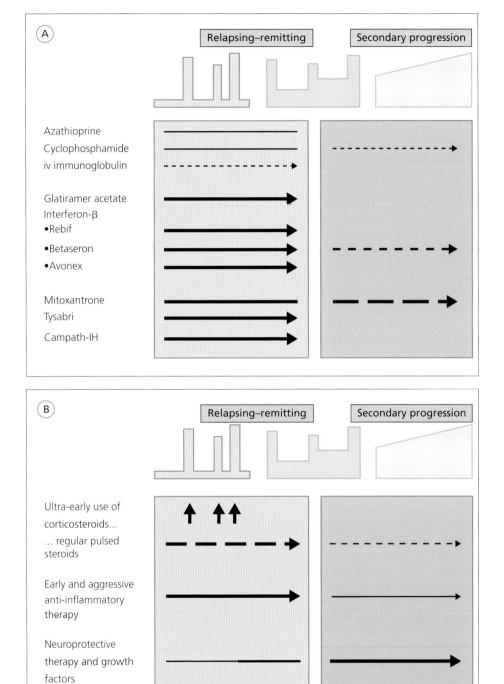

Figure 19.1 (A) In 2005, the available treatments for multiple sclerosis reduce inflammation and the number of new episodes but, almost without exception, have no effect on disease progression. (B) In the years ahead, redefinition of therapeutic strategies based on theoretical not empirical considerations is set to improve prospects for limiting and repairing the damage. The width of the line mirrors the strength of the published evidence for each outcome.

- Is there a critical period when the naked axon can be rescued by reclothing it in myelin?
- How much axonal loss can be tolerated before attempting to remyelinate 'open space' becomes illogical?
- How many axons must be remyelinated to achieve useful conduction through a critical pathway?
- Can axon outgrowth be promoted in order to increase the 'theatre' of remyelinaton?
- Which intervention provides the best 'medicine'?
- How can the treatment most effectively be delivered and distributed?
- Which lesion(s) should be targeted?
- How should remyelination be measured in clinical studies?
- What is needed to protect *neo*-myelin?

The relationship between suppression of the inflammatory response and remyelination is complex. Experimental therapies increasingly need to be considered in the context of their relative impact on injury and repair. The weight of the evidence might be taken as indicating that the suppression of inflammation is a bad thing. As we discuss in Chapter 10, remyelination is most active, experimentally and perhaps also in the clinical context, during the phase of active inflammation. But that is not the whole story. M. Rodriguez and Lindsley (1992) showed enhanced remyelination in animals with Theiler's virus demyelination treated with cyclophosphamide, or monoclonal antibodies directed against CD8 and CD4 cells; methylprednisolone increases the rate but not the extent of remyelination in a non-immune model of demyelination (Pavelko *et al* 1998); glatiramer acetate, which we presume mainly to suppress the inflammatory process in multiple sclerosis, increases growth factor production (Ziemssen *et al* 2002) and thereby possibly enhances repair.

But before investing wholesale in strategies for remyelination, it may yet be too early to conclude that effective anti-inflammatory treatment will not do enough to prevent all aspects of the natural history in multiple sclerosis, making repair an essential further part of the strategy for comprehensive management of the disease, and one that must be instituted sufficiently early in the course to save axons. Nor can we provide any evidence to sustain the hope expressed by many patients in the clinic as 'Might I be someone with a better than average capacity for remyelination and repair?' or can we support the clinical evidence that structure and function do recover over time by showing that genetic factors determine good and poor responders. As we discuss in Chapter 3, there is no confirmation of the single report, itself indirect, that a ciliary neurotrophic factor polymorphism confers poor regenerative potential following disease activity. Standing back from these dilemmas of neurobiological reasoning and clinical science timing, we do anticipate that clinical and neurobiological programmes of research will soon converge to the point where it is appropriate to attempt clinical trials aimed at directly restoring structure and function of strategically placed demyelinating lesions, displacing the passive attitude that treating the disease process is sufficient and may (or may not) carry the added value of improved remyelination.

Hints that endogenous repair might proceed better if only the environment of stubborn lesions could be altered, were originally provided by the observation that spontaneous remyelination is much enhanced in animals with Theiler's murine (demyelinating) encephalomyelitis virus treated with immune serum raised by immunization with spinal cord homogenate. A decade later, the best analysis is that a family of naturally present, autoreactive, IgM antibodies acts to promote the normal reparative potential of the central nervous system. As we discuss in Chapter 18, the earliest attempts to induce remyelination using commercially prepared immunoglobulin failed to demonstrate clinical improvement as a marker of successful remyelination. These trials did not combine immunoglobulin administration with aggressive efforts to stabilize the inflammatory process, and may partly have failed on that account. Addressing the possibility of enhancing remyelination through increased availability of growth promoting molecules, Cannella *et al* (1998) reported that glial growth factor 2 (GGF2) enhances myelin repair in experimental model systems; this compound is currently being tested in preclinical studies for a possible human trial. Butzkueven *et al* (2002) have shown that leukaemia inhibitory factor promotes oligodendrocyte survival and reduces immune-mediated demyelination; and J.L. Mason *et al* (2003) reported that insulin-like growth factor promotes oligodendrocyte survival and enhances remyelination. Considering the complexity of myelination, it seems unlikely that the application of a single growth factor will ever solve the problem, as we discuss in Chapter 10 with respect to the experimental literature. To us, it seems unlikely that the complex task of recoating axons with a myelin sheath could be accomplished better or more easily by anything other than a member of the oligodendrocyte lineage even if, pragmatically, intermediates that stimulate endogenous cells prove easier to administer and deliver.

Remyelination requires juxtaposing cells that have the ability to re-form compact myelin close to intact naked axons. In practice, this will involve access to a cell that is proliferative and migratory because the available experimental evidence indicates that the fully differentiated oligodendrocyte is incapable of division, and intrinsically immobile. This is not surprising in view of the enormous structural complexity of oligodendrocytes, each having multiple processes anchoring the cell to several axons. It seems that only the more streamlined glial progenitor can circumvent these navigational problems; but, even then, inhibitions created physically and biologically by astrocyte scars may prove problematic. As we discuss in Chapter 10, the need somehow to enhance mobility of the remyelinating cell, perhaps through modification of integrins and other cell surface adhesion molecules that determine migration, or manipulation of the environment through which migration is set to occur, is already identified and the problem partly characterized.

When the notion that remyelination might be promoted in multiple sclerosis first arose, it was in the wake of experimental studies using gliotoxins to create focal demyelinating lesions, and their repair by cell implantation. It followed that transplantation became the paradigm for assisted repair in multiple sclerosis. The many limitations and problems that later emerged from the experimental literature made it difficult to suggest a preferred strategy or clinical protocol. Soon after, the arrival of techniques for identifying and manipulating cells of the glial lineage *in vitro* and *in vivo* led to the recognition that adult nervous systems contain oligodendrocyte precursors; and, subsequently, that these accumulate around the edge of persistently demyelinated lesions. There followed a change in emphasis whereby it became simpler and more practical to consider a strategy that exploited this availability, and had as its aims harnessing the potential for endogenous repair, with all the ethical and immunological advantages so conferred, rather than continuing to debate the problems of which cell type and how this might be delivered as the formula for success. But to come full circle, the apparent sluggish behaviour of endogenous oligodendrocyte precursors, and the delays in identifying the environmental conditions needed to coax them into activity, have to some extent been parked by the advent of stem cell biology. As we discuss in Chapter 10, the two features that suggest new possibilities are the evidence for transdifferentiation, whereby cells harvested from one source (skin or bone marrow) can be used to supply another (the nervous system), and the discovery that intravenous delivery of stem cells achieves widespread distribution to the sites of tissue injury. For all these reasons, we keep an open mind on whether the cell needed to enhance remyelination will be provided by host (local or surrogate) or donor tissue.

We do not know whether there is a critical period during which the recently demyelinated axon must be rescued by new myelin, and whether later it loses molecular arrangements that make remyelination possible. Nor is it clear how much percentage loss can be tolerated in a given pathway before function is irreversibly sacrificed, and the opening up of alternative routes or tolerating persistent disabilities become the only options. There are no firm ideas on how many fibres must be repaired in order to achieve sufficient increase in electrical activity to restore function. These issues need answers before clinical strategies are declared, but the thinking has begun. Clearly, it makes no sense to attempt remyelination in a situation where there is already extensive axon degeneration, as is now thought to be the case in patients well established in the progressive phase. For this reason, it could be argued that attempts to repair the lesions of advanced chronic progressive multiple sclerosis are futile. In Chapter 10, we discuss the mechanisms of axon degeneration and regeneration. The message is clear. Fibres in the peripheral nervous system regenerate, those in the central nervous system do not. The difference is in the environment, not the intrinsic capacity for regeneration. Already, some of the molecules that inhibit and facilitate axon growth in the central nervous system are identified; others will no doubt be added to the list – such as brain-derived neurotrophic factor (BDNF), which appears to prevent myelin-associated glycoprotein from inhibiting nerve regeneration (Cai *et al* 1999) – opening other therapeutic mechanisms in due course. Even now, we can speculate that the problems of progressive multiple sclerosis, attributable to axonopathy, might be improved by the use of chondroitin sulfatase, which digests extracellular matrix, and anti-Nogo antibodies, which inhibit the molecules present on myelin that limit axon outgrowth – both soon to be evaluated in the context of spinal cord injury. Trials in multiple sclerosis seem logical and appropriate.

So what are the possibilities, based on contemporary experimental evidence, for repairing demyelinated pathways? Before starting such trials, consideration must be given to how it can be proved that enhancing remyelination stabilizes tissue integrity, re-establishes saltatory conduction and restores neurological function. There is some progress in differentiating demyelinated from remyelinated lesions in the brain by imaging techniques:

the magnetization transfer ratio (MTR) is significantly higher in lesions that are remyelinated (Barkhof *et al* 2003; Schmierer *et al* 2004). In some patients and some lesions, oligodendrocyte progenitor cells are lost, whereas in others the axon is degenerate or not permissive for remyelination. Any strategy for stimulating remyelination depends critically on knowing whether the key problem resides in the axon or the oligodendrocyte. Whatever decisions are ultimately taken on choice of the intervention, and the method of its delivery, an informative lesion is needed in which to assess outcomes. Clinical, imaging and other biomarkers, selected for their sensitivity and specificity in this particular context, are needed. We favour attention to a sentinel lesion rather than general measures of brain structure and constitution. Our view is that, notwithstanding the dilemma posed above, any attempts to enhance remyelination would need to be combined with adequate suppression of disease activity. We conclude that immunological processes, as they occur in the person with multiple sclerosis, do more harm than good; and we find no evidence that the short- or longer-term course of the disease has been adversely affected by immunological treatments, as would by now have become apparent were these systematically compromising repair processes and thereby advancing rates of disability and progression.

Most is known about the spinal cord and this might appear the obvious choice for a first clinical intervention. The symptoms are a major cause of disability, and can to some extent be measured using physiological and imaging techniques. Magnetic resonance imaging usually shows many lesions in series within the corticospinal tracts so that remyelinating any one would be of limited value. Cord atrophy indicating axon degeneration is usually present in patients with stable or progressive deficits. The optic nerve is attractive because the symptoms are clinically eloquent; physiological assessment and imaging are well developed. However, the natural history of optic neuritis is usually for recovery occurring over many months, making it difficult to demonstrate that intervention has altered the natural history of visual recovery. Timing would need fine judgment – waiting for the establishment of persistent visual deficits but avoiding manipulation of a nerve with degenerate axons, because the evidence is that atrophy occurs after unilateral optic neuritis despite recovery of vision (Hickman *et al* 2002a). The cerebellar peduncle gives rise to symptoms that can be measured, and at a site where remyelination is known to occur and can be imaged. The typical severe proximal tremor is usually unilateral. It presents early and rarely recovers spontaneously. The responsible lesion can often be identified, although the presence of multiple infratentorial abnormalities may make identification of the sentinel lesion difficult, and it has spectroscopic features consistent with preserved axons with near normal tissue integrity (Charlotte Brierley, unpublished observations).

If there is a commitment to applying advances in neurobiology to the management of disability and progression in multiple sclerosis, it is not too early to be planning the clinical science strategy. We are sensitive to the needs and aspirations of people with multiple sclerosis for whom remyelination seems to be the missing element in a comprehensive strategy for managing the disorder. At the same time, the application of new knowledge in neurobiology needs to be targeted at individuals in whom the dividend from novel interventions is most likely to be present and detectable – in the interests of the many others for whom this may represent an important adjunct to presently available (or future) therapies that successfully limit ongoing disease activity. Planning for these applications requires a sophisticated infrastructure and needs to be no less rigorous than the programme of neurobiology on which much preclinical work depends. To summarize much that has gone before, the planning must address:

- *Goals*: the prospect for combining existing treatments for modifying the course of multiple sclerosis with interventions that aim to restore structure and function is timely given the advances in knowledge relating to the processes of tissue damage and repair. Patients have long expected that clinical science can deliver strategies that both limit and repair the damage.
- *Therapy*: candidates are likely either to be cell based – sacrificing detailed knowledge of the elements needed to replace myelin sheaths and protect the underlying axons in the interests of using 'something that works' – or factors that act to engage host tissues and realize the potential for endogenous remyelination.
- *Delivery*: intravenous or intrathecal administration results in widespread delivery throughout the inflammatory neuraxis, with axonal protection and functional improvement, obviating the need for multiple stereotactic transplants – an important practical consideration and one that has (reasonably) proved a conceptual stumbling block for those asked to evaluate the possibility of cell-based therapies in recent years.
- *Recipient*: timing matters, selecting an epoch when the nervous system is irreversibly injured but not so degenerate as to leave no tissue amenable for repair and the restoration of function.
- *Treatment of ongoing disease activity*: it seems certain that disease-modifying treatment will be needed in order to maximize prospects that the intervention gains a foothold, and protects functional new myelin from further waves of tissue destruction.
- *Outcomes*: detailed protocols must be developed for screening the outcome of remyelination therapy, extrapolating the experience of a sentinel lesion to the disease as a whole, and selecting the anatomically defined lesion on the basis that this has objectively measurable clinical and paraclinical outcomes; assessments will include neurophysiological, imaging and clinical disability/functional measurements.

TAILORING TREATMENT TO DEFINED GROUPS

Throughout, we have discussed future prospects on the basis that multiple sclerosis is one disease. In Chapter 14, we debate the issue of complexity and heterogeneity. The existence of several disease mechanisms would imply that subtle or radical differences in approach might be needed for separate groups of patients. At present, we are not in a position to stratify subgroups of patients in a way that is reliable enough to justify 'bespoke' treatments. But the pharmacogenetics agenda, and the implications of dissecting the pathology so as to separate disease mechanisms, make it likely that these choices will eventually emerge. Microarray techniques are clarifying how currently available therapies impact on gene expression in patients and may ultimately provide insight into what determines which patients will respond favourably to a medication ('responder status'; Koike *et al* 2003; Stürzebecher *et al* 2003). Increasingly, biomarkers are becoming available that provide signatures for variations on a single theme or different works in the one repertoire (Lassmann *et al* 2003; Lennon *et al* 2004; Lucchinetti *et al* 2000).

POSTSCRIPT

With each visit, we update our patients on recent progress, reviewing particularly the advances that pertain to their case. We remind them of the fundamental importance of the basic and clinical science research efforts needed to identify better treatments and ultimately to eliminate this disease. Although our ability to affect the long-term course of multiple sclerosis is unpredictable, we do now have a greater range of symptomatic and disease-modifying treatments than was hitherto available. We also recognize the need for experience and thoroughness in providing evidence-based advice on treatment so as to optimize the care of individual patients. We ended the previous edition of this book acknowledging that patients often ask 'when will the problem of multiple sclerosis be solved?' This has not changed. Again, we cannot guess, but continue to offer encouragement that the pace of research has never been more active, the orientation of that research never more coherent, and the prospects for a dividend from the vast investment of resources and hope in solving this difficult disease never better.

References

Abb L, Schaltenbrand G 1956 Statistische Untersuchung zum Problem der multiplen Sklerose II. *Dtsch Z Nervenheilk* **174**: 199–218

Abbas AK, Murphy KM, Sher A 1996 Functional diversity of helper T lymphocytes. *Nature* **383**: 787–793

Abbott NJ 2002 Astrocyte–endothelial interactions and blood-brain barrier permeability. *J Anat* **200**: 629–638

Abbott RJ, Howe JG, Currie S, Holland J 1982 Multiple sclerosis plaque mimicking tumour on computed tomography. *Br Med J* **285**: 1616–1617

Abbruzzese G, Gandolfo C, Loeb C 1983 Bolus methylprednisolone vs ACTH in the treatment of multiple sclerosis. *Ital J Neurol Sci* **2**: 169–172

Abdul-Majid K-B, Stefferl A, Bourquin C et al 2002 Fc receptors are critical for autoimmune inflammatory damage to the central nervous system in experimental autoimmune encephalomyelitis. *Scand J Immunol* **55**: 70–81

Abecasis GR, Cherny SS, Cookson WO, Cardon LR 2002 Merlin – rapid analysis of dense genetic maps using sparse gene flow trees. *Nature Genet* **30**: 97–101

Abele M, Schols L, Schwartz S, Klockgether T 2003 Prevalence of antigliadin antibodies in ataxia patients. *Neurology* **60**: 1566–1568

Abernethy J 1809 *Surgical Observations on the Constitutional Origin and Treatment of Local Disease; and on Aneurisms*. London: Longman, Hurst, Rees & Orme, pp. 91–94

Ablashi DV, Lapps W, Kaplan M et al 1998 Human herpesvirus-6 (HHV-6) infection in multiple sclerosis: a preliminary report. *Mult Scler* **4**: 490–496

Aboul-Enein F, Lassmann H 2005 Mitochondrial damage and histotoxic hypoxia: a pathway of tissue injury in inflammatory brain disease? *Acta Neuropathol* **109**: 49–55

Aboul-Enein F, Rauschka H, Kornel B et al 2003 Preferential loss of myelin associated glycoprotein reflects hypoxia-like white matter damage in stroke and inflammatory brain diseases. *J Neuropath Exp Neurol* **62**: 25–33

Abraham S, Scheinberg LC, Smith CR, La Rocca NG 1997 Neurologic impairment and disability status in outpatients with multiple sclerosis reporting dysphagia symptomatology. *J Neurolog Rehab* **11**: 7–13

Abramsky O 1994 Pregnancy and multiple sclerosis. *Ann Neurol* **36 (Suppl)**: 39–41

Abramsky O, Teitelbaum D, Arnon R 1977 Effect of a synthetic polypeptide (Cop 1) on patients with multiple sclerosis and acute disseminated encephalomyelitis: preliminary report. *J Neurol Sci* **31**: 433–438

Academy of Medical Sciences 2004 *Restoring Neurological Function: Putting the Neurosciences to Work in Neurorehabilitation*. London: Academy of Medical Sciences, p. 71

Acar G, Idiman F, Idiman E et al 2003 Nitric oxide as an activity marker in multiple sclerosis. *J Neurol* **250**: 588–592

Acarin N, Rio J, Fernandez AL et al 1996 Different antiganglioside antibody pattern between relapsing–remitting and progressive multiple sclerosis. *Acta Neurol Scand* **93**: 99–103

Acha-Orbea H, Mitchell DJ, Timmermann L et al 1988 Limited heterogeneity of T cell receptors from lymphocytes mediating autoimmune encephalomyelitis allows specific immune intervention. *Cell* **54**: 263–273

Acheson ED, Bachrach CA, Wright FM 1960 Some comments on the relationship of the distribution of multiple sclerosis to latitude, solar radiation and other variables. *Acta Neurol Scand* **35**: 132–47

Achiron A, Ziv A, Djaldetti R et al 1992a Aphasia in multiple sclerosis: clinical and radiologic correlations. *Neurology* **42**: 2195–2197

Achiron A, Pras E, Gilad R et al 1992b Open controlled therapeutic trial of intravenous immune globulin in relapsing–remitting multiple sclerosis. *Arch Neurol* **49**: 1233–1236

Achiron A, Gabbay U, Gilad R et al 1998 Intravenous immunoglobulin in multiple sclerosis: a double-blind, placebo-controlled trial. *Neurology* **50**: 398–402

Achiron A, Barak Y, Rotstein Z 2003 Longitudinal disability curves for predicting the course of relapsing–remitting multiple sclerosis. *Mult Scler* **9**: 486–491

Achiron A, Edelstein S, Viev-Ner Y et al 2004a Bone strength in multiple sclerosis: cortical midtibial speed-of-sound assessment. *Mult Scler* **10**: 488–493

Achiron A, Kishner I, Dolev M et al 2004b Effect of intravenous immunoglobulin treatment on pregnancy and postpartum-related relapses in multiple sclerosis. *J Neurol* **251**: 1133–1137

Achiron A, Polliack M, Rao SM et al 2005 Cognitive patterns and progression in

multiple sclerosis: construction and validation of percentile curves. *J Neurol Neurosurg Psychiatry* **76**: 744–749

Ackerman KD, Heyman R, Rabin BS et al 2002 Stressful life events precede exacerbations of multiple sclerosis. *Psychosom Med* **64**: 916–920

Ackerman KD, Stover A, Heyman R et al 2003 Relationship of cardiovascular reactivity, stressful life events, and multiple sclerosis disease activity. *Brain Behav Immun* **17**: 141–151

Ackerman R, Rehse-Küpper B, Gollmer E, Schmidt R 1988 Chronic neurologic manifestations of erythema migrans borreliosis. *Ann NY Acad Sci* **539**: 16–23

ACR Ad Hoc Committee on Neuropsychiatric Lupus Nomenclature 1999 The American College of Rheumatology nomenclature and case definitions for neuropsychiatric lupus syndromes. *Arthritis Rheum* **42**: 599–668

Adam AM 1989 Multiple sclerosis: epidemic in Kenya. *East Afr Med J* **66**: 503–506

Adams CW 1977 Pathology of multiple sclerosis: progression of the lesion. *Br Med Bull* **33**:15–20

Adams CW, Poston RN 1990 Macrophage histology in paraffin-embedded multiple sclerosis plaques is demonstrated by the monoclonal pan-macrophage marker HAM-56: correlation with chronicity of the lesion. *Acta Neuropathol* **80**: 208–211

Adams CW, Abdulla YH, Torres EM, Poston RN 1987 Periventricular lesions in multiple sclerosis: their perivenous origin and relationship to granular ependymitis. *Neuropathol Appl Neurobiol* **13**: 141–152

Adams CW, Poston RN, Buk SJ 1989 Pathology, histochemistry and immunocytochemistry of lesions in acute multiple sclerosis. *J Neurol Sci* **92**: 291–306

Adams DK, Sutherland JM, Fletcher WB 1950 Early clinical manifestations of disseminated sclerosis. *Br Med J* **2**: 431–436

Adams RD, Kubik CS 1952 The morbid anatomy of the demyelinating diseases. *Am J Med* **12**: 510–546

Adelman B, Sandrock A, Panzara MA 2005 Natalizumab and progressive multifocal leukoencephalopathy. *N Engl J Med* **353**: 432–433

Ader M, Schachner M, Bartsch U 2001 Transplantation of neural precursor cells into the dysmyelinated CNS of mutant mice deficient in the myelin-associated glycoprotein and Fyn tyrosine kinase. *Eur J Neurosci* **14**: 561–566

Adie WJ 1930 Acute retrobulbar neuritis in disseminated sclerosis. *Trans Ophthalmol Soc UK* **103**: 262–267

Afshar G, Muraro PA, McFarland HF, Martin R 1998 Lack of over-expression of T cell receptor Vβ5.2 in myelin basic protein-specific T cell lines derived from HLA-DR2 positive multiple sclerosis patients and controls. *J Neuroimmunol* **84**: 7–13

Agresti C, Bernardo A, Del Russo N et al 1998 Synergistic stimulation of MHC class I and IRF-1 gene expression by IFN-γ and TNF-α in oligodendrocytes. *Eur J Neurosci* **10**: 2975–2983

Agresti C, Meomartini ME, Amadio S et al 2005 ATP regulates oligodendrocyte progenitor migration, proliferation, and differentiation: involvement of metabotropic P2 receptors. *Brain Res Rev* **48**: 157–165

Agundez JAG, Arroyo R, Ledesma MC et al 1995 Frequency of CYP2D6 allelic variants in multiple sclerosis. *Acta Neurol Scand* **92**: 464–467

Aharoni R, Teitelbaum D, Sela M, Arnon R 1997 Copolymer 1 induces T cells of the T helper type 2 that crossreact with myelin basic protein and suppress experimental autoimmune encephalomyelitis. *Proc Natl Acad Sci USA* **94**: 10821–10826

Aharoni R, Teitelbaum D, Sela M, Arnon R 1998 Bystander suppression of experimental autoimmune encephalomyelitis by T cell lines and clones of the Th2 type induced by copolymer 1. *J Neuroimmunol* **91**: 135–146

Aharoni R, Kayhan B, Eilam R et al 2003 Glatiramer acetate-specific T cells in the brain express T helper 2/3 cytokines and brain-derived neurotrophic factor *in situ*. *Proc Natl Acad Sci USA* **100**: 14157–14162

Ahern GP, Hsu S-F, Jackson MB 1999 Direct actions of nitric oxide on rat neurohypophysial K+ channels. *J Physiol* **520**: 165–176

Ahern GP, Hsu S-F, Klyachko VA, Jackson MB 2000 Induction of persistent sodium current by exogenous and endogenous nitric oxide. *J Biol Chem* **275**: 28810–28815

Ahlgren C, Anderson O 2005 No major birth order effect on the risk of multiple sclerosis. *Neuroepidemiology* **24**: 38–41

Ahmed I 1988 Survival after herpes simplex type II myelitis. *Neurology* **38**: 1500

Aisen M, Arlt G, Foster S 1990 Diaphragmatic paralysis without bulbar or limb paralysis in multiple sclerosis. *Chest* **98**: 499–501

Aisen ML, Arnold A, Baiges I, Maxwell S, Rosen M 1993 The effect of mechanical damping loads on disabling action tremor. *Neurology* **43**: 1346–1350

Aisen M, Sevilla D, Fox N 1996 Inpatient rehabilitation for multiple sclerosis. *J Neurol Rehab* **10**: 43–46

Akassoglou K, Bauer J, Kassiotis G et al 1998 Oligodendrocyte apoptosis and primary demyelination induced by local TNF/p55TNF receptor signaling in the central nervous system of transgenic mice: models for multiple sclerosis with primary oligodendrogliopathy. *Am J Pathol* **153**: 801–813

Akassoglou K, Douni E, Bauer J et al 2003 Exclusive tumor necrosis factor (TNF) signaling by the p75TNF receptor triggers inflammatory ischemia in the CNS of transgenic mice. *Proc Natl Acad Sci USA* **100**: 709–714

Akassoglou K, Adams RA, Bauer J et al 2004 Fibrin depletion decreases inflammation and delays the onset of demyelination in a tumor necrosis factor transgenic mouse model for multiple sclerosis. *Proc Natl Acad Sci USA* **101**: 6698–6703

Akenami FO, Siren V, Koskiniemi M, Siimes MA, Teravainen H, Vaheri A 1996 Cerebrospinal fluid activity of tissue plasminogen activator in patients with neurological diseases. *J Clin Pathol* **49**: 577–580

Åkesson E, Oturai A, Berg J et al 2002 A genome-wide screen for linkage in Nordic sib-pairs with multiple sclerosis. *Genes Immun* **3**: 279–285

Åkesson E, Coraddu F, Marrosu M et al 2003 Refining the linkage analysis on chromosome 10 in 449 sib-pairs with multiple sclerosis. *J Neuroimmunol* **143**: 31–38

Akira S, Takeda K, Kaisho T 2001 Toll-like receptors: critical proteins linking innate and acquired immunity. *Nat Immunol* **2**: 675–680

Akiyama Y, Honmou O, Kato T et al 2001 Transplantation of clonal neural precursor cells derived from adult human brain established functional peripheral myelin in the rat spinal cord. *Exp Neurol* **167**: 27–39

Akiyama Y, Radtke C, Kocsis JD 2002 Remyelination of the rat spinal cord by transplantation of identified bone marrow stromal cells. *J Neurosci* **22**: 6623–6630

Akman-Demir G, Bahar S, Coban O et al 2003 Cranial MRI in Behcet's disease: 134 examinations of 98 patients. *Neuroradiology* **45**: 851–859

Alajouanine T, Thurel T, Papaioanou C 1949 La douleur à type de décharge électrique provoquée par la flexion de la tête et parcourant le corps de haut en bas. *Rev Neurol* **81**: 89–97

Alam SM, Kyriakides T, Lawden M, Newman PK 1993 Methylprednisolone in multiple sclerosis: a comparison of oral with intravenous therapy at equivalent high dose. *J Neurol Neurosurg Psychiatry* **56**: 1219–1220

Albani C, Albani G 1997 A case of cutaneous necrosis during interferon-β 1b (β-IFN) therapy in multiple sclerosis. *J Neurol Neurosurg Psychiatry* **62**: 418–428

Albers JW, Kelly JJ 1989 Acquired inflammatory demyelinating polyneuropathies: clinical and electrodiagnostic features. *Muscle Nerve* **12**: 435–451

Albina JE, Henry WL Jr 1991 Suppression of lymphocyte proliferation through the nitric oxide synthesizing pathway. *J Surg Res* **50**: 403–409

Albrecht PJ, Murtie JC, Ness JK et al 2003 Astrocytes produce CNTF during the remyelination phase of viral-induced spinal cord demyelination to stimulate FGF-2 production. *Neurobiol Dis* **13**: 89–101

Al Deeb SM, Yaqub BA, Bruyn GW, Biary NM 1997 Acute transverse myelitis. A localized form of postinfectious encephalomyelitis. *Brain* **120**: 115–1122

Alderton WK, Cooper CE, Knowles RG 2001 Nitric oxide synthases: structure, function and inhibition. *Biochem J* **357**: 593–615

Al-Din ASN 1986 Multiple sclerosis in Kuwait: clinical and epidemiological study. *J Neurol Neurosurg Psychiatry* **49**: 928–931

Al-Din ASN, Al-Saffar M, Siboo R, Behbehani K 1986 Association between HLA-D region epitopes and multiple sclerosis. *Tissue Antigens* **27**: 196–200

Al-Din ASN, Khogali M, Poser CM et al 1990 Epidemiology of multiple sclerosis in Arabs in Kuwait: a comparative study between Kuwaitis and Palestinians. *J Neurol Sci* **100**: 137–141

Aladro Y, Alemany MJ, Perez-Vieitez MC et al 2005 Prevalence and incidence of multiple sclerosis in Las Palmas, Canary Islands, Spain. *Neuroepidemiology* **24**: 70–75

Al-Araji A, Mohammed AI 2005 Multiple sclerosis in Iraq: does it have the same features encountered in Western countries? *J Neurol Sci* **234**: 67–71

Al-Araji AH, Oger J 2005 Reappraisal of Lhermitte's sign in multiple sclerosis. *Mult Scler* **11**: 398–402

Alehan FK, Kahveci S, Uslu Y et al 2004 Acute disseminated encephalomyelitis associated with hepatitis A virus infection. *Ann Trop Paediatr* **24**: 141–144

Alessandri-Haber N, Paillart C, Arsac C et al 1999 Specific distribution of sodium channels in axons of rat embryo spinal motoneurones. *J Physiol* **518**: 203–214

Alexander EL, Malinow K, Lejewski JE, Jerdan ME, Provost TT, Alexander GE 1986 Primary Sjögren's syndrome with central nervous system disease mimicking multiple sclerosis. *Ann Intern Med* **104**: 323–330

Alexander L, Loman J, Lesses HF, Green I 1950 Blood groups and multiple sclerosis. *Assoc Res Nerv Ment Disease* **28**: 179–200

Alexander WS 2002 Suppressors of cytokine signalling (SOCS) in the immune system. *Nature Rev Immunol* **2**: 410–416

Alizadeh M, Babron M-C, Birebent B et al 2003a Genetic interaction of CTLA-4 with HLA-DR15 in multiple sclerosis patients. *Ann Neurol* **54**: 119–122

Alizadeh M, Génin E, Babron MC et al 2003b Genetic analysis of multiple sclerosis in Europeans: French data. *J Neuroimmunol* **143**: 74–78

Allarmargot C, Pouplard-Barthelaix A, Fressinaud C 2001 A single intracerebral microinjection of platelet-derived growth factor (PDGF) accelerates the rate of remyelination in vivo. *Brain Res* **918**: 28–39

Allbutt TC 1871 *On the Use of the Ophthalmoscope in Disease of the Nervous*

System and the Kidneys. London: Macmillan

Allcock RJ, de la Concha EG, Fernandez-Arguero M *et al* 1999 Susceptibility to multiple sclerosis mediated by HLA-DRB1 is influenced by a second gene telomeric of the TNF cluster. *Hum Immunol* **60**: 1266–1273

Allegretta M, Nicklas JA, Sriram S, Albertini RJ 1990 T cells responsive to myelin basic protein in patients with multiple sclerosis. *Science* **247**: 718–721

Allen IV 1991 Pathology of multiple sclerosis. In: Matthews WB (ed.) *McAlpine's Multiple Sclerosis*, 2nd edn. Edinburgh: Churchill Livingstone, pp. 341–378

Allen IV, Millar JH, Hutchinson MJ 1978 General disease in 120 necropsy-proven cases of multiple sclerosis. *Neuropathol Appl Neurobiol* **4**: 279–284

Allen IV, Glover G, McKeown SR, McCormick D 1979 The cellular origin of lysosomal enzymes in the plaque in multiple sclerosis. A histochemical study with combined demonstration of myelin and acid phosphatase. *Neuropathol Appl Neurobiol* **5**: 197–210

Allen IV, Glover G, Anderson R 1981 Abnormalities in the macroscopically normal white matter in cases of mild or spinal multiple sclerosis (MS). *Acta Neuropathol* **7 (Suppl)**: 176–178

Allen IV, McQuid S, Miradkhur M, Nevin G 2001 Pathological abnormalities in the normal-appearing white matter in multiple sclerosis. *Neurol Sci* **22**:141–144

Allen KW 1994 The prevalence of multiple sclerosis in the health district of Bassetlaw. In: Firnhaber W, Lauer K (eds) *Multiple Sclerosis in Europe: An Epidemiological Update*. Darmstadt: Leuchtturm-Verlag/LTV Press, pp. 104–112

Allen M, Sandberg-Wollheim M, Sjogren K *et al* 1994 Association of susceptibility to multiple sclerosis in Sweden with HLA class II DRB1 and DQB1 alleles. *Hum Immunol* **39**: 41–48

Allen RK, Sellars RE, Sandstrom PA 2003 A prospective study of 32 patients with neurosarcoidosis. *Sarcoidosis Vasc Diffuse Lung Dis* **20**: 149–151

Allison RS 1931 Disseminated sclerosis in North Wales: an inquiry into its incidence, frequency, distribution and other etiological factors. *Brain* **53**: 391–430

Allison RS 1943 *Sea Diseases*. London: Bale

Allison RS 1950 Survival in disseminated sclerosis: a clinical study of a series of cases first seen twenty years ago. *Brain* **73**: 103–120

Allison RS 1963 Some neurologic aspects of medical geography. *Proc R Soc Med* **56**: 71–76

Allison RS, Millar JHD 1954 Prevalence and familial incidence of disseminated sclerosis (a report to the Northern Ireland Hospitals Authority on the results of a three year survey). Prevalence of disseminated sclerosis in Northern Ireland. *Ulster Med J* **23 (Suppl 2)**: 91

Allison TJ, Garboczi DN 2002 Structure of γδ T cell receptors and their recognition of non-peptide antigens. *Mol Immunol* **38**: 1051–1061

Almazan G, Liu HN, Khorchid A *et al* 2000 Exposure of developing oligodendrocytes to cadmium causes HSP72 induction, free radical generation, reduction of glutathione levels, and cell death. *Free Radic Biol Med* **29**: 858–869

Almeras L, Meresse B, Seze J *et al* 2002 Interleukin-10 promoter polymorphism in multiple sclerosis: association with disease progression. *Eur Cytokine Netw* **13**: 200–206

Aloisi F, Giampaolo A, Russo G *et al* 1992 Developmental appearance, antigenic profile and proliferation of glial cells of the human embryonic spinal cord. *Glia* **5**: 171–181

Alonso G 2000 Prolonged corticosterone treatment of adult rats inhibits the proliferation of oligodendrocyte progenitors present throughout white and gray matter regions of the brain. *Glia* **31**: 219–231

Alonso-Valle H, Munoz R, Hernandez JL, Matorras P 2001 Acute disseminated encephalomyelitis following *Leptospira* infection. *Eur Neurol* **46**:104–105

Alotaibi S, Kennedy J, Tellier R *et al* 2004 Epstein–Barr virus in pediatric multiple sclerosis. *J Am Med Assoc* **291**: 1875–1879

Alperovitch A, LaCanuet P, Marteau R 1981 Birth order and risk of multiple sclerosis: are they associated and how? *Acta Neurol Scand* **63**: 136–138

Alpini D, Pugnetti L, Caputo D *et al* 2004 Vestibular evoked myogenic potentials in multiple sclerosis: clinical and imaging correlations. *Mult Scler* **10**: 316–321

Alsalameh S, Manger B, Kern P, Kalden J 1998 New onset of rheumatoid arthritis during interferon beta-1b treatment in a patient with multiple sclerosis: comment on the case report by Jabaily and Thompson. *Arthritis Rheum* **41**: 754

Al-Shammri S, Nelson RF, Voevodin A 2003 HHV-6 DNAemia in patients with multiple sclerosis in Kuwait. *Acta Neurol Scand* **107**: 122–124

Al-Shammri S, Nelson RF, Al-Muzairi I, Akanji AO 2004 HLA determinants of susceptibility to multiple sclerosis in an Arabian Gulf population. *Mult Scler* **10**: 381–386

Alshubaili AF, Alramzy K, Ayyad, YM, Gerish Y 2005 Epidemiology of multiple sclerosis in Kuwait: new trends in incidence and prevalence. *Eur Neurol* **53**: 125–131

Alter M, Speer J 1968 Clinical evaluation of possible etiologic factors in multiple sclerosis. *Neurology* **18**: 109–115

Alter M, Halpern L, Kurland LT *et al* 1962 Multiple sclerosis in Israel: prevalence among immigrants and native inhabitants. *Arch Neurol* **7**: 253–263

Alter M, Okihiro M, Rowley W, Morris T 1971 Multiple sclerosis among orientals and caucasians in Hawaii. *Neurology* **21**: 122–130

Alter M, Harshe M, Anderson E *et al* 1976 Genetic association of multiple sclerosis and HLA determinants. *Neurology* **26**: 31–36

Alter M, Kahana E, Loewenson R 1978 Migration and risk of multiple sclerosis. *Neurology* **28**: 1089–1093

Althaus HH, Kloppner S, Schmidt-Schultz T, Schwartz P 1992 Nerve growth factor induces proliferation and enhances fiber regeneration in oligodendrocytes isolated from adult pig brain. *Neurosci Lett* **135**: 219–223

Althaus J 1877 *Diseases of the Nervous System*. London: Smith Elder & Co, pp. 330–335

Altintas A, Cai Z, Pease LR, Rodriguez M 1993 Differential expression of H-2K and H-2D in the central nervous system of mice infected with Theiler's virus. *J. Immunol* **151**: 2803–2812

Altintas A, Alici Y, Melikoglu M, Siva A 2002 Arthritis during interferon beta-1b treatment in multiple sclerosis. *Mult Scler* **8**: 534–536

Altrocchi PH 1963 Acute transverse myelopathy. *Arch Neurol* **9**: 111–119

Alusi SH, Glickman S, Aziz TZ, Bain PG 1999 Tremor in multiple sclerosis. *J Neurol Neurosurg Psychiatry* **66**: 131–134

Alusi SH, Worthington J, Glickman S, Bain PG 2001a A study of tremor in multiple sclerosis. *Brain* **124**: 720–730

Alusi SH, Aziz TZ, Glickman S *et al* 2001b Stereotactic lesional surgery for the treatment of tremor in multiple sclerosis: a prospective case-controlled study. *Brain* **124**: 1576–1589

Alvarado-de la Barrera C, Zuniga-Ramos J *et al* 2000 HLA class II genotypes in Mexican Mestizos with familial and non-familial multiple sclerosis. *Neurology* **55**: 1897–1900

Alvarez G, Castillo JL, Ruiz F *et al* 1992 Multiple sclerosis in Chile. *Acta Neurol Scand* **85**: 1–4

Alvarez-Dolado M, Pardal R, Garcia-Verdugo JM *et al* 2003 Fusion of bone-marrow-derived cells with Purkinje neurons, cardiomyocytes and hepatocytes. *Nature* **425**: 968–973

Alves D, Pires MM, Guimarès A, Miranda MC 1986 Four cases of late onset metachromatic leukodystrophy in a family: clinical, biochemical and neuropathological studies. *J Neurol Neurosurg Psychiatry* **49**: 1417–1422

Alvord EC 1985 Disseminated encephalomyelitis: its variations in form and their relationships to other diseases of the nervous system. In: Koetsier JC (ed.) *Handbook of Clinical Neurology*, Vol 47. Amsterdam: Elsevier, pp. 467–502

Alvord EC, Kies MW 1959 Clinico-pathological correlations in experimental allergic encephalomyelitis II Development of an index for quantitative assay of encephalitogenic activity of antigens. *J Neuropath Exp Neurol* **18**: 447–457

Alvord EC, Shaw CM, Hruby S, Kies MW 1965 Encephalitogen-induced inhibition of experimental allergic encephalomyelitis: prevention, suppression and therapy. *Ann NY Acad Sci* **122**: 333–345

Amato MP, Ponziani G 2000 A prospective study on the prognosis of multiple sclerosis. *Neurol Sci* **21 (Suppl)**: 831–838

Amato MP, Fratiglioni L, Groppi C et al 1988 Interrater reliability in assessing functional systems and disability on Kurtzke scale in multiple sclerosis. *Arch Neurol* **45**: 746–748

Amato MP, Pracucci G, Ponziano G et al 1993 Long term safety of azathioprine therapy in multiple sclerosis. *Neurology* **43**: 831–833

Amato MP, Ponziani G, Pracucci G et al 1995 Cognitive impairment in early-onset multiple sclerosis. Pattern, predictors, and impact on everyday life in a 4-year follow-up. *Arch Neurol* **52**: 168–172

Amato MP, Ponziani G, Bartolozzi ML, Siracusa G 1999 A prospective study on the natural history of multiple sclerosis: clues to the conduct and interpretation of clinical trials. *J Neurol Sci* **168**: 96–106

Amato MP, Ponziani G, Siracusa G, Sorbi S 2001 Cognitive dysfunction in early-onset multiple sclerosis: a reappraisal after 10 years. *Arch Neurol* **58**: 1602–1606

Amato MP, Battaglia MA, Caputo D et al 2002 The costs of multiple sclerosis: a cross-sectional, multicenter cost-of-illness study in Italy. *J Neurol* **249**: 152–163

Amato MP, Grimaud J, Achiti I et al 2004 European validation of a standardized clinical description of multiple sclerosis. *J Neurol* **251**: 1472–1480

Ambrosini E, Columba-Cabezas S, Serafini B et al 2003 Astrocytes are the major intracerebral source of macrophage inflammatory protein-3alpha/CCL20 in relapsing experimental autoimmune encephalomyelitis and in vitro. *Glia* **41**: 290–300

Amela-Peris R, Aladro Y, Conde-Sendin MA et al 2004 Familial multiple sclerosis in Canary Islands. *Rev Neurol* **39**: 911–914

American PVO 1999 *Multiple Sclerosis Clinical Practice Guidelines: Fatigue And Multiple Sclerosis – evidence-based management strategies for fatigue in multiple sclerosis.* Washington, DC: Paralyzed Veterans of America

Ames FR, Louw S 1977 Multiple sclerosis in coloured South Africans. *J Neurol Neurosurg Psychiatry* **40**: 729–735

Aminoff MJ, Logue V 1974 Clinical features of spinal vascular malformations. *Brain* **97**: 197–210

Amirzargar A, Mytilineos J, Yousefipour A et al 1998 HLA class II (DRB1, DQA1 and DQB1) associated genetic susceptibility in Iranian multiple sclerosis (MS) patients. *Eur J Immunogenet* **25**: 297–301

Amor S, Groome N, Linington C et al 1994 Identification of epitopes of myelin oligodendrocyte glycoprotein for the induction of experimental allergic encephalomyelitis in SJL and Biozzi AB/H mice. *J Immunol* **153**: 4349–4356

An SF, Groves M, Martinian L et al 2002 Detection of infectious agents in brain of patients with acute hemorrhagic leukoencephalitis. *J Neurovirol* **8**: 439–446

Andermann F, Cosgrove JBR, Lloyd-Smith D, Walters AM 1959 Paroxysmal dysarthria and ataxia in multiple sclerosis. A report of two unusual cases. *Neurology* **9**: 211–216

Andermann F, Cosgrove JBR, Lloyd-Smith DL et al 1961 Facial myokymia in multiple sclerosis. *Brain* **84**: 31–44

Andersen O, Lygner P-E, Bergstrom T et al 1993 Viral infections trigger multiple sclerosis relapses: a prospective seroepidemiological study. *J Neurol* **240**: 417–422

Andersen O, Lycke J, Tollesson PO et al 1996 Linomide reduces the rate of active lesions in relapsing–remitting multiple sclerosis. *Neurology* **47**: 895–900

Anderson AC, Nicholson LB, Legge KL et al 2000 High frequency of autoreactive myelin proteolipid protein-specific T cells in the periphery of naive mice: mechanisms of selection of the self-reactive repertoire. *J Exp Med* **191**: 761–770

Anderson CM, Nedergaard M 2003 Astrocyte-mediated control of cerebral microcirculation. *Trends Neurosci* **26**: 340–344

Anderson DW, Ellenberg JH, Leventhal CM et al 1992 Revised estimate of the prevalence of multiple sclerosis in the United States. *Ann Neurol* **31**: 333–336

Anderson MS, Venanzi ES, Klein L et al 2002 Projection of an immunological self shadow within the thymus by the AIRE protein. *Science* **298**: 1395–1401

Anderson SA, Shukaliak-Quandt J, Jordan EK et al 2004 Magnetic resonance imaging of labelled T-cells in a mouse model of multiple sclerosis. *Ann Neurol* **55**: 654–659

Anderson UG, Bjork L, Skansen-Saphir U, Anderson JP 1993 Down-regulation of cytokine production and interleukin-2 receptor expression by pooled human IgG. *Immunology* **79**: 211–216

Andersson M, Alvarez-Cermeno J, Bernardi G et al 1994 Cerebrospinal fluid in the diagnosis of multiple sclerosis: a consensus report. *J Neurol Neurosurg Psychiatry* **57**: 897–902

Andersson PB, Perry VH, Gordon S 1992 The acute inflammatory response to lipopolysaccharide in CNS parenchyma differs from that in other body tissues. *Neuroscience* **48**: 169–186

Andersson PB, Waubant E, Gee L, Goodkin DE 1999 Multiple sclerosis that is progressive from the time of onset. Clinical characteristics and progression of disability. *Arch Neurol* **56**: 1138–1142

Andjelkovic AV, Pachter JS 1998 Central nervous system endothelium in neuroinflammatory, neuroinfectious, and neurodegenerative disease. *J Neurosci Res* **51**: 423–430

Andler W, Roosen K 1980 Multiple Sklerose im ersten Lebensjahrzehnt. *Klin Pädiatr* **192**: 365–369

Ando DG, Clayton J, Kono D et al 1989 Encephalitogenic T cells in the B10.PL model of experimental allergic encephalomyelitis (EAE) are of the Th1 lymphokine subtype cell. *Immunology* **124**: 132–143

de Andres C, Guillem A, Rodriguez-Mahou M, Lopez Longo FJ 2001 Frequency and significance of anti-Ro (SS-A) antibodies in multiple sclerosis patients. *Acta Neurol Scand* **104**: 83–87

Andrews JM 1972 The ultrastructural neuropathology of multiple sclerosis. In: Wolfgram F, Ellison GW, Stevens JG (eds) *Multiple Sclerosis. Immunology, Virology and Ultrastructure.* New York: Academic Press, pp. 23–52

Andrews KL, Husmann DA 1997 Bladder dysfunction and management in multiple sclerosis. *Mayo Clin Proc* **72**: 1176–1183

von Andrian UH, Engelhardt B 2003 Alpha4 integrins as therapeutic targets in autoimmune disease. *N Engl J Med* **348**: 68–72

von Andrian UH, Mackay CR 2000 T cell function and migration: two sides of the same coin. *N Engl J Med* **343**: 1020–1034

Andrianokos AA, Duffy J, Suzuki M, Sharp JT 1976 Transverse myelopathy in systemic lupus erythematosus. Report of three cases and review of literature. *Ann Intern Med* **83**: 616–624

Andriezen WL 1893 The neuroglial elements of the brain. *Br Med J* **2**: 227–230

Anema JR, Heijenbrok MW, Faes TJC et al 1991 Cardiovascular autonomic function in multiple sclerosis. *J Neurol Sci* **104**: 129–134

Annunziata P, D'Ettorre M, Menchini U et al 1988 Frequency of blood–retina and blood–brain barrier changes in multiple sclerosis. *Ital J Neurol Sci* **9**: 345–349

Annunziata P, Morana P, Giorgio A et al 2003 High frequency psoriasis in relatives is associated with early onset in an Italian multiple sclerosis cohort. *Acta Neurol Scand* **108**: 327–331

Annunziata P, Marroni M, Francisci D, Stagni G 2005 Acute transverse myelitis and hepatitis C virus. *Infez Med* **13**: 45–47

Anon 1873 Guys' Hospital. Case of insular sclerosis of the brain and spinal cord (under the care of Dr Moxon). *Lancet* **i**: 236

Anon 1875a Guys' Hospital. Two cases of insular sclerosis of the brain and spinal cord. *Lancet* **i**: 471–473

Anon 1875b Guys' Hospital. Two cases of insular sclerosis of the brain and spinal cord. *Lancet* **i**: 609

Anon 1875c Report on Clinical Society of London. *Lancet* **i**: 545

Anon 1948 Streptomycin treatment of pulmonary tuberculosis. A Medical Research Council investigation. *Br Med J* **ii**: 769–782

Anon 1950 Die multiple Sklerose des Menschen (book review). *Arch Neurol Psychiatry* **63**: 190

Anon 1992 Diagnosis of Sjögren's syndrome. *Lancet* **340**: 150–151

Anon 1994 Biogen's IFN-β-1a reduces progression of disability in multiple sclerosis. *Clin Courier* **12**: 1–4

Anon 1995 *Morbidity Statistics from General Practice. Fourth National Study 1991–2,*

OPCS series MB5 no. 3. London: HMSO (full version available in electronic format)

Anon 1998 Burden of illness of multiple sclerosis. Part I: Cost of illness. The Canadian Burden of Illness Study Group. *Can J Neurol Sci* **25**: 23–30

Ansari KA 1976 Olfaction in multiple sclerosis. *Eur Neurol* **14**: 138–145

Antel JP, Arnason BGW, Medof ME 1979 Suppressor cell function in multiple sclerosis: correlation with clinical disease severity. *Ann Neurol* **5**: 338–342

Antel JP, Reder AT, Noronha AB 1985 Cellular immunity and immune regulation in multiple sclerosis. *Semin Hematol* **5**: 117–126

Anthony DC, Ferguson B, Matyzak MK et al 1997 Differential matrix and metalloproteinase expression in cases of multiple sclerosis and stroke. *Neuropathol Appl Neurobiol* **23**: 406–415

Anthony DC, Miller KM, Fearn S et al 1998 Matrix metalloproteinase expression in an experimentally induced DTH model of multiple sclerosis. *J Neuroimmunol* **87**: 62–72

Antonovsky A, Leibowitz U, Medalie JM et al 1968 Reappraisal of possible etiologic factors in multiple sclerosis. *Am J Pub Health* **58**: 836–848

Antony JM, van Marle G, Opii W et al 2004 Human endogenous retrospective glycoprotein-mediated induction of redox reactants causes oligodendrocyte death and demyelination. *Nat Neurosci* **7**: 1021–1023

Appay V, Rowland-Jones SL 2002 The assessment of antigen-specific CD8+ T cells through the combination of MHC class I tetramer and intracellular staining. *J Immunol Meth* **268**: 9–19

Apple D, Keinees K, Biehl JP 1978 The syndrome of inappropriate antidiuretic hormone secretion in multiple sclerosis. *Arch Int Med* **138**: 1713–1714

Appleby MW, Ramsdell F 2003 A forward-genetic approach for analysis of the immune system. *Nat Rev Immunol* **3**: 463–471

Araki I, Matsui M Ozawa K et al 2003 Relationship of bladder dysfunction to lesion site in multiple sclerosis. *J Urol* **169**: 1384–1387

Archelos JJ, Hartung HP 2000 Pathogenetic role of autoantibodies in neurological disease. *Trends Neurosci* **23**: 317–327

Archelos JJ, Trotter J, Previtali S et al 1998 Isolation and characterisation of an oligodendrocyte precursor-derived B-cell epitope in multiple sclerosis. *Ann Neurol* **43**: 15–24

Archelos JJ, Storch MK, Hartung HP 2000 The role of B cells and autoantibodies in multiple sclerosis. *Ann Neurol* **47**: 694–706

Archibald CJ, Wei X, Scott JN et al 2004 Posterior fossa lesion volume and slowed information processing in multiple sclerosis. *Brain* **127**: 1526–1534

Arcos-Burgos M, Palacio G, Sanchez JL et al 1999 Multiple sclerosis: association to HLA DQalpha in a tropical population. *Exp Clin Immunogenet* **16**: 131–138

Ardissone P, Rota E, Durelli L et al 2002 Effects of high doses of corticosteroids on bone metabolism. *J Endocrin Invest* **25**: 129–133

Arevalo-Martin A, Vela JM, Molina-Holgado E et al 2003 Therapeutic action of cannabinoids in a murine model of multiple sclerosis. *J Neurosci* **23**: 2511–2516

Ariga T, Miyatake T, Yu RK 2001 Recent studies on the roles of antiglycosphingolipids in the pathogenesis of neurological disorders. *J Neurosci Res* **65**: 363–370

Aring CD 1965 Observations on multiple sclerosis and conversion hysteria. *Brain* **88**: 663–674

Armstrong MA, McDonnell GV, Graham CA et al 1999 Relationship between tumour necrosis factor-alpha (TNFalpha) production and a specific multiple sclerosis (MS) associated TNF gene haplotype. *Mult Scler* **5**: 165–170

Armstrong RC, Dorn HH, Kufta CV et al 1992 Pre-oligodendrocytes from adult human CNS. *J Neurosci* **12**: 1538–1547

Armutlu K, Karabudak R, Nurlu G 2001 Physiotherapy approaches in the treatment of ataxic multiple sclerosis: a pilot study. *Neurorehab Neural Repair* **15**: 203–211

Arnason BGW, Davis FA, Dean G et al 1982 Round the World. *Lancet* **112**: 734

Arnason BGW, Dayal A, Qu ZX et al 1996 Mechanisms of action of interferon-beta in multiple sclerosis. *Springer Semin Immunopathol* **18**: 125–148

Arnason BGW, Jacobs G, Hanlon M et al 1999 TNF neutralization in MS – results of a randomized, placebo-controlled multicenter study. *Neurology* **53**: 457–465

Arnett HA, Mason J, Marino M et al 2001 TNF alpha promotes proliferation of oligodendrocyte progenitors and remyelination. *Nat Neurosci* **4**: 1116–1122

Arnett HA, Fancy SPJ, Alberta JA et al 2004 bHLH transcription factor Olig1 is required to repair demyelinated lesions in the CNS. *Science* **306**: 2111–2115

Arnold AC, Pepose JS, Hepler RS, Foos RY 1984 Retinal periphlebitis and retinitis in multiple sclerosis I. Pathological characteristics. *Ophthalmology* **91**: 255–261

Arnold AC, Baloh RW, Yee RD, Hepler RS 1990 Internuclear ophthalmoplegia in the Chiari type II malformation. *Neurology* **40**: 1850–1854

Arnold B, Schönrich G, Hämmerling GJ 1993 Multiple levels of peripheral tolerance. *Immunol Today* **14**: 12–14

Arnouts C 1959 La sclérose en plaques chez l'enfant: une observation anatomoclinique et une observation clinique nouvelle. *Acta Neurol Belg* **59**: 796–814

Arroyo EJ, Scherer SS 2000 On the molecular architecture of myelinated fibers *Histochem Cell Biol* **113**: 1–18

Arroyo EJ, Xu Y-T, Zhou L et al 1999 Myelinating Schwann cells determine the internodal localization of Kv1.1, Kv1.2, Kvbeta2, and Caspr. *J Neurocytol* **28**: 333–347

Arroyo EJ, Xu T, Grinspan J et al 2002 Genetic dysmyelination alters the molecular architecture of the nodal region. *J Neurosci* **22**: 1726–1737

Arruda WO, Scola RH, Teive HA, Werneck LC 2001 Multiple sclerosis: report on 200 cases from Curitiba, southern Brazil, and comparison with other Brazilian series. *Arq Neuropsiquiatr* **59**: 165–170

Arsenijevic Y, Weiss S, Schneider B, Aebischer P 2001 Insulin-like growth factor-I is necessary for neural stem cell proliferation and demonstrates distinct actions of epidermal growth factor and fibroblast growth factor-2. *J Neurosci* **21**: 7194–7202

Arvanitis DN, Wang H, Bagshaw RD et al 2004 Membrane-associated estrogen receptor and caveolin-1 are present in central nervous system myelin and oligodendrocyte plasma membranes. *J Neurosci Res* **75**: 603–613

Arya SC 2001 Acute disseminated encephalomyelitis associated with poliomyelitis vaccine. *Pediatr Neurol* **24**: 325

Asakura K, Rodriguez M 1998 A unique population of circulating autoantibodies promotes central nervous system remyelination. *Mult Scler* **4**: 217–221

Asakura K, Miller D, Murray K et al 1996 Monoclonal autoantibody SCH94.03, which promotes central nervous system remyelination, recognizes an antigen on the surface of oligodendrocytes. *J Neurosci Res* **43**: 273–281

Ascherio A, Munch M 2001 Epstein Barr virus and multiple sclerosis. *Epidemiology* **11**: 220–224

Ascherio A, Zhang SM, Hernán MA et al 2001b Hepatitis B vaccination and the risk of multiple sclerosis. *New Engl J Med* **344**: 327–332

Ascherio A, Munger KL, Lennette ET et al 2001a Epstein-Barr virus antibodies and risk of multiple sclerosis. A prospective study. *J Amer Med Assoc* **286**: 3083–3088

Aschoff JC, Conrad B, Kornhuber HH 1974 Acquired pendular nystagmus with oscillopsia in multiple sclerosis. *J Neurol Neurosurg Psychiatry* **37**: 570–577

Ashburner J, Friston K 2000 Voxel-based morphometry – the methods. *NeuroImage* **11**: 805–821

Ashworth B 1957 Chronic retrobulbar and chiasmal neuritis. *Br J Ophthalmol* **51**: 698–702

Asselman P, Chadwick DW, Marsden CD 1975 Visual evoked responses in the diagnosis and management of multiple sclerosis. *Brain* **98**: 261–282

van Assen S, Bosma F, Staals LME et al 2004 Acute disseminated encephalomyelitis associated with *Borrelia burgdorferi*. *J Neurol* **251**: 626–629

Attar A, Lemann M, Ferguson A et al 1999 Comparison of a low dose polyethylene glycol electrolyte solution with lactulose for treatment of chronic constipation. *Gut* **44**: 226–230

Atwood A, Poser C 1961 Neurologic complications of Sjögren's syndrome. *Neurology* **11**: 1034–1041

Au WY, Lie AK, Cheung RT et al 2002 Acute disseminated encephalomyelitis after para-influenza infection post bone marrow transplantation. *Leuk Lymphoma* **43**: 455–457

Aubourg P, Feil R, Guidoux S 1990 The red-green visual pigment gene region in adrenoleucodystrophy. *Am J Hum Genet* **46**: 459–469

Auer DP, Schumann EM, Kumpfel T et al 2000 Seasonal fluctuations of gadolinium-enhancing magnetic resonance imaging lesions in multiple sclerosis. *Ann Neurol* **47**: 276–277

Auff E, Budka H 1980 Immunohistologische Methoden in der Neuropathologie. In: Jellinger K (ed.) *Curr Topics Neuropathol Facult Wien* **6**: 21–29

Aulkemeyer P, Hausner G, Brinkmeier H et al 2000 The small sodium-channel blocking factor in the cerebrospinal fluid of multiple sclerosis patients is probably an oligopeptide. *J Neurol Sci* **172**: 49–54

AUSTIMS Research Group 1989 Interferon-α and transfer factor in the treatment of multiple sclerosis: a double blind, placebo-controlled trial. *J Neurol Neurosurg Psychiatry* **52**: 566–574

Austin SG, Zee CS, Waters C 1992 The role of magnetic resonance imaging in acute transverse myelitis. *Can J Neurol Sci* **19**: 508–511

Averbuch-Heller L, Steiner I, Abramsky O 1992 Neurological manifestations of progressive systemic sclerosis. *Arch Neurol* **49**: 1292–1295

Averbuch-Heller L, Stahl JS, Rottach KG, Leigh RJ 1995 Gabapentin as treatment of nystagmus. *Ann Neurol* **38**: 972

Averbuch-Heller L, Tusa RJ, Fuhry L et al 1997 A double-blind controlled study of gabapentin and baclofen as treatment for acquired nystagmus. *Ann Neurol* **41**: 818–825

Avis SP, Pryse-Phillips WE 1995 Sudden death in multiple sclerosis associated with sun exposure: a report of two cases. *Can J Neurol Sci* **22**: 305–307

Axelson O, Landtblom AM, Flodin U 2001 Multiple sclerosis and ionizing radiation. *Neuroepidemiology* **20**: 175–178

Axtell RC, Webb MS, Barnum SR, Raman C 2004 Cutting edge: critical role for CD5 in experimental autoimmune encephalomyelitis: inhibition of engagement reverses disease in mice. *J Immunol* **173**: 2928–2932

Azouvi P, Mane M, Thiebaut JB et al 1996 Intrathecal baclofen administration for control of severe spinal spasticity: functional improvement and long-term follow-up. *Arch Phys Med Rehab* **77**: 35–39

Baas D, Legrand C, Samarut J, Flamant F 2002 Persistence of oligodendrocyte precursor cells and altered myelination in optic nerve associated to retina degeneration in mice devoid of all thyroid hormone receptors. *Proc Natl Acad Sci USA* **99**: 2907–2911

Baba H, Akita H, Ishibashi T et al 1999 Completion of myelin compaction, but not the attachment of oligodendroglial processes triggers K+ channel clustering. *J Neurosci Res* **58**: 752–764

Babbe H, Roers A, Waisman A et al 2000 Clonal expansion of CD8+ T cells dominate the T cell infiltrate in active multiple sclerosis lesions as shown by micromanipulation and single cell polymerase chain reaction. *J Exp Med* **192**: 393–404

Babinski J 1885a *Étude anatomique et clinique sur la sclérose en plaques.* Paris: Masson

Babinski J 1885b Recherches sur l'anatomie pathologique de la sclérose en plaques et etude comparative des diverses varietes de la scléroses de la moelle. *Arch Physiol (Paris)* **2–6**:186–207

Babinski J, Dubois R 1918 Douleurs à forme décharge électrique consécutives aux traumatismes de la nuque. *Presse Méd* **26**: 64

Bach J-F 2003 Regulatory T cells under scrutiny. *Nat Rev Immunol* **3**: 189–198

Bachman DS, Laó-Velez C, Estanol B 1976 Dystonia and choreoathetosis in multiple sclerosis. *Arch Neurol* **33**: 590

Bachmann MF, Kopf M 2001 On the role of the innate immunity in autoimmune disease. *J Exp Med* **193**: F47–F50

Bachmann R, Eugster HP, Frei K et al 1999 Impairment of TNF-receptor 1 signalling but not Fas signalling diminishes T-cell apoptosis in MOG-peptide induced chronic demyelinating autoimmune encephalomyelitis in mice. *Am J Pathol* **154**: 1417–1422

Back SA, Luo NL, Borenstein NS et al 2002 Arrested oligodendrocyte lineage progression during human cerebral white matter development: dissociation between the timing of progenitor differentiation and myelinogenesis. *J Neuropathol Exp Neurol* **61**: 197–211

Bagasra O, Michaels FH, Zheng YM et al 1995 Activation of the inducible form of nitric oxide synthase in the brains of patients with multiple sclerosis. *Proc Natl Acad Sci USA* **92**: 12041–12045

Bagnato F, Jeffries N, Richert ND et al 2003 Evolution of T1 black holes in patients with multiple sclerosis imaged monthly for four years. *Brain* **126**: 1782–1789

Baig S, Olsson T, Yu-Ping J et al 1991 Multiple sclerosis: cells secreting antibodies against myelin-associated glycoprotein are present in the cerebrospinal fluid. *Scand J Immunol* **33**: 73–79

Bailey P 1950 Letter to the editor. *Arch Neurol Psychiatry* **63**: 790

Baillie 1820 Some observations upon paraplegia in adults. *Med Trans R Coll Phys Lond* **6**: 16–26

Bains JS, Ferguson AV 1997 Nitric oxide depolarizes type II paraventricular nucleus neurons in vitro. *Neuroscience* **79**: 149–159

Bajaj NP, Waldman A, Orrell R et al 2002 Familial adult onset of Krabbe's disease resembling hereditary spastic paraplegia with normal neuroimaging. *J Neurol Neurosurg Psychiatry* **72**: 635–638

Bajramovic JJ, Lassmann H, van-Noort JM 1997 Expression of alpha-β-crystallin in glia cells during lesional development in multiple sclerosis. *J Neuroimmunol* **78**: 143–151

Bakchine S, Duyckaerts Ch, Hassine L et al 1991 Lésions neurologiques centrales et périphériques au cours d'un syndrome de Gougerot-Sjögren primitif. *Rev Neurol* **147**: 368–375

Baker DG 2002 Multiple sclerosis and thermoregulatory dysfunction. *J Appl Physiol* **92**: 1779–1780

Baker D, Pryce G 2003 The therapeutic potential of cannabis in multiple sclerosis. *Expert Opin Invest Drugs* **12**: 561–567

Baker D, Rosenwasser OA, O'Neill JK, Turk JL 1995 Genetic analysis of experimental allergic encephalomyelitis in mice. *J Immunol* **155**: 4046–4051

Baker D, Adamson P, Greenwood J 2003 Potential of statins for the treatment of multiple sclerosis. *Lancet Neurol* **2**: 9–10

Baker JB, Larson SJ, Sances A, White PT 1968 Evoked potentials as an aid to the diagnosis of multiple sclerosis. *Neurology* **18**: 286

Baker MD 2000 Axonal flip-flops and oscillators. *Trends Neurosci* **23**: 514–519

Baker MD, Bostock H 1992 Ectopic activity in demyelinated spinal root axons of the rat. *J Physiol* **451**: 539–552

Baker MD, Bostock H 1999 The pH dependence of late sodium current in large sensory neurons. *Neuroscience* **92**: 1119–1130

Bakke A, Myhr KM, Gronning M, Nyland H 1996 Bladder, bowel and sexual dysfunction in patients with multiple sclerosis—a cohort study. *Scand J Urol Nephrol* **179**: 61–66

Bakshi R, Mazziotta JC 1996 Acute transverse myelitis after influenza vaccination: magnetic resonance imaging findings. *J Neuroimag* **6**: 248–250

Bakshi R, Kinkel PR, Mechtler LL et al 1998 Magnetic resonance imaging findings in 22 cases of myelitis: comparison between patients with and without multiple sclerosis. *Eur J Neurol* **5**: 35–48

Bakshi R, Miletich RS, Henschel K et al 1999 Fatigue in multiple sclerosis: cross-sectional correlation with brain MRI findings in 71 patients. *Neurology* **53**: 1151–1153

Bakshi R, Dmochowski J, Shaikh ZA, Jacobs L 2001 Gray matter T2 hypointensity is related to plaques and atrophy in the brains of multiple sclerosis patients. *J Neurol Sci* **185**: 19–26

Bakshi R, Benedict RHB, Bermel RA et al 2002 T2 hypointensity in the deep gray matter of patients with multiple sclerosis. *Arch Neurol* **59**: 62–68

Balashov KE, Olek MJ, Smith DR et al 1998 Seasonal variation of interferon-gamma production in progressive multiple sclerosis. *Ann Neurol* **44**: 824–828

Balashov KE, Rottman JB, Weiner HL, Hancock WW 1999 CCR5(+) and CXCR3(+) T cells are increased in multiple sclerosis and their ligands MIP-1alpha and IP-10 are expressed in demyelinating brain lesions. *Proc Natl Acad Sci USA* **96**: 6873–6878

Ballerini C, Campani D, Rombola G et al 2000 Association of apolipoprotein E polymorphism to clinical heterogeneity of multiple sclerosis. *Neurosci Lett* **296**: 174–176

Ballerini C, Roasati E, Salvetti M et al 2002 Protein tyrosine phosphatase receptor-type C exon 4 gene mutation distribution in an Italian multiple sclerosis population. *Neurosci Lett* **328**: 325–327

Ballerini C, Guerini FR, Rombola G et al 2004 HLA-multiple sclerosis association in continental Italy and correlation with disease prevalence in Europe. *J Neuroimmunol* **150**: 178–185

Balo J 1928 Encephalitis periaxialis concentrica. *Arch Neurol* **19**: 242–264

Balomenos D, Balderas RS, Mulvany KP et al 1995 Incomplete T cell receptor Vb allelic exclusion and dual Vb-expressing cells. *J Immunol* **155**: 3308–3312

Bal-Price A, Brown GC 2001 Inflammatory neurodegeneration mediated by nitric oxide from activated glia-inhibiting neuronal respiration, causing glutamate release and excitotoxicity. *J Neurosci* **21**: 6480–6491

Bamford CR, Sibley W, Laguna JF 1978a Anesthesia in multiple sclerosis. *Can J Neurol Sci* **5**: 41–44

Bamford CR, Sibley WA, Laguna JF 1978b Swine influenza vaccination in patients with multiple sclerosis. *Arch Neurol* **35**: 242–243

Bamford CR, Ganley JP, Sibley WA, Laguna JF 1978c Uveitis, perivenous sheathing and multiple sclerosis. *Neurology* **28**: 119–124

Bamford CR, Smith MS, Sibley WA 1980 Horner's syndrome: an unusual manifestation of multiple sclerosis. *Can J Neurol Sci* **7**: 65–66

Bamford CR, Sibley WA, Thies C et al 1981 Trauma as an etiologic and aggravating factor in multiple sclerosis. *Neurology* **31**: 1229–1234

Bamford CR, Sibley WA, Thies C 1983 Seasonal variation of multiple sclerosis exacerbations in Arizona. *Neurology* **33**: 697–701

Bamji SX, Majdan M, Pozniak CD et al 1998 The p75 neurotrophin receptor mediates neuronal apoptosis and is essential for naturally occurring sympathetic neuron death. *J Cell Biol* **140**: 911–923

Bammer HG, Schaltenbrand G, Solcher H 1960 Zwillingsunter-suchungen bei Multipler Sklerose. *Dtsch Z Nervenheilk* **181**: 261–279

Bammer HG, Hofman A, Zick R 1965 Aderhautentzündungen bei Multipler Sklerose und die sogenannten Uveoenzephalomeningitis. *Dtsch Z Nervenheilk* **187**: 300–316

Ban M, Stewart GJ, Bennetts BH et al 2002 A genome screen for linkage in Australian sibling-pairs with multiple sclerosis. *Genes Immun* **3**: 464–469

Ban M, Sawcer SJ, Heard R et al 2003 A genome wide screen for linkage

disequilibrium in Australian HLA-DRB1*1501 positive multiple sclerosis patients. *J Neuroimmunol* **143**: 60–64

Ban M, Maranian M, Yeo TW et al 2005 No evidence for association of the protein kinase C alpha gene with multiple sclerosis. *J Neurol* **252**: 619–620

Banati RB, Newcombe J, Gunn RN et al 2000 The peripheral benzodiazepine binding site in the brain in multiple sclerosis: quantitative in vivo imaging of microglia as a measure of disease activity. *Brain* **123**: 2321–2337

Bandini F, Castello E, Mazzella L et al 2001 Gabapentin but not vigabatrin is effective in the treatment of acquired nystagmus in multiple sclerosis: how valid is the GABAergic hypothesis? *J Neurol Neurosurg Psychiatry* **71**: 107–110

Bandini F, Beronio A, Ghiglione E et al 2004 The diagnostic value of vestibular evoked myogenic potentials in multiple sclerosis: a comparative study with MRI and visually evoked potentials. *J Neurol* **251**: 617–621

Banerji NK, Millar JHD 1974 Chiari malformation presenting in adult life. *Brain* **97**: 157–168

Bangham CRM, Nightingale S, Cruickshank JK, Daenke S 1989 PCR analysis from multiple sclerosis patients for the presence of HTLV-1. *Science* **246**: 821

Banik NL 1992 Pathogenesis of myelin breakdown in demyelinating diseases: role of proteolytic enzymes. *Crit Rev Neurobiol* **6**: 257–271

Banik NL, Mauldin LB, Hogan EL 1979 Activity of 2′,3′-cyclic nucleotide 3′-phosphorylase in human cerebrospinal fluid. *Ann Neurol* **5**: 539–541

Bansal R, Pfeiffer SE 1997 FGF-2 converts mature oligodendrocytes to a novel phenotype. *J Neurosci Res* **50**: 215–228

Bansal A, van den Boom D, Kammerer S et al 2002 Association testing by DNA pooling: an effective initial screen. *Proc Natl Acad Sci USA* **99**: 16871–16874

Banwell B, Tremlett H 2005 Coming of age: the use of immunomodulatory therapy in children with multiple sclerosis. *Neurology* **64**: 778–779

Baoxun Z, Xuiqin I, Yupu G et al 1981 Multiple sclerosis: a clinical study from Beijing, China. *Eur Neurol* **20**: 394–400

Baranano DE, Ferris CD, Snyder SH 2001 Atypical neural messengers. *Trends Neurosci* **24**: 99–106

Baranzini SE, Jeong MC, Butunoi C et al 1999 B cell repertoire diversity and clonal expansion in multiple sclerosis brain lesions. *J Immunol* **163**: 5133–5144

Barbellion WNP 1919 *The Journal of a Disappointed Man*. London: Chatto & Windus

Barcellos LF, Klitz W, Field LL et al 1997a Association mapping of disease loci using a pooled DNA genomic screen. *Am J Hum Gen* **61**: 734–747

Barcellos LF, Thomson G, Carrington M et al 1997b Chromosome 19 single-locus and

multilocus haplotype associations with multiple sclerosis. evidence of a new susceptibility locus in Caucasian and Chinese patients. *J Am Med Assoc* **278**: 1256–1261

Barcellos LF, Schito AM, Rimmler JB et al 2000 Chemokine receptor Δ5 polymorphism and age of onset in familial multiple sclerosis. Multiple Sclerosis Genetics Group. *Immunogenetics* **51**: 281–288

Barcellos LF, Caillier S, Dragone L et al 2001 PTPRC (CD45) is not associated with the development of multiple sclerosis in US patients. *Nature Genet* **29**: 23–24

Barcellos LF, Oksenberg JR, Green AJ et al 2002 Genetic basis for clinical expression in multiple sclerosis. *Brain* **125**: 150–158

Barcellos LF, Oksenberg JR, Begovich AB et al 2003 HLA-DR2 dose effect on susceptibility to multiple sclerosis and influence on disease course. *Am J Hum Genet* **72**: 710–716

Barcellos LF, Begovich AB, Reynolds RL et al 2004 Linkage and association with the NOS2A locus on chromosome 17q11 in multiple sclerosis. *Ann Neurol* **55**: 793–800

Baretz RM, Stephenson GR 1981 Emotional responses to multiple sclerosis. *Psychosoms* **22**: 117–127

Barger SW, Hörster D, Furukawa K et al 1995 Tumor necrosis factors a and b protect neurons against amyloid b-peptide toxicity: Evidence for involvement of a kB-binding factor and attenuation of peroxide and Ca^{2+} accumulation. *Proc Natl Acad Sci USA* **92**: 9328–9332

Bari F, Errico RA, Louis TM, Busija DW 1996 Interaction between ATP-sensitive K+ channels and nitric oxide on pial arterioles in piglets. *J Cereb Blood Flow Metab* **16**: 1158–1164

Barile L, Lavalle C 1992 Transverse myelitis in systemic lupus erythematosus: the effect of IV pulse methylprednisolone and cyclophosphamide. *J Rheumatol* **19**: 370–372

Barker AT, Jalinous R, Freeeston IL 1985 Non-invasive magnetic stimulation of the human motor cortex. *Lancet* **i**: 1106–1107

Barker AT, Freeston IL, Jalinous R, Jarratt JA 1986 Clinical evaluation of conduction time measurement in central motor pathways using magnetic stimulation of the human brain. *Lancet* **i**: 1325–1326

Barker CF, Billingham RE 1977 Immunologically privileged sites. *Adv Immunol* **25**: 1–54

Barker LF 1922 Exogenous causes of multiple sclerosis. In: *Multiple Sclerosis [Disseminated Sclerosis]*. New York: P.B. Hoeber and the Association for Research in Nervous and Mental Diseases, pp. 22–26, 48

Barkhof F, Polman C 1997 Oral or intravenous methylprednisolone for acute relapses of MS? *Lancet* **349**: 893–894

Barkhof F, Hommes OR, Scheltens P, Valk J 1991 Quantitative MRI changes in gadolinium-DPTA enhancement after high-dose intravenous methylprednisolone in multiple sclerosis. *Neurology* **41**: 1219–1222

Barkhof F, Freguin STFM, Hommes OR et al 1992 A correlative triad of gadolinium-DTPA MRI, EDSS and CSF-MBP in relapsing multiple sclerosis patients treated with high dose intravenous methylprednsiolone. *Neurology* **42**: 63–67

Barkhof F, Tas MW, Frequin ST et al 1994 Limited duration of the effect of methylprednisolone on changes on MRI in multiple sclerosis. *Neuroradiology* **36**: 382–387

Barkhof F, Filippi M, Miller DH et al 1997a Comparison of MR imaging criteria at first presentation to predict conversion to clinically definite multiple sclerosis. *Brain* **120**: 2059–2069

Barkhof F, Filippi M, Miller DH et al 1997b Strategies for optimizing MRI techniques aimed at monitoring disease activity in multiple sclerosis treatment trials. *J Neurol* **244**: 76–84

Barkhof F, Bruck W, De Groot CJ et al 2003a Remyelinated lesions in multiple sclerosis: magnetic resonance image appearance. *Arch Neurol* **60**: 1073–1081

Barkhof F, Rocca M, Francis G et al 2003b Validation of diagnostic magnetic resonance imaging criteria for multiple sclerosis and response to interferon β1a. *Ann Neurol* **53**: 718–724

Barnard RO, Jellinek EH 1967 Multiple sclerosis with amyotrophy complicated by oligodendroglioma: history of recurrent herpes zoster. *J Neurol Sci* **5**: 441–455

Barned S, Goodman AD, Mattson DH 1995 Frequency of antinuclear antibodies in multiple sclerosis. *Neurology* **45**: 384–385

Barnes D, Hughes R 1997 Oral versus intravenous corticosteroids in acute relapses of multiple sclerosis. Authors response. *Lancet* **349**: 1697

Barnes D, McDonald WI 1992 The ocular manifestations of multiple sclerosis. 2. Abnormalities of eye movements. *J Neurol Neurosurg Psychiatry* **55**: 863–868

Barnes D, McDonald WI, Landon DN, Johnson G 1988 The characterization of experimental gliosis by quantitative nuclear magnetic resonance imaging. *Brain* **111**: 83–94

Barnes D, Munro PM, Youl BD et al 1991 The longstanding MS lesion: a quantitative MRI and electron microscopic study. *Brain* **114**: 1271–1280

Barnes D, Hughes RAC, Morris RW et al 1997 Randomised trial of oral and intravenous methylprednisolone in acute relapses of multiple sclerosis. *Lancet* **349**: 902–906

Barnes MP, Bateman DE, Cleland PG et al 1985 Intravenous methylprednisolone for multiple sclerosis in relapse. *J Neurol Neurosurg Psychiatry* **48**: 157–159

Barnett MH, Prineas JW 2004 Relapsing and remitting multiple sclerosis: pathology of the newly forming lesion. *Ann Neurol* **55**: 458–468

Barnett MH, Williams DB, Day S et al 2003 Progressive increase in incidence and prevalence of multiple sclerosis in Newcastle, Australia: a 35-year study. *J Neurol Sci* **213**: 1–6

Barnett SC, Alexander CL, Iwashita Y et al 2000 Identification of a human olfactory ensheathing cell that can effect transplant-mediated remyelination of demyelinated CNS axons. *Brain* **123**: 1581–1588

Baron JL, Madri JA, Ruddle NH et al 1993 Surface expression of α4 integrin by CD4 T cells is required for their entry into brain parenchyma. *J Exp Med* **177**: 57–68

Baron W, Shattil SJ, ffrench-Constant C 2002 The oligodendrocyte precursor mitogen PDGF stimulates proliferation by activation of alpha(v)beta3 integrens. *EMBO J* **21**: 1957–1966

Baron W, Decker L, Colognato H, ffrench-Constant C 2003 Regulation of integrin growth factor interactions in oligodendrocytes by lipid raft microdomains. *Curr Biol* **13**: 151–155

Baron W, Colognato H, ffrench-Constant C 2005 Integrin-growth factor interactions as regulators of oligodendroglial development and function. *Glia* **49**: 467–479

Baron-Van Evercooren A, Avellana-Adalid V, Lachapelle F, Liblau R 1997 Schwann cell transplantation and myelin repair of the CNS. *Mult Scler* **3**: 157–161

Barr D, Kupersmith MJ, Turbin R et al 2000 Isolated sixth nerve palsy: an uncommon presenting sign of multiple sclerosis. *J Neurol* **247**: 701–704

Barratt BJ, Payne F, Rance HE et al 2002 Identification of the sources of error in allele frequency estimations from pooled DNA indicates an optimal experimental design. *Ann Hum Genet* **66**: 393–405

Barratt HJ, Miller D, Rudge P 1988 The site of the lesion causing deafness in multiple sclerosis. *Scand Audiol* **17**: 67–71

Barres BA, Raff MC 1993 Proliferation of oligodendrocyte precursor cells depends on electrical activity in axons. *Nature* **361**: 258–260

Barres BA, Hart IK, Coles HSR et al 1992 Cell death and control of cell survival in the oligodendrocyte lineage. *Cell* **70**: 31–46

Barth KA, Kishimoto Y, Rohr KB et al 1999 Bmp activity establishes a gradient of positional information throughout the entire neural plate. *Development* **126**: 4977–4987

Bartholdi D, Zumsteg D, Verrips A et al 2004 Spinal phenotype of cerebrotendinous xanthomatosis: a pitfall in the diagnosis of multiple sclerosis. *J Neurol* **251**: 105–107

Bartlett PF, Noble MD, Pruss RM et al 1981 Rat neural antigen-2 (RAN-2): a cell surface antigen on astrocytes, ependymal cells, Müller cells and lepto-meninges defined by a monoclonal antibody. *Brain Res* **204**: 339–351

Barton A, Woolmore JA, Ward D et al 2004 Association of protein kinase C alpha (PRKCA) gene with multiple sclerosis in a UK population. *Brain* **127**: 1717–1722

Barton JJS, Cox TA 1993 Acquired pendular nystagmus in multiple sclerosis: clinical observations and the role of optic neuropathy. *J Neurol Neurosurg Psychiatry* **56**: 262–267

Bartosik-Psujek H, Archelos JJ 2004 Tau protein and 14–3–3 are elevated in the cerebrospinal fluid of patients with multiple sclerosis and correlate with intrathecal synthesis of IgG. *J Neurol* **251**: 414–420

Bartsch U, Peshava P, Raff M, Schachner M 1993 Expression of janusin (J1–160/180) in the retina and optic nerve of the developing and adult mouse. *Glia* **9**: 57–69

Bashir R, Okano M, Kleveland et al 1991 SCID/human mouse model of central nervous system lymphoproliferative disease. *Lab Invest* **65**: 702–709

Baskett PJF, Armstrong R 1970 Anaesthetic problems in multiple sclerosis. *Anaesthesia* **25**: 397–401

Bass B, Weinshenker B, Rice GPA et al 1988 Tizanidine versus baclofen in the treatment of spasticity in patients with multiple sclerosis. *Can J Neurol Sci* **15**: 15–19

Basso O, Campi R, Frydenberg M et al 2004 Multiple sclerosis in women having children with multiple partners: a population based study in Denmark. *Mult Scler* **10**: 621–625

Bassoe P, Grinker RR 1930 Human rabies and rabies vaccine encephalomyelitis. *Arch Neurol Psychiatry* **23**: 1138–1160

Bastian HC 1882 Special diseases of the spinal cord. In: R Quain (ed.) *A Dictionary of Medicine: Including General Pathology, General Therpaeutics, Hygiene, and the Diseases Peculiar to Women and Children*, by various writers. London: Longmans Green & Co, pp 1479–1483

Bastian HC 1910 Thrombotic softening of the spinal cord: a case of so-called acuter myelitis. *Lancet* **ii**: 1531–1534

Bateman DE, White JE, Elrington G et al 1987 Three further cases of Lyme disease. *Br Med J* **294**: 548–549

Bates D, Fawcett PRW, Shaw DA, Weightman D 1978 Polyunsaturated fatty acids in treatment of acute remitting multiple sclerosis. *Br Med J* **2**: 1390–1391

Battistini L, Selmaj K, Kowal C et al 1995 Multiple sclerosis: limited diversity of the Vδ2-Jδ3 T-cell receptor in chronic active lesions. *Ann Neurol* **37**: 198–203

Baud O, Greene AE, Li J et al 2004 Gutathione peroxidase-catalase cooperativity is required for resistance to hydrogen peroxide by mature rat oligodendocytes. *J Neurosci* **24**: 1531–1540

Bauer H 1953 Über die Bedutung der Papier-Elektrophorese des Liquors fur die clinische Forschung. *Dtsch Z Nervenheilk* **170**: 381–401

Bauer HJ 1987 Multiple sclerosis in Europe. Symposium report. *J Neurol* **234**: 195–206

Bauer HJ, Hanefeld FA 1993 *Multiple Sclerosis, Its Impact from Childhood to Old Age*. London: Saunders

Bauer HJ, Firnhaber W, Winkler W 1965 Prognostic criteria in multiple sclerosis. *Ann NY Acad Sci* **122**: 542–551

Bauer HJ, Poser S, Ritter G (eds) 1980 *Progress in Multiple Sclerosis Research*. Berlin: Springer-Verlag, p. 677

Bauer J, Wekerle H, Lassmann H 1995 Apoptosis in brain-specific autoimmune disease. *Curr Opin Immunol* **7**: 839–843

Bauer J, Bradl M, Hickey WF *et al* 1998 T cell apoptosis in inflammatory brain lesions: destruction of T-cells does not depend on antigen recognition. *Am J Pathol* **153**: 715–724

Bauer J, Stadelmann C, Bancher C *et al* 1999 Apoptosis of T-lymphocytes in acute disseminated encephalomyelitis. *Acta Neuropathol* **97**: 543–546

Baumann N, Turpin J-C 2000 Adult-onset leukodystrophies. *J Neurol* **247**: 751–759

Baumhackl U 1995 Multiple sclerosis in lower Austria, prevalence in the city and district of St Poelten. *J Neuroimmunol* **Suppl I**: S57

Baumhackl U, Eibl G, Ganzinger U *et al* 2002 Prevalence of multiple sclerosis in Austria: results of a nationwide survey. *Neuroepidemiology* **21**: 226–234

Baumhefner RW, Tourtellotte WW, Syndulkok P *et al* 1987 Effects of intravenous natural beta interferon on clinical neurofunction, magnetic resonance imaging plaque burden, intrablood-brain barrier IgG synthesis, blood and cerebrospinal fluid cellular immunology and visual evoked responses. *Ann Neurol* **22**: 171

Beall SS, Concannon P, Charmley P *et al* 1989 The germline repertoire of T cell receptor beta chain genes in patients with chronic progressive multiple sclerosis. *J Neuroimmunol* **21**: 59–66

Beall SS, Biddison WE, McFarlin DE *et al* 1993 Susceptibility for multiple sclerosis is determined, in part, by inheritance of a 175-kb region of the TCR Vbeta locus and HLA class II genes. *J Neuroimmunol* **45**: 53–60

Beardsley TL, Brown SVL, Sydnor CF, Grimson BS, Klintworth GK 1984 Eleven cases of sarcoidosis of the optic nerve. *Am J Ophthalmol* **97**: 62–77

Beatty WW, Monson N 1996 Problem solving by patients with multiple sclerosis: comparison of performance on the Wisconsin and California Card Sorting Tests. *J Int Neuropsychol Soc* **2**:134–140.

Beatty WW, Goodkin DE, Monson N *et al* 1988 Anterograde and retrograde amnesia in patients with chronic progressive multiple sclerosis. *Arch Neurol* **45**: 611–619

Beatty WW, Goodkin DE, Beatty PA, Monson N 1989 Frontal lobe dysfunction and memory impairment in patients with chronic progressive multiple sclerosis. *Brain Cogn* **11**: 73–86

Beaudouin E, Kanny G, Gueant JL *et al* 1992 Anaphylaxie à la carboxymethylcellulose: à propos de deux cas de chocs a des corticoides injectables. *Allerg Immunol* **24**: 333–335

Beaudoin L, Laloux V, Novak J *et al* 2002 NKT cells inhibit the onset of diabetes by impairing the development of pathogenic T cells specific for pancreatic cells. *Immunity* **17**: 725–736

Becchetti A, Gamel K, Torre V 1999 Cyclic nucleotide-gated channels: pore topology studied through the accessibility of reporter cysteines. *J Gen Physiol* **114**: 377–392

Bech E, Lycke J, Gadeberg P *et al* 2002 A randomized, double-blind, placebo-controlled MRI study of anti-herpes virus therapy in MS. *Neurology* **58**: 31–36

Becher B, Durell BG, Noelle RJ 2002 Experimental autoimmune encephalitis and inflammation in the absence of interleukin-12. *J Clin Invest* **110**: 493–497

Becher B, Durell BG, Noelle RJ 2003 IL-23 produced by CNS-resident cells controls T cell encephalitogenicity during the effector phase of experimental autoimmune encephalomyelitis. *J Clin Invest* **112**: 1186–1191

Bechmann I, Steiner B, Gimsa U *et al* 2002 Astrocyte-induced T cell elimination is CD95 ligand dependent. *J Neuroimmunol* **132**: 60–65

Bechtold DA, Smith KJ 2005 Sodium-mediated axonal degeneration in inflammatory demyelinating disease. *J Neurol Sci* **233**: 27–35

Bechtold DA, Davies M, Kapoor R, Smith KJ 2004a Axonal protection in a model of MS: comparison of efficacy of different anticonvulsants. *J Neurol Neurosurg Psychiatry* **75**: 1214

Bechtold DA, Kapoor R, Smith KJ 2004b Axonal protection using flecainide in experimental autoimmune encephalomyelitis. *Ann Neurol* **55**: 607–616

Bechtold DA, Yue X, Evans RM *et al* 2005 Axonal protection in experimental autoimmune neuritis by the sodium channel blocking agent flecainide 1. *Brain* **128**: 18–28

Beck RW, the Optic Neuritis Study Group 1992 Corticosteroid treatment of optic neuritis: a need to change treatment practices. *Neurology* **42**: 1133–1135

Beck RW 1995 The Optic Neuritis Treatment Trial: three-year follow-up results. *Arch Ophthalmol* **113**: 136–137

Beck RW, Cleary PA, Anderson MM *et al* 1992 A randomized controlled trial of corticosteroids in the treatment of acute optic neuritis. *N Engl J Med* **326**: 581–588

Beck RW, Cleary PA, the Optic Neuritis Study Group 1993a Optic neuritis treatment trial. *Arch Ophthalmol* **111**: 773–775

Beck RW, Cleary PA, Trobe JD *et al* 1993b The effect of corticosteroids for acute optic neuritis on the subsequent development of multiple sclerosis. *N Engl J Med* **329**: 1764–1769

Beck RW, Chandler DL, Cole SR *et al* 2002 Interferon beta-1a for early multiple sclerosis: CHAMPS trial subgroup analyses. *Ann Neurol* **51**: 481–490

Beck RW, Trobe JD, Moke PS *et al* 2003 High- and low-risk profiles for the development of multiple sclerosis within 10 years after optic neuritis: experience of the optic neuritis treatment trial. *Arch Opthalmol* **121**: 944–949

Beck S, Trowsdale J 2000 The human major histocompatability complex: lessons from the DNA sequence. *Annu Rev Genomics Hum Genet* **1**: 117–137

Becker KG, Simon RM, Bailey-Wilson JE 1998 Clustering of non-major histocompatibility complex susceptibility candidate loci in human autoimmune disease. *Proc Natl Acad Sci USA* **95**: 9979–9984

Beebe GW, Kurtzke JF, Kurland LT *et al* 1967 Studies in the natural history of multiple sclerosis. III Epidemiological analysis of the army experience in World War II. *Neurology* **17**: 1–17

Beenakker EA, Oparina TI, Hartgring A *et al* 2001 Cooling garment treatment in MS: clinical improvement and decrease in leukocyte NO production. *Neurology* **57**: 892–894

Beer M, Sandstede J, Weilbach F *et al* 2001 Cardiac metabolism and function in patients with multiple sclerosis: a combined 31P-MR-spectroscopy and MRI study. *Rofo Fortschr Geb Rontgenstr Neuen Bildgeb Verfahr* **173**: 399–404

Beer S, Kesselring J 1994 High prevalence of multiple sclerosis in Switzerland. *Neuroepidemiology* **13**: 14–18

Beer S, Rösler KM, Hess CW 1995 Diagnostic value of paraclinical tests in multiple sclerosis: relative sensitivities and specificities for reclassification according to the Poser criteria. *J Neurol Neurosurg Psychiatry* **59**: 152–159

Begovich AB, Helmuth RC, Oksenberg JR *et al* 1990 HLA-DP beta and susceptibility to multiple sclerosis: an analysis of Caucasoid and Japanese patient populations. *Hum Immunol* **28**: 365–372

Behan PO 1977 Diffuse myelitis associated with rubella vaccination. *Br Med J* **1**: 166

Behan PO, Chaudhuri A, Roep BO 2003 The pathogenesis of multiple sclerosis revisited. *J Roy Coll Phys (Edin)* **32**: 244–265

Bejar JM, Ziegler DK 1984 Onset of multiple sclerosis in a 24-month-old child. *Arch Neurol* **41**: 881–882

Belachew S, Aguirre AA, Wang H *et al* 2002 Cyclin-dependent kinase-2 controls oligodendrocyte progenitor cell cycle progression and is downregulated in adult oligodendrocyte progenitors. *J Neurosci* **22**: 8553–8562

Bell MD, Taub DD, Perry VH 1996 Overriding the brain's intrinsic resistance to leucocyte recruitment with intraparenchymal injections of recombinant chemokines. *Neuroscience* **74**: 283–292

Bell RB, Ramachandran S 1995 The relationship of TAP1 and TAP2 dimorphisms to multiple sclerosis susceptibility. *J Neuroimmunol* **59**: 210–214

Bellomi F, Scagnolari C, Tomassini V *et al* 2003 Fate of neutralizing and binding antibodies to IFN beta in MS patients treated with IFN beta for 6 years. *J Neurol Sci* **215**: 3–8

Belopitova L, Guergueltcheva PV, Bojinova V 2001 Definite and suspected multiple sclerosis in children: long-term follow-up and magnetic resonance imaging findings. *J Child Neurol* **16**: 317–324

Ben Hamida M 1977 La sclérose en plaques en Tunisie: étude clinique de 100 observations. *Rev Neurol (Paris)* **33**: 109–117

Bencsik K, Rajda C, Klivenyi P et al 1998 The prevalence of multiple sclerosis in the Hungarian city of Szeged. *Acta Neurol Scand* **97**: 315–319

Bencsik K, Rajda C, Fuvesi J et al 2001 The prevalence of multiple sclerosis, distribution of clinical forms of the disease and functional status of patients in Csongrad County, Hungary. *Eur Neurol* **46**: 206–209

Ben-Dov N, Hallevy C, Almog Y 2002 Cervical cord syndrome complicating pneumococcal pneumonia. *J Neurol* **249**: 1309–1310

Benedikz JG, Magnusson H, Poser CM et al 1991 Multiple sclerosis in Iceland 1900–1985. *J Trop Geogr Neurol* **1**: 16–22

Benedikz JG, Magnusson H, Gudmundsson G 1994 Multiple sclerosis in Iceland, with observations on the alleged epidemic in the Faroe Islands. *Ann Neurol* **36 (Suppl 2)**: S175–S179

Benedikz JG, Stefansson M, Gudmundsson J et al 2002 The natural history of untreated multiple sclerosis in Iceland. A total population-based 50 year prospective study. *Clin Neurol Neurosurg* **104**: 208–210

Ben-Hur T, Einstein O, Mizrachi-Kol R et al 2003 Transplanted multipotential neural precursor cells migrate into the inflamed white matter in response to experimental autoimmune encephalomyelitis. *Glia* **41**: 73–80

Benito-Leon J, Martin E, Vela L et al 1998 Multiple sclerosis in Mostoles, central Spain. *Acta Neurol Scand* **98**: 238–242

Benito-Leon J, Morales JM, Rivera-Navarro J 2002 Health-related quality of life and its relationship to cognitive and emotional functioning in multiple sclerosis patients. *Eur J Neurol* **9**: 497–502

Benjelloun N, Charriaut-Marlangue C, Hantaz-Ambroise D et al 2002 Induction of cell death in rat brain by a gliotoxic factor from cerebrospinal fluid in multiple sclerosis. *Cell Mol Biol* **48**: 205–212

Benn T, Halfpenny C, Scolding N 2001 Glial cells as targets for cytotoxic immune mediators. *Glia* **36**: 200–211

Bennett L, Hamilton R, Neutel CI et al 1977 Survey of persons with multiple sclerosis in Ottawa, 1974–1975. *Can J Public Health* **68**: 141–147

Bennett V, Lambert S 1999 Physiological roles of axonal ankyrins in survival of premyelinated axons and localization of voltage-gated sodium channels. *J Neurocytol* **28**: 303–318

Bennetto L, Totham A, Healy P et al 2004 Plasma exchange in episodes of severe inflammatory demyelination of the central nervous system. A report of six cases. *J Neurol* **251**: 1515–1521

Bennetts BH, Teutsch SM, Heard RN et al 1995 TAP2 polymorphisms in Australian multiple sclerosis patients. *J Neuroimmunol* **59**: 111–121

Bennetts BH, Teutsch SM, Buhler MM et al 1997 The CCR5 deletion mutation fails to protect against multiple sclerosis. *Hum Immunol* **58**: 52–59

Bennetts BH, Teutsch SM, Buhler MM et al 1999 HLA-DMB gene and HLA-DRA promoter region polymorphisms in Australian multiple sclerosis patients. *Hum Immunol* **60**: 886–893

Ben-Nun A, Cohen IR 1982 Experimental autoimmune encephalomyelitis (EAE) mediated by T cell lines: process of selection of lines and characterization of the cells. *J Immunol* **129**: 303–308

Ben-Nun A, Wekerle H, Cohen IR 1981a The rapid isolation of clonable antigen-specific T lymphocyte lines capable of mediating autoimmune encephalomyelitis. *Eur J Immunol* **11**: 195–199

Ben-Nun A, Wekerle H, Cohen IR 1981b Vaccination against autoimmune encephalomyelitis using attenuated cells of a T lymphocyte line reactive against myelin basic protein. *Nature* **292**: 60–61

Ben-Nun A, Liblau RS, Cohen L et al 1991 Restricted T-cell receptor Vβ gene by myelin basic protein-specific T-cell clones in multiple sclerosis: predominant genes vary in individuals. *Proc Natl Acad Sci USA* **88**: 2466–2470

Ben-Nun A, Mendel I, Bakimer R et al 1996 The autoimmune reactivity to myelin oligodendrocyte glycoprotein (MOG) in multiple sclerosis is potentially pathogenic: effect of copolymer 1 on MOG-induced disease. *J Neurol* **243**: S14–S22

Benoit P, Douron E, Destel A, Warot P 1986 Spirochaetes and Lyme disease. *Lancet* **ii**: 1223

Benson JM, Campbell KA, Guan Z et al 2000 T-cell activation and receptor down-modulation precede deletion induced by mucosally administered antigen. *J Clin Invest* **106**: 1031–1038

van den Berg JS, van Eikema Hommes OR, Wuis EW et al 1997 Anaphylactoid reaction to intravenous methylprednisolone in a patient with multiple sclerosis. *J Neurol Neurosurg Psychiatry* **63**: 813–814

Berg D, Maurer M, Warmuth-Metz M et al 2000 The correlation between ventricular diameter measured by transcranial sonography and clinical disability and cognitive dysfunction in patients with multiple sclerosis. *Arch Neurol* **57**: 1289–1292

Berg O, Hanley J 1963 Narcolepsy in two cases of multiple sclerosis. *Acta Neurol Scand* **39**: 252–257

Bergamaschi R, Romani A, Tonietti S et al 2000 Usefulness of Bayesian graphical models for early prediction of disease progression in multiple sclerosis. *Neurol Sci* **21(Suppl)**: 819–823

Bergamaschi R, Berzuini C, Romani A et al 2001 Predicting secondary progression in relapsing–remitting multiple sclerosis: a Bayesian analysis. *J Neurol Sci* **189**: 13–21

Berger BC, Leopold IH 1968 The incidence of uveitis in multiple sclerosis. *Am J Ophthalmol* **62**: 540

Berger JR, Sheremata WA 1983 Persistent neurological deficit precipitated by hot bath test in multiple sclerosis. *J Am Med Assoc* **249**: 1751–1753

Berger JR, Sheremata WA 1985 Reply to letter by F.A Davis. *J Am Med Assoc* **253**: 203

Berger JR, Koralnik IJ 2005 Progressive multifocal leukoencephalopathy and natalizumab – unforeseen consequences. *N Engl J Med* **353**: 414–416

Berger JR, Sheremata WA, Resnick L et al 1989 Multiple sclerosis-like illness occurring with human immunodeficiency virus infection. *Neurology* **39**: 324–328

Berger T, Weerth S, Kojima K et al 1997 Experimental autoimmune encephalomyelitis: the antigen specificity of T-lymphocytes determines the topography of lesions in the central and peripheral nervous system. *Lab Invest* **76**: 355–364

Berger T, Rubner P, Schautzer F et al 2003 Antimyelin antibodies as a predictor of clinically definite multiple sclerosis after the first demyelinating event. *New Engl J Med* **349**: 139–145

Bergerin H, Bakouche P, Chaquat D, Nicolle MH, Reignier A, Nick J 1980 L'atteinte du système nerveux central au cours de la maladie de Behçet. *Semaine Hôpitaux* **56**: 533–538

Bergh FT, Dayyani F, Ziegler-Heitbrock L 2004 Impact of type-I-interferon on monocyte subsets and their differentiation to dendritic cells. An in vivo and ex vivo study in multiple sclerosis patients treated with interferon-beta. *J Neuroimmunol* **146**: 176–188

Bergin JD 1957 Rapidly progressive dementia in disseminated sclerosis. *J Neurol Neurosurg Psychiatry* **20**: 285–292

Bergkvist M, Sandberg-Wolheim M 2001 Serological differences in monozygotic twin pairs discordant for multiple sclerosis. *Acta Neurol Scand* **104**: 262–265

Bergkvist M, Martinsson T, Aman P, Sandberg-Wollheim M 1996 No genetic linkage between multiple sclerosis and the interferon α/β locus. *J Neuroimmunol* **65**: 163–165

Bergkvist M, Olsson M, Sandberg-Wollheim M 2004 No evidence for genetic linkage between development of multiple sclerosis and components of the IFN system and the JAK-STAT pathway. *Mult Scler* **10**: 87–88

Berk C, Constantoyannis C, Honey CR 2003 The treatment of trigeminal neuralgia in patients with multiple sclerosis using percutaneous radiofrequency rhizotomy. *Can J Neurol Sci* **30**: 220–223

Berkman N, Benzarti T, Dhaoui R et al 1996 Neuropapillite bilatérale avec décollement séreux du neuroépithélium, au décours d'une vaccination contre l'hépatite B. *Bull Soc Ophtalmol Fr* **96**: 187–189

Berkowitz BW 1985 Matutinal vertigo: clinical characteristics and possible management. *Arch Neurol* **41**: 874–877

Berman M, Feldmann S, Alter M, Zilber N, Kahana E 1981 Acute transverse myelitis:

incidence and aetiologic considerations. *Neurology* **31**: 966–971

Bernardi S, Grasso MG, Bertollini R et al 1991 The influence of pregnancy on relapses in multiple sclerosis: a cohort study. *Acta Neurol Scand* **84**: 403–406

Bernheimer H, Budka H, Müller P 1983 Brain tissue immunoglobulins in adrenoleukodystrophy: a comparison with multiple sclerosis and systemic lupus erythematosus. *Acta Neuropathol* **59**: 95–102

Berr C, Dogoujon JM, Clanet M et al 1989 A possible new genetic marker associated with a severe course of multiple sclerosis located on chromosome 2: Km. *N Engl J Med* **320**: 467

Berry GT, Kaplan PB, Lichtenstein GR 2000 Hyperammonia possibly due to corticosteroids. *Arch Neurol* **57**: 1085

Bertolene K, Coyle PK, Krupp LB, Doscher CA 1993 Cytokine correlates of fatigue in MS. *Neurology* **43**: A356

Bertolotto A, Malucchi S, Sala A et al 2002 Differential effects of three interferon betas on neutralising antibodies in patients with multiple sclerosis: a follow up study in an independent laboratory. *J Neurol Neurosurg Psychiatry* **73**: 148–153

Bertolotto A, Deisenhammer F, Gallo P, Sorensen P 2004 Immunogenicity of interferon beta: differences among products. *J Neurol* **251**: II15–II24

Bertrams J, Kuwert E, Liedtke U 1972 HL-A antigens and multiple sclerosis. *Tissue Antigens* **2**: 405–408

Besser M, Wank R 1999 Clonally restricted production of the neurotrophins brain-derived neurotrophic factor and neurotrophin-3 mRNA by human immune cells and Th1/Th2-polarized expression of their receptors. *J Immunol* **162**: 6303–6306

Bethoux F, Miller DM, Kinkel RP 2001 Recovery following acute exacerbations of multiple sclerosis: from impairment to quality of life. *Mult Scler* **7**: 137–142

Betelli E, Prabhu Das MR, Howard ED et al 1998 IL-10 is critical in the regulation of autoimmune encephalomyelitis as demonstrated by studies of IL-10- and IL-4-deficient and transgenic mice. *J Immunol* **161**: 3299–3306

Bettelli E, Pagany M, Weiner HL et al 2003 Myelin oligodendrocyte glycoprotein-specific T cell receptor transgenic mice develop spontaneous autoimmune optic neuritis. *J Exp Med* **197**: 1073–1081

Betts CD, D'Mellow MT, Fowler CJ 1993 Urinary symptoms and the neurological features of bladder dysfunction in multiple sclerosis. *J Neurol Neurosurg Psychiatry* **56**: 245–250

Betts CD, Jones SJ, Fowler CG, Fowler CJ 1994 Erectile dysfunction in multiple sclerosis: associated neurological and neurophysical deficits, and treatment of the condition. *Brain* **117**: 1303–1310

Beutler E, Sipe JC, Romine JS et al 1996 The treatment of chronic progressive multiple sclerosis with cladribine. *Proc Natl Acad Sci USA* **93**: 1716–1720

Bevan Lewis W 1897 The structure of the first or outermost layer of the cerebral cortex. *Edinb Med J* **1**: 573–592

Bever CT 1994 The current status of studies of aminopyridines in patients with multiple sclerosis. *Ann Neurol* **36**: S118–S121

Bever CT, Leslie J, Camenga D, Panitch HS, Johnson KP 1990 Preliminary trial of 3,4-aminopyridine in patients with multiple sclerosis. *Ann Neurol* **27**: 421–427

Bever CT, Young D, Anderson PA et al 1994 The effects of 4-aminopyridine in multiple sclerosis patients: results of a randomised, placebo-controlled, double-blind, concentration-controlled, crossover trial. *Neurology* **44**: 1504–1509

Bezman L, Moser AB, Raymond GV et al 2001 Adrenoleucodystrophy: incidence, new mutation rate and results of extended family screening. *Ann Neurol* **49**: 512–517

Bhakoo KK, Pearce D 2000 In vitro expression of N-acetyl aspartate by oligodendrocytes: implications for proton magnetic resonance spectroscopy signal in vivo. *J Neurochem* **74**: 254–262

Bharucha NE, Bharucha EP, Wadia HN et al 1988 Prevalence of multiple sclerosis in the Parsis of Bombay. *Neurology* **38**: 727–729

Bhatia KP, Brown P, Gregory R et al 1995 Progressive myoclonic ataxia associated with coeliac disease. The myoclonus is of cortical origin but the pathology is in the cerebellum. *Brain* **118**: 1087–1093

Bhatti MT, Newman NJ 1999 A multiple sclerosis-like illness in a man harboring the mtDNA 14484 mutation. *J Neuroophthalmol* **19**: 28–33

Bhigjee AI 1987 Multiple sclerosis in a black patient: a case report. *S Afr Med J* **72**: 873–875

Bianchi M, Sacerdote P, Ricciardi-Castagnoli P et al 1992 Central effects of tumor necrosis factor alpha and interleukin-1 alpha on nociceptive thresholds and spontaneous locomotor activity. *Neurosci Lett* **148**: 76–80

Bickerstaff ER, Small JM, Guest IA 1958 The relapsing course of certain meningiomas in relation to pregnancy and menstruation. *J Neurol Neurosurg Psychiatry* **21**: 89–91

Biddison WE, Taub DD, Cruikshank WW, Center SM, Connor EW, Honma K 1997 Chemokine and matrix metalloproteinase secretion by myelin proteolipid protein-specific CD8+ T cells: potential roles in inflammation. *J Immunol* **158**: 3046–3053

Bieber AJ, Warrington A, Pease LR, Rodriguez M 2001 Humoral autoimmunity as a mediator of CNS repair. *Trends Neurosci* **24**: S39–S44

Bieber AJ, Warrington A, Asakura K et al 2002 Human antibodies accelerate the rate of remyelination following lysolecithin-induced demyelination in mice. *Glia* **37**: 241–249

Bieber AJ, Kerr S, Rodriguez M 2003 Efficient central nervous system remyelination requires T cells. *Ann Neurol* **53**: 680–684

Bielecki B, Mycko M, Tronczyńska E et al 2003 A whole genome screen for association in Polish multiple sclerosis patients. *J Neuroimmunol* **143**: 107–111

Bielefeldt K, Whiteis CA, Chapleau MW, Abboud FM 1999 Nitric oxide enhances slow inactivation of voltage-dependent sodium currents in rat nodose neurons. *Neurosci Lett* **271**: 159–162

Bielekova B, Martin R 2004 Development of biomarkers in multiple sclerosis. *Brain* **27**: 1463–1478

Bielekova B, Goodwin B, Richert N et al 2000 Encephalitogenic potential of the myelin basic protein peptide (amino acids 83–99) in multiple sclerosis: results of a phase II clinical trial with an altered peptide ligand. *Nature Med* **6**: 1167–1175

Bielekova B, Richert N, Howard T et al 2004 Humanized anti-CD25 (daclizumab) inhibits disease activity in multiple sclerosis patients failing to respond to interferon β. *Proc Natl Acad Sci USA* **101**: 8705–8708

Bielschowsky M 1903 Zür Histologie der multiplen Sklerose. *Neurolisches Zentralblatt* **22**: 770–777

Bien CG, Bauer J, Deckwerth TL et al 2002 Destruction of neurons by cytotoxic T cells: a new pathogenic mechanism in Rasmussen's encephalitis. *Ann Neurol* **51**: 311–318

Bienfang DC, Kantrowitz FG, Noble JL, Raynor AM 1977 Ocular abnormalities after influenza immunization. *Arch Ophthalmol* **95**: 1649

Bignami A, Gherardi D, Gallo D 1961 Sclerosi a placche acuta a localizzazone ipotalamica con sintomalogia psichica di tip malincolinco. *Riv Neurol* **31**: 240–268

Bilinska M, Frydecka I, Noga L et al 2004 Progression of multiple sclerosis is associated with exon 1 CTLA-4 gene polymorphism. *Acta Neurol Scand* **110**: 67–71

Billiau A, Heremans H, Vanderkerckhove F et al 1988 Enhancement of experimental allergic encephalomyelitis in mice by antibodies against IFN-gamma. *J Immunol* **140**: 1506–1510

Billiau A, Kieseier BC, Hartung HP 2004 Biologic role of interferon beta in multiple sclerosis. *J Neurol* **251**: II10–II14

Billon N, Terrinoni A, Jolicoeur C et al 2004 Roles for p53 and p73 during oligodendrocyte development. *Development* **131**: 1211–1220

Bing R, Reese H 1926 Die MultipleSclerose in der nord west Schwiez. *Schweiz Med Wochenschr* **56**: 30–34

Binzer M, Forsgren L, Holmgren G et al 1994 Familial clustering of multiple sclerosis in a northern Swedish rural district. *J Neurol Neurosurg Psychiatry* **57**: 497–499

Biousse V, Trichet C, Bloch-Michel E, Roullet E 1999 Multiple sclerosis associated with uveitis in two large clinic-based series. *Neurology* **52**: 179–181

Birk K, Rudick R 1986 Pregnancy and multiple sclerosis. *Arch Neurol* **43**: 719–726

Birk K, Ford C, Smeltzer S et al 1990 The clinical course of multiple sclerosis during pregnancy and the puerperium. *Arch Neurol* 47: 738–742

Birkhead R, Friedmam JH 1987 Hiccups and vomiting as initial manifestations of multiple sclerosis. *J Neurol Neurosurg Psychiatry* 50: 232–233

Birnbaum G, van Ness B 1992 Quantitation of T-cell receptor V beta chain expression on lymphocytes from blood, brain, and spinal fluid in patients with multiple sclerosis and other neurological diseases. *Ann Neurol* 32: 24–30

Bishop A, Anderson JE 2005 NO signaling in the CNS: from the physiological to the pathological. *Toxicology* 208: 193–205

Bitar D, Whitacre CC 1988 Suppression of experimental autoimmune encephalomyelitis by the oral administration of myelin basic protein. *Cell Immunol* 112: 364–370

Bitsch A, Wegener C, da Costa C et al 1999 Lesion development in Marburg's type of acute multiple sclerosis: from inflammation to demyelination. *Mult Scler* 5: 138–146

Bitsch A, KuhlmannT, Da Costa C et al 2000a Tumour necrosis factor alpha mRNA expression in early multiple sclerosis lesions: correlation with demyelinating activity and oligodendrocyte pathology. *Glia* 29: 366–375

Bitsch A, Schuchardt J, Bunkowski S et al 2000b Acute axonal injury in multiple sclerosis: correlation with demyelination and inflammation. *Brain* 123: 1174–1183

Bitsch A, Kuhlmann T, Stadelmann C et al 2001 A longitudinal MRI study of histopathologically defined hypointense multiple sclerosis lesions. *Ann Neurol* 49: 793–796

Bitti PP, Murgia BS, Ticca A et al 2001 Association between the ancestral haplotype HLA A30B18DR3 and multiple sclerosis. *Genet Epidemiol* 20: 271–283

Bizzi A, Ulug AM, Crawford TO et al 2001 Quantitative proton MR spectroscopic imaging in acute disseminated encephalomyelitis. *Am J Neuroradiol* 22: 1125–1130

Bizzozero OA, DeJesus G, Bixler HA et al 2005 Evidence of nitrosative damage in the brain white matter of patients with multiple sclerosis. *Neurochem Res* 30: 139–149

Bjartmar C, Kidd G, Mork S et al 2000 Neurological disability correlates with spinal cord axonal loss and reduced N-acetyl aspartate in chronic multiple sclerosis patients. *Ann Neurol* 48: 893–901

Bjartmar C, Kinkel RP, Kidd G et al 2001 Axonal loss in normal-appearing white matter in a patient with acute MS. *Neurology* 57: 1248–1252

Bjartmar C, Wujek JR, Trapp BD 2003 Axonal loss in the pathology of MS: consequences for understanding the progressive phase of the disease. *J Neurol Sci* 206: 165–171

Bjerrum OW, Bach FW, Zeeberg I 1988 Increased level of cerebrospinal fluid beta 2-microglobulin is related to neurologic impairment in multiple sclerosis. *Acta Neurol Scand* 78: 72–75

Björkman PJ 1997 MHC restriction in three dimensions: a view of T cell receptor/ligand interactions. *Cell* 89: 167–170

Björkman PJ, Saper MA, Samraoui B et al 1987 Structure of the human class I histocompatibility antigen. *Nature* 329: 506–512

Björnson CRR, Rietze RL, Reynolds BA et al 1999 Turning brain into blood: a hematopoietic fate adopted by adult neural stem cells in vivo. *Science* 283: 534–537

Black JA, Waxman SG 1996 Sodium channel expression: a dynamic process in neurons and non-neuronal cells. *Dev Neurosci* 18: 139–152

Black JA, Felts P, Smith KJ et al 1991 Distribution of sodium channels in chronically demyelinated spinal cord axons: immuno-ultrastructral localization and electrophysiological observations. *Brain Res* 544: 59–70

Black JA, Sontheimer H, Waxman SG 1993 Spinal cord astrocytes *in vitro*: phenotypic diversity and sodium channel immunoreactivity. *Glia* 7: 272–285

Black JA, Cummins TR, Plumpton C et al 1999a Upregulation of a silent sodium channel after peripheral, but not central, nerve injury in DRG neurons. *J Neurophysiol* 82: 2776–2785

Black JA, Fjell J, Dib-Hajj S et al 1999b Abnormal expression of SNS/PN3 sodium channel in cerebellar Purkinje cells following loss of myelin in the taiep rat. *NeuroReport* 10: 913–918

Black JA, Dib-Hajj S, Baker D et al 2000 Sensory neuron-specific sodium channel SNS is abnormally expressed in the brains of mice with experimental allergic encephalomyelitis and humans with multiple sclerosis. *Proc Natl Acad Sci USA* 97: 11598–11602

Blackburn-Munro G, Fleetwood-Walker SM 1999 The sodium channel auxiliary subunits beta1 and beta2 are differentially expressed in the spinal cord of neuropathic rats. *Neuroscience* 90: 153–164

Blake G, Murphy S 1997 Onset of myasthenia gravis in a patient with multiple sclerosis during interferon-1b treatment. *Neurology* 49: 1747–1748

Blakemore WF 1976 Invasion of Schwann cells into the spinal cord of the rat following local injections of lysolecithin. *Neuropathol Appl Neurobiol* 2: 21–39

Blakemore WF 2000 Olfactory glia and CNS repair: a step in the road from proof of principle to clinical application. *Brain* 123: 1543–1544

Blakemore WF, Franklin RJM 2000 Transplantation options for therapeutic central nervous system remyelination. *Cell Transplantation* 9: 289–294

Blakemore WF, Smith KJ 1983 Node-like axonal specializations along demyelinated central nerve fibres: ultrastructural observations. *Acta Neuropathol* 60: 291–296

Blakemore WF, Eames RA, Smith KJ, McDonald WI 1977 Remyelination in the spinal cord of the cat following intraspinal injections of lysolecithin. *J Neurol Sci* 33: 31–43

Blakemore WF, Gilson JM, Crang AJ 2000 Transplanted glial cells migrate over a greater distance and remyelinate demyelinated lesions more rapidly than endogenous remyelinating cells. *J Neurosci Res* 61: 288–294

Blakemore WF, Chari DM, Gilson JM, Crang AJ 2002 Modelling large areas of demyelination in the rat reveals the potential and possible limitations of transplanted glial cells for remyelination in the CNS. *Glia* 38: 155–168

Blakemore WF, Gilson JM, Crang AJ 2003 The presence of astrocytes in areas of demyelination influences remyelination following transplantation of oligodendrocyte progenitors. *Exp Neurol* 184: 955–963

Blanc M, Clanet M, Berr C et al 1986 Immunoglobulin allotypes and susceptibility to multiple sclerosis. *J Neurol Sci* 75: 1–5

Blanco Y, Yague J, Graus F, Saiz A 2003 No association of inducible nitric oxide synthase gene (NOS2A) to multiple sclerosis. *J Neurol* 250: 598–600

Blanco Y, Saiz A, Carreras E, Graus F 2005 Autologous haematopoietic-stem-cell transplantation for multiple sclerosis. *Lancet Neurol* 4: 54–63

Blankenhorn EP, Butterfield RJ, Rigby R et al 2000 Genetic analysis of the influence of pertussis toxin on experimental allergic encephalomyelitis susceptibility: an environmental agent can override genetic checkpoints. *J Immunol* 164: 3420–3425

Blasko I, Stampfer-Kountchev M, Robatscher P et al 2004 How chronic inflammation can affect the brain and support the development of Alzheimer's disease in old age: the role of microglia and astrocytes. *Aging Cell* 3: 169–176

Blenow K, Fredman P, Wallin A et al 1994 Formulas for the quantitation of intrathecal IgG production: their validity in the presence of blood-brain barrier damage and their utility in multiple sclerosis. *J Neurol Sci* 121: 90–96

Blight AR, Toombs JP, Bauer MS, Widmer WR 1991 The effects of 4-aminopyridine on neurological deficits in chronic cases of traumatic spinal cord injury in dogs: a phase I clinical trial. *J Neurotrauma* 8: 103–119

Blinkenberg M, Rune K, Jemsen CV et al 2000 Cortical cerebral metabolism correlates with MRI lesion load and cognitive dysfunction in MS. *Neurology* 54: 558–564

Blocq P, Londe A 1890 Anatomie pathologique de la moelle épinière. *Nouv Iconographie Salpétrière* 3: 309–312

Bloor JW, Johnson RJ, Canales L, Dunn DP 1974 Reversible paralysis of automatic respiration. *Arch Neurol* 34: 686–689

Bluestone JA, Khattri R, Sciammas R, Sperling AI 1995 TCRγδ cells: a specialized T-cell subset in the immune system. *Annu Rev Cell Biol* 11: 307–353

Blumberg BM, Mock DJ, Powers JM et al 2000 The HHV6 paradox: ubiquitous commensal or insidious pathogen? A two step in situ PCR approach. *J Clin Virol* **16**: 159–178

Blumen SC, Bevan S, Abu-Mouch S et al 2003 A locus for complicated hereditary spastic paraplegia maps to chromosome 1q24–1q32. *Ann Neurol* **54**: 796–203

Blumhardt LD, Barrett G, Halliday AM 1982 The pattern visual evoked potential in the clinical assessment of undiagnosed spinal cord disease. *Adv Neurol* **37**: 463–471

Bo L, Mork S, Kong PA et al 1994 Detection of MHC class II-antigens on macrophages and microglia, but not on astrocytes and endothelia in active multiple sclerosis lesions. *J Neuroimmunol* **51**: 135–146

Bo L, Vedeler CA, Nyland HI et al 2003a Subpial demyelination in the cerebral cortex of multiple sclerosis patients. *J Neuropathol Exp Neurol* **62**: 723–732

Bo L, Vedeler CA, Nyland H et al 2003b Intracortical multiple sclerosis lesions are not associated with increased lymphocyte infiltration. *Mult Scler* **9**: 323–331

Bobowick AR, Kurtzke JF, Brody JA et al 1978 Twin study of multiple sclerosis: an epidemiologic inquiry. *Neurology* **28**: 978–987

Bocko D, Bilinska M, Dobosz T et al 2003 Lack of association between an exon 1 CTLA-4 gene polymorphism A(49)G and multiple sclerosis in a Polish population of the Lower Silesia region. *Arch Immunol Ther Exp* **51**: 201–205

Bode MK, Tikkakoski T, Tuisku S et al 2001 Isolated neurosarcoidosis – MR findings and pathological correlation. *Acta Radiol* **42**: 563–567

Boden G 1948 Radiation myelitis of the cervical spinal cord. *Br J Radiol* **21**: 464–469

Boehm T, Scheu S, Pfeffer K, Bleul CC 2003 Thymic medullary epithelial cell differentiation, thymocyte emigration, and the control of autoimmunity require lympho-epithelial cross talk via LTbR. *J Exp Med* **198**: 757–769

von Boehmer H 1992 Thymic selection: a matter of life and death. *Immunol Today* **13**: 454–458

von Boehmer H, Teh HS, Kisielow P 1989 The thymus selects the useful, neglects the useless and destroys the harmful. *Immunol Today* **10**: 57–61

Boggild MD, Williams R, Haq N, Hawkins CP 1996 Cortical plaques visualised by fluid-attenuated inversion recovery imaging in relapsing multiple sclerosis. *Neuroradiology* **38**: S10–S13

Boghen D, Sebag M, Michaud J 1988 Paraneoplastic optic neuritis and encephalomyelitis: report of a case. *Arch Neurol* **45**: 353–356

Bogousslavsky J, Hungerbüler JP, Regli F, Graf HJ 1982 Subacute myelopathy as the presenting manifestation of sarcoidosis. *Acta Neurochir* **65**: 193–197

Bogue M, Candéias S, Benoist C, Mathis D 1991 A special repertoire of a:b T cells in neonatal mice. *EMBO J* **10**: 3647–3654

Boiko AN 1994 Multiple sclerosis prevalence in Russia and other countries of the former USSR. In: Firnhaber W, Lauer K (eds) *Multiple Sclerosis in Europe: An Epidemiological Update*. Darmstadt: Leuchtturm-Verlag/LTV Press, pp. 219–230

Boiko AN, Deomina T, Favorava O et al 1995 Epidemiology of multiple sclerosis in Russia and other countries of the former Soviet Union: investigations of environmental and genetic factors. *Acta Neurol Scand* **161 (Suppl)**: 71–76

Boiko AN, Gusev EI, Sudomoina MA et al 2002 Association and linkage of juvenile MS with HLA-DR2(15) in Russians. *Neurology* **58**: 658–660

Boiko T, Rasband MN, Levinson SR et al 2001 Compact myelin dictates the differential targeting of two sodium channel isoforms in the same axon. *Neuron* **30**: 91–104

Bolanos JP, Peuchen S, Heales SJ et al 1994 Nitric oxide-mediated inhibition of the mitochondrial respiratory chain in cultured astrocytes. *J Neurochem* **63**: 910–916

Bolanos JP, Almeida A, Stewart V et al 1997 Nitric oxide-mediated mitochondrial damage in the brain: mechanisms and implications for neurodegenerative diseases. *J Neurochem* **68**: 2227–2240

Bolger C, Bojanic S, Sheahan N et al 2000 Ocular microtremor (OMT): a new neurophysiological approach to multiple sclerosis. *J Neurol Neurosurg Psychiatry* **68**: 639–642

Bolotina VM, Najibi S, Palacino JJ et al 1994 Nitric oxide directly activates calcium-dependent potassium channels in vascular smooth muscle. *Nature* **368**: 850–853

Bolviken B, Celius EG, Nilsen R, Strand T 2003 Radon: a possible risk factor in multiple sclerosis. *Neuroepidemiology* **22**: 87–94

Boman J, Roblin PM, Sundstrom P et al 2000 Failure to detect *Chlamydia pneumoniae* in the central nervous system of patients with MS. *Neurology* **54**: 265

Bombardier CH, Blake KD, Ehde DM et al 2004 Alcohol and drug abuse among persons with multiple sclerosis. *Mult Scler* **10**: 35–40

Bon CL, Garthwaite J 2003 On the role of nitric oxide in hippocampal long-term potentiation. *J Neurosci* **23**: 1941–1948

Bonduelle M 1967 Les formes bénignes de la sclérose en plaques. *Presse Med* **75**: 2023–2026

Bonduelle M, Albaranès R 1962 Etude statistique de 145 cas de la sclérose en plaques. *Semaine Hôpitaux* **38**: 3762–3773

Bonduelle M, Bouygues P, Sallou C 1954 La sclérose en plaques chez l'enfant. *Presse Med* **62**: 563–564

Bonduelle M, Bouygues P, Chaumont P 1964 Amyotrophies et abolition des réflexes dans la sclérose en plaques. *Sémaine Hôpitaux* **40**: 814–821

Bonetti B, Raine CS 1997 Multiple sclerosis: oligodendrocytes display cell death-related molecules *in situ* but do not undergo apoptosis. *Ann Neurol* **42**: 74–84

Bonetti B, Stegagno C, Cannella B et al 1999 Activation of NF-kappaB and c-jun transcription factors in multiple sclerosis lesions: implications for oligodendrocyte pathology. *Am J Pathol* **155**: 1433–1438

Bonilla S, Alarcon P, Villaverde R et al 2002 Haematopoietic progenitor cells from adult bone marrow differentiate into cells that express oligodendroglial antigens in the neonatal mouse brain. *Eur J Neurosci* **15**: 575–582

Boon M, Nolte IM, Bruinenberg M et al 2001 Mapping of a susceptibility gene for multiple sclerosis to the 51 kb interval between G511525 and D6S1666 using a new method of haplotype sharing analysis. *Neurogenetics* **3**: 221–230

Booss J, Esiri MM, Tourtellotte WW, Mason DY 1983 Immunohistological analysis of T lymphocyte subsets in the central nervous system in chronic progressive multiple sclerosis. *J Neurol Sci* **62**: 219–232

Borello-France D, Leng W, O'Leary M et al 2004 Bladder and sexual function among women with multiple sclerosis. *Mult Scler* **10**: 455–461

Borg-Stein J, Pine ZM, Miller JR, Brin MF 1993 Botulinum toxin for the treatment of spasticity in multiple sclerosis. *Am J Phys Med Rehab* **72**: 364–368

Bornstein MB, Appel SH 1961 The application of tissue culture to the study of experimental 'allergic' encephalomyelitis. I. Patterns of demyelination. *J Neuropathol Exp Neurol* **20**: 141–147

Bornstein MB, Crain SM 1965 Functional studies of cultured brain tissues as related to 'demyelinative disorders'. *Science* **148**: 1242–1244

Bornstein MB, Miller A, Teitelbaum D et al 1982 Multiple sclerosis: trial of a synthetic polypeptide. *Ann Neurol* **11**: 317–319

Bornstein MB, Miller A, Slagle S et al 1987 A pilot trial of Cop 1 in exacerbating-remitting multiple sclerosis. *N Engl J Med* **317**: 408–414

Bornstein MB, Miller A, Slagle S et al 1991 A placebo-controlled double-blind randomised two-center, pilot trial of Cop-1 in chronic progressive multiple sclerosis. *Neurology* **41**: 533–539

Borodic GE, Ferrante R, Wiegener AW, Young RR 1992 Treatment of spasticity with botulinum toxin. *Ann Neurol* **31**: 113

Borrás C, Rio J, Porcel J et al 1999 Emotional state of patients with relapsing–remitting MS treated with interferon beta-1b. *Neurology* **52**: 1636–1639

Borst M 1903 Die multiple Sklerose des Zentralnervensystem. *Ergebn allg Path Menschen Tieres* **9**: 67–187

Boskovich SA, Lowder CY, Meisler DM, Gutman FA 1993 Systemic diseases associated with intermediate uveitis. *Cleveland Clin J Med* **60**: 460–465

Bosma R, Wynia K, Havlikova E et al 2005 Efficacy of desmopressin in patients with multiple sclerosis suffering from bladder dysfunction: a meta-analysis. *Acta Neurol Scand* **112**: 1–5

Bostock H 1984 Internodal conduction along undissected nerve fibers in experimental neuropathy. In: Dyck PJ, Thomas PK, Lambert EH, Bunge R (eds) *Peripheral Neuropathy*. Philadelphia: W.B Saunders, pp. 900–910

Bostock H 1993 Impulse propagation in experimental neuropathy. In: Dyck PJ, Thomas PK, Griffin JW *et al* (eds) *Peripheral Neuropathy*. Philadelphia: W.B Saunders, pp. 109–120

Bostock H 1994 The pathophysiology of demyelination. In: Herndon RM, Seil FJ (eds) *Multiple Sclerosis: Current Status of Research and Treatment*. New York: Demos Publications, pp. 89–112

Bostock H, Grafe P 1985 Activity-dependent excitability changes in normal and demyelinated rat spinal root axons. *J Physiol* **365**: 239–257

Bostock H, Rothwell JC 1997 Latent addition in motor and sensory fibres of human peripheral nerve. *J Physiol* **498**: 277–294

Bostock H, Sears 1976 Continuous conduction in demyelinated mammalian nerve fibres. *Nature* **263**: 786–787

Bostock H, Sears 1978 The internodal axon membrane: electrical excitability and continuous conduction in segmental demyelination. *J Physiol* **280**: 273–301

Bostock H, Sherratt RM, Sears TA 1978 Overcoming conduction failure in demyelinated nerve fibres by prolonging action potentials. *Nature* **274**: 385–387

Bostock H, Hall SM, Smith KJ 1980 Demyelinated axons can form 'nodes' prior to remyelination. *J Physiol* **308**: 21–23

Bostock H, Sears TA, Sherratt RM 1981 The effects of 4-aminopyridine and tetraethylammonium ions on normal and demyelinated mammalian nerve fibres. *J Physiol* **313**: 301–315

Bostock H, Cikurel K, Burke D 1998 Threshold tracking techniques in the study of human peripheral nerve. *Muscle Nerve* **21**: 137–158

Bot JCJ, Barkhof F, Lycklama G *et al* 2000 Comparison of a conventional cardiac-triggered dual spin-echo and a fast STIR sequence in detection of spinal cord lesions in multiple sclerosis. *Eur Radiol* **10**: 753–758

Bot JCJ, Barkhof F, Lycklama G *et al* 2002 Differentiation of multiple sclerosis from other inflammatory disorders and cerebrovascular disease: value of spinal MR imaging. *Radiology* **223**: 46–56

Bot JCJ, Barkhof F, Polman CH *et al* 2004 Spinal cord abnormalities in newly diagnosed MS patients: added value of spinal MRI examination. *Neurology* **62**: 226–233

Botstein DR, Risch N 2003 Discovering genotypes underlying human phenotypes: past successes for mendelian disease, future approaches for complex disease. *Nature Genet* **33**: 228–237

Botstein DR, White RL, Skolnick MH, Davis R 1980 Construction of a genetic map in humans. *Am J Hum Genet* **32**: 314–331

Boudouresques J, Khalil R, Cherif AA *et al* 1975 Epilepsie et sclérose en plaques. *Rev Neurol* **131**: 729–735

Bourneville DM, Guerard L 1869 *De la sclérose en plaques disséminées*. Paris: Delahaye

Bourneville DM, Regnard PML 1876–1880 *Iconographie photographique de la Salpétrière*. Service de M. Charcot, 3 vols

Bourquin C, Schubart A, Tobollik S *et al* 2003 Selective unresponsiveness to conformational B cell epitopes of the myelin oligodendrocyte glycoprotein in H-2(b) mice. *J Immunol* **171**: 455–461

Bouslama-Oueghlani L, Wehrle R, Sotelo C, Dusart I 2003 The developmental loss of the ability of Purkinje cells to regenerate their axons occurs in the absence of myelin: an in vitro model to prevent myelination. *J Neurosci* **23**: 8318–81329

Bousso P, Bhakta NR, Lewis RS, Robey E 2002 Dynamics of thymocyte-stromal cell interactions visualized by two-photon microscopy. *Science* **296**: 1876–1880

Boutin B, Esquivel E, Mayer M *et al* 1988 Multiple sclerosis in children: report of clinical and paraclinical features of 19 cases. *Neuropediatrics* **19**: 118–123

Bowden AN, Bowden PMA, Friedman AL, Perkin GD, Rose FC 1974 A trial of cortocotrophin gelatin injection in acute optic neuritis. *J Neurol Neurosurg Psychiatry* **37**: 869–873

Bowe CM, Kocsis JD, Targ EF, Waxman SG 1987 Physiological effects of 4-aminopyridine on demyelinated mammalian motor and sensory fibers. *Ann Neurol* **22**: 264–268

Boyd JG, Lee J, Skihar V *et al* 2004 LacZ-expressing olfactory ensheathing cells do not associate with myelinated axons after implantation into the compressed spinal cord. *Proc Natl Acad Sci USA* **101**: 2162–2166

Boylan KK, Takahashi N, Diamond M *et al* 1987 DNA length polymorphism located 5' to the human myelin basic protein gene. *Am J Hum Genet* **40**: 387–400

Boylan KK, Takahashi N, Paty D *et al* 1990 DNA length polymorphism 5' to the myelin basic protein gene is associated with multiple sclerosis. *Ann Neurol* **27**: 291–297

Boyle EA, McGeer PL 1990 Cellular immune response in multiple sclerosis plaques. *Am J Pathol* **137**: 575–584

Boyle ME, Berglund EO, Murai KK *et al* 2001 Contactin orchestrates assembly of the septate-like junctions at the paranode in myelinated peripheral nerve. *Neuron* **30**: 385–397

Boz C, Velioglu S, Ozmenoglu M 2003 Acute disseminated encephalomyelitis after bee sting. *Neurol Sci* **23**: 313–315

Bozek CB, Kastrukoff CF, Wright JM, Perry TL, Larsen TA 1987 A controlled trial of isoniazid therapy for action tremor in multiple sclerosis. *J Neurol* **234**: 36–39

Bozzali M, Cercignani M, Sormani MP *et al* 2002 Quantification of brain grey matter damage in different MS phenotypes by use of diffusion tensor MR imaging. *Am J Neuroradiol* **23**: 985–988

Bradbury EJ, Moon LDF, Popat RJ *et al* 2002 Chondroitinase ABC promotes functional recovery after spinal cord injury. *Nature* **416**: 636–640

Bradbury M 1979 *The Concept of the Blood Brain Barrier*. New York: John Wiley

Bradbury M, Cserr HF 1985 Drainage of cerebral interstitial fluid of cerebrospinal fluid into lymphatics. In: Johnston MG (ed.) *Experimental Biology of the Lymphatic Circulation*. Amsterdam: Elsevier, pp. 355–394

Bradley WG, Whitty CWM 1967 Acute optic neuritis: its clinical features and their relation to prognosis for recovery of vision. *J Neurol Neurosurg Psychiatry* **30**: 531–538

Bradley WG, Whitty CWM 1968 Acute optic neuritis: prognosis for development of multiple sclerosis. *J Neurol Neurosurg Psychiatry* **31**: 10–18

Brady CM, DasGupta R, Dalton C *et al* 2004 An open-label pilot study of cannabis-based extracts for bladder dysfunction in advanced multiple sclerosis. *Mult Scler* **10**: 425–433

Brady ST, Witt AS, Kirkpatrick LL *et al* 1999 Formation of compact myelin is required for maturation of the axonal cytoskeleton. *J Neurosci* **19**: 7278–7288

Brahic M, Bureau J-F 1997 Multiple sclerosis and retroviruses. *Ann Neurol* **42**: 984–985

Brain WR 1930 Critical review: disseminateed sclerosis. *Q J Med* **23**: 343–391

Brain WR 1933 *Diseases of the Nervous System*, 1st edn. London: Oxford University Press, pp. 350–361, 366–369, 389–402

Brain WR 1936 Prognosis of disseminated sclerosis. *Lancet* **2**: 866–867

Brain WR 1940 *Diseases of the Nervous System*, 2nd edn. London: Oxford University Press, pp. 469–505

Brain WR, Wilkinson M 1957 The association of cervical spondylosis and disseminated sclerosis. *Brain* **80**: 456–478

Bramanti P, Sessa E, Rifici C *et al* 1998 Enhanced spasticity in primary progressive MS patients treated with interferon beta-1b. *Neurology* **51**: 1720–1723

Bramwell B 1903 On the relative frequency of disseminated sclerosis in this country (Scotland and the North of England) and in America. *Rev Neurol Psych Edinb* i: 12–17

Bramwell B 1917 The prognosis in disseminated sclerosis; duration in two hundred cases of disseminated sclerosis. *Edinb Med J* **18**: 15–23

Brand A, Richter-Landsberg C, Leibfritz D 1993 Multinuclear NMR studies on the energy metabolism of glial and neuronal cells. *Dev Neurosci* **15**: 289–298

Brandt JT, Triplett DA, Alving B, Scharrer I 1995 Criteria for the diagnosis of lupus anticoagulants: an update. *Thromb Hemost* **74**: 1185–1190

824

Brandt S, Gyldensted C, Offner H, Melchior JC 1981 Multiple sclerosis with onset in a two-year-old boy. *Neuropediatrics* **12**: 75–82

Brard F, Shannon M, Luning Prak E *et al* 1999 Somatic mutation and light chain rearrangement generate autoimmunity in anti-single-stranded DNA transgenic MRL/*lpr* mice. *J Exp Med* **190**: 691–704

Brass SD, Caramanos Z, Santos C *et al* 2003 Multiple sclerosis vs acute disseminated encephalomyelitis in childhood. *Pediatr Neurol* **29**: 227–231

Brassat D, Azais-Vuillemin C, Yaounag J *et al* 1999 Familial factors influence disability in MS multiplex families. French Multiple Sclerosis Genetics Group. *Neurology* **52**: 1632–1636

Brassat D, Recher C, Waubant E *et al* 2002 Therapy-related acute myeloblastic leukemia after mitoxantrone treatment in a patient with MS. *Neurology* **59**: 954–955

Brassington JC, Marsh NV 1998 Neuropsychological aspects of multiple sclerosis. *Neuropsychol Rev* **8**: 43–77

Bräuer AU, Savaskan NE, Kühn H *et al* 2003 A new phospolipid phosphatase, PRG-1, is involved in axon growth and regenerative sprouting. *Nat Neurosci* **6**: 572–578

Braun N, Michel U, Ernst BP *et al* 1996 Gene polymorphism at position -308 of the tumor necrosis factor-alpha (TNF-α) in multiple sclerosis and its influence on the regulation of TNF-α production. *Neurosci Lett* **215**: 75–78

Brautbar C, Alter M, Kahana E 1976 HLA antigens in multiple sclerosis. *Neurology* **26**: 50–56

Bregman BS, Kunkel-Bagden E, Schnell L *et al* 1995 Recovery from spinal cord injury mediated by antibodies to neurite growth inhibitors. *Nature* **378**: 498–501

Brehm U, Piddlesden SJ, Gardinier MV, Linington C 1999 Epitope specificity of demyelinating monoclonal autoantibodies directed against the human myelin oligodendrocyte glycoprotein (MOG). *J Neuroimmunol* **97**: 9–15

Breij ECW, van der Pol W-L, van Winsen L *et al* 2003 No association of FcγRIIa, FcγRIIIa and FcγRIIIb polymorphisms with MS. *J Neuroimmunol* **140**: 210–215

Breithaupt C, Schubart A, Zander H *et al* 2003 Structural insights into the antigenicity of myelin oligodendrocyte glycoprotein. *Proc Natl Acad Sci USA* **100**: 9446–9451

Breland AE, Currier RD 1983 Scorpion venom and multiple sclerosis. *Lancet* ii: 1021

Brenner RE, Munro PM, Williams SC *et al* 1993 The proton NMR spectrum in acute EAE: the significance of the change in the Cho:Cr ratio. *Magn Reson Med* **29**: 737–745

Brenner T, Arnon R, Sela M *et al* 2001 Humoral and cellular immune responses to Copolymer 1 in multiple sclerosis patients treated with Copaxone. *J Neuroimmunol* **115**: 152–160

Brewis M, Poskanzer DC, Rolland C, Miller H 1966 Neurological disease in an English city. *Acta Neurol Scand* **42** (Suppl 24): 1–89

Brex PA, Jenkins R, Fox NC *et al* 2000 Detection of ventricular enlargement in patients at the earliest clinical stage of MS. *Neurology* **54**: 1689–1691

Brex PA, Miszkiel KA, O'Riordan JI *et al* 2001a Assessing the risk of early multiple sclerosis in patients with clinically isolated syndromes: the role of a follow up MRI. *J Neurol Neurosurg Psychiatry* **70**: 390–393

Brex PA, Molyneux PD, Smiddy P *et al* 2001b The effect of interferon beta-1b on the size and evolution of enhancing lesions in secondary progressive MS. *Neurology* **57**: 2185–2190

Brex PA, Ciccarelli O, O'Riordan JI *et al* 2002 A longitudinal study of abnormalities on MRI and disability from multiple sclerosis. *N Engl J Med* **346**: 158–164

Brey RL, Holliday SL, Saklad AR *et al* 2002 Neuropsychiatric syndromes in lupus: prevalence using standardised definitions. *Neurology* **58**: 1214–1220

Briant L, Avoustin P, Clayton J *et al* 1993 Multiple sclerosis susceptibility: population and twin study of polymorphisms in the T cell receptor beta and gamma genes region. French Group on Multiple Sclerosis. *Autoimmunity* **15**: 67–73

Brickner RM 1935 Quinine therapy in cases of multiple sclerosis over a five year period. *Arch Neurol Psychiatry* **33**: 1235–1254

Brickner RM 1936 A critique of therapy in multiple sclerosis. *Bull Neurol Inst NY* **4**: 665–698

Brickner RM 1950 The significance of localised vasoconstrictions in multiple sclerosis. *Res Publ Assoc Res Nerv Mental Dis* **28**: 236–244

Brierley CM, Crang AJ, Iwashita Y *et al* 2001 Remyelination of demyelinated CNS axons by transplanted human Schwann cells: the deleterious effect of contaminating fibroblasts. *Cell Transplant* **10**: 305–315

Brightman M 1991 Implication of astroglia in the blood-brain barrier. *Ann NY Acad Sci* **633**: 343–347

Bril V, Ilse WK, Pearce R *et al* 1996 Pilot trial of immunoglobulin versus plasma exchange in patients with Guillain-Barre syndrome. *Neurology* **46**: 100–103

Brindley GS 1994 Impotence and ejaculatory failure. *The Handbook of Neuro-Urology*. New York, Dekker: pp. 31–348

Brindley GS 1970 *Physiology of the Retina and Visual Pathway*. London, Edward Arnold

Brindley GS, Polkey CE, Rushton DN 1982 Sacral anterior root stimulation for bladder control in paraplegia. *Paraplegia* **20**: 365–381

Brink BP, Veerhuis R, Breij EC *et al* 2005 The pathology of multiple sclerosis is location dependent: no significant complement activation is detected in purely cortical lesions. *J Neuropathol Exp Neurol* **64**: 147–155

Brinkmeier H, Wollinsky KH, Seewald MJ *et al* 1993 Factors in the cerebrospinal fluid of multiple sclerosis patients interfering with voltage-dependent sodium channels. *Neurosci Lett* **156**: 172–175

Brinkmeier H, Seewald MJ, Wollinsky KH, Rudel R 1996 On the nature of endogenous antiexcitatory factors in the cerebrospinal fluid of patients with demyelinating neurological disease. *Muscle Nerve* **19**: 54–62

Brinkmeier H, Aulkemeyer P, Wollinsky KH, Rudel R 2000 An endogenous pentapeptide acting as a sodium channel blocker in inflammatory autoimmune disorders of the central nervous system. *Nature Med* **6**: 808–811

Brisman R, Mooij R 2000 Gamma knife radiosurgery for trigeminal neuralgia: dose-volume histograms of the brainstem and trigeminal nerve. *J Neurosurg* **93**: 155–158

Brismar T 1981a Electrical properties of isolated demyelinated rat nerve fibres. *Acta Physiol Scand* **113**: 161–166

Brismar T 1981b Specific permeability properties of demyelinated rat nerve fibres. *Acta Physiol Scand* **113**: 167–176

Brismar T, Frankenhaeuser B 1981 Potential clamp analysis of mammalian myelinated fibres. *Trends Neurosci* **4**: 68–70

Britton CB, Meas-Tejada R, Fenoglio CM, Hays AP, Garvey GG, Miller JR 1985 A new complication of AIDS: thoracic myelitis caused by herpes simplex virus. *Neurology* **35**: 1071–1074

British and Dutch Multiple Sclerosis Azathioprine Trial Group 1988a Histocompatibility antigens in multiple sclerosis patients participating in a multicentre trial of azathioprine. *J Neurol Neurosurg Psychiatry* **51**: 412–415

British and Dutch Multiple Sclerosis Azathioprine Trial Group 1988b Double masked trial of azathioprine in multiple sclerosis. *Lancet* ii: 179–183

Broadley SA, Deans J, Sawcer SJ *et al* 2000 Autoimmune disease in first degree relatives of patients with multiple sclerosis in the United Kingdom. *Brain* **123**: 1102–1111

Broadley SA, Sawcer S, D'Alfonso S *et al* 2001a A genome screen for multiple sclerosis in Italian families. *Genes Immun* **2**: 205–210

Broadley SA, Sawcer SJ, Chataway SJ *et al* 2001b No association between multiple sclerosis and the notch3 gene responsible for cerebral autosomal dominant arteriopathy with subcortical infarcts and leukoencephalopathy (CADASIL). *J Neurol Neurosurg Psychiatry* **71**: 97–99

Broadwell RD, Salcman M 1981 Expanding the definition of the blood-brain barrier to protein. *Proc Natl Acad Sci USA* **78**: 7820–7824

Brocke S, Gaur A, Piercy C *et al* 1993 Induction of relapsing paralysis in experimental autoimmune encephalomyelitis by bacterial superantigen. *Nature* **365**: 642–644

Brocke S, Piercy C, Steinman L *et al* 1999 Antibodies to CD44 and integrin α4, but not L-selectin, prevent central nervous system inflammation and experimental encephalomyelitis by blocking secondary leukocyte recruitment. *Proc Natl Acad Sci USA* **96**: 6896–6901

Brockmann K, Dechent P, Wilken B et al 2003 Proton MRS profile of cerebral metabolic abnormalities in Krabbe disease. *Neurology* **60**: 819–825

Brod SA, Marshall GD, Henninger EM et al 1996 Interferon-β1b treatment decreases tumor necrosis factor-α and increases interleukin-6 production in multiple sclerosis. *Neurology* **46**: 1633–1638

Brod SA, Lindsey JW, Vriesendorp FS et al 2001 Ingested IFN-alpha: results of a pilot study in relapsing–remitting MS. *Neurology* **57**: 845–852

Broggi G, Ferroli P, Franzini A et al 2000 Microvascular decompression for trigeminal neuralgia: comments on a series of 250 cases, including 10 patients with multiple sclerosis. *J Neurol Neurosurg Psychiatry* **68**: 59–64

Broholm H, Andersen B, Wanscher B et al 2004 Nitric oxide synthase expression and enzymatic activity in multiple sclerosis. *Acta Neurol Scand* **109**: 261–269

Broman T 1964 Blood brain barrier damage in multiple sclerosis. Supra-vital test observations. *Acta Neurol Scand* **10**: 21–24

Broman T, Bergmann L, Fog T et al 1965 Aspects of classification methods in multiple sclerosis. *Acta Neurol Scand* **41 (Suppl 13)**: 543–548

Broman T, Andersen O, Bergmann L 1981 Clinical studies on multiple sclerosis. I. Presentation of an incidence material from Gothenburg. *Acta Neurol Scand* **63**: 6–33

Brønnum-Hansen H, Koch-Henriksen N, Hyllested K 1994 Survival of patients with multiple sclerosis in Denmark: a nationwide, long term epidemiologic survey. *Neurology* **44**: 1901–1907

Brønnum-Hansen H, Koch-Henriksen N, Stenager E 2004 Trends in survival and cause of death in Danish patients with multiple sclerosis. *Brain* **127**: 844–850

Bronstein AM, Morris J, du Boulay GH et al 1990a Abnormalities of horizontal gaze: clinical oculographic and magnetic resonance imaging findings. I. Abducens palsy. *J Neurol Neurosurg Psychiatry* **53**: 194–199

Bronstein AM, Rudge P, Morris P et al 1990b Abnormalities of horizontal gaze: clinical oculographic and magnetic resonance imaging findings. II. Gaze palsy and internuclear ophthalmoplegia. *J Neurol Neurosurg Psychiatry* **53**: 200–207

Bronstein JM, Popper P, Micevych PE, Farber DB 1996 Isolation and characterisation of a novel oligodendrocyte-specific protein. *Neurology* **47**: 772–778

Brooks DJ, Leenders KL, Head G et al 1984 Studies on regional oxygen utilisation and cognitive function in multiple sclerosis. *J Neurol Neurosurg Psychiatry* **47**: 1182–1191

Brophy B 1987 *Baroque-n'-Roll*. London: Hamilton, pp. 1–27

Brorson JR, Schumacker PT, Zhang H 1999 Nitric oxide acutely inhibits neuronal energy production. *J Neurosci* **19**: 147–158

Brorson O, Brorson SH, Henriksen TH et al 2001 Association between multiple sclerosis and cystic structures in cerebrospinal fluid. *Infection* **29**: 315–319

Brosnan CF, Raine CS 1996 Mechanisms of immune injury in multiple sclerosis. *Brain Pathol* **6**: 243–257

Brosnan CF, Stoner GL, Bloom BR, Wisniewski HM 1977 Studies on demyelination by activated lymphocytes in the rabbit eye. II. Antibody dependent cell mediated demyelination. *J Immunol* **118**: 2103–2110

Brosnan CF, Cammer W, Norton WT, Bloom BR 1980 Proteinase inhibitors suppress the development of experimental allergic encephalomyelitis. *Nature* **285**: 235–237

Brosnan CF, Bornstein MB, Bloom BR 1981 The effects of macrophage depletion on the clinical and pathologic expression of experimental allergic encephalomyelitis. *J Immunol* **126**: 614–620

Brosnan CF, Litwak MS, Schroeder CE et al 1989 Preliminary studies of cytokine-induced functional effects on the visual pathways in the rabbit. *J Neuroimmunol* **25**: 227–239

Brown AM, Westenbroek RE, Catterall WA, Ransom BR 2001 Axonal L-type Ca2+ channels and anoxic injury in rat CNS white matter. *J Neurophysiology* **85**: 900–911

Brown DL, Login IS, Borish L, Powers PL 2001 An urticarial IgE-mediated reaction to interferon beta-1b. *Neurology* **56**: 1416–1417

Brown GC 1999 Nitric oxide and mitochondrial respiration. *Biochim Biophys Acta* **1411**: 351–369

Brown GC, Borutaite V 2001 Nitric oxide, mitochondria, and cell death. *IUBMB Life* **52**: 189–195

Brown GC, Bolanos JP, Heales SJ, Clark JB 1995 Nitric oxide produced by activated astrocytes rapidly and reversibly inhibits cellular respiration. *Neurosci Lett* **193**: 201–204

Brown J, Jardetzky T, Saper M et al 1993 Three dimensional structure of the human class II histocompatibility antigen. *Nature* **332**: 845–850

Brown JR, Beebe GW, Kurtzke JF et al 1979 The design of clinical studies to assess therapeutic efficacy in multiple sclerosis. *Neurology* **29**: 3–23

Brown MM, Swash M 1989 Polyarteritis nodosa and other systemic vasculitides. In: Toole JF (ed.) *Handbook of Clinical Neurology*. Amsterdam: Elsevier, Vol. 55 (part III), pp. 353–367

Brown P 1994 Pathophysiology of spasticity. *J Neurol Neurosurg Psychiatry* **57**: 773–777

Brown WF, Ebers GC, Hudson AJ, Pringle CE, Veitch J 1992 Motor evoked responses in primary lateral sclerosis. *Muscle Nerve* **15**: 626–629

Brown WJ 1978 The capillaries in acute and subacute multiple sclerosis plaques: a morphometric analysis. *Neurology* **28**: 84–92

Brownell B, Hughes JT 1962 The distribution of plaques in the cerebrum in multiple sclerosis. *J Neurol Neurosurg Psychiatry* **25**: 315–320

Bruce AJ, Boling W, Kindy MS et al 1996 Altered neuronal and microglial responses to excitotoxic and ischemic brain injury in mice lacking TNF receptors. *Nature Med* **2**: 788–794

Brück W, Schmied M, Suchanek G et al 1994 Oligodendrocytes in the early course of multiple sclerosis. *Ann Neurol* **35**: 65–73

Brück W, Porada P, Poser S et al 1995 Monocyte/macrophage differentiation in early multiple sclerosis lesions. *Ann Neurol* **38**: 788–796

Brück W, Bitsch A, Kolenda H et al 1997 Inflammatory central nervous system demyelination: correlation of magnetic resonance imaging findings with lesion pathology. *Ann Neurol* **42**: 783–793

Brück W, Lucchinetti CF, Lassmann H 2003 The pathology of primary progressive multiple sclerosis. *Mult Scler* **8**: 93–97

Brumlik J, Means ED 1969 Tremorine-tremor, shivering and acute cerebellar ataxia in the adult and child – a comparative study. *Brain* **92**: 157–190

Brundin L, Morcos E, Olsson T et al 1999 Increased intrathecal nitric oxide formation in multiple sclerosis: cerebrospinal fluid nitrite as activity marker. *Eur J Neurol* **6**: 585–590

Brundula V, Rewcastle NB, Metz LM et al 2002 Targeting leukocyte MMPs and transmigration: minocycline as a potential therapy for multiple sclerosis. *Brain* **125**: 1297–1308

Brunner C, Lassmann H, Waehneldt TV et al 1989 Differential ultrastructural localization of myelin basic protein, myelin/oligodendroglial glycoprotein, and 2',3'-cyclic nucleotide 3'-phosphodiesterase in the CNS of adult rats. *J Neurochem* **52**: 296–304

Brusa A, Jones SJ, Plant GT 2001 Long term remyelination after optic neuritis: a 2 year visual evoked potential and psychophysical serial study. *Brain* **124**: 468–479

Brustle O, Spiro AC, Karram K et al 1997 In vitro-generated neural precursors participate in mammalian brain development. *Proc Natl Acad Sci USA* **94**: 14809–14814

Brustle O, Jones KN, Learish RD et al 1999 Embryonic stem cell-derived glial precursors: a source of myelinating transplants. *Science* **285**: 754–756

Bsibsi M, Ravid R, Gveric D, van Noort JM 2003 Broad expression of Toll-like receptors in the human central nervous system. *J Neuropathol Exp Neurol* **61**: 1013–1021

Buchanan RJ, Martin RA, Zuniga M et al 2004 Nursing home residents with multiple sclerosis: comparisons of African American residents to white residents at admission. *Mult Scler* **10**: 660–667

Buckley C, Kennard C, Swash M 1982 Treatment of acute exacerbations of multiple sclerosis with intravenous methylprednisolone. *J Neurol Neurosurg Psychiatry* **45**: 179–180

Buddeberg BS, Kerschensteiner M, Merkler D et al 2004 Behavioural testing in a localised animal model of multiple sclerosis. *J Neuroimmunol* 153: 158–170

von Büdingen H-C, Tanuma N, Villoslada P et al 2001 Immune responses against the myelin/oligodendrocyte glycoprotein in experimental autoimmune demyelination. *J Clin Immunol* 21: 155–170

von Büdingen HC, Hauser SL, Fuhrmann A et al 2002 Molecular characterization of antibody specificities against myelin/oligodendrocyte glycoprotein in autoimmune demyelination. *Proc Natl Acad Sci USA* 99: 8207–8212

Bufill E, Blesa R, Galan I, Dean G 1995 Prevalence of multiple sclerosis in the region of Osano, Catalonia, northern Spain. *J Neurol Neurosurg Psychiatry* 58: 577–581

Buhler MMcW, Bennetts BH, Heard RNS, Stewart GJ 2000 T cell receptor β chain genotyping in Australian relapsing–remitting multiple sclerosis patients. *Mult Scler* 6: 140–147

Buhmann C, Gbadomosi J, Heeson C 2002 Visual recovery in a man with the rare combination of mtDNA 11778 LHON mutation and a MS-like disease after mitoxantrone therapy. *Acta Neurol Scand* 196: 236–239

Buljevac D, Flach HZ, Hop WCJ et al 2002 Prospective study on the relationship between infections and multiple sclerosis exacerbations. *Brain* 125: 952–960

Buljevac D, Verkooyen RP, Jacobs BC et al 2003a *Chlamydia pneumoniae* and the risk for exacerbation in multiple sclerosis patients. *Ann Neurol* 54: 828–831

Buljevac D, Hop WC, Reedeker W et al 2003b Self-reported stressful life events and exacerbations in multiple sclerosis: prospective study. *Brit Med J* 327: 646

Bulman DE, Ebers GC 1992 The geography of multiple sclerosis reflects genetic susceptibility. *J Trop Geogr Neurol* 2: 66–72

Bulman DE, Sadovnick AD, Cripps J, Ebers GC 1991a Age of onset in siblings concordant for multiple sclerosis. *Brain* 114: 937–950

Bulman DE, Armstrong H, Ebers GC 1991b Allele frequencies of the third component of complement (C3) in MS patients. *J Neurol Neurosurg Psychiatry* 54: 554–555

Bundey S 1991 Uses and limitations of twin studies. *J Neurol* 238: 360–364

Bunge MB, Bunge RP, Ris H 1961 Ultrastructural study of remyelination in an experimental lesion in adult cat spinal cord. *J Biophys Biochem Cytol* 10: 67–94

Bunge MB, Bunge RP, Pappas GD 1962 Electron microscopic demonstration of connections between glia and myelin sheaths in the developing mammalian central nervous system. *J Cell Biol* 12: 448–453

Burchiel KJ 1980 Abnormal impulse generation in focally demyelinated trigeminal roots. *J Neurosurg* 53:674–683

Burchiel KJ 1981 Ectopic impulse generation in demyelinated axons: effects of Pa$_{CO_2}$, pH, and disodium edetate. *Ann Neurol* 9: 378–383

Bureau JF, Montagutelli X, Bihl F et al 1993 Mapping loci influencing the persistence of Theiler's virus in the murine central nervous system. *Nature Genet* 5: 87–91

Burgerman R, Rigamonti D, Randle JM, Fishman P, Panitch HS, Johnson KP 1992 The association of cervical spondylosis and multiple sclerosis. *Surg Neurol* 38: 265–270

Burguera JA, Catalá J, Casanova B 1991 Thalamic demyelination and paroxysmal dystonia in multiple sclerosis. *Mov Disord* 6: 379–381

Burk K, Abele M, Fetter M et al 1996 Autosomal dominant cerebellar ataxia type 1 clinical features and MRI in families with SCA1, SCA2 and SCA3. *Brain* 119: 1497–1505

Burke D 1993 Microneurography, impulse conduction, and paresthesias. *Muscle Nerve* 16: 1025–1032

Burke D, Mogyoros I, Vagg R, Kiernan MC 1998 Quantitative description of the voltage dependence of axonal excitability in human cutaneous afferents. *Brain* 121: 1975–1983

Burke D, Kiernan MC, Bostock H 2001 Excitability of human axons. *Clin Neurophysiol* 112: 1575–1585

Burne J, Staple JK, Raff MC 1996 Glial cells are increased proportionally in transgenic optic nerves with increased numbers of axons. *J Neurosci* 16: 2064–2073

Burnet FM 1959 *The Clonal Selection Theory of Acquired Immunity*. Cambridge: Cambridge University Press

Burnfield A 1985 *Multiple Sclerosis: A Personal Exploration*. London: Souvenir Press

Burnham JA, Wright RP, Driesbach J, Murray RS 1991 The effect of high-dose steroids on MRI gadolinium enhancement in acute demyelinating lesions. *Neurology* 41: 1349–1354

Burns FR, Li X, Shen N et al 1989 Both rat and mouse T cell receptors specific for the encephalitogenic determinant of myelin basic protein use similar Vα and Vβ chain genes even though the major histocompatibility complex and encephalitogenic determinants being recognized are different. *J Exp Med* 169: 27–39

Burns J, Rosenzweig A, Zweiman B, Lisak RP 1983 Isolation of myelin basic protein-reactive T cell lines from normal human blood. *Cell Immunol* 81: 435–440

Burns J, Littlefield K, Gill J, Trotter J 1991 Autoantigen-induced self lysis of human myelin basic protein-specific T lymphocytes. *J Neuroimmunol* 35: 227–236

Burt R 1997 BMT for severe autoimmune diseases: an idea whose time has come. *Oncology* 11: 1001–1017

Burt R, Burns W, Hess A 1995 Bone marrow transplantation for multiple sclerosis. *Bone Marrow Transplant* 16: 1–6

Burt RK, Burns WH, Miller SD 1997 Bone marrow transplantation for multiple sclerosis: returning to Pandora's box. *Immunol Today* 18: 559–561

Burt RK, Cohen BA, Russell E et al 2003 Hematopoietic stem cell transplantation for progressive multiple sclerosis: failure of a total body irradiation-based conditioning regimen to prevent disease progression in patients with high disability scores. *Blood* 102: 2373–2378

Burt RK, Cohen B, Rose J et al 2005 Hematopoietic stem cell transplantation for multiple sclerosis. *Arch Neurol* 62: 860–864

Burwick RM, Ramsay PP, Haines JL et al 2005 APOE in multiple sclerosis susceptibility and severity: meta- and pooled analyses (submitted)

Bush TG, Puvanachandra N, Horner CH et al 1999 Leukocyte infiltration, neuronal degeneration, and neurite outgrowth after ablation of scar-forming, reactive astrocytes in adult transgenic mice. *Neuron* 23: 297–308

Butcher EC, Picker LJ 1996 Lymphocyte homing and homeostasis. *Science* 272: 60–66

Butt AM, Jenkins HG 1994 Morphological changes in oligodendrocytes in the intact mouse optic nerve following intravitreal injection of tumour necrosis factor. *J Neuroimmunol* 51: 27–33

Butt AM, Ransom BR 1989 Visualisation of oligodendrocytes and astrocytes in the intact rat optic nerve by intracellular injection of lucifer yellow and horseradish peroxidase. *Glia* 2: 470–475

Butt AM, Duncan A, Hornby MF et al 1999 Cells expressing the NG2 antigen contact nodes of Ranvier in adult CNS white matter. *Glia* 26: 84–91

Butt AM, Kiff J, Hubbard P, Berry M 2002 Synantocytes: new functions for novel NG2 expressing glia. *J Neurocytol* 31: 551–565

Butter C, Baker D, O'Neill JK, Turk JL 1991 Mononuclear cell trafficking and plasma protein extravasation into the CNS during chronic relapsing experimental allergic encephalomyelitis in Biozzi AB/H mice. *J Neurol Sci* 104: 9–12

Butterfield RJ, Sudweeks JD, Blakenhorn EP et al 1998 New genetic loci that control susceptibility and symptoms of experimental allergic encephalomyelitis in inbred mice. *J Immunol* 161: 1860–1867

Butterfield RJ, Blankenhorn EP, Roper RJ et al 1999 Genetic analysis of disease subtypes and sexual dimorphisms in mouse experimental allergic encephalomyelitis (EAE): relapsing/remitting and monophasic remitting/nonrelapsing EAE are immunogenetically distinct. *J Immunol* 162: 3096–3102

Butterfield RJ, Blankenhorn EP, Roper RJ et al 2000 Identification of genetic loci controlling the characteristics and severity of brain and spinal cord lesions in experimental allergic encephalomyelitis. *Am J Pathol* 157: 637–645

Butzkueven H, Zhang JG, Soilu-Hanninen M et al 2002 LIF receptor signaling limits immune-mediated demyelination by enhancing oligodendrocyte survival. *Nature Med* 8: 613–619

Bye AME, Kendall B, Wilson J 1985 Multiple sclerosis in childhood: a new look. *Dev Med Child Neurol* 27: 215–222

Cabarrocas J, Bauer J, Piaggio E *et al* 2003 Effective and selective immune surveillance of the brain by MHC class I-restricted cytotoxic T lymphocytes. *Eur J Immunol* 33: 1174–1182

Cabre P, Heinzlef O, Merle H *et al* 2001 MS and neuromyelitis optica in Martinique (French West Indies). *Neurology* 56: 507–514

Cabre P, Signate A, Olindo S *et al* 2005 Role of return migration in the emergence of multiple sclerosis in the French West Indies. *Brain* 128: 899–910

Cabrera-Gomez JA, Echazabal-Santana N, Real-Gonzalez Y *et al* 2005 Hereditary Melkersson–Rosenthal syndrome and multiple sclerosis. *Mult Scler* 11: 364–366

Cai D, Shen Y, De Bellard M *et al* 1999 Prior exposure to neurotrophins blocks inhibition of axonal regeneration by MAG and myelin via a cAMP-dependent mechanism. *Neuron* 22: 89–101

Caillier S, Barcellos LF, Baranzini SE *et al* 2003 Osteopontin polymorphisms and disease course in multiple sclerosis. *Genes Immun* 4: 312–315

Caine ED, Schwid SR 2002 Multiple sclerosis, depression, and the risk of suicide. *Neurology* 59: 662–663

Cajal SR 1894 *Les nouvelles ideés sur la structure du système nerveux*. Paris: Reinwald

Cajal SR 1899–1904 *Textura del sistema nervioso del hombre y de los vertebrados*. 3 volumes. Madrid 1899–1904 [*Texture of the Nervous System of Man and Vertebrates*, Pasik P, Pasik T (trans.), Vienna: Springer, 1999–2002]

Cajal SR 1913 Contribucion al conocmiento de la neuroglia del cerebra humano. *Trab Lab de Invest Biol* 11: 255–315

Cala LA, Mastaglia FL 1976 Computerised axial tomography in multiple sclerosis. *Lancet* i: 689

Calabrese V, Bella R, Testa D *et al* 1998 Increased cerebrospinal fluid and plasma levels of ultraweak chemiluminescence are associated with changes in the thiol pool and lipid-soluble fluorescence in multiple sclerosis: the pathogenic role of oxidative stress. *Drugs Exp Clin Res* 24: 125–131

Calabrese V, Scapagnini G, Ravagna A *et al* 2002 Nitric oxide synthase is present in the cerebrospinal fluid of patients with active multiple sclerosis and is associated with increases in cerebrospinal fluid protein nitrotyrosine and S-nitrosothiols and with changes in glutathione levels. *J Neurosci Res* 70: 580–587

Calabresi PA, Pelfrey CM, Tranquill LR *et al* 1997a VLA-4 expression on peripheral blood lymphocytes is downregulated after treatment of multiple sclerosis with interferon beta. *Neurology* 49: 1111–1116

Calabresi PA, Stone LA, Bash CN *et al* 1997b Interferon beta results in immediate reduction of contrast-enhanced MRI lesions in multiple sclerosis patients followed by weekly MRI. *Neurology* 48: 1446–1448

Calabresi PA, Tranquill LR, Dambrosia JM *et al* 1997c Increases in soluble VCAM-1 correlate with a decrease in MRI lesions in multiple sclerosis treated with interferon beta-1b. *Ann Neurol* 41: 669–674

Calabresi PA, Austin H, Racke MK *et al* 2002a Impaired renal function in progressive multiple sclerosis. *Neurology* 59:1799–1801

Calabresi PA, Wilterdink JL, Rogg JM *et al* 2002b An open-label trial of combination therapy with interferon beta-1a and oral methotrexate in MS. *Neurology* 58: 314–317

Calaora V, Rogister B, Bismuth K *et al* 2001 Neuregulin signaling regulates neural precursor growth and the generation of oligodendrocytes in vitro. *J Neurosci* 21: 4740–4751

Calcagno P, Ruoppolo G, Grasso MG *et al* 2002 Dysphagia in multiple sclerosis – prevalence and prognostic factors. *Acta Neurol Scand* 105: 40–43

Caldwell JH, Schaller KL, Lasher RS *et al* 2000 Sodium channel Na(v)1.6 is localized at nodes of Ranvier, dendrites, and synapses. *Proc Natl Acad Sci USA* 97: 5616–5620

Callanan MM, Logsdail SJ, Ron MA, Warrington EK 1989 Cognitive impairment in patients with clinically isolated lesions of the type seen in multiple sclerosis. *Brain* 1123: 361–374

Callegaro D, de Lolio CA, Radvany J *et al* 1992 Prevalence of multiple sclerosis in the city of Sao Paolo, Brazil in 1990. *Neuroepidemiology* 11: 11–14

Callegaro D, Goldbaum M, Morais L *et al* 2001 The prevalence of multiple sclerosis in the city of Sao Paulo, Brazil 1997. *Acta Neurol Scand* 104: 208–213

Calvin WH, Loeser JD, Howe JF 1977 A neurophysiological theory for the pain mechanism of tic douloureux. *Pain* 3: 147–154

Calvin WH, Devor M, Howe JF 1982 Can neuralgias arise from minor demyelination? Spontaneous firing, mechanosensitivity, and after discharge from conducting axons. *Exp Neurol* 75: 755–763

Calza L, Fernandez M, Giuliani A *et al* 2002 Thyroid hormone activates oligodendrocyte precursors and increases a myelin-forming protein and NGF content in the spinal cord during experimental allergic encephalomyelitis. *Proc Natl Acad Sci USA* 99: 3258–3263

Camenga DL, Johnson KP, Alter M *et al* 1986 Systemic recombinant α-2 therapy in relapsing multiple sclerosis. *Arch Neurol* 43: 1239–1246

Cameron RS, Rakic P 1991 Glial cell lineage in the cerebral cortex: a review and synthesis. *Glia* 4: 124–137

Cammer W 2002 Apoptosis of oligodendrocytes in secondary cultures from neonatal rat brains. *Neurosci Lett* 327: 123–127

Cammer W, Zhang H 1999 Maturation of oligodendrocytes is more sensitive to TNFα than is survival of precursors and immature oligodendrocytes. *J Neuroimmunol* 97: 37–42

Camp SJ, Stevenson VL, Thompson AJ *et al* 1999 Cognitive function in primary progressive and transitional progressive multiple sclerosis: a controlled study with MRI correlates. *Brain* 122: 1341–1348

Campbell AMG, Daniel P, Porter RJ *et al* 1947 Disease of the nervous system occurring among research workers on swayback in lambs. *Brain* 70: 50–58

Campbell AMG, Herdan G, Tatlow WF, Whittle EG 1950 Lead in relation to disseminated sclerosis. *Brain* 73: 52–70

Campbell IL, Stalder AK, Akwa Y *et al* 1998 Transgenic models to study the actions of cytokines in the central nervous system. *Neuroimmunomodulation* 5: 126–135

Campi A, Filippi M, Comi G *et al* 1995 Acute transverse myelopathy: spinal and cranial MR study with clinical follow-up. *Am J Neuroradiol* 16: 115–123

Campi A, Benndorf G, Filippi M *et al* 2001 Primary angiitis of the central nervous system: serial MRI of brain and spinal cord. *Neuroradiology* 43: 599–607

Campuzano V, Montermini L, Molto MD *et al* 1996 Friedreich's ataxia: autosomal recessive disease caused by an intronic GAA triplet repeat expansion. *Science* 271: 1423–1427

Canadian Burden of Illness Study Group 1998 Burden of illness of multiple sclerosis. Part I: Cost of illness. *Can J Neurol Sci* 25: 23–30

Canadian Co-operative Multiple Sclerosis Study Group 1991 The Canadian co-operative trial of cyclophosphamide and plasma exchange in progressive multiple sclerosis. *Lancet* 337: 441–446

Canadian MS Research Group 1987 A randomised controlled trial of amantidine in fatigue associated with multiple sclerosis. *Can J Neurol Sci* 14: 273–278

Cangemi FE, Bergen RL 1980 Optic atrophy following swine flu vaccination. *Ann Ophthalmol* 12: 857–863

Cannella B, Raine CS 1995 The adhesion molecule and cytokine profile of multiple sclerosis lesions. *Ann Neurol* 37: 424–435

Cannella B, Raine CS 2004 Multiple sclerosis: cytokine receptors on oligodendrocytes predict innate regulation. *Ann Neurol* 55: 46–57

Cannella B, Cross AH, Raine CS 1991 Adhesion-related molecules in the central nervous system. Upregulation correlates with inflammatory cell influx during relapsing experimental autoimmune encephalomyelitis. *Lab Invest* 65: 23–31

Cannella B, Hoban CJ, Gao YL *et al* 1998 The neuregulin, glial growth factor 2, diminishes autoimmune demyelination and enhances remyelination in a chronic relapsing model for multiple sclerosis. *Proc Natl Acad Sci USA* 95: 10100–10105

Cannella B, Pitt D, Marchionni M, Raine CS 1999 Neuregulin and erbB receptor expression in normal and diseased human white matter. *J Neuroimmunol* **100**: 233–242

Cannella B, Pitt D, Capello E, Raine CS 2000 Insulin-like growth factor-1 fails to enhance central nervous system meylin repair during autoimmune demyelination. *Am J Pathol* **157**: 933–943

Canoll PD, Musacchia JM, Hardy R *et al* 1996 GGF/neuregulin is a neuronal signal that promotes the proliferation and survival and inhibits the differentiation of oligodendrocyte progenitors. *Neuron* **17**: 229–243

Cao L, Liu L, Chen ZY *et al* 2004 Olfactory ensheathing cells genetically modified to secrete GDNF to promote spinal cord repair. *Brain* **127**: 535–549

Caplan LR, Nadelson T 1980 Multiple sclerosis and hysteria: lessons learnt from their association. *J Am Med Assoc* **243**: 2418–2420

Cappelen-Smith C, Kuwabara S, Lin CSY *et al* 2000 Activity-dependent hyperpolarization and conduction block in chronic inflammatory demyelinating polyneuropathy. *Ann Neurol* **48**: 826–832

Caraccio N, Dardano A, Manfredonia F *et al* 2005 Long-term follow-up of 106 multiple sclerosis patients undergoing IFN-β1a or 1b therapy: predictive factors of thyroid disease development and duration. *J Clin Endocrinol Metab* **90**: 4133–4137

Caramalho I, Lopes-Carvalho T, Ostler D *et al* 2003 Regulatory T cells selectively express Toll-like receptors and are activated by lipopolysaccharide. *J Exp Med* **197**: 403–411

Caramanos Z, Arnold DL 2005 Evidence for use of glatiramer acetate in multiple sclerosis. *Lancet Neurol* **4**: 74–75; discussion 76–77

Carboni S, Aboul-Enein F, Waltzinger C *et al* 2003 CD134 plays a crucial role in the pathogenesis of EAE and is upregulated in the CNS of patients with multiple sclerosis. *J Neuroimmunol* **145**: 1–11

Cardon T, Wyremblewski P, Lesoin F, Brunaud V, Destée A 1992 Angiome caverneux de la moelle cervicale. *Rev Neurol* **148**: 152–154

Carey RG, Seibert JH, Posavac EJ 1988 Who makes the most progress in inpatient rehabilitation? An analysis of functional gain. *Arch Phys Med Rehab* **69**: 337–343

Carlander B, Dauvilliers Y, Billiard M 2001 Immunological aspects of narcolepsy. *Rev Neurol* **157**: S97–S100

Carlson CS, Eberle M, Kruglyak L, Nickerson D 2004 Mapping complex disease loci in whole-genome association studies. *Nature* **429**: 446–452

Carmichael EA 1931 The aetiology of disseminated sclerosis: some criticisms of recent work, especially to the 'spherula insularis'. *Proc R Soc Med* **34**: 591–606

Carmody RJ, Hilliard B, Maguschak K *et al* 2002 Genomic scale profiling of autoimmune inflammation in the central nervous system: the nervous response to inflammation. *J Neuroimmunol* **133**: 95–107

Caroll WM, Jennings AR, Ironside LJ 1998 Identification of the adult resting progenitor cell by autoradiographic tracking of oligodendrocyte precursors in experimental CNS demyelination. *Brain* **121**: 293–302

Carp RI, Licursi PC, Merz PA, Merz GS 1972 Decreased percentage of polymorphonuclear neutrophils in mouse peripheral blood after inoculation with material from multiple sclerosis patients. *J Exp Med* **136**: 618–629

Carp RI, Licursi PL, Merz PA *et al* 1977 Multiple sclerosis – associated agent. *Lancet* **ii**: 814

Carrieri PB, Provitera V, De Rosa T *et al* 1998 Profile of cerebrospinal fluid and serum cytokines in patients with relapsing–remitting multiple sclerosis: a correlation with clinical activity. *Immunopharmacol Immun* **20**: 373–382

Carrington M, Colonna M, Spies T *et al* 1993 Haplotypic variation of the transporter associated with antigen processing (TAP) genes and their extension of HLA class II region haplotypes. *Immunogenetics* **37**: 266–273

Carrithers MD, Visintin I, Kang SJ, Janeway CA 2000 Differential adhesion molecule requirements for immune surveillance and inflammatory recruitment. *Brain* **123**: 1092–1101

Carrithers MD, Visintin I, Viret C, Janeway CS Jr 2002 Role of genetic background in P selectin-dependent immune surveillance of the central nervous system. *J Neuroimmunol* **129**: 51–57

Carrizosa AM, Nicholson LB, Farzan M *et al* 1998 Expansion by self antigen is necessary for the induction of experimental autoimmune encephalomyelitis by T cells primed with a cross-reactive environmental antigen. *J Immunol* **161**: 3307–3314

Carroll CB, Zajicek JP 2004 The 'harlequin' sign in association with multiple sclerosis. *J Neurol* **251**: 1145–1146

Carswell R 1838 *Pathological Anatomy: Illustrations of the Elementary Forms of Disease.* London: Orme, Brown, Green & Longman

Carter JL, Noseworthy JH 1994 Ventilatory dysfunction in multiple sclerosis. *Clin Chest Med* **15**: 693–703

Carter S, Sciarra D, Merritt HH 1950 The course of multiple sclerosis as determined by autopsy proven cases. *Res Publ Assoc Res Nerv Mental Dis* **28**: 471–511

Cartlidge NEF 1972 Autonomic function in multiple sclerosis. *Brain* **95**: 661–664

Cartlidge NEF, Hudgson P, Weightman D 1974 A comparison of baclofen and diazepam in the treatment of spasticity. *J Neurol Sci* **23**: 17–24

Carton H, Vlietinck R, Debruyne J *et al* 1997 Recurrence risks of multiple sclerosis in relatives of patients in Flanders, Belgium. *J Neurol Neurosurg Psychiatry* **62**: 329–333

Casaccia-Bonnefil P, Carter BD, Dobrowsky RT, Chao MV 1996 Death of oligodendrocytes mediated by the interaction of nerve growth factor with its receptor p75. *Nature* **383**: 716–719

Cascino I, Galeazzi M, Salvetti M *et al* 1994 HSP70–1 promoter polymorphism tested in three autoimmune diseases. *Immunogenet* **39**: 291–293

Cascino I, Ballerini C, Audino S *et al* 1998 Fas gene polymorphisms are not associated with systemic lupus erythematosus, multiple sclerosis and HIV infection. *Disease Markers* **13**: 221–225

Casellas R, Shih T, Kleinewietfeld M *et al* 2001 Contribution of receptor editing to the antibody repertoire. *Science* **291**: 1541–1544

Cash E, Minty A, Ferrara P *et al* 1994 Macrophage-inactivating IL-13 suppresses experimental autoimmune encephalomyelitis in rats. *J Immunol* **153**: 4258–4267

Casquero P, Villoslada P, Montalban X, Torrent M 2001 Frequency of multiple sclerosis in Menorca, Balearic Islands, Spain. *Neuroepidemiology* **20**: 129–133

Cassetta I, Granieri E, Marchi D *et al* 1998 An epidemiological study of multiple sclerosis in central Sardinia, Italy. *Acta Neurol Scand* **98**: 391–394

Cassetta I, Invernizzi M, Granieir E 2001 Multiple sclerosis and dental amalgam: case-control study in Ferrara, Italy. *Neuroepidemiology* **20**: 134–137

Castaigne P, Escourolle R, Laplane D, Augustin P 1966 Comas transitoires avec hyperthermie au cours de la sclérose en plaques. *Rev Neurol* **114**: 147–150

Castaigne P, Cambier J, Masson M *et al* 1970 Les manifestations motrices paroxystiques de la sclérose en plaques. *Presse Med* **78**: 1921–1924

Castaigne P, Lhermitte F, Escurolle R *et al* 1981 Les scléroses en plaques asymptomatiques. *Rev Neurol* **137**: 729–739

Casula FC (undated) *The History of Sardinia.* Cagliari: Editrice Mediterranea

Caton R 1875 The electric currents of the brain. *Br Med J* **2**: 278

Cattaneo C, Almici C, Borlenghi E *et al* 2003 A case of acute promyelocytic leukaemia following mitoxantrone treatment of multiple sclerosis. *Leukemia* **17**: 985–986

Cavalli-Sforza LL, Menozzi P, Piazza A 1994 *The History and Geography of Human Genes.* Princeton, NJ: Princeton Universty Press

Cecconi F, Alvarez-Bolado G, Meyer BI *et al* 1998 Apaf1 (CED-4 homolog) regulates programmed cell death in mammalian development. *Cell* **94**: 727–737

Celesia GG, Kaufman DI, Brigell M *et al* 1990 Optic neuritis: a prospective study. *Neurology* **40**: 919–923

Celius EG, Vandvik B 2001 Multiple sclerosis in Oslo, Norway: prevalence on 1 January 1995 and incidence over a 25-year period. *Eur J Neurol* **8**: 463–469

Celius EG, Harbo HF, Egeland T *et al* 2000 Sex and age at diagnosis are correlated with the HLA-DR2, DQ6 haplotype in multiple sclerosis. *J Neurol Sci* **178**: 132–135

Cella DF, Dineen K, Arnason B *et al* 1996 Validation of the functional assessment of multiple sclerosis quality of life instrument. *Neurology* **47**: 129–139

829

Cella M, Jabrossay F, Alebardi O et al 1999 Plasmacytoid monocytes migrate to inflamed lymph nodes and produce large amounts of type I interferon. *Nature Med* **5**: 919–923

Ceman S, Rudersdorf R, Long E, Demars R 1992 MHC class II deletion mutant expresses normal levels of transgene encoded class II molecules that have abnormal conformation and impaired antigen presentation ability. *J Immunol* **149**: 754–761

Cendrowski WS 1968 Multiple sclerosis: discordance of three dizygotic twin pairs. *J Med Genet* **5**: 266–268

Cendrowski WS, Makowski J 1972 Epilepsy in multiple sclerosis. *J Neurol Sci* **17**: 389–398

Cendrowski WS, Wender M, Dominik W et al 1969 Epidemiological study of multiple sclerosis in Western Poland. *Eur Neurol* **2**: 90–108

Cengiz N, Ozbenli T, Onar L et al 2002 Adult metachromatic leukodystrophy: three cases with normal nerve conduction velocities in a family. *Acta Neurol Scand* **105**: 454–457

Centonze D, Rossi S, Boffa L et al 2005 CSF from MS patients can induce acute conduction block in the isolated optic nerve. *Eur J Neurol* **12**: 45–48

Cepok S, Jacobsen M, Schock S et al 2001 Patterns of cerebrospinal fluid pathology correlate with disease progression in multiple sclerosis. *Brain* **124**: 2169–2176

Cepok S, Rosche B, Grummel V et al 2005a Short-lived plasma blasts are the main B cell effector subset during the course of multiple sclerosis. *Brain* **128**: 1667–1676

Cepok S, Zhou D, Srivastava S et al 2005b Identification of Epstein–Barr virus proteins as putative targets of the immune response in multiple sclerosis. *J Clin Invest* **115**: 1352–1360

Cercignani M, Bozzali M, Iannucci G et al 2001a Magnetisation transfer ratio and mean diffusivity of normal appearing white and grey matter from patients with multiple sclerosis. *J Neurol Neurosurg Psychiatry* **70**: 311–317

Cercignani M, Inglese M, Pagani E et al 2001b Mean diffusivity and fractional anisotropy histograms of patients with multiple sclerosis. *Am J Neuroradiol* **22**: 952–958

Cerf JA, Carels G 1966 Multiple sclerosis: serum factor producing reversible alterations in bioelectric responses. *Science* **152**: 1066–1068

Cerizza M, Nemni R, Tamma F 1987 Adult metachromatic leukodystrophy: an underdiagnosed disease. *J Neurol Neurosurg Psychiatry* **50**: 1710–1712

Cestan R, Guillain G 1900 Le paraplegie spasmodique familiale et la sclérose en plaques familiale. *Rev Med* **20**: 813–836

Chabas D, Baranzini SE, Mitchell D et al 2001 The influence of the proinflammatory cytokine, osteopontin, on autoimmune demyelinating disease. *Science* **294**: 1731–1735

Chabriat H, Chen QM, Poisson M, Delattre JY 1994 Dégénérescence cérébelleuse paranéoplastique. *Rev Neurol* **150**: 105–114

Chagnac Y, Martinovits G, Tadmor R, Goldhammer Y 1986 Paroxysmal atrial fibrillation associated with an attack of multiple sclerosis. *Postgrad Med J* **62**: 385–387

Chajek T, Fainaru M 1975 Behçet's disease: report of 41 cases and review of literature. *Medicine* **54**: 179–196

Chakraborty R, Kamboh, MI, Nwankwo M, Ferrell RE 1992 Caucasian genes in American blacks: new data. *Am J Hum Genet* **50**: 145–155

Chalk JB, McCombe PA, Pender MP 1994 Conduction abnormalities are restricted to the central nervous system in experimental autoimmune encephalomyelitis induced by inoculation with proteolipid protein but not with myelin basic protein. *Brain* **117**: 975–986

Chalk JB, McCombe PA, Pender MP 1995 Restoration of conduction in the spinal roots correlates with clinical recovery from experimental autoimmune encephalomyelitis. *Muscle Nerve* **18**: 1093–1100

Challoner PB, Smith KT, Parker JD et al 1995 Plaque-associated expression of human herpesvirus 6 in multiple sclerosis. *Proc Natl Acad Sci USA* **92**: 7440–7444

Chalmers RM, Robertson NP, Kellar-Wood H et al 1995 Sequence of the human homologue of a mitochondrially encoded murine transplantation antigen in patients with multiple sclerosis. *J Neurol* **242**: 332–334

Chalmers RM, Robertson NP, Compston DAS, Harding AE 1996 Sequence of mitochondrial DNA in patients with multiple sclerosis. *Ann Neurol* **40**: 239–243

CHAMPS Study Group 2002 MRI predictors of early conversion to clinically definite MS in the CHAMPS placebo group. *Neurology* **59**: 998–1005

Chancellor AM, Addidle M, Dawson K 2003 Multiple sclerosis is more prevalent in northern New Zealand than previously reported. *Intern Med J* **33**: 79–83

Chandler BJ 1999 Impact of neurologic disability on sex and relationships. In: Fowler C (ed.) *Neurology of Bladder, Bowel, and Sexual Dysfunction*. Boston, MA: Butterworth-Heinemann, pp. 69–93

Chandran SC, Svendsen C, Compston A, Scolding N 1998 Regional potential for oligodendrocyte generation in the rodent embryonic spinal cord following exposure to EGF and FGF-2. *Glia* **24**: 382–389

Chandran SC, Kato H, Gerreli D et al 2003 FGF dependent generation of oligodendrocytes by a hedgehog independent pathway. *Development* **30**: 6599–6609

Chandran SC, Compston DAS, Jauniaux E et al 2004 Differential generation of oligodendrocytes from human and rodent embryonic spinal cord neural precursors. *Glia* **47**: 314–324

Chang A, Nishiyama A, Peterson J et al 2000 NG2-positive oligodendrocyte progenitor cells in adult human brain and multiple sclerosis lesions. *J Neurosci* **20**: 6404–6412

Chang A, Tourtellotte WW, Rudick R, Trapp BD 2002 Premyelinating oligodendrocytes in chronic lesions of multiple sclerosis. *New Engl J Med* **346**: 165–173

Chang T 1971 Recurrent viral infection (reinfection). *New Engl J Med* **284**: 765–773

Chang Y-Y, Wu H-S, Tsai T-C, Liu J-S 1994 Intractable hiccup due to multiple sclerosis: MR imaging of medullary plaque. *Can J Neurol Sci* **21**: 271–272

Chao CC, Hu S, Peterson PK 1995 Glia, cytokines, and neurotoxicity. *Crit Rev Neurobiol* **9**: 189–205

Chapenko SD, Milers A, Nora Z et al 2003 Correlation between HHV-6 reactivation and multiple sclerosis disease activity. *J Med Virol* **69**: 111–117

Chapman J, Sylantiev C, Nisipeanu P, Korczyn AD 1999 Preliminary observations on APOE epsilon4 allele and progression of disability in multiple sclerosis. *Arch Neurol* **56**: 1484–1487

Chapman J, Vinokurov S, Achiron A et al 2001 APOE is a major predictor of long term progression of disability in MS. *Neurology* **56**: 312–316

Charcot JM 1865 Sclérose du cordons lateraux del la moelle épiniere chez une femme hysterique atteinte de contracture permaneste des quatres membres. *L' Union Med* **25**: 451–457, 467–472

Charcot JM 1868a [Seance du 14 mars]. *Comptes rendus des seances et memoires lus a la societe de Biologie* **20**: 13–14

Charcot JM 1868b Histologie de la sclérose en plaques. *Gazette Hôpitaux* **41**: 554, 557–558, 566

Charcot JM 1868c Leçons sur les maladies chroniques du système nerveux. I: Des scléroses de la moelle épinière. *Gazette Hôpitaux* **41**: 405–406, 409

Charcot JM 1872 *Leçons sur les Maladies du Systeme Nerveux faites a la Salpêtrière*. Paris: A. Delahaye and E. Lecrosnier, Progres Medicale, pp. 1–495 and 1–504 [*Lectures on the Diseases of the Nervous System Delivered at the Salpétrière, Sigerson G (trans.)*. London: The New Sydenham Society, 1877, pp. 157–222]

Charcot JM 1875 *Leçons sur les maladies du système nerveux faites a la Salpetrière*, 2nd edn. Paris: A. Delahaye

Charcot JM 1877 *Lectures on Diseases of the Nervous System*. London: New Sydenham Society

Charcot JM 1886 *Ouevres complètes de J.-M. Charcot. Leçons sur les maladies du système nerveux recueilles et publiées par Bourneville*. Paris: Bureau du Progres Medical and A Delahaye, Tome 1

Charcot JM 1887 *Leçons du mardi a la Salpétrière. Professeur Charcot. Polycliniques*. Paris: Bureaux du Progres Medical and A Delahaye, pp. 398–422

Chard DT, Griffin CM, Parker GJM et al 2002a Brain atrophy in clinically early relapsing–remitting multiple sclerosis. *Brain* 125: 327–337

Chard DT, Griffin CM, McLean MA *et al* 2002b Brain metabolite changes in cortical grey matter and normal appearing white matter in clinically early relapsing remitting multiple sclerosis. *Brain* 125: 2342–2352

Chard DT, Parker GJM, Griffin CM *et al* 2002c The reproducibility and sensitivity of brain tissue volume measurements derived from an SPM-based segmentation methodology. *JMRI* 15: 259–267

Chard DT, Brex PA, Ciccarelli O *et al* 2003 The longitudinal relation between brain lesion load and atrophy in multiple sclerosis: a 14 year follow up study. *J Neurol Neurosurg Psychiatry* 74: 1551–1554

Chard DT, Griffin CM, Rashid W *et al* 2004 Progressive grey matter atrophy in clinically early relapsing–remitting multiple sclerosis. *Mult Scler* 10: 387–391

Chari DM, Blakemore WF 2002a Efficient recolonisation of progenitor-depleted areas of the CNS by adult oligodendrocyte progenitor cells. *Glia* 37: 307–313

Chari DM, Blakemore WF 2002b New insights into remyelination failure in multiple sclerosis: implications for glial cell transplantation. *Mult Scler* 8: 271–277

Chari DM, Crang AJ, Blakemore WF 2003a Decline in rate of colonization of oligodendrocyte progenitor cell (OPC)-depleted tissue by adult OPCs with age. *J Neuropathol Exp Neurol* 62: 908–916

Chari DM, Huang WL, Blakemore WF 2003b Dysfunctional oligodendrocyte progenitor cell (OPC) populations may inhibit repopulation of OPC depleted tissue. *J Neurosci Res* 73: 787–793

Charles P, Hernandez MP, Stankoff B *et al* 2000 Negative regulation of central nervous system myelination by polysialylated-neural cell adhesion molecule. *Proc Natl Acad Sci USA* 97: 7585–7590

Charles P, Reynolds R, Seilhean D *et al* 2002a Re-expression of PSA-NCAM by demyelinated axons: an inhibitor of remyelination in multiple sclerosis? *Brain* 125: 1972–1979

Charles P, Tait S, Faivre-Sarrailh C *et al* 2002b Neurofascin is a glial receptor for the paranodin-caspr-contactin axonal complex at the axoglial junction. *Current Biol* 12: 217–220

Charmley P, Beall SS, Concannon P *et al* 1991 Further localisation of a multiple sclerosis susceptibility gene on chromosome 7q using a new T cell receptor beta-chain DNA polymorphism. *J Neuroimmunol* 32: 231–241

Charpentier B, Hiesse C, Lantz O *et al* 1992 Evidence that antihuman tumor necrosis factor monoclonal antibody prevents OKT3-induced acute syndrome. *Transplantation* 54: 997–1002

Chartier-Kastler EJ, Mozer P, Denys P *et al* 2002 Neurogenic bladder management and cutaneous non-continent ileal conduit. *Spinal Cord* 40: 443–448

Chase WMA 1959 A critique of attempts at passive transfer of sensitivity to nervous tissue. In: Kies MW, Alvord EC (eds) *Allergic Encephalomyelitis*. Springfield, IL: Thomas, pp. 348–374

Chataway SJS, Feakes R, Coraddu F *et al* 1998 The genetics of multiple sclerosis: principles, background and updated results of the United Kingdom systematic genome screen. *Brain* 121: 1869–1887

Chataway SJS, Sawcer SJ, Coraddu F *et al* 1999a Evidence that allelic variants of the spinocerebellar ataxia type 2 gene influence susceptibility to multiple sclerosis. *Neurogenetics* 2: 91–96

Chataway SJS, Sawcer S, Feakes R *et al* 1999b A screen of candidates from peaks of linkage: evidence for the involvement of myeloperoxidase in multiple sclerosis. *J Neuroimmunol* 98: 208–213

Chataway SJS, Sawcer S, Sherman D *et al* 1999c No evidence for association of multiple sclerosis with the complement factors C6 and C7. *J Neuroimmunol* 99: 150–156

Chataway SJS, Mander A, Robertson N *et al* 2001 Multiple sclerosis in sibling pairs: an analysis of 250 families. *J Neurol Neurosurg Psychiatry* 71: 757–761

Chaudhuri A, Behan PO 2001 Acute cervical hyperextension-hyperflexion injury may precipitate and/or exacerbate symptomatic multiple sclerosis. *Eur J Neurol* 8: 659–664

Chen C, Nagy Z, Luning Prak E, Weigert M 1995a Immunoglobulin heavy chain gene replacement: a mechanism of receptor editing. *Immunity* 3: 747–755

Chen C, Nagy Z, Radic MZ *et al* 1995b The site and stage of anti-DNA B cell deletion. *Nature* 373: 252–255

Chen C-H, Houchi H, Ohnaka M *et al* 1998 Nitric oxide activates Ca2+-activated K+ channels in cultured bovine adrenal chromaffin cells. *Neurosci Lett* 248: 127–129

Chen M, Gran B, Costello K *et al* 2001 Glatiramer acetate induces a Th2-biased response and crossreactivity with myelin basic protein in patients with MS. *Mult Scler* 7: 209–219

Chen MS, Huber AB, van der Haar ME *et al* 2000 Nogo-A is a myelin-associated neurite outgrowth inhibitor and an antigen for monoclonal antibody IN-1. *Nature* 403: 434–439

Chen R, Cohen LG, Hallett M 2002 Nervous system reorganization following injury. *Neuroscience* 111: 761–773

Chen S, Luo D, Streit WJ, Harrison JK 2002 TFG-β1 upregulates CX3CR1 expression and inhibits fractalkine-stimulated signaling in rat microglia. *J Neuroimmunol* 133: 46–55

Chen SJ, De Vries GH 1989 The mitogenic effect of the axolemma-enriched fraction on cultured oligodendrocytes. *J Neurochem* 52: 325

Chen W, Frank ME, Jin W, Wahl SM 2001 TGF-β released by apoptotic T cells contributes to an immunosuppressive milieu. *Immunity* 14: 715–725

Chen Y, Devor M 1998 Ectopic mechanosensitivity in injured sensory axons arises from the site of spontaneous electrogenesis. *Eur J Pain* 2: 165–178

Chen Y, Kuchroo VK, Inobe J *et al* 1994 Regulatory T cell clones induced by oral tolerance: suppression of autoimmune encephalomyelitis. *Science* 265: 1237–1240

Chen Y, Inobe J, Marks R *et al* 1995 Peripheral depletion of antigen-reactive T cells in oral tolerance. *Nature* 376: 177–180

Chen ZJ, Ughrin Y, Levine JM 2002 Inhibition of axon growth by oligodendrocyte precursor cells. *Mol Cell Neurosci* 20: 125–139

Cheng B, Christakos S, Mattson MP 1994 Tumor necrosis factors protect neurons against metabolic-excitotoxic insults and promote maintenance of calcium homeostasis. *Neuron* 12: 139–153

Chevassut K 1930 The aetiology of disseminated sclerosis. *Lancet* i: 552–560

Chia Y-W, Fowler CF, Kamm MA *et al* 1995 Prevalence of bowel dysfunction in patients with multiple sclerosis and bladder dysfunction. *J Neurol* 242: 105–108

Chiappa KH 1980 Pattern shift visual, brainstem auditory, and short latency somatosensory evoked potentials in multiple sclerosis. *Neurology* 30: 110–123

Chiappa KH, Harrison JL, Brooks EB, Young RR 1980 Brainstem auditory evoked responses in 200 patients with multiple sclerosis. *Ann Neurol* 7: 135–143

Chiara T, Carlos J, Martin D *et al* 1998 Cold effect on oxygen uptake, perceived exertion, and spasticity in patients with multiple sclerosis. *Arch Phys Med Rehab* 79: 523–528

Chien Y-H, Jores R, Crowley MP 1996 Recognition by γ/δ T cells. *Annu Rev Immunol* 14: 511–532

Chin RL, Latov N 2005 Peripheral neuropathy and celiac disease. *Curr Treat Options Neurol* 7: 43–48

Ching W, Zanazzi G, Levinson SR, Salzer JL 1999 Clustering of neuronal sodium channels requires contact with myelinating Schwann cells. *J Neurocytol* 28: 295–301

Chiocchetti A, Comi C, Indelicato M *et al* 2005 Osteopontin gene haplotypes correlate with multiple sclerosis development and progression. *J Neuroimmunol* 163: 172–178

Chitnis T, Najafian N, Abdallah KA *et al* 2001 CD28-independent induction of experimental autoimmune encephalomyelitis. *J Clin Invest* 107: 575–583

Chiu SY, Ritchie JM 1980 Potassium channels in nodal and internodal axonal membrane of mammalian myelinated fibres. *Nature* 284: 170–171

Chiu SY, Ritchie JM 1981 Evidence for the presence of potassium channels in the paranodal region of acutely demyelinated mammalian single nerve fibres. *J Physiol* 313: 415–437

Chluba J, Steeg C, Becker A *et al* 1989 T cell receptor β chain usage in myelin basic protein-specific rat T lymphocytes. *Eur J Immunol* 19: 279–284

Chmielewska-Badora J, Cisak E, Dutkiewicz J 2000 Lyme borreliosis and multiple sclerosis: any connection? A seroepidemic study. *Ann Agric Environ Med* **7**: 141–143

Chofflon M, Juillard C, Juillard P, Gauthier G, Grau GE 1992 Tumor necrosis factor α production as a possible predictor of relapse in patients with multiple sclerosis. *Eur Cytokine Netw* **3**: 523–531

Choi YB, Lipton SA 2000 Redox modulation of the NMDA receptor. *Cell Mol Life Sci* **57**: 1535–1541

Chong HT, Li PCK, Ong B et al 2002 Severe spinal cord involvement is a universal feature of Asians with multiple sclerosis: a joint Asian study. *Neurol J Southeast Asia* **7**: 35–40

Chopra JS, Radhakrishnan K, Sawhney BB et al 1980 Multiple sclerosis in north-west India. *Acta Neurol Scand* **62**: 312–321

Chou YK, Buenafe AC, Dedrick R et al 1994 T cell receptor Vβ gene usage in the recognition of myelin basic protein by cerebrospinal fluid- and blood-derived T cells from patients with multiple sclerosis. *J Neurosci Res* **37**: 169–181

Christensen T, Sorensen PD, Hansen HJ, Moller-Larsen A 2003 Antibodies against a human endogenous retrovirus and the preponderance of env splice variants in multiple sclerosis patients. *Mult Scler* **9**: 6–15

Christopher V, Scolding N, Przemioslo RT 2005 Acute hepatitis secondary to interferon beta-1a in multiple sclerosis. *J Neurol* **252**: 855–856

Chrousos GA, Kattah JC, Beck RW, Cleary PA, the Optic Neuritis Study Group 1993 Side effects of glucocorticoid treatment. Experience of the Optic Neuritis Treatment Trial. *J Am Med Assoc* **269**: 2110–2112

Chu CQ, Wittmer S, Dalton DK 2000 Failure to suppress the expansion of the activated CD4 T cell population in interferon gamma-deficient mice leads to exacerbation of experimental autoimmune encephalomyelitis. *J Exp Med* **192**: 123–128

Chun SJ, Rasband MN, Sidman RL et al 2003 Integrin-linked kinase is required for laminin-2-induced oligodendrocyte cell spreading and CNS myelination. *J Cell Biol* **163**: 397–408

Cianchetti C, Zuddas A, Randazzo AP et al 1999 Lamotrigine adjunctive therapy in painful phenomena in MS: preliminary observations. *Neurology* **53**: 433

Ciccarelli O, Werring DJ, Wheeler-Kingshott CA et al 2001 Investigation of MS normal-appearing brain using diffusion tensor MRI with clinical correlations. *Neurology* **56**: 926–933

Ciccarelli O, Parker GJM, Toosy AT et al 2003a From diffusion tractography to quantitative white matter tract measures: a reproducibility study. *NeuroImage* **18**: 348–359

Ciccarelli O, Toosy AT, Parker GJM et al 2003b Diffusion tractography based group mapping of major white-matter pathways in the human brain. *Neuroimage* **19**: 1545–1555

Ciccarelli O, Toosy AT, Hickman SJ et al 2005 Optic radiation changes after optic neuritis detected by tractography-based group mapping. *Hum Brain Mapping* **25**: 308–316

Cid C, Alcazar A, Regidor I et al 2002 Neuronal apoptosis induced by cerebrospinal fluid from multiple sclerosis patients correlates with hypointense lesions on T1 magnetic resonance imaging. *J Neurol Sci* **193**: 103–109

Cid C, Alvarez-Cermeno JC, Regidor I et al 2003 Caspase inhibitors protect against neuronal apoptosis induced by cerebrospinal fluid from multiple sclerosis patients. *J Neuroimmunol* **136**: 119–124

Cifelli A, Matthews PM 2002 Cerebral plasticity in multiple sclerosis. *Mult Scler* **8**: 193–199

Cifelli A, Arridge M, Jezzard P et al 2002 Thalamic neurodegeneration in multiple sclerosis. *Ann Neurol* **52**: 650–653

Ciric B, Howe CL, Paz Soldan M et al 2003 Human monoclonal IgM antibody promotes CNS myelin repair independent of Fc function. *Brain Pathol* **13**: 608–616

Ciric B, Van Keulen V, Paz Soldan M et al 2004 Antibody-mediated remyelination operates through mechanism independent of immunomodulation. *J Neuroimmunol* **146**: 153–161

Ciusani E, Allen M, Sandberg-Wollheim M et al 1995 Analysis of HLA-class II DQA1, DQB1, DRB1 and DPB1 in Italian multiple sclerosis patients. *Eur J Immunogenet* **22**: 171–178

Ciusani E, Gelati M, Frigerio S et al 2001 Modulation of experimental allergic encephalomyelitis in Lewis rats by administration of a peptide of Fas ligand. *J Autoimmun* **17**: 273–280

Clanet M, Radue EW, Kappos L et al 2002 A randomized, double-blind, dose-comparison study of weekly interferon beta-1a in relapsing MS. *Neurology* **59**: 1507–1517

Clanet M, Kappos L, Hartung HP et al 2004 Interferon beta-1a in relapsing multiple sclerosis: four-year extension of the European IFNbeta-1a Dose-Comparison Study. *Mult Scler* **10**: 139–144

Clark AJ, Ware MA, Yazer E et al 2004 Patterns of cannabis use among patients with multiple sclerosis. *Neurology* **62**: 2098–2100

Clark EA, Lane PJL 1991 Regulation of human B cell activation and adhesion. *Ann Rev Immunol* **9**: 97–128

Clark RB, Lingenheld EG 1998 Adoptively transferred EAE in γδ T cell knock-out mice. *J Autoimmun* **11**: 105–110

Clark VA, Detels R, Visscher BR et al 1982 Factors associated with a malignant or benign course of multiple sclerosis. *J Am Med Assoc* **248**: 856–860

Clear D 1999 Anaphylactoid reaction to methyl prednisolone developing after starting treatment with interferon beta-1b. *J Neurol Neurosurg Psychiatry* **66**: 690

Clegg A, Bryant J 2001 Immunomodulatory drugs for multiple sclerosis: a systematic review of clinical and cost effectiveness. *Expert Opin Pharmacother* **2**: 623–639

Clemen CS, Spottke EA, Lütjohann D et al 2005 Cerebrotendinous xanthomatosis: at treatable ataxia. *Neurology* **64**: 1476

Clements JM, Cossins JA, Wells GM et al 1997 Matrix metalloproteinase expression during experimental autoimmune encephalomyelitis and effects of a combined matrix metalloproteinase and tumour necrosis factor-alpha inhibitor. *J Neuroimmunol* **74**: 85–94

Clerget-Darpoux F, Govaerts A, Feingold N 1984 HLA and susceptibility to multiple sclerosis. *Tissue Antigens* **24**: 160–169

Clerici M, Fernandez M 1992 Restriction fragment length polymorphism analysis of HLA-DR and DQ-linked alleles in multiple sclerosis in Spain. *J Neuroimmunol* **41**: 245–248

Clerici M, Shearer GM 1993 A Th1 to Th2 switch is a critical step in the etiology of HIV infection. *Immunol Today* **14**: 107–111

Clerici M, Fusi ML, Caputo D et al 1999 Immune responses to antigens of human endogenous retroviruses in patients with acute or stable multiple sclerosis. *J Neuroimmunol* **99**: 173–182

Clifford DB 1983 Tetrahydro-cannabinol for treatment of multiple sclerosis. *Ann Neurol* **13**: 669–671

Clifford DB, Trotter JL 1984 Pain in multiple sclerosis. *Arch Neurol* **41**: 1270–1272

Clifford-Jones RE, Cunningham K, Halliday AM et al 1985a Visual evoked potentials in meningiomas compressing the anterior visual pathways. *Electroencephalography and Clin Neurophysiol* **61**: S52

Clifford-Jones RE, McDonald WI, Landon DN 1985b Chronic optic nerve compression: an experimental study. *Brain* **108**: 241–262

Cocco E, Mancosu C, Fadda E et al 2002 Lack of evidence for a role of the myelin basic protein gene in multiple sclerosis susceptibility in Sardinian patients. *J Neurol* **249**: 1552–1555

Cocco E, Sardu C, Lai M et al 2004a Anticipation of age at onset in multiple sclerosis: a Sardinian cohort study. *Neurology* **62**: 1794–1798

Cocco E, Murru MR, Melis C et al 2004b PTPRC (CD45) C77G mutation contribution to multiple sclerosis susceptibility in Sardinian patients. *J Neurol* **251**: 1085–1088

Cock H, Mandler R, Ahmed W, Schapira AHV 1997 Neuromyelitis optica (Devic's syndrome): no association with the primary mitochondrial DNA mutations found in Leber hereditary optic neuropathy. *J Neurol Neurosurg Psychiatry* **62**: 85–87

Coffey RJ, Cahill D, Steers W et al 1993 Intrathecal baclofen for intractable spasticity of spinal origin: results of a long term multicenter study. *J Neurosurg* **78**: 226–232

Coffman RL, von der Weid T 1997 Multiple pathways for the initiation of T helper 2 (Th2) responses. *J Exp Med* **185**: 373–375

Cogan MS, Kline LB, Duvall ER 1987 Bilateral internuclear ophthalmoplegia in systemic lupus erythematosus. *J Clin Neuroophthalmol* 7: 69–73

Cogle CR, Yachnis AT, Laywell ED *et al* 2004 Bone marrow transdifferentiation in brain after transplantation: a retrospective study. *Lancet* 363: 1432–1437

Cohen D, Cohen O, Marcadet A *et al* 1984 Class II HLA-DC beta-chain DNA restriction fragments differentiate among HLA-DR2 individuals in insulin-dependent diabetes and multiple sclerosis. *Proc Natl Acad Sci USA* 81: 1774–1778

Cohen IR 1992 The cognitive paradigm and the immunological homunculus. *Immunol Today* 13: 490–494

Cohen IR, Miller A (eds) 1994 *Autoimmune Disease Models: A Guidebook.* New York: Academic Press

Cohen IR, Young DB 1991 Autoimmunity, microbial immunity and the immunological homunculus. *Immunol Today* 12: 105–110

Cohen JA, Cutter GR, Fischer JS *et al* 2002 Benefit of interferon beta-1a on MSFC progression in secondary progressive MS. *Neurology* 59: 679–687

Cohen L 1965 Disturbance of taste as a symptom of multiple sclerosis. *Br J Oral Surg* 2: 184–185

Cohen L, Macrae D 1962 Tumors in the region of the foramen magnum. *J Neurosurg* 19: 462–469

Cohen MM, Lessell S, Wolf PA 1979 A prospective study of the risk of developing multiple sclerosis in uncomplicated optic neuritis. *Neurology* 29: 208–213

Cohen O, Biran I, Steiner I 2000 Cerebrospinal fluid oligoclonal IgG bands in patients with spinal arteriovenous malformation and structural central nervous system lesions. *Arch Neurol* 57: 553–557

Cohen O, Steiner-Birmanns B, Biran I *et al* 2001 Recurrence of acute disseminated encephalomyelitis at the previously affected brain site. *Arch Neurol* 58: 797–801

Cohen RA, Fisher M 1989 Amantadine treatment of fatigue associated with multiple sclerosis. *Arch Neurol* 46: 676–680

Cohen SR, Brune MJ, Herndon RM, McKhann GM 1978 Cerebrospinal fluid myelin basic protein and multiple sclerosis. *Adv Exp Med Biol* 100: 513–519

Cole GF, Auchterlonie LA, Best PV 1995 Very early onset multiple sclerosis. *Dev Med Child Neurol* 37: 667–672

Colello RJ, Pott U, Schwab ME 1994 The role of oligodendrocytes and myelin on axon maturation in the developing rat retinofugal pathway. *J Neurosci* 14: 2594–2605

Colello RJ, Devey RL, Imperato E, Pott U 1995 The chronology of oligodendrocyte differentiation in the rat optic nerve: evidence for a signalling step initiating myelination in the CNS. *J Neurosci* 15: 7665–7672

Coleman RJ, Quinn NP, Marsden CD 1988 Multiple sclerosis presenting as adult onset dystonia. *Mov Disord* 3: 329–332

Coles AJ, Paolili A, Molyneux P *et al* 1999a Monoclonal antibody treatment exposes three mechanisms underlying the clinical course in multiple sclerosis. *Ann Neurol* 46: 296–304

Coles AJ, Wing M, Smith S *et al* 1999b Pulsed monoclonal antibody treatment and autoimmune thyroid disease in multiple sclerosis. *Lancet* 354: 1691–1695

Coles AJ, Le Page E, Cox AL *et al* 2005 The window of therapeutic opportunity in multiple sclerosis: evidence from monoclonal antibody therapy in relapsing–remitting and secondary progressive disease. *J Neurol* 253: 98–108

Collard RC, Koehler RPM, Mattson DH 1997 Frequency and significance of antinuclear antibodies in multiple sclerosis. *Neurology* 49: 857–861

Collins M, Goodfellow P, Spurr N *et al* 1985 The human T cell receptor alpha chain gene maps to chromosome 14. *Nature* 314: 273–274

Colognato H, Baron W, Avellana-Adalid V *et al* 2002 CNS integrins switch growth factor signalling to promote target-dependent survival. *Nat Cell Biol* 4: 833–841

Colombo B, Boneschi FM, Rossi P *et al* 2000 MRI and motor evoked potential findings in nondisabled multiple sclerosis patients with and without symptoms of fatigue. *J Neurol* 247: 506–509

Colosimo C, Pozzilli C, Frontoni M *et al* 1997 No increase of serum autoantibodies during therapy with recombinant human interferon-beta1a in relapsing-remitting multiple sclerosis. *Acta Neurol Scand* 96: 372–374

Columba-Cabezas S, Serafini B, Ambrosini E, Aloisi F 2003 Lymphoid chemokines CCL19 and CCL21 are expressed in the central nervous system during experimental autoimmune encephalomyelitis: implications for the maintenance of chronic neuroinflammation. *Brain Pathol* 13: 38–51

Comabella M, Altet L, Peris F *et al* 2004 Genetic analysis of SLCI IAI polymorphisms in multiple sclerosis patients. *Mult Scler* 10: 618–620

Comi G, Hartung H 2005 Evidence for use of glatiramer acetate in multiple sclerosis.[comment]. *Lancet Neurol* 4: 75–76; discussion 76–77

Comi G, Martinelli V, Giuliani G *et al* 1989 Incidence of multiple sclerosis in Italy: a multicenter study. In: Bataglia MA (ed.) *Multiple Sclerosis Research*. Amsterdam: Elsevier, pp. 159–163

Comi G, Filippi M, Martenelli V *et al* 1995 Brain MRI correlates of cognitive impairment in primary and secondary progressive multiple sclerosis. *J Neurol Sci* 132: 222–227

Comi G, Rovaris M, Falautano M *et al* 1999 A multiparametric MRI study of frontal lobe dementia in multiple sclerosis. *J Neurol Sci* 171:135–144

Comi G, Kappos L, Clanet M *et al* 2000 Guidelines for autologous blood and marrow stem cell transplantation in multiple sclerosis: a consensus report written on behalf of the European Group for Blood and Marrow Transplantation and the European Charcot Foundation. BMT-MS Study Group. *J Neurol* 247: 376–382

Comi G, Filippi M, Barkhof F *et al* 2001a Effect of early interferon treatment on conversion to definite multiple sclerosis. *Lancet* 357: 1576–1582

Comi G, Filippi M, Wolinsky JS 2001b European/Canadian multicenter, double-blind, randomized, placebo-controlled study of the effects of glatiramer acetate on magnetic resonance imaging-measured disease activity and burden in patients with relapsing multiple sclerosis. *Ann Neurol* 49: 290–297

Comi G, Leocani L, Colombo B, Rossi P 2002 Pathophysiology and treatment of fatigue in multiple sclerosis. In: Abramsky O, Compston DAS, Miller A, Said G (eds) *Brain Disease – Therapeutic Strategies and Repair*. London: Martin Dunitz, pp. 389–394

Compston DAS 1981 Multiple sclerosis in the Orkneys. *Lancet* ii: 98

Compston DAS 1988 The 150th anniversary of the first depiction of the lesions of multiple sclerosis. *J Neurol Neurosurg Psychiatry* 51: 1249–1252

Compston DAS 1990a The dissemination of multiple sclerosis. *J R Coll Physicians Lond* 24: 207–218

Compston DAS 1990b Risk factors for multiple sclerosis: race or place? *J Neurol Neurosurg Psychiatry* 53: 821–823

Compston DAS 1995 Brain repair. *J Intern Med* 237: 127–134

Compston DAS 1997 Remyelination in multiple sclerosis: a challenge for therapy. The Charcot Lecture for 1996: European Charcot Foundation. *Mult Scler* 3: 51–70

Compston DAS 2003 Revisiting The pathogenesis of multiple sclerosis revisited. *The International MS Journal* 10: 29–31

Compston DAS 2004 The marvellous harmony of the nervous parts: the origins of multiple sclerosis. *Clin Med* 4: 346–354

Compston DAS, Coles AJ 2002 Multiple sclerosis. *Lancet* 359: 1221–1231

Compston DAS, Howard S 1982 HLA typing in multiple sclerosis. *Lancet* ii: 661

Compston DAS, Swingler RJ 1989 Life expectancy in multiple sclerosis. *J Neurol Neurosurg Psychiatry* 52: 1312

Compston DAS, Batchelor JR, McDonald WI 1976 B lymphocyte alloantigens associated with multiple sclerosis. *Lancet* ii: 1261–1265

Compston DAS, Batchelor JR, Earl CJ, McDonald WI 1978 Factors influencing the risk of multiple sclerosis in patients with optic neuritis. *Brain* 101: 495–512

Compston DAS, Vakarelis BN, Paul E *et al* 1986 Viral infection in patients with multiple sclerosis and HLA-DR matched controls. *Brain* 109: 325–344

Compston DAS, Hughes PJ, Morgan BP, Gibbs J, Milligan NM 1987 High dose methylprednisolone in the treatment of multiple sclerosis. 2. Immunological effects. *J Neurol Neurosurg Psychiatry* **50**: 517–522

Compston DAS, Morgan BP, Campbell AK et al 1989 Immunocytochemical localisation of the terminal complement complex in multiple sclerosis. *Neuropathol Appl Neurobiol* **15**: 307–316

Compston ND 1953 Disseminated sclerosis: assessment of the effect of treatment on the course of the disease. *Lancet* ii: 271–275

de la Concha EG, Arroyo R, Crusius JBA et al 1997 Combined effect of HLA-DRB1*1501 and interleukin-1 receptor antagonist gene allele 2 in susceptibility to relapsing/remitting multiple sclerosis. *J Neuroimmunol* **80**: 172–178

Confavreux C 1977 *L'histoire naturelle de la sclérose en plaques. Etude par informatique de 349 observations.* Thèse de Médecine, Université Claude Bernard, Lyon 184 pp.

Confavreux C 1994 Establishment and use of multiple sclerosis registers – EDMUS. *Ann Neurol* **36 (Suppl)**: 136–139

Confavreux C 2002 Relapses, progression, inflammation and neurodegeneration in multiple sclerosis: a changing view. *Adv Clin Neurosci Rehab* **2**: 7–9

Confavreux C, Paty DW 1995 Current status of computerization of multiple sclerosis clinical data for research in Europe and North America: the EDMUS / MS – COSTAR connection. *Neurology* **45**: 573–576

Confavreux C, Vukusic S 2002 Natural history of multiple sclerosis: implications for counselling and therapy. *Curr Opin Neurol* **15**: 257–266

Confavreux C, Vukusic S 2004 Non-specific immunosuppressants in the treatment of multiple sclerosis. *Clin Neurol Neurosurg* **106**: 263–269

Confavreux C, Vukusic S 2006a Age at disability milestones in multiple sclerosis. *Brain* **129**: 595–605

Confavreux C, Vukusic S 2006b Natural history of multiple sclerosis: a unifying concept. *Brain* **129**: 606–616

Confavreux C, Wolfson C 1989 Mathematical models and individualized outcome estimates in multiple sclerosis. *Biomed Pharmacother* **43**: 675–680

Confavreux C, Aimard D, Devic M 1980 Course and prognosis of multiple sclerosis assessed by the computerised data processing of 349 patients. *Brain* **103**: 281–300

Confavreux C, Chapuis-Cellier C, Arnaud P et al 1986 Oligoclonal 'fingerprint' of CSF IgG in multiple sclerosis patients is not modified following intrathecal administration of natural beta-interferon. *J Neurol Neurosurg Psychiatry* **49**: 1308–1312

Confavreux C, Darchy P, Alperovitch A et al 1987 Le Sud-Est francais, zone à haut risque de sclérose en plaques? *Presse Medicale* **16**: 622–623

Confavreux C, Compston DAS, Hommes OR et al 1992 EDMUS, an European database for multiple sclerosis. *J Neurol Neurosurg Psychiatry* **55**: 671–676

Confavreux C, Moreau T, Jouvet A et al 1993 Association sclérose latérale amyotrophique et sclérose en plaques. *Rev Neurol* **149**: 351–353

Confavreux C, Hours M, Moreau T et al 1996 Clinical databasing in multiple sclerosis: EDMUS and the European effort. In: Abramsky O (ed.) *Frontiers in Multiple Sclerosis: Clinical Research and Therapy.* London: Martin Dunitz, pp. 299–312

Confavreux C, Grimaud J, Vukusic S, Moreau T 1998a Peut-on prédire l'évolution de la sclérose en plaques? *Rev Neurol* **154**: 624–628

Confavreux C, Hutchinson M, Hours M et al 1998b Rate of pregnancy-related relapse in multiple sclerosis. *N Engl J Med* **339**: 285–291

Confavreux C, Vukusic S, Moreau T, Adeleine P 2000 Relapses and progression of disability in multiple sclerosis. *N Engl J Med* **343**: 1430–1438

Confavreux C, Suissa S, Saddier P et al 2001 Vaccinations and the risk of relapse in multiple sclerosis. Vaccines in Multiple Sclerosis Study Group. *New Engl J Med* **344**: 319–326

Confavreux C, Vukusic S, Adeleine P 2003 Early clinical predictors and progression of irreversible disability in multiple sclerosis: an amnesic process. *Brain* **126**: 770–782

Conférence de Consensus sur la sclérose en plaques. Paris, 7 et 8 juin 2001 Recommandations du jury. *Rev Neurol* **157**: 1184–1192

Consroe P, Musty R, Rein J et al 1997 The perceived effects of smoked cannabis on patients with multiple sclerosis. *Eur Neurol* **38**: 44–48

Constant SL, Bottomly K 1997 Induction of the Th1 and Th2 CD4+ T cell response: alternative approaches. *Annu Rev Immunol* **15**: 297–322

Constantinescu CS, Raps EC, Cohen JA et al 1994 Olfactory disturbances as the initial or most prominent symptom of multiple sclerosis. *J Neurol Neurosurg Psychiatry* **57**: 1011–1012

Constantinescu CS, Whiteley A, Blumhardt LD 2000 Long term azathioprine fails to prevent onset of multiple sclerosis: report of two cases. *Mult Scler* **6**: 362–363

Contini C, Cultrera R, Seraceni S et al 2004 Cerebrospinal fluid molecular demonstration of *Chlamydia pneumoniae* DNA is associated to clinical and brain magnetic resonance imaging activity in a subset of patients with relapsing–remitting multiple sclerosis. *Mult Scler* **10**: 360–369

Cook JH, Arden GB 1977 Unilateral retrobulbar neuritis: a comparison of evoked potentials and psychophysical measurements. In: Desmedt JE (ed.) *Visual Evoked Potentials in Man: New Development.* Oxford, Clarendon Press, pp. 450–457

Cook SD 2000 Trauma does not precipitate multiple sclerosis. *Arch Neurol* **57**: 1077–1078

Cook SD, Dowling PC 1982 MS in Iceland revisited. *Neurology* 32: 1204–1205

Cook SD, Dowling PC, Russell WC 1978 Multiple sclerosis and canine distemper. *Lancet* i: 605–606

Cook SD, Gudmundsson G, Benedikz J, Dowling PC 1980 Multiple sclerosis and distemper in Iceland, 1966–1978. *Acta Neurol Scand* **61**: 244–251

Cook SD, Cromarty MB, Tapp W et al 1985 Declining incidence of multiple sclerosis in the Orkney Islands. *Neurology* **35**: 545–551

Cook SD, Devereux C, Triano R et al 1986 Effect of total lymphoid irradiation in chronic progressive multiple sclerosis. *Lancet* i: 1405–1409

Cook SD, Blumberg B, Dowling PC et al 1987 Multiple sclerosis and canine distemper on Key West, Florida. *Lancet* i: 1426–1427

Cook SD, MacDonald J, Tapp W et al 1988 Multiple sclerosis in the Shetland Islands: an update. *Acta Neurol Scand* **77**: 148–151

Cook SD, Triano R, Rohowsky-Kochan C et al 1992 Gamma globulin in progressive multiple sclerosis. *Acta Neurol Scand* **86**: 171–175

Cook SD, Devereux C, Triano R et al 1995 Combination total lymphoid irradiation and low dose corticosteroid therapy for progressive multiple sclerosis. *Acta Neurol Scand* **91**: 22–27

Cooke RG 1990 MS in the Faroe Islands and the possible protective effect of ealy childhood exposure to the 'MS agent'. *Acta Neurol Scand* **82**: 230–233

Cooke WT, Smith WT 1966 Neurological disorders associated with adult celiac disease. *Brain* **89**: 683–722

Cooney BS, Grossman RI, Farber RE 1996 Frequency of magnetic resonance abnormalities in patients with migraine. *Headache* **36**: 616–621

Copolymer 1 Multiple Sclerosis Study Group. *Neurology* **50**: 701–708

Coppin H, Ribouchon M-T, Bausero P et al 2000 No evidence for transmission disequilibrium between a new marker at the myelin basic protein locus and multiple sclerosis in French patients. *Genes Immun* **1**: 478–482

Coraddu F, Reyes-Yanez MP, Aladro Y et al 1998a HLA associations with multiple sclerosis in the Canary Islands. *J Neuroimmunol* **87**: 130–135

Coraddu F, Sawcer S, Feakes R et al 1998b HLA typing in the United Kingdom multiple sclerosis genome screen. *Neurogenetics* **2**: 24–33

Coraddu F, Sawcer S, D'Alfonso S et al 2001 A genome screen for multiple sclerosis in Sardinian multiplex families. *Eur J Hum Gen* **9**: 621–626

Coraddu F, Lai M, Mancosu C et al 2003 A genome-wide screen for linkage disequilibrium in Sardinian multiple sclerosis. *J Neuroimmunol* **143**: 120–123

Cordier AC, Haumont SM 1980 Development of thymus, parathyroids, and ultra-branchial bodies in NMRI and nude mice. *Am J Anat* **157**: 227–263

Cordonnier C, De Sèze J, Breteau G et al 2003 Prospective study of patients presenting with acute partial transverse myelopathy. *J Neurol* **250**: 1447–1452

Corley SM, Ladiwala U, Besson A, Yong VW 2001 Astrocytes attenuate oligodendrocyte death in vitro through an alpha(6) integrin-laminin-dependent mechanism. *Glia* **36**: 281–294

Cornblath WT, Quint DJ 1997 MRI in optic nerve enlargement in optic neuritis. *Neurology* **48**: 821–825

Corona T, Leon C, Ostrosky-Zeichner L 1999 Severe anaphylaxis with recombinant interferon beta. *Neurology* **52**: 425

Correale J, Gilmore W, McMillan M et al 1995a Patterns of cytokine secretion by autoreactive proteolipid protein-specific T cell clones during the course of multiple sclerosis. *J Immunol* **154**: 2959–2968

Correale J, McMillan M, Le T, Weiner LP 1995b Isolation and characterization of autoreactive proteolipid protein peptide specific T cell clones from multiple sclerosis patients. *Neurology* **45**: 1370–1378

Corrette BJ, Repp H, Dreyer F, Schwarz JR 1991 Two types of fast K+ channels in rat myelinated nerve fibres and their sensitivity to dendrotoxin. *Pflugers Arch Eur J Physiol* **418**: 408–416

Corsini E, Gelati M, Dufour A et al 1997 Effects of β-interferon-1b treatment in MS patients on adhesion between PBMNCs, HUVECs and MS-HBECs: an *in vivo* and *in vitro* study. *J Neuroimmunol* **79**: 76–83

Cortese I, Tafi R, Grimaldi LME et al 1996 Identification of peptides specific for cerebrospinal fluid antibodies in multiple sclerosis by using phage libraries. *Proc Natl Acad Sci USA* **93**: 11063–11067

Cortese I, Capone S, Luchetti S et al 1998 CSF-enriched antibodies do not share specificities among MS patients. *Mult Scler* **4**: 118–123

Cortese I, Capone S, Luchetti S et al 2001 Cross-reactive phage-displayed mimotopes lead to the discovery of mimicry between HSV-1 and a brain-specific protein. *J Neuroimmunol* **113**: 119–128

Cosby SL, McQuaid S, Taylor MJ et al 1989 Examination of eight cases of multiple sclerosis and 56 neurological and non-neurological controls for genomic sequences of measles virus, canine distemper virus, simian virus 5 and rubella virus. *J Gen Virol* **70**: 2027–2036

Cosnett JE 1973 Neurological disease in Natal. In: JD Spillane (ed.) *Tropical Neurology*. London: Oxford University Press, pp. 259–272

Cosnett JE 1981a Multiple sclerosis and neuromyelitis optica. Case report and speculation. *S Afr Med J* **60**: 249–251

Cosnett JE 1981b Multiple sclerosis and neuromyelitis optica in tropical and subtropical countries. *Med Hypotheses* **7**: 61–63

Cossins JA, Clements JM, Ford J et al 1997 Enhanced expression of MMP-7 and MMP-9 in demyelinating multiple sclerosis lesions. *Acta Neuropathol* **94**: 590–598

Costa JL, Diazgranados JA 1994 Ivermectin for spasticity in spinal cord injury. *Lancet* **343**: 739

Cotton F, Weiner HL, Jolesz FA et al 2003 MRI contrast uptake in new lesions in relapsing–remitting MS followed at weekly intervals. *Neurology* **60**: 640–646

Cottrell DA, Kremenchutzky M, Rice GPA et al 1999a The natural history of multiple sclerosis: a geographically based study. 5. The clinical features and natural history of primary progressive multiple sclerosis. *Brain* **122**: 625–639

Cottrell DA, Kremenchutzky M, Rice GPA et al 1999b The natural history of multiple sclerosis: a geographically based study. 6. Applications to planning and interpretation of clinical therapeutic trials in primary progressive multiple sclerosis. *Brain* **122**: 641–647

Cottrell SS, Wilson SAK 1926 The affective symptomatology of disseminated sclerosis. *J Neurol Psychopathol* **7**: 1–50

Cournu-Rebeix I, Genin E, Lesca G et al 2003 Intercellular adhesion molecule-1: a protective haplotype against multiple sclerosis. *Genes Immun* **4**: 518–523

Courville CB 1968 Acute lesions of multiple sclerosis – possible significance of vascular changes. *J Neuropathol Exp Neurol* **27**: 159 (abstract)

Courville CB 1970 Concentric sclerosis. In: Vinken PJ, Bruyn GW (eds) *Handbook of Clinical Neurology*. Amsterdam: Elsevier, Vol 9, pp. 437–451

Coustans M, Leray E, Le Page E et al 2004 Both relapsing–remitting and primary progressive multiple sclerosis are a two-stage disease, suggesting two consecutive mechanisms underlying the progression of disability in multiple sclerosis. *Mult Scler* **10 (Suppl)**: S111

Cowan EP, Pierce ML, MacFarland HF, McFarlin DE 1991a HLA-DR and DQ allelic sequences in multiple sclerosis patients are identical to those found in the general population. *Hum Immunol* **32**: 203–210

Cowan EP, Pierce M, Dhib-Jalbut S 1991b Interleukin 1 downregulates HLA class I expression on a human glioblastoma cell line. *J Neuroimmunol* **33**: 17–28

Cowan J, Ormerod IEC, Rudge P 1990 Hemiparetic multiple sclerosis. *J Neurol Neurosurg Psychiatry* **53**: 675–680

Cowan JM, Dick JPR, Day BL, Rothwell JC, Thompson PD, Marsden CD 1984 Abnormalities in central motor pathway conduction in multiple sclerosis. *Lancet* **ii**: 304–307

Coward DM 1994 Tizanidine: neuropharmacology and mechanism of action. *Neurology* **44 (Suppl 9)**: S6–S11

Cox AL, Coles AJ, Antoun N et al 2005 Recurrent myelitis and optic neuritis in a 29-year-old woman. *Lancet Neurol* **4**: 510–516

Cox DR 1972 Regression models and life tables. *J R Stat Soc Series B* **34**: 187–220

Coyle PK 1989 Borrelia burgdorferi antibodies in multiple sclerosis patients. *Neurology* **39**: 760–761

Coyle PK 2002 Lyme disease. *Cur Neurol Neurosci Rep* **2**: 479–487

Coyle PK, Krupp LB, Doscher C 1993 Significance of reactive Lyme serology in multiple sclerosis. *Ann Neurol* **34**: 745–747

Craelius W, Migdal MW, Luessenhop CP et al 1982 Iron deposits surrounding multiple sclerosis plaques. *Arch Pathol Lab Med* **106**: 397–399

Craig J, Young CA, Ennis M et al 2003 A randomised controlled trial comparing rehabilitation against standard therapy in multiple sclerosis patients receiving intravenous steroid treatment. *J Neurol Neurosurg Psychiatry* **74**: 1225–1230

Craner MJ, Zajicek JP 2001 Immunosuppressive treatments in MS – side effects from azathioprine. *J Neurol* **248**: 625–626

Craner MJ, Lo AC, Black JA et al 2003a Annexin II/p11 is up-regulated in Purkinje cells in EAE and MS. *NeuroReport* **14**: 555–558

Craner MJ, Lo AC, Black JA, Waxman SG 2003b Abnormal sodium channel distribution in optic nerve axons in a model of inflammatory demyelination. *Brain* **126**: 1552–1561

Craner MJ, Hains BC, Lo AC et al 2004a Co-localization of sodium channel Nav1.6 and the sodium-calcium exchanger at sites of axonal injury in the spinal cord in EAE. *Brain* **127**: 294–303

Craner MJ, Newcombe J, Black JA et al 2004b Molecular changes in neurons in multiple sclerosis: altered axonal expression of Nav1.2 and Nav1.6 sodium channels and Na+/Ca2+ exchanger. *Proc Natl Acad Sci USA* **101**: 8168–8173

Craner MJ, Damarjian TG, Liu S et al 2005 Sodium channels contribute to microglia/macrophage activation in EAE and MS. *Glia* **49**: 220–229

Crang AJ, Gilson J, Blakemore WF 1998 The demonstration by transplantation of the very restricted remyelinating potential of post-mitotic oligodendrocytes. *J Neurocytol* **27**: 541–553

Crang AJ, Gilson JM, Li WW, Blakemore WF 2004 The remyelinating potential and in vitro differentiation of MOG-expressing oligodendrocyte precursors isolated from the adult rat CNS. *Eur J Neurosci* **20**: 1445–1460

Craven RA, Totty N, Harnden P et al 2002 Laser capture microdissection and two-dimensional polyacrylamide gel electrophoresis: evaluation of tissue preparation and sample limitations. *Am J Pathol* **160**: 815–822

Crawley F, Saddeh I, Barker S, Katifi H 2001 Acute pulmonary oedema: presenting symptoms of multiple sclerosis. *Mult Scler* **7**: 71–72

Crecelius W 1928 Uber Antimonbehandlung der multiplen Sklerose. *Deutsche Medizinische Wochenschrift* **54**: 1332–1334

Cree BAC, Goodin DS, Hauser SL 2002 Neuromyelitis optica. *Semin Neurol* **22**: 105–122

Cree BAC, Khan O, Bourdette D et al 2004 Clinical characteristics of African Americans vs Caucasian Americans with multiple sclerosis. *Neurology* **63**: 2039–2045

Cree BA, Lamb S, Morgan K et al 2005 An open label study of the effects of rituximab in neuromyelitis optica. *Neurology* **64**: 1270–1272

Cripps J, Rudd A, Ebers GC 1982 Birth order and multiple sclerosis. *Acta Neurol Scand* **66**: 342–346

Critchley M 1969 Four illustrious neuroluetics. *Proc R Soc Med* **62**: 669–673

Crockard AD, Treacy MT, Droogan AG et al 1995 Transient immunomodulation by intravenous methylprednisolone treatment of multiple sclerosis. *Mult Scler* **1**: 20–24

Crockard AD, Treacy MT, Droogan AG, Hawkins SA 1996 Methylprednisolone attenuates interferon-beta induced expression of HLA-DR on monocytes. *J Neuroimmunol* **70**: 29–35

Cross AH, Cannella B, Brosnan CF, Raine CS 1990 Homing to central nervous system vasculature by antigen-specific lymphocytes. I. Localization of ^{14}C-labelled cells during acute, chronic, and relapsing experimental allergic encephalomyelitis. *Lab Invest* **63**: 162–170

Cross AH, Cannella B, Brosnan CF, Raine CS 1991 Hypothesis: antigen-specific T cells prime central nervous system endothelium for recruitment of nonspecific inflammatory cells to effect autoimmune demyelination. *J Neuroimmunol* **33**: 237–244

Cross AH, Tuohy VK, Raine CS 1993 Development of reactivity to new myelin antigens during chronic relapsing autoimmune demyelination. *Cell Immunol* **146**: 261–269

Cross AH, Manning PT, Keeling RM et al 1998 Peroxynitrite formation within the central nervous system in active multiple sclerosis. *J Neuroimmunol* **88**: 45–56

Cross AH, San M, Stern MK et al 2000 A catalyst of peroxynitrite decomposition inhibits murine experimental autoimmune encephalomyelitis. *J Neuroimmunol* **107**: 21–28

Cross SA, Salomao DR, Parisi JE et al 2003 Paraneoplastic autoimmune optic neuritis with retinitis defined by CRMP-5-Ig. *Ann Neurol* **54**: 38–50

Croxford JL, Miller SD 2003 Immunoregulation of a viral model of multiple sclerosis using the synthetic cannabinoid R+WIN55,212. *J Clin Invest* **111**: 1231–1240

Cruikshank EK 1973 Neurological disorders in Jamaica. In: Spillane JD (ed.) *Tropical Neurology*. London: Oxford University Press, pp. 421–434

Cruikshank EK, Montgomery RD, Spillane JD 1961 Obscure neurological disorders in Jamaica. *World Neurol* **2**: 199–211

Cruickshank JK, Rudge P, Dalgleish AG et al 1989 Tropical spastic paraplegia and human T cell lymphotropic virus type 1 in the United Kingdom. *Brain* **112**: 1057–1090

Crusius JBA, Pena AS, van Oosten BW et al 1995 Interleukin-1 receptor antagonist gene polymorphism and multiple sclerosis. *Lancet* **346**: 979–980

Cruveilhier J 1829–42 *Anatomie pathologique du corps humain; descriptions avec figures lithographiées et coloriées; des diverses alterations morbides dont le corps humain est susceptible*. Paris: J.B. Baillière, 40 livraisons

Cruz BA, Queiroz ED, Nunes SV et al 2000 Severe Raynaud's phenomenon associated with interferon-beta therapy for multiple sclerosis: case report. *Arq Neuropsiquiatr* **58**: 556–559

Cserr HF 1984 Convection of brain interstitial fluid. In: Shapiro K, Marmarou A, Portnoy H (eds) *Hydrocephalus*. New York: Raven Press, pp. 59–68

Cserr HF, Harling-Berg CJ, Knopf PM 1992 Drainage of brain extracellular fluid into blood and deep cervical lymph and its immunological significance. *Brain Pathol* **2**: 269–276

Cua DJ, Sherlock J, Chen Y et al 2003 Interleukin-23 rather than interleukin-12 is the critical cytokine for autoimmune inflammation of the brain. *Nature* **421**: 744–748

Cuadrado MJ, Khamashta MA, Ballesteros A et al 2000 Can neurologic manifestations of Hughes (antiphospholipid) syndrome be distinguished from multiple sclerosis? Analysis of 27 patients and review of the literature. *Medicine* **79**: 57–68

Cuddigan J, Frantz RA 1998 Pressure ulcer research: pressure ulcer treatment. A monograph from the National Pressure Ulcer Advisory Panel. Review. *Adv Wound Care* **11**: 294–300; quiz, 302.

Cui XY, Hu QD, Tekaya M et al 2004 NB-3/notch1 pathway via Deltex1 promotes neural progenitor cell differentiation into oligodendrocytes. *J Biol Chem* **279**: 25858–25865

Culican SM, Baumrind NL, Yamamoto M, Pearlman AL 1990 Cortical radial glia: identification in tissue culture and evidence for their transformation to astrocytes. *J Neurosci* **10**: 684–692

Cullen CG, Middleton D, Savage DA, Hawkins S 1991 HLA-DR and DQ DNA genotyping in multiple sclerosis patients in Northern Ireland. *Hum Immunol* **30**: 1–6

Cumings JN 1953 The examination of the cerebrospinal fluid and cerebral cyst fluid by paper strip electrophoresis. *J Neurol Neurosurg Psychiatry* **16**: 152–157

Cummins TR, Waxman SG 1997 Downregulation of tetrodotoxin-resistant sodium currents and upregulation of a rapidly repriming tetrodotoxin-sensitive sodium current in small spinal sensory neurons after nerve injury. *J Neurosci* **17**: 3503–3514

Cummins TR, Black JA, Dib-Hajj SD, Waxman SG 2000 Glial-derived neurotrophic factor upregulates expression of functional SNS and NaN sodium channels and their currents in axotomized dorsal root ganglion neurons. *J Neurosci* **20**: 8754–8761

Cummins TR, Renganathan M, Stys PK et al 2003 The pentapeptide QYNAD does not block voltage-gated sodium channels. *Neurology* **60**: 224–229

Cunningham S, Patterson CC, McDonnell G et al 2005 Haplotype analysis of the preprotachykinin-1 (TAC1) gene in multiple sclerosis. *Genes Immun* **6**: 265–270

Cupples LA, Risch N, Farrer LA, Myers RH 1991 Estimation of morbid risk and age at onset with missing information. *Am J Hum Genet* **49**: 76–87

Currie S, Urich H 1974 Concurrence of multiple sclerosis and glioma. *J Neurol Neurosurg Psychiatry* **37**: 598–605

Currier RD, Haerer AF, Maydrech EF 1993 Low dose oral methotrexate treatment of multiple sclerosis: a pilot study. *J Neurol Neurosurg Psychiatry* **56**: 1217–1218

Curtius F 1933 *Multiple Sklerose und Erbanlage* Leipzig: Thieme

Curtius F, Speer H 1937 Multiple Sklerose und Erbanlage II Mittelung. *Z Neurol Psychiatr* **160**: 226–245

Custer AW, Kazarinova-Noyes K, Sakurai T et al 2003 The role of the ankyrin-binding protein NrCAM in node of Ranvier formation. *J Neurosci* **23**: 10032–10039

Cutter GR, Baier ML, Rudick RA et al 1999 Development of a multiple sclerosis functional composite as a clinical trial outcome measure. *Brain* **122**: 871–882

Cutter NC, Scott DD, Johnson JC, Whiteneck G 2000 Gabapentin effect on spasticity in multiple sclerosis: a placebo-controlled, randomized trial. *Arch Phys Med Rehab* **81**: 164–169

Cuzner ML, Hayes GM, Newcombe J, Woodroofe MN 1988 The nature of inflammatory components during demyelination in multiple sclerosis. *J Neuroimmunol* **20**: 203–209

Cuzner ML, Gveric D, Strand C et al 1996 The expression of tissue-type plasminogen-activator, matrix metalloproteinases and endogenous inhibitors in the central nervous system in multiple sclerosis: comparison of stages of lesion evolution. *J Neuropathol Exp Neurol* **55**: 1194–1204

Cuzner ML, Opdenakker G 1999 Plasminogen activators and matrix metalloproteinases, mediators of extracellular proteolysis in inflammatory demyelination of the central nervous system. *J Neuroimmunol* **94**: 1–14

Dahl D, Perides G, Bignami A 1989 Axonal regeneration in old multiple sclerosis plaques: immunohistochemical study with monoclonal antibodies to phosphorylated and non-phosphorylated neurofilament proteins. *Acta Neuropathol* **79**: 154–159

Dahl OP, Aarseth JH, Myhr KM et al 2004 Multiple sclerosis in Nord-Trondelag County, Norway: a prevalence and incidence study. *Acta Neurol Scand* **109**: 378–384

Dai KZ, Harbo HF, Celius EG et al 2001 The T cell regulator gene SH2D2A contributes to the genetic susceptibility of multiple sclerosis. *Genes Immun* **2**: 263–268

Dai X, Lercher LD, Clinton PM et al 2003 The trophic role of oligodendrocytes in the basal forebrain. *J Neurosci* **23**: 5846–5853

Dai Y, Xu C, Holmberg M et al 2001a Linkage analysis suggests a region of importance for multiple sclerosis in 3p14–13. *Genes Immun* **2**: 451–454

Dai Y, Masterman T, Huang WX et al 2001b Analysis of an interferon-gamma gene dinucleotide-repeat polymorphism in Nordic multiple sclerosis patients. *Mult Scler* **7**: 157–163

Dai Y, Masterman T, Huang W, Hillert J 2002 Analysis of a CD40 ligand dinucleotide microsatellite in multiple sclerosis. *Eur J Immunogenet* **29**: 81–85

Dale RC, de Sousa C, Chong WK et al 2000 Acute disseminated encephalomyelitis, multiphasic disseminated encephalomyelitis and multiple sclerosis in children. *Brain* **123**: 2407–2422

Dale RC, Church AJ, Cardosa F et al 2001 Post-streptococcal acute disseminated encephalomyelitis with basal ganglia involvement and auto-reactive anti-basal ganglia antibodies. *Ann Neurol* **50**: 588–595

Daley D, Code C, Andersen H 1962 Disturbances of swallowing and esophageal motility in patients with multiple sclerosis. *Neurology* **12**: 250–256

D'Alfonso S, Nistico L, Zavattari P et al 1999 Linkage analysis of multiple sclerosis with candidate region markers in Sardinian and Continental Italian families. *Eur J Hum Genet* **7**: 377–385

D'Alfonso S, Mellai M, Giordano M et al 2002 Identification of single nucleotide variations in the coding and regulatory regions of the myelin-associated glycoprotein gene and study of their association with multiple sclerosis. *J Neuroimmunol* **126**: 196–204

Dalton CM, Brex PA, Jenkins R et al 2002a Application of the new McDonald criteria in patients with clinically isolated syndromes suggestive of multiple sclerosis. *Ann Neurol* **52**: 47–53

Dalton CM, Brex PA, Jenkins R et al 2002b Progressive ventricular enlargement in patients with clinically isolated syndromes is associated with the early development of multiple sclerosis. *J Neurol Neurosurg Psychiatry* **73**: 141–147

Dalton CM, Brex PA, Miszkiel KA et al 2003a New T2 lesions to enable an earlier diagnosis of multiple sclerosis in clinically isolated syndromes. *Ann Neurol* **53**: 673–676

Dalton CM, Brex PA, Miszkiel KM et al 2003b Spinal cord MRI in optic neuritis. *J Neurol Neurosurg Psychiatry* **74**: 1577–1580

Dalton CM, Chard DT, Davies GR et al 2004a Early development of multiple sclerosis is associated with progressive grey matter atrophy in patients presenting with clinically isolated syndromes. *Brain* **127**: 1101–1107

Dalton CM, Miszkiel KA, Barker GJ et al 2004b Effect of natalizumab on conversion of gadolinium enhancing lesions to T1 hypointense lesions in relapsing multiple sclerosis. *J Neurol* **251**: 407–413

Daly MJ, Rioux JD, Schaffner SF et al 2001 High-resolution haplotype structure in the human genome. *Nature Genet* **29**: 229–232

Danilov AI, Andersson M, Bavand N et al 2003 Nitric oxide metabolite determinations reveal continuous inflammation in multiple sclerosis. *J Neuroimmunol* **136**: 112–118

D'Arcangelo G, Grassi F, Ragozzino D et al 1991 Interferon inhibits synaptic potentiation in rat hippocampus. *Brain Res* **564**: 245–248

Dargent B, Paillart C, Carlier E et al 1994 Sodium channel internalization in developing neurons. *Neuron* **13**: 683–690

Darragh TM, Simon RP 1985 Nucleus tractus solitarius lesions elevate pulmonary arterial pressure and lymph flow. *Ann Neurol* **17**: 565–569

Das TK, Park DM 1989 Effect of treatment with botulinum toxin on spasticity. *Postgrad Med J* **65**: 208–210

DasGupta P, Haslam C, Goodwin R, Fowler CJ 1997 The 'Queen Square bladder stimulator': a device for assisting emptying of the neurogenic bladder. *Br J Urol* **80**: 234–237

DasGupta R, Wiseman O, Kanabar G, Fowler C 2004 Efficacy of sildenafil in the treatment of female sexual dysfunction due to multiple sclerosis. *J Urol* **171**: 1189–1193

Dastur OK, Singhal BS 1976 Eales' disease with neurological involvement Part II Pathology and pathogenesis. *J Neurol Sci* **27**: 323–345

Daugherty WT, Lederman RJ, Nodar RH, Conomy JP 1983 Hearing loss in multiple sclerosis. *Arch Neurol* **40**: 33–35

Davalos D, Grutzendler J, Yang G et al 2005 ATP mediates rapid microglial response to local brain injury *in vivo*. *Nature Neurosci* **8**: 752–758

Davenport CB 1921 Multiple sclerosis from the standpoint of geographic distribution and race. In: *Association for Research in Nervous and Mental Diseases (ARNMD)*, Vol 2. New York: Hoeber, pp. 8–19

Davenport CB 1922 Multiple sclerosis from the standpoint of geographic distribution and race. *Arch Neurol* **8**: 51–58

David E 2004 Competency, power of attorney, informed consent, wills. In: Rizzo M, Eslinger P (eds) *Principles and Practice of Behavioral Neurology and Neuropsychology*. Philadelphia, PA, WB Saunders, pp. 1071–1076

Davidoff F, DeAngelis CD, Drazen JM et al 2001 Sponsorship, authorship, and accountability. *N Engl J Med* **345**: 825–827

Davie CA, Hawkins CP, Barker GJ et al 1994 Serial proton magnetic resonance spectroscopy in acute multiple sclerosis. *Brain* **117**: 49–58

Davie CA, Barker GJ, Webb S et al 1995 Persistent functional deficit in multiple sclerosis and autosomal dominant cerebellar ataxia is associated with axon loss. *Brain* **118**: 1583–1592

Davie CA, Barker GJ, Webb S et al 1996 A proton spectroscopy study of disability in multiple sclerosis. *J Neurol* **243 (Suppl 2)**: S33

Davie CA, Barker GJ, Thompson AJ et al 1997 ^{1}H magnetic resonance spectroscopy of chronic cerebral white matter lesions and normal appearing white matter in multiple sclerosis. *J Neurol Neurosurg Psychiatry* **63**: 736–742

Davies GR, Ramio-Torrenta LI, Hadjiprocopis A et al 2004 Evidence for grey matter MTR abnormality in relapsing remitting MS in patients with short disease duration and minimal disability. *J Neurol Neurosurg Psychiatry* **75**: 998–1002

Davies GR, Altmann DR, Hadjiprocopis A et al 2005 Increasing normal appearing grey and white matter magnetisation transfer ratio abnormality in early relapsing remitting MS. *J Neurol* **252**: 1037 1044

Davies J 1982 Selective depression of synaptic transmission of spinal neurones in the cat by a new centrally acting muscle relaxant 5-chloro-4-(2-imidazolin-2-yl-amino)-2,1,3-benzothiadazole (DS 103–282). *Br J Pharmacol* **76**: 473–481

Davies JL, Kawaguchi Y, Bennett ST et al 1994 A genome-wide search for human type 1 diabetes susceptibility genes. *Nature* **371**: 130–136

Davies M, Björkman P 1988 T cell antigen receptor genes and T cell recognition. *Nature* **344**: 395–402

Davies MB, Weatherby SJ, Haq N, Ellis SJ 2000 A multiple sclerosis-like syndrome associated with glue-sniffing. *J Roy Soc Med* **93**: 313–314

Davies SE, Newcombe J, Williams SR et al 1995 High resolution proton NMR spectroscopy of multiple sclerosis lesions. *J Neurochem* **64**: 742–748

Davies SJ, Fitch MT, Memberg SP et al 1997 Regeneration of adult axons in white matter tracts of the central nervous system. *Nature* **390**: 680–683

Davis FA 1985 Neurological deficits following the hot bath test in multiple sclerosis. *J Am Med Assoc* **253**: 203

Davis FA, Jacobson S 1971 Altered thermal sensitivity in injured and demyelinated nerve: a possible model of temperature effects in multiple sclerosis. *J Neurol Neurosurg Psychiatry* **34**: 551–561

Davis FA, Schauf CL 1981 Approaches to the development of pharmacological interventions in multiple sclerosis. *Adv Neurol* **31**: 505–510

Davis FA, Becker FO, Michael JA, Sorensen E 1970 Effect of intravenous sodium bicarbonate, disodium edetate (Na$_2$EDTA), and hyperventilation on visual and oculomotor signs in multiple sclerosis. *J Neurol Neurosurg Psychiatry* **33**: 723–732

Davis FA, Michael JA, Tomaszewski JS 1973 Fluctuation of motor function in multiple sclerosis related to circadian temperature variations. *Dis Nerv Syst* **34**: 33–36

Davis FA, Schauf CL, Reed BJ, Kesler RL 1975 Experimental studies of the effects of

837

extrinsic factors on conduction in normal and demyelinated nerve. *J Neurol Neurosurg Psychiatry* **39**: 442–448

Davis FA, Bergen D, Schauf C et al 1976 Movement phosphenes in optic neuritis: a new clinical sign. *Neurology* **26**: 1100–1104

Davis FA, Stefoski D, Rush J 1990 Orally administered 4-aminopyridine improves clinical signs in multiple sclerosis. *Ann Neurol* **27**: 186–192

Davis JL, Kawaguchi Y, Bennett ST et al 1994 A genome-wide search for human type 1 diabetes susceptibility genes. *Nature* **371**: 130–136

Davis LE, Hersh EM, Curtis JE et al 1972 Immune status of patients with multiple sclerosis: analysis of primary and established immune responses in 24 patients. *Neurology* **22**: 989–997

Davis MM 2002 A new trigger for T cells. *Cell* **110**: 285–287

Davison C, Goodhart SP, Lander J 1934 Multiple sclerosis and amyotrophies. *Arch Neurol Psychiatry* **31**: 270–289

Davison K, Bagley CR 1969 Schizophrenia-like psychoses associated with organic disorders of the central nervous system: a review of the literature. *Br J Psychiatry Special Publication* **4**: 113–184

Davodeau F, Peyrat M-A, Romagné F et al 1995 Dual T cell receptor β chain expression on human T lymphocytes. *J Exp Med* **181**: 1391–1398

Dawson GD 1947a Cerebral responses to electrical stimulation of peripheral nerve in man. *J Neurol Neurosurg Psychiatry* **10**: 134–140

Dawson GD 1947b Investigations on a patient subject to myoclonic seizures after sensory stimulation. *J Neurol Neurosurg Psychiatry* **10**: 141–162

Dawson J 1916 The histology of disseminated sclerosis. *Trans R Soc Edinb* **50**: 517–740

Dawson MR, Polito A, Levine JM, Reynolds R 2003 NG2-expressing glial progenitor cells: an abundant and widespread population of cycling cells in the adult rat CNS. *Mol Cell Neurosci* **24**: 476–488

Day AL, Sypert GW 1976 Spinal cord sarcoidosis. *Ann Neurol* **1**: 79–85

Deacon WE, Alexander L, Siedler HD, Kurland LT 1959 Multiple sclerosis in a small New England community. *N Engl J Med* **261**: 1059–1061

Dean G 1949 Disseminated sclerosis in South Africa: its relationship to swayback and suggested treatment. *Br Med J* **1**: 842–845

Dean G 1967 Annual incidence, prevalence and mortality of MS in white South African-born and in white immigrants to South Africa. *Br Med J* **2**: 724–730

Dean G 2002 *The Turnstone*. Liverpool: Liverpool University Press

Dean G, Elian M 1997 Age at immigration to England of Asian and Caribbean immigrants and the risk of developing multiple sclerosis. *J Neurol Neurosurg Psychiatry* **63**: 565–568

Dean G, Gray R 1990 Do nurses or doctors have an increased risk of developing

multiple sclerosis? *J Neurol Neurosurg Psychiatry* **53**: 899–902

Dean G, Kurtzke JF 1971 On the risk of multiple sclerosis according to age at immigration to South Africa. *Br Med J* **3**: 725–729

Dean G, McLoghlin H, Brady R et al 1976 Multiple sclerosis amongst immigrants in Greater London. *Br Med J* **1**: 861–864

Dean G, Grimaldi G, Kelly R, Karhausen L 1979 Multiple sclerosis is southern Europe I: Prevalence in Sicily in 1975. *J Epidemiol Community Health* **33**: 107–110

Dean G, Goodall J, Downie A 1981a The prevalence of multiple sclerosis in the Outer Hebrides compared with north-east Scotland and the Orkney and Shetland Islands. *J Epidemiol Community Health* **35**: 110–113

Dean G, Savettieri G, Giordano D et al 1981b The prevalence of multiple sclerosis in Sicily. II. Agrigento city. *J Epidemiol Community Health* **35**: 118–122

Dean G, McDougall EI, Elian M 1985 Multiple sclerosis in research workers studying swayback in lambs: an updated report. *J Neurol Neurosurg Psych* **48**: 859–865

Dean G, Bhigjee AIG, Bill PLA et al 1994 Multiple sclerosis in black South Africans and Zimbabweans. *J Neurol Neurosurg Psychiatry* **57**: 1064–1069

Dean G, Aksoy H, Akalin T et al 1997 Multiple sclerosis in the Turkish- and Greek-speaking communities of Cyprus. A United Nations (UNHCR) bicommunal project. *J Neurol Sci* **145**: 163–168

Dean G, Elian M, de Bono AG et al 2002 Multiple sclerosis in Malta in 1999: an update. *J Neurol Neurosurg Psych* **73**: 256–260

De Angelis CD, Drazen JM, Frizelle FA et al 2005 Is this clinical trial fully registered?A statement from the International Committee of Medical Journal Editors. *N Engl J Med* **352**: 2436–2438

DeBroff DM, Donahue SP 1993 Bilateral optic neuropathy as the initial manifestation of systemic sarcoidosis. *Am J Ophthalmol* **116**: 108–110

Debruyne JC, Versijpt J, van Laere KJ et al 2003 PET visualization of microglia in multiple sclerosis patients using [¹¹C]PK11195. *Eur J Neurol* **10**: 257–264

De Castro S, Cartoni D, Millifiorini F et al 1995 Non-invasive assessment of mitoxantrone cardiotoxicity in relapsing–remitting multiple sclerosis. *J Clin Pharmacol* **35**: 627–632

Decker L, ffrench-Constant C 2004 Lipid rafts and integrin activation regulate oligodendrocyte survival. *J Neurosci* **24**: 3816–3825

Deckert-Schluter M, Schluter D, Hof H et al 1994 Differential expression of ICAM-1, VCAM-1 and their ligands LFA-1, Mac-1, CD43, VLA-4, and MHC class II antigens in murine Toxoplasma encephalitis: a light microscopic and ultrastructural immunohistochemical study. *J Neuropathol Exp Neurol* **53**: 457–468

D'Costa DF, Vania AK, Millac PA 1990 Multiple sclerosis associated with trismus. *Postgrad Med J* **66**: 853–854

Defer G-L, Barre J, Ladudal P et al 1995 Methylprednisolone infusion during acute exacerbation of MS: plasma and CSF concentrations. *Eur Neurol* **35**: 143–148

De Graaf AS 1974 Multiple sclerosis in northern Norway. *Eur Neurol* **11**: 281–295

De Groot CJ, Bergers E, Kamphorst W et al 2001 Post-mortem MRI-guided sampling of multiple sclerosis brain lesions: increased yield of active demyelinating and (p)reactive lesions. *Brain* **124**: 1635–1645

Deguchi K, Takeuchi H, Miki H et al 1992 Electrophysiological follow-up of acute and chronic experimental allergic encephalomyelitis in the Lewis rat. *Eur Arch Psych Clin Neurosci* **242**: 1–5

Dehmeshki J, Chard DT, Leary SM et al 2003 The normal appearing grey matter in primary progressive multiple sclerosis: a magnetisation transfer imaging study. *J Neurol* **250**: 67–74

D'Hooghe MB, Warshawski F, Ebers GS 1989 Neurogenic pulmonary edema: brain stem localization of responsible lesions. *Neurology* **39 (Suppl 1)**: 244 (abstract)

Deisenhammer F, Schellekens H, Bertolotto A 2004 Measurement of neutralizing antibodies to interferon beta in patients with multiple sclerosis. *J Neurol* **251**: II31–II39

Dejaegher L, de Bruyere M, Ketelaer P, Carton H 1983 HLA antigens and prognosis of multiple sclerosis. Part II. *J Neurol* **229**: 167–174

Dejerine J 1894 Etude sur la sclérose en plaques cerebro-spinale. A forme de sclérose laterale amyotrophique. *Rev Med (Paris)* **iv**: 193–212

De Keyser J 1988 Autoimmunity in multiple sclerosis. *Neurology* **38**: 371–374

De Keyser J, Zwanikken C, Boon M 1998 Effects of influenza vaccination and influenza illness on exacerbations in multiple sclerosis. *J Neurol Sci* **159**: 51–53

Dekker JW, Easteal S, Jakobsen IB et al 1993 HLA-DPB1 alleles correlate with risk for multiple sclerosis in Caucasoid and Cantonese patients lacking the high risk DQB1*0602 allele. *Tissue Antigens* **41**: 31–36

Delalande S, De Sèze J, Fauchais AL et al 2004 Neurologic manifestations in primary Sjögren's syndrome: a study of 82 patients. *Medicine* **83**: 280–291

De la Monte SM, Ropper AH, Dickersin GR et al 1986 Relapsing central and peripheral demyelinating diseases: unusual pathologic features. *Arch Neurol* **43**: 626–629

Delarasse C, Daubas P, Mars LT et al 2003 Myelin/oligodendrocyte glyoprotein-deficient (MOG-deficient) mice reveal lack of immune tolerance to MOG in wild-type mice. *J Clin Invest* **112**: 544–553

Delasnerie-Laupretre N, Alperovitch A 1992 Migration and age at onset of multiple sclerosis: some pitfalls of migrant studies. *Acta Neurol Scand* **85**: 408–411

De Leersnyder H, Burstin J, Ponsot G et al 1981 Névrites optiques chez l'enfant. *Arch Fr Pediatr* **38**: 563–572

Deloulme JC, Raponi E, Gentil BJ et al 2004 Nuclear expression of S100B in oligodendrocyte progenitor cells correlates with differentiation toward the oligodendroglial lineage and modulates oligodendroyctes maturation. *Mol Cell Neurosci* **27**: 453–465

DeLuca GC, Ebers GC, Esiri MM 2004 Axonal loss in multiple sclerosis: a pathological survey of the corticospinal and sensory tracts. *Brain* **127**: 1009–1018

De March AK, De Bouwerie M, Kolopp-Sarda MN et al 2003 Anti-myelin oligodendrocyte glycoprotein B-cell responses in multiple sclerosis. *J Neuroimmunol* **135**: 117–125

Demaree HA, DeLuca J, Gaudino EA, Diamond BJ 1999 Speed of information processing as a key deficit in multiple sclerosis: implications for rehabilitation. *J Neurol Neurosurg Psychiatry* **67**: 661–663

Deng W, Wang H, Rosenberg PA et al 2004 Role of metabotropic glutamate receptors in oligodendrocyte excitotoxicity and oxidative stress. *Proc Natl Acad Sci USA* **101**: 7751–7756

Denny-Brown D 1952 Multiple sclerosis: the clinical problems. *Am J Med* **12**: 501–509

Denny-Brown D, Brenner C 1944 Lesion in peripheral nerve resulting from compression by spring clip. *Arch Neurol and Psychiatry* **52**: 1–19

De Pauw A, Dejaeger E, D'hooghe B, Carton H 2002 Dysphagia in multiple sclerosis. *Clin Neurol Neurosurg* **104**: 345–351

Derbinski J, Schulte A, Kyewski B, Klein L 2001 Promiscuous gene expression in medullary thymic epithelial cells mirrors the peripheral self. *Nat Immunol* **2** 1032–1039

Derbinski J, Gäbler J, Brors B et al 2005 Promiscuous gene expression in thymic epithelial cells is regulated at multiple levels. *J Exp Med* **202**: 33–45

Derfuss T, Gurkov R, Bergh FT et al 2001 Intrathecal antibody production against *Chlamydia pneumoniae* in multiple sclerosis is part of a polyspecific immune response. *Brain* **124**: 1325–1335

De Sèze J, Stojkovic T, Destee M et al 2000a Paroxysmal kinesigenic choreoathetosis as a presenting symptom of multiple sclerosis. *J Neurol* **247**: 487–80

De Sèze J, Stojkovic T, Gauvrit JY et al 2000b Cardiac repolarization abnormalities in multiple sclerosis: spinal cord MRI correlates. *Muscle Nerve* **23**: 1284–1286

De Sèze J, Stojkovic T, Gauvrit JY et al 2001a Autonomic dysfunction in multiple sclerosis: cervical spinal cord atrophy correlates. *J Neurol* **248**: 297–303

De Sèze J, Devos D, Castelnovo G et al 2001b The prevalence of Sjogren's syndrome in patients with primary progressive multiple sclerosis. *Neurology* **57**: 1359–1363

De Sèze J, Stojkovic T, Breteau G et al 2001c Acute myelopathies: clinical, laboratory and outcome profiles in 79 cases. *Brain* **124**: 1509–1521

De Sèze J, Peoc'h K, Ferriby D et al 2002 14–3–3 protein in the cerebrospinal fluid of patients with acute transverse myelitis and multiple sclerosis. *J Neurol* **249**: 626–627

De Sèze J, Chapelotte M, Delalande D et al 2004 Intravenous corticosteroids in the postpartum period for reduction of acute exacerbations in multiple sclerosis. *Mult Scler* **10**: 596–597

Desmedt JE, Noel P 1973 Average somatosensory evoked potentials in the evaluation of lesions of the sensory nerves and of the central somatosensory pathway. *New Dev Electromyogr Clin Neurophysiol* **2**: 352–371

Desmond AD, Shuttleworth KED 1977 The results of urinary diversion in multiple sclerosis. *Br J Urol* **49**: 495–502

De Sousa EA, Albert RH, Kalman B 2002 Cognitive impairments in multiple sclerosis: a review. *Am J Alzheimers Dis Demen* **17**: 23–29

De Souza LH, Ashburn A 1996 Assessment of motor function in people with multiple sclerosis. *Physiother Res Int* **1**: 98–111

D'Souza SD, Antel JP, Freedman MS 1994 Cytokine induction of heat shock protein expression in human oligodendrocytes: an interleukin-1 mediated mechanism. *J Neuroimmunol* **50**: 17–24

D'Souza SD, Alinauskas KA, McCrea E et al 1995 Differential susceptibility of human CNS-derived cell populations to TNF-dependent and independent immune mediated injury. *J Neurosci* **15**: 7293–7300

D'Souza SD, Bonetti B, Balasingam V et al 1996a Multiple sclerosis: Fas signaling in oligodendrocyte cell death. *J Exp Med* **184**: 2361–2370

D'Souza SD, Alinauskas KA, Antel JP 1996b Ciliary neurotrophic factor selectively protects human oligodendrocytes from tumor necrosis factor-mediated injury. *J Neurosci Res* **43**: 289–298

DeStefano N, Matthews PM, Antel JP et al 1995 Chemical pathology of acute demyelinating lesions and its correlation with disability. *Ann Neurol* **38**: 901–909

DeStefano N, Matthews PM, Narayanan S et al 1997 Axonal dysfunction and disability in a relapse of multiple sclerosis: longitudinal study of a patient. *Neurology* **49**: 1138–1141

DeStefano N, Narayanan S, Matthews P et al 1999 In vivo evidence for axonal dysfunction remote from focal cerebral demyelination of the type seen in multiple sclerosis. *Brain* **122**: 1933–1939

DeStefano N, Dotti MT, Mortilla M et al 2000 Evidence of diffuse brain pathology and unspecific genetic characterization in a patient with an atypical form of adult-onset Krabbe disease. *J Neurol* **247**: 226–228

DeStefano N, Matthews PM, Filippi M et al 2003a Evidence of early cortical atrophy in MS: relevance to white matter changes and disability. *Neurology* **60**: 1157–1162

DeStefano F, Verstraeten T, Jackson LA et al 2003b Vaccinations and risk of central nervous system demyelinating diseases in adults. *Arch Neurol* **60**: 504–509

Detels R, Brody JF, Edgar AH 1972 Multiple sclerosis among American, Japanese and Chinese migrants to California and Washington. *J Chron Dis* **25**: 3–10

Detels R, Visscher B, Malmgrem RM et al 1977 Evidence for lower susceptibility to multiple sclerosis in Japanese-Americans. *Am J Epidemiol* **105**: 303–310

Detels R, Clark VA, Valdiviezo NL et al 1982 Factors associated with a rapid course of multiple sclerosis. *Arch Neurol* **39**: 337–341

Deuschl G, Bain P, Brin M 1998 Consensus statement of the Movement Disorder Society on Tremor. *Mov Disord* **13** (Suppl 3). 2–23

Devaux JJ, Alcaraz G, Grinspan J et al 2003a Kv3.1b is a novel component of CNS nodes. *J Neurosci* **23**: 4509–4518

Devaux JJ, Forni C, Beeton C et al 2003b Myelin basic protein-reactive T cells induce conduction failure *in vivo* but not *in vitro*. *NeuroReport* **14**: 317–320

Devaux JJ, Kleopa KA, Cooper EC, Scherer SS 2004 KCNQ2 is a nodal K+ channel. *J Neurosci* **24**: 1236–1244

Devey ME, Major PJ, Bleasdale-Barr KM et al 1990 Experimental allergic encephalomyelitis (EAE) in mice selectively bred to produce high affinity (HA) or low affinity (LA) antibody responses. *Immunology* **69**: 519–524

Devic E 1894 Myélite subaiguë compliquée de névrite optique. *Bull Med* **8**: 1033

Devinsky O, Cho E-S, Petito K, Price RW 1991 Herpes zoster myelitis. *Brain* **114**: 1181–1196

Devor M, Amir R, Rappaport ZH 2002 Pathophysiology of trigeminal neuralgia: the ignition hypothesis. *Clin J Pain* **18**: 4–13

Devos P, Destée A, Prin L, Warot P 1984 Sclérose en plaques et maladie lupique. *Rev Neurol* **140**: 513–515

Dhib-Jalbut S 2002 Mechanisms of action of interferons and glatiramer acetate in multiple sclerosis. *Neurology* **58**: S3–S9

Dhopesh VP, Weinstein JD 1977 Spinal arteriovenous malformation simulating multiple sclerosis: importance of early diagnosis. *Dis Nerv Syst* **38**: 848–851

Di Bello IC, Dawson MR, Levine JM, Reynolds R 1999 Generation of oligodendroglial progenitors in acute inflammatory demyelinating lesions of the rat brain stem is associated with demyelination rather than inflammation. *J Neurocytol* **28**: 365–381

Di Fabio RP, Soderberg J, Choi T et al 1998 Extended outpatient rehabilitation: its influence on symptom frequency, fatigue, and functional status for persons with progressive multiple sclerosis. *Arch Phys Med Rehabil* **79**: 141–146

Di Majo L, Bisceglia M, Lanzillo R et al 2002 Aphasia as a rare presentation of monosymptomatic demyelinating disease: case report and review of the literature. *Neurol Sci* 23: 79–82

Di Santo JP 2001 Lung Krüppel-like factor: a quintessential player in T cell quiescence. *Nature Immunol* 2: 667–668

Dib C, Faure S, Fizames C et al 1996 A comprehensive genetic map of the human genome based on 5,264 microsatellites. *Nature* 380: 152–154

Dib-Hajj SD, Fjell J, Cummins TR et al 1999 Plasticity of sodium channel expression in DRG neurons in the chronic constriction injury model of neuropathic pain. *Pain* 83: 591–600

Dichgans M, Mayer M, Uttner I et al 1998 The phenotypic spectrum of CADASIL: clinical findings in 102 cases. *Ann Neurol* 44: 731–739

Diem R, Hobom M, Maier K et al 2003 Methylprednisolone increases neuronal apoptosis during autoimmune CNS inflammation by inhibition of an endogenous neuroprotective pathway. *J Neurosci* 23: 6993–7000

Diemel LT, Copelman CA, Cuzner ML 1998 Macrophages in the CNS: friends of foe? *Neurochem Res* 23: 341–347

van Diemen HA, van Dongen MM, Dammers JW, Polman CH 1992 Increased visual impairment after exercise (Uhthoff's phenomenon) in multiple sclerosis: therapeutic possibilities. *Eur Neurol* 32: 231–234

van Diemen HA, Polman CH, van Dongen MM et al 1993 4-aminopyridine induces functional improvement in multiple sclerosis patients: a neurophysiological study. *J Neurol Sci* 116: 220–226

DiMario FJ, Berman PH 1987 Multiple sclerosis presenting at 4 years of age: clinical and MRI correlations. *Clin Pediatr* 27: 32–37

Dimayuga FO, Ding Q, Keller JN et al 2003 The neuregulin GGF2 attenuates free radical release from activated microglial cells. *J Neuroimmunol* 136: 67–74

Ding JW, Dickie J, O'Brodovich H et al 1998 Inhibition of amiloride-sensitive sodium-channel activity in distal lung epithelial cells by nitric oxide. *Am J Physiol – Lung Cell Mol Physiol* 274: L378–L387

Dinkler 1904 Zur Kasuistik der multiplen Herdsklerose des Gehirns und Rückenmarks. *Dtsch Z Nervenheilk* 26: 233–247

Disability Committee of the Royal College of Physicians 1991 *National Concepts of Rehabilitation.* London: Royal College of Physicians Publications

Dittel BN, Stefanova I, Germain RN, Janeway CA 1999 Cross-antagonism of a T cell clone expressing two distinct T cells receptors. *Immunity* 11: 289–298

Ditunno JF Jr, Formal CS 1994 Chronic spinal cord injury. *N Engl J Med* 330: 550–556

Djaldetti R, Ziv I, Achiron A, Melamed E 1996 Fatigue in multiple sclerosis compared with chronic fatigue syndrome: a quantitative assessment. *Neurology* 46: 632–635

DMKG Study Group 2003 Misoprostol in the treatment of trigeminal neuralgia associated with multiple sclerosis. *J Neurol* 250: 542–545

Doetsch F 2003 The glial identity of neural stem cells. *Nat Neurosci* 6: 1127–1134

Doetsch F, Caille I, Lim DA, Garcia-Verdugo JM, Alvarez-Buylla A 1999 Subventricular zone astrocytes are neural stem cells in the adult mammalian brain. *Cell* 97: 703–716

Dogulu CF, Kansu T 1997 Upside-down reversal of vision in multiple sclerosis. *J Neurol* 244: 461–462

Dolei A, Serra C, Mameli G et al 2002 Multiple sclerosis-associated retrovirus (MSRV) in Sardinian MS patients. *Neurology* 58: 471–473

Domeniconi M, Cao Z, Spencer T et al 2002 Myelin-associated glycoprotein interacts with the Nogo66 receptor to inhibit neurite outgrowth. *Neuron* 35: 283–290

Doncel AM, Rubio A, Arroyo R et al 2002 Interleukin-10 polymorphisms in Spanish multiple sclerosis patients. *J Neuroimmunol* 131: 168–172

Dong C, Juedes AE, Temann U-A et al 2001 ICOS co-stimulatory receptor is essential for T-cell activation and function. *Nature* 409: 70–101

Dong-Si T, Weber J, Liu YB et al 2004 Increased prevalence of and gene transcription by *Chlamydia pneumoniae* in cerebrospinal fluid of patients with relapsing–remitting multiple sclerosis. *J Neurol* 251: 542–547

Donnadieu E, Revy P, Trautmann A 2001 Imaging T cell antigen recognition and comparing immunological and neuronal synapses. *Immunol* 103: 417–425

Donnan PT, Parratt JDE, Wilson SV et al 2005 Multiple sclerosis in Tayside, Scotland: detection of clusters using a spatial scan statistic. *Mult Scler* 11: 403–408

Dooley JM, Wright BA 1985 Adrenoleukodystrophy mimicking multiple sclerosis. *Can J Neurol Sci* 12: 73–74

Doolittle TH, Myers RH, Lehrich JR et al 1990 Multiple sclerosis sibling pairs: clustered onset and familial predisposition. *Neurology* 40: 937–950

Doraiswamy PM, Rao SM 2004 Treating cognitive deficits in multiple sclerosis: are we there yet? *Neurology* 63: 1552–1553

Dore-Duffy P, Donaldson JO, Rothman BL, Zurier RB 1982 Antinuclear antibodies in multiple sclerosis. *Arch Neurol* 39: 504–506

Dore-Duffy P, Ho SY, Donovan C 1991 Cerebrospinal fluid eicosanoid levels: endogenous PGD2 and LTC4 synthesis by antigen-presenting cells that migrate to the central nervous system. *Neurology* 41: 322–324

Dore-Duffy P, Washington R, Dragovic L 1993 Expression of endothelial cell activation antigens in microvessels from patients with multiple sclerosis. *Adv Exper Med Biol* 331: 243–248

Dore-Duffy P, Newman W, Balabanov R et al 1995 Circulating, soluble adhesion proteins in cerebrospinal fluid and serum of patients with multiple sclerosis: correlation with clinical activity. *Ann Neurol* 37: 55–62

Dornmair K, Goebels N, Weltzien H-U et al 2003 T cell-mediated autoimmunity: novel techniques to characterize autoreactive T cell receptors. *Am J Pathol* 163: 1215–1226

Dorr J, Bechmann I, Waiczies S et al 2002 Lack of tumor necrosis factor-related apoptosis-inducing ligand but presence of its receptors in the human brain. *J Neurosci* 22: RC209

Doty RL, Li C, Mannon LJ, Yousem DM 1998 Olfactory dysfunction in multiple sclerosis: relation to plaque load in inferior frontal and temporal lobes. *Ann N Y Acad Sci* 855: 781–786

Doty RL, Li C, Mannon LJ, Yousem DM 1999 Olfactory dysfunction in multiple sclerosis: relation to longitudinal changes in plaque numbers in central olfactory structures. *Neurology* 53: 880–882

Douglass LH, Jorgensen CL 1948 Pregnancy and multiple sclerosis. *Am J Obstetr Gynecol* 55: 332–336

Dousset V, Rosman R, Ramer KN et al 1992 Experimental allergic encephalomyelitis and multiple sclerosis lesion characterization with magnetization transfer imaging. *Radiology* 182: 483–491

Dousset V, Brochet B, Vital F, Nagem F, Bonnet J, Caille JM 1994 Imaging including diffusion and magnetization transfer of chronic relapsing experimental encephalomyelitis – correlation with immunological and pathological data. *Proc Soc Magn Reson* 2: 1401 (abstract)

Dousset V, Brochet B, Vital A et al 1995 Lysolecithin-induced demyelination in primates: preliminary *in vivo* study with MR and magnetization transfer. *Am J Neuroradiol* 16: 225–231

Dousset V, Delalande C, Ballarino L et al 1999 In vivo macrophage activity imaging in the central nervous system detected by magnetic resonance. *Magn Reson Med* 41: 329–333

Dousset V, Brochet B, Cailee J-M, Petry K 2000 MS lesions enhancement with ultrasmall particle iron oxide: the first phase II study. *Rev Neurol* 156: 3S40

Dowling PC, Bosch VV, Cook SD 1980 Possible beneficial effect of high dose intravenous steroid therapy in acute demyelinating disease and transverse myelitis. *J Neurol Neurosurg Psychiatry* 30: 33–36

Dowling P, Shang G, Raval S et al 1996 Involvement of the CD95 (APO-1/Fas) receptor/ligand system in multiple sclerosis brain. *J Exp Med* 184: 1513–1518

Downie AW 1984 The Chief Scientist Report. Multiple sclerosis in North East Scotland. *Health Bull Edinb* 42: 151–156

Drazen JM 2005 Patients at risk. *N Engl J Med* 353: 417

Dressnandt J, Conrad B 1996 Lasting reduction of severe spasticity after ending chronic treatment with intrathecal baclofen. *J Neurol Neurosurg Psychiatry* 60: 168–173

Dreyfus GL, Mayer K 1929 Vier Jähne Malariabehandlung der multiplen Sklerose. *Dtsch Z Nervenheilk* 111: 68–98

Droogan AG, Kirk CW, Hawkins SA et al 1996 T-cell receptor alpha, beta, gamma, and delta chain gene microsatellites show no association with multiple sclerosis. *Neurology* **47**: 1049–1053

Droogan AG, Crockard AD, McMillan SA, Hawkins SA 1998 Effects of intravenous methylprednisolone therapy on leukocyte and soluble adhesion molecule expression in MS. *Neurology* **50**: 224–229

Drouin E, Nataf S, Lande G, Louboutin JP 1998 Abnormalities of cardiac repolarization in multiple sclerosis: relationship with a model of allergic encephalomyelitis in rat. *Muscle & Nerve* **21**: 940–942

Drulovic B, Ribaric-Jankes K, Kostic VE, Sternic N 1993 Sudden hearing loss as the initial monosymptom of multiple sclerosis. *Neurology* **43**: 2703–2705

Drulovic J, Dozic S, Levic Z et al 1998 Unusual association of multiple sclerosis and tomaculous neuropathy. *J Neurol Sci* **157**: 217–222

Du C, Yao S, Ljunggren-Rose Å, Sriram S 2002 *Chlamydia pneumoniae* infection of the central nervous system worsens experimental allergic encephalitis. *J Exp Med* **196**: 1639–1644

Dubois BD, Masure S, Hurtenbach U et al 1999 Resistance of young gelatinase B-deficient mice to experimental autoimmune encephalomyelitis and necrotizing tail lesions. *J Clin Invest* **104**: 1507–1515

Dubois BD, Keenan E, Porter BE et al 2003 Interferon beta in multiple sclerosis: experience in a British specialist multiple sclerosis centre. *J Neurol Neurosurg Psychiatry* **74**: 946–949

Dubois-Dalcq M, Niedieck B, Buyse M 1970 Action of anti-cerebroside sera on myelinated nervous tissue cultures. *Patol Eur* **5**: 331–347

Dubois-Dalcq M, Schumacher G, Sever JL 1973 Acute multiple sclerosis: electron-microscopic evidence for and against a viral agent in the plaques. *Lancet* **ii**: 1408–1411

Duchen MR 2000 Mitochondria and calcium: from cell signalling to cell death. *J Physiol* **529**: 57–68

Duckworth D 1885 Disseminated cerebro-spinal sclerosis in an early stage affecting exclusively the right extremities. *Lancet* **i**: 879–880

Duclos P 1992 Adverse events after hepatitis B vaccination. *Can Med Assoc J* **147**: 1023–1026

Duclos P 2003 Safety of immunization and adverse events following vaccination against hepatitis B. *Expert Opin Drug Safety* **2**: 225–231

Duda PW, Schmied MC, Cook SL et al 2000 Glatiramer acetate (Copaxone) induces degenerate, Th2-polarized immune responses in patients with multiple sclerosis. *J Clin Invest* **105**: 967–976

Dufour A, Corsini E, Gelati M et al 2000 In vitro glatiramer acetate treatment of brain endothelium does not reduce adhesion phenomena. *Ann Neurol* **47**: 680–682

Dugandzija-Novakovic S, Koszowski AG, Levinson SR, Shrager P 1995a Clustering of Na+ channels and node of Ranvier formation in remyelinating axons. *J Neurosci* **15**: 492–503

Dugandzija-Novakovic S, Shrager P 1995b Survival, development, and electrical activity of central nervous system myelinated axons exposed to tumor necrosis factor in vitro. *J Neurosci Res* **40**: 117–126

Dukart G, JS B 1984 An overview of cardiac episodes following mitoxantrone administration. *Cancer Treat Symp* **3**: 35–41

Dumas M, Jauberteau-Marchan MO 2000 The protective role of Langerhans' cells and sunlight in multiple sclerosis. *Med Hypotheses* **55**: 517–520

Duncan SR, Scott S, Duncan CJ 2005 Reappraisal of the historical selective pressures for the CCR5-Δ32 mutation. *J Med Genet* **42**: 205–208

Dunn V, Bale JF, Zimmerman RA et al 1986 MRI in children with postinfectious disseminated encephalomyelitis. *Mag Reson Imag* **4**: 25–32

Dupont B (ed.) 1992 Nomenclature for the factors of the HLA system, 1991. *Tissue Antigens* **39**: 1–13

Dupont B, Lisak RP, Jersild C et al 1977 HLA antigens in black Americans with multiple sclerosis. *Transplantation Proc* **9 (Suppl 1)**: 181–185

Dupont RM, Jernigan TL, Butters N et al 1990 Subcortical abnormalities detected in bipolar affective disorder using magnetic resonance imaging: clinical and neuropsychological significance. *Arch Gen Psychiatry* **47**: 55–59

Dupree JL, Girault J-A, Popko B 1999 Axo-glial interactions regulate the localization of axonal paranodal proteins. *J Cell Biol* **147**: 1145–1151

Duquette P, Decary F, Pleines J et al 1985 Clinical sub-groups of multiple sclerosis in relation to HLA: DR alleles as possible markers of disease progression. *Can J Neurol Sci* **12**: 106–110

Duquette P, Murray TJ, Pleines J et al 1987 Multiple sclerosis in childhood: clinical profile in 125 patients. *J Pediatr* **111**: 359–363

Durelli L, Cocito D, Riccio A et al 1986 High-dose intravenous methylprednisolone in the treatment of multiple sclerosis: clinical-immunological correlations. *Neurology* **36**: 238–243

Durelli L, Bongioanni MR, Cavallo R et al 1994 Chronic systemic high-dose recombinant interferon alfa-2a reduces exacerbation rate, MRI signs of disease activity, and lymphocyte interferon gamma production in relapsing–remitting multiple sclerosis. *Neurology* **44**: 406–413

Durelli L, Bongioanni MR, Ferrero B et al 1996 Interferon alpha-2a treatment of relapsing–remitting multiple sclerosis: disease activity resumes after stopping treatment. *Neurology* **47**: 123–129

Durelli L, Bongioanni MR, Ferrero B et al 1998 Interferon treatment for multiple sclerosis: autoimmune complications may be lethal. *Neurology* **50**: 570–571

Durelli L, Ferrero B, Oggero A et al 1999 Autoimmune events during interferon beta-1b treatment for multiple sclerosis. *J Neurol Sci* **162**: 74–83

Durelli L, Verdun E, Barbero P et al 2002 Every-other-day interferon beta-1b versus once-weekly interferon beta-1a for multiple sclerosis: results of a 2-year prospective randomised multicentre study (INCOMIN). *Lancet* **359**: 1453–1460

Dustin ML, Colman DR 2002 Neural and immunological synaptic relations. *Science* **298**: 785–789

Dutton RW, Bradley LM, Swain SL 1998 T cell memory. *Annu Rev Immunol* **16**: 201–223

DuVall MD, Zhu S, Fuller CM, Matalon S 1998 Peroxynitrite inhibits amiloride-sensitive Na+ currents in Xenopus oocytes expressing alpha beta gamma-rENaC. *Am J Physiol* **274**: C1417–C1423

Duvefelt K, Anderson M, Fogdell-Hahn A, Hillert J 2004 A NOTCH4 association with multiple sclerosis is secondary to HLA-DR*1501. *Tissue Antigens* **63**: 13–20

Dworkin RH, Bates D, Millar JHD, Paty DW 1984 Linoleic acid and multiple sclerosis: a reanalysis of three double blind trials. *Neurology* **34**: 1441–1445

Dyment DA, Ebers GC 2002 An array of sunshine in multiple sclerosis. *N Engl J Med* **347**: 1445–1447

Dyment DA, Willer CJ, Scott B et al 2001 Genetic susceptibility to MS: a second stage analysis in Canadian MS families. *Neurogenetics* **3**: 145–151

Dyment DA, Cader MZ, Wiler CJ et al 2002a A multigenerational family with multiple sclerosis. *Brain* **125**: 1474–1482

Dyment DA, Steckley JL, Willer CJ et al 2002b No evidence to support CTLA-4 as a susceptibility gene in MS families: the Canadian collaborative study. *J Neuroimmunol* **123**: 193–198

Dyment DA, Steckley JL, Morrison K et al 2004a TCR beta polymorphisms and multiple sclerosis. *Genes Immun* **5**: 337–342

Dyment DA, Sadovnick AD, Willer CJ et al 2004b An extended genome scan in 442 Canadian multiple sclerosis-affected sibships: a report from the Canadian collaborative Study Group. *Hum Mol Genet* **13**: 1005–1015

Dyment DA, Herrera BM, Cader MZ et al 2005 Complex interactions among MHC haplotypes in multiple sclerosis: susceptibility and resistance *Hum Mol Genet* **14**: 2019–2026

Dziembowska M, Tham TN, Lau P et al 2005 A role for CXCR4 signaling in survival and migration of neural and oligodendrocyte precursors. *Glia* **50**: 258–269

Earl CJ 1964 Some aspects of optic atrophy. *Trans Ophthalmol Soc UK* **84**: 215–226

Earl CJ, Martin B 1967 Prognosis in optic neuritis related to age. *Lancet* **i**: 74–76

Eastman R, Sheridan J, Poskanzer DC 1973 Multiple sclerosis clustering in a small

Massachusetts community, with possible common exposure 23 years before onset. *New Engl J Med* **289**: 793–794

Eaves IA, Merriman TR, Barber RA *et al* 2000 The genetically isolated populations of Finland and Sardinia may not be a panacea for linkage disequilibrium mapping of common disease genes. *Nature Genet* **25**: 320–323

Ebers G 2000 The natural history of multiple sclerosis. *Neurol Sci* **21 (Suppl)**: 815–817

Ebers GC 1985a Osler and neurology. *Can J Neurol Sci* **12**: 236–242

Ebers GC 1985b Optic neuritis and multiple sclerosis. *Arch Neurol* **42**: 702–704

Ebers GC 1998 Natural history of multiple sclerosis. In: Compston A, Ebers G, Lassmann H *et al* (eds) *McAlpine's Multiple Sclerosis, 3rd edn.* London: Churchill Livingstone, pp. 191–221

Ebers GC, Cripps J, Rudd A 1982a Birth order and multiple sclerosis. *Acta Neurol Scand* **66**: 342–346

Ebers GC, Paty DW, Stiller CR *et al* 1982b HLA typing and sibling pairs with multiple sclerosis. *Lancet* **ii**: 88–90

Ebers GC, Bulman DE, Sadovnick AD *et al* 1986 A population based study of multiple sclerosis in twins. *N Engl J Med* **315**: 1638–1642

Ebers GC, Sadovnick AD, Risch NJ 1995 A genetic basis for familial aggregation in multiple sclerosis. *Nature* **377**: 150–151

Ebers GC, Kukay K, Bulman D *et al* 1996 A full genome search in multiple sclerosis. *Nature Genet* **13**: 472–476

Ebers GC, Yee IM, Sadovnick AD, Duquette P 2000a Conjugal multiple sclerosis: population-based prevalence and recurrence risks in offspring. Canadian Collaborative Study Group. *Ann Neurol* **48**: 927–931

Ebers GC, Koopman WJ, Hader W *et al* 2000b The natural history of multiple sclerosis: a geographically based study. *Brain* **123**: 641–649

Ebers GC, Sadovnick AD, Dyment DA *et al* 2004 Parent-of-origin effect in multiple sclerosis: observations in half-siblings. *Lancet* **363**: 1773–1774

Edan G, Miller DH, Clanet M *et al* 1997 Therapeutic effect of mitoxantrone combined with methylprednisolone in multiple sclerosis: a randomised multi-center study of active disease using MRI and clinical criteria. *J Neurol Neurosurg Psychiatry* **62**: 112–118

Eddleston M, Mucke L 1993 Molecular profile of reactive astrocytes – implications for their role in neurologic disease. *Neuroscience* **54**: 15–36

Edgley K, Sullivan M, Dehoux E 1991 A survey of multiple sclerosis: determinants of employment status. *Can J Rehab* **4**: 127–132

Edland A, Nyland H, Riise T, Larsen JP 1996 Epidemiology of multiple sclerosis in the county of Vestfold, eastern Norway: incidence and prevalence calculations. *Acta Neurol Scand* **93**: 104–109

Edmund J, Fog T 1955 Visual and motor instability in multiple sclerosis. *Arch Neurol Psychiatry* **73**: 316–323

Edwards BA 1889 *De l'hemiplegie dans quelques affections nerveuses.* Paris: Bureaux du Progres & A. Delahaye et Lecrosnier

Edwards LJ, Constantinescu CS 2004 A prospective study of conditions associated with multiple sclerosis in a cohort of 658 consecutive outpatients attending a multiple sclerosis clinic. *Mult Scler* **10**: 575–581

Edwards S, Zvartau M, Clarke H *et al* 1998 Clinical relapses and disease activity on magnetic resonance imaging associated with viral upper respiratory tract infections in multiple sclerosis. *J Neurol Neurosurg Psychiatry* **64**: 736–741

Egen JG, Kuhns MS, Allison JP 2002 CTLA-4: new insights into its biological function and use in tumor immunotherapy. *Nat Immunol* **3**: 611–618

Eglitis MA, Mezey E 1997 Hematopoietic cells differentiate into both microglia and macroglia in the brains of adult mice. *Proc Natl Acad Sci USA* **94**: 4080–4085

Ehde D, Gibbons L, Chwastiak L *et al* 2003 Chronic pain in a large community sample of persons with multiple sclerosis. *Mult Scler* **9**: 605–611

Ehling R, Gassner Ch, Lutterotti A *et al* 2004 Genetic variants in the tumor necrosis factor receptor II gene in patients with multiple sclerosis. *Tissue Antigens* **63**: 28–33

Ehrhard PB, Erb P, Graumann U, Otten U 1993 Expression of nerve growth factor and nerve growth factor receptor tyrosine kinase Trk in activated CD4-positive T-cell clones. *Proc Natl Acad Sci USA* **90**: 10984–10988

Ehrlich P, Morgenroth J 1901 Über Hämolysine: Fünfte Mitteilung. Berlin. *Klin Wschr* **38**: 251–256

Eichler FS, Barker PB, Cox C *et al* 2002 Proton MR spectroscopic imaging predicts lesion progression on MRI in X-linked adrenoleucodystrophy. *Neurology* **58**: 901–907

Eichorst H 1896 Über infantile und hereditare multiple Sklerose. *Virchow's Arch Pathologie Anat Berl* **146**: 173–192

Eickhoff K, Heipertz R 1979 The activity of 2′, 3′-cyclic nucleotide 3′-phosphohydrolase in human cerebrospinal fluid. *Clin Chim Acta* **92**: 303–305

Eidelberg D, Newton MR, Johnson G *et al* 1988 Chronic unilateral optic neuropathy: a magnetic resonance study. *Ann Neurol* **24**: 3–11

Eikelenboom MJ, Petzold A, Lazeron RH *et al* 2003 Multiple sclerosis: neurofilament light chain antibodies are correlated to cerebral atrophy. *Neurology* **60**: 219–223

Eisen A, Odusote K 1980 Central and peripheral conduction times in multiple sclerosis. *Electroencephalogr Clin Neurophysiol* **48**: 253–265

Ekbom K 1966 Familial multiple sclerosis associated with narcolepsy. *Arch Neurol* **15**: 337–344

Eldridge R, McFarland H, Sever J *et al* 1978 Familial multiple sclerosis: clinical, histocompatibility, and viral serological studies. *Ann Neurol* **3**: 72–80

Eldridge R, Anayiotos CP, Schlesinger S *et al* 1984 Hereditary adult-onset leukodystrophy simulating chronic progressive multiple sclerosis. *N Engl J Med* **311**: 948–953

Elian M, Dean G 1977 Multiple sclerosis and epilepsy. In: Perry JK (ed.) *Epilepsy, the 8th International Symposium.* New York: Raven Press, pp. 341–344

Elian M, Dean G 1987 Multiple sclerosis among United Kingdom born children of immigrants from the West Indies. *J Neurol Neurosurg Psychiatry* **50**: 327–332

Elian M, Alonso A, Awad J *et al* 1987 HLA associations with multiple sclerosis in Sicily and Malta. *Disease Markers* **5**: 89–99

Elian M, Nightingale S, Dean G 1990 Multiple sclerosis among United Kingdom-born children of immigrants from the Indian subcontinent, Africa and the West Indies. *J Neurol Neurosurg Psychiatry* **53**: 906–911

Elliott JI, Douek DC, Altmann DM 1996 Mice lacking $\alpha\beta^+$ T cells are resistant to the induction of experimental autoimmune encephalomyelitis. *J Neuroimmunol* **70**: 139–144

Ellis H 1998 MS. *Lancet* **351**: 1295

Ellison GW, Myers LW, Mickey MR *et al* 1989 A placebo-controlled, randomised, double-masked, variable dosage, clinical trial of azathioprine with and without methylprednisolone in multiple sclerosis. *Neurology* **39**: 1018–1026

Elovaara I, Lällä M, Spåre E *et al* 1998 Methylprednisolone reduces adhesion molecules in blood and cerebrospinal fluid in patients with MS. *Neurology* **51**: 1703–1708

Elovaara I, Ukkonen M, Leppakynnas M *et al* 2000 Adhesion molecules in multiple sclerosis: relation to subtypes of disease and methylprednisolone therapy. *Arch Neurol* **57**: 546–551

Elrington GM, Bateman DE, Jeffrey MJ, Lawton NF 1989 Adrenoleukodystrophy: heterogeneity in two brothers. *J Neurol Neurosurg Psychiatry* **52**: 310–313

Encinas JA, Lees MB, Sobel RA *et al* 1996 Genetic analysis of susceptibility to experimental autoimmune encephalomyelitis in a cross between SJL/J and B10.S mice. *J Immunol* **157**: 2186–2192

Encinas JA, Wicker LS, Peterson LB *et al* 1999 QTL influencing autoimmune diabetes and encephalomyelitis map to a 0.15-cM region containing *IL2*. *Nature Genet* **21**: 158–160

Encinas JA, Lees MB, Sobel RA *et al* 2001 Identification of genetic loci associated with paralysis, inflammation and weight loss in mouse experimental autoimmune encephalomyelitis. *Int Immunol* **13**: 257–264

Eng LF, Ghirnikar RS 1994 GFAP and astrogliosis. *Brain Pathol* **4**: 229–237

Engel U, Wolswijk G 1996 Oligodendrocyte-type-2 astrocyte (0–2a) progenitor cells derived from adult-rat spinal-cord – in-vitro characteristics and response to PDGF, bFGF and NT-3. *Glia* 16: 16–26

van Engelen BGM, Hommes OR, Pinckers A *et al* 1992 Improved vision after intravenous immunoglobulin in stable demyelinating optic neuritis. *Ann Neurol* 32: 835–836

Engelhardt B, Wolburg H 2004 Transendothelial migration of leukocytes: through the front door or around the side of the house? *Eur J Immunol* 34: 2955–2963

Engelhardt B, Laschinger M, Schulz M *et al* 1998 The development of experimental autoimmune encephalomyelitis in the mouse requires alpha4-integrin but not alpha4beta7-integrin. *J Clin Invest* 102: 2096–2105

Engelken JD, Yuh WTC, Carter KD, Nerad JA 1992 Optic nerve sarcoidosis: MR findings. *Am J Neuroradiol* 13: 228–230

Engell T 1986 Neurological disease activity in multiple sclerosis patients with periphlebitis retinae. *Acta Neurol Scand* 73: 168–172

Engell T 1988 A clinico-pathoanatomical study of multiple sclerosis diagnosis. *Acta Neurol Scand* 78: 29–44

Engell T 1989 A clinical patho-anatomical study of clinically silent multiple sclerosis. *Acta Neurol Scand* 79: 428–430

Engell T, Andersen PK 1982 The frequency of periphlebitis retinae in multiple sclerosis. *Acta Neurol Scand* 65: 601–608

Engell T, Raus NE, Thompsen M, Platz M 1982 HLA and heterogeneity of multiple sclerosis. *Neurology* 32: 1043–1046

Engell T, Hvidberg A, Uhrenholdt A 1984 Multiple sclerosis: periphlebitis retinalis et cerebrospinalis. A correlation between periphlebitis retinalis and abnormal technetium brain scintigraphy. *Acta Neurol Scand* 69: 293–297

Engell T, Jensen OA, Klinken L 1985 Periphlebitis retinae in multiple sclerosis: a histopathological study of 2 cases. *Acta Ophthalmol* 68: 83–88

England JD, Gamboni F, Levinson SR, Finger TE 1990 Changed distribution of sodium channels along demyelinated axons. *Proc Natl Acad Sci USA* 87: 6777–6780

England JD, Gamboni F, Levinson SR 1991 Increased numbers of sodium channels form along demyelinated axons. *Brain Res* 548: 334–337

England JD, Levinson SR, Shrager P 1996 Immunocytochemical investigations of sodium channels along nodal and internodal portions of demyelinated axons. *Microsc Res Techn* 34: 445–451

England S, Bevan S, Docherty RJ 1996 PGE2 modulates the tetrodotoxin-resistant sodium current in neonatal rat dorsal root ganglion neurones via the cyclic AMP-protein kinase A cascade. *J Physiol* 495: 429–440

Enzinger C, Ropele S, Smith S *et al* 2004a Accelerated evolution of brain atrophy and 'black holes' in MS patients with *APOE-ε4*. *Ann Neurol* 55: 563–569

Enzinger C, Ropele S, Strasser-Fuchs S *et al* 2004b Lower levels of N-acetylaspartate in multiple sclerosis patients with the apolipoprotein E epsilon4 allele. *Arch Neurol* 61: 296

Eoli M, Wood NW, Kellar-Wood H *et al* 1994a No linkage between multiple sclerosis and the T cell receptor alpha chain locus. *J Neurol Sci* 14: 32–37

Eoli M, Pandolfo M, Milanese C *et al* 1994b The myelin basic protein gene is not a major susceptibility locus for multiple sclerosis in Italian patients. *J Neurol* 241: 615–619

Epplen C, Jackel S, Santos EJM *et al* 1997 Genetic predisposition to multiple sclerosis as revealed by immunoprinting. *Ann Neurol* 41: 341–352

Eraksoy M, Kürtüncü M, Akman-Demir G *et al* 2003a A whole genome screen for linkage in Turkish multiple sclerosis. *J Neuroimmunol* 143: 17–24

Eraksoy M, Hensiek A, Kürtüncü M *et al* 2003b A genome screen for linkage disequilibrium in Turkish multiple sclerosis. *J Neuroimmunol* 143: 129–132

Erben S 1898 Zur Histologie und Pathologie der inselförmigen Sklerose. *Neurol Centralb* 14: 626–635

Erdem E, Carlier R, Idir ABC *et al* 1993a Gadolinium-enhanced MRI in central nervous system Behçet's disease. *Neuroradiology* 35: 142–144

Erdem E, Carlier R, Delvalle A, Caquet R, Etienne JP, Doyon D 1993b Gadolinium enhanced MRI in Whipple's disease. *Neuroradiology* 35: 581–583

Erdemli G, Krnjevic K 1995 Nitric oxide tonically depresses a voltage- and Ca-dependent outward current in hippocampal slices. *Neurosci Lett* 201: 57–60

Eriksson M, Ben-Menachem E, Andersen O 2002 Epileptic seizures, cranial neuralgias and paroxysmal symptoms in remitting and progressive multiple sclerosis. *Mult Scler* 8: 495–499

Eriksson M, Andersen O, Runmarker B 2003 Long-term follow-up of patients with clinically isolated syndromes, relapsing–remitting and secondary progressive multiple sclerosis. *Mult Scler* 9: 260–274

Eriksson PS, Perfilieva E, Bjork-Eriksson T *et al* 1998 Neurogenesis in the adult human hippocampus. *Nature Med* 4: 1313–1317

Esiri MM 1977 Immunoglobulin-containing cells in multiple sclerosis plaques. *Lancet* ii: 478–480

Esiri MM 1980 Multiple sclerosis: a quantitative and qualitative study of immunoglobulin-containing cells in the central nervous system. *Neuropathol Appl Neurobiol* 6: 9–21

Esiri MM, Reading MC 1987 Macrophage populations associated with multiple sclerosis plaques. *Neuropathol Appl Neurobiol* 13: 451–465

Esiri MM, Reading MC, Squier MV, Hughes JT 1989 Immunocytochemical characterization of the macrophage and lymphocyte infiltrate in the brain in six cases of human encephalitis. *Neuropathol Appl Neurobiol* 15: 289–305

Espey MG, Chernyshev ON, Reinhard JF *et al* 1997 Activated human microglia produce the excitotoxin quinolinic acid. *NeuroReport* 8: 431–434

Estes ML, Rudick RA, Barnett GH, Ransohoff RM 1990 Stereotactic biopsy of an active multiple sclerosis lesion: immunocytochemical analysis and neuropathologic correlation with magnetic resonance imaging. *Arch Neurol* 47: 1299–1303

Etus V, Akansel G, Ilbay K *et al* 2002 Multiple sclerosis and coexisting extramedullary spinal cord tumour: a case report. *Neurol Sci* 23: 119–122

Eugster HP, Frei K, Kopf M *et al* 1998 IL-6-deficient mice resist myelin oligodendrocyte glycoprotein-induced autoimmune encephalomyelitis. *Eur J Immunol* 28: 2178–2187

Eugster HP, Frei K, Bachmann R *et al* 1999 Severity of symptoms and demyelination in MOG-induced EAE depends on TNFR1. *Eur J Immunol* 29: 626–632

European Study Group in Interferon Beta-1b in Secondary Progressive MS 1998 Placebo-controlled multicentre randomised trial of interferon beta-1b in treatment of secondary progressive multiple sclerosis. *Lancet* 352: 1491–1497

Evangelou N, Jackson M, Beeson D, Palace J 1999 Association of the APOE e4 allele with disease activity in multiple sclerosis. *J Neurol Neurosurg Psych* 67: 203–205

Evangelou N, Konz D, Esiri MM *et al* 2000a Regional axonal loss in the corpus callosum correlates with cerebral white matter lesion volume and distribution in multiple sclerosis. *Brain* 123: 1845–1849

Evangelou N, Esiri MM, Smith S *et al* 2000b Quantitative pathological evidence for axonal loss in normal appearing white matter in multiple sclerosis. *Ann Neurol* 47: 391–395

Evangelou N, Konz D, Esiri MM *et al* 2001 Size-selective neuronal changes in the anterior optic pathways suggest a differential susceptibility to injury in multiple sclerosis. *Brain* 124: 1813–1820

Evangelou N, DeLuca GC, Owens T, Esiri MM 2005 Pathological study of spinal cord atrophy in multiple sclerosis suggests limited role of focal lesions. *Brain* 128: 29–34

Evans AC, Frank JA, Antel JP, Miller DH 1997 The role of MRI in clinical trials of multiple sclerosis: comparison of image processing techniques. *Ann Neurol* 41: 125–132

Evans AR, Vasko MR, Nicol GD 1999 The cAMP transduction cascade mediates the PGE2-induced inhibition of potassium currents in rat sensory neurones. *J Physiol* 516: 163–178

Evans CF, Horwitz MB, Hobbs MV, Oldstone MB 1996 Viral infection of transgenic mice expressing a viral protein in oligodendrocytes leads to chronic central nervous system autoimmune disease. *J Exp Med* **184**: 2371–2384

Evans M, Kaufman M 1981 Establishment in culture of pluripotent cells from mouse embryos. *Nature* **292**: 154–156

Evron S, Brenner T, Abramsky O 1984 Suppressive effect of pregnancy on the development of experimental allergic encephalomyelitis in rabbits. *Am J Reprod Immunol* **5**: 109–113

Expanded Programme on Immunization (EPI) 1997 Lack of evidence that hepatitis B vaccine causes multiple sclerosis. *Wkly Epidemiol Rec* **72**: 149–152

Eyssette M, Rohmer F, Serratrice G, Warter JM, Boisson D 1988 Multi-centre, double-blind trial of a novel antispastic agent, tizanidine, in spasticity associated with multiple sclerosis. *Curr Med Res Opin* **10**: 699–708

Fabry Z, Raine CS, Hart MN 1994 Nervous tissue as an immune compartment: the dialect of the immune response in the CNS. *Immunol Today* **15**: 218–224

Falcone M, Rajan AJ, Bloom BR, Brosnan CF 1998 A critical role for IL-4 in regulating disease severity in experimental allergic encephalomyelitis as demonstrated in IL-4-deficient C57BL/6 mice and BALB/c mice. *J Immunol* **160**: 4822–4830

Fallis RJ, McFarlin DE 1989 Chronic relapsing experimental allergic encephalomyelitis: cytotoxicity effected by a class II-restricted T cell line specific for an encephalitogenic epitope. *J Immunol* **143**: 2160–2165

Fallis RJ, Powers ML, Sy M-S, Weiner HL 1987 Adoptive transfer of murine chronic relapsing autoimmune encephalomyelitis: analysis of basic protein-reactive cells in lymphoid organs and nervous system of donor and recipient animals. *J Neuroimmunol* **14**: 205–219

Fallowfield L, Jenkins V 2004 Communicating sad, bad, and difficult news in medicine. *Lancet* **363**: 312–319

Fancy SP, Zhao C, Franklin RJ 2004 Increased expressionh of Nkx2.2 and Olig2 identifies reactive oligodendrocyte progenitor cells responding to demyelination in the adult CNS. *Mol Cell Neurosci* **27**: 247–254

Farina C, Then Bergh F, Albrecht H *et al* 2001 Treatment of multiple sclerosis with Copaxone (COP): Elispot assay detects COP-induced interleukin-4 and interferon-gamma response in blood cells. *Brain* **124**: 705–719

Farina C, Vargas V, Heydari N *et al* 2002 Treatment with glatiramer acetate induces specific IgG4 antibodies in multiple sclerosis patients. *J Neuroimmunol* **123**: 188–192

Farina L, Bizzi A, Finochiarro G *et al* 2000 MR imaging and proton MR spectroscopy in adult Krabbe disease. *Am J Neuroradiol* **21**: 1478–1482

Fassas A, Kimiskidis V 2003 Stem cell transplantation for multiple sclerosis: what is the evidence? *Blood Rev* **17**: 233–240

Fassas A, Anagnostopoulos A, Kazis A *et al* 2000 Autologous stem cell transplantation in progressive multiple sclerosis—an interim analysis of efficacy. *J Clin Immunol* **20**: 24–30

Fassas A, Passweg JR, Anagnostopoulos A *et al* 2002 Hematopoietic stem cell transplantation for multiple sclerosis: a retrospective multicenter study. *J Neurol* **249**: 1088–1097

Fatemi A, Barker PB, Ulu AM *et al* 2003 MRI and proton MRSI in women heterozygous for X-linked adrenoleucodystrophy. *Neurology* **60**: 1301–1307

Fatigue Guidelines Development Panel of the Multiple Sclerosis Council for Clinical Practice Guidelines 1998 *Fatigue and Multiple Sclerosis: Evidence-based Management Strategies for Fatigue in Multiple Sclerosis*. Washington, DC: Paralyzed Veterans of America

Faulkner JR, Herrmann JE, Wood MJ *et al* 2004 Reactive astrocytes protect tissue and preserve function after spinal cord injury. *J Neurosci* **24**: 2143–2155

Favorova OO, Andreewski TV, Boiko AN *et al* 2002 The chemokine receptor CCR5 deletion mutation is associated with MS in HLA-DR4-positive Russians. *Neurology* **59**: 1652–1655

Fawcett J, Skegg DCG 1988 Geographic distribution of MS in New Zealand. *Neurology* **38**: 416–418

Fawcett JW, Asher RA 1999 The glial scar and central nervous system repair. *Brain Res Bull* **49**: 377–391

Fazekas F, Offenbacher H, Fuchs S *et al* 1988 Criteria for an increased specificity of MRI interpretation in elderly subjects with suspected multiple sclerosis. *Neurology* **38**: 1822–1825

Fazekas F, Deisenhammer F, Strasser-Fuchs S *et al* and the Austrian Immunoglobulin in Multiple Sclerosis Study Group 1997 Randomised placebo-controlled trial of monthly intravenous immunoglobulin therapy in relapsing–remitting multiple sclerosis. *Lancet* **349**: 589–593

Fazekas F, Barkhof F, Filippi M *et al* 1999 The contribution of magnetic resonance imaging to the diagnosis of multiple sclerosis. *Neurology* **53**: 448–456

Fazekas F, Strasser Fuchs S, Schmidt H *et al* 2000 Apolipoprotein E genotype related differences in brain lesions of multiple sclerosis. *J Neurol Neurosurg Psychiatry* **69**: 25–28

Fazekas F, Strasser-Fuchs S, Kollegger H *et al* 2001 Apolipoprotein E epsilon 4 is associated with rapid progression of multiple sclerosis. *Neurology* **57**: 853–857

Fazzone HE, Lefton DR, Kupersmith MJ 2003 Optic neuritis: correlation of pain and magnetic resonance imaging. *Ophthalmology* **110**: 1646–1649

Feakes R, Chataway J, Sawcer S *et al* 1998 Susceptibility to multiple sclerosis and the immunoglobulin heavy chain gene cluster. *Ann Neurol* **44**: 984

Feakes R, Sawcer S, Chataway J *et al* 1999 Exploring the dense mapping of a region of potential linkage in complex disease: an example in multiple sclerosis. *Genet Epidemiol* **17**: 51–63

Feakes R, Sawcer S, Broadley S *et al* 2000a Interleukin 1 receptor antagonist (IL-1ra) in multiple sclerosis. *J Neuroimmunol* **105**: 96–101

Feakes R, Sawcer S, Smillie B *et al* 2000b No evidence for the involvement of interleukin-2 or the immunoglobulin heavy chain cluster in determining genetic susceptibility to multiple sclerosis. *J Neurol Neurosurg Psych* **68**: 679

Fedetz M, Matezanz F, Pascual M *et al* 2001 The −174/-597 promoter polymorphisms in the interleukin-6 gene are not associated with susceptibility to multiple sclerosis. *J Neurol Sci* **190**: 69–72

Fedetz M, Alcina A, Fernandez O *et al* 2002 Analysis of −631 and -475 interleukin-2 promoter single nucleotide polymorphisms in multiple sclerosis. *Eur J Immunogenet* **29**: 389–390

Feigenson JS, Scheinberg L, Catalano M *et al* 1981 The cost-effectiveness of multiple sclerosis rehabilitation: a model. *Neurology* **31**: 1316–1322

Feigin I, Ogata J 1971 Schwann cells and peripheral myelin within human central nervous tissues: the mesenchymal character of Schwann cells. *J Neuropathol Exp Neurol* **30**: 603–612

Feigin I, Popoff N 1966 Regeneration of myelin in multiple sclerosis. *Neurology* **16**: 364–372

Feinstein A 2002 An examination of suicidal intent in patients with multiple sclerosis. *Neurology* **59**: 674–678

Feinstein A, Ron MA 1990 Psychosis associated with demonstrable brain disease. *Psych Med* **20**: 793–803

Feinstein A, Youl B, Ron M 1992a Acute optic neuritis: a cognitive and magnetic resonance imaging study. *Brain* **115**: 1403–1415

Feinstein A, Kartsounis LD, Miller DH *et al* 1992b Clinically isolated lesions of the type seen in multiple sclerosis: a cognitive, psychiatric, and MRI follow up study. *J Neurol Neurosurg Psychiatry* **55**: 869–876

Feinstein A, Ron M, Thompson A 1993a A serial study of psychometric and magnetic resonance imaging changes in multiple sclerosis. *Brain* **116**: 569–602

Feinstein A, du Boulay G, Ron MA 1993b Psychotic illness in multiple sclerosis: a clinical and MRI study. *Br J Psychiatry* **161**: 680–685

Feinstein A, O'Connor P, Gray T, Feinstein K 1999 Pathological laughing and crying in multiple sclerosis: a preliminary report suggesting a role for the prefrontal cortex. *Mult Scler* **5**: 69–73

Feinstein A, Levine B, Protzner A 2000 Confabulation and multiple sclerosis: a rare association. *Mult Scler* **6**: 186–191

Feldman RG, Kelly-Hayes M, Conomy JP, Foley JM 1978 Baclofen for spasticity in multiple sclerosis: double-blind crossover and three year study. *Neurology* **28**: 1094–1098

Felgenhauer K 1971 *Vergleichende Disc-elektrophorese von Serum un Liquor cerebrospinalis*, Stuttgart: Thieme

Felgenhauer K 1974 Protein size and cerebrospinal fluid composition. *Klin Wochenschr* **52**: 1158–1164

Felgenhauer K 1990 Psychiatric disorders in the encephalitic form of multiple sclerosis. *J Neurol* **237**: 11–18

Felts PA, Smith KJ 1992 Conduction properties of central nerve fibres remyelinated by Schwann cells. *Brain Res* **574**: 178–192

Felts PA, Smith KJ 1993 Segmental demyelinated central axons: the morphology of conducting axons. *Neuropathol Appl Neurobiol* **19**: 449–450

Felts PA, Smith KJ 1994 The use of potassium channel blocking agents in the therapy of demyelinating diseases. *Ann Neurol* **36**: 454

Felts PA, Kapoor R, Smith KJ 1995 A mechanism for ectopic firing in central demyelinated axons. *Brain* **118**: 1225–1231

Felts PA, Baker TA, Smith KJ 1997 Conduction in segmentally demyelinated mammalian central axons. *J Neurosci* **17**: 7267–7277

Felts PA, Deerinck TJ, Ellisman MH et al 1998 Sodium and potassium channel immunolocalisation in demyelinated and remyelinated central axons. *Neuropathol Appl Neurobiol* **24**: 154–155

Fenichel GM 1982 Neurological complications of immunisation. *Ann Neurol* **12**: 119–128

Fenichel GM 1999 Assessment: Neurologic risk of immunization. Report of the Therapeutics and Technology Assessment Subcommittee of the American Academy of Neurology. *Neurology* **52**: 1546–1552

Fenyk-Melody JE, Garrison AE, Brunnert SR et al 1998 Experimental autoimmune encephalomyelitis is exacerbated in mice lacking the NOS2 gene. *J Immunol* **160**: 2940–2946

Ferguson B, Matyszak MK, Esiri MM, Perry VH 1997 Axonal damage in acute multiple sclerosis lesions. *Brain* **120**: 393–399

Ferguson FR, Liversedge LA 1959 A clinical aphorism in the diagnosis of multiple sclerosis. *Lancet* **i**: 1159–1160

Ferini-Strambi L, Filippi M, Martinelli V et al 1994 Nocturnal sleep study in multiple sclerosis: correlations with clinical and brain magnetic resonance imaging findings. *J Neurol Sci* **125**: 194–197

Fernandes-Filho F, Vedeler CA, Myhr KM et al 2002 TNF-alpha and -beta gene polymorphisms in multiple sclerosis: a highly significant role for determinants in the first intron of the TNF-beta gene. *Autoimmunity* **35**: 377–380

Fernandez O, Bufill E 1994 Prevalence of multiple sclerosis in Spain: validation of an epidemiological protocol in two geographically separated areas. In: Firnhaber W, Lauer K (eds) *Multiple Sclerosis in Europe: An Epidemiological Update*. Darmstadt: Leuchtturm-Verlag/LTV Press, pp. 184–189

Fernandez O, Luque G, San Roman C et al 1994 The prevalence of multiple sclerosis in the Sanitary district of Velez-Malaga, southern Spain. *Neurology* **44**: 425–429

Fernandez O, Fernandez V, Alonso A et al 2004 DQB1*0602 allele shows a strong association with multiple sclerosis in patients in Malaga, Spain. *J Neurol* **251**: 440–444

Fernandez PA, Tang DG, Cheng L et al 2000 Evidence that axon-derived neuregulin promotes oligodendrocyte survival in the developing rat optic nerve. *Neuron* **28**: 81–90

Fernandez-Arquero M, Arroyo R, Rubio A et al 1999 Primary association of a TNF gene polymorphism with susceptibility to multiple sclerosis. *Neurology* **53**: 1361–1363

Fernando KTM, McLean MA, Chard DT et al 2004 Elevated white matter myo-inositol in clinically isolated syndromes suggestive of multiple sclerosis. *Brain* **127**:1361–1369

Ferrari MD, Hilkens PHE, Kremer B et al 1988 Intermittent pyramidal claudication as presenting and sole symptom in multiple sclerosis. *J Neurol Neurosurg Psychiatry* **51**: 147–148

Ferri C, Sciacca FL, Veglia F et al 1999 APOEε2–4 and –491 polymorphisms are not associated with MS. *Neurology* **53**: 888–889

Ferri C, Sciacca FL, Grimaldi L et al 2000 Lack of association between IL-1A and IL-1B promoter polymorphisms and multiple sclerosis. *J Neurol Neurosurg Psychiatry* **69**: 564–5

Ferriby D, De Sèze J, Stojkovic T et al 2001 Long-term follow-up of neurosarcoidosis. *Neurology* **57**: 927–929

Fewster ME, Kies B 1984 HLA antigens in multiple sclerosis in coloured South Africans. *J Neurol Sci* **66**: 175–181

Feys P, Helsen W, Liu X et al 2005 Effects of peripheral cooling on intention tremor in multiple sclerosis. *J Neurol Neurosurg Psychiatry* **76**: 373–379

ffrench Constant C, Raff MC 1986 Proliferating bipotential glial progenitor cells in adult rat optic nerve. *Nature* **319**: 499–502

Fiebich BL, Lieb K, Engels S, Heinrich M 2002 Inhibition of LPS-induced p42/44 MAP kinase activation and iNOS/NO synthesis by parthenolide in rat primary microglial cells. *J Neuroimmunol* **132**: 18–24

Field EJ 1979 Multiple sclerosis: recent advances in aethiopathogenesis. In: Smith WT, Cavanagh JB (eds) *Recent Advances in Neuropathology I*. London: Churchill Livingstone, pp. 277–298

Field EJ 1989 *Multiple Sclerosis. A Conceptual Reappraisal with Heuristic Implications*. Springfield, IL: C.C. Thomas

Fielder AHL, Batchelor JR, Vakarelis BN, Compston DAS, McDonald WI 1981 Optic neuritis and multiple sclerosis: do factor B alleles influence progression of disease? *Lancet* **ii**: 1246–1248

Fiette L, Aubert C, Brahic M, Rossi CP 1993 Theiler's virus infection of b2-microglobulin deficient mice. *J Virol* **67**: 589–592

Fife BT, Huffnagle GB, Kuziel WA, Karpus WJ 2000 CC chemokine receptor 2 is critical for induction of experimental autoimmune encephalomyelitis. *J Exp Med* **192**: 899–906

Fife C, Otto G, Capsuto EG et al 2001 Incidence of pressure ulcers in a neurologic intensive care unit. *Crit Care Med* **29**: 283–290

Filipovic R, Jakovcevski I, Zecevic N 2003 GRO-alpha and CXCR2 in the human fetal brain and multiple sclerosis lesions. *Dev Neurosci* **25**: 279–290

Filipovic SR, Drulovic J, Stojsavljevic N, Levic Z 1997 The effects of high-dose intravenous methylprednisolone on event-related potentials in patients with multiple sclerosis. *J Neurol Sci* **152**: 147–153

Filippi M, Horsfield MA, Morrissey SP et al 1994 Quantitative brain MRI lesion load predicts the course of clinically isolated syndromes suggestive of multiple sclerosis. *Neurology* **44**: 635–641

Filippi M, Paty DW, Kappos L et al 1995a Correlations between changes in disability and T$_2$-weighted brain MRI activity in multiple sclerosis: a follow-up study. *Neurology* **45**: 255–260

Filippi M, Campi A, Martinelli V et al 1995b Comparison of triple dose versus standard dose gadolinium-DTPA for detection of MRI enhancing lesions in patients with primary progressive multiple sclerosis. *J Neurol Neurosurg Psychiatry* **59**: 540–544

Filippi M, Horsfield MA, Tofts PS et al 1995c Quantitative assessment of MRI lesion load in monitoring the evolution of multiple sclerosis. *Brain* **118**: 1601–1612

Filippi M, Campi A, Martinelli V et al 1995d A brain MRI study of different types of chronic-progressive multiple sclerosis. *Acta Neurol Scand* **91**: 231–233

Filippi M, Campi A, Martinelli V et al 1995e Transitional progressive multiple sclerosis: MRI and MTI findings. *Acta Neurol Scand* **92**: 178–182

Filippi M, Yousry T, Baratti C et al 1996 Quantitative assessment of MRI lesion load in multiple sclerosis. A comparison of conventional spin echo with fast fluid-attenuated inversion recovery. *Brain* **119**: 1349–1355

Filippi M, Horsfield MA, Ader HJ et al 1998a Guidelines for using quantitative measures of brain magnetic resonance imaging abnormalities in monitoring the treatment of multiple sclerosis. *Ann Neurol* **43**: 499–506

Filippi M, Rocca MA, Martino G, Horsfield MA, Comi G 1998b Magnetization transfer changes in the normal appearing white matter precede the appearance of enhancing lesions in patients with multiple sclerosis. *Ann Neurol* **43**: 809–814

Filippi M, Rocca MA, Rizzo G et al 1998c Magnetization transfer ratios in multiple sclerosis lesions enhancing after different doses of gadolinium. *Neurology* **50**: 1289–1293

Filippi M, Iannucci G, Tortorella C et al 1999a Comparison of MS clinical phenotypes using conventional and magnetization transfer MRI. *Neurology* **52**: 588–594

Filippi M, Rocca MA, Moiola L *et al* 1999b MRI and magnetization transfer imaging changes in the brain and cervical cord of patients with Devic's neuromyelitis optica. *Neurology* **53**: 1705–1710

Filippi M, Rovaris M, Iannucci G *et al* 2000a Whole brain volume changes in patients with progressive MS treated with cladribine. *Neurology* **55**: 1714–1718

Filippi M, Rovaris M, Rice GP *et al* 2000b The effect of cladribine on T1 'black hole' changes in progressive MS. *J Neurol Sci* **176**: 42–44

Filippi M, Rovaris M, Rocca MA *et al* 2001a Glatiramer acetate reduces the proportion of new MS lesions evolving into 'black holes'. *Neurology* **57**: 731–733

Filippi M, Wolinsky JS, Sormani MP, Comi G for the European/Canadian Glatiramer Acetate Study Group 2001b Enhancement frequency decreases with increasing age in relapsing–remitting multiple sclerosis. *Neurology* **56**: 422–423

Filippi M, Rocca MA, Colombo B *et al* 2002a Functional magnetic resonance imaging correlates of fatigue in multiple sclerosis. *Neuroimage* **15**: 559–567

Filippi M, Rocca MA, Falini A *et al* 2002b Correlations between structural CNS damage and functional MRI changes in primary progressive MS. *Neuroimage* **15**: 537–546

Filippi M, Sormani MP, Wolinsky J *et al* 2002c Glatiramer acetate reduces the proportion of new MS lesions evolving into 'black holes'. *Neurology* **58**: 1440–1441

Filippi M, Bozzali M, Rovaris M *et al* 2003 Evidence for widespread axonal damage at the earliest clinical stage of multiple sclerosis. *Brain* **126**: 433–437

Filippi M, Rovaris M, Inglese M *et al* 2004a Interferon beta-1a for brain tissue loss in patients at presentation with syndromes suggestive of multiple sclerosis: a randomised, double-blind, placebo-controlled trial. *Lancet* **364**: 1489–1496

Filippi M, Rocca MA, Mezzapesa DM *et al* 2004b Simple and complex movement-associated functional MRI changes in patients at presentation with clinically isolated syndromes suggestive of multiple sclerosis. *Hum Brain Mapping* **21**: 108–117

Filippini G, Munari L, Incorvaia B *et al* 2003a Interferons in relapsing remitting multiple sclerosis: a systematic review. *Lancet* **361**: 545–552

Filippini G, Munari L, Ebers G *et al* 2003b Interferons in relapsing remitting multiple sclerosis (letter). *Lancet* **361**: 1823

Filippini G, Munari L, Ebers G *et al* 2003c Interferons in relapsing remitting multiple sclerosis (letter) *Lancet* **361**: 1824–1825

Fillmore PD, Brace M, Troutman SA *et al* 2003 Genetic analysis of the influence of neuroantigen-complete Freund's adjuvant emulsion structures on the sexual dimorphism and susceptibility to experimental allergic encephalomyelitis. *Am J Pathol* **163**: 1623–1632

Finelli PF 1991 Conjugal multiple sclerosis: a clinical and laboratory study. *Neurology* **41**: 1320–1321

Fink JK 2002 Hereditary spastic paraplegia: the pace quickens. *Ann Neurol* **51**: 669–672

Finkel MJ, Halperin JJ 1992 Nervous system Lyme borreliosis: revisited. *Arch Neurol* **49**: 102–107

Finkelman FD 1995 Relationships among antigen presentation, cytokines, immune deviation and autoimmune disease. *J Exp Med* **182**: 279–282

Finsen BR, Tönder N, Xavier GF *et al* 1993 Induction of microglial immunomolecules by anterogradely degenerating mossy fibers in the rat hippocampal formation. *J Chem Neuroanat* **6**: 276–275

Finsterer J, Grass R, Stollberger C, Mamoli B 1998 Immunoglobulins in acute, parainfectious, disseminated encephalo-myelitis. *Clin Neuropharmacol* **21**: 258–261

Fiorentino DF, Bond MW, Mosmann TR 1989 Two types of mouse T helper cell. IV. Th2 clones secrete a factor that inhibits cytokine production by Th1 clones. *J Exp Med* **170**: 2081–2095

Fiotti N, Zivadinov R, Altamura N *et al* 2004 MMP-9 microsatellite polymorphism and multiple sclerosis. *J Neuroimmunol* **152**: 147–153

Firnhaber W, Lauer K (eds) 1994 *Multiple Sclerosis in Europe: An Epidemiological Update*. Darmstadt: Leuchtturm-Verlag/LTV Press

Firouzi R, Rolland A, Michel M *et al* 2003 Multiple sclerosis associated retrovirus particles cause T-lymphocyte-dependent death with brain hemorrhage in humanized SCID mice model. *J Neurovirol* **9**: 79–93

Firth D 1948 *The Case of Augustus D'Este*. Cambridge: Cambridge University Press

Fischer BH, Marks M, Reith T 1983 Hyperbaric oxygen treatment of multiple sclerosis: a randomised, placebo controlled double-blind study. *N Engl J Med* **308**: 181–186

Fischer C, Joyeux O, Haguenauer JP *et al* 1984 Surdité et acouphènes lors de poussées dans 10 cas de sclérose en plaques. *Rev Neurol* **140**: 117–125

Fischer D, He Z, Benowitz LI 2004 Counteracting the Nogo receptor enhances optic nerve regeneration if retinal ganglion cells are in an active growth state. *J Neurosci* **24**: 1646–1651

Fischer JS, LaRocca NG, Miller DM *et al* 1999 Recent developments in the assessment of quality of life in multiple sclerosis. *Mult Scler* **5**: 251–259

Fischer JS, Priore RL, Jacobs LD *et al* 2000 Neuropsychological effects of interferon beta-1a in relapsing multiple sclerosis. Multiple Sclerosis Collaborative Research Group. *Ann Neurol* **48**: 885–892

Fisher A, Gresty M, Chambers B, Rudge P 1983 Primary position upbeating nystagmus. *Brain* **106**: 949–964

Fisher D, He Z, Benowitz Li 2004 Counteracting the Nogo receptor enhances optic nerve regeneration if retinal ganglion cells are in an active growth state. *J Neurosci* **24**: 1646–1651

Fisher E, Rudick RA, Cutter G *et al* 2000 Relationship between brain atrophy and disability: an 8-year follow-up study of multiple sclerosis patients. *Mult Scler* **6**: 373–377

Fisher E, Rudick RA, Simon JH *et al* 2002 Eight-year follow up study of brain atrophy in patients with MS. *Neurology* **59**: 1412–1420

Fisher M, Long RR, Drachman DA 1985 Hand muscle atrophy in multiple sclerosis. *Arch Neurol* **40**: 811–815

Fishman RA 1992 *Cerebrospinal Fluid in Diseases of the Nervous System*, Philadephia: W.B. Saunders

Fisk JD, Pontefract A, Ritvo PG *et al* 1994 The impact of fatigue on patients with multiple sclerosis. *Can J Neurol Sci* **21**: 9–14

Fiten P, Vandenbroeck K, Dubois B *et al* 1999 Microsatellite polymorphisms in the gene promotor of monocyte chemotactic protein-3 and analysis of the association between monocyte chemotactic protein-3 alleles and multiple sclerosis development. *J Neuroimmunol* **95**: 195–201

Flachenecker P, Wolf, A, Krauser M *et al* 1999 Cardiovascular autonomic dysfunction in multiple sclerosis: correlation with orthostatic intolerance. *J Neurol* **246**: 578–586

Flachenecker P, Reiners K, Krauser M *et al* 2001 Autonomic dysfunction in multiple sclerosis is related to disease activity and progression of disability. *Mult Scler* **7**: 327–334

Flashman JF, Latham O 1915 A contribution to the study of the aetiology of disseminated sclerosis. *Med J Aust* **2**: 265–269

Flensner G, Lindencrona C 2002 The cooling-suit: case studies of its influence on fatigue among eight individuals with multiple sclerosis. *J Adv Nurs* **37**: 541–550

Flechter S, Vardi J, Pollak L, Rabey JM 2002 Comparison of glatiramer acetate (Copaxone) and interferon beta-1b (Betaferon) in multiple sclerosis patients: an open-label 2-year follow-up. *J Neurol Sci* **197**: 51–55

Flügel A, Willem M, Berkowicz T, Wekerle H 1999 Gene transfer into CD4+ T lymphocytes: green fluorescent protein engineered, encephalitogenic T cells used to illuminate immune responses in the brain. *Nature Med* **5**: 843–847

Flügel A, Schwaiger F-W, Neumann H *et al* 2000 Neuronal FasL induces cell death of encephalitogenic T lymphocytes. *Brain Pathol* **10**: 353–364

Flügel A, Berkowicz T, Ritter T *et al* 2001a Migratory activity and functional changes of green fluorescent effector T cells before and during experimental autoimmune encephalomyelitis. *Immunity* **14**: 547–560

Flügel A, Matsumoro K, Neumann H *et al* 2001b Anti inflammatory activity of nerve growth factor in experimental autoimmune encephalomyelitis: inhibition of monocyte transendothelial migration. *Eur J Immunol* **31**: 11–22

Fog T 1950 Topographic distribution of plaques in the spinal cord in multiple sclerosis. *Arch Neurol* **63**: 382–414

Fog T 1951 ACTH behandling ved sclerosis disseminata. *Nordisk Medicin* **46**: 1742–1748

Fog T 1965 The topography of plaques in multiple sclerosis with special reference to cerebral plaques. *Acta Neurol Scand* **41 (Suppl 15)**: 1–161

Fog T 1966 The course of multiple sclerosis. *Acta Neurol Scand* **42**: 608–611

Fog T 1980 Interferon treatment of multiple sclerosis patients: a pilot study. In: Boese A (ed.) *Search for the Cause of Multiple Sclerosis and other Chronic Diseases of the Nervous System*. Weinheim: Verlag Chemie, pp. 491–493

Fog T, Hyllested K 1966 Prevalence of disseminated sclerosis in the Faroes, the Orkneys, and Shetland. *Acta Neurol Scand* **42 (Suppl 19)**: 9–11

Fog T, Linnemann F 1970 The course of multiple sclerosis in 73 cases with computer-designed curves. *Acta Neurol Scand* **46 (Suppl)**: 1–175

Fogarty M, Richardson WD, Kessaris N 2005 A subset of oligodendrocytes generated from radial glia in the dorsal spinal cord. *Development* **132**: 1951–1959

Fogdell A, Olerup O, Vrethem M, Hillert J 1997 Linkage analysis of HLA class II genes in Swedish multiplex families with multiple sclerosis. *Neurology* **48**: 758–762

Fogdell-Hahn A, Ligers A, Gronning M et al 2000 Multiple sclerosis: a modifying influence of HLA class I genes in an HLA class II associated autoimmune disease. *Tissue Antigens* **55**: 140–148

Foix C, Alajouanine T 1926 La myelité necrotique subaigue. *Rev Neurol* **2**: 1–42

Fok-Seang J, DiProspero NA, Meiners S et al 1998 Cytokine-induced changes in the ability of astrocytes to support migration of oligodendrocyte precursors and axon growth. *Eur J Neurosci* **10**: 2400–2415

Folgar S, Gatto EM, Raina G, Micheli F 2003 Parkinsonism as a manifestation of multiple sclerosis. *Mov Disord* **18**: 108–110

Fontaine B, Seilhean D, Tourbah A et al 1994 Dementia in two histologically confirmed cases of multiple sclerosis: one case with isolated dementia and one case associated with psychiatric symptoms. *J Neurol Neurosurg Psychiatry* **57**: 353–359

Fontaine B, Cournu I, Arnaud I et al 1999 Chromosome 17q22-q24 and multiple sclerosis genetic susceptibility. *Genes Immun* **1**: 149–150

Fontana A, Grieder A, Arrenbrecht ST, Grob P 1980 *In vitro* stimulation of glia cells by a lymphocyte produced factor. *J Neurol Sci* **46**: 55–62

Foong J, Ron MA 2003 Neuropsychiatry: cognition and mood disorders. In: McDonald WI, Noseworthy JH (eds) *Multiple Sclerosis*, 2nd edn. London: Butterworth Heinemann, pp. 115–124

Foong J, Rozewicz L, Quaghebeur G et al 1997 Executive function in multiple sclerosis: the role of frontal lobe pathology. *Brain* **120**: 15–26

Foong J, Davie CA, Thompson AJ et al 1999 Correlates of executive function in multiple sclerosis: use of MRS as an index of focal pathology. *J Neuropsychiatry Clin Neurosci* **11**: 45–50

Foong J, Rozewicz L, Chong WK et al 2000 A comparison of neuropsychological deficits in primary and secondary progressive multiple sclerosis. *J Neurol Sci* **247**: 97–101

Foote AK, Blakemore WF 2005 Inflammation stimulates remyelination in areas of chronic demyelination. *Brain* **128**: 528–539

Forbes RB, Swingler RJ 1999 Estimating the prevalence of multiple sclerosis in the United Kingdom by using capture–recapture methodology. *Am J Epidemiol* **149**: 1016–1024

Forbes RB, Wilson SV, Swingler RJ 1999 The prevalence of multiple sclerosis in Tayside, Scotland: do latitudinal gradients really exist? *J Neurol* **246**: 1033–1040

Ford AL, Foulcher E, Lemckert FA, Sedgwick JD 1996 Microglia induce CD4 T lymphocyte final effector function and death. *J Exp Med* **184**: 1737–1745

Ford B, Tampieri D, Francis G 1992 Long-term follow-up of acute partial transverse myelopathy. *Neurology* **42**: 250–252

Ford HL, Gerry E, Airey CM et al DR 1998a The prevalence of multiple sclerosis in the Leeds Health Authority. *J Neurol Neurosurg Psych* **64**: 605–610

Ford HL, Trigwell P, Johnson M 1998b The nature of fatigue in multiple sclerosis. *J Psychosom Res* **45**: 33–38

Ford HL, Tennant GE, Whalley A et al 2001 Developing a disease-specific quality of life measure for people with multiple sclerosis. *Clin Rehabil* **15**: 247–258

Ford HL, Gerry E, Johnson M, Williams R 2002 A prospective study of the incidence, prevalence and mortality of multiple sclerosis in Leeds. *J Neurol* **249**: 260–265

Ford ML, Onami TM, Sperling AI et al 2003 CD43 modulates severity and onset of experimental autoimmune encephalomyelitis. *J Immunol* **171**: 6527–6533

Forrester K, Ambs S, Lupold SE et al 1996 Nitric oxide-induced p53 accumulation and regulation of inducible nitric oxide synthase expression by wild-type p53. *Proc Natl Acad Sci USA* **93**: 2442–2447

Forsthuber T, Yip HC, Lehmann PV 1996 Induction of Th1 and Th2 immunity in neonatal mice. *Science* **271**: 1728–1730

Fossati G, Cooke A, Papafio RQ et al 1999 Triggering a second T cell receptor on diabetogenic T cells can prevent induction of diabetes. *J Exp Med* **190**: 577–583

Fossier P, Blanchard B, Ducrocq C et al 1999 Nitric oxide transforms serotonin into an inactive form and this affects neuro-modulation. *Neuroscience* **93**: 597–603

Foster RM, Harries JR 1970 Multiple sclerosis in the African. *Br Med J* **3**: 628

Fourrier A, Touzé E, Alpérovitch A, Bégaud B 1999 Association between hepatitis B vaccine and multiple sclerosis: a case-control study. *Pharmacoepidemiology and Drug Safety* **8 (Suppl)**: S140–S141

Fourrier A, Bégaud B, Alpérovitch A et al 2001 Hepatitis B vaccination and first episodes of central nervous system demyelinating disorders: a comparison between reported and expected number of cases. *Br J Clin Pharmacol* **51**: 489–490

Fowler CJ 1997 The cause and management of bladder, sexual and bowel symptoms in multiple sclerosis. *Baillières Clin Neurol* **6**: 447–466

Fowler CJ, van Kerrbroeck P, Nordenbo A, van Poppel H 1992a Treatment of lower urinary tract dysfunction in patients with multiple sclerosis. *J Neurol Neurosurg Psychiatry* **55**: 986–969

Fowler CJ, Jewkes D, McDonald WI, Lynn B, de Groat WC 1992b Intravesical capsaicin for neurogenic bladder dysfunction. *Lancet* **339**: 1239

Fowler CJ, Beck RO, Gerrard S, Betts CD, Fowler CG 1994 Intravesical capsaicin for treatment of detrusor hyperreflexia. *J Neurol Neurosurg Psychiatry* **57**: 169–173

Fowler CJ, Miller JR, Sharief M 1999 Viagra (sildenafil citrate) for the treatment of erectile dysfunction in men with multiple sclerosis. *Ann Neurol* **46**: 497

Fowler CJ, Miller JR, Sharief MK et al 2005 A double blind, randomised study of sildenafil citrate for erectile dysfunction in men with multiple sclerosis. *J Neurol Neurosurg Psychiatry* **76**: 700–705

Fox CM, Bensa S, Bray I, Zajicek JP 2004 The epidemiology of multiple sclerosis in Devon: a comparison of the new and old classification criteria. *J Neurol Neurosurg Psychiatry* **75**: 56–60

Fox NC, Jenkins R, Lary SM et al 2000 Progressive cerebral atrophy in MS: a serial study using registered, volumetric MRI. *Neurology* **54**: 807–812

Fraenkel M, Jakob A 1913 Zur Pathologie der multiplen Sklerose mit besonderer Berücksichtigung der akuten Formen. *Z Neurol Psychiatr* **14**: 565–603

Fraker PJ, Lill Elghanian DA 2004 The many roles of apoptosis in immunity as modified by aging and nutritional status. *J Nutr Health Aging* **8**: 56–63

Francabandera F, Holland N, Wiesel-Levison P, Scheinberg L 1988 Multiple sclerosis rehabilitation: inpatient versus outpatient. *Rehab Nursing* **13**: 251–253

Franciotta DM, Grimaldi LM, Martino GV et al 1989 Tumor necrosis factor in serum and cerebrospinal fluid of patients with multiple sclerosis. *Ann Neurol* **26**, 787–789

Franciotta D, Dondi E, Bergamaschi R et al 1995 HLA complement gene polymorphisms in multiple sclerosis: a study on 80 Italian patients. *J Neurol* **242**: 64–68

Franciotta D, Bergamashi R, Piccolo G et al 2000 Multiple secondary Leber's hereditary optic neuropathy mutations in Italian patients with multiple sclerosis. *J Neurol* **247**: 304–305

Franciotta D, Martino G, Zardini E *et al* 2001 Serum and CSF levels of MCP-1 and IP-10 in multiple sclerosis patients with acute and stable disease and undergoing immunomodulatory therapies. *J Neuroimmunol* **115**: 192–198

Francis DA, Heron JR 1985 Ocular flutter in suspected multiple sclerosis: a presenting paroxysmal manifestation. *Postgrad Med J* **61**: 333–334

Francis DA, Brazier DM, Batchelor JR *et al* 1986 GM allotypes in multiple sclerosis influence susceptibility in HLA DQ1 positive patients from the north east of Scotland. *Clin Immunol Immunopathol* **41**: 409–416

Francis DA, Batchelor JR, McDonald WI 1987a Multiple sclerosis in north east Scotland. An association with HLA DQw 1. *Brain* **110**: 181–196

Francis DA, Compston DAS, Batchelor JR, McDonald WI 1987b A reassessment of the risk of multiple sclerosis developing in patients with optic neuritis after extended follow-up. *J Neurol Neurosurg Psychiatry* **50**: 758–765

Francis DA, Bain P, Swan AV, Hughes RAC 1991a An assessment of disability rating scales used in multiple sclerosis. *Arch Neurol* **48**: 299–301

Francis DA, Thompson AJ, Brookes P *et al* 1991b Multiple sclerosis and HLA: is the susceptibility gene really HLA-DR or -DQ? *Hum Immunol* **32**: 119–124

Francis GS, Freedman MS, Antel JP 1997 Failure of intravenous immunoglobulin to arrest progression of multiple sclerosis: a clinical and MRI based study. *Mult Scler* **3**: 370–376

Francis GS, Rice GP, Alsop JC 2005 Interferon beta-1a in MS: results following development of neutralizing antibodies in PRISMS. *Neurology* **65**: 48–55

Frank JA, Miller BR, Arbab AS *et al* 2003 Clinically applicable labeling of mammalian and stem cells by combining superparamagnetic iron oxides and transfection agents. *Radiology* **228**: 480–487

Frank JA, Richert N, Bash C *et al* 2004 Interferon-β-1b slows progression of atrophy in RRMS: three-year follow-up in NAb– and NAb+ patients. *Neurology* **62**: 719–725

Frank MM, Basta M, Fries LF 1992 The effect of intravenous immune globulin on complement-dependent immune damage of cells and tissues. *Clin Immunol Immunopathol* **62**: S82–S86

Franklin GM, Nelson LM, Heaton RK *et al* 1988 Stress and its relationship to acute exacerbations in multiple sclerosis. *J Neurol Rehab* **2**: 7–11

Franklin GM, Nelson LM, Filley CM, Heaton RK 1989 Cognitive loss in multiple sclerosis: case reports and review of literature. *Arch Neurol* **46**: 162–167

Franklin RJ 2002 Why does remyelination fail in multiple sclerosis? *Nat Rev Neurosci* **3**: 705–714

Franklin RJ, Bayley SA, Blakemore WF 1996 Transplanted CG-4 cells (an oligodendrocyte progenitor cell line) survive, migrate and contribute to repair of areas of demyelination in X-irradiated and damaged spinal cord but not in normal spinal cord. *Exp Neurol* **137**: 263–276

Frasson E, Polo A, di Summa A *et al* 1997 Multiple sclerosis associated with duplicated CMT1A: a report of two cases. *J Neurol Neurosurg Psychiatry* **63**: 413–414

Freal JE, Kraft GH, Coryell JK 1984 Symptomatic fatigue in multiple sclerosis. *Arch Phys Med Rehab* **65**: 135–138

Frederick TJ, Wood TL 2004 IGF-I and FGF-2 coordinately enhance cyclin D1 and cyclin E-cdk2 association and activity to promote G1 progression in oligodendrocyte progenitor cells. *Mol Cell Neurosci* **25**: 480–492

Frederiksen JL 1999 *A Prospective Study of Acute Optic Neuritis: Clinical, MRI, CSF, Neurophysiological and HLA Findings.* Copenhagen: FADL Publishers, p. 83

Frederiksen JL, Larsson HBW, Ottovay E *et al* 1991a Acute optic neuritis with normal visual acuity. *Acta Ophthalmol* **69**: 357–366

Frederiksen JL, Larsson HBW, Olesen J, Stigsby B 1991b MRI, VEP, SEP and biothesiometry suggest monosymptomatic acute optic neuritis to be a first manifestation of multiple sclerosis. *Acta Neurol Scand* **83**: 343–350

Fredrikson S 1996 Nasal spray desmopressin treatment of bladder dysfunction in patients with multiple sclerosis. *Acta Neurol Scand* **94**: 31–34

Fredrikson S, Kam-Hansen S 1989 The 150-year anniversary of multiple sclerosis: does its early history give an etiological clue? *Perspect Biol Med* **32**: 237–243

Fredrikson S, Eneroth P, Link H 1987 Intrathecal production of neopterin in aseptic meningo-encephalitis and multiple sclerosis. *Clin Exp Immunol* **67**: 76–81

Fredrikson S, Michelsberg J, Hillert J *et al* 1992 Conjugal multiple sclerosis: immunogenetic characterisation and analysis of T- and B-cell reactivity to myelin antigens. *Neurology* **42**: 577–582

Fredrikson S, Cheng Q, Jiang GX, Wasserman D 2003 Elevated suicide risk among patients with multiple sclerosis in Sweden. *Neuroepidemiology* **22**: 146–152

Freeborough PA, Fox NC 1997 The boundary shift integral: an accurate and robust measure of cerebral volume changes from registered repeat MRI. *IEEE Trans Med Imag* **16**: 623–629

Freeborough PA, Fox NC 1998 Modeling brain deformations in Alzheimer disease by fluid registration of serial 3D MR images. *J Comput Assist Tomogr* **22**: 838–843

Freedman DM, Dosemeci M, Alavanja MC 2000 Mortality from multiple sclerosis and exposure to residential and occupational solar radiation: a case-control study based on death certificates. *Occup Environ Med* **57**: 418–421

Freedman MS, Atkins HL 2004 Suppressing immunity in advancing MS. Too much too late, or too late for much? *Neurology* **62**: 168–169

Freedman MS, Gray TA 1989 Vascular headache: a presenting symptom of multiple sclerosis. *Can J Neurol Sci* **16**: 63–66

Freedman MS, Ruijs TCG, Selin LK, Antel JP 1991 Peripheral blood γδ T cells lyse fresh human brain-derived oligodendrocytes. *Ann Neurol* **30**: 794–800

Freedman MS, King J, Oger J *et al* 2003 Interferons in relapsing remitting multiple sclerosis. *Lancet* **361**: 1822–1823; author reply 1823–1824

Freedman MS, Murzeniok P, Wang W *et al* 2004 Human gamma-delta T cells block conduction in a novel xenogeneic *in vitro* model for studying CNS-immune interactions. *J Neuroimmunol* [abstracts]

Freedman MS, Thompson EJ, Deisenhammer F *et al* 2005a Recommended standard of cerebrospinal fluid analysis in the diagnosis of multiple sclerosis. A consensus statement. *Arch Neurol* **62**: 865–870

Freedman MS, Francis GS, Sanders EA *et al* 2005b Randomized study of once-weekly interferon beta-1a therapy in relapsing multiple sclerosis: three-year data from the OWIMS study. *Mult Scler* **11**: 41–45

Freeman JA, Thompson A 2000 Community services in multiple sclerosis: still a matter of chance. *J Neurol Neurosurg Psychiatry* **69**: 728–732

Freeman JA, Thompson AJ 2003 Rehabilitation in multiple sclerosis. In: McDonald WI, Noseworthy JH (eds) *Multiple Sclerosis, 2nd edn*, Philadelphia: Butterworth-Heinemann, pp. 317–328

Freeman JA, Langdon DW, Hobart JC, Thompson AJ 1997 The impact of inpatient rehabilitation on progressive multiple sclerosis. *Ann Neurol* **42**: 236–244

Freeman JA, Langdon DW, Hobart JC, Thompson AJ 1999 Inpatient rehabilitation in multiple sclerosis: do the benefits carry over into the community? *Neurology* **52**: 50–56

Frei K, Siepl C, Groscurth P *et al* 1987 Antigen presentation and tumor cytotoxicity by interferon-gamma-treated microglial cells. *Eur J Immunol* **17**: 1271–1278

French Research Group on Multiple Sclerosis 1992 Multiple sclerosis in 54 twinships: concordance rate is independent of zygosity. *Ann Neurol* **32**: 724–727

Frerichs FT 1849 Ueber Hirnsklerose. *Arch Gesammte Med* **10**: 334–350

Frese A, Bethke F, Ludemann P, Stogbauer F 1999 Enhanced spasticity in primary progressive MS patients treated with interferon beta-1b. *Neurology* **53**: 1892–1893

Fridkis-Hareli M, Strominger JL 1998 Promiscuous binding of synthetic copolymer 1 to purified HLA-DR molecules. *J Immunol* **160**: 4386–4397

Fridkis-Hareli M, Teitelbaum D, Gurevich E *et al* 1994 Direct binding of myelin basic protein and synthetic copolymer 1 to class II major histocompatibility complex molecules on living antigen-presenting cells

– specificity and promiscuity. *Proc Natl Acad Sci USA* **91**: 4872–4876

Friede RL 1961 Enzyme histochemical studies in multiple sclerosis. *Arch Neurol* **5**: 433–443

Friedlander AH, Zeff S 1974 Atypical trigeminal neuralgia in patients with multiple sclerosis. *J Oral Surg* **32**: 301–303

Friedman GD 1987 *Primer of Epidemiology*. New York: McGraw-Hill International

Friedman JE, Lyons MJ, Cu G et al 1999 The association of the human herpesvirus-6 and MS. *Mult Scler* **5**: 355–362

Friedman JE, Zabriskie JB, Plank C et al 2005 A randomized clinical trial of valacyclovir in multiple sclerosis. *Mult Scler* **11**: 286–295

Friese MA, Fugger L 2005 Autoreactive CD8$^+$ T cells in multiple sclerosis: a new target for therapy? *Brain* **128**: 1747–1763

Frisén L, Hoyt WF 1974 Insidious atrophy and retinal nerve fibres in multiple sclerosis: fundoscopic identification in patients with and without visual complaint. *Arch Ophthalmol* **92**: 91–97

Frisén L, Hoyt WF, Bird AC, Weale RA 1973 Diagnostic uses of the Pulfrich phenomenon. *Lancet* **ii**: 385–386

Frith JA 1988 History of multiple sclerosis: an Australian persepctive. *Clin Exp Neurol* **25**: 7–16

Frith JA, McLeod JG 1988 Pregnancy and multiple sclerosis. *J Neurol Neurosurg Psychiatry* **51**: 495–498

Frith JA, McLeod JG, Basten A et al 1986 Transfer factor as a therapy for multiple sclerosis: a follow-up study. *Clin Exp Neurol* **22**: 149

Frith JA, McLeod JG, Hely M 2000 Acute optic neuritis in Australia: a 13 year prospective study. *J Neurol Neurosurg Psychiatry* **68**: 246

Fritz RB, Zhao ML 2001 Regulation of experimental autoimmune encephalomyelitis in the C57BL/6J mouse by NK1.1, DX5+, ab+ T cells. *J Immunol* **166**: 4209–4215

Fritz RB, Russell JP, Zhao M-L 1998 Persistence of an encephalitogenic T cell clone in the spinal cord during chronic, relapsing experimental autoimmune encephalomyelitis. *J Neuroimmunol* **89**: 1–9

Frohman EM, Frohman TC 2003 Horizontal monocular saccadic failure: an unusual clinically isolated syndrome progressing to multiple sclerosis. *Mult Scler* **9**: 55–58

Frohman EM, Zhang H, Dewey RB et al 2000 Vertigo in MS: utility of positional and particle repositioning maneuvers. *Neurology* **55**: 1566–1569

Frohman EM, Frohman TC, Fleckenstein J et al 2001 Ocular contrapulsion in multiple sclerosis: clinical features and pathophysiological mechanisms. *J Neurol Neurosurg Psychiatry* **70**: 688–692

Frohman EM, Frohman TC, Moreault AM 2002 Acquired sexual paraphilia in patient with multiple sclerosis. *Arch Neurol* **59**: 1006–1010

Frohman EM, Goodin DS, Calabresi PA et al 2003 The utility of MRI in suspected MS. Report of the Therapeutics and Technology

Assessment Subcommittee of the American Academy of Neurology. *Neurology* **61**: 602–611

Frohman EM, Dewey RB, Frohman TC 2004 An unusual variant of the dorsal midbrain syndrome in MS: clinical characteristics and pathophysiologic mechanisms. *Mult Scler* **10**: 322–325

Frohman EM, Frohman TC, Zee DS et al 2005 The neuro-ophthalmology of multiple sclerosis. *Lancet Neurol* **4**: 111–121

Frohman LP, Giurgis M, Turbin RE, Bielory L 2003 Sarcoidosis of the anterior visual pathways: 24 new cases. *J Neuroophthalmol* **23**: 190–197

Fromann C 1864 *Untersuchungen über die normale und pathologische Amatomie des Ruckenmarks, zweiter Theil.* Jena: Fromann

Fromann C 1878 *Untersuchungen über die Gewebsveränderungen bei der multiplen Sklerose des Gehirns und Rückenmarks.* Jena: Fromann

Frost EE, Buttery PC, Milner R, ffrench-Constant C 1999 Integrins mediate a neuronal survival signal for oligodendrocytes. *Curr Biol* **9**: 1251–1254

Frost EE, Nielsen JA, Le TQ, Armstrong RC 2003 PDGF and FGF2 regulate oligodendrocyte progenitor responses to demyelination. *J Neurobiol* **54**: 457–472

Früh K, Yang Y 1999 Antigen presentation by MHC class I and its regulation by interferon-γ. *Curr Opin Immunol* **11**: 76–81

Fruttiger M, Karlsson L, Hall AC et al 1999 Defective oligodendrocyte development and severe hypomyelination in PDGF-A knockout mice. *Development* **126**: 457–467

Frzovic D, Morris ME, Vowels L 2000 Clinical tests of standing balance: performance of persons with multiple sclerosis. *Arch Phys Med Rehab* **81**: 215–221

Fu L, Matthews PM, DeStefano N et al 1998 Imaging axonal damage of normal-appearing white matter in multiple sclerosis. *Brain* **121**: 103–113

Fugger L, Ryder LP, Morling N et al 1990a DNA typing for HAL-DPB1.02 and -DPB1.04 in multiple sclerosis and juvenile rheumatoid arthritis. *Immunogenetics* **32**: 150–156

Fugger L, Sandberg-Wollheim M, Morling N et al 1990b The germline repertoire of T-cell receptor beta chain genes in patients with relapsing remitting multiple sclerosis or optic neuritis. *Immunogenetics* **31**: 278–280

Fuhr P, Borggrefe-Chappuis A, Schindler C, Kappos L 2001 Visual and motor evoked potentials in the course of multiple sclerosis. *Brain* **124**: 2162–2168

Fujimoto S, Kondoh H, Yamamoto Y et al 1990 Holter electrocardiogram monitoring in nephrotic patients during methylprednisolone pulse therapy. *Am J Nephrol* **10**: 231–236

Fujinami RS, Oldstone MBA 1985 Amino acid homology between the encephalitogenic site of myelin basic protein (MBP) and virus: mechanism for autoimmunity. *Science* **230**: 1043–1046

Fukazawa T, Moriwaka F, Sugiyama K et al 1993 Cerebrospinal fluid IgG profiles and multiple sclerosis in Japan. *Acta Neurol Scand* **88**: 178–183

Fukazawa T, Moriwaka F, Hamada K et al 1997a Facial palsy in multiple sclerosis. *J Neurol* **244**: 483–488

Fukazawa T, Sasaki H, Kikuchi S, Hamada K, Hamada T, Tashiro K 1997b Dominantly inherited leukodystrophy showing cerebellar deficits, and spastic paraparesis: a new entity? *J Neurol* **244**: 446–449

Fukazawa T, Yanagawa T, Kikuchi S et al 1999a CTLA-4 gene polymorphism may modulate disease in Japanese multiple sclerosis patients. *J Neurol Sci* **171**: 49–55

Fukazawa T, Yabe I, Kikuchi S et al 1999b Association of vitamin D receptor gene polymorphism with multiple sclerosis in Japanese. *J Neurol Sci* **166**: 47–52

Fukazawa T, Kikuchi S, Sasaki H et al 2000a Genomic HLA profiles of MS in Hoikkaido, Japan: important role of DPB1*0501 allele. *J Neurol* **247**: 175–178

Fukazawa T, Yamasaki K, Ito H et al 2000b Both the HLA-DPB1 and -DRB1 alleles correlate with risk for multiple sclerosis in Japanese: clinical phenotypes and gender as important factors. *Tissue Antigens* **55**: 199–205

Fukazawa T, Kikuchi S, Niino M et al 2003 Multiphasic demyelinating disorder with acute transverse myelitis in Japanese. *J Neurol* **250**: 624–626

Fukazawa T, Kikuchi S, Miyagishi R et al 2005 CTLA-4 gene polymorphism is not associated with conventional multiple sclerosis in Japanese. *J Neuroimmunol* **159**: 225–229

Fukushima T, Mayanagi Y 1975 Neurophysiological examination (SEP) for the objective diagnosis of spinal lesions. In: Klug W, Brock M, Klinger M, Spoerri O (eds) *Adv Neurosurg* **2**: 158–168

Fulford KWM, Caterall RD, Delhanty JJ, Doniach D, Kremer M 1972 A collagen disorder of the nervous system presenting as multiple sclerosis. *Brain* **95**: 373–386

Fulton BP, Burne JF, Raff MC 1992 Visualisation of O-2A progenitor cells in developing and adult rat optic nerve by quisqualate-stimulated cobalt uptake. *J Neurosci* **12**: 4816–4833

Fulton JC, Grossman RI, Mannon LJ et al 1999 Familial multiple sclerosis: volumetric assessment in clinically symptomatic and asymptomatic individuals. *Mult Scler* **5**: 74–77

Funakawa I, Terao A 1998 Intractable hiccups and syncope in multiple sclerosis. *Acta Neurol Scand* **98**: 136–139

Funakawa I, Hara K, Yasuda T, Terao A 1993 Intractable hiccups and sleep apnea syndrome in multiple sclerosis: report of two cases. *Acta Neurol Scand* **88**: 401–405

Furlan R, Martino G, Galbiati F et al 1999 Caspase-1 regulates the inflammatory process leading to autoimmune demyelination. *J Immunol* **163**: 2403–2409

849

Furlan R, Brambilla E, Ruffini F *et al* 2001 Intrathecal delivery of IFN-gamma protects C57BL/6 mice from chronic-progressive experimental autoimmune encephalomyelitis by increasing apoptosis of central nervous system-infiltrating lymphocytes. *J Immunol* **167**: 1821–1829

Furtado GD, Olivares-Villagomez D, de Lafaille MAC *et al* 2001 Regulatory T cells in spontaneous autoimmune encephalomyelitis. *Immunol Rev* **182**: 122–134

Furukawa K, Barger SW, Blalock EM, Mattson MP 1996 Activation of K+ channels and suppression of neuronal activity by secreted beta-amyloid-precursor protein. *Nature* **379**: 74–78

Fux CA, Pfister S, Nohl F, Zimmerli S 2003 Cytomegalovirus-associated acute transverse myelitis in immunocompetent adults. *Clin Microbiol Infect* **9**: 1187–1190

Gabay L, Lowell S, Rubin LL, Anderson DJ 2003 Deregulation of dorsoventral patterning by FGF confers trilineage differentiation capacity on CNS stem cells in vitro. *Neuron* **40**: 485–499

Gabriel SB, Schaffner SF, Nguyen H *et al* 2002 The structure of haplotype blocks in the human genome. *Science* **296**: 2225–2229

Gade-Andavolu R, MacMurray JP, Blake H *et al* 1998 Association between the gamma-aminobutyric acid A3 receptor gene and multiple sclerosis. *Arch Neurol* **55**: 513–516

Gade-Andavolu R, Comings DE, MacMurray J *et al* 2004 RANTES: a genetic risk marker for multiple sclerosis. *Mult Scler* **10**: 536–539

Gaertner S, De Graaf KL, Greve B, Weissert R 2004 Antibodies against glycosylated native MOG are elevated in patients with multiple sclerosis. *Neurology* **63**: 2381–2383

Gaines AR, Varricchio F 1998 Interferon beta-1b injection site reactions and necroses. *Mult Scler* **4**: 70–73

Gaiser CN, Johnson MJ, de Lange G *et al* 1987 Susceptibility to multiple sclerosis associated with an immunoglobulin gamma 3 restriction length polymorphism. *J Clin Invest* **79**: 309–313

Galer BS, Lipton RB, Weinstein S *et al* 1990 Apoplectic headache and oculomotor nerve palsy: an unusual presentation of multiple sclerosis. *Neurology* **40**: 1465–1466

Galetta S, Schatz NJ, Glaser JS 1989 Acute sarcoid optic neuropathy with spontaneous recovery. *J Clin Neuroophthalmol* **9**: 27–32

Gall JC, Hayles AB, Siekert RG, Keith HM 1958 Multiple sclerosis in children. *Pediatrics* **21**: 703–709

Gallo A, Rovaris M, Riva R *et al* 2005 Diffusion-tensor magnetic resonance imaging detects normal appearing white matter damage unrelated to short-term disease activity in patients at the earliest clinical stage of multiple sclerosis. *Arch Neurol* **62**: 803–808

Gallo P, Piccinno M, Pagni S, Tavolato B 1988 Interleukin-2 levels in serum and cerebrospinal fluid of multiple sclerosis patients. *Ann Neurol* **24**: 795–797

Gallo P, Piccinno MG, Tavaloto B, Siden A 1991 A longitudinal study on IL-2, sIL-2R, IL-4 and IFN-gamma in multiple sclerosis CSF and serum. *J Neurol Sci* **101**: 227–232

Gallo P, Chiusole P, Sanzari M *et al* 1994 Effect of high dose steroid therapy on T cell subpopulations: a longitudinal study in MS patients. *Acta Neurol Scand* **89**: 95–101

Gallou M, Madigand M, Masse L *et al* 1983 Epidemiologie de la sclérose en plaques en Bretagne. *Presse Med* **12**: 995–999

Gambardella A, Valentino P, Labate A *et al* 2003 Temporal lobe epilepsy as a unique manifestation of multiple sclerosis. *Can J Neurol Sci* **30**: 228–232

GAMES and the Transatlantic Multiple Sclerosis genetics cooperative 2003 A meta-analysis of whole genome linkage screens in multiple sclerosis. *J Neuroimmunol* **143**: 39–46

GAMES Collaborative Group 2005 Linkage disequilibrium screening for multiple sclerosis implicates *JAG1* and *POU2AF1* as susceptibility genes in Europeans. *J Immunol* (in press)

Gammon G, Klotz J, Ando D, Sercarz EE 1990 The T cell response to a multideterminant antigen: clonal heterogeneity of the T cell response, variation between syngeneic individuals and *in vitro* selection of T cell specificities. *J Immunol* **144**: 1571–1577

Gandevia SC, Allen GM, Butler JE, Taylor JL 1996 Supraspinal factors in human muscle fatigue: evidence for suboptimal output from the motor cortex. *J Physiol* **490**: 529–536

Ganter P, Prince C, Esiri MM 1999 Spinal cord axonal loss in multiple sclerosis: a post-mortem study. *Neuropathol Appl Neurobiol* **25**: 459–467

Garbern JY, Yool DA, Moore GJ *et al* 2002 Patients lacking the major CNS myelin protein, proteolipid protein 1, develop length-dependent axonal degeneration in the absence of demyelination and inflammation. *Brain* **125**: 551–561

Garcia JR, Rodriguez S, Henriquez MS *et al* 1989 Prevalence of multiple sclerosis in Lanzarote (Canary Islands). *Neurology* **39**: 265–567

Garcin R 1936 Sclérose en plaques familiale et paraplegie spasmodique familiale a forme de sclérose en plaques. *Rev Neurol* **65**: 58–60

Garcin R, Godlewski S, Lapresle J 1960 Névralgie du trijumau et sclérose en plaques (à propos d'une observation anatomo-clinique). *Rev Neurol* **102**: 441–451

Garcin R, Lapresle J, Fardeau M 1962 Documents pour servir a l'étude des amyotrophies et des abolitions durable des réflexes tendineux observeés dans la sclérose en plaques. *Rev Neurol* **107**: 417–431

Gard AL, Pfeiffer SE 1990 Two proliferative stages of the oligodendrocyte lineage (A2B5+O4− and O4+GalC−) under different mitogenic control. *Neuron* **5**: 615–625

Gardinier MV, Amiguet P, Linington C, Matthieu J-M 1992 Myelin/oligodendrocyte glycoprotein is a unique member of the immunoglobulin superfamily. *J Neurosci Res* **33**: 177–187

Garson JA, Tuke PW, Giraud P *et al* 1998 Detection of virion-associated MSRV-RNA in serum of patients with multiple sclerosis. *Lancet* **351**: 33

Garthwaite G, Goodwin DA, Garthwaite J 1999 Nitric oxide stimulates cGMP formation in rat optic nerve axons, providing a specific marker of axon viability. *Eur J Neurosci* **11**: 4367–4372

Garthwaite G, Goodwin DA, Batchelor AM *et al* 2002 Nitric oxide toxicity in CNS white matter: an in vitro study using rat optic nerve. *Neuroscience* **109**: 145–155

Gasperini C, Grasso MG, Fiorelli M *et al* 1995 A controlled study of potential risk factors preceding exacerbation in multiple sclerosis. *J Neurol Neurosurg Psychiatry* **59**: 303–305

Gasperini C, Pozzilli CD, Bastianelli S *et al* 1998 Effect of steroids on Gd-enhancing lesions before and during recombinant beta interferon 1α treatment in relapsing remitting multiple sclerosis. *Neurology* **50**: 403–406

Gasperini C, Paolillo A, Giugni E *et al* 2002 MRI brain volume changes in relapsing remitting multiple sclerosis patients treated with interferon beta-1a. *Mult Scler* **8**: 119–123

Gass A, Barker GJ, Kidd D *et al* 1994 Correlation of magnetisation transfer ratio with clinical disability in multiple sclerosis. *Ann Neurol* **36**: 62–67

Gass A, Moseley IF, Barker GJ *et al* 1996 Lesion discrimination in optic neuritis using high-resolution fat-suppressed fast spin-echo MRI. *Neuroradiology* **38**: 317–321

Gass A, Kitchen N, MacManus DCR *et al* 1997 Trigeminal neuralgia in patients with multiple sclerosis: lesion localization with MRI. *Neurology* **49**: 1142–1144

Gaudet JPC, Hashimoto L, Sadovnick AD, Ebers GC 1995a Is sporadic MS caused by an infection of adolescence and early adulthood? A case-control study of birth order position. *Acta Neurol Scand* **91**: 19–21

Gaudet JPC, Hashimoto L, Sadovnick AD, Ebers GC 1995b A study of birth order and multiple sclerosis in multiplex families. *Neuroepidemiology* **14**: 188–192

Gault F 1894 *De la neuromyélite optique aigue*. Lyon: Thèse de Lyon

Gaupp S, Pitt D, Kuziel WA *et al* 2003 Experimental autoimmune encephalomyelitis (EAE) in CCR2(−/−) mice: susceptibility in multiple strains. *Am J Pathol* **162**: 139–150

Gausas J, Paterson PY, Day ED, Dal Canto MC 1982 Intact B-cell activity is essential for complete expression of experimental allergic encephalomyelitis in Lewis rats. *Cell Immunol* **72**: 360–366

Gautam AM, Lock CB, Smilek DE *et al* 1994 Minimum structural requirements for peptide presentation by major histocompatibility complex class II molecules: implications in induction of autoimmunity. *Proc Natl Acad Sci USA* **91**: 767–771

Gautam AM, Liblau R, Chelvanayagam G et al 1998 A viral peptide with limited homology to a self peptide can induce clinical signs of experimental autoimmune encephalomyelitis. *J Immunol* **161**: 60–64

Gauthier S, Bharanidharan P, Stazzone L et al 2003 Treatment of relapsing remitting interferon/glatiramer acetate unresponsive patients with pulse cyclophosphamide. *Neurology* **60**: A148

Gautier-Smith PC 1973 Lhermitte's sign in subacute combined degeneration of the cord. *J Neurol Neurosurg Psychiatry* **36**: 861–863

Gawne-Cain M, O'Riordan JI, Thompson AJ et al 1997 Multiple sclerosis lesion detection in the brain: a comparison of fast fluid-attenuated inversion recovery and conventional T_2 weighted dual spin echo. *Neurology* **49**: 364–370

Gay D, Esiri M 1991 Blood-brain barrier damage in acute multiple sclerosis plaques: an immunocytochemical study. *Brain* **114**: 557–572

Gay FW, Drye TJ, Dick GW, Esiri MM 1997 The application of multifactorial cluster analysis in the staging of plaques in early multiple sclerosis: identification and characterization of primary demyelinating lesion. *Brain* **120**: 1461–1483

Gayou A, Brochet B, Dousset V 1997 Transitional progressive multiple sclerosis: a clinical and imaging study. *J Neurol Neurosurg Psychiatry* **63**: 396–398

Gbadamosi J, Munchau A, Weiller C, Schafer H 2003a Severe heart failure in a young multiple sclerosis patient. *J Neurol* **250**: 241–242

Gbadamosi J, Buhmann C, Tessmer W et al 2003b Effects of mitoxantrone on multiple sclerosis patients' lymphocyte subpopulations and production of immunoglobulin, TNF-alpha and IL-10. *Eur Neurol* **49**: 137–141

Ge Y, Grossman RI, Udupa JK et al 2000 Brain atrophy in relapsing–remitting multiple sclerosis and secondary progressive multiple sclerosis: longitudinal data analysis. *Radiology* **214**: 665–670

Gean-Marton AD, Venzia LG, Marton KL et al 1991 Abnormal corpus callosum: a sensitive and specific indicator of multiple sclerosis. *Radiology* **180**: 215–221

Geisler MW, Sliwinski M, Coyle PK et al 1996 The effects of amantadine and pemoline on cognitive functioning in multiple sclerosis. *Arch Neurol* **53**: 185–188

Gelati M, Corsini E, De Rossi M et al 2002 Methylprednisolone acts on peripheral blood mononuclear cells and endothelium in inhibiting migration phenomena in patients with multiple sclerosis. *Arch Neurol* **59**: 774–780

Genain CP, Lee-Parritz D, Nguyen M-H et al 1994 In healthy primates, circulating autoreactive T cells mediate autoimmune disease. *J Clin Invest* **94**: 1339–1345

Genain CP, Abel K, Belmar N et al 1996 Late complications of immune deviation therapy in a nonhuman primate. *Science* **274**: 2054–2057

Genain CP, Cannella B, Hauser SL, Raine CS 1999 Identification of autoantibodies associated with myelin damage in multiple sclerosis. *Nature Med* **5**: 170–175

Genoud S, Lappe-Siefke C, Goebbels S et al 2002 Notch1 control of oligodendrocyte differentiation in the spinal cord. *J Cell Biol* **158**: 709–718

Gentiloni N, Schiavino D, Della Corte F et al 1992 Neurogenic pulmonary edema: a presenting symptom in multiple sclerosis. *Ital J Neurol Sci* **13**: 435–438

Geny C, Pradat P F, Yulis J et al 1992 Hypothermia, Wernicke encephalopathy and multiple sclerosis. *Acta Neurol Scand* **86**: 632–634

Georgi W 1961 Multiple sklerose: pathologisch-anatomische Befund multipler sklerose bei klinisch nicht diagnostizierten Krankheiten. *Schweizer Med Wochenschr* **91**: 605–607

Georgiev D, Milanov I 1994 Epidemiological survey of multiple sclerosis in Bulgaria. In: Firnhaber W, Lauer K (eds) *Multiple Sclerosis in Europe: An Epidemiological Update*. Darmstadt: Leuchtturm-Verlag/LTV Press, pp. 184–189

Geren BB 1954 The formation from the Schwann cell surface of myelin in the peripheral nerves of chick embryos. *Exp Cell Res* **7**: 558–562

Germain RN 1994 MHC-dependent antigen processing and peptide presentation: providing ligands for T lymphocyte activation. *Cell* **76**: 287–299

Gerritse K, Deen C, Fasbender M et al 1994 The involvement of specific anti myelin basic protein antibody-forming cells in multiple sclerosis immunopathology. *J Neuroimmunol* **49**: 153–159

Gerritse K, Laman JD, Noelle RJ et al 1996 CD40-CD40 ligand interactions in experimental allergic encephalomyelitis and multiple sclerosis. *Proc Natl Acad Sci USA* **93**: 2499–2504

Gervais A, Gaillard O, Plassart E et al 1998 Apolipoprotein E polymorphism in multiple sclerosis. *Ann Clin Biochem* **35**: 135–136

Gessain A, Gout O 1992 Chronic myelopathy associated with human T-lymphotropic virus type 1 (HTLV-1). *Ann Intern Med* **117**: 933–946

Geurts JJG, Wolswijk G, Bo L et al 2003 Altered expression patterns of group I and II metabotropic glutamate receptors in multiple sclerosis. *Brain* **126**: 1755–1766

Geurts JJ, Bo L, Pouwels PJ et al 2005a Cortical lesions in multiple sclerosis: combined postmortem MR imaging and histopathology. *Am J Neuroradiol* **26**: 572–577

Geurts JJ, Pouwels PJ, Uitdehaag BM et al 2005b Intracortical lesions in multiple sclerosis: improved detection with 3D double inversion–recovery MR imaging. *Radiology* **236**: 254–260

Geuze HJ 1998 The role of endosomes and lysosomes in MHC class II functioning. *Immunol Today* **19**: 282–287

Ghabanbasani MZ, Gu XX, Spaaaepen M et al 1995 Importance of HLA-DRB1 and DQA1 genes and of the amino acid polymorphisms in the functional domain of DRB1 chain in multiple sclerosis. *J Neuroimmunol* **59**: 77–82

Ghadirian P, Dadgostar B, Azani R, Maisonneuve P 2001 A case-control study of the association between socio-economic, lifestyle and medical history factors and multiple sclerosis. *Can J Public Health* **92**: 281–285

Ghalie RG, Mauch E, Edan G et al 2002 A study of therapy-related acute leukemia after mitoxantrone therapy for multiple sclerosis. *Mult Scler* **8**: 441–445

Ghatak NR 1992 Occurrence of oligodendrocytes within astrocytes in demyelinating lesions. *J Neuropathol Exp Neurol* **51**: 40–46

Ghatak NR, Hirano A, Doron Y, Zimmerman HM 1973 Remyelination in multiple sclerosis with peripheral type myelin. *Arch Neurol* **29**: 262–267

Ghatak NR, Hirano A, Lijtmaer H, Zimmerman HM 1974 Asymptomatic demyelinated plaque in the spinal cord. *Arch Neurol* **30**: 484–486

Ghawche F, Destée A 1990 Hypothermie et sclérose en plaques. Un cas avec trois épisodes d'hypothermie transitoire. *Rev Neurol* **146**: 767–769

Ghezzi A 1999 Sexuality and multiple sclerosis. *Scand J Sexol* **2**: 125–140

Ghezzi A, Caputo D 1981 Pregnancy: a factor influencing the course of multiple sclerosis? *Eur Neurol* **20**: 115–117

Ghezzi A, Di Falco M, Locatelli C et al 1989 Clinical controlled randomized trial of azathioprine in multiple sclerosis. In: Gonsette RE, Delmotte P (eds) *Recent Advances in Multiple Sclerosis Therapy*. Amsterdam: Elsevier.

Ghezzi A, Montanini R, Basso PF et al 1990 Epilepsy in multiple sclerosis. *Eur Neurol* **30**: 218–223

Ghezzi, A, Deplano V, Faroni J et al 1997 Multiple sclerosis in childhood: clinical features of 149 cases. *Mult Scler* **3**: 43–46

Ghezzi A, Martinelli V, Torri V et al 1999 Long term follow up of optic neuritis: the risk of developing multiple sclerosis, its outcome and the prognostic role of paraclinical tests. *J Neurol* **246**: 770–775

Ghezzi A, Martinelli V, Rodegher M et al 2000 The prognosis of idiopathic optic neuritis. *Neurol Sci* **21(Suppl)**: 865–869

Ghezzi A, Pozzilli C, Liguori M, Marrosu MG 2002 Prospective study of multiple sclerosis with early onset. *Mult Scler* **8**: 115–118

Ghezzi A, Bergamaschi R, Martinelli V et al 2004 Clinical characteristics, course and prognosis of relapsing Devic's Neuromyelitis Optica. *J Neurol* **251**: 47–52

Ghezzi A, Amato MP, Capobianco M et al 2005 Disease-modifying drugs in childhood–juvenile multiple sclerosis: results of an Italian co-operative study. *Mult Scler* **11**: 420–424

Giang DW, Poduri KR, Eskin TA *et al* 1992 Multiple sclerosis masquerading as a mass lesion. *Neuroradiology* **34**: 150–154

Gianola S, Rossi F 2004 GAP-43 overexpression in adult mouse Purkinje cells overrides myelin-derived inhibition of neurite growth. *Eur J Neurosci* **19**: 819–830

Gibson J, Frank A 2002 Supporting individuals with disabling multiple sclerosis. *J R Soc Med* **95**: 580–586

Gideon P, Henriksen O, Sperling B *et al* 1992 Early time course of N-acetylaspartate, creatine and phosphocreatine, and compounds containing choline in the brain after acute stroke: a proton magnetic resonance spectroscopy study. *Stroke* **23**: 1566–1572

Giedraitis V, Modin H, Callander M *et al* 2003 Genome-wide TDT analysis in a localized population with a high prevalence of multiple sclerosis indicates the importance of a region on chromosome 14q. *Genes Immun* **4**: 559–563

Gieffers J, Pohl D, Treib J *et al* 2001 Presence of *Chlamydia pneumoniae* DNA in the cerebral spinal fluid is a common phenomenon in a variety of neurological diseases and not restricted to multiple sclerosis. *Ann Neurol* **49**: 585–589

Giegerich G, Pette M, Meinl E *et al* 1992 Diversity of T cell receptor α and β chain genes expressed by human T cells specific for similar myelin basic protein peptide/major histocompatibility complexes. *Eur J Immunol* **22**: 753–758

Giess R, Maurer M, Linker R *et al* 2002a Association of a null mutation in the CNTF gene with early onset of multiple sclerosis. *Arch Neurol* **59**: 407–409

Giess R, Maurer M, Pohl D 2002b A null mutation in the CNTF gene is associated with early onset of multiple sclerosis. *Arch Neurol* **59**: 407–409

Gijbels K, Masure S, Carton H, Opdennakker G 1992 Gelatinase in the cerebrospinal fluid of patients with multiple sclerosis and other inflammatory neurological disorders. *J Neuroimmunol* **41**: 29–34

Gijbels K, Galardy RE, Steinman L 1994 Reversal of experimental autoimmune encephalomyelitis with a hydroxamate inhibitor of matrix metalloproteases. *J Clin Invest* **94**: 2177–2182

Gilbert JJ, Sadler M 1983 Unsuspected multiple sclerosis. *Arch Neurol* **40**: 533–536

Gilden DH 2002 A search for virus in multiple sclerosis. *Hybrid Hybridomics* **21**: 93–97

Gilden DH, Burgoon MP, Kleinschmidt-DeMasters BK *et al* 2001 Molecular immunological strategies to identify antigens and B-cell responses unique to multiple sclerosis. *Arch Neurol* **58**: 43–48

Gilgun-Sherki Y, Panet H, Melamed E, Offen D 2003 Riluzole suppresses experimental autoimmune encephalomyelitis: implications for the treatment of multiple sclerosis. *Brain Res* **989**: 196–204

Gilgun-Sherki Y, Melamed E, Offen D 2004 The role of oxidative stress in the pathogenesis of multiple sclerosis: the need for effective antioxidant therapy. *J Neurol* **251**: 261–268

Gill KP, Chia YW, Henry MM Shorvon PJ 1994 Defecography in multiple sclerosis patients with severe constipation. *Radiology* **191**: 553–556

Gillespie JW, Ahram M, Best CJ *et al* 2002 The role of tissue microdissection in cancer research. *Cancer J* **7**: 32–39

Gilli F, Bertolotto A, Sala A *et al* 2004 Neutralizing antibodies against IFN-beta in multiple sclerosis: antagonization of IFN-beta mediated suppression of MMPs. *Brain* **127**: 259–268

Gilliatt RW 1982 Electrophysiology of peripheral neuropathies – an overview. *Muscle Nerve* **5**: S108–S116

Gilmore M, Grennan E, 2003 A pilot study of the relationship between multiple sclerosis and the physical environment in northwest Ireland. *Environ Geochem Health* **25**: 157–163

Giobbia M, Carniato A, Scotton PG *et al* 1999 Cytomegalovirus-associated transverse myelitis in a non-immunocompromised patient. *Infection* **27**: 228–230

Giordana MT, Richiardi P, Trevisan E *et al* 2003 Abnormal ubiquitination of axons in normally myelinated white matter in multiple sclerosis brain. *Neuropath Appl Neurobiol* **28**: 35–41

Giovannoni G 1998 Cerebrospinal fluid and serum nitric oxide metabolites in patients with multiple sclerosis. *Mult Scler* **4**: 27–30

Giovannoni G, Goodman A 2005 Neutralizing anti-IFN-beta antibodies: how much more evidence do we need to use them in practice? *Neurology* **65**: 6–8

Giovannoni G, Heales SJR, Silver NC *et al* 1997 Raised serum nitrate and nitrite levels in patients with multiple sclerosis. *Journal of Neurological Science* **145**: 77–81

Giovannoni G, Heales SJ, Land JM, Thompson EJ 1998 The potential role of nitric oxide in multiple sclerosis. *Mult Scler* **4**: 212–216

Giovannoni G, Miller DH, Lossef NA *et al* 2001a Serum inflammatory markers and clinical/MRI markers of disease progression in multiple sclerosis. *J Neurol* **248**: 487–495

Giovannoni G, Thompson AJ, Miller DH, Thompson EJ 2001b Fatigue is not associated with raised inflammatory markers in multiple sclerosis. *Neurology* **57**: 676–681

Giraudon P, Vincent P, Vuaillat C *et al* 2004 Semaphorin CD100 from activated T lymphocytes induces process extension collapse in oligodendrocytes and death of immature neural cells. *J Immunol* **172**: 1246–1255

Girgrah N, Letarte M, Becker LE *et al* 1991 Localisation of CD44 glycoprotein to fibrous astrocytes in normal appearing white matter and to reactive astrocytes in active lesions in multiple sclerosis. *J Neuropath Exp Neurol* **50**: 779–792

Giroud M, Guard O, Dumas R 1988 Anomalies cardio-respiratoires dans la sclérose en plaques. *Rev Neurol* **14**: 284–288

Giubilei F, Antonini G, Di Legge S *et al* 2002 Blood cholesterol and MRI activity in first clinical episode suggestive of multiple sclerosis. *Acta Neurol Scand* **106**: 109–112

Giulian D, Johnson B, Krebs JF *et al* 1991 A growth factor from neuronal cell lines stimulates myelin protein synthesis in mammalian brain. *J Neurosci* **11**: 327–336

Giunti D, Borsellino G, Benelli R *et al* 2003 Phenotypic and functional analysis of T cells homing into the CSF of subjects with inflammatory diseases of the CNS. *J Leukoytec Biol* **73**: 584–590

Givogri MI, Costa RM, Schonmann V *et al* 2002 Central nervous system myelination in mice with deficient expression of Notch1 receptor. *J Neurosci* **67**: 309–320

Glaser GH, Merritt HH 1952 Effects of corticotrophin (ACTH) and cortisone on disorders of the nervous system. *J Am Med Assoc* **148**: 898–904

Gledhill RF, McDonald WI 1977 Morphological characteristics of central demyelination and remyelination: a single-fiber study. *Ann Neurol* **1**: 552–560

Gledhill RF, Harrison BM, McDonald WI 1973 Pattern of remyelination in the CNS. *Nature* **244**: 443–444

Glick ME, Meshkinpour H, Haldeman S *et al* 1982 Colonic dysfunction in multiple sclerosis. *Gastroenterology* **83**: 1002–1007

Global Advisory Committee on Vaccine Safety, 20–21 June 2002. *Wkly Epidemiol Rec* **77**: 389–394

Gneiss C, Reindl M, Lutterotti A *et al* 2004 Interferon-beta: the neutralizing antibody (NAb) titre predicts reversion to NAb negativity. *Mult Scler* **10**: 507–510

Go T, Imai T 2000 A residual cystic lesion in acute disseminated encephalomyelitis. *Neuroradiology* **42**: 682–684

Goas JY, Marion JL, Missoum A 1983 High dose intravenous methyl prednisolone in acute exacerbations of multiple sclerosis. *J Neurol Neurosurg Psychiatry* **46**: 99

Gobbini MI, Smith ME, Richert ND *et al* 1999 Effect of open label pulse cyclophosphamide therapy on MRI measures of disease activity in five patients with refractory relapsing–remitting multiple sclerosis. *J Neuroimmunol* **99**: 142–149

Goddard DR, Berry M, Butt AM 1999 In vivo actions of fibroblast growth factor-2 and insulin-like growth factor-I on oligodendrocyte development and myelination in the central nervous system. *J Neurosci Res* **57**: 74–85

Goddard DR, Berry M, Kirvell SL, Butt AM 2001 Fibroblast growth factor-2 inhibits myelin production by oligodendrocytes in vivo. *Mol Cell Neurosci* **18**: 557–569

Godfrey DI, Hammond KJL, Poulton LD *et al* 2000 NKT cells: facts, functions and fallacies. *Immunol Today* **21**: 573–583

Goebels N, Hofstetter H, Schmidt S *et al* 2000 Repertoire dynamics of autoreactive T cells in multiple sclerosis patients and healthy subjects: epitope spreading versus clonal persistence. *Brain* **123**: 508–518

Goebels N, Helmchen C, Abel-Horn M *et al* 2001 Extensive myelitis associated with *Mycoplasma pneumoniae* infection: magnetic resonance imaging and clinical long term follow up. *J Neurol* 248: 204–208

Goedde R, Sawcer S, Boehringer S *et al* 2002 A genome screen for linkage disequilibrium in HLA-DRB1*15-positive Germans with multiple sclerosis based on 4666 microsatellite markers. *Hum Genet* 111: 270–277

Goertsches R, Villoslada P, Comabella M *et al* 2003 A genomic screen of Spanish multiple sclerosis patients reveals multiple loci associated with the disease. *J Neuroimmunol* 143: 124–128

Goertsches R, Comabella M, Navarro A *et al* 2005 Genetic association between polymorphisms in the ADAMTS14 gene and multiple sclerosis. *J Neuroimmunol* 164: 140–147

van der Goes A, Brouwer J, Hoekstra K *et al* 1998 Reactive oxygen species are required for the phagocytosis of myelin by macrophages. *J Neuroimmunol* 92: 67–75

van der Goes A, Kortekaas M, Hoekstra K *et al* 1999 The role of anti-myelin (auto)-antibodies in the phagocytosis of myelin by macrophages. *J Neuroimmunol* 101: 61–67

Goffette S, van Pesch V, Vanoverschelde JL *et al* 2005 Severe delayed heart failure in three multiple sclerosis patients previously treated with mitoxantrone. *J Neurol* 252: 1217–1222

Gogate N, Verma L, Min Zhau J *et al* 1994 Plasticity in the adult human oligodendrocyte lineage. *J Neurosci* 14: 4571–4587

Gogolin KJ, Kolaga VJ, Baker L *et al* 1989 Subtypes of HLA-DQ and -DR defined by DQB1 and DRB1 RFLPs: allele frequency in the general population and in insulin dependent diabetes (IDMM) and multiple sclerosis patients. *Ann Hum Genet* 353: 357–360

Gold DP, Offner H, Sun D *et al* 1991 Analysis of T cell receptor β chains in Lewis rats with experimental allergic encephalomyelitis: conserved complementary determining region 3. *J Exp Med* 174: 1467–1476

Gold MS, Zhang L, Wrigley DL, Traub RJ 2002 Prostaglandin E(2) modulates TTX-R I(Na) in rat colonic sensory neurons. *J Neurophysiol* 88: 1512–1522

Gold R, Linington C 2002 Devic's disease: bridging the gap between laboratory and clinic. *Brain* 125: 1425–1427

Gold R, Schmied M, Giegerich G *et al* 1994 Differentiation between cellular apoptosis and necrosis by combined use of *in situ* tailing and nick translation techniques. *Lab Invest* 71: 219–225

Gold R, Schmied M, Tontsch U *et al* 1996 Antigen presentation by astrocytes primes rat T lymphocytes for apoptotic cell death: a model for T-cell apoptosis *in vivo*. *Brain* 119: 651–659

Gold R, Buttgereit F, Toyka KV 2001 Mechanism of action of glucocorticosteroid hormones: possible implications for therapy of neuroimmunological disorders. *J Neuroimmunol* 117: 1–8

Goldacre MJ, Wotton CJ, Seagroatt V, Yeates D 2004 Multiple sclerosis after infectious mononucleosis: record linkage study. *J Epidemiol Commun Hlth* 58: 1032–1035

Goldberg ID, Kurland LT 1962 Mortality in 33 countries for diseases of the nervous system. *World Neurol* 3: 444–465

Goldberg JL, Barnes BA 2000 Nogo in nerve regeneration. *Nature* 403: 369–370

Goldberg SH, van der Meer P, Hesselgesser J *et al* 2001 CXCR3 expression in human central nervous system diseases. *Neuropathol Appl Neurobiol* 27: 127–138

Golde S, Chandran S, Brown GC, Compston DAS 2002 Different pathways for iNOS-mediated toxicity *in vitro* dependent on neuronal maturation and NMDA-receptor expression. *J Neurochem* 82: 269–282

Golde S, Coles AJ, Lindquist JA, Compston DAS 2003 Decreased iNOS-synthesis mediates dexamethasone induced protection of neurones from inflammatory injury in vitro. *Eur J Neurosci* 18: 2527–2537

Golden GS, Woody RC 1987 The role of nuclear magnetic imaging in the diagnosis of MS in children. *J Neurol* 37: 689–693

Goldstein B 1946 Two cases of disseminated sclerosis in African natives. *East Afr Med J* 23: 170–173

Goldstein I, Lue TF, Padma-Nathan H *et al* 1998 Oral sildenafil in the treatment of erectile dysfunction. Sildenafil Study Group. *N Engl J Med* 338: 1397–404

Golgi C 1894 *Untersuchungen über den Feineren bau des Centralen und Peripherischen nervensystems*. Jena: von Gustav Fischer

Gollan L, Salomon D, Salzer J, Peles E 2003 Caspr regulates the processing of contactin and inhibits its binding to neurofascin. *J Cell Biol* 163: 1213–1218

Gomaa A, Shalaby M, Osman M *et al* 1996 Topical treatment of erectile dysfunction: randomised double blind placebo controlled trial of cream containing aminophylline, isosorbide dinitrate, and co-dergocrine mesylate. *Br Med J* 312: 1512–1515

Gombert J-M, Herbelin A, Tancrède-Bohin E *et al* 1996 Early quantitative and functional deficiency of NK1+-like thymocytes in the NOD mouse. *Eur J Immunol* 26: 2989–2998

Gomes WA, Mehler MF, Kessler JA 2003 Transgenic overexpression of BMP4 increases astroglial and decreases oligodendroglial lineage commitment. *Dev Biol* 255: 164–177

Gomez-Lira M, Moretto G, Bonamini D *et al* 2002 Myelin oligodendrocyte glycoprotein polymorphisms and multiple sclerosis. *J Neuroimmunol* 133: 241–243

Gomez-Lira M, Liguouri M, Magnani C *et al* 2003 CD45 and multiple sclerosis: the exon 4 C77G polymorphism (additional studies and meta-analysis) and new markers. *J Neuroimmunol* 140: 216–221

Gondim FdeA, Thomas FP 2001 Episodic hyperlibidinism in multiple sclerosis. *Mult Scler* 7: 67–70

Gonen O, Catalaa I, Babb JS *et al* 2000 Total brain N-acetylaspartate: a new measure of disease load in MS. *Neurology* 54: 15–19

Gonsette R, Andre-Balisaux G, Delmotte P 1966 La permeabilité des vaisseaux cerebraux VI Demyelinisation experimentale provoquée par des substances agissant sur la barrière hematoencephalique. *Acta Neurol Belg* 66: 247–262

Gonsette RE 2004 Combination therapy for multiple sclerosis. *The International MS Journal* 11: 10–21

Gonzalez CF, Swirsky-Sacchetti T, Mitchell D *et al* 1994 Distributional patterns of multiple sclerosis brain lesions. Magnetic resonance imaging clinical correlation. *Journal of Neuroimaging* 4: 188–195

Gonzalez-Scarano F, Grossman RI, Galetta S *et al* 1987 Multiple sclerosis disease activity correlates with gadolinium-enhanced magnetic resonance imaging. *Ann Neurol* 21: 300–306

Good K, Clark CM, Oger J *et al* 1992 Cognitive impairment and depression in mild multiple sclerosis. *J Nerv Mental Disease* 180: 730–732

Goodin DS 2003 Interferons in relapsing remitting multiple sclerosis. *Lancet* 361: 1821; author reply 1823–1824

Goodin DS, Ebers GC, Johnson KP *et al* 1999 The relationship of MS to physical trauma and psychological stress – Report of the Therapeutics and Technology Assessment Subcommittee of the American Academy of Neurology. *Neurology* 52: 1737–1745

Goodin DS, Frohman EM, Garmany GP Jr *et al* 2002 Disease modifying therapies in multiple sclerosis: report of the Therapeutics and Technology Assessment Subcommittee of the American Academy of Neurology and the MS Council for Clinical Practice Guidelines. *Neurology* 58: 169–178

Goodin DS, Arnason B, Coyle P *et al* 2003 The use of mitoxantrone (Novantrone) for the treatment of multiple sclerosis – Report of the Therapeutics and Technology Assessment Subcommittee of the American Academy of Neurology. *Neurology* 61: 1332–1338

Goodkin DE 1991 Inter and intra observer variablity for grades 1.0–3.5 of the Kurtzke Expanded Disability Status Scale (EDSS). *Neurology* 42: 859–863

Goodkin DE 1994 Interferon beta-1b. *Lancet* 344: 1057–1060

Goodkin DE 2000 Interferon beta-1b in secondary progressive MS: clinical and MRI results of a 3-year randomized controlled trial (abstract) 54: 2352

Goodkin DE, Hertsgaard D 1989 Seasonal variation of multiple sclerosis exacerbations in North Dakota. *Arch Neurol* 46: 1015–1018

Goodkin DE, Hertsgaard D, Rudick RA 1989 Exacerbation notes and adherence to disease type in a prospectively followed-up population with multiple sclerosis: implications for clinical trials. *Arch Neurol* 46: 1107–1112

Goodkin DE, Bailly PC, Teetzen ML et al 1991 The efficacy of azathioprine in relapsing remitting multiple sclerosis. *Neurology* 41: 20–25

Goodkin DE, Cookfair D, Wende K et al 1992 Inter- and intra-rater scoring agreement using grades 1.0 to 3.5 of the Kurtzke Expanded Disability Status Scale (EDSS). Multiple Sclerosis Collaborative Research Group. *Neurology* 42: 859–863

Goodkin DE, Rudick RA, VanderBrug Medendorp S et al 1995 Low-dose (7.5 mg) oral methotrexate reduces the rate of progression in chronic progresssive multiple sclerosis. *Ann Neurol* 37: 30–40

Goodkin DE, Rudick RA, VanderBrug Medendorp S et al 1996 Low-dose oral methotrexate in chronic progressive multiple sclerosis: analyses of serial MRIs. *Neurology* 47: 1153–1157

Goodkin DE, Shulman M, Winkelhake J et al 2000 A phase I trial of solubilized DR2:MBP84–102 (AG284) in multiple sclerosis. *Neurology* 54: 1414–1420

Goodman AD, Miller DH 2002 Infections and MS: clinical trials move to center stage. *Neurology* 58: 7–8

Goodman AD, Mock DJ, Powers JM et al 2003 Human herpesvirus 6 genome and antigen in acute multiple sclerosis lesions. *J Infect Dis* 187: 1365–1376

Goodnow CC 1992 Transgenic mice and analysis of B-cell tolerance. *Ann Rev Immunol* 10: 489–518

Gore J 2003 Out of the shadows – MRI and the Nobel Prize. *N Engl J Med* 349: 2290–2292

Goris A, Epplen C, Fiten P et al 1999 Analysis of an IFN gamma gene (IFNγ) polymorphism in multiple sclerosis in Europe: effect of population structure on association with disease. *J Interferon Cytokine Res* 19: 1037–1046

Goris A, Heggarty S, Marrosu MG et al 2002 Linkage disequilibrium analysis of chromosome 12q14–15 in multiple sclerosis: delineation of a 118-kb interval around interferon-gamma (IFNG) that is involved in male versus female differential susceptibility. *Genes Immun* 3: 470–476

Goris A, Sawcer SJ, Vandenbroeck K et al 2003 New candidate loci for multiple sclerosis susceptibility revealed by a whole genome association screen in a Belgian population. *J Neuroimmunol* 143: 65–69

Gorodetsky C, Najera R, Rangel BE et al 1986 Immunogenetic profile of multiple sclerosis in Mexicans. *Hum Immunol* 16: 364–374

Gosselink R, Kovacs L, Ketelaer P et al 2000 Respiratory muscle weakness and respiratory muscle training in severely disabled multiple sclerosis patients. *Arch Phys Med Rehab* 81: 747–751

Goswami KKA, Randall RE, Lange LS, Russell WC 1987 Antibodies against the paramyxovirus SV5 in cerebrospinal fluids

of some multiple sclerosis patients. *Nature* 327: 244–247

Gottschalk M, Kumpfel T, Flachenecker P et al 2005 Fatigue and regulation of the hypothalamo–pituitary–adrenal axis in multiple sclerosis. *Arch Neurol* 62: 277–280

Gould E, Tanapat P, McEwen BS et al 1998 Proliferation of granule cell precursors in the dentate gyrus of adult monkeys is diminished by stress. *Proc Natl Acad Sci USA* 95: 3168–3171

Gould ES, Bird AC, Leaver PK, McDonald WI 1977 Treatment of optic neuritis by retrobulbar injection of triamcinolone. *Br Med J* i: 1495–1497

Gould HJ 1982 Disabilities and how to live with them: multiple sclerosis. *Lancet* ii: 1208–1210

Gould HJ, England JD, Liu ZP, Levinson SR 1998 Rapid sodium channel augmentation in response to inflammation induced by complete Freund's adjuvant. *Brain Res* 802: 69–74

Goureau O, Amiot F, Dautry F, Courtois Y 1997 Control of nitric oxide production by endogenous TNF-alpha in mouse retinal pigmented epithelial and Muller glial cells. *Biochem Biophys Res Commun* 240: 132–135

Gourie-Devi M, Nagaraja D 1982 Multiple sclerosis in south India. In: Kuroiwa Y, Kurland L (ed.) *Multiple Sclerosis East and West.* Fukoka: Kyushu University Press, pp. 135–148

Gout O, Théodorou I, Liblau R, Lyon-Caen O 1997 Central nervous system demyelination after recombinant hepatitis B vaccination: report of 25 cases. *Neurology* 48 (Suppl): A424

Govaerts A, Gony J, Martin-Mondiere C et al 1985 HLA in multiple sclerosis: population family studies. *Tissue Antigens* 25: 187–199

Goverman J, Woods A, Larson L et al 1993 Transgenic mice that express a myelin basic protein-specific T cell receptor develop spontaneous autoimmunity. *Cell* 72: 551–560

Gowers WR 1888 *A Manual of Disease of the Nervous System.* London: J. & A. Churchill, pp. 507–519

Gowers WR 1893 *A Manual of Disease of the Nervous System.* 2nd edn. London: J. & A. Churchill, Vol II, p. 1069

Graesser D, Solowiej A, Bruckner M et al 2002 Altered vascular permeability and early onset of experimental autoimmune encephalomyelitis in PECAM-1-deficient mice. *J Clin Invest* 109: 383–392

Graff-Radford NR, Rizzo M 1987 Neglect in a patient with multiple sclerosis. *Eur Neurol* 26: 100–103

Grafman J, Rao S, Bernardin L, Leo GJ 1991 Automatic memory processes in patients with multiple sclerosis. *Arch Neurol* 48: 1072–1075

Graham C, Kirk C, Nevin N et al 1993 Lack of association between myelin basic protein gene microsatellite and multiple sclerosis. *Lancet* 341: 1596

Graham EM, Ellis CJK, Sanders MD, McDonald WI 1986 Optic neuropathy in sarcoidosis. *J Neurol Neurosurg Psychiatry* 49: 756–763

Gran B, Bielekova B, McFarland H et al 2000a Development of multiple sclerosis after hepatitis B vaccination: an immunologic case report. *Neurology* 54 (suppl 3): A164

Gran B, Tranquill LR, Chen M et al 2000b Mechanisms of immunomodulation by glatiramer acetate. *Neurology* 55: 1704–1714

Gran B, Zhang G-X, Yu S et al 2002 IL-12p35-deficient mice are susceptible to experimental autoimmune encephalomyelitis: evidence for redundancy in the IL-12 system in the induction of central nervous system autoimmune demyelination. *J Immunol* 169: 7104–7110

GrandPré T, Nakamura F, Vartanian T, Strittmatter SM 2000 Identification of the Nogo inhibitor of axon regeneration as a Reticulon protein. *Nature* 403: 439–444

Granieri E, Casetta I 1997 Common childhood and adolescent infections and multiple sclerosis. *Neurology* 49 (Suppl 2): S42–S54

Granieri E, Rosati G 1982 Italy: a medium- or high-risk area for multiple sclerosis? An epidemiological study in Barbagia, Sardinia, southern Italy. *Neurology* 32: 466–472

Granieri E, Tola MR 1994 Experience in multiple sclerosis epidemiology in Italy. In: Firnhaber W, Lauer K (eds) *Multiple Sclerosis in Europe: An Epidemiological Update.* Darmstadt: Leuchtturm-Verlag/LTV Press, pp. 184–189

Granieri E, Rosati G, Tola R et al 1983 The frequency of multiple sclerosis in Mediterranean Europe: an incidence and prevalence study in Barbagia, Sardinia, insular Italy. *Acta Neurol Scand* 68: 84–89

Granieri E, Tola R, Paolino E et al 1985 The frequency of multiple sclerosis in Italy: a descriptive study in Ferrara. *Ann Neurol* 17: 80–84

Granieri E, Casetta I, Tola M et al 1993 Multiple sclerosis: does epidemiology contribute to providing etiological clues? *J Neurol Sci* 115 (Suppl): S16–S23

Granieri E, Malagu S, Casetta I et al 1996 Multiple sclerosis in Italy: a reappraisal of incidence and prevalence in Ferrara. *Arch Neurol* 53: 793–798

Granieri E, Casetta I, Govoni V et al 2000 The increasing incidence and prevalence of MS in a Sardinian province. *Neurology* 55: 842–848

Grant I, McDonald WI, Trimble MR et al 1984 Deficient learning and memory in early and middlé phases of multiple sclerosis. *J Neurol Neurosurg Psychiatry* 47: 250–255

Grant I, Brown GW, Harris T et al 1989 Severely threatening events and marked life difficulties preceding onset or exacerbation of multiple sclerosis. *J Neurol Neurosurg Psych* 52: 8–13

Grant RM, Carver AD, Sloan RL 1998 Multiple sclerosis in Fife. *Scot Med J* 43: 44–47

Grasso MG, Lubich S, Guidi L et al 2000 Cerebellar deficit and respiratory impairment: a strong association in multiple sclerosis? *Acta Neurol Scand* **101**: 98–103

Graumann U, Reynolds R, Steck AJ, Schaeren-Wiemers, N 2003 Molecular changes in normal appearing white matter in multiple sclerosis are characteristic of neuroprotective mechanisms against hypoxic insult. *Brain Pathol* **13**: 554–573

Graves MC 1981 Gastric outlet obstruction in a patient with multiple sclerosis. *Ann Neurol* **10**: 397–398

Graveson GS 1950 Syphilitic optic neuritis. *J Neurol Neurosurg Psychiatry* **13**: 216–224

Gray F, Chimelli L, Mohr M et al 1991 Fulminating multiple sclerosis-like leukoencephalopathy revealing human immunodeficiency virus infection. *Neurology* **41**: 105–109

Greco A, Minghetti L, Sette G et al 1999 Cerebrospinal fluid isoprostane shows oxidative stress in patients with multiple sclerosis. *Neurology* **53**: 1876–1879

Green AJ, Barcellos LF, Rimmler JB et al 2001 Sequence variation in the transforming growth factor-beta 1 (TGFβ1) gene and multiple sclerosis susceptibility. The Multiple Sclerosis Genetics Group. *J Neuroimmunol* **116**: 116–124

Green DR, Beere HM 2000 Gone but not forgotten. *Nature* **405**: 28–29

Greenberg HS, Werness SAS, Pugh JE, Andrews RO, Anderson DJ, Domino EF 1994 Short term effects of smoking marijuana on balance in patients with multiple sclerosis and normal volunteers. *Clin Pharmacol Ther* **51**: 292–296

Greenberg SJ, Ehrlich GD, Abbott MA et al 1989 Detection of sequences homologous to human retroviral DNA in multiple sclerosis by gene amplification. *Proc Natl Acad Sci USA* **86**: 2878–2882

Greenfield JG, Carmichael EA 1925 *The Cerebrospinal Fluid in Clinical Diagnosis.* London: Macmillan

Greenfield JG, King LS 1936 Histopathology of the cerebral lesions in disseminated sclerosis. *Brain* **59**: 445–458

Greenspun B, Stineman M, Agri R 1987 Multiple sclerosis and rehabilitation outcome. *Arch Phys Med Rehab* **68**: 434–437

Greenstein JL, McFarland HF, Mingioli ES, McFarlin DE 1984 The lymphoproliferative response to measles virus in twins with multiple sclerosis. *Ann Neurol* **15**: 79–84

Greenwood K, Butt AM 2003 Evidence that perinatal and adult NG2-glia are not conventional oligodendrocyte progenitors and do not depend on axons for their survival. *Mol Cell Neurosci* **23**: 544–558

Greer JM, Pender MP 2005 The presence of glutamic acid at positions 71 or 74 in pocket 4 of the HLA-DRbeta1 chain is associated with the clinical course of multiple sclerosis. *J Neurol Neurosurg Psychiatry* **76**: 656–662

Greer JM, Sobel RA, Sette A et al 1996 Immunogenic and encephalitogenic epitope clusters of myelin proteolipid protein. *J Immunol* **156**: 371–379

Greer JM, Csurhes PA, Cameron KD et al 1997 Increased immunoreactivity to two overlapping peptides of myelin proteolipid protein in multiple sclerosis. *Brain* **120**: 1447–1460

Gregori N, Proschel C, Noble M, Mayer-Proschel M 2002 The tripotential glial-restricted precursor (GRP) cell and glial development in the spinal cord: generation of bipotential oligodendrocyte-type-2 astrocyte progenitor cells and dorsal-ventral differences in GRP cell function. *J Neurosci* **22**: 248–256

Grenman R 1985 Involvement of the audiovestibular system in multiple sclerosis. *Acta Oto-Laryngologica* **420 (Suppl)**: 1–95

Gresty MA, Eli JJ, Findley LJ 1982 Acquired pendular nystagmus: its characteristics, localising value and pathophysiology. *J Neurol Neurosurg Psychiatry* **45**: 431–439

Greter M, Heppner FL, Lemos MP et al 2005 Dendritic cells permit immune invasion of the CNS in an animal model of multiple sclerosis. *Nature Med* **11**: 328–334

Grewal IS, Foellmer HG, Grewal KD et al 1996 Requirement for CD40 ligand in costimulation induction, T cell activation, and experimental allergic encephalomyelitis. *Science* **273**: 1864–1867

Grewal IS, Foellmer HG, Grewal KD et al 2001 CD62L is required on effector cells for local interactions in the CNS to cause myelin damage in experimental allergic encephalomyelitis. *Immunity* **14**: 291–302

Grewel RP, Petronas N, Barton NW 1991 Late onset globoid cell leukodystrophy. *J Neurol Neurosurg Psychiatry* **54**: 1011–1012

Grieb P, Ryba M, Stelmasiak Z et al 1994 Cladribine and multiple sclerosis (letter). *Lancet* **344**: 538

Griffin CM, Chard DT, Parker GJM et al 2002a The relationship between lesion and normal appearing brain tissue abnormalities in early relapsing remitting MS. *J Neurol* **249**: 193–199

Griffin CM, Dehmeshki J, Chard DT et al 2002b TI histograms of normal-appearing brain tissue are abnormal in early relapsing–remitting multiple sclerosis. *Mult Scler* **8**: 211–216

Griffin JW, Goren E, Schaumberg H, Engel WK, Loriaux L 1977 Adrenomyeloneuropathy: a probable variant of adrenoleukodystrophy. *Neurology* **27**: 1107–1113

Griffin JW, Li CY, Macko C et al 1996 Early nodal changes in the acute motor axonal neuropathy pattern of the Guillain–Barre syndrome. *J Neurocytology* **25**: 33–51

Grigoresco D 1932 Contribution à l'étude des troubles dûs à des lésions des noyaux gris dans la sclérose en plaques. *Rev Neurol* **58**: 27–45

Grima B, Zelenika D, Pessac B 1992 A novel transcript overlapping the myelin basic protein gene. *J Neurochem* **59**: 2318–2323

Grima DT, Torrance GW, Francis G et al 2000 Cost and health related quality of life consequences of multiple sclerosis. *Mult Scler* **6**: 91–98

Grimaldi LM, Salemi G, Grimaldi G et al 2001 High incidence and increasing prevalence of MS in Enna (Sicily), southern Italy. *Neurology* **57**: 1891–1893

Grimaldi LM, Pincherle A, Martinelli-Boneschi F et al 2003 An MRI study of *Chlamydia pneumoniae* infection in Italian multiple sclerosis patients. *Mult Scler* **9**: 467–471

Grimaud J, Millar J, Thorpe JW et al 1995 Signal intensity on MRI of basal ganglia in multiple sclerosis. *J Neurol Neurosurg Psychiatry* **59**: 306–308

Grinspan JB, Stern JL, Franceschini B, Pleasure D 1993 Trophic effects of basic fibroblast growth factor (bFGF) on differentiated oligodendroglia: a mechanism for regeneration of the oligodendroglial lineage. *J Neurosci Res* **36**: 672–680

Grisold W, Lutz D, Wolf D 1980 Necrotising myelopathy associated with acute lymphoblastic leukaemia. *Acta Neuropathol* **49**: 231–235

Gronlie SA, Myrvoll E, Hansen G, Grønning M, Mellgren SI 2000 Multiple sclerosis in north Norway, and its first appearance in an indigenous population. *J Neurol* **247**: 129–133

Grønning M 1994 The epidemiology of multiple sclerosis in Norway: a 50 year follow-up in a stable population. In: Firnhaber W, Lauer K (eds) *Multiple Sclerosis in Europe: An Epidemiological Update.* Darmstadt: Leuchtturm-Verlag/LTV Press, pp. 62–66

Grønning M, Mellgren SI 1985 Multiple sclerosis in the two northernmost counties of Norway. *Acta Neurol Scand* **72**: 321–327

Grønning M, Riise T, Kvåle G et al 1991 Incidence of multiple sclerosis in Hordaland, western Norway: a fluctuating pattern. *Neuroepidemiology* **10**: 53–61

Gronseth GS, Ashman EJ 2000 Practice parameter: the usefulness of evoked potentials in identifying clinically silent lesions in patients with suspected multiple sclerosis (an evidence-based review). Report of the Quality Standards Subcommittee of the American Academy of Neurology. *Neurology* **54**: 1720–1725

Gross K, Kokk A, Kaasik AE 1993 Prevalence of MS in south Estonia. Evidence of a new border of the Fennoscandian focus. *Acta Neurol Scand* **88**: 241–246

Grossman M, Robinson KM, Onishi K et al 1995 Sentence comprehension in multiple sclerosis. *Acta Neurol Scand* **92**: 324–331

Grossman RI 1994 Magnetization transfer in multiple sclerosis. *Ann Neurol* **36**: 97–99

Grossman RI, Gonzalez-Scarano F, Atlas SW et al 1986 Multiple sclerosis: gadolinium enhancement in MR imaging. *Radiology* **161**: 721–725

Grossman RI, Braffman BH, Brorson JR et al 1988 Multiple sclerosis: serial study of gadolinium-enhanced MR imaging. *Radiology* **169**: 117–122

Grossman RI, Lenkinski RE, Ramer KN et al 1992 MR proton spectroscopy in multiple sclerosis. *Am J Neuroradiol* **13**: 1535–1543

Grosz K 1924 Malaria behandlung der multipler Sklerose. *Jahrbucher Psychiatr Neurol* **43**: 198–214

Grouard G, Rissoan M-C, Filgueira L *et al* 1997 The enigmatic plasmacytoid T cells develop into dendritic cells with interleukin (IL)-3 and CD40-ligand. *J Exp Med* **185**: 1101–1111

Groves AK, Barnett SC, Franklin RJM *et al* 1993 Repair of demyelinated lesions by transplantation of purified O-2A progenitor cells. *Nature* **362**: 453–455

Grufferman S, Barton JW, Eby NL 1987 Increased sex concordance of sibling pairs with Behcet's disease, Hodgkin's disease, multiple sclerosis and sarcoidosis. *Am J Epidemiol* **126**: 365–369

Gudmundsson KR 1971 Clinical studies of multiple sclerosis in Iceland. *Acta Neurol Scand* **47 (Suppl 48)**: 1–78

Gudnardottir M, Helgedottir H, Bjarnason O, Jonsdottir K 1964 Virus isolated from the brain of a patient with multiple sclerosis. *Exp Neurol* **9**: 85–95

Guenard V, Frisch G, Wood PM 1996 Effects of axonal injury on astrocyte proliferation and morphology *in vitro*: implications for astrogliosis. *Exp Neurol* **137**: 175–190

Guerini FR, Losciale L, Mediati M *et al* 2000 A polymorphism in the repetitive (TGGA) sequence 5' to the human myelin basic protein gene in Italian multiple sclerosis patients. *J Neurovirol* **6 (Suppl 2)**: S28–S32

Guerini FR, Ferrante P, Losciale L *et al* 2003 Myelin basic protein gene is associated with MS in DR4- and DR5- positive Italians and Russians. *Neurology* **61**: 520–526

Guilhoto LM, Osorio CA, Machado LR *et al* 1995 Pediatric multiple sclerosis: report of 14 cases. *Brain Dev* **17**: 9–12

Guilian D, Johnson B, Krebs JF *et al* 1991 A growth factor from neuronal cell lines stimulates myelin protein synthesis in mammalian brain. *J Neurosci* **11**: 327–336

Guillain G, Bize R 1933 Sur un cas de sclérose en plaques avec torticollis spasmodique. *Rev Neurol* **40**: 133–138

Guillain G, Barré JA, Strohl A 1916 Sur un syndrôme de radiculonervite avec hyperalbuminose du liqid cephalorachidien sans reaction cellulaire, remarqués sur les charactères cliniques et graphiques des reflexes tendineux. *Bull Soc Med Hôpital (Paris)* **40**: 1462–1470

Günther, Schön 1840 Versuche und Bemerkungen über Regeneration der Nerven und Abhängigkeit der peripherischen Nerven von den Centralorganen. *Müllers Arch Anat Physiol Wissenschaftl Med*: 270–286

Guo YP, Gao SF 1983 Concentric sclerosis. In: Tyrer JH, Eadie MJ (eds) *Clinical and Experimental Neurology. Proceedings of the Australian Association of Neurologists.* Sydney: Adis Health Science Press, Vol 19, pp. 67–76

Gupta MK 1987 Myelin basic protein and demyelinating diseases. *Crit Rev Clin Lab Sci* **24**: 287–314

Gupta YK 1984 Gastroparesis with multiple sclerosis. *J Am Med Assoc* **252**: 42

Gupte G, Stonehouse M, Wassmer E *et al* 2003 Acute disseminated encephalomyelitis: a review of 18 cases in childhood. *J Paediatr Child Health* **39**: 336–342

Guseo A, Jellinger K 1975 The significance of perivascular infiltrations in multiple sclerosis. *J Neurol* **211**: 51–60

Guseo A, Jofeju E, Kocsis A 1994 Epidemiology of multiple sclerosis in western Hungary 1957–1992. In: Firnhaber W, Lauer K (eds) *Multiple Sclerosis in Europe: An Epidemiological Update.* Darmstadt: Leuchtturm-Verlag/LTV Press, pp. 279–286

Gusev E, Boiko A, Lauer K *et al* 1996 Environmental risk factors in MS: a case control study in Moscow. *Acta Neurol Scand* **94**: 386–394

Guthikonda P, Baker J, Mattson DH 1998 Interferon-beta-1-b (IFN-β) decreases induced nitric oxide (NO) production by a human astrocytoma cell line. *J Neuroimmunol* **82**: 133–139

Guthrie TC 1951 Visual and motor changes in patients with multiple sclerosis. *Arch Neurol Psychiatry* **65**: 437–451

Guttmann L 1952 Principles of rehabilitation in disseminated sclerosis. *Br J Phys Med* **15**: 189–191

Guzman NJ, Fang MZ, Tang SS *et al* 1995 Autocrine inhibition of Na+/K(+)-ATPase by nitric oxide in mouse proximal tubule epithelial cells. *J Clin Invest* **95**: 2083–2088

Gveric D, Hanemaaijer R, Newcombe J *et al* 2001 Plasminogen activators in multiple sclerosis lesions: implications for the inflammatory response and axonal damage. *Brain* **124**: 1978–1999

Gveric D, Herrera B, Petzold A *et al* 2003 Impaired fibrinolysis in multiple sclerosis: a role for tissue plasminogen activator inhibitors. *Brain* **126**: 1590–1598

Gyapay G, Morissette J, Vignal A *et al* 1994 The 1993–94 Genethon human genetic linkage map. *Nature Genet* **7**: 246–339

Haahr S, Koch-Henriksen N, Moller-Larsen A *et al* 1995 Increased risk of multiple sclerosis after late Epstein–Barr virus infection: a historical prospective study. *Mult Scler* **1**: 73–77

Haahr S, Munch M, Christensen T *et al* 1997 Cluster of multiple sclerosis patients from a Danish community. *Lancet* **349**: 923

Haarr M 1963 Retinal periphlebitis in multiple sclerosis. *Acta Neurol Scand* **39 (Suppl 4)**: 270–272

Haase AT, Ventura P, Gibbs CJ, Tourtellotte WW 1981 Measles virus nucleotide sequences: detection by hybridization *in situ*. *Science* **212**: 672–675

Haase CG, Guggenmos J, Brehm U *et al* 2001 The fine specificity of the myelin oligodendrocyte glycoprotein autoantibody response in patients with multiple sclerosis and normal healthy controls. *J Neuroimmunol* **114**: 220–225

Haase CG, Schmidt S, Faustmann PM 2002 Frequencies of the G-protein beta3 subunit C825T polymorphism and the delta32 mutation of the chemokine receptor-5 in patients with multiple sclerosis. *Neurosci Lett* **330**: 293–295

Hachem S, Aguirre A, Vives V *et al* 2005 Spatial and temporal expression of S100B in cells of oligodendrocyte lineage. *Glia* **52**: 81–97

Hachinski VC, Potter P, Merskey H 1987 Leuko-araiosis. *Arch Neurol* **44**: 21–23

Hackett J, Swanson P, Leahy D *et al* 1996 Search for retrovirus in patients with multiple sclerosis. *Ann Neurol* **40**: 805–809

Hackstein H, Bitsch A, Bohnert A *et al* 2001 Analysis of interleukin-4 receptor alpha chain variants in multiple sclerosis. *J Neuroimmunol* **15**: 240–248

Hadden JW, Speafico F 1985 New strategies of immunotherapy. *Springer Semin Immunopathol* **8**: 139–152

Hader WJ 1982 Prevalence of multiple sclerosis in Saskatoon. *Can Med Assoc J* **127**: 295–297

Hader WJ, Feasby TE, Noseworthy JH *et al* 1985 Multiple sclerosis in Canadian native people. *Neurology* **35 (Suppl 1)**: 300 (abstract)

Hader WJ, Rozdilsky B, Nair CP 1986 The concurrence of multiple sclerosis and amyotrophic lateral sclerosis. *Can J Neurol Sci* **13**: 66–69

Hader WJ, Elliot M, Ebers GC 1988 Epidemiology of multiple sclerosis in London and Middlesex County, Ontario, Canada. *Neurology* **38**: 617–621

Hader WJ, Irvine DG, Schiefer HB 1990 A cluster-focus of multiple sclerosis at Henribourg, Saskatchewan. *Can J Neurol Sci* **17**: 391–394

Hader WJ, Seland TP, Hader MB *et al* 1996 The occurrence of multiple sclerosis in the Hutterites of North America. *Can J Neurol Sci* **23**: 291–295

Hadjivassiliou M, Grunewald RA, Chattopadhyay AK *et al* 1998 Clinical, radiological, neurophysiological and neuropathological characteristics of gluten ataxia. *Lancet* **352**: 1582–1585

Hadjivassiliou M, Grunewald R, Sharrack B *et al* 2003 Gluten ataxia in perspective: epidemiology, genetic susceptibility and clinical characteristics. *Brain* **126**: 685–691

Haegert DG, Francis GS 1992 Contribution of a single DQ beta chain residue to multiple sclerosis in French Canadians. *Hum Immunol* **34**: 85–90

Haegert DG, Francis GS 1993 HLA-DQ polymorphisms do not explain HLA class II associations with multiple sclerosis in two Canadian patient groups. *Neurology* **43**: 1207–1210

Haegart DG, Michaud M, Schwab C, Francis GS 1990 Multiple sclerosis and HLA class II susceptibility and resistance genes. *J Neurosci Res* **26**: 66–73

Haegert DG, Muntoni DG, Murru MR *et al* 1993 HAL-DQA1 and -DQB1 associations with multiple sclerosis in Sardinia and French Canada: evidence for immunogenetically distinct patient groups. *Neurology* **43**: 548–552

Haegert DG, Swift FV, Benedikz J 1996 Evidence for a complex role of HLA class II genotypes in susceptibility to multiple sclerosis in Iceland. *Neurology* **46**: 1107–1111

Hafer-Macko C, Hsieh ST, Li CY *et al* 1996 Acute motor axonal neuropathy: an antibody-mediated attack on axolemma. *Ann Neurol* **40**: 635–644

Hafler DA, Buchsbaum M, Johnson D, Weiner HL 1985a Phenotypic and functional analysis of T cells cloned directly from the blood and cerebrospinal fluid of patients with multiple sclerosis. *Ann Neurol* **18**: 451–458

Hafler DA, Fox DA, Manning ME *et al* 1985b *In vivo* activated T lymphocytes in the peripheral blood and cerebrospinal fluid of patients with multiple sclerosis. *N Engl J Med* **312**: 1405–1411

Hafler DA, Fallis RJ, Dawson DM *et al* 1986 Immunologic responses of progressive multiple sclerosis patients treated with an anti-T-cell monoclonal antibody, anti-T12. *Neurology* **36**: 777–784

Hafler DA, Ritz F, Schlossman SF, Weiner HL 1988 Anti-CD4 and anti-CD2 monoclonal antibody infusions in subjects with multiple sclerosis: immunosuppressive effect and human anti-mouse responses. *J Immunol* **141**: 131–138

Hafler DA, Saadeh MG, Kuchroo VK *et al* 1996 TCR usage in human and experimental demyelinating disease. *Immunol Today* **17**: 152–159

Hageman ATH, Gabreels FJM, de Jong JGN *et al* 1995 Clinical symptoms of adult metachromatic leukodystrophy and arylsulfatase A pseudo deficiency. *Arch Neurol* **52**: 408–413

Haghighi S, Andersen O, Rosengren L *et al* 2000 Incidence of CSF abnormalities in siblings of multiple sclerosis patients and unrelated controls. *J Neurol* **247**: 616–622

Hahn CD, Shroff MM, Blaser SI, Banwell BL 2004 MRI criteria for multiple sclerosis. Evaluation in a pediatric cohort. *Neurology* **62**: 806–808

Hahn JS, Siegler DJ, Enzmann D 1996 Intravenous gammaglobulin therapy in recurrent acute disseminated encephalomyelitis. *Neurology* **46**: 1173–1174

Haile RW, Iselius L, Hodge S *et al* 1981 Segregation and linkage of 40 multiplex multiple sclerosis families. *Hum Heredity* **31**: 252–258

Hailman E, Burack WR, Shaw AS *et al* 2002 Immature CD4⁺CD8⁺ thymocytes form a multifocal immunological synapse with sustained tyrosine phosphorylation. *Immunity* **16**: 839–848

Haimanot R 1985 MS – a case report on an Ethiopian. *Ethiopian Med J* **23**: 27

Haines JL, Ter-Minassian M, Bazyk A *et al* 1996 A complete genomic screen for multiple sclerosis underscores a role for the major histocompatibility complex. *Nature Genet:* **13**: 469–471

Haines JL, Terwedow HA, Burgess K *et al* 1998 Linkage of the MHC to familial multiple sclerosis suggests genetic heterogeneity. The Multiple Sclerosis Genetics Group. *Hum Mol Genet* **7**: 1229–1234

Haines JL, Bradford Y, Garcia ME *et al* 2002 Multiple susceptibility loci for multiple sclerosis. *Hum Mol Genet* **11**: 2251–2256

Hajihosseini M, Tham TN, Dubois-Dalcq M 1996 Origin of oligodendrocytes within the human spinal cord. *J Neurosci* **16**: 7981–7994

Halawa I, Lolli F, Link H 1989 Terminal component of complement C9 in CSF and plasma of patients with MS and aseptic meningitis. *Acta Neurol Scand* **80**: 130–135

Hale G, Xia MQ, Tighe HP *et al* 1990 The Campath-1 antigen (CDw52). *Tissue Antigens* **35**: 1–10

Halfpenny CA, Scolding NJ 2003 Immune modifying agents do not impair the survival, migration or proliferation of oligodendrocyte progenitors (CG-4) in vitro. *J Neuroimmunol* **139**: 9–16

Hall A, Giese NA, Richardson WD 1996 Spinal cord oligodendrocytes develop from ventrally derived progenitor cells that express PDGF alpha-receptors. *Development* **122**: 4085–4094

Hall GL, Compston DAS, Scolding NJ 1997a Beta-interferon and multiple sclerosis. *Trends Neurosci* **20**: 63–67

Hall GL, Wing MG, Compston DAS, Scolding NJ 1997b Beta-interferon regulates the immunoregulatory activity of neonatal rodent microglia. *J Neuroimmunol* **72**: 11–19

Hall GL, Girdlestone J, Compston DAS, Wing MG 1999 Recall antigen presentation by gamma interferon activated microglia results in T cell proliferation, cytokine release and propagation of the immune response. *J Neuroimmunol* **98**: 105–111

Hall JI 1967 Studies on demyelinated peripheral nerves in guinea-pigs with experimental allergic neuritis: a histological and electrophysiological study. II Electrophysiological observations. *Brain* **90**: 313–332

Hall M 1841 *On Diseases and Derangements of the Nervous System in their Primary Forms and in their Modifications by Age, Sex, Constitution, Hereditary Predisposition, Excesses, General Disorder and Organic Disease.* London: Ballière

Hall SM, Redford EJ, Smith KJ 2000 Tumour necrosis factor-alpha has few morphological effects within the dorsal columns of the spinal cord, in contrast to its effects in peripheral nervous system. *J Neuroimmunol* **106**: 130–136

Haller P, Patzold U 1979 Die Optikusneuritis im Kindesalter. *Forschr Neurol Psychiatr* **47**: 209–216

Hallervorden J 1940 Die zentralen Entmarkungserkrankungen. *Dtsch Z Nervenheilk* **150**: 201–239

Hallervorden J, Spatz H 1933 Über die konzentrische Sklerose und die physikalisch-chemischen Faktoren bei der Ausbreitung von Entmarkungsprozessen. *Arch Psychiatr Nervenkr* **98**: 641–701

Hallet M, Londsey JW, Adelstein BD, Riley PO 1985 Controlled trial of isoniazid therapy for severe postural cerebellar tremor in multiple sclerosis. *Neurology* **35**: 1374–1377

Halliday AM 1993 The visual evoked potential in the investigation of diseases of the optic nerve. In: Halliday AM (ed.) *Evoked Potentials in Clinical Testing.* Edinburgh: Churchill Livingstone, pp. 195–278

Halliday AM, Wakefield GS 1963 Cerebral evoked potentials in patients with associated sensory loss. *J Neurol Neurosurg Psychiatry* **26**: 211–219

Halliday AM, McDonald WI, Mushin J 1972 Delayed visual evoked response in optic neuritis. *Lancet* i: 982–985

Halliday AM, McDonald WI, Mushin J 1973a Visual evoked response in diagnosis of multiple sclerosis. *Br Med J* **4**: 661–664

Halliday AM, McDonald WI, Mushin J 1973b Delayed pattern-evoked responses in optic neuritis in relation to visual acuity. *Trans Ophthalmol Soc UK* **93**: 315–324

Halliday AM, Halliday E, Kriss A *et al* 1976 The pattern-evoked potential in compression of the anterior visual pathways. *Brain* **99**: 357–374

Hallpike JF, Adams CW, Bayliss OB 1970a Histochemistry of myelin: proteolytic activity around multiple sclerosis plaques. *Histochem J* **2**: 199–208

Hallpike JF, Adams CW, Bayliss OB 1970b Histochemistry of myelin: loss of basic protein in early myelin breakdown and multiple sclerosis plaques. *Histochem J* **2**: 323–328

Hamdi T 1975 Multiple sclerosis in Iraq: a clinical and geomedical survey. *J Postgrad Med* **21**: 1–9

Hamidon BB, Raymond AA 2003 Acute disseminated encephalomyelitis (ADEM) presenting as seizures secondary to anti-tetanus toxin vaccination. *Med J Malaysia* **58**: 780–782

Hammarberg H, Lidman O, Lundberg H *et al* 2000 Neuroprotection by encephalomyelitis: rescue of mechanically injured neurons and neurotrophin production by CNS-infiltrating T and natural killer cells. *J Neurosci* **20**: 5283–5291

Hammarstrom AKM, Gage PW 1998 Inhibition of oxidative metabolism increases persistent sodium current in rat CA1 hippocampal neurons. *J Physiol* **510**: 735–741

Hammarstrom AKM, Gage PW 1999 Nitric oxide increases persistent sodium current in rat hippocampal neurons. *J Physiology* **520**: 451–461

Hammond SR, De Wytt C, Maxwell IC *et al* 1987 The epidemiology of multiple sclerosis in Queensland, Australia. *J Neurol Sci* **80**: 185–204

Hammond SR, English D, de Wytt C *et al* 1988a The clinical profile of MS in Australia: a comparison between medium- and high-frequency prevalence zones. *Neurology* **38**: 980–986

857

Hammond SR, McLeod JG, Millingen KS et al 1988b The epidemiology of multiple sclerosis in 3 Australian cities: Perth, Newcastle and Hobart. *Brain* 111: 1–25

Hammond SR, McLeod JG, Macaskill P, English D 1996 Multiple sclerosis in Australia: socio-economic factors. *J Neurol Neurosurg Psychiatry* 61: 311–313

Hammond SR, English DR, McLeod JG 2000a The age-range of risk of developing multiple sclerosis: evidence from a migrant population in Australia. *Brain* 123: 968–974

Hammond SR, McLeod JG, Macaskill P, English DR 2000b Multiple sclerosis in Australia: prognostic factors. *J Clin Neurosci* 7: 16–19

Hammond WA 1871 *A Treatise on Diseases of the Nervous System.* New York: Appleton, pp. 278–300

Hammondeh M, Kahn MA 1982 Clinical variant of systemic lupus erythematosus resembling multiple sclerosis. *J Rheumatol* 9: 336–337

Hanahan D 1999 Peripheral-antigen-expressing cells in thymic medulla: factors in self-tolerance and autoimmunity. *Curr Opin Immunol* 10: 656–662

Handa R, Sahota P, Kumar M et al 2003 In vivo proton magnetic resonance spectroscopy (MRS) and single photon emission computerized tomography (SPECT) in systemic lupus erythematosus (SLE). *Magn Reson Med* 21: 1033–1037

Hanefeld F, Bauer HJ, Christen HJ et al 1991 Multiple sclerosis in childhood: report of 15 cases. *Brain Dev* 13: 410–416

Hanrahan PS, Russel AS, McLean DR 1988 Ankylosing spondylitis and multiple sclerosis: a possible association. *J Rheumatol* 15: 1512–1514

Hansen C, Hopf HC, Treede RD 1996 Paradoxical heat sensation in patients with multiple sclerosis: evidence for a supraspinal integration of temperature sensation. *Brain* 119: 1729–1736

Hao Q, Saida T, Kawakami H et al 1992 HLAs and genes in Japanese patients with multiple sclerosis: evidence for increased frequencies of HLA-Cw3, HLA-DR2 and HLA-DQB1*0602. *Hum Immunol* 35: 116–124

Hao Q, Miyashita N, Matsui M et al 2002 *Chlamydia pneumoniae* infection associated with enhanced MRI spinal lesions in multiple sclerosis. *Mult Scler* 8: 436–440

Haran MJ, Jenney AW, Keenan RJ et al 2001 Paraplegia secondary to *Burkholderia pseudomallei* myelitis: a case report. *Arch Phys Med Rehabil* 82: 1630–1632

Harbison JW, Calabrese VP, Edlich RF 1989 A fatal case of sun exposure in a multiple sclerosis patient. *J Emerg Med* 7: 465–467

Harbo HF, Celius EG, Vardtdal F, Spurkland A 1999 CTLA4 promoter and exon 1 dimorphisms in multiple sclerosis. *Tissue Antigens* 53: 106–110

Harbo HF, Datta P, Oturai A et al 2003 Two genome-wide linkage disequilibrium screens in Scandinavian multiple sclerosis patients. *J Neuroimmunol* 143: 101–106

Harbo HF, Lie BA, Sawcer S et al 2004 Genes in the HLA class I region may contribute to the HLA class II-associated genetic susceptibility to multiple sclerosis. *Tissue Antigens* 63: 237–247

Hardesty I 1904 On the development and nature of the neuroglia. *Am J Anat* 3: 229–268

Harding AE 1984 *The Hereditary Ataxias and Related Disorders.* Edinburgh: Churchill Livingstone

Harding AE, Sweeney MG, Miller DH et al 1992 Occurrence of a multiple sclerosis-like illness in women who have a Leber's hereditary optic neuropathy mitochondrial DNA mutation. *Brain* 115: 979–989

Hardy RJ, Friedrich VL 1996 Oligodendrocyte progenitors are generated throughout the embryonic mouse brain, but differentiate in restricted foci. *Development* 122: 2059–2069

Hargreaves ER 1969 Epidemiological studies in Cornwall. *Proc R Soc Med* 54: 209–216

Haring JS, Perlman S 2003 Bystander CD4 T cells do not mediate demyelination in mice infected with a neurotropic coronavirus. *J Neuroimmunol* 137: 42–50

Haring JS, Pewe LL, Perlman S 2002 Bystander CD8 T cell-mediated demyelination after viral infection of the central nervous system. *J Immunol* 169: 1550–1555

Harris JO, Frank JA, Patronas N et al 1991 Serial gadolinium-enhanced magnetic resonance imaging scans in patients with early, relapsing–remitting multiple sclerosis: implications for clinical trials and natural history. *Ann Neurol* 29: 548–555

Harris W 1940 An analysis of 1,433 cases of paroxysmal trigeminal neuralgia (trigeminal tic) and the end results of Gasserian alcohol injection. *Brain* 63: 209–224

Harris W 1950 Rare forms of paroxysmal trigeminal neuralgia and their relation to disseminated sclerosis. *Br Med J* 2: 1015–1019

Harrison AC, Becker WJ, Stell WK 1987 Colour vision abnormalities in multiple sclerosis. *Can J Neurol Sci* 14: 279–285

Harrison BM, McDonald WI, Ochoa J 1972 Remyelination in the central diphtheria toxin lesion. *J Neurol Sci* 17: 293–302

Hart MN, Earle KM 1975 Haemorrhagic and perivenous encephalitis: a clinical-pathological review of 38 cases. *J Neurol Neurosurg Psychiatry* 38: 585–591

Hartelius L, Runmarker B, Andersen O 2000 Prevalence and characteristics of dysarthria in a multiple-sclerosis incidence cohort: relation to neurological data. *Folia Phoniatr Logop* 52: 160–177

Hartmann M, Rottach KG, Wohlgemuth WA, Pfadenhauer K 1999 Trigeminal neuralgia triggered by auditory stimuli in multiple sclerosis. *Arch Neurol* 56: 731–733

Hartung HP, Grossman RI 2001 ADEM: distinct disease or part of the MS spectrum? *Neurology* 56: 1257–1260

Hartung HP, Kieseier BC 2000 The role of matrix metalloproteinases in autoimmune damage to the central and peripheral nervous system. *J Neuroimmunol* 107: 140–147

Hartung HP, Munschauer FE 2004 Assessment and management of neutralizing antibodies in patients with multiple sclerosis. *J Neurol* 251: II40–II42

Hartung HP, Gonsette R, Konig N et al 2002 Mitoxantrone in progressive multiple sclerosis: a placebo-controlled, double-blind, randomised, multicentre trial. *Lancet* 360: 2018–2025

Hartung HP, Schellekens H, Munschauer III F 2004 Neutralizing antibodies to interferon beta patients with multiple sclerosis: scientific background and clinical implications. *J Neurol* 251: II1–II3

van Haver H, Lissoir F, Droissart C et al 1986 Transfer factor therapy in multiple sclerosis: a three year prospective double-blind clinical trial. *Neurology* 36: 1399–1402

Harzheim M, Schlegel U, Urbach H et al 2004 Discriminatory features of acute transverse myelitis: a retrospective analysis of 45 patients. *J Neurol Sci* 217: 217–223

Hashimoto LL, Mak T, Ebers GC 1992 T-cell receptor alpha-chain polymorphisms in multiple sclerosis. *J Neuroimmunol* 40: 41–48

Hashimoto LL, Walter M, Cox D, Ebers GC 1993 Immunoglobulin heavy chain variable region polymorphisms in multiple sclerosis susceptibility. *J Neuroimmunol* 44: 77–83

Haskell CA, Hancock WW, Salant DJ et al 2001 Targeted deletion of CX(3)CR1 reveals a role for fractalkine in cardiac allograft rejection. *J Clin Invest* 108: 679–688

Hassler R, Bronisch F, Mandringer F, Riechert T 1975 Intention myoclonus of multiple sclerosis, its patho-anatomical basis and stereotaxic relief. *Neurochirurgica* 18: 90–106

Hasson J, Terry RD, Zimmermann HM 1958 Peripheral neuropathy in multiple sclerosis. *Neurology* 8: 503–510

Hatten ME, Liem, RKH, Mason CA 1991 Astroglia in CNS injury. *Glia* 4: 233–243

Hauben E, Butovsky O, Nevo U et al 2000a Passive or active immunization with myelin basic protein promotes recovery from spinal cord contusion. *J Neurosci* 20: 6421–6430

Hauben E, Nevo U, Yoles E et al 2000b Autoimmune T cells as potential neuroprotective therapy for spinal cord injury. *Lancet* 354: 286–287

Hauben E, Agranov E, Gothilf A et al 2001 Posttraumatic therapeutic vaccination with modified myelin self antigen prevents complete paralysis while avoiding autoimmune disease. *J Clin Invest* 108: 591–599

Haupts M, Schejbal P, Pohlau D, Malin J, Przuntek H, Gehlen W 1994 Epidemiological data on multiple sclerosis from an industrial area in north-west Germany. In: Firnhaber W, Lauer K (eds) *Multiple Sclerosis in Europe: An Epidemiological Update.* Darmstadt: Leuchtturm-Verlag/LTV Press, pp. 143–146

Hauser ER, Boehnke M, Guo SW, Risch N 1996 Affected-sib-pair interval mapping and exclusion for complex genetic traits: sampling considerations. *Genet Epidemiol* **13**: 117–137

Hauser SL, Bresnan MJ, Reinherz EL, Weiner HL 1982 Childhood multiple sclerosis: clinical features and demonstration of changes in T cell subsets with disease activity. *Ann Neurol* **11**: 463–468

Hauser SL, Dawson DM, Lehrich JR *et al* 1983 Intensive immunosuppression in progressive multiple sclerosis. *N Engl J Med* **308**: 173–180

Hauser SL, Aubert C, Burks JS *et al* 1986 Analysis of human T-lymphotropic virus sequences in multiple sclerosis tissue. *Nature* **322**: 176–177

Hauser SL, Fleischnick E, Weiner HL *et al* 1989 Extended major histocompatibility complex haploptypes in patients with multiple sclerosis. *Neurology* **39**: 275–277

Hauser SL, Doolittle TH, Lincoln R, Brown RH, Dinarello CA 1990 Cytokine accumulations in CSF of multiple sclerosis patients: frequent detection of interleukin-1 and tumor necrosis factor but not interleukin-6. *Neurology* **40**: 1735–1739

Hauser SL, Doolittle TH, Lopez-Bresnahan M *et al* 1992 Antispasticity effect of threonine in multiple sclerosis. *Arch Neurol* **49**: 923–926

Hauser SL, Oksenberg JR, Lincoln R *et al* 2000 Interaction between HLA-DR2 and abnormal brain MRI in optic neuritis and early MS. Optic Neuritis Study Group. *Neurology* **54**: 1859–1861

van Haver H, Lissoir F, Droissart C *et al* 1986 Transfer factor therapy in multiple sclerosis: a three year prospective double-blind clinical trial. *Neurology* **36**: 1399–1402

Hawkes CH 2002 Is multiple sclerosis a sexually transmitted infection? *J Neurol Neurosurg Psych* **73**: 439–443

Hawkins CP, Munro PMG, MacKenzie F *et al* 1990a Duration and selectivity of blood-brain barrier breakdown in chronic relapsing experimental allergic encephalomyelitis studied using gadolinium-DTPA and protein markers. *Brain* **113**: 365–378

Hawkins CP, MacKenzie F, Tofts PS *et al* 1990b Patterns of blood-brain barrier breakdown in inflammatory demyelination. *Brain* **114**: 801–810

Hawkins SA, Kee F 1988 Updated epidemiological studies of multiple sclerosis in Northern Ireland. *J Neurol* **235** (Suppl): S86

Hawkins SA, McDonnell GV 1999 Benign multiple sclerosis? Cliical course, long term follow up, and asessment of prognostic factors. *J Neurol Neurosurg Psych* **67**: 148–152

Hawley RJ 2000 Hyperammonia possibly due to corticosteroids. *Arch Neurol* **57**: 1085–1086

Hayashi T, Morimoto C, Burks JS *et al* 1988 Dual-labeled immunocytochemistry of the active multiple sclerosis lesion: major histocompatibility complex and activation antigens. *Ann Neurol* **24**: 523–531

Hayday AC 2000 γδ T cells: a right time and a right place for a conserved third way of protection. *Annu Rev Immunol* **18**: 975–1026

Hayes CE, Nashold FE, Spach KM, Pedersen LB 2003 The immunological functions of the vitamin D endocrine system. *Mol Cell Biol* **49**: 277–300

He B, Navikas V, Lundahl J *et al* 1995 Tumor necrosis factor α-308 alleles in multiple sclerosis and optic neuritis. *J Neuroimmunol* **63**: 143–147

He B, Xu C, Yang B *et al* 1998 Linkage and association analysis of genes encoding cytokines and myelin proteins in multiple sclerosis. *J Neuroimmunol* **86**: 13–19

He B, Giedraitis V, Ligers A *et al* 2002a Sharing of a conserved haplotype suggests a susceptibility gene for multiple sclerosis at chromosome 17p11. *Eur J Hum Genet* **10**: 271–275

He B, Wen W, Strong MJ 2002b Activated microglia (BV-2) facilitation of TNF-α-mediated motor neuron death in vitro. *J Neuroimmunol* **128**: 31–38

He W, Ingraham C, Rising L *et al* 2001 Multipotent stem cells from the mouse basal forebrain contribute GABAergic neurons and oligodendrocytes to the cerebral cortex during embryogenesis. *J Neurosci* **21**: 8854–8862

Heales SJR, Barker JE, Stewart VC *et al* 1997 Nitric oxide, energy metabolism and neurological disease. *Biochem Soc Trans* **25**: 939–943

Heard RN, McDonald WI, Batchelor JR *et al* 1989a An RFLP study of HLA-D gene polymorphism in multiple sclerosis. *Immunobiology of HLA* **1**: 913–915

Heard RN, Cullen C, Middleton D *et al* 1989b An allelic cluster of DQ alpha restriction fragments is associated with multiple sclerosis: evidence that a second haplotype may influence disease susceptibility. *Hum Immunol* **25**: 111–123

Heath WR, Miller JFAP 1993 Expression of two α chains on the surface of T cells in T cell receptor transgenic mice. *J Exp Med* **178**: 1807–1811

Heaton RK, Nelson LM, Thompson DS *et al* GM 1985 Neuropsychological findings in relapsing–remitting and chronic-progressive multiple sclerosis. *J Consult Clin Psychol* **53**: 103–110

Heber-Katz E, Acha-Orbea H 1989 The V-region disease hypothesis: evidence from autoimmune encephalomyelitis. *Immunol Today* **10**: 164–169

Hedera P, Fink JK, Bockenstedt PL, Brewer GJ 2003 Myeloneuropathy and pancytopenia due to copper deficiency and high zinc levels of unknown origin. *Arch Neurol* **60**: 1303–1306

Hedlund G, Sandberg-Wollheim M, Sjögren HO 1989 Increased proportion of CD4$^+$CDw29$^+$CD45R$^-$UCHL-1$^+$ lymphocytes in the cerebrospinal fluid of both multiple sclerosis patients and healthy individuals. *Cell Immunol* **118**: 406–412

Heesen C, Kolbeck J, Gold SM *et al* 2003 Delivering the diagnosis of MS – results of a survey among patients and neurologists. *Acta Neurol Scand* **107**: 363–368

Heggarty S, Sawcer SJ, Hawkins S *et al* 2003 A genome wide scan for association with multiple sclerosis in a N. Irish case control population. *J Neuroimmunol* **143**: 93–96

Hein T, Hopfenmuller W 2000 Projection of the number of multiple sclerosis patients in Germany. *Nervenartz* **71**: 288–294

Heininger K, Fierz W, Schafer B *et al* 1989 Electrophysiological investigations in adoptively transferred experimental autoimmune encephalomyelitis in the Lewis rat. *Brain* **112**: 537–552

Heinrich M, Gorath M, Richter-Landsberg C 1999 Neurotrophin-3 (NT-1) modulates early differentiation of oligodendrocytes in rat brain cortical cultures. *Glia* **28**: 244–255

Heins N, Malatesta P, Cecconi F *et al* 2002 Glial cells generate neurons: the role of the transcription factor Pax6. *Nature Neurosci* **5**: 308–315

Heinzlef O, Alamowitch S, Sazdovitch V *et al* 1999 Autoimmune disease in families of French patients with multiple sclerosis. *Acta Neurol Scand* **100**: 1–5

Heinzlef O, Weill B, Johanet C *et al* 2002 Anticardiolipin antibodies in patients with multiple sclerosis do not represent a subgroup of patients according to clinical, familial, and biological characteristics. *J Neurol Neurosurg Psychiatry* **72**: 647–649

Heltberg A 1987 Twin studies in multiple sclerosis. *Ital J Neurol Sci* **6**: 35–39

Heltberg A, Holm NV 1982 Concordance in twins and recurrence in sibships in multiple sclerosis. *Lancet* **i**: 1068

Hely MA, McManus PG, Doran TJ *et al* 1986a Acute optic neuritis: a prospective study of risk factors for multiple sclerosis. *J Neurol Neurosurg Psychiatry* **49**: 1125–1130

Hely MA, McManus PG, Walsh JC, McLeod JG 1986b Visual evoked responses and ophthalmological examination in optic neuritis: a follow-up study. *J Neurol Sci* **75**: 275–283

Hemmer B, Gran B, Zhao Y *et al* 1999 Identification of candidate T cell epitopes and molecular mimics in chronic Lyme disease. *Nature Med* **5**: 1346–1349

Hench PS 1938 The ameliorating effect of pregnancy on chronic atrophic (infectious rheumatoid) arthritis, fibrositis, and intermittent hydrarthrosis. *Proc Staff Meet Mayo Clin* **13**: 161–167

Henderson RD, Bain CJ, Pender MP 2000 The occurrence of autoimmune diseases in patients with multiple sclerosis and their families. *J Clin Neurosci* **7**: 434–437

Henke AF, Cohle SD, Cottingham SL 2000 Fatal hyperthermia secondary to sunbathing in a patient with multiple sclerosis. *Am J Forensic Med Pathol* **21**: 204–206

Hennessey A, Swingler RJ, Compston DAS 1989 The incidence and mortality of multiple sclerosis in South East Wales. *J Neurol Neurosurg Psychiatry* **52**: 1085–1089

Hennessey A, Robertson NP, Swingler R, Compston DAS 1999 Urinary, faecal and sexual dysfunction in patients with multiple sclerosis. *J Neurol* **246**: 1027–1032

Hensiek AE, Sawcer SJ, Feakes R et al 2002 HLA-DR 15 is associated with female gender and younger age at diagnosis in multiple sclerosis. *J Neurol Neurosurg Psych* **72**: 184–187

Hensiek AE, Roxburgh R, Smilie B et al 2003a Updated results of the United Kingdom linkage based genome screen in multiple sclerosis. *J Neuroimmunol* **143**: 25–30

Hensiek AE, Roxburgh R, Meranian M et al 2003b Osteopontin gene and clinical severity of multiple sclerosis. *J Neurol* **250**: 943–947

Hensiek AE, Seaman S, Barcellos L et al 2005 Familial effects on the clinical course in multiple sclerosis (submitted)

Henson RA, Urich H 1982 *Cancer and the Nervous System: The Neurological Manifestations of Systemic Malignant Disease*. Oxford: Blackwell Scientific Publications

Herishanu Y, Louzoun Z 1986 Trihexyphenidyl treatment of vertical pendular nystagmus. *Neurology* **36**: 82–84

Herishanu YO, Badarna S, Sarov B et al 1989 A possible harmful late effect of methylprednisolone therapy on a time cluster of optic neuritis. *Acta Neurol Scand* **80**: 163–170, 569–574

Herman A, Kappler JW, Marrack P, Pullen AM 1991 Superantigens: mechanisms of T cell stimulation and role in immune responses. *Annu Rev Immunol* **9**: 745–772

Hermans G, Stinissen P, Hauben L et al 1997 Cytokine profile of myelin basic protein reactive T cells in multiple sclerosis and healthy individuals. *Ann Neurol* **42**: 18–27

Hermanson O, Jepsen K, Rosenfeld M 2002 N-CoR controls differentiation of neural stem cells into astrocytes. *Nature* **419**: 934–939

Hernán MA, Olek MJ, Ascherio A 1999 Geographic variation of MS incidence in two prospective studies of US women. *Neurology* **53**: 1711–1718

Hernán MA, Zhang SM, Lipworth L et al 2001a Multiple sclerosis and age at infection with common viruses. *Epidemiology* **12**: 301–306

Hernán MA, Olek MJ, Ascherio A 2001b Cigarette smoking and incidence of multiple sclerosis. *Amer J Epidem* **154**: 69–74

Hernán MA, Jick SS, Olek MJ, Jick H 2004 Recombinant hepatitis B vaccine and the risk of multiple sclerosis: a prospective study. *Neurology* **63**: 838–842

Hernán MA, Jick SS, Logroscino G et al 2005 Cigarette smoking and the progression of multiple sclerosis. *Brain* **128**: 1461–1465

Hernandez MA 2002 Epidemiology of multiple sclerosis in the Canary Islands (Spain): a study on the island of La Palma. *J Neurol* **249**: 1378–1381

Herndon RM, Brooks B 1985 Misdiagnosis of multiple sclerosis. *Semin Neurol* **5**: 94–98

Herndon RM, Rubinstein LJ, Freeman JM, Mathieson G 1970 Light and electron microscopic observations on Rosenthal fibers in Alexander's disease and in multiple sclerosis. *J Neuropathol Exp Neurol* **29**: 524–551

Herrera DG, Garcia-Verdugo JM, Alvarez-Buylla A 1999 Adult-derived neural precursors transplanted into multiple regions in the adult brain. *Ann Neurol* **46**: 867–877

Herrnstadt C, Elson JL, Fahy E et al 2002 Reduced-median-network analysis of complete mitochondrial DNA coding-region sequences for the major African, Asian, and European haplogroups. *Am J Hum Genet* **70**: 1152–1171

Herroelen L, de Keyser J, Eginger G 1991 Central-nervous-system demyelination after immunisation with recombinant hepatitis B vaccine. *Lancet* **338**: 1174–1175

Hess CW, Mills KR, Murray NMF 1986 Measurement of central motor conduction in multiple sclerosis by magnetic brain stimulation. *Lancet* **ii**: 355–358

Hess CW, Mills KR, Murray NMF, Schriefer TN 1987 Magnetic brain stimulation: central motor conduction studies in multiple sclerosis. *Ann Neurol* **22**: 744–752

Heun R, Sliwka U, Ruttinger H, Schimrigk 1992 Intrathecal versus systemic corticosteroids in the treatment of multiple sclerosis: results of a pilot study. *J Neurol* **239**: 31–35

Heyer E 1995 Mitochondrial and nuclear genetic contribution of female founders to a contemporary population in northeast Quebec. *Am J Hum Genet* **56**: 1450–1455

Heyes MP, Achim CL, Wiley CA et al 1996 Human microglia convert l-tryptophan into the neurotoxin quinolinic acid. *Biochem J* **320**: 595–597

Hickey WF 1991 Migration of hematogenous cells through the blood brain barrier and the initiation of CNS inflammation. *Brain Pathol* **1**: 97–105

Hickey WF 2001 Basic principles of immunological surveillance of the normal central nervous system. *Glia* **36**: 118–124

Hickey WF, Gonatas NK 1984 Suppressor T-lymphocytes in the spinal cord of Lewis rats recovered from acute experimental allergic encephalomyelitis. *Cell Immunol* **85**: 284–288

Hickey WF, Kimura H 1988 Perivascular microglial cells of the CNS are bone-marrow derived and present antigen *in vivo*. *Science* **239**: 290–293

Hickey WF, Osborn JP, Kirby WM 1985 Expression of Ia molecules by astrocytes during acute experimental allergic encephalomyelitis in the Lewis rat. *Cell Immunol* **91**: 528–535

Hickey WF, Hsu BL, Kimura H 1991 T-lymphocyte entry into the central nervous system. *J Neurosci Res* **28**: 254–260

Hickey WF, Vass K, Lassmann H 1992 Bone marrow-derived elements in the central nervous system: an immunohistochemical and ultrastructural survey of rat chimeras. *J Neuropathol Exp Neurol* **51**: 246–256

Hickman SJ, Brex PA, Brierley CMH et al 2001 Detection of optic nerve atrophy following a single episode of unilateral optic neuritis by MRI using a fat-saturated short-echo fast FLAIR sequence. *Neuroradiology* **43**: 123–128

Hickman SJ, Brierley CM, Brex PA et al 2002a Continuing optic nerve atrophy following optic neuritis: a serial MRI study. *Mult Scler* **8**: 339–342

Hickman SJ, Dalton CM, Miller DH, Plant GT 2002b Management of acute optic neuritis. *Lancet* **360**: 1953–1962

Hickman SJ, Kapoor R, Jones SJ et al 2003 Corticosteroids do not prevent optic nerve atrophy following optic neuritis. *J Neurol Neurosurg Psychiatry* **74**: 1139–1141

Hickman SJ, Toosy AT, Miszkiel KA et al 2004a Visual recovery following acute optic neuritis: a clinical, electrophysiological and magnetic resonance imaging study. *J Neurol* **251**: 996–1005

Hickman SJ, Toosy AT, Jones SJ et al 2004b A serial MRI study following optic nerve mean area in acute optic neuritis. *Brain* **127**: 2498–2505

Hickman SJ, Toosy AT, Jones SJ et al 2004c Serial magnetization transfer imaging in acute optic neuritis. *Brain* **127**: 692–700

Hierons R, Lyle TK 1959 Bilateral retrobulbar neuritis. *Brain* **82**: 56–67

Hietaharju A, Peltola J, Seppa J et al 2001 The coexistence of systemic lupus erythematosus and multiple sclerosis in a mother and daughter. *Scand J Rheumatol* **30**: 120–122

Higgins PJ, Weiner HL 1988 Suppression of experimental autoimmune encephalomyelitis by oral administration of myelin basic protein and its fragments. *J Immunol* **140**: 440–445

Hill AB 1952 Assessment of therapeutic trials. *Trans Med Soc* **68**: 128–147

Hill KE, Zollinger LV, Watt HE et al 2004 Inducible nitric oxide synthase in chronic active multiple sclerosis plaques: distribution, cellular expression and association with myelin damage. *J Neuroimmunol* **151**: 171–179

Hillary FG, Chiaravalloti ND, Ricker JH et al 2003 An investigation of working memory rehearsal in multiple sclerosis using fMRI. *J Clin Exp Neuropsychol* **25**: 965–978

Hille B 1992 *Ionic Channels of Excitable Membranes*, 2nd edn. Sunderland, MA: Sinauer Associates

Hillert J 1993 Immunoglobulin constant region gene polymorphisms in multiple sclerosis. *J Neuroimmunol* **43**: 9–14

Hillert J 1994 Human leucocyte antigen studies in multiple sclerosis. *Ann Neurol* **36** **(Suppl)**: S15–S17

Hillert J, Olerup O 1993 Multiple sclerosis is associated with genes within or close to the HLA-DR-DQ sub-region on a normal DR15 DQ6, Dw2 haplotype. *Neurology* **43**: 163–168

Hillert J, Leng C, Olerup O 1991 No association with germline T cell receptor beta chain alleles or haplotypes in Swedish patients with multiple sclerosis. *J Neuroimmunol* **31**: 141–147

Hillert J, Gronnig M, Nyland H et al 1992a Immunogenetic heterogeneity in multiple sclerosis. *J Neurol Neurosurg Psychiatry* **55**: 887–890

Hillert J, Leng C, Olerup O 1992b T-cell receptor alpha-chain gene germline polymorphisms in multiple sclerosis. *Neurology* **42**: 80–84

Hillert J, Kall T, Vrethem M et al 1994 The HLA-Dw2 haplotype segregates closely with multiple sclerosis in multiplex families. *J Neuroimmunol* **50**: 95–100

Hilliard B, Samoilova EB, Liu TS et al 1999 Experimental autoimmune encephalomyelitis in NF-kappa B-deficient mice: roles of NF-kappa B in the activation and differentiation of autoreactive T cells. *J Immunol* **163**: 2937–2943

Hilton AA, Slavin AJ, Hilton DJ, Barnard CCA 1995 Characterisation of cDNA and genomic clones encoding human myelin oligodendrocyte glycoprotein. *J Neurochem* **65**: 309–318

Hilton J 1876 *On Rest and Pain. A course of lectures on the influence of mechanical and physiological rest in the treatment of accidents and surgical diseases and the diagnostic value of pain.* London: Bell & Sons

Hilton P, Hertogs, Stanton SL 1983 The use of desmopressin (DDAVP) for nocturia in women with multiple sclerosis. *J Neurol Neurosurg Psychiatry* **46**: 854–855

Hindley DT, Newton RW, Clarke MA et al 1993 Steroid-responsive relapsing encephalopathy presenting in young children. *Neuropediatrics* **24**: 182

Hinds J, Eidelman B, Wald A 1990 Prevalence of bowel dysfunction in multiple sclerosis. *Gastroenterology* **98**: 1538–1542

Hinks GL, Franklin RJ 2000 Delayed changes in growth factor gene expression during slow remyelination in the CNS of aged rats. *Mol Cell Neurosci* **16**: 542–556

Hinks LJ, Price SE, Mason CR et al 1995 Single strand conformation analysis of two genes within the first intron of the neurofibromatosis type I gene in patients with multiple sclerosis. *Neuropathol Appl Neurobiol* **21**: 201–207

Hinrichs DJ, Humphres RC 1983 The response of the nude (athymic) rat to actively induced and transferred experimental allergic encephalomyelitis. *J Immunol* **131**: 4–5

Hirschberg DL, Schwartz M 1995 Macrophage recruitment to acutely injured central nervous system is inhibited by a resident factor: a basis for an immune-brain barrier. *J Neuroimmunol* **61**: 89–96

Hirschbiegel H 1967 Remittierende Verlaüfe bei Spinaltumoren. *Dtsch Z Nervenheilk* **190**: 74–82

Hisahara S, Shoji S, Okano H, Miura M 1997 ICE-CED-3 family executes oligodendrocyte apoptosis by tumor necrosis factor. *J Neurochem* **69**: 10–20

Hjalgrim H, Rasmussen S, Rostgaard K et al 2004 Familial clustering of Hodgkin lymphoma and multiple sclerosis. *J Ntal Cancer Inst* **96**: 780–784

Hjelmström P, Juedes AE, Fjell J, Ruddle NH 1998a B cell deficient mice develop experimental allergic encephalomyelitis with demyelination after myelin oligodendrocyte glycoprotein immunization. *J Immunol* **161**: 4480–4483

Hjelmström P, Juedes AE, Ruddle NH 1988b Cytokines and antibodies in myelin oligodendrocyte glycoprotein-induced experimental allergic encephalomyelitis. *Res Immunol* **149**: 794–804; 847–848; 855–860

Hjorth RJ, Willison RG 1973 The electromyogram in facial myokymia and hemifacial spasm. *J Neurol Sci* **20**: 117–126

Ho H-Z, Tiwari JL, Haile RW, Terasaki PI, Morton NE 1982 HLA-linked and unlinked determinants of multiple sclerosis. *Immunogenetics* **15**: 509–517

Ho KL, Wolfe DE 1981 Concurrence of multiple sclerosis and primary intracranial neoplasms. *Cancer* **47**: 2913–2919

Hobart JC 2002 Measuring disease impact in disabling neurological conditions: are patients' perspectives and scientific rigor compatible? *Curr Opin Neurol* **15**: 721–724

Hobart JC, Thompson AJ 2002 Measurement of neurological outcomes. In: Asbury AK, McKhann G, McDonald WI et al (eds) *Diseases of the Nervous System*, 3rd edn, 2 vols. Cambridge: Cambridge University Press, pp. 105–117

Hobart JC, Lamping DL, Thompson AJ 1996 Evaluating neurological outcome measures: the bare essentials. *J Neurol Neurosurg Psychiatry* **60**: 127–130

Hobart JC, Freeman JA, Thompson AJ 2000 Kurtzke scales revisited: the application of psychometric methods to clinical intuition. *Brain* **123**: 1027–1040

Hobart JC, Lamping D, Fitzpatrick R et al 2001 The Multiple Sclerosis Impact Scale (MSIS-29): a new patient-based outcome measure. *Brain* **124**: 962–973

Hobart JC, Riazi A, Lampling DL et al 2003 Measuring the impact of MS on walking ability: the 12-item MS Walking Scale (MSWS-12). *Neurology* **60**: 31–36

Hochberg MC 1997 Updating the American College of Rheumatology revised criteria for the classification of systemic lupus erythematosus. *Arthritis Rheum* **40**: 1725

Hockertz MK, Paty DW, Beall SS 1998 Susceptibility to relapsing progressive multiple sclerosis is associated with inheritance of a gene linked to the variable region of the TcR beta chain locus: use of affected family-based controls. *Am J Hum Genet* **62**: 373–385

Hoefsmit ECM, Duijvestijn AM, Kamperdijk EWA 1982 Relation between Langerhans cells, veiled cells, and interdigitating cells. *Immunobiology* **161**: 255–265

Hoek RM, Ruuls SR, Murphy CA et al 2000 Down-regulation of the macrophage lineage through interaction with OX2 (CD200). *Science* **290**: 1768–1771

Hofbauer M, Wiesener S, Babbe H et al 2003 Clonal tracking of autoaggressive T cells in polymyositis by combining laser microdissection, single-cell PCR, and CDR3- spectratype analysis. *Proc Natl Acad Sci USA* **100**: 4090–4095

Hoffman HI 1955 Acute necrotic myelopathy. *Brain* **78**: 377–393

Hoffman RE, Zack MM, Davis LE, Burchfiel CM 1981 Increased incidence and prevalence of multiple sclerosis in Los Alamos County, New Mexico. *Neurology* **31**: 1489–1492

Hoffmann JA, Kafatos FC, Janeway CA, Ezekowitz RAB 1999 Phylogenetic perspectives in innate immunity. *Science* **284**: 1313–1318

Hoffmann V, Pohlau D, Przuntek H et al 2002 A null mutation within the ciliary neurotrophic factor (CNTF) gene: implications for susceptibility and disease severity in patients with multiple sclerosis. *Genes Immun* **3**: 53–55

Hofman FM, Hinton DR, Johnson K, Merrill JE 1989 Tumour necrosis factor identified in multiple sclerosis brain. *J Exp Med* **170**: 607–612

Höfteberger R, Aboul-Enein F, Brueck W et al 2004 Expression of major histocompatibiltiy complex Class I molecules on the different cell types in multiple sclerosis lesions. *Brain Pathol* **14**: 43–50

Hogan EL, Krigman MNL 1973 Herpes zoster myelitis. *Arch Neurol* **29**: 309–313

Hogg N 2002 The biochemistry and physiology of s-nitrosothiols. *Ann Rev Pharmacol Toxicol* **42**: 585–600

Hogh P, Oturai A, Schreiber K et al 2000 Apoliprotein E and multiple sclerosis: impact of the epsilon-4 allele on susceptibility, clinical type and progression rate. *Mult Scler* **6**: 226–230

Hohlfeld R 1997 Biotechnological agents for the immunotherapy of multiple sclerosis: principles, problems and perspectives. *Brain* **120**: 865–916

Hohlfeld R, Wekerle H 2004 Autoimmune concepts of multiple sclerosis as a basis for selective immunotherapy: from pipe dreams to (therapeutic) pipelines. *Proc Natl Acad Sci USA* **101**: 14599–14606

Hohlfeld R, Wekerle H 2005 Drug Insight: Using monoclonal antibodies to treat multiple sclerosis. *Nature Clin Pract* **1**: 34–44

Hohlfeld R, Wiendl H 2001 The ups and downs of multiple sclerosis therapeutics. *Ann Neurol* **49**: 281–284

Hohlfeld R, Kerschensteiner M, Stadelmann C et al 2000 The neuroprotective effect of inflammation: implications for the therapy of multiple sclerosis. *J Neuroimmunol* **107**: 161–166

Hohol MJ, Guttmann CR, Orav J et al 1997 Serial neuropsychological assessment and magnetic resonance imaging analysis in multiple sclerosis. *Arch Neurol* **54**: 1018–1025

Hohol MJ, Olek MJ, Orav EJ et al 1999 Treatment of progressive multiple sclerosis

861

with pulse cyclophosphamide/ methylprednisolone: response to therapy is linked to the duration of progressive disease. *Mult Scler* **5**: 403–409

Hoitsma E, Faber CG, Drent M, Sharma OP 2004 Neurosarcoidosis: a clinical dilemma. *Lancet Neurol* **3**: 397–407

Hoke A, Silver J 1994 Heterogeneity among astrocytes in reactive gliosis. *Pers Dev Neurobiol* **2**: 269–274

Hollinger P, Sturzenegger M, Mathis J *et al* 2002 Acute disseminated encephalomyelitis in adults: a reappraisal of clinical, CSF, EEG and MRI findings. *J Neurol* **249**: 320–329

Holmans P 1993 Asymptotic properties of affected sib-pair linkage analysis. *Am J Hum Genet* **52**: 362–374

Holmes FF, Stubbs DW, Larsen WE 1967 Systemic lupus erythematosus and multiple sclerosis in identical twins. *Arch Int Med* **119**: 302–304

Holmes G 1906 On the relation between loss of function and structural change in focal lesions of the central nervous system, with special reference to secondary degeneration. *Brain* **29**: 514–523

Holmes G 1922 Clinical symptoms of cerebellar disease and their interpretation. Lancet i: 1177–82, 1231–37; ii: 59–65, 111–115

Holscher C 1997 Nitric oxide, the enigmatic neuronal messenger: its role in synaptic plasticity. *Trends Neurosci* **20**: 298–303

Holt GR, Koch C 1999 Electrical interactions via the extracellular potential near cell bodies. *J Computational Neurosci* **6**: 169–184

Holt S, Hudgins D, Krishnan KR, Critchley EM 1976 Diffuse myelitis associated with rubella vaccination. *Br Med J* **2**: 1037–1038

Hommes OR, Sorensen PS, Fazekas F *et al* for the European Study on Immunoglobulin in multiple sclerosis trialists 2004 Intravenous immunoglobulin in secondary progressive multiple sclerosis: randomised placebo-controlled trial. *Lancet* **364**: 1149–1156

Honan WP, Heron JR, Foster DH *et al* 1990 Visual loss in multiple sclerosis and its relation to previous optic neuritis, disease duration and clinical classification. *Brain* **113**: 975–987

Hong S, Scherer DC, Singh N *et al* 1999 Lipid antigen presentation in the immune system: lessons learned from CD1d knock-out mice. *Immunol Rev* **169**: 44

Hong S, Wilson MT, Serizawa I *et al* 2001 The natural killer T-cell ligand α-galactosyl-ceramide prevents autoimmune diabetes in non-obese diabetic mice. *Nature Med* **7**: 1052–1056

Honig LS 1992 Paroxysmal kinesigenic choreoathetosis. *J Neurol Neurosurg Psychiatry* **55**: 982

Honkaniemi J, Dastidar P, Kahara V, Haapasalo H 2001 Delayed MR imaging changes in acute disseminated encephalomyelitis. *Am J Neuroradiol* **22**:1117–1124

Honmou O, Utzschneider DA, Rizzo MA *et al* 1994 Delayed depolarization and slow sodium currents in cutaneous afferents. *J Neurophysiol* **71**: 1627–1637

Honmou O, Felts PA, Waxman SG, Kocsis JD 1996 Restoration of normal conduction properties in demyelinated spinal cord axons in the adult rat by transplantation of exogenous Schwann cells. *J Neurosci* **16**: 3199–3208

Honnorat J, Saiz A, Giometto B *et al* 2001 Cerebellar ataxia with anti-glutamic acid decarboxylase antibodies: study of 14 patients. *Arch Neurol* **58**: 225–230

Hooge JP, Redekop WK 1992 Multiple sclerosis with very late onset. *Neurology* **42**: 1907–1910

Hooge JP, Redekop WK 1995 Trigeminal neuralgia in multiple sclerosis. *Neurology* **45**: 1294–1296

Hoogervorst ELJ, Kalkers NF, van Winsen LML *et al* 2001 Differential treatment effect on measures of neurologic exam, functional impairment and patient self-report in multiple sclerosis. *Mult Scler* **7**: 335–339

Hoogervorst ELJ, Polman CH, Barkhof F 2002 Cerebral volume changes in multiple sclerosis patients treated with high-dose intravenous methylprednisolone. *Mult Scler* **8**: 415–419

Hoogervorst ELJ, Zwemmer JNP, Jelles B *et al* 2004 Multiple Sclerosis Impact Scale (MSIS-29): relation to established measures of impairment and disability. *Mult Scler* **10**: 569–574

Hoogstraten MC, Minderhoud JM 1990 Long term effect of ACTH treatment of relapse in multiple sclerosis. *Acta Neurol Scand* **82**: 74–77

Hoogstraten MC, Cats A, Minderhoud JM 1987 Bed rest and ACTH in the treatment of exacerbations in multiple sclerosis patients. *Acta Neurol Scand* **76**: 346–350

Hoogstraten MC, van der Ploeg RJO, Burg W vd, Vreeling A, van Marle S, Minderhoud JM 1988 Tizanidine versus baclofen in the treatment of spasticity in multiple sclerosis patients. *Acta Neurol Scand* **77**: 224–230

Hooper DC, Bagasra O, Marini JC *et al* 1997 Prevention of experimental allergic encephalomyelitis by targeting nitric oxide and peroxynitrite: implications for the treatment of multiple sclerosis. *Proc Natl Acad Sci USA* **94**: 2528–2533

Hooper DC, Scott GS, Zborek A *et al* 2000 Uric acid, a peroxynitrite scavenger, inhibits CNS inflammation, blood–CNS barrier permeability changes, and tissue damage in a mouse model of multiple sclerosis. *J Fed Am Soc Exp Biol* **14**: 691–698

Hooper J, Whittle IR 1998 Long-term outcome after thalamotomy for movement disorders in multiple sclerosis. *Lancet* **352**: 1984

Hooper R 1826 *The Morbid Anatomy of the Human Brain, illustrated by coloured engravings of the most frequent and important organic diseases to which that viscus is the subject.* London: Longman, Rees, Orme, Brown & Longman

Hooper-van Veen T, Schrijver HM, Zwiers A *et al* 2003 The interleukin-1 gene family in multiple sclerosis susceptibility and disease course. *Mult Scler* **9**: 535–539

Hopf HC, Stamatovic AM, Wahren W 1970 Die cerebralen Anfällen bei der multiplen Sklerose. *J Neurol* **198**: 256–279

Hopkins RS, Indian RW, Pinnow E, Conomy J 1991 Multiple sclerosis in Galion, Ohio: prevalence and results of a case-control study. *Neuroepidemiology* **10**: 192–199

Hopkins SJ, Rothwell NJ 1995 Cytokines and the nervous system. 1: Expression and recognition. *Trends Neurosci* **18**: 83–88

Hopper CL, Matthews CG, Cleeland CS 1972 Symptom instability and thermoregulation in multiple sclerosis. *Neurology* **22**: 142–148

Hornabrook RSL, Miller DH, Newton MR *et al* 1992 Frequent involvement of the optic radiation in patients with acute isolated optic neuritis. *Neurology* **42**: 77–79

Hornabrook RW 1971 The prevalence of multiple sclerosis in New Zealand. *Acta Neurol Scand* **47**: 426–438

Horner PJ, Power AE, Kempermann G *et al* 2000 Proliferation and differentiation of progenitor cells throughout the intact adult rat spinal cord. *J Neurosci* **20**: 2218–2228

Horton BT, Wagener HP 1948 Retrobulbar neuritis treatment with histamine. *J Lab Clin Med* **33**: 1611–1612

Horton BT, Wagener HP Aiat JA, Woltman HW 1944 Treatment of multiple sclerosis by the intravenous administration of histamine. *J Am Med Assoc* **124**: 800–801

Horton R, Wilming L, Rand V *et al* 2004 Gene map of the extended human MHC. *Nature Rev Genet* **5**: 889–899

Horvath R, Abicht A, Shoubridge EA *et al* 2000 Leber's hereditary optic neuropathy presenting as multiple sclerosis-like disease of the CNS. *J Neurol* **247**: 65–67

Hosokawa M, Klegeris A, Maguire J, McGeer PL 2003 Expression of complement messenger RNAs and proteins by human oligodendroglial cells. *Glia* **42**: 417–423

Hostetler JA 1974 *The Hutterite Society.* Baltimore, MD: Johns Hopkins University Press

Hostettler ME, Knapp PE, Carlson SL 2002 Platelet-activating factor induces cell death in cultured astrocytes and oligodendrocytes: involvement of caspase-3. *Glia* **38**: 228–239

Hotopf MH, Pollock S, Lishman WA 1994 An unusual presentation of multiple sclerosis. *Psychol Med* **24**: 525–528

Hou JB, Zhang ZX 1992 Prevalence of multiple sclerosis: a door to door survey in Lan Cang La Hu Zu autonomous county, Yunnan Province of China. *Neuroepidemiology* **11**: 52

Houshmand M, Sanati MH, Rashedi I *et al* 2004 Lack of association between Leber's hereditary optic neuropathy primary point mutations and multiple sclerosis in Iran. *Eur Neurol* **51**: 68–71

Houtchens MK, Richert JR, Sami A, Rose JW 1997 Open label gabapentin treatment for pain in multiple sclerosis. *Mult Scler* **3**: 250–253

Houzen H, Niino M, Kikuchi S *et al* 2003 The prevalence and clinical characteristic of MS in northern Japan. *J Neurol Sci* **211**: 49–53

Hoverd PA, Fowler CJ 1998 Desmopressin in the treatment of daytime urinary frequency in patients with multiple sclerosis. *J Neurol Neurosurg Psychiatry* **65**: 778–780

Howard AK, Li DKB, Oger J 2003 MRI contributes to the differentiation between MS and HTLV-1 associated myelopathy in British Columbian coastal natives. *Can J Neurol Sci* **30**: 41–48

Howard RS, Wiles CM, Hirsch NP, Loh L, Spencer GT, Newsom-Davis J 1992 Respiratory involvement in multiple sclerosis. *Brain* **115**: 479–494

Howard RS, Greenwood R, Gawler J et al 1993 A familial disorder associated with palatal myoclonus, other brainstem signs, tetraparesis, ataxia and Rosenthal fibre formation. *J Neurol Neurosurg Psychiatry* **56**: 977–981

Howe JF, Calvin WH, Loeser JD 1976 Impulses reflected from dorsal root ganglia and from focal nerve injuries. *Brain Res* **116**: 139–144

Howell MD, Winters ST, Olee T et al 1989 Vaccination against experimental allergic encephalomyelitis with T cell receptor peptides. *Science* **246**: 668–670

Howell WM, Sage DA, Evans PR et al 1991 No association between susceptibility to multiple sclerosis and HLA-DPB1 alleles in the French Canadian population. *Tissue Antigens* **37**: 156–160

Hsieh J, Aimone JB, Kaspar BK et al 2004 IGF-I instructs multipotent adult neural progenitor cells to become oligodendrocytes. *J Cell Biol* **164**: 111–122

Hu S, Sheng WS, Ehrlich LC et al 2000 Cytokine effects on glutamate uptake by human astrocytes. *Neuroimmunomodulation* **7**: 153–159

Hua LL, Liu JSH, Brosnan CF, Lee SC 1998 Selective inhibition of human glial inducible nitric oxide synthase by interferon-beta: implications for multiple sclerosis. *Ann Neurol* **43**: 384–387

Huang C-C, Chu N-S, Chen T-J, Shaw M-S 1988 Acute haemorrhagic leucoencephalitis with a prolonged clinical course. *J Neurol Neurosurg Psychiatry* **51**: 870–874

Huang D, Han Y, Rani MR et al 2000 Chemokines and chemokine receptors in inflammation of the nervous system: manifold roles and exquisite regulation. *Immunol Rev* **177**: 52–67

Huang E, The BS, Zeck O et al 2002 Gamma knife radiosurgery for treatment of trigeminal neuralgia in multiple sclerosis patients. *Stereotactic Funct Neurosurg* **79**: 44–50

Huang QR, Teutsch SM, Buhler MMcW et al 2000 Evaluation of the Apo-1/Fas promoter Mva 1 polymorphism in multiple sclerosis. *Mult Scler* **6**: 14–18

Huang W-X, He B, Hillert J 1996 An interleukin-1 receptor antagonist gene polymorphism is not associated with multiple sclerosis. *J Neuroimmunol* **67**: 143–144

Huang YM, Hussien Y, Jin YP et al 2001a Multiple sclerosis: deficient in vitro responses of blood mononuclear cells to IFN-beta. *Acta Neurol Scand* **104**: 249–256

Huang YM, Hussien Y, Yarilin D et al 2001b Interferon-beta induces the development of type 2 dendritic cells. *Cytokine* **13**: 264–271

Huang YM, Kouwenhoven M, Jin YP et al 2001c Dendritic cells derived from patients with multiple sclerosis show high CD1a and low CD86 expression. *Mult Scler* **7**: 95–99

Huang YM, Stoyanova N, Jin YP et al 2001d Altered phenotype and function of blood dendritic cells in multiple sclerosis are modulated by IFN-beta and IL-10. *Clin Exp Immunol* **124**: 306–314

Hübbe P, Dam AM 1973 Spastic paraplegia of unknown origin: a follow-up of 32 patients. *Acta Neurol Scand* **49**: 536–542

Huber M, Bamborschke S, Assheuer J, Heib WD 1988 Intravenous natural beta interferon treatment of chronic exacerbating-remitting multiple sclerosis: clinical response and MRI/CSF findings. *J Neurol* **235**: 171–173

Huber O 1895 Zur patholischen Anatomie der multiplen Sklerose der Ruckenmarks. *Arch pathologische Anat* **140**: 396–410

Huber S, Kappos L, Fuhr P et al 1999 Combined acute disseminated encephalomyelitis and acute motor axonal neuropathy after vaccination for hepatitis A and infection with *Campylobacter jejuni*. *J Neurol* **246**: 1204–1206

Hughes GRV 1983 Thrombosis, abortion, cerebral disease and the lupus anticoagulant. *Br Med J* **287**: 1088–1089

Hughes GRV 2003 Migraine, memory loss, and 'multiple sclerosis': neurological features of the antiphospholipid (Hughes) syndrome. *Postgrad Med J* **79**: 81–83

Hughes JC, Enderby PM, Langton HR 1994 Dysphagia and multiple sclerosis: a study and discussion of its nature and impact. *Clin Rehab* **8**: 18–26

Hughes JT 1978 *Pathology of the Spinal Cord*, 2nd edn. London: Lloyd-Luke

Hughes PJ, Kirk PF, Dyas J et al 1988 Factors influencing circulating OKT8 cell phenotypes in patients with multiple sclerosis. *J Neurol Neurosurg Psychiatry* **50**: 1156–1159

Hughes RAC, Mair WGP 1977 Acute necrotic myelopathy with pulmonary tuberculosis. *Brain* **100**: 223–238

Huh GS, Boulanger LM, Du H et al 2000 Functional requirement for class I MHC in CNS development and plasticity. *Science* **290**: 2155–2159

Huitinga I, Van Rooijen N, De Groot CJA et al 1990 Suppression of experimental allergic encephalomyelitis in Lewis rats after elimination of macrophages. *J Exp Med* **172**: 1025–1033

Huitinga I, Ruuls SR, Jung S et al 1995 Macrophages in T cell line mediated, demyelinating, and chronic-relapsing experimental autoimmune encephalomyelitis in Lewis rats. *Clin Exp Immunol* **100**: 344–351

Huitinga I, Erkut ZA, van Beurden D, Swabb DF 2004 Impaired hypothalamus-pituitary-adrenal axis activity and more severe multiple sclerosis with hypothalamic lesions. *Ann Neurol* **55**: 37–45

Huizar P, Kuno M, Miyata Y 1975 Electrophysiological properties of spinal motoneurones of normal and dystrophic mice. *J Physiol* **248**: 231–246

Huizinga TWJ, Westendorp RGJ, Bollen ELEM et al 1997 TNF-α promotor polymorphisms, production and susceptibility to multiple sclerosis in different groups of patients. *J Neuroimmunol* **72**: 149–153

Hull TP, Bates JH 1997 Optic neuritis after influenza vaccination. *Am J Ophthalmol* **124**: 703–704

Hulshof S, Montagne L, DeGroot CJ, Van der Valk P 2002 Cellular localization and expression patterns of interleukin-10, interleukin-4 and their receptors in multiple sclerosis lesions. *Glia* **38**: 24–35

Hulter BM, Lundberg PO 1995 Sexual function in women with advanced multiple sclerosis. *J Neurol Neurosurg Psychiatry* **59**: 83–86

Hume AL, Waxman SG 1988 Evoked potentials in suspected multiple sclerosis: diagnostic value and prediction of clinical course. *J Neurol Sci* **83**: 191–210

Hung T-P 1982 MS in Taiwan – a reappraisal. In: Kuroiwa Y, Kurland L (eds) *Multiple Sclerosis: East and West*. Fukuoka, Japan: Kyuhu University Press, pp. 83–96

Hunter KE, Sporn MB, Davies AM 1993 Transforming growth factor-betas inhibit mitogen-stimulated proliferation of astrocytes. *Glia* **7**: 203–211

Hunter MI, Nlemadim BC, Davidson DL 1985 Lipid peroxidation products and antioxidant proteins in plasma and cerebrospinal fluid from multiple sclerosis patients. *Neurochem Res* **10**: 1645–1652

Hunter SB, Ballinger WE, Rubin JJ 1987 Multiple sclerosis mimicking primary brain tumour. *Arch Pathol Lab Med* **111**: 464–468

Hunter SF, Hafler DA 2000 Ubiquitous pathogens: links between infection and autoimmunity in MS? *Neurology* **55**:164–165

Huntley GW, Benson DL, Colman DR 2002 Structural remodeling of the synapse in response to physiological activity. *Cell* **108**: 1–4

Hupperts R, Broadley S, Mander A et al 2001 Patterns of disease in concordant parent-child pairs with multiple sclerosis. *Neurology* **57**: 290–295

Hurst EW 1941 Acute haemorrhagic leuco-encephalitis, a previously undefined entity. *Med J Aust* **2**: 1–6

Huseby ES, Liggitt D, Brabb T et al 2001 A pathogenic role for myelin-specific CD8+ T-cells in a model for multiple sclerosis. *J Exp Med* **194**: 669–676

Hussien Y, Sanna A, Soderstrom M et al 2001 Glatiramer acetate and IFN-beta act on dendritic cells in multiple sclerosis. *J Neuroimmunol* **121**: 102–110

Hutchins M, Weller RO 1986 Anatomical relationships of the pia mater to cerebral blood vessels in man. *Neurosurgery* **65**: 316–325

Hutchinson M 1993 Pregnancy in multiple sclerosis. *J Neurol Neurosurg Psychiatry* **56**: 1043–1045

Hutchinson M, Bresnihan B 1983 Neurological lupus erythematosus with tonic seizures simulating multiple sclerosis. *J Neurol Neurosurg Psychiatry* **46**: 583–585

Hutchinson WM 1976 Acute optic neuritis and the prognosis for multiple sclerosis. *J Neurol Neurosurg Psychiatry* **39**: 283–289

Hutter CDD, Laing P 1996 Multiple sclerosis: sunlight, diet, immunology and aetiology. *Med Hypotheses* **46**: 67–74

Huynh HK, Oger J, Dorovini-Zis K 1995 Interferon-β down-regulates interferon-γ induced class II molecule expression and morphological changes in primary cultures of human brain microvessel endothelial cells. *J Neuroimmunol* **60**: 63–73

Hwang JM, Chang BL, Park SS 2001 Leber's hereditary optic neuropathy mutations in Korean patients with multiple sclerosis. *Ophthalmologica* **215**: 398–400

Hyllested K 1956 *Disseminated Sclerosis in Denmark: Prevalence and Geographical Distribution*, Copenhagen: J Jorgensen

Hyllested K 1961 Lethality, duration, and mortality of disseminated sclerosis in Denmark. *Acta Psychiatr Scand* **36**: 553–564

Hyllested K 1966 On the prognosis of retrobulbar neuritis. *Acta Ophthalmol* **44**: 246–252

Hyman N, Barnes M, Bhakta B *et al* 2000 Botulinum toxin (Dysport) treatment of hip adductor spasticity in multiple sclerosis: a prospective, randomised, double blind, placebo controlled, dose ranging study. *J Neurol Neurosurg Psychiatry* **68**: 707–712

Hynson JL, Kornberg AJ, Coleman LT *et al* 2001 Clinical and neuroradiological features of acute disseminated encephalomyelitis in children. *Neurology* **56**: 1308–1312

Iannucci G, Mascalchi M, Salvi F, Filippi M 2000a Vanishing Balo-like lesions in multiple sclerosis. *J Neurol Neurosurg Psychiatry* **69**: 399–400

Iannucci G, Tortorella C, Rovaris M *et al* 2000b Prognostic value of MR and magnetization transfer imaging findings in patients with clinically isolated syndromes suggestive of multiple sclerosis at presentation. *Am J Neuroradiol* **21**: 1034–1038

Ibrahim MZM, Adams CWM 1963 The relationship between enzyme activity and neuroglia in plaques of multiple sclerosis. *J Neurol Neurosurg Psychiatry* **26**: 101–110

Ibrahim MZM, Adams CWM 1965 The relation between enzyme activity and neuroglia in early plaques of multiple sclerosis. *J Pathol Bacteriol* **90**: 239–243

Ibsen SJ, Clausen J 1995 Genetic susceptibility to multiple sclerosis may be linked to polymorphism of the myelin basic protein gene. *J Neurol Sci* **131**: 96–98

Idrissova ZhR, Boldyreva MN, Dekonenko EP *et al* 2003 Acute disseminated encephalomyelitis in children: clinical features and HLA-DR linkage. *Eur J Neurol* **10**: 537–546

IFNB Multiple Sclerosis Study Group 1993 Interferon beta-1b is effective in relapsing–remitting multiple sclerosis. 1. Clinical results of a multicenter, randomized, double-blind, placebo-controlled trial. *Neurology* **43**: 655–661

IFNB Multiple Sclerosis Study Group and the University of British Columbia MS/MRI Analysis Group 1995 Interferon beta-1b in the treatment of multiple sclerosis: final outcome of the randomised controlled trial. *Neurology* **45**: 1277–1285

IFNB Multiple Sclerosis Study Group and the University of British Columbia MS/MRI Analysis Group 1996 Neutralising antibodies during treatment of multiple sclerosis with interferon beta-1b: experience during the first three years. *Neurology* **47**: 889–894

Igarashi M, Schaumburg HH, Powers I *et al* 1976 Fatty acid abnormalities in adrenoleukodystrophy. *J Neurochem* **26**: 851–860

Ijdo JW, Conti-Kelly AM, Greco P *et al* 1999 Anti-phospholipid antibodies in patients with multiple sclerosis and MS-like illnesses: MS or APS? *Lupus* **8**: 109–115

Ikuta F, Zimmerman HM 1976 Distribution of plaques in seventy autopsy cases of multiple sclerosis in the United States. *Neurology* **26**: 26–28

Ikuta K, Ogura T, Shimizu A, Honjo T 1985 Low frequency of somatic mutation in β-chain variable region genes of human T cell receptors. *Proc Natl Acad Sci USA* **82**: 7701–7705

Illés Z, Kondo T, Newcombe J *et al* 2000 Differential expression of NK T cells Va24JaQ invariant TCR chain in the lesions of multiple sclerosis and chronic inflammatory demyelinating polyneuropathy. *J Immunol* **164**: 4375–4381

Ilonen J, Herva E, Reunanen M *et al* 1977 HLA antigens and antibody responses to measles and rubella viruses in multiple sclerosis. *Acta Neurol Scand* **55**: 299–309

Ilyas AA, Chen ZW, Cook SD 2003 Antibodies to sulfatides in the cerebrospinal fluid of patients with multiple sclerosis. *J Neuroimmunol* **139**: 76–80

Imaizumi T, Lankford KL, Waxman SG *et al* 1998 Transplanted olfactory ensheathing cells remyelinate and enhance axonal conduction in the demyelinated dorsal columns of the rat spinal cord. *J Neuroscience* **18**: 6176–6185

Imaizumi T, Lankford KL, Kocsis JD 2000 Transplantation of olfactory ensheathing cells or Schwann cells restores rapid and secure conduction across the transected spinal cord. *Brain Res* **854**: 70–78

Ingalls TH, Huguenin I, Ghent T 1989 Clustering of multiple sclerosis in Galion, Ohio, 1982–1985. *Am J Forensic Med Pathol* **10**: 213–215

Ingle GT, Stevenson VL, Miller DH, Thompson AJ 2003 Primary progressive multiple sclerosis: a 5-year clinical and MR study. *Brain* **126**: 2528–2536

Ingle GT, Sastre-Garriga J, Miller DH, Thompson AJ 2005 Is inflammation important in early PPMS? A longitudinal MRI study. *J Neurol Neurosurg Psychiatry* **76**: 1255–1258

Inglese M, Salvi F, Iannucci G *et al* 2002a Magnetization transfer and diffusion tensor MR imaging of acute disseminated encephalomyelitis. *Am J Neuradiol* **23**: 267–272

Inglese M, Ghezzi A, Bianchi S *et al* 2002b Irreversible disability and tissue loss in multiple sclerosis: a conventional and magnetization transfer magnetic resonance imaging study of the optic nerves. *Arch Neurol* **59**: 250–255

Inglese M, van Waesberghe JHTM, Rovaris M *et al* 2003 The effect of interferon β-1b on quantities derived from MT MRI in secondary progressive MS. *Neurology* **60**: 853–860

Inglese M, Mancardi GL, Pagani E *et al* 2004 Brain tissue loss occurs after suppression of enhancement in patients with multiple sclerosis treated with autologous haematopoietic stem cell transplantation. *J Neurol Neurosurg Psychiatry* **75**: 643–644

Ingram DA, Swash M, Thompson AJ 1987 Clinical evaluation of magnetic brain stimulation in degenerative and demyelinating disorders of the CNS. *Electroencephalogr Clin Neurophysiol* **66**: S122

Innes JRM, Kurland LT 1952 Is multiple sclerosis caused by a virus? *Am J Med* **12**: 574–585

International HapMap Consortium 2005 A haplotype map of the human genome. *Nature* **437**: 1299–1320

International Human Genome Sequencing Consortium 2001 Initial sequencing and analysis of the human genome. *Nature* **40**: 860–921

International Multiple Sclerosis Genetics Consortium 2005 A high density screen for linkage in multiple sclerosis. *Am J Hum Genet* **77**: 454–467

International Study Group for Behcet's Disease 1990 Criteria for diagnosis of Behcet's disease. *Lancet* **335**: 1078–1080

Ipsen J 1950 Life expectancy and probable disability in multiple sclerosis. *N Engl J Med* **243**: 909–913

Irani DN, Kerr DA 2000 14–3–3 protein in the cerebrospinal fluid of patients with acute transverse myelitis. *Lancet* **355**: 901

Iriarte J, De Castro P 2002 Fatigue is not associated with raised inflammatory markers in multiple sclerosis. *Neurology* **58**: 1134–1135

Iriarte J, Subira ML, Castro P 2000 Modalities of fatigue in multiple sclerosis: correlation with clinical and biological factors. *Mult Scler* **6**: 124–130

Isaac C, Li DK, Genton M *et al* 1988 Multiple sclerosis: a serial study using MRI in relapsing patients. *Neurology* **38**: 1511–1515

Isaacs JD, Watts RA, Hazleman BL *et al* 1992 Humanised monoclonal antibody therapy for rheumatoid arthritis. *Lancet* **340**: 748–752

Isager H, Anderson k, Hyllested K 1980 Risk of multiple sclerosis inversely associated with birth-order position. *Acta Neurol Scand* **61**: 393–396

Isayama Y, Takahashi T, Shimoyoma T, Yamadori A 1982 Acute optic neuritis and multiple sclerosis. *Neurology* **32**: 73–76

Isbister CM, Mackenzie PJ, Anderson D *et al* 2003 Co-occurrence of multiple sclerosis and myasthenia gravis in British Columbia. *Mult Scler* **9**: 550–553

Ishibashi M, McMahon AP 2002 A sonic hedgehog-dependent signaling relay regulates growth of diencephalic and mesencephalic primordia in the early mouse embryo. *Development* **129**: 4807–4819

Ishigami T, White CA, Pender MP 1998 Soluble antigen therapy induces apoptosis of autoreactive T cells preferentially in the target organ rather than in the peripheral lymphoid organs. *Eur J Immunol* **28**: 1626–1635

Ishikawa K, Tanaka M, Black JA, Waxman SG 1999 Changes in expression of voltage-gated potassium channels in dorsal root ganglion neurons following axotomy. *Muscle Nerve* **22**: 502–507

Isler W 1961 Multiple Sklerose im Kindersalter. *Helvetica Pediatrica Acta* **16**: 412–431

Issazadeh S, Ljungdahl Å, Höjeberg B *et al* 1995a Cytokine production in the central nervous system of Lewis rats with experimental autoimmune encephalomyelitis: dynamics of mRNA expression for interleukin-10, interleukin-12, cytolysin, tumor necrosis factor α and tumor necrosis factor β. *J Neuroimmunol* **61**: 205–212

Issazadeh S, Mustafa M, Ljungdahl Å *et al* 1995b Interferon γ, interleukin 4 and transforming growth factor β in experimental autoimmune encephalomyelitis in Lewis rats: dynamics of cellular mRNA expression in the central nervous system and lymphoid cells. *J Neurosci Res* **40**: 579–590

Issazadeh S, Navikas V, Schaub M *et al* 1998 Kinetics of expression of costimulatory molecules and their ligands in murine relapsing experimental autoimmune encephalomyelitis in vivo. *J Immunol* **161**: 1104–1112

Ito M, Blumberg BM, Mock DJ *et al* 2001 Potential environmental and host participants in the early white matter lesion of adreno-leukodystrophy: morphologic evidence for CD8 cytotoxic T cells, cytolysis of oligodendrocytes and CD1 mediated lipid antigen presentation. *J Neuropath Exp Neurol* **60**: 1004–1019

Itoh T, Aizawa H, Hashimoto K *et al* 2003 Prevalence of multiple sclerosis in Asahikawa, a city in northern Japan. *J Neurol Sci* **214**: 7–9

Itoyama Y, Sternberger NH, Webster HdeF *et al* 1980 Immunocytochemical observation on the distribution of myelin-associated glycoprotein and myelin basic protein in multiple sclerosis lesions. *Ann Neurol* **7**: 167–177

Itoyama Y, Webster HD, Sternberger NH *et al* 1982 Distribution of papovavirus, myelin associated glycoprotein, and myelin basic protein in progressive multifocal leukoencephalopathy lesions. *Ann Neurol* **11**: 396–404

Itoyama Y, Webster Hde F, Richardson EP Jr, Trapp BD 1983 Schwann cell remyelination of demyelinated axons in spinal cord multiple sclerosis lesions. *Ann Neurol* **14**: 339–346

Itoyama Y, Ohnishi A, Tateishi J *et al* 1985 Spinal cord multiple sclerosis lesions in Japanese patients: Schwann cell remyelination occurs in areas that lack glial fibrillary acidic protein. *Acta Neuropathol* **65**: 217–223

Ivanova A, Nakahira E, Kagawa T *et al* 2003 Evidence for a second wave of oligodendrogenesis in the postnatal cerebral cortex of the mouse. *J Neurosci Res* **73**: 581–92

Iversen L 2003 Cannabis and the brain. *Brain* **126**: 1252–1270

Ivnik RJ 1978 Neuropsychological test performance as a function of the duration of MS-related symptomatology. *J Clin Psychiatry* **39**: 304–307

Izikson L, Klein RS, Charo IF *et al* 2000 Resistance to experimental autoimmune encephalomyelitis in mice lacking the CC chemokine receptor (CCR)2. *J Exp Med* **192**: 1075–1080

Izquierdo G, Lyon-Caen O, Marteau R *et al* 1986 Early onset multiple sclerosis: clinical study of 12 pathologically proven cases. *Acta Neurol Scand* **73**: 493–497

Jabaily J, Thompson J 1997 Effects of interferon beta-1B in rheumatoid arthritis: a case report. *Arthritis Rheum* **40**: 1370

Jabs DA, Mill NR, Newman SA, Johnson MA, Stevens MB 1986 Optic neuropathy in systemic lupus erythematosus. *Arch Ophthalmol* **104**: 564–568

Jackson G, Miller M, Littlejohn G, Helme R, King R 1986 Bilateral internuclear ophthalmoplegia in systemic lupus erythematosus. *J Rheumatol* **13**: 1151–1162

Jacobs LD, O'Malley J, Freeman A, Ekes R 1981 Intrathecal interferon reduces exacerbations of multiple sclerosis. *Science* **214**: 1026–1028

Jacobs LD, O'Malley J, Freeman A, Ekes R 1982 Intrathecal interferon in multiple sclerosis. *Arch Neurol* **39**: 609–615

Jacobs LD, Kinkel PR, Kinkel WR 1986a Silent brain lesions in patients with isolated optic neuritis: a clinical and nuclear magnetic resonance imaging study. *Arch Neurol* **43**: 452–455

Jacobs LD, Salazar AM, Herndon R *et al* 1986b Multicenter double-blind study of effect of intrathecally administered natural human fibroblast interferon on exacerbations of multiple sclerosis. *Lancet* **ii**: 1411–1414

Jacobs LD, Salazar AM, Herndon R *et al* 1987 Intrathecally administered natural human fibroblast interferon reduces exacerbations of multiple sclerosis: results of a multicenter double-blind study. *Arch Neurol* **44**: 589–595

Jacobs LD, Munschauer FE, Kaba SE 1991 Clinical and magnetic resonance imaging in optic neuritis. *Neurology* **41**: 15–19

Jacobs LD, Kaba S, Pullicino P 1994 The lesion causing continuous facial myokymia in multiple sclerosis. *Arch Neurol* **51**: 1115–1119

Jacobs LD, Cookfair DL, Rudick RA *et al* 1995 A phase III trial of intramuscular recombinant interferon beta for exacerbating–remitting multiple sclerosis: design and conduct of study; baseline characteristics of patients. *Mult Scler* **1**: 118–135

Jacobs LD, Cookfair DL, Rudick RA *et al* 1996 Intramuscular interferon beta-1a for disease progression in relapsing multiple sclerosis. The Multiple Sclerosis Collaborative Research Group (MSCRG). *Ann Neurol* **39**: 285–294

Jacobs LD, Kaba SE, Miller CM *et al* 1997 Correlation of clinical, magnetic resonance imaging, and CSF findings in optic neuritis. *Ann Neurol* **41**: 392–398

Jacobs LD, Beck RW, Simon JH *et al* and the CHAMPS Study Group 2000 Intramuscular interferon beta-1a therapy initiated during a first demyelinating event in multiple sclerosis. *N Engl J Med* **343**: 898–904

Jacobsen M, Schweer D, Ziegler *et al* 2000 A point mutation in *PTPRC* is associated with the development of multiple sclerosis. *Nature Genet* **26**: 495–499

Jacobsen M, Cepok S, Quak E *et al* 2002 Oligoclonal expansion of memory CD8+ T cells in cerebrospinal fluid from multiple sclerosis patients. *Brain* **125**: 538–550

Jacobson DM, Thompson HS, Corbett JJ 1988 Optic neuritis in the elderly: prognosis for visual recovery and long-term follow up. *Neurology* **38**: 1834–1837

Jacobson DM, Marx JJ, Dlesk A 1991 Frequency and clinical significance of Lyme seropositivity in patients with isolated optic neuritis. *Neurology* **41**: 706–711

Jacobson DM, Moster ML Eggenberger ER *et al* 1999 Isolated trochlear nerve palsy in patients with multiple sclerosis. *Neurology* **53**: 877–879

Jacobson S, Flerlage ML, McFarland HF 1985 Impaired measles virus-specific cytotoxic T cell responses in multiple sclerosis. *J Exp Med* **162**: 839–850

Jacôme DE 1985 La toux diabolique: neurogenic tussive crises. *Postgrad Med J* **61**: 515–516

Jacôme DE 2001 Blepharoclonus in multiple sclerosis. *Acta Neurol Scand* **104**: 380–384

Jahng AW, Maricic I, Pedersen B *et al* 2001 Activation of natural killer T cells potentiates or prevents experimental autoimmune encephalomyelitis. *J Exp Med* **194**: 1789–1799

Jahnke U, Fischer EH, Alvord EC 1985 Sequence homology between certain viral proteins and proteins related to encephalomyelitis and neuritis. *Science* **229**: 282–284

865

Jain KK 2000 Evaluation of mitoxantrone for the treatment of multiple sclerosis. *Expert Opin Invest Drugs* **9**: 1139–1149

Jain S, Maheshwari M 1985 Multiple sclerosis: Indian experience in the last thirty years. *Neuroepidemiology* **4**: 96–107

Jain S, Proudlock F, Constantinescu CS, Gottlob I 2002 Combined pharmacologic and surgical approach to acquired nystagmus due to multiple sclerosis. *Am J Ophthalmol* **134**: 780–782

Jaing TH, Lin KL, Chiu CH et al 2001 Acute disseminated encephalomyelitis in autoimmune hemolytic anemia. *Pediatr Neurol* **24**: 303–305

James PB 1982 Evidence for subacute fat embolism as the cause of multiple sclerosis. *Lancet* i: 380–386

Jameson SC, Hogquist KA, Bevan MJ 1995 Positive selection in the thymus. *Ann Rev Immunol* **13**: 93–126

Jamieson J 1886 Cases of multiple neuritis. *Aust Med J* **8**: 295–302

Jander S, Stoll G 1998 Differential induction of interleukin-12, interleukin-18, and interleukin-1-beta converting enzyme mRNA in experimental autoimmune encephalomyelitis of the Lewis rat. *J Neuroimmunol* **91**: 93–99

Jander S, Heidenreich F, Stoll G 1993 Serum and CSF levels of solule intercellular adhesion molecule-1 (ICAM-1) in inflammatory neurologic diseases. *Neurology* **43**: 1809–1813

Janeway CA 1992 The T cell receptor as a multicomponent signalling machine: CD4/CD8 coreceptors and CD45 in T cell activation. *Ann Rev Immunol* **10**: 645–674

Jankovic BD, Waksman BH, Arnason BG 1962 Role of the thymus in response to bovine serum immune reactions in rats. The immunologic response to bovine serum albumin (antibody formation, Arthus reactivity, and delayed hypersensitivity) in rats thymectomised or splenectomised at various times after birth. *J Exp Med* **116**: 159–176

Jans H, Heltberg A, Zeeberg I, Kristensen JH, Fog T, Raun NE 1984 Immune complexes and the complement factors C4 and C3 in cerebrospinal fluid and serum from patients with chronic progressive multiple sclerosis. *Acta Neurol Scand* **69**: 34–38

Janssen RS, Kaplan JE, Khabbaz RF et al 1991 HTLV-1-associated myelopathy/tropical spastic paraparesis in the United States. *Neurology* **41**: 1355–1357

Jansson M, Panoutsakopoulos V, Baker J et al 2002 Cutting edge: attenuated experimental autoimmune encephalomyelitis in eta-1/osteopontin-deficient mice. *J Immunol* **168**: 2096–2099

Janzer RC, Raff MC 1987 Astrocytes induce blood brain barrier properties in endothelial cells. *Nature* **325**: 253–257

Jarrett L, Nandi P, Thompson AJ 2002 Managing severe lower limb spasticity in multiple sclerosis: does intrathecal phenol have a role? *J Neurol Neurosurg Psych* **73**: 705–709

Jean I, Allamargot C, Barthelaix-Pouplard A, Fressinaud C 2002 Axonal lesions and PDGF-enhanced remyelination in the rat corpus callosum after lysolecithin demyelination. *NeuroReport* **13**: 627–631

Jean I, Lavialle C, Barthelaix-Pouplard A, Fressinaud C 2003 Neurotrophin-3 specifically increases mature oligodendrocyte population and enhances remyelination after chemical demyelination of adult rat CNS. *Brain Res* **972**: 110–118

Jedlicka P, Benes B, Hron B et al 1994 Epidemiology of MS in the Czech Republic. In: Firnhaber W, Lauer K (eds) *Multiple Sclerosis in Europe: An Epidemiological Update*. Darmstadt: Leuchtturm-Verlag/LTV Press, pp. 261–265

Jeffery ND, Blakemore WF 1997 Locomotor deficits induced by experimental spinal cord demyelination are abolished by spontaneous remyelination. *Brain* **120**: 27–37

Jeffrey DR, Mandler RN, Davis LE 1993 Transverse myelitis: retrospective analysis of 33 cases with differentiation of cases associated with multiple sclerosis and parainfectious events. *Arch Neurol* **50**: 532–535

Jeffrey DR, Absher J, Pfeiffer FE, Jackson H 2000 Cortical deficits in multiple sclerosis on the basis of subcortical lesions. *Mult Scler* **6**: 50–55

Jeffreys AJ, Kauppi L, Neumann R 2001 Intensely punctate meiotic recombination in the class II region of the major histocompatibility complex. *Nature Genet* **29**: 217–22

Jellinek EH 1990 Heine's illness: the case for multiple sclerosis. *J R Soc Med* **83**: 516–519

Jellinger K 1969 Einige morphologïsche Aspekte der Multiplen Sklerose. *Wiener Z Nervenheilk* **Suppl II**: 12–37

Jenkins HG, Ikeda H 1992 Tumour necrosis factor causes an increase in axonal transport of protein and demyelination in the mouse optic nerve. *J Neurol Sci* **108**: 99–104

Jenkins MK, Khoruts A, Ingulli E et al 2001 In vivo activation of antigen specific CD4 T cells. *Annu Rev Immunol* **19**: 23–45

Jennekens-Schinkel A, van der Velde EA, Sanders EACM, Lanser JBK 1989 Visuospatial problem solving, conceptual reasoning and sorting behaviour in multiple sclerosis out-patients. *J Neurol Sci* **90**: 187–202

Jennekens-Schinkel A, Laboyrie PM, Lanser JBK, van der Velde EA 1990 Cognition in patients with multiple sclerosis after 4 years. *J Neurol Sci* **99**: 229–247

Jennett B 1996 Epidemiology of head injury. *J Neurol Neurosurg Psych* **60**: 362–369

Jennings AR, Kirilak Y, Carroll WM 2002 In situ characterisation of oligodendrocyte progenitor cells in adult mammalian optic nerve. *J Neurocytol* **31**: 27–39

Jensen PS, Rasmussen P, Reske-Nielsen E 1982 Association of trigeminal neuralgia with multiple sclerosis: clinical and pathological features. *Acta Neurol Scand* **65**: 182–185

Jepson RG, Mihaljevic L, Craig J 2004 Cranberries for preventing urinary tract infections. *Cochrane Database Syst Rev* 1: CD001321 and CD001321

Jersild C, Svejgaard A, Fog T 1972 HL-A antigens and multiple sclerosis. *Lancet* i: 1240–1241

Jersild C, Fog T, Hansen GS et al 1973 Histocompatibility determinants in multiple sclerosis, with special reference to clinical course. *Lancet* ii: 1221–1225

Jersild C, Kurtzke JF, Riisom K et al 1993 Multiple sclerosis in the Faroe Islands. VI Studies of HLA markers. *Tissue Antigens* **42**: 105–110

Jiang F, Frederick TJ, Wood TL 2001 IGF-I synergizes with FGF-2 to stimulate oligodendrocyte progenitor entry into the cell cycle. *Dev Biol* **232**: 414–423

Jiang GX, Cheng Q, Fredrikson S, Link H 1999 First hospital-admission rate as an epidemiological indicatotor for patients with multiple sclerosis in Stockholm 1984–1993. *Acta Neurol Scand* **100**: 64–68

Jiang H, Zhang S-L, Pernis B 1992 Role of CD8+ T cells in murine experimental allergic encephalomyelitis. *Science* **256**: 1213–1215

Jiang H, Milo R, Swoveland P et al 1995 Interferon β-1b reduces interferon γ-induced antigen-presenting capacity of human glial and B cells. *J Neuroimmunol* **61**: 17–25

Jiang H, Braunstein NS, Yu B et al 2001 CD8+ T cells control the TH phenotype of MBP-reactive CD4+ T cells in EAE mice. *Proc Natl Acad Sci USA* **98**: 6301–6306

Jiang Y, Jahagirdar BN, Reinhardt RL et al 2002 Pluripotency of mesenchymal stem cells derived from adult marrow. *Nature* **418**: 41–49

Jiang Y, Henderson D, Blackstad M et al 2003 Neuroectodermal differentiation from mouse multipotent adult progenitor cells. *Proc Natl Acad Sci USA* **100**: 11854–11860

Jimenez-Jimenez FJ, Zurdo JM, Hernanz A et al 2002 Tau protein concentrations in cerebrospinal fluid of patients with multiple sclerosis. *Acta Neurol Scand* **106**: 351–354

Jimi T, Wakayama 1993 Mexiletine for the treatment of spasticity due to neurological disorders. *Muscle Nerve* **16**: 885

Jin J-P, de Pedro-Cuesta J, Soderstrom M et al 1998 Incidence of optic neuritis in Stockholm, Sweden 1990–1995: I. Age, sex birth and ethnic-group related patterns. *J Neurol Sci* **159**: 107–114

Jin YP, de Pedro-Cuesta J, Soderstrom M, Link H 1999 Incidence of optic neuritis in Stockholm, Sweden, 1990–1995: II. Time and space patterns. *Arch Neurol* **56**: 975–980

Jin YP, de Pedro-Cuesta J, Soderstrom M et al 2000 Seasonal patterns in optic neuritis and multiple sclerosis: a meta-analysis. *J Neurol Sci* **181**: 56–64

Jin YP, de Pedro-Cuesta J, Huang YH, Soderstrom M 2003 Predicting multiple sclerosis at optic neuritis onset. *Mult Scler* 9: 135–141

Jing W, Patel M, Nathanson M et al 1998 Acute transverse myelitis associated with tuberculin skin test (PPD). *Neurology* 50: 1921–1922

Jirholt J, Lindqvist A, Karlsson J et al 2002 Identification of susceptibility genes for experimental autoimmune encephalomyelitis that overcome the effect of protective alleles at the eae2 locus. *Int Immunol* 14: 79–85

Joannides A, Gaughwin P, Scott M et al 2003 Postnatal astrocytes promote neural induction from adult human bone marrow-derived stem cells. *J Hematother Stem Cell Res* 12: 681–688

Joannides A, Gaughwin P, Schwicning C et al 2004 Efficient generation of neural precursors from adult human skin: astrocytes promote neurogenesis from skin-derived stem cells. *Lancet* 364: 172–178

Joensen P 1992 Parts of Faroese neuroepidemiology. *Ann Soci Sci Faeroensis* Suppl XVII: 32

Joffe RT, Lippert GP, Gray TA et al 1987 Mood disorder and multiple sclerosis. *Arch Neurol* 44: 376–378

Johansson CB, Momma S, Clarke DL et al 1999 Identification of a neural stem cell in the adult mammalian central nervous system. *Cell* 96: 25–34

John GR, Shankar SL, Shafit-Zagardo B et al 2002 Multiple sclerosis: re-expression of a developmental pathway that restricts oligodendrocyte maturation. *Nature Med* 8: 1115–1121

Johns CD, Flanders KC, Ranges GE, Sriram S 1991 Successful treatment of experimental allergic encephalomyelitis with transforming growth factor beta 1. *J Immunol* 147: 1792–1796

Johns LD, Sriram S 1993 Experimental allergic encephalomyelitis: neutralizing antibody to TGF beta 1 enhances the clinical severity of the disease. *J Neuroimmunol* 47: 1–7

Johns TG, Kerlero de Rosbo N, Menon KK et al 1995 Myelin oligodendrocyte glycoprotein induces a demyelinating encephalomyelitis resembling multiple sclerosis. *J Immunol* 154: 5536–5541

Johns TG, Bernard CC 1997 Binding of complement component Clq to myelin oligodendrocyte glycoprotein: a novel mechanism for regulating CNS inflammation. *Mol Immunol* 34: 33–38

Johnson GC, Esposito L, Barratt BJ et al 2001 Haplotype tagging for the identification of common disease genes. *Nature Genet* 29: 233–237

Johnson J 2003 On receiving the diagnosis of multiple sclerosis: managing the transition. *Mult Scler* 9: 82–88

Johnson KP, Knobler RL, Greenstein JL et al 1990 Recombinant human beta interferon treatment of relapsing–remitting multiple sclerosis: pilot study results. *Neurology* 40 (Suppl 1): 261 (abstract)

Johnson KP, Brooks BR, Cohen JA et al 1995 Copolymer 1 reduces relapse rate and improves disability in relapsing–remitting multiple sclerosis: results of a phase III multicenter, double-blind placebo-cxontrolled trial. *Neurology* 45: 1268–1276

Johnson KP, Brooks BR, Cohen JA et al 1998 Extended use of glatiramer acetate (Copaxone) is well tolerated and maintains its clinical effect on multiple sclerosis relapse rate and degree of disability. Copolymer 1 Multiple Sclerosis Study Group. *Neurology* 50: 701–708

Johnson KP, Brooks BR, Ford CC et al 2000 Sustained clinical benefits of glatiramer acetate in relapsing multiple sclerosis patients observed for 6 years. *Mult Scler* 6: 255–266

Johnson KP, Brooks BR, Cohen JA et al 2001 Extended use of glatiramer acetate (Copaxone) is well tolerated and maintains its clinical effect on multiple sclerosis relapse rate and degree of disability. 1998. *Neurology* 57: S46–S53

Johnson KP, Brooks BR, Ford CC et al 2003 Glatiramer acetate (Copaxone): comparison of continuous versus delayed therapy in a six-year organized multiple sclerosis trial. *Mult Scler* 9: 585–591

Johnson MR, Ferner RE, Bobrow M et al 2000 Detailed analysis of the oligodendrocyte myelin glycoprotein gene in four patients with neurofibromatosis 1 and primary progressive multiple sclerosis. *J Neurol Neurosurg Psychiatry* 68: 643–646

Johnson RT 1982 *Viral Infections of the Nervous System.* New York: Raven Press

Johnson RT 1994 The virology of demyelinating diseases. *Ann Neurol* 36 (Suppl): 54–60

Johnston JB, Silva C, Holden J et al 2001 Monocyte activation and differentiation augment human endogenous retrovirus expression: implications for inflammatory brain diseases. *Ann Neurol* 50: 434–442

Jolivet Reynaud C, Perron H, Ferrante P et al 1999 Specificities of multiple sclerosis cerebrospinal fluid and serum antibodies against mimotopes. *Clin Immunol* 93: 283–293

Jonasdottir A, Thorlacius T, Fossdal R et al 2003 A whole genome association study in Icelandic multiple sclerosis patients with 4804 markers. *J Neuroimmunol* 143: 88–92

Jones CK, Riddehough A, Li DKB et al 2001 MRI cerebral atrophy in relapsing remitting MS: results of the PRISMS trial. *Neurology* 56(Suppl 3): A379

Jones J, Frith S, Piddlesden S et al 1991 Imaging calcium changes in individual oligodendrocytes attacked by T cell derived perforin. *Immunology* 74: 572–577

Jones RE, Heron JR, Foster DH et al 1983 Effects of 4-aminopyridine in patients with multiple sclerosis. *J Neurol Sci* 60: 353–362

Jones RF, Burke D, Marosszeky JE, Gillies JD 1970 A new agent for the control of spasticity. *J Neurol Neurosurg Psychiatry* 33: 464–468

Jones SJ 1993 Somatosensory evoked potentials. II: Clinical observations and applications.

In: Halliday AM (ed.) *Evoked Potentials in Clinical Testing.* Edinburgh: Churchill Livingstone, pp. 421–466

Jones SJ, Sprague L, Vaz Pato M 2002 Electrophysiological evidence for a defect in the processing of temporal sound patterns in multiple sclerosis. *J Neurol Neurosurg Psychiatry* 73: 561–567

de Jong BA, Huizinga TW, Zanelli E et al 2002a Evidence for additional genetic risk indicators of relapse-onset MS within the HLA region. *Neurology* 59: 549–555

de Jong BA, Huizinga TWJ, Bollen ELEM et al 2002b Production of IL-1β and IL-1Ra as risk factors for susceptibility and progression of relapse-onset multiple sclerosis. *J Neuroimmunol* 126: 172–179

de Jong BA, Engelen M, van Schaik IN, Vermeulen M 2005 Confusing Cochrane reviews on treatment in multiple sclerosis. *Lancet Neurol* 4: 330–331

Jonsson A, Korfitzen EM, Heltberg A et al 1993 Effects of neuropsychological treatment in patients with multiple sclerosis. *Acta Neurol Scand* 88: 394–400

Jonsson L, Thomas K-A, Stenquist M et al 1991 Acute peripheral facial palsy simulating Bell's palsy in a case of probable multiple sclerosis with a clinically correlated transient pontine lesion on magnetic resonance imaging. *J Otorhinolaryngol Rel Specialt* 53: 362–365

Jordan CA, Friedrich VL Jr, Godfraind C et al 1989 Expression of viral and myelin gene transcripts in a murine CNS demyelinating disease caused by a coronavirus. *Glia* 2: 318–329

Josien E, Lefebvre V, Vermesch P, Pasquier F, Petit H 1993 Adrénoleucomyéloneuropathy de l'adulte. *Rev Neurol* 149: 230–232

Joutel A, Corpechot C, Ducros A et al 1996 Notch3 mutations in cadasil, a hereditary adult-onset condition causing stroke and dementia. *Nature* 383: 707–710

Joyce KA, Rees JE 1995 Transverse myelitis after measles, mumps, and rubella vaccination. *Br Med J* 311: 422

Juhler M, Barry DI, Offner H et al 1984 Blood-brain barrier and blood-spinal cord barrier permeability during the course of experimental allergic encephalomyelitis *Brain Res* 302: 347–355

Jung M, Pesheva P, Schachner M, Trotter J 1993 Astrocytes and neurons regulate the expression of the neural recognition molecule janusin by cultured oligodendrocytes. *Glia* 9: 163–175

Jung S, Siglienti I, Grauer O et al 2004 Induction of IL-10 in rat peritoneal macrophages and dendritic cells by glatiramer acetate. *J Neuroimmunol* 148: 63–73

Jungi TW, Brcic M, Kuhnert P et al 1990 Effect of IgG for intravenous use on Fc receptor mediated phagocytosis by human monocytes. *Clin Exp Immunol* 82: 163–169

Jurewicz A, Matysiak M, Tybor K, Selmaj K 2003 TNF-induced death of adult human oligodendrocytes is mediated by c-jun

NH₂-terminal kinase-3. *Brain* **126**: 1358–1370

Kääb G, Haarmann I, Wekerle H, Bradl M 1998 The myelin basic protein specific T cell repertoire in Lewis rats: T cell receptor diversity is influenced both by intrathymic milieu and by extrathymic peptide presentation. *Eur J Immunol* **28**: 1499–1506

Kabat EA, Moore DH, Landow H 1942 An electrophoretic study of the protein components in cerebrospinal fluid and their relationship to the serum proteins. *J Clin Invest* **21**: 571–577

Kaeser HE 1962 Funktionsprüfungen peripherer Nerven bei experimentellen Polyneuritiden und bei der Wallerschen Degeneration. *Dtsch Z Nervenheilk* **183**: 268–304

Kaeser HE, Lambert EH 1962 Nerve function studies in experimental polyneuritis. *Electroencephalogr Clin Neurophysiol* **22** (**Suppl**): 29–35

Kahana E, Leibowitz U, Alter M 1971 Cerebral multiple sclerosis. *Neurology* **21**: 1179–1185

Kahana E, Leibowitz U, Fishback M, Alter M 1973 Slowly progressive and acute visual impairment in multiple sclerosis. *Neurology* **23**: 729–723

Kahana E, Zilber N, Abramson JH et al 1994 Multiple sclerosis: genetic versus environmental aetiology: epidemiology in Israel updated. *J Neurol* **241**: 341–346

Kahn MA, Kusher I 1979 Ankylosing spondylitis and multiple sclerosis: a possible association. *Arthritis Rheum* **22**: 784–786

Kaiboriboon K, Olsen TJ, Hayat GR 2005 Cauda equine and conus medullaris syndrome in sarcoidosis. *Neurologist* **11**: 179–198

Kaiserling E, SteinH, Müller-Hermelink HK 1974 Interdigitating reticulum cells in the human thymus. *Cell Tiss Res* **155**: 47–55

Kaji R, Suzumura A, Sumner AJ 1988 Physiological consequences of antiserum-mediated experimental demyelination in CNS. *Brain* **111**: 675–694

Kaji R, Sumner AJ 1989a Effect of digitalis on central demyelinative conduction block in vivo. *Ann Neurol* **25**: 159–165

Kaji R, Sumner AJ 1989b Ouabain reverses conduction disturbances in single demyelinated nerve fibers. *Neurology* **39**: 1364–1368

Kaji R, Happel L, Sumner AJ 1990 Effect of digitalis on clinical symptoms and conduction variables in patients with multiple sclerosis. *Ann Neurol* **28**: 582–584

Kaji R, Bostock H, Kohara N et al 2000 Activity-dependent conduction block in multifocal motor neuropathy. *Brain* **123**: 1602–1611

Kakigi R, Kuroda Y, Neshige R et al 1992 Physiological study of the spinothalamic tract conduction in multiple sclerosis. *J Neurol Sci* **107**: 205–209

Kalanie H, Tabatabai SS 1998 Combined immunoglobulin and azathioprine in multiple sclerosis. *Eur Neurol* **39**: 178–181

Kalanie H, Kamgooyan M, Sadeghian H, Kalanie AR 2000 Histocompatibility antigen (HLA) associations with multiple sclerosis in Iran. *Mult Scler* **6**: 317–319

Kalita J, Misra UK, Mandal SK 1998 Prognostic predictors of acute transverse myelitis. *Acta Neurol Scand* **98**: 60–63

Kalkers NF, Bergers E, Castelijns JA et al 2001 Optimizing the association between disability and biological markers in MS. *Neurology* **57**: 1253–1258

Kalkers NF, Barkhof F, Bergers E et al 2002a The effect of the neuroprotective agent riluzole on MRI parameters in primary progressive multiple sclerosis. *Mult Scler* **8**: 532–533

Kalkers NF, Vrenken H, Uitdehaag BM et al 2002b Brain atrophy in multiple sclerosis: impact of lesions and of damage of whole brain tissue. *Mult Scler* **8**: 410–414

Källen B, Nilsson O 1986 Dissociation between histological and clinical signs of experimental autoimmune encephalomyelitis. *Acta Pathol Microbiol Immunol Scand* **94**: 159–164

Kallmann B-A, Sauer J, Schliesser M et al 2004 Determination of ventricular diameters in multiple sclerosis patients with transcranial sonography: a two year follow up study. *J Neurol* **251**: 30–34

Kalman B, Leist TP 2003 A mitochondrial component of neurodegeneration in multiple sclerosis. *Neuromol Med* **3**: 147–158

Kalman B, Mandler RN 2002 Studies of mitochondrial DNA in Devic's disease revealed no pathogenic mutations, but polymorphisms also found in association with multiple sclerosis. *Ann Neurol* **51**: 661–662

Kalman B, Takacs K, Gyodin E et al 1991 Sclerosis multiplex in gypsies. *Acta Neurol Scand* **84**: 181–185

Kalman B, Lublin FD, Alder H 1996 Characterisation of the mitochondrial DNA in patients with multiple sclerosis. *J Neurol Sci* **140**: 75–89

Kalman B, Rodriguez-Valdez JL, Bosch U, Lublin FD 1997 Screening for Leber's hereditary optic neuropathy associated mitochondrial DNA mutations in patients with prominent optic neuritis. *Mult Scler* **2**: 279–282

Kalman B, Li S, Chatterjee D et al 1999 Large scale screening of the mitochondrial DNA reveals no pathogenic mutations but a haplotype associated with multiple sclerosis in Caucasians. *Acta Neurol Scand* **99**: 16–25

Kamalian N, Keesey RE, ZuRhein GM 1975 Lateral hypothalamic demyelination and cachexia in a case of 'malignant' multiple sclerosis. *Neurology* **25**: 25–30

Kamme F, Salunga R, Yu JX et al 2003 Single-cell microarray analysis in hippocampus CA1: demonstration and validation of cellular heterogeneity. *J Neurosci* **23**: 3607–3615

Kanchandani R, Howe JG 1982 Lhermitte's sign in multiple sclerosis: a clinical survey and review of the literature. *J Neurol Neurosurg Psychiatry* **45**: 308–312

Kanda T, Iwasaki T, Yamawaki M et al 2000 Anti-GM1 antibody facilitates leakage in an in vitro blood–nerve barrier model. *Neurology* **55**: 585–587

Kandel ER, Schwartz JH 1985 *Principles of Neural Science*. New York: Elsevier

Kane M 1995 Global programme for control of hepatitis B infection. *Vaccine* **13** (**Suppl 1**): S47–S49

Kankonkar S, Jeyanti G, Singhal BS, Shankarkumar U 2003 Evidence for novel DRB1*15 allele association among clinically definite multiple sclerosis patients from Mumbai, India. *Hum Immunol* **64**: 478–482

Kanpolat Y, Berk C, Savas A, Bekar A 2000 Percutaneous controlled radiofrequency rhizotomy in the management of patients with trigeminal neuralgia due to multiple sclerosis. *Acta Neurochir* **142**: 685–689; discussion 689–690

Kansu T, Kirkali P, Kansu E, Zileli T 1989 Optic neuropathy in Behçet's disease. *J Clin Neuroophthalmol* **9**: 277–280

Kantarci O, Siva A, Eraksoy M et al 1998 Survival and predictors of disability in Turkish MS patients. Turkish Multiple Sclerosis Study Group (TUMSSG). *Neurology* **51**: 765–772

Kantarci OH, Atkinson EJ, Hebrink DD et al 2000a Association of two variants in IL-1beta and IL-1 receptor antagonist genes with multiple sclerosis. *J Neuroimmunol* **106**: 220–227

Kantarci OH, Hebrink DD, Atkinson EJ et al 2000b A comprehensive screen for genetic variation in the IFNgamma gene in multiple sclerosis. *Neurology* **56**: A95

Kantarci OH, Atkinson EJ, Hebrink DD et al 2000c Association of a myeloperoxidase promoter polymorphism with multiple sclerosis. *J Neuroimmunol* **105**: 189–194

Kantarci OH, de Andrade M, Weinshenker BG 2002 Identifying disease modifying genes in multiple sclerosis. *J Neuroimmunol* **123**: 144–159

Kantarci OH, Hebrink DD, Achenbach SJ et al 2003a CLTA4 is associated with susceptibility to multiple sclerosis. *J Neuroimmunol* **134**: 133–141

Kantarci OH, Schaefer-Klein JL, Hebrink DD et al 2003b A population-based study of IL4 polymorphisms in multiple sclerosis. *J Neuroimmunol* **137**: 134–139

Kantarci OH, Hebrink DD, Achenbach SJ et al 2004a Association of APOE polymorphisms with disease severity in MS is limited to women. *Neurology* **62**: 811–814

Kantarci OH, Hebrink DD, Achenbach SJ et al 2004b CD95 polymorphisms are associated with susceptibility to MS in women: a population-based study of CD95 and CD95L in MS. *J Neuroimmunol* **146**: 162–170

Kantarci OH, Goris A, Hebrink DD et al 2005 IFNG polymorphisms are associated with gender differences in susceptibility to multiple sclerosis. *Genes Immun* **6**: 153–161

Kanter DS, Horensky D, Sperling RA et al 1995 Plasmapheresis in fulminant acute disseminated encephalomyelitis. *Neurology* **45**: 824–827

Kantor AB, Herzenberg LA 1993 Origin of murine B cell lineages. *Ann Rev Immunol* **11**: 501–538

Kantor R, Bakhanashvili M, Achiron A 2003 A mutated CCR5 gene may have favourable prognostic implications in MS. *Neurology* **61**: 238–240

Kanwar JR, Harrison JEB, Wang D *et al* 2000 Beta7 integrins contribute to demyelinating disease of the central nervous system. *J Neuroimmunol* **103**: 146–152

Kanyerezi BR, Kiire CF, Obace A 1980 Multiple sclerosis in Mulago Hospital, Uganda. *East Afr Med J* **57**: 262–266

Kaplan EL, Meier P 1958 Non-parametric estimation from incomplete observations. *J Am Stat Assoc* **53**: 457–481

Kaplan MR, Meyer-Franke A, Lambert S *et al* 1997 Induction of sodium channel clustering by oligodendrocytes. *Nature* **386**: 724–728

Kaplan MR, Cho MH, Ullian EM *et al* 2001 Differential control of clustering of the sodium channels Na(v)1.2 and Na(v)1.6 at developing CNS nodes of Ranvier. *Neuron* **30**: 105–119

Kaplan SA, Reis RB, Kohn IJ *et al* 1999 Safety and efficacy of sildenafil in postmenopausal women with sexual dysfunction. *Urology* **53**: 481–486

Kaplanski G, Retornaz F, Durand J, Soubeyrand J 1995 Central nervous system demyelination after vaccination against hepatitis B and HLA haplotype. *J Neurol Neurosurg Psychiatry* **58**: 758–759

Kaplin AI, Krishnan C, Deshpande DM *et al* 2005 Diagnosis and management of acute myelopathies. *Neurologist* **11**: 2–18

Kapoor R, Miller DH, Jones SJ *et al* 1988 Effects of intravenous methylprednisolone on outcome in MRI-based prognostic subgroups in acute optic neuritis. *Neurology* **50**: 230–237

Kapoor R, Brown P, Thompson PD, Miller DH 1992 Propriospinal myoclonus in multiple sclerosis. *J Neurol Neurosurg Psychiatry* **55**: 1086–1088

Kapoor R, Smith KJ, Felts PA, Davies M 1993 Internodal potassium currents can generate ectopic impulses in mammalian myelinated axons. *Brain Res* **611**: 165–169

Kapoor R, Li YG, Smith KJ 1997 Slow sodium-dependent potential oscillations contribute to ectopic firing in mammalian demyelinated axons. *Brain* **120**: 647–652

Kapoor R, Miller DH, Jones SJ *et al* 1998 Effects of intravenous methylprednisolone on outcome in MRI based prognostic subgroups in acute optic neuritis. *Neurology* **50**: 230–237

Kapoor R, Davies M, Smith KJ 1999 Temporary axonal conduction block and axonal loss in inflammatory neurological disease: a potential role for nitric oxide? *Ann NY Acad Sci* **893**: 304–308

Kapoor R, Blaker PA, Hall SM *et al* 2000 Protection of axons from degeneration resulting from exposure to nitric oxide. *Rev Neurol (Paris)* **156**: 367

Kapoor R, Davies M, Blaker PA *et al* 2003 Blockers of sodium and calcium entry protect axons from nitric oxide-mediated degeneration. *Ann Neurol* **53**: 174–180

Kappos L, Duda P 2002 The Janus face of CNS-directed autoimmune response: a therapeutic challenge. *Brain* **125**: 2379–2380

Kappos L, Kesselring J 2003 Interferons in relapsing remitting multiple sclerosis. *Lancet* **361**:1821–2; author reply 1823–1824

Kappos L, Patzold U, Dommasch D *et al* 1988 Cyclosporine versus azathioprine in the long term treatment of multiple sclerosis – results of the German multicentre study. *Ann Neurol* **23**: 56–63

Kappos L, Heun R, Mertens H-G 1990 A 10-year matched-pairs study comparing azathioprine and no immunosupppression in multiple sclerosis. *Eur Arch Psychiatry Clin Neurosci* **240**: 34–38

Kappos L, Radu EW, Haas J *et al* 1994 European multicenter trial of deoxyspergualin (DSG) versus placebo: results of the first interim analysis. *J Neurol* **241 (Suppl 1)**: S27

Kappos L, Moeri D, Radue EW *et al* 1999 Predictive value of gadolinium-enhanced magnetic resonance imaging for relapse rate and changes in disability or impairment in multiple sclerosis: a meta-analysis. *Lancet* **353**: 964–969

Kappos L, Comi G, Panitch H *et al* 2000 Induction of a non-encephalitogenic type 2 T helper-cell autoimmune response in multiple sclerosis after administration of an altered peptide ligand in a placebo-controlled, randomized phase II trial. *Nature Med* **6**: 1176–1182

Kappos L, Polman C, Pozzilli C *et al* 2001 Final analysis of the European multicenter trial on IFNβ-1b in secondary-progressive MS. *Neurology* **57**: 1969–1975

Kappos L, Clanet M, Sandberg-Wollheim M *et al* 2005 Neutralizing antibodies and efficacy of interferon beta-1a: a 4-year controlled study. *Neurology* **65**: 40–47

Kara P, Friedlander MJ 1998 Dynamic modulation of cerebral cortex synaptic function by nitric oxide. *Prog Brain Res* **118**: 183–198

Karabudak R, Kurne A, Guc D *et al* 2004 Effect of interferon beta-1a on serum matrix metalloproteinase – 9(MMP-9) and tissue inhibitor of matrix metalloproteinase (TIMP-1) in relapsing remitting multiple sclerosis patients: one year follow-up results. *J Neurol* **251**: 279–283

Karacostas D, Christodoulou C, Drevelengas A *et al* 2002 Cytomegalovirus-associated transverse myelitis in a non-immunocompromised patient. *Spinal Cord* **40**: 145–149

Karandikar NJ, Vanderlugt CL, Walunas TL *et al* 1996 CTLA-4: a negative regulator of autoimmune disease. *J Exp Med* **184**: 783–788

Karandikar NJ, Crawford MP, Yan X *et al* 2002 Glatiramer acetate (Copaxone) therapy induces CD8(+) T cell responses in patients with multiple sclerosis. *J Clin Invest* **109**: 641–649

Karlsson J, Zhao X, Lonskaya I *et al* 2003 Novel quantitative trait loci controlling development of experimental autoimmune encephalomyelitis and proportion of lymphocyte subpopulations. *J Immunol* **170**: 1019–1026

Karnezis T, Mandemakers W, McQualter JL *et al* 2004 The neurite outgrowth inhibitor Nogo A is involved in autoimmune-mediated demyelination. *Nat Neurosci* **7**: 736–744

Karni A, Kohn Y, Safirman C *et al* 1999a Evidence for the genetic role of human leukocyte antigens in low frequency of DRB1*0501 multiple sclerosis patients in Israel. *Mult Scler* **5**: 410–415

Karni A, Bakimer-Kleiner R, Abramsky O, Ben-Nun A 1999b Elevated levels of antibody to myelin-oligodendrocyte glycoprotein is not specific for patients with multiple sclerosis. *Arch Neurol* **56**: 311–315

Karni A, Kahana E, Zilber N *et al* 2003 The frequency of multiple sclerosis in Jewish and Arab populations in greater Jerusalem. *Neuroepidemiology* **22**: 82–86

Karp CL, van Boxel-Dezaire AH, Byrnes AA, Nagelkerken L 2001 Interferon-beta in multiple sclerosis: altering the balance of interleukin-12 and interleukin-10? *Curr Opin Neurol* **14**: 361–368

Karpas A, Kampft U, Siden A *et al* 1986 Lack of evidence for involvement of known human retroviruses in multiple sclerosis. *Nature* **322**: 177–178

Karpus WJ, Lukacs NW, McRae BL *et al* 1995 An important role for the chemokine macrophage inflammatory protein-1a in the pathogenesis of the T cell-mediated autoimmune disease, experimental autoimmune encephalomyelitis. *J Immunol* **155**: 5003–5010

Karpusas M, Whitty A, Runkel L, Hochman P 1998 The structure of human interferon-beta: implications for activity. *Cell Mol Life Sci* **54**: 1203–1216

Kartje GL, Schulz MK, Lopez-Yunez A *et al* 1999 Corticostriatal plasticity is restricted by myelin-associated neurite growth inhibitors in the adult rat. *Ann Neurol* **45**: 778–786

Karussis DM, Leker RR, Ashkenazi A, Abramsky O 1998 A subgroup of multiple sclerosis patients with anticardiolipin antibodies and unusual clinical manifestations: do they represent a new nosological entity? *Ann Neurol* **44**: 629–634

Karussis DM, Meiner Z, Lehmann D *et al* 1996 Treatment of secondary progressive multiple sclerosis with the immunomodulator linomide: a double-blind, placebo-controlled pilot study with monthly magnetic resonance imaging evaluation. *Neurology* **47**: 341–346

Kaspar A, Brinkmeier H, Rudel R 1994 Local anaesthetic-like effect of interleukin-2 on muscular Na+ channels: no evidence for involvement of the IL-2 receptor. *Pflugers Arch* **426**: 61–67

869

Kassiotis G, Pasparakis M, Kollias G, Probert L 1999 TNF accelerates the onset but does not alter the incidence and severity of myelin basic protein-induced experimental autoimmune encephalomyelitis. *Eur J Immunol* **29**: 774–780

Kassubek J, Tumani H, Ecker D *et al* 2003 Age-related brain parenchymal fraction is significantly decreased in young multiple sclerosis patients: a quantitative MRI study. *NeuroReport* **14**: 427–430

Kastenbauer S, Koedel U, Wick M *et al* 2003 CSF and serum levels of soluble fractalkine (CX3CL1) in inflammatory diseases of the nervous system. *J Neuroimmunol* **137**: 210–217

Kastrup O, Stude P, Limmroth V 2002 Balo's concentric sclerosis: evolution of active demyelination demonstrated by serial contrast-enhanced MRI. *J Neurol* **249**: 811–814

Katz D, Taubenberger JK, Cannella B *et al* 1993 Correlation between MRI findings and lesion development in chronic active multiple sclerosis. *Ann Neurol* **34**: 661–669

Katz JD, Ropper AH 2000 Progressive necrotic myelopathy: clinical course in 9 patients. *Arch Neurol* **57**: 355–361

Kaufman DL, Clare-Salzler M, Tian J *et al* 1993 Spontaneous loss of T-cell tolerance to glutamic acid decarboxylase in murine insulin-dependent diabetes. *Nature* **366**: 69–72

Kaufman JM, Fam B, Jacobs SC *et al* 1977 Bladder cancer and squamous metaplasia in spinal cord injury patients. *J Urology* **118**: 967–971

Kaufman M 1997 Treatment of multiple sclerosis with high-dose corticosteroids may prolong the prothrombin time to dangerous levels in patients taking warfarin. *Mult Scler* **3**: 248–249

Kaufman M, Gaydos CA, Sriram S *et al* 2002 Is *Chlamydia pneumoniae* found in spinal fluid samples from multiple sclerosis patients? Conflicting results. *Mult Scler* **8**: 289–294

Kaufmann SHE 1990 Heat shock proteins and the immune response. *Immunol Today* **11**: 129–136

Kaur C, Singh J, Lim MK *et al* 1995 The response of neurons and microglia to blast injury in the rat brain. *Neuropathol Appl Neurobiol* **21**: 369–377

Kawakami N, Lassmann S, Li Z *et al* 2004 The activation status of neuroantigen-specific T cells in the target organ determines the clinical outcome of autoimmune encephalomyelitis. *J Exp Med* **199**: 185–197

Kawakami N, Nägerl UV, Odoardi F *et al* 2005 Live imaging of effector cell trafficking and autoantigen recognition within the unfolding autoimmune encephalomyelitis lesion. *J Exp Med* **201**: 1805–1814

Kawamata T, Akiyama H, Yamada T, McGeer PL 1992 Immunologic reactions in amyotrophic lateral sclerosis brain and spinal cord. *Am J Pathol* **140**: 691–707

Kazarian EL, Gager WE 1978 Optic neuritis complicating measles, mumps, and rubella vaccination. *Am J Ophthalmol* **86**: 544–547

Kazarinova-Noyes K, Shrager P 2002 Molecular constituents of the node of Ranvier. *Mol Neurobiol* **26**: 167–182

Keane AH 1920 *Man Past and Present*. Cambridge: Cambridge University Press

Keane JR 1974 Periodic alternating nystagmus with downward beating nystagmus. *Arch Neurol* **30**: 399–402

Keane JR 2005 Internuclear ophthalmoplegia: unusual causes in 114 of 410 patients. *Arch Neurol* **62**: 714–717

Keegan M, Pineda AA, McClelland RL *et al* 2002 Plasma exchange for severe attacks of CNS demyelination: predictors of response. *Neurology* **58**: 143–146

Keegan M, Konig F, Bitsch A *et al* 2004 Multiple sclerosis pathological subtype predicts response to therapeutic plasma exchange. *Neurology* **62**: 259–260

Keirstead HS, Blakemore WF 1999 The role of oligodendrocytes and oligodendrocyte progenitors in CNS remyelination. *Adv Exp Med Biol* **468**: 183–197

Keitner JL, Johnson CA, Spurn JO, Beck RW, Optic Neuritis Study Group 1993 Baseline visual field profile of optic neuritis. *Arch Ophthalmol* **111**: 231–234

Keles MS, Taysi S, Sen N *et al* 2001 Effect of corticosteroid therapy on serum and CSF malondialdehyde and antioxidant proteins in multiple sclerosis. *Can J Neurol Sci* **28**: 141–143

Kellar-Wood H, Powys S, Gray J, Compston DAS 1994a MHC in coded TAP1 and TAP2 dimorphisms in multiple sclerosis. *Tissue Antigens* **43**: 129–132

Kellar-Wood H, Robertson N, Govan GG *et al* 1994b Leber's hereditary optic neuropathy mitochondrial DNA mutations in multiple sclerosis. *Ann Neurol* **36**: 109–112

Kellar-Wood H, Wood NW, Hoilmans P *et al* 1995 Multiple sclerosis and the HLA-D region: linkage and association studies. *J Neuroimmunol* **58**: 183–190

Keller G, Snodgrass HR 1999 Human embryonic stem cells: the future is now. *Nature Med* **5**: 151–152

Kelles A, Janssens J, Tack J 2000 IL-1beta and IL-6 excite neurones and suppress cholinergic neurotransmission in the myenteric plexus of the guinea pig. *Neurogastroenterol Motil* **12**: 531–538

Kelly BJ, Cronin M, Curran JJ 1989 Anticardiolipin syndrome resembling multiple sclerosis. *Arthritis Rheum* **32**: S71 (B126)

Kelly MA, Cavan DA, Penny MA *et al* 1993 The influence of HLA-DR and -DQ alleles on progression to multiple sclerosis following a clinically isolated syndrome. *Hum Immunol* **37**: 185–191

Kelly MA, Zhang Y, Penny MA *et al* 1995a Genetic susceptibility to multiple sclerosis in a Shanghai Chinese population. *Hum Immunol* **42**: 203–208

Kelly MA, Jacobs KH, Penny MA *et al* 1995b An investigation of HLA-encoded genetic susceptibility to multiple sclerosis in subjects of Asian Indian and Afro-Caribbean ethnic origin. *Tissue Antigens* **45**: 197–202

Kelly R 1985 In: Vinken PJ, Bruyn G, Klawans JHL (eds) *Handbook of Clinical Neurology*. Amsterdam: Elsevier, Vol 47, pp. 49–78

Kelsoe G 1996 Life and death in germinal centers (Redux). *Immunity* **4**: 107–111

Kemp K, Lion JR, Magram G 1977 Lithium in the case of a manic patient with multiple sclerosis: a case report. *Dis Nerv Syst* **38**: 210–211

Kenealy SJ, Babron MC, Bradford Y *et al* 2004 A second-generation genomic screen for multiple sclerosis. *Am J Hum Genet* **75**: 1070–1078

Kennedy C, Carroll FD 1960 Optic neuritis in children. *Arch Ophthalmol* **63**: 747–755

Kennedy C, Carter S 1961 Relation of optic neuritis to multiple sclerosis in children. *Pediatrics* **28**: 377–387

Kennedy MK, Torrance DS, Picha KS, Mohler KM 1992 Analysis of cytokine mRNA expression in the central nervous system of mice with experimental autoimmune encephalomyelitis reveals that IL-10 mRNA expression correlates with recovery. *J Immunol* **149**: 2496–2505

Kennedy PGE, Fok-Seang J 1986 Studies on the development, antigenic phenotype, and function of human glial cells in tissue culture. *Brain* **109**: 1261–1277

Kennedy PGE, Steiner I 1994 On the possible viral aetiology of multiple sclerosis. *Q J Med* **87**: 523–528

Kennedy PGE, Narayan O, Ghotbi Z *et al* 1985 Persistent expression of Ia antigen and viral genome in visna-maedi virus-induced inflammatory cells: possible role of lentivirus-induced interferon. *J Exp Med* **162**: 1970–1982

Kent-Braun JA, Sharma KR, Weiner MW, Miller RG 1994 Effects of exercise on muscle activation and metabolism in multiple sclerosis. *Muscle Nerve* **17**: 1162–1169

Kepes JJ 1993 Large focal tumor-like demyelinating lesions of the brain: intermediate entity between multiple sclerosis and acute disseminated encephalomyelitis? A study of 31 patients. *Ann Neurol* **33**: 18–27

Kerlero de Rosbo N, Bernard CC *et al* 1985 Concomitant detection of changes in myelin basic protein and permeability of blood-spinal cord barrier in acute experimental autoimmune encephalomyelitis by electroimmunoblotting. *J Neuroimmunol* **9**: 349–361

Kerlero de Rosbo N, Milo R, Lees MB *et al* 1993 Reactivity to myelin antigens in multiple sclerosis. *J Clin Invest* **92**: 2602–2608

Kerlero de Rosbo N, Mendel I, Ben-Nun A 1995 Chronic relapsing experimental autoimmune encephalomyelitis with a delayed onset and an atypical course, induced on PL/J mice by myelin oligodendrocyte glycoprotein (MOG)-derived peptide: preliminary analysis of MOG T cell epitopes. *Eur J Immunol* 25: 985–993

Kerlero de Rosbo N, Hoffman M *et al* 1997 Predominance of the autoimmune response to myelin oligodendrocyte glycoprotein (MOG) in multiple sclerosis: reactivity to the extracellular domain of MOG is directed against three main regions. *Eur J Immunol* 27: 3059–3069

Kermode AG, Plant GT, MacManus DG *et al* 1989 Behçet's disease with slowly enlarging midbrain mass on MRI: resolution following steroid therapy. *Neurology* 39: 1251–1252

Kermode AG, Thompson AJ, Tofts P *et al* 1990 Breakdown of the blood-brain barrier precedes symptoms and other MRI signs of new lesions in multiple sclerosis: pathogenetic and clinical implications. *Brain* 113: 1477–1489

Keros S, McBain CJ 1997 Arachidonic acid inhibits transient potassium currents and broadens action potentials during electrographic seizures in hippocampal pyramidal and inhibitory interneurons. *J Neurosci* 17: 3476–3487

Kerschensteiner M, Gallmeier E, Behrens L *et al* 1999 Activated human T cells, B cells, and monocytes produce brain-derived neurotrophic factor in vitro and in inflammatory brain lesions: a neuroprotective role of inflammation? *J Exp Med* 189: 865–870

Kerschensteiner M, Stadelmann C, Dechant G *et al* 2003 Neurotrophic cross-talk between the nervous and immune systems: implications for neurological diseases. *Ann Neurol* 53: 292–304

Kersh EN, Shaw AS, Allen PM 1998 Fidelity of T cell activation through multistep T cell receptor zeta-phosphorylation. *Science* 281: 572–575

Kerschensteiner M, Bareyre FM, Buddeberg BS *et al* 2004 Remodeling of axonal connections contributes to recovery in an animal model of multiple sclerosis 1. *J Exp Med* 200: 1027–1038

Kessaris N, Jamen F, Rubin LL, Richardson WD 2004 Cooperation between sonic hedgehog and fibroblast growth factor/MAPK signalling pathways in neocortical precursors. *Development* 131: 1289–1298

Kesselring J, Miller DH, MacManus DG *et al* 1989 Quantitative magnetic resonance imaging in multiple sclerosis: the effect of high dose intravenous methylprednisolone. *J Neurol Neurosurg Psychiatry* 52: 14–17

Kesselring J, Miller DH, Robb SA *et al* 1990 Acute disseminated encephalomyelitis: magnetic resonance imaging findings and the distinction from multiple sclerosis. *Brain* 113: 291–302

Khan AA, Bose C, Yam LS *et al* 2001 Physiological regulation of the immunological synapse by agrin. *Science* 292, 1681–1686

Khan OA, Xia Q, Bever CT, Johnson KP, Panitch HS, Dhib-Jalbut SS 1996 Interferon beta-1b serum levels in multiple sclerosis

following subcutaneous administration. *Neurology* 46: 1639–1643

Khan OA, Bauserman SC, Rothman MI *et al* 1997 Concurrence of multiple sclerosis and brain tumor: clinical considerations. *Neurology* 48: 1330–1333

Khan OA, Zvartau-Hind M, Caon C *et al* 2001a Effect of monthly intravenous cyclophosphamide in rapidly deteriorating multiple sclerosis patients resistant to conventional therapy. *Mult Scler* 7: 185–188

Khan OA, Caon C, Zvartau-Hind M *et al* 2001b Clinical course and before and after change of immunomodulating therapy in relapsing–remitting MS. *Neurology* 56: A355

Khan OA, Tselis AC, Kamholz JA *et al* 2001c A prospective, open-label treatment trial to compare the effect of IFNbeta-1a (Avonex), IFNbeta-1b (Betaseron), and glatiramer acetate (Copaxone) on the relapse rate in relapsing–remitting multiple sclerosis: results after 18 months of therapy. *Mult Scler* 7: 349–353

Khan S, Yakub BA, Poser CM *et al* 1995 Multiphasic disseminated encephalomyelitis presenting as alternating hemiplegia. *J Neurol Neurosurg Psychiatry* 58: 467–470

Khatri BO, McQuillen P, Harrington GJ *et al* 1985 Chronic progressive multiple sclerosis: double blind controlled trial of plasmapheresis in patients taking immunosuppressive treatment. *Neurology* 35: 312–319

Khatri BO, McQuillen P, Hoffman RG 1991 Plasma exchange in chronic progressive multiple sclerosis: a long term study. *Neurology* 41: 409–414

Kheradvar A, Tabassi AR, Nikbin B *et al* 2004 Influence of HLA on progression of optic neuritis to multiple sclerosis: results of a four-year follow-up study. *Mult Scler* 10: 526–531

Khorchid A, Fragoso G, Shore G, Almazan G 2002 Catecholamine-induced oligodendrocyte cell death in culture is developmentally regulated and involves free radical generation and differential activation of caspase-3. *Glia* 40: 283–299

Khoury SJ, Hancock WW, Weiner HL 1992 Oral tolerance to myelin basic protein and natural recovery from experimental autoimmune encephalomyelitis are associated with downregulation of inflammatory cytokines and differential upregulation of transforming growth factor β, interleukin 4, and prostaglandin E expression in the brain. *J Exp Med* 176: 1355–1364

Khoury SJ, Akalin E, Chandraker A *et al* 1995 CD28-B7 costimulatory blockade by CTLA4Ig prevents actively induced experimental autoimmune encephalomyelitis and inhibits Th1 but spares Th2 cytokines in the central nervous system. *J Immunol* 155: 4521–4524

Khun P, Steiner G 1917 Über die Ursache der multiplen Sklerose. *Med Klin* 13: 1007–1014

Kibler RF, Fritz RB, Chou FC-H *et al* 1977 Immune response of Lewis rats to peptide

C1 (residues 68–88) of guinea pig and rat myelin basic proteins. *J Exp Med* 146: 1323–1331

Kidd D, Thompson AJ 1997 Prospective study of neurorehabilitation in multiple sclerosis. *J Neurol Neurosurg Psychiatry* 62: 423–424

Kidd D, Thorpe JW, Thompson *et al* 1993 Spinal cord MRI using multi-array coils and fast spin echo. II: Findings in multiple sclerosis. *Neurology* 43: 2632–2637

Kidd D, Thompson AJ, Kendall BE *et al* 1994 Benign form of multiple sclerosis: MRI evidence for less frequent and less inflammatory disease activity. *J Neurol Neurosurg Psychiatry* 57: 1070–1072

Kidd D, Thorpe JW, Kendall BE *et al* 1996 MRI dynamics of brain and spinal cord in progressive multiple sclerosis. *J Neurol Neurosurg Psychiatry* 60: 15–19

Kidd D, Thompson PD, Day BL *et al* 1998 Central motor conduction time in progressive multiple sclerosis: correlations with MRI and disease activity. *Brain* 121: 1109–1116

Kidd D, Barkhof F, McConnell R *et al* 1999a Cortical lesions in multiple sclerosis. *Brain* 122: 17–26

Kidd D, Steuer A, Denman AM, Rudge P 1999b Neurological complications in Behçet's syndrome. *Brain* 122: 2183–2194

Kidd D, Burton B, Plant GT, Graham EM 2003 Chronic relapsing inflammatory optic neuropathy (CRION). *Brain* 126: 278–284

Kiernan BW, ffrench Constant C 1993 Oligodendrocyte precursor (O-2A progenitor cell) migration: a model system for the study of cell migration in the developing central nervous system. *Development* 119 (Suppl): S219–S225

Kiernan MC, Hales JP, Gracies JM *et al* 1997 Paraesthesiae induced by prolonged high frequency stimulation of human cutaneous afferents. *J Physiology* 501: 461–471

Kiernan MC, Lin CS, Andersen KV *et al* 2001 Clinical evaluation of excitability measures in sensory nerve. *Muscle Nerve* 24: 883–892

Kiernan MC, Guglielmi JM, Kaji R *et al* 2002 Evidence for axonal membrane hyperpolarization in multifocal motor neuropathy with conduction block. *Brain* 125: 664–675

Kierstead HS, Levine JM, Blakemore WF 1998 Response of the oligodendrocyte progenitor cell population (defined by NG2 labelling) to demyelination of the adult spinal cord. *Glia* 22: 161–170

Kies B 1989 An epidemiological study of multiple sclerosis in Cape Town, South Africa. *XIVth World Congress of Neurology, New Delhi, India*, abstract 612B05

Kies MW, Murphy JB, Alvord EC 1960 Fractionation of guinea pig brain proteins with encephalitogenic activity. *Federation Proc (Bethesda)* 19: 207

Kies MW, Alvord EC Jr, Martenson RE, LeBaron FN 1966 Encephalitogenic activity of bovine basic proteins. *Science* 151: 821–822

Kikuchi S, Fukazawa T, Niino M *et al* 2002a Estrogen receptor gene polymorphism and multiple sclerosis in Japanese patients: interaction with HLA-DRB1*1501 and disease modulation. *J Neuroimmunol* **128**: 77–81

Kikuchi S, Niino M, Fukazawa T et al 2002b An assessment of the association between IL-2 gene polymorphisms and Japanese patients with multiple sclerosis. *J Neurol Sci* **205**: 47–50

Kikuchi S, Fukazawa T, Niino M et al 2003 HLA-related subpopulations of MS in Japanese with and without oligoclonal bands. *Neurology* **60**: 647–651

Kilbinger H 1996 Modulation of acetylcholine release by nitric oxide. *Prog Brain Res* **109**: 219–224

Killestein J, Hoogervorst EL, Reif M et al 2002a Safety, tolerability, and efficacy of orally administered cannabinoids in MS. *Neurology* **58**: 1404–1407

Killestein J, Olsson T, Wallstrom E et al 2002b Antibody-mediated suppression of Vbeta5.2/5.3(+) T cells in multiple sclerosis: results from an MRI-monitored phase II clinical trial. *Ann Neurol* **51**: 467–474

Killestein J, Rep MHG, Meilof JF et al 2002c Seasonal variation in immune measurements and MRI markers of disease activity in MS. *Neurology* **58**: 1077–1080

Killestein J, Hoogervorst EL, Reif M et al 2003 Immunomodulatory effects of orally administered cannabinoids in multiple sclerosis. *J Neuroimmunol* **137**: 140–143

Killian JM, Bressler RB, Armstrong RM, Huston DP 1988 Controlled pilot trial of monthly intravenous cyclophosphamide in multiple sclerosis. *Arch Neurol* **45**: 27–30

Kim G, Tanuma N, Kojima T et al 1998 CDR3 size spectratyping and sequencing of spectratype-derived TCR of spinal cord T cells in autoimmune encephalomyelitis. *J Immunol* **160**: 509–513

Kim HJ, Ifergan I, Antel J et al 2004 Type-2 monocyte and microglia differentiation mediated by glatiramer acetate therapy in patients with multiple sclerosis. *J Neuroimmunol* **172**: 7144–7153

Kim JH, Auerbach JM, Rodriguez-Gomez JA et al 2002 Dopamine neurons derived from embryonic stem cells function in an animal model of Parkinson's disease. *Nature* **418**: 50–56

Kim JH, Lee SI, Park SI, Yoo WH 2003 Recurrent transverse myelitis in primary antiphospholipid syndrome: case report and literature review. *Rheumatol Int* **24**: 244–246

Kim JY, Sun Q, Oglesbee M, Yoon SO 2003 The role of ErbB2 signaling in the onset of terminal differentiation of oligodendrocytes in vivo. *J Neurosci* **23**: 5561–5571

Kim KK 2003 Idiopathic recurrent transverse myelitis. *Arch Neurol* **60**: 1290–1294

Kim SU, Murray MR, Tourtellotte WW 1970 Demonstration in tissue culture of myelino-toxicity in cerebrospinal fluid and brain extracts from multiple sclerosis patients. *J Neuropathol Exp Neurol* **29**: 420–431

Kim SU, McMorris FA, Sprinkle T 1984 Immunofluorescence demonstration of

2',3'-cyclic nucleotide phosphodiesterase in cultured oligodendrocytes of mouse, rat, calf and human. *Brain Res* **300**: 195–199

Kim YS, Kim SU 1991 Oligodendroglial cell death induced by oxygen radicals and its protection by catalase. *J Neurosci Res* **29**: 100–106

Kimiskidis V, Tsimourtou VSP et al 2002 Autologous stem cell transplantation in multiple sclerosis: the MRI study. *J Neurol* **249**: I61

Kimura K, Hunter SF, Thollander MS et al 2000 Concurrence of inflammatory bowel disease and multiple sclerosis. *Mayo Clin Proc* **75**: 802–806

Kinlen LJ 1985 Incidence of cancer in rheumatoid arthritis and other disorders after immunosuppressive treatment. *Am J Med* **78**: 44–49

Kinnman J, Link H 1984 Intrathecal production of oligoclonal IgM and IgG in CNS sarcoid. *Acta Neurol Scand* **69**: 97–106

Kinnunen E 1983 The incidence of optic neuritis and its prognosis for multiple sclerosis. *Acta Neurol Scand* **68**: 371–377

Kinnunen E 1984 Multiple sclerosis in Finland: evidence of increasing frequency and uneven geographic distribution. *Neurology* **34**: 457–461

Kinnunen E, Wikström J 1986 Prevalence and prognosis of epilepsy in patients with multiple sclerosis. *Epilepsia* **27**: 729–733

Kinnunen E, Koskenvuo M, Kaprio J, Aho K 1987 Multiple sclerosis in a nationwide series of twins. *Neurology* **37**: 1627–1629

Kinnunen E, Juntunen J, Ketonen L et al 1988 Genetic susceptibility to multiple sclerosis: a co-twin study of a nation-wide series. *Arch Neurol* **45**: 1108–1111

Kinnunen E, Müller K, Keto P et al 1993 Cerebrospinal fluid and MRI findings in three patients with multiple sclerosis and systemic lupus erythematosus. *Acta Neurol Scand* **87**: 356–360

Kioy PG 2001 Emerging picture of multiple sclerosis in Kenya. *East Afr Med J* **78**: 93–96

Kipnis J, Yoles E, Cohen A et al 2000 T cell immunity to copolymer 1 confers neuroprotection on the damaged optic nerve: possible therapy for optic neuropathies. *Proc Natl Acad Sci USA* **97**: 7446–7451

Kira JI 2003 Multiple sclerosis in the Japanese population. *Lancet Neurol* **2**: 117–126

Kira JI, Kanai T, Nishimura Y et al 1996 Western versus Asian types of multiple sclerosis: immunogenetically and clinically distinct disorders. *Ann Neurol* **40**: 569–574

Kira JI, Yamasaki K, Horiuchi I et al 1999 Changes in the clinical phenotypes of multiple sclerosis during the past 50 years in Japan. *J Neurol Sci* **166**: 53–57

Kirk CW, Droogan AG, Hawkins SA et al 1997 Tumour necrosis factor microsatellites show association with multiple sclerosis. *J Neurol Sci* **147**: 21–25

Kirk CW, Graham CA, McDonnell GV, Hawkins SA 2000 Chromosome 10 locus

apolipoprotein C-11 association with multiple sclerosis. *Mult Scler* **6**: 291–292

Kirk J 1979 The fine structure of the CNS in multiple sclerosis: vesicular demyelination in an acute case. *Neuropathol Appl Neurobiol* **5**: 289–294

Kirk J, Hutchinson WM 1978 The fine structure of the CNS in multiple sclerosis: interpretation of cytoplasma papovavirus-like and paramyxovirus-like inclusions. *Neuropathol Appl Neurobiol* **4**: 343–356

Kirk PF, Compston DAS 1990 The effect of methylprednisolone on lymphocyte phenotype and function in patients with multiple sclerosis. *J Neuroimmunol* **26**: 1–8

Kirk PF, Williams J, Petersen M, Compston DAS 1994 The effect of methylprednisolone on monocyte eicosanoid production in patients with multiple sclerosis. *J Neurol* **241**: 427–431

Kirkpatrick JB, Hayman LA 1987 White matter lesions in MR imaging of clinically healthy brains of elderly subjects: possible pathological basis. *Radiology* **162**: 509–511

Kiss JP, Vizi ES 2001 Nitric oxide: a novel link between synaptic and nonsynaptic transmission. *Trends Neurosci* **24**: 211–215

Kivisäkk P, Alm GV, Tian WZ et al 1997 Neutralising and binding anti-interferon-β-1b treatment of multiple sclerosis. *Mult Scler* **3**: 184–190

Kivisäkk P, Tian W, Matusevicius D et al 1998a Optic neuritis and cytokines: no relation to MRI abnormalities and oligoclonal bands. *Neurology* **50**: 217–223

Kivisäkk P, Matusevicius D, He B et al 1998b IL-15 mRNA expression is up-regulated in blood and cerebrospinal fluid mononuclear cells in multiple sclerosis (MS). *Clin Exp Immunol* **111**: 193–197

Kivisäkk P, Lundahl, J, von Heigl Z, Fredrikson S 1998c No evidence for increased frequency of autoantibodies during interferon-beta1b treatment of multiple sclerosis. *Acta Neurol Scand* **97**: 320–323

Kivisäkk P, Trebst C, Liu Z et al 2002 T-cells in the cerebrospinal fluid express a similar repertoire of inflammatory chemokine receptors in the absence or presence of CNS inflammation: implications for CNS trafficking. *Clin Exp Immunol* **129**: 510–518

Kivisäkk P, Mahad D, Callahan MK et al 2003 Human cerebrospinal fluid central memory CD4+ T cells: evidence for trafficking through choroid plexus and meninges via P-selectin. *Proc Natl Acad Sci USA* **100**: 8389–8394

Klapper JA 1994 Interferon beta treatment of multiple sclerosis. *Neurology* **44**: 188; author reply 188–190

Klausner I 1901 Ein Beitrag zür Aetiologie der multiplen Sklerose. *Arch Psychiat* **34**: 841–869

Kleijnen J, Knipschild P 1995 Hyperbaric oxygen for multiple sclerosis: review of controlled trials. *Acta Neurol Scand* **91**: 330–334

Klein GM, Rose MS, Seland TP 1994 A prevalence study of multiple sclerosis in the

Crowsnest Pass region of southern Alberta. *Can J Neurol Sci* **21**: 262–265

Klein L, Klugmann M, Nave K-A et al 2000 Shaping of the autoreactive T cell repertoire by a splice variant of self protein expressed in thymic epithelial cells. *Nature Med* **6**: 56–61

Klein RS, Izikson L, Means T et al 2004 IFN-inducible protein 10/CXC chemokine ligand 10-independent induction of experimental autoimmune encephalomyelitis. *J Immunol* **112**: 550–559

Kleine TO, Albrecht J, Zofel F 1999 Flow cytometry of cerebrospinal fluid (CSF) lymphocytes: alterations of blood/CSF ratios of lymphocyte subsets in inflammatory disorders of the human central nervous system. *Clin Chem Lab Med* **37**: 231–241

Kleinman M, Brunquell P 1995 Acute disseminated encephalomyelitis: response to intravenous immunoglobulin? *J Child Neurol* **10**: 481–483

Kleinschmidt-Demasters BK, Tyler KL 2005 Progressive multifocal leukoencephalopathy complicating treatment with natalizumab and interferon beta-1a for multiple sclerosis. *N Engl J Med* **353**: 369–374

Kleyweg RP, van der Meche FG, Meulstee J 1988 Treatment of Guillain-Barre syndrome with high-dose gammaglobulin. *Neurology* **38**: 1639–1641

Klie LB, Margulies SL, Oh SJ 1982 Optic neuritis and myelitis following rubella vaccination. *Arch Neurol* **39**: 443–444

Klitz W, Maiers M, Spellman S et al 2003 New HLA haplotype frequency reference standards: high-resolution and large sample typing of HLA DR-DQ haplotypes in a sample of European Americans. *Tissue Antigens* **62**: 296–307

Klostermann W, Vieregge P, Köpf D 1993 Spamodic torticollis in multiple sclerosis: significance of an upper cervical spinal cord lesion. *Mov Disord* **8**: 234–236

van der Knaap MAA, Kamphorst W, Barth PG et al 1998 Phenotypic variation in leucoencephalopathy with vanishing white matter. *Neurology* **51**: 540–547

van der Knaap MAA, Leegwater PAJ, Konst AAM et al 2002 Mutations in each of the 5 subunits of translation initiation factor eIF2B can cause leucoencephalopathy with vanishing white matter. *Ann Neurol* **51**: 264–270

van der Knaap MS, Valk J 1995 *Magnetic Resonance of Myelin, Myelination and Myelin Disorders*. Berlin: Springer

Knobler RL, Panitch HS, Braheny JC et al 1984 Systemic alpha interferon therapy of multiple sclerosis. *Neurology* **34**: 1273–1279

Knox KK, Brewer JH, Henry JM et al 2000 Human herpesvirus 6 and multiple sclerosis: systemic active infections in patients with early disease. *Clin Infect Dis* **31**: 894–903

Kobayashi K, Kobayashi H, Ueda M, Honda Y 1996 Monoclonal antibody, KK1, recognises

human retinal astrocytes and distinguishes a sub-type of astrocyte in mouse brain. *Brain Res* **740**: 57–65

Koch MJ, Reed D, Stern R, Brody JA 1974 Multiple sclerosis: a cluster in a small northwestern United States community. *J Am Med Assoc* **228**: 1555–1557

Koch-Henriksen N 1989 An epidemiological study of multiple sclerosis: familial aggregation, social determinants and exogenous factors. *Acta Neurol Scand* **80** (Suppl 124): 123

Koch-Henriksen N 1995 Multiple sclerosis in Scandinavia and Finland. *Acta Neurol Scand suppl* **161**: 55–59

Koch-Henriksen N 1999 The Danish multiple sclerosis register: a 50-year follow-up. *Mult Scler* **5**: 293–296

Koch-Henriksen N, Bronnum-Hansen H, Hyllested K 1992 Incidence of multiple sclerosis in Denmark 1948–1982: a descriptive nationwide study. *Neuroepidemiology* **11**: 1–10

Koch-Henriksen N, Bronnum-Hansen H, Hyllested K 1994 The Danish multiple sclerosis registry: a 44 year review. In: Firnhaber W, Lauer K (eds) *Multiple Sclerosis in Europe: An Epidemiological Update*. Darmstadt: Leuchtturm-Verlag/LTV Press, pp. 79–86

Koch-Henriksen N, Bronnum-Hansen H, Stenager E 1998 Underlying cause of death in Danish patients with multiple sclerosis: results from the Danish Multiple Sclerosis registry. *J Neurol Neurosurg Psych* **65**: 56–59

Koh CS, Gausas J, Paterson PY 1993 Neurovascular permeability and fibrin deposition in the central nervous system of Lewis rats with cell-transferred experimental allergic encephalomyelitis in relationship to clinical and histopathological features of the disease. *J Neuroimmunol* **47**: 141–146

Koh D-R, Fung-Leung W-P, Ho A et al 1992 Less mortality but more relapses in experimental allergic encephalomyelitis in CD8$^{-/-}$ mice. *Science* **256**: 1210–1213

Kohama I, Lankford KL, Preiningerova J et al 2001 Transplantation of cryopreserved adult human Schwann cells enhances axonal conduction in demyelinated spinal cord. *J Neurosci* **21**: 944–950

Kohji T, Matsumoto Y 2000 Coexpression of Fas/FasL and Bax on brain and infiltrating T cells in the central nervous system is closely associated with apoptotic cell death during autoimmune encephalomyelitis. *J Neuroimmunol* **106**: 165–171

Kohler J, Kasper J, Kern U, Thoden U, Rehse-Küpper B 1986 Borrelia encephalomyelitis. *Lancet* **ii**: 35

Koibuchi T, Nakamura T, Miura T et al Acute disseminated encephalomyelitis following *Plasmodium vivax* malaria. *J Infect Chemother* **9**: 254–256

Koike F, Satoh J-I, Miyake S et al 2003 Microarray analysis identifies interferon beta regulated genes in multiple sclerosis. *J Neuroimmunol* **139**: 109–118

Kojima A, Tanaka-Kojima Y, Sakakura T, Nishizuka Y 1976 Prevention of post-thymectomy autoimmune thyroiditis in mice. *Lab Invest* **34**: 601–605

Kojima K, Berger Th, Lassmann H et al 1994 Experimental autoimmune panencephalitis and uveoretinitis transfered to the Lewis rat by T-lymphocytes specific for the S100β molecule, a calcium binding protein of astroglia. *J Exp Med* **180**: 817–829

Kojima K, Lassmann H, Wekerle H, Linington C 1997 The thymus and self tolerance: co-existence of encephalitogenic S-100 beta-specific T cells and their nominal autoantigen, in the normal adult rat thymus. *Int Immunol* **9**: 897–904

Kolb SJ, Costello F, Lee AG et al 2003 Distinguishing ischaemic stroke from the stroke-like lesions of MELAS using apparent diffusion coefficient mapping. *J Neurol Sci* **216**: 11–15

Koldovsky V, Koldovsky P, Henle G, Henle W, Ackerman R, Haase G 1975 Multiple sclerosis-associated agent: transmission to animals and some properties of the agent. *Infect Immunol* **12**: 1355–1366

Koles AJ, Rasminsky M 1972 A computer simulation of conduction in demyelinated nerve fibres. *J Physiol* **227**: 351–364

Köller H, Siebler M, Pekel M, Müller HW 1993 Depolarization of cultured astrocytes by leukotriene B$_4$: evidence for the induction of a K$^+$ concuctance inhibitor. *Brain Res* **612**: 28–44

Köller H, Thiem K, Siebler M 1996 Tumour necrosis factor-alpha increases intracellular Ca2+ and induces a depolarization in cultured astroglial cells. *Brain* **119**: 2021–2027

Köller H, Siebler M, Hartung H-P 1997 Immunologically induced electrophysiological dysfunction: implications for inflammatory diseases of the CNS and PNS. *Progr Neurobiol* **52**: 1–26

Köller H, Allert N, Oel D et al 1998 TNF alpha induces a protein kinase C-dependent reduction in astroglial K+ conductance. *NeuroReport* **9**: 1375–1378

Komoly S, Hudson LD, Webster HD, Bondy CA 1992 Insulin-like growth factor I gene expression is induced in astrocytes during experimental demyelination. *Proc Natl Acad Sci USA* **89**: 1894–1898

Koncan-Vracko B 1994 Epidemiological investigations of multiple sclerosis in Slovenia. In: Firnhaber W, Lauer K (eds) *Multiple Sclerosis in Europe: An Epidemiological Update*. Darmstadt: Leuchtturm-Verlag/LTV Press, pp. 294

Kondo T, Raff M 2000 Oligodendrocyte precursor cells reprogrammed to become multipotential CNS stem cells. *Science* **289**: 1754–1757

Kondo T, Raff MC 2004 A role for Noggin in the development of oligodendrocyte precursor cells. *Dev Biol* **267**: 242–251

Kondo T, Yamamura T, Inobe J-I et al 1996 TCR repertoire to proteolipid protein (PLP) in

873

multiple sclerosis (MS): homologies between PLP-specific T cells and MS associated T cells in TCR junctional sequences. *Int Immunol* **8**: 123–130

Konno H, Yamamoto T, Suzuki H *et al* 1990 Targeting of adoptively transferred experimental allergic encephalomyelitis lesion at the site of Wallerian degeneration. *Acta Neuropathol* **80**: 521–526

Koprowski H, De Freitas EC, Harper ME *et al* 1985 Multiple sclerosis and human T-cell lymphotrophic retroviruses. *Nature* **318**: 154–160

Kornek B, Lassmann H 1999 Axonal pathology in multiple sclerosis: a historical note. *Brain Pathol* **9**: 651–656

Kornek B, Storch M, Weissert R *et al* 2000 Multiple sclerosis and chronic autoimmune encephalomyelitis: a comparative quantitative study of axonal injury in active, inactive and remyelinated lesions. *Am J Pathol* **157**: 267–276

Kornek B, Storch MK, Bauer J *et al* 2001 Distribution of calcium channel subunit in dystrophic axons in multiple sclerosis and experiemntal autoimmune encephalomyelitis. *Brain* **124**: 1114–1124

Körner H, Lemckert FA, Chaudhri G *et al* 1997 Tumor necrosis factor blockade in actively induced experimental autoimmune encephalomyelitis prevents clinical disease despite activated T cell infiltration to the central nervous system. *Eur J Immunol* **27**: 1973–1981

Kornhuber HH, Schutz A 1990 Efficient treatment of neurogenic bladder disorders in multiple sclerosis with initial intermittent catheterisation and ultrasound-controlled training. *Eur Neurol* **30**: 260–267

Korn-Lubetzki I, Kahana E, Cooper G, Abramsky O 1984 Activity of multiple sclerosis during pregnancy and puerperium. *Ann Neurol* **16**: 229–231

Kotter MR, Setzu A, Sim FJ *et al* 2001 Macrophage depletion impairs oligodendrocyte remyelination following lysolecithin-induced demyelination. *Glia* **35**: 204–212

Kotzin BL, Karuturi S, Chou YK *et al* 1991 Preferential T-cell receptor β-chain variable gene use in myelin basic protein-reactive T-cell clones from patients with multiple sclerosis. *Proc Natl Acad Sci USA* **88**: 9161–9165

Koudriavtseva T, Thompson AJ, Fiorelli M *et al* 1997 Gadolinium enhanced MRI predicts clinical and MRI disease activity in relapsing–remitting multiple sclerosis. *J Neurol Neurosurg Psychiatry* **62**: 285–287

Kovacs GG, Hoeftberger R, Majtenyi K *et al* 2005 Neuropathology of white matter disease in Leber's hereditary optic neuropathy associated with the T14484C mutation. *Brain* **128**: 35–41

Kowalzick L 1997 Psoriasis flare caused by recombinant interferon beta injections. *J Am Acad Dermatol* **36**: 501

Kozak T, Havrdova E, Pitha J *et al* 2002 Immunoablative therapy with PBPC support with in vitro or in vivo T-cell depletion in patients with poor risk multiple sclerosis. *Bone Marrow Transplantation* **29**: S15

Kozin F, Haughton V, Bernhard GC 1977 Neuro-Behçet-disease: two cases and neuroradiologic findings. *Neurology* **17**: 1148–1152

Koziol JA, Feng AC 2004 Seasonal variations in exacerbations and MRI parameters in relapsing–remitting multiple sclerosis. *Neuroepidemiology* **23**: 217–223

Kozlowski PB, Schuller-Levis GB, Wisniewski HM 1987 Induction of synchronized relapses in SJL/J mice with chronic relapsing experimental allergic encephalomyelitis. *Acta Neuropathol* **74**: 163–168

Kozovska ME, Hong J, Zang YC *et al* 1999 Interferon beta induces T-helper 2 immune deviation in MS. *Neurology* **53**: 1692–1697

Kraft GH 1998 Rehabilitation principles for patients with multiple sclerosis. *J Spinal Cord Med* **21**: 117–120

Kraft GH, Freal JE, Coryell JK *et al* 1981 Multiple sclerosis: early prognostic guidelines. *Arch Phys Med Rehab* **62**: 54–58

Krakowski M, Owens T 1996 Interferon-gamma confers resistance to experimental allergic encephalomyelitis. *Eur J Immunol* **26**: 1641–1646

Krakowski ML, Owens T 2000 Naive T lymphocytes traffic to inflamed central nervous system, but require antigen recognition for activation. *Eur J Immunol* **30**: 1002–1009

Kral MG, Xiong Z, Study RE 1999 Alteration of Na+ currents in dorsal root ganglion neurons from rats with a painful neuropathy. *Pain* **81**: 15–24

Kramer R, Zhang Y, Gehrmann J *et al* 1995 Gene transfer through the blood-nerve barrier: nerve growth factor engineered neuritogenic T lymphocytes attenuate experimental autoimmune neuritis. *Nature Med* **1**: 1162–1166

Krametter D, Niederweiser G, Berghold A *et al* 2001 *Chlamydia pneumoniae* in multiple sclerosis: humoral immune responses in serum and cerebrospinal fluid and correlation with disease activity marker. *Mult Scler* **7**: 13–18

Kranz JMS, Kurland LT, Schuman LM, Layton D 1983 Multiple sclerosis in Olmsted and Mower Counties, Minnesota. *Neuroepidemiology* **2**: 206–218

Kraus J, Oschmann P, Engelhardt B *et al* 2000a CD45RA+ ICAM3+ lymphocytes in cerebrospinal fluid and blood as markers of disease activity in patients with multiple sclerosis. *Acta Neurol Scand* **102**: 326–332

Kraus J, Oschmann P, Engelhardt B *et al* 2000b Soluble and cell surface ICAM-3 in blood and cerebrospinal fluid of patients with multiple sclerosis: influence of

methylprednisolone treatment and relevance as markers for disease activity. *Acta Neurol Scand* **101**: 135–139

Krauscher MF, Miller EM 1982 Central serous choroidoretinopathy misdiagnosed as a manifestation of multiple sclerosis. *Ann Ophthalmol* **14**: 215–218

Kreisler A, De Sèze J, Stojkovic T *et al* 2003 Multiple sclerosis, interferon beta, and clinical thyroid dysfunction. *Acta Neurol Scand* **107**: 154–157

Krellmann H 1980 Egk, Werner In: Sadie S (ed.) *New Grove Dictionary of Music and Musicians.* London: Macmillan, Vol 6, p. 68

Kremenchutzky M, Cottrell D, Rice G *et al* 1999 The natural history of multiple sclerosis: a geographically based study 7. Progressive-relapsing and relapsing-progressive multiple sclerosis: a re-evaluation. *Brain* **122**: 1941–1949

Kriesel JD, White A, Hayden F *et al* 2004 Multiple sclerosis attacks are associated with picornavirus infections. *Mult Scler* **10**: 145–148

Krishnan C, Kerr DA 2005 Idiopathic transverse myelitis. *Arch Neurol* **62**: 1011–1013

Kriss A, Francis DA, Cuendet F *et al* 1988 Recovery after optic neuritis in childhood. *J Neurol Neurosurg Psychiatry* **51**: 1253–1258

Kroencke DC, Lynch SG, Denney DR 2000 Fatigue in multiple sclerosis: relationship to depression, disability, and disease pattern. *Mult Scler* **6**: 131–136

Kroepfl JF, Viise LR, Charron AJ *et al* 1996 Investigation of myelin/oligodendrocyte glycoprotein membrane topology. *J Neurochem* **67**: 2219–2122

Kroner A, Mehling M, Hemmer B *et al* 2005a A PD-1 polymorphism is associated with disease progression in multiple sclerosis. *Ann Neurol* **58**: 50–57

Kroner A, Vogel F, Kolb-Mäurer *et al* 2005b Impact of the Asp299Gly polymorphism in the toll-like receptor 4 (*TLR4*) gene on disease course of multiple sclerosis. *J Neuroimmunol* **165**: 161–165

Krücke W 1973 On the histopathology of acute hemorrhagic leucoencephalitis, acute disseminated encephalitis and concentric sclerosis. In: Shiraki H, Yonezawa T, Kuroiwa Y (eds) *International Symposium on Aetiology and Pathogenesis of the Demyelinating Diseases*, Kyoto, pp. 1–27

Kruglyak L 1999 Prospects for whole-genome linkage disequilibrium mapping of common disease genes. *Nature Genetics* **22**: 139–144

Kruglyak L, Lander ES 1995 Complete multipoint sib-pair analysis of qualitative and quantitative traits. *Am J Hum Genet* **57**: 439–454

Kruglyak L, Daly MJ, Reeve-Daly MP, Lander ES 1996 Parametric and nonparametric linkage analysis: a unified multipoint approach. *Am J Hum Genet* **58**: 1347–1363

Krumbholz M, Theil D, Derfuss T *et al* 2005 BAFF is produced by astrocytes and upregulated in multiple sclerosis lesions and primary central nervous system lymphoma. *J Exp Med* **201**: 195–200

Krupp LB 2003 Fatigue in multiple sclerosis: definition, pathophysiology and treatment. *CNS Drugs* **17**: 225–234

Krupp LB, Elkins LE 2000 Fatigue and declines in cognitive functioning in multiple sclerosis. *Neurology* **55**: 934–939

Krupp LB, Pollina DA 1996 Mechanisms and management of fatigue in progressive neurological disorders. *Curr Opin Neurol* **9**: 456–460

Krupp LB, Rizvi SA 2002 Symptomatic therapy for underrecognized manifestations of multiple sclerosis. *Neurology* **58**: S32–S39

Krupp LB, Alvarez LA, LaRocca NG, Scheinberg LC 1988 Fatigue in multiple sclerosis. *Arch Neurol* **45**: 435–437

Krupp LB, Coyle PK, Doscher C *et al* 1995 Fatigue therapy in multiple sclerosis: results of a double-blind, randomised, parallel trial of amantidine, pemoline and placebo. *Neurology* **45**: 1956–1961

Krupp LB, Christodoulou C, Melville P *et al* 2004a Effects of donepezil on memory and cognition in multiple sclerosis: comprehensive analysis of the AIMS Study. *Neurology* **62**: A179–A180

Krupp LB, Christodoulou C, Melville P *et al* 2004b Donepezil improved memory in multiple sclerosis in a randomized clinical trial. *Neurology* **63**: 1579–1585

Ksiazek SM, Repka MX, Maguire A *et al* 1989 Divisional oculomotor nerve paresis caused by intrinsic brainstem disease. *Ann Neurol* **26**: 714–718

Ku B, Lee K 1998 Acute transverse myelitis caused by Coxsackie virus B4 infection: a case report. *J Korean Med Sci* **13**: 449–453

Kubes P, Suzuki M, Granger DN 1991 Nitric oxide: an endogenous modulator of leukocyte adhesion. *Proc Natl Acad Sci USA* **88**: 4651–4655

Kuchroo VK, Sobel RA, Laning JC *et al* 1992 Experimental allergic encephalomyelitis mediated by cloned T cells specific for a synthetic peptide of myelin proteolipid protein: fine specificity and T cell receptor Vβ usage. *J Immunol* **148**: 3776–3782

Kuhlmann T, Glas M, zum Bruch C *et al* 2002a Investigation of bax, bcl-2, bcl-x and p53 gene polymorphisms in multiple sclerosis. *J Neuroimmunol* **129**: 154–160

Kuhlmann T, Lingfield G, Bitsch A *et al* 2002b Acute axonal damage in multiple sclerosis is most extensive in early disease stages and decreases over time. *Brain* **125**: 2202–2212

Kujala P, Portin R, Ruutiainen J 1997 The progress of cognitive decline in multiple sclerosis: a controlled 3-year follow-up. *Brain* **120**: 289–297

Kukekov VG, Laywell ED, Suslov ON *et al* 1999 Multipotent stem/progenitor cells with similar properties arise from two neurogenic regions of adult human brain. *Exp Neurol* **156**: 333–344

Kuker W, Nagěle T, Korfel A *et al* 2005 Primary central nervous system lymphoma (PCNSL): MRI features at presentation in 100 patients. *J Neuro-oncol* **72**:169–77

Kumar N, Low PA 2004 Myeloneuropathy and anaemia due to copper malabsorption. *J Neurol* **251**: 747–749

Kumar N, McEvoy KM, Ahlskog JE 2003 Myelopathy due to copper deficiency following gastric surgery. *Arch Neurol* **60**: 1782–1785

Kumar N, Gross JB jr, Ahlskog JE 2004 Copper deficiency myelopathy produces a picture like subacute combined degeneration. *Neurology* **63**: 33–39

Kunkel EJ, Butcher EC 2002 Chemokines and the tissue-specific migration of lymphocytes. *Immunity* **16**: 1–4

Kuokkanen S, Sundvall M, Terwilliger JD *et al* 1996 A putative vulnerability locus to multiple sclerosis maps to 5p14-p12 in a region syntenic to the murine locus Eae2. *Nature Genet* **13**: 477–480

Kuokkanen S, Gschwend M, Rioux JD *et al* 1997 Genomewide scan of multiple sclerosis in Finnish multiplex families. *Am J Hum Genet* **61**: 1379–1387

Kupersmith MJ, Alban T, Zeiffer B, Lefton D 2002 Contrast-enhanced MRI in acute optic neuritis: relationship to visual performance. *Brain* **125**: 812–822

Kupfer H, Monks CRF, Kupfer A 1994 Small splenic B cells that bind to antigen-specific T helper (Th) cells and face the site of cytokine production in the Th cells selectively proliferate: immunofluorescence microscopic studies of Th-B antigen-presenting cell interactions. *J Exp Med* **179**: 1507–1515

Kurdi A, Abdallat A, Ayesh I *et al* 1977 Different B lymphocyte alloantigens associated with multiple sclerosis in Arabs and Northern Europeans. *Lancet* **i**: 1123–1125

Kurenny DE, Moroz LL, Turner RW *et al* 1994 Modulation of ion channels in rod photoreceptors by nitric oxide. *Neuron* **13**: 315–324

Kurland LT 1952 The frequency and geographic distribution of multiple sclerosis as indicated by mortality statistics and morbidity surveys in the United States and Canada. *Am J Hyg* **55**: 457–476

Kurland LT 1994 Trauma and multiple sclerosis. *Ann Neurol* **36 (Suppl)**: S33–S37

Kurland LT, Beebe GW, Kurtzke JF *et al* 1966 Studies on the natural history of multiple sclerosis. 2. The progression of optic neuritis to multiple sclerosis. *Acta Neurol Scand* **42 (Suppl 19)**: 157–176

Kurland LT, Molgaard CA, Kurland EM *et al* 1984 Swine flu vaccine and multiple sclerosis. *J Am Med Assoc* **251**: 2672–2675

Kuroiwa Y 1985 Concentric sclerosis. In: Koetsier JC (ed) *Handbook of Clinical Neurology*. Amsterdam: Elsevier, Vol 47, pp. 409–417

Kuroiwa Y, Igata A, Itahara K *et al* 1975 Nationwide survey of multiple sclerosis in Japan: clinical analysis of 1,084 cases. *Neurology* **25**: 845–51

Kuroiwa Y, Shibasaki S, Tabira T, Itoyama Y 1982 Clinical picture of multiple sclerosis in Asia. In: Kuroiwa Y, Kurland LT (eds) *Multiple Sclerosis East and West*. Kyushu: Kyushu University Press, pp. 31–47

Kuroiwa Y, Shibasaki H, Ikeda M 1983 Prevalence of multiple sclerosis and its north-south gradient in Japan. *Neuroepidemiology* **2**: 62–69

Kurtzke JF 1956 Course of exacerbations of multiple sclerosis hospitalised patients. *Arch Neurol Psychiatry* **76**: 175–184

Kurtzke JF 1961 On the evaluation of disability in multiple sclerosis. *Neurology* **11**: 686–694

Kurtzke JF 1965a Further notes on disability evaluation in multiple sclerosis, with scale modifications. *Neurology* **15**: 654–661

Kurtzke JF 1965b On the time of onset in multiple sclerosis. *Acta Neurol Scand* **41**: 140–158

Kurtzke JF 1967 Further considerations on the geographic distribution of multiple sclerosis. *Acta Neurol Scand* **43**: 283–297

Kurtzke JF 1970 Clinical manifestations of multiple sclerosis. In: Vinken PJ, Bruyn GW (eds) *Handbook of Clinical Neurology*. Amsterdam: Elsevier, Vol 9, pp. 161–216

Kurtzke JF 1974 Further features of the Fennoscandian focus of multiple sclerosis. *Acta Neurol Scand* **50**: 478–502

Kurtzke JF 1975 A reassessment of the distribution of multiple sclerosis. *Acta Neurol Scand* **51**: 110–157

Kurtzke JF 1977 Geography in multiple sclerosis. *J Neurol* **215**: 1–26

Kurtzke JF 1980a The geographic distribution of multiple sclerosis: an update with special reference to Europe and the Mediterranean region. *Acta Neurol Scand* **62**: 65–80

Kurtzke JF 1980b Epidemiologic contributions to multiple sclerosis – an overview. *Neurology* **30 (Part 2)**: 61–79

Kurtzke JF 1983a Rating neurologic impairment in multiple sclerosis: an expanded disability status scale (EDSS). *Neurology* **33**: 1444–1452

Kurtzke JF 1983b Epidemiology of multiple sclerosis. In: Hallpike JF, Adams CWM, Tourtellotte WW (eds) *Multiple Sclerosis: Pathology, Diagnosis and Management*. London: Chapman & Hall, pp. 47–95

Kurtzke JF 1985a Optic neuritis or multiple sclerosis. *Arch Neurol* **42**: 704–710

Kurtzke JF 1985b Epidemiology of multiple sclerosis. In: Vinken PJ, Bruyn GW, Klawans HL (eds) *Handbook of Clinical Neurology*, revised series, *Demyelinating Diseases*. Amsterdam: Elsevier, Vol 3, pp. 259–287

Kurtzke JF 1988 Multiple sclerosis: what's in a name? *Neurology* **38**: 309–316

Kurtzke JF 1989 On estimating survival: a tale of two censors. *J Clin Epidemiol* **42**: 169–175

Kurtzke JF 1991 Multiple sclerosis: changing times. *Neuroepidemiology* **10**: 1–8

Kurtzke JF 1993 Epidemiologic evidence for multiple sclerosis as an infection. *Clin Microbiol Rev* **6**: 382–427

Kurtzke JF 1996 An introduction to neuroepidemiology. *Neuroepidemiology* **14**: 255–272

Kurtzke JF 2000 Epidemiology of multiple sclerosis: does this really point toward an etiology? Lectio Doctoralis. *Neurol Sci* **21**: 383–403

Kurtzke JF 2004 Origin of DSS: to present the plan. *Newsletter VA Special Interest Group Consortium MS Centers* **3**: 1–4

Kurtzke JF 2005 Epidemiology and etiology of multiple sclerosis. *Phys Med Rehab Clin N Am* **16**: 327–349

Kurtzke JF, Bui QH 1980 Multiple sclerosis in a migrant population: 2. Half Orientals immigrating in childhood. *Ann Neurol* **8**: 256–260

Kurtzke JF, Heltberg A 2001 Multiple sclerosis in the Faroe Islands: an epitome. *J Clin Epidemiol* **54**: 1–22

Kurtzke JF, Hyllested K 1979 Multiple sclerosis in the Faroe islands: 1. Clinical and epidemiological features. *Ann Neurol* **5**: 6–21

Kurtzke JF, Hyllested K 1986 Multiple sclerosis in the Faroe Islands. II. Clinical update, transmission, and the nature of MS. *Neurology* **36**: 307–328

Kurtzke JF, Hyllested K 1987 Multiple sclerosis in the Faroe Islands. III. An alternative assessment of the three epidemics. *Acta Neurol Scand* **76**: 317

Kurtzke JF, Hyllested K 1988 Validity of the epidemics of multiple sclerosis in the Faroe islands. *Neuroepidemiology* **7**: 190–227

Kurtzke JF, Page 1997 Epidemiology of multiple sclerosis in US veterans. VII. Risk factors for MS. *Neurology* **48**: 204–213

Kurtzke JF, Beebe GW, Nagler B, Auth TL, Kurland LT, Nefzger MD 1968a Studies on natural history of multiple sclerosis. 4: Clinical features of the onset bout. *Acta Neurol Scand* **44**: 467–499

Kurzke JF, Park CS, Oh SJ 1968b Multiple sclerosis in Korea: clinical features and prevalence. *J Neurol Sci* **6**: 463–481

Kurtzke JF, Auth TL, Beebe GW et al 1969 Survival in multiple sclerosis. *Trans Am Neurol Assoc* **94**: 134–139

Kurtzke JF, Beebe GW, Nagler B, Nefzger MD, Auth TL, Kurland LT 1970a Studies on the natural history of multiple sclerosis 5: long-term survival in young men. *Arch Neurol* **22**: 215–225

Kurtzke JF, Dean G, Botha DPJ 1970b A method of estimating the age at immigration of white immigrants to South Africa with an example of its importance. *S Afr Med J* **44**: 663–669

Kurtzke JF, Kurland LT, Goldberg ID 1971 Mortality and migration in multiple sclerosis. *Neurology* **21**: 1186–1197

Kurtzke JF, Beebe GW, Nagler B et al 1973 Studies on the natural history of multiple sclerosis. 7: Correlates of clinical changes in an early bout. *Acta Neurol Scand* **49**: 379–395

Kurtzke JF, Beebe GW, Nagler B, Kurland LT, Auth TL 1977 Studies on the natural history of multiple sclerosis. 8. Early

prognostic features of the later course of the illness. *J Chroni Dis* **30**: 819–830

Kurtzke, JF, Beebe GW, Norman Jr JE 1979 Epidemiology of multiple sclerosis in US veterans. 1. Race, sex, and geographic distribution. *Neurology* **29**: 1228–1235

Kurtzke JF, Gudmundsson KR, Bergmann S 1982 Multiple sclerosis in Iceland. 1. Evidence of a post-war epidemic. *Neurology* **32**: 143–150

Kurtzke JF, Beebe GW, Norman JE 1985 Epidemiology of multiple sclerosis in US veterans. III. Migration and the risk of MS. *Neurology* **35**: 672–678

Kurtzke JF, Hyllested K, Arbuckle JD et al 1988 Multiple sclerosis in the Faroe Islands. IV. The lack of a relationship between canine distemper and the epidemics of MS. *Acta Neurol Scand* **78**: 484–500

Kurtzke JF, Page WF, Murphy FM et al 1992 Epidemiology of multiple sclerosis in veterans. 4. Age at onset. *Neuroepidemiology* **11**: 226–235

Kurtzke JF, Hyllested K, Heltberg A, Olsen A 1993 Multiple sclerosis in the Faroe Islands. V. The occurrence of the fourth epidemic as validation of transmission. *Acta Neurol Scand* **88**: 161–173

Kurtzke JF, Hyllested K, Heltberg A 1995 Multiple sclerosis in the Faroe Islands: transmission across four epidemics. *Acta Neurol Scand* **91**: 321–325

Kurtzke JF, Hyllested K, Arbuckle JD et al 1997 Multiple sclerosis in the Faroe Islands. 7. Results of a case control questionnaire with multiple controls. *Acta Neurol Scand* **96**: 149–157

Kurtzke JF, Delasnerie-Laupretre N, Wallin MT 1998 Multiple sclerosis in North African migrants to France. *Acta Neurol Scand* **98**: 302–309

Kusuhara T, Nakajima M, Inoue H et al 2002 Parainfectious encephalomyeloradiculitis associated with herpes simplex virus 1 DNA in cerebrospinal fluid. *Clin Infect Dis* **34**: 1199–1205

Kutzelnigg A, Lucchinetti CF, Stadelmann C et al 2005 Cortical demyelination and diffuse white matter injury in multiple sclerosis. *Brain* **128**: 2705–2712

Kuwabara S, Cappelen-Smith C, Lin CSY et al 2000 Excitability properties of median and peroneal motor axons. *Muscle Nerve* **23**: 1365–1373

Kuwabara S, Cappelen-Smith C, Lin CS et al 2001 Differences in accommodative properties of median and peroneal motor axons. *J Neurol Neurosurg Psychiatry* **70**: 372–376

Kuwabara S, Ogawara K, Sung JY et al 2002 Differences in membrane properties of axonal and demyelinating Guillain-Barre syndromes. *Ann Neurol* **52**: 180–187

Kwon EE, Prineas JW 1994 Blood brain barrier abnormalities in longstanding multiple sclerosis lesions: an immunohistochemical study. *J Neuropathol Exp Neurol* **53**: 625–636

Kwon OJ, Karni A, Israel S et al 1999 HLA class II susceptibility to multiple sclerosis

among Ashkenazi and non-Ashkenazi Jews. *Arch Neurol* **56**: 555–560

Laaksonen M, Pastinen T, Sjoroos M et al 2002 HLA class II associated risk and protection against multiple sclerosis – a Finnish family study. *J Neuroimmunol* **122**: 140–145

Laaksonen M, Jonasdittir A, Fossdal R et al 2003 A whole genome association study in Finish multiple sclerosis patients with 3669 markers. *J Neuroimmunol* **143**: 70–73

van der Laan LJW, Ruuls SR, Weber KS et al 1996 Macrophage phagocytosis of myelin *in vitro* determined by flow cytometry: phagocytosis is mediated by CR3 and induces production of tumor necrosis factor-α and nitric oxide. *J Neuroimmunol* **70**: 45–152

van der Laan LJ, van der Goes A, Wauben MH et al 2002 Beneficial effect of modified peptide inhibitor of alpha4 integrins on experimental allergic encephalomyelitis in Lewis rats. *J Neurosci Res* **67**: 191–199

Laan M, Wiebe V, Khusnutdinova E et al 2005 X-chromosome as a marker for population history: linkage disequilibrium and haplotype study in Eurasian populations. *Eur J Hum Genet* **13**: 452–462

LaBan MM, Martin T, Pechur J, Sarnacki S 1998 Physical and occupational therapy in the treatment of patients with multiple sclerosis. *Phys Med Rehab Clin N Am* **9**: 603–614

Lacour A, De Seze J, Revenco E et al 2004 Acute aphasia in multiple sclerosis: a multicenter study of 22 patients. *Neurology* **62**: 974–977

Ladd H, Oist C, Jonnson B 1974 The effect of Dantrium® on spasticity in multiple sclerosis. *Acta Neurol Scand* **50**: 397–408

Ladiwala U, Lachance C, Simoneau SJ et al 1998 p75 neurotrophin receptor expression on adult human oligodendrocytes: signaling without cell death in response to NGF. *J Neurosci* **18**: 1297–1304

Ladiwala U, Li H, Antel JP, Nalbantoglu J 1999 Induction by tumor necrosis factor-alpha and involvement of p53 in cell death of human oligodendrocytes. *J Neurochem* **73**: 605–611

Lafaille JJ, Nagashima K, Katsuki M, Tonegawa S 1994 High incidence of spontaneous autoimmune encephalomyelitis in immunodeficient anti-myelin basic protein T cell receptor mice. *Cell* **78**: 399–408

Lafaille JJ, Keere FV, Hsu AL et al 1997 Myelin basic protein-specific T helper 2 (Th2) cells cause experimental autoimmune encephalomyelitis in immunodeficient hosts rather than protect them from disease. *J Exp Med* **186**: 307–312

Laguemy A, Arnaud A, Le Masson G et al 1998 Study of central and peripheral conductions to the diaphragm in 22 patients with definite multiple sclerosis. *Electromyogr Clin Neurophysiol* **38**: 333–342

Lai HM, Hodgson T, Gawne-Cain M et al 1996 A preliminary study into the sensitivity of disease activity detection by serial weekly magnetic resonance imaging in multiple sclerosis. *J Neurol Neurosurg Psychiatry* **60**: 339–341

Lai K, Kaspar BK, Gage FH, Schaffer DV 2003 Sonic hedgehog regulates adult neural progenitor proliferation in vitro and in vivo. *Nat Neurosci* **6**: 21–27

Lai MM, Kerrison JB, Miller NF 2004 Reversible bilateral internuclear ophthalmoplegia associated with FK506. *J Neurol Neurosurg Psychiatry* **75**: 776–778

Lakatos A, Smith PM, Barnett SC, Franklin RJ 2003 Meningeal cells enhance limited CNS remyelination by transplanted olfactory ensheathing cells. *Brain* **126**: 598–609

La Mantia L, Illeni MT, Milanese C et al 1990 HLA and multiple sclerosis in Italy: a review of the literature. *J Neurol* **237**: 441–444

La Mantia L, Eoli M, Milanese C, Salmaggi A, Dufour A, Torri V 1994 Double-blind trial of dexamethasone versus methylprednisolone in multiple sclerosis acute relapses. *Eur Neurol* **34**: 199–203

La Mantia L, Milanese C, Mascoli N et al 2002 Cyclophosphamide for multiple sclerosis. *Cochrane Database Syst Rev* **4**: CD002819

van Lambalgen R, Sanders EACM, D'Amaro J 1986 Sex distribution, age of onset and HLA profiles in two types of multiple sclerosis: a role for sex hormones and microbial infections in the development of autoimmunity. *J Neurol Sci* **76**: 13–21

Lambert S, Davis JQ, Bennett V 1997 Morphogenesis of the node of Ranvier: co-clusters of ankyrin and ankyrin-binding integral proteins define early developmental intermediates. *J Neurosci* **17**: 7025–7036

Lamers KH, van Engelen BG, Gabreels FJ, Hommes OR, Borm GF, Wevers RA 1995 Cerebrospinal neuron-specific enolase, S-100 and myelin basic protein in neurological disorders. *Acta Neurol Scand* **92**: 247–251

Lamers KJ, de-Reus HP, Jongen PJ 1998 Myelin basic protein in CSF as indicator of disease activity in multiple sclerosis. *Mult Scler* **4**: 124–126

Lammens M, Lissoir F, Carton H 1989 Hypothermia in three patients with multiple sclerosis. *Clin Neurol Neurosurg* **91**: 117–121

Lamoureux G, Duquette P, Lapiuerre Y et al 1983 HLA antigens-linked genetic control in multiple sclerosis patients resistant and susceptible to infection. *J Neurol* **230**: 91–104

Lampasona V, Franciotta D, Furlan R et al 2004 Similar low frequency of anti-MOG IgG and IgM in MS patients and healthy subjects. *Neurology* **62**: 2092–2094

Lampert PW, Carpenter S 1965 Electron microscopic studies on the vascular permeability and the mechanism of demyelination in experimental allergic encephalomyelitis. *J Neuropathol Exp Neurol* **24**: 11–24

Lana-Peixoto MA, Lana-Peixoto MI 1992 Is multiple sclerosis in Brazil and Asia alike? *Arq Neuropsiquiatr* **50**: 419–425

Lana-Peixoto MA, Teixeira A, The Brazilian Committee for Treatment and Research in Multiple Sclerosis (BCTRIMS) 2002 Simple phonic tic in multiple sclerosis. *Mult Scler* **8**: 510–511

Lander E, Krugylak L 1995 Genetic dissection of complex traits: guidelines for interpreting and reporting linkage results. *Nature Genet* **11**: 241–224

Landtblom AM, Riise T, Boiko A, Soderfeldt B 2002 Distribution of multiple sclerosis in Sweden based on mortality and disability compensation statistics. *Neuroepidemiology* **21**: 167–179

Landtblom AM, Wastenson M, Ahmadi A, Soderkvist P 2003 Multiple sclerosis and exposure to organic solvents, investigated by genetic polymorphisms of the GSTM1 and CYP2D6 enzyme systems. *Neurol Sci* **24**: 248–251

Landtblom AM, Riise T, Kurtzke JF 2005 Further considerations on the distribution of multiple sclerosis in Sweden. *Acta Neurol Scand* **111**: 238–246

Landy PJ 1983 A prospective study of the risk of developing multiple sclerosis in optic neuritis in a tropical and subtropical area. *J Neurol Neurosurg Psychiatry* **46**: 659–661

Lang HLE, Jacobsen H, Ikemizu S et al 2002 A functional and structural basis for TCR cross-reactivity in multiple sclerosis. *Nature Immunol* **3**: 940–943

Lange KFA 1913 Die Ausflockung kolloidalen Goldes dürch Zerebrospinalflüssigkeit bei luetischen Affektion des Zentralnervensystems. *Z Chemother* **1**: 44–78

Langer-Gould A, Atlas SW, Bollen AW, Pelletier D 2005 Progressive multifocal leukoencephalopathy in a patient treated with natalizumab. *N Engl J Med* **353**: 375–381

Langrish CL, Chen Y, Blumenschein WM et al 2005 IL-23 drives a pathogenic T cell population that induces autoimmune inflammation. *J Exp Med* **201**: 233–240

Lannes-Vieira J, Goudable B, Drexler K et al 1995 Encephalitogenic, myelin basic protein specific T cells from naive rat thymus: preferential use of the T cell receptor gene Vb8.2 and expression of the CD4⁻CD8⁻ phenotype. *Eur J Immunol* **25**: 611–616

Lapierre Y, Bouchard S, Tansey C, Gendron D, Barkas WJ, Francis GS 1987 Treatment of spasticity with tizanidine in multiple sclerosis. *Can J Neurol Sci* **14**: S13–S17

Lappe-Siefke C, Goebbels S, Gravel M et al 2003 Disruption of Cnp1 uncouples oligodendroglial functions in axonal support and myelination. *Nature Genet* **33**: 366–374

Largo C, Cuevas P, Somjen GG et al 1996 The effect of depressing glial function in rat brain *in situ* on ion homeostasis, synaptic transmission and neuron survival. *J Neurosci* **16**: 1219–1229

Larsen F, Oturai A, Ryder LP et al 2000 A linkage analysis of a candidate region in Scandinavian sib pairs with multiple sclerosis reveals linkage to chromosome 17q. *Genes Immun* **1**: 456–459

Larsen JP, Aarli JA, Riise T 1984 Western Norway, a high risk area for multiple sclerosis: a prevalence/incidence study in the county of Hordaland. *Neurology* **34**: 1202–1207

Larsson HBW, Frederiksen J, Kjaer L et al 1988 *In vivo* determination of T_1 and T_2 in the brain of patients with severe but stable multiple sclerosis. *Magn Reson Med* **7**: 43–55

Lassmann H 1983 Comparative neuropathology of chronic experimental allergic encephalomyelitis and multiple sclerosis. *Schrift Neurol* **25**: 1–135

Lassmann H 2003a Axonal injury in multiple sclerosis. *J Neurol Neurosurg Psychiatry* **74**: 695–697

Lassmann H 2003b Brain damage when multiple sclerosis is diagnosed clinically. *Lancet* **361**: 1317–1318

Lassmann H, Vass K 1995 Are current immunological concepts of multiple sclerosis reflected by the immunopathology of its lesions? *Springer Semin Immunopathol* **17**: 77–87

Lassmann H, Wisniewski HM 1979a Chronic relapsing experimental allergic encephalomyelitis: clinicopathological comparison with multiple sclerosis. *Arch Neurol* **36**: 490–497

Lassmann H, Wisniewski HM 1979b Chronic relapsing experimental allergic encephalomyelitis: effect of age at the time of sensitization on clinical course and pathology. *Acta Neuropathol* **47**: 111–116

Lassmann H, Wisniewski HM 1979c Chronic relapsing experimental allergic encephalomyelitis: morphological sequence of myelin degradation. *Brain Res* **169**: 357–368

Lassmann H, Kitz K, Wisniewski HM 1980 Structural variability of demyelinating lesions in different models of subacute and chronic experimental allergic encephalomyelitis. *Acta Neuropathol* **51**: 191–201

Lassmann H, Budka H, Schnaberth G 1981a Inflammatory demyelinating polyradiculitis in a patient with multiple sclerosis. *Arch Neurol* **38**: 99–102

Lassmann H, Kitz K, Wisniewski HM 1981b *In vivo* effect of sera from animals with chronic relapsing experimental allergic encephalomyelitis on central and peripheral myelin. *Acta Neuropathol* **55**: 297–306

Lassmann H, Kitz K, Wisniewski HM 1981c The development of periventricular lesions in chronic relapsing experimental allergic encephalomyelitis in guinea pigs: a light and scanning electron microscope study. *Neuropathol Appl Neurobiol* **7**: 1–11

Lassmann H, Brunner C, Bradl M, Linington C 1988 Experimental allergic encephalomyelitis: the balance between encephalitogenic T lymphocytes and demyelinating antibodies determines size and structure of demyelinated lesions. *Acta Neuropathol* **75**: 566–576

Lassmann H, Zimprich F, Vass K, Hickey WF 1991a Microglial cells are a component of the perivascular glia limitans. *J Neurosci Res* **28**: 236–243

Lassmann H, Rössler K, Zimprich F, Vass K 1991b Expression of adhesion molecules and histocompatibility antigens at the blood-brain barrier. *Brain Pathol* **1**: 115–123

Lassmann H, Schmied M, Vass K, Hickey WF 1993 Bone marrow derived elements and resident microglia in brain inflammation. *Glia* **7**: 19–24

Lassmann H, Bartsch U, Montag D, Schachner M 1997 Dying back oligodendrogliopathy: a late sequel of myelin-associated glycoprotein deficiency. *Glia* **19**: 104–110

Lassmann H, Brück W, Lucchinetti C 2001 Heterogeneity of multiple sclerosis pathogenesis: implications for diagnosis and therapy. *Trends Mol Med* **7**: 115–121

Lassmann H, Reindl M, Rauschka H *et al* 2003 A new paraclinical CSF marker for hypoxia-like tissue damage in multiple sclerosis lesions. *Brain* **126**: 1347–1357

Lataste X, Emre M, Davis C, Groves L 1994 Comparative profile of tizanidine in the management of spasticity. *Neurology* **44 (Suppl 9)**: S53–S59

Lauer K 1994 The risk of multiple sclerosis in the USA in relation to sociogeographic features: a factor-analytic study. *J Clin Epidemiol* **47**: 43–48

Lauer K, Firnhaber W 1987 Epidemiological investigations into multiple sclerosis in southern Hesse. V. Course and prognosis. *Acta Neurol Scand* **76**: 12–17

Lauer K, Firnhaber W 1994 Descriptive and analytical epidemiological data on multiple sclerosis from a long-term study in southern Hesse, Germany. In: Firnhaber W, Lauer K (eds) *Multiple Sclerosis in Europe: An Epidemiological Update.* Darmstadt: Leuchtturm-Verlag/LTV Press, pp. 147–158

Lauer K, Firnhaber W, Reining R, Leuchtweis B 1984 Epidemiological investigations into multiple sclerosis in Southern Hesse. I. Methodological problems and basic epidemiological characteristics. *Acta Neurol Scand* **70**: 257–265

Laughlin MJ, Barker J, Bambach B *et al* 2001 Hematopoietic engraftment and survival in adult recipients of umbilical-cord blood from unrelated donors. *N Engl J Med* **344**: 1815–1822

Laule C, Vavasour IM, Moore GR et al 2004 Water content and myelin water fraction in multiple sclerosis. A T2 relaxation study. *J Neurol* **251**: 284–293

Lavalle C, Pizarro S, Drenkard C, Sanchez-Guarro J, Alarcón-Segoria D 1990 Transverse myelitis: a manifestation of systemic lupus erythematosus strongly associated with antiphospholipid antibodies. *J Rheumatol* **17**: 34–37

Lawrence N, Oger J, Aziz T *et al* 2003 A sensitive radioimmunoprecipitation assay for assessing the clinical relevance of antibodies to IFN beta. *J Neurol Neurosurg Psychiatry* **74**: 1236–1239

Lawthom C, Durey P, Hughes T 2003 Constipation as a presenting symptom. *Lancet* **362**: 958

Laywell ED, Rakic P, Kukekov VG *et al* 2000 Identification of a multipotent astrocytic stem cell in the immature and adult mouse brain. *Proc Natl Acad Sci* **97**: 13883–13888

Lazarte JA 1950 Multiple sclerosis: prognosis for ambulatory and nonambulatory patients. *Assoc Res Nerv Ment Dis Proc* **28**: 512–523

Lazeron RH, Langdon DW, Filippi M *et al* 2000 Neuropsychological impairment in multiple sclerosis patients: the role of (juxta)cortical lesion on FLAIR. *Mult Scler* **6**: 280–285

Leandri M, Lundardi G, Inglese M *et al* 2000 Lamotrigine in trigeminal neuralgia secondary to multiple sclerosis. *J Neurol* **247**: 556–558

Leao RN, Oikawa T, Rosa ES *et al* 2002 Isolation of dengue 2 virus from a patient with central nervous system involvement (transverse myelitis). *Rev Soc Bras Med Trop* **35**: 401–404

Leary SM, Davie CA, Parker GJ *et al* 1999 1H magnetic resonance spectroscopy of normal appearing white matter in primary progressive multiple sclerosis. *J Neurol* **246**: 1023–1026

Leary SM, McLean BN, Thompson EJ *et al* 2002 Local synthesis of IgA in the cerebrospinal fluid of patients with neurological diseases. *J Neurol* **247**: 609–615

Leary SM, Miller DH, Stevenson VL *et al* 2003 Interferon beta-1a in primary progressive MS: an exploratory, randomized, controlled trial. *Neurology* **60**: 44–51

Leary SM, Porter B, Thompson AJ 2005 Multiple sclerosis: diagnosis and the management of acute relapses. *J Postgrad Med J* **81**:302–308

Lebar R, Lubetzki C, Vincent C *et al* 1986 The MS autoantigen of central nervous system myelin, a glycoprotein present in oligodendrocyte membranes. *Clin Exp Immunol* **66**: 423–434

Lee AG, Tang RA, Wong GG *et al* 2000 Isolated inferior rectus muscle palsy resulting from a nuclear third nerve lesion as the initial manifestation of multiple sclerosis. *J Neuroophthalmol* **20**: 246–247

Lee J, Elston J, Vickers S *et al* 1988 Botulinum toxin therapy for squint. *Eye* **2**: 24–28

Lee JC 1972 Evolution in the concept of the blood brain barrier phenomenon. In: Zimmermann HM (ed.) *Progress in Neuropathology.* New York: Grune & Stratton, pp. 84–145

Lee KH, Hashimoto SA, Hooge JP *et al* 1991 Magnetic resonance imaging of the head in the diagnosis of multiple sclerosis: a prospective 2-year follow-up with comparison of clinical evaluation, evoked potentials, oligoclonal banding, and CT. *Neurology* **41**: 657–660

Lee MA, Smith S, Palace J *et al* 1999 Spatial mapping of T2 and gadolinium-enhancing T1 lesion volumes in multiple sclerosis: evidence for distinct mechanisms of lesion genesis? *Brain* **122**: 1261–1270

Lee MA, Reddy H, Johansen-Berg H *et al* 2000 The motor cortex shows adaptive functional changes to brain injury from multiple sclerosis. *Ann Neurol* **47**: 606–613

Lee MA, Blamire AM, Pendlebury S *et al* 2000 Axonal injury or loss in the internal capsule and motor impairment in multiple sclerosis. *Arch Neurol* **57**: 65–70

Lee SC, Raine CS 1989 Multiple sclerosis: oligodendrocytes in active lesions do not express class II major histocompatibility complex molecules. *J Neuroimmunol* **25**: 261–266

Lee SC, Moore GR, Golensky G, Raine CS 1990 Multiple sclerosis: a role for astroglia in active demyelination suggested by class II MHC expression and ultrastructural study. *J Neuropathol Exp Neurol* **49**: 122–136

Lee SC, Dickson DW, Brosnan CF 1995 Interleukin-1, nitric oxide and reactive astrocytes. *Brain Behav Immun* **9**: 345–354

Lee SJ, Benveniste EN 1999 Adhesion molecule expression and regulation on cells of the central nervous system. *J Neuroimmunol* **98**: 77–88

Lee WB, Berger JR, O'Halloran HS 2003 Parinaud syndrome heralding MS. *Neurology* **60**: 322

Lees G 1998 Effects of pyrethroid molecules on rat nerves in vitro: potential to reverse temperature-sensitive conduction block of demyelinated peripheral axons. *Br J Pharmacol* **123**: 487–496

Legras A 1934 Multiple Sclerose bij Tweelingen. *Ned Tijdschr Geneeskd* **78**: 174–177

Le Hir M, Bluethmann H, Kosco-Vilbois MH *et al* 1996 Differentiation of follicular dendritic cells and full antibody responses require tumor necrosis factor receptor-1 signalling. *J Exp Med* **183**: 2367–2372

Lehman RAW, Fieger HG 1978 Arachnoid cyst producing recurrent neurological disturbances. *Surg Neurol* **10**: 134–136

Lehmann PV, Forsthuber T, Miller A, Sercarz EE 1992 Spreading of T-cell autoimmunity to cryptic determinants of an autoantigen. *Nature* **358**: 155–157

Lehmann PV, Sercarz EE, Forsthuber T *et al* 1993 Determinant spreading and the dynamics of the autoimmune T cell repertoire. *Immunol Today* **14**: 203–208

Lehnardt S, Lachance C, Patrizi S *et al* 2002 The toll-like receptor TLR4 is necessary for lipopolysaccharide-induced oligodendrocyte injury in the CNS. *J Neurosci* **22**: 2478–2486

Lehrmann E, Molinari A, Speciale C, Schwarcz R 2001 Immunohistochemical visualization of newly formed quinolinate in the normal and excitotoxically lesioned rat striatum. *Exp Brain Res* **141**: 389–397

Lehoczky T, Halasy-Lehoczky M 1963 Forme 'bénigne' de la sclérose en plaques. *La Presse Médicale* **71**: 2294–2296

LeHuen A, Lantz O, Beaudoin L *et al* 1998 Over-expression of natural killer T cells protects Va14-Ja281 transgenic nonobese mice against diabetes. *J Exp Med* **188**: 1831–1839

Leibowitz U, Alter M 1968 Optic nerve involvement as initial manifestation of multiple sclerosis. *Acta Neurol Scand* **44**: 70–80

Leibowitz U, Alter M 1970 Clinical factors associated with increased disability in multiple sclerosis. *Acta Neurol Scand* **46**: 53–70

Leibowitz U, Alter M 1973 *Multiple Sclerosis: Clues to its Cause*. Amsterdam: North Holland

Leibowitz U, Alter M, Halpern L 1964a Clinical studies of multiple sclerosis in Israel. III. Clinical course and prognosis related to age at onset. *Neurology* **14**: 926–932

Leibowitz U, Halpern L, Alter M 1964b Clinical studies of multiple sclerosis in Israel. I. A clinical analysis based on a country-wide survey. *Arch Neurol* **10**: 502–512

Leibowitz U, Antonovsky A, Kats R, Alter M 1967 Does pregnancy increase the risk of multiple sclerosis ? *J Neurol Neurosurg Psychiatry* **30**: 354–357

Leibowitz U, Kahana E, Alter M 1969 Survival and death in multiple sclerosis. *Brain* **92**: 115–130

Leibowitz U, Kahana E, Alter M 1970 Multiple sclerosis in immigrant and native populations of Israel. *Lancet* **i**: 1323–1325

Leibowitz U, Kahana E, Alter M 1972 Population studies of multiple sclerosis in Israel. In: Field EJ, Bell TM, Carnegie PRK (eds) *Multiple Sclerosis: Progress and Research*. Amsterdam: North Holland, pp. 179–196

Leidtke W, Edelmann W, Bieri PL et al 1996 GFAP is necessary for the integrity of CNS white matter architecture and long-term maintenance of myelination. *Neuron* **17**: 607–615

Leigh RJ, Zee DS 1999 *The Neurology of Eye Movements*, 3rd edn. New York: Oxford University Press

Leigh RJ, Burnstine TH, Ruff RL, Kasmer RJ 1991 The effect of anti-cholinergic agents upon acquired nystagmus: a double-blind study of trihexiphenidyl and trihexethyl chloride. *Neurology* **41**: 1737–1741

Lenman AJ, Tulley FM, Vrbova G et al 1989 Muscle fatigue in some neurological disorders. *Muscle Nerve* **12**: 938–942

Lennon VA, Wingerchuk DM, Kryzer TJ et al 2004 A serum autoantibody marker of neuromyelitis optica: distinction from multiple sclerosis. *Lancet* **364**: 2106–2112

Lennon VA, Kryzer TJ, Pittock SJ et al 2005 IgG marker of optic-spinal multiple sclerosis binds to the aquaporin-4 water channel. *J Exp Med* **202**: 473–477

Lenschow DJ, Walunas TL, Bluestone JA 1996 CD28/B7 system of T cell costimulation. *Ann Rev Immunol* **14**: 233–258

Leocani L, Colombo B, Magnani G et al 2001 Fatigue in multiple sclerosis is associated with abnormal cortical activation to voluntary movement – EEG evidence. *Neuroimage* **13**: 1186–1192

Leonard JP, Waldburger KE, Goldman SJ 1995 Prevention of experimental autoimmune encephalomyelitis by antibodies against interleukin 12. *J Exp Med* **181**: 381–386

Lepore FE 1991 The origin of pain in optic neuritis. *Arch Neurol* **48**: 748–749

Lepore FE 1994 Uhthoff's symptom in disorders of the anterior visual pathways. *Neurology* **44**: 1036–1038

Leppert D, Waubant E, Burk M et al 1996 Interferon beta-1b inhibits gelatinase secretion and *in vitro* migration of human T cells: a possible mechanism for treatment efficacy in multiple sclerosis. *Ann Neurol* **40**: 846–852

Lesca G, Deschamps R, Lubetski C et al 2002 Acute myelitis in early *Borrelia burgdorferi* infection. *J Neurol* **249**: 1472–1474

Le Souef PN, Goldblatt J, Lynch NR 2000 Evolutionary adaptation of inflammatory immune responses in human beings. *Lancet* **356**: 242–244

Lester E, Feld E, Kinzie J, Wollmann R 1979 Necrotising myelopathy complicating Hodgkin's disease. *Arch Neurol* **36**: 583–585

Letournel F, Etcharry-Bouyx F, Verny C et al 2003 Two clinicopathological cases of a dominantly inherited, adult onset orthochromatic leucodystrophy. *J Neurol Neurosurg Psychiatry* **74**: 671–673

Leussink VI, Jung S, Merschdorf U et al 2001 High-dose methylprednisolone therapy in multiple sclerosis induces apoptosis in peripheral blood leukocytes. *Arch Neurol* **58**: 91–97

Leuzzi V, Lyon G, Cilio MR et al 1999 Childhood demyelinating diseases with a prolonged remitting course and their relation to Schilder's disease: report of two cases. *J Neurol Neurosurg Psychiatry* **66**: 407–408

Levesque M 1999 Interferon-beta 1 A-induced polyarthritis in a patient with the HLA-DRB1*0404 allele. *Arthritis Rheum* **42**: 569–573

Levin LI, Munger KL, Ruberstone MV et al 2005 Temporal relationship between elevation of Epstein–Barr virus antibody titers and initial onset of neurological symptoms in multiple sclerosis. *J Amer Med Assoc* **293**: 2496–2500

Levin MC, Lee SM, Kalume F et al 2002 Autoimmunity due to molecular mimicry as a cause of neurological disease. *Nature Med* **8**: 509–513

Levine JM, Stincome F, Lee Y-S 1993 Development and differentiation of glial precursor cells in the rat cerebellum. *Glia* **7**: 307–321

Levine RA, Gardner JC, Fullerton BC et al 1994 Multiple sclerosis lesions of the auditory pons are not silent. *Brain* **117**: 1127–1141

Levine S, Hoenig EM 1968 Induced localization of allergic adrenalitis and encephalomyelitis at sites of thermal injury. *J Immunol* **100**: 1310–1318

Levine S, Sowinski R 1980 Experimental allergic encephalomyelitis: inhibition of clinical signs and paradoxical enhancement of lesions in second attacks. *Am J Pathol* **101**: 375–386

Levine S, Wenk EJ 1965 A hyperacute form of allergic encephalomyelitis. *Am J Path* **47**: 61–88

Levy-Bruhl D, Rebière I, Desenclos JC, Drucker J 1999 Comparaison entre les risques de premières atteintes démyélinisantes centrales aiguës et les bénéfices de la vaccination contre l'hépatite B. *Bull Epidemiol hebdomadaire* **9**: 33–35

Lewis RA, Sumner AJ, Brown MJ, Asbury AK 1982 Multifocal demyelinating neuropathy with persistent conduction block. *Neurology* **32**: 958–964

Lexa FJ, Grossman RI 1994 MR of sarcoidosis of the head and spine: spectrum of manifestations and radiographic response to steroid therapy. *Am J Neuroradiol* **15**: 973–982

Leyden E 1863 Über graue Degeneration des Ruckenmarks. *Dtsch Klin* **15**: 121–128

Lhermitte F, Marteau R, Gazengel J et al 1973 The frequency of relapse in multiple sclerosis: a study based on 245 cases. *J Neurol* **205**: 47–59

Lhermitte F, Guillaumat L, Lyon-Caen O 1984 Monocular blindness with preserved direct and consensual pupillary reflex in multiple sclerosis. *Arch Neurol* **41**: 993–994

Lhermitte J, Bollak, Nicholas M 1924 Les douleurs à type de décharge électrique consécutives à la flexion céphalique dans la sclérose en plaques. *Rev Neurol* **42**: 56–62

Li DK, Paty DW 1999 Magnetic resonance imaging results of the PRISMS trial: a randomized, double-blind, placebo-controlled study of interferon-beta1a in relapsing–remitting multiple sclerosis. Prevention of Relapses and Disability by Interferon-beta1a Subcutaneously in Multiple Sclerosis. *Ann Neurol* **46**: 197–206

Li DK, Zhao GJ, Paty DW, and The University of British Columbia MS MRI Analysis Research Group The Spectrims Study Group 2001 Randomized controlled trial of interferon-beta-1a in secondary progressive MS: MRI results. *Neurology* **56**: 1505–1513

Li H, Newcombe J, Groome NP, Cuzner ML 1993 Characterization and distribution of phagocytic macrophages in multiple sclerosis plaques. *Neuropathol Appl Neurobiol* **19**: 214–223

Li H, Jiang Y, Luning Prak E et al 2001 Editors and editing of anti-DNA receptors. *Immunity* **15**: 947–957

Li J, Hansen D, Mortensen PB, Olsen J 2002a Myocardial infarction in parents who lost a child: a nationwide prospective cohort study in Denmark. *Circulation* **106**: 1634–1639

Li J, Johansen C, Hansen D, Olsen J 2002b Cancer incidence in parents who lost a child: a nationwide study in Denmark. *Cancer* **95**: 2237–2242

Li J, Johnsen SP, Olsen J 2003a Stroke in parents who lost a child: a nationwide follow-up study in Denmark. *Neuroepidemiology* **22**: 211–216

Li J, Precht DH, Mortensen PB, Olsen J 2003b Mortality in parents after death of a child in Denmark: a nationwide follow-up study. *Lancet* **361**: 363–367

Li J, Johansen C, Bronnum-Hansen H et al 2004a The risk of multiple sclerosis in bereaved parents: a nationwide cohort study in Denmark. *Neurology* **62**: 726–729

Li J, Norgard B, Precht DH, Olsen J 2004b Psychological stress and inflammatory bowel disease: a follow-up study in parents who lost a child in Denmark. *Am J Gastroenterol* 99: 1129–1133

Li S, Stys PK 2001 Na(+)-K(+)-ATPase inhibition and depolarization induce glutamate release via reverse Na(+)-dependent transport in spinal cord white matter. *Neuroscience* 107: 675–683

Li S, Mealing GA, Morley P, Stys PK 1999 Novel injury mechanism in anoxia and trauma of spinal cord white matter: glutamate release via reverse Na+-dependent glutamate transport. *J Neurosci* 19: RC16

Li S, Jiang Q, Stys PK 2000 Important role of reverse Na+-Ca2+ exchange in spinal cord white matter injury at physiological temperature. *J Neurophysiol* 84: 1116–1119

Li Y, Li H, Martin R, Mariuzza RA 2000 Structural basis for the binding of an immunodominant peptide from myelin basic protein in different registers by two HLA-DR2 proteins. *J Mol Biol* 304: 177–188

Li Y, Li H, Dimasi N et al 2001 Crystal structure of a superantigen bound to the high-affinity, zinc-dependent site on MHC class II. *Immunity* 14: 93–114

Li Z, Chapleau MW, Bates JN et al 1998 Nitric oxide as an autocrine regulator of sodium currents in baroreceptor neurons. *Neuron* 20: 1039–1049

Liang L, Bickenbach JR 2002 Somatic epidermal stem cells can produce multiple cell lineages during development. *Stem Cells* 20: 21–31

Liblau RS, van Endert P, Sandberg-Wollheim M et al 1993 Antigen processing gene polymorphisms in HLA-DR2 multiple sclerosis. *Neurology* 43: 1192–1197

Liblau RS, Singer SM, McDevitt HO 1995 Th1 and Th2 CD4+ T cells in the pathogenesis of organ-specific autoimmune diseases. *Immunol Today* 16: 34–38

Lider O, Reshef T, Beraud E et al 1988 Anti-idiotypic network induced by T-cell vaccination against experimental autoimmune encephalomyelitis. *Science* 239: 181–183

Lider O, Santos LMB, Lee CSY et al 1989 Suppression of experimental autoimmune encephalomyelitis by oral administration of myelin basic protein. II. Suppression of disease and *in vitro* immune responses is mediated by antigen specific CD8+ T lymphocytes. *J Immunol* 142: 748–752

Lieberman AP, Pitha PM, Shin HS, Shin ML 1989 Production of tumor necrosis factor and other cytokines by astrocytes stimulated with lipopolysaccharide or a neurotropic virus. *Proc Natl Acad Sci USA* 86: 6348–6352

Liem KFJ, Jessell TM, Briscoe J 2000 Regulation of the neural patterning activity of sonic hedgehog by secreted BMP inhibitors expressed by notochord and somites. *Development* 127: 4855–4866

Ligers A, Xu C, Saarinen S et al 1999 The CTLA-4 gene is associated with multiple sclerosis. *J Neuroimmunol* 97: 182–190

Ligers A, Dyment DA, Willer CJ et al 2001a Evidence of linkage with HLA-DR in

DRB1*1501-negative families with multiple sclerosis. *Am J Hum Genet* 69: 900–903

Ligers A, Teleshova N, Masterman T et al 2001b CTLA-4 gene expression is influenced by promoter and exon-1 polymorphisms. *Genes Immun* 2: 145–152

Lightman S, McDonald WI, Bird AC et al 1987 Retinal venous sheathing in optic neuritis: its significance for the pathogenesis of multiple sclerosis. *Brain* 110: 405–414

Liguori M, Sawcer S, Setakis E et al 2003 A whole genome screen for linkage disequilibrium in multiple sclerosis performed in a continental italian population. *J Neuroimmunol* 143: 97–100

Liguori M, Cittadella R, Manna I et al 2004 Association between synapsin III gene promoter polymorphisms and multiple sclerosis. *J Neurol* 251: 165–170

Likosky WH, Fireman B, Elmore R et al 1991 Intense immunosuppression in chronic progressive multiple sclerosis: the Kaiser study. *J Neurol Neurosurg Psychiatry* 54: 1055–1060

Lillien LE, Sendtner M, Raff MC 1990 Extracellular matrix-associated molecules collaborate with ciliary neurotrophic factor to induce type-2 astrocyte development. *J Cell Biol* 111: 635–644

Lily O, Palace J, Vincent A 2004 Serum autoantibodies to cell surface determinants in multiple sclerosis: a flow cytometric study. *Brain* 127: 269–279

Lim ET, Grant D, Pashenkov M et al 2004 Cerebrospinal fluid levels of brain specific proteins in optic neuritis. *Mult Scler* 10: 261–265

Lim ET, Berger T, Reindl M et al 2005 Anti-myelin antibodies do not allow an earlier diagnosis of multiple sclerosis. *Mult Scler* 11: 492–494

Lim KE, Hsu YY, Hsu WC, Chan CY 2003 Multiple complete ring-shaped enhanced MRI lesions in acute disseminated encephalomyelitis. *Clin Imaging* 27: 281–284

Lima MASD, Bica RBS, Araujo AQC 2004 Gender influence on the progression of HTLV-I associated myelopathy/tropical spastic paraparesis. *J Neurol Neursurg Psychiatry* 76: 294–296

Limburg CC 1950 The geographic distribution of multiple sclerosis and its estimated prevalence in the US. *Assoc Res Nerv Mental Dis* 28: 15–24

Lin X, Turner B, Constantinescu CS et al 2002 Cerebral volume change in secondary progressive multiple sclerosis: effect of intravenous immunoglobulins (IVIG). *J Neurology* 249: I169–I170

Lin X, Tench CR, Turner B et al 2003 Spinal cord atrophy and disability in multiple sclerosis over four years: application of a reproducible automated technique in monitoring disease progression in a cohort of the interferon β-1a (Rebif) treatment trial. *J Neurol Neurosurg Psychiatry* 74: 1090–1094

Lincoln MR, Montpetit A, Cader MZ et al 2005 A predominant role for the HLA class II region in the association of the MHC region

with multiple sclerosis. *Nat Genet* 37: 1108–1112

Lincoln NB, Dent A, Harding J et al 2002 Evaluation of cognitive assessment and cognitive intervention for people with multiple sclerosis. *J Neurol Neurosurg Psychiatry* 72: 93–98

Lindå H, Hammarberg H, Cullheim S et al 1998 Expression of MHC class I and β2-microglobulin in rat spinal motoneurons: regulatory influences of IFN-gamma and axotomy. *Exp Neurol* 150: 282–295

Lindberg C, Andersen O, Vahlne A et al 1991 Epidemiological investigation of the association between infectious mononucleosis and multiple sclerosis. *Neuroepidemiology* 10: 62–65

Lindberg RLP, De Groot CJA, Montagne L et al 2001 The expression profile of matrix metalloproteinases (MMPs) and their inhibitors (TIMPs) in lesions and normal appearing white matter of multiple sclerosis. *Brain* 124: 1743–1753

Linden D 1998a Autonomic evaluation by means of standard tests and power spectral analysis in multiple sclerosis. Reply. *Muscle Nerve* 20: 679

Linden D 1998b Severe Raynaud's phenomenon associated with interferon-beta treatment for multiple sclerosis. *Lancet* 352: 878–879

Linden D, Diehl RR, Kretzschmar A, Berlit P 1997 Autonomic evaluation by means of standard tests and power spectral analysis in multiple sclerosis. *Muscle Nerve* 20: 809–814

Lindert R-B, Haase CG, Brehm U et al 1999 Multiple sclerosis: B- and T-cell responses to the extracellular domain of the myelin oligodendrocyte glycoprotein. *Brain* 122: 2089–2099

Lindquist S, Schott BH, Ban M et al 2005 The BDNF-Val66Met polymorphism: implications for susceptibility to multiple sclerosis and severity of disease. *J Neuroimmunol* 67: 183–185

Lindsberg PJ, Ohman J, Lehto T et al 1996 Complement activation in the central nervous system following blood-brain barrier damage in man. *Ann Neurol* 40: 587–596

Lindsey JW 2005 Familial recurrence rates and genetic models of multiple sclerosis. *Am J Med Genet A* 135: 53–58

Lindsey JW, Hodgkinson S, Mehta R et al 1994a Phase 1 clinical trial of chimeric monoclonal anti-CD4 antibody in multiple sclerosis. *Neurology* 44: 413–419

Lindsey JW, Hodgkinson S, Mehta R et al 1994b Repeated treatment with chimeric anti-CD4 antibody in multiple sclerosis. *Ann Neurol* 36: 183–189

Lindstedt M 1991 Multiple sclerosis – is research on the wrong track? *Med Hypotheses* 34: 69–72

Linington C, Lassmann H 1987 Antibody responses in chronic relapsing experimental allergic encephalomyelitis: correlation of serum demyelinating activity with antibody titer to myelin/oligodendrocyte glycoprotein (MOG). *J Neuroimmunol* 17: 61–70

Linington C, Webb M, Woodhams PL 1984 A novel myelin associated glycoprotein defined by a mouse monoclonal antibody. *J Neuroimmunol* **6**: 387–396

Linington C, Bradl M, Lassmann H et al 1988 Augmentation of demyelination in rat acute allergic encephalomyelitis by circulating mouse monoclonal antibodies directed against a myelin/oligodendrocyte glycoprotein. *Am J Pathol* **130**: 443–454

Linington C, Lassmann H, Morgan BP, Compston DAS 1989 Immunohistochemical localization of terminal complement component C9 in experimental allergic encephalomyelitis. *Acta Neuropathol* **79**: 78–85

Linington C, Engelhardt B, Kapocs G, Lassmann H 1992 Induction of persistently demyelinating lesions in the rat following the repeated adoptive transfer of encephalitogenic T cells and demyelinating antibodies. *J Neuroimmunol* **40**: 219–224

Link H 1967 Immunoglobulin G and low molecular weight proteins in human cerebrospinal fluid – chemical and immunological characterisation with special reference to multiple sclerosis. *Acta Neurol Scand* **43**: 1–136

Link H, Cruz M, Gessain A et al 1989 Chronic progressive myelopathy associated with HTLV-1: oligoclonal IgG and anti-HTLV-1 antibodies in cerebrospinal fluid and serum. *Neurology* **39**: 1566–1572

Link H, Baig S, Olsson O et al 1990 Persistent anti-myelin basic protein IgG antibody response in multiple sclerosis cerebrospinal fluid. *J Neuroimmunol* **28**: 237–248

Link J, Söderström M, Olsson T et al 1994 Increased transforming growth factor-α, interleukin-4 and interferon-γ in multiple sclerosis. *Ann Neurol* **36**: 379–386

Linker RA, Maurer M, Gaupp S et al 2002 CNTF is a major protective factor in demyelinating CNS disease: a neurotrophic cytokine as modulator in neuroinflammation. *Nature Med* **8**: 620–624

Linnebank M, Kesper K, Jeub M et al 2003 Hereditary elevation of angiotensin converting enzyme suggesting neurosarcoidosis. *Neurology* **61**: 1819–1820

Liour SS, Yu RK 2003 Differentiation of radial glia-like cells from embryonic stem cells. *Glia* **42**: 109–117

Lipton HL, Teasdell RD 1973 Acute transverse myelopathy in adults. *Arch Neurol* **28**: 252–257

Lipton MM, Freund J 1953 The transfer of experimental allergic encephalomyelitis in the rat by means of parabiosis. *J Immunol* **71**: 380–384

Lipton SA 1998 Neuronal injury associated with HIV-1: approaches and treatment. *Annu Rev Pharmacol Toxicol* **38**: 159–177

Lisak RP, Hirayama M, Kuchmy D et al 1983 Cultured human and rat oligodendrocytes and rat Schwann cells do not have immune response gene associated antigen (Ia) on their surface. *Brain Res* **289**: 285–292

Lisk D 1991 Multiple sclerosis in a west African. *Afr J Neurol Sci* **10**: 10–12

Litvan I, Grafman J, Vendell P et al 1988 Multiple memory defects in patients with multiple sclerosis. *Arch Neurol* **45**: 607–610

Litzenburger T, Fässler R, Bauer J et al 1998 B lymphocytes producing demyelinating autoantibodies: development and function in gene-targeted transgenic mice. *J Exp Med* **188**: 169–180

Litzenburger T, Blüthmann H, Morales P et al 2000 Development of MOG autoreactive transgenic B lymphocytes: receptor editing in vivo following encounter of a self-antigen distinct from MOG. *J Immunol* **165**: 5360–5366

Liu A, Stadelmann C, Moscarello M et al 2005 Expression of stathmin, a developmentally controlled cytoskeleton regulating molecule, in demyelinating disorders. *J Neurosci* **25**: 737–747

Liu C, Blumhardt LD 2000 Disability outcome measures in therapeutic trials of relapsing remitting multiple sclerosis: effects of heterogeneity of disease course in placebo cohorts. *J Neurol Neurosurg Psychiatry* **68**: 450–457

Liu C, Playford ED, Thompson AJ 2003 Does neurorehabilitation have a role in relapsing–remitting multiple sclerosis? *J Neurol* **250**: 1214–1218

Liu H, Loo KK, Palaszynski K et al 2003 Estrogen receptor alpha mediates estrogen's immune protection in autoimmune disease. *J Immunol* **171**: 6936–6940

Liu J, Marino MW, Wong G et al 1998 TNF is a potent anti-inflammatory cytokine in autoimmune-mediated demyelination. *Nature Med* **4**: 78–83

Liu JS, Zhao ML, Brosnan CF, Lee SC 2001 Expression of inducible nitric oxide synthase and nitrotyrosine in multiple sclerosis lesions. *Am J Pathol* **158**: 2057–2066

Liu Q-S, Jia Y-S, Ju G 1997 Nitric oxide inhibits neuronal activity in the supraoptic nucleus of the rat hypothalamic slices. *Brain Res Bull* **43**: 121–125

Liu R, Cai J, Hu X et al 2003 Region-specific and stage-dependent regulation of Olig gene expression and oligodendrogenesis by Nkx6.1 homeodomain transcription factor. *Development* **130**: 6221–6231

Liu S, Qu Y, Stewart TJ et al 2000 Embryonic stem cells differentiate into oligodendrocytes and myelinate in culture and after spinal cord transplantation. *Proc Natl Acad Sci USA* **97**: 6126–6131

Liu Y, Rao MS 2004 Olig genes are expressed in a heterogeneous population of precursor cells in the developing spinal cord. *Glia* **45**: 67–74

Liu Z, Pelfrey CM, Cotleur A et al 2001 Immunomodulatory effects of interferon beta-1a in multiple sclerosis. *J Neuroimmunol* **112**: 153–162

Liuzzi GM, Trojano M, Fanelli M et al 2002 Intrathecal synthesis of matrix metalloproteinase-9 in patients with multiple sclerosis: implication for pathogenesis. *Mult Scler* **9**: 222–228

Llewellyn-Smith N, Lai M, Miller DH et al 1997 Effects of anti-CD4 antibody treatment on lymphocyte subsets and stimulated tumor necrosis factor alpha production: a study of 29 multiple sclerosis patients entered into a clinical trial of cM-T412. *Neurology* **48**: 810–816

Llorca J, Guerrero-Alonso P, Prieto-Salceda D 2005 Mortality trends of multiple sclerosis in Spain, 1951–1997: an age–period–cohort analysis. *Neuroepidemiology* **24**: 129–134

Lo AC, Black JA, Waxman SG 2002 Neuroprotection of axons with phenytoin in experimental allergic encephalomyelitis. *NeuroReport* **13**: 1909–1912

Lo AC, Saab CY, Black JA, Waxman SG 2003 Phenytoin protects spinal cord axons and preserves axonal conduction and neurological function in a model of neuroinflammation in vivo. *J Neurophysiol* **90**: 3566–3571

Lobnig BM, Chantelau E 2002 Multiple sclerosis and type 1 diabetes in Sardinia. *Lancet* **360**: 1253

Lock C, Hermans G, Pedotti R et al 2002 Gene-microarray analysis of multiple sclerosis lesions yields new targets validated in autoimmune encephalomyelitis. *Nature Med* **8**: 500–508

Lockwood CM, Thiru S, Isaacs JD et al 1993 Long-term remission of untreatable systemic vasculitis with monoclonal antibody therapy. *Lancet* **341**: 1620–1622

Lockyer MJ 1991 Prevalence of multiple sclerosis in five rural Suffolk practices. *Br Med J* **303**: 347–348

Loddenkemper T, Grote K, Evers S et al 2002 Neurological manifestations of the oculodentodigital dysplasia syndrome. *J Neurol* **249**: 584–595

Lodge PA, Allegretta M, Steinman L, Sriram S 1995 Myelin basic protein peptide specificity and T-cell receptor gene usage of HPRT mutant T-cell clones in patients with multiple sclerosis. *Ann Neurol* **36**: 734–740

Loers G, Aboul-Enein F, Bartsch U, Lassmann H 2004 Comparison of myelin, axon, lipid, and immunopathology in the central nervous system of differentially myelin-compromised mutant mice: a morphological and biochemical study. *Mol Cell Neurosci* **27**: 175–189

Loes DJ, Fatemi A, Melhem ER et al 2003 Analysis of MRI patterns aids prediction of progression in X-linked adrenoleucodystrophy. *Neurology* **61**: 369–374

Logan A, Frautschy SA, Gonzalez AM et al 1992 Enhanced expression of transforming growth factor beta1 in the rat brain after a localised cerebral injury. *Brain Res* **587**: 216–225

Logan A, Berry M, Gonzalez AM et al 1994 Effects of transforming growth factor beta1 on scar production in the injured central nervous system of the rat. *Eur J Neurosci* **6**: 355–363

Logigian EL, Kaplan RF, Steere AC 1990 Chronic neurologic manifestations of Lyme disease. *N Engl J Med* **323**: 1438–1444

Lopez Larrea C, Uria DF, Coto E 1990 HLA antigens in multiple sclerosis of northern Spanish population. *J Neurol Neurosurg Psychiatry* **53**: 434–435

Lord D, O'Farrell AGO, Staunton H, Keelan E 1990 The inheritance of MS susceptibility. *Irish J Med Sci* **159**: 1–20

Lord SE, Halligan PW, Wade DT 1998a Visual gait analysis: the development of a clinical assessment and scale. *Clinical Rehab* **12**: 107–119

Lord SE, Wade DT, Halligan PW 1998b A comparison of two physiotherapy treatment approaches to improve walking in multiple sclerosis: a pilot randomized controlled study. *Clinical Rehab* **12**: 477–486

Lorentzen JC, Issazadeh S, Storch M et al 1995 Protracted, relapsing and demyelinating experimental autoimmune encephalomyelitis in DA rats immunized with syngeneic spinal cord and incomplete Freund's adjuvant. *J Neuroimmunol* **63**: 193–205

Losseff NA, Wang L, Lai HM et al 1996a Progressive cerebral atrophy in multiple sclerosis: a serial MRI study. *Brain* **119**: 2009–2020

Losseff NA, Webb SL, O'Riordan JI et al 1996b Spinal cord atrophy and disability in multiple sclerosis: a new reproducible and sensitive MRI method with potential to monitor disease progression. *Brain* **119**: 701–708

Lossinsky AS, Badmajew V, Robson J, Moretz C, Wisniewski HM 1989 Sites of egress of inflammatory cells and horse radish peroxidase transport across the blood brain barrier in a murine model of chronic relapsing experimental allergic encephalomyelitis. *Acta Neuropathol* **78**: 359–371

Losy J, Niezgoda A 2001 IL-18 in patients with multiple sclerosis. *Acta Neurol Scand* **104**: 171–173

Lou J, Gasche Y, Zheng L et al 1999 Interferon-beta inhibits activated leukocyte migration through human brain microvascular endothelial cell monolayer. *Lab Invest* **79**: 1015–1025

Louis J-C, Magal E, Takayama S, Varon S 1993 CNTF protection of oligodendrocytes against natural and tumor necrosis factor-induced death. *Science* **259**: 689–692

Louis PCA 1825 *Recherches anatomico-pathologiques sur la phthisie.* Paris: Gabon

Lovas G, Szilagyi N, Majtenyi K et al 2000 Axonal changes in chronic demyelinated cervical spinal cord plaques. *Brain* **123**: 308–317

Love S, Gradidge T, Coakham HB 2001 Trigeminal neuralgia due to multiple sclerosis: ultrastructural findings in trigeminal rhizotomy specimens. *Neuropathol Appl Neurobiol* **27**: 238–244

Lovett-Racke AE, Martin R, McFarland HF et al 1997 Longitudinal study of myelin basic protein-specific T-cell receptors during the course of multiple sclerosis. *J Neuroimmunol* **78**: 162–171

Low NL, Carter S 1956 Multiple sclerosis in children. *Pediatrics* **18**: 24–39

Lowenthal A 1964 *Agar Gel Electrophoresis in Neurology.* Amsterdam: Elsevier

Lowenthal A, Van Sande M, Karcher D 1960 The differential diagnosis of neurological diseases by fractionating electrophoretically the CSF gamma globulins. *J Neurochem* **6**: 51–56

Lu F, Selak M, O'Connor J et al 2000 Oxidative damage to mitochondrial DNA and activity of mitochondrial enzymes in chronic active lesions of multiple sclerosis. *J Neurol Sci* **177**: 95–103

Lu JL, Sheikh KA, Wu HS et al 2000 Physiologic-pathologic correlation in Guillain-Barre syndrome in children. *Neurology* **54**: 33–39

Lu M, Zhang N, Maruyama M, Hawley RG, Ho AD 1996 Retrovirus-mediated gene expression in hematopoietic cells correlates inversely with growth factor stimulation. *Hum Gene Ther* **7**: 2263–2271

Lu QR, Yuk D, Alberta JA et al 2000 Sonic hedgehog-regulated oligodendrocyte lineage genes encoding bHLH proteins in the mammalian central nervous system. *Neuron* **25**: 317–329

Lu QR, Cai L, Rowitch D et al 2001 Ectopic expression of Olig1 promotes oligodendrocyte formation and reduces neuronal survival in developing mouse cortex. *Nat Neurosci* **4**: 973–974

Lu QR, Sun T, Zhu Z et al 2002 Common developmental requirement for Olig function indicates a motor neuron/oligodendrocyte connection. *Cell* **109**: 75–86

Lu W, Bhasin M, Tsirka SE 2002 Involvement of tissue plasminogen activator in onset and effector phases of experimental allergic encephalomyelitis. *J Neurosci* **22**: 10781–10789

Lublin FD, Reingold SC 1996 Defining the clinical course of multiple sclerosis: results of an international survey. National Multiple Sclerosis Society (USA) Advisory Committee on Clinical Trials of New Agents in Multiple Sclerosis. *Neurology* **46**: 907–911

Lublin FD, Whitaker JN, Eidelman BH, Miller AE, Arnason BGW, Burks JS 1996 Management of patients receiving interferon beta-1b for multiple sclerosis: report of a consensus conference. *Neurology* **46**: 12–18

Lublin FD, Reingold SC, the National Multiple Sclerosis Society (USA) Advisory Committee on Clinical Trials of New Agents in Multiple Sclerosis 1997 Guidelines for clinical trials of new therapeutic agents in multiple sclerosis. *Neurology* **48**: 572–574

Lublin FD and the Hu 23F2G MS Study Group 1999 A Phase II trial of anti-cd11/cd18 monoclonal antibody in acute exacerbations of multiple sclerosis. *Neurology* **52**: A290

Lublin FD, Cutter G, Elfont R et al 2001 A trial to assess the safety of combining therapy with interferon beta-1a and glatiramer acetate in patients with relapsing MS. *Neurology* **56**: A148

Lublin FD, Baier M, Cutter G et al 2002 Results of the extension of a trial to assess the longer term safety of combining interferon beta-1a and glatiramer acetate. *Neurology* **58**: A85

Lublin FD, Baier M, Cutter G 2003 Effect of relapses on development of residual deficit in multiple sclerosis. *Neurology* **61**: 1528–1532

Lucas J 1790 An account of uncommon symptoms succeeding the measles, with some additional remarks on the infection of measles and smallpox. *Lond Med J* **XI**: 325–331

Lucas M, Sanchez-Solino O, Solano F et al 1998 Interferon beta-1b inhibits reactive oxygen species production in peripheral blood monocytes of patients with relapsing–remitting multiple sclerosis. *Neurochem Int* **33**: 101–102

Lucchinetti CF, Brueck W, Rodriguez M, Lassmann H 1996 Distinct patterns of multiple sclerosis pathology indicates heterogeneity in pathogenesis. *Brain Pathol* **6**: 259–274

Lucchinetti CF, Kiers L, O'Duffy A et al 1997 Risk factors for developing multiple sclerosis after childhood optic neuritis. *Neurology* **49**: 1413–1418

Lucchinetti CF, Brück W, Parisi J et al 1999 A quantitative analysis of oligodendrocytes in multiple sclerosis lesions: a study of 117 cases. *Brain* **122**: 2279–2295

Lucchinetti CF, Brück W, Parisi J et al 2000 Heterogeneity of multiple sclerosis lesions: implications for the pathogenesis of demyelination. *Ann Neurol* **47**: 707–717

Lucchinetti CF, Mandler R, McGavern D et al 2002 A role for humoral mechanisms in the pathogenesis of Devic's neuromyelitis optica. *Brain* **125**: 1450–1461

Lucotte GL, Bathelier C, Mercier G 2000 TNF-alpha polymorphisms in multiple sclerosis: no association with −238 and −308 promoter alleles, but the microsatellite allele a11 is associated with the disease in French patients. *Mult Scler* **6**: 78–80

Lucotte GL, French MS Consortium 2002 Confirmation of a gene for multiple sclerosis (MS) to chromosome region 19q13.3. *Genet Couns* **13**: 133–138

Ludwin SK 1980 Chronic demyelination inhibits remyelination in the central nervous system: an analysis of contributing factors. *Lab Invest* **43**: 382–387

Ludwin SK 1990 Oligodendrocyte survival in Wallerian degeneration. *Acta Neuropathol* **80**: 184–191

Ludwin SK 1997 The pathobiology of the oligodendrocyte. *J Neuropathol Exp Neurol* **56**: 111–124

Ludwin SK, Johnson ES 1981 Evidence for a 'dying-back' gliopathy in demyelinating disease. *Ann Neurol* **9**: 301–305

Ludwin SK, Henry JM, McFarland H 2001 Vascular proliferation and angiogenesis in multiple sclerosis: clinical and pathogenetic implications. *J Neuropathol Exp Neurol* **60**: 505

Lueck CJ, Pires M, Cartney ACE, Graham EM 1993 Ocular and neurological Behçet's disease without orogenital ulceration. *J Neurol Neurosurg Psychiatry* **56**: 505–508

Lugaresi A, Uncini A, Gambi D 1993 Basal ganglia involvement in multiple sclerosis with alternating side paroxysmal dystonia. *J Neurol* **240**: 257–261

Lujan S, Masjuan J, Roldan E et al 1998 The expression of integrins on activated T-cells in multiple sclerosis: effect of intravenous methylprednisolone treatment. *Mult Scler* **4**: 239–242

Lumsden CE 1970 The neuropathology of multiple sclerosis. In: Vinken PJ, Bruyn GW, *Handbook of Clinical Neurology*. Amsterdam: Elsevier, Vol 9, pp. 217–309

Lunardi G, Leandri M, Albano C et al 1997 Clinical effectiveness of lamotrigine and plasma levels in essential and symptomatic trigeminal neuralgia. *Neurology* **48**: 1714–1717

Lundberg PO 1981 Sexual dysfunction in women with multiple sclerosis. *Int Rehab Med* **3**: 32–34

Lunding J, Midgard R, Vedeler CA 2002 Oligoclonal bands in cerebrospinal fluid: a comparative study of isoelectric focusing, agarose gel electrophoresis and IgG index. *Acta Neurol Scand* **102**: 322–325

Luo L, Salunga RC, Guo H et al 1999 Gene expression profiles of laser-captured adjacent neuronal cell types. *Nature Med* **1**: 122

Luomala M, Elovaara I, Koivula T, Lehtimaki T 1999 Intercellular adhesion molecule-1 K/E 469 polymorphism and multiple sclerosis. *Ann Neurol* **45**: 546–547

Luomala M, Elovaara I, Ukkonen M et al 2000 Plasminogen activator inhibitor 1 gene and the risk of MS in women. *Neurology* **54**: 1862–1864

Luomala M, Elovaara L, Ukkonen M et al 2001a The combination of HLA-DR1 and HLA-DR53 protects against MS. *Neurology* **56**: 383–385

Luomala M, Lehtimaka T, Elovaara I et al 2001b A study of interleukin-1 cluster genes in susceptibility to and severity of multiple sclerosis. *J Neurol Sci* **185**: 123–127

Luomala M, Lehtimaki T, Huhtala H et al 2003 Promoter polymorphism of IL-10 and severity of multiple sclerosis. *Acta Neurol Scand* **108**: 396–400

Lus G, Romano F, Scuotto A et al 2004 Azathioprine and interferon beta 1a in relapsing–remitting multiple sclerosis patients: increasing efficacy of combined treatment. *Eur Neurol* **51**: 15–20

Luster AD 1998 Chemokines – chemotactic cytokines that mediate inflammation. *N Engl J Med* **338**: 436–445

Luxton RW, Zeman A, Holzel H et al 1995 Affinity to antigen-specific IgG distinguishes multiple sclerosis from encephalitis. *J Neurol Sci* **132**: 11–19

Luys JB 1873 *Iconographie photographique des centres nerveux*. Paris: Baillière

Luyt K, Varadi A, Molnar E 2003 Functional metabotropic glutamate receptors are expressed in oligodendrocyte progenitor cells. *J Neurochem* **84**: 1452–1464

Lycke J, Wikkelso C, Bergh AC et al 1993 Regional cerebral blood flow in multiple sclerosis measured by single photon emission tomography with technetium-99mhexamethylpropyleneamine oxime. *Eur Neurol* **33**: 163–167

Lycke J, Svennerholm B, Hjelmquist E et al 1996 Acyclovir treatment of relapsing–remitting multiple sclerosis: a randomised, placebo-controlled, double-blind study. *J Neurol* **243**: 214–224

Lycke JN, Karlsson J-E, Andersen O, Rosengren LE 1998 Neurofilament protein in cerebrospinal fluid: a potential marker of activity in multiple sclerosis. *J Neurol Neurosurg Psychiatry* **64**: 402–404

Lycklama GT Nijeholt GJ, van Walderveen MA, Castelijns PA et al 1998 Brain and spinal cord abnormalities in multiple sclerosis: correlation between MRI parameters, clinical subtypes and symptoms. *Brain* **121**: 687–697

Lycklama GT, Thompson A, Filippi M et al 2003 Spinal-cord MRI in multiple sclerosis. *Lancet Neurol* **2**: 555–562

Lyman WD, Kadish AS, Raine CS 1981 Experimental allergic encephalomyelitis in the guinea pig: variation in peripheral blood lymphocyte responsiveness to myelin basic protein during disease development. *Cell Immunol* **63**: 409–416

Lynch JP 2003 Neurosarcoidosis: how good are the diagnostic tests? *J Neuroophthalmol* **23**: 187–189

Lynch SG, Rose JW, Smoker W, Petajan JH 1990 MRI in familial multiple sclerosis. *Neurology* **40**: 900–903

Lynch SG, Rose JW, Petagan JH et al 1991 Discordance of T-cell receptor beta-chain genes in familial multiple sclerosis. *Ann Neurol* **30**: 402–410

Lynch SG, Rose JW, Petagan JH, Leppert M 1992 Discordance of the T-cell receptor alpha-chain gene in familial multiple sclerosis. *Neurology* **42**: 839–844

Lynch SG, Peter K, LeVine SM 1996 Desferroxamine in chronic progressive multiple sclerosis: a pilot study. *Mult Scler* **2**: 157–160

Lynn B 1959 Retrobulbar neuritis: a survey of the present condition of cases occurring over the last fifty six years. *Trans Ophthalmol Soc UK* **50**: 262–267

Lyon-Caen O, Izquierdo G, Marteau R, Lhermitte F, Castaigne P, Hauw JJ 1985 Late onset multiple sclerosis: a clinical study of 16 pathologically proven cases. *Acta Neurol Scand* **72**: 56–60

Lyon-Caen O, Jouvert R, Hauser S et al 1986 Cognitive function in recent-onset demyelinating disease. *Arch Neurol* **43**: 1138–1141

Lyons J-A, San M, Happ MP, Cross AH 1999 B cells are critical to induction of

experimental allergic encephalomyelitis by protein but not by a short encephalitogenic peptide. *Eur J Immunol* **29**: 3432–3439

Lyons PR, Newman PK, Saunders M 1988 Methylprednisolone therapy in multiple sclerosis: a profile of adverse effects. *J Neurol Neurosurg Psychiatry* **51**: 285–287

Ma JJ, Nishimura M, Mine H et al 1998 HLA-DRB1 and tumor necrosis factor gene polymorphisms in Japanese patients with multiple sclerosis. *J Neuroimmunol* **92**: 109–112

Ma RLZ, Gao JF, Meeker ND et al 2002 Identification of Bphs, an autoimmune disease locus, as histamine receptor H1. *Science* **297**: 620–623

MacAllister WS, Belman AL, Milazzo M et al 2005 Cognitive functioning in children and adolescents with multiple sclerosis. *Neurology* **64**: 1422–1425

McAlpine D 1931 Acute disseminated encephalomyelitis; its sequelae and relationship to disseminated sclerosis. *Lancet* i: 846–852

McAlpine D 1946 The problem of multiple sclerosis. *Brain* **69**: 233–250

McAlpine D 1957 Familial incidence and role of hereditary factors in multiple sclerosis. 6th Congres international de neurologie: rapports et discussions. *Acta Med Belg* **(Suppl)**: 107–121

McAlpine D 1961 The benign form of multiple sclerosis: a study based on 241 cases seen within three years of onset and followed up until the tenth year or more of the disease. *Brain* **84**: 186–203

McAlpine D 1964 The benign form of multiple sclerosis: results of a long-term follow up. *Br Med J* **2**: 1029–1032

McAlpine D, Compston ND 1952 Some aspects of the natural history of disseminated sclerosis: incidence, course and prognosis: factors affecting onset and course. *Q J Med* **21**: 135–167

McAlpine D, Compston ND, Lumsden CE 1955 *Multiple Sclerosis*. Edinburgh: Livingstone

McAlpine D, Lumsden CE, Acheson ED 1965 *Multiple Sclerosis: a Re-appraisal*. Edinburgh: E. & S. Livingstone

McAlpine D, Lumsden CE, Acheson ED 1972 *Multiple Sclerosis: A Reappraisal*, 2nd edn. Edinburgh: Churchill Livingstone

McArthur JB 1987 Neurologic manifestations of AIDS. *Medicine* **66**: 407–437

McArthur JC, Young F 1986 Multiple sclerosis and pregnancy. In: Goldstein RJ (ed.) *Neurological Disorders of Pregnancy*. New York: Futura Publishing, pp. 197–211

McArthur JC, Haughey N, Gartner S et al 2003 Human immunodeficiency virus associated dementia: an evolving disease. *J Neurovirol* **9**: 205–221

McCall MG, Brereton T, Lee G et al 1968 Frequency of multiple sclerosis in 3 Australian cities – Perth, Newcastle and Hobart. *J Neurol Neurosurg Psychiatry* **31**: 1–9

McCarthy KD, De Vellis J 1980 Preparation of separate astroglial and oligodendroglial cell cultures from rat cerebral tissue. *J Cell Biol* **85**: 890–902

McCombe PA, Nickson I, Tabi Z, Pender MP 1996 Corticosteroid treatment of experimental autoimmune encephalomyelitis in the Lewis rat results in the loss of Vβ8.2$^+$ and myelin basic protein-reactive cells from the spinal cord, with increased total T-cell apoptosis but reduced apoptosis of Vβ8.2$^+$ cells. *J Neuroimmunol* **70**: 93–101

McCoubrie M, Shuttleworth D 1978 The prevalence of multiple sclerosis in west Yorkshire. *Br Med J* **2**: 570

McDermott CJ, Grierson AJ, Wood JD *et al* 2003 Hereditary spastic paraparesis: disrupted intracellular transport associated with the spastin mutation. *Ann Neurol* **54**: 748–759

MacDonald BK, Cockerell OC, Sander JWAS, Shorvon SD 2000 The incidence and prevalence of neurological disorders in a prospective community-based study in the UK. *Brain* **123**: 665–676

MacDonald JL, Roberts DF, Shaw DA, Saunders M 1976 Blood groups and other polymorphisms in multiple sclerosis. *J Med Genet* **13**: 30–33

McDonald JW, Liu X-Z, Qu Y *et al* 1999 Transplanted embryonic stem cells survive, differentiate and promote recovery in injured rat spinal cord. *Nature Med* **5**: 1410–1412

MacDonald SC, Simcoff R, Jordan LM *et al* 2002 A population of oligodendrocytes derived from multipotent neural precursor cells expresses a cholinergic phenotype in culture and responds to ciliary neurotrophic factor. *J Neurosci Res* **68**: 255–264

McDonald WI 1961 Conduction velocity of cutaneous afferent fibres during experimental demyelination. *Proc University Otago Med Schl* **39**: 29–30

McDonald WI 1962 Conduction in muscle afferent fibres during experimental demyelination in cat nerve. *Acta Neuropathol* I: 425–432

McDonald WI 1963 The effects of experimental demyelination on conduction in peripheral nerve: a histological and electrophysiological study. II. Electrophysiological observations. *Brain* **86**: 501–524

McDonald WI 1975 Mechanisms of functional loss and recovery in spinal cord damage. In: *Outcome of Severe Damage to the Central Nervous System, Ciba Foundation Symposium.* pp. 23–33

McDonald WI 1982 Clinical consequences of conduction defects produced by demyelination. In: Culp WJ, Ochoa J (eds) *Abnormal Nerves and Muscles as Impulse Generators.* Oxford: Oxford University Press, pp. 253–270

McDonald WI 1983 Attitudes to the treatment of multiple sclerosis. *Arch Neurol* **40**: 667–670

McDonald WI 1986 The pathophysiology of multiple sclerosis. In: McDonald WI, Silberberg DH (eds) *Multiple Sclerosis.* London: Butterworths, pp. 112–133

McDonald WI 1994 The pathological and clinical dynamics of multiple sclerosis. *J Neuropathol Exp Neurol* **53**: 338–343

McDonald WI 1998 Pathophysiology of multiple sclerosis. In: Compston A, Ebers G, Lassmann H *et al* (eds) *McAlpine's Multiple Sclerosis*, 3rd edn. London: Churchill Livingstone, pp. 359–378

McDonald WI 2002 Multiple sclerosis in its European matrix. *Mult Scler* **8**: 181–191

McDonald WI 2004 Multiple sclerosis in its European matrix: some aspects of history, mechanisms and treatment. *Can J Neurol Sci* **31**: 37–47

McDonald WI, Barnes D 1989 Lessons from magnetic resonance imaging in multiple sclerosis. *Trends Neurosci* **12**: 376–379

McDonald WI, Barnes D 1992 The ocular manifestations of multiple sclerosis. 1 Abnormalities of the afferent visual system. *J Neurol Neurosurg Psychiatry* **55**: 747–752

McDonald WI, Halliday AM 1977 Diagnosis and classification of multiple sclerosis. *Br Med Bull* **33**: 4–9

McDonald WI, Sears TA 1969 Effect of demyelination on conduction in the central nervous system. *Nature* **221**: 182–183

McDonald WI, Sears TA 1970 The effects of experimental demyelination on conduction in the central nervous system. *Brain* **93**: 583–598

McDonald WI, Silberberg DH 1986 The diagnosis of multiple sclerosis. In: McDonald WI, Silberberg DH (eds) *Multiple Sclerosis.* London: Butterworths, pp. 1–10

McDonald WI, Miller DH, Thompson AJ 1994 Are magnetic resonance findings predictive of clinical outcome in therapeutic trials in multiple sclerosis? The dilemma of interferon-β. *Ann Neurol* **36**: 14–18

McDonald WI, Compston A, Edan G *et al* 2001 Recommended diagnostic criteria for multiple sclerosis: guidelines from the International Panel on the diagnosis of multiple sclerosis. *Ann Neurol* **50**: 121–127

McDonnell GV, Hawkins SA 1996 Primary progressive multiple sclerosis: a distinct syndrome? *Mult Scler* **2**: 137–141

McDonnell GV, Hawkins SA 1998a An epidemiological study of multiple sclerosis in Northern Ireland. *Neurology* **50**: 423–428

McDonnell GV, Hawkins SA 1998b Clinical study of primary progressive multiple sclerosis in Northern Ireland, UK. *J Neurol Neurosurg Psychiatry* **64**: 451–454

McDonnell GV, Hawkins SA 1999 High incidence and prevalence of multiple sclerosis in south-east Scotland: evidence of a genetic predisposition (letter). *J Neurol Neursurg Psychiatry* **66**: 411

McDonnell GV, Hawkins SA 2000 Multiple sclerosis in northern Ireland: a historical and global perspective. *Ulster Med J* **69**: 97–105

McDonnell GV, Hawkins SA 2002 Primary progressive multiple sclerosis: increasing clarity but many unanswered questions. *J Neurol Sci* **199**: 1–15

McDonnell GV, Kirk CW, Middleton D *et al* 1999a Genetic association studies of tumour necrosis factor α and β and tumour necrosis factor receptor 1 and 2 polymorphisms across the clinical spectrum of multiple sclerosis. *J Neurol* **246**: 1051–1058

McDonnell GV, Mawhinney H, Graham CA *et al* 1999b A study of the HLA-DR region in clinical subgroups of multiple sclerosis and its influence on prognosis. *J Neurol Sci* **165**: 77–83

McDonnell GV, Kirk CW, Hawkins SA, Graham CA 1999c Lack of association of transforming growth factor (TGF)beta1 and beta2 gene polymorphisms with multiple sclerosis (MS) in northern Ireland. *Mult Scler* **5**: 105–109

McDonnell GV, Kirk CW, Hawkins SA, Graham CA 2000 An evaluation of interleukin genes as susceptibility loci for multiple sclerosis. *J Neurol Sci* **176**: 4–12

McDonnell GV, Cabrera-Gomez J, Calne DB *et al* 2003 Clinical presentation of primary progressive multiple sclerosis 10 years after the incidental finding of typical magnetic resonance imaging brain lesions: the subclinical stage of primary progressive multiple sclerosis may last 10 years. *Mult Scler* **9**: 210–212

McDonough J, Dutta R, Gudz T *et al* 2003 Decreases in GABA and mitochondrial genes are implicated in MS cortical pathology through microarray analysis of postmortem MS cortex. *Soc Neurosci Abstr* **213**: 212

McDougall AJ, McLeod JG 2003 Autonomic nervous system function in multiple sclerosis. *J Neurol Sci* **215**: 79–85

McFarland HF 1992 Twin studies and multiple sclerosis. *Ann Neurol* **32**: 722–723

McFarland HF, Frank J, Albert P *et al* 1992 Using gadolinium-enhanced magnetic resonance imaging lesions to monitor disease activity in multiple sclerosis. *Ann Neurol* **32**: 758–766

McFarling DA, Susac JO 1979 Hoquet diabolique: intractable hiccups as a manifestation of multiple sclerosis. *Neurology* **26**: 797–801

McGavern DB, Murray PD, Rivera-Quinones C *et al* 2000 Axonal loss results in spinal cord atrophy, electrophysiological abnormalities and neurological deficits following demyelination in a chronic inflammatory model of multiple sclerosis. *Brain* **123**: 519–531

McGeer PL, Itagaki S, Boyes BE, McGeer EG 1988 Reactive microglia are positive for HLA-DR in the substantia nigra of Parkinson's and Alzheimer's disease brains. *Neurology* **38**: 1285–1291

McGeoch DJ 2001 Molecular evolution of the γ-Herpesvirinae. *Phil Trans R Soc Lond* **356**: 421–435

MacGregor HS 1991 Multiple sclerosis clusters in Florida. *J Epidemiol Commun Hlth* **45**: 88

McGrother CW, Dugmore C, Phillips MJ *et al* 1999 Multiple sclerosis, dental caries and fillings: a case-control study. *Brit Dent J* **187**: 261–264

McGuigan C, McCarthy A, Quigley C et al 2004 Latitudinal variation in the prevalence of multiple sclerosis in Ireland, an effect of genetic diversity. *J Neurol Neurosurg Psychiatry* **75**: 572–576

McHenry L 1969 *Garrison's History of Neurology*. Springfield, IL: C.C. Thomas, pp. 253–254

McHugh K, McMenamin JB 1987 Acute disseminated encephalomyelitis in childhood. *Irish Med J* **80**: 412–414

McIntosh-Michaelis SA, Roberts MH, Wilkinson SM et al 1991 The prevalence of cognitive impairment in a community survey of multiple sclerosis. *Br J Clin Psychol* **30**: 333–348

McIvor GP, Riklan M, Reznikoff M 1984 Depression in multiple sclerosis as a function of length and severity of illness, age, remissions and perceived social support. *J Neuropsychol* **40**: 1028–1033

MacKarell P 1990 *Depictions of an Odyssey*. Corsham, Wiltshire: National Society for Education in Art and Design

MacKay A, Whittall K, Adler J et al 1994 In vivo visualization of myelin water in brain by magnetic resonance. *Magn Reson Med* **31**: 673–677

MacKay JR, Goldstein G 1967 Thymus and muscle (letter to editor). *Clin Exp Immunol* **2**: 139–140

McKay RD 1999 Brain stem cells change their identity. *Nature Med* **5**: 261–262

Mackay RP 1950 The familial recurrence of multiple sclerosis. In: *Multiple Sclerosis and the Demyelinating Diseases. Proc Assoc Res Nerv Mental Dis* **28**: 150–177

Mackay RP 1953 Multiple sclerosis: its onset and duration. *Med Clin N Am* **37**: 511–521

Mackay RP, Hirano A 1967 Forms of benign multiple sclerosis: report of two 'clinically silent' cases discovered at autopsy. *Arch Neurol* **17**: 588–600

Mackay RP, Myrianthopoulous NC 1958 Multiple sclerosis in twins: preliminary report in twins and their relatives. *Arch Neurol Psychiatry* **80**: 667–674

Mackay RP, Myrianthopoulous NC 1966 Multiple sclerosis in twins and their relatives: final report. *Arch Neurol* **15**: 449–462

MacKenzie W 1840 *A Practical Treatise on Diseases of the Eye*, 3rd edn. London: Longman

MacKenzie-Graham A, Pribyl TM, Kim S et al 1997 Myelin protein expression is increased in lymph nodes of mice with relapsing experimental autoimmune encephalomyelitis. *J Immunol* **159**: 4602–4610

McKeown LP, Porter-Armstrong AP, Baxter GD 2004 Caregivers of people with multiple sclerosis: experiences of support. *Mult Scler* **10**: 219–230

McKeown SR, Allen IV 1978 The cellular origin of lysosomal enzymes in the plaque of multiple sclerosis: a combined histological and biochemical study. *Neuropath Appl Neurobiol* **4**: 471–482

McKerracher L, David S, Jackson DL et al 1994 Identification of myelin associated glycoprotein as a major myelin-derived inhibitor of neurite growth. *Neuron* **13**: 805–811

McKinnon PJ, Margolskee RF 1996 SC1: a marker for astrocytes in the adult rodent brain is upregulated during reactive astrocytosis. *Brain Res* **709**: 27–36

McKinnon RD, Dubois-Dalcq M 1990 Fibroblast growth factor blocks myelin basic protein gene expression in differentiating O-2A glial progenitor cells. *Ann NY Acad Sci* **605**: 358–359

McKinnon RD, Piras G, Ida JA, Dubois-Dalcq M 1993 A role for TGF-beta in oligodendrocyte differentiation. *J Cell Biol* **121**: 1397–1407

McKinnon RD, Waldron S, Kiel ME 2005 PDGF alpha-receptor signal strength controls an RTK rheostat that integrates phosphoinositol 3′-kinase and phospholipase gamma pathways during oligodendrocyte maturation. *J Neurosci* **25**: 3499–3508

McLarnon JG, Michikawa M, Kim SU 1993 Effects of tumor necrosis factor on inward potassium current and cell morphology in cultured human oligodendrocytes. *Glia* **9**: 120–126

MacLaurin H 1873 Case of amblyopia from partial neuritis, treated with subcutaneous injections of strychnia. *NSW Med Gazette* **3**: 214

McLean AR, Berkson J 1951 Mortality and disability in multiple sclerosis: a statistical estimate of prognosis. *J Am Med Assoc* **146**: 1367–1369

MacLean AR, Berkson J, Woltmnan HW, Schionneman L 1950 Multiple sclerosis in a rural community. *Arch Res Nerv Mental Dis Proc* **28**: 25–27

McLean BN, Luxton RW, Thompson EJ 1990 A study of immunoglobulin G in the cerebrospinal fluid of 1007 patients with suspected neurological disease using isoelectric focusing and the log IgG-index: a comparison and diagnostic applications. *Brain* **113**: 1269–1289

McLean BN, Zeman AZ, Barnes D, Thompson EJ 1993 Patterns of blood brain barrier impairment and clinical features in multiple sclerosis. *J Neurol Neurosurg Psychiatry* **56**: 356–360

MacLennan ICM 1994 Germinal centers. *Annu Rev Immunol* **12**: 117–139

McLeod J, Hammond SR, Hallpike JF 1994 Epidemiology of multiple sclerosis in Australia. *Med J Aust* **160**: 117–119, 121–122

McLuckie A, Savage R 1993 Atrial fibrillation following methylprednisolone pulse therapy in an adult. *Chest* **104**: 622–623

Maclure M 1991 The case-crossover design: a method for studying transient effects on the risk of acute events. *Am J Epidemiol* **133**: 144–153

McMahon BJ, Helminiak C, Wainwright RB et al 1992 Frequency of adverse reactions to hepatitis B vaccine in 43,618 persons. *Am J Med* **92**: 254–256

McMahon JA, Takada S, Zimmerman LB et al 1998 Noggin-mediated antagonism of BMP signaling is required for growth and patterning of the neural tube and somite. *Genes Dev* **12**: 1438–1452

McManus C, Berman JW, Brett FM et al 1998 MCP-1, MCP-2 and MCP-3 expression in multiple sclerosis lesions: an immunohistochemical and in situ hybridization study. *J Neuroimmunol* **86**: 20–29

McMenamin PG 1999 Distribution and phenotype of dendritic cells and resident tissue macrophages in the dura mater, leptomeninges, and choroid plexus of the rat brain as demonstrated in wholemount preparations. *J Comp Neurol* **405**: 553–562

McNatt SA, Yu C, Giannotta SL et al 2005 Gamma knife radiosurgery for trigeminal neuralgia. *Neurosurgery* **56**: 1295–301; discussion 1301–1303

McPherson D, Starr A 1993 Auditory evoked potentials in the clinic. In: Halliday AM (ed.) *Evoked Potentials in Clinical Testing*. Edinburgh: Churchill Livingstone, pp. 359–381

McQualter JL, Darwiche R, Ewing C et al 2001 Granulocyte macrophage colony-stimulating factor: a new putative therapeutic target in multiple sclerosis. *J Exp Med* **194**: 873–882

McRae BL, Semnani RT, Hayes MP, van Seventer GA 1998 Type I IFNs inhibit human dendritic cell IL-12 production and Th1 cell development. *J Immunol* **160**: 4298–4304

McTigue DM, Horner PJ, Stokes BT, Gage FH 1998 Neurotrophin-3 and brain-derived neurotrophic factor induce oligodendrocyte proliferation and myelination of regenerating axons in the contused adult rat spinal cord. *J Neurosci* **18**: 5354–5365

Madigand DM, Oger JJ-F, Fauchet R et al 1982 HLA profiles in multiple sclerosis suggest two forms of disease and the existence of protective haplotypes. *J Neurol Sci* **53**: 519–529

Madsen LS, Andersson EC, Jansson L et al 1999 A humanized model for multiple sclerosis using HLA DR2 and a human T cell receptor. *Nature Genet* **23**: 343–347

Maeda A, Sobel RA 1996 Matrix metalloproteinases in the normal human central nervous system, microglia nodules and multiple sclerosis lesions. *J Neuropathol Exp Neurol* **55**: 300–309

Maeda Y, Solansky M, Menonna J et al 2001 Platelet-derived growth factor-alpha receptor-positive oligodendroglia are frequent in multiple sclerosis lesions. *Ann Neurol* **49**: 776–785

Maehlen J, Olsson T, Zachau A, Klareskog L 1989 Local enhancement of major histocompatibility complex (MHC) class I and class II expression and cell infiltration in experimental allergic encephalomyelitis around axotomized motor neurons. *J Neuroimmunol* **23**: 125–132

Maglivi SS, Leavitt BR, Macklis JD 2000 Induction of neurogenesis in the neocortex of adult mice. *Nature* **405**: 951–955

Magnus T, Chan A, Grauer O et al 2001 Microglial phagocytosis of apoptotic inflammatory T cells leads to down-regulation of microglial immune activation. *J Immunol* **167**: 5004–5010

Magnus T, Chan A, Linker RA et al 2002 Astrocytes are less efficient in the removal of apoptotic lymphocytes than microglia cells: implications for the role of glial cells in the inflamed central nervous system. *J Neuropathol Exp Neurol* **61**: 760–766

Magy L, Mertens C, Avellana-Adalid V et al 2003 Inducible expression of FGF2 by a rat oligodendrocyte precursor cell line promotes CNS myelination in vitro. *Exp Neurol* **184**: 912–922

Mahad DJ, Howell SJ, Woodroofe MN 2002 Expression of chemokines in the CSF and correlation with clinical disease activity in patients with multiple sclerosis. *J Neurol Neurosurg Psychiatry* **72**: 498–502

Mahad DJ, Trebst C, Kivisäkk P et al 2004 Expression of chemokine receptors CCR1 and CCR5 reflects differential activation of mononuclear phagocytes in pattern II and pattern III multiple sclerosis lesions. *J Neuropath Exp Neurol* **63**: 262–273

Mahassin F, Algayres JP, Valmary J et al 1993 Myélite aigüe après vaccination contre l'hépatite B. *Presse Med* **22**: 1997–1998

Maier K, Rau CR, Storch MK et al 2004 Ciliary neurotrophic factor protects retinal ganglion cells from secondary cell death during acute autoimmune optic neuritis in rats. *Brain Pathol* **14**: 378–387

Maimone D, Reder AT, Finocchiaro F, Recupero E 1991a Internal capsule plaque and tonic spasms in multiple sclerosis. *Arch Neurol* **48**: 427–429

Maimone D, Gregor S, Arnason BG, Reder AT 1991b Cytokine levels in the cerebrospinal fluid and serum of patients with multiple sclerosis. *J Neuroimmunol* **32**: 67–74

Mainero C, Faroni J, Gasperini C et al 1999 Fatigue and magnetic resonance imaging activity in multiple sclerosis. *J Neurol* **246**: 454–458

Majed H, Chandran SC, Niclou S et al 2005 A novel role for Sema3A in neuroprotection from injury mediated by activated microglia. *J Neurosci* **24**: 1730–1738

Majid A, Galetta SL, Sweeney CJ et al 2002 Epstein–Barr virus myeloradiculitis and encephalomyeloradiculitis. *Brain* **125**: 159–165

Malcus-Vocanson C, Giraud P, Broussolle E, Perron H, Mandrand B, Chazot G 1998 A urinary marker for multiple sclerosis. *Lancet* **351**: 1330

Malcus-Vocanson C, Giraud P, Micoud F et al 2001 Glial toxicity in urine and multiple sclerosis. *Mult Scler* **7**: 383–388

Male DK, Pryce G, Hughes CCW 1987 Antigen presentation in brain: MHC induction on brain endothelium and astrocyte compared. *Immunology* **60**: 453–459

Male DK, Pryce G, Rahman J 1990 Comparison of the immunological properties of rat cerebral and aortic endothelium. *J Neuroimmunol* **30**: 161–168

Male DK, Rahman J, Pryce G et al 1994 Lymphocyte migration into the CNS modelled in vitro: roles of LFA-1, ICAM-1 and VLA-4. *Immunology* **81**: 366–372

Malferrari G, Stella A, Monferini E et al 2005 CTLA4 and multiple sclerosis in the Italian population. *Exp Mol Pathol* **78**: 55–57

Malhotra AS, Goren H 1981 The hot bath test in the diagnosis of multiple sclerosis. *J Am Med Assoc* **246**: 1113–1114

Malik O, Compston DAS, Scolding NJ 1998 Interferon-beta inhibits astrocyte proliferation in vitro. *J Neuroimmunol* 1998 **86**: 155–162

Malipiero U, Frei K, Spanaus K-S et al 1997 Myelin oligodendrocyte glycoprotein-induced autoimmune encephalomyelitis is chronic/relapsing in perforin knockout mice, but monophasic in Fas- and Fas ligand-deficient lpr and gld mice. *Eur J Immunol* **27**: 3151–3160

Malmgren RM, Valdiviezo NL, Visscher BR et al 1983 Underlying cause of death as recorded for multiple sclerosis patients: associated factors. *J Chronic Dis* **36**: 699–705

Malone PR, Stanton SL, Riddle PR 1985 Urinary diversion for incontinence – a beneficial procedure? *Ann R Coll Surg Engl* **76**: 349–352

Malucchi S, Sala A, Gilli F et al 2004 Neutralizing antibodies reduce the efficacy of IFN during treatment of multiple sclerosis. *Neurology* **62**: 2031–2037

Manabe Y, Sasaki C, Warita H et al 2000 Sjogren's syndrome with acute transverse myelopathy as the initial manifestation. *J Neurol Sci* **176**: 158–161

Management of Multiple Sclerosis in Primary and Secondary Care. Clinical Guideline 8, November 2003. www.nice.org.uk

Mancall EL, Rosales RK 1964 Necrotising myelopathy associated with visceral carcinoma. *Brain* **87**: 639–656

Mancardi GL, Saccardi R, Filippi M et al 2001 Autologous hematopoietic stem cell transplantation suppresses Gd-enhanced MRI activity in MS. *Neurology* **57**: 62–68

Mancini J, Chabrol B, Moulene E, Pinsard N 1996 Relapsing acute encephalopathy: a complication of diphtheria-tetanus-poliomyelitis immunization in a young boy. *Eur J Pediatr* **155**: 135–138

Mandler RN, Davis LE, Jeffrey DR, Kormfield M 1993 Devic's neuromyelitis optica: a clinicopathological study of 8 patients. *Ann Neurol* **34**: 162–168

Mandler RN, Ahmed W, Dencoff JE 1998 Devic's neuromyelitis optica: a prospective study of seven patients treated with prednisone and azathioprine. *Neurology* **51**: 1219–1220

Manitt C, Colicos MA, Thompson KM et al 2001 Widespread expression of netrin-1 by neurons and oligodendrocytes in the adult mammalian spinal cord. *J Neurosci* **21**: 3911–3922

Manley NR 2000 Thymus organogenesis and molecular mechanisms of thymic epithelial cell differentiation. *Semin Immunol* **12**: 421–428

Mann CLA, Davies MB, Boggild MD et al 2000 Glutathione S-transferase polymorphisms in multiple sclerosis and their relationship to disability. *Neurology* **54**: 552–557

Mann CLA, Davies MB, Stevenson VL et al 2002 Interleukin 1 genotypes in multiple sclerosis and relationship to disease severity. *J Neuroimmunol* **129**: 197–204

Mann MB, Wu S, Rostamkhani M et al 2002 Association between the phenylethanol-amine N-methyltransferase gene and multiple sclerosis. *J Neuroimmunol* **124**: 101–105

Mao CC, Gancher ST, Herndon RM 1988 Movement disorders in multiple sclerosis. *Mov Disord* **3**: 109–116

Mao Z, Bonni A, Xia F et al 1999 Neuronal activity-dependent cell survival mediated by transcription factor MEF2. *Science* **286**: 785–790

Mao-Draayer Y, Panitch H 2004 Alexia without agraphia in multiple sclerosis: case report with magnetic resonance imaging localization. *Mult Scler* **10**: 705–707

Marburg O 1906 Die sogennante 'akute multiple sklerose'. *Jahrb Psychiatr Neurol* **27**: 211–312

Marburg O 1936 Multiple Sklerose. In: Bumke, Förster (eds) *Handbuch der Neurologie*, Vol 13, p. 546–693

Marcao AM, Wiest R, Schindler K et al 2005 Adult onset metachromatic leukodystrophy without electroclinical peripheral nervous system involvement: a new mutation in the ARSA gene. *Arch Neurol* **62**: 309–313

Marchioni E, Marinou-Aktipi K, Uggetti C et al 2002 Effectiveness of intravenous immunoglobulin treatment in adult patients with steroid-resistant monophasic or recurrent acute disseminated encephalomyelitis. *J Neurol* **249**: 100–104

Marcos MM, Walsh EC, Ke X et al 2005 A high resolution linkage disequilibrium map of the human major histocompatibility complex and first generation of tag single nucleotide polymorphisms. *Am J Hum Genet* **76**: 634–646

Mariani C, Farina E, Cappa SF et al 1991 Neuropsychological assessment in multiple sclerosis: a follow-up study with magnetic resonance imaging. *J Neurol* **238**: 395–400

Marie P 1884 Sclérose en plaques et maladies infectieuses. *Progrès Med* **12**: 287–289, 305–307, 349–351, 365–366

Marie P 1895 *Lectures on Diseases of the Spinal Cord*. London: New Sydenham Society, pp. 102–153

Marie P, Chatelin C 1917 Sur certains symptômes d'origine vraisemblablement radiculaire, chez les blessés du crâne. *Rev Neurol* **24ii**: 336

Marine J-C, Topham DJ, Mckay C et al 1999 SOCS1 deficiency causes a lymphocyte dependent perinatal lethality. *Cell* 98: 609–616

Marinesco G 1919 Etude sur l'origine et la nature de la sclérose en plaques. *Rev Neurol* 26: 481–488

Markovic M, Trajkovic V, Drulovic J *et al* 2003 Antibodies against myelin oligodendrocyte glycoprotein in the cerebrospinal fluid of multiple sclerosis patients. *J Neurol Sci* 211: 67–73

Markovic-Plese S, Fukaura H, Zhang J *et al* 1995 T cell recognition of immunodominant and cryptic proteolipid protein epitopes in humans. *J Immunol* 155: 982–992

Markovic-Plese S, Bielekova B, Kadom N *et al* 2002 Longitudinal magnetic resonance imaging study on the effect of azathioprine in relapsing–remitting multiple sclerosis patients refractory to the treatment with interferon beta-1b. *Neurology* 58: A492

Marrie RA, Wolfson C 2001 Multiple sclerosis and varicella zoster virus infection: a review. *Epidemiol Infect* 127: 315–325

Marrie RA, Wolfson C, Sturkenboom MC *et al* 2000 Multiple sclerosis and antecedent infections: a case–control study. *Neurology* 54: 2307–2310

Marrosu MG, Muntoni F, Murru MR *et al* 1988 Sardinian multiple sclerosis is associated with HLA-DR4: a serologic and molecular analysis. *Neurology* 38: 1749–1753

Marrosu MG, Muntoni F, Murru MR *et al* 1992 HLA-DQB1 genotype in Sardinian multiple sclerosis: evidence for a key role of DQB1.0201 and DQB1.0302 alleles. *Neurology* 42: 883–886

Marrosu MG, Fadda E, Mancosu C *et al* 2000a The contribution of HLA to multiple sclerosis susceptibility in Sardinian affected sibling pairs. *Ann Neurol* 47: 411–412

Marrosu MG, Schirru L, Fadda E *et al* 2000b ICAM-1 gene is not associated with multiple sclerosis in Sardinian patients. *J Neurol* 247: 677–680

Marrosu MG, Murru R, Murru MR *et al* 2001 Dissection of the HLA association with multiple sclerosis in the founder isolated population of Sardinia. *Hum Mol Genet* 10: 2907–2916

Marrosu MG, Lai M, Cocco E *et al* 2002a Genetic factors and the founder effect explain familial MS in Sardinia. *Neurology* 58: 283–288

Marrosu MG, Cocco E, Lai M *et al* 2002b Patients with multiple sclerosis and risk of type-1 diabetes mellitus in Sardinia, Italy: a cohort study. *Lancet* 349: 1461–1465

Marrosu MG, Sardu C, Cocco E *et al* 2004 Bias in parental transmission of the HLA-DR3 allele in Sardinian multiple sclerosis. *Neurology* 63: 1084–1086

Mars LT, Laloux V, Goude K *et al* 2002 Va14-Ja281 NKT cells naturally regulate experimental autoimmune encephalomyelitis in nonobese diabetic mice. *J Immunol* 168: 6007–6011

Marsden CD, Merton PA, Morton HB 1980 Maximal twitches from stimulation of the motor cortex in man. *J Physiol* 312: 5P

Marsden CD, Obeso JA, Lang AE 1982 Adrenoleukomyeloneuropathy presenting as spinocerebellar degeneration. *Neurology* 32: 1031–1032

Marsh SGE, Albert ED, Bodmer WF *et al* 2002 Nomenclature for factors of the HLA system, 2002. *Tissue Antigens* 60: 407–464

Marshall EK 1948 Clinical therapeutic trial of the new drug. *Bull Johns Hopkins Hosp* 85: 221–230

Marshall J 1955 Spastic paraplegia of middle age. *Lancet* i: 643–646

Martell M, Marcadet A, Strominger J *et al* 1987 T cell receptor alpha genes might be involved in multiple sclerosis genetic susceptibility. *CR Acad Sci* 304: 105–110

Martin D, Near SL 1995 Protective effect of the interleukin-1 receptor antagonist (IL-1ra) on experimental allergic encephalomyelitis in rats. *J Neuroimmunol* 61: 241–245

Martin R, Jaraquemada D, Flerlage M *et al* 1990 Fine specificity and HLA restriction of myelin basic protein-specific cytotoxic T cell lines from multiple sclerosis patients and healthy individuals. *J Immunol* 145: 540–548

Martin R, Howell MD, Jaraquemada D *et al* 1991 A myelin basic protein peptide is recognized by cytotoxic T cells in the context of four HLA-DR types associated with multiple sclerosis. *J Exp Med* 173: 19–24

Martin R, McFarland HF, McFarlin DE 1992a Immunological aspects of demyelinating diseases. *Annu Rev Immunol* 10: 153–187

Martin R, Utz U, Coligan JE *et al* 1992b Diversity in fine specificity and T cell receptor usage of the human CD4+ cytotoxic T cell response specific for the immunodominant myelin basic protein peptide 87–106. *J Immunol* 148: 1359–1366

Martinelli V, Comi G, Filippi M *et al* 1991 Paraclinical tests in acute-onset optic neuritis: basal data and results of a short follow-up. *Acta Neurol Scand* 84: 231–236

Martiney JA, Rajan AJ, Charles PC *et al* 1998 Prevention and treatment of experimental autoimmune encephalomyelitis by CNI-1493, a macrophage-deactivating agent. *J Immunol* 160: 5588–5595

Martinez-Caceres EM, Barrau MA, Brieva L *et al* 2002 Treatment with methylprednisolone in relapses of multiple sclerosis patients: immunological evidence of immediate and short-term but not long-lasting effects. *Clin Exp Immunol* 127: 165–171

Martinez-Naves E, Victoria-Gutierrez M, Lopez-Larrea C 1993 The germline repertoire of T cell receptor beta chain genes in multiple sclerosis patients from Spain. *J Neuroimmunol* 47: 9–14

Martinez-Yelamos A, Saiz A, Sanchez-Valle R *et al* 2001 14–3–3 protein in the CSF as a prognostic marker in early multiple sclerosis. *Neurology* 57: 722–724

Martins Silva B, Thorlacius T, Benediktsson K *et al* 2003 A whole genome association study in multiple sclerosis patients from north Portugal. *J Neuroimmunol* 143: 116–119

Martyn CN, Kean D 1988 The one-and-a-half syndrome: clinical correlation with a pontine lesion demonstrated by nuclear magnetic resonance imaging in a case of multiple sclerosis. *Br J Ophthalmol* 72: 515–517

Martyn CN, Cruddas M, Compston DAS 1993 Symptomatic Epstein–Barr virus infection and multiple sclerosis. *J Neurol Neurosurg Psychiatry* 56: 167–168

Masdeu JC, Quinto C, Olivera C *et al* 2000 Open-ring imaging sign: highly specific for atypical brain demyelination. *Neurology* 54: 1427–1433

Mason D 1991 Genetic variation in the stress response: susceptibility to experimental allergic encephalomyelitis and implications for human inflammatory disease. *Immunol Today* 12: 57–60

Mason JL, Goldman JE 2002 A2B5+ and O4+ Cycling progenitors in the adult forebrain white matter respond differentially to PDGF-AA, FGF-2, and IGF-1. *Mol Cell Neurosci* 20: 30–42

Mason JL, Suzuki K, Chaplin DD, Matsushima GK 2001 Interleukin-1beta promotes repair of the CNS. *J Neurosci* 21: 7046–7052

Mason JL, Xuan S, Dragatsis I *et al* 2003 Insulin-like growth factor (IGF) signaling through type 1 IGF receptor plays an important role in remyelination. *J Neurosci* 23: 7710–7718

Mason JL, Toews A, Hostettler JD *et al* 2004 Oligodendrocytes and progenitors become progressively depleted within chronically demyelinated lesions. *Am J Pathol* 164: 1673–1682

Mason JL, Angelastro JM, Ignatovoa TN *et al* 2005 ATF5 regulates the proliferation and differentiation of oligodendrocytes. *Mol Cell Neurosci* 29: 372–380

Mason WP, Graus F, Lang B *et al* 1997 Small cell lung cancer, paraneoplastic cerebellar degeneration and the Lambert–Eaton myasthenic syndrome. *Brain* 120: 1279–1300

Massacesi L, Parigi A, Barilaro A *et al* 2000 MRI Evaluation of azathioprine activity on encephalic lesions in relapsing–remitting multiple sclerosis. *Neurology* 54: A16–A17

Massaro AR, Michetti F, Laudison A, Bergonzi P 1985 Myelin basic protein and S-100 antigen in cerebrospinal fluid of patients with multiple sclerosis in the acute phase. *Ital J Neurol Sci* 6: 53–56

Massaro AR, Albrechtsen M, Bock E 1987 N-CAM in cerebrospinal fluid: a marker of synaptic remodelling after acute phases of multiple sclerosis? *Ital J Neurol Sci* 6: 85–88

Massey JM 2003 Domestic violence in neurological practice. In: Noseworthy JH (ed.) *Neurological Therapeutics: Principles and Practice.* London: Martin Dunitz, pp. 65–68

Masterman T, Ligers A, Olsson T *et al* 2000 HLA-DR15 is associated with lower age at onset in multiple sclerosis. *Ann Neurol* 48: 211–219

Masterman T, Ligers A, Zhang Z *et al* 2002a CTLA4 polymorphisms and the multiple

887

sclerosis phenotype. *J Neuroimmunol* **131**: 208–212

Masterman T, Zhang Z, Hellgren D *et al* 2002b APOE genotypes and disease severity in multiple sclerosis. *Mult Scler* **8**: 98–103

Mastrostefano R, Occhipinti E, Bigotti G, Pompili A 1987 Multiple sclerosis plaque simulating cerebral tumour: case report and review of the literature. *Neurosurgery* **21**: 244–246

Masucci EF, Saini N, Kurtzke JF 1989 Bilateral ballism in multiple sclerosis. *Neurology* **39**: 1941–1942

Matesanz F, Fedetz M, Collado-Romero M *et al* 2001 Allelic expression and interleukin-2 polymorphisms in multiple sclerosis. *J Neuroimmunol* **119**: 101–105

Mather FJ, Simon RM, Clark GM, Von Hoff DD 1987 Cardiotoxicity in patients treated with mitoxantrone: Southwest Oncology Group Phase II studies. *Cancer Treat Rep* **71**: 609–613

Mathew NT, Mathai KV, Abraham J, Taori GM 1971 Incidence and pattern of demyelinating disease in India. *J Neurol Sci* **13**: 27–38

Mathewson AJ, Berry M 1985 Observations on the astrocyte response to a cerebral stab wound in adult rats. *Brain Res* **327**: 61–69

Mathis C, Denisenko-Nehrbass N, Girault JA, Borrelli E 2001 Essential role of oligodendrocytes in the formation and maintenance of central nervous system nodal regions. *Development* **128**: 4881–4890

Mathisen PM, Pease S, Garvey J *et al* 1993 Identification of an embryonic isoform of myelin basic protein that is expressed widely in the mouse embryo. *Proc Natl Acad Sci USA* **90**: 10125–10129

Matias-Guiu J, Boulmar F, Martin R *et al* 1990 Multiple sclerosis in Spain: an epidemiological study of the Alcoy health region, Valencia. *Acta Neurol Scand* **81**: 479–483

Matias-Guiu J, Galiano L, Ribera C *et al* 1994 In: Firnhaber W, Lauer K (eds) *Multiple Sclerosis in Europe: An Epidemiological Update*. Darmstadt: Leuchtturm-Verlag/LTV Press, p. 190

Matsuda M, Tabata K, Miki J *et al* 2001 Multiple sclerosis with secondary syringomyelia: an autopsy report. *J Neurol Sci* **184**: 189–196

Matsumoto J, Morrow D, Kaufman K *et al* 2001 Surgical therapy for tremor in multiple sclerosis – an evaluation of outcome measures. *Neurology* **57**: 1876–1882

Matsumoto Y, Abo T 1994 Lack of 'determinant spread' to the minor encephalitogenic epitope in myelin basic protein-induced acute experimental autoimmune encephalomyelitis in the rat. *Cell Immunol* **155**: 517–523

Matsumoto Y, Fujiwara M 1987 Absence of donor-type major histocompatibility complex class I antigen-bearing microglia in the rat central nervous systsem of radiation bone marrow chimeras. *J Neuroimmunol* **17**: 71–82

Matsumoto Y, Fujiwara M 1988 Adoptively transfered experimental allergic encephalomyelitis in chimeric rats: identification of transfered cells in the lesions of the central nervous system. *Immunology* **65**: 23–29

Matsumoto Y, Fujiwara M 1993 Immunomodulation of experimental autoimmune encephalomyelitis by staphylococcal enterotoxin D. *Cell Immunol* **149**: 268–278

Matsumoto Y, Kohyama K, Aikawa Y *et al* 1998 Role of natural killer cells and TCR-gd T cells in acute autoimmune encephalomyelitis. *Eur J Immunol* **28**: 1681–1688

Matsumoto Y, Yoon WK, Jee Y *et al* 2003 Complementarity-determining region 3 spectratyping analysis of the TCR repertoire in multiple sclerosis. *J Immunol* **170**: 4846–4853

Matthews JN 1995 Small clinical trials: are they all bad? *Stat Med* **14**:115–126

Matthews JR 1995 *Quantification and the Quest for Medical Certainty*. Princeton, NJ: Princeton University Press

Matthews WB 1958 Tonic seizures in disseminated sclerosis. *Brain* **81**: 193–206

Matthews WB 1962 Epilepsy and disseminated sclerosis. *Q J Med* **31**: 141–155

Matthews WB 1966 Facial myokymia. *J Neurol Neurosurg Psychiatry* **29**: 35–39

Matthews WB 1968 The neurological complications of ankylosing spondylitis. *J Neurol Sci* **6**: 561–573

Matthews WB 1975 Paroxysmal symptoms in multiple sclerosis. *J Neurol Neurosurg Psychiatry* **38**: 617–623

Matthews WB 1979 Multiple sclerosis presenting with acute remitting psychiatric symptoms. *J Neurol Neurosurg Psychiatry* **42**: 859–863

Matthews WB 1998 Symptoms and signs of multiple sclerosis. In: Compston A, Ebers G, Lassmann H *et al* (eds) *McAlpine's Multiple Sclerosis*, 3rd edn. London: Churchill Livingstone, pp. 145–190

Matthews WB, Esiri M 1983 The migrant sensory neuritis of Wartenberg. *J Neurol Neurosurg Psychiatry* **46**: 1–4

Matthews WB, Small DG 1979 Serial recordings of visual and somatosensory evoked potentials in multiple sclerosis. *J Neurol Sci* **40**: 11–21

Matthews WB, Small DG, Small M, Pountney E 1977 Pattern evoked visual potential in the diagnosis of multiple sclerosis. *J Neurol Neurosurg Psychiatry* **40**: 1009–1014

Matthews WB, Acheson ED, Batchelor JR, Weller RO 1985 *McAlpine's Multiple Sclerosis*, 1st edn. London: Churchill Livingstone

Matthews WB, Compston DAS, Allen IV, Martyn CN 1991 *McAlpine's Multiple Sclerosis*, 2nd edn. Edinburgh: Chuchill Livingstone

Matute C 1998 Characteristics of acute and chronic kainate excitotoxic damage to the optic nerve. *Proc Natl Acad Sci USA* **95**: 10229–10234

Matute C, Alberdi E, Domercq M *et al* 2001 The link between excitotoxic oligodendroglial death and demyelinating diseases. *Trends Neurosci* **24**: 224–230

Matysiak M, Jurewicz A, Jaskolski D, Selmaj K 2002 TRAIL induces death of human oligodendrocytes isolated from adult brain. *Brain* **125**: 2469–2480

Matyszak MK, Perry VH 1996a A comparison of leucocyte responses to heat-killed bacillus Calmette–Guerin in different CNS compartments. *Neuropathol Appl Neurobiol* **22**: 44–53

Matyszak MK, Perry VH 1996b The potential role of dendritic cells in immune-mediated inflammatory diseases in the central nervous system. *Neuroscience* **74**: 599–608

Matyszak MK, Perry VH 1996c Delayed-type hypersensitivity lesions in the central nervous system are prevented by inhibitors of matrix metalloproteinases. *J Neuroimmunol* **69**: 141–149

Matyszak MK, Townsend MJ, Perry VH 1997 Ultrastructural studies of an immune-mediated inflammatory response in the CNS parenchyma directed against a nn-CNC antigen. *Neuroscience* **78**: 549–560

Mauch E, Kornhuber HH, Knapf H, Fetzer V, Laufer H 1992 Treatment of multiple sclerosis with mitoxantrone. *Eur Arch Psychiatry Clin Neurosci* **242**: 96–102

Mauerhoff T, Pujol-Borrell R, Mirakian R, Bottazzo GF 1988 Differential expression and regulation of major histocompatibility complex (MHC) products in neural and glial cells of the human foetal brain. *J Neuroimmunol* **18**: 271–289

Maurer M, Kruse N, Giess R *et al* 1999 Gene polymorphism at position −308 of the tumor necrosis factor alpha promotor is not associated with disease progression in multiple sclerosis patients. *J Neurol* **246**: 949–954

Maurer M, Kruse N, Giess R *et al* 2000 Genetic variation at position −1082 of the interleukin 10 (IL10) promotor and the outcome of multiple sclerosis. *J Neuroimmunol* **104**: 98–100

Maurer M, Ponath A, Kruse N, Rieckmann P 2002 CTLA4 exon 1 dimorphism is associated with primary progressive multiple sclerosis. *J Neuroimmunol* **131**: 213–215

Mayr WT, Pittock SJ, McClelland RL *et al* 2003 Incidence and prevalence of multiple sclerosis in Olmsted County, Minnesota 1985–2000. *Neurology* **61**: 1373–1377

Mayr-Wohlfart U, Paulus C, Hennenberg A, Rodel G 1996 Mitochondrial DNA mutations in multiple sclerosis patients with severe optic involvement. *Acta Neurol Scand* **94**: 167–171

Mazza G, Ponsford M, Lowrey P *et al* 2002 Diversity and dynamics of the T-cell response to MBP in DR2+ve individuals. *Clin Exp Immunol* **128**: 538–547

Mazzarello P, Poloni M, Piccolo G, Cosi V, Pinelli P 1983 Intrathecal methylprednisolone acetate in multiple sclerosis treatment. *Clinical evaluation.* *Acta Neurolo Belg* **83**: 190–196

Mbonda E, Larnaout A, Maertens A *et al* 1990 Multiple sclerosis in a black Cameroonian woman. *Acta Neurol Belg* **90**: 218–222

Mead RJ, Singhrao SK, Neal JW *et al* 2002 The membrane attack complex of complement causes severe demyelination associated with acute axonal injury. *J Immunol* **168**: 458–465

Mead SH, Proukakis C, Wood NW *et al* 2001 A large family with hereditary spastic paraparesis due to a frame shift mutation of the spastin (SPG4) gene: association with multiple sclerosis in two affected siblings and epilepsy in other affected family members. *J Neurol Neurosurg Psychiatry* **71**: 788–791

Meadows SP 1969 Retrobulbar and optic neuritis in childhood and adolescence. *Trans Ophthalmol Soc UK* **89**: 603–638

Meca-Lallana JE, Martin JJ, Lucas C *et al* 1999 Susac syndrome: clinical and diagnostic approach: a new case report. *Rev Neurol* **29**: 1027–1032

van der Meche FG, Schmitz PI 1992 A randomized trial comparing intravenous immune globulin and plasma exchange in Guillain-Barré syndrome. Dutch Guillain-Barré Study Group. *N Engl J Med* **326**: 1123–1129

Medaer R 1979 Does the history of multiple sclerosis go back as far as the 14th century? *Acta Neurol Scand* **60**: 189–192

Medaer R, Stinissen P, Truyen L *et al* 1995 Depletion of myelin basic protein autoreactive T cells by T-cell vaccination: pilot trial in multiple sclerosis. *Lancet* **346**: 807–808

Medana IM, Esiri MM 2003 Axonal damage: a key predictor of outcome in human CNS diseases. *Brain* **126**: 515–530

Medana IM, Gallimore A, Oxenius A *et al* 2000 MHC class I-restricted killing of neurons by virus specific CD8+ T lymphocytes is effected through the Fas/FasL, but not the perforin pathway. *Eur J Immunol* **30**: 3623–3633

Medana IM, Li ZX, Flügel A *et al* 2001a Fas ligand (CD95L) protects neurons against perforin-mediated T lymphocyte cytotoxicity. *J Immunol* **167**: 674–681

Medana IM, Martinic MA, Wekerle H, Neumann H 2001b Transection of major histocompatibility complex class I-induced neurites by cytotoxic T lymphocytes. *Am J Pathol* **159**: 809–815

Meh D, Denislic M 1998 Autonomic evaluation by means of standard tests and power spectral analysis in multiple sclerosis. *Muscle Nerve* **21**: 678–680

van der Mei IA, Ponsonby AL, Blizzard L, Dwyer T 2001 Regional variation in multiple sclerosis prevalence in Australia and its association with ambient ultraviolet radiation. *Neuroepidemiology* **20**: 168–174

van der Mei IA, Ponsonby AL, Dwyer T *et al* 2003 Past exposure to sun, skin phenotype, and the risk of multiple sclerosis: case-control study. *Br Med J* **327**: 316

Meier P, Finch A, Evan G 2000 Apoptosis in development. *Nature* **407**: 796–801

Meinl E, Weber F, Drexler K *et al* 1993 Myelin basic protein specific T lymphocyte repertoire in multiple sclerosis: complexity of response and dominance of nested epitopes due to recruitment of multiple T cell clones. *J Clin Invest* **92**: 2633–2643

Meinl E, Hoch RM, Dornmair K *et al* 1997 Encephalitogenic potential of myelin basic protein-specific T cells isolated from normal rhesus macaques. *Am J Pathol* **150**: 445–453

Mekki-Dauriac S, Agius E, Kan P, Cochard P 2002 Bone morphogenetic proteins negatively control oligodendrocyte precursor specification in the chick spinal cord. *Development* **129**: 5117–5130

Melamed D, Nemazee D 1997 Self antigen does not accelerate immature B cell apoptosis, but stimulates receptor editing as a consequence of developmental arrest. *Proc Natl Acad Sci USA* **94**: 9267–9272

Melin J, Usenius JP, Fogelholm R 1996 Left ventricular failure and pulmonary edema in acute multiple sclerosis. *Acta Neurol Scand* **93**: 315–317

Mellai M, Giordano M, D'Alfonso S *et al* 2003 Prolactin and prolactin receptor gene polymorphisms in multiple sclerosis and systemic lupus erythematosus. *Hum Immunol* **64**: 274–284

Mellars P 2004 Neanderthals and the modern human colonization of Europe. *Nature* **432**: 461–465

Mellins E, Kempin S, Smith L *et al* 1991 A gene required for class 2 restricted antigen presentation maps to the major histocompatibility complex. *J Exp Med* **174**: 1607–1615

Ménage P, de Toffol B, Degenne D, Saudeau D, Bardos P, Autret A 1993 Syndrome de Gougerot-Sjögren primitif. Atteinte neurologique centrale évoluant par poussées. *Rev Neurol* **149**: 554–556

Ménage P, Carreau V, Tourbah A *et al* 1994 Les adrénoleucodystrophies hétérozygotes symptomatiques de l'adulte: 10 cas. *Rev Neurol* **149**: 445–454

Menard A, Paranhos-Baccala G, Pelletier J *et al* 1997 A cytotoxic factor for glial cells: a new avenue of research for multiple sclerosis? *Cell Mol Biol* **43**: 889–901

Mendel I, Kerlero de Rosbo N, Ben-Nun A 1995 A myelin oligodendrocyte glycoprotein peptide induces typical chronic experimental autoimmune encephalomyelitis in H-2b mice: fine specificity and T cell receptor Vb expression of encephalitogenic T cells. *Eur J Immunol* **25**: 1951–1959

Mendel I, Kerlero de Rosbo N, Ben-Nun A 1996 Delineation of the minimal encephalitogenic epitope within the immunodominant region of myelin oligodendrocyte glycoprotein: diverse V beta gene usage by T-cells recognizing the core epitope encephalitogenic for T-cell receptor V beta b and T cell receptor V

beta a H-2b mice. *Eur J Immunol* **26**: 2470–2479

Mendel I, Katz A, Kozak N *et al* 1998 Interleukin-6 functions in autoimmune encephalomyelitis: a study in gene-targeted mice. *Eur J Immunol* **28**: 1727–1737

Mendell JR, Kolkin S, Kissel JT *et al* 1987 Evidence for central nervous system demyelination in chronic inflammatory demyelinating polyradiculoneuropathy. *Neurology* **37**: 1291–1294

Menkes JH 1990 The leucodystrophies. *N Engl J Med* **322**: 54–55

Menon GJ, Thaller VT 2002 Therapeutic external ophthalmoplegia with bilateral retrobulbar botulinum toxin: an effective treatment for acquired nystagmus with oscillopsia. *Eye* **16**: 804–806

Menozzi P, Piazza A, Cavalli-Sforza L 1978 Synthetic maps of human gene frequencies in Europeans. *Science* **201**: 786–792

Menuhin Y 1996 Du Pre, Jacqueline Mary. In: CS Nicholls (ed.) *Dictionary of National Biography 1986–1990*. Oxford: Oxford University Press, pp. 114–116

Merelli E, Casoni F 2000 Prognostic factors in multiple sclerosis: role of intercurrent infections and vaccinations against influenza and hepatitis B. *Neurol Sci* **21 (Suppl)**: 853–856

Merelli E, Bedin R, Sola P *et al* 1997 Human herpes virus 6 and human herpes virus 8 DNA sequences in brains of multiple sclerosis patients, normal adults and children. *J Neurol* **244**: 450–454

Merle H, Smadja D, Merle S *et al* 2005 Visual phenotype of multiple sclerosis in the Afro-Caribbean population and the influence of migration to metropolitan France. *Eur J Ophthalmol* **15**: 392–399

Merrill JE 1992 Proinflammatory and antiinflammatory cytokines in multiple sclerosis and central nervous system acquired immunodeficiency syndrome. *J Immunother* **12**: 167–170

Merrill JE, Benveniste EN 1996 Cytokines in inflammatory brain lesions: helpful and harmful. *Trends Neurosci* **19**: 331–338

Merrill JE, Ignarro LJ, Sherman MP *et al* 1993 Microglial cell cytotoxicity of oligodendrocytes is mediated through nitric oxide. *J Immunol* **151**: 2132–2141

Merriman A, Cordell HJ, Eaves IA *et al* 2001 Suggestive evidence for association of human chromosome 18q12-q21 and its orthologue on rat and mouse chromosome 18 with several autoimmune diseases. *Diabetes* **50**: 184–194

Mertens C, Brassat D, Reboul J *et al* 1998 A systematic study of oligodendrocyte growth factors as candidates for genetic susceptibility to MS. *Neurology* **51**: 748–753

Mertin J, Rudge P, Kremer M *et al* 1982 Double blind controlled trial of immunosuppression in the treatment of multiple sclerosis: final report. *Lancet* **ii**: 351–354

Merton PA, Morton HB 1980a Stimulation of the cerebral cortex in the intact human subject. *Nature* **285**: 227

889

Merton PA, Morton HB 1980b Electrical stimulation of human motor and visual cortex through the scalp. *J Physiol* **305**: 9–10

Merton PA, Morton HB, Hill DK, Marsden CD 1982 Scope of a technique for electrical stimulation of the human brain, spinal cord and muscle. *Lancet* **2**: 597–600

Messersmith DJ, Murtie JC, Le TQ *et al* 2000 Fibroblast growth factor 2 (FGF2) and FGF receptor expression in an experimental demyelinating disease with extensive remyelination. *J Neurosci Res* **62**: 241–256

Metz L, Page S 2003 Oral cannabinoids for spasticity in multiple sclerosis: will attitude continue to limit use? *Lancet* **362**: 1513

Metz LM, Fritzler MJ, Seland TP 1988 Sjögren's syndrome infrequently mimics multiple sclerosis. *Can J Neurol Sci* **15**: 198

Metz LM, Sabuda D, Hilsden RJ *et al* 1999 Gastric tolerance of high-dose pulse oral prednisone in multiple sclerosis. *Neurology* **53**: 2093–2096

Metz LM, Zhang Y, Yeung M *et al* 2004 Minocycline reduces gadolinium-enhancing magnetic resonance imaging lesions in multiple sclerosis. *Ann Neurol* **55**: 756

Meuth SG, Budde T, Duyar H *et al* 2003 Modulation of neuronal activity by the endogenous pentapeptide QYNAD. *Eur J Neurosci* **18**: 2697–2706

Mews I, Bergmann M, Bunkowski S *et al* 1998 Oligodendrocyte and axon pathology in clinically silent multiple sclerosis lesions. *Mult Scler* **4**: 55–62

Meyer-Franke A, Kaplan MR, Pfeiger FW, Barres BA 1995 Characterisation of the signalling interactions that promote the survival and growth of developing retinal ganglion cells in culture. *Neuron* **15**: 805–819

Meyer-Rienecker H 1994 Epidemiological analyses on multiple sclerosis in the region of Rostock, north-East Germany. In: Firnhaber W, Lauer K (eds) *Multiple Sclerosis in Europe: An Epidemiological Update*. Darmstadt: Leuchtturm-Verlag/LTV Press, pp. 134–142

Meyer-Rienecker H, Buddenhagen F 1988 Incidence of multiple sclerosis: a periodic or stable phenomenon. *J Neurol* **235**: 241–244

MHC Sequencing Consortium 1999 Complete sequence and gene map of a human major histocompatibility complex. *Nature* **401**: 921–923

Mi S, Lee X, Shao Z *et al* 2004 LINGO-1 is a component of the Nogo-66 receptor/p75 signaling complex. *Nature Neurosci* **7**: 221–228

Mi S, Miller RH, Lee X *et al* 2005 LINGO-1 negatively regulates myelination by oligodendrocytes. *Nature Neurosci* **8**: 745–751

Micera A, Lambiase A, Rama P, Aloe L 1999 Altered nerve growth factor level in the optic nerve of patients affected by multiple sclerosis. *Mult Scler* **5**: 389–394

Michielsens B, Wilms G, Marchal G, Carton H 1990 Serial magnetic resonance imaging studies with paramagnetic contrast medium: assessment of disease activity in patients with multiple sclerosis before and after influenza vaccination. *Eur Neurol* **30**: 258–259

Middleton D, Savage DA, Cullen C *et al* 1992 Frequency of HLA-DP1 alleles in multiple sclerosis patients from northern Ireland. *Eur J Immunogenet* **19**: 323–326

Middleton D, Megaw G, Cullen C *et al* 1994 TAP1 and TAP2 polymorphisms in multiple sclerosis patients. *Hum Immunol* **40**: 131–134

Middleton LT, Dean G 1991 Multiple sclerosis in Cyprus. *J Neurol Sci* **103**: 29–36

Midgard R, Riise T, Nyland H 1991 Epidemiologic trends in multiple sclerosis in More and Romsdal, Norway: a prevalence/incident study in a stable population. *Neurology* **41**: 887–892

Midgard R, Albrektsen G, Riise T *et al* 1995 Prognostic factors for survival in multiple sclerosis: a longitudinal, population-based study in More and Romsdal, Norway. *J Neurol Neurosurg Psychiatry* **58**: 417–421

Midgard R, Riise T, Svanes C *et al* 1996a Incidence of multiple sclerosis in More and Romsdal, Norway from 1950–1991. *Brain* **119**: 203–211

Midgard R, Gronning M, Riise T *et al* 1996b Multiple sclerosis and chronic inflammatory diseases: a case-control study. *Acta Neurol Scand* **93**: 322–328

Miethke T, Wahl C, Heeg K *et al* 1992 T cell-mediated lethal shock triggered in mice by the superantigen staphylococcal enterotoxin B: critical role of tumor necrosis factor. *J Exp Med* **175**: 91–98

Mikaeloff Y, Adamsbaum C, Husson B *et al* 2004a MRI prognostic factors for relapse after acute CNS inflammatory demyelination in childhood. *Brain* **127**: 1942–1947

Mikaeloff Y, Suissa S, Vallée L *et al* 2004b First episode of acute CNS inflammatory demyelination in childhood: prognostic factors for multiple sclerosis and disability. *J Pediatrics* **144**: 246–252

Milanese C, Salmaggi A, La Mantia L *et al* 1988a Intrathecal beta-interferon in multiple sclerosis (letter). *Lancet* **ii**: 563–564

Milanese C, La Mantia L, Salmagi A *et al* 1988b Double blind controlled randomised study on azathioprine efficacy in multiple sclerosis: preliminary results. *Ital J Neurol Sci* **9**: 53–57

Milanese C, Salmaggi A, La Mantia L *et al* 1990 Double blind controlled study of intrathecal beta-interferon in multiple sclerosis: clinical and laboratory results. *J Neurol Neurosurg Psychiatry* **53**: 554–557

Milanese C, La Mantia L, Salmaggi A, Eoli M 1993 A double blind study on azathioprine efficacy in multiple sclerosis: final report. *J Neurol* **240**: 295–298

Milanov I, Topalov N, Kmetski T 1999 Prevalence of multiple sclerosis in Gypsies and Bulgarians. *Neuroepidemiology* **18**: 218–222

Milea D, Napolitano M, Dechy M *et al* 2001 Complete bilateral horizontal gaze paralysis disclosing multiple sclerosis. *J Neurol Neurosurg Psychiatry* **70**: 252–255

Millar JHD, Allison RS 1971 *Multiple Sclerosis, A Disease Acquired in Childhood*. Springfield, IL: C.C. Thomas

Millar JHD, Allison RS, Cheeseman EA, Merrett JD 1959 Pregnancy as a factor influencing relapse in disseminated sclerosis. *Brain* **82**: 417–426

Millar JHD, Vas CJ, Noronha MJ *et al* 1967 Long-term treatment of multiple sclerosis with corticotropin. *Lancet* **2**: 429–431

Millar JHD, Zilkha KJ, Langman MJS *et al* 1973 Double-blind trial of linolate supplementation of the diet in multiple sclerosis. *Br Med J* **1**: 765–768

Millefiorini E, Gasperini C, Possillie C *et al* 1997 Randomized placebo-controlled trial of mitoxantrone in relapsing–remitting multiple sclerosis: 24 month clinical and MRI outcome. *J Neurol* **244**: 153–159

Miller A, Lider O, Roberts AB *et al* 1992 Suppressor T cells generated by oral tolerization to myelin basic protein suppress both the *in vitro* and *in vivo* immune responses by the release of transforming growth factor β after antigen-specific triggering. *Proc Natl Acad Sci USA* **89**: 421–425

Miller A, Lanir N, Shapiro S *et al* 1996 Immunoregulatory effects of interferon-β and interacting cytokines on human vascular endothelial cells: implications for multiple sclerosis and other autoimmune diseases. *J Neuroimmunol* **64**: 151–161

Miller AE, Morgante RN, Buchwald LY *et al* 1997 A multicentre, randomised, double-blind, placebo-controlled trial of influenza immunisation in multiple sclerosis. *Neurology* **48**: 312–314

Miller DH 1988 MRI: sensitive and safe in diagnosing multiple sclerosis. *MRI Decisions* **2**: 17–24

Miller DH 2004a Brain atrophy, interferon beta, and treatment trials in multiple sclerosis. *Lancet* **364**: 1463–1464

Miller DH 2004b Biomarkers and surrogate outcomes in neurodegenerative disease: lessons from multiple sclerosis. *NeuroRx* **1**: 284–294

Miller DH, Hornabrook RW, Dagger J, Fong R 1986a Ethnic and HLA patterns related to multiple sclerosis in Wellington, New Zealand. *J Neurol Neurosurg Psychiatry* **49**: 43–46

Miller DH, Johnson G, McDonald WI *et al* 1986b Detection of optic nerve lesions in optic neuritis with magnetic resonance imaging. *Lancet* **1**: 1490–1491

Miller DH, McDonald WI, Blumhardt LD *et al* 1987a Magnetic resonance imaging in isolated noncompressive spinal cord syndromes. *Ann Neurol* **22**: 714–723

Miller DH, Ormerod IEC, Gibson A *et al* 1987b MR brain scanning in patients with vasculitis: differentiation from multiple sclerosis. *Neuroradiology* **29**: 226–231

Miller DH, Ormerod IEC, McDonald WI et al 1988a The early risk of multiple sclerosis after optic neuritis. *J Neurol Neurosurg Psychiatry* **51**: 1569–1571

Miller DH, Rudge P, Johnson G et al 1988b Serial gadolinium enhanced magnetic resonance imaging in multiple sclerosis. *Brain* **111**: 927–939

Miller DH, Newton MR, van der Poel JC et al 1988c Magnetic resonance imaging of the optic nerve in optic neuritis. *Neurology* **38**: 175–179

Miller DH, Kendall BE, Barter S et al 1988d Magnetic resonance imaging in central nervous system sarcoidosis. *Neurology* **38**: 378–383

Miller DH, Hornabrook RW, Dagger J, Fong R 1989a Class 2 antigens in multiple sclerosis. *J Neurol Neurosurg Psychiatry* **52**: 575–577

Miller DH, Ormerod IEC, Rudge P et al 1989b The early risk of multiple sclerosis following acute syndromes of the brainstem and spinal cord. *Ann Neurol* **26**: 635–639

Miller DH, Hammond SR, McCloud JG, Skegg DCG 1990a Multiple sclerosis in Australia and New Zealand: are the determinants genetic or environmental? *J Neurol Neurosurg Psychiatry* **53**: 903–905

Miller DH, Robb SA, Ormerod IEC et al 1990b Magnetic resonance imaging of inflammatory and demyelinating white matter diseases of childhood. *Dev Med Child Neurol* **32**: 97–107

Miller DH, Barkhof F, Berry I et al 1991 Magnetic resonance imaging in monitoring the treatment of multiple sclerosis. *J Neurol Neurosurg Psychiatry* **54**; 683–688

Miller DH, Hornabrook PW, Purdie G 1992a The natural history of multiple sclerosis: a regional study with some longitudinal data. *J Neurol Neurosurg Psychiatry* **55**: 341–346

Miller DH, Buchanan N, Barker G et al 1992b Gadolinium enhanced magnetic resonance imaging in systemic lupus erythematosus. *J Neurol* **239**: 460–464

Miller DH, Thompson AJ, Morrissey SP et al 1992c High dose steroids in acute relapses of multiple sclerosis: MRI evidence for a possible mechanism of therapeutic effect. *J Neurol Neurosurg Psychiatry* **55**: 450–453

Miller DH, Albert PS, Barkhof F et al 1996 Guidelines for using magnetic resonance techniques in monitoring the treatment of multiple sclerosis. *Ann Neurol* **39**: 6–16

Miller DH, Kesselring J, McDonald WI, Paty DW, Thompson AJ 1997 *Magnetic Resonance in Multiple Sclerosis*. Cambridge: Cambridge University Press

Miller DH, Grossman RI, Reingold SC, McFarland HF 1998 The role of magnetic resonance techniques in understanding and managing multiple sclerosis. *Brain* **121**: 3–24

Miller DH, Molyneux PD, Barker GJ et al 1999 Effect of interferon-beta1b on magnetic resonance imaging outcomes in secondary progressive multiple sclerosis: results of a European multicenter, randomized, double-blind, placebo-controlled trial. European Study Group on Interferon-beta1b in secondary progressive multiple sclerosis. *Ann Neurol* **46**: 850–859

Miller DH, Barkhof F, Frank JA et al 2002 Measurement of atrophy in multiple sclerosis: pathological basis, methodological aspects and clinical relevance. *Brain* **125**: 1676–1695

Miller DH, Khan OA, Sheremata WA et al 2003a A controlled trial of natalizumab for relapsing multiple sclerosis. *N Engl J Med* **348**: 15–23

Miller DH, Thompson AJ, Filippi M 2003b Magnetic resonance studies of abnormalities in the normal appearing white matter and grey matter in multiple sclerosis. *J Neurol* **250**: 1407–1419

Miller DH, Filippi M, Fazekas F et al 2004 The role of MRI within diagnostic criteria for multiple sclerosis: a critique. *Ann Neurol* **56**: 273–278

Miller DH, Barkhof F, Montalban X et al 2005 Clinically isolated syndromes suggestive of MS: part 2: non-conventional MRI, recovery processes, and management. *Lancet Neurol* **4**:341–348

Miller DJ, Asakura K, Rodriguez M 1996 Central nervous system remyelination: clinical application of basic neuroscience principles. *Brain Pathol* **6**: 331–344

Miller DM, Weinstock-Guttman B, Bethoux F et al 2000 A meta-analysis of methylprednisolone in recovery from multiple sclerosis exacerbations. *Mult Scler* **6**: 267–723

Miller HG, Evans MJ 1953 Prognosis in acute disseminated encephalomyelitis: with a note on neuromyelitis optica. *Q J Med* **22**: 347–379

Miller HG, Gibbons JL 1953 Acute disseminated encephalomyelitis and acute multiple sclerosis: results of treatment with ACTH. *Br Med J* **2**: 1345–1348

Miller HG, Stanton JB, Gibbons JL 1956 Parainfectious encephalomyelitis and related syndromes. *Q J Med* **25**: 427–505

Miller HG, Newell DJ, Ridley A et al 1961a Therapeutic trials in multiple sclerosis: preliminary report of the effects of intrathecal injection of tuberculin (PPD). *J Neurol Neurosurg Psychiat* **24**: 118–120

Miller HG, Newell DJ, Ridley A 1961b Multiple sclerosis: treatment of acute exacerbations with corticotrophin (ACTH). *Lancet* **ii**: 1120–1122

Miller HG, Simpson CA, Yeates WK 1965 Bladder dysfunction in multiple sclerosis. *Br Med J* **1**: 1265–1269

Miller HG, Cendrowski W, Shapira K 1967 Multiple sclerosis and vaccination. *Br Med J* **2**: 210–213

Miller JFAP 1961 Immunological function of the thymus. *Lancet* **2**: 748–749

Miller LG, Fahey JM 1994 Interleukin-1 modulates GABAergic and glutamatergic function in brain. *Ann NY Acad Sci* **739**: 292–298

Miller RA, Gralow 1984 The induction of Leu-1 antigen expression in human malignant and normal B cells by phorbol myristic acetate (PMA). *J Immunol* **133**: 3408–3414

Miller RH, Dinsio K, Wang R et al 2004 Patterning of spinal cord oligodendrocyte development by dorsally derived BMP4. *J Neurosci Res* **76**: 9–19

Miller SD, McRae BL, Vanderlugt CL et al 1995a Evolution of the T-cell repertoire during the course of experimental immune-mediated demyelinating diseases. *Immunol Rev* **144**: 225–244

Miller SD, Vanderlugt C, Lenschow DJ et al 1995b Blockade of CD28/B7–1 interaction prevents epitope spreading and clinical relapses of murine EAE. *Immunity* **3**: 739–745

Milligan NM, Compston DAS 1994 A placebo controlled trial of isoprinosine (immunovir) in the treatment of patients with multiple sclerosis. *J Neurol Neurosurg Psychiatry* **57**: 164–168

Milligan NM, Newcombe R, Compston DAS 1987 A double blind controlled trial of high dose methylprednisolone in patients with multiple sclerosis. I. Clinical effects. *J Neurol Neurosurg Psychiatry* **50**: 511–516

Mills KR, Murray NMR 1985 Corticospinal tract conduction time in multiple sclerosis. *Ann Neurol* **18**: 601–605

Milner BA, Regan D, Heron JR 1974 Differential diagnosis of multiple sclerosis by visual evoked potential recording. *Brain* **97**: 755–772

Milner MM, Ebner F, Justich E, Urban C 1990 Multiple sclerosis in chidhood: contribution of serial MRI to earlier diagnosis. *Dev Med Child Neurol* **32**: 769–777

Milner R, ffrench Constant C 1994 A developmental analysis of oligodendroglial integrins in primary cells: changes in *av* associated B subunits during differentiation. *Development* **120**: 3497–3506

Milonas I 1994 Epidemiological data of multiple sclerosis in Northern Greece. In: Firnhaber W, Lauer K (eds) *Multiple Sclerosis in Europe: An Epidemiological Update*. Darmstadt: Leuchtturm-Verlag/LTV Press, pp. 332–333

Mimura Y, Gotow T, Nishi T, Osame M 1994 Mechanisms of hyperpolarization induced by two cytokines, hTNF alpha and hIL-1 alpha in neurons of the mollusc, *Onchidium. Brain Res* **653**: 112–118

Minagar A, Sheremata WA 2000 Glossopharyngeal neuralgia and MS. *Neurology* **54**: 1368–1370

Minagar A, Jy W, Jimenez JJ et al 2001 Elevated plasma endothelial microparticles in multiple sclerosis. *Neurology* **56**: 1319–1324

Minagar A, Sheremata WA, Weiner WJ 2002 Transient movement disorders and multiple sclerosis. *Parkinsonism Relat Disord* **9**: 111–113

Minden SL, Schiffer RB 1990 Affective disorders in multiple sclerosis. *Arch Neurol* **47**: 98–104

Minden SL, Orav J, Schildkraut JJ 1988 Hypomanic reactions to ACTH and prednisone treatment for multiple sclerosis. *Neurology* **38**: 1631–1634

Minderhoud JM, Zwanniken CP 1994 Increasing prevalence and incidence of multiple sclerosis: an epidemiological study in the province of Groningen, The Netherlands. In: Firnhaber W, Lauer K (eds) *Multiple Sclerosis in Europe: An Epidemiological Update*. Darmstadt: Leuchtturm-Verlag/LTV Press, pp. 113–121

Minderhoud JM, Leemhuis JG, Kremer J, Laban E, Smits PML 1984 Sexual disturbances arising from multiple sclerosis. *Acta Neurol Scand* **70**: 299–306

Minderhoud JM, van der Hoeven JH, Prange AJA 1988 Course and prognosis of chronic progressive multiple sclerosis. *Acta Neurol Scand* **78**: 10–15

Minneboo A, Barkhof F, Polman CH *et al* 2004 Infratentorial lesions predict long-term disability in patients with initial findings suggestive of multiple sclerosis. *Arch Neurol* **61**: 217–221

Minton K 2001 Immune mechanisms in neurological disorders: protective or destructive? *Trends Immunol* **22**: 655–657

Minuk GY, Lewkonia RM 1986 Possible familial association of multiple sclerosis and inflammatory bowel disease. *N Engl J Med* **314**: 586

Miosge LA, Blasioli J, Blery M, Goodnow CC 2002 Analysis of an ethylnitrosourea-generated mouse mutation defines a cell intrinsic role of nuclear factor kappaB2 in regulating circulating B cell numbers. *J Exp Med* **196**: 1113–1119

Miravalle A, Roos KL 2003 Encephalitis following smallpox vaccination. *Arch Neurol* **60**: 925–928

Miretti MM, Walsh EC, Ke X *et al* 2005 A high-resolution linkage-disequilibrium map of the human major histocompatibility complex and first generation of tag single-nucleotide polymorphisms. *Am J Hum Genet* **76**: 634–646

Miró J, Peña-Sagredo JL, Beriano J, Insúa S, Leno C, Velarde R 1990 Prevalence of primary Sjögren's syndrome in patients with multiple sclerosis. *Ann Neurol* **27**: 582–584

Mirowska D, Wicha W, Czlonkowski A *et al* 2004 Increase of matrix metalloproteinase-9 in peripheral blood of multiple sclerosis patients treated with high doses of methylprednisolone. *J Neuroimmunol* **146**: 171–175

Mirsattari SM, Johnston JB, McKenna R *et al* 2001 Aboriginals with multiple sclerosis: HLA types and predominance of neuromyelitis optica. *Neurology* **56**: 317–123

Misu T, Onodera H, Fujihara K *et al* 2001 Chemokine receptor expression on T cells in blood and cerebrospinal fluid at relapse and remission of multiple sclerosis: imbalance of Th1/Th2-associated chemokine signaling. *J Neuroimmunol* **114**: 207–212

Miterski B, Jaeckel S, Epplen JT *et al* 1999 The interferon gene cluster: a candidate region for MS predisposition? *Genes Immun* **1**: 37–44

Miterski B, Eppelen JT, Poehlau D *et al* 2000 SCA2 alleles are not general predisposition factors for multiple sclerosis. *Neurogenetics* **2**: 235–236

Miterski B, Bohringer S, Klein W *et al* 2002a Inhibitors in the NfkappaB cascade comprise prime candidate genes predisposing to multiple sclerosis, especially in selected combinations. *Genes Immun* **3**: 211–219

Miterski B, Sindern E, Haupts M *et al* 2002b PTPRC (CD45) is not associated with multiple sclerosis in a large cohort of German patients. *BMC Med Genet* **16**: 3–5

Mitome M, Low HP, van den Pol A *et al* 2001 Towards the reconstruction of central nervous system white matter using neural precursor cells. *Brain* **124**: 2147–2161

Mitsunaga Y, Ciric B, VanKeulen V *et al* 2002 Direct evidence that a human antibody derived from a patient serum can promote myelin repair in a mouse model of chronic progressive demyelinating disease. *FASEB J* **16**: 1325–1327

Miura K 1911 [Discussion of paper by Nonne pp. 123–145] *Dtsch Z Nervenheilk* **41**: 146

Mix E, Olsson T, Correales J *et al* 1990 B cells expressing CD5 are increased in cerebrospinal fluid of patients with multiple sclerosis. *Clin Exp Immunol* **79**: 21–27

Miyagishi R, Niino M, Fukazawa T *et al* 2003 C-C chemokine receptor 2 gene polymorphism in Japanese patients with multiple sclerosis. *J Neuroimmunol* **145**: 135–138

Miyamoto K, Miyake S, Yamamura T 2001 A synthetic glycolipid prevents autoimmune encephalomyelitis by inducing Th2 bias of natural killer T cells. *Nature* **413**: 531–534

Miyazawa I, Fujihara K, Itoyama Y 2002 Eugène Devic (1858–1930). *J Neurol* **249**: 351–352

Miyazawa R, Hikima A, Takano Y *et al* 2001 Plasmapheresis in fulminant acute disseminated encephalomyelitis. *Brain Dev* **23**: 424–426

Moalem G, Leibowitz-Amit R, Yoles E *et al* 1999 Autoimmune T cells protect neurons from secondary degeneration after central nervous system axotomy. *Nature Med* **5**: 49–55

Moalem G, Gdalyahu A, Shani Y *et al* 2000 Production of neurotrophins by activated T cells: implications for neuroprotective autoimmunity. *J Autoimmun* **15**: 331–345

Modi G, Mochan A, Modi M, Saffer D 2001 Demyelinating disorder of the central nervous system occurring in black South Africans. *J Neurol Neurosurg Psychiatry* **70**: 500–505

Modin H, Dai Y, Masterman T *et al* 2001 No linkage or association of the nitric oxide synthase genes to multiple sclerosis. *J Neuroimmunol* **119**: 95–100

Modin H, Masterman T, Thorlacius T *et al* 2003 Genome-wide linkage screen of a consanguineous multiple sclerosis kinship. *Mult Scler* **9**: 128–134

Modrego Pardo PJ, Pina Latorre MA, Lopez A, Errea JM 1997 Prevalence of multiple sclerosis in the province of Teruel, Spain. *J Neurol* **244**: 182–185

Modrego Pardo PJ, Pina MA 2003 Trends in prevalence and incidence of multiple sclerosis in Bajo Aragon, Spain. *J Neurol Sci* **216**: 89–93

Moen T, Stein R, Bratlie A, Bindervik E 1984 Distribution of HLA SB antigens in multiple sclerosis. *Tissue Antigens* **24**: 126–127

Moffie D 1966 De geografische vervreiding van multipele scleros. *Nederlands Tijdschr Geneeskd* **110**: 1454–1457

Mogenet I, Simiand-Erdociain E, Canonge JM, Pris J 2003 Acute myelogenous leukemia following mitoxantrone treatment for multiple sclerosis. *Ann Pharmacother* **37**: 747–748

Mogensen S (ed.) 1997 Proceedings of the 4th International Symposium on Retrovirus in Multiple Sclerosis and Related Diseases, Copenhagen, Denmark, 26 September 1996. *Acta Neurol Scand* **95 (Suppl 169)**: 1–98

Mogyoros I, Kiernan MC, Burke D, Bostock H 1997 Excitability changes in human sensory and motor axons during hyperventilation and ischaemia. *Brain* **120**: 317–325

Mogyoros I, Bostock H, Burke D 2000 Mechanisms of paresthesias arising from healthy axons. *Muscle Nerve* **23**: 310–320

Mohan N, Edwards ET, Cupps TR *et al* 2001 Demyelination occurring during anti-tumor necrosis factor alpha therapy for inflammatory arthritides. *Arthritis Rheum* **44**: 2862–2869

Mohlke KL, Erdos MR, Scott LJ *et al* 2002 High-throughput screening for evidence of association by using mass spectrometry genotyping on DNA pools. *Proc Natl Acad Sci USA* **99**:16928–16933

Mohr DC, Goodkin DE, Bacchetti P *et al* 2000 Psychological stress and the subsequent appearance of new brain MRI lesions in MS. *Neurology* **55**: 55–61

Mohr DC, Hart SL, Julian L *et al* 2004 Association between stressful life events and exacerbation in multiple sclerosis: a meta-analysis. *Br Med J* **328**: 731

Mohr PD, Strang FA, Sambrook MA, Boddie HG 1977 The clinical and surgical features in 40 patients with primary cerebellar ectopia (adult Chiari malformation). *Q J Med* **46**: 85–96

Moins-Teisserenc H, Semana G, Alizadeh M *et al* 1995 TAP2 gene polymorphism contributes to genetic susceptibility to multiple sclerosis. *Hum Immunol* **42**: 195–202

Mojon DS, Herbert J, Sadiq SA *et al* 1999a Leber's hereditary optic neuropathy mitochondrial DNA mutations at nucleotides 11778 and 3460 in multiple sclerosis. *Ophthalmologica* **213**: 171–175

Mojon DS, Fujihara K, Hirano M *et al* 1999b Leber's hereditary optic neuropathy mitochondrial DNA mutations in familial multiple sclerosis. *Graefes Arch Clin Exp Ophthalmol* **237**: 348–350

Mokhtarian F, McFarlin DE, Raine CS 1984 Adoptive transfer of myelin basic protein-sensitized T cells produces chronic relapsing demyelinating disease in mice. Nature 309: 356–358

Mokri B, Weinshenker BG, Goudreau JL et al 1998 Long-tract myelopathy: a novel paraneoplastic syndrome. Ann Neurol 44: 486

Molina-Holgado E, Vela JM, Arevalo-Martin A, Guaza C 2001 LPS/IFN-gamma cytotoxicity in oligodendroglial cells: role of nitric oxide and protection by the anti-inflammatory cytokine IL-10. Eur J Neurosci 13: 493–502

Moll C, Mourre C, Lazdunski M, Ulrich J 1991 Increase of sodium channels in demyelinated lesions of multiple sclerosis. Brain Res 556: 311–316

Møller P, Hammerberg P 1963 Retinal periphlebitis in multiple sclerosis. Acta Neurol Scand 39 (Suppl 4): 263–270

Mollgard K, Saunders NR 1986 The development of the human blood brain and blood CSF barriers. Neuropathol Appl Neurobiol 12: 337–358

Mollnes TE, Vandvik B, Lea T, Vartdal F 1987 Intrathecal complement activation in neurological disease evaluated by analysis of the terminal complement complex. J Neurol Sci 78: 17–28

Molofsky AV, Pardal R, Iwashita T et al 2003 Bmi-1 dependence distinguishes neural stem cell self-renewal from progenitor proliferation. Nature 425: 962–967

Moloney JBM, Masterson JG 1982 Detection of adrenoleucodystrophy carriers by means of evoked potentials. Lancet ii: 852–853

Molyneux PD, Kappos L, Polman C et al 2000 The effect of interferon beta-1b treatment on MRI measures of cerebral atrophy in secondary progressive multiple sclerosis. European Study Group on Interferon beta-1b in secondary progressive multiple sclerosis. Brain 123: 2256–2263

Molyneux PD, Barker GJ, Barkhof F et al 2001 Clinical MRI correlations in a European trial of interferon beta-1b in secondary progressive MS. Neurology 57: 2191–2197

Montag D, Giese KP, Bartsch V et al 1994 Mice deficient for the myelin associated glycoprotein gene show subtle abnormalities in myelin. Neuron 13: 229–246

Montalban X 2004 Overview of European pilot study of interferon β-1b in primary progressive multiple sclerosis. Mult Scler 10: S62–S64

Monteiro J, Hingorani R, Peroglizzi R et al 1996 Oligoclonality of CD8+ T cells in multiple sclerosis. Autoimmunity 23: 127–138

Montgomery SM, Lambe M, Olsson T, Ekbom A 2004 Parental age, family size, and risk of multiple sclerosis. Epidemiology 15: 717–723

Montomoli C, Allemani C, Solinas G et al 2002a An ecologic study of geographical variation in multiple sclerosis risk in central Sardinia, Italy. Neuroepidemiology 21: 187–193

Montomoli C, Prokopenko I, Caria A et al 2002b Multiple sclerosis recurrence risk for siblings in an isolated population of Central Sardinia, Italy. Genet Epidemiol 22: 265–271

Monzani F, Caraccio N, Meucci G et al 1999 Effect of 1-year treatment with interferon-beta-1b on thyroid function and autoimmunity in patients with multiple sclerosis. Eur J Endocrinol 141: 325–331

Monzani F, Caraccio N, Casolaro A et al 2000 Long-term interferon β-1b therapy for MS: is routine thyroid assessment always useful? Neurology 55: 549–552

Moody DB, Porcelli SA 2001 CD1 trafficking: Invariant chain gives a new twist to the tale. Immunity 15: 861–865

Moon LDF, Asher RA, Rhodes KE, Fawcett JW 2001 Regeneration of CNS axons back to their original target following treatment of adult rat brain with chondroitinase ABC. Nat Neurosci 4: 465–466

Moore CEG, Lees AJ, Schady W 1996 Multiple sclerosis leading to blepharospasm and dystonia in a sibling pair. J Neurol 243: 667–670

Moore FG, Andermann F, Richardson J et al 2001 The role of MRI and nerve root biopsy in the diagnosis of neurosarcoidosis. Can J Neurol Sci 28: 349–353

Moore GR, Raine CS 1988 Immunogold localization and analysis of IgG during immune-mediated demyelination. Lab Invest 59: 641–648

Moore GR, Neumann PE, Suzuki K et al 1985 Balo's concentric sclerosis: new observations on lesion development. Ann Neurol 17: 604–611

Moore GR, Leung E, MacKay AL 2000 A pathology-MRI study of the short-T2 component in formalin-fixed multiple sclerosis brain. Neurology 55: 1506–1510

Moore PM, Lisak RP 1990 Multiple sclerosis and Sjögren's syndrome: a problem of diagnosis or in definition of two disorders of unknown aetiology. Ann Neurol 27: 595–596

Mor F, Cohen IR 1993 Shifts in the epitopes of myelin basic protein recognized by Lewis rat T cells before, during and after the induction of experimental autoimmune encephalomyelitis. J Clin Invest 92: 2199–2206

Mor F, Cohen IR 1995 Pathogenicity of T cells responsive to diverse cryptic epitopes of myelin basic protein in the Lewis rat. J Immunol 155: 3693–3699

Moreau T, Thorpe J, Miller D et al 1994 Preliminary evidence from magnetic resonance imaging for reduction in disease activity after lymphocyte depletion in multiple sclerosis. Lancet 344: 298–301

Moreau T, Coles A, Wing M et al 1996 Transient increase in symptoms associated with cytokine release in patients with multiple sclerosis. Brain 119: 225–237

Moreau T, Manceau E, Lucas B et al 2000 Incidence of multiple sclerosis in Dijon, France: a population-based ascertainment. Neurol Res 22: 156–159

Moreau T, Blanc S, Riche G et al 2001 A pilot safety and tolerability study of interferon beta 1a in combination with azathioprine in multiple sclerosis. Neurology 56: A353

Morell P 1984 Myelin, 2nd edn. New York: Plenum Press

Moreno H, Bueno E, Hernandez Cruz A et al 1995 Nitric oxide and cGMP modulate a presynaptic K+ channel in vitro. Soc Neurosci Meeting Abstr 209.10

Moretti R, Torre P, Antonello RM et al 2000 Recurrent atrial fibrillation associated with pulse administration of high doses of methylprednisolone: a possible prophylactic treatment. Eur J Neurol 7: 130

Morgan BP, Campbell AK, Compston DAS 1984 Terminal component of complement (C9) in cerebrospinal fluid of patients with multiple sclerosis. Lancet ii: 251–254

Morgan BP, Gasque P, Singhrao S, Piddlesden SJ 1997 The role of complement in disorders of the nervous system. Immunopharmacology 38: 43–50

Morganti G, Naccarato S, Elian M et al 1984 Multiple sclerosis in the Republic of San Marino. J Epidemiol Commun Hlth 38: 23–28

Morgello S 1995 Pathogenesis and classification of primary central nervous system lymphoma: an update. Brain Pathol 5: 383–393

Moriabadi NF, Niewiesk S, Kruse N et al 2001 Influenza vaccination in MS: absence of T-cell response against white matter proteins. Neurology 56: 938–943

Moriarty DM, Blackshaw AJ, Talbot PR et al 1999 Memory dysfunction in multiple sclerosis corresponds to juxtacortical lesion load on fast fluid-attenuated inversion-recovery MR images. Am J Neuroradiol 20: 1956–1962

Morling N, Sandberg-Wollheim M, Fugger L et al 1992 Immunogenetics of multiple sclerosis and optic neuritis: DNA polymorphism of HLA class II genes. Immunogenetics 35: 391–394

Morris JC 1868 Case of the late Dr CVW Pennock. Am J Med Sci 56: 138–144

Morrissey SP, Miller DH, Kendall BE et al 1993a The significance of brain magnetic resonance imaging abnormalities at presentation with clinically isolated syndromes suggestive of multiple sclerosis: a five year follow-up study. Brain 116: 135–146

Morrissey SP, Miller DH, Hermazewski R et al 1993b Magnetic resonance imaging of the central nervous system in Behcet's Disease. Eur Neurol 33: 287–293

Morrissey SP, Borruat FX, Miller DH et al 1995 Bilateral simultaneous optic neuritis in adults: clinical, imaging, serological and genetic studies. J Neurol Neurosurg Psychiatry 58: 70–74

Mortensen JT, Bronnum-Hansen H, Rasmussen K 1998 Multiple sclerosis and organic solvents. Epidemiology 9: 168–171

Moser AB, Kreiter N, Bezman L et al 1999 Plasma very long chain fatty acids in 3,000 peroxisome disease patients and 29,000 controls. Ann Neurol 45: 100–110

Moser HW 1995 Adenoleukodystrophy. *Curr Opin Neurol* 8: 221–226

Moser HW 1997 Adrenoleukodystrophy: phenotype, genetics, pathogenesis, and therapy. *Brain* 120: 1485–1508

Moser HW, Suzuki K 2002 In: Asbury AK, McKhann GM, McDonald WI *et al* (eds) *Diseases of the Nervous System, Clinical Neuroscience and Therapeutic Principles*, 3rd edn. Cambridge: Cambridge University Press

Moser HW, Moser AE, Singh I, O'Neill BP 1984 Adrenoleucodystrophy: survey of 303 cases: biochemistry, diagnosis and therapy. *Ann Neurol* 16: 628–641

Moser HW, Moser AB, Naidu S, Bergin A 1991 Clinical aspects of adrenoleukodystrophy and adrenomyeloneuropathy. *Dev Neurosci* 13: 254–261

Mosmann TR, Coffman RL 1989 Th1 and Th2 cells: different patterns of lymphokine secretion lead to different functional properties. *Ann Rev Immunol* 7: 145–173

Mosmann TR, Sad S 1996 The expanding universe of T-cell subsets: Th1, Th2 and more. *Immunol Today* 17: 138–145

Mossmann SS, Bronstein AM, Rudge P, Gresty MA 1985 Acquired pendular nystagmus suppressed by alcohol. *Neuroophthalmology* 13: 99–106

Mosser J, Douar AM, Sarde CO *et al* 1993 Putative X-linked adrenoleukodystrophy gene shares unexpected homology with ABC transporters. *Nature* 361: 726–730

Mosser J, Lutz Y, Stoeckel ME *et al* 1994 The gene responsible for adrenoleucodystrophy encodes a peroxisomal membrane protein. *Hum Mol Genet* 3: 265–271

Mossner R, Fassbender K, Kuhnen J, Schwartz A, Hennerici M 1996 Vascular cell adhesion molecule – a new approach to detect endothelial cell activation in MS and encephalitis *in vivo*. *Acta Neurol Scand* 93: 118–122

Moster ML, Savino PJ, Sergott RC, Bosley TM, Schatz NJ 1984 Isolated sixth nerve palsies in younger adults. *Arch Ophthalmol* 102: 1328–1330

Motomura S, Tabira T, Kuroiwa Y 1980 A clinical comparative study of multiple sclerosis and neuro-Behçet's syndrome. *J Neurol Neurosurg Psychiatry* 43: 210–213

Mottershead JP, Schmierer K, Clemence M *et al* 2003 High field MRI correlates of myelin content and axonal density in multiple sclerosis – a post-mortem study of the spinal cord. *J Neurol* 250: 1293–1301

Moulin DE, Foley KM, Ebers GC 1988 Pain syndromes in multiple sclerosis. *Neurology* 38: 1830–1834

Mouren P, Tatossian A, Toga M *et al* 1966 Etude critique du syndrome hémiballique. *Encéphale* 55: 212–274

Moxon W 1875 Eight cases of insular sclerosis of the brain and spinal cord. *Guys' Hosp Rep* 20: 437–478

Muir D, Compston DAS 1996 Growth factor stimulation triggers apoptotic cell death in mature rat oligodendrocytes. *J Neurosci Res* 44: 1–11

Mukherjee A, Vogt RF, Linthicum DS 1985 Measurement of myelin basic protein by radioimmunoassay in closed head trauma, multiple sclerosis and other neurological diseases. *Clin Biochem* 18: 304–307

Mukhopadhyay G, Doherty P, Walsh FS *et al* 1994 A novel role for myelin associated glycoprotein as an inhibitor of axonal regeneration. *Neuron* 13: 757–767

Mullen KT, Plant GT 1986 Colour and luminance vision in human optic neuritis. *Brain* 109: 1–13

Müller E 1904 Pathologische Anatomie und Pathogenese. In: *Die Multiple Sklerose des Gehirns und Rückenmarks*. Jena: Gustav Fischer, pp. 300–344

Müller E 1910 Uber sensible Reizerscheinungen bei beginnender multipler sklerose. *Neurolisch Centralblatt* 29: 17–20

Müller R 1949 Studies on disseminated sclerosis with special reference to symptomatology: course and prognosis. *Acta Med Scand* 222 (Suppl): 1–214

Müller R 1951 Course and prognosis of disseminated sclerosis in relation to age at onset. *Arch Neurol Psychiatry* 66: 561–570

Müller R 1953 Genetic aspects of multiple sclerosis. *Arch Neurol Psychiatry* 70: 733–740

Multiple Sclerosis. Hope through research. www.ninds.nih.gov/health_and_medical/pubs/multiple_sclerosis.htm

Multiple Sclerosis Genetics Group 1998 Clinical demographics of multiplex families with multiple sclerosis. *Ann Neurol* 43: 530–534

Multiple Sclerosis Study Group 1990 Efficacy and toxicity of cyclosporine in chronic progressive multiple sclerosis: a randomised, double blinded, placebo controlled clinical trial. *Ann Neurol* 27: 591–605

Mumford CJ, Compston DAS 1993 Problems with rating scales for multiple sclerosis: a novel solution – the CAMBS score. *J Neurol* 240: 209–215

Mumford CJ, Fraser MB, Wood NW, Compston DAS 1992 Multiple sclerosis in the Cambridge health district of East Anglia. *J Neurol Neurosurg Psychiatry* 55: 881–882

Mumford, CJ, Wood NW, Kellar-Wood HF, Thorpe J, Miller D, Compston DAS 1994 The British Isles survey of multiple sclerosis in twins. *Neurology* 44: 11–15

Munari LM, Filippini G 2004 Lack of evidence for use of glatiramer acetate in multiple sclerosis. *Lancet Neurol* 3: 641

Munari L, Filippini G 2005 Evidence for use of glatiramer acetate in multiple sclerosis. *Lancet Neurol* 4: 76–77

Munari L, Lovati R, Boiko A 2004 Therapy with glatiramer acetate for multiple sclerosis. *Cochrane Database Syst Rev* 1: CD004678

Munch M, MollerLarsen A, Christensen T *et al* 1995 B-lymphoblastoid cell lines from multiple sclerosis patients and a healthy control producing a putative new human retrovirus and Epstein–Barr virus. *Mult Scler* 1: 78–81

Munch M, Hvas J, Christensen T *et al* 1998 A single subtype of Epstein-Barr virus in

members of multiple sclerosis clusters. *Acta Neurol Scand* 98: 395–399

Mungall AJ, Palmer SA, Sims SK *et al* 2003 The DNA sequence and analysis of human chromosome 6. *Nature* 425: 805–811

Munger KL, Peeling RW, Hernan MA *et al* 2003 Infection with *Chlamydia pneumoniae* and risk of multiple sclerosis. *Epidemiology* 14: 141–147

Munger KL, Zhang SM, O'Reilly E *et al* 2004 Vitamin D intake and incidence of multiple sclerosis. *Neurology* 62: 60–65

Murakami M, Honjo T 1995 Involvement of B-1 cells in mucosal immunity and autoimmunity. *Immunol Today* 16: 534–539

Muramatsu M, Honjo T 2001 Complex layers of genetic alteration in the generation of antibody diversity. *Trends Immunol* 22: 66–68

Muraro PA, Leist T, Bielekova B, McFarland HF 2000 VLA-4/CD49d downregulated on primed T lymphocytes during interferon-beta therapy in multiple sclerosis. *J Neuroimmunol* 111: 186–194

Muraro PA, Wandinger KP, Bielekova B *et al* 2003 Molecular trafficking of antigen-specific T cell clones in neurological immune-mediated disorders. *Brain* 126: 20–31

Muraro PA, Liberati L, Bonanni L *et al* 2004 Decreased integrin gene expression in patients with MS responding to interferon-β treatment. *J Immunol* 150: 123–131

Muraro PA, Douek DC, Packer A *et al* 2005 Thymic output generates a new and diverse TCR repertoire after autologous stem cell transplantation in multiple sclerosis patients. *J Exp Med* 201: 805–816

Murata Y, Inada K, Negi A 2000 Susac syndrome. *Am J Ophthalmol* 129: 682–684

Muri RM, Weinberg O 1985 The clinical spectrum of internuclear ophthalmoplegia in multiple sclerosis. *Arch Neurol* 42: 851–855

Murphy KM, Reiner SL 2003 The lineage decisions of helper T cells. *Nature Rev Immunol* 2: 933–944

Murphy N, Confavreux C, Haas J *et al* 1998 Quality of life in multiple sclerosis in France, Germany and the United Kingdom. *J Neurol Neurosurg Psych* 65: 460–466

Murray BJ, Apetauerova D, Scammell TE 2000 Severe acute disseminated encephalomyelitis with normal MRI at presentation. *Neurology* 55: 1237–1238

Murray J 2005 *Multiple Sclerosis: The History of a Disease*. New York: Demos

Murray K, Dubois Dalcq M 1997 Emergence of oligodendrocytes from human neural spheres. *J Neurosci Res* 50: 146–156

Murray NMF 1991 Magnetic stimulation of cortex: clinical applications. *J Clin Neurophysiol* 8: 66–76

Murray PD, McGavern DB, Lin X *et al* 1998 Perforin-dependent neurologic injury in a viral model of multiple sclerosis. *J Neurosci* 18: 7306–7314

Murray PD, McGavern DB, Sathornsumetee S, Rodriguez M 2001 Spontaneous remyelination following extensive demyelination is associated with improved neurological function in a viral model of multiple sclerosis. *Brain* **124**: 1403–1416

Murray RS, Brown B, Brian D, Cabirac GF 1992 Detection of coronavirus RNA and antigen in multiple sclerosis brain. *Ann Neurol* **31**: 525–533

Murray S, Bashir K, Penrice G, Womersley SJ 2004 Epidemiology of multiple sclerosis in Glasgow. *Scot Med J* **49**: 100–104

Murray TJ 1976 An unusual occurrence of multiple sclerosis in a small rural community. *Can J Neurol Sci* **3**: 192–194

Murray TJ 1985 Amantadine therapy for fatigue in multiple sclerosis. *Can J Neurol Sci* **12**: 251–254

Murray TJ, Murray SJ 1984 Characteristics of patients found not to have multiple sclerosis. *Can Med Assoc J* **131**: 336–337

Murthy SNK, Faden HS, Cohen ME, Bakshi R 2002 Acute disseminated encephalomyelitis in children. *Pediatrics* **110**: e21

Musette P, Bequet D, Delarbre C *et al* 1996 Expansion of a recurrent Vβ5.3$^+$ T cell population in newly diagnosed and untreated HLA-DR2 multiple sclerosis patients. *Proc Natl Acad Sci USA* **93**: 12461–12466

Mushlin AI, Mooney C, Grow V *et al* 1994 The value of diagnostic information to patients with suspected multiple sclerosis. *Arch Neurol* **51**: 67–72

Musial A, Eissa NT 2001 Inducible nitric-oxide synthase is regulated by the proteasome degradation pathway. *J Biol Chem* **276**: 24268–24273

Mussini JM, Hauw JJ, Escourolle R 1977 Immunofluorescence studies of intra cytoplasmatic immunoglobulin binding lymphoid cells in the central nervous system: report of 32 cases including 19 multiple sclerosis. *Acta Neuropathol* **40**: 227–232

Mutsaers SE, Carroll WM 1998 Focal accumulation of intra-axonal mitochondria in demyelination of the cat optic nerve. *Acta Neuropathol* **96**: 139–143

Mycko MP, Kowalski W, Kwinkowski M *et al* 1998a Multiple sclerosis: the frequency of allelic forms of tumor necrosis factor and lymphotoxin-α. *J Neuroimmunol* **84**: 198–206

Mycko MP, Kwinkowski M, Tronczynska E *et al* 1998b Multiple sclerosis: the increased frequency of the ICAM-1 exon 6 gene point mutation genetic type K469. *Ann Neurol* **44**: 70–75

Mycko MP, Papoian R, Boschert U *et al* 2003 cDNA microarray analysis in multiple sclerosis lesions: detection of genes associated with disease activity. *Brain* **126**: 1048–1057

Myers KJ, Sprent J, Dougherty JP, Ron Y 1992 Synergy between encephalitogenic T cells and myelin basic protein-specific antibodies in the induction of experimental autoimmune encephalomyelitis. *J Neuroimmunol* **41**: 1–8

Myers LW, Ellison GW, Lucia M *et al* 1977 Swine influenza virus vaccination in patients with multiple sclerosis. *J Infect Dis* **136 (Suppl)**: S546–S554

Myers LW, Fahey JL, Moody DJ *et al* 1987 Cyclophosphamide 'pulses' in chronic progressive multiple sclerosis. *Arch Neurol* **44**: 828–832

Myers LW, Ellison GW, Merrill JE *et al* 1995 Pentoxyfilline not a promising treatment for multiple sclerosis. *Neurology* **45 (Suppl 4)**: A419

Myers LW, Ellison GW, Merrill JE *et al* 1998 Pentoxifylline is not a promising treatment for multiple sclerosis in progression phase. *Neurology* **51**: 1483–1486

Myhr KM, Raknes G, Nyland H, Vedeler C 1999a Immunoglobulin G Fc receptor (FcγR) IIA and IIB polymorphisms related to disability in MS. *Neurology* **52**: 1771–1776

Myhr KM, Riise T, Green Lilleas FE *et al* 1999b Interferon-alpha2a reduces MRI disease activity in relapsing–remitting multiple sclerosis. Norwegian Study Group on Interferon-alpha in Multiple Sclerosis. *Neurology* **52**: 1049–1056

Myhr KM, Riise T, Vedeler C *et al* 2001 Disability and prognosis in multiple sclerosis: demographic and clinical variables important for the ability to walk and awarding of disability pension. *Mult Scler* **7**: 59–65

Myhr KM, Vagnes KS, Maroy TH *et al* 2002 Interleukin-10 promoter polymorphism in patients with multiple sclerosis. *J Neurol Sci* **202**: 93–97

Nadler JP 1993 Multiple sclerosis and hepatitis B vaccination. *Clin Infect Dis* **17**: 928–929

Nagata S, Goldstein P 1995 The Fas death factor. *Science* **167**: 1449–1456

Nagra RM, Becher B, Tourtellotte WW *et al* 1997 Immunohistochemical and genetic evidence of myeloperoxidase involvement in multiple sclerosis. *J Neuroimmunol* **78**: 97–107

Naismith RT, Cross AH 2004 Does the hepatitis B vaccine cause multiple sclerosis? *Neurology* **63**: 772–773

Naito S, Namerow N, Mickey MR, Terasaki PI 1972 Multiple sclerosis: association with HL-A3. *Tissue Antigens* **2**: 1–4

Naito S, Kuroiwa T, Itoyama T *et al* 1978 HLA and Japanese MS. *Tissue Antigens* **12**: 19–24

Nakahara J, Seiwa C, Shibuya A *et al* 2003 Expression of Fc receptor for immunoglobulin M in oligodendrocytes and myelin of mouse central nervous system. *Neurosci Lett* **337**: 73–76

Nakamine H, Okano M, Taguchi Y *et al* 1991 Hematopathologic features of Epstein-Barr virus-induced human B-lymphoproliferation in mice with severe combined immunodeficiency. A model of lymphoproliferative diseases in immunocompromised patients. *Lab Invest* **65**: 389–399

Nakamura N, Nokura K, Zettsu T *et al* 2003 Neurologic complications associated with influenza vaccination: two adult cases. *Intern Med* **42**: 191–194

Nakashima I, Fujihara K, Okita N *et al* 1999 Clinical and MRI study of brain stem and cerebellar involvement in Japanese patients with multiple sclerosis. *J Neurol Neurosurg Psychiatry* **67**: 153–157

Nakashima I, Fujihara K, Misu T *et al* 2000 Significant correlation between IL-10 levels and IgG indices in the cerebrospinal fluid of patients with multiple sclerosis. *J Neuroimmunol* **111**: 64–67

Nakazato T, Sato T, Nakamura T *et al* 1989 Adrenoleukodystrophy presenting as spinocerebellar degeneration. *Eur Neurol* **29**: 229–234

Namekawa M, Takiyama Y, Aoki Y *et al* 2002 Identification of GFAP gene mutation in hereditary adult-onset Alexander's disease. *Ann Neurol* **52**: 779–785

Namerow NS 1968a Circadian temperature rhythm and vision in multiple sclerosis. *Neurology* **18**: 417–422

Namerow NS 1968b Somatosensory evoked responses in multiple sclerosis patients with varying sensory loss. *Neurology* **18**: 1197–1204

Namerow NS 1972 The pathophysiology of multiple sclerosis. In: Wolfgram F, Ellison GW, Stevens JG *et al* (eds) *Multiple Sclerosis: Immunology, Virology and Ultrastructure*. New York: Academic Press, pp. 143–172

Namerow NS, Enns N 1972 Visual evoked responses in patients with multiple sclerosis. *J Neurol Neurosurg Psychiatry* **35**: 829–833

Namerow NS, Thompson LR 1969 Plaques, symptoms, and the remitting course of multiple sclerosis. *Neurology* **19**: 765–774

Nance PW, Shears AH, Nance DM 1989 Reflex changes induced by clonidine in spinal cord injured patients. *Paraplegia* **27**: 296–301

Narang HK, Field EJ 1973 Paramyxovirus like tubules in multiple sclerosis biopsy material. *Acta Neuropathol* **25**: 281–290

Narayana PA, Doyle TJ, Lai D, Wolinsky JS 1998 Serial proton magnetic resonance spectroscopic imaging, contrast enhanced magnetic resonance imaging, and quantitative lesion volumetry in multiple sclerosis. *Ann Neurol* **43**: 56–71

Narayanan S, Fu L, Pioro E *et al* 1997 Imaging of axonal damage in multiple sclerosis: spatial distribution of magnetic resonance imaging lesions. *Ann Neurol* **41**: 385–391

Narayanan S, DeStefano N, Francis GS *et al* 2001 Axonal metabolic recovery in multiple sclerosis patients treated with interferon beta-1b. *J Neurol* **249**: 979–986

Narciso P, Galgani S, Del Grosso B *et al* 2001 Acute disseminated encephalomyelitis as manifestation of primary HIV infection. *Neurology* **57**: 1493–1496

Narikawa K, Misu T, Fujihara K *et al* 2004 CSF chemokine levels in relapsing neuromyelitis optica and multiple sclerosis. *J Neuroimmunol* **149**: 182–186

Narod S, Johnson-Lussenburg CM, Zheng Q, Nelson R 1985 Clinical viral infections and multiple sclerosis. *Lancet* 165–166

Nash RA, Bowen JD, McSweeney PA et al 2003 High-dose immunosuppressive therapy and autologous peripheral blood stem cell transplantation for severe multiple sclerosis. *Blood* **102**: 2364–2372

Nasseri K, TenVoorde BJ, Ader HJ et al 1998 Longitudinal follow-up of cardiovascular reflex tests in multiple sclerosis. *J Neurol Sci* **155**: 50–54

Nataf S, Carroll SL, Wetsel RA et al 2000 Attenuation of experimental autoimmune demyelination in complement-deficient mice. *J Immunol* **165**: 5867–5873

Nathan MPR, Chase PH, Elguezabel A, Weinstein M 1976 Spinal cord sarcoidosis. *NY State J Med* **76**: 748–752

Nauta JJP, Thompson AJ, Barkhof F, Miller DH 1994 Magnetic resonance imaging in monitoring the treatment of multiple sclerosis patients: statistical power of parallel groups and cross-over designs. *J Neurol Sci* **122**: 6–14

Navikas V, Link H 1996 Review: cytokines and the pathogenesis of multiple sclerosis. *J Neurosci Res* **45**: 322–333

Navikas V, Link H, Palasik W et al 1995 Increased mRNA expression of IL-10 in mononuclear cells in multiple sclerosis and optic neuritis. *Scand J Immunol* **41**: 171–178

Navikas V, He B, Link J et al 1996a Augmented expression of tumour necrosis factor-α and lymphotoxin in mononuclear cells in multiple sclerosis and optic neuritis. *Brain* **119**: 213–223

Navikas V, Matusevicius D, Söderström M et al 1996b Increased interleukin 6 mRNA expression in blood and cerebrospinal fluid mononuclear cells in multiple sclerosis. *J Neuroimmunol* **64**: 63–69

Ndhlovu LC, Ishii N, Murata K et al 2001 Critical involvement of OX40 ligand signals in the T cell priming events during experimental autoimmune encephalomyelitis. *J Immunol* **167**: 2991–2999

Nedergaard M 1994 Direct signaling from astrocytes to neurons in cultures of mammalian brain cells. *Science* **263**: 1768–1771

Nehls M, Kyewski B, Messerle M et al 1996 Two genetically separable steps in the differentiation of thymic epithelium. *Science* **272**: 886–889

Neilley LK, Goodin DS, Goodkin DE, Hauser SL 1996 Side effect profile of interferon beta-1b in MS: results of an open label trial. *Neurology* **46**: 552–554

Nelissen I, Fiten P, Vandenbroeck K et al 2000 PECAM1, MPO and PRKAR1A at chromosome 17q21-q24 and susceptibility for multiple sclerosis in Sweden and Sardinia. *J Neuroimmunol* **108**: 153–159

Nelissen I, Dubois B Goris A et al 2002 Gelatinase B, PECAM-1 and MCP-3 gene polymorphisms in Belgian multiple sclerosis. *J Neurol Sci* **200**: 43–48

Nellerman LJ, Frederiksen J, Morling N 1995 PCR typing of two short tandem repeat (STR) structures upstream of the human myelin basic protein (MBP) gene: the genetic susceptibility in multiple sclerosis and monosymptomatic idiopathic optic neuritis in Danes. *Mult Scler* **1**: 186–198

Nelson DA, Jeffries WH, McDowell F 1958 Effects of induced hyperthermia on some neurological diseases. *Arch Neurol Psychiatry* **79**: 31–39

Nelson LM, Anderson DW 1995 Case finding for epidemiological surveys of multiple sclerosis in United States communities. *Mult Scler* **1**: 48–55

Nelson LM, Hamman RF, Thompson HM et al 1986 Higher than expected prevalence of multiple sclerosis (MS) in northern Colorado: dependence on methodologic issues. *Neuroepidemiology* **5**: 17–28

Nelson LM, Franklin GM, Jones MC, and the Multiple Sclerosis Study Group 1988 Risk of multiple sclerosis exacerbation during pregnancy and breast-feeding. *J Am Med Assoc* **259**: 3441–3443

Nemazee D 2000 Receptor selection in B and T lymphocytes. *Annu Rev Immunol* **18**: 19–51

Nepom GT 2002 Therapy of autoimmune diseases: clinical trials and new biologics. *Curr Opin Immunol* **14**: 812–815

Nery S, Wichterle H, Fishell G 2001 Sonic hedgehog contributes to oligodendrocyte specification in the mammalian forebrain. *Development* **128**: 527–540

Nesbit GM, Forbes GS, Scheithauer BW et al 1991 Multiple sclerosis: histopathologic and MR and/or CT correlation in 37 cases at biopsy and three cases at autopsy. *Radiology* **180**: 467–474

Ness JK, Mitchell NE, Wood TL 2002 IGF-1 and NT-3 signaling pathways in developing oligodendroctyes: differential regulation and activation of receptors and the downstream effector Akt. *Dev Neurosci* **24**: 437–445

Ness JK, Scaduto RC Jr, Wood TL 2004 IGF-I prevents glutamate-mediated bax translocation and cytochrome C release in O4+ oligodendrocyte progenitors. *Glia* **46**: 183–194

Neu I, Mallinger J, Wildfeuer A, Mehlber L 1992 Leukotriene in the cerebrospinal fluid of multiple sclerosis patients. *Acta Neurol Scand* **86**: 586–587

Neuhaus O, Hartung HP 2001 In search of a disease marker: the cytokine profile of primary progressive multiple sclerosis. *Mult Scler* **7**: 143–144

Neuhaus O, Farina C, Yassouridis A et al 2000 Multiple sclerosis: comparison of copolymer-1- reactive T cell lines from treated and untreated subjects reveals cytokine shift from T helper 1 to T helper 2 cells. *Proc Natl Acad Sci USA* **97**: 7452–7457

Neuhaus O, Farina C, Wekerle H, Hohlfeld R 2001 Mechanisms of action of glatiramer acetate in multiple sclerosis. *Neurology* **56**: 702–708

Neuhaus O, Strasser-Fuchs S, Fazekas F et al 2002 Statins as immunomodulators: comparison with interferon-beta 1b in MS. *Neurology* **59**: 990–997

Neuhaus O, Stuve O, Zamvil SS, Hartung H 2004 Are statins a treatment option for multiple sclerosis? *Lancet* **3**: 369–371

Neumann H, Cavalie A, Jenne DE, Wekerle H 1995 Induction of MHC class I genes in neurons. *Science* **269**: 549–552

Neumann H, Boucraut J, Hahnel C et al 1996 Neuronal control of MHC class II inducibility in rat astrocytes and microglia. *Eur J Neurosci* **8**: 2582–2590

Neumann H, Schmidt H, Cavalie A et al 1997 MHC class I gene expression in single neurons of the central nervous system: differential regulation by interferon-γ and tumor necrosis factor-α. *J Exp Med* **185**: 305–316

Neumann H, Medana I, Bauer J, Lassmann H 2002 Cytotoxic T lymphocytes in autoimmune and degenerative CNS diseases. *Trends Neurosci* **25**: 313–319

Neumann JW, Ziegler DK 1972 Therapeutic trial of immunosuppressive agents in multiple sclerosis. *Neurology* **22**: 1268–1271

Neusch C, Rozengurt N, Jacobs RE et al 2001 Kir4.1 potassium channel subunit is crucial for oligodendrocyte development and in vivo myelination. *J Neurosci* **21**: 5429–5438

Newcombe J, Cuzner ML 1993 Organization and research applications of the UK Multiple Sclerosis Society tissue bank. *J Neural Transm* **39 (Suppl)**: 155–163

Newcombe J, Hawkins CP, Henderson CL et al 1991 Histopathology of multiple sclerosis lesions detected by magnetic resonance imaging in unfixed postmortem central nervous system tissue. *Brain* **114**: 1013–1023

Newcombe J, Li H, Cuzner ML 1994 Low density lipoprotein uptake by macrophages in multiple sclerosis plaques: implications for pathogenesis. *Neuropathol Appl Neurobiol* **20**: 152–162

Newman AK 1875 On insular sclerosis of the brain and spinal cord. *Aust Med J* **20**: 369–374

Newman EA 1986 High potassium conductance in astrocyte endfeet. *Science* **233**: 453–454

Newman PK, Saunders M 1989 Clinical aspects of methylprednisolone in multiple sclerosis. In: Capildeo R (ed.) *Steroids in Diseases of the Central Nervous System*. Chichester: Wiley, pp. 197–206

Newman PK, Saunders M, Tilley PJB 1982 Methylprednisolone therapy in multiple sclerosis. *J Neurol Neurosurg Psychiatry* **45**: 941–942

Newman TA, Woolley ST, Hughes PM et al 2001 T-cell- and macrophage-mediated axon damage in the absence of a CNS-specific immune response: involvement of metalloproteinases. *Brain* **124**: 2203–2214

Ng J, Frith R 2002 Nanging. *Lancet* **360**: 384

Nguyen D, Stangel M 2001 Expression of the chemokine receptors CXCR1 and CXCR2 in rat oligodendroglial cells. *Devl Brain Res* **128**: 77–81

Nguyen JP, Degos JD 1993 Thalamic stimulation and proximal tremor: a specific target in the nucleus ventromedialis thalami. *Arch Neurol* **50**: 498–500

Nguyen KB, McCombe PA, Pender MP 1994 Macrophage apoptosis in the central nervous system in experimental autoimmune encephalomyelitis. *J Autoimmun* **7**: 145–152

Nguyen KB, Pender MP 1998 Phagocytosis of apoptotic lymphocytes by oligodendrocytes in experimental autoimmune encephalomyelitis. *Acta Neuropathol* **95**: 40–46

Nguyen KB, McCombe PA, Pender MP 1997 Increased apoptosis of T lymphocytes and macrophages in the central and peripheral nervous systems of Lewis rats with experimental autoimmune encephalomyelitis treated with dexamethasone. *J Neuropathol Exp Neurol* **56**: 58–69

Nicholas RS, Wing MG, Compston A 2001a Nonactivated microglia promote oligodendrocyte precursor survival and maturation through the transcription factor NF-kappa B. *Eur J Neurosci* **13**: 959–967

Nicholas RS, Compston DAS, Brown DR 2001b Inhibition of TNFα-induced NF-kB converts the metabolic effects of microglial-derived TNF-α on mouse cerebellar neurones to neurotoxicity. *J Neurochemistry* **76**: 1431–1438

Nicholas RS, Stevens S, Wing MG, Compston DAS 2002 Microglia-derived IGF-2 and CNTF prevent TNFα induced death of mature oligodendrocytes *in vitro*. *J Neuroimmunol* **124**: 36–44

Nicholas RS, Stevens S, Wing M, Compston DAS 2003a Oligodendrocyte-derived stress signals can recruit microglia *in vitro*. *NeuroReport* **14**: 1001–1005

Nicholas RS, Partridge J, Donn RP et al 2003b The role of the PTPRC (CD45) mutation in the development of multiple sclerosis in the North West region of the United Kingdom. *J Neurol Neurosurg Psych* **74**: 944–945

Nicholl JA, Kinrade E, Love S 1993 PCR-mediated search for herpes simplex virus DNA in sections of brain from patients with multiple sclerosis and other neurological disorders. *J Neurol Sci* **113**: 144–151

Nicholson LB, Greer JM, Sobel RA et al 1995 An altered peptide ligand mediates immune deviation and prevents autoimmune encephalomyelitis. *Immunity* **3**: 397–405

Nick S, Pileri P, Tongiani S et al 1995 T cell receptor γδ repertoire is skewed in cerebrospinal fluid of multiple sclerosis patients: molecular and functional analyses of γδ antigen-reactive clones. *Eur J Immunol* **25**: 355–363

Nico B, Frigeri A, Nicchia GP et al 2001 Role of aquaporin-4 water channel in the development and integrity of the blood-brain barrier. *J Cell Sci* **114**: 1297–1307

Nicoletti A, lo Bartolo ML, Lo Fermo S et al 2001 Prevalence and incidence of multiple sclerosis in Catania, Sicily. *Neurology* **56**: 62–66

Nicoletti A, Sofia V, Biondi R et al 2003 Epilepsy and multiple sclerosis in Sicily: a population-based study. *Epilepsia* **44**: 1445–1448

Nicolson M, Lowis GW 2002 The early history of the Multiple Sclerosis Society of Great Britain and Northern Ireland: a socio-historical study of lay/practitioner interaction in the context of a medical charity. *Med Hist* **46**: 141–174

Niederwieser G 2000 Lethal capillary leak syndrome after a single administration of interferon beta-1b. *Neurology* **54**: 1545–1546

Niederwieser G, Bonelli RM, Kammerhuber F et al 2001 Intracerebral haemorrhage under interferon-beta therapy. *Eur J Neurol* **8**: 363–364

Niehaus A, Shi J, Grzenkowski M et al 2000 Patients with active relapsing–remitting multiple sclerosis synthesize antibodies recognizing oligodendrocyte progenitor cell surface protein: implications for remyelination. *Ann Neurol* **48**: 362–371

Nielsen JF, Sinkjaer T, Jakobsen J 1996 Treatment of spasticity with repetitive magnetic stimulation: a double-blind placebo-controlled study. *Mult Scler* **2**: 227–232

Nieto M, Schuurmans C, Britz O, Guillemot F 2001 Neural bHLH genes control the neuronal versus glial fate decision in cortical progenitors. *Neuron* **29**: 401–413

Niino M, Kikuchi S, Fukazawa T et al 2000a Estrogen receptor gene polymorphism in Japanese patients with multiple sclerosis. *J Neurol Sci* **179**: 70–75

Niino M, Fukazawa T, Yabe T et al 2000b Vitamin D receptor gene polymorphism in multiple sclerosis and the association with HLA class II alleles. *J Neurol Sci* **177**: 65–71

Niino M, Kikuchi S, Fukazawa T et al 2001a Heat shock protein 70 gene polymorphism in Japanese patients with multiple sclerosis. *Tissue Antigens* **58**: 93–96

Niino M, Kikuchi S, Fukazawa T et al 2001b Genetic polymorphisms of IL-1β and IL-1 receptor antagonist in association with multiple sclerosis in Japanese patients. *J Neuroimmunol* **118**: 295–299

Niino M, Kikuchi S, Miyagishi R et al 2002a An examination of the association between β2 adrenergic receptor polymorphisms and multiple sclerosis. *Mult Scler* **8**: 475–478

Niino M, Kikuchi S, Fukazawa T et al 2002b No association of vitamin D-binding protein gene polymorphisms in Japanese patients with MS. *J Neuroimmunol* **127**: 177–179

Niino M, Kikuchi S, Fukazawa T et al 2003a Genetic polymorphisms of osteopontin in association with multiple sclerosis in Japanese patients. *J Neuroimmunol* **136**: 125–129

Niino M, Kikuchi S, Fukazawa T et al 2003b Polymorphisms of apolipoprotein E and Japanese patients with multiple sclerosis. *Mult Scler* **9**: 382–386

Nikoskelainen E 1975 Symptoms, signs and early course of optic neuritis. *Acta Ophthalmol* **53**: 254–272

Nikoskelainen E, Riekkenen P 1974 Optic neuritis: a sign of multiple sclerosis or other diseases of the central nervous system. *Acta Neurol Scand* **50**: 690–710

Nikoskelainen E, Sogg RL, Rosenthal AR, Friberg TR, Dorfman LJ 1977 The early phase in Leber hereditary optic atrophy. *Arch Ophthalmol* **95**: 969–978

Nilsson P, Larsson EM, Maly-Sundgren P et al 2005 Predicting the outcome of optic neuritis: evaluation of risk factors after 30 years of follow-up. *J Neurol* **252**: 396–402

Nimmerjahn A, Kirchhoff F, Helmchen F 2005 Resting microglial cells are highly dynamic surveillants of brain parenchyma in vivo. *Science* **308**: 1314–1318

Ninfo V, Rizzutto N, Terzian H 1967 Assoziazione anatomo-clinical di nevrite ipertrofica e sclerosi a placche. *Acta Neurol* **22**: 228–237

Nishimura M, Obayashi H, Ohta M et al 1995 No association of the 11778 mitochondrial DNA mutation and multiple sclerosis in Japan. *Neurology* **45**: 1333–1334

Nishiyama A, Lin XH, Giese N et al 1996 Co-localization of NG2 proteoglycan and PDGF alpha-receptor on O2A progenitor cells in the developing rat brain. *J Neurosci Res* **43**: 299–314

Nisipeanu P, Korczyn AD 1993 Psychological stress as risk factor for exacerbations in multiple sclerosis. *Neurology* **43**: 1311–1312

Nistor GI, Totoiu MO, Haque N et al 2005 Human embryonic stem cells differentiate into oligodendrocytes in high purity and myelinate after spinal cord transplantation. *Glia* **49**: 385–396

Nitsch R, Pohl EE, Smorodchenko A et al 2004 Direct impact of T cells on neurons revealed by two-photon microscopy in living brain tissue. *J Neurosci* **24**: 2458–2464

Niu MT, Davis DM, Ellenberg S 1996 Recombinant Hepatitis B vaccination of neonates and infants: emerging safety data from the Vaccine Adverse Event Reporting System. *Pediatr Infect Dis J* **15**: 771–776

Nixon C, McSweeny 1893 Diffuse cerebro-spinal sclerosis. *Dublin J Med Sci* **95**: 71–72

Nobile-Orazio E, Cappellari A, Meucci N et al 2002 Multifocal motor neuropathy: clinical and immunological features and response to IVIg in relation to the presence and degree of motor conduction block. *J Neurol Neurosurg Psychiatry* **72**: 761–766

Noble PG, Antel JP, Yong VW 1994 Astrocytes and catalase prevent the toxicity of catecholamines to oligodendrocytes. *Brain Res* **633**: 83–90

Nonaka T, Honmou O, Sakai J et al 2000 Excitability changes of dorsal root axons following nerve injury: implications for injury-induced changes in axonal Na+ channels. *Brain Res* **859**: 280–285

Nonne M, Holzmann W 1911 Seroligisches zür multiplen Sklerose Speziel uber die Cobrareaktion bei der multiplen Sklerose. *Dtsch Z Nerven* **41**: 123–145 van den Noort S, Eidelman B, Rammohan K et al 1998 National MS Society Clinical Bulletin: Disease Management Consensus Statement. New York: National MS Society

Nordenbo AM, Andersen JR, Andersen JT 1996 Disturbances of ano-rectal function in multiple sclerosis. J Urol 243: 445–451

Nordin M, Nyström B, Wallin U, Hagbarth K-E 1984 Ectopic sensory discharges and paraesthesiae in patients with disorders of peripheral nerves, dorsal roots and dorsal columns. Pain 20: 231–245

Norman JE, Kurtzke JF, Beebe GW 1983 Epidemiology of multiple sclerosis in US veterans. 2. Latitude, climate and the risk of MS. J Chron Dis 36: 551–559

Noronha A, Toscas A, Jensen MA 1993 Interferon beta-1b decreases T cell activation and interferon γ production in multiple sclerosis. Neurology 43: 655–661

Noronha ABC, Richman DP, Arnason BGW 1980 Detection of in vivo stimulated cerebrospinal fluid lymphocytes by flow cytometry in patients with multiple sclerosis. N Engl J Med 303: 713–717

Noronha MJ, Vas CJ, Aziz H 1968 Autonomic dysfunction (sweating responses) in multiple sclerosis. J Neurol Neurosurg Psychiatry 31: 19–22

Norstrand IF, Craelius 1989 A trial of deforoxamine (Desferl) in the treatment of multiple sclerosis: a pilot study. Clin Trials J 26: 365–369

Norton WT, Cammer W 1984 Chemical pathology of diseases involving myelin. In: Morrell P (ed.) Myelin. New York: Plenum Press, pp. 369–404

Nos C, Comabella M, Tintore M et al 1996 High dose intravenous immunoglobulin does not improve abnormalities in the blood-brain barrier during acute relapse of multiple sclerosis. J Neurol Neurosurg Psychiatry 61: 418

Nos C, Sastre-Garriga J, Borràs C et al 2004 Clinical impact of intravenous methylprednisolone in attacks of multiple sclerosis. Mult Scler 10: 413–416

Noseworthy JH, Hartung HP 2003 Multiple sclerosis and related conditions. In: Noseworthy JH (ed.) Neurological Therapeutics: Principles and Practice. London: Martin Dunitz

Noseworthy JH, Paty D, Wonnacott T et al 1983 Multiple sclerosis after age of 50. Neurology 33: 1537–1544

Noseworthy JH, Bass BH, Vandervoort MK et al 1989a The prevalence of primary Sjögren's syndrome in a multiple sclerosis population. Ann Neurol 25: 195–198

Noseworthy JH, Vandervoort MK, Hopkins M, Ebers GC 1989b A referendum on clinical trial research in multiple sclerosis: the opinion of the participants at the Jekyll Island workshop. Neurology 39: 977–981

Noseworthy JH, Vandenvoort MK, Wong CJ, Ebers GC 1990 Interrater variability with the Expanded Disability Status Scale (EDSS) and Functional Systems (FS) in a multiple sclerosis clinical trial. The Canadian Cooperation MS Study Group. Neurology 40: 971–975

Noseworthy JH, Hopkins MB, Vandervoort MK et al 1993 An open-trial evaluation of mitoxantrone in the treatment of progressive MS. Neurology 43: 1401–1406

Noseworthy JH, Ebers GC, Vandervoort MK et al 1994 The impact of blinding on the results of a randomised, placebo-controlled multiple sclerosis clinical trial. Neurology 44: 16–20

Noseworthy JH, O'Brien P, the Mayo Clinic–Canadian Cooperative MS Study Group 1998 The Mayo Clinic–Canadian Cooperative Trial of sulfasalazine in active multiple sclerosis. Neurology 51: 1342–1352

Noseworthy JH, Lucchinetti C, Rodriguez M et al 2000a Multiple sclerosis. N Engl J Med 343: 938–952

Noseworthy JH, O'Brien PC, Weinshenker BG et al 2000b IV immunoglobulin does not reverse established weakness in MS. Neurology 55: 1135–1143

Noseworthy JH, Wolinsky JS, Lublin FD et al 2000c Linomide in relapsing and secondary progressive MS: part I: trial design and clinical results. North American Linomide Investigators. Neurology 54: 1726–1733

Noseworthy JH, O'Brien PC, Petterson TM et al 2001 A randomized trial of intravenous immunoglobulin in inflammatory demyelinating optic neuritis. Neurology 56: 1514–1522

Noseworthy JH, Kappos L, Daumer M 2003 Competing interest in multiple sclerosis research. Lancet 361: 350

Nossal GJV 2001 A purgative mastery. Nature 412: 685–686

Novakovic SD, Deerinck TJ, Levinson SR et al 1996 Clusters of axonal Na+ channels adjacent to remyelinating Schwann cells. J Neurocytol 25: 403–412

Novakovic SD, Levinson SR, Schachner M, Shrager P 1998 Disruption and reorganization of sodium channels in experimental allergic neuritis. Muscle Nerve 21: 1019–1032

Nowak DA, Widenka DC 2001 Neurosarcoidosis: a review of its intracranial manifestations. J Neurol 248: 363–372

Nyffeler T, Stabba A, Sturzenegger M 2003 Progressive myelopathy with selective involvement of the lateral and posterior columns after inhalation of heroin vapour. J Neurol 250: 496–498

Nyland H, Mork S, Matre R 1982 In-situ characterization of mononuclear cell infiltrates in lesions of multiple sclerosis. Neuropathol Appl Neurobiol 8: 403–411

Nyquist PA, Cascino G, Rodriguez M 2001 Seizures in patients with multiple sclerosis seen at Mayo Clinic, Rochester, MN, 1990–1998. Mayo Clin Proc 76: 983–986

Nyquist PA, Cascino GD, McClelland RL et al 2002 Incidence of seizures in patients with multiple sclerosis: a population-based study. Mayo Clin Proc 77: 910–912

O'Brien CF 2002 Treatment of spasticity with botulinum toxin. Clin J Pain 18: S182–S190

Ochs G, Struppler A, Meyerson BA et al 1989 Intrathecal baclofen for long-term treatment of spasticity: a multi-centre study. J Neurol Neurosurg Psychiatry 52: 933–939

O'Connor KC, Appel H, Bregoli L et al 2005 Antibodies from inflamed central nervous system tissue recognize myelin oligodendrocyte glycoprotein. J Immunol 175: 1974–1982

O'Connor PW, Goodman A, Willmer-Hulme AJ et al 2004 Randomized multicenter trial of natalizumab in acute MS relapses: clinical and MRI effects. Neurology 62: 2038–2043

O'Duffy JD, Goldstein NP 1976 Neurologic involvement in seven patients with Behçet's syndrome. Am J Med 61: 170–178

Odum N, Hyldig-Nielsen JJ, Morling N et al 1988 HLA-DP antigens are involved in the susceptibility to multiple sclerosis. Tissue Antigens 31: 235–237

Odum N, Saida T, Ohta M, Svejgaard A 1989 HLA-DP antigens and HTLV-1 antibody status among Japanese with multiple sclerosis: evidence for an increased frequency of HLA-DPw4. J Immunogenet 16: 467–473

Oehmichen M, Gruninger H, Wietholter H, Gencic M 1979 Lymphatic efflux of intracerebrally injected cells. Acta Neuropathol 45: 61–65

Oehmichen M, Domasch D, Wietholter H 1982 Origin, proliferation, and fate of cerebrospinal fluid cells: a review on cerebrospinal fluid cell kinetics. J Neurol 227: 145–150

Offenbacher H, Fazekas F, Schmidt R et al 1993 Assessment of MRI criteria for a diagnosis of MS. Neurology 43: 905–909

Offner H, Vainiene M, Gold DP et al 1992 Characterization of the immune response to a secondary encephalitogenic epitope of basic protein in Lewis rats. I. T cell receptor peptide regulation of T cell clones expressing cross-reactive Vβ genes. J Immunol 149: 1706–1711

Offner H, Buenafe AC, Vainiene M et al 1993 Where, when, and how to detect biased expression of disease-relevant Vβ genes in rats with experimental autoimmune encephalomyelitis. J Immunol 151: 506–517

Ogasawara N 1965 Multiple sclerosis with Rosenthal's fibers. Acta Neuropathol 5: 61–68

Ogata J, Feigin I 1975 Schwann cells and regenerated peripheral myelin in multiple sclerosis: an ultrastructural study. Neurology 25: 713–716

Ogawa G, Mochizuki H, Kanzaki M et al 2004 Seasonal variation of multiple sclerosis exacerbations in Japan. Neurol Sci 24: 417–419

Oger J, Vorobeychick G, Al-Fahim A et al 1997 Neutralizing antibodies in Betaseron-treated MS patients and in vitro immune function before treatment. Neurology 48: A80

Oh LY, Larsen PH, Krekoski CA et al 1999 Matrix metalloproteinase-9/gelatinase B is required for process outgrowth by oligodendrocytes. J Neurosci 19: 8464–8475

Oh LY, Denninger A, Colvin JS et al 2003 Fibroblast growth factor receptor 3 signaling regulates the onset of oligodendrocyte terminal differentiation. *J Neurosci* 23: 883–894

Oh S, Huang X, Chiang C 2005 Specific requirements of sonic hedgehog signaling during oligodendrocyte development. *Dev Dyn* [eub ahead of print]

Ohashi T, Yamamura T, Inobe J-I et al 1995 Analysis of proteolipid lipoprotein (PLP)-specific T cells in multiple sclerosis: identification of PLP 95–116 as an HLA-DR2, w15-associated determinant. *Int Immunol* 7: 1771–1778

Ohe Y, Ishikawa K, Itoh Z, Tatemoto K 1996 Cultured leptomeningeal cells secrete cerebrospinal fluid proteins. *J Neurochem* 67: 964–971

Ohgoh M, Hanada T, Smith T et al 2002 Altered expression of glutamate transporters in experimental autoimmune encephalomyelitis. *J Neuroimmunol* 125: 170–178

Ohkoshi N, Komatsu Y, Mizusawa H, Kanazawa I 1998 Primary position upbeat nystagmus increased on downward gaze: clinicopathologic study of a patient with multiple sclerosis. *Neurology* 50: 551–553

Ohlenbusch A, Wilichowski E, Hanefeld F 1998a Characterisation of the mitochondrial genome in childhood multiple sclerosis. III Optic neuritis and LHON mutations. *Neuropaediatrics* 29: 175–179

Ohlenbusch A, Wilichowski E, Hanefeld F 1998b Characterisation of the mitochondrial genome in childhood multiple sclerosis. III Multiple sclerosis without optic neuritis and the non-LHON associated genes. *Neuropaediatrics* 29: 313–319

Ohlenbusch A, Pohl D, Hanefeld F 2002 Myelin oligodendrocyte gene polymorphisms and childhood multiple sclerosis. *Paediatr Res* 52: 175–179

Oikonen M, Laaksonen M, Laippapa P et al 2003 Ambient air quality and occurrence of multiple sclerosis relative risk. *Neuroepidemiology* 22: 95–99

Ojeda V 1984 Necrotising myelopathy associated with malignancy. *Cancer* 53: 1115–1123

Oka Y, Kanbayashi T, Mezaki T et al 2004 Low CSF hypocretin-1/orexin-A associated with hypersomnia secondary to hypothalamic lesion in a case of multiple sclerosis. *J Neurol* 251: 855–886

Oken BS, Kishiyama S, Zajdel D et al 2004 Randomized controlled trial of yoga and exercise in multiple sclerosis. *Neurology* 62: 2058–2064

Okinaka S, Tsubaki T, Kuroiwa Y et al 1958 Multiple sclerosis and allied diseases in Japan: clinical characteristics. *Neurology* 8: 756–763

Oksanen V, Gröngagen-Riska C, Fyhrquist F, Somer H 1985 Systemic manifestations and enzyme studies in sarcoidosis with neurologic involvement. *Acta Med Scand* 218: 123–127

Oksenberg JR, Gaiser CN, Cavalli-Sforza L, Steinman L 1988 Polymorphic markers of human T cell receptor alpha and beta genes: family studies and comparison of frequencies in healthy individuals and patients with multiple sclerosis and myasthenia gravis. *Hum Immunol* 22: 111–121

Oksenberg JR, Sherritt M, Begovich AB et al 1989 T cell receptor V alpha and C alpha alleles associated with multiple sclerosis and myasthenia gravis. *Proc Natl Acad Sci USA* 86: 988–992

Oksenberg JR, Panzara MA, Begovich AB et al 1993 Selection for T-cell receptor vβ-Dβ-Jβ gene rearrangements with specificity for a myelin basic protein peptide in brain lesions of multiple sclerosis. *Nature* 362: 68–70

Oksenberg JR, Barcellos LF, Cree BA et al 2004 Mapping multiple sclerosis susceptibility to the HLA-DR locus in African Americans. *Am J Hum Genet* 74: 160–167

Okuda Y, Nakatsuji Y, Fujimura H et al 1995 Expression of the inducible isoform of nitric oxide synthase in the central nervous system of mice correlates with the severity of actively induced experimental allergic encephalomyelitis. *J. Neuroimmunol* 62: 103–112

Okuda Y, Sakoda S, Fujimura H, Yanagihara T 1997 Nitric oxide via an inducible isoform of nitric oxide synthase is a possible factor to eliminate inflammatory cells from the central nervous system of mice with experimental allergic encephalomyelitis. *J Neuroimmunol* 73: 107–116

Olafson RA, Rushton JG, Sayre GP 1966 Trigeminal neuralgia in a patient with multiple sclerosis: an autopsy report. *J Neurosurg* 24: 755–759

Olafsson E, Benedikz J, Hauser WA 1999 Risk of epilepsy in patients with multiple sclerosis: a population-based study in Iceland. *Epilepsia* 40: 745–747

Oldberg A, Franzen A, Heinegård D 1986 Cloning and sequence analysis of rat bone sialoprotein (osteopontin) cDNA reveals an Arg-Gly-Asp cell-binding sequence. *Proc Natl Acad Sci USA* 83: 8819–8823

Oldstone MB, Southern PJ 1993 Trafficking of activated cytotoxic T-lymphocytes into the central nervous system: use of a transgenic model. *J Neuroimmunol* 46: 25–31

Olek MJ, Hohol MJ, Weiner HL 1996 Methotrexate in the treatment of multiple sclerosis. *Ann Neurol* 39: 684

Olerup O, Hillert J 1991 HLA class II-associated genetic susceptibility in multiple sclerosis: a critical evaluation. *Tissue Antigens* 38: 1–15

Olerup O, Wallin J, Carlsson B et al 1987 Genomic HLA typing by RFLP analysis, using DR beta and DQ cDNA beta probes reveals normal DR-DQ linkages in patients with multiple sclerosis. *Tissue Antigens* 30: 135–138

Olerup O, Hillert J, Fredrikson S et al 1989 Primarily chronic progressive and relapsing/remitting multiple sclerosis: two immunogenetically distinct disease entities. *Proc Natl Acad Sci USA* 86: 7113–7117

Olerup O, Hillert J, Fredrikson S 1990 The HLA-D region associated MS susceptibility genes may be located telomeric to the HLA-DP sub-region. *Tissue Antigens* 35: 37–39

Oleson CV, Sivalingam JJ, O'Neill BJ, Staas WE Jr 2003 Transverse myelitis secondary to coexistent Lyme disease and babesiosis. *J Spinal Cord Med* 26: 168–171

Oleszak EL, Zaczynska E, Bhattacharjee M et al 1998 Inducible nitric oxide synthase and nitrotyrosine are found in monocytes/macrophages and/or astrocytes in acute, but not in chronic, multiple sclerosis. *Clin Diagn Lab Immunol* 5: 438–445

Olgiati R, Jacquet J, Di Prampero PE 1986 Energy cost of walking and exertional dyspnoea in multiple sclerosis. *Am Rev Respir Dis* 134: 1005–1010

Olindo S, Guillon B, Helias J et al 2002 Decrease in heart ventricular ejection fraction during multiple sclerosis. *Eur J Neurol* 9: 287–291

Olitsky PK, Yager RH 1949 Experimental disseminated encephalomyelitis in white mice. *J Exp Med* 90: 213–224

Oliveras De Lariva C, Aragones OJM, Mercadet Sobreques J 1968 Estudio de la esclerosis multiple en Asturias. *Neurologia* 6: 41–45

Oliveri RL, Sibilia G, Valentino P et al 1998 Pulsed methylprednisolone induces a reversible impairment of memory in patients with relapsing–remitting multiple sclerosis. *Acta Neurol Scand* 97: 366–369

Oliverio PJ, Restrepo L, Mitchell SA et al 2000 Reversible tacrolimus-induced neurotoxicity isolated to the brain stem. *Am J Neuroradiol* 21: 1251–1254

Ollivier CP d'Angers 1824 *De la Moelle Epinière et de ses Maladies*. Paris: Crevot

Ollivier CP d'Angers 1827 *Traité de la Moelle Epinière et de ses Maladies*, 2nd edn. Paris: Crevot

Olsen NK, Hansen AW, Nørby S et al 1995 Leber's hereditary optic neuropathy with a disorder indistinguishable from multiple sclerosis in a male harbouring the mitochondrial DNA 11778 mutation. *Acta Neurol Scand* 91: 326–329

Olsson JE, Moller E, Link H 1976 HLA haplotypes in families with high frequency of multiple sclerosis. *Arch Neurol* 33: 808–812

Olsson T 1992 Immunology of multiple sclerosis. *Curr Opin Neurol Neurosurg* 5: 195–202

Olsson T 1994 Role of cytokines in multiple sclerosis and experimental autoimmune encephalomyelitis. *Eur J Neurol* 1: 7–19

Olsson T, Baig S, Hogeberg B, Link H 1990a Anti-myelin basic protein and anti-myelin antibody-producing cells in multiple sclerosis. *Ann Neurol* 47: 132–136

Olsson T, Zhi WW, Hojeberg B et al 1990b Autoreactive T lymphocytes in multiple sclerosis determined by antigen-induced secretion of interferon-γ. *J Clin Invest* **86**: 981–985

Olsson Y 1974 Mast cells in plaques of multiple sclerosis. *Acta Neurol Scand* **50**: 611–618

O'Malley PP 1966 Severe mental symptoms in disseminated sclerosis: a neuropathological study. *J Irish Med Assoc* **55**: 115–127

Omari KM, John GR, Sealfon SC, Raine CS 2005 CXC chemokine receptors on human oligodendrocytes: implications for multiple sclerosis. *Brain* **128**: 1003–1015

Ombredane A 1929 *Sur les troubles mentaux de la sclérose en plaques*. Paris: Thèse de Paris

Once Weekly Interferon for MS Study Group (OWIMS) 1999 Evidence of interferon beta-1a dose response in relapsing–remitting MS. *Neurology* **53**: 679–686

Onda A, Hamba M, Yabuki S, Kikuchi S 2002 Exogenous tumor necrosis factor-alpha induces abnormal discharges in rat dorsal horn neurons. *Spine* **27**: 1618–1624

O'Neill BP, Moser HW, Saxena KM 1982 Familial X-linked Addison disease as an expression of adrenoleukodystrophy (ALD): elevated C26 fatty acids in cultured skin fibroblasts. *Neurology* **32**: 543–547

O'Neill BP, Marber JR, Forbes GS, Moser HW 1983 Adrenoleucodystrophy: clinical and computerised tomography features of a childhood variant form. *Neurology* **33**: 1203–1205

Ono T, Zambenedetti MR, Yamasaki K *et al* 1998 Molecular analysis of class I (HLA-A and -B) and HLA class II (HLA-DRB1) genes in Japanese patients with multiple sclerosis (Western type and Asian type). *Tissue Antigens* **52**: 539–542

van Oosten BW, Lai M, Barkhof F *et al* 1996a A phase II trial of anti-CD4 antibodies in the treatment of multiple sclerosis. *Mult Scler* **1**: 339–342

van Oosten BW, Rep MHG, van Lier RAW *et al* 1996b A pilot study investigating the effects of orally administered pentoxifylline on selected immune variables in patients with multiple sclerosis. *J Neuroimmunol* **66**: 49–55

van Oosten BW, Lai M, Hodgkinson S *et al* 1997 Treatment of multiple sclerosios with the monoclonal anti-CD4 antibody cM-T412: results of a randomised, double-blind, placebo-controlled, MR monitored phase II trial. *Neurology* **49**: 351–357

van Ooteghem P, De Hooghe MB, Vlietinck R, Carton H 1994 Prevalence of multiple sclerosis in Flanders, Belgium. *Neuroepidemiology* **13**: 220–225

Opal P, Zoghbi HY 2002 The hereditary ataxias. In: Asbury AK, McKhann GM, McDonald WI *et al* (eds) *Diseases of the Nervous System: Clinical Neuroscience and Therapeutic Principles*, 3rd edn. Cambridge: Cambridge University Press, pp. 1880–1895

Opdenakker G, Van-Damme J 1994 Cytokine-regulated proteases in autoimmune diseases. *Immunol Today* **15**:103–107

Opdenakker G, Nelissen I, Van Damme J 2003 Functional roles and therapeutic targeting of gelatinase B and chemokines in multiple sclerosis (review). *Lancet* **2**: 747–756

Openshaw H, Stuve O, Antel JP *et al* 2000a Multiple sclerosis flares associated with recombinant granulocyte colony-stimulating factor. *Neurology* **54**: 2147–2150

Openshaw H, Lund BT, Kashyap A *et al* 2000b Peripheral blood stem cell transplantation in multiple sclerosis with busulfan and cyclophosphamide conditioning: report of toxicity and immunological monitoring. *Biol Blood Marrow Transplant* **6**: 563–575

Operskalski EA, Visscher BR, Malgren RM, Detels R 1989 A case control study of multiple sclerosis. *Neurology* **39**: 825–829

Oppel G 1963 Mikroskopische Untersuchungen über die Anzahl und Kaliber der markhaltige Nervenfasern im Fasiculus opticus des Menschen. *Graefes Arch Ophthalmol* **160**: 19–27

Oppenheim C, Galanaud D, Samson Y *et al* 2000 Can diffusion weighted magnetic resonance imaging help differentiate stroke from stroke-like events in MELAS? *J Neurol Neurosurg Psychiatry* **69**: 248–250

Oppenheim H 1894 *Lehrbuch der Nervenkrankheiten*. Berlin: S. Karger

Oppenheim H 1911 *Textbook of Nervous Diseases for Physicians and Students* (translated from the 5th edition by A. Bruce). Edinburgh: A Schulze & Co, pp. 332–350

Oppenheim H 1914 Der Formenreichtum der multiplen Sklerose. *Dtsch Z Nervenheilk* **52**: 169–239

Oppenheim H 1917 Über den facialen Typus der multiplen Sklerose. *Neurol Zentralblatt* **36**: 142–143

Oppenheimer D 1978 The cervical cord in multiple sclerosis. *Neuropathol Appl Neurobiol* **4**: 151–162

Oppenheimer DR 1962 *Observations on the Pathology of Demyelinating Disease*. Thesis, University of Oxford

Oppenheimer S, Hoffbrand BI 1986 Optic neuritis and myelopathy in systemic lupus erythematosus. *Can J Neurol Sci* **13**: 129–132

Optic Neuritis Study Group 1991 The clinical profile of optic neuritis. *Arch Ophthalmol* **109**: 1673–1678

Optic Neuritis Study Group 1997a The 5-year risk of MS after optic neuritis: experience of the Optic Neuritis Treatment Trial. *Neurology* **49**: 1404–1413

Optic Neuritis Study Group 1997b Visual function 5 years after optic neuritis. *Arch Ophthalmol* **115**: 1544–1552

Optic Neuritis Study Group 2003 High- and low-risk profiles for the development of multiple sclerosis within 10 years after optic neuritis. *Arch Ophthalmol* **121**: 944–949

Orban T 1955 Beitrag zu dem Augenhinter-grundsveranderungen bei Sklerosis multiplex. *Ophthalmolgica* **30**: 387–396

Ordenstein L 1868 *Sur la paralysie agitante et la sclérose en plaques generalisées*. Paris: Delahaye

Orentas DM, Hayes JE, Dyer KL, Miller RH 1999 Sonic hedgehog signaling is required during the appearance of spinal cord oligodendrocyte precursors. *Development* **126**: 2419–2429

O'Riordan JI, Gallagher HL, Thompson AJ *et al* 1996 Clinical, CSF, and MRI findings in Devic's neuromyelitis optica. *J Neurol Neurosurg Psychiatry* **60**: 382–387

O'Riordan JI, Losseff NA, Phatouros C *et al* 1998a Asymptomatic spinal cord lesions in clinical isolated optic nerve, brain stem and spinal cord syndromes suggestive of demyelination. *J Neurol Neurosurg Psychiatry* **64**: 353–357

O'Riordan JI, Thompson AJ, Kingsley DPE *et al* 1998b The prognostic value of brain MRI in clinically isolated syndromes of the CNS: a 10-year follow-up. *Brain* **121**: 495–503

O'Riordan JI, Gomez-Anson B, Moseley IF, Miller DH 1999 Long term MRI follow-up of patients with post infectious encephalomyelitis: evidence of a monophasic disease. *J Neurol Sci* **167**:132–136

O'Riordan S, Nor AM, Hutchinson M 2002 CADASIL imitating multiple sclerosis: the importance of MRI markers. *Mult Scler* **8**: 430–432

Ormerod IEC, McDonald WI 1984 Multiple sclerosis presenting with progressive visual failure. *J Neurol Neurosurg Psychiatry* **47**: 943–946

Ormerod IEC, Miller DH, McDonald WI *et al* 1987 The role of NMR imaging in the assessment of multiple sclerosis and isolated neurological lesions: a quantitative study. *Brain* **110**: 1579–1616

Ormerod IEC, Waddy HM, Kermode AG *et al* 1992 Involvement of the central nervous system in chronic inflammatory demyelinating polyneuropathy: a clinical, electrophysiological and magnetic resonance imaging study. *J Neurol Neurosurg Psychiatry* **53**: 789–793

Ormerod IEC, Harding AE, Miller DH *et al* 1994 Magnetic resonance imaging in degenerative ataxic disorders. *J Neurol Neurosurg Psychiatry* **57**: 51–57

Oro AS, Guarino TJ, Driver R *et al* 1996 Regulation of disease susceptibility: decreased prevalence of IgE-mediated allergic disease in patients with multiple sclerosis. *J Allergy Clin Immunol* **97**: 1402–1408

Orr D, McKendrick MM, Sharrack B 2004 Acute disseminated encephalomyelitis temporally associated with campylobacter gastroenteritis. *J Neurol Neurosurg Psychiatry* **75**: 792–793

Ortiz-Ortiz L, Weigle WO 1976 Cellular events in the induction of experimental allergic encephalomyelitis in rats. *J Exp Med* **144**: 604–616

Oski J, Kalimo H, Marttlila RJ *et al* 1996 Inflammatory brain changes in Lyme borreliosis: a report on three patients and review of the literature. *Brain* **119**: 2143–2154

Osler W 1880 Cases of insular sclerosis. *Can Med Surg J* **9**: 1–11

Osler W 1929 *Bibliotecha Osleriana*. A catalogue of books illustrating the history of medicine and science collected, arranged, and annotated by Sir William Osler, Bt and bequeathed to McGill University. Oxford: Clarendon Press, pp. 675–676

Osoegawa M, Niino M, Ochi H et al 2004 Platelet-activating factor acetylhydrolase gene polymorphism and its activity in Japanese patients with multiple sclerosis. J Neuroimmunol 150: 150–156

Osoegawa M, Miyagishi R, Ochi II et al 2005 Platelet-activating factor receptor gene polymorphism in Japanese patients with multiple sclerosis. J Neuroimmunol 161: 195–198

Osterhout DJ, Marin-Husstege M, Abano P, Casaccia-Bonnefil P 2002 Molecular mechanisms of enhanced susceptibility to apoptosis in differentiating oligodendrocytes. J Neurosci Res 69: 24–29

Osterman PO 1976 Paroxysmal itching in multiple sclerosis. Br J Dermatol 95: 555–558

O'Sullivan M, Jarosz JM, Martin RJ et al 2001 MRI hyperintensities of the temporal lobe and external capsule in patients with CADASIL. Neurology 56: 628–634

Osuntokun BO 1973 Neurological disorders in Nigeria. In: Spillane JD (ed.) Tropical Neurology. London: Oxford University Press, pp. 161–190

Ota K, Matsui M, Milford EL et al 1990 T-cell recognition of an immunodominant myelin basic protein epitope in multiple sclerosis. Nature 346: 183–187

Otaegui D, Saenz A, Martinez-Zabaleta M et al 2004 Mitochondrial haplogroups in Basque multiple sclerosis patients. Mult Scler 10: 532–535

Ott M, Demisch L, Engelhardt W, Fischer PA 1993 Interleukin-2, soluble interleukin-2-receptor, neopterin, L-tryptophan and beta 2-microglobulin levels in CSF and serum of patients with relapsing–remitting or chronic–progressive multiple sclerosis. J Neurol 241: 108–114

Oturai AB, Larsen F, Ryder LP et al 1999 Linkage and association analysis of susceptibility regions on chromosomes 5 and 6 in 106 Scandinavian sibling pair families with multiple sclerosis. Ann Neurol 46: 612–616

Oturai AB, Ryder LP, Fredrikson S et al 2004 Concordance for disease course and age of onset in Scandinavian multiple sclerosis coaffected sib pairs. Mult Scler 10: 5–8

Ouardouz M, Nikolaeva MA, Coderre E et al 2003 Depolarization-induced Ca2+ release in ischemic spinal cord white matter involves L-type Ca2+ channel activation of ryanodine receptors. Neuron 40: 53–63

Owen JJT, Jenkinson EJ 1984 Early events in T lymphocyte genesis in the fetal thymus. Am J Anat 170: 301–310

Owens GP, Kraus H, Burgoon MP et al 1998 Restricted use of V$_H$4 germline segments in an acute multiple sclerosis brain. Ann Neurol 43: 236–243

Owens GP, Burgoon MP, Anthony J et al 2001 The immunoglobulin G heavy chain repertoire in multiple sclerosis plaques is distinct from the heavy chain repertoire in peripheral blood lymphocytes. Clin Immunol 98: 258–263

Owens T 2003 The enigma of multiple sclerosis: inflammation and neurodegeneration causes heterogenous dysfunction and damage. Curr Opin Neurol 16: 259–265

Owens T, Renno T, Taupin V, Krakowski M 1994 Inflammatory cytokines in the brain: does the CNS shape immune responses? Immunol Today 15: 566–571

Owens T, Wekerle H, Antel J 2001 Genetic models of CNS inflammation. Nature Med 7: 161–165

Ozawa K, Suchanek G, Breitschopf H et al 1994 Patterns of oligodendroglia pathology in multiple sclerosis. Brain 117: 1311–1322

Ozenci V, Kouwenhoven M, Teleshova N et al 2000 Multiple sclerosis: pro- and anti-inflammatory cytokines and metalloproteinases are affected differentially by treatment with IFN-beta. J Neuroimmunol 108: 236–243

Ozturk V, Idiman E, Sengun IS, Yulsel Z 2002 Multiple sclerosis and parkinsonism: a report. Funct Neurol 17: 145–147

Pachner AR 2003 Anti-IFNβ antibodies in IFNβ-treated MS patients: summary. Neurology 61: S1–S5

Pachner AR, Steere AC 1985 The triad of neurologic manifestations of Lyme disease: meningitis, cranial neuritis and radiculoneuritis. Neurology 35: 47–53

Pachner AR, Duray P, Steere AC 1989 Central nervous system manifestations of Lyme disease. Arch Neurol 46: 790–795

Padberg F, Haase CG, Feneberg W et al 2001 No association between anti-myelin oligodendrocyte glycoprotein antibodies and serum/cerebrospinal fluid levels of the soluble interleukin-6 receptor complex in multiple sclerosis. Neurosci Lett 305: 13–16

Padmashri R, Chakrabarti KS, Sahal D et al 2004 Functional characterization of the pentapeptide QYNAD on rNav1.2 channels and its NMR structure. Pflugers Arch 447: 895–907

Padovan E, Casorati G, Dellabona P et al 1993 Expression of two T cell receptor alpha chains: dual receptor T cells. Science 262: 422–424

Padovan E, Giachino C, Cella M, Valitutti S, Acuto O, Lanzavecchia A 1995 Normal T lymphocytes can express two different T cell receptor beta chains: implications for the mechanism of allelic exclusion. J Exp Med 181: 1587–1591

Page SA, Verhoef MJ, Stebbins RA et al 2003 Cannabis use as described by people with multiple sclerosis. Can J Neurol Sci 30: 201–205

Page WF, Kurtzke JF, Murphy FM, Norman JE 1993 Epidemiology of multiple sclerosis in US veterans: V. Ancestry and the risk of multiple sclerosis. Ann Neurol 33: 632–639

Page WF, Mack TM, Kurtzke JF, Murphy FM, Norman JE 1995 Epidemiology of multiple sclerosis in US veterans: 6. Population ancestry and surname ethnicity as risk factors for multiple sclerosis. Neuroepidemiology 14: 286–296

Paintal AS 1966 The influence of diameter of medullated nerve fibres of cats on the rising and falling phases of the spike and its recovery. J Physiol 184: 791–811

Palace J, Rothwell P 1997 New treatments and azathioprine in multiple sclerosis. Lancet 350: 261

Palacio LG, Rivera D, Builes JJ et al 2002 Multiple sclerosis in the tropics: genetic association to STR's loci spanning the HLA and TNF. Mult Scler 8: 249–255

Palffy G 1982 MS in Hungary, including the Gypsy population. In: Kuroiwa Y, Kurland LT (eds) Multiple Sclerosis: East and West. Kyushu: Kyushu University Press, pp. 149–157

Palffy G, Merei FT 1961 The possible role of vaccines and sera in the pathogenesis of multiple sclerosis. World Neurol 2: 167–172

Palffy G, Czopf J, Kuntar L, Gyodi E 1994 Multiple sclerosis in Baranya County in Hungarians and in Gypsies. In: Firnhaber W, Lauer K (eds) Multiple Sclerosis in Europe: An Epidemiological Update. Darmstadt: Leuchtturm-Verlag/LTV Press, pp. 274–278

Pambakian AL, Kennard C 1997 Can visual function be restored in patients with homonymous hemianopia? Br J Ophthalmol 81: 324–328

Pamir MN, Kansu T, Erbengi A, Zileli T 1981 Papilloedema in Behçet syndrome. Arch Neurol 38: 643–645

Pandey JP, Goust JM, Salier JP 1981 Immunoglobulin G heavy chain (Gm) allotypes in multiple sclerosis. J Clin Invest 67: 1797–1800

Panelius M 1969 Studies on epidemiological, clinical and etiological aspects of multiple sclerosis. Acta Neurol Scand 45 (Suppl 39): 1–82

Pang Y, Cai Z, Rhodes PG 2005 Effect of tumor necrosis factor-alpha on developing optic nerve oligodendrocytes in culture. J Neurosci Res 80: 226–234

Panitch HS 1987 Systemic α-interferon in multiple sclerosis. Arch Neurol 44: 61–63

Panitch HS 1994 Influence of infection on exacerbations of multiple sclerosis. Ann Neurol 36 (Suppl.): S25–S28

Panitch HS, Hirsch RI, Schindler J, Johnson KP 1987a Treatment of multiple sclerosis with gamma-interferon: exacerbation associated with activation of the immune system. Neurology 37: 1097–1102

Panitch HS, Hirsch RL, Haley AS, Johnson KP 1987b Exacerbations of multiple sclerosis in patients treated with gamma interferon. Lancet i: 893–895

Panitch HS, Bever T, Katz E, Johnson KP 1991 Upper respiratory tract infections trigger attacks of multiple sclerosis in patients treated with interferon. J Neuroimmunol (Suppl 1): 125

Panitch HS, Goodin DS, Francis G et al 2002 Randomized, comparative study of interferon beta-1a treatment regimens in MS: the EVIDENCE Trial. *Neurology* **59**: 1496–1506

Pannetier C, Even J, Kourilsky P 1995 T-cell repertoire diversity and clonal expansions in normal and clinical samples. *Immunol Today* **16**: 176–181

Pantano P, Iannetti GD, Caramia F et al 2002 Cortical motor reorganization after a single clinical attack of multiple sclerosis. *Brain* **125**: 1607–1615

Paolillo A, Coles AJ, Molyneux PD et al 1999 Quantitative MRI in patients with secondary progressive MS treated with monoclonal antibody Campath 1H. *Neurology* **53**: 751–757

Paolillo A, Buzzi MG, Giugni E et al 2003 The effect of Bacille Calmette–Guérin on the evolution of new enhancing lesions to hypointense T1 lesions in relapsing remitting MS. *J Neurol* **250**: 247–248

Papadopoulos CM, Tsai S-Y, Alsbiei T et al 2002 Functional recovery and neuroanatomical plasticity following middle cerebral artery occlusion and IN-1 antibody treatment in the adult rat. *Ann Neurol* **51**: 433–441

Papadopoulos V, Micheli A, Nikiforidis D, Mimidis K 2005 Primary biliary cirrhosis complicated by transverse myelitis in a patient without Sjogren's syndrome. *J Postgrad Med* **51**: 43–44

Papais-Alvarenga RM, Miranda-Santos CM, Puccioni-Sohler M et al 2002 Optic neuromyelitis syndrome in Brazilian patients. *J Neurol Neurosurg Psychiatry* **73**: 429–435

Papiha SS, Duggan KM, Roberts DF 1991 Factor B (Bf) allotypes and multiple sclerosis in north east England. *Hum Heredity* **41**: 397–402

Parinaud H 1884 Troubles oculaires de la sclérose en plaques. *J Santé Publique* **3**: 3–5

Parisi A, Filice G 2001 Transverse myelitis associated with *Mycoplasma pneumoniae* pneumonitis: a report of two cases. *Infez Med* **9**: 39–42

Parisi, V, Manni G, Spadaro M et al 1999 Correlation between morphological and functional retinal impairment in multiple sclerosis patients. *Invest Ophthalmol Vis Sci* **40**: 2520–2527

Park CS 1966 Multiple sclerosis in Korea. *Neurology* **16**: 919–926

Park HJ, Won CK, Pyun KH, Shin HC 1995 Interleukin 2 suppresses afferent sensory transmission in the primary somatosensory cortex. *NeuroReport* **6**: 1018–1020

Park RM 2002 Letter to the editor. *Arch Environ Health* **57**: 383

Park S-K, Miller R, Krane I, Vartanian T 2001a The erbB2 gene is required for the development of terminally differentiated spinal cord oligodendrocytes. *J Cell Biol* **154**: 1245–1258

Park S-K, Solomon D, Vartanian T 2001b Growth factor control of CNS myelination. *Dev Neurosci* **23**: 327–337

Parker GJ, Wheeler-Kingshott CA, Barker GJ 2002 Estimating distributed anatomical brain connectivity using fast marching methods and diffusion tensor imaging. *IEEE Trans Med Imaging* **21**: 505–512

Parker HL 1928 Trigeminal neuralgic pain associated with multiple sclerosis. *Brain* **51**: 46–62

Parker HL 1946 Periodic ataxia. *Collected Papers Mayo Clin* **38**: 642–645

Parkin PJ, Hierons R, McDonald WI 1984 Bilateral optic neuritis: a long-term follow up. *Brain* **107**: 951–964

Parmley VC, Schiffman JS, Maitland CG, Miller NR, Dreyer RF, Hoyt WF 1987 Does neuroretinitis rule out multiple sclerosis? *Arch Neurol* **44**: 1045–1048

Parry AM, Corkill R, Blamire AM et al 2003a Beta-interferon does not always slow the progression of axonal injury in multiple sclerosis. *J Neurol* **250**: 171–178

Parry AM, Scott RB, Palace J et al 2003b Potentially adaptive functional changes in cognitive processing for patients with multiple sclerosis and their acute modulation by rivastigmine. *Brain* **126**: 2750–2760

Pasare C, Medzhitov R 2003 Toll pathway-dependent blockade of CD4+CD25+ T cell-mediated suppression by dendritic cells. *Science* **299**: 1033–1036

Pascual-Leone A, Altafullah I, Dhuna A 1991 Hemiageusia: an unusual presentation of multiple sclerosis. *J Neurol Neurosurg Psychiatry* **54**: 657

Pashenkov M, Huang YM, Kostulas V et al 2001 Two subsets of dendritic cells are present in human cerebrospinal fluid. *Brain* **124**: 480–492

Pashenkov M, Söderström M, Link H 2003a Secondary lymphoid organ chemokines are elevated in the cerebrospinal fluid during central nervous system inflammation. *J Neuroimmunol* **135**: 154–160

Pashenkov M, Teleshova N, Link H 2003b Inflammation in the central nervous system: the role for dendritic cells. *Brain Pathol* **13**: 23–33

Pasternak JF, De Vivo DC, Prensky AL 1980 Steroid-responsive encephalomyelitis in childhood. *Neurology* **30**: 481–486

Patarca R, Freeman GJ, Singh RR et al 1989 Structural and functional studies of the early T lymphocyte activation 1 (*ETA1*) gene: definition of a novel T cell dependent response associated with genetic resistance to bacterial infection. *J Exp Med* **170**: 145–161

Paterson PY 1960 Transfer of allergic encephalomyelitis in rats by means of lymph node cells. *J Exp Med* **111**: 119–135

Pathak R, Khare KC 1967 Disseminated sclerosis syndrome following antirabic vaccination. *J Indian Med Assoc* **49**: 484–485

Patten SB, Metz LM, and Group SS 2002 Interferon beta1a and depression in secondary progressive MS: data from the SPECTRIMS Trial. *Neurology* **59**: 744–746

Patten SB, Beck CA, Williams JV et al 2003 Major depression in multiple sclerosis: a population-based perspective. *Neurology* **61**: 1524–1527

Patterson DL, Yunginger JW, Dunn WF et al 1995 Anaphylaxis induced by the carboxymethylcellulose component of injectable triamcinolone acetonide suspension (Kenalog). *Ann Allergy Asthma Immunol* **74**: 163–166

Patterson VH, Heron JR 1980 Visual field abnormalities in multiple sclerosis. *J Neurol Neurosurg Psychiatry* **43**: 205–208

Patti F, Cataldi ML, Nicoletti F et al 2001 Combination of cyclophosphamide and interferon-beta halts progression in patients with rapidly transitional multiple sclerosis. *J Neurol Neurosurg Psychiatry* **71**: 404–407

Patti F, Ciancio MR, Reggio E et al 2002 The impact of outpatient rehabilitation on quality of life in multiple sclerosis. *J Neurol* **249**: 1027–1033

Paty DW, Ebers GC 1998 *Multiple Sclerosis*. Philadelphia: F.A. Davis

Paty DW, Poser C 1984 *The Diagnosis of Multiple Sclerosis*. New York: Thieme-Stratton

Paty DW, Cousin HK, Read S, Adlakha K 1978 Linoleic acid in multiple sclerosis: failure to show any therapeutic benefit. *Acta Neurol Scand* **58**: 53–58

Paty DW, Blume WT, Brown WF, Jaatoul N, Kertesz A, McInnis W 1979 Chronic progressive myelopathy: investigation with CSF electrophoresis, evoked potentials and CT scan. *Ann Neurol* **6**: 419–424

Paty DW, Oger JJ, Kastrukoff LF et al 1988 MRI in the diagnosis of MS: a prospective study with comparison of clinical evaluation, evoked potentials, oligoclonal banding and CT. *Neurology* **38**: 180–185

Paty DW, Li DKB, The IFNB Multiple Sclerosis Study Group 1993 Interferon beta-1b is effective in relapsing–remitting multiple sclerosis: MRI results of a multicenter, randomized, double-blind, placebo-controlled trial. *Neurology* **43**: 662–667

Paty DW, Studney D, Redekop K, Lublin F 1994 MS COSTAR: a computerised patient record adapted for clinical research purposes. *Ann Neurol* **36 (Suppl)**: S134–S135

Paty DW, Arnason B, Li D, Traboulsee A 2003 Interferons in relapsing remitting multiple sclerosis. *Lancet* **361**: 1822; author reply 1823–1824.

Patzold T, Schwengelbeck M, Ossege LM et al 2002 Changes of the MS functional composite and EDSS during and after treatment of relapses with methylprednisolone in patients with multiple sclerosis. *Acta Neurol Scand* **105**: 164–168

Patzold U, Pocklington PR 1982 Course of multiple sclerosis: first results of a prospective study carried out of 102 MS patients from 1976–1980. *Acta Neurol Scand* **65**: 248–266

Patzold U, Hecker H, Pocklington P 1982 Azathioprine in treatment of multiple sclerosis. *J Neurol Sci* **54**: 377–394

Pavelko KD, van Engelen BGM, Rodriguez M 1998 Acceleration in the rate of CNS remyelination in lysolecithin-induced demyelination. *J Neurosci* **18**: 2498–2505

Payami H, Thomson G, Motro U, Louis E, Hudes E 1985 The affected sib method IV. Sib trios. *Ann Hum Genet* **49**: 303–314

Pazmany T, Kosa JP, Tomasi TB *et al* 2000 Effect of transforming growth factor-β₁ on microglial MHC-class II expression. *J Neuroimmunol* **103**: 122–130

Peces R, Urra JM, Escalada P *et al* 1993 High dose of methyl-prednisolone inhibits the OKT3-induced cytokine related syndrome (letter). *Nephron* **63**: 118

Pedersen L, Trojaborg W 1981 Visual, auditory and somatosensory pathway involvement in hereditary cerebellar ataxia, Friedreich's ataxia and familial spastic paraplegia. *Electroencephalogr Clin Neurophysiol* **52**: 283–297

Pedersen RA, Troost BT, Abel LA, Zorub D 1980 Intermittent downbeat nystagmus and oscillopsia reversed by suboccipital craniectomy. *Neurology* **30**: 1239–1242

Pedotti R, Mitchell D, Wedemeyer J *et al* 2001 An unexpected version of horror autotoxicus: anaphylactic shock to a self peptide. *Nature Med* **2**: 216–222

Pehl U, Schmid HA 1997 Electrophysiological response of neurons in the rat spinal cord to nitric oxide. *Neuroscience* **77**: 563–573

Pekmezovic T, Jarebinski M, Drulovic J *et al* 2001 Prevalence of multiple sclerosis in Belgrade, Yugoslavia. *Acta Neurol Scand* **104**: 353–357

Pekmezovic T, Jarebinski M, Drulovic J *et al* 2002 Survival of multiple sclerosis patients in the Belgrade population. *Neuroepidemiology* **21**: 235–240

Pekny M, Leveen P, Pekna M *et al* 1995 Mice lacking glial fibrillary acidic protein display astrocytes devoid of intermediate filaments but develop and reproduce normally. *EMBO J* **14**: 1590–1598

Pelanda R, Schwers S, Sonoda E *et al* 1997 Receptor editing in a transgenic mouse model: site, efficiency, and role in cell tolerance and antibody diversification. *Immunity* **7**: 765–775

Peles E, Salzer JL 2000 Molecular domains of myelinated axons. *Curr Opin Neurobiol* **10**: 558–565

Peletier D, Nelson SJ, Oh J *et al* 2003 MRI lesion volume heterogeneity in primary progressive MS in relation with axonal damage and brain atrophy. *J Neurol Neurosurg Psychiatry* **74**: 950–952

Pelletier J, Habib M, Brouchon M *et al* 1992 Etude du transfert interhémisphérique dans la sclérose en plaques. Corrélations morpho-fonctionelles. *Rev Neurol* **148**: 672–679

Pelosi L, Geesken JM, Holly M *et al* 1997 Working memory impairment in early multiple sclerosis: evidence from an event-related potential study of patients with clinically isolated myelopathy. *Brain* **120**: 2039–2058

Pena-Rossi C, McAllister A, Fiette L, Brahic M 1991 Theiler's virus infection induces a specific cytotoxic T lymphocytic response. *Cell Immunol* **138**: 341–348

Pencek TL, Schauf CL, Low PA *et al* 1980 Disruption of the perineurium in amphibian peripheral nerve: morphology and physiology. *Neurology* **30**: 593–599

Pender MP 1988a The pathophysiology of myelin basic protein-induced acute experimental allergic encephalomyelitis in the Lewis rat. *J Neurol Sci* **86**: 277–289

Pender MP 1988b The pathophysiology of acute experimental allergic encephaolmyelitis induced by whole spinal cord in the Lewis rat. *J Neurol Sci* **84**: 209–222

Pender MP 1989 Recovery from acute experimental allergic encephalomyelitis in the Lewis rat: early restoration of nerve conduction and repair by Schwann cells and oligodendrocytes. *Brain* **112**: 393–416

Pender MP 1998 Genetically determined failure of activation-induced apoptosis of autoreactive T cells as a cause of multiple sclerosis. *Lancet* **351**: 978–981

Pender MP 1999 Activation-induced apoptosis of autoreactive and alloreactive T lymphocytes in the target organ as a major mechanism of tolerance. *Immunol Cell Biol* **77**: 216–223

Pender MP, Chalk JB 1989 Connective tissue disease mimicking multiple sclerosis. *Aust NZ J Med* **19**: 469–472

Pender MP, Sears TA 1984 The pathophysiology of acute experimental allergic encephalomyelitis in the rabbit. *Brain* **107**: 699–726

Pender MP, Nguyen KB, McCombe PA, Kerr JFR 1991 Apoptosis in the nervous system in experimental allergic encephalomyelitis. *J Neurol Sci* **104**: 81–87

Penderis J, Shields SA, Franklin RJ 2003a Impaired remyelination and depletion of oligodendrocyte progenitors does not occur following repeated episodes of focal demyelination in the rat central nervous system. *Brain* **126**: 1382–1391

Penderis J, Woodruff RH, Lakatos A *et al* 2003b Increasing local levels of neuregulin (glial growth factor-2) by direct infusion into areas of demyelination does not alter remyelination in the rat CNS. *Eur J Neurosci* **18**: 2253–2264

Penfield W 1924 Oligodendroglia and its relation to classical neuroglia. *Brain* **47**: 430–452

Penfield W 1932 Neuroglia, normal and pathological. In: Penfield W, Paul B (eds) *Cytology and Cellular Pathology of the Nervous System*. New York: Hoeber, pp. 421–481

Penn RD, Kroin JS 1985 Continuous intrathecal baclofen for severe spasticity. *Lancet* **ii**: 125–127

Penn RD, Savoy SM, Corcos D *et al* 1989 Intrathecal baclofen for severe spinal spasticity. *N Engl J Med* **320**: 1517–1521

Pennypacker KR, Hong J-S, Mullis SB *et al* 1996 Transcription factors in primary glial cultures: changes with neuronal interactions. *Mol Brain Res* **37**: 224–230

Penrose LS 1935 The detection of autosomal linkage in data which consists of pairs of brothers and sisters of unspecified parentage. *Ann Eugen* **6**: 133–138

Pentland B, Ewing DJ 1987 Cardiovascular reflexes in multiple sclerosis. *Eur Neurol* **26**: 46–50

Pépin B, Goldstein B, Man HX *et al* 1978 Maldie de Eales avec manifestations neurologiques. *Rev Neurol* **134**: 427–436

Percy AK, Nobrega FT, Ozaki H *et al* 1971 Multiple sclerosis in Rochester, Minnesota: a 60-year appraisal. *Arch Neurol* **25**: 105–111

Percy AK, Nobrega FT, Kurland LT 1972 Optic neuritis and multiple sclerosis. *Arch Ophthalmol* **87**: 135–139

Peress NS, Perillo E, Seidman RJ 1996 Glial transforming growth factor (TGF)-β isotypes in multiple sclerosis: differential expression of TGF-β1, 2 and 3 isotypes in multiple sclerosis. *J Neuroimmunol* **71**: 115–123

Perez L, Alvarez-Cermeno JC, Rodriguez C *et al* 1995 B cells capable of spontaneous IgG secretion in cerebrospinal fluid from patients with multiple sclerosis: dependency on local IL-6 production. *Clin Exp Immunol* **101**: 449–452

Pericak-Vance MA, Rimmler JB, Martin ER *et al* 2001 Linkage and association analysis of chromosome 19q13 in multiple sclerosis. *Neurogenetics* **3**: 195–201

Pericak-Vance MA, Rimmler JB, Haines JL *et al* 2004 Investigation of seven proposed regions of linkage in multiple sclerosis: an American and French collaborative study. *Neurogenetics* **5**: 45–48

Pericot I, Brieva L, Tintore M *et al* 2003 Myelopathy in seronegative Sjogren syndrome and/or primary progressive multiple sclerosis. *Mult Scler* **9**: 256–259

Perier O, Gregoire A 1965 Electron microscopic features of multiple sclerosis. *Brain* **88**: 937–952

Perini P, Gallo P 2001 The range of multiple sclerosis associated with neurofibromatosis type 1. *J Neurol Neurosurg Psychiatry* **71**: 679–681

Perini P, Tagliaferri C, Belloni M *et al* 2001 The HLA-DR13 haplotype is associated with 'benign' multiple sclerosis in northeast Italy. *Neurology* **57**: 158–159

Perkin GD, Rose FC 1979 *Optic Neuritis and its Differential Diagnosis*. Oxford: Oxford University Press

Perks WH, Lascelles RG 1976 Paroxysmal brain stem dysfunction as presenting feature of multiple sclerosis. *Br Med J* **2**: 1175–1176

Perlin MW, Lancia G, Ng SK 1995 Toward fully automated genotyping: genotyping microsatellite markers by deconvolution. *Am J Hum Genet* **57**: 1199–1210

Perrin PJ, Maldonado JH, Davis TA *et al* 1996 CTLA-4 blockade enhances clinical disease and cytokine production during experimental allergic encephalomyelitis. *J Immunol* **157**: 1333–1336

Perron H, Geny C, Laurent A *et al* 1989 Leptomeningeal cell line from multiple sclerosis with reverse transcriptase activity and viral particles. *Res Virol* **140**: 551–561

Perron H, Lalande B, Gratacap B *et al* 1991 Isolation of retrovirus from patients with multiple sclerosis. *Lancet* **337**: 862–863

Perron H, Gratacap B, Lalande B et al 1992 In vitro transmission and antigenicity of a retrovirus isolated from a multiple sclerosis patient. Res Virol 143: 337–350

Perron H, Garson JA, Bedin F et al 1997 Molecular identification of a novel retrovirus repeatedly isolated from patients with multiple sclerosis. The Collaborative Research Group on Multiple Sclerosis. Proc Natl Acad Sci USA 94: 7583–7588

Perron H, Jouvin-Marche E, Michel M et al 2001 Multiple sclerosis retrovirus particles and recombinant envelope trigger an abnormal immune response in vitro, by inducing polyclonal Vβ16 T-lymphocyte activation. Virology 287: 321–332

Perron H, Lazarini F, Ruprecht K et al 2005 Human endogenous retrovirus (HERV)-W ENV and GAG proteins: physiological expression in human brain and pathological modulation in multiple sclerosis lesions. J Neurovirol 11: 22–33

Perry LL, Barzaga-Gilbert E, Trotter JL 1991 T cell sensitization to proteolipid protein in myelin basic protein-induced relapsing experimental allergic encephalomyelitis. J Neuroimmunol 33: 7–15

Perry VH 1998 A revised view of the central nervous system microenvironment and major histocompatibility complex class II antigen presentation. J Neuroimmunol 90: 113–121

Perry VH, Tsao JW, Feam S, Brown MC 1995 Inflammation in the nervous system. Curr Opin Neurobiol 5: 636–641

Persson HE, Sachs C 1981 Visual evoked potentials elicited by pattern reversal during provoked visual impairment in multiple sclerosis. Brain 104: 369–382

Pertschuk LP, Cook AW, Gupta J 1976 Measles antigen in multiple sclerosis: identification in the jejunum by immunofluorescence. Life Sci 19: 1603–1608

Peselow ED, Fieve RR, Deutsch SI, Kaufman M 1981 Coexistent manic symptoms and multiple sclerosis. Psychosomatics 22: 824–825

Petajan JH, White AT 2000 Motor-evoked potentials in response to fatiguing grip exercise in multiple sclerosis patients. Clin Neurophysiol 111: 2188–2195

Petajan JH, Gappmaier E, White AT et al 1996 Impact of aerobic training on fitness and quality of life in multiple sclerosis. Ann Neurol 39: 432–441

Peter JB, Boctor FN, Tourtellottee WW 1991 Serum and CSF levels of IL-2, sIL-2R, TNF-alpha, and IL-1-beta: expected lack of clinical utility. Neurology 41: 121–123

Petereit HF, Bamborschke S, Esse AD, Heiss WD 1997 Interferon gamma producing blood lymphocytes are decreased by interferon beta therapy in patients with multiple sclerosis. Mult Scler 3: 180–183

Petereit HF, Lindemann H, Schoppe S 2003 Effect of immunomodulatory drugs on in vitro production of brain-derived neurotrophic factor. Mult Scler 9: 16–20

Peters A, Proskauer CC 1969 The ratio between myelin segments and oligodendrocytes in the optic nerve of adult rats. Anat Rec 163: 243–251

Peters A, Palay SL, Webster HF 1976 The Fine Structure of the Nervous System: The Neurones and Supporting Cells. Philadephia: W.B. Saunders

Peters GB, Bakri SJ, Krohel GB 2002 Cause and prognosis of nontraumatic sixth nerve palsies in young adults. Ophthalmology 109: 1925–1928

Petersen P, Kastrup J, Zeeberg I, Boysen G 1986 Chronic pain treatment with intravenous lidocaine. Neurol Res 8: 189–190

Peterson JW, Bo L, Mork S et al 2001 Transsected neurites, apoptotic neurons and reduced inflammation in cortical multiple sclerosis lesions. Ann Neurol 50: 389–400

Peterson JW, Bo L, Mork S et al 2002 VCAM-1 positive microglia target oligodendrocytes at the border of multiple sclerosis lesions. J Neuropathol Exp Neurol 61: 539–546

Petito CK, Navia BA, Cho E-S, Jordon BD, George DC, Price RW 1986 Vacuolar myelopathy pathologically resembling subacute combined degeneration in patients with acquired immunodeficiency syndrome. N Engl J Med 312: 874–879

Petkau AJ 2003 Statistical approaches to assessing the effects of neutralizing antibodies: IFNβ-1b in the pivotal trial of relapsing–remitting multiple sclerosis. Neurology 61 (Suppl 5): S35–S37

Petkau AJ, White RA, Ebers GC et al 2004 Longitudinal analyses of the effects of neutralizing antibodies on interferon beta-1b in relapsing–remitting multiple sclerosis. Mult Scler 10: 126–138

Petrescu A 1994 Epidemiology of multiple sclerosis in Rumania. In: Firnhaber W, Lauer K (eds) Multiple Sclerosis in Europe: An Epidemiological Update. Darmstadt: Leuhtturm-Verlag/LTV Press, pp. 287–293

Petro DJ, Ellenberger C 1981 Treatment of human spasticity with delta-9 tetrahydrocannibinol. J Clin Pharmacol 21: 4135–4165

Pette H 1928 Über die Pathogenese der multiplen Sklerose. Dtsch Z Nervenheilk 105: 76–132

Pette M, Fujita K, Kitze B et al 1990a Myelin basic protein-specific T lymphocyte lines from MS patients and healthy individuals. Neurology 40: 1770–1776

Pette M, Fujita K, Wilkinson D et al 1990b Myelin autoreactivity in multiple sclerosis: recognition of myelin basic protein in the context of HLA-DR2 products by T lymphocytes of multiple sclerosis patients and healthy donors. Proc Natl Acad Sci USA 87: 7968–7972

Pette M, Pette DF, Muraro PA et al 1997 Interferon-β interferes with the proliferation but not the cytokine secretion of myelin basic protein-specific, T-helper type 1 lymphocytes. Neurology 49: 385–392

Petty GW, Matteson EL, Younge BR et al 2001 Recurrence of Susac syndrome (retinocochleocerebral vasculopathy) after remission of 18 years. Mayo Clin Proc 76: 958–960

Petty MA, Lo EH 2002 Junctional complexes of the blood-brain barrier: permeability changes in neuroinflammation. Progr Neurobiol 68: 311–323

Petzold A, Eikelenboom MJ, Gveric D et al 2002 Markers for different glial cell responses in multiple sclerosis: clinical and pathological correlations. Brain 125: 1462–1473

Petzold A, Eikelenboom MJ, Keir GJ et al 2005 Axonal damage accumulates in the progressive stage of multiple sclerosis: a 3-year follow up study. J Neurol Neurosurg Psychiatry 76: 206–211

Peyser JM, Edwards JR, Poser CM, Filskov SB 1980 Cognitive function in patients with multiple sclerosis. Arch Neurol 37: 577–579

Peyser JM, Rao SM, LaRocca NG, Kaplan E 1990 Guidelines for neuropsychologic research in multiple sclerosis. Arch Neurol 47: 94–97

Pfausler B, Engelhardt K, Kampfl A et al 2002 Post-infectious central and peripheral nervous system diseases complicating Mycoplasma pneumoniae infection: report of three cases and review of the literature. Eur J Neurol 9: 93–96

Phadke JG 1987 Survival patterns and cause of death in patients with multiple sclerosis: results from an epidemiological survey in north east Scotland. J Neurol Neurosurg Psychiatry 50: 523–531

Phadke JG 1990 Clinical aspects of multiple sclerosis in north-east Scotland with particular reference to its course and prognosis. Brain 113: 1597–1628

Phadke JG, Best PV 1983 Atypical and clinically silent multiple sclerosis: a report of 12 cases discovered unexpectedly at necropsy. J Neurol Neurosurg Psychiatry 46: 414–420

Phadke JG, Downie AW 1987 Epidemiology of multiple sclerosis in the North East (Grampian Region) of Scotland – an update. J Epidemiol Commun Hlth 41: 5–13

Pham DL, Prince JL 1999 An adaptive fuzzy C-means algorithm for image segmentation in the presence of intensity in homogeneities. Patt Recog Lett 20: 57–68

Pham DL, Xu C, Prince JL 2000 Current methods in medical image segmentation. Annu Rev Biomed Engl 2: 315–337

Pham-Dinh D, Mattei M-G, Nussbaum J-L et al 1993 Myelin/oligodendrocyte glycoprotein is a member of a subset of the immunoglobulin superfamily encoded within the major histocompatibility complex. Proc Natl Acad Sci USA 90: 7990–7994

Phokeo V, Ball AK 2000 Transection of dysmyelinated optic nerve axons in adult rats lacking myelin basic protein. NeuroReport 11: 3375–3379

Piani D, Frei K, Do K et al 1991 Murine brain macrophages induce NMDA receptor mediated neurotoxicity in vitro by secreting glutamate. Neurosci Lett 133: 159–162

Pichichero ME, Cernichiari E, Lopreiato J, Treanor J 2002 Mercury concentrations and metabolism in infants receiving vaccines containing thiomersal: a descriptive study. *Lancet* **360**: 1737–1741

Pickard C, Mann C, Sinnott P et al 1999 Interleukin-10 (IL10) promoter polymorphisms and multiple sclerosis. *J Neuroimmunol* **101**: 207–210

Pickett GE, Bisnaire D, Ferguson GG 2005 Percutaneous retrogasserian glycerol rhizotomy in the treatment of tic douloureux associated with multiple sclerosis. *Neurosurgery* **56**: 537–45; discussion 537–545

Pickuth D, Heywang-Kobrunner SH 2000 Neurosarcoidosis: evaluation with MRI. *J Neuroradiol* **27**: 185–188

Piddlesden SJ, Morgan BP 1993 Killing of rat glial cells by complement: deficiency of the rat analogue of CD59 is the cause of oligodendrocyte susceptibility to lysis. *J Neuroimmunol* **48**: 169–176

Piddlesden S, Lassmann H, Laffafian I et al 1991 Antibody-mediated demyelination in experimental allergic encephalomyelitis is independent of complement membrane attack complex formation. *Clin Exp Immunol* **83**: 245–250

Piddlesden S, Lassmann H, Zimprich F et al 1993 The demyelinating potential of antibodies to myelin oligodendrocyte glycoprotein is related to their ability to fix complement. *Am J Pathol* **143**: 555–564

Piddlesden SJ, Storch MK, Hibbs M et al 1994 Soluble recombinant complement receptor 1 inhibits inflammation and demyelination in antibody-mediated demyelinating experimental allergic encephalomyelitis. *J Immunol* **152**: 5477–5484

Pierani A, Brenner-Morton S, Chiang C, Jessell TM 1999 A sonic hedgehog-independent, retinoid-activated pathway of neurogenesis in the ventral spinal cord. *Cell* **97**: 903–915

Pierig R, Belliveau J, Amouri R et al 2002 Association of a gliotoxic activity with active multiple sclerosis in US patients. *Cell Mol Biol* **48**: 199–203

Piéron R, Coulaud J M, Debure A et al 1979 Nevrite optique et sarcoidose. *Semaine Hôpitaux* **55**: 137–139

Pihlaja H, Rantamaki T, Wikstrom T et al 2003 Linkage disequilibrium between the MBP tetranucleotide repeat and multiple sclerosis is restricted to a geographically-defined subpopulation in Finland. *Genes Immun* **4**: 138–146

Pina MA, Ara JR, Modrego PJ et al 1998 Prevalence of multiple sclerosis in the sanitary district of Calatayud, Northern Spain: is Spain a zone of high risk for this disease? *Neuroepidemiology* **17**: 258–264

Pina MA, Ara JR, Lasierra P et al 1999 Study of HLA as a predisposing factor and its possible influence on the outcome of multiple sclerosis in the sanitary district of Calatayud, northern Spain. *Neuroepidemiology* **18**: 203–209

Pinching A 1977 Clinical testing of olfaction reassessed. *Brain* **100**: 377–388

Piperidou HN, Heliopoulos IN, Maltezos ES, Milonas IA 2003 Epidemiological data of multiple sclerosis in the province of Evros, Greece. *Eur Neurol* **49**: 8–12

Pirttila T, Nurmikko T 1995 CSF oligoclonal bands, MRI, and the diagnosis of multiple sclerosis. *Acta Neurol Scand* **92**: 468–471

Pirttila T, Haanpaa M, Mehta PD, Lehtimaki T 2000 Apolipoprotein E (APOE) phenotype and APOE concentrations in multiple sclerosis and acute herpes zoster. *Acta Neurol Scand* **102**: 94–98

Pitt D, Werner P, Raine CS 2000 Glutamate excitotoxicity in a model of multiple sclerosis. *Nature Med* **6**: 67–70

Pittock SJ, Keir G, Alexander M et al 2001 Rapid clinical and CSF response to intravenous gamma globulin in acute disseminated encephalomyelitis. *Eur J Neurol* **8**: 725

Pittock SJ, Mayr WT, McClelland RL et al 2004a Change in MS-related disability in a population-based cohort: a 10-year follow-up study. *Neurology* **62**: 51–59

Pittock SJ, Mayr WT, McClelland RL et al 2004b Disability profile of MS did not change over 10 years in a population-based prevalence cohort. *Neurology* **62**: 601–606

Pittock SJ, McClelland RL, Mayr WT et al 2004c Clinical implications of benign multiple sclerosis: a 20-year population-based follow-up study. *Ann Neurol* **56**: 303–306

Pittock SJ, McClelland RL, Mayr WT et al 2004d Prevalence of tremor in multiple sclerosis and associated disability in the Olmsted County population. *Mov Disord* **19**: 1482–1485

Pitzalis C, Sharrack B, Gray IA et al 1997 Comparison of the effects of oral versus intravenous methylprednisolone regimens on peripheral blood T lymphocyte adhesion molecule expression, T cell subsets distribution and TNF alpha concentrations in multiple sclerosis. *J Neuroimmunol* **74**: 62–68

Pizzi M, Sarnico I, Boroni F et al 2004 Prevention of neuron and oligodendrocyte degeneration by interleukin-6 (IL-6) and IL-6 receptor/IL6 fusion protein in organotypic hippocampal slices. *Mol Cell Neurosci* **25**: 301–311

Plant GT, Kermode AG, du Boulay EPGH, McDonald WI 1989 Spasmodic torticollis due to a midbrain lesion in a case of multiple sclerosis. *Mov Disord* **4**: 359–362

Plant GT, Kermode AG, Turano G et al 1992 Symptomatic retrochiasmal lesions in multiple sclerosis: clinical features, visual evoked potentials, and magnetic resonance imaging. *Neurology* **42**: 68–76

Plasma Exchange/Sandoglobulin Guillain–Barré Syndrome Trial Group 1997 Randomised trial of plasma exchange, intravenous immunoglobulin, and combined treatments in Guillain–Barré syndrome. *Lancet* **349**: 225–230

Plata-Salamán CR, ffrench-Mullen JM 1992 Interleukin-1 beta depresses calcium currents in CA1 hippocampal neurons at pathophysiological concentrations. *Brain Res Bull* **29**: 221–223

Plata-Salamán CR, ffrench-Mullen JMH 1993 Interleukin-2 modulates calcium currents in dissociated hippocampal CAI neurons. *NeuroReport* **4**: 579–581

Plata-Salamán CR, Oomura Y, Kai Y 1988 Tumor necrosis factor and interleukin-1beta suppression of food intake by direct action in the central nervous system. *Brain Res* **448**: 106–114

Platz P, Ryder LP, Staub Nielson L et al 1975 HL-A and idiopathic optic neuritis. *Lancet* **i**: 520–521

Plohmann AM, Kappos L, Ammann W et al 1998 Computer assisted retraining of attentional impairments in patients with multiple sclerosis. *J Neurol Neurosurg Psychiatry* **64**: 455–462

Pluchino S, Quattrini A, Brambilla E et al 2003 Injection of adult neurospheres induces recovery in a chronic model of multiple sclerosis. *Nature* **422**: 688–694

Pluchino S, Zanotti L, Rossi B et al 2005 Neurosphere-derived multipotent precursors promote neuroprotection by an immunomodulatory mechanism. *Nature* **436**: 266–271

Plumb J, McQuaid S, Mirakhur M, Kirk J 2002 Abnormal endothelial tight junctions in active lesions and normal appearing white matter in multiple sclerosis. *Brain Pathol* **12**: 199–211

Plumb J, Armstrong MA, Duddy M et al 2003 CD83-positive dendritic cells are present in occasional perivascular cuffs in multiple sclerosis lesions. *Mult Scler* **9**: 142–147

Poeck K, Markus P 1964 Gibt es eine gutartige Verlaufsform der multiplen Sklerose. *Münchener Med Wochenschr* **106**: 2190–2197

Pohl D, Rostasy K, Gartner J, Hanefeld F 2005 Treatment of early onset multiple sclerosis with subcutaneous interferon beta-1a. *Neurology* **64**: 888–890

Poisson M 1984 Sex hormone receptors in human meningiomas. *Clin Neuropharmacol* **7**: 320–324

Polanczyk M, Zamora A, Subramanian S et al 2003 The protective effect of 17beta-estradiol on experimental autoimmune encephalomyelitis is mediated through estrogen receptor-alpha. *Am J Pathol* **163**: 1599–1605

Poland GA, Jacobson RM 2004 Prevention of hepatitis B with the hepatitis B vaccine. *N Engl J Med* **351**: 2832–2838

Pollock M, Calder C, Allpress S 1977 Peripheral nerve abnormality in multiple sclerosis. *Ann Neurol* **2**: 41–48

Polman CH, Matthaei I, De Groot CJA et al 1988 Low-dose cyclosporin A induces relapsing remitting experimental allergic encephalomyelitis in the Lewis rat. *J Neuroimmunol* **17**: 209–216

Polman CH, Bertelsmann FW, de Waal R et al 1994a 4-Aminopyridine is superior to 3,4-diaminopyridine in the treatment of patients with multiple sclerosis. *Arch Neurol* 51: 1136–1139

Polman CH, Bertelsmann FW, van Loenen AC, Koetsier JC 1994b 4-Aminopyridine in the treatment of patients with multiple sclerosis. *Arch Neurol* 51: 292–296

Polman CH, Kappos L, White R et al 2003 Neutralizing antibodies during treatment of secondary progressive MS with interferon beta-1b. *Neurology* 60: 37–43

Polman C, Barkhof F, Sandberg-Wollheim M et al 2005a Treatment with laquinimod reduces development of active MRI lesions in relapsing MS. *Neurology* 64: 987–991

Polman CH, Wolinsky JS, Reingold SC 2005b Multiple sclerosis diagnostic criteria: three years later. *Mult Scler* 11: 5–12

Polman CH, Reingold SC, Edan G et al 2005c Diagnostic criteria for multiple sclerosis: 2005 revisions to the 'McDonald' criteria. *Ann Neurol* 58: 840–846

Pompidou A, Rancurel G, Delsaux MC et al 1986 Clinical and immunological improvement of active multiple sclerosis by isoprinosine treatment: a randomised pilot study. *Presse Med* 15: 930–931

Pon RA, Freedman MS 2003 Study of Herpesvirus saimiri immortalization of γδ T cells derived from peripheral blood and CSF of multiple sclerosis patients. *J Neuroimmunol* 139: 119–132

Ponsonby A-L, van der Mei I, Dwyer T et al 2005 Exposure to infant siblings during early life and risk of multiple sclerosis. *J Am Med Assoc* 293: 463–469

Popko B, Corbin JG, Baerwald KD et al 1997 The effects of interferon-gamma on the central nervous system. *Mol Neurobiol* 14: 19–35

Popov VS 1983 Clinical picture and epidemiology of disseminated sclerosis. *Z Nevropatol Psikhiatr Imeni SS Korsakora* 83: 1330–1334

Popovich PG, Jones TB 2003 Manipulating neuroinflammatory reactions in the injured spinal cord: back to basics. *Trends Pharmacol Sci* 24: 13–17

Popovic N, Schubart A Goetz BD et al 2002 Inhibition of autoimmune encephalomyelitis by a tetracycline. *Ann Neurol* 51: 215–223

Porrini AM, Gambi D, Reder AT 1995 Interferon effects on interleukin-10 secretion: mononuclear cell response to interleukin-10 is normal in multiple sclerosis patients. *J Neuroimmunol* 61: 27–34

Porst H 1997 Transurethral alprostadil with MUSE (medicated urethral system for erection) vs intra-cavernous alprostadil: a comparative study in 103 patients with erectile dysfunction. *Int J Impotence Res* 9: 187–192

Porter B, Keenan E 2003 Nursing at a specialist diagnostic clinic for multiple sclerosis. *Br J Nursing* 12: 650–656

Porter S 2004 An historical whodunit. *Biologist* 51: 109–113

Poser CM 1965 Clinical diagnostic criteria in epidemiological studies of multiple sclerosis. *Ann NY Acad Sci* 122: 506–519

Poser CM 1982 Neurological complications of swine influenza vaccination. *Acta Neurol Scand* 66: 413–431

Poser CM 1987a The peripheral nervous system in multiple sclerosis: a review and pathogenetic hypothesis. *J Neurol Sci* 79: 83–90

Poser CM 1987b Trauma and multiple sclerosis: an hypothesis. *J Neurol* 234: 155–159

Poser CM 1994 The dissemination of multiple sclerosis: a Viking saga? A historical essay. *Ann Neurol* 36 (Suppl 2): S231–S243

Poser CM 1995 Viking voyages: the origin of multiple sclerosis? *Acta Neurol Scand* 161 (Suppl): 11–22

Poser CM 2000 Trauma to the central nervous system may result in formation or enlargement of multiple sclerosis plaques. *Arch Neurol* 57: 1074–1076

Poser CM, Brinar VV 2003 Epilepsy and multiple sclerosis. *Epilepsy Behav* 4: 6–12

Poser CM, Hibberd PL 1988 Analysis of the 'epidemic' of multiple sclerosis in the Faroe Islands. II. Biostatistical aspects. *Neuroepidemiology* 7: 181–189

Poser CM, Vernant J 1993 La sclérose en plaques dans le race noire. *Bull Soc Pathol Exotique* 86: 1–5

Poser CM, Presthus J, Hörsdal O 1966 Clinical characteristics of autopsy-proven multiple sclerosis. *Neurology* 16: 791–798

Poser CM, Paty DW, Scheinberg L et al 1983 New diagnostic criteria for multiple sclerosis: guidelines for research protocols. *Ann Neurol* 13: 227–231

Poser CM, Hibberd PL, Benedicz J, Gudmundsson G 1988 Analysis of the 'epidemic' of multiple sclerosis in the Faroe Islands. I. Clinical and epidemiological aspects. *Neuroepidemiology* 7: 168–180

Poser CM, Roman GC, Vernant J-C 1990 Multiple sclerosis or HTLV-1 myelitis. *Neurology* 40: 1020–1022

Poser CM, Benedikz J, Hibberd PL 1992 The epidemiology of multiple sclerosis: the Iceland model. Onset-adjusted prevalence rate and other methodological considerations. *J Neurol Sci* 111: 143–152

Poser S 1978 Multiple sclerosis. In: *An Analysis of 812 Cases by Means of Electronic Data Processing.* Berlin: Springer-Verlag

Poser S 1994 The epidemiology of multiple sclerosis in southern Lower Saxony. In: Firnhaber W, Lauer K (eds) *Multiple Sclerosis in Europe: An Epidemiological Update.* Darmstadt: Leuchtturm-Verlag/LTV Press: pp. 130–133

Poser S, Hauptvogel H 1973 Clinical data from 418 MS patients in relation to the diagnosis: first experiences with an optical mark reader documentation system. *Acta Neurol Scand* 49: 473–479

Poser S, Kurtzke JF 1991 Epidemiology of MS (letter to the editor). *Neurology* 41: 157–158

Poser S, Poser W 1983 Multiple sclerosis and gestation. *Neurology* 33: 1422–1427

Poser S, Hermann-Grevels I, Wikstrom J, Poser W 1978 Clinical features of the spinal form of multiple sclerosis. *Acta Neurol Scand* 57: 151–158

Poser S, Raun NE, Wikstrom J, Poser W 1979a Pregnancy, oral contraceptives and multiple sclerosis. *Acta Neurol Scand* 59: 108–118

Poser S, Wikström J, Bauer HJ 1979b Clinical data and identification of special forms of multiple sclerosis with a standardised documentation system. *J Neurol Sci* 40: 159–168

Poser S, Bauer HJ, Poser W 1982a Prognosis of multiple sclerosis: results from an epidemiological area in Germany. *Acta Neurol Scnad* 65: 347–354

Poser S, Raun NE, Poser W 1982b Age of onset, initial symptomatology and the course of multiple sclerosis. *Acta Neurol Scand* 66: 355–362

Poser S, Poser W, Schlaf G et al 1986 Prognostic indicators in multiple sclerosis. *Acta Neurol Scand* 74: 387–392

Poser S, Kurtzke JF, Schlaf G 1989a Survival in multiple sclerosis. *J Clin Epidemiol* 42: 159–168

Poser S, Stickel B, Krtsch U et al 1989b Increasing incidence of multiple sclerosis in south Lower Saxony, Germany. *Neuroepidemiology* 8: 207–213

Poser S, Luer W, Bruhn H et al 1992 Acute demyelinating disease: classification and non invasion diagnosis. *Acta Neurol Scand* 86: 597–585

Poskanzer DC, Schapira K, Miller H 1963 Epidemiology of multiple sclerosis in the counties of Northumberland and Durham. *J Neurol Neurosurg Psychiatry* 26: 368–376

Poskanzer DC, Walker AM, Yon Kondi J, Sheridan JL 1976 Studies in the epidemiology of multiple sclerosis in the Orkney and Shetland Islands. *Neurology* 26: 14–17

Poskanzer DC, Prenney LP, Sheridan JL, Yon Kondy J 1980a Multiple sclerosis in the Orkney and Shetland Islands. 1. Epidemiology, clinical factors and methodology. *J Epidemiol Commun Hlth* 34: 229–239

Poskanzer DC, Terasaki PI, Prenney LP et al 1980b Multiple sclerosis in the Orkney and Shetland Islands. III. Histocompatibility determinants. *J Epidemiol Commun Hlth* 34: 253–257

Posner JB 1986 Paraneoplastic syndromes. In: Asbury AK, McKhann GM, McDonald MI (eds) *Diseases of the Nervous System.* Philadephia: W.B. Saunders, pp. 1105–1120

Potemkowski A, Walczak A, Nocon D et al 1994 Epidemiological analysis of multiple sclerosis in the Szczecin Region, north-western part of Poland. In: Firnhaber W, Lauer K (eds) *Multiple Sclerosis in Europe: An Epidemiological Update.* Darmstadt: Leuchtturm-Verlag/LTV Press, pp. 249–254

Powell T, Sussman JG, Davies-Jones GA 1992 MR imaging in acute multiple sclerosis: ringlike appearance in plaques suggesting the presence of paramagnetic free radicals. *Am J Neuroradiol* 13: 1544–1546

Powers JM, Liu Y, Moser AB, Moser HW 1992 The inflammatory myelinopathy of adreno-leukodystrophy: cells, effector molecules, and pathogenetic implications. *J Neuropath Exp Neurol* 51: 630–643

Powers JM, DeCiero DP, Ito M et al H 2000 Adrenomyeloneuropathy: a neuropathologic review featuring its noninflammatory myelopathy. *J Neuropath Exp Neurol* **59**: 89–102

Pozza M, Bettelli C, Aloe L et al 2000 Further evidence for a role of nitric oxide in experimental allergic encephalomyelitis: aminoguanidine treatment modifies its clinical evolution. *Brain Res* **855**: 39–46

Pozzilli C, Passafiume D, Bernardi S et al 1991 SPECT, MRI and cognitive functions in multiple sclerosis. *J Neurol Neurosurg Psychiatry* **54**: 110–115

Pozzilli C, Bastianello S, Koudriavtseva T et al 1996 Magnetic resonance imaging changes with recombinant human interferon-β-1a: a short term study in relapsing–remitting multiple sclerosis. *J Neurol Neurosurg Psychiatry* **61**: 251–258

Pozzilli C, Brunetti M, Amicosante AM et al 2002 Home based management in multiple sclerosis: results of a randomised controlled trial. *J Neurol Neurosurg Psychiatry* **73**: 250–255

Pozzilli C, Palmisano L, Mainero C et al 2004 Relationship between emotional distress in caregivers and health status in persons with multiple sclerosis. *Mult Scler* **10**: 442–446

van Praag H, Schinder AF, Christie BR et al 2002 Functional neurogenesis in the adult hippocampus. *Nature* **415**: 1030–1034

Pradhan S, Mishra VN 2004 A central demyelinating disease with atypical features. *Mult Scler* **10**: 308–315

Pradhan S, Gupta RP, Shashank S, Pandey N 1999 Intravenous immunoglobulin therapy in acute disseminated encephalomyelitis. *J Neurol Sci* **165**: 56–61

Prange AJA, Lauer K, Poser S et al 1986 Epidemiological aspects of multiple sclerosis: a comparative study of four centres in Europe. *Neuroepidemiology* **5**: 71–79

Prasad DV, Nguyen T, Li Z et al 2004 Murine B7-H3 is a negative regulator of T cells. *J Immunol* **173**: 2500–2506

Prasad RS, Smith SJ, Wright H 2003 Lower abdominal pressure versus external bladder stimulation to aid bladder emptying in multiple sclerosis: a randomized controlled study. *Clin Rehab* **17**: 42–47

Prat A, Al-Asmi A, Duquette P, Antel JP 1999 Lymphocyte migration and multiple sclerosis: relation with disease course and therapy. *Ann Neurol* **46**: 253–256

Pratt RTC 1951 An investigation of the psychiatric aspects of disseminated sclerosis. *J Neurol Neurosurg Psychiatry* **14**: 326–336

Pratt RTC, Compston ND, McAlpine D 1951 The familial incidence of multiple sclerosis and its significance. *Brain* **74**: 191–232

Prelog K, Blome S, Dennis C 2003 Neurosarcoidosis of the conus medullaris and cauda equina. *Australas Radiol* **47**: 295–297

Preston SD, Steart PV, Wilkinson A et al 2003 Capillary and arterial cerebral amyloid angiopathy in Alzheimer's disease: defining the perivascular route for the elimination of amyloid beta from the human brain. *Neuropathol Appl Neurobiol* **29**: 106–117

Previdi P, Buzzi P 1992 Paroxysmal dystonia due to a lesion of the cervical cord: case report. *Ital J Neurosci* **13**: 521–523

Pribyl TM, Campagnoni CW, Kampf K et al 1993 The human myelin basic protein gene is included within a 179-kilobase transcription unit: expression in the immune and central nervous system. *Proc Natl Acad Sci USA* **90**: 10695–10699

Pribyl TM, Campagnoni CW, Kampf K et al 1996 Expression of the myelin proteolipid protein gene in human fetal thymus. *J Neuroimmunol* **67**: 125–130

Price P, Cuzner ML 1979 Proteinase inhibitors in cerebrospinal fluid in multiple sclerosis. *J Neurol Sci* **42**: 251–259

Priller J, Flügel A, Wehner T et al 2001 Targeting gene-modified hematopoietic cells to the central nervous system: use of green fluorescent protein uncovers microglial engraftment. *Nature Med* **7**: 1356–1361

Prineas JW 1975 Pathology of the early lesion in multiple sclerosis. *Hum Pathol* **6**: 531–554

Prineas JW 1979 Multiple sclerosis: presence of lymphatic capillaries and lymphoid tissue in the brain and spinal cord. *Science* **203**: 1123–1125

Prineas JW 1985 The neuropathology of multiple sclerosis. In: Koetsier JC (ed.) *Handbook of Clinical Neurology: Demyelinating Diseases*. Amsterdam: Elsevier, Vol 47, pp. 337–395

Prineas JW, Connell F 1979 Remyelination in multiple sclerosis. *Ann Neurol* **5**: 22–31

Prineas JW, Graham JS 1981 Multiple sclerosis: capping of surface immunoglobulin G on macrophages engaged in myelin breakdown. *Ann Neurol* **10**: 149–158

Prineas JW, McDonald WI 1997 Demyelinating disease. In: Graham DI, Lantos PL. *Greenfield's Neuropathology*, 6th edn. London: Arnold, pp. 813–896

Prineas JW, Wright RG 1978 Macrophages, lymphocytes, and plasma cells in the perivascular compartment in chronic multiple sclerosis. *Lab Invest* **38**: 409–421

Prineas JW, Kwon EE, Cho ES, Sharer LR 1984 Continual breakdown and regeneration of myelin in progressive multiple sclerosis plaques. *Ann NY Acad Sci* **436**: 11–32

Prineas JW, Kwon EE, Sharer LR, Cho E-S 1987 Massive early remyelination in acute multiple sclerosis. *Neurology* **37**: 109

Prineas JW, Kwon EE, Goldenberg PZ et al 1989 Multiple sclerosis: oligodendrocyte proliferation and differentiation in fresh lesions. *Lab Invest* **61**: 489–503

Prineas JW, Kwon EE, Goldenberg PZ et al 1990 Interaction of astrocytes and newly formed oligodendrocytes in resolving multiple sclerosis lesions. *Lab Invest* **63**: 624–636

Prineas JW, Barnard RO, Revesz T et al 1993a Multiple sclerosis: pathology of recurrent lesions. *Brain* **116**: 681–693

Prineas JW, Barnard RO, Kwon EE et al 1993b Multiple sclerosis: remyelination of nascent lesions. *Ann Neurol* **33**: 137–151

Prineas JW, Kwon EE, Cho ES et al 2001 Immunopathology of secondary–progressive multiple sclerosis. *Ann Neurol* **50**: 646–657

Pringle CE, Hudson AJ, Munoz DG, Kiernan JA, Brown WF, Ebers GC 1992 Primary lateral sclerosis: clinical features, neuropathology and diagnostic criteria. *Brain* **115**: 495–520

Pringle NP, Richardson WD 1993 A singularity of PDGF alpha receptor expression in the dorsoventral axis of the neural tube may define the origin of the oligodendrocyte lineage. *Development* **117**: 525–533

Pringle NP, Mudhar HS, Collarini EJ, Richardson WD 1992 PDGF receptors in the rat CNS: during late neurogenesis, PDGF alpha-receptor expression appears to be restricted to glial cells of the oligodendrocyte lineage. *Development* **115**: 535–551

Pringle NP, Guthrie S, Lumsden A, Richardson WD 1998 Dorsal spinal cord neuroepithelium generates astrocytes but not oligodendrocytes. *Neuron* **20**: 883–893

Pringle NP, Yu WP, Howell M et al 2003 FGFR3 expression by astrocytes and their precursors: evidence that astrocytes and oligodendrocytes originate in distinct neuroepithelial domains. *Development* **130**: 93–102

Prinjha R, Moore SE, Vinson M, Blake 2000 Inhibitor of neurite outgrowth in humans. *Nature* **403**: 383–384

PRISMS (Prevention of Relapses and Disability by Interferon-beta 1a Subsequently in Multiple Sclerosis) Study Group 1998 Randomised, double-blind, placebo-controlled study of interferon-beta 1a in relapsing–remitting multiple sclerosis: clinical results. *Lancet* **352**: 1498–1504

PRISMS Study Group and University of British Columbia MS MRI Analysis Group 2001 PRISMS-4: long-term efficacy of interferon-beta-1a in relapsing MS. *Neurology* **56**: 1628–1636

Probert L, Akassoglou K, Pasparakis M et al 1995 Spontaneous inflammatory demyelinating disease in transgenic mice showing central nervous system-specific expression of tumor necrosis factor. *Proc Natl Acad Sci USA* **92**: 11294–11298

Probert L, Eugster HP, Akassoglou K et al 2000 TNFR1 signalling is critical for the development of demyelination and the limitation of T-cell responses during immune-mediated CNS disease. *Brain* **123**: 2005–2019

Probst-Cousin S, Kowolik D, Kuchelmeister K et al 2002 Expression of annexin-1 in multiple sclerosis plaques. *Neuropath Appl Neurobiol* **28**: 292–300

Prochazka A, Gorassini M 1998 Ensemble firing of muscle afferents recorded during normal locomotion in cats. *J Physiol* **507**: 293–304

Proescholdt MA, Jacobson S, Tresser N et al 2003 Vascular endothelial growth factor is expressed in multiple sclerosis plaques and can induce inflammatory lesions in experimental allergic encephalomyelitis rats. *J Neuropathol Exp Neurol* **61**: 914–925

907

Propert DN, Bernard CCA, Simons MJ 1982 Gm allotypes in multiple sclerosis. *J Immunogenet* **9**: 359–361

Proudfoot AE 2002 Chemokine receptors: multifaceted therapeutic targets. *Nat Rev Immunol* **2**: 215

Proulx NL, Freedman MS, Chan JW et al 2003 Acute disseminated encephalomyelitis associated with *Pasteurella multocida* meningitis. *Can J Neurol Sci* **30**: 155–158

Provencale J, Bouldin TW 1992 Lupus-related myelopathy: report of three cases and review of literature. *J Neurol Neurosurg Psychiatry* **55**: 830–835

Provencher SW 1993 Estimation of metabolite concentrations from localized in vivo proton NMR spectra. *Magn Reson Med* **30**: 672–679

Pryce G, Ahmed Z, Hankey D et al 2003 Cannabinoids inhibit neurodegeneration in models of multiple sclerosis. *Brain* **126**: 2191–2202

Pryor W (ed.) 2004 *Virginia Woolf and the Raverats: A different sort of friendship.* Bath: Clear Books

Pryse-Phillips WEM 1986 The incidence and prevalence of multiple sclerosis in Newfoundland and Labrador, 1960–1984. *Ann Neurol* **20**: 323–328

Pryse-Phillips WEM, Chandra RK, Rose B 1984 Anaphylactoid reaction to methylprednisolone pulsed therapy for multiple sclerosis. *Neurology* **34**: 1119–1121

Pugliatti M, Sotgiu S, Solinas G et al 2001a Multiple sclerosis epidemiology in Sardinia: evidence for a true increasing risk. *Acta Neurol Scand* **103**: 20–26

Pugliatti M, Solinas G, Sotgiu S et al 2001b Multiple sclerosis distribution in northern Sardinia: spatial cluster analysis of prevalence. *Neurology* **58**: 277–282

Pujol J, Bello J, Deus J et al 1997 Lesions in the left arcuate fasciculus region and depressive symptoms in multiple sclerosis. *Neurology* **49**: 1105–1110

Pulfrich von C 1922 Die Stereoskopie im Dienste der isochromen ünd heterochromen Photometrie. *Naturwissenschaften* **10**: 553–564, 569–574, 596–601, 714–722, 735–743, 751–761

Pulkkinen K, Luomala M, Kuusisto H et al 2004 Increase in CCR5 Delta32/Delta32 genotype in multiple sclerosis. *Acta Neurol Scand* **109**: 342–347

Purba JS, Raadsheer FC, Hofman MA et al 1995 Increased number of corticotrophin releasing hormone (CRH) neurons in the hypothalamic paraventricular nucleus of patients with multiple sclerosis. *Neuroendocrinology* **62**: 62–70

Purves Stewart J 1930 A specific vaccine treatment in disseminated sclerosis. *Lancet* i: 560–564

Putnam TJ 1935 Studies in multiple sclerosis. IV. Encephalitis and sclerotic plaques produced by venular obstruction. *Arch Neurol* **33**: 929–940

Putnam TJ 1936 Studies in multiple sclerosis VII: similarities between some forms of encephalomyelitis and multiple sclerosis. *Arch Neurol Psychiatry* **35**: 1289–1308

Putnam TJ 1938 The centenary of multiple sclerosis. *Arch Neurol Psychiatry* **40**: 806–813

Putnam TJ 1939 Criteria of effective treatment in multiple sclerosis. *J Am Med Assoc* **112**: 2488–2491

Putnam TJ, Adler A 1937 Vascular architecture of the lesions of multiple sclerosis. *Arch Neurol Psychiatry* **38**: 1–15

Qi Y, Cai J, Wu Y et al 2001 Control of oligodendrocyte differentiation by the Nkx2.2 homeodomain transcription factor. *Development* **128**: 2723–2733

Qi Y, Tan M, Hui CC, Qiu M 2003 Gli2 is required for normal Shh signaling and oligodendrocyte development in the spinal cord. *Mol Cell Neurosci* **23**: 440–450

Qin S, Cobbold SP, Pope H et al 1993 'Infectious' transplantation tolerance. *Science* **259**: 974–977

Qin Y, Duquette P, Zhang Y et al 1998 Clonal expansion and somatic hypermutation of V_H genes of B cells from cerebrospinal fluid in multiple sclerosis. *J Clin Invest* **102**: 1045–1050

Qin Y, Zhang DQ, Prat A et al 2000 Characterization of T cell lines derived from glatiramer-acetate-treated multiple sclerosis patients. *J Neuroimmunol* **108**: 201–206

Qiu J, Cai D, Dai H et al 2002 Spinal axon regeneration induced by elevation of cyclic AMP. *Neuron* **34**: 895–903

Quagliariello V, Scheld WM 1992 Bacterial meningitis: pathogenesis, pathophysiology and progress. *N Engl J Med* **327**: 864–872

Quan D, Pelak V, Tanabe J et al 2005 Spinal and cranial hypertrophic neuropathy in multiple sclerosis. *Muscle Nerve* **31**: 772–779

Quarles RH 1989 Glycoproteins of myelin and myelin forming cells. In: Margolis RU, Margolis RK (eds) *Neurobiology of Glycoconjugates.* New York: Plenum Press, pp. 243–275

Quasthoff S, Pojer C, Mori A et al 2003 No blocking effects of the pentapeptide QYNAD on Na+ channel subtypes expressed in Xenopus oocytes or action potential conduction in isolated rat sural nerve. *Neurosci Lett* **352**: 93–96

Quelvennec E, Bera O, Cabre P et al 2003 Genetic and functional studies in multiple sclerosis patients from Martinique attest for a specific and direct role of the HLA-DR locus in the syndrome. *Tissue Antigens* **61**: 166–171

Quesnel S, Feinstein A 2004 Multiple sclerosis and alcohol: a study of problem drinking. *Mult Scler* **10**: 197–201

Raabe TD, Suy S, Welcher A, DeVries GH 1997 Effect of neu differentiation factor isoforms on neonatal oligodendrocyte function. *J Neurosci Res* **50**: 755–768

Rabin J 1973 Hazard of influenza vaccine in neurologic patients. *J Am Med Assoc* **225**: 63–64

Rabins PV, Brooks BR, O'Donnell P et al 1986 Structural brain correlates of emotional disorder in multiple sclerosis. *Brain* **109**: 585–597

Racadot E, Rumbach L, Bataillard M et al 1993 Treatment of multiple sclerosis with anti-CD4 monoclonal antibody. *J Autoimmun* **6**: 771–786

Racke MK, Dhib-Jalbut S, Cannella B et al 1991 Prevention and treatment of chronic relapsing experimental allergic encephalomyelitis by transforming growth factor-β1. *J Immunol* **146**: 3012–3017

Racke MK, Cannella B, Albert P et al 1992 Evidence of endogenous regulatory function of transforming growth factor-beta 1 in experimental allergic encephalomyelitis. *Int Immunol* **4**: 615–620

Racke MK, Bonomo A, Scott DE et al 1994 Cytokine-induced immune deviation as a therapy for inflammatory autoimmune disease. *J Exp Med* **180**: 1961–1966

Radhakrishnan K, Ashok PP, Sridharan R, Mousa ME 1985 Prevalence and pattern of multiple sclerosis in Benghazi, North-Eastern Libya. *J Neurol Sci* **70**: 39–46

Radic MZ, Zouali M 1996 Receptor editing, immune diversification, and self-tolerance. *Immunity* **5**: 505–511

Rafalowska J, Krajewski S, Dolinska E, Dziewulska D 1992 Does damage to perivascular astrocytes in multiple sclerosis participate in blood brain barrier permeability. *Neuropathol Polska* **30**: 73–80

Raff MC 1992 Social controls on cell survival and cell death. *Nature* **356**: 397–400

Raff MC, Miller RH, Noble M 1983 A glial progenitor that develops *in vitro* into an astrocyte or an oligodendrocyte depending on culture medium. *Nature* **303**: 390–396

Raff MC, Williams BP, Miller RH 1984 The *in vitro* differentiation of a bipotential glial progenitor cell. *EMBO J* **3**: 1857–1864

Raff MC, Whitmore AV, Finn JT 2002 Axonal self-destruction and neurodegeneration. *Science* **296**: 868–871

Raine CS 1984 The neuropathology of myelin diseases. In: Morrell P (ed.) *Myelin.* New York: Plenum Press, pp. 259–310

Raine CS 1997 The Norton lecture: a review of the oligodendrocyte in the multiple sclerosis lesion. *J Neuroimmunol* **77**: 135–152

Raine CS, Wu E 1993 Multiple sclerosis: remyelination in acute lesions. *J Neuropathol Exp Neurol* **52**: 199–204

Raine CS, Powers JM, Suzuki K 1974a Acute multiple sclerosis: confirmation of paramyxovirus-like intranuclear inclusions. *Arch Neurol* **30**: 39–46

Raine CS, Snyder DH, Valsamis MP, Stone SH 1974b Chronic experimental encephalomyelitis in inbred guinea pigs: an ultrastructural study. *Lab Invest* **31**: 369–380

Raine CS, Scheinberg L, Waltz JM 1981 Multiple sclerosis: oligodendrocyte survival and proliferation in an active established lesion. *Lab Invest* **45**: 534–546

Raine CS, Cannella B, Dujivestijn AM, Cross AH 1990a Homing to central nervous vasculature by antigen specific lymphocytes. II. Lymphocyte-endothelial cell adhesion during the initial stage of autoimmune demyelination. *Lab Invest* **63**: 476–489

Raine CS, Lee SC, Scheinberg LC et al 1990b Adhesion molecules on endothelial cells in the central nervous system: an emerging area in the neuroimmunology of multiple sclerosis. *Clin Immunol Immunopathol* **57**: 173–187

Raivich G, Bohatschek M, Kloss CUA et al 1999 Neuroglial activation repertoire in the injured brain: graded response, molecular mechanisms and cues to physiological function. *Brain Res Rev* **30**: 77–105

Rajan AJ, Gao Y-L, Raine CS, Brosnan CF 1996 A pathogenic role for γδ-1 cells in relapsing–remitting experimental allergic encephalomyelitis in the SJL mouse. *J Immunol* **157**: 941–949

Rajan AJ, Klein JDS, Brosnan CF 1999 The effect of gamma-delta T cell depletion on cytokine gene expression. *J Immunol* **160**: 5955–5962

Rajda C, Bencsik K, Seres E et al 2003 A genome-wide screen for association in Hungarian multiple sclerosis. *J Neuroimmunol* **143**: 84–87

Rajewsky K 1996 Clonal selection and learning in the antibody system. *Nature* **381**: 751–758

Raknes G, Fernandes Filho JA, Pandey JP et al 2000 IgG allotypes and subclasses in Norwegian patients with multiple sclerosis. *J Neurol Sci* **175**: 111–115

Ramanathan M, Weinstock-Guttman B, Nguyen LT et al 2001 In vivo gene expression revealed by cDNA arrays: the pattern in relapsing–remitting multiple sclerosis patients compared with normal subjects. *J Neuroimmunol* **116**: 213–219

Ramer MS, Priestley JV, McMahon SB 2000 Functional regeneration of sensory axons into the adult spinal cord. *Nature* **403**: 312–316

Ramirez-Lassepas M, Tulloch JW, Quinones MR, Snyder BD 1992 Acute radicular pain as a presenting symptom in multiple sclerosis. *Arch Neurol* **49**: 255–258

Rammohan KW, Rosenberg JH, Lynn DJ et al 2002 Efficacy and safety of modafinil (Provigil) for the treatment of fatigue in multiple sclerosis: a two centre phase 2 study. *J Neurol Neurosurg Psychiatry* **72**: 179–183

Ranscht B, Clapshaw PA, Price J et al 1982 Development of oligodendrocytes and Schwann cells studied with a monoclonal antibody against galactocerebroside. *Proc Natl Acad Sci USA* **79**: 2709–2713

Ransohoff RM 1999 Mechanisms of inflammation in MS tissue: adhesion molecules and chemokines. *J Neuroimmunol* **98**: 57–68

Ransohoff RM, Estes ML 1991 Astrocyte expression of major histocompatibility complex gene products in multiple sclerosis brain tissue obtained by stereotactic biopsy. *Arch Neurol* **48**: 1244–1246

Ransohoff RM, Kivisäkk P, Kidd G 2003 Three or more routes for leukocyte migration into the central nervous system. *Nature Rev Immunol* **3**: 569–581

Ranzato F, Perini P, Tzintzeva E et al 2003 Increasing frequency of multiple sclerosis in Padova, Italy: a 30 year epidemiological survey. *Mult Scler* **9**: 387–392

Rao AB, Richert N, Howard T et al 2002 Methylprednisolone effect on brain volume and enhancing lesions in MS before and during IFNbeta-1b. *Neurology* **59**: 688–694

Rao MS, Noble M, Mayer-Proschel M 1998 A tripotential glial precursor cell is present in the developing spinal cord. *Proc Natl Acad Sci USA* **95**: 3996–4001

Rao SM, Leo GJ 1988 Mood disorder and multiple sclerosis. *Arch Neurol* **45**: 247–248

Rao SM, Hammeke TA, McQuillen MP et al 1984 Memory disturbance in chronic progressive multiple sclerosis. *Arch Neurol* **41**: 625–631

Rao SM, Leo GJ, Haughton VM et al 1989a Correlation of magnetic resonance imaging with neuropsychological testing in multiple sclerosis. *Neurology* **39**: 161–166

Rao SM, Bernardin L, Leo GJ et al 1989b Cerebral disconnection in multiple sclerosis: relationship to atrophy of the corpus callosum. *Arch Neurol* **46**: 918–920

Rao SM, Leo GJ, Bernardin L, Unverzagt F 1991a Cognitive dysfunction in multiple sclerosis. I. Frequency, patterns and predictions. *Neurology* **41**: 685–691

Rao SM, Leo GJ, Ellington L et al 1991b Cognitive dysfunction in multiple sclerosis. II Impact on employment and social functioning. *Neurology* **41**: 692–696

Rao SM, Grafman J, DiGiulio D et al 1993 Memory disturbance in multiple sclerosis: its relation to working memory, semantic encoding and implicit learning. *Neuropsychology* **7**: 364–374

Rapalino O, Lazarov-Spiegler O, Agranov E et al 1998 Implantation of stimulated homologous macrophages results in partial recovery of paraplegic rats. *Nature Med* **4**: 814–821

Rasband MN, Shrager P 2000 Ion channel sequestration in central nervous system axons. *J Physiol* **525**: 63–73

Rasband MN, Trimmer JS 2001 Subunit composition and novel localization of K+ channels in spinal cord. *J Comp Neurol* **429**: 166–176

Rasband MN, Trimmer JS, Schwarz TL et al 1998 Potassium channel distribution, clustering, and function in remyelinating rat axons. *J Neurosci* **18**: 36–47

Rasband MN, Peles E, Trimmer JS et al 1999a Dependence of nodal sodium channel clustering on paranodal axoglial contact in the developing CNS. *J Neurosci* **19**: 7516–7528

Rasband MN, Trimmer JS, Peles E et al 1999b K+ channel distribution and clustering in developing and hypomyelinated axons of the optic nerve. *J Neurocytol* **28**: 319–331

Rasche D, Kress B, Schwark C et al 2004 Treatment of trigeminal neuralgia associated with multiple sclerosis: case report. *Neurology* **63**: 1714–1715

Rashid W, Parkes LM, Ingle GT et al 2004 Abnormalities of cerebral perfusion in multiple sclerosis. *J Neurol Neurosurg Psychiatry* **75**: 1288–1293

Rasminsky M 1973 The effects of temperature on conduction in demyelinated single nerve fibers. *Arch Neurol* **28**: 287–292

Rasminsky M 1978 Ectopic generation of impulses and cross-talk in spinal nerve roots of 'dystrophic' mice. *Ann Neurol* **3**: 351–357

Rasminsky M 1980 Ephaptic transmission between single nerve fibres in the spinal nerve roots of dystrophic mice. *J Physiol* **305**: 151–169

Rasminsky M 1987 Spontaneous activity and cross-talk in pathological nerve fibers. *Res Publ Assoc Res Nerv Mental Dis* **65**: 39–49

Rasminsky M, Sears TA 1972 Internodal conduction in undissected demyelinated nerve fibres. *J Physiol* **227**: 323–350

Rasmussen HB, Geny C, Deforges L et al 1995 Expression of endogenous retroviruses in blood mononuclear cells and brain tissue from multiple sclerosis patients. *Mult Scler* **1**: 82–87

Rasmussen HB, Kelly MA, Francis DA, Clausen J 2000 Association between the endogenous retrovirus HRES-1 and multiple sclerosis in the United Kingdom – evidence of genetically different disease subsets? *Disease Markers* **16**: 101–104

Rasmussen HB, Kelly MA, Clausen J 2001a Additive effect of the HLA-DR15 haplotype on susceptibility to multiple sclerosis. *Mult Scler* **7**: 91–93

Rasmussen HB, Kelly MA, Clausen J 2001b Genetic susceptibility to multiple sclerosis: detection of polymorphic nucleotides and an intron in the 3' untranslated region of the major histocompatibility complex class II transactivator gene. *Hum Immunol* **63**: 371–377

Rasmussen HB, Kelly MA, Francis DA, Clausen J 2001c CTLA4 in multiple sclerosis: lack of genetic association in a European Caucasian population but evidence of interaction with HLA-DR2 among Shaghai Chinese. *J Neurol Sci* **184**: 143–147

Ravaglia S, Ceroni M, Moglia A et al 2004 Post-infectious and post-vaccinal acute disseminated encephalomyelitis occurring in the same patients. *J Neurol* **251**: 1147–1150

Rawson MD, Liversedge LA 1969 Treatment of retrobulbar neuritis with corticotrophin. *Lancet* **ii**: 222

Rawson MD, Liversedge LA, Goldfarb G, McGill BA 1966 Treatment of acute retrobulbar neuritis with corticotrophin. *Lancet* **ii**: 1044–1046

Ray CL, Dreizin IJ 1996 Bilateral optic neuropathy associated with influenza vaccination. *J Neuroophthalmol* **16**: 182–184

Raymond GV 2002 Progressive cerebral degeneration of childhood. In: Asbury AK, McKann GM, McDonald WI et al (eds)

Diseases of the Nervous System, 3rd edn. Cambridge: Cambridge University Press, pp. 1911–1921

Read CF 1932 Multiple sclerosis and Lhermitte's sign. *Arch Neurol Psychiatry* **27**: 227–228

Reboul J, Mertens C, Levillayer F et al 2000 Cytokines in genetic susceptibility to multiple sclerosis: a candidate gene approach. *J Neuroimmunol* **102**: 107–112

de Recondo A, Guichard JP 1997 Acute disseminated encephalomyelitis presenting as multiple cystic lesions. *J Neurol Neurosurg Psychiatry* **63**: 15

Reddy EP, Sandberg-Wollheim M, Mettus RV et al 1989 Amplification and molecular cloning of HTLV-1 sequences from DNA of multiple sclerosis patients. *Science* **243**: 529–533

Reddy H, Narayanan S, Arnoutelis R et al 2000 Evidence for adaptive functional changes in the cerebral cortex with axonal injury from multiple sclerosis. *Brain* **123**: 2314–2320

Reddy H, Narayanan S, Woolrich M et al 2002 Functional brain reorganization for hand movement in patients with multiple sclerosis: defining distinct effects of injury and disability. *Brain* **125**: 2646–2657

Reder AT, Arnason BGW 1985 Immunology of multiple sclerosis. In: Koetsier JC (ed.) *Handbook of Clinical Neurology: Demyelinating Diseases*. Amsterdam: Elsevier, Vol 47, pp. 337–395

Reder AT, Arnason BG 1995 Trigeminal neuralgia in multiple sclerosis relieved by a prostraglandin E analogue. *Neurology* **45**: 1097–1100

Reder AT, Makowiec RL, Lowy MT 1994 Adrenalin size is increased in multiple sclerosis. *Arch Neurol* **51**: 151–154

Redford EJ, Hall SM, Smith KJ 1995 Vascular changes and demyelination induced by the intraneural injection of tumour necrosis factor. *Brain* **118**: 869–878

Redford EJ, Kapoor R, Smith KJ 1997 Nitric oxide donors reversibly block axonal conduction: demyelinated axons are especially susceptible. *Brain* **120**: 2149–2157

Reding M, La Rocca N 1987 Acute hospital care versus rehabilitation hospitalization for management of nonemergent complications in multiple sclerosis. *J Neurol Rehab* **1**: 13–17

Redlich E 1896 Zur Pathologie der multiplen Sklerose. *Arbeit Neurol Inst (Obersteiner Arbeit)* **IV**: 1–34

Rees LH, Grant DB, Wilson J 1975 Plasma corticotrophin levels in Addison–Schilder's disease. *Br Med J* **3**: 201–202

Regan D, Silver R, Murray JT 1977 Visual acuity and contrast sensitivity in multiple sclerosis: hidden visual loss. *Brain* **100**: 563–579

Reich D, Patterson N, De Jager PL et al 2005 A whole-genome admixture scan finds a candidate locus for multiple sclerosis susceptibility. *Nat Genet* **37**: 1113–1118

Reichert F, Rotshenker S 1996 Deficient activation of microglia during optic nerve degeneration. *J Neuroimmunol* **70**: 153–161

Reichert F, Rotshenker S 2003 Complement-receptor-3 and scavenger-receptor-AI/II mediated myelin phagocytosis in microglia and macrophages. *Neurobiol Dis* **12**: 65–72

Reidel MA, Stippich C, Heiland S et al 2003 Differentiation of multiple sclerosis plaques, subacute cerebral ischaemic infarcts, focal vasogenic oedema and lesions of subacute arteriosclerotic encephalopathy using magnetisation transfer measurements. *Neuroradiology* **45**: 289–294

Reik L 2002 *Neurosyphilis*. In: Asbury AK, McKann GM, McDonald WI et al (eds) *Diseases of the Nervous System*, 3rd edn. Cambridge: Cambridge University Press, pp. 1766–1776

Reik L, Burgdorfer W, Donaldson JO 1986 Neurologic abnormalities in Lyme disease without erythema chronicum migrans. *Am J Med* **81**: 73–78

Reimers D, Lopez-Toledano MA, Mason I et al 2001 Developmental expression of fibroblast growth factor (FGF) receptors in neural stem cell progeny: modulation of neuronal and glial lineages by basic FGF treatment. *Neurol Res* **23**: 612–621

Reindl M, Linington C, Brehm U et al 1999 Antibodies against the myelin oligodendrocyte glycoprotein and the myelin basic protein in multiple sclerosis and other neurological diseases: a comparative study. *Brain* **122**: 2047–2056

Reindl M, Khantane S, Ehling R et al 2003 Serum and cerebrospinal fluid antibodies to Nogo-A in patients multiple sclerosis and acute neurological disorders. *J Neuroimmunol* **145**: 139–147

Reingold SC 1990 Fatigue and multiple sclerosis. *MS News Mult Scler Soc Gt Br N Ireland* **142**: 30–31

Reinherz EL, Weiner HL, Hauser SL et al 1980 Loss of suppressor cells in active multiple sclerosis. *N Engl J Med* **303**: 125–129

Reis e Sousa C 2001 Dendritic cells as sensors of infection. *Immunity* **14**: 495–498

Reiser H, Stadecker MJ 1996 Costimulatory B7 molecules in the pathogenesis of infectious and autoimmune diseases. *N Engl J Med* **335**: 1369–1377

Reith KG, DiChiro G, Cromwell LD et al 1981 Primary demyelinating disease simulating glioma of the corpus callosum. *J Neurosurg* **55**: 620–624

Relvas JB, Setzu A, Baron W et al 2001 Expression of dominant-negative and chimeric subunits reveals an essential role for beta1 integrin during myelination. *Curr Biol* **11**: 1039–1043

Remlinger P 1928 Les paralysies due traitement antirabique. *Ann Inst Pasteur* **55 (Suppl)**: 35–68

Renfrew C 2002 Genetics and language in contemporary archaelogy. In: Cunliffe B, Davies W, Renfrew C. *Archaeology: The Widening Debate*. London: Oxford University Press, pp. 43–76

Renganathan M, Cummins TR, Hormuzdiar WN et al 2000 Nitric oxide is an autocrine regulator of Na^+ currents in axotomized C-type DRG neurons. *J Neurophysiol* **83**: 2431–2442

Renganathan M, Cummins TR, Waxman SG 2002 Nitric oxide blocks fast, slow, and persistent Na+ channels in C-type DRG neurons by S-nitrosylation. *J Neurophysiol* **87**: 761–775

Renganathan M, Gelderblom M, Black JA, Waxman SG 2003 Expression of Nav1.8 sodium channels perturbs the firing patterns of cerebellar Purkinje cells. *Brain Res* **959**: 235–242

Renno T, Zeine R, Girard JM, Gillani S, Dodelet V, Owens T 1994 Selective enrichment of Th1 CD45RB[low] CD4[+] T cells in autoimmune infiltrates in experimental allergic encephalomyelitis. *Int Immunol* **6**: 347–354

Renno T, Krakowski M, Piccirillo C et al 1995 TNF-alpha expression by resident microglia and infiltrating leukocytes in the central nervous system of mice with experimental allergic encephalomyelitis. Regulation by Th1 cytokines. *J Immunol* **154**: 944–953

Rep MH, Hintzen RQ, Polman CH, van Lier RA 1996 Recombinant interferon-beta blocks proliferation but enhances interleukin-10 secretion by activated human T-cells. *J Neuroimmunol* **67**: 111–118

Requena I, Arias M, López-Ibor L et al 1991 Cavernomas of the central nervous system: clinical and neuroimaging manifestations in 47 patients. *J Neurol Neurosurg Psychiatry* **54**: 590–594

Reth M 1989 Antigen receptor tail clue. *Nature* **338**: 383–384

Reubinoff BE, Itsykson P, Turetsky T et al 2001 Neural progenitors from human embryonic stem cells. *Nat Biotechnol* **19**: 1134–1140

Reulen JPH, Sanders EACM, Hogenhuis LAH 1983 Eye movement disorders in multiple sclerosis and optic neuritis. *Brain* **106**: 121–140

Reunanen K, Finnila S, Laaksonen M et al 2002 Chromosome 19q13 and multiple sclerosis susceptibility in Finland: a linkage and two-stage association study. *J Neuroimmunol* **126**: 134–142

Revel M, Chebath J, Mangelus M et al 1995 Antagonsim of interferon beta in interferon gamma: inhibition of signal transduction *in vitro* and reduction of serum levels in multiple sclerosis patients. *Mult Scler* **1**: S5–S11

Revel MP, Valiente E, Gray F et al 1993 Concentric MR patterns in multiple sclerosis: report of two cases. *J Neuroradiol* **20**: 252–257

Revesz T, Kidd D, Thompson AJ et al 1994 A comparison of the pathology of primary and secondary progressive multiple sclerosis. *Brain* **117**: 759–765

Revol A, Vighetto A, Confavreux C et al 1990 Myoclonies oculo-velo-palatines et sclérose en plaques. *Rev Neurol* **146**: 518–521

Revy P, Sospedra M, Barbour B, Trautmann A 2001 Functional antigen-independent synapses formed between T cells and dendritic cells. *Nat Immunol* **2**: 925–931

Reynier P, Penisson-Besnier I, Moreau C et al 1999 mtDNA haplotyping J: a contributing factor of optic neuritis. *Eur J Hum Genet* **7**: 404–406

Reynolds ES 1904 Some cases of family disseminated sclerosis. *Brain* **27**: 163–169

Reynolds JR (ed.) 1868 *A System of Medicine*, Vol 2. London: Macmillan

Reynolds R, Dawson M, Papadopoulos D et al 2002 The response of NG2-expressing oligodendrocyte progenitors to demyelination in MOG-EAE and MS. *J Neurocytol* **31**: 523–536

Reznik M, Franck G, Flandroy P, Lenelle J 1994 Syndrome médullaire pseudo-tumorale rélévant une sclérose en plaques probable débutante. Corrélations cliniques radiologiques et neuropathologiques. *Acta Neurol Belg* **94**: 8–16

Ribeton J 1919 *Etude clinique des douleurs à forme de décharge electrique consécutives aux traumatismes de la nuque*, Thèse de la Faculté de Médicine de l'Université de Paris, pp. 9–68

Ricard D, Stankoff B, Bagnard D et al 2000 Differential expression of collapsin response mediator proteins (CRMP/ULIP) in subsets of oligodendrocytes in the postnatal rodent brain. *Mol Cell Neurosci* **16**: 324–337

Rice CL, Vollmer TL, Bigland-Ritchie B 1992 Neuromuscular responses of patients with multiple sclerosis. *Muscle Nerve* **15**: 1123–1132

Rice CM, Scolding NJ 2004 Adult stem cells – reprogramming neurological repair? *Lancet* **364**: 193–199

Rice GP, Dickey C, Lesaux J, Vandervoort P, MacEwan L, Ebers GC 1995 Ondanestron for disabling cerebellar tremor. *Ann Neurol* **38**: 973

Rice GP, Ebers GC, Lublin FD, Knobler RL 1999 Ibuprofen treatment versus gradual introduction of interferon beta-1b in patients with MS. *Neurology* **52**: 1893–1895

Rice GP, Filippi M, Comi G 2000 Cladribine and progressive MS: clinical and MRI outcomes of a multicenter controlled trial. Cladribine MRI Study Group. *Neurology* **54**: 1145–1155

Rice GP, Incorvaia B, Munari L et al 2001 Interferon in relapsing-remitting multiple sclerosis. *Cochrane Database Syst Rev* **4**: CD002002

Rice-Oxley M, Rees JR, Williams ES 1995 A prevalence survey of multiple sclerosis in Sussex. *J Neurol Neurosurg Psychiatry* **58**: 27–30

Rich MM, Pinter MJ, Kraner SD, Barchi RL 1998 Loss of electrical excitability in an animal model of acute quadriplegic myopathy. *Ann Neurol* **43**: 171–179

Richards M, Corte-Real H, Forster P et al 1996 Paleolithic and neolithic lineages in the European mitochondrial gene pool. *Am J Hum Genet* **59**: 185–203

Richards PT, Cuzner ML 1978 Proteolytic activity in CSF. *Adv Exper Med Biol* **100**: 521–527

Richardson JH, Wucherpfennig KW, Endo N et al 1989 PCR analysis of DNA from multiple sclerosis patients for the presence of HTLV-1. *Science* **246**: 821–823

Richert JR, Robinson ED, Deibler GE et al 1989 Human cytotoxic T-cell recognition of a synthetic peptide of myelin basic protein. *Ann Neurol* **26**: 342–346

Richert ND, Ostuni JL, Bash CN et al 2001 Interferon beta-1b and intravenous methylprednisolone promote lesion recovery in multiple sclerosis. *Mult Scler* **7**: 49–58

Richey ET, Kooi KA, Tourtellotte WW 1971 Visually evoked responses in multiple sclerosis. *J Neurol Neurosurg Psychiatry* **34**: 275–280

Richie LI, Ebert PJR, Wu LC et al 2002 Imaging synapse formation during thymocyte selection: inability of CD3 to form a stable central accumulation during negative selection. *Immunity* **16**: 595–606

Ridet JL, Malhotra SK, Privat A, Gage FH 1997 Reactive astrocytes: cellular and molecular cues to biological function. *Trends Neurosci* **20**: 570–577

Ridley A, Schapira K 1961 Influence of surgical procedures on the course of multiple sclerosis. *Neurology* **11**: 81–92

Rieckmann P, Toyka KV 1999 Escalating immunotherapy of multiple sclerosis. Austrian–German–Swiss Multiple Sclerosis Therapy Consensus Group [MSTCG]. *Eur Neurol* **42**: 121–127

Rieckmann P, Nunke K, Burchhardt M et al 1993 Soluble intercellular adhesion molecule-1 in cerebrospinal fluid: an indicator for the inflammatory impairment of the blood-cerebrospinal fluid barrier. *J Neuroimmunol* **47**: 133–140

Rieckmann P, Michel U, Albrecht M et al 1995 Soluble forms of intercellular adhesion molecule-1 (ICAM-1) block lymphocyte attachment to cerebral endothelial cells. *J Neuroimmunol* **60**: 9–15

Rieckmann P, Weber F, Gunther A et al 1996 Pentoxyfilline, a phosphodiesterase inhibitor, induces immune deviation in patients with multiple sclerosis. *J Neuroimmunol* **64**: 193–200

Riedel K, Kempf VA, Bechtold A, Klimmer M 2001 Acute disseminated encephalomyelitis (ADEM) due to *Mycoplasma pneumoniae* infection in an adolescent. *Infection* **29**: 240–242

Rietberg MB, Brooks D, Uitdehaag BM, Kwakkel G 2005 Exercise therapy for multiple sclerosis. *Cochrane Database Syst Rev* **1**: CD003980

Riikonen R 1989 The role of infection and vaccination in the genesis of optic neuritis and multiple sclerosis in children. *Acta Neurol Scand* **80**: 425–431

Riikonen R, Donner M, Erkkilä H 1988 Optic neuritis in children and its relationship to multiple sclerosis: a clinical study of 21 children. *Dev Med Child Neurol* **30**: 349–359

Riise T 1997 Cluster studies in multiple sclerosis. *Neurology* **49 (Suppl 2)**: S27–S32

Riise T, Klauber MR 1992 Relationship between the degree of individual space-time clustering and the age at onset of disease among multiple sclerosis patients. *Int J Epidemiol* **21**: 528–532

Riise T, Gronning M, Aarli JA et al 1988 Prognostic factors for life expectancy in multiple sclerosis analysed by Cox-models. *J Clin Epidemiol* **41**: 1031–1036

Riise T, Gronning M, Klauber MR et al 1991 Clustering of residence of multiple sclerosis patients at age 13–20 years in Hordaland, Norway. *Am J Epidemiol* **133**: 932–939

Riise T, Gronning M, Fernández O et al 1992 Early prognostic factors for disability in multiple sclerosis, a European multicenter study. *Acta Neurol Scand* **85**: 212–218

Riise T, Nortdedt MW, Ascherio A 2003 Smoking is a risk factor for multiple sclerosis. *Neurology* **61**: 1122–1124

Riley D, Lang AE 1988 Hemiballismus in multiple sclerosis. *Mov Disord* **3**: 88–94

Rindfleisch E 1863 Histologisches Detail zur grauen Degeneration von Gehirn und Rückenmark. *Arch Pathol Anat Physiol Klin Med (Virchow)* **26**: 474–483

Ringel RA, Riggs JE, Brick JF 1988 Reversible coma with prolonged absence of pupillary and brainstem reflexes: an unusual response to a hypoxic-ischemic event in MS. *Neurology* **38**: 1275–1278

Rinne UK 1980 Tizanidine treatment of spasticity in multiple sclerosis and chronic myelopathy. *Curr Ther Res* **28**: 827–836

Rio J, Montalban X 2000 Ibuprofen treatment versus gradual introduction of interferon beta-1b in patients with MS. *Neurology* **54**: 1710

Rio J, Nos C, Marzo ME et al 1998 Low-dose steroids reduce flu-like symptoms at the initiation of IFNbeta-1b in relapsing–remitting MS. *Neurology* **50**: 1910–1912

del Río Hortega H 1939 The microglia. *Lancet* **1**: 1023–1026

del Río Hortega P 1921 Estudios sobre la neuroglia. La glia de escasas radiaciones (oligodendroglia). *Boletin Real Soc Esp Hist Nat* **21**: 63–92

Riordan-Eva P, Sanders MD, Govan GG et al 1995 The clinical features of Leber's hereditary optic neuropathy defined by the presence of a pathogenic mitochondrial DNA mutation. *Brain* **118**: 319–337

Risau W 1991 Induction of blood-brain barrier endothelial cell differentiation. *Ann NY Acad Sci* **633**: 405–419

Risch NJ 1990a Linkage strategies for genetically complex traits. I. Multilocus models. *Am J Hum Genet* **46**: 222–228

Risch NJ 1990b Linkage strategies for genetically complex traits. II. The power of affected relative pairs. *Am J Hum Genet* **46**: 229–241

Risch NJ 1990c Linkage strategies for genetically complex traits. III. The effect of marker polymorphism on the analysis of affected relative pairs. *Am J Hum Genet* **46**: 242–253

Risch NJ 2000 Searching for genetic determinants in the new millennium. *Nature* **405**: 847–856

Risch NJ, Merikangas K 1996 The future of genetic studies of complex human diseases. *Science* **273**: 1516–1517

911

Risch NJ, Teng J 1998 The relative power of family-based and case-control designs for linkage disequilibrium studies of complex human diseases I. DNA pooling. *Genome Res* 8: 1273–1288

Rischbieth RHC 1968 Retrobulbar neuritis in the State of South Australia. *Proc Aust Soc Neurologists* 5: 573–575

Riser M, Géraud G, Rascol A *et al* 1971 L'évolution de la sclérose en plaques: Etude de 203 observations suivies au-delà de 10 ans. *Rev Neurol* 124: 479–486

Risien Russell JS 1899 Disseminate sclerosis. In: Clifford Allbutt T (ed.) *A System of Medicine*, Vol VII. London: Macmillan, pp. 50–96

Rissoan M-C, Soumelis V, Kadowaki N *et al* 1999 Reciprocal control of T helper cell and dendritic cell differentiation. *Science* 283: 1183–1186

Ristori G, Carcassi C, Lai S *et al* 1997 HLA-DM polymorphisms do not associate with multiple sclerosis: an association study with analysis of myelin basic protein T cell specificity. *J Neuroimmunol* 77: 181–184

Ristori G, Buzzi MG, Sabatini U *et al* 1999 Use of Bacille Calmette-Guérin (BCG) in multiple sclerosis. *Neurology* 53: 1588–1589

Ristori G, Giunti D, Perna A *et al* 2000 Myelin basic protein intramolecular spreading without disease progression in a patient with multiple sclerosis. *J Neuroimmunol* 110: 240–243

Ritchie AM, Gilden DH, Williamson AR *et al* 2004 Comparative analysis of the CD19+ and CD138+ cell antibody repertoires in the cerebrospinal fluid of patients with multiple sclerosis. *J Immunol* 173: 649–656

Ritchie JM, Rang HP, Pellegrino R 1981 Sodium and potassium channels in demyelinated and remyelinated mammalian nerve. *Nature* 294: 257–259

Ritter G, Poser S 1974 Epilepsie ünd multiple Sklerose. *Münchener Med Wochenschr* 116: 1984–1986

Rivera-Quinones C, MacGavern D, Schmelzer JD *et al* 1998 Absence of neurological deficits following extensive demyelination in a class I-deficient murine model of multiple sclerosis. *Nature Med* 4: 187–193

Rivers TM, Schwentker FF 1935 Encephalomyelitis accompanied by myelin destruction experimentally produced in monkeys. *J Exp Med* 61: 689–702

Rivers TM, Sprunt DH, Berry GP 1933 Observations on attempts to produce acute disseminated encephalomyelitis in monkeys. *J Exp Med* 58: 39–53

Rivkin MJ, Flax J, Mozell R *et al* 1995 Oligodendroglial development in human fetal cerebrum. *Ann Neurol* 38: 92–101

Rizzo JF, Lessell S 1988 Risk of developing multiple sclerosis after uncomplicated optic neuritis: a long term prospective study. *Neurology* 38: 185–190

Rizzo JF, Lessell S 1991 Optic neuritis and ischemic optic neuropathy: overlapping clinical profiles. *Arch Ophthalmol* 109: 1668–1672

Rizzo M, Kellison IL 2004 Eyes, brains, and autos. *Arch Ophthalmol* 122: 641–647

Rizzo MA, Kocsis JD, Waxman SG 1996 Mechanisms of paresthesiae, dysesthesiae, and hyperesthesiae: role of Na channel heterogeneity. *Eur Neurol* 36: 3–12

Roberts DF 1986 Who are the Orcadians? *Anthrop Anzeiger* 44: 93–104

Roberts DF 1991 Consanguinity and multiple sclerosis in Orkney. *Genet Epidemiol* 8: 147–151

Roberts DF, Bates D 1982 The genetic contribution to multiple sclerosis: evidence from north east England. *J Neurol Sci* 54: 287–293

Roberts DF, Papiha SS 1979 Polymorphisms and multiple sclerosis in Orkney. *J Epidemiol Commun Hlth* 33: 236–242

Roberts DF, Roberts MJ 1979 Genetic analysis of multiple sclerosis in Orkney. *J Epidemiol Commun Hlth* 33: 229–235

Roberts DF, Roberts MJ, Poskanser DC 1983 Genetic analysis of multiple sclerosis in Shetland. *J Epidemiol Commun Hlth* 37: 281–285

Roberts MHW, Martin JP, McLelland L *et al* 1991 The prevalence of multiple sclerosis in the Southampton South West Hampshire Health Authority. *J Neurol Neurosurg Psychiatry* 54: 55–59

Robertson NP, Deans J, Fraser M, Compston DAS 1995 Multiple sclerosis in the north Cambridgeshire districts of East Anglia. *J Neurol Neurosurg Psychiatry* 59: 71–76

Robertson NP, Deans J, Fraser M, Compston DAS 1996a The south Cambridgeshire multiple sclerosis register: a three year update. *J Epidemiol Commun Hlth* 50: 274–279

Robertson NP, Fraser M, Deans J *et al* 1996b Age adjusted recurrence risks for relatives of patients with multiple sclerosis. *Brain* 119: 449–455

Robertson NP, Clayton D, Fraser MB *et al* 1996c Clinical concordance in sibling pairs with multiple sclerosis. *Neurology* 47: 347–352

Robertson NP, O'Riordan JI, Chataway J *et al* 1997 Clinical characteristics and offspring recurrence rates of conjugal multiple sclerosis. *Lancet* 349: 1587–1590

Robertson WF 1897 The normal histology and pathology of the neuroglia (in relation specially to mental diseases). *J Mental Sci* 43: 733–752

Robertson WF 1899 On a new method of obtaining a black reaction in certain tissue elements of the central nervous system (platinum method). *Scot Med Surg J* 4: 23–30

Robey E, Itano A, Fanslow WC, Fowlkes BJ 1994 Constitutive CD8 expression allows inefficient maturation of CD4 helper T cells in class II major histocompatibility complex mutant mice. *J Exp Med* 179: 1997–2004

Robinson K, Rudge P 1977 Abnormalities of the auditory evoked potentials in patients with multiple sclerosis. *Brain* 100: 19–40

Robinson WH, Fontoura P, Lee BJ *et al* 2003 Protein microarrays guide tolerizing DNA vaccine treatment of autoimmune encephalomyelitis. *Nat Biotechnol* 21: 1033–1039

Rocca MA, Colombo B, Pratesi A *et al* 2000 A magnetization transfer imaging study of the brain in patients with migraine. *Neurology* 54: 507–509

Rocca MA, Filippi M, Herzog J *et al* 2001 A magnetic resonance imaging study of the cervical cord in patients with CADASIL. *Neurology* 56: 1392–1394

Rocca MA, Falini A, Colombo B *et al* 2002a Adaptive functional changes in the cerebral cortex of patients with nondisabling multiple sclerosis correlate with the extent of brain structural damage. *Ann Neurol* 51: 330–339

Rocca MA, Matthews PM, Caputo D *et al* 2002b Evidence for widespread movement-associated functional MRI changes in patients with PPMS. *Neurology* 58: 866–872

Rocca MA, Gavazzi C, Mezzapesa DM *et al* 2003a A functional magnetic resonance imaging study of patients with secondary progressive multiple sclerosis. *Neuroimage* 19: 1770–1777

Rocca MA, Mezzapesa DM, Falini A *et al* 2003b Evidence for axonal pathology and adaptive cortical reorganization in patients at presentation with clinically isolated syndromes suggestive of multiple sclerosis. *Neuroimage* 18: 847–855

Rocca MA, Iannucci G, Rovaris M *et al* 2003c Occult tissue damage in patients with primary progressive multiple sclerosis is independent of T2 visible lesions – a diffusion tensor MR study. *J Neurol* 250: 456–460

Rocca MA, Pagani E, Ghezzi A *et al* 2003d Functional cortical changes in patients with multiple sclerosis and nonspecific findings on conventional magnetic resonance imaging scans of the brain. *Neuroimage* 19: 826–836

Rocca MA, Falini A, Colombo B *et al* 2004 Is an altered pattern of cortical activations in patients at presentation with clinically isolated syndromes suggestive of MS influence the subsequent evolution to definite MS? *J Neurol* 251: 51

Rocca MA, Mezzapesa DM, Ghezzi A *et al* 2005 A widespread pattern of cortical activations in patients at presentation with clinically isolated syndromes is associated with evolution to definite multiple sclerosis. *Am J Neuroradiol* 26: 1136–1139

Rodewald H-R, Paul S, Haller C *et al* 2001 Thymus medulla consisting of epithelial islets each derived from a single progenitor. *Nature* 414: 763–768

Rodgers MM, Mulcare JA, King DL *et al* 1999 Gait characteristics of individuals with multiple sclerosis before and after a 6-month aerobic training program. *J Rehab Res Development* 36: 183–188

Rodgers JR, Cook RG 2005 MHC class Ib molecules bridge innate and acquired immunity. *Nature Rev Immunol* 5: 459–471

Rodriguez D, Della Gaspera B, Zalc B *et al* 1997 Identification of a Val 145 Ile substitution in the human myelin oligodendrocyte glycoprotein: lack of association with multiple sclerosis. *Mult Scler* **3**: 377–381

Rodriguez M 1992 Central nervous system demyelination and remyelination in multiple sclerosis and viral models of disease. *J Neuroimmunol* **40**: 255–263

Rodriguez M 2003 A function of myelin is to protect axons from subsequent injury: implications for deficits in multiple sclerosis. *Brain* **126**: 751–752

Rodriguez M, Lennon VA 1990 Immunoglobulins promote remyelination in the central nervous system. *Ann Neurol* **27**: 12–17

Rodriguez M, Lindsley MD 1992 Immunosuppression promotes CNS remyelination in chronic virus-induced demyelinating disease. *Neurology* **42**: 348–357

Rodriguez M, Miller DJ 1994 Immune promotion of central nervous system remyelination. *Prog Brain Res* **103**: 343–355

Rodriguez M, Scheithauer B 1994 Ultrastructure of multiple sclerosis. *Ultrastruct Pathol* **18**: 3–13

Rodriguez M, Sriram S 1988 Successful therapy of Theiler's virus-induced demyelination (DA strain) with monoclonal anti-Lyt-2 antibody. *J Immunol* **140**: 2950–2955

Rodriguez M, Lafuse WP, Leibowitz J, David CS 1986 Partial suppression of Theiler's virus induced demyelination *in vivo* by administration of monoclonal antibodies to immune-response gene products (Ia antigens). *Neurology* **36**: 964–970

Rodriguez M, Lennon VA, Benviste EN, Merrill JE 1987 Remyelination by oligodendrocytes stimulated by antiserum to spinal cord. *J Neuropathol Exp Neurol* **46**: 84–95

Rodriguez M, Wynn DR, Kimlinger TK, Katzmann JA 1990 Terminal component of complement (C9) in the cerebrospinal fluid of patients with multiple sclerosis and neurologic controls. *Neurology* **40**: 855–857

Rodriguez M, Karnes W, Bartleson JD, Pineda AA 1993a Plasma-pheresis in acute episodes of fulminant CNS inflammatory demyelination. *Neurology* **43**: 1100–1104

Rodriguez M, Scheithauer BW, Forbes G, Kelly PJ 1993b Oligodendrocyte injury is an early event in lesions of multiple sclerosis. *Mayo Clin Proc* **68**: 627–636

Rodriguez M, Prayoonwiwat N, Howe C, Sanborn K 1994a Proteolipid protein gene expression in demyelination and remyelination of the central nervous system: a model for multiple sclerosis. *J Neuropathol Exp Neurol* **53**: 136–143

Rodriguez M, Siva A, Ward J et al 1994b Impairment, disability, and handicap in multiple sclerosis: a population-based study in Olmsted County, Minnesota. *Neurology* **44**: 28–33

Rodriguez M, Siva A, Cross SA et al 1995 Optic neuritis: a population-based study in Olmsted County, Minnesota. *Neurology* **45**: 244–250

Rodriguez M, Miller DJ, Lennon VA 1996 Immunoglobulins reactive with myelin basic

protein promote CNS remyelination. *Neurology* **46**: 538–545

Roed HG, Langkilde A, Sellebjerg F 2005 A double-blind, randomized trial of IV immunoglobulin treatment in acute optic neuritis. *Neurology* **64**: 804–810

Rogers CL, Shetter AG, Ponce FA et al 2002 Gamma knife radiosurgery for trigeminal neuralgia associated with multiple sclerosis. *J Neurosurg* **97**: 529–532

Rokitansky K 1857 Uber Bindegewebswucherungen im Nervensysteme. Sitzungsberichte der mathematisch – naturwissenschaftlichen. *Klass Kaiserlichen Akad Wiessenschaften Wien* **24**: 517–536

Rolak LA, Brown S 1990 Headaches and multiple sclerosis: a clinical study and review of the literature. *J Neurol* **237**: 300–302

Rollin H 1976 Geschmackstorungen bei multipler Sklerose [Gustatory disturbances in multiple sclerosis]. *Laryng Rhinol* **55**: 678–681

Romagnani S 1994 Lymphokine production by human T cells in disease states. *Annu Rev Immunol* **12**: 227–257

Romani A, Bergamaschi R, Versino M et al 2000 Circadian and hypothermia-induced effects on visual and auditory evoked potentials in multiple sclerosis. *Clin Neurophysiol* **111**: 1602–1606

Romberg A, Virtanen A, Aunola S et al 2004 Exercise capacity, disability and leisure physical activity of subjects with multiple sclerosis. *Mult Scler* **10**: 212–218

Romi F, Krakenes J, Aarli JA, Tysnes OB 2004 Neuroborreliosis with vasculitis causing stroke-like manifestations. *Eur Neurol* **51**: 49–50

Romine J, Sipe J, Koziol J et al 1999 A double-blind, placebo-controlled, randomized trial of Cladribine in relapsing–remitting multiple sclerosis. *Proc Assoc Am Phys* **111**: 35–44

Ron MA, Feinstein A 1992 Multiple sclerosis and the mind. *J Neurol Neurosurg Psychiatry* **55**: 1–3

Ron MA, Logsdail SJ 1989 Psychiatric morbidity in multiple sclerosis: a clinical and MRI study. *Psychol Med* **19**: 887–895

Ron MA, Callanan MM, Warrington EK 1991 Cognitive abnormalities in multiple sclerosis: a psychometric and MRI study. *Psychol Med* **21**: 59–68

Roos RA, Wintzen AR, Vielvoye G, Polder TW 1991 Paroxysmal kinesigenic choreoathetosis as presenting symptom of multiple sclerosis. *J Neurol Neurosurg Psychiatry* **54**: 657–658

Ropele S, Filippi M, Valsasina P et al 2005 Assessment and correction of B_1-induced errors in magnetization transfer ratio measurements. *Magn Reson Med* **53**: 134–140

Roper J, Schwarz JR 1989 Heterogeneous distribution of fast and slow potassium channels in myelinated rat nerve fibres. *J Physiol* **416**: 93–110

Rosati G 1989 The infectious hypothesis of multiple sclerosis in epidemiology. The time trend of the disease in Sardinia, Italy. In: Battaglia M (ed.) *Multiple Sclerosis Research*. Amsterdam: Elsevier, pp. 137–146

Rosati G 1994 Descriptive epidemiology of multiple sclerosis in Europe in the 1980s: a critical overview. *Ann Neurol* **36 (Suppl 2)**: S164–S174

Rosati G 2001 The prevalence of multiple sclerosis in the world: an update. *Neurol Sci* **22**: 117–139

Rosati G, Granieri E, Carreres M, Tola R 1980 Multiple sclerosis in southern Europe: a prevalence study in the socio-sanitary district of Copparo, northern Italy. *Acta Neurol Scand* **62**: 244–249

Rosati G, Granieri E, Carreras L et al 1981 Multiple sclerosis in northern Italy: prevalence in the province of Ferrara in 1978. *Ital J Neurol Sci* **2**: 17–23

Rosati G, Aiello I, Granieri E et al 1986 Incidence of multiple sclerosis in Macomer, Sardinia, 1912–1981: onset of the disease after 1950. *Neurology* **36**: 14–19

Rosati G, Aiello I, Pirastru MI et al 1987 Sardinia, a high-risk area for multiple sclerosis: a prevalence and incidence study in the district of Alghero. *Ann Neurol* **21**: 190–194

Rosati G, Aiello I, Mannu L et al 1988 Incidence of multiple sclerosis in the town of Sassari, Sardinia, 1965 to 1985: evidence for increasing occurrence of the disease. *Neurology* **38**: 384–388

Rose AS, Kuzma JW, Kurtzke JF et al 1970 Cooperative study in the evaluation of therapy in multiple sclerosis: ACTH vs placebo: Final report. *Neurology* **20**: 1–19

Rose AS, Ellison GW, Myers LW, Tourtellotte WW 1976 Criteria for the clinical diagnosis of multiple sclerosis. *Neurology* **26**: 20–22

Rose FC 1970 The aetiology of optic neuritis. *Clin Sci* **39**: 17P

Rose J, Gerken S, Lynch S et al 1993 Genetic susceptibility in familial multiple sclerosis not linked to the myelin basic protein gene. *Lancet* **341**: 1179–1181

Rose JW, Watt HE, White AT, Carlson NG 2004 Treatment of multiple sclerosis with an anti-interleukin-2 receptor monoclonal antibody. *Ann Neurol* **56**: 864–867

Rosen JA 1965 Pseudo-isochromatic visual testing in the diagnosis of disseminated sclerosis. *Trans Am Neurol Assoc* **98**: 283–284

Rosen JA 1979 Prolonged azathioprine treatment of non-remitting multiple sclerosis. *J Neurol Neurosurg Psychiatry* **42**: 338–344

Rosenberg GA 1970 Meningoencephalitis following an influenza vaccination. *N Engl J Med* **283**: 1209

Rosenberg GA, Dencoff JE, Correa N, Reiners M, Ford CC 1996 Effect of steroids on CSF matrix metalloproteinases in multiple sclerosis: relation to blood-brain barrier injury. *Neurology* **46**: 1626–1632

Rosenberg JH, Shafor R 2005 Fatigue in multiple sclerosis: a rational approach to evaluation and treatment. *Curr Neurol Neurosci Rep* **5**: 140–146

Rosenbluth J, Blakemore WF 1984 Structural specializations in cat of chronically demyelinated spinal cord axons as seen in freeze-fracture replicas. *Neurosci Lett* **48**: 171–177

Rosenbluth J, Tao-Cheng J-H, Blakemore WF 1985 Dependence of axolemmal differentiation on contact with glial cells in chronically demyelinated lesions of cat spinal cord. *Brain Res* **358**: 287–302

Rosengren LE, Lycke J, Andersen O 1995 Glial fibrillary acidic protein in CSF of multiple sclerosis patients: relation to neurological deficit. *J Neurol Sci* **133**: 61–65

Rösener M, Muraro PA, Riethmüller A *et al* 1997 2',3'-cyclic nucleotide 3'-phosphodiesterase: a novel candidate autoantigen in demyelinating autoimmune diseases. *J Neuroimmunol* **75**: 28–34

Ross C, Clemmesen KM, Svenson M *et al* 2000 Immunogenicity of interferon-beta in multiple sclerosis patients: influence of preparation, dosage, dose frequency, and route of administration. Danish Multiple Sclerosis Study Group. *Ann Neurol* **48**: 706–712

Rosse RB 1989 Fatigue in multiple sclerosis. *Arch Neurol* **46**: 841–842

Rossini PM, Di Stefano E, Boatta M, Basciani M 1985 Evaluation of sensory-motor 'central' conduction in normal subjects and in patients with multiple sclerosis. In: Morocutti C, Risso PA (eds) *Evoked Potentials: Neurophysiological and Clinical Aspects*. Amsterdam: Elsevier, pp. 115–130

Rossini PM, Pasqualetti P, Pozzilli C *et al* 2001 Fatigue in progressive multiple sclerosis: results of a randomized, double-blind, placebo-controlled, crossover trial of oral 4-aminopyridine. *Mult Scler* **7**: 354–358

Roström B, Link H 1981 Oligoclonal immunoglobulins in cerebrospinal fluid in acute cerebrovascular disease. *Neurology* **31**: 590–596

Roth M-P, Ballivet S, Descoins P *et al* 1994a Multiple sclerosis in the Pyrenees-Atlantiques: a case-control study conducted in the southwest of France. In: Firnhaber W, Lauer K (eds) *Multiple Sclerosis in Europe: An Epidemiological Update*. Darmstadt: Leuchtturm-Verlag/LTV Press, pp. 177–178

Roth M-P, Clayton J, Patois E, Alperovitch A 1994b Gender distributions in parents and children concordant for multiple sclerosis. *Neuroepidemiology* **13**: 211–215

Roth M-P, Nogueira L, Coppin H *et al* 1994c Tumour necrosis factor polymorphisms in multiple sclerosis: no additional association independent of HLA. *J Neuroimmunol* **51**: 93–99

Roth M-P, Riond J, Champagne E *et al* 1994d CRB-V gene usage in monozygotic twins discordant for multiple sclerosis. *Immunogenetics* **39**: 281–285

Roth M-P, Dolbois L, Borot N *et al* 1995 Myelin oligodendrocyte glycoprotein (MOG) gene polymorphisms and multiple sclerosis: no

evidence of disease association with MOG. *J Neuroimmunol* **61**: 117–122

Roth NI, Coppin H, Descoins P *et al* 1991 HLA-DPB1 gene polymorphism and multiple sclerosis: a large case–control study in the southwest of France. *J Neuroimmunol* **34**: 215–222

Rothwell NJ, Luheshi G, Toulmond S 1996 Cytokines and their receptors in the central nervous system: physiology, pharmacology, and pathology. *Pharmacol Ther* **69**: 85–95

Rothwell PM, Charlton D 1998 High incidence and prevalence of multiple sclerosis in south-east Scotland: evidence of a genetic predisposition. *J Neurol Neurosurg Psychiatry* **64**: 730–735

Rothwell PM, McDowell Z, Wong, CK, Dorman PJ 1997 Doctors and patients don't agree: cross-sectional study of patients' and doctors' perceptions and assessments of disability in multiple sclerosis. *Br Med J* **314**: 1580–1583

Rotola A, Merlotti I, Caniatti L *et al* 2004 Human herpesvirus 6 infects the central nervous system of multiple sclerosis patients in the early stages of the disease. *Mult Scler* **10**: 348–354

Rotondi M, Oliviero A, Profice P *et al* 1998 Occurrence of thyroid autoimmunity and dysfunction throughout a nine-month follow-up in patients undergoing interferon-beta therapy for multiple sclerosis. *J Endocrinol Invest* **21**: 748–752

Rotondi M, Mazziotti G, Biondi B *et al* 2000 Long-term treatment with interferon-beta therapy for multiple sclerosis and occurrence of Graves' disease. *J Endocrinol Invest* **23**: 321–324

Rott O, Wekerle H, Fleischer B 1992 Protection from experimental allergic encephalomyelitis by application of a bacterial superantigen. *Int Immunol* **4**: 347–354

Rouher F, Plane C, Sole P 1969 Intérêt des potentiels évoqués visuels dans les affections du nerf optique. *Arch Ophtalmol (Paris)* **29**: 555–564

Roullet E, Verdier-Taillefer M-H, Amarenco P *et al* 1993 Pregnancy and multiple sclerosis: a longitudinal study of 125 remittent patients. *J Neurol Neurosurg Psychiatry* **56**: 1062–1065

Rousseau JJ, Lust C, Zangerle PF, Bigaignon G 1986 Acute transverse myelitis as presenting symptom of Lyme disease. *Lancet* **2**: 1222–1223

Roussel V, Yi F, Jauberteau MO *et al* 2000 Prevalence and clinical significance of anti-phopholipid antibodies in multiple sclerosis: a study of 89 patients. *J Autoimmun* **14**: 259–265

Rovaris M, Barnes D, Woodrofe N *et al* 1996 Patterns of disease activity in multiple sclerosis patients: a study with quantitative gadolinium enhanced brain MRI and cytokine measurements in different clinical subgroups. *J Neurol* **243**: 536–542

Rovaris M, Fillipi M, Minicucci L *et al* 2000a Cortical/subcortical disease burden and cognitive impairment in patients with

multiple sclerosis. *Am J Neuroradiol* **21**: 402–408

Rovaris M, Viti B, Ciboddo C *et al* 2000b Brain involvement in systemic immune-mediated diseases: a magnetic resonance and magnetization transfer imaging study. *J Neurol Neurosurg Psychiatry* **68**:170–177

Rovaris M, Viti B, Ciboddo G *et al* 2000c Cervical cord magnetic resonance imaging findings in systemic immune-mediated diseases. *J Neurol Sci* **176**: 128–130

Rovaris M, Bozzali M, Rocca MA *et al* 2001a An MR study of tissue damage in the cervical cord of patients with migraine. *J Neurol Sci* **183**: 43–46

Rovaris M, Bozzali M, Santuccio G *et al* 2001b In vivo assessment of the brain and cervical cord pathology of patients with primary progressive multiple sclerosis. *Brain* **124**: 2540–2549

Rovaris M, Comi G, Rocca M *et al* and the European/Canadian Glatiramer Acetate Study Group 2001c Short term brain volume change in relapsing–remitting multiple sclerosis: effect of glatiramer acetate and implications. *Brain* **124**: 1803–1812

Rovaris M, Comi G, Sormani MP *et al* 2001d Effects of seasons on magnetic resonance imaging-measured disease activity in patients with multiple sclerosis. *Ann Neurol* **49**: 415–417

Rovaris M, Bozzali M, Iannucci G *et al* 2002a Assessment of normal-appearing white and gray matter in patients with primary progressive multiple sclerosis: a diffusion-tensor magnetic resonance imaging study. *Arch Neurol* **59**: 1406–1412

Rovaris M, Codella M, Moiola L *et al* 2002b Effect of glatiramer acetate on MS lesions enhancing at different gadolinium doses. *Neurology* **59**: 1429–1432

Rovaris M, Holtmannspotter M, Rocca MA *et al* 2002c Contribution of cervical cord MRI and brain magnetization transfer imaging in the assessment of individual patients with multiple sclerosis: a preliminary study. *Mult Scler* **8**: 52–58

Rowe VD, Wang D, John HA *et al* 2003 Rescue therapy with high dose intravenous methotrexate in MS patients worsening despite Avonex therapy. *Neurology* **60**: A149–A150

Rowen L, Koop BF, Hood L 1996 The complete 685-kilobase DNA sequence of the human b T cell receptor locus. *Science* **272**: 1755–1762

Roxburgh RH, Seaman SR, Masterman T *et al* 2005a Multiple sclerosis severity score: ranking disability at similar duration to rate disease severity. *Neurology* **64**: 1144–1151

Roxburgh RH, Sawcer SJ, Meranian M *et al* 2005b Multiple sclerosis and CTLA-4: different polymorphisms of this gene may predispose to different autoimmune diseases. *J Neuroimmunol* **171**: 193–197

Rozza L, Bortolotti P, Sica A *et al* 1993 Kinesigenic dystonia as the first manifestation of multiple sclerosis with cervical and brainstem lesions. *Eur Neurol* **33**: 331–332

Rubio JP, Bahlo M, Butzkueven H et al 2002 Genetic dissection of the HLA region using haplotypes of Tasmanian with multiple sclerosis. *Am J Hum Genet* **70**: 1125–1137

Rubio JP, Bahlo M, Tubridy N et al 2004 Extended haplotype analysis in the HLA complex reveals an increased frequency of the HFE-C282Y mutation in individuals with multiple sclerosis. *Hum Genet* **114** : 573–580

Rubio N, Rodriguez R, Arevalo MA 2004 In vitro myelination by oligodendrocyte precursor cells transfected with the neurotrophin-3 gene. *Glia* **47**: 78–87

Rucker CW 1944a Sheathing of the retinal veins in multiple sclerosis. *Mayo Clin Proc* **19**: 176–178

Rucker CW 1944b Sheathing of the retinal veins in multiple sclerosis. *J Am Med Assoc* **127**: 970–973

Rucker CW 1947 Retinopathy of multiple sclerosis. *Trans Am Ophthalmol Soc* **45**: 564–570

Rucker CW 1972 Sheathing of the retinal veins in multiple sclerosis: review of pertinent literature. *Mayo Clin Proc* **47**: 335–340

Rudd Bosch JLR, Groen J 1996 treatment of refractory urge urinary incontinence with sacral spinal nerve stimulation in multiple sclerosis patients. *Lancet* **348**: 717–719

Rudge JS, Silver J 1990 Inhibition of neurite outgrowth on astroglial scars *in vitro*. *J Neurosci* **10**: 3594–3603

Rudge PR 1973 Optic neuritis as a complication of carcinoma of the breast. *Proc R Soc Med* **66**: 106–107

Rudge PR 1999 Are clinical trials of therapeutic agents for MS long enough? *Lancet* **353**: 1033–1034

Rudge PR, Koetsier JC, Mertin J et al 1989 Randomised double blind controlled trial of cyclosporin in multiple sclerosis. *J Neurol Neurosurg Psychiatry* **52**: 559–565

Rudge PR, Ali A, Cruickshank JK 1991 Multiple sclerosis, tropical spastic paraplegia and HTLV-1 infection in Afro-Caribbean patients in the United Kingdom. *J Neurol Neurosurg Psychiatry* **54**: 689–694

Rudge PR, Miller DH, Crimlisk H, Thorpe J 1995 Does interferon beta cause initial exacerbation of multiple sclerosis? *Lancet* **345**: 580

Rudick RA 1995 Pregnancy and multiple sclerosis. *Arch Neurol* **52**: 849–850

Rudick RA, Barna BP 1990 Serum interleukin 2 and soluble interleukin 2 receptor in patients with multiple sclerosis who are experiencing severe fatigue. *Arch Neurol* **47**: 254–255

Rudick RA, Bidlack JM, Knutson SW 1985 Multiple sclerosis: cerebrospinal fluid immune complexes that bind C1q. *Arch Neurol* **42**: 856–858

Rudick RA, Schiffer RB, Schwetz KM, Herndon RM 1986 Multiple sclerosis: the problem of incorrect diagnosis. *Arch Neurol* **43**: 578–583

Rudick RA, Breton D, Krall RL 1987 The GABA-agonist progabide for spasticity in multiple sclerosis. *Arch Neurol* **44**: 1033–1036

Rudick RA, Antel J, Confavreux C et al 1996a Clinical outcomes assessment in multiple sclerosis. *Ann Neurol* **40**: 469–479

Rudick RA, Ranschoff RM, Peppler R et al 1996b Interferon beta induces interleukin-10 expression: relevance to multiple sclerosis. *Ann Neurol* **40**: 618–627

Rudick RA, Antel J, Confavreax C et al 1997a Recommendations from the National Multiple Sclerosis Society Clinical Outcomes Assessment Task Force. *Ann Neurol* **42**: 379–382

Rudick RA, Cohen JA, Weinstock-Guttman B et al 1997b Management of multiple sclerosis. *N Engl J Med* **337**: 1604–1611

Rudick RA, Goodkin DE, Jacobs LD et al 1997c Impact of interferon beta-1a on neurologic disability in relapsing multiple sclerosis. *Neurology* **49**: 358–363

Rudick RA, Simonian NA, Alam JA et al 1998a Incidence and significance of neutralizing antibodies to interferon beta-1a in multiple sclerosis. Multiple Sclerosis Collaborative Research Group (MSCRG). *Neurology* **50**: 1266–1272

Rudick RA, Ranschoff RM, Lee JC et al 1998b In vivo effects of interferon beta-1a on immunosuppressive cytokines in multiple sclerosis *Neurology* **50**: 1294–300

Rudick RA, Fischer E, Lee JC et al 1999 Use of the brain parenchymal fraction to measure whole brain atrophy in relapsing–remitting MS. Multiple Sclerosis Collaborative Research Group. *Neurology* **53**: 1698–1704

Rudick RA, Cutter G, Reingold S 2002 The Multiple Sclerosis Functional Composite: a new clinical outcome measure for multiple sclerosis trials. *Mult Scler* **8**: 359–365

Rudick RA, Cookfair DL, Griffin J et al 2003 Interferons in relapsing remitting multiple sclerosis. *Lancet* **361**: 1824; author reply 1824–1825

Ruegg SJ, Buhlmann M, Renaud S et al 2004 Cervical dystonia as first manifestation of multiple sclerosis. *J Neurol* **251**: 1408–1410

Ruge D, Brochner R, Daris L 1958 A study of the treatment of 637 patients with trigeminal neuralgia. *J Neurosurg* **15**: 528–536

Ruggieri M, Polizzi A, Pavone L, Grimaldi LME 1999 Multiple sclerosis in children under 6 years of age. *Neurology* **53**: 478–484

Rush JA 1980 Retrobulbar optic neuritis in sarcoidosis. *Ann Ophthalmol* **12**: 390–394

Ruiz P, Garren H, Hirschberg DL et al 1999 Microbial epitopes act as altered peptide ligands to prevent experimental autoimmune encephalomyelitis. *J Exp Med* **189**: 1275–1283

Rumsby MG 1978 Organization and structure in central nerve myelin. *Biochem Soc Trans* **6**: 448–462

Runmarker B, Andersen O 1993 Prognostic factors in a multiple sclerosis incident cohort with twenty-five years of follow-up. *Brain* **116**: 117–134

Runmarker B, Andersen O 1995 Pregnancy is associated with a lower risk of onset and a better prognosis in multiple sclerosis. *Brain* **118**: 253–261

Runmarker B, Martinsson T, Wahlstrom J, Andersen O 1994a HLA and prognosis in multiple sclerosis. *J Neurol* **241**: 385–390

Runmarker B, Andersson C, Oden A, Andersen O 1994b Prediction of outcome in multiple sclerosis based on multivariate models. *J Neurol* **241**: 597–604

Ruprecht K, Warmuth-Metz M, Waespe W, Gold R 2002 Symptomatic hyperekplexia in a patient with multiple sclerosis. *Neurology* **58**: 503–504

Rush JA, Younge BR 1981 Paralysis of cranial nerves III, IV and VI. *Arch Ophthalmol* **99**: 76–79

Rushton D 1975 Use of Pulfrich pendulum for detecting abnormal delay in the visual pathway in multiple sclerosis. *Brain* **98**: 283–296

Rushton JG, Olafson RA 1965 Trigeminal neuralgia associated with multiple sclerosis. *Arch Neurol* **13**: 383–386

Rushton WAH 1937 Initiation of the propagated disturbance. *Proc R Soc Lond Series B: Biol Sci* **124**: 210–243

Rusin JA, Vezina G, Chadduck WM, Chandra RS 1995 Tumoral multiple sclerosis of the cerebellum in a child. *Am J Neuroradiol* **16**: 1164–1166

Russell DS 1955 The nosological unity of acute haemorrhagic leucoencephalitis and acute disseminated encephalomyelitis. *Brain* **78**: 369–376

Russo R, Tenenbaum S, Morena M, Battagliotti C 2000 Interferon-beta 1a induced juvenile chronic arthritis in genetically predisposed young patient with multiple sclerosis: comment on the case report by Levesque et al. *Arthritis Rheum* **43**: 1190

Rutschmann OT, McCrory DC, Matchar DB et al 2002 Immunization and MS: a summary of published evidence and recommendations. *Neurology* **59**: 1837–1843

Ruutianen J, Salonen R, Halonen P et al 1991 Treatment of acute exacerbations in early multiple sclerosis: cyclosporin A or prednisolone. *Acta Neurol Scand* **83**: 52–54

Ryder LP, Anderson E, Svejgaard A 1978 An HLA map of Europe. *Hum Heredity* **28**: 171–200

Saab CY, Craner MJ, Kataoka Y, Waxman SG 2004 Abnormal Purkinje cell activity in vivo in experimental allergic encephalomyelitis. *Exp Brain Res* **158**: 1–8

Saarela J, Schoenberg Fejzo M, Chen D et al 2002 Fine mapping of a multiple sclerosis locus to 2.5 Mb on chromosome 17q22-q24. *Hum Mol Gen* **11**: 2257–2267

Saarela J, Chen D, Chi WS et al 2003 The physical map of the multiple sclerosis susceptibility on chromosome 17q22–24 exposes blocks of segmental duplication. *Am J Hum Genet* **71** (Suppl): 151 (abstract)

Sacconi S, Salviati L, Merelli E 2001 Acute disseminated encephalomyelitis associated with hepatitis C virus infection. *Arch Neurol* **58**: 1679–1681

Sachidanandam R, Weissman D, Schmidt SC *et al* 2001 A map of human genome sequence variation containing 1.42 million single nucleotide polymorphisms. *Nature* **409**: 928–933

Sackett DL, Haynes RB, Tugwell P 1985 *Clinical Epidemiology: A Basic Science for Clinical Medicine.* Boston: Little, Brown, pp. 161–162

Sackett DL, Straus SE, Richardson WS *et al* 2000 *Evidence-Based Medicine. How to Practice and Teach EBM*, 2nd edn. Toronto: Churchill Livingstone

Sacks JG, Melen O 1975 Bitemporal visual field defects in presumed multiple sclerosis. *J Am Med Assoc* **234**: 69–72

Sadatipour BT, Greer JM, Pender MP 1998 Increased circulating antiganglioside antibodies in primary and secondary progressive multiple sclerosis. *Ann Neurol* **44**: 980–983

Sadeghi-Nejad A, Senior B 1990 Adrenomyeloneuropathy presenting as Addison's disease in childhood. *N Engl J Med* **322**: 13–16

Sadeh M, Shacked I, Rappaport ZH, Tadmor R 1982 Surgical extirpation of a venous angioma of the medulla oblongata simulating multiple sclerosis. *Surg Neurol* **17**: 334–335

Sadeh M, Kuritzky A, Ben-David E, Goldhammer Y 1992 Adult metachromatic leukodystrophy with an unusual relapsing–remitting course. *Postgrad Med J* **68**: 192–195

Sadlack B, Merz H, Schorle H *et al* 1993 Ulcerative colitis-like disease in mice with a disrupted interleukin-2 gene. *Cell* **75**: 253–261

Sadovnick AD 1982 Concordance in twins and recurrence in siblings of multiple sclerosis. *Lancet* **i**: 1068

Sadovnick AD 1994 Genetic epidemiology of multiple sclerosis: a survey. *Ann Neurol* **36 (Suppl 2)**: S194–S203

Sadovnick AD, Baird PA 1988 The familal nature of multiple sclerosis: age-corrected empiric recurrence risks for children and siblings of patients. *Neurology* **38**: 990–991

Sadovnick AD, Ebers GC 1993 Epidemiology of multiple sclerosis: a critical overview. *Can J Neurol Sci* **20**: 17–29

Sadovnick AD, Scheifele DW 2000 School-based hepatitis B vaccination programme and adolescent multiple sclerosis. *Lancet* **355**: 549–550

Sadovnick AD, Yee IM 1994 Season of birth in multiple sclerosis. *Acta Neurol Scand* **89**: 190–191

Sadovnick AD, Baird PA, Ward RH 1988 Multiple sclerosis; updated risks for relatives. *Am J Med Genet* **29**: 533–541

Sadovnick AD, Paty DW, Yannakoulias G 1989 Concurrence of multiple sclerosis and inflammatory bowel disease. *N Engl J Med* **321**: 763–764

Sadovnick AD, Bulman D, Ebers GC 1991a Parent child concordance in multiple sclerosis. *Ann Neurol* **29**: 252–255

Sadovnick AD, Eisen K, Ebers GC, Paty DW 1991b Cause of death in patients attending multiple sclerosis clinics. *Neurology* **41**: 1193–1196

Sadovnick AD, Ebers GC, Wilson RW, Paty DW 1992 Life expectancy in patients attending multiple sclerosis clinics. *Neurology* **42**: 991–994

Sadovnick AD, Armstrong H, Rice GPA *et al* 1993 A population-based study of multiple sclerosis in twins: update. *Ann Neurol* **33**: 281–285

Sadovnick AD, Eisen K, Hashimoto SA *et al* 1994 Pregnancy and multiple sclerosis: a prospective study. *Arch Neurol* **51**: 1120–1124

Sadovnick AD, Ebers GC, Dyment DA, Risch N, the Canadian Collaborative Study Group 1996a Evidence for genetic basis of multiple sclerosis. *Lancet* **347**: 1728–1730

Sadovnick AD, Remick RA, Allen J *et al* 1996b Depression and multiple sclerosis. *Neurology* **46**: 628–632

Sadovnick AD, Yee IM, Ebers GC, Risch N 1998 Effect of age at onset and parental disease status on sibling risks for MS. *Neurology* **50**: 719–723

Sadovnick AD, Yee IM, Ebers GC, Canadian Collaborative Study Group 2000 Factors influencing sib risks for multiple sclerosis. *Clin Genet* **58**: 431–435

Sadovnick AD, Yee IM, Ebers GC, Canadian Collaborative Study Group 2001 Recurrence risks to sibs of MS index cases: impact of consanguineous matings. *Neurology* **56**: 784–785

Safronov BV, Kampe K, Vogel W 1993 Single voltage-dependent potassium channels in rat peripheral nerve membrane. *J Physiol* **460**: 675–691

Sagar HJ, Warlow CP, Sheldon PWE, Esiri MM 1982 Multiple sclerosis with clinical and radiological features of cerebral tumour. *J Neurol Neurosurg Psychiatry* **45**: 802–808

Sahlas DJ, Miller SP, Guerin M *et al* 2000 Treatment of acute disseminated encephalomyelitis with intravenous immunoglobulin. *Neurology* **54**: 1370–1372

Sahrbacher UC, Lechner F, Eugster H-P *et al* 1998 Mice with an inactivation of the inducible nitric oxide synthase gene are susceptible to experimental autoimmune encephalomyelitis. *Eur J Immunol* **28**: 1332–1338

Said G, Lacroix C, Plante-Bordeneuve V *et al* 2002 Nerve granulomas and vasculitis in sarcoid peripheral neuropathy: a clinicopathological study of 11 patients. *Brain* **125**: 264–275

Saida T, Tashiro K, Itoyama Y *et al* 2005 Interferon beta-1b is effective in Japanese RRMS patients: a randomized, multicenter study. *Neurology* **64**: 621–630

Saini HS, Gorse KM, Boxer LM, Sato-Bigbee C 2004 Neurotrophin-3 and CREB-mediated signaling pathway regulate Bc1–2

expression in oligodendrocyte progenitor cells. *J Neurochem* **89**: 951–961

Saito S, Naito S, Kawanami S, Kuroiwa Y 1976 HLA studies on multiple sclerosis in Japan. *Neurology* **26 (Part 2)**: 49

Saiz A, Marcos MA, Graus F *et al* 2001 No evidence of CNS infection with *Chlamydia pneumoniae* in patients with multiple sclerosis. *J Neurol* **248**: 617–618

Saiz A, Blanco Y, Carreras E *et al* 2004 Clinical and MRI outcome after autologous hematopoietic stem cell transplantation in MS. *Neurology* **62**: 282–284

Sajantila A, Lahermo P, Anttinen T *et al* 1995 Genes and language in Europe: an analysis of mitochondrial lineages. *Genome Res* **5**: 42–52

Sajantila A, Salem AH, Savolainen P *et al* 1996 Paternal and maternal DNA lineages reveal a bottleneck in the founding of the Finnish population. *Proc Natl Acad Sci USA* **93**: 12035–12039

Sakaguchi S 2000 Regulatory T cells: key controllers of immunological self tolerance. *Cell* **101**: 455–458

Sakaguchi S, Sakaguchi N 2000 Role of genetic factors in organ specific autoimmune diseases induced by manipulating the thymus or T cells, and not self-antigens. *Rev Immunogenet* **2**: 147–153

Sakaguchi S, Sakaguchi N, Asano M *et al* 1995 Immunologic self-tolerance maintained by activated T cells expressing IL-2 receptor a-chains (CD25): breakdown of a single mechanism of self-tolerance causes various autoimmune diseases. *J Immunol* **155**: 1151–1164

Sakurai M, Kanazawa I 1999 Positive symptoms in multiple sclerosis: their treatment with sodium channel blockers, lidocaine and mexiletine. *J Neurol Sci* **162**: 162–168

Salama HH, Hong J, Zang YC *et al* 2003 Blocking effects of serum reactive antibodies induced by glatiramer acetate treatment in multiple sclerosis. *Brain* **126**: 2638–2647

Salemi G, Ragonese P, Aridon P *et al* 2000a Incidence of multiple sclerosis in Bagheria City, Sicily, Italy. *Neurol Sci* **21**: 361–365

Salemi G, Ragonese P, Aridon P *et al* 2000b Is season of birth associated with multiple sclerosis? *Acta Neurol Scand* **101**: 381–383

Salemi G, Callari G, Gammino M *et al* 2004 The relapse rate of multiple sclerosis changes during pregnancy: a cohort study. *Acta Neurol Scand* **110**: 23–26

Salier JP, Sesboue R, Martin-Mondiere C *et al* 1986 Combined influences of Gm and HLA phenotypes upon multiple sclerosis susceptibility and severity. *J Clin Invest* **78**: 533–538

Sallstom T 1942 Occurrence and distribution of multiple sclerosis in Sweden: geographic pathology of multiple sclerosis. *Acta Med Scand* **137 (Suppl)**: 1–14

Sallusto F, Lanzavecchia A, Mackay CR 1998 Chemokines and chemokine receptors in T cell priming and Th1/Th2 mediated responses. *Immunol Today* **19**: 568–574

Sallusto F, Lenig D, Förster R *et al* 1999 Two subsets of memory T lymphocytes with distinct homing potentials and effector functions. *Nature* **401**: 708–712

Salmaggi A, Sandberg-Wollheim M 1993 Monocyte phenotype in blood and cerebrospinal fluid: compartment specific pattern is unrelated to neurological disease. *J Neurol Sci* **120**: 201–207

Salmaggi A, Corsini E, La Mantia L *et al* 1997 Immunological monitoring of azathioprine treatment in multiple sclerosis patients. *J Neurol* **244**: 167–174

Salmi A, Reunanen M, Ilonen J, Panelius M 1983 Intrathecal antibody synthesis to virus antigens in multiple sclerosis. *Clin Exp Immunol* **52**: 241–249

Salomon B, Bluestone JA 2001 Complexities of CD28/B7: CTLA-4 costimulatory pathways in autoimmunity and transplantation. *Annu Rev Immunol* **19**: 225–252

Salonen R, Ilonen J, Reunanen M, Salmi A 1982 Defective production of interferon-alpha associated with HLA-DW2 antigen in stable multiple sclerosis. *J Neurol Sci* **55**: 197–206

Salvetti M, Ristori G, D'Amato M *et al* 1993 Predominant and stable T-cell responses to regions of myelin basic protein can be detected in individual patients with multiple sclerosis. *Eur J Immunol* **23**: 1232–1239

Salvetti M, Pisani A, Bastianello S *et al* 1995 Clinical and MRI assessment of disease activity in patients with multiple sclerosis after influenza vaccination. *J Neurol* **242**: 143–146

Salvi F, Mascalchi M, Plasmati R *et al* 1992 Multiple lesions in cerebral white matter in two young adults with thoracic extramedullary tumours. *J Neurol Neurosurg Psychiatry* **55**: 216–218

Samkoff LM, Daras M, Tuchman AJ, Koppel BS 1997 Amelioration of refractory dysestheic limb pain in multiple sclerosis by gabapentin. *Neurology* **49**: 304–305

Samoilova EB, Horton JL, Hilliard B *et al* 1998a IL-6-deficient mice are resistant to experimental autoimmune encephalomyelitis: roles of IL-6 in the activation and differentiation of autoreactive T cells. *J Immunol* **161**: 6480–6486

Samoilova EB, Horton JL, Chen YH 1998b Experimental autoimmune encephalomyelitis in intercellular adhesion molecule-1-deficient mice. *Cell Immunol* **190**: 83–89

Sanai N, Tramontin AD, Quinones-Hinojosa E *et al* 2004 Unique astrocyte ribbon in adult human brain contains neural stem cells but lacks chain migration. *Nature* **427**: 740–744

Sanchez T, Hassinger L, Paskevich PA *et al* 1996 Oligodendroglia regulate the regional expansion of axon calibre and local accumulation of neurofilaments during development independent of myelin formation. *J Neurosci* **16**: 5095–5105

Sanchez-Ramos J, Song S, Cardozo-Pelaez F *et al* 2000 Adult bone marrow stromal cells

differentiate into neural cells in vitro. *Exp Neurol* **164**: 247–256

Sandberg-Wollheim M 1975 Optic neuritis: studies on the cerebrospinal fluid in relation to clinical course in 61 patients. *Acta Neurol Scand* **52**: 167–178

Sandberg-Wollheim M 1983 Lymphocyte populations in the cerebrospinal fluid and peripheral blood of patients with multiple sclerosis and optic neuritis. *Neurology* **17**: 575–581

Sandberg-Wollheim M, Baird L, Schanfield M *et al* 1984 Association of CSF IgG concentration and immunoglobulin allotype in multiple sclerosis and optic neuritis. *Clin Immunol Immunopathol* **31**: 212–221

Sandberg-Wollheim M, Bynke H, Cronqvist S *et al* 1990 A long term prospective study of optic neuritis: evaluation of risk factors. *Ann Neurol* **27**: 386–393

Sandberg-Wollheim M, Axell T, Hansen BU *et al* 1992 Primary Sjögren's syndrome in patients with multiple sclerosis. *Neurology* **42**: 845–847

Sandberg-Wollheim M, Ciusani E, Salmaggi A, Pociot F 1995 An evaluation of tumour necrosis factor microsatellite alleles in genetic susceptibility to multiple sclerosis. *Mult Scler* **1**: 181–185

Sandberg-Wollheim M, Bever C, Carter J *et al* 2005 Comparative tolerance of IFN beta-1a regimens in patients with relapsing multiple sclerosis. The EVIDENCE study. *J Neurol* **252**: 8–13

Sander M 1898 Hirnrindenbefunde bei multipler Sklerose. *Monatsschr Psychol Neurol* **4**: 429–436

Sanders EACM, Arts RJHM 1986 Paraesthesiae in multiple sclerosis. *J Neurol Sci* **74**: 297–305

Sanders ME, Koski CL, Robbins D *et al* 1986 Activated terminal complement in cerebrospinal fluid in Guillain–Barré syndrome and multiple sclerosis. *J Immunol* **136**: 4456–4459

Sanders V, Conrad AJ, Tourtellotte WW 1993 On classification of post-mortem multiple sclerosis plaques for neuroscientists. *J Neuroimmunol* **46**: 207–216

Sandroni P, Walker C, Starr A 1992 'Fatigue' in patients with multiple sclerosis: motor pathway conduction and event-related potentials. *Arch Neurol* **49**: 517–524

Santiago E, Perez-Mediavilla LA, Lopez-Moratalla N 1998 The role of nitric oxide in the pathogenesis of multiple sclerosis. *J Physiol Biochem* **54**: 229–237

Santos M, Pinto-Basto J, Rio ME *et al* 2003 A whole genome screen for association with multiple sclerosis in Portuguese patients. *J Neuroimmunol* **143**: 112–115

Santos M, Costa M, Rio ME *et al* 2004 Genotypes at the APOE and SCA2 loci do not predict the course of multiple sclerosis in patients of Portugese origin. *Mult Scler* **10**: 153–157

Sarasoja T, Wikstrom J, Paltamaa J 2004 Occurrence of multiple sclerosis in central Finland: a regional and temporal

comparison during 30 years. *Acta Neurol Scand* **110**: 331–336

Sarchielli P, Presciutti O, Pelliccioli GP *et al* 1999 Absolute quantification of brain metabolites by proton magnetic resonance spectroscopy in normal appearing white matter of multiple sclerosis patients. *Brain* **122**: 513–522

Sarkari NBS 1968 Involuntary movements in multiple sclerosis. *Br Med J* **2**: 738–740

Sarkari NBS, Bickerstaff ER 1969 Relapses and remissions in brain stem tumours. *Br Med J* **2**: 21–23

Saruhan-Direskeneli G, Weber F, Meinl E *et al* 1993 Human T cell autoimmunity against myelin basic protein: CD4+ cells recognising epitopes of the T cell receptor β chain from a myelin basic protein-specific T cell clone. *Eur J Immunol* **23**: 530–536

Saruhan-Direskeneli G, Esin S, Baykan-Kurt B *et al* 1997 HLA-DR and -DQ associations with multiple sclerosis in Turkey. *Hum Immunol* **55**: 59–65

Sastre-Garriga J, Reverter JC, Font J *et al* 2001 Anticardiolipin antibodies are not a useful screening tool in a nonselected large group of patients with multiple sclerosis. *Ann Neurol* **49**: 408–411

Sastre-Garriga J, Tintore M, Rovira A *et al* 2003 Conversion to multiple sclerosis after a clinically isolated syndrome of the brainstem: cranial magnetic resonance imaging, cerebrospinal fluid and neurophysiological findings. *Mult Scler* **9**: 39–43

Sastre-Garriga J, Tintore M, Rovira A *et al* 2004a Specificity of Barkhof criteria in predicting conversion to multiple sclerosis when applied to clinically isolated brainstem syndromes. *Ann Neurol* **61**: 222–224.

Sastre-Garriga J, Ingle GT, Chard DT *et al* 2004 Grey and white matter atrophy in early clinical stages of primary progressive multiple sclerosis. *Neuroimage* **22**: 353–359

Sastre-Garriga J, Ingle GT, Chard DT *et al* 2005 Grey and white matter volume changes in early primary progressive multiple sclerosis: a longitudinal study. *Brain* **128**: 1454–1460

Sato T, Kamata Y, Irifune M, Nishikawa T 1995 Inhibition of purified (Na+,K+)-ATPase activity from porcine cerebral cortex by NO generating drugs. *Brain Res* **704**: 117–120

Satoh J, Kim SU 1994 Proliferation and differentiation of fetal human oligodendrocytes *in vitro*. *J Neurosci Res* **39**: 260–272

Satoh J, Paty DW, Kim SU 1996 Counteracting effect of IFN-β on IFN-γ-induced proliferation of human astrocytes in culture. *Mult Scler* **1**: 279–287

Satoh JI, Tokumoto H, Kurohara K *et al* 1997 Adult-onset Krabbe disease with homozygous T1853C mutation in the galactocerebrosidase gene: unusual MRI findings of corticospinal tract demyelination. *Neurology* **49**:1203–1204

Sauter MK, Panitch HS, Kristt DA 1991 Myelopathic neurosarcoidosis: diagnostic value of enhanced MRI. *Neurology* **41**: 150–157

Savettieri G, Daricello B, Giordano D et al 1981 The prevalence of multiple sclerosis in Sicily. I. Monreale City. *J Epidemiol Community Health* **35**: 114–117

Savettieri G, Elian M, Giordano D et al 1986 A further study on the prevalence of multiple sclerosis in Sicily: Caltanissetta city. *Acta Neurol Scand* **73**: 71–75

Savettieri G, Castiglione MG, D'Arpa A et al 1991 Are multiple domicile changes a risk factor for multiple sclerosis? A case-control study. *Neuroepidemiology* **10**: 24–26

Savettieri G, Salemi G, Ragonese P et al 1998 Prevalence and incidence of multiple sclerosis in the city of Monreale, Italy. *J Neurol* **245**: 40–43

Savettieri G, Cittadella R, Valentino P et al 2002 Lack of an association between estrogen receptor 1 gene polymorphisms and multiple sclerosis in southern Italy in humans. *Neurosci Lett* **327**: 115–118

Savettieri G, Andreoli V, Bonavita S et al 2003 Apolipoprotein E genotype does not influence the progression of multiple sclerosis. *J Neurol* **250**: 1094–1098

Savettieri G, Messina D, Andreoli V et al 2004 Gender-related effect of clinical and genetic variables on the cognitive impairment in multiple sclerosis. *J Neurol* **251**: 1208–1214

Sawa GM, Paty DW 1979 The use of baclofen in treatment of spasticity in multiple sclerosis. *J Neurol Sci* **6**: 351–356

Sawada M, Hara N, Maeno T 1990 Extracellular tumor necrosis factor induces a decreased K^+ conductance in an identified neuron of *Aplysia kurodai*. *Neurosci Lett* **115**: 219–225

Sawada M, Hara N, Maeno T 1991 Analysis of a decreased Na^+ conductance by tumor necrosis factor in identified neurons of *Aplysia kurodai*. *J Neurosci Res* **28**: 466–473

Sawada M, Ichinose M, Hara N 1995 Nitric oxide induces an increased Na+ conductance in identified neurons of *Aplysia*. *Brain Res* **670**: 248–256

Sawcer SJ, Jones HB, Feakes R et al 1996 A genome screen in multiple sclerosis reveals susceptibility loci on chromosome 6p21 and 17q22. *Nature Genet* **13**: 464–468

Sawcer SJ, Jones HB, Judhe D et al 1997 Empirical genomewide significance levels established by whole genome simulations. *Genetic Epidemiology* **14**: 223–229

Sawcer SJ, Meranian M, Setakis E et al 2002 A whole genome screen for linkage disequilibrium in multiple sclerosis confirms disease associations with regions previously linked to susceptibility. *Brain* **125**: 1337–1347

Sawcer SJ, Maranian M, Singlehurst S et al 2004 Enhancing linkage analysis of complex disorders: an evaluation of high-density genotyping. *Hum Mol Genet* **13**: 1943–1949

Scarisbrick IA, Blaber SI, Lucchinetti CF et al 2002 Activity of a newly identified serine

protease in CNS demyelination. *Brain* **125**: 1283–1296

Scarpini E, Galimberti D, Baron P et al 2002 IP-10 and MCP-1 levels in CSF and serum from multiple sclerosis patients with different clinical subtypes of the disease. *J Neurol Sci* **195**: 41–46

Schachter M 1933 Un illustré malade: le poete Henri Heine. *Paris Med* **1 (Suppl)**: 415–417

Schafer DP, Bansal R, Hedstrom KL et al 2004 Does paranode formation and maintenance require partitioning of neurofascin 155 into lipid rafts? *J Neurosci* **24**: 3176–3185

Schaltenbrand G 1943 *Die Multiple Sklerose des Menschen*. Leipzig: Thieme

Schapira K 1959 The seasonal incidence of onset and exacerbations in multiple sclerosis. *J Neurol Neurosurg Psychiatry* **22**: 285–286

Schapira K, Poskanzer DC, Millar H 1963 Familial and conjugal multiple sclerosis. *Brain* **86**: 315–332

Schapira K, Poskanzer DC, Newell DJ, Miller H 1966 Marriage, pregnancy and multiple sclerosis. *Brain* **89**: 419–428

Schauf CL, Davis FA 1981 Circulating toxic factors in multiple sclerosis: a perspective. *Adv Neurol* **31**: 267–280

Schauf CL, Smith KJ 1981 Segregation of ionic channels at amphibian nodes of Ranvier. *J Physiol* **320**: 114P–115P

Schaumburg HH, Powers JM, Suzuki K, Raine CS 1974 Adrenoleukodystrophy (sex-linked Schilder disease). *Arch Neurol* **31**: 210–213

Schaumburg HH, Powers JM, Raine CS et al 1975 Adrenoleukodystrophy. *Arch Neurol Psychiatry* **32**: 577–591

Schechter SL 1986 Lyme disease associated with optic neuropathy. *Am J Med* **81**: 143–145

Schellekens H, Casadevall N 2004 Immunogenicity of recombinant human proteins: causes and consequences. *J Neurol* **251**: II4–9

Scherb G 1905 Sclérose en plaques fruste ou syndrome cérébelleux de Babinski. *Nouv Iconographie Salpétrière* **18**: 31–35

Scherer SS, Arroyo EJ 2002 Recent progress on the molecular organization of myelinated axons. *J Peripher Nerv Syst* **7**: 1–12

Scherokman BJ, Selhorst JB, Waybright EA et al 1985 Improved optic nerve conduction with ingestion of ice water. *Ann Neurol* **17**: 418–419

Schierle G, Hansson O, Leist M et al 1999 Caspase inhibition reduces apoptosis and increase survival of nigral transplants. *Nature Med* **5**: 97–100

Schiffenbauer J, Johnson HM, Butfiloski EJ et al 1993 Staphylococcal enterotoxins can reactivate experimental allergic encephalomyelitis. *Proc Natl Acad Sci USA* **90**: 8543–8546

Schiffer RB, Caine ED, Bamford KA, Levy S 1983 Depressive episodes in patients with multiple sclerosis. *Am J Psychiatry* **140**: 1498–1500

Schiffer RB, Wineman NM, Weitkamp LR 1986 Association between bipolar affective

disorder and multiple sclerosis. *Am J Psychiatry* **143**: 94–95

Schiffer RB, Weitkamp LR, Ford C, Hall WJ 1994 A genetic marker and family history study of the upstate New York multiple sclerosis cluster. *Neurology* **44**: 329–333

Schiffer RB, McDermott MP, Copley C 2001 A multiple sclerosis cluster associated with a small, north-central Illinois community. *Arch Environ Health* **56**: 389–395

Schiffmann R, van der Knaap MA 2004 The latest on leukodystrophies. *Curr Opin Neurol* **17**: 187–192

Schilder P 1912 Zur Kenntnis der sogenannten diffusen Sklerose (über Encephalitis periaxialis diffusa). *Z Neurol Psychiatr* **10**: 1–60

Schimmel MS, Schlesinger Y, Berger I et al 2002 Transverse myelitis: unusal sequelae of neonatal group B streptococcus disease. *J Perinatol* **22**: 580–581

Schleper B, Stuerenburg HJ 2001 Copper deficiency-associated myelopathy in a 46-year-old woman. *J Neurol* **248**: 705–706

Schlesinger H 1909 Zür Frage der akuten multiplen Sklerose und der encephalomyelitis disseminata im Kindesalter. *Arbeit Neurologish Inst (Wien)* **17**: 410–432

Schlüsener HJ, Meyermann R 1993 Intercrines in brain pathology: expression of intercrines in a multiple sclerosis and Morbus Creutzfeldt–Jacob lesion. *Acta Neuropathol* **86**: 393–396

Schlüsener HJ, Wekerle H 1985 Autoaggressive T lymphocyte lines recognizing the encephalitogenic region of myelin basic protein: *in vitro* selection from unprimed rat T lymphocyte populations. *J Immunol* **135**: 3128–3133

Schlüsener HJ, Sobel RA, Linington C, Weiner HL 1987 A monoclonal antibody against a myelin oligodendrocyte glycoprotein induces relapses and demyelination in central nervous system autoimmune disease. *J Immunol* **139**: 4016–4021

Schlüter D, Meyer T, Kwok LY et al 2002 Phenotype and regulation of persistent intracerebral T cells in murine *Toxoplasma* encephalitis. *J Immunol* **169**: 315–322

Schmidt J, Gold R, Schönrock L et al 2000 T-cell apoptosis in situ in experimental autoimmune encephalomyelitis following methylprednisolone pulse therapy. *Brain* **123**: 1431–1441

Schmidt R, Fazekas F, Offenbacher H et al 1991 Magnetic resonance imaging white matter lesions and cognitive impairment in hypertensive individuals. *Arch Neurol* **48**: 417–420

Schmidt RT, Lee RH, Spehlemann R 1976 Comparison of dantrolene sodium and diazepam in the treatment of spasticity. *J Neurol Neurosurg Psychiatry* **39**: 350–356

Schmidt S, Hertfelder HJ, von Spiegel T et al 1999 Lethal capillary leak syndrome after a single administration of interferon beta-1b. *Neurology* **53**: 220–222

Schmidt S, Barcellos LF, DeSombre K et al 2002 Association of polymorphisms in the apolipoprotein E region with susceptibility to and progression of multiple sclerosis. *Am J Hum Genet* **70**: 708–717

Schmidt S, Passotiropoulos A, Sotgiu S *et al* 2003 Investigation of a genetic variation of a variable number tandem repeat polymorphism of interleukin-6 gene in patients with multiple sclerosis. *J Neurol* **250**: 607–611

Schmied M, Breitschopf H, Gold R *et al* 1993 Apoptosis of T lymphocytes – a mechanism to control inflammation in the brain. *Am J Pathol* **143**: 446–452

Schmierer K, Irlbacher K, Grosse P *et al* 2002 Correlates of disability in multiple sclerosis detected by transcranial magnetic stimulation. *Neurology* **59**: 1218–1224

Schmierer K, Scaravilli F, Altmann DR *et al* 2004 Magnetization transfer ratio and myelin content in *post mortem* multiple sclerosis brain. *Ann Neurol* **56**: 407–415

Schmucker J, Ader M, Brockschnieder D *et al* 2003 erbB3 is dispensable for oligodendrocyte development in vitro and in vivo. *Glia* **44**: 67–75

Schmutzhardt E, Pohl P, Stanek G 1988 *Borrelia burgdorferi* antibodies in patients with relapsing/remitting form and chronic progressive form of multiple sclerosis. *J Neurol Neurosurg Psychiatry* **51**: 1215–1218

Schnadelbach O, Blaschuk OW, Symonds M *et al* 2000 N-cadherin influences migration of oligodendrocytes on astrocyte monolayers. *Mol Cell Neurosci* **15**: 288–302

Schneider C, Gold R, Dalakas MC *et al* 1996 MHC class I mediated cytotoxicity does not induce apoptosis in muscle fibers nor in inflammatory T cells: studies in patients with polymyositis, dermatomyositis and inclusion body myositis. *J Neuropathol Exp Neurol* **55**: 1205–1209

Schneider RD, Ong BH, Moran MJ, Greenhouse AH 1969 Multiple sclerosis in early childhood: case report with notes of frequency. *Clin Pediatr* **8**: 115–118

Schnell L, Fearn S, Schwab ME *et al* 1999 Cytokine-induced acute inflammation in the brain and spinal cord. *J Neuropathol Exp Neurol* **58**: 245–254

Schnider A, Benson FD, Rosner LJ 1993 Callosal disconnection in multiple sclerosis. *Neurology* **43**: 1243–1245

Schob F 1907 Ein Beitrag zür pathologischen Anatomie der multiplen Sklerose. *Monataschr Psychiat Neurol* **22**: 62–87

Schob F 1923 Über Wurzelfibromatose bei multipler Sklerose. *Z Neurol Psychiatr* **83**: 481–496

Scholl GB, Song H-S, Wray SH 1991 Uhthoff's symptom in optic neuritis: relationship to magnetic resonance imaging and development of multiple sclerosis. *Ann Neurol* **30**: 180–184

Scholz A, Reid G, Vogel W, Bostock H 1993 Ion channels in human axons. *J Neurophysiol* **70**: 1274–1279

Schon F, Hart PE, Hodgson TL *et al* 1999 Suppression of pendular nystagmus by smoking cannabis in a patient with multiple sclerosis. *Neurology* **53**: 2209–2210

Schon F, Hodgson TL, Mort D, Kennard C 2001 Ocular flutter associated with a localized lesion in the paramedian pontine reticular formation. *Ann Neurol* **50**: 413–416

Schonrock LM, Kuhlmann T, Adler S *et al* 1998 Identification of glial cell proliferation in early multiple sclerosis lesions. *Neuropathol Appl Neurobiol* **24**: 320–330

Schori H, Kipnis J, Yoles E *et al* 2001 Vaccination for protection of retinal ganglion cells against death from glutamate cytotoxicity and ocular hypertension: implications for glaucoma. *Proc Natl Acad Sci USA* **98**: 3398–3403

Schorlemmer HU, Seiler FR 1991 15-deoxyspergualin (15-DOS) for therapy in an animal model of multiple sclerosis (MS): disease modifying activity on acute and chronic relapsing experimental allergic encephalomyelitis (EAE). *Agents Actions* **34**: 156–160

Schrader H, Gotlibsen OB, Skomedal GN 1980 Multiple sclerosis and narcolepsy/cataplexy in a monozygotic twin. *Neurology* **30**: 105–108

Schreiber K, Oyurai AB, Ryder LP *et al* 2002 Disease severity in Danish multiple sclerosis patients evaluated by MRI and three genetic markers (HLA-DRB1*1501, CCR5 deletion mutation, apolipoprotein E). *Mult Scler* **8**: 295–298

Schrijver HM, Crusius JB, Uitehaag BM *et al* 1999 Association of interleukin-1beta and interleukin-1 receptor antagonist genes with disease severity in MS. *Neurology* **52**: 595–599

Schrijver HM, van As J, Crusius JB *et al* 2003 Interleukin (IL)-1 gene polymorphisms: relevance of disease severity associated alleles with IL-1beta and IL-1ra production in multiple sclerosis. *Mediators Inflamm* **12**: 89–94

Schrijver HM, Crusius JB, Garcia-Gonzalez MA *et al* 2004 Gender-related association between the TGFB1+869 polymorphism and multiple sclerosis. *J Interferon Cytokine Res* **24**: 536–542

Schrijver IA, van Meurs M, Melief M-J *et al* 2001 Bacterial peptidoglycan and immune reactivity in the central nervous system in multiple sclerosis. *Brain* **124**: 1544–1554

Schroder R, Zander H, Andreas A, Mauff G 1983 Multiple sclerosis: immunogenetic analyses of sib-pair double case families. II Studies on the association of multiple sclerosis with C2, C4, BF, C3, C6 and GLO polymorphisms. *Immunobiol* **164**: 160–170

Schroth WS, Tenner SM, Rappaport BA, Mani R 1992 Multiple sclerosis as a cause of atrial fibrillation and electrocardiographic changes. *Arch Neurol* **49**: 422–424

Schuele SU, Kellinghaus C, Shook SJ *et al* 2005 Incidence of seizures in patients with multiple sclerosis treated with intrathecal baclofen. *Neurology* **64**: 1086–1087

Schuller E, Govaerts A 1983 First results of immunotherapy with immunoglobulin-γ in multiple sclerosis. *Eur Neurol* **22**: 205–212

Schulz T-J, Parkes A, Mizogouchi E *et al* 1996 Development of CD4⁻CD8⁻abTCR+NK1.1+ T lymphocytes: thymic selection by self antigen. *J Immunol* **157**: 4379–4389

Schumacher GA, Beebe G, Kibler RF *et al* 1965 Problems of experimental trials of therapy in multiple sclerosis: report by the panel on the evaluation of experimental trials of therapy in multiple sclerosis. *Ann NY Acad Sci* **122**: 552–568

Schumacher TNM 2003 T-cell-receptor gene therapy. *Nature Rev Immunol* **2**: 512–519

Schumann EM, Kumpfel T, Bergh FT *et al* 2002 Activity of the hypothalamic-pituitary-adrenal axis in multiple sclerosis: correlations with gadolinium-enhancing lesions and ventricular volume. *Ann Neurol* **51**: 763–767

Schurch B, De Sèze M, Denys P et al 2005 Botulinum toxin type A is a safe and effective treatment for neurogenic urinary incontinence: results of a single treatment, randomized, placebo-controlled 6-month study. *J Urol* **174**: 196–200

Schuurman PR, Bosch DA, Bossuyt PM *et al* 2000 A comparison of continuous thalamic stimulation and thalamotomy for suppression of severe tremor. *N Engl J Med* **342**: 461–468

Schwab C, McGeer PL 2002 Complement activated C4d immunoreactive oligodendrocytes delineate small cortical plaques in multiple sclerosis. *Exp Neurol* **174**: 81–88

Schwankhaus JD, Patronas N, Dorwart R, Eldridge R, Schlesinger S, McFarland H 1988 Computed tomography and magnetic resonance imaging in a newly described adult-onset leukodystrophy. *Arch Neurol* **45**: 1004–1008

Schwankhaus JD, Katz DA, Eldridge R, Schlesinger S, McFarland H 1994 Clinical and pathological features of an autosomal dominant, adult-onset leukodystrophy simulating chronic progressive multiple sclerosis. *Arch Neurol* **51**: 757–766

Schwankhaus JD, Parisi JE, Gulledge WR *et al* 1995 Hereditary adult-onset Alexander's disease with palatal myoclonus, spastic paraparesis and cerebellar ataxia. *Neurology* **45**: 2226–2271

Schwartz M 2001 Physiological approaches to neuroprotection: boosting of protective autoimmunity. *Survey Ophthalmol* **45**: S256–S260; discussion S273–S276

Schwartz M, Kipnis J 2001 Protective autoimmunity: regulation and prospects for vaccination after brain and spinal cord injuries. *Trends Mol Med* **7**: 252–258

Schwartz M, Moalem G, Leibowitz-Amit R, Cohen IR 1999 Innate and adaptive immune responses can be beneficial for CNS repair. *Trends Neurosci* **22**: 295–299

Schwartzberg C, le Goff P, le Menn C 1981 Complications neuro-ophthalmologique de lupus erythémateux disséminé. *Semaine Hôpitaux* 57: 1292–1300

Schwarz JR, Grigat G 1989 Phenytoin and carbamazepine: potential- and frequency-dependent block of Na currents in mammalian myelinated nerve fibers. *Epilepsia* 30: 286–294

Schwarz JR, Corrette BJ, Mann K, Wietholter H 1991 Changes of ionic channel distribution in myelinated nerve fibres from rats with experimental allergic neuritis. *Neurosci Lett* 122: 205–209

Schwarz S, Knauth M, Schwab S et al 2000 Acute disseminated encephalomyelitis after parenteral therapy with herbal extracts: a report of two cases. *J Neurol Neurosurg Psychiatry* 69: 516–518

Schwarz S, Mohr A, Knauth M et al 2001 Acute disseminated encephalomyelitis: a follow up study of 40 adult patients. *Neurology* 56: 1313–1318

Schweer D, Jacobsen M, Ziegler A et al 2001 No association of three polymorphisms in the alpha-2-macroglobulin and lipoprotein related receptor genes with multiple sclerosis. *J Neuroimmunol* 118: 300–303

Schwid SR, Bever CT Jr 2001 The cost of delaying treatment in multiple sclerosis: what is lost is not regained. *Neurology* 56: 1620

Schwid SR, Noseworthy JH 1999 Targeting immunotherapy in multiple sclerosis: a near hit and a clear miss. *Neurology* 53: 444–445

Schwid SR, Murray TJ 2005 Treating fatigue in patients with MS: one step forward, one step back. *Neurology* 64: 1111–1112

Schwid SR, Goodman AD, Puzas JE et al 1996 Sporadic corticosteroid pulses and osteoporosis in multiple sclerosis. *Arch Neurol* 53: 753–757

Schwid SR, Goodman AD, Mattson DH 1997a Autoimmune hyperthyroidism in patients with multiple sclerosis treated with interferon beta-1b. *Arch Neurol* 54: 1169–1190

Schwid SR, Petrie MD, McDermott MP et al 1997b Quantitative assessment of sustained-release 4-aminopyridine for symptomatic treatment of multiple sclerosis. *Neurology* 48: 817–821

Schwid SR, Petrie MD, Murray R et al 2003 A randomized controlled study of the acute and chronic effects of cooling therapy for MS. *Neurology* 60: 1955–1960

Schwob VS, Clark HB, Agrawal D, Agrawal HC 1985 Electron microscopic immunocytochemical localization of myelin proteolipid protein and myelin basic protein to oligodendrocytes in rat brain during myelination. *J Neurochem* 45: 559–571

Sciacca FL, Ferr C, Vandenbroeck K et al 1999 Relevance of interleukin 1 receptor antagonist intron 2 polymorphism in Italian MS patients. *Neurology* 52: 1896–1898

Sciacca FL, Ferri C, D'Alfonso S et al 2000 Association study of a new polymorphism in the PECAM-1 gene in multiple sclerosis. *J Neuroimmunol* 104: 174–178

Scolding NJ 2001 New cells from old. *Lancet* 357: 329–330

Scolding NJ, Compston DAS 1991 Oligo-dendrocyte susceptibility to injury by specific antibodies. *Immunology* 72: 127–132

Scolding N, Compston DAS 1995 Growth factors fail to protect rat oligodendrocytes against humoral injury *in vitro*. *Neurosci Lett* 183: 75–78

Scolding NJ, Morgan BP, Houston A et al 1989a Normal rat serum cytotoxicity against syngeneic oligodendrocytes: complement activation and attack in the absence of anti-myelin antibodies. *J Neurol Sci* 89: 289–300

Scolding NJ, Morgan BP, Houston WAJ et al 1989b Vesicular removal by oligodendrocytes of membrane attack complexes formed by complement. *Nature* 339: 620–622

Scolding N, Jones J, Compston DAS, Morgan BP 1990 Oligodendrocyte susceptibility to injury by T-cell perforin. *Immunology* 70: 6–10

Scolding NJ, Morgan BP, Campbell AK, Compston DAS 1992 The role of calcium in rat oligodendrocyte injury and repair. *Neurosci Lett* 135: 95–97

Scolding NJ, Rayner PJ, Sussman J et al 1995 A proliferative adult human oligodendrocyte progenitor. *NeuroReport* 6: 441–445

Scolding NJ, Jayne DRW, Zajicek JP, Meyer PAR, Wriaght EP, Lockwood CM 1997 Cerebral vasculitis – recognition, diagnosis and management. *Q J Med* 90: 61–73

Scolding NJ, Morgan BP, Compston DAS 1998a The expression of complement regulatory proteins by adult human oligodendrocytes. *J Neuroimmunol* 84: 69–75

Scolding NJ, Franklin R, Stevens S et al 1998b Oligodendrocyte progenitors are present in the normal adult human CNS and in the lesions of multiple sclerosis. *Brain* 121: 2221–2228

Scott FB, Bradley WE, Timm GW 1973 Treatment of urinary incontinence by an implantable prosthetic sphincter. *Urology* 1: 252–259

Scott TF 1993 Neurosarcoidosis: progress and clinical aspects. *Neurology* 43: 8–12

Scott TF, Hess D, Brillman J 1994 Antiphospholipid antibody syndrome mimicking multiple sclerosis clinically and by magnetic resonance imaging. *Arch Int Med* 154: 917–920

Scott TF, Bhagavatula K, Snyder PJ, Chieffe C 1998 Transverse myelitis: comparison with spinal cord presentations of multiple sclerosis. *Neurology* 50: 429–433

Scott TF, Schramke CJ, Novero J, Chieffe C 2000 Short-term prognosis in early relapsing–remitting multiple sclerosis. *Neurology* 55: 689–693

Scotti G, Gerevini S 2001 Diagnosis and differential diagnosis of acute transverse myelopathy: the role of neuroradiological investigations and review of the literature. *Neurol Sci* 22: S69–S73

Sean Riminton D, Körner H, Strickland DH et al 1998 Challenging cytokine

redundancy: inflammatory cell movement and clinical course of experimental autoimmune encephalomyelitis are normal in lymphotoxin-deficient, but not tumor necrosis factor-deficient, mice. *J Exp Med* 187: 1517–1528

Sears TA, Bostock H 1981 Conduction failure in demyelination: is it inevitable? *Adv Neurol* 31: 357–375

Sears TA, Bostock H, Sheratt M 1978 The pathophysiology of demyelination and its implications for the symptomatic treatment of multiple sclerosis. *Neurology* 28: 21–26

Seboun E, Robinson MA, Doolittle TH et al 1989 A susceptibility locus for multiple sclerosis is linked to the T cell receptor beta chain complex. *Cell* 57: 1095–1100

Seboun E, Oksenberg JR, Rombos A et al 1999 Linkage analysis of candidate myelin genes in familial multiple sclerosis. *Neurogenetics* 2: 155–162

Secondary Progressive Efficacy Clinical Trial of Recombinant Interferon-beta-1a in MS (SPECTRIMS) Study Group 2001 Randomized controlled trial of interferon-beta-1a in secondary progressive MS: clinical results. *Neurology* 56: 1496–1504

Sedano MJ, Trejo JM, Macarron JL et al 2000 Continuous facial myokymia in multiple sclerosis: treatment with botulinum toxin. *Eur Neurol* 43: 137–140

Seddon B, Zamoyska R 2003 Regulation of peripheral T-cell homeostasis by receptor signalling. *Curr Opin Immunol* 15: 321–324

Sedgwick JD 1988 Long-term depletion of CD8+ T cells in vivo in the rat: no observed role for CD8+ (cytotoxic/suppressor) cells in the immunoregulation of experimental allergic encephalomyelitis. *Eur J Immunol* 18: 495–502

Seeldrayers PA, Borenstein S, Gerard J-M, Flament-Durand J 1987 Reversible capsulo-tegmental locked-in state as first manifestation of multiple sclerosis. *J Neurol Sci* 80: 153–160

Segal BM, Klinman DM, Shevach EM 1997 Microbial products induce autoimmune disease by an IL-2 dependent pathway. *J Immunol* 158: 5087–5090

Segal BM, Dwyer BK, Shevach EM 1998 An interleukin (IL)-10/IL-12 immunoregulatory circuit controls susceptibility to autoimmune disease. *J Exp Med* 187: 537–546

Seguin EC 1880 On the coincidence of optic neuritis and subacute transverse myelitis. *J Nerv Mental Dis* 5: 281–293

Seguin EC, Shaw JC, van Derveer A 1878 A contribution to the pathological anatomy of disseminated cerebro-spinal sclerosis. *J Nerv Mental Dis* 5: 281–293

Seiffer W 1905 Über psychische, inbesondere Intelligenzstörungen bei multipler Sklerose. *Arch Psychiatr Nervenkr* 40: 252–303

Seil FJ, Smith ME, Leiman AL, Kelly JM 1975 Myelination inhibiting and neuroelectric blocking factors in experimental allergic encephalomyelitis. *Science* 187: 951–953

Seil FJ, Leiman AL, Kelly JM 1976 Neuroelectric blocking factors in multiple sclerosis and normal human sera. *Arch Neurol* 33: 418–422

Seilhean D, Gansmuller A, Baron-van Evercooren A et al 1996 Myelination by transplanted human and mouse central nervous system tissue after long-term cryopreservation. *Acta Neuropathol* 91: 82–88

Seitelberger F 1960 Histochemistry of demyelinating diseases proper including allergic encephalomyelitis and Pelizaues-Merzbacher's disease. In: Cumings JN (ed.) *Modern Scientific Aspects of Neurology*. London: Arnold, pp. 146–185

Seitelberger F 1967 Autoimmunologic aspects of demyelinating encephalitides. *Nervenarzt* 38: 525–535

Seitelberger F 1973 Pathology of multiple sclerosis. *Ann Clin Res* 5: 337–344

Seitelberger F, Jellinger K, Tschabitscher H 1958 Zür Genese der akuten Entmarkungsenzephalitis. *Wien Klin Wochenschr* 70: 453–459

Selcen D, Anlar B, Renda Y 1996 Multiple sclerosis in childhood: report of 16 cases. *Eur Neurol* 36: 79–84

Self SG, Longton G, Kopecky KG, Liang KY 1991 On estimating HLA/diseases association with application to a study of aplastic anaemia. *Biometrics* 47: 53–61

Selhorst JB, Saul RF 1995 Uhthoff and his symptom. *J Neuroophthalmol* 15: 63–69

Sellebjerg FT, Fredriksen JL, Olssson T 1994 Anti-myelin basic protein and anti-proteolipid protein antibody-secreting cells in the cerebrospinal fluid of patients with acute optic neuritis. *Arch Neurol* 51: 1032–1036

Sellebjerg F, Christiansen M, Nielsen PM, Frederiksen JL 1998a Cerebrospinal fluid measures of disease activity in patients with multiple sclerosis. *Mult Scler* 4: 475–479

Sellebjerg F, Frederiksen JL, Nielsen PM, Olesen J 1998b Double-blind, randomized, placebo-controlled study of oral, high-dose methylprednisolone in attacks of MS. *Neurology* 51: 529–534

Sellebjerg F, Jaliashvili I, Christiansen M, Garred P 1998c Intrathecal activation of the complement system and disability in multiple sclerosis. *J Neurol Sci* 157: 168–174

Sellebjerg F, Frederiksen JL, Nielsen PM, Olesen J 1999 [Randomized controlled trial of high-dose peroral methylprednisolone in attacks of multiple sclerosis]. *Ugeskrift Laeger* 161: 6625–6629

Sellebjerg F, Madsen HO, Jensen CV et al 2000a CCR5 delta32, matrix metalloproteinase-9 and disease activity in multiple sclerosis. *J Neuroimmunol* 102: 98–106

Sellebjerg F, Christiansen M, Jensen J, Frederiksen JL 2000b Immunological effects of oral high-dose methylprednisolone in acute optic neuritis and multiple sclerosis. *Eur J Neurol* 7: 281–289

Sellebjerg F, Giovannoni G, Hand A et al 2002 Cerebrospinal fluid levels of nitric oxide metabolites predict response to methylprednisolone treatment in multiple

sclerosis and optic neuritis. *J Neuroimmunol* 125: 198–203

Selmaj K, Raine CS 1988 Tumour necrosis factor mediates myelin and oligodendrocyte damage *in vitro*. *Ann Neurol* 23: 339–346

Selmaj KW, Raine CS 1995 Experimental autoimmune encephalomyelitis: immunotherapy with anti-tumor necrosis factor antibodies and soluble tumor necrosis factor receptors. *Neurology* 45: S44–S49

Selmaj K, Farooq M, Norton WT et al 1990 Proliferation of astrocytes *in vitro* in response to cytokines: a primary role for tumor necrosis factor. *J Immunol* 144: 129–135

Selmaj K, Brosnan CF, Raine CS 1991a Colocalization of lymphocytes bearing γδ T-cell receptor and heat shock protein hsp65+ oligodendrocytes in multiple sclerosis. *Proc Natl Acad Sci USA* 88: 6452–6456

Selmaj K, Raine C, Cannella B, Brosnan C 1991b Identification of lymphotoxin and tumour necrosis factor in multiple sclerosis lesions. *J Clin Invest* 87: 949–954

Selmaj K, Raine CS, Farooq M et al 1991c Cytokine cytotoxicity against oligodendrocytes: apoptosis induced by lymphotoxin. *J Immunol* 147: 1522–1529

Selmaj K, Brosnan CF, Raine CS 1992 Expression of heat shock protein-65 by oligodendrocytes *in vivo* and *in vitro*: implications for multiple sclerosis. *Neurology* 42: 795–800

Semana G, Yaouang J, Alizadeh M et al 1997 Interleukin-1 receptor antagonist gene in multiple sclerosis. *Lancet* 349: 476

Semra YK, Seidi OA, Sharief MK 2002 Heightened intrathecal release of axonal cytoskeletal proteins in multiple sclerosis is associated with progressive disease and clinical disability. *J Neuroimmunol* 122: 132–139

Senaratne MPJ, Carroll D, Warren KG, Kappagoda T 1984 Evidence for cardiovascular autonomic nerve dysfunction in multiple sclerosis. *J Neurol Neurosurg Psychiatry* 47: 947–952

Senejoux A, Roulot D, Belin C, Tsakiris L 1996 Myélite aiguë après immunisation contre l'hépatite B par un vaccin recombinant. *Gastroenterol Clin Biol* 20: 401–402

Sepcic J, Antonelli L, Materljan E, Sepic-Grahovac D 1989 Multiple sclerosis cluster in Gorski Kotar, Croatia, Yugoslavia. In: Battaglia M (ed.) *Multiple Sclerosis Research*. Amsterdam: Elsevier, pp. 165–169

Septien L, Bourgois M, Altaba A et al 1991 La sclérose en plaques chez l'enfant. L'impact des troubles de la mémoire. *Arch Fr Pediatr* 48: 263–265

Serafini B, Rosicarelli B, Magliozzi R, Stigliano E, Aloisi F 2004 Detection of ectopic B-cell follicles with germinal centers in the meninges of patients with secondary progressive multiple sclerosis. *Brain Pathol* 14: 164–174

Serjeantson SW, Gao X, Hawkins BR et al 1992 Novel HLA-DR2 related haplotypes in

Hong Kong Chinese implicate the DQB1.0602 allele in susceptibility to multiple sclerosis. *Eur J Immunol* 19: 11–19

Sesboue R, Daveau M, Degos J et al 1985 IgG (Gm) allotypes and multiple sclerosis in a French population: phenotype distribution and quantitative abnormalities in CSF with respect to sex, disease severity and presence of intrathecal antibodies. *Clin Immunol Immunopathol* 37: 143–153

Setakis E 2003 Statistical analysis of the GAMES studies. *J Neuroimmunol* 143: 47–52

Setzu A, ffrench-Constant C, Franklin RJ 2004 CNS axons retain their competence for myelination throughout life. *Glia* 45: 307–311

Shaby JA 1958 Multiple sclerosis in Iraq. *Wein Z Nervenheilk* 15: 267–283

Shafit-Zagardo B, Kress Y, Zhao ML, Lee SC 1999 A novel microtubule-associated protein-2 expressed in oligodendrocytes in multiple sclerosis lesions. *J Neurochem* 73: 2531–2537

Shah BS, Stevens EB, Gonzalez MI et al 2000 beta3, a novel auxiliary subunit for the voltage-gated sodium channel, is expressed preferentially in sensory neurons and is upregulated in the chronic constriction injury model of neuropathic pain. *Eur J Neurosci* 12: 3985–3990

Shahrokhi F, Chiappa KH, Young RR 1978 Pattern shift visual evoked responses. *Arch Neurol* 35: 65–71

Shakespeare DT, Boggild M, Young C 2003 Anti-spasticity agents for multiple sclerosis (Cochrane Review). *Cochrane Library* 3: update software

Shakir RA, Sulaiman RA, Rudman M 1990 Neurological presentation of neuro-Behçet's syndrome: clinical categories. *Eur Neurol* 30: 249–253

Sham P, Bader JS, Craig I et al 2002 DNA pooling: a tool for large-scale association studies. *Nature Rev Genet* 3: 862–871

Shao Y, McCarthy KD 1994 Plasticity of astrocytes. *Glia* 11: 147–155

Shapiro S, Galboiz Y, Lahat N et al 2003 The 'immunological-synapse' at its APC side in relapsing and secondary-progressive multiple sclerosis: modulation by interferon-beta. *J Neuroimmunol* 144: 116–124

Sharief MK Hentges R 1991 Association between tumor necrosis factor-alpha and disease progression in patients with multiple sclerosis. *N Engl J Med* 325: 467–472

Sharief MK, Thompson EJ 1992 *In vivo* relationship of tumor necrosis factor-alpha to blood brain barrier damage in patients with active multiple sclerosis. *J Neuroimmunol* 38: 27–33

Sharief MK, Thompson EJ 1993 Correlation of interleukin-2 and soluble interleukin-2 receptor with clinical activity of multiple sclerosis. *J Neurol Neurosurg Psychiatry* 56: 169–174

Sharief MK, Noori MA, Ciardi M, Cirelli A, Thompson EJ 1993 Increased levels of circulating ICAM-1 in serum and cerebrospinal fluid of patients with active multiple sclerosis: correlation with TNF-alpha and blood–brain barrier damage. *J Neuroimmunol* **43**: 15–21

Sharpe G, Price SE, Last A, Thompson RJ 1995 Multiple sclerosis in island populations – prevalence in the Bailiwicks of Guernsey and Jersey. *J Neurol Neurosurg Psychiatry* **58**: 22–26

Sharpe JA 2003 Gaze disorders. In: Noseworthy JH (ed.) *Neurological Therapeutics: Principles and Practice*. London: Martin Dunitz, pp.1799–1816

Sharpe JA, Sanders MD 1975 Atrophy of myelinated nerve fibres in the retina in optic neuritis. *Br J Ophthalmol* **59**: 229–232

Sharpe JA, Hoyt WF, Rosenberg MA 1975 Convergence evoked nystagmus: congenital and acquired. *Arch Neurol* **32**: 191–194

Sharrack B, Hughes RAC 1999 The Guy's Neurological Disability Scale (GNDS): a new disability measure for multiple sclerosis. *Mult Scler* **5**: 223–233

Sharrack B, Hughes RAC, Soudain S, Dunn G 1999 The psychometric properties of clinical rating scales used in multiple sclerosis. *Brain* **122**: 141–159

Sharrack B, Hughes RA, Morris RW *et al* 2000 The effect of oral and intravenous methylprednisolone treatment on subsequent relapse rate in multiple sclerosis. *J Neurolog Sci* **173**: 73–77

Shaw AS 2001 FERMing up the synapse. *Immunity* **15**: 683–686

Shaw CE, Dunbar PR, Macaulay HA, Neale TJ 1995 Measurement of immune markers in the serum and cerebrospinal fluid of multiple sclerosis patients during clinical remission. *J Neurol* **242**: 53–58

Shaw CE, Milner RM, Compston DAS, ffrench Constant C 1996 Integrin expression during axo-glial interactions: a developmental comparison of oligodendrocytes and Schwann cells. *J Neurosci* **16**: 1163–1172

Shaw CM, Alvord EC 1987 Multiple sclerosis beginning in infancy. *J Child Neurol* **2**: 252–256

Shaw FE, Graham DJ, Guess HA, Milstein JB 1988 Postmarketing surveillance for neurologic adverse events reported after hepatitis B vaccination. *Am J Epidemiol* **127**: 337–352

Shaw PJ, Smith NM, Ince PG, Bates D 1987 Chronic periphlebitis retinae in multiple sclerosis: a histological study. *J Neurol Sci* **77**: 147–152

Sheean GL, Murray NMF, Rothwell JC *et al* 1997 An electrophysiological study of the mechanism of fatigue in multiple sclerosis. *Brain* **120**: 299–315

Sheffner JM, Mackin GA, Dawson DM 1992 Lower motor dysfunction in patients with multiple sclerosis. *Muscle Nerve* **15**: 1265–1270

Sheikh KA, Sun J, Liu Y *et al* 1999 Mice lacking complex gangliosides develop Wallerian degeneration and myelination defects. *Proc Natl Acad Sci USA* **96**: 7532–7537

Shepherd DI 1979 Clinical features of multiple sclerosis in north-east Scotland. *Acta Neurol Scand* **60**: 218–230

Shepherd DI, Downie AW 1978 Prevalence of multiple sclerosis in North East Scotland. *Br Med J* **2**: 314–316

Shepherd DI, Downie AW 1980 A further prevalence study of multiple sclerosis in North East Scotland. *J Neurol Neurosurg Psychiatry* **43**: 310–315

Shepherd DI, Summers A 1996 The prevalence of multiple sclerosis in Rochdale. *J Neurol Neurosurg Psychiatry* **61**: 415–417

Sheremata WA, Poskanzer DC, Withum DG *et al* 1985 Unusual occurrence on a tropical island of multiple sclerosis (letter). *Lancet* **2**: 618

Sherratt RM, Bostock H, Sears TA 1980 Effects of 4-aminopyridine on normal and demyelinated mammalian nerve fibres. *Nature* **283**: 570–572

Sherrington CS 1906 *The Integrative Action of the Nervous System*. New York: Charles Scribner's Sons

Sherritt MA, Oksensberg JR, Kerlero de Rosbo N, Bernard CCA 1992 Influence of HLA-DR2, HLA-DPw4 and the T cell receptor alpha chain genes on the susceptibility to multiple sclerosis. *Int Immunol* **4**: 177–181

Sherwin AL 1957 Multiple sclerosis in historical perspective. *McGill Med J* **26**: 39–48

Shevell MI, Bradley BK 1994 The 'Schaltenbrand experiment', Wurzburg, 1940: scientific, historical, and ethical perspectives. *Neurology* **44**: 350–356

Shi Y, Lie DC, Taupin P *et al* 2004 Expression and function of orphan nuclear receptor TLX in adult neural stem cells. *Nature* **427**: 78–83

Shibasaki H, Kuroiwa Y 1974 Painful tonic seizure in multiple sclerosis. *Arch Neurol* **30**: 437–451

Shibasaki H, McDonald WI, Kuroiwa Y 1981 Racial modification of clinical picture of multiple sclerosis: comparison between British and Japanese patients. *J Neurol Sci* **49**: 253–271

Shields GS, Castillo M 2002 Myelitis caused by *Cladophialophora bantiana*. *Am J Roentgenol* **179**: 278–279

Shimizu T, Kagawa T, Wada T *et al* 2005 Wnt signaling controls the timing of oligodendrocyte development in the spinal cord. *Dev Biol* **282**: 397–410

Shimizu Y, Newman W, Tanaka Y, Shaw S 1992 Lymphocyte interaction with endothelial cells. *Immunol Today* **13**: 106–112

Shimonkevitz R, Colburn C, Burnham JA *et al* 1993 Clonal expansion of activated γ/δ T cells in recent-onset multiple sclerosis. *Proc Natl Acad Sci USA* **90**: 923–927

Shin T, Kim S, Moon C *et al* 2000 Aminoguanidine-induced amelioration of autoimmune encephalomyelitis is mediated by reduced expression of inducible nitric oxide synthase in the spinal cord. *Immunol Invest* **29**: 233–241

Shinar Y, Pras E, Siev-Ner I *et al* 1998 Analysis of allelic association between D6S461 marker and multiple sclerosis in Ashkenazi and Iraqi Jewish patients. *J Mol Neurosci* **11**: 265–269

Shinar Y, Livneh A, Villa Y *et al* 2003 Common mutations in the familial Mediterranean fever gene associated with rapid progression to disability in non-Ashkenazi Jewish multiple sclerosis patients. *Genes Immun* **4**: 197–203

Shinder V, Amir R, Devor M 1998 Cross-excitation in dorsal root ganglia does not depend on close cell-to-cell apposition. *NeuroReport* **9**: 3997–4000

Shintaku M, Hirano A, Llena JF 1988 Increased diameter of demyelinated axons in chronic multiple sclerosis of the spinal cord. *Neuropathol Appl Neurobiol* **14**: 505–510

Shiraishi K, Higuchi Y, Ozawa K 2004 Dystonia in a 13 year old boy with secondary progressive multiple sclerosis. *Brain Dev* **26**: 539–541

Shirazi Y, Rus HG, Macklin WB, Shin ML 1993 Enhanced degradation of messenger RNA encoding myelin proteins by terminal complement complexes in oligodendrocytes. *J Immunol* **150**: 4581–4590

Shores EW, Van Ewijk W, Singer A 1991 Disorganization and restoration of thymic medullary epithelial cells in T cell receptor-negative SCID mice: evidence that receptor-bearing lymphocytes influence maturation of the thymic microenvironment. *Eur J Immunol* **21**: 1657–1661

Shortman K, LiuY-J 2002 Mouse and human dendritic cell subtypes. *Nature Rev Immunol* **2**: 151–161

Shrager P 1977 Slow sodium inactivation in nerve after exposure to sulhydryl blocking reagents. *J Gen Physiol* **69**: 183–202

Shrager P 1993 Axonal coding of action potentials in demyelinated nerve fibers. *Brain Res* **619**: 278–290

Shrager P, Rubinstein CT 1990 Optical measurement of conduction in single demyelinated axons. *J Gen Physiol* **95**: 867–890

Shrager P, Custer AW, Kazarinova K *et al* 1998 Nerve conduction block by nitric oxide that is mediated by the axonal environment. *J Neurophysiol* **79**: 529–536

Sibley JT, Olszynski WP, De Coteau WE, Sundaram MB 1992 The incidence and prognosis of central nervous system disease in systemic lupus erythematosus. *J Rheumatol* **19**: 47–52

Sibley WA, Foley J 1965a Seasonal variation in multiple sclerosis and retrobulbar neuritis in Northeastern Ohio. *Trans Am Neurol Assoc* **90**: 295–297

Sibley WA, Foley JM 1965b Infection and immunization in multiple sclerosis. *Ann NY Acad Sci* **122**: 457–466

Sibley WA, Bamford CR, Laguna JF 1976 Influenza vaccination in patients with multiple sclerosis. *J Am Med Assoc* **236**: 1965–1966

Sibley WA, Bamford CR, Clark K 1984 Triggering factors in multiple sclerosis. In: Poser CM (ed.) *The Diagnosis of Multiple Sclerosis*. New York: Thieme-Stratton, pp. 14–24

Sibley, WA, Bamford CR, Clark K 1985 Clinical viral infections and multiple sclerosis. *Lancet* i: 1313–1315

Sibley WA, Bamford CR, Clark K et al 1991 A prospective study of physical trauma and multiple sclerosis. *J Neurol Neurosurg Psychiatry* **54**: 584–589

Sichel J 1837 *Traité de l'Ophthalmie, la cataracte et l'amaurose*. Paris: Baillière

Sichel J 1852–1859 *Iconographie ophthalmologique ou description avec figures coloriées des maladies de l'organe de la vue comprenant l'anatomie pathologique, le pathologie et le therapeutique medico-chirurgicales*. Texte et atlas. Paris: Baillière

Sicotte NL, Liva SM, Klutch R et al 2002 Treatment of multiple sclerosis with the pregnancy hormone estriol. *Ann Neurol* **52**: 421–428

Siegal FP, Kadowaki N, Shodell M et al 1999 The nature of the principal type 1 interferon producing cells in human blood. *Science* **284**: 1835–1837

Siemerling E 1924 Multiple Sklerose (Pathogenese, Aetiologie, Therapie). *Klin Woschenschr* **3**: 609–612

Siemerling E, Raecke J 1911 Zür pathologisdien Anatomie und Pathogenense der multiple on Sklerose. *Arch Psychiatr Nervenkr* **48**: 824

Siemerling E, Raecke E 1914 Beitrag zur Klinik und Pathologie der multiplen Sklerose mit besonderer Berücksichtigung ihrer Pathogenese. *Arch Psychiatr Nervenkr* **53**: 385–564

Siemkowicz E 1976 Multiple sclerosis and surgery. *Anaesthesia* **31**: 1211–1216

Silber E, Semra YK, Gregson NA, Sharief MK 2002 Patients with progressive multiple sclerosis have elevated antibodies to neurofilament subunit. *Neurology* **58**: 1372–1381

Silber MH, Willcox PA, Bowen RM, Unger A 1990 Neuromyelitis optica (Devic's syndrome) and pulmonary tuberculosis. *Neurology* **40**: 934–938

Silberberg, DH, Stuart, WH, van den Noort, S, Therapeutics Technology Assessment Subcommittee of the American Academy of Neurology, The Multiple Sclerosis Council for Clinical Practice Guidelines 2002 Disease modifying therapies in multiple sclerosis: report of the Therapeutics and Technology Assessment Subcommittee of the American Academy of Neurology and the Multiple Sclerosis Council for Clinical Practice Guidelines. *Neurology* **58**: 169–178

Silfverskiöld BP 1947 Retinal periphlebitis with paraplegia. *Arch Neurol Psychiatry* **57**: 351–357

Siller MH 1989 Syphilitic myelopathy. *Genitourin Med* **65**: 338–341

Silver NC, Good CD, Barker GJ et al 1997 Sensitivity of contrast enhanced MRI in multiple sclerosis: effective gadolinium dose, magnetisation transfer contrast and delayed imaging. *Brain* **120**: 1149–1161

Silver NC, Good CD, Sormani MP et al 2001 A modified protocol to improve the detection of enhancing brain and spinal cord lesions in multiple sclerosis. *J Neurol* **248**: 215–224

Silverman N, Maniatis T 2001 NF-kappaB signaling pathways in mammalian and insect innate immunity. *Genes Dev* **15**: 2321–2342

Silversides JA, Heggarty SV, McDonnell GV et al 2004 Influence of CCR5 δ32 polymorphism on multiple sclerosis susceptibility and disease course. *Mult Scler* **10**: 149–152

Sim FJ, Zhao C, Li WW et al 2002a Expression of the POU-domain transcription factors SCIP/Oct-6 and Brn-2 is associated with Schwann cell but not oligodendrocyte remyelination in the CNS. *Mol Cell Neurosci* **20**: 669–682

Sim FJ, Zhao C, Penderis J, Franklin RJ 2002b The age-related decrease in CNS remyelination efficiency is attributable to an impairment of both oligodendrocyte progenitor recruitment and differentiation. *J Neurosci* **22**: 2451–2459

Simeon-Aznar CP, Tolosa-Vilella C, Cuenca-Luque R et al 1992 Transverse myelitis in systemic lupus erythematosus: two cases with magnetic resonance imaging. *Br J Rheumatol* **31**: 555–558

Simmons ML, Frondoza CG, Coyle JT 1991 Immunocytochemical localization of N-acetyl-aspartate with monoclonal antibodies. *Neuroscience* **45**: 37–45

Simmons RD, Willenborg DO 1990 Direct injection of cytokine into the spinal cord causes autoimmune encephalomyelitis-like inflammation. *J Neurol Sci* **100**: 37–42

Simmons RD, Bernard CC, Singer G, Carnegie PR 1982 Experimental autoimmune encephalomyelitis: an anatomically-based explanation of clinical progression in rodents. *J Neuroimmunol* **3**: 307–318

Simmons RD, Hall CA, Gleeson P et al 2001 Prevalence survey of multiple sclerosis in the Australian Capital Territory. *Intern Med J* **31**: 161–167

Simon JH, Jacobs LD, Campion M et al 1997 Magnetic resonance studies of intramuscular interferon β-1a for relapsing multiple sclerosis. *Ann Neurol* **43**: 79–87

Simon JH, Jacobs L, Kinkel RP 2001 Transcallosal bands: a sign of neuronal tract degeneration in early MS? *Neurology* **57**: 1888–1890

Simon RP, Gean-Marton AD, Sander JE 1991 Medullary lesion inducing pulmonary edema: a magnetic resonance imaging study. *Ann Neurol* **30**: 727–730

Simone IL, Carrara D, Tortorella C et al 2002 Course and prognosis in early-onset MS: comparison with adult onset forms. *Neurology* **59**: 1922–1928

Simpson CA, Vejjajiva A, Caspary EA, Miller H 1965 ABO blood groups in multiple sclerosis. *Lancet* i: 1366–1367

Simpson JE, Newcombe J, Cuzner ML, Woodroofe MN 1998 Expression of monocyte chemoattractant protein-1 and other beta-chemokines by resident glia and inflammatory cells in multiple sclerosis lesions. *J Neuroimmunol* **84**: 238–249

Simpson JE, Rezaie P, Newcombe J et al 2000a Expression of the beta-chemokine receptors CCR2, CCR3 and CCR5 in multiple sclerosis central nervous system tissue. *J Neuroimmunol* **108**: 192–200

Simpson JE, Newcombe J, Cuzner ML, Woodroofe MN 2000b Expression of the interferon-gamma-inducible chemokines IP-10 and Mig and their receptor, CXCR3, in multiple sclerosis lesions. *Neuropathol Appl Neurobiol* **26**: 133–142

Sims TJ, Gilmore SA, Waxman SG 1991 Radial glia give rise to perinodal processes. *Brain Res* **549**: 25–35

Sinclair C, Mirakhur M, Kirk J et al 2005 Up-regulation of osteopontin and alphaBeta.crystalline in the normal-appearing white matter of multiple sclerosis: an immunohistochemical study utilizing tissue microarrays. *Neuropath Appl Neurobiol* **31**: 292–303

Sindern E, Haas J, Stark E, Wurster U 1992 Early onset MS under the age of 16: clinical and paraclinical features. *Acta Neurol Scand* **86**: 280–284

Sindic CJ, Monteyne P, Laterre EC 1994 The intrathecal synthesis of virus-specific oligoclonal IgG in multiple sclerosis. *J Neuroimmunol* **54**: 75–80

Singer M, Yakovlev PI 1954 *The Human Brain in Saggital Section*. Springfield, IL: C.C. Thomas

Singh AK, Wilson MT, Hong S et al 2001 Natural killer T cell activation protects mice against experimental autoimmune encephalomyelitis. *J Exp Med* **194**: 1801–1811

Singh S, Alexander M, Korah IP 1999 Acute disseminated encephalomyelitis: MR imaging features. *Am J Roentgenol* **172**: 1101–1107

Singh VK, Mehrotra S, Narayan P et al 2000 Modulation of autoimmune diseases by nitric oxide. *Immunol Res* **22**: 1–19

Singhal BS 1985 Multiple sclerosis – Indian experience. *Ann Acad Med Singapore* **14**: 32–36

Singhal BS, Wadia NH 1975 Profile of multiple sclerosis in the Bombay region on the basis of critical clinical appraisal. *J Neurol Sci* **26**: 259–270

Sinha AA, Bell RB, Steinman L, McDevitt HO 1991 Oligonucleotide dot-blot analysis of HLA-DQbeta alleles associated with multiple sclerosis. *J Neuroimmunol* **32**: 61–65

Sipe JC, Knobler RL, Braheny SL et al 1984 A neurologic rating scale (NRS) for use in multiple sclerosis. *Neurology* **34**: 1368–1372

Sipe JC, Romine JS, Kotziol JA et al 1994 Cladribine in treatment of chronic progressive multiple sclerosis. *Lancet* **344**: 9–13

923

Sipski ML, Rosen RC, Alexander CJ, Hamer RM 2000 Sildenafil effects on sexual and cardiovascular responses in women with spinal cord injury. *Urology* **55**: 812–815

Sironi A, Mamoli A, d'Alessandro G *et al* 1991 Frequency of multiple sclerosis in Valle d'Aosta, 1971–1985. *Neuroepidemiology* **10**: 66–69

Siva A, Radhakrishnan K, Kurland LT *et al* 1993 Trauma and multiple sclerosis: a population based cohort study from Olmsted County, Minnesota. *Neurology* **43**: 1878–1882

Siva A, Kantarci OH, Saip S *et al* 2001 Behcet's disease: diagnostic and prognostic aspects of neurological involvement. *J Neurol* **248**: 95–103

Sivasankaran R, Pei J, Wang KC *et al* 2004 PKC mediates inhibitory effects of myelin and chondroitin sulfate proteoglycans on axonal regeneration. *Nat Neurosci* **7**: 261–268

Skegg DCG, Corwin PA, Craven RS *et al* 1987 Occurrence of multiple sclerosis at the north and south of New Zealand. *J Neurol Neurosurg Psychiatry* **50**: 134–139

Skinner PJ, Haase AT 2002 *In situ* tetramer staining. *J Immunol Meth* **268**: 29–34

Skoff R, Price D, Stocks A 1976 Electron microscope autoradiographic studies of gliogenesis in rat optic nerve. I. Cell proliferation. *J Comp Neurol* **169**: 291–312

Skoog B, Runmarker B, Andersen O 2004 A 37–50 year follow-up of the Gothenburg multiple sclerosis cohort. *Mult Scler* **10** (**Suppl**): S156

Skundric DS, Huston K, Shaw M *et al* 1994 Experimental allergic encephalomyelitis: T cell trafficking to the central nervous system in a resistant Thy-1 congenic mouse strain. *Lab Invest* **71**: 671–679

Slamovits TL, Rosen CE, Cheny KP, Striph GG 1991 Visual recovery in patients with optic neuritis and visual loss to no light perception. *Am J Ophthalmol* **111**: 209–214

Sleeper AA, Cummins TR, Dib-Hajj SD *et al* 2000 Changes in expression of two tetrodotoxin-resistant sodium channels and their currents in dorsal root ganglion neurons after sciatic nerve injury but not rhizotomy. *J Neurosci* **20**: 7279–7289

Sliwa JA, Bell HK, Mason KD *et al* 1996 Upper urinary tract abnormalities in multiple sclerosis patients with urinary symptoms. *Arch Phys Med Rehab* **77**: 247–251

Sloan JB, Berk M, Gebel HM, Fretzin DF 1987 Multiple sclerosis and systemic lupus erythematosus: occurrence in two generations of the same family. *Arch Int Med* **147**: 1317–1320

Sloka JS, Pryse-Phillips WE, Stefanelli M 2005a Incidence and prevalence of multiple sclerosis in Newfoundland and Labrador. *Can J Neurol Sci* **32**: 37–42

Sloka JS, Pryse-Phillips WE, Stefanelli M 2005b Multiple sclerosis in Newfoundland and Labrador – a model for disease prevalence. *Can J Neurol Sci* **32**: 43–49

Small DG 1976 Peripherally evoked spinal cord potentials in neurological diagnosis. In: Nicholson JP (ed.) *Scientific Aids in Hospital Diagnosis.* New York: Plenum Press, pp. 155–163

Small DG, Matthews WB, Small M 1978 The cervical somatosensory evoked potential in the diagnosis of multiple sclerosis. *J Neurol Sci* **35**: 211–224

Small RK, Riddle P, Noble M 1987 Evidence for migration of oligodendrocyte-type 2 astrocyte progenitor cells into the developing rat optic nerve. *Nature* **328**: 155–157

Smeltzer SC, Utell MJ, Rudick RA, Herndon RM 1988 Pulmonary function and dysfunction in multiple sclerosis. *Arch Neurol* **45**: 1245–1249

Smith AJF, Jackson MW, Neufing P *et al* 2004 A functional autoantibody in narcolepsy. *Lancet* **364**: 2122–2124

Smith CP, Nishiguchi J, O'Leary M *et al* 2005 Single-institution experience in 110 patients with botulinum toxin A injection into bladder or urethra. *J Urol* **65**: 37–41

Smith CR, Scheinberg L 1990 Coincidence of myoclonus and multiple sclerosis: dramatic response to clonazepam. *Neurology* **40**: 1633

Smith CR, LaRocca NG, Giesser BS, Scheinberg LA 1991 High-dose oral baclofen: experience in patients with multiple sclerosis. *Neurology* **41**: 1829–1831

Smith CR, Birnbaum G, Carter JL, Greenstein J, Lublin FD, the US Tizanidine Study Group 1994 Tizanidine treatment of spasticity caused by multiple sclerosis. *Neurology* **44** (**Suppl 9**): S34–S43

Smith DR, Balashov KE, Hafler DA *et al* 1997 Immune deviation following pulse cyclophosphamide/methylprednisolone treatment of multiple sclerosis: increased interleukin-4 production and associated eosinophilia. *Ann Neurol* **42**: 313–318

Smith HB, Espir MLE, Whitty CWM *et al* 1957 Abnormal immunological reaction in disseminated sclerosis: a preliminary report. *J Neurol Neurosurg Psychiatry* **20**: 1–10

Smith KJ 1994 Conduction properties of central demyelinated and remyelinated axons, and their relation to symptom production in demyelinating disorders. *Eye* **8**: 224–237

Smith KJ, Hall SM 1980 Nerve conduction during peripheral demyelination and remyelination. *J Neurol Sci* **48**: 201–219

Smith KJ, Hall SM 2001 Factors directly affecting impulse transmission in inflammatory demyelinating disease: recent advances in our understanding. *Curr Opin Neurol* **14**: 289–298

Smith KJ, Lassmann H 2002 The role of nitric oxide in multiple sclerosis. *Lancet Neurol* **1**: 232–241

Smith KJ, McDonald WI 1980 Spontaneous and mechanically evoked activity due to central demyelinating lesion. *Nature* **286**: 154–155

Smith KJ, McDonald WI 1982 Spontaneous and evoked electrical discharges from a central demyelinating lesion. *J Neurol Sci* **55**: 39–47

Smith KJ, McDonald WI 1999 The pathophysiology of multiple sclerosis: the mechanisms underlying the production of symptoms and the natural history of the disease. *Phil Trans R Soc Lond* **354**: 1649–1673

Smith KJ, Schauf CL 1981a Effects of gallamine triethiodide on membrane currents in amphibian and mammalian peripheral nerve. *J Pharmacol Exp Ther* **217**: 719–726

Smith KJ, Schauf CL 1981b Gallamine triethiodide (flaxedil): tetraethylammonium- and pancuronium-like effects in myelinated nerve fibers. *Science* **212**: 1170–1172

Smith KJ, Schauf CL 1981c Size-dependent variation of nodal properties in myelinated nerve. *Nature* **293**: 297–299

Smith KJ, Blakemore WF, McDonald WI 1979 Central remyelination restores secure conduction. *Nature* **280**: 395–396

Smith KJ, Blakemore WF, McDonald WI 1981 The restoration of conduction by central remyelination. *Brain* **104**: 383–404

Smith KJ, Bostock H, Hall SM 1982 Saltatory conduction precedes remyelination in axons demyelinated with lysophosphatidylcholine. *J Neurol Sci* **54**: 13–31

Smith KJ, Felts PA, Baker TA 1994 Conduction properties of glial-ensheathed and sparsely ensheathed central demyelinated axons. *Ann Neurol* **36**: 287

Smith KJ, Felts PA, Kapoor R 1997 Axonal hyperexcitability: mechanisms and role in symptom production in demyelinating diseases. *Neuroscientist* **3**: 237–246

Smith KJ, Pyrdol J, Gauthier L *et al* 1998 Crystal structure of HLA-DR2 (DRA*0101, DRB*1501) complexed with a peptide from human myelin basic protein. *J Exp Med* **188**: 1511–1520

Smith KJ, Kapoor R, Felts PA 1999 Demyelination: the role of reactive oxygen and nitrogen species. *Brain Pathol* **9**: 69–92

Smith KJ, Felts PA, John GR 2000 Effects of 4-aminopyridine on demyelinated axons, synapses and muscle tension. *Brain* **123**: 171–184

Smith KJ, Kapoor R, Hall SM, Davies M 2001a Electrically active axons degenerate when exposed to nitric oxide. *Ann Neurol* **49**: 470–476

Smith KJ, Kapoor R, Hall SM, Davies M 2001b Partial sodium channel blockade protects axons from degeneration caused by the combination of impulse activity and exposure to nitric oxide. *Soc Neurosci Meeting Abstr* 103.12

Smith MB, Brar SP, Nelson LM, Franklin GM 1992 Baclofen effect on quadriceps strength in multiple sclerosis. *Arch Phys Med Rehab* **73**: 237–240

Smith ME, Stone LA, Alpert PS *et al* 1993 Clinical worsening in multiple sclerosis is associated with increased frequency and area of gadopentetate dimeglumine-enhancing magnetic resonance imaging lesions. *Ann Neurol* **33**: 480–489

Smith ME, Eller NL, McFarland HF *et al* 1999 Age dependence of clinical and pathological manifestations of autoimmune demyelination: implications for multiple sclerosis. *Am J Pathol* **155**: 1147–1161

Smith MW, Patterson N, Lautenberger JA 2004 A high-density admixture map for disease gene discovery in african americans. *Am J Hum Genet* **74**: 1001–1013

Smith PF 2002 Cannabinoids in the treatment of pain and spasticity in multiple sclerosis. *Curr Opin Invest Drugs* **3**: 859–864

Smith PM, Blakemore WF 2000 Porcine neural progenitors require commitment to the oligodendrocyte lineage prior to transplantation in order to achieve significant remyelination of demyelinated lesions in the adult CNS. *Eur J Neurosci* **12**: 2414–2424

Smith PM, Franklin RJM 2001 The effect of immunosuppressive protocols on spontaneous CNS remyelination following toxin-induced demyelination. *J Neuroimmunol* **119**: 261–268

Smith S, DeStefano N, Jenkinson M, Matthews P 2001 Normalised accurate measurement of longitudinal brain change. *J Comput Assist Tomog* **25**: 466–475

Smith SL, Otis TS 2003 Persistent changes in spontaneous firing of Purkinje neurons triggered by the nitric oxide signaling cascade. *J Neurosci* **23**: 367–372

Smith T, Cuzner ML 1994 Neuroendocrine-immune interactions in homeostasis and autoimmunity. *Neuropathol Appl Neurobiol* **20**: 413–422

Smith T, Zeeberg I, Sjo O 1986 Evoked potentials in multiple sclerosis before and after high-dose methylprednisolone infusion. *Eur Neurol* **25**: 67–73

Smith T, Schmied M, Hewson AK, Lassmann H, Cuzner ML 1996 Apoptosis of T cells and macrophages in the central nervous system of intact and adrenalectomized Lewis rats during experimental allergic encephalomyelitis. *J Autoimmunity* **9**: 167–174

Smith T, Groom A, Zhu B, Turski L 2000 Autoimmune encephalomyelitis ameliorated by AMPA antagonists. *Nature Med* **6**: 62–66

Snider BJ, Choi J, Turetsky DM *et al* 2000 Nitric oxide reduces Ca2+ and Zn2+ influx through voltage-gated Ca2+ channels and reduces Zn2+ neurotoxicity. *Neuroscience* **100**: 651–661

Snow BJ, Tsui JKC, Bhatt MH, Varelas M, Hashimoto SA, Calne DB 1990 Treatment of spasticity with Botulinum toxin: a double-blind study. *Ann Neurol* **28**: 512–515

Sobel RA 2001 The extracellular matrix in multiple sclerosis: an update. *Braz J Med Biol Res* **34**: 603–609

Sobel RA, Ames MB 1988 Major histocompatibility complex molecule expression in the human central nervous system: immunohistochemical analysis of 40 patients. *J Neuropath Exp Neurol* **47**: 19–28

Sobel RA, Mitchell ME 1989 Fibronectin in multiple sclerosis lesions. *Am J Pathol* **135**: 161–168

Sobel RA, Hafler DA, Castro EE *et al* 1988 The 2H4 (CD45R) antigen is selectively decreased in multiple sclerosis lesions. *J Immunol* **140**: 2210–2214

Sobel RA, Mitchell ME, Fondren G 1990 Intercellular adhesion molecule-1 (ICAM-1) in cellular immune reactions in the human central nervous system. *Am J Pathol* **136**: 1309–1316

Söderström M, Lindqvist M, Hillert J *et al* 1994a Optic neuritis: findings on MRI, CSF examination and HLA class II typing in 60 patients and results of short term follow up. *J Neurol* **241**: 391–397

Söderström M, Link H, Sun J B *et al* 1994b Autoimmune T cell repertoire in optic neuritis and multiple sclerosis: T cells recognizing multiple myelin proteins are accumulated in cerebrospinal fluid. *J Neurol Neurosurg Psychiatry* **57**: 544–551

Söderström M, Hillert J, Link J *et al* 1995 Expression of IFN-γ, IL-4 and TGF-α in multiple sclerosis in relation to HLA-Dw2 phenotype and stage of disease. *Mult Scler* **1**: 173–180

Söderström M, Ya-Ping J, Hillert J, Link H 1998 Optic neuritis: prognosis for multiple sclerosis from MRI, CSF and HLA findings. *Neurology* **50**: 708–714

Sohal RS, Weindruch R 1996 Oxidative stress, caloric restriction, and aging. *Science* **273**: 59–63

Soilu-Hanninen M, Salmi A, Salonen R 1995 Interferon-beta downregulates expression of VLA-4 antigen and antagonizes interferon-gamma-induced expression of HLA-DQ on human peripheral blood monocytes. *J Neuroimmunol* **60**: 99–106

Sokic DV, Stojsavljevic N, Drulovic J *et al* 2001 Seizures in multiple sclerosis. *Epilepsia* **42**: 72–79

Solansky M, Maeda Y, Ming X *et al* 2001 Proliferating oligodendrocytes are present in both active and chronic inactive multiple sclerosis plaques. *J Neurosci Res* 15. **65**: 308–317

Solaro C, Tanganelli P 2004 Tiagabine for treating painful tonic spasms in multiple sclerosis: a pilot study. *J Neurol Neurosurg Psychiatry* **75**: 341

Solaro C, Lunardi GL, Capello E *et al* 1998 An open-label trial of gabapentin treatment of paroxysmal symptoms in multiple sclerosis patients. *Neurology* **51**: 609–611

Solaro C, Uccelli MM, Guglieri P *et al* 2000 Gabapentin is effective in treating nocturnal painful spasms in multiple sclerosis. *Mult Scler* **6**: 192–193

Solaro C, Brichetto G, Amato MP *et al* 2004 The prevalence of pain in multiple sclerosis: a multicenter cross-sectional study. *Neurology* **63**: 919–921

Solaro C, Allemani C, Messmer-Ucelli M *et al* 2005 The prevalence of multiple sclerosis in the north-west Italian province of Genoa. *J Neurol* **252**: 436–440

Soldan SS, Berti R, Salem N *et al* 1997 Association of human herpes virus 6 (HHV-6) with multiple sclerosis: increased IgM response to HHV-6 early antigen and detection of serum HHV-6 DNA. *Nature Med* **3**: 1394–1397

Soldan SS, Leist TP, Juhng KN *et al* 2000 Increased lymphoproliferative response to human herpesvirus type 6A variant in multiple sclerosis patients. *Ann Neurol* **47**: 306–313

Soliven B, Albert J 1992 Tumor necrosis factor modulates Ca²⁺ currents in cultured sympathetic neurons. *J Neurosci* **123**: 2665–2671

Sommer C, Schmidt C, George A 1998 Hyperalgesia in experimental neuropathy is dependent on the TNF receptor 1. *Exp Neurol* **151**: 138–142

Sommerlund M, Pallesen G, Moller-Larsen A *et al* 1993 Retrovirus-like particles in an Epstein–Barr virus producing cell line derived from a patient with chronic progressive myelopathy. *Acta Neurol Scand* **87**: 71–76

Song H, Stevens CF, Gage FH 2002 Astroglia induce neurogenesis from adult neural stem cells. *Nature* **417**: 39–44

Song M-R, Ghosh A 2004 FGF2-induced chromatin remodeling regulates CNTF-mediated gene expression and astrocyte differentiation. *Nat Neurosci* **7**: 229–235

Song P, Lie-Cheng W, Wang GD *et al* 2002 Interleukin-2 regulates membrane potentials and calcium channels via mu opioid receptors in rat dorsal root ganglion neurons. *Neuropharmacology* **43**: 1324–1329

Sonnenberg B 1991 *Lost Property: Memoirs and Confessions of a Bad Boy*. London: Faber & Faber

Soos JM, Ashley TA, Morrow J *et al* 1999 Differential expression of B7 co-stimulatory molecules by astrocytes correlates with T cell activation and cytokine production. *Int Immunol* **11**: 1169–1179

Sorensen PS, Wanscher B, Szpirt W *et al* 1996 Plasma exchange combined with azathioprine in multiple sclerosis using serial gadolinium-enhanced MRI to monitor disease activity: a randomized single-masked cross-over pilot study. *Neurology* **46**: 1620–1625

Sorensen PS, Wanscher B, Jensen C *et al* 1998 Intravenous immunoglobulin G reduces MRI activity in relapsing multiple sclerosis. *Neurology* **50**: 1273–1281

Sorenson PS, Ross C, Clemmesen K *et al* 2003 Clinical importance of neutralising antibodies against interferon beta in patients with relapsing–remitting multiple sclerosis. *Lancet* **362**: 1184–1191

Sorensen PS, Haas J, Sellebjerg F *et al* 2004 IV immunoglobulins as add-on treatment to methylprednisolone for acute relapses in MS. *Neurology* **63**: 2028–2033

Sorensen PS, Koch-Henriksen N, Ross C *et al* 2005 Appearance and disappearance of neutralizing antibodies during interferon-beta therapy. *Neurology* **65**: 33–39

Sorensen TL, Tani M, Jensen J *et al* 1999 Expression of specific chemokines and chemokine receptors in the central nervous system of multiple sclerosis patients. *J Clin Invest* **103**: 807–815

Sorensen TL, Roed H, Sellebjerg F 2002a Chemokine receptor expression on B cells and effect of interferon-beta in multiple sclerosis. *J Neuroimmunol* **122**: 125–131

Sorensen TL, Trebst C, Kivisäkk P et al 2002b Multiple sclerosis: a study of CXCL10 and CXCR3 co-localization in the inflamed central nervous system. *J Neuroimmunol* **127**: 59–68

Sorkin LS, Doom CM 2000 Epineurial application of TNF elicits an acute mechanical hyperalgesia in the awake rat. *J Periph Nerv Syst* **5**: 96–100

Sorkin LS, Xiao WH, Wagner R, Myers RR 1997 Tumour necrosis factor-alpha induces ectopic activity in nociceptive primary afferent fibres. *Neuroscience* **81**: 255–262

Sormani MP, Molyneux PD, Gasperini C et al 1999 Statistical power of MRI monitored trials in multiple sclerosis: new data and comparison with previous results. *J Neurol Neurosurg Psychiatry* **66**: 465–469

Sornas R, Ostlund H 1972 The cytology of the cerebrospinal fluid. *Acta Neurol Scand* **48**: 81–89

Sosa Enriquez M, Leon Betancor P, Rosas C, Navarro MC 1983 La esclerosis multiple en la provincia de Las Palmas. *Arch Neurobiol* **46**: 161–166

Sospedra M, Martin R 2005 Immunology of multiple sclerosis. *Annu Rev Immunol* **23**: 683–747

Sotgiu S, Serra C, Marrosu MG et al 1999 Cytokine production in patients carrying multiple sclerosis-linked HLA-DR alleles. *J Neurol* **246**: 1194–1196

Sotgiu S, Piana A, Pugliatti M et al 2001a *Chlamydia pneumoniae* in the cerebrospinal fluid of patients with multiple sclerosis and neurological controls. *Mult Scler* **7**: 371–374

Sotgiu S, Pugliatti M, Solinas G et al 2001b Imunogenetic heterogeneity of multiple sclerosis in Sardinia. *Neurol Sci* **22**: 167–170

Sotgiu S, Pugliatti M, Rosati G, Sechi GP 2001c Which syringomyelia is truly associated with multiple sclerosis? *J Neurol Sci* **190**: 99–100

Sotgiu S, Serra C, Mameli G et al 2002 Multiple sclerosis-associated retrovirus and MS prognosis: an observational study. *Neurology* **59**: 1071–1073

Souberbielle BE, Martin-Mondiere C, O'Brien ME et al 1990 A case–control epidemiological study of MS in the Paris area with particular reference to past disease history and profession. *Acta Neurol Scand* **82**: 303–310

Soula C, Danesin C, Kan P et al 2001 Distinct sites of origin of oligodendrocytes and somatic motoneurons in the chick spinal cord: oligodendrocytes arise from Nkx2 2-expressing progenitors by a Shh-dependent mechanism. *Development* **128**: 1369–1379

Southwood C, He C, Garbern J et al 2004 CNS myelin paranodes require Nkx6–2 homeoprotein transcriptional activity for

normal structure. *J Neurosci* **24**: 11215–11225

Sozzi G, Marotta P, Piatti L et al 1987 Paroxysmal sensory-motor attacks due to a spinal cord lesion identified by MRI. *J Neurol Neurosurg Psychiatry* **50**: 490–492

Spalding F 2001 *Gwen Raverat. Friends, family and affections.* London: Harvill Press

Spassky N, de Castro F, Le Bras BI et al 2002 Directional guidance of oligodendroglial migration by class 3 semaphorins and netrin-1. *J Neurosci* **22**: 5992–6004

Spatt J, Goldenberg G, Mamoli B 1995 Epilepsia partialis continua in multiple sclerosis. *Lancet* **345**: 658–659

Spector RH, Glaser JS, Schatz NJ 1980 Demyelinative chiasmal lesions. *Arch Neurol* **37**: 757–762

Spiegel J, Hansen C, Baumgartner U et al 2003 Sensitivity of laser-evoked potentials versus somatosensory evoked potentials in patients with multiple sclerosis. *Clin Neurophysiol* **114**: 992–1002

Spielman RS, McGinnis RE, Ewens WJ 1993 Transmission test for linkage disequilibrium: the insulin gene region and insulin-dependent diabetes mellitus (IDMM). *Am J Hum Genet* **52**: 506–516

Spielmeyer W 1922 *Histopathologie des Nervensystems.* Berlin: Springer

Spies T, Bresnahan M, Bahram S et al 1990 A gene in the human histocompatibility complex class II region controlling the class I antigen presentation pathway. *Nature* **348**: 744–747

Spillane JD 1981 *The Doctrine of the Nerves: Chapters in the History of Neurology.* Oxford: Oxford University Press

Spillane JD, Wells CEC 1964 The neurology of Jennerian vaccination. *Brain* **87**: 1–44

Spissu A, Cannas A, Ferrigno P et al 1999 Anatomic correlates of painful tonic spasms in multiple sclerosis. *Mov Disord* **14**: 331–335

Spitsin SV, Hooper DC, Mikheeva T, Koprowski H 2001 Uric acid levels in patients with multiple sclerosis: analysis in mono- and dizygotic twins. *Mult Scler* **7**: 165–166

Spitsin SV, Scott GS, Kean RB et al 2000 Protection of myelin basic protein immunized mice from free-radical mediated inflammatory cell invasion of the central nervous system by the natural peroxynitrite scavenger uric acid. *Neurosci Lett* **292**: 137–141

Spitzer NC 1999 New dimensions of neuronal plasticity. *Nat Neurosci* **2**: 489–491

Spoor TC, Rockwell DL 1988 Treatment of optic neuritis with intravenous megadose corticosteroids. *Ophthalmology* **95**: 131–134

Sprawson CA 1927 Disseminated sclerosis in India. *Trans 7th Congress Far East Assoc Trop Med* **1**: 5 (abstract)

Sprent J, Surh CD 2002 T cell memory. *Annu Rev Immunol* **20**: 551–579

Springer TA 1994 Traffic signals for lymphocyte recirculation and leukocyte emigration: the multistep paradigm. *Cell* **76**: 301–314

Sprinkle T, Wells M, Garver F, Smith D 1980 Studies on Wolfgram high molecular weight CNS proteins: relationship to 2'-3'-cyclic nucleotide 3'-phosphohydrolase. *J Neurochem* **35**: 1200–1208

Spuler S, Yousry T, Scheller A et al 1996 Multiple sclerosis: prospective analysis of TNF-alpha and 55 kDa TNF receptor in CSF and serum in correlation with clinical and MRI activity. *J Neuroimmunol* **66**: 57–64

Spurkland A, Ronningen KS, Vandvik B et al 1991a HLA-DQA1 and HLA-DQB1 genes may jointly determine susceptibility to develop multiple sclerosis. *Hum Immunol* **30**: 69–75

Spurkland A, Tabira T, Ronningen KS et al 1991b HLA-DRB1, -DQA1, -DQB1, -DPA1, -DPA1 and -DPB1 genes in Japanese multiple sclerosis patients. *Tissue Antigens* **37**: 171–173

Spurkland A, Knutsen I, Undlien DE, Vardtal F 1994 No association of multiple sclerosis to alleles at the TAP2 locus. *Hum Immunol* **39**: 299–301

Srinivasan R, Sailasuta N, Hurd R et al 2005 Evidence of elevated glutamate in multiple sclerosis using magnetic resonance spectroscopy at 3T. *Brain* **128**: 1016–1025

Sriram S, Stratton CWQ, Yao S-Y et al 1999 *Chlamydia pneumoniae* infection of the central nervous system in multiple sclerosis. *Ann Neurol* **46**: 6–14

Sriram U, Barcellos LF, Villoslada P et al 2003 Pharmacogenomic analysis of interferon receptor polymorphisms in multiple sclerosis. *Genes Immun* **4**: 147–152

Stadelmann C, Kerschensteiner M, Misgeld T et al 2002 BDNF and gp145trkB in multiple sclerosis brain lesions: neuroprotective interactions between immune cells and neuronal cells? *Brain* **125**: 75–85

Stadelmann C, Ludwin S, Tabira T et al 2005 Tissue preconditioning may explain concentric lesions in Baló's type of multiple sclerosis. *Brain* **128**: 979–987

Staffen W, Mair A, Zauner H et al 2002 Cognitive function and fMRI in patients with multiple sclerosis: evidence for compensatory cortical activation during an attention task. *Brain* **125**: 1275–1282

Stahl JS, Rottach KG, Averbuch-Heller L et al 1996 A pilot study of gabapentin as treatment for acquired nystagmus. *Neuroophthalmology* **16**: 107–113

Stahl SM, Johnson KP, Malamud N 1980 The clinical and pathological spectrum of brain-stem vascular malformations: long term course simulates multiple sclerosis. *Arch Neurol* **37**: 25–29

Stalder AK, Carson MJ, Pagenstecher A et al 1998 Late-onset chronic inflammatory encephalopathy in immune-competent and severe combined immune-deficient (SCID) mice with astrocyte-targeted expression of tumor necrosis factor. *Am J Pathol* **153**: 767–783

Stamler JS, Simon DI, Osborne JA et al 1992 S-nitrosylation of proteins with nitric oxide:

synthesis and characterization of biologically active compounds. *Proc Natl Acad Sci USA* 89: 444–448

Stammers M, Rowen L, Rhodes D et al 2000 BTL-II: a polymorphic locus with homology to the butyrophilin gene family, located at the border of the major histocompatibility complex class II and class III regions in human and mouse. *Immunogenetics* 51: 373–382

Stangel M, Compston A 2001 Polyclonal immunoglobulins (IVIg) modulate nitric oxide production and microglial functions in vitro via Fc receptors. *J Neuroimmunol* 112: 63–71

Stangel M, Hartung HP 2002 [Intravenous immunoglobulins in multiple sclerosis: studies and mechanisms of action – an update]. *Nervenarzt* 73: 119–124

Stangel M, Compston A, Scolding NJ 1999 Polyclonal immunoglobulins for intravenous use do not influence the behaviour of cultured oligodendrocytes. *J Neuroimmunol* 96: 228–233

Stangel M, Boegner F, Klatt CH et al 2000a Placebo controlled pilot trial to study the remyelinating potential of intravenous immunoglobulins in multiple sclerosis. *J Neurol Neurosurg Psychiatry* 68: 89–92

Stangel M, Joly E, Scolding NJ, Compston DAS 2000b Normal polyclonal immunoglobulins ('ivIG') inhibit microglial phagocytosis *in vitro. J Neuroimmunol* 106: 137–144

Stanislaus R, Singh AK, Singh I 2001 Lovastatin treatment decreases mononuclear cell infiltration into the CNS of Lewis rats with experimental allergic encephalomyelitis. *J Neurosci Res* 66: 155–162

Stankoff B, Aigrot MS, Noel F et al 2002a Ciliary neurotrophic factor (CNTF) enhances myelin formation: a novel role for CNTF and CNTF-related molecules. *J Neurosci* 22: 9221–9227

Stankoff B, Barron S, Allard J et al 2002b Oligodendroglial expression of Edg-2 receptor: developmental analysis and pharmacological responses to lysophosphatidic acid. *Mol Cell Neurosci* 20: 415–28

Stankoff B, Waubant E, Confavreux C et al 2005 Modafinil for fatigue in MS: a randomized placebo-controlled double-blind study. *Neurology* 64: 1139–1143

Stanley GP, Pender MP 1991 The pathophysiology of chronic relapsing experimental allergic encephalomyelitis in the Lewis rat. *Brain* 114: 1827–1853

Staples D, Lincoln NB 1979 Intellectual impairment in multiple sclerosis and its relation to functional abilities. *Rheumatol Rehab* 18: 153–160

Starck M, Albrecht H, Pollmann W et al 1997 Drug therapy for acquired pendular nystagmus in multiple sclerosis. *J Neurol* 244: 9–16

Staugaitis SD, Roberts JK, Sacco RL, Miller JR 1998 Devic type multiple sclerosis in an 81 year old woman. *J Neurol Neurosurg Psychiatry* 64: 417

Stazi MA, Cotichini R, Patriarca V et al 2002 The Italian twin project: from the personal identification number to a national twin registry. *Twin Res* 5: 382–386

Stazio A, Kurland LT, Bell GL et al 1964 Multiple sclerosis in Winnipeg, Manitoba. Methodological consideration of epidemiologic survey: ten-year follow-up of a community-wide study and population re-survey. *J Chronic Disease* 17: 415–438

Steck B Amsler F, Kappos L, Burgin D 2001 Gender-specific differences in the process of coping in families with a parent affected by a chronic somatic disease (e.g multiple sclerosis). *Psychopathology* 34: 236–244

Steckley JL, Dyment DA, Sadovnick et al 2000 Genetic analysis of vitamin D related genes in Canadian multiple sclerosis patients. Canadian Collaborative Study Group. *Neurology* 54: 729–732

Stefferl A, Brehm U, Storch M et al 1999 Myelin oligodendrocyte glycoprotein induces experimental autoimmune encephalomyelitis in the resistant Brown Norway rat: disease susceptibility is determined by MHC and MHC-linked effects on the B-cell response. *J Immunol* 163: 40–49

Stefferl A, Schubart A, Storch M et al 2000 Butyrophilin, a milk protein, modulates the encephalitogenic T cell response to myelin oligodendrocyte glycoprotein in experimental autoimmune encephalomyelitis. *J Immunol* 165: 2859–2865

Stefoski D, Davis FA, Faut M, Schauf CL 1987 4-aminopyridine in patients with multiple sclerosis. *Ann Neurol* 21: 71–81

Stefoski D, Davis FA, Fitzsimmons WE, Luskin SS, Rush J, Parkhurst GW 1991 4-aminopyridine in multiple sclerosis: prolonged administration. *Neurology* 41: 1344–1348

Stein EC, Schiffer RB, Hall WJ, Young N 1987 Multiple sclerosis and the workplace: report of an industry-based cluster. *Neurology* 37: 1672–1677

Stein R, Nordal HJ, Oftedal, Slettebo M 1987 The treatment of spasticity in multiple sclerosis: a double blind clinical trial of a new anti-spastic drug tizanidine compared with baclofen. *Acta Neurol Scand* 75: 190–194

Steindler DA, Pincus DW 2002 Stem cells and neuropoiesis in the adult human brain. *Lancet* 359: 1047–1054

Steiner G 1931 Regionale Verteilung der Entmarkungsherde in ihrer Bedeutung für die Pathogenese der multiplen Sklerose. *Krankheitserreger und Gewebsbefund bei multipler Sklerose*. Berlin: Springer, pp. 108–120

Steiner I, Nisipianu P, Wirguin I 2001 Infection and the etiology and pathogenesis of multiple sclerosis. *Curr Neurol Neurosci Rep* 1: 271–276

Steiniger B, Van der Meide PH 1988 Rat ependyma and microglia cells express class II MHC antigens after intravenous infusion of recombinant gamma interferon. *J Neuroimmunol* 19: 111–118

Steinman L 2003 Optic neuritis, a new variant of experimental encephalomyelitis, a durable model for all seasons, now in its seventieth year. *J Exp Med* 197: 1065–1071

Steinman L 2005 Blocking adhesion molecules as therapy for multiple sclerosis: natalizumab. *Nat Rev Drug Discov* 4: 510–508

Steinman RM, Cohn ZA 1973 Identification of a novel cell type in peripheral lymphoid organs of mice. I. Morphology, quantitation, tissue distribution. *J Exp Med* 137: 1142–1162

Stenager E, Knudsen L, Jensen K 1991 Acute and chronic pain syndromes in multiple sclerosis. *Acta Neurol Scand* 84: 197–200

Stenager E, Stenager EN, Jensen K 1996 Sexual function in multiple sclerosis: a 5-year follow-up study. *Ital J Neurol Sci* 17: 67–69

Stenager E, Bronnum-Hansen H, Koch-Henriksen N 2003 The risk of multiple sclerosis in nurses: a population-based epidemiological study. *Mult Scler* 9: 299–301

Stenager EN, Stenager E, Koch-Henriksen N et al 1992 Suicide and multiple sclerosis. *J Neurol Neurosurg Psychiatry* 55: 542–545

Stendahl L, Link H, Moller E, Norrby E 1976 Relation between genetic markers and oligoclonal IgG in CSF in optic neuritis. *J Neurol Sci* 27: 93–98

Stendahl-Brodin L, Link H 1983 Optic neuritis: oligoclonal bands increase the risk of multiple sclerosis. *Acta Neurol Scand* 67: 301–304

Stephanova DI, Chobanova M 1997 Action potentials and ionic currents through paranodally demyelinated human motor nerve fibres: computer simulations. *Biol Cybernetics* 76: 311–314

Sterman AB, Coyle PK, Panesci DJ, Grimson R 1985 Disseminated abnormalities of cardiovascular autonomic functions in multiple sclerosis. *Neurology* 35: 1665–1668

Steultjens EM, Dekker J, Bouter LM et al 2003 Occupational therapy for multiple sclerosis. *Cochrane Database Syst Rev* 3: CD003608

Stevens B, Porta S, Haak LL et al 2002 Adenosine: a neuron-glial transmitter promoting myelination in the CNS in response to action potentials. *Neuron* 36: 855–868

Stevenson VL, Acheson JF, Ball J, Plant GT 1996 Optic neuritis following measles/rubella vaccination in two 13-year-old children. *Br J Ophthalmol* 80: 1110–1111

Stevenson VL, Gawne-Cain ML, Barker GJ, Thompson AJ, Miller DH 1997 Imaging of the spinal cord and brain in multiple sclerosis: a comparison study between fast flair and fast spin echo. *J Neurol* 244: 119–124

Stevenson VL, Miller DH, Rovaris M et al 1999 Primary and transitional progressive MS: a clinical and MRI cross-sectional study. *Neurology* 52: 839–845

Stevenson VL, Miller DH, Leary SM et al 2000 One year follow up study of primary and transitional progressive multiple sclerosis. *J Neurol Neurosurg Psychiatry* **68**: 713–718

Stewart GJ, Basten A, Bashir HV et al 1977 HLA-DW2, viral immunity and family studies in multiple sclerosis. *J Neurol Sci* **32**: 153–167

Stewart GJ, McLeod JG, Basten A, Bashir HE 1981 HLA family studies in multiple sclerosis: a common gene, dominantly expressed. *Hum Immunol* **3**: 13–29

Stewart GJ, Teutsch SM, Castle M, Heard RNS, Bennetts BH 1997 HLA-DR, -DQA1 and DQB1 associations in Australian multiple sclerosis patients. *Eur J Immunogenet* **24**: 81–92

Stewart VC, Giovannoni G, Land JM et al 1997 Pretreatment of astrocytes with interferon-alpha/beta impairs interferon-gamma induction of nitric oxide synthase. *J Neurochem* **68**: 2547–2551

Stewart VC, Land JM, Clark JB, Heales SJR 1998 Pretreatment of astrocytes with interferon-α/β prevents neuronal mitochondrial respiratory chain damage. *J Neurochem* **68**: 2547–2551

Stewart WA, Hall LD, Berry K 1986 Magnetic resonance imaging (MRI) in multiple sclerosis (MS): pathological correlation studies in eight cases. *Neurology* **36**: 320

Stidworthy MF, Genoud S, Li WW et al 2004 Notch1 and Jagged1 are expressed after CNS demyelination, but are not a major rate-determining factor during remyelination. *Brain* **127**: 1928–1941

Stinissen P, Vandevyver C, Medaer R et al 1995 Increased frequency of γδ T cells in cerebrospinal fluid and peripheral blood of patients with multiple sclerosis: reactivity, cytotoxicity, and T cell receptor V gene rearrangements. *J Immunol* **154**: 4883–4849

Stohl W, Gonatas NK 1978 Chronic permeability of the central nervous system to mononuclear cells in experimental allergic encephalomyelitis in the Lewis rat. *J Immunol* **120**: 844–850

Stolp-Smith KA 1998 Lifetime care needs of individuals with multiple sclerosis. *J Spinal Cord Med* **21**: 121–123

Stolp-Smith KA, Carter JL, Rohe DE, Knowland DP 1997 Management of impairment, disability, and handicap due to multiple sclerosis. *Mayo Clin Proc* **72**: 1184–1196

Stolt CC, Lommes P, Sock E et al 2003 The Sox9 transcription factor determines glial fate choice in the developing spinal cord. *Genes Dev* **17**: 1677–1689

Stone J, Sharpe M, Carson A et al 2002 Are functional motor and sensory symptoms really more frequent on the left? A systematic review. *J Neurol Neurosurg Psychiatry* **73**: 578–581

Stone J, Sharpe M, Rothwell PM, Warlow CP 2003 The 12 year prognosis of unilateral functional weakness and sensory disturbance. *J Neurol Neurosurg Psychiatry* **74**: 591–596

Stone LA, Frank JA, Albert PS et al 1995 The effect of interferon-β on blood brain barrier disruptions demonstrated by contrast-enhanced magnetic resonance imaging in relapsing–remitting multiple sclerosis. *Ann Neurol* **37**: 611–619

Stone LA, Frank JA, Albert PS et al 1997 Characterisation of MRI response to treatment with interferon beta-1b: contrast-enhancing MRI lesion frequency as a primary outcome measure. *Neurology* **49**: 862–869

Stone SH, Lerner EM 1965 Chronic disseminated allergic encephalomyelitis in guinea pigs. *Ann NY Acad Sci* **122**: 227–241

Storch MK, Piddlesden S, Haltia M et al 1998a Multiple sclerosis: *in situ* evidence for antibody and complement mediated demyelination. *Ann Neurol* **43**: 465–471

Storch MK, Stefferl A, Brehm U et al 1998b Autoimmunity to myelin oligodendrocyte glycoprotein in rats mimics the spectrum of multiple sclerosis pathology. *Brain Pathol* **8**: 681–694

Strachan JR, Pryor JP 1987 Diagnostic intracorporeal papaverine and erectile dysfunction. *Br J Urol* **59**: 264–266

Stransky E 1903 Über diskontinuierliche Zerfallsprozesse an der peripheren Nervenfaser. *J Psychol Neurol (Leipzig)* **1**: 169–199

Strasser-Fuchs S, Fazekas F, Flooh E et al 1997 Die Einstellung von Patienten mit multipler Sklerose zur Krankheitsaufklärung. *Nervenarzt* **68**: 963–966

Stratton K, Almario DA, McCormick MC (eds) 2002 *Immunization Safety Review: Hepatitis B Vaccine and Demyelinating Neurological Disorders*. Washington, DC: National Academies Press

Striano P, Striano S, Carrieri PB, Boccella P 2003 Epilepsia partialis continua as a first symptom of multiple sclerosis: electrophysiological study of one case. *Mult Scler* **9**: 199–203

Strijbos PJ, Leach MJ, Garthwaite J 1996 Vicious cycle involving Na+ channels, glutamate release, and NMDA receptors mediates delayed neurodegeneration through nitric oxide formation. *J Neurosci* **16**: 5004–5013

Strober W, Ehrhardt RO 1993 Chronic intestinal inflammation: an unexpected outcome in cytokine or T cell receptor mutant mice. *Cell* **75**: 203–205

Strumpell A 1896 Zür pathologie den multiplen Sklerose. *Neurolisches Zentralblatt* **15**: 961–964

Strumpell A 1931 *A Practice of Medicine* (ranslated from the 30th German edition by C.F. Marshall and C.M. Ottley). London: Baillière, Tindall & Cox, pp. 1833–1844

Sturkenboom MCJM, Abenhaim L, Wolfson C et al 1999 Vaccinations, demyelination and multiple sclerosis study (VDAMS): a population-based study in the UK. *Pharmacoepidemiol Drug Safety* **8(Suppl)**: S170–S171

Sturkenboom MC, Wolfson C, Roullet E et al 2000 Demyelination, multiple sclerosis, and hepatitis B vaccination: a population-based study in the UK. *Neurology* **54 (Suppl 3)**: A166

Stürzebecher S, Wandinger KP, Rosenwald A et al 2003 Expression profiling identifies responder and non-responder phenotypes to interferon-beta in multiple sclerosis. *Brain* **126**: 1419–1429

Stuve O, Dooley NP, Uhm JH et al 1996 Interferon β-1b decreases the migration of T lymphocytes *in vitro*: effects on matrix metalloproteinase-9. *Ann Neurol* **40**: 853–863

Stuve O, Chabot S, Jung SS et al VW 1997 Chemokine-enhanced migration of human peripheral blood mononuclear cells is antagonized by interferon beta-1b through an effect on matrix metalloproteinase-9. *J Neuroimmunol* **80**: 38–46

Stys P 2004 Axonal degeneration in multiple sclerosis: is it time for neuroprotective strategies? *Ann Neurol* **55**: 601–603

Stys PK, LoPachin RM 1997 Mechanisms of calcium and sodium fluxes in anoxic myelinated central nervous system axons. *Neuroscience* **82**: 21–32

Stys PK, Waxman SG, Ransom BR 1991 Na(+)-Ca2+ exchanger mediates Ca2+ influx during anoxia in mammalian central nervous system white matter. *Ann Neurol* **30**, 375–380

Stys PK, Sontheimer H, Ransom BR, Waxman SG 1993 Noninactivating, tetrodotoxin-sensitive Na+ conductance in rat optic nerve axons. *Proc Natl Acad Sci USA* **90**: 6976–6980

Su Y, Ganea D, Peng X, Jonakait M 2003 Galanin down-regulates microglial tumor necrosis factor-α production by a post-transcriptional mechanism. *J Neuroimmunol* **134**: 52–60

Suarez B, Hodge S 1979 A simple method to detect linkage for rare recessive diseases: an application to juvenile diabetes. *Clin Genet* **15**: 126–136

Subramaniam A, Harris A, Pignatelli E et al 2003 Metastasis to and from the central nervous system – the 'relatively protected site'. *Lancet Oncol* **3**: 498–507

Subramanian G, Adams MD, Venter JC, Broder S 2001 Implications of the human genome for understanding human biology and medicine. *J Am Med Assoc* **286**: 2296–2307

Suda H, Hosokawa T, Ohno R, Hamaguchi K, Tsukada Y 1984 2',3'-Cyclic nucleotide 3'-phosphodiesterase activity in the cerebrospinal fluid of patients with demyelinating diseases. *Neurochem Pathol* **2**: 85–102

Sudomoina MA, Boiko AN, Demina TL et al 1998 Association of multiple sclerosis in the Russian population with HLA-DRB1 gene alleles. *Mol Biol* **32**: 255–260

Sudweeks JD, Todd JA, Blankenhorn EP et al 1993 Locus controlling *Bordetella pertussis*-induced histamine sensitization (*Bphs*), and autoimmune disease susceptibility gene, maps to T-cell receptor β-chain gene on mouse chromosome 6. *Proc Natl Acad Sci USA* **90**: 3700–3704

Suen WE, Bergman CM, Hjelmström P, Ruddle NH 1997 A critical role for lymphotoxin in experimental allergic encephalomyelitis. *J Exp Med* **186**: 1233–1240

Sugano M, Hirayama K, Saito T et al 1992 Necrotic plaque formation in a case of frontal lobe multiple sclerosis. *Rinsho Shinkeigaku* **32**: 621–625

Sugawa M, Sakurai Y, Ishikawa-Ieda Y et al 2002 Effects of erythropoietin on glial cell development: oligodendrocyte maturation and astrocyte proliferation. *Neurosci Res* **44**: 391–403

Sullivan F, Hutchinson M, Bahandeka S, Moore RE 1987 Chronic hypothermia in multiple sclerosis. *J Neurol Neurosurg Psychiatry* **50**: 813–815

Sullivan PG, Bruce-Keller AJ, Rabchevsky AG et al 1999 Exacerbation of damage and altered NF-kB activation in mice lacking tumor necrosis factor receptors after traumatic brain injury. *J Neurosci* **19**: 6248–6256

Sumelahti M-L, Tienari PJ, Wikstrom J et al 2000 Regional and temporal variation in the incidence of multiple sclerosis in Finland 1979–1993. *Neuroepidemiology* **19**: 67–75

Sumelahti M-L, Tienari PJ, Wikstrom J et al 2001 Increasing prevalence of multiple sclerosis in Finland. *Acta Neurol Scand* **103**: 153–158

Sumelahti M-L, Tienari PJ, Wikstrom J et al 2002 Survival of multiple sclerosis in Finland between 1964–1993. *Mult Scler* **8**: 350–355

Summerfield R, Tubridy N, Sirker A et al 2002 Pulmonary oedema with multiple sclerosis. *J R Soc Med* **95**: 401–402

Sumner AJ, Saida K, Saida T et al 1982 Acute conduction block associated with experimental antiserum-mediated demyelination of peripheral nerve. *Ann Neurol* **11**: 469–477

Sun D, Wekerle H 1986 Ia-restricted encephalitogenic T-lymphocytes mediating EAE lyse autoantigen presenting astrocytes. *Nature* **320**: 70–72

Sun D, Qin Y, Chluba J, Epplen JT, Wekerle H 1988 Suppression of experimentally induced autoimmune encephalomyelitis by cytolytic T-T-cell interactions. *Nature* **332**: 843–845

Sun D, Gold DP, Smith L et al 1992 Characterization of rat encephalitogenic T cells bearing non-Vβ8 T cell receptors. *Eur J Immunol* **22**: 591–594

Sun D, Hu X-Z, Coleclough C 1995 The clonal composition of myelin basic protein-reactive encephalitogenic T cell populations is influenced both by the structure of relevant antigens and the nature of antigen-presenting cells. *Eur J Immunol* **25**: 69–74

Sun D, Whitaker JN, Huang Z et al 2001 Myelin antigen specific CD8+ T cells are encephalitogenic and produce severe disease in C57Bl/6 mice. *J Immunol* **166**: 7579–7587

Sun J, Olsson T, Wang W-Z et al 1991a Autoreactive T and B cells responding to myelin proteolipid protein in multiple sclerosis and controls. *Eur J Immunol* **21**: 1461–1468

Sun J, Link H, Olsson H et al 1991b T and B cell responses to myelin-oligodendrocyte glycoprotein in multiple sclerosis. *J Immunol* **146**: 1490–1495

Sun T, Pringle NP, Hardy AP et al 1998 Pax6 influences the time and site of origin of glial precursors in the ventral neural tube. *Mol Cell Neurosci* **12**: 228–239

Sun Y, Goderie SK, Temple S 2005 Asymmetric distribution of EGFR recptor during mitosis generates diverse CNS progenitor cells. *Neuron* **45**: 873–886

Sundström P, Nystrom L, Forsgren L 2003 Incidence (1988–97) and prevalence (1997) of multiple sclerosis in Vasterbotten County in northern Sweden. *J Neurol Neurosurg Psychiatry* **74**: 29–32

Sundström P, Juto P, Wadell G et al 2006 An altered immune response to Epstein–Barr virus in multiple sclerosis. A prospective study. *Neurology* **62**: 2277–2282

Sundvall M, Jirholt J, Yang HT et al 1995 Identification of murine loci associated with susceptibility to chronic experimental autoimmune encephalomyelitis. *Nature Genet* **10**: 313–317

Sunku J, Kurland LT 1994 Multiple sclerosis and trauma (letter). *Neurology* **44**: 2416

Suppiah V, Alloza I, Heggarty S et al 2005 The CTLA4 +49 A/G*G-CT60*G haplotype is associated with susceptibility to multiple sclerosis in Flanders. *J Neuroimmunol* **164**: 148–153

Surridge D 1969 An investigation into some psychiatric aspects of multiple sclerosis. *Br J Psychiatry* **115**: 749–764

Susac JO, Murtagh FR, Egan RA et al 2003 MRI findings in Susac's syndrome. *Neurology* **61**: 1783–1787

Sussman CR, Vartanian T, Miller RH 2005 The ErbB4 neuregulin receptor mediates suppression of oligodendrocyte maturation. *J Neurosci* **25**: 5757–5762

Sussmuth SD, Reiber H, Tumani H 2001 Tau protein in cerebrospinal fluid (CSF): a blood-CSF barrier related evaluation in patients with various neurological diseases. *Neurosci Lett* **300**: 95–98

Sutherland JM 1956 Observations on the prevalence of multiple sclerosis in northern Scotland. *Brain* **79**: 635–654

Sutherland JM 1989 *A Far Off Sunlit Place*, Brisbane: Amphion Press

Sutherland JM, Tyrer JH, Eadie MJ et al 1966 The prevalence of multiple sclerosis in Queensland, Australia: a field survey. *Acta Neurol Scand* **42 (Suppl 19)**: 57–67

Sutkowski N, Conrad B, Thorley-Lawson DA, Huber BT 2001 Epstein–Barr virus transactivates the human endogenous retrovirus HERV-K18 that encodes a superantigen. *Immunity* **15**: 579–589

Suzuki K, Andrews JM, Waltz JM, Terry RD 1969 Ultrastructural studies of multiple sclerosis. *Lab Invest* **20**: 444–454

Svendsen KB, Jensen TS, Overvad K et al 2003 Pain in patients with multiple sclerosis: a population-based study. *Arch Neurol* **60**: 1089–1094

Svenningsson A, Runmarker B, Lycke J, Andersen O 1990 Incidence of MS during two fifteen-year periods in the Gothenburg region of Sweden. *Acta Neurol Scand* **82**: 161–168

Svenningsson A, Hansson GK, Andersen O et al 1993 Adhesion molecule expression on cerebrospinal fluid T lymphocytes: evidence for common recruitment mechanisms in multiple sclerosis, aseptic meningitis and normal controls. *Ann Neurol* **34**: 155–161

Svenningsson A, Petersson AS, Andersen O, Hansson GK 1999 Nitric oxide metabolites in CSF of patients with MS are related to clinical disease course. *Neurology* **53**: 1880–1882

Swanborg RH, Whittum-Hudson JA, Hudson AP 2003 Infectious agents and multiple sclerosis – are *Chlamydia pneumoniae* and human herpes virus 6 involved? *J Neuroimmunol* **136**: 1–8

Swank RL 1953 Treatment of multiple sclerosis with low fat diet. *Arch Neurol Psychiatry* **69**: 91–103

Swanton JK, Fernando K, Dalton CM et al 2005 Modification of MRI criteria for MS in patients with clinically isolated syndromes. *J Neurol Neurosurg Psychiatry* [epub ahead of print]

Sweeney VP, Sadovnick AD, Brandejs V 1986 Prevalence of multiple sclerosis in British Columbia. *Can J Neurol Sci* **13**: 47–51

Sweeney WJ 1955 Pregnancy and multiple sclerosis. *Am J Obstet Gynecol* **66**: 124–130

Swinburn WR, Liversedge LA 1973 Long-term treatment of multiple sclerosis with azathioprine. *J Neurol Neurosurg Psychiatry* **36**: 124–126

Swingler RJ, Compston DAS 1986 The distribution of multiple sclerosis in the United Kingdom. *J Neurol Neurosurg Psychiatry* **49**: 1115–1124

Swingler RJ, Compston DAS 1988 The prevalence of multiple sclerosis in South East Wales. *J Neurol Neurosurg Psychiatry* **51**: 1520–1524

Swingler RJ, Compston DAS 1992 The clinical features of multiple sclerosis in south east Wales. *Q J Med* **83**: 325–337

Sykes B 1999 The molecular genetics of European ancestry. *Phil Trans R Soc Lond* **354**: 131–139

Symon L, Kuyama H, Kendall B 1984 Dural arteriovenous malformations of the spine: clinical features and surgical results in 55 cases. *J Neurosurg* **60**: 238–247

Tabi Z, McCombe PA, Pender MP 1994 Apoptotic elimination of Vβ8.2+ cells from the central nervous system during recovery from experimental autoimmune encephalomyelitis induced by passive transfer of Vβ8.2+ encephalitogenic T cells. *Eur J Immunol* **24**: 2609–2617

Tabira T, Itoyama Y, Kuroiwa Y et al 1983 Delayed type skin response to myelin basic protein in chronic relapsing experimental allergic encephalomyelitis. *J Neuroimmunol* **5**: 295–304

Tabira T, Itoyama Y, Kuroiwa Y 1984 The role of locally retained antigens in chronic relapsing experimental allergic encephalomyelitis in guinea pigs. In: Alvord EC, Kies MW, Suckling AJ (eds) *Experimental Allergic Encephalomyelitis: A Useful Model for Multiple Sclerosis?* New York: Allan Liss, pp. 43–48

Tachibana N, Howard RS, Hirsch NO, Miller DH, Moseley IF, Fish D 1994 Sleep problems in multiple sclerosis. *Eur Neurol* **34**: 320–323

Tagawa A, Ono S, Inoue K et al 2001 A new familial adult-onset leucodystrophy manifesting as cerebellar ataxia and dementia. *J Neurol Sci* **183**: 47–55

Taguchi O, Nishizuka Y 1980 Autoimmune oophoritis in thymectomized mice: T cell requirement in adoptive cell transfer. *Clin Exp Immunol* **42**: 324–331

Taguchi O, Nishizuka Y 1981 Experimental autoimmune orchitis after neonatal thymectomy in the mouse. *Clin Exp Immunol* **46**: 425–434

Taguchi O, Nishizuka Y 1987 Self tolerance and localized autoimmunity: mouse models of autoimmune disease that suggest tissue-specific suppressor T cells are involved in self tolerance. *J Exp Med* **165**: 146–156

Tahmoush AJ, Amir MS, Connor WW et al 2002 CSF-ACE activity in probable CNS neurosarcoidosis. *Sarcoidosis Vasc Diffuse Lung Dis* **19**: 191–197

Tajouri L, Mellick A, Ashton K et al 2003 Quantitative and qualitative changes in gene expression patterns characterize the activity of plaques in multiple sclerosis. *Mol Brain Res* **119**: 170–183

Tajouri L, Ferreira L, Ovcaric M et al 2004 Investigation of a neuronal nitric oxide synthase gene (NOS1) polymorphism in a multiple sclerosis population. *J Neurol Sci* **218**: 25–28

Tajouri L, Mellick AS, Tourtellotte A et al 2005 An examination of MS candidate genes identified as differentially regulated in multiple sclerosis plaque tissue, using absolute and comparative real-time Q-PCR analysis. *Brain Res Brain Res Protoc* **15**: 79–91

Takacs M, Kalman B, Gyodi E et al 1990 Association between the lack of HLA-DQw6 and the low incidence of multiple sclerosis in Hungarian Gypsies. *Immunogenetics* **31**: 383–385

Takahashi JL, Giuliani F, Power C et al 2003 Interleukin-1β promotes oligodendrocyte death through glutamate excitotoxicity. *Ann Neurol* **53**: 588–595

Takahashi PY, Kiemele LJ, Jones JP 2004 Wound care for elderly patients: advances and clinical applications for practicing physicians. *Mayo Clin Proc* **79**: 260–267

Takano R, Hisahara S, Namikawa K et al 2000 Nerve growth factor protects oligodendrocytes from tumor necrosis factor-alpha-induced injury through Akt-mediated signaling mechanisms. *J Biol Chem* **275**: 16360–16365

Takata T, Hirakawa M, Sakurai M, Kanazawa I 1999 Fulminant form of acute disseminated encephalomyelitis: successful treatment with hypothermia. *J Neurol Sci* **165**: 94–97

Takebayashi H, Yoshida S, Sugimori M et al 2000 Dynamic expression of basic helix-loop-helix Olig family members: implication of Olig2 in neuron and oligodendrocyte differentiation and identification of a new member, Olig3. *Mech Dev* **99**: 143–148

Takebayashi H, Nabeshima Y, Yoshida S et al 2002 The basic helix-loop-helix factor olig2 is essential for the development of motoneuron and oligodendrocyte lineages. *Curr Biol* **12**: 1157–1163

Talley CL 2005 The emergence of multiple sclerosis 1870–1950: a puzzle of historical epidemiology. *Perspect Biol Med* **48**: 383–395

Tan C-T 1988 Multiple sclerosis in Malaysia. *Arch Neurol* **45**: 624–627

Tan EM, Cohen AS, Fries JF et al 1982 The 1982 revised criteria for the diagnosis of systemic lupus erythematosus. *Arthritis Rheum* **25**: 1271–1277

Tan H, Kilicaslan B, Onbas O, Buyukavci M 2004 Acute disseminated encephalomyelitis following hepatitis A virus infection. *Pediatr Neurol* **30**: 207–209

Tan IL, Lycklama a Nijeholt GJ, Polman CH et al 2000 Linomide in the treatment of multiple sclerosis: MRI results from prematurely terminated phase-III trials. *Mult Scler* **6**: 99–104

Tan J, Town T, Paris D et al 1999 Activation of microglial cells by the CD40 pathway: relevance to multiple sclerosis. *J Neuroimmunol* **97**: 77–85

Tancredi V, D'Arcangelo G, Grassi F et al 1992 Tumor necrosis factor alters synaptic transmission in rat hippocampal slices. *Neurosci Lett* **146**: 176–178

Tanne D, D'Ohlaberriague L, Schultz L et al 1999 Anticardiolipin antibodies and their associations with cerebrovascular risk factors. *Neurology* **52**: 1368–1373

Tanuma N, Shin T, Matsumoto Y 2000 Characterization of acute versus chronic relapsing autoimmune encephalomyelitis in DA rats. *J Neuroimmunol* **108**: 171–180

Tao-Cheng JH, Brightman MW 1988 Development of membrane interactions between brain endothelial cells and astrocytes *in vitro*. *Int J Dev Neurosci* **6**: 5–37

Taphoorn MJ, van Someron E, Snoek FJ et al 1993 Fatigue, sleep disturbances and circadian rhythm in multiple sclerosis. *J Neurol* **240**: 446–448

Targ EF, Kocsis JD 1985 4-Aminopyridine leads to restoration of conduction in demyelinated rat sciatic nerve. *Brain Res* **328**: 358–361

Targ EF, Kocsis JD 1986 Action potential characteristics of demyelinated rat sciatic nerve following application of 4-aminopyridine. *Brain Res* **363**: 1–9

Targett MP, Sussman J, Scolding NJ et al 1996 Failure to remyelinate rat axons following transplantation of glial cells obtained from the adult human brain. *Neuropathol Appl Neurobiol* **22**: 199–206

Targoni OS, Lehmann PV 1998 Endogenous myelin basic protein inactivates the high avidity T cell repertoire. *J Exp Med* **187**: 2055–2063

Tartaglia MC, Narayanan S, Francis SJ et al 2004 The relationship between diffuse axonal damage and fatigue in multiple sclerosis. *Arch Neurol* **61**: 201–207

Tas MW, Barkhof F, Van den Walderveen MAA et al 1995 The effect of gadolinium on the sensitivity and specificity of MR imaging in the initial diagnosis of multiple sclerosis. *Am J Neuroradiol* **16**: 259–264

Tasaki I 1953 *Nervous Transmission*. Springfield, IL: C.C. Thomas

Tassinari T, Parodi S, Badino R, Vercelli M 2001 Mortalilty trend for multiple sclerosis in Italy (1974–1993). *Eur J Epidemiol* **17**: 105–110

Taub RG, Rucker CW 1954 The relationship of retrobulbar neuritis to multiple sclerosis. *Am J Ophthalmol* **32**: 488–497

Taupin V, Renno T, Bourbonniere L et al 1997 Increased severity of experimental autoimmune encephalomyelitis, chronic macrophage/microglia reactivity and demyelination in transgenic mice producing tumor necrosis factor-alpha in the central nervous system. *Eur J Immunol* **27**: 905–913

Tavolato B 1975 Immunoglobulin G distribution in multiple sclerosis brain: an immunofluorescence study. *J Neurol Sci* **24**: 1–11

Tazi-Ahnini R, Henry J, Offer C et al 1997 Cloning, localization, and structure of new members of the butyrophilin gene family in the juxta-telomeric region of the major histocompatibility complex. *Immunogenetics* **47**: 55–63

Teesalu T, Hinkkanen AE, Vaheri A 2001 Coordinated induction of extracellular proteolysis systems during experimental autoimmune encephalomyelitis in mice. *Am J Pathol* **159**: 2227–2237

Teitelbaum D, Webb C, Meshorer A et al 1973 Suppression by several synthetic polypeptides of experimental allergic encephalomyelitis induced in guinea pigs and rabbits with bovine and human basic encephalitogen. *Eur J Immunol* **3**: 273–279

Teitelbaum D, Aharoni R, Sela M, Arnon R 1991 Cross-reactions and specificities of monoclonal antibodies against myelin basic protein and against the synthetic copolymer 1. *Proc Natl Acad Sci USA* **88**: 9528–9532

Teitelbaum D, Fridkis-Hareli M, Arnon R, Sela M 1996 Copolymer 1 inhibits chronic relapsing experimental allergic encephalomyelitis induced by proteolipid protein (PLP) peptides in mice and interferes with PLP-specific T cell responses. *J Neuroimmunol* **64**: 209–217

Teitelbaum D, Brenner T, Abramsky O et al 2003 Antibodies to glatiramer acetate do not interfere with its biological functions and therapeutic efficacy. *Mult Scler* **9**: 592–599

Tejada-Simon MV, Zang YCQ, Hong J et al 2003 Cross-reactivity with myelin basic protein and human herpes virus-6 in multiple sclerosis. *Ann Neurol* **53**: 189–197

Tekki-Kessaris N, Woodruff R, Hall AC et al 2001 Hedgehog-dependent oligodendrocyte lineage specification in the telencephalon. *Development* **128**: 2545–2554

Telischi FF, Grobman LR, Sheremata WA et al 1991 Hemifacial spasm: occurrence in multiple sclerosis. *Arch Otolaryngol Head Neck Surg* **117**: 554–556

Templeton AR 2002 Out of Africa again and again. *Nature* **316**: 45–51

Tenembaum S, Chamoles N, Fejerman N 2002 Acute disseminated encephalomyelitis: a long-term follow-up study of 84 pediatric patients. *Neurology* **59**: 1224–1231

Tenser RB, Hay KA, Aberg JA 1993 Immunoglobulin G immunosuppression of multiple sclerosis. *Arch Neurol* **50**: 417–420

Ter Braak JGW, van Herwaarden A 1933 Ophthalmo-encephalo-myelitis mit ungewönlichen Augenerscheinungen. *Klin Monatsbl Augenheilkd* **91**: 316–343

Ter Meulen V, Koprowski H, Iwasaki Y et al 1972 Fusion of cultured multiple sclerosis brain cells with indicator cells: presence of nucleocapsids and virions and isolation of parainfluenza-type virus. *Lancet* **ii**: 1–5

Terasaki PI, Park MS, Opelz G, Ting A 1976 Multiple sclerosis and high frequency of a B lymphocyte alloantigen. *Science* **193**: 1245–1247

Terwilliger JD, Zollner S, Laan M, Paabo S 1998 Mapping genes through the use of linkage disequilibrium generated by genetic drift: 'drift mapping' in small populations with no demographic expansion. *Hum Hered* **48**: 138–154

Tesar JT, McMillan V, Molina R, Armstrong J 1992 Optic neuropathy and central nervous system disease associated with primary Sjögren's syndrome. *Am J Med* **92**: 686–692

Teunissen CE, Dijkstra C, Polman C 2005 Biological markers in CSF and blood for axonal degeneration in multiple sclerosis. *Lancet Neurol* **4**: 32–41

Teutsch SM, Bennetts BH, Buhler MM et al 1999 The DRB1 Val86/Val86 genotype associates with multiple sclerosis in Australian patients. *Hum Immunol* **60**: 715–722

Teutsch SM, Booth DR, Bennetts BH et al 2003 Identification of 11 novel and common single nucleotide polymorphisms in the interleukin-7 receptor-alpha gene and their associations with multiple sclerosis. *Eur J Hum Genet* **11**: 509–515

Teutsch SM, Booth DR, Bennetts BH et al 2004 Association of common T cell activation gene polymorphisms with multiple sclerosis in Australian patients. *J Neuroimmunol* **148**: 218–230

Tharakan J, Ranganath PR, Jacob PC 2005 Multiple sclerosis in Oman. *Neurol J SE Asia* (in press)

Theien BE, Vanderlugt CL, Eagar TN et al 2001 Discordant effects of anti-VLA-4 treatment before and after onset of relapsing experimental autoimmune encephalomyelitis. *J Clin Invest* **107**: 995–1006

Thery C, Zitvogel L, Amigorena S 2002 Exosomes: composition, biogenesis and function. *Nat Rev Immunol* **2**: 569–579

Thiery E, de Reuck J 1974 Monoballism in multiple sclerosis. *Acta Neurol Belg* **74**: 241–249

Thomaides TN, Zoukos Y, Chaudhuri KR, Mathias CJ 1993 Physiological assessment of aspects of autonomic function in patients with secondary progressive multiple sclerosis. *J Neurol* **240**: 139–143

Thomas FJ, Wiles CM 1999 Dysphagia and nutritional status in multiple sclerosis. *J Neurol* **246**: 677–682

Thomas FJ, Hughes TA, Anstey A 2001 Azathioprine treatment in multiple sclerosis: pretreatment assessment of metaboliser status. *J Neurol Neurosurg Psychiatry* **70**: 815

Thomas PK, Walker RWH, Rudge PR et al 1987 Chronic demyelinating peripheral neuropathy associated with multifocal central nervous system demyelination. *Brain* **110**: 53–76

Thomke F, Lensch E, Ringel K, Hopf HC 1997 Isolated cranial nerve palsies in multiple sclerosis. *J Neurol Neurosurg Psychiatry* **63**: 682–685

Thompson AJ 1998 Multiple sclerosis: rehabilitation measures. *Semin Neurol* **18**: 397–403

Thompson AJ 2002a Developing clinical outcome measures in multiple sclerosis: an evolving process. *Mult Scler* **8**: 357–358

Thompson AJ 2002b Progress in neurorehabilitation in multiple sclerosis. *Curr Opin Neurol* **15**: 267–270

Thompson AJ, Brazil J, Feighery C et al 1985 CSF myelin basic protein in multiple sclerosis. *Acta Neurol Scand* **72**: 577–583

Thompson AJ, Hutchinson M, Brazil J et al 1986 A clinical and laboratory study of benign multiple sclerosis. *Q J Med* **58**: 69–80

Thompson AJ, Kennard C, Swash M et al 1989 Relative efficacy of intravenous methylprednisolone and ACTH in the treatment of acute relapse in MS. *Neurology* **39**: 969–971

Thompson AJ, Smith I, Brenton D et al 1990a Neurological deterioration in young adults with phenylketonuria. *Lancet* **336**: 602–605

Thompson AJ, Kermode AG, Macmanus DG et al 1990b Patterns of disease activity in multiple sclerosis: clinical and magnetic resonance imaging study. *Br Med J* **300**: 631–634

Thompson AJ, Kermode AG, Wicks D et al 1991 Major differences in the dynamics of primary and secondary progressive multiple sclerosis. *Ann Neurol* **29**: 53–62

Thompson AJ, Miller D, Youl B et al 1992 Serial gadolinium-enhanced MRI in relapsing/remitting multiple sclerosis of varying disease duration. *Neurology* **42**: 60–63

Thompson AJ, Kermode AG, Moseley IF et al 1993a Seizures due to multiple sclerosis:

seven patients with MRI correlation. *J Neurol Neurosurg Psychiatry* **56**: 1317–1320

Thompson AJ, Tillotson S, Smith I et al 1993b Brain MRI changes in phenylketonuria. *Brain* **116**: 811–821

Thompson AJ, Polman CH, Miller DH et al 1997 Primary progressive multiple sclerosis (review). *Brain* **120**: 1085–1096

Thompson AJ, Montalban X, Barkhof F et al 2000 Diagnostic criteria for primary progressive MS: a position paper. *Ann Neurol* **47**: 831–835

Thompson DS, Nelson LM, Burns A et al 1986 The effects of pregnancy in multiple sclerosis: a retrospective study. *Neurology* **36**: 1097–1099

Thompson EJ 1995 Cerebrospinal fluid. *J Neurol Neurosurg Psychiatry* **59**: 349–357

Thompson PD, Day BL, Rothwell JC et al 1987 The interpretation of electromyographic responses to electrical stimulation of the motor cortex in diseases of the upper motor neurone. *J Neurol Sci* **80**: 91–110

Thompson RJ, Mason CR, Douglas AJ et al 1996 Analysis of polymorphisms of the 2',3'-cyclic nucleotide-3'-phosphodiesterase gene in patients with multiple sclerosis. *Mult Scler* **2**: 215–221

Thomson CE, Vouyiouklis DA, Barrie JA et al 2005 Plp gene regulation in the developing murine optic nerve: correlation with oligodendroglial process alignment along the axons. *Dev Neurosci* **27**: 27–36

Thomson JA, Itskovitz-Eldor J, Shapiro SS et al 1998 Embryonic stem cell lines derived from human blastocysts. *Science* **282**: 1145–1147

Thorpe JW, Kidd D, Kendall BE 1993 Spinal cord MRI using multi-array coils and fast spin echo. I: Technical aspects and findings in healthy adults. *Neurology* **43**: 2625–2631

Thorpe JW, Mumford CJ, Compston DAS et al 1994a The British Isles survey of multiple sclerosis in twins: MRI findings. *J Neurol Neurosurg Psychiatry* **57**: 491–496

Thorpe JW, Moseley IF, Hawkes CH et al 1994b Brain and spinal cord magnetic resonance imaging in motor neurone disease. *J Neurol Neurosurg Psychiatry* **57**: 1298

Thorpe JW, Barker GJ, Jones SJ et al 1995 Magnetisation transfer ratios and transverse magnetisation decay curves in optic neuritis: correlation with clinical findings and electrophysiology. *J Neurol Neurosurg Psychiatry* **59**: 487–492

Thorpe JW, Kidd D, Moseley IF et al 1996a Serial gadolinium-enhanced MRI of the brain and spinal cord in early relapsing–remitting multiple sclerosis. *Neurology* **46**: 373–378

Thorpe JW, Kidd D, Moseley IF et al 1996b Spinal MRI in patients with suspected multiple sclerosis and negative brain MRI. *Brain* **119**: 709–714

Thorpe JW, Moseley IF, Hawkes CH et al 1996c Brain and spinal cord MRI in motor neuron disease. *J Neurol Neurosurg Psychiatry* **61**: 314–317

Thums K 1951 Einelige Zwillinge mit koncordanter multiplen Sklerose. *Wiener Z Nervenheilk* **4**: 173–203

Thygesen P 1949 Prognosis in initial stage of disseminated primary demyelinating disease of central nervous system. *Arch Neurol Psychiatry* **61**: 339–351

Thygesen P 1955 Disseminated sclerosis: influence of age on the different modes of progression. *Acta Psychiatr Neurol Scand* **30**: 365–374

Tiberio M, Chard DT, Altmann DR *et al* 2005 Gray and white matter volume change in early RRMS: a 2 year longitudinal study. *Neurology* **64**: 1001–1007

Tienari PJ, Salonen O, Wikstrom J *et al* 1992a Familial multiple sclerosis: MRI findings in clinically affected and unaffected siblings. *J Neurol Neurosurg Psychiatry* **55**: 883–886

Tienari PJ, Wikstrom J, Sajantila A *et al* 1992b Genetic susceptibility to multiple sclerosis linked to myelin basic protein gene. *Lancet* **340**: 987–991

Tienari PJ, Wikstrom J, Koskimies S *et al* 1993 Reappraisal of HLA in multiple sclerosis: close linkage in multiplex families. *Eur J Hum Genet* **1**: 257–268

Tienari PJ, Terwilliger JD, Ott J *et al* 1994 Two-locus linkage analysis in multiple sclerosis (MS). *Genomics* **19**: 320–325

Tienari PJ, Sumelahti ML, Rantamaki T, Wikstrom J 2004 Multiple sclerosis in western Finland: evidence for a founder effect. *Clin Neurol Neurosurg* **106**: 175–179

Tietjen I, Rihel JM, Cao YX *et al* 2003 Single-cell transcriptional analysis of neuronal progenitors. *Neuron* **38**: 161–175

Tillman AJB 1950 The effect of pregnancy on multiple sclerosis and its management. *Assoc Res Nerv Mental Dis* **28**: 548–582

Tilney F, Riley HA 1938 *The Form and Functions of the Central Nervous System*, 3rd edn. New York: Hoeber

Timme W and the Commission 1922 *Assoc Res Nerv Mental Dis* **2**: 47–48

Timsit S, Martinez S, Allinquant B *et al* 1995 Oligodendrocytes originate in a restricted zone of the embryonic ventral neural tube defined by DM-20 mRNA expression. *J Neurosci* **15**012–1024

Tincani A, Balestrieri G, Faden D, Di Mario C 1991 Systemic lupus eythematosus in pregnancy. *Lancet* **338**: 756–757

Tindall RSA, Walker JE, Ehle AL *et al* 1982 Plasmapheresis in multiple sclerosis: prospective trial of pheresis and immunosuppression versus immunosuppression alone. *Neurology* **32**: 739–743

Tintoré M, Rovira A, Martinez MJ *et al* 2000 Isolated demyelinating syndromes: comparison of different MR imaging criteria to predict conversion to clinically definite multiple sclerosis. *Am J Neuroradiol* **21**: 702–706

Tintoré M, Rovira A, Brieva L *et al* 2001 Isolated demyelinating syndromes: comparison of CSF oligoclonal bands and different imaging criteria to predict conversion to CDMS. *Mult Scler* **7**: 359–363

Tintoré M, Rovira A, Rio J *et al* 2003 New diagnostic criteria for multiple sclerosis: application in first demyelinating episode. *Neurology* **60**: 27–30

Tintoré M, Rovira A, Rio J *et al* 2005 Is optic neuritis more benign than other first attacks in multiple sclerosis? *Ann Neurol* **57**: 210–215

Tippett DS, Fishman PS, Panitch HS 1991 Relapsing transverse myelitis. *Neurology* **41**: 703–706

Tisch R, Yang Y-D, Singer SM *et al* 1993 Immune response to glutamic acid decarboxylase correlates with insulitis in non-obese diabetic mice. *Nature* **366**: 72–75

Titcombe AF, Willison RG 1961 Flicker fusion in multiple sclerosis. *J Neurol Neurosurg Psychiatry* **24**: 260–265

Tivol EA, Borriello F, Schweitzer AN *et al* 1995 Loss of CTLA-4 leads to massive lymphoproliferation and fatal multiorgan tissue destruction, revealing a critical negative regulatory role of CTLA-4. *Immunity* **3**: 541–547

Tjoa CW, Benedict RH, Winstock-Guttman B *et al* 2005 MRI T2 hypointensity of the dentate nucleus is related to ambulatory impairment in multiple sclerosis. *J Neurol Sci* **234**: 17–24

Todman DH 1988 A paroxysmal ocular motility disorder in multiple sclerosis. *Aust NZ J Med* **18**: 785–787

Toivanen AL, Valanne L, Tatlisumak T 2002 Acute disseminated encephalomyelitis following nephropathia epidemica. *Acta Neurol Scand* **105**: 333–336

Tola MA, Yugueros MI, Fernandez-Buey N, Fernandez-Herranz R 1999 Prevalence of multiple sclerosis in Valladolid, Spain. *J Neurol* **246**: 170–174

Tola MR, Granieri E, Caniatti L *et al* 1992 Systemic lupus erythematosus presenting with neurological disorders. *J Neurol* **239**: 61–64

Toma JG, Akhavan M, Fernandus KJ *et al* 2001 Isolation of multipotent adult stem cells from dermis of mammalian skin. *Nat Cell Biol* **3**: 778–784

Toms R, Weiner HL, Johnson D 1990 Identification of IgE-positive cells and mast cells in frozen sections of multiple sclerosis brains. *J Neuroimmunol* **30**: 169–177

Tonegawa S 1983 Somatic generation of antibody diversity. *Nature* **302**: 575–581

Toosy AT, Werring DJ, Bullmore ET *et al* 2002 Functional magnetic resonance imaging of the cortical response to photic stimulation in humans following optic neuritis recovery. *Neurosci Lett* **330**: 255–259

Toosy AT, Hickman SJ, Miszkiel KA *et al* 2005 Adaptive cortical plasticity in higher visual areas after acute optic neuritis. *Ann Neurol* **57**: 622–633

Tooyama I, Kimura H, Akiyama H, McGeer PL 1990 Reactive microglia express class I and class II major histocompatibility complex antigens in Alzheimer's disease. *Brain Res* **523**: 273–280

Topaloglu H, Berker M, Kansu T *et al* 1992 Optic neuritis and myelitis after booster tetanus toxoid vaccination. *Lancet* **339**: 178–179

Torrey EF, Miller J, Rawlings R, Yolken RH 2000 Seasonal birth patterns of neurological disorders. *Neuroepidemiology* **19**: 177–185

Tosti ME, Traversa G, Bianco E, Mele A 1999 Multiple sclerosis and vaccination against hepatitis B: analysis of risk benefit profile. *Ital J Gastroenterol Hepatol* **31**: 388–391

Totaro R, Marini C, Cialfi A *et al* 2000 Prevalence of multiple sclerosis in the L'Aquila district, central Italy. *J Neurol Neurosurg Psychiatry* **68**: 349–352

Totoiu MO, Nistor GI, Lane TE, Keirstead HS 2004 Remyelination, axonal sparing, and locomotor recovery following transplantation of glial-committed progenitor cells into the MHV model of multiple sclerosis. *Exp Neurol* **187**: 254–265

Tourbah A, Gout O, Liblau R *et al* 1999 Encephalitis after hepatitis B vaccination: recurrent disseminated encephalitis or MS? *Neurology* **53**: 396–401

de la Tourette G 1886 *Etudes cliniques et physiologiques sur la marché*. Paris: Progrès Médicale and Delahaye et Lecrosnier

Tournier-Lasserve E, Cashman N, Roullet E, Lyoncean O, Degos JD, Bach MA 1987 T-cell markers in cerebrospinal fluid of patients with multiple sclerosis and other neurological diseases. In: Lowenthal A, Raus J (eds) *Cellular and Humoral Immunological Components of Cerebrospinal Fluid in Multiple Sclerosis*. New York: Plenum Press, pp. 237–248

Tourtellotte WW 1985 The cerebrospinal fluid in multiple sclerosis. *Handbook of Clinical Neurology, Vol 3*. Amsterdam: Elsevier, pp. 79–130

Tourtellotte WW, Parker JA 1966 Multiple sclerosis: correlation between immunoglobulin G in cerebrospinal fluid and brain. *Science* **154**: 1044–1046

Tourtellotte WW, Potvin AR, Baumhefner RW *et al* 1980 Multiple sclerosis de novo CNS IgG synthesis. *Arch Neurol* **37**: 620–624

Tourtellotte WW, Baumhefner RW, Syndulko K *et al* 1988 The long march of the cerebrospinal fluid profile indicative of clinical definite multiple sclerosis; and still marching. *J Neuroimmunol* **20**: 217–227

Touzé E, Gout O, Verdier-Taillefer MH *et al* 2000 Premier épisode de démyélinisation du système nerveux central et vaccination contre l'hépatite B. Etude cas-témoins pilote *Rev Neurol* **156**: 242–246

Touzé E, Fourrier A, Rue-Fenouche C *et al* 2002 Hepatitis B vaccination and first central nervous system demyelinating event: a case-control study. *Neuroepidemiology* **21**: 180–186

Toyonaga B, Yoshikai Y, Vadasz V *et al* 1985 Organisation and sequences of the diversity, joining and constant regions of the human T cell receptor beta chain. *Proc Natl Acad Sci USA* **82**: 8624–8628

Trabattoni D, Ferrante P, Fusi ML et al 2000 Augmented type 1 cytokines and human endogenous retroviruses specific immune responses in patients with acute multiple sclerosis. J Neurovirol 6: S38–S41

Traboulsee A, Dehmeshki J, Brex PA et al 2002 Normal-appearing brain tissue MTR histograms in clinically isolated syndromes suggestive of MS. Neurology 59: 126–128

Traboulsee A, Dehmeshki J, Peters KR et al 2003 Disability in multiple sclerosis is related to normal appearing brain tissue MTR histogram abnormalities. Mult Scler 9: 566–573

Traccis S, Rosati G, Monaco M, Aiello I, Agnetti V 1990 Successful treatment of acquired pendular elliptical nystagmus in multiple sclerosis with isoniazid and base-out prisms. Neurology 40: 492–494

Tran EH, Hoekstra K, Van Rooijen N et al 1998 Immune invasion of the central nervous system parenchyma and experimental allergic encephalomyelitis, but not leukocyte extravasation from blood, are prevented in macrophage-depleted mice. J Immunol 161: 3767–3775

Tran EH, Prince EN, Owens T 2000a IFN-gamma shapes immune invasion of the central nervous system via regulation of chemokines. J Immunol 164: 2759–2768

Tran EH, Kuziel WA, Owens T 2000b Induction of experimental autoimmune encephalomyelitis in C57BL/6 mice deficient in either the chemokine macrophage inflammatory protein-1alpha or its CCR5 receptor. Eur J Immunol 30: 1410–1415

Tran GT, Hodgkinson SJ, Carter N et al 2002 Attenuation of experimental allergic encephalomyelitis in complement component 6-deficient rats is associated with reduced complement C9 deposition, P-selectin expression, and cellular infiltrate in spinal cords. J Immunol 168: 4293–4300

Tran M, Bhargava R, MacDonald IM 2001 Leber hereditary optic neuropathy, progressive visual loss, and multiple-sclerosis-like symptoms. Am J Ophthalmol 132: 591–593

Tranchant C, Bhatia KP, Marsden CD 1995 Movement disorders in multiple sclerosis. Mov Disord 10: 418–423

Transatlantic Multiple Sclerosis Genetics Cooperative 2001 A meta-analysis of genome screens in multiple sclerosis. Mult Scler 7: 3–11

Transverse Myelitis Consortium Working Group 2002 Proposed diagnostic criteria and nosology of acute transverse myelitis. Neurology 59: 499–505

Trapp BD 2004 Pathogenesis of multiple sclerosis: the eyes only see what the mind is prepared to comprehend. Ann Neurol 55: 455–457

Trapp BD, Peterson J, Ransohof RM et al 1998 Axonal transection in the lesions of multiple sclerosis. N Engl J Med 338: 278–285

Trapp BD, Ransohoff R, Rudick R 1999 Axonal pathology in multiple sclerosis: relationship to neurologic disability. Curr Opin Neurol 12: 295–302

Traugott U, Lebon P 1988a Multiple sclerosis: involvement of interferons in lesion pathogenesis. Ann Neurol 24: 243–251

Traugott U, Lebon P 1988b Demonstration of alpha, beta, and gamma interferon in active chronic multiple sclerosis lesions. Ann NY Acad Sci 540: 309–311

Traugott U, Lebon P 1988c Interferon-γ and Ia antigen are present on astrocytes in active chronic multiple sclerosis lesions. J Neurol Sci 84: 257–264

Traugott U, Reinherz EL, Raine CS 1983a Multiple sclerosis: distribution of T cells, T cell subsets and Ia-positive macrophages in lesions of different ages. J Neuroimmunol 4: 201–221

Traugott U, Reinherz EL, Raine CS 1983b Multiple sclerosis: distribution of T cell subsets within active chronic lesions. Science 219: 308–310

Trebst C, Sorensen TL, Kivisäkk P et al 2001 CCR1+/CCR5+ mononuclear phagocytes accumulate in the central nervous system of patients with multiple sclerosis. Am J Pathol 159: 1701–1710

Treib J, Haas A, Stille W et al 2000 Multiple sclerosis and Chlamydia pneumoniae. Ann Neurol 47: 408

Tremlett HL, Luscombe DK, Wiles CM 1998 Use of corticosteroids in multiple sclerosis by consultant neurologists in the United Kingdom. J Neurol Neurosurg Psychiatry 65: 362–365

Trevisani F, Gattinara GC, Caraceni P et al 1993 Transverse myelitis following hepatitis B vaccination. J Hepatol 19: 317–318

Trinchieri G 2003 Interleukin-12 and the regulation of innate resistance and adaptive immunity. Nature Rev Immunol 3: 133–146

Trinka E, Unterberger I, Spiegel M et al 2002 De novo aphasic status epilepticus as presenting symptom of multiple sclerosis. J Neurol 249: 782–783

Trip SA, Schlottmann P, Jones SJ et al 2005 Retinal nerve fibre layer axonal loss and visual dysfunction in optic neuritis. Ann Neurol 58: 383–391

Tröhler U 2000 To Improve the Evidence of Medicine. The eighteenth-century British origins of a critical approach. Edinburgh: Royal College of Physicians

Troiano R, Hafstein M, Ruderman M et al 1984 Effect of high-dose intravenous steroid administration on contrast-enhancing computed tomographic scan lesions in multiple sclerosis. Ann Neurol 15: 257–263

Troiano R, Jotkowitz A, Cook SD et al 1992 Rate and types of fractures in corticosteroid-treated multiple sclerosis patients. Neurology 42: 1389–1391

Trojaborg W, Petersen E 1979 Visual and somatosensory evoked cortical potentials in multiple sclerosis. J Neurol Neurosurg Psychiatry 42: 323–330

Trojano M, Avolio C, Manzari C et al 1995 Multivariate analysis of predictive factors of multiple sclerosis with a validated method to assess clinical events. J Neurol Neurosurg Psychiatry 58: 300–306

Trojano M, Avolio C, Simone IL et al 1996 Soluble intercellular adhesion molecule 1 in serum and cerebrospinal fluid of clinically active relapsing–remitting multiple sclerosis: correlation with Gd-TPA magnetic resonance imaging-enhancement and cerebrospinal fluid findings. Neurology 47: 1535–1541

Trojano M, Liguori M, De Robertis F et al 1999 Comparison of clinical and demographic features between affected pairs of Italian multiple sclerosis multiplex families; relation to tumour necrosis factor genomic polymorphisms. J Neurol Sci 162: 194–200

Trojano M, Liguori M, Zimatore GB et al 2002 Age-related disability in multiple sclerosis. Ann Neurol 51: 475–480

Trooster WJ, Teelken AW, Kampinga J et al 1993 Suppression of acute experimental allergic encephalomyelitis by the synthetic sex hormone 17-alpha-ethinylestradiol: an immunological study in the Lewis rat. Int Arch Allergy Immunol 102: 133–140

Trooster WJ, Teelken AW, Lijnema TH et al 1994 Treatment of acute experimental allergic encephalomyelitis in the Lewis rat with the sex hormone progesterone. Int J Immunopath Pharmacol 7: 183–192

Trostle DC, Helfrich D, Medsger TA 1986 Systemic sclerosis (scleroderma) and multiple sclerosis. Arthritis Rheum 29: 124–127

Trotter J, Schachner M 1989 Cells positive for the 04 surface antigen isolated by cell sorting are able to differentiate into astrocytes or oligodendrocytes. Dev Brain Res 46: 115–122

Trotter JL, Garvey WF 1980 Prolonged effects of large-dose methylprednisolone infusion in multiple sclerosis. Neurology 30: 702–708

Trouillas P, Courjon L 1972 Epilepsy with multiple sclerosis. Epilepsia 13: 325–333

Trousse F, Giess MC, Soula C et al 1995 Notochord and floor plate stimulate oligodendrocyte differentiation in cultures of the chick dorsal neural tube. J Neurosci Res 41: 552–560

Trowsdale J, Hanson I, Mockridge I et al 1990 Sequences encoded in the class II region of the MHC related to the ABC superfamily of transporters. Nature 348: 741–744

Trubo R 2001 Courage. The story of the mighty effort to end the devastating effects of multiple sclerosis, Chicago: Ivan Dee

Truelle JL, Pallison E, LeGall D et al 1987 Troubles intellectuels et thymiques dans la sclérose en plaques. Rev Neurol 143: 595–601

Truyen L, van Waesberghe JHTM, van Walderveen MAA et al 1996 Accumulation of hypointense lesion ('black holes') on T1 SE MRI in multiple sclerosis correlates with disease progression. Neurology 47: 1469–1476

Tsai CP, Yuan CL, Yu HY et al 2004 Multiple sclerosis in Taiwan. J Chin Med Assoc 67: 500–505

Tsai HH, Frost E, To V *et al* 2002 The chemokine receptor CXCR2 controls positioning of oligodendrocyte precursors in developing spinal cord by arresting their migration. *Cell* **110**: 373–383

Tsai HH, Tessier-Lavigne M, Miller RH 2003 Netrin 1 mediates spinal cord oligodendrocyte precursor dispersal. *Development* **130**: 2095–2105

Tschabitscher H 1958 Die klinischen und experimentellen Forschungen der multiplen Sklerose. *Wiener Z Nervenheilk* **14**: 381

Tselis A 2001 Acute disseminated encephalomyelitis. *Curr Treat Options Neurol* **3**: 537–542

Tselis AC, Lisak RP 1995 Acute disseminated encephalomyelitis and isolated central nervous system demyelinative syndromes. *Curr Opin Neurol* **8**: 227–229

Tsuchida T, Parker KC, Turner RV *et al* 1995 Autoreactive CD8$^+$ T cell responses to human myelin protein-derived peptides. *Proc Natl Acad Sci USA* **91**: 10859–10863

Tsukada N, Miyagi K, Matsuda M *et al* 1991 Tumor necrosis factor and interleukin-1 in the CSF and sera of patients with multiple sclerosis. *J Neurol Sci* **104**: 230–234

Tsukada N, Matsuda M, Miyagi K, Yanagisawa N 1993 Increased levels of intercellular adhesion molecule-1 (ICAM-1) and tumor necrosis factor receptor in the cerebrospinal fluid of patients with multiple sclerosis. *Neurology* **43**: 2679–2682

Tsukada N, Matsuda M, Miyagi K, Yanagisawa N 1994 *In vitro* intercellular adhesion molecule-1 expression on brain endothelial cells in multiple sclerosis. *J Neuroimmunol* **49**: 181–187

Tsukada N, Miyagi K, Matsuda M, Yanagisawa N 1995 Soluble E-selectin in the serum and cerebrospinal fluid of patients with multiple sclerosis and human T-lymphocyte virus type 1-associated myelopathy. *Neurology* **45**: 1914–1918

Tsunoda I, Kuang LQ, Theil DJ, Fujinami RS 2000 Antibody association with a novel model for primary progressive multiple sclerosis: induction of relapsing–remitting and progressive forms of EAE in H2s mouse strains. *Brain Pathol* **10**: 402–418

Tubridy N, Ader HJ, Barkhof F *et al* 1998a Exploratory treatment trials in multiple sclerosis using MRI: sample size calculations for relapsing remitting and secondary progressive subgroups using placebo controlled parallel groups. *J Neurol Neurosurg Psychiatry* **64**: 50–55

Tubridy N, Coles AJ, Molyneux P *et al* 1998b Secondary progressive multiple sclerosis: the relationship between short-term MRI activity and clinical features. *Brain* **121**: 225–231

Tubridy N, Behan PO, Capildeo R *et al* 1999 The effect of anti-alpha4 integrin antibody on brain lesion activity in MS. The UK Antegren Study Group. *Neurology* **53**: 466–472

Tuke PW, Hawke S, Griffiths PD, Clark DA 2004 Distribution and quantification of human herpesvirus 6 in multiple sclerosis and control brains. *Mult Scler* **10**: 355–359

Tullman MJ, Delman BN, Lublin FD, Weinberger J 2003 Magnetic resonance imaging in early disseminated Lyme disease. *J Neuroimaging* **13**: 264–268

Tuohy VK, Yu M, Yin L *et al* 1998 The epitope spreading cascade during experimental autoimmune encephalomyelitis and multiple sclerosis. *Immunol Rev* **164**: 93–100

Tuohy VK, Yu M, Yin L *et al* 2000 Modulation of the IL-10/IL-12 cytokine circuit by interferon-beta inhibits the development of epitope spreading and disease progression in murine autoimmune encephalomyelitis. *J Neuroimmunol* **111**: 55–63

Turnley AM, Faux CH, Rietze RL *et al* 2002 Suppressor of cytokine signaling 2 regulates neuronal differentiation by inhibiting growth hormone signaling. *Nat Neurosci* **5**: 1155–1162

Tuzun E, Akman-Demir G, Eraksoy M 2001 Paroxysmal attacks in multiple sclerosis. *Mult Scler* **7**: 402–404

Tuzun S, Altintas A, Karacan I *et al* 2003 Bone status in multiple sclerosis: beyond corticosteroids. *Mult Scler* **9**: 600–604

Tweedy HC 1894 Note on a case of insular sclerosis. *Dublin J Med Sci* **98**: 10–13

Twomey JA, Espir MLE 1980 Paroxysmal symptoms as the first manifestation of multiple sclerosis. *J Neurol Neurosurg Psychiatry* **43**: 269–304

Tyler KL, Gross RA, Cascino GD 1986 Unusual viral causes of transverse myelitis: hepatitis A virus and cytomegalovirus. *Neurology* **36**: 855–858

Tyndall A, Koike T 2002 High-dose immunoablative therapy with hematopoietic stem cell support in the treatment of severe autoimmune disease: current status and future direction. *Intern Med* **41**: 608–612

Ubogu EE, Lindenberg JR, Werz MA 2003 Transverse myelitis associated with *Acinetobacter baumanii* intrathecal pump catheter-related infection. *Reg Anesth Pain Med* **28**: 470–474

Uccelli M, Mohr LM, Battaglia M *et al* 2004 Peer support groups in multiple sclerosis: current effectiveness and future directions. *Mult Scler* **10**: 80–84

Uchimura I, Shiraki H 1957 A contribution to the classification and pathogenesis of demyelinating encephalomyelitis. *J Neuropathol Exp Neurol* **16**: 139–208

Ueda H, Howson JMM, Esposito L *et al* 2003 Association of the T-cell regulatory gene CTLA4 with susceptibility to autoimmune disease. *Nature* **423**: 506–511

Ueda N, Yoshikawa T, Chihara M *et al* 1988 Atrial fibrillation following methylprednisolone pulse therapy. *Pediatr Nephrol* **2**: 29–31

Ueno M, Tokunaga Y, Terachi S *et al* 2000 Asymmetric sweating in a child with multiple sclerosis. *Pediatr Neurol* **23**: 74–76

Uhlenbrock D, Sehlen S 1989 The value of T1-weighted images in the differentiation between MS, white matter lesions and subcortical arteriosclerotic encephalopathy (SAE). *Neuroradiology* **31**: 203–212

Uhthoff W 1890 Untersuchungen über die bei der multiplen Herdsklerose vorkommenden Augenstörungen. *Arch Psychiatr Nervenkrankeiten* **21**: 55–116

Uitdehaag BMJ, Polman CH, Valk J, Koetsier JC, Lucas CJ 1989 Magnetic resonance imaging studies in multiple sclerosis twins. *J Neurol Psychiatry* **52**:1417–1419

Uitdehaag BMJ, Ader HJ, Roosma TJA *et al* 2002 Multiple sclerosis functional composite: impact of reference population and interpretation of change. *Mult Scler* **8**: 366–371

Uitdehaag BMJ, Kappos L, Bauer L *et al* 2005 Discrepancies in the interpretation of clinical symptoms and signs in the diagnosis of multiple sclerosis. A proposal for standardization. *Mult Scler* **11**: 227–231

Uitti RJ, Rajput AH 1986 Multiple sclerosis presenting as isolated oculomotor palsy. *Can J Neurol Sci* **13**: 270–272

Uldry PA, Regli F 1992 Syndrome pseudo-radiculaire au cours de la sclérose en plaques: quartre cas avec imagerie par résonance magnétique. *Rev Neurol* **148**: 692–695

Ulrich J, Groebke-Lorenz W 1983 The optic nerve in multiple sclerosis: a morphological study with retrospective clinico-pathological correlations. *Neuroophthalmology* **3**: 149–159

Ulvestad E, Williams K, Vedeler C *et al* 1994 Reactive microglia in multiple sclerosis lesions have an increased expression of receptors for the Fc part of IgG. *J Neurol Sci* **121**: 125–131

Uncini A, Di Muzio A, Di Guglielmo G *et al* 1999 Effect of rhTNF-alpha injection into rat sciatic nerve. *J Neuroimmunol* **94**: 88–94

United Kingdom Tizanidine Trial Group 1994 A double-blind, placebo-controlled trial of tizanidine in the treatment of spasticity caused by multiple sclerosis. *Neurology* **44 (Suppl 9)**: S70–S78

Urban JL, Kumar V, Kono DH *et al* 1988 Restricted use of T cell receptor V genes in murine autoimmune encephalomyelitis raises possibilities for antibody therapy. *Cell* **54**: 577–592

Ure DR, Rodriguez M 2002 Polyreactive antibodies to glatiramer acetate promote myelin repair in murine model of demyelinating disease. *FASEB J* **16**: 1260–1262

Urenjak J, Williams SR, Gadian DG, Noble M 1993 Proton nuclear magnetic resonance spectroscopy unambiguously identifies different neural cell types. *J Neurosci* **13**: 981–989

Uria DF, Gutierrez V, Menes BB *et al* 1993 HLA class 2 susceptibility and resistance genes in patients with multiple sclerosis from northern Spain, by DNA-RFLP genotyping. *J Neurol Neurosurg Psychiatry* **56**: 722–723

Uria DF, Abad P, Calatayud MT *et al* 1997 Multiple sclerosis in Gijon health district,

Asturias, northern Spain *Acta Neurol Scand* **96**: 375–379

Us O, Lolli F, Baig S, Link H 1989 Intrathecal synthesis of beta-2-microglobulin in multiple sclerosis and aseptic meningoencephalitis. *Acta Neurol Scand* **80**: 598–602

Utz U, Biddison WE, McFarland HF *et al* 1993 Skewed T-cell receptor repertoire in genetically identical twins correlates with multiple sclerosis. *Nature* **364**: 243–247

Utzschneider DA, Thio C, Sontheimer H *et al* 1993 Action potential conduction and sodium channel content in the optic nerve of the myelin-deficient rat. *Proc R Soc Lond B* **254**: 245–250

Utzschneider DA, Archer DR, Kocsis JD *et al* 1994 Transplantation of glial cells enhances action potential conduction of amyelinated spinal cord axons in the myelin-deficient rat. *Proc Natl Acad Sci USA* **91**: 53–57

Vagg R, Mogyoros I, Kiernan MC, Burke D 1998 Activity-dependent hyperpolarization of human motor axons produced by natural activity. *J Physiol* **507**: 919–925

Vahtera T, Haaranen M, Viramo-Koskela AL, Ruutiainen J 1997 Pelvic floor rehabilitation is effective in patients with multiple sclerosis. *Clin Rehab* **11**: 211–219

Vajkoczy P, Laschinger M, Engelhardt B 2001 α4-integrin-VCAM binding mediates G protein independent capture of encephalitogenic T cell blasts to CNS white matter microvessels. *J Clin Invest* **108**: 557–565

Valdo P, Stegagno C, Mazzucco S *et al* 2003 Enhanced expression of NGF receptors in multiple sclerosis lesions. *J Neuropathol Exp Neurol* **61**: 91–98

Valentiner W 1856 Über die sklerose des Gehirns und Ruckenmarks. *Dtsch Klin* **8**: 147–151, 158–162, 167–169

Valiquette G, Adams GM, Herbert J 1992 DDAVP in the management of nocturia in multiple sclerosis. *Ann Neurol* **31**: 577

Valiquette G, Herbert J, Maede-D'Alisera P 1996 Desmopressin in the management of nocturia in patients with multiple sclerosis: a double-blind, crossover trial. *Arch Neurol* **53**. 1270–1275

Valli A, Sette A, Kappos L *et al* 1993 Binding of myelin basic protein peptides to human histocompatibility leukocyte antigen class II molecules and their recognition by T cells from multiple sclerosis patients. *J Clin Invest* **91**: 616–628

Van Assche G, Van Ranst M, Sciot R *et al* 2005 Progressive multifocal leukoencephalopathy after natalizumab therapy for Crohn's disease. *N Engl J Med* **353**: 362–368

Vandenbark AA, Offner H, Reshef T *et al* 1985 Specificity of T lymphocyte lines for peptides of myelin basic protein. *J Immunol* **139**: 229–233

Vandenbark AA, Hashim G, Offner H 1989 Immunization with a synthetic T-cell receptor V-region peptide protects against experimental autoimmune encephalomyelitis. *Nature* **341**: 541–544

Vandenbark AA, Chou YK, Whitham R *et al* 1996a Treatment of multiple sclerosis with T-cell receptor peptides: results of a double-blind pilot trial. *Nature Med* **2**: 1109–1115

Vandenbark AA, Hashim GA, Offner H 1996b T cell receptor peptides in treatment of autoimmune disease: rationale and potential. *J Neurosci Res* **43**: 391–402

Vandenbark AA, Morgan E, Bartholomew R *et al* 2001 TCR peptide therapy in human autoimmune diseases. *Neurochem Res* **26**: 713–730

Vandenbroeck K, Martino G, Marrosu MG *et al* 1997 Occurrence and clinical relevance of an interleukin-4 gene polymorphism in patients with multiple sclerosis. *J Neuroimmunol* **76**: 189–192

Vandenbroeck K, Goris A, Murru R *et al* 1999 A dinucleotide repeat polymorphism located in the IFNalpha/beta chain cluster at chromosome 9p22 is not associated with multiple sclerosis in Sardinia. *Exp Clin Immunogenet* **16**: 26–29

Vandenbroeck K, Fiten P, Ronsse I *et al* 2000a High-resolution analysis of IL6 minisatellite polymorphism in Sardinian multiple sclerosis: effect on onset and course of disease. *Genes Immun* **1**: 460–463

Vandenbroeck K, Hardt C, Louage J *et al* 2000b Lack of association between the interferon regulatory factor-1 (IRF1) locus at 5q31.1 and multiple sclerosis in Germany, northern Italy, Sardinia and Sweden. *Genes Immun* **1**: 290–294

Vandenbroeck K, Fiten P, Heggarty S *et al* 2002 Chromosome 7q21–22 and multiple sclerosis: evidence for a genetic susceptibility effect in vicinity to the protachykinin-1 gene. *J Neuroimmunol* **125**: 141–148

Van den Burg W, van Zomeren EA, Minderhoud JM *et al* 1987 Cognitive impairment in patients with multiple sclerosis and mild physical disability. *Arch Neurol* **44**: 494–501

Van der Aa A, Hellings N, Bernard CCA *et al* 2003 Functional properties of myelin oligodendrocyte glycoprotein-reactive T cells in multiple sclerosis patients and controls. *J Neuroimmunol* **137**: 164–176

Van der Knaap MS, van der Voorn P, Barkhof F *et al* 2003 A new leukodystrophy with brainstem and spinal cord involvement and high lactate. *Ann Neurol* **53**: 252–258

Vanderlugt CL, Miller SD 2002 Epitope spreading in immunemediated diseases: implications for immunotherapy. *Nature Rev Immunol* **2**: 85–95

Vanderlugt CL, Karandikar NJ, Lenschow DJ *et al* 1997 Treatment with intact anti-B7–1 mAb during disease remission enhances epitopes spreading and exacerbates relapses in R-EAE. *J Neuroimmunol* **79**: 113–118

Vandevyver C, Stinissen P, Cassiman J-J, Raus J 1994a TAP1 and TAP2 transporter gene polymorphisms in multiple sclerosis: no evidence for disease association with TAP. *J Neuroimmunol* **54**: 35–40

Vandevyver C, Buyse I, Philippaerts L *et al* 1994b HLA and T-cell receptor polymorphisms in Belgian multiple sclerosis patients: no evidence for disease association with the T-cell recpetor. *J Neuroimmunol* **52**: 25–32

Van Ewijk W 1991 T cell differentiation is influenced by thymic microenvironments. *Ann Rev Immunol* **9**: 591–616

Van Ewijk W, Shores EW, Singer A 1994 Crosstalk in the mouse thymus. *Immunol Today* **15**: 214–217

Vaney C, Henzel-Gutenbrunner M, Jobin P *et al* 2004 Efficacy, safety and tolerability of an orally administered cannabis extract in the treatment of spasticity in patients with multiple sclerosis: a randomized, double-blind, placebo-controlled, crossover study. *Mult Scler* **10**: 417–424

Van Geel BM, Bezman L, Loes DJ *et al* 2001 Evolution of phenotypes in adult male patients with X-linked adreno-leucodystrophy. *Ann Neurol* **49**: 186–194

Van Gehuchten P 1966 Lesions de ganglions spineaux dans la sclérose en plaques. *Acta Neurol Belg* **66**: 331–340

Van Lieshout HBM, Van Engelen BGM, Sanders EACM, Renier WA 1993 Diagnosing multiple sclerosis in childhood. *Acta Neurol Scand* **88**: 339–343

Van Noort J, van Sechel AC, Bajramovic JJ *et al* 1995 The small heat-shock protein αβ crystallin as candidate autoantigen in multiple sclerosis. *Nature* **375**: 798–810

Vanopdenbosch L, Dubos B, D'Hooghe MB *et al* 2000 Mitochondrial mutations of Leber's hereditary optic neuropathy: a risk factor for multiple sclerosis. *J Neurol* **247**: 535–543

Van Waesberghe JHTM, Kamphorst W, De Groot CRA *et al* 1999 Axonal loss in multiple sclerosis lesions: magnetic resonance imaging insights into substrates of disability. *Ann Neurol* **46**: 747–754

Van Walderveen MAA, Tas MW, Barkhof F *et al* 1994 Magnetic resonance evaluation of disease activity during pregnancy in multiple sclerosis. *Neurology* **44**: 327–332

Van Walderveen MA, Barkhof F, Tas MW *et al* 1998a Patterns of brain magnetic resonance abnormalities on T2-weighted spin echo images in clinical subgroups of multiple sclerosis: a large cross-sectional study. *Eur Neurol* **40**: 91–98

Van Walderveen MAA, Kamphorst W, Scheltens P *et al* 1998b Histopathologic correlate of hypointense lesions on T1-weighted spin-echo MRI in multiple sclerosis. *Neurology* **50**: 1282–1288

Van Walderveen MAA, Barkhof F, Pouwels PJW *et al* 1999a Neuronal damage in T1-hypointense multiple sclerosis lesions demonstrated in vivo using proton magnetic resonance spectroscopy. *Ann Neurol* **46**: 79–87

Van Walderveen MAA, Truyen L, van Oosten BW *et al* 1999b Development of hypointense lesions on T1-weighted spin-echo magnetic resonance images in multiple sclerosis: relation to inflammatory activity. *Arch Neurol* **56**: 345–351

Vartanian T, Fischbach G, Miller R 1999 Failure of spinal cord oligodendrocyte development in mice lacking neuregulin. *Proc Natl Acad Sci USA* **96**: 731–735

Vartanian T, Sorensen PS, Rice G 2004 Impact of neutralizing antibodies on the clinical efficacy of interferon beta in multiple sclerosis. *J Neurol* **251**: II25–II30

Vartdal F, Sollid LM, Vandevik B et al 1989 Patients with multiple sclerosis carry DQb1 genes which encode shared polymorphic amino acid sequences. *Hum Immunol* **25**: 103–110

Vas CJ 1969 Sexual impotence and some autonomic disturbances in men with multiple sclerosis. *Acta Neurol Scand* **45**: 166–183

Vass K, Lassmann H 1990 Intrathecal application of interferon gamma: progressive appearance of MHC antigens within the rat nervous system. *Am J Pathol* **137**: 789–800

Vass K, Lassmann H, Wisniewski HM, Iqbal K 1984 Ultracytochemical distribution of myelin basic protein after injection into the cerebrospinal fluid. *J Neurol Sci* **63**: 423–433

Vass K, Lassmann H, Wekerle H, Wisniewski HM 1986 The distribution of Ia antigen in the lesions of rat acute experimental allergic encephalomyelitis. *Acta Neuropathol* **70**: 149–160

Vass K, Heininger K, Schäfer B et al 1992 Interferon-γ potentiates antibody-mediated demyelination *in vivo*. *Ann Neurol* **32**: 198–206

Vassallo L, Elian M, Dean G 1978 Multiple sclerosis in southern Europe. II. Prevalence in Malta in 1978. *J Epidemiol Commun Hlth* **33**: 111–113

Vaughan JH, Riise T, Rhodes GH et al 1996 An Epstein Barr virus-related cross reactive autoimmune response in multiple sclerosis in Norway. *J Neuroimmunol* **69**: 95–102

van Veen T, Crusius JBA, Schrijver HM et al 2001 Interleukin-12p40 genotype plays a role in the susceptibility to multiple sclerosis. *Ann Neurol* **50**: 275

van Veen T, Kalkers NF, Crusius JBA et al 2002 The FAS-670 polymorphism influences susceptibility to multiple sclerosis. *J Neuroimmunol* **128**: 95–100

van Veen T, Crusius JBA, van Winsen L et al 2003a CTLA-4 and CD28 gene polymorphisms in susceptibility, clinical course and progression of multiple sclerosis. *J Neuroimmunol* **140**: 188–193

van Veen T, van Winsen L, Crusius JB et al 2003b [Alpha]B-crystallin genotype has impact on the multiple sclerosis phenotype. *Neurology* **61**: 1245–1249

Vejjajiva A 1982 Some clinical aspects of multiple sclerosis. In: Kuroiwa Y, Kurland L (eds) *Multiple Sclerosis: East and West*. Fukoka, Japan: Kyushu University Press, pp. 117–122

Vela JM, Molina-Holgado E, Arevalo-Martin A et al 2002 Interleukin-1 regulates proliferation and differentiation of oligodendrocyte progenitor cells. *Mol Cell Neurosci* **20**: 489–502

Ventner JC, Adams MD, Myers EW et al 2001 The sequence of the human genome. *Science* **291**: 1304–1351

Verdru P, Theys P, D'Hooghe MB, Carton H 1994 Pregnancy and multiple sclerosis: the influence on long term disability. *Clin Neurol Neurosurg* **96**: 38–41

Verheul GAM, Tyssen CC 1990 Multiple sclerosis occurring with paroxysmal unilateral dystonia. *Mov Disord* **5**: 352–353

Vernant J-C, Cabre P, Smadja D et al 1997 Recurrent optic neuromyelitis with endocrinopathies: a new syndrome. *Neurology* **48**: 58–64

Verrips A, Nijeholt GJ, Barkhof F et al 1999 Spinal xanthomatosis: a variant of cerebrotendinous xanthomatosis. *Brain* **122**: 1589–1595

Ververken D, Carton H, Billiau A 1979 Intrathecal administration of interferon in MS patients. In: Karcher D, Lowenthal A, Strosberg AD (eds) *Humoral Immunology on Neurological Disease*. New York: Plenum, pp. 625–627

Vervliet G, Claeys H, van Haver H et al 1983 Interferon production and natural killer (NK) activity in leukocyte cultures from multiple sclerosis patients. *J Neurol Sci* **60**: 137–150

Vesalius A 1543 *De humani corporis fabrica libri septum*, Basel: Oporini

Vicari AM, Ciceri F, Folli F et al 1998 Acute promyelocytic leukemia following mitoxantrone as single agent for the treatment of multiple sclerosis. *Leukemia* **12**: 441–442

Vicari AP, Zlotnik A 1996 Mouse NK1.1⁺ T cells: a new family of T cells. *Immunol Today* **17**: 71–76

Vickrey BG, Hays RD, Harooni R et al 1995 A health-related quality of life measure for multiple sclerosis. *Qual Life Res* **4**: 187–206

Viehover A, Miller RH, Park SK et al 2001 Neuregulin: an oligodendrocyte growth factor absent in active multiple sclerosis lesions. *Dev Neurosci* **23**: 377–386

Vieregge P, Klostermann W, Brückmann H 1992 Parkinsonism in multiple sclerosis. *Mov Disord* **7**: 380–382

Viglietta V, Baecher-Allan C, Weiner HL, Hafler DA 2004 Loss of functional suppression by CD4⁺CD25⁺ regulatory T cells in patients with multiple sclerosis. *J Exp Med* **199**: 971–979

Vilar LM, Masjuan J, Gonzales-Porque P et al 2003 Intrathecal IgM synthesis is a prognostic factor in multiple sclerosis. *Ann Neurol* **53**: 222–226

Villadangos JA, Ploegh HL 2000 Proteolysis in MHC class II antigen presentation: Who's in charge? *Immunity* **12**: 233–239

Villar LM, Sádaba MC, Roldán E et al 2005 Intrathecal synthesis of oligoclonal IgM against myelin lipids predicts an aggressive disease course in MS. *J Clin Invest* **115**: 187–194

Villard-Mackintosh L, Vessey MP 1993 Oral contraceptives and reproductive factors in multiple sclerosis incidence. *Contraception* **47**: 161–168

Villoslada P, Barcellos LF, Rio J et al 2002 The HLA locus and multiple sclerosis in Spain: role in disease susceptibility, clinical course and response to interferon-B. *J Neuroimmunol* **130**: 194–201

Villoslada P, Barcellos LF, Oksenberg JR 2004 Chromosome 7q21–22 and multiple sclerosis. *J Neuroimmunol* **150**: 1–2

Vinas FC, Rengachary S 2001 Diagnosis and management of neurosarcoidosis. *J Clin Neurosci* **8**: 505–513

Vinuela FV, Fox AJ, Debrun GM et al 1982 New perspectives in computed tomography of multiple sclerosis. *Am J Radiol* **139**: 123–127

Vinuesa CG, Goodnow CC 2004 Illuminating autoimmune regulators through controlled variation of the mouse genome sequence. *Immunity* **20**: 669–679

Virchow R 1854 Über eine im Gehirn und Rückenmark des Menschen aufgefundene Substanz mit der chemischen Reaction der Cellulose. *Arch Pathol Anat Physiol Klin Med* **15**: 217–236

Virchow R 1858 *Cellularpathologie in ihre Begrundung auf Physiologïsche und Pathologïsche Gewebelehre*. Berlin: A. Hirschwald

Visentin S, Levi G 1997 Protein kinase C involvement in the resting and interferon-gamma-induced K⁺ channel profile of microglial cells. *J Neurosci Res* **47**: 233–241

Visscher BR, Detels R, Dudley JP et al 1979 Genetic susceptibility to multiple sclerosis. *Neurology* **29**: 1354–1360

Visscher BR, Liu KS, Clark VA et al 1984 Onset symptoms as predictors of mortality and disability in multiple sclerosis. *Acta Neurol Scand* **70**: 321–328

Visser L, de Vos AF, Hamann J et al 2002 Expression of the EGF-TM7 receptor CD97 and its ligand CD55 (DAF) in multiple sclerosis. *J Neuroimmunol* **132**: 156–163

Visser LH, Beekman R, Tijssen CC et al 2004 A randomized, double-blind, placebo-controlled pilot study of i.v. immune globulins in combination with i.v. methylprednisolone in the treatment of relapses in patients with MS. *Mult Scler* **10**: 89–91

Vitale E, Cook S, Sun R et al 2002 Linkage analysis conditional on HLA status in a large North American pedigree supports the presence of a multiple sclerosis susceptibility locus on chromosome 12p12. *Hum Mol Genet* **11**: 295–300

Vitali C, Bombardieri S, Moutsopoulos HM et al 1996 Assessment of the European classification criteria for Sjogren's syndrome in a series of clinically defined cases: results of a prospective multicentric study. *Ann Rheum Dis* **55**: 116–121

Vitali C, Bombardieri S, Jonsson R et al 2002 Classification criteria for Sjogren's syndrome: a revised version of the European criteria proposed by the European-American Consensus Group. *Ann Rheum Dis* **61**: 554–558

Vogt MHJ, Lopatinskaya L, Smits M et al 2003 Elevated osteopontin levels in active relapsing–remitting multiple sclerosis. *Ann Neurol* **53**: 819–822

Vollenweider R, Lennert K 1983 Plasmacytoid T-cell clusters in non-specific lymphadenitis. *Virchows Arch B* **44**: 1–14

Vollmer TL, Key L, Durkalski V et al 2004a Oral simvastatin treatment in relapsing–remitting multiple sclerosis. *Lancet* **363**: 1607–1608

Vollmer TL, Phillips JT, Goodman AD et al 2004b An open-label safety and drug interaction study of natalizumab (Antegren™) in combination with interferon-beta (Avonex®) in patients with multiple sclerosis. *Mult Scler* **10**: 511–520

Voltz R, Starck M, Zingler V et al 2004 Mitoxantrone therapy in multiple sclerosis and acute leukaemia: a case report out of 644 treated patients. *Mult Scler* **10**: 472–474

Von Leden H, Horton BT 1948 The auditory nerve in multiple sclerosis. *Arch Otolaryngol* **48**: 51–57

Vorechovsky I, Kralovicova J, Tchiloian E et al 2001 Does 77C-G in PTPRC modify autoimmune disorders linked to major histocompatibility locus? *Nature Genet* **29**: 22–23

de Vos AF, van Meurs M, Brok HP et al 2002 Transfer of central nervous system autoantigens and presentation in secondary lymphoid organs. *J Immunol* **169**: 5415–5423

Vos CMP, van Haastert ES, de Groot CJA et al 2003 Matrix metalloproteinase-12 is expressed in phagocytotic macrophages in active multiple sclerosis lesions. *J Neuroimmunol* **138**: 106–114

Voskuhl RR, Martin R, Bergman C et al 1993 T helper 1 (Th1) functional phenotype of human myelin basic protein-specific T lymphocytes. *Autoimmunity* **15**: 137–143

Voskuhl RR, Goldstein AM, Simonis T et al 1996 DR2/DQw1 inheritance and haplotype sharing in affected siblings from multiple sclerosis families. *Ann Neurol* **39**: 804–807

Voudris KA, Vagiakou EA, Skardoutsou A 2002 Acute disseminated encephalomyelitis associated with parainfluenza virus infection in childhood. *Brain Dev* **24**: 112–114

Vrethem M, Dahle C, Ekerfeld C et al 1998 CD4 and CD8 lymphocyte subsets in cerebrospinal fluid and peripheral blood from patients with multiple sclerosis, meningitis and normal controls. *Acta Neurol Scand* **97**: 215–220

de Vries E 1960 *Postvaccinial Perivenous Encephalitis*. Amsterdam: Elsevier

de Vries RR, Khan M, Bernini LF et al 1979 Genetic control of survival in epidemics. *J Immunogenet* **6**: 271–287

Vukusic S, Confavreux C 2003a Primary and secondary progressive multiple sclerosis. *J Neurol Sci* **206**: 153–155

Vukusic S, Confavreux C 2003b Prognostic factors for progression of disability in the secondary progressive phase of multiple sclerosis. *J Neurol Sci* **206**: 135–137

Vukusic S, Hutchinson M, Hours M et al 2004 Pregnancy and multiple sclerosis (the PRIMS study): clinical predictors of post-partum relapse. *Brain* **127**: 1353–1360

Vulpian A 1866 Note sur la sclerose en plaques de la moelle épinière. *L'Union Med* **30**: 459–465, 475–482, 507–512, 541–548

Vyshkina T, Leist TP, Shugart YY, Kalman B 2004 CD45 (PTPRC) as a candidate gene in multiple sclerosis. *Mult Scler* **10**: 614–617

Vyshkina T, Banisor I, Shugart YY et al 2005a Genetic variants of Complex I in multiple sclerosis. *J Neurol Sci* **228**: 55–64

Vyshkina T, Shugart YY, Birnbaum G et al 2005b Association of haplotypes in the beta-chemokine locus with multiple sclerosis. *Eur J Hum Genet* **13**: 240–247

Waage A, Halstensen A, Shalaby R, Brandtzaeg P, Kierulf P, Espevik T 1989 Local production of tumor necrosis factor α, interleukin 1 and interleukin 6 in meningococcal meningitis. Relation to the inflammatory response. *J Exp Med* **170**: 1559–1568

Wada T, Kagawa T, Ivanova A et al 2000 Dorsal spinal cord inhibits oligodendrocyte development. *Dev Biol* **227**: 42–55

Wade DT, Makela P, Robson P et al 2004 Do cannabis-based medicinal extracts have general or specific effects on symptoms in multiple sclerosis? A double-blind, randomized, placebo-controlled study on 160 patients. *Mult Scler* **10**: 434–441

Wadia NH, Bhatia K 1990 Multiple sclerosis is prevalent in the Zoroastrians (Parsis) of India. *Ann Neurol* **28**: 177–179

Wadia NH, Trikannad VS, Krishnaswamy PR 1980 Association of HLA-B12 with multiple sclerosis in India. *Tissue Antigens* **15**: 90–93

van Waesberghe JH, van Walderveen MA, Castelijns JA et al 1998 Patterns of lesion development in multiple sclerosis: longitudinal observations with T1-weighted spin-echo and magnetization transfer MR. *Am J Neuroradiol* **19**: 675–683

Wagner H 2001 Toll meets bacterial CpG DNA. *Immunity* **14**: 499–502

Wagner HJ, Hennig H, Jabs WT et al 2000 Altered prevalence and reactivity of anti-Epstein Barr virus antibodies in patients with multiple sclerosis. *Viral Immunol* **13**: 497–502

Wagner J 1956 Devic's disease. *S Afr Med J* **30**: 489–492

Waisbren BA 1982 Swine-influenza vaccine. *Ann Intern Med* **97**: 149

Wajgt A, Gorny MK, Jenek R 1983 The influence of high-dose prednisolone medication on auto-antibody specific activity and on circulating immune complex level in cerebrospinal fluid of multiple sclerosis patients. *Acta Neurol Scand* **68**: 378–385

Wakatsuki T, Miyata M, Shishido S et al 2000 Sjogren's syndrome with primary biliary cirrhosis, complicated by transverse myelitis and malignant lymphoma. *Intern Med* **39**: 260–265

Wakayama T, Tabar V, Rodriguez I et al 2001 Differentiation of embryonic stem cell lines generated from adult somatic cells by nuclear transfer. *Science* **292**: 740–742

Wakefield AJ, More LJ, Difford J, McLaughlin JE 1994 Immunohistochemical study of vascular injury in acute multiple sclerosis. *J Clin Pathol* **47**: 129–133

Waksman BH, Porter H, Lees MB, Adams RD 1954 A study of the chemical nature and components of bovine white matter effective in producing allergic encephalomyelitis in the rabbit. *J Exp Med* **100**: 451–471

Waldner H, Whitters MJ, Sobel RA et al 2000 Fulminant spontaneous autoimmunity of the central nervous system in mice transgenic for the myelin proteolipid protein-specific T cell receptor. *Proc Natl Acad Sci USA* **97**: 3412–3417

Walker G, Pfeilschifter J, Kunz D 1997 Mechanisms of suppression of inducible nitric-oxide synthase (iNOS) expression in Interferon (IFN)-γ-stimulated RAW 264.7 cells by dexamethasone. *J Biol Chem* **272**: 16679–16687

Walker G, Pfeilschifter J, Otten U, Kunz D 2001 Proteolytic cleavage of inducible nitric oxide synthase (iNOS) by calpain I. *Biochim Biophys Acta* **1568**: 216–224

Wallace DC, Singh G, Lott MT et al 1988 Mitochondrial DNA mutation associated with Leber's hereditary optic neuropathy. *Science* **242**: 486–491

Wallace VC, Cottrell DF, Brophy PJ, Fleetwood-Walker SM 2003 Focal lysolecithin-induced demyelination of peripheral afferents results in neuropathic pain behavior that is attenuated by cannabinoids. *J Neurosci* **23**: 3221–3233

Waller A 1850 Experiments on the section of glossopharyngeal and hypoglossal nerves of the frog and observations of the alternatives produced thereby in the structure of their primitive fibres. *Phil Trans R Soc Lond* **140**: 423–429

Walley T, Barton S 1995 A purchaser perspective of managing new drugs: interferon beta as a case study. *Br Med J* **311**: 796–799

Wallin MT, Page WF, Kurtzke JF 2000 Epidemiology of multiple sclerosis in US veterans. VIII. Long term survival after onset of multiple sclerosis. *Brain* **123**: 1677–1687

Wallin MT, Page WF, Kurtzke JF 2004 Multiple sclerosis in United States veterans of Vietnam era and later military service. 1. Race, sex and geography. *Ann Neurol* **55**: 65–71

Wallstrom E, Diener P, Ljungdahl A et al 1996 Memantine abrogates neurological deficits,

937

but not CNS inflammation, in Lewis rat experimental autoimmune encephalomyelitis. *J Neurol Sci* **137**: 89–96

Walsh EC, Mather KA, Schaffner SF *et al* 2003 An integrated haplotype map of the human major histocompatibility complex. *Am J Hum Genet* **73**: 580–590

Walter MA, Gibson WT, Ebers GC, Cox DW 1991 Susceptibility to multiple sclerosis is associated with the proximal immunoglobulin heavy chain region. *J Clin Invest* **87**: 1266–1273

Waltereit R, Kuker W, Jurgens S *et al* 2002 Acute transverse myelitis associated with *Coxiella burnetii* infection. *J Neurol* **249**: 1459–1461

Walther EU, Hohlfeld R 1999 Multiple sclerosis: side effects of interferon beta therapy and their management. *Neurology* **53**: 1622–1627

Wanders RJA, van Roermund CWT, van Wijland MJA *et al* 1988 X linked adrenoleukodystrophy: identification of the primary defect at the level of a deficient peroxisomal very long chain fatty acyl CoA synthetase using a newly developed method for the isolation of peroxisomes from skin fibroblasts. *J Inherited Metab Dis* **11** (Suppl 2): 173–177

Wandinger KP, Wessel K, Trillenberg P *et al* 1998 Effect of high-dose methylprednisolone administration on immune functions in multiple sclerosis patients. *Acta Neurol Scand* **97**: 359–365

Wandinger KP, Jabs W, Siekhaus A *et al* 2000 Association between clinical disease activity and Epstein-Barr virus reactivation in MS. *Neurology* **55**:178–184

Wandinger KP, Sturzebecher CS, Bielekova B *et al* 2001 Complex immunomodulatory effects of interferon-beta in multiple sclerosis include the upregulation of T helper 1-associated marker genes. *Ann Neurol* **50**: 349–357

Wang B, Geng Y-B, Wang C-R 2001 CD1-restricted NK T cells protect nonobese diabetic mice from developing diabetes. *J Exp Med* **194**: 313–320

Wang CY, Kawashima H, Takami T *et al* 1998 A case of multiple sclerosis with initial symptoms of narcolepsy. *No To Hattatsu* **30**: 300–306

Wang H, Allen ML, Grigg JJ *et al* 1995 Hypomyelination alters K+ channel expression in mouse mutants shiverer and trembler. *Neuron* **15**: 1337–1347

Wang KC, Koprivica V, Kim JA *et al* 2002 Oligodendrocyte-meylin glycoprotein is a Nogo receptor ligand that inhibits neurite outgrowth. *Nature* **417**: 941–944

Wang L-C, Baird DH, Hatten ME, Mason CA 1994 Astroglial differentiation is required for support of neurite outgrowth. *J Neurosci* **14**: 3195–3207

Wang S, Sdrulla AD, diSibio G *et al* 1998 Notch receptor activation inhibits oligodendrocyte differentiation. *Neuron* **21**: 63–75

Wang S, Cheng Q, Malik S, Yang J 2000 Interleukin-1beta inhibits gamma-aminobutyric acid type A (GABA(A)) receptor current in cultured hippocampal neurons. *J Pharmacol Exp Ther* **292**: 497–504

Wang S, Sdrulla A, Johnson JE *et al* 2001 A role for the helix-loop-helix protein ID2 in the control of oligodendrocyte development. *Neuron* **29**: 603–614

Wang W-Z, Olsson T, Kostulas V, Hojeberg B, Ekre H-P, Link H 1992 Myelin antigen reactive T cells in cerebrovascular diseases. *Clin Exp Immunol* **88**: 157–162

Wansen K, Pastinen T, Kuokkanen S *et al* 1997 Immune system genes in multiple sclerosis: genetic association and linkage analysis on TCR-β, IGH, IFN-γ and IL-1ra/IL-1B loci. *J Neuroimmunol* **79**: 29–36

Warf BC, Fok-Seang J, Miller RH 1991 Evidence for the ventral origin of oligodendrocyte precursors in the rat spinal cord. *J Neurosci* **11**: 2477–2488

Warren KG, Catz I, Jeffrey VM, Carrol DJ 1986 Effect of methylprednisolone on CSF IgG parameters, myelin basic protein and anti-myelin basic protein in multiple sclerosis exacerbations. *Can J Neurol Sci* **13**: 25–30

Warren KG, Catz I, Johnson E, Mielke B 1994 Anti-myelin basic protein and anti-proteolipid protein specific forms of multiple sclerosis. *Ann Neurol* **35**: 280–289

Warren KG, Catz I, Steinman L 1995 Fine specificity of the antibody-response to myelin basic protein in the central nervous system in multiple sclerosis: the minimal B-cell epitope and a model of its features. *Proc Natl Acad Sci USA* **92**: 11061–11065

Warren S, Warren KG 1982 Multiple sclerosis and diabetes mellitus: further evidence of a relationship. *Can J Neurol Sci* **9**: 415–419

Warren S, Warren KG 1992 Prevalence of multiple sclerosis in Barrhead County, Alberta, Canada. *Can J Neurol Sci* **19**: 72–75

Warren S, Warren KG 1993 Prevalence of multiple sclerosis in Westlock County, Alberta. *Neurology* **43**: 1760–1763

Warren S, Warren KG 1994 A population based study of parent gender effect in familial multiple sclerosis. *Neurology* **44** (Suppl 2): A194

Warren S, Greenhill S, Warren KG 1982 Emotional stress and the development of multiple sclerosis: case-control evidence of a relationship. *J Chronic Dis* **35**: 821–831

Warren S, Cockerill R, Warren KG 1991a Risk factors by onset age in multiple sclerosis. *Neuroepidemiology* **10**: 9–17

Warren S, Warren KG, Cockerill R 1991b Emotional stress and coping in multiple sclerosis (MS) exacerbations. *J Psychosom Res* **35**: 37–47

Warren S, Warren KG, Svenson LW *et al* 2003 Geographic and temporal distribution of mortality rates for multiple sclerosis in Canada, 1965–1994. *Neuroepidemiology* **22**: 75–81

Warren WR 1956 Encephalopathy due to influenza vaccine. *Arch Int Med* **97**: 803–805

Warrington AE, Pfeiffer SE 1992 Proliferation and differentiation of O4+ oligodendrocytes in postnatal cerebellum: analysis in unfixed tissue slices using anti-glycolipid antibodies. *J Neurosci Res* **33**: 338–353

Warrington AE, Barbarese E, Pfeiffer SE 1993 Differential myelinogenic capacity of specific developmental stages of the oligodendrocyte lineage upon transplantation into hypomyelinating hosts. *J Neurosci Res* **34**: 1–13

Warrington AE, Asakura K, Bieber AJ *et al* 2000 Human monoclonal antibodies reactive to oligodendrocytes promote remyelination in a model of multiple sclerosis. *Proc Natl Acad Sci USA* **97**: 6820–6825

Washington R, Burton J, Todd RF *et al* 1994 Expression of immunologically relevant endothelial cell activation antigens on isolated central nervous system microvessels from patients with multiple sclerosis. *Ann Neurol* **35**: 89–97

Watanabe I, Okazaki H 1973 Virus-like structure in multiple sclerosis. *Lancet* **ii**: 569–570

Watanabe M, Hadzic T, Nishiyama A 2004 Transient upregulation of Nkx2.2 expression in oligodendrocyte lineage cells during remyelination. *Glia* **46**: 311–322

Watanabe R, Wege H, Ter Meulen V 1983 Adoptive transfer of EAE-like lesions from rats with coronavirus-induced demyelinating encephalomyelitis. *Nature* **305**: 150–151

Waterhouse J (ed.) 1976 Cancer incidence in five continents. *Int Agency Res Cancer Lyon* **3**: 456

Waterston JA, Gilligan BS 1986 Paraneoplastic optic neuritis and external ophthalmoplegia. *Aust NZ J Med* **16**: 703–704

Watkins SM, Espir M 1966 Migraine and multiple sclerosis. *J Neurol Neurosurg Psychiatry* **32**: 35–37

Watts R 2000 Musculoskeletal and systemic reactions to biological therapeutic agents. *Curr Opin Rheumatol* **12**: 49–52

Waubant E, Alize P, Tourbah A, Agid Y 2001 Paroxysmal dystonia (tonic spasm) in multiple sclerosis. *Neurology* **57**: 2320–2321

Waxman SG 1981 Clinicopathological correlations in multiple sclerosis and related diseases. *Adv Neurol* **31**: 169–182

Waxman SG 1989 Demyelination in spinal cord injury. *J Neurol Sci* **91**: 1–14

Waxman SG 1992 Demyelination in spinal cord injury and multiple sclerosis: what can we do to enhance functional recovery? *J Neurotrauma* **9**: S105–S117

Waxman SG 1995 Sodium channel blockade by antibodies: a new mechanism of neurological disease? *Ann Neurol* **37**: 421–423

Waxman SG 2001 Acquired channelopathies in nerve injury and MS. *Neurology* **56**: 1621–1627

Waxman SG 2002 Sodium channels as molecular targets in multiple sclerosis. *J Rehab Res Dev* **39**: 233–242

Waxman SG 2005a Sodium channel blockers and axonal protection in neuroinflammatory disease. *Brain* **128**: 5–6

Waxman SG 2005b Cerebellar dysfunction in multiple sclerosis: evidence for an acquired channelopathy. *Prog Brain Res* **148**: 353–365

Waxman SG, Brill MH 1978 Conduction through demyelinated plaques in multiple sclerosis: computer simulations of facilitation by short internodes. *J Neurol Neurosurg Psychiatry* **41**: 408–416

Waxman SG, Foster RE 1980 Ionic channel distribution and heterogeneity of the axon membrane in myelinated fibers. *Brain Res* **203**: 205–234

Waxman SG, Geschwind N 1983 Major morbidity related to hyperthermia in multiple sclerosis. *Ann Neurol* **13**: 348

Waxman SG, Ritchie JM 1993 Molecular dissection of the myelinated axon. *Ann Neurol* **33**: 121–136

Waxman SG, Black JA, Ransom BR, Stys PK 1994a Anoxic injury of rat optic nerve: ultrastructural evidence for coupling between Na+ influx and Ca(2+)-mediated injury in myelinated CNS axons. *Brain Res* **644**: 197–204

Waxman SG, Utzschneider DA, Kocsis JD 1994b Enhancement of action potential conduction following demyelination: experimental approaches to restoration of function in multiple sclerosis and spinal cord injury. *Prog Brain Res* **100**: 233–243

Waxman SG, Dib-Hajj S, Cummins TR, Black JA 2000 Sodium channels and their genes: dynamic expression in the normal nervous system, dysregulation in disease states. *Brain Res* **886**: 5–14

Waybright EA, Gutmann L, Chou SM 1979 Facial myokymia: pathological features. *Arch Neurol* **36**: 244–245

Weatherby SJ, Mann CLA, Davies MB et al 2000a Polymorphisms of apolipoprotein E: outcome and susceptibility in multiple sclerosis. *Mult Scler* **6**: 32–36

Weatherby SJ, Mann CL, Fryer AA et al 2000b No association between the APOE epsilon4 allele and outcome and susceptibility in primary progressive multiple sclerosis. *J Neurol Neurosurg Psychiatry* **68**: 532

Weatherby SJ, Thomson W, Pepper L et al 2001 HLA-DRB1 and disease outcome in multiple sclerosis. *J Neurol* **248**: 304–310

Webb A, Clark P, Skepper J et al 1995 Guidance of oligodendrocytes and their progenitors by substratum topography. *J Cell Sci* **108**: 2747–2760

Weber A, Infante-Duarte C, Sawcer S et al 2003 A genome-wide German screen for linkage disequilibrium in multiple sclerosis. *J Neuroimmunol* **143**: 79–83

Weber A, Wandinger K-P, Mueller W et al 2004 Identification and functional characterization of a highly polymorphic region in the human TRAIL promoter in multiple sclerosis. *J Neuroimmunol* **149**: 195–201

Weber F, Rudel R, Aulkemeyer P, Brinkmeier H 2002 The endogenous pentapeptide QYNAD induces acute conduction block in the isolated rat sciatic nerve. *Neurosci Lett* **317**: 33–36

Weber H, Pfadenhauer K, Stohr M, Rosler A 2002 Central hyperacusis with phonophobia in multiple sclerosis. *Mult Scler* **8**: 505–509

Weber J, Delanger T, Hannequin D et al 1990 Anorectal manometric anomalies in seven patients with frontal lobe brain damage. *Dig Dis Sci* **35**: 225–230

Weber JL, May PE 1989 Abundant class of human DNA polymorphisms which can be typed using the polymerase chain reaction. *Am J Hum Genet* **44**: 388–396

Weber MS, Starch M, Wagenpfeil S et al 2004 Multiple sclerosis: glatiramer acetate inhibits monocyte reactivity *in vitro* and *in vivo*. *Brain* **127**: 1370–1378

Weber P, Bartsch U, Rasband MN et al 1999 Mice deficient for tenascin-R display alterations of the extracellular matrix and decreased axonal conduction velocities in the CNS. *J Neurosci* **19**: 4245–4262

Webster G, Knobler R, Lublin F et al 1996 Cutaneous ulcerations and pustular psoriasis flare caused by recombinant interferon beta injections in patients with multiple sclerosis. *J Am Acad Dermatol* **34**: 365–367

Wechsler IS 1922 Statistics of multiple sclerosis including a study of the infantile, congenital, familial, hereditary forms and the mental and psychic symptoms. *Arch Neurol Psychiatry* **8**: 59–75

Weder B, Wiedersheim P, Matter L, Steck A, Otto F 1987 Chronic progressive neurological involvement in *Borrelia burgdorferi* infection. *J Neurol* **234**: 40–43

Weese D, Roskamp D, Leach G, Zimmern P 1993 Intravesical oxybutinin chloride: experience with 42 patients. *Urology* **41**: 527–530

Wegmann TG, Lin H, Guilbert L, Mosmann TR 1993 Bidirectional cytokine interactions in the maternal-fetal relationship: is successful pregnancy a TH2 phenomenon? *Immunol Today* **14**: 353–356

Wei R, Jonakait GM 1999 Neurotrophins and the anti-inflammatory agents interleukin-4 (IL-4), IL-10, IL-11, and transforming growth factor-β1 (TGF-β1) down-regulate T cell costimulatory molecules B7 and CD40 on cultured rat microglia. *J Neuroimmunol* **95**: 8–18

Wei S, Charmley P, Birchfield RI, Cancannon P 1994 Human T cell receptor V beta gene polymorphisms in multiple sclerosis. *Am J Hum Genet* **56**: 963–969

Wei TY, Baumann RJ 1999 Acute disseminated encephalomyelitis after Rocky Mountain spotted fever. *Pediatr Neurol* **21**: 503–505

Weidenheim KM, Epshteyn I, Rashbaum WK, Lyman WD 1994 Patterns of glial development in the human foetal spinal cord during the late first and second trimester. *J Neurocytol* **23**: 343–353

Weinberg AD, Wyrick G, Celnik B et al 1993 Lymphokine mRNA expression in the spinal cord of Lewis rats with experimental autoimmune encephalomyelitis is associated with a host recruited CD45Rhi/CD4+ population during recovery. *J Neuroimmunol* **48**: 105–118

Weiner HL 2000 Oral tolerance, an active immunologic process mediated by multiple mechanisms. *J Clin Invest* **106**: 935–937

Weiner HL, Ellison GW 1983 A working protocol to be used as a guideline for trials in multiple sclerosis. *Arch Neurol* **40**: 704–710

Weiner HL, Dau PC, Khatri BO et al 1989 Double-blind study of true versus sham plasma exchange in patients treated with immunosuppression for acute attacks of multiple sclerosis. *Neurology* **39**: 1143–1149

Weiner HL, Mackin GA, Orav EJ et al 1993a Intermittent cyclophosphamide pulse therapy in progressive multiple sclerosis: final report of the Northeast Cooperative Multiple Sclerosis treatment group. *Neurology* **43**: 910–918

Weiner HL, Mackin GA, Matsui M et al 1993b Double-blind pilot trial of oral tolerisation with myelin antigens in multiple sclerosis. *Science* **259**: 1321–1324

Weinshenker BG 1997 Natural history of multiple sclerosis in randomized clinical trials. *Int Mult Scler J* **4**: 7–11

Weinshenker BG 1999 Databases in MS research: pitfalls and promises. *Mult Scler* **5**: 206–211

Weinshenker BG, Ebers GC 1987 The natural history of multiple sclerosis. *Can J Neurol Sci* **14**: 255–261

Weinshenker BG, Rodriguez M 1995 Epidemiology of multiple sclerosis. In: Gorelick PB, Alter M (eds) *Handbook of Neuroepidemiology*. New York: Marcel Decker, pp. 533–564

Weinshenker BG, Bass B, Rice GP et al 1989a The natural history of multiple sclerosis: a geographically based study. 1. Clinical course and disability. *Brain* **112**: 133–146

Weinshenker BG, Bass B, Rice GP et al 1989b The natural history of multiple sclerosis: a geographically based study. 2. Predictive value of the early clinical course. *Brain* **112**: 1419–1428

Weinshenker BG, Hader W, Carriere W et al 1989c The influence of pregnancy on disability from multiple sclerosis: a population-based study in Middlesex County, Ontario. *Neurology* **39**: 1438–1440

Weinshenker BG, Bulman D, Carriere W et al 1990 A comparison of sporadic and familial multiple sclerosis. *Neurology* **40**: 1354–1358

Weinshenker BG, Rice GPA, Noseworthy JH et al 1991a The natural history of multiple sclerosis: a geographically based study. 3: Multivariate analysis of predictive factors and models of outcome. *Brain* **114**: 1045–1056

Weinshenker BG, Rice GPA, Noseworthy JH et al 1991b The natural history of multiple sclerosis: a geographically based study. 4: Applications to planning and interpretation of clinical therapeutic trials. *Brain* **114**: 1057–1067

Weinshenker BG, Bass B, Karlik S, Ebers GC, Rice GPA 1991c An open trial of OKT3 in patients with multiple sclerosis. *Neurology* **41**: 1047–1052

Weinshenker BG, Penman M, Bass B 1992 A double-blind, randomised controlled trial of pemoline in fatigue associated with multiple sclerosis. *Neurology* **42**: 1468–1471

Weinshenker BG, Issa M, Baskerville J 1996 Long-term and short-term outcome of multiple sclerosis: a 3-year follow-up study. *Arch Neurol* **53**: 353–358

Weinshenker BG, Wingerchuk DM, Liu Q *et al* 1997 Genetic variation in the tumor necrosis factor (α) gene and the outcome of multiple sclerosis. *Neurology* **49**: 378–385

Weinshenker BG, Santrach P, Bissonet AS *et al* 1998 Major histocompatibility complex class II alleles and the course and outcome of MS: a population-based study. *Neurology* **51**: 742–747

Weinshenker BG, Hebrink D, Wingerchuk DM *et al* 1999a Genetic variants in the tumor necrosis factor receptor 1 gene in patients with MS. *Neurology* **52**: 1500–1503

Weinshenker BG, O'Brien PC, Petterson TM *et al* 1999b A randomised trial of plasma exchange in acute central nervous system inflammatory demyelinating disease. *Ann Neurol* **46**: 878–886

Weinshenker BG, Hebrink DD, Klein C *et al* 2000 Genetic variation in the B7–1 gene in patients with multiple sclerosis. *J Neuroimmunol* **105**: 184–188

Weinshenker BG, Hebrink D, Kantarci O *et al* 2001 Genetic variation in the transforming growth factor β1 gene in multiple sclerosis. *J Neuroimmunol* **120**: 138–145

Weinshilboum RM, Sladek SL 1980 Mercaptopurine pharmacogenetics: monogenic inheritance of erythrocyte thiopurine methyltransferase activity. *Am J Hum Genet* **32**: 651–662

Weinstein A, Schwid SI, Schiffer RB *et al* 1999 Neuropsychologic status in multiple sclerosis after treatment with glatiramer. *Arch Neurol* **56**: 319–324

Weinstock-Guttman B, Ransohoff RM *et al* 1995 The interferons: biological effects, mechanisms of action, and use in multiple sclerosis. *Ann Neurol* **37**: 7–15

Weinstock-Guttman B, Kinkel R, Cohen J *et al* 1997 Treatment of fulminant multiple sclerosis with intravenous cyclophosphamide. *Neurologist* **3**: 178–185

Weinstock-Guttman B, Jacobs LD, Brownscheidle CM *et al* 2003a Multiple sclerosis characteristics in African American patients in the New York State Multiple Sclerosis Consortium. *Mult Scler* **9**: 293–298

Weinstock-Guttman B, Badgett D, Patrick K *et al* 2003b Genomic effects of IFN-beta in multiple sclerosis patients. *J Immunol* **171**: 2694–2704

Weinstock-Guttman B, Gallagher E, Baier M *et al* 2004 Risk of bone loss in men with multiple sclerosis. *Mult Scler* **10**: 170–175

Weishaupt A, Gold R, Gaupp S *et al* 1997 Antigen therapy eliminates T cell inflammation by apoptosis: effective treatment of experimental autoimmune neuritis with recombinant myelin protein P2. *Proc Natl Acad Sci USA* **94**: 1338–1343

Weiss W, Dambrosia JM 1983 Common problems in designing therapeutic trials in multiple sclerosis. *Arch Neurol* **40**: 678–680

Weissman IL 1993 Developmental switches in the immune system. *Cell* **76**: 207–218

Weitkamp LR 1983 Multiple sclerosis susceptibility: interaction between sex and HLA. *Arch Neurol* **40**: 399–401

Wekerle H 1993 Lymphocyte traffic to the brain. In: Pardridge WM (ed.) *Cellular and Molecular Biology of the Blood–Brain Barrier*. New York: Raven Press, pp. 67–85

Wekerle H 1994 Antigen presentation by CNS glia. In: Kettenmann H, Ransom B (eds) *Neuroglial Cells*. Oxford: Oxford University Press, pp. 685–699

Wekerle H, Ketelsen U-P 1977 Intrathymic pathogenesis and dual genetic control of myasthenia gravis. *Lancet* **i**: 678–680

Wekerle H, Linington C, Lassmann H, Meyermann R 1986 Cellular immune reactivity within the CNS. *Trends Neurosci* **9**: 271–277

Wekerle H, Kojima K, Lannes-Vieira J *et al* 1994 Animal models. *Ann Neurol* **36**: S47–S53

Wekerle H, Bradl M, Linington C *et al* 1996 The shaping of the brain-specific T lymphocyte repertoire in the thymus. *Immunol Rev* **149**: 231–243

Weller M, Stevens A, Sommer N *et al* 1991 Cerebrospinal fluid interleukins, immunoglobulins, and fibronectin in neuroborreliosis. *Arch Neurol* **48**: 837–841

Weller M, Constam DB, Malipiero U, Fontana A 1994 Transforming growth factor-β2 induces apoptosis of murine T cell clones without down-regulating *bcl-2* mRNA expression. *Eur J Immunol* **24**: 1293–1300

Weller RO, Kida S, Zhang E-T 1992 Pathways of fluid drainage for the brain – morphological aspects and immunological significance in rat and man. *Brain Pathol* **2**: 277–362

Weller RO, Engelhardt B, Phillips MJ 1996 Lymphocyte targeting of the central nervous system: a review of afferent and efferent CNS immune pathways. *Brain Pathol* **6**: 275–188

Wender M, Pruchnik-Grabowska D, Hertmanowska H *et al* 1985 Epidemiology of multiple sclerosis in western Poland – a comparison between prevalence rates in 1965 and 1981. *Acta Neurol Scand* **72**: 210–217

Werner FC, Vischer TL, Wohlwend D, Zubler RH 1989 Cell surface antigen CD5 is a marker for activated human B cells. *Eur J Immunol* **19**: 1209–1213

Werner K, Bitsch A, Bunkowski S *et al* 2002 The relative number of macrophages / microglia expressing macrophage colony stimulating factor and its receptor decreases in multiple sclerosis. *Glia* **40**: 121–129

Werner P, Pitt D, Raine CS 2000 Glutamate excitotoxicity – a mechanism for axonal damage and oligodendrocyte death in multiple sclerosis? *J Neural Transmission* **60 (Suppl)**: 375–380

Werner P, Pitt P, Raine CS 2001 Multiple sclerosis: altered glutamate homeostasis in

lesions correlates with oligodendrocyte and axonal damage. *Ann Neurol* **50**: 169–180

Werring DJ, Brassat D, Droogan AG *et al* 2000a The pathogenesis of lesions and normal-appearing white matter changes in multiple sclerosis: a serial diffusion MRI study *Brain* **123**: 1667–1676

Werring DJ, Bullmore ET, Toosy AT *et al* 2000b Recovery from optic neuritis is associated with a change in the distribution of cerebral response to visual stimulation: a functional magnetic resonance imaging study. *J Neurol Neurosurg Psychiatry* **68**: 441–449

Westergaard E, Brightman MW 1973 Transport of proteins across normal cerebral arterioles. *J Comp Neurol* **152**: 17–44

Westlund KB 1970 Distribution and mortality time trend of multiple sclerosis and some other diseases in Norway. *Acta Neurol Scand* **46**: 455–483

Westlund KB, Kurland LT 1953 Studies on multiple sclerosis in Winnipeg, Manitoba and New Orleans, Louisiana. I. Prevalence. Comparison between the patient groups in Winnipeg and New Orleans. *Am J Hygiene* **57**: 380–396

Whitaker JN for the Advisory Committee on Clinical Trials of New Agents in Multiple Sclerosis, National Multiple Sclerosis Society 1993 Expanded clinical trials of treatment for multiple sclerosis. *Ann Neurol* **34**: 755–756

Whitaker JN 1998 Myelin basic protein in cerebrospinal fluid and other body fluids. *Mult Scler* **4**: 16–21

Whitaker JN, Lisak RP, Bashir RM *et al* 1980 Immunoreactive myelin basic protein in the cerebrospinal fluid in neurological disorders. *Ann Neurol* **7**: 58–64

Whitaker JN, Gupta M, Smith OF 1986 Epitopes of immunoreactive myelin basic protein in human cerebrospinal fluid. *Ann Neurol* **20**: 329–336

Whitaker JN, Benveniste EN, Zhou S 1990 Cerebrospinal fluid. In: Cook SD (ed.) *Handbook of Multiple Sclerosis*. New York: Marcel Dekker, pp. 251–270

Whitaker JN, Williams PH, Layton BA *et al* 1994 Correlation of clinical features and findings on cranial magnetic resonance imaging with urinary myelin basic protein-like material in patients with multiple sclerosis. *Ann Neurol* **35**: 577–585

Whitaker JN, McFarland HF, Rudge P, Reingold SC 1995a Outcome assessment in multiple sclerosis clinical trials: a critical analysis. *Mult Scler* **1**: 37–47

Whitaker JN, Kachelhofer RD, Bradley EL *et al* 1995b Urinary myelin basic protein-like material as a correlate of the progression of multiple sclerosis. *Ann Neurol* **38**: 625–632

White AT, Wilson TE, Davis SL, Petajan JH 2000 Effect of precooling on physical performance in multiple sclerosis. *Mult Scler* **6**: 176–180

White CA, McCombe PA, Pender MP 1998 Microglia are more susceptible than macrophages to apoptosis in the central nervous system in experimental autoimmune encephalomyelitis through a mechanism not involving Fas (CD95). *Int Immunol* **10**: 935–941

White RHR 1961 The aetiology and neurological complications of retinal vasculitis. *Brain* **84**: 601–608

Whitlock FA, Siskind MM 1980 Depression as a major symptom of multiple sclerosis. *J Neurol Neurosurg Psychiatry* **43**: 861–865

Whitney LW, Becker KG, Tresser NJ *et al* 1999 Analysis of gene expression in multiple sclerosis lesions using cDNA microarrays. *Ann Neurol* **46**: 425–428

Whittemore SR, Sanon HR, Wood PM 1993 Concurrent isolation and characterisation of oligodendrocytes, microglia and astrocytes from adult human spinal cord. *Int J Dev Neurosci* **11**: 755–764

Whittle IR, Hooper J, Pentland B 1998 Thalamic deep-brain stimulation for movement disorders due to multiple sclerosis. *Lancet* **351**: 109–110

Whytt R 1765 Observations on the nature, causes and cure of those disorders which have been commonly called nervous hypochondriac or hysteric to which are prefixed some remarks on the sympathy of the nerves. London: Becket, Du Hondt & Balfour

Wiberg M, Templer DI 1994 Season of birth in multiple sclerosis in Sweden: replication of Denmark findings. *J Orthomol Med* **9**: 7–74

Wiesel PH, Norton C, Glickman S, Kamm MA 2001 Pathophysiology and management of bowel dysfunction in multiple sclerosis. *Eur J Gastroenterol Hepatol* **13**: 441–448

Wiesemann E, Klatt J, Sonmez D *et al* 2001 Glatiramer acetate (GA) induces IL-13/IL-5 secretion in naive T cells. *J Neuroimmunol* **119**: 137–144

Wiesner W, Wetzel SG, Kappos L *et al* 2002 Swallowing abnormalities in multiple sclerosis: correlation between videofluoroscopy and subjective symptoms. *Eur Radiol* **12**: 789–792

Wikstrom J, Tienari PJ, Sumelahti ML *et al* 1994 Multiple sclerosis in Finland: evidence of uneven geographic distribution, increasing frequency and high familial occurrence. In: Firnhaber W, Lauer K (eds) *Multiple Sclerosis in Europe: An Epidemiological Update*. Darmstadt: Leuchtturm-Verlag/LTV Press, pp. 73–78

Wilcox CE, Ward AMV, Evans A, Baker D, Rothlein R, Turk JL 1990 Endothelial cell expression of the intercellular adhesion molecule-1 (ICAM-1) in the central nervous system of guinea pigs during acute and chronic relapsing experimental allergic encephalomyelitis. *J Neuroimmunol* **30**: 43–50

Wilczak N, De Keyser J 1997 Insulin like growth factor-1 receptors in normal appearing white matter and chronic plaques in multiple sclerosis. *Brain Res* **772**: 243–246

Wildbaum G, Youssef S, Grabie N, Karin N 1998 Neutralizing antibodies to IFN-gamma-inducing factor prevent experimental autoimmune encephalomyelitis. *J Immunol* **161**: 6368–6374

Wildin RS, Smyk-Pearson S, Filipovich AH 2003 Clinical and molecular features of the immunodysregulation, polyendocrinopathy, enteropathy, X linked (IPEX) syndrome. *J Med Genet* **39**: 537–545

Wiles CM, Clarke CRA, Irwin HP *et al* 1986 Hyperbaric oxygen in multiple sclerosis. *Br Med J* **292**: 367–371

Wiles CM, Omar L, Swan AV *et al* 1994 Total lymphoid irradiation in multiple sclerosis. *J Neurol Neurosurg Psychiatry* **57**: 154–163

Wiles CM, Newcombe RG, Fuller KJ *et al* 2001 Controlled randomised crossover trial of the effects of physiotherapy on mobility in chronic multiple sclerosis. *J Neurol Neurosurg Psychiatry* **70**: 174–179

Wiles CM, Brown P, Chapel H *et al* 2002 Intravenous immunoglobulin in neurological disease: a specialist review. *J Neurol Neurosurg Psychiatry* **72**: 440–448

Wiley CA, van Patten PD, Carpenter PM *et al* 1987 Acute ascending necrotising myelopathy caused by herpes simplex virus type 2. *Neurology* **37**: 1791–1794

Wilichowski E, Ohlenbusch A, Hanefeld F 1998 Characterisation of the mitochondrial genome in childhood multiple sclerosis II Multiple sclerosis without optic neuritis and LHON associated genes. *Neuropaediatrics* **29**: 307–312

Wilkin GP, Marriott DR, Cholewinski AJ 1990 Astrocyte heterogeneity. *Trends Neurosci* **13**: 43–46

Wilkins A, Compston DAS 2005 Trophic factors attenuate nitric oxide mediated neuronal and axonal injury *in vitro*: roles and interactions of MAPkinase signaling pathways. *J Neurochem* **92**: 1487–1496

Wilkins A, Chandran S, Compston A 2001 A role for oligodendrocyte-derived IGF-1 in trophic support of cortical neurons. *Glia* **36**: 48–57

Wilkins A, Majed H, Layfield R *et al* 2003 Oligodendrocytes promote neuronal survival and axonal length by distinct intracellular mechanisms: a novel role for oligodendrocyte-derived glial cell line-derived neurotrophic factor. *J Neurosci* **23**: 4967–4974

Wilks S 1878 *Lectures on Diseases of the Nervous System*. London: Churchill

Willenborg DO, Fordham SA, Cowden WB, Ramshaw IA 1995 Cytokines and murine autoimmune encephalomyelitis: inhibition or enhancement of disease with antibodies to select cytokines, or by delivery of exogenous cytokines using a recombinant vaccinia virus system. *Scand J Immunol* **41**: 31–41

Willenborg DO, Fordham SA, Bernard CC *et al* 1996 IFN-gamma plays a critical down-regulatory role in the induction and effector phase of myelin oligodendrocyte glycoprotein-induced autoimmune encephalomyelitis. *J Immunol* **157**: 3223–3227

Willenborg DO, Staykova MA, Cowden WB 1999 Our shifting understanding of the role of nitric oxide in autoimmune

encephalomyelitis: a review. *J Neuroimmunol* **100**: 21–35

Willer CJ, Sadovnick AD, Ebers GC 2002 Microchimerism in autoimmunity and transplantation: potential relevance to multiple sclerosis. *J Neuroimmunol* **126**: 126–133

Willer CJ, Dyment DA, Risch NJ *et al* 2003 Twin concordance and sibling recurrence rates in multiple sclerosis. The Canadian collaborative study. *Proc Natl Acad Sci USA* **100**: 12877–12882

Willer CJ, Dyment DA, Sadovnick AD *et al* 2005 Timing of birth and risk of multiple sclerosis: population based study. *Br Med J* **330**: 120

Williams A, Eldridge R, McFarland H *et al* 1980 Multiple sclerosis in twins. *Neurology* **30**: 1139–1147

Williams ES, McKeran RO 1986 Prevalence of multiple sclerosis in a South London borough. *Br Med J* **293**: 237–239

Williams ES, Jones DR, McKeran RO 1991 Mortality rates from multiple sclerosis: geographical and temporal variations revisited. *J Neurol Neurosurg Psychiatry* **54**: 104–109

Williams KE, Ulvestad E, Antel JP 1994 B7/BB-1 antigen expression on adult human microglia studied *in vitro* and *in situ*. *Eur J Immunol* **24**: 3031–3037

Williams MH, Bowie C 1993 Evidence of unmet need in the care of severely physically disabled adults.[retraction in BMJ. 1998 Jun 6;316(7146):1700; PMID: 9652920] *Br Med J* **306**: 95–98

Williams RM, Lees MB, Cambi F, Macklin WB 1982 Chronic allergic encephalomyelitis induced in rabbits with bovine white matter proteolipid apoprotein. *J Neuropathol Exp Neurol* **41**: 508–521

Williamson RA, Burgoon MP, Owens GP *et al* 2001 Anti-DNA antibodies are a major component of the intrathecal B cell response in multiple sclerosis. *Proc Natl Acad Sci USA* **98**: 1793–1798

Williamson RT 1894 The early pathological changes in disseminated sclerosis. *Med Chronicle (Manchester)* **19**: 373–379

Williamson RT 1908 *Diseases of the Spinal Cord*. Oxford, Oxford University Press and Hodder & Stoughton

Willis T 1684 *Dr Willis's Practice of Physick*. London: Dring, Harper & Leigh

Willison HJ, Yuki N 2002 Anti-ganglioside antibodies and peripheral neuropathy. *Brain* **125**: 2591–2625

Willoughby EW, Paty DW 1988 Scales for rating impairment in multiple sclerosis: a critique. *Neurology* **38**: 1793–1798

Willoughby EW, Grochowski E, Li DKB *et al* 1989 Serial magnetic resonance scanning in multiple sclerosis: a second prospective study in relapsing patients. *Ann Neurol* **25**: 43–49

Wilson HC, Onischke C, Raine CS 2003 Human oligodendrocyte precursor cells in vitro: phenotypic analysis and differential response to growth factors. *Glia* **44**: 153–165

Wilson IGH 1927 Disseminated sclerosis: the rat as possible carrier of infection. *Lancet* **ii**: 1220–1223

Wilson SAK 1906 A case of disseminated sclerosis with weakness of each internal rectus and nystagmus on lateral deviation limited to the outer eye. *Brain* **29**: 297–298

Wilson SAK 1924 Pathological laughing and crying. *J Neurol Psychopathol* **4**: 299–333

Wilson SAK 1940 Disseminated sclerosis. In: *Neurology*. London: Edward Arnold, pp. 148–178

Wilson SAK, McBride HJ 1925 Epilepsy as a symptom of disseminated sclerosis. *J Neurol Psychopathology* **6**: 91–103

Wilson WA, Ghavari AE, Koike T et al 1999 International consensus statement on preliminary classification criteria for definite antiphospholipid syndrome. *Arthritis Rheum* **42**: 1309–1311

Winchester RJ, Ebers GC, Fu SM, Espinosa L, Zabriskie J, Kunkel HG 1975 B-cell allo-antigen Ag7a in multiple sclerosis. *Lancet* **ii**: 814

Windhagen A, Newcombe J, Dangond F et al 1995 Expression of costimulatory molecules B7–1 (CD80), B7–2 (CD86), and interleukin 12 cytokine in multiple sclerosis lesions. *J Exp Med* **182**: 1985–1986

Windhagen A, Maniak S, Marckmann S et al 2001 Lymphadenopathy in patients with multiple sclerosis undergoing treatment with glatiramer acetate. *J Neurol Neurosurg Psychiatry* **70**: 415–416

Windrem MS, Nunes MC, Rashbaum WK et al 2004 Fetal and adult human oligodendrocyte progenitor cell isolates myelinate the congenitally dysmyelinated brain. *Nature Med* **10**: 93–97

Winfield JB, Shaw M, Silverman LM, Eisenberg RA, Wilson HA, Koffler D 1983 Intrathecal IgG synthesis and blood-brain barrier impairment in patients with systemic lupus erythematosus and central nervous system dysfunction. *Am J Med* **74**: 837–844

Wing MG, Zajicek JP, Seilly DJ et al 1992 Inhibition of antibody-dependent classical pathway activation by oligodendrocytes using CD59. *Immunology* **76**: 140–145

Wing MG, Moreau T, Greenwood J et al 1996 Mechanism of first-dose cytokine-release syndrome by Campath 1-H: involvement of CD16 (FcgammaRIII) and CD11a/CD18 (LFA-1) on NK cells. *J Clin Invest* **98**: 2819–2826

Wingerchuk DM, Weinshenker BG 2003 Neuromyelitis optica: clinical predictors of a relapsing course and survival. *Neurology* **60**: 848–853

Wingerchuk D, Liu Q, Sobell J et al 1997 A population-based case-control study of the tumor necrosis factor alpha-308 polymorphism in multiple sclerosis. *Neurology* **49**: 626–628

Wingerchuk DM, Benarroch E, Rodriguez M 1998 Treatment of multiple sclerosis-related fatigue with aspirin. *Can J Neurosci* **25**: S32

Wingerchuk DM, Hogancamp WF, O'Brien PC, Weinshenker BG 1999 The clinical course of neuromyelitis optica (Devic's syndrome). *Neurology* **53**: 1107–1114

Wingerchuk DM, Benarroch EE, O'Brien PC et al 2005 A randomized controlled crossover trial of aspirin for fatigue in multiple sclerosis. *Neurology* **64**: 1267–1269

Winter G, Milstein M 1991 Man-made antibodies. *Nature* **349**: 293–299

Winyard KE, Smith JL, Culbertson WW, Paris-Hamelin A 1989 Ocular Lyme borreliosis. *Am J Ophthalmol* **108**: 651–657

Wise CM, Agudelo CA 1988 Optic neuropathy as an initial manifestation of Sjögren's syndrome. *J Rheumatol* **15**: 799–802

Wise LH, Lanchbury JS, Lewis CM 1999 Meta-analysis of genome searches. *Ann Hum Genet* **63**: 263–272

Wisniewski HM, Lossinsky AS 1991 Structural and functional aspects of the interaction of inflammatory cells with the blood-brain barrier in experimental brain inflammation. *Brain Pathol* **1**: 89–96

Wisniewski HM, Oppenheimer D, McDonald WI 1976 Relation between myelination and function in MS and EAE. *J Neuropathol Exp Neurol* **35**: 327

Wolfson C, Confavreux C 1985 A Markov model of the natural history of multiple sclerosis. *Neuroepidemiology* **4**: 227–239

Wolfson C, Confavreux C 1987 Improvements to a simple Markov model of natural history of multiple sclerosis: I. Short term prognosis. *Neuroepidemiology* **6**: 101–115

Wolinsky JS, for the PROMiSe Study Group 2004 The PROMiSe trial: baseline data review and progress report. *Mult Scler* **10**: S65–S72

Wolinsky JS, Narayana PA, Noseworthy JH et al 2000 Linomide in relapsing and secondary progressive MS. Part II: MRI results. MRI Analysis Center of the University of Texas-Houston, Health Science Center, and the North American Linomide Investigators. *Neurology* **54**: 1734–1741

Wolinsky JS, Narayana PA, Johnson KP and Multiple Sclerosis Study Group and the MRI Analysis Center 2001 United States open-label glatiramer acetate extension trial for relapsing multiple sclerosis: MRI and clinical correlates. Multiple Sclerosis Study Group and the MRI Analysis Center. *Mult Scler* **7**: 33–41

Wolinsky JS, Comi G, Filippi M et al 2002 Copaxone's effect on MRI-monitored disease in relapsing MS is reproducible and sustained. *Neurology* **59**: 1284–1286

Wolinsky J, Pardo L, Stark Y et al 2003 Toward an improved understanding of primary progressive MS. *ACTRIMS 2003, Eighth Annual Meeting of the Americas Committee for Research and Treatment in Multiple Sclerosis, San Francisco, CA*, pp. 5–6

Wolswijk G 1998 Chronic stage multiple sclerosis lesions contain a relatively quiescent population of oligodendrocyte precursor cells. *J Neurosci* **18**: 601–609

Wolswijk G 2000 Oligodendrocyte survival, loss and birth in lesions of chronic-stage multiple sclerosis. *Brain* **123**: 105–115

Wolswijk G 2002 Oligodendrocyte precursor cells in the demyelinated multiple sclerosis spinal cord. *Brain* **125**: 338–349

Wolswijk G, Balesar R 2003 Changes in the expression and localization of the paranodal protein Caspr on axons in chronic multiple sclerosis. *Brain* **126**: 1638–1649

Wolswijk G, Noble M 1989 Identification of an adult specific glial progenitor cell. *Development* **105**: 387–400

Wolswijk G, Noble M 1992 Co-operation between PDGF and FGF converts slowly dividing 0–2A (adult) progenitor cells to rapidly dividing cells with characteristics of O-2A (perinatal) progenitor cells. *J Cell Biol* **118**: 889–900

Wood A, Wing MG, Benham CD, Compston DAS 1993 Specific induction of intracellular calcium oscillations by complement membrane attack on oligodendroglia. *J Neurosci* **13**: 3319–3332

Wood DD, Bilbao JM, O'Connors P, Moscarello MA 1996 Acute multiple sclerosis (Marburg type) is associated with developmentally immature myelin basic protein. *Ann Neurol* **40**: 18–24

Wood NW, Holmans P, Clayton D et al 1994 No linkage or association between multiple sclerosis and the myelin basic protein gene in affected sibling pairs. *J Neurol Neurosurg Psychiatry* **57**: 1191–1194

Wood NW, Kellar-Wood HF, Holmans P et al 1995a The T-cell receptor beta locus and susceptibility to multiple sclerosis. *Neurology* **45**: 1859–1863

Wood NW, Sawcer SJ, Kellar-Wood H et al 1995b A susceptibility gene for multiple sclerosis linked to the immunoglobulin heavy chain variable region. *J Neurol* **242**: 677–682

Wood PM, Bunge RP 1991 The origin of remyelinating cells in the adult central nervous system: the role of the mature oligodendrocyte. *Glia* **4**: 225–232

Wood PM, Williams AK 1984 Oligodendrocyte proliferation and CNS myelination in cultures containing dissociated embryonic neuroglia and dorsal root ganglion neurons. *Dev Brain Res* **12**: 225–241

Woodland DL 2002 Immunity and retroviral superantigens in humans. *Trends Immunol* **23**: 57–58

Woodroofe MN, Cuzner ML 1993 Cytokine mRNA expression in inflammatory multiple sclerosis lesions: detection by non-radioactive *in situ* hybridization. *Cytokine* **5**: 583–588

Woodroofe MN, Hayes GM, Cuzner ML 1989 Fc receptor density, MHC antigen expression and superoxide production are increased in interferon-γ-treated microglia isolated from adult rat brain. *Immunology* **68**: 421–426

Woodruff RH, Fruttiger M, Richardson WD, Franklin RJ 2004 Platelet-derived growth factor regulates oligodendrocyte progenitor numbers in adult CNS and their response following CNS demyelination. *Mol Cell Neurosci* **25**: 252–262

Woods AH 1929 The nervous disease of the Chinese. *Arch Neurol Psychiatry* **21**: 542–570

Woolf CJ, Allchorne A, Safieh-Garabedian B, Poole S 1997 Cytokines, nerve growth factor and inflammatory hyperalgesia: the contribution of tumour necrosis factor alpha. *Br J Pharmacol* **121**: 417–424

Worthington J, Jones R, Crawford M, Forti A 1994 Pregnancy and multiple sclerosis – a 3 year prospective study. *J Neurol* **241**: 228–233

Wosik K, Antel J, Kuhlmann T et al 2003 Oligodendrocyte injury in multiple sclerosis: a role for p53. *J Neurochem* **85**: 635–644

Wren D, Wolswijk G, Noble M 1992 *In vitro* analysis of the origin and maintenance of O-2A^adult progenitor cells. *J Cell Biol* **116**: 167–176

Wroe SJ, Pires M, Harding B, Youl BD, Shorvon SD 1991 Whipple's disease confined to the CNS presenting with multiple intercerebral mass lesions. *J Neurol Neurosurg Psychiatry* **54**: 989–992

Wu E, Raine CS 1992 Multiple sclerosis: interactions between oligodendrocytes and hypertrophic astrocytes and their occurrence in other, nondemyelinating conditions. *Lab Invest* **67**: 88–99

Wu E, Brosnan CF, Raine CS 1993 SP-40/40 immunoreactivity in inflammatory CNS lesions displaying astrocyte/oligodendrocyte interactions. *J Neuropathol Exp Neurol* **52**: 129–134

Wu JV, Shrager P 1994 Resolving three types of chloride channels in demyelinated Xenopus axons. *J Neurosci Res* **38**: 613–620

Wu JV, Rubinstein CT, Shrager P 1993 Single channel characterization of multiple types of potassium channels in demyelinated Xenopus axons. *J Neurosci* **13**: 5153–5163

Wu V, Schwartz JP 1998 Cell culture models for reactive gliosis: new perspectives. *J Neurosci Res* **51**: 675–681

Wucherpfennig KW 2001 Mechanisms for the induction of autoimmunity by infectious agents. *J Clin Invest* **108** 1097–1104

Wucherpfennig KW, Strominger JL 1995 Molecular mimicry in T cell-mediated autoimmunity: viral peptides activate human T cell clones specific for myelin basic protein. *Cell* **80**: 695–705

Wucherpfennig KW, Ota K, Endo N et al 1990 Shared human T cell receptor Vβ usage to immunodominant regions of myelin basic protein. *Science* **248**: 1016–1019

Wucherpfennig KW, Newcombe J, Li H et al 1992a T-cell receptor V alpha-V beta repertoire and cytokine gene expression in active multiple sclerosis lesions. *J Exp Med* **175**: 993–1002

Wucherpfennig KW, Newcombe J, Li H et al 1992b γδ T cell receptor repertoire in acute multiple sclerosis lesions. *Proc Natl Acad Sci USA* **89**: 4588–4592

Wucherpfennig KW, Sette A, Southwood S et al 1994a Structural requirements for binding of an immunodominant myelin basic protein peptide to DR2 isotypes and for its recognition by human T cells clones. *J Exp Med* **179**: 279–290

Wucherpfennig KW, Zhang J, Witek C et al 1994b Clonal expansion and persistence of human T cells specific for an immunodominant myelin basic protein peptide. *J Immunol* **152**: 5581–5592

Wuerfel J, Bellmann-Strobl J, Brunecker P et al 2004 Changes in cerebral perfusion precede plaque formation in multiple sclerosis. *Brain* **127**: 111–119

von Wussow P, von Wussow D, Jakschies HK et al 1990 The human intracellular Mx-homologous protein is specifically induced by type I interferons. *Eur J Immunol* **20**: 2015–2019

Wuthrich R, Rieder HP 1970 The seasonal incidence of multiple sclerosis in Switzerland. *Eur Neurol* **3**: 257–264

www.agmed.sante.gouv.fr [2004] Vaccins contre l'hépatite B: résumé des débats de la Commission Nationale de Pharmacovigilance du 21 septembre 2004

www.anaes.fr [2003] Réunion de consensus. Vaccination contre le virus de l'hépatite B. 10 et 11 septembre 2003, Paris. Texte des recommandations

www.nmss.org [2001] Research/clinical update 2 February 2001

www.who.int [2004] Global Advisory Committee on Vaccine Safety, Final Statement, September 2004

Wybar KC 1952 Ocular manifestations of disseminated sclerosis. *Proc R Soc Med* **45**: 315–320

Wynn DR, Rodriguez M, O'Fallon MM, Kurland LT 1990 A reappraisal of the epidemiology of multiple sclerosis in Olmsted County, Minnesota. *Neurology* **40**: 780–786

Wyss-Coray T, Borrow P, Brooker MJ, Mucke L 1997 Astroglial overproduction of TGF-beta 1 enhances inflammatory central nervous system disease in transgenic mice. *J Neuroimmunol* **77**: 45–50

Wyss-Coray T, Yan F, Lin AHT et al 2002 Prominent neurodegeneration and increased plaque formation in complement-inhibited Alzheimer's mice. *Proc Natl Acad Sci USA* **99**: 10837–10842

Xia MQ, Hale G, Lifely MR et al 1993 Structure of the Campath-1 antigen, a glycosylphosphotidylinated-anchored glycoprotein which is an exceptionally good target for complement lysis. *Biochem J* **293**: 633–640

Xiao B, Linington C, Link H 1991 Antibodies to myelin-oligodendrocyte glycoprotein in cerebrospinal fluid from patients with multiple sclerosis and controls. *J Neuroimmunol* **31**: 91–96

Xiao B, Zhang GX, Ma CG, Link H 1996 The cerebrospinal fluid from patients with multiple sclerosis promotes neuronal and oligodendrocyte damage by delayed production of nitric oxide in vitro. *J Neurol Sci* **142**: 114–120

Xin M, Yue T, Ma Z et al 2005 Myelinogenesis and axonal recognition by oligodendrocytes in brain are uncoupled in Olig1-null mice. *J Neurosci* **25**: 1354–1365

Xu C, Dai Y, Fredrickson S et al 1999 Association and linkage analysis of candidate chromosomal regions in multiple sclerosis: indication of disease genes in 12q23 and 7ptr-15. *Eur J Hum Gen* **7**: 110–116

Xu C, Dai Y, Lorentzen JC 2001 Linkage analysis in multiple sclerosis of chromosomal regions syntenic to experimental autoimmune disease loci. *Eur J Hum Gen* **9**: 458–463

Xu GY, Hughes MG, Ye Z et al 2004 Concentrations of glutamate released following spinal cord injury kill oligodendrocytes in the spinal cord. *Exp Neurol* **187**: 329–336

Xu X-H, McFarlin DE 1984 Oligoclonal bands in CSF: twins with MS. *Neurology* **34**: 769–774

Yabuki S, Hayabara T 1979 Paroxysmal dysesthesia in multiple sclerosis. *Folia Psychiatr Neurol Jpn* **33**: 97–104

Yahr MD, Lobo-Antunes J 1972 Relapsing encephalomyelitis following the use of influenza vaccine. *Arch Neurol* **27**: 182–183

Yamada S, DePasquale M, Patlak CS, Cserr HF 1991 Albumin outflow into deep cervical lymph from different regions of rabbit brain. *Am J Physiol* **261**: H1197–H1204

Yamamoto M 1986 Recurrent transverse myelitis associated with collagen disease. *J Neurol* **233**: 185–187

Yamamoto T, Imai T, Yamasaki M 1989 Acute ventilatory failure in multiple sclerosis. *J Neurol Sci* **89**: 313–324

Yamamoto T, Kawamura J, Hashimoto S, Nakamura M 1991 Extensive proliferation of peripheral type myelin in necrotic spinal cord lesions of multiple sclerosis. *J Neurol Sci* **102**: 163–169

Yamanouchi N, Okada S, Kodama K et al 1995 White matter changes caused by chronic solvent abuse. *Am J Neuroradiol* **16**: 1643–1649

Yamasaki K, Horiuchi I, Minohara M et al 1999 HLA-DPB1*0501-associated opticospinal multiple sclerosis: clinical, neuroimaging and immunogenetic studies. *Brain* **122**: 1689–1696

Yamashita T, Ando Y, Obayashi K et al 1997 Changes in nitrite and nitrate (NO2-/NO3-) levels in cerebrospinal fluid of patients with multiple sclerosis. *J Neurol Sci* **153**: 32–34

Yan H, Rivkees SA 2002 Hepatocyte growth factor stimulates the proliferation and migation of oligodendrocyte precursor cells. *J Neurosci* **22**: 597–606

Yang D, Biragyn A, Kwak LW, Oppenheim JJ 2002 Mammalian defensins in immunity: more than just microbicidal. *Trends Immunol* **23**: 291–296

Yao D-L, Webster HdeF, Hudson LD et al 1994 Concentric sclerosis (Balo): morphometric and *in situ* hybridization study of lesions in six patients. *Ann Neurol* **35**: 18–30

Yao D-L, Liu X, Hudson LD, Webster H deF 1995 Insulin-like growth factor 1 treatment reduces demyelination and up-regulates gene expression of myelin related proteins in experimental autoimmune encephalomyelitis. *Proc Natl Acad Sci USA* **92**: 6190–6194

Yao S, Stratton CW, Mitchell WM, Sriram S 2001 CSF oligoclonal bands in MS include antibodies against *Chlamydia* antigens. *Neurology* **56**: 1168–1176

Yapici Z, Eraksoy M 2002 Bilateral demyelinating tumefactive lesions in three children with hemiparesis. *J Child Neurol* **17**: 655–660

Yaquib BA, Daif AK 1988 Multiple sclerosis in Saudi Arabia. *Neurology* **38**: 621–623

Yarom Y, Naparstek Y, Lev-Ram V et al 1983 Immunospecific inhibition of nerve conduction by T lymphocytes reactive to basic protein of myelin. *Nature* **303**: 246–247

Ye P, D'Ercole AJ 1999 Insulin-like growth factor I protects oligodendrocytes from tumor necrosis factor-alpha-induced injury. *Endocrinology* **140**: 3063–3072

Ye P, Li L, Richards RG et al 2002 Myelination is altered in insulin-like growth factor-I null mutant mice. *J Neurosci* **22**: 6041–6051

Ye P, Bagnell R, D'Ercole AJ 2003 Mouse NG2+ oligodendrocyte precursors express mRNA for proteolipid protein but not its DM-20 variant: a study of laser microdissection-captured NG2+ cells. *J Neurosci* **23**: 4401–4405

Yednock TA, Cannon C, Fritz LC et al 1992 Prevention of experimental autoimmune encephalomyelitis by antibodies against α4β1 integrin. *Nature* **356**: 63–66

Yeh EA, Collins A, Cohen ME et al 2004 Detection of coronavirus in the central nervous system of a child with acute disseminated encephalomyelitis. *Pediatrics* **113**: 73–76

Yeo TW, Roxburgh R, Maranian M et al 2003 Refining the analysis of a whole genome linkage disequilibrium association map: the United Kingdom. *J Neuroimmunol* **143**: 53–59

Yeo TW, Maranian M, Singlehurst S et al 2004 Four single nucleotide polymorphisms from the Vitamin D receptor gene in UK multiple sclerosis. *J Neurol* **251**: 753–754

Yiannoutsos CT, Major EO, Curfman B et al 1999 Relation of JC virus DNA in the cerebrospinal fluid to survival in acquired immunodeficiency syndrome patients with biopsy-proven progressive multifocal leucoencephalopathy. *Ann Neurol* **45**: 816–821

Yong VW 2002 Differential mechanisms of action of interferon-beta and glatiramer aetate in MS. *Neurology* **59**: 802–808

Yoshida EM, Rasmussen SL, Steinbrecher UP et al 2001 Fulminant liver failure during interferon beta treatment of multiple sclerosis. *Neurology* **56**: 1416

Yoshida T, Tanaka M, Sotomatsu A, Okamoto K 1999 Effect of methylprednisolone-pulse

therapy on superoxide production of neutrophils. *Neurol Res* **21**: 509–512

Youl BD, Kermode AG, Thompson AJ et al 1991a Destructive lesions in demyelinating disease. *J Neurol Neurosurg Psychiatry* **54**: 288–292

Youl BD, Turano G, Miller DH et al 1991b The pathophysiology of acute optic neuritis: an association of gadolinium leakage with clinical and electrophysiological deficits. *Brain* **114**: 2437–2450

Younes-Mhenni S, Janier MF, Cinotti L et al 2004 FDG-PET improves tumour detection in patients with paraneoplastic neurological syndromes. *Brain* **127**: 2331–2338

Young AC, Saunders J, Ponsford JR 1976 Mental change as an early feature of multiple sclerosis. *J Neurol Neurosurg Psychiatry* **39**: 1008–1013

Young IR, Hall AS, Pallis CA et al 1981 Nuclear magnetic resonance imaging of the brain in multiple sclerosis. *Lancet* **ii**: 1063–1066

Young RB 1976 Fluorescein angiography and retinal venous sheathing in multiple sclerosis. *Can J Ophthalmol* **11**: 31–36

Young RR, Delwade PJ 1981a Drug therapy: spasticity (part 1). *N Engl J Med* **304**: 28–33

Young RR, Delwade PJ 1981b Drug therapy: spasticity (part 2). *N Engl J Med* **304**: 96–99

Young W, Rosenbluth J, Wojak JC et al 1989 Extracellular potassium activity and axonal conduction in spinal cord of the myelin-deficient mutant rat. *Exp Neurol* **106**: 41–51

Younger DS, Pedley TA, Thorpy MJ 1991 Multiple sclerosis and narcolepsy: possible similar genetic susceptibility. *Neurology* **41**: 447–448

Youssef S, Wildbaum G, Maor G et al 1998 Long-lasting protective immunity to experimental autoimmune encephalomyelitis following vaccination with naked DNA encoding C-C chemokines. *J Immunol* **161**: 3870–3879

Youssef S, Stuve O, Patarroyo JC et al 2002 The HMG-CoA reductase inhibitor, atorvastatin, promotes a Th2 bias and reverses paralysis in central nervous system autoimmune disease. *Nature* **420**: 78–84

Yu JS, Hayashi T, Seboun E et al 1991 Fos RNA accumulation in multiple sclerosis white matter tissue. *J Neurol Sci* **103**: 209–215

Yu JS, Pandey JP, Massacesi L et al 1993 Segregation of immunoglobulin heavy chain constant region genes in multiple sclerosis sibling pairs. *J Neuroimmunol* **42**: 113–116

Yu WP, Collarini EJ, Pringle NP, Richardson WD 1994 Embryonic expression of myelin genes: evidence for a focal source of oligodendrocyte precursors in the ventricular zone of the neural tube. *Neuron* **12**: 1353–1362

Yu YL, Woo E, Hawkins BR et al 1989 Multiple sclerosis among Chinese in Hong Kong. *Brain* **112**: 1445–1467

Yuan J, Yankner B 2000 Apoptosis in the nervous system. *Nature* **407**: 802–809

Yudkin PL, Ellison GW, Ghezzi A et al 1991 Overview of azathioprine treatment in multiple sclerosis. *Lancet* **338**: 1051–1055

Yung SY, Gokhan S, Jurcsak J et al 2002 Differential modulation of BMP signaling promotes the elaboration of cerebral cortical GABAergic neurons or oligodendrocytes from a common sonic hedgehog-responsive ventral forebrain progenitor species. *Proc Natl Acad Sci USA* **99**: 16273–16278

Yushchenko M, Mader M, Elitok E et al 2003 Interferon-beta-1b decreased matrix metalloproteinase-9 serum levels in primary progressive multiple sclerosis. *J Neurol* **250**: 1224–1228

Zaffaroni M, Ghezzi A 2000 The prognosis value of age, gender, pregnancy and endocrine factors in multiple sclerosis. *Neurol Sci* **21 (Suppl)**: 857–860

Zajicek JP 1990 Sarcoidosis of the cauda equina: a report of three cases. *J Neurol* **237**: 244–246

Zajicek JP, Compston DAS 1994 Myelination *in vitro* of dorsal root ganglia by glial progenitor cells. *Brain* **117**: 1333–1350

Zajicek JP, Compston DAS 1995 Human oligodendrocytes are not sensitive to complement – a study of CD59 expression in the human central nervous system. *Lab Invest* **73**: 128–138

Zajicek JP, Wing M, Scolding NJ, Compston DAS 1992 Interactions between oligodendrocytes and microglia, a major role for complement and tumour necrosis factor in oligodendrocyte adherence and killing. *Brain* **115**: 1611–1631

Zajicek JP, Scolding NJ, Foster O et al 1999 Central nervous system sarcoidosis – diagnosis and management based on a large series. *Q J Med* **92**: 103–117

Zajicek JP, Fox P, Sanders H et al 2003 Cannabinoids for treatment of spasticity and other symptoms related to multiple sclerosis (CAMS study): multicentre randomised placebo-controlled trial. *Lancet* **362**: 1517–1526

Zakrzewska-Pniewska B, Styczynska M, Podlecka A et al 2004 Association of apolipoprotein E and myeloperoxidase genotypes to clinical course of familial and sporadic multiple sclerosis. *Mult Scler* **10**: 266–271

Zamvil SS, Steinman L 1990 The T lymphocyte in experimental allergic encephalomyelitis. *Ann Rev Immunol* **8**: 579–622

Zamvil SS, Steinman L 2003 Diverse targets for intervention during inflammatory and neurodegenerative phases of multiple sclerosis. *Neuron* **38**: 685–688

Zamvil SS, Nelson PA, Trotter J et al 1985 T-cell clones specific for myelin basic protein induce chronic relapsing paralysis and demyelination. *Nature* **317**: 355–358

Zander H, Kuntz B, Scholz S, Albert ED 1976 Analysis for joint segregation of HLA and multiple sclerosis in families (abstract). In: Dausset J (ed.) *HLA and Disease*. Paris

Zander H, Abb J, Kaudewitz O, Riethmuller G 1982 Natural killing activity and interferon production in multiple sclerosis. *Lancet* **i**: 280

Zandman-Goddard G, Levy Y, Weiss P et al 2003 Transverse myelitis associated with chronic hepatitis C. *Clin Exp Rheumatol* **21**: 111–113

Zang YC, Samanta AK, Halder JB et al 2000a Aberrant T cell migration toward RANTES and MIP-1 alpha in patients with multiple sclerosis: overexpression of chemokine receptor CCR5. *Brain* **123**: 1874–1882

Zang YC, Yang D, Hong J et al 2000b Immunoregulation and blocking antibodies induced by interferon beta treatment in MS. *Neurology* **55**: 397–404

Zang YC, Halder JB, Samanta AK et al 2001 Regulation of chemokine receptor CCR5 and production of RANTES and MIP-1alpha by interferon-beta. *J Neuroimmunol* **112**: 174–180

Zang YC, Hong J, Robinson R et al 2003a Immune regulatory properties and interactions of copolymer-I and beta-interferon 1a in multiple sclerosis. *J Neuroimmunol* **137**: 144–153

Zang YC, Hong J, Rivera VM et al 2003b Human anti-idiotypic T cells induced by TCR peptides corresponding to a common CDR3 sequence motif in myelin basic protein-reactive T cells. *Int Immunol* **15**: 1073–1080

Zarei M, Chandran S, Compston A, Hodges J 2003 Cognitive presentation of multiple sclerosis: evidence for a cortical variant. *J Neurol Neurosurg Psychiatry* **74**: 872–877

Zayas MD, Lucas M, Solano F et al 2001 Association of a CA repeat polymorphism upstream of the Fas ligand gene with multiple sclerosis. *J Neuroimmunol* **116**: 238–241

Zee DS, Leigh JR 2002 Oculomotor control: normal and abnormal. In: Asbury AK, McKhann GM, McDonald WI et al (eds) *Diseases of the Nervous System: Clinical Neuroscience and Therapeutic Principles.* Vol 1. pp. 634–657

Zeine R, Owens T 1992 Direct demonstration of the infiltration of murine central nervous system by Pgp-1/CD44^high CD45RB^low CD4^+ T cells that induce experimental allergic encephalomyelitis. *J Neuroimmunol* **40**: 57–70

Zeine R, Cammer W, Barbarese E et al 2001 Structural dynamics of oligodendrocyte lysis by perforin in culture: relevance to multiple sclerosis. *J Neurosci* **64**: 380–391

Zelenika D, Grima B, Pessac B 1993 A new family of transcripts of the myelin basic protein gene: expression in brain and in immune system. *J Neurochem* **60**: 1574–1577

Zeman AZJ, Kidd D, McLean BN et al 1996 A study of oligoclonal band negative multiple sclerosis. *J Neurol Neurosurg Psychiatry* **60**: 27–30

Zenker W, Bankoul S, Braun JS 1994 Morphological indications for considerable diffuse reabsorption of cerebrospinal fluid in spinal meninges particularly in the areas of meningeal funnels: an electron-microscopical study including tracing experiments in rats. *Anat Embryol* **189**: 243–258

Zenzola A, De Mari M, De Blasi R et al 2001 Paroxysmal dystonia with thalamic lesion in multiple sclerosis. *Neurol Sci* **22**: 391–394

Zettl UK, Gold R, Hartung H-P, Toyka KV 1994 Apoptotic death of T-lymphocytes in experimental autoimmune neuritis of the Lewis rat. *Neurosci Lett* **176**: 75–79

Zettl UK, Gold R, Toyka KV, Hartung H-P 1995 Intravenous glucocorticosteroid treatment augments apoptosis of inflammatory T cells in experimental autoimmune neuritis (EAN) of the Lewis rat. *J Neuropathol Exp Neurol* **54**: 540–547

Zettl UK, Mix E, Zielasek J et al 1997 Apoptosis of myelin-reactive T cells induced by reactive oxygen and nitrogen intermediates in vitro. *Cell Immunol* **178**: 1–8

Zhang J, Medaer R, Hashim GA et al 1992 Myelin basic protein-specific T lymphocytes in multiple sclerosis: precursor frequency, fine specificity, and cytotoxicity. *Ann Neurol* **32**: 330–338

Zhang J, Medaer R, Stinsson P et al 1993 MHC-restricted depletion of human myelin basic protein-reactive T cells by T cell vaccination. *Science* **261**: 1451–1454

Zhang J, Markovic-Plese S, Lacet B et al 1994 Increased frequency of interleukin 2-responsive T cells specific for myelin basic protein and proteolipid protein in peripheral blood and cerebrospinal fluid of patients with multiple sclerosis. *J Exp Med* **179**: 973–984

Zhang J, Vandevyver C, Stinissen P, Raus J 1995 *In vivo* clonotypic regulation in human myelin basic protein-reactive T cells by T cell vaccination. *J Immunol* **155**: 5865–5877

Zhang J, Hutton G, Zang Y 2002 A comparison of the mechanisms of action of interferon beta and glatiramer acetate in the treatment of multiple sclerosis. *Clin Ther* **24**: 1998–2021

Zhang X, Izikson L, Liu L, Weiner HL 2001 Activation of CD25^+CD4^+ regulatory T cells by oral antigen administration. *J Immunol* **167**: 4245–4253

Zhang X-M, Heber-Katz E 1992 T cell receptor sequences from encephalitogenic T cells in adult Lewis rats suggest an early ontogenic origin. *J Immunol* **148**: 746–752

Zhang X, Cai J, Klueber KM et al 2005 Induction of oligodendrocyte from adult human olfactory epithelial-derived progenitors by transcription factors. *Stem Cells* **23**: 442–453

Zhang Z, Duvefelt K, Svensson F et al 2005 Two genes encoding immune-regulatory molecules (LAG3 and IL7R) confer susceptibility to multiple sclerosis. *Genes Immun* **6**: 145–152

Zhou L, Messing A, Chiu SY 1999 Determinants of excitability at transition zones in Kv1.1-deficient myelinated nerves. *J Neurosci* **19**: 5768–5781

Zhou Q, Anderson DJ 2002 The bHLH transcription factors OLIG2 and OLIG1 couple neuronal and glial subtype specification. *Cell* **109**: 61–73

Zhou Q, Wang S, Anderson DJ 2000 Identification of a novel family of oligodendrocyte lineage-specific basic helix-loop-helix transcription factors. *Neuron* **25**: 331–343

Zhou Q, Rammohan K, Lin S et al 2003 CD24 is a genetic modifier for risk and progression of multiple sclerosis. *Proc Natl Acad Sci USA* **100**: 15041–15046

Ziemssen T, Kumpfel T, Klinkert WEF et al 2002 Glatiramer acetate-specific T-helper 1- and 2-type cell lines produce BDNF: implications for multiple sclerosis therapy. *Brain* **125**: 2381–2391

Zihl J, Werth R 1984 Contributions to the study of 'blind sight'. II The role of specific practice for saccadic localisation in patients with postgeniculate visual field defects. *Neuropsychologia* **22**: 13–22

Zipp F, Weber F, Huber S et al 1995 Genetic control of multiple sclerosis: increased production of lymphotoxin and TNFα by HLA-DR2+ T cells. *Ann Neurol* **38**: 723–730

Zipp F, Kerschensteiner M, Dornmair K et al 1998 Complexity of the anti-T cell receptor immune response: implications for T cell vaccination therapy of multiple sclerosis. *Brain* **121**: 1395–1407

Zipp F, Weil JG, Einhaupl KM 1999 No increase in demyelinating disease after hepatitis B vaccination. *Nature Med* **5**: 964–965

Zipp F, Windemuth C, Pankow H et al 2000a Multiple sclerosis associated aminoacids of polymorphic regions relevant for the HLA antigen binding are confined to HLA-DR'. *Hum Immunol* **61**: 1021–1030

Zipp F, Wendling U, Beyer M et al 2000b Dual effect of glucocorticoids on apoptosis of human autoreactive and foreign antigen-specific T cells. *J Neuroimmunol* **110**: 214–222

Zivadinov R, Rudick RA, De Masi R et al 2001a Effects of IV methylprednisolone on brain atrophy in relapsing–remitting MS. *Neurology* **57**: 1239–1247

Zivadinov R, Sepcic J, Nasuelli D et al 2001b A longitudinal study of brain atrophy and cognitive disturbances in the early phase of relapsing–remitting multiple sclerosis. *J Neurol Neurosurg Psychiatry* **70**: 773–780

Zivadinov R, Uxa L, Zacchi T et al 2003a HLA genotypes and disease severity assessed by magnetic resonance imaging findings in patients with multiple sclerosis. *J Neurol* **250**: 1099–1106

Zivadinov R, Iona L, Monti-Bragadin L et al 2003b The use of standardized incidence and prevalence rates in epidemiological studies on multiple sclerosis: a meta-analysis study. *Neuroepidemiology* **22**: 65–74

Zivadinov R, Zorzon M, Locatelli L et al 2003c Sexual dysfunction in multiple sclerosis: a MRI, neurophysiological and urodynamic study. *J Neurol Sci* **210**: 73–76

945

Zorgdrager A, De Keyser J 1998 Premenstrual exacerbations of multiple sclerosis. *J Neurol Neurosurg Psychiatry* **65**: 279–280

Zorzon M, Zivadinov R, Bosco A *et al* 1999 Sexual dysfunction in multiple sclerosis: a case-control study. 1. Frequency and comparison of groups. *Mult Scler* **5**: 418–427

Zorzon M, Ukmar M, Bragadin LM *et al* 2000 Olfactory dysfunction and extent of white matter abnormalities in multiple sclerosis: a clinical and MR study. *Mult Scler* **6**: 386–390

Zorzon M, Zivadinov R, Bragadin LM *et al* 2001 Sexual dysfunction in multiple sclerosis: a 2-year follow up study. *J Neurol Sci* **187**: 1–5

Zorzon M, Zivadinov R, Locatelli L *et al* 2003a Correlation of sexual dysfunction and brain magnetic resonance imaging in multiple sclerosis. *Mult Scler* **9**: 108–110

Zorzon M, Zivadinov R, Nasuelli D *et al* 2003b Risk factors of multiple sclerosis: a case-control study. *Neurol Sci* **24**: 242–247

Zorzon M, Zivadinov R, Locatelli L *et al* 2005 Long-term effects of intravenous high dose methylprednisolone pulses on bone mineral density in patients with multiple sclerosis. *Eur J Neurol* **12**: 550–556

Zouali H, Faure-Delanef L, Lucotte G 1999 Chromosome 19 locus apolipoprotein C-II association with multiple sclerosis. *Mult Scler* **5**: 134–136

Zoukos Y, Kidd D, Woodroofe MN *et al* 1994 Increased expression of high affinity IL-R receptors and β-adrenoceptors on peripheral blood mononuclear cells is associated with clinical and MRI activity in MS. *Brain* **117**: 307–315

Zsombok A, Schrofner S, Hermann A, Kerschbaum HH 2000 Nitric oxide increases excitability by depressing a calcium activated potassium current in snail neurons. *Neurosci Lett* **295**: 85–88

Zucchi I, Bini L, Valaperta R *et al* 2001 Proteomic dissection of dome formation in a mammary cell line: role of tropomyosin-5b and maspin. *Proc Natl Acad Sci USA* **98**: 5608–5613

Zwemmer JNP, van Veen T, van Winsen L *et al* 2004 No major association of ApoE genotype with disease characteristics and MRI findings in multiple sclerosis. *Mult Scler* **10**: 272–277

Index

973